Staff

Executive Publisher
Judith A. Schilling McCann, RN, MSN

Editorial Director
H. Nancy Holmes

Clinical Director
Joan M. Robinson, RN, MSN

Art Director
Elaine Kasmer

Clinical Managers
Eileen Cassin Gallen, RN, BSN;
Collette Bishop Hendler, RN, BS, CCRN

Electronic Project Manager
John Macalino

Editorial Project Manager
Christiane L. Brownell, ELS

Editor
Rita M. Doyle

Clinical Editors
Christine M. Damico, RN, MSN, CPNP;
Kimberly A. Zalewski, RN, MSN

Copy Editor
Tom Wolf

Digital Composition Services
Diane Paluba (manager),
Joyce Rossi Biletz, Donald G. Knauss

Manufacturing
Beth J. Welsh

Editorial Assistants
Karen Kirk, Jeri O'Shea, Linda Ruhf

Indexer
Deborah K. Tourtlotte

The clinical procedures described and recommended in this publication are based on research and consultation with nursing, medical, pharmaceutical, and legal authorities. To the best of our knowledge, these procedures reflect currently accepted practice; nevertheless, they can't be considered absolute and universal recommendations. For individual application, all recommendations must be considered in light of the patient's clinical condition and, before the administration of new or infrequently used drugs, in light of the latest package-insert information. The authors and publisher disclaim responsibility for adverse effects resulting directly or indirectly from the suggested procedures, from undetected errors, or from the reader's misunderstanding of the text.

 Printed in Colombia. For information, write Lippincott Williams & Wilkins, 323 Norristown Road, Suite 200, Ambler, PA 19002-2758.

Visit our Web site at NDHnow.com

NDH28010507
ISSN 0273-320X
ISBN-13: 978-1-58255-683-3
ISBN-10: 1-58255-683-0

midazolam HCl	morphine sulfate	nalbuphine HCl	pentazocine lactate	pentobarbital Na	perphenazine	phenobarbital Na	prochlorperazine edisylate	promazine HCl	promethazine HCl	ranitidine HCl	scopolamine HBr	secobarbital Na	sodium bicarbonate	thiethylperazine mal	thiopental Na	
Y	P	Y	P	P	Y		P	P	P	Y	P					atropine sulfate
Y	Y		Y	N	Y		Y		Y		Y			Y		butorphanol tartrate
Y	P		P	N	Y		P	P	P	N*	P				N	chlorpromazine HCl
Y	Y	Y	Y	N	Y		Y	Y	Y		Y	N				cimetidine HCl
																codeine phosphate
										Y						dexamethasone sodium phosphate
N	P		P	N	Y		N	N	N	Y	P				N	dimenhydrinate
Y	P	Y	P	N	Y		P	P	P	Y	P				N	diphenhydramine HCl
Y	P	Y	P	N	Y		P	P	P		P					droperidol
Y	P		P	N	Y		P	P	P	Y	P					fentanyl citrate
Y	Y	Y	N	N			Y	Y	Y	Y	Y	N	N		N	glycopyrrolate
	N*		N			P(5)			N							heparin Na
Y			Y	Y		N	N*		Y	Y	Y			Y		hydromorphone HCl
Y	P	Y	P	N	Y		P	P	P	N	P					hydroxyzine HCl
Y	N		P	N	Y		P	P	P	Y	P				N	meperidine HCl
Y	P		P		P*		P	P	P*	Y	P		N			metoclopramide HCl
	Y	Y		N	N		N	Y	Y	N	Y			Y		midazolam HCl
Y			P	N*	Y		P*	P	P*	Y	P				N	morphine sulfate
Y				N			Y		N*	Y	Y			Y		nalbuphine HCl
	P			N	Y		P	P*	P*	Y	P					pentazocine lactate
N	N*	N	N		N		N	N	N	N	P		Y		Y	pentobarbital Na
N	Y		Y	N			Y		Y	Y	Y			N		perphenazine
										N						phenobarbital Na
N	P*	Y	P	N	Y			P	P	Y	P				N	prochlorperazine edisylate
Y	P		P*	N			P		P		P					promazine HCl
Y	P*	N*	P*	N	Y		P	P		Y	P				N	promethazine HCl
N	Y	Y	Y	N	Y	N	Y		Y		Y			Y		ranitidine HCl
Y	P	Y	P	P	Y		P	P	P	Y					Y	scopolamine HBr
																secobarbital Na
				Y											N	sodium bicarbonate
Y		Y			N					Y						thiethylperazine maleate
	N			Y			N		N		Y		N			thiopental Na

28th Edition

Nursing2008® DRUG HANDBOOK®

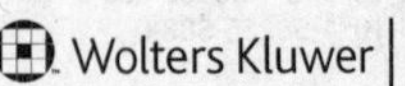

Wolters Kluwer | Lippincott Williams & Wilkins

Health

Philadelphia • Baltimore • New York • London

Buenos Aires • Hong Kong • Sydney • Tokyo

Contents

General Information

Anti-infectives

Cardiovascular System Drugs

Central Nervous System Drugs

Drugs for Fluid and Electrolyte Balance

Hematologic Drugs

Antineoplastics

Immunomodulators

Ophthalmic, Otic, and Nasal Drugs

Topical Drugs

Nutritional Drugs

Miscellaneous Categories

Appendices and Index

Contributors and consultants

At the time of publication, the contributors and consultants held the following positions.

Steven R. Abel, PharmD, FASHP
Professor and Head
Department of Pharmacy Practice
Purdue University
Indianapolis

Lynn Marie Antonawich, BSN, RN
Staff Nurse
Good Samaritan Hospital Medical Center
West Islip, N.Y.

Fatima Ahmad, MSc, PharmD
Drug Information Specialist
AstraZeneca
Wilmington, Del.

Lawrence Carey, PharmD
Assistant Professor
Philadelphia University

Kim Cooper, RN, MSN
Nursing Department Chair
Ivy Tech Community College of Indiana
Terre Haute

Lillian Craig, RN, MSN, FNP-C
Nursing Adjunct Faculty
Oklahoma Panhandle State University
Goodwell

Michele A. Danish, RPh, PharmD
Pharmacy Clinical Manager
St. Joseph Health Services
North Providence, R.I.

Melissa Devlin, PharmD
Clinical Pharmacist
Excellrx Inc.
Philadelphia

Camille Dieudonne, PharmD
Clinical Pharmacist
Mercy Hospital
Philadelphia

Laurie Donaghy, RN, CEN
Staff Nurse
Frankford Hospital
Philadelphia

Christopher A. Fausel, PharmD, BCPS, BCOP
Clinical Pharmacist
Indiana University Hospital
Indianapolis

Valerie Gillis, RN, BScN, CPAN
PeriAnesthesia Educator
University of Washington Medical Center
Seattle, Wasg.

Tatyana Gurvich, PharmD
Clinical Pharmacologist
Glendale (Calif.) Adventist Family Practice Residency Program

Julie Hixson-Wallace, Pharm.D., BCPS
Dean, College of Pharmacy
Harding University
Searcy, Ark.

Mary Kate Kelly, RPh, PharmD
President
Health Content Consultants
Pottstown, Pa.

Julia N. Kleckner, PharmD
Clinical Pharmacist
Concord Pharmacy
Glen Mills, Pa

Michelle Kosich, PharmD
Clinical Pharmacist
Mercy Fitzgerald Hospital
Darby, Pa.

Terri Ann Polesky, RPh
Consultant
Aliquippa, Pa.

Dawn Pollitt, PharmD
Clinical Pharmacist
Keystone Mercy Health Plan
Philadelphia

Joanne Whitney, PhD, PharmD
Director, Drug Product Services Laboratory
Associate Clinical Professor
Department of Clinical Pharmacy
University of California
San Francisco

How to use *Nursing2008 Drug Handbook*

Nursing2008 Drug Handbook, created by pharmacists and nurses, focuses on drug information that nurses need to know. *Nursing2008 Drug Handbook* emphasizes nursing aspects of drugs without trying to replace detailed pharmacology texts. The unique book design makes the content readily accessible and applicable in any clinical setting. this edition also emphasizes safety to help you avoid medication errors.

Features in this edition

The 28th edition offers features that enhance nursing knowledge and skills and promote drug safety:

- New monographs for over 20 new, FDA-approved drugs
- "Safety Alert!" label for drugs that present an avoidable danger for you or your patient and the sidesteps for you to take
- A symbol in the drug monographs (✐) indicating that the drug is illustrated in the color photoguide
- A symbol that shows off-label uses at a glance (♦)
- "Adjust-a-dose" logos to highlight dosage adjustments that may be needed in certain patient populations
- New to this edition: Pharmacologic class is listed for each drug entry.
- "I.V. administration" section that gives step-by-step guidance on safely preparing, giving, and storing I.V. drugs
- "Incompatibilities" section to highlight drugs which shouldn't be given together
- Tables that show the route, onset, peak, and duration of each drug
- An "Alert" logo that signals cautionary tips to help you avoid common medication errors, with a special "look alike–sound alike" logo for drug names easily confused with a similar name
- New to this edition: Half-life listed for each drug entry
- An "Effects on lab test results" section in every monograph
- New to this edition: In the "Interactions" section, drugs that cause a rapid- and delayed-onset interaction highlighted
- A guide to common abbreviations approved by the Joint Commission as safe to use throughout the book with an appendix on which ones to avoid
- Three new appendices (detailed entries including dosages and a quick guide) on combination drugs and a guide to vitamins and minerals, including dosages
- An appendix on drugs affected by cytochrome P-450 enzymes
- An appendix on drugs that affect the QTc interval, as well as appendices on herbal medicines, sound-alike and look-alike drugs, dialyzable drugs, drugs that shouldn't be crushed, normal lab test values, therapeutic drug monitoring guidelines, combination pain management drugs, and adverse reactions misinterpreted as age-related changes
- Free NDH2008*Plus!* CD-ROM (inside the back cover) that lets you view and print complete drug monographs and customizable patient-teaching instructions for 200 commonly used drugs
- A link from NDH2008*Plus!* to NDHnow.com, the *Nursing2008 Drug Handbook* Web site, which provides monthly drug updates, important drug news, new drug warnings and indications, patient-teaching aids, 10 continuing-education tests, and more.

Introductory chapters

Chapter 1 explains generally how drugs work. It includes drug actions, interactions, and reactions. Chapter 2 gives general guidelines about drug use in pregnancy and the presence of drugs in breast milk. It also covers the unique problems of giving drugs to children and elderly patients and offers suggestions to minimize problems in these areas. Chapter 3 discusses techniques and provides guidelines for safe drug administration.

Therapeutic class chapters

Chapters 4 to 94 classify all drugs according to their approved therapeutic uses. Drugs with more than one therapeutic use are classified according to their most common use; they're also listed (with a cross-reference to the major drug entry) in drug groups that share their secondary applications. For example, nadolol, a beta blocker, is described in the chapter that covers antianginals because its major therapeutic application is the management of angina pectoris. Less commonly, nadolol is used to treat hypertension, so it's also listed among the generic drugs grouped as antihypertensives, with a cross-reference to Chapter 20, Antianginals.

Such classification by therapeutic use offers several advantages. It helps you identify an unknown drug by its clinical application alone. It also identifies all other drugs that share the same use and provides easy comparison of their dosages and effects. In this way, it quickly lets you refer to similar drugs for patients who can't tolerate or don't respond to a particular drug.

Each chapter, representing a major therapeutic use, begins with an alphabetical list of the generic drugs described in the chapter. Specific information on each drug is arranged under the following headings: *Pregnancy risk category, Controlled substance schedule*, *Available forms, Indications & dosages, I.V. administration (*with *Incompatibilities)*, *Action* (with quick-reference table), *Adverse reactions, Interactions, Effects on lab test results, Contraindications & cautions, Nursing considerations,* and *Patient teaching.* (See *Pregnancy risk categories* and *Controlled substance schedules*.)

In each drug entry, drugs may have received a "Safety Alert!" label. This label is reserved for drugs, designated by the Institute for Safe Medication Practices, that are dangerous to you or your patient, either because they are powerful and hazardous or prone to accidental error.

Further into the entry, the generic name is followed by an alphabetized list of its brand names. A brand name followed by an open diamond (◊) indicates an OTC drug. Canadian brands are designated with a dagger (†); and Australian brands are followed by a double dagger (‡). Brand names that appear in the Photoguide to Tablets and Capsules are highlighted with a capsule symbol (💊). A brand name with no symbol is available in the United States, Canada, and possibly Australia. The mention of a brand name in no way implies endorsement of that product or guarantees its legality.

Available forms

This section lists the preparations available for each drug (for example, tablets, capsules, solutions for injection) and specifies available dosage forms and strengths. Dosage strengths specifically available in Canada are designated with a dagger (†), and those in Australia with a double dagger (‡). Preparations that don't require a prescription are marked with an open diamond (◊).

Indications & dosages

This section lists general dosage information for adults, children, and elderly patients. Dosage instructions reflect current trends in therapeutics and can't be considered absolute or universal. For individual patients, dosage instructions must be considered in light of the patient's condition.

Indications for dosages that aren't approved by the FDA are followed by a closed diamond (♦). The logo for "Adjust-a-dose" indicates dosage adjustments for certain patients, such as those with renal impairment.

I.V. administration

This section provides guidelines for reconstituting and mixing I.V. drugs, giving them safely, and storing them properly.

Incompatibilities

This new section lists drugs incompatible with the I.V. solution being discussed, detailing all of the known information.

Action

This section succinctly describes the mechanism of action—that is, how the drug provides its therapeutic effect. For example, although all antihypertensives lower blood pressure, they don't all do so by the same process.

Also included, in table form, are the onset, peak (described in terms of effect or peak blood level), and duration of drug action for each route of administration, if data are available or applicable. Values listed are for patients with normal renal function, unless specified otherwise.

Adverse reactions

This section lists adverse reactions to each drug by body system. The most common adverse reactions (those experienced by at least 10% of people taking the drug in clinical trials) appear in *italic* type; less common reactions are in roman type; life-threatening reactions are in ***bold italic*** type; and reactions that are common *and* life-threatening are in **BOLD CAPITAL LETTERS.**

Interactions

This section lists each drug's confirmed, clinically significant interactions with other drugs (additive effects, potentiated effects, and antagonistic effects); herbs; foods; beverages; and lifestyle behaviors. Rapid-onset interactions are highlighted in color in this section.

Drug interactions are listed under the drug that is adversely affected. For example, because magnesium trisilicate, an antacid ingredient, interacts with tetracycline to decrease tetracycline absorption, this interaction is listed under tetracycline. To check on the possible effects of using two or more drugs simultaneously, refer to the interaction entry for each drug in question.

Effects on lab test results

This section lists increased and decreased levels, counts, and other values in laboratory test results, which may be caused by the drug's systemic effects. It also indicates false-positive, false-negative, and otherwise altered results of laboratory tests a drug may cause.

Contraindications & cautions

This section lists any conditions, especially diseases, in which the use of the drug is undesirable, as well as those for which the drug should be given with caution.

Nursing considerations

This section provides information useful to nurses, such as monitoring techniques and suggestions for prevention and treatment of adverse reactions. Also included are suggestions for ensuring patient comfort and for preparing, giving, and storing the drug.

An "Alert" logo gives important advice about life-threatening effects of the drug and its administration.

A special "lookalike–soundalike" alert provides infomation to avoid medication errors that may occur when drug names that sound or look alike are confused.

Patient teaching

This section gives the nurse guidelines on teaching the patient about each drug. It includes instructions for explaining the drug's purpose, promoting compliance, ensuring proper use and storage of the drug, and preventing or minimizing adverse reactions.

Photoguide to tablets and capsules

To make drug identification easier and to enhance patient safety, *Nursing2008 Drug Handbook* offers a 32-page full-color photoguide to the most commonly prescribed tablets and capsules. Shown in actual size, the drugs are arranged alphabetically for quick reference, along with their most common dosage strengths. Below the name of each drug, you'll find a cross-reference to information on the drug. Brand names of drugs that appear in the photoguide are shown in the text with a special capsule symbol (💊). Page references to the drug photos appear in boldface type in the index (for example, **C12**).

Guide to abbreviations

ACE	angiotensin-converting enzyme
ADH	antidiuretic hormone
AIDS	acquired immunodeficiency syndrome
ALT	alanine transaminase
AST	aspartate transaminase
AV	atrioventricular
b.i.d.	twice daily
BPH	benign prostatic hypertrophy
BSA	body surface area
BUN	blood urea nitrogen
cAMP	cyclic 3′, 5′ adenosine monophosphate
CBC	complete blood count
CK	creatine kinase
CMV	cytomegalovirus
CNS	central nervous system
COPD	chronic obstructive pulmonary disease
CSF	cerebrospinal fluid
CV	cardiovascular
D_5W	dextrose 5% in water
DIC	disseminated intravascular coagulation
dl	deciliter
DNA	deoxyribonucleic acid
ECG	electrocardiogram
EEG	electroencephalogram
EENT	eyes, ears, nose, throat
FDA	Food and Drug Administration
g	gram
G	gauge
GABA	gamma-aminobutyric acid
GFR	glomerular filtration rate
GGT	gamma-glutamyltransferase
GI	gastrointestinal
gtt	drops
GU	genitourinary
G6PD	glucose-6-phosphate dehydrogenase
H_1	histamine_1
H_2	histamine_2
HDL	high-density lipoprotein
HIV	human immunodeficiency virus
HMG-CoA	3-hydroxy-3-methylglutaryl coenzyme A
I.D.	intradermal
I.M.	intramuscular
INR	International Normalized Ratio
IPPB	intermittent positive-pressure breathing
I.V.	intravenous
kg	kilogram
L	liter
lb	pound
LDH	lactate dehydrogenase
LDL	low-density lipoprotein
M	molar
m^2	square meter
MAO	monoamine oxidase
mcg	microgram
mEq	milliequivalent
mg	milligram
MI	myocardial infarction
min	minute
ml	milliliter
mm^3	cubic millimeter
mo	month

msec	millisecond
NSAID	nonsteroidal anti-inflammatory drug
OTC	over-the-counter
PABA	para-aminobenzoic acid
PCA	patient-controlled analgesia
P.O.	by mouth
P.R.	by rectum
p.r.n.	as needed
PT	prothrombin time
PTT	partial thromboplastin time
PVC	premature ventricular contraction
q	every
q.i.d.	four times daily
RBC	red blood cell
RDA	recommended daily allowance
REM	rapid eye movement
RNA	ribonucleic acid
RSV	respiratory syncytial virus
SA	sinoatrial
SubQ	subcutaneous
sec	second
SIADH	syndrome of inappropriate antidiuretic hormone
S.L.	sublingual
SSRI	selective serotonin reuptake inhibitor
T_3	triiodothyronine
T_4	thyroxine
t.i.d.	three times daily
tsp	teaspoon
USP	United States Pharmacopeia
UTI	urinary tract infection
WBC	white blood cell
wk	week

1

Drug actions, interactions, and reactions

Any drug a patient takes causes a series of physical and chemical events in his body. The first event, when a drug combines with cellular drug receptors, is the drug action. What happens next is the drug effect. Depending on the type of cellular drug receptors affected by a given drug, an effect can be local, systemic, or both. A systemic drug effect can follow a local effect. For example, when you apply a drug to the skin, it causes a local effect. But transdermal absorption of that drug can then produce a systemic effect. A local effect can also follow systemic absorption. For example, the peptic ulcer drug cimetidine produces a local effect after it's swallowed by blocking histamine receptors in the stomach's parietal cells. Diphenhydramine, on the other hand, causes a systemic effect by blocking histamine receptors throughout the body.

Drug properties

Drug absorption, distribution, metabolism, and excretion make up a drug's pharmacokinetics. These parts also describe a drug's onset of action, peak level, duration of action, and bioavailability.

Absorption

Before a drug can act in the body, it must be absorbed into the bloodstream—usually after oral administration, the most common route. Before an oral drug can be absorbed, it must disintegrate into particles small enough to dissolve in gastric juices. Only after dissolving can the drug be absorbed. Most absorption of orally given drugs occurs in the small intestine because the mucosal villi provide extensive surface area. Once absorbed and circulated in the bloodstream, the drug is bioavailable, or ready to produce a drug effect. The speed of absorption and whether absorption is complete or partial depend on the drug's effects, dosage form, administration route, interactions with other substances in the GI tract, and various patient characteristics. Oral solutions and elixirs bypass the need for disintegration and dissolution and are usually absorbed faster. Some tablets have enteric coatings to prevent disintegration in the acidic environment of the stomach; others have coatings of varying thickness that simply delay release of the drug.

Drugs given I.M. must first be absorbed through the muscle into the bloodstream. Rectal suppositories must dissolve to be absorbed through the rectal mucosa. Drugs given I.V. are injected directly into the bloodstream and are bioavailable completely and immediately.

Distribution

After absorption, a drug moves from the bloodstream into the fluids and tissues in the body, a movement known as distribution. All of the area to which a drug is distributed is known as volume of distribution. Individual patient variations can change the amount of drug distributed throughout the body. For example, in an edematous patient, a given dose must be distributed to a larger volume than in a nonedematous patient. Occasionally, a dose is increased to account for this difference. In this case, the dose should be decreased after the edema is corrected. Conversely, a dose given to a dehydrated patient must be decreased to allow for its distribution to a much smaller volume. Patients who are very obese may present another problem when considering drug distribution. Some drugs—such as digoxin, gentamicin, and tobramycin—aren't well-distributed to fatty tissue. Sometimes, doses based on actual body weight may lead to overdose and serious toxicity. In these cases, doses must be based on lean body weight, or adjusted body weight, which may be estimated from actuarial tables that give average weight range for height.

Metabolism

Most drugs are metabolized in the liver. Hepatic diseases may affect the liver's metabolic functions and may increase or decrease a drug's usual metabolism.

Closely monitor all patients with hepatic disease for drug effect and toxicity.

The rate at which a drug is metabolized varies from person to person. Some patients metabolize drugs so quickly that the drug levels in their blood and tissues prove therapeutically inadequate. In other patients, the rate of metabolism is so slow that ordinary doses can produce toxicity.

Excretion

The body eliminates drugs by metabolism (usually hepatic) and excretion (usually renal). Drug excretion is the movement of a drug or its metabolites from the tissues back into circulation and from the circulation into the organs of excretion, where they're removed from the body. Most drugs are excreted by the kidneys, but some can be eliminated through the lungs, exocrine glands (sweat, salivary, or mammary), liver, skin, and intestinal tract. Drugs also may be removed artificially by direct mechanical intervention, such as peritoneal dialysis or hemodialysis.

Other modifying factors

One important factor influencing a drug's action and effect is its tendency to bind to plasma proteins, especially albumin, and other tissue components. Because only a free, unbound drug can act in the body, protein binding greatly influences the amount and duration of effect. Malnutrition, renal failure, and other protein-bound drugs can influence protein binding. When protein binding changes, the drug dose may need to be changed also.

The patient's age is another important factor. Elderly patients usually have decreased hepatic function, less muscle mass, diminished renal function, and lower albumin levels. These patients need lower doses and sometimes longer dosage intervals to avoid toxicity. Neonates have underdeveloped metabolic enzyme systems and inadequate renal function, so they need highly individualized dosages and careful monitoring.

Underlying disease also may affect drug action and effect. For example, acidosis may cause insulin resistance. Genetic diseases, such as G6PD deficiency and hepatic porphyria, may turn drugs into toxins, with serious consequences. Patients with G6PD deficiency may develop hemolytic anemia when given certain drugs, such as sulfonamides. A genetically susceptible patient can develop acute porphyria if given a barbiturate. A patient with a highly active hepatic enzyme system, such as a rapid acetylator, can develop hepatitis when treated with isoniazid because of the quick intrahepatic buildup of a toxic metabolite.

Drug administration issues

How a drug is given can also influence a drug's action in the body. The dosage form of a drug is important. Some tablets and capsules are too large to be easily swallowed by sick patients. An oral solution may be substituted, but it will produce higher drug levels than a tablet because the liquid is more easily and completely absorbed. When a potentially toxic drug (such as digoxin) is given, its increased absorption can cause toxicity. Sometimes a change in dosage form also requires a change in dosage.

Routes of administration aren't interchangeable. For example, diazepam is readily absorbed P.O. but is slowly and erratically absorbed I.M. On the other hand, gentamicin must be given parenterally because oral administration results in drug levels too low for systemic infections.

Improper storage can alter a drug's potency. Store most drugs in tight containers protected from direct sunlight and extremes in temperature and humidity that can cause them to deteriorate. Some drugs require special storage conditions, such as refrigeration. Caution patients not to store drugs in a bathroom because of the constantly changing environment.

The timing of drug administration can be important. Sometimes, giving an oral drug during or shortly after a meal decreases the amount of drug absorbed. In most drugs, this isn't significant and may even be desirable with irritating drugs such as aspirin. But penicillins and tetracyclines shouldn't be taken at mealtimes because certain foods can inactivate them. If in doubt about the effect of food on a certain drug, check with a pharmacist.

Consider the patient's age, height, and weight. The prescriber will need this information when calculating the dosage for many drugs. Record all information accurately on the patient's chart. The chart should also include all current laboratory data, especially renal and liver function studies, so the prescriber can adjust the dosage as needed.

Watch for metabolic changes and physiologic changes (depressed respiratory function, acidosis, or alkalosis) that might alter drug effect.

Know the patient's medical history. Whenever possible, obtain a comprehensive family history from the patient or his family. Ask about past reactions to drugs, possible genetic traits that might affect drug response, and the current use of other drugs, herbal remedies, and vitamin supplements. Multiple drug therapies can cause serious and fatal drug interactions and dramatically change many drugs' effects.

Drug interactions

A drug interaction occurs when a drug given with or shortly after another drug alters the effect of either or both drugs. Usually the effect of one drug is increased or decreased. For instance, one drug may inhibit or stimulate the metabolism or excretion of the other or free it for further action by releasing the drug from protein-binding sites.

Combination therapy is based on drug interaction. One drug may be given to complement the effects of another. Probenecid, which blocks the excretion of penicillin, is sometimes given with penicillin to maintain an adequate level of penicillin for a longer time. In many cases, two drugs with similar actions are given together precisely because of the additive effect. For instance, aspirin and codeine are commonly given in combination because together they provide greater pain relief than if either is given alone.

Drug interactions are sometimes used to prevent or antagonize certain adverse reactions. The diuretics hydrochlorothiazide and spironolactone are often given together because the former is potassium-depleting and the latter potassium-sparing.

Not all drug interactions are beneficial: many drugs interact and decrease efficacy or increase toxicity. An example of decreased efficacy occurs when a tetracycline is given with drugs or foods that contain calcium or magnesium (such as antacids or milk). These bind with tetracycline in the GI tract and cause inadequate drug absorption. An example of increased toxicity can be seen in a patient taking a diuretic and lithium. The diuretic may increase the lithium level, causing lithium toxicity. This drug effect is known as *antagonism*. Avoid drug combinations that produce these effects, if possible.

Adverse reactions

Drugs cause adverse *effects*; patients have adverse *reactions*. An adverse reaction may be tolerated to obtain a therapeutic effect, or it may be hazardous and unacceptable. Some adverse reactions subside with continued use. For example, the drowsiness caused by paroxetine and the orthostatic hypotension caused by prazosin usually subside after several days when the patient develops tolerance. But many adverse reactions are dosage related and lessen or disappear only if the dosage is reduced. Most adverse reactions aren't therapeutically desirable, but a few can be put to clinical use. An outstanding example of this is the drowsiness caused by diphenhydramine, which makes it useful as a mild sedative.

Drug hypersensitivity, or drug allergy, is the result of an antigen–antibody immune reaction that occurs in the body when a drug is given to a susceptible patient. One of the most dangerous of all drug hypersensitivities is penicillin allergy. In its most severe form, penicillin anaphylaxis can rapidly become fatal.

Rarely, idiosyncratic reactions occur. These reactions are highly unpredictable and unusual. One of the best-known idiosyncratic adverse reactions is aplastic anemia caused by the antibiotic chloramphenicol. This reaction appears in only 1 of 40,000 patients, but when it does occur, it can be fatal. A more common idiosyncratic reaction is extreme sensitivity to very low doses of a drug or insensitivity to higher-than-normal doses.

To deal with adverse reactions correctly, you need to be alert to even minor changes in the patient's clinical status. Such minor changes may be an early warning of pending toxicity. Listen to the patient's complaints about his reactions to a drug, and consider each objectively. You may be able to reduce adverse reactions in several ways. Obviously, dosage reduction can help. But, in many cases, so does a simple rescheduling of the dose. For example, pseudoephedrine may produce stimulation that will be no problem if it's given early in the day. Similarly, drowsiness from antihistamines or tranquilizers can be harmless if these drugs are given at bedtime. Most important, your patient needs to be told which adverse reactions to expect so that he won't become worried or even stop taking the drug on his own. Always advise the patient to report adverse reactions to the prescriber immediately.

Your ability to recognize signs and symptoms of drug allergies or serious idiosyncratic reactions may save your patient's life. Ask each patient about the drugs he's taking currently or has taken in the past and whether he experienced any unusual reactions from taking them. If a patient claims to be allergic to a drug, ask him to tell you exactly what happens when he takes it. He may be calling a harmless adverse reaction, such as upset stomach, an allergic reaction, or he may have a true tendency toward anaphylaxis. In either case, you and the prescriber need to know this. Of course, you must record and report clinical changes throughout the patient's hospital stay. If you suspect a severe adverse reaction, withhold the drug until you can check with the pharmacist and the prescriber.

Toxic reactions

Chronic drug toxicities are usually caused by the cumulative effect and resulting buildup of the drug in the body. These effects may be extensions of the desired therapeutic effect. For example, normal doses of glyburide normalize the glucose level, but higher doses can produce hypoglycemia.

Drug toxicities occur when a drug level rises as a result of impaired metabolism or excretion. For example, hepatic dysfunction impairs the metabolism of theophylline, raising its levels. Similarly, renal dysfunction may cause digoxin toxicity because this drug is eliminated from the body by the kidneys. Of course, excessive dosage can cause toxic levels also. For instance, tinnitus is usually a sign that the safe dose of aspirin has been exceeded.

Most drug toxicities are predictable, dosage-related, and reversible upon dosage adjustment. So, monitor patients carefully for physiologic changes that might alter drug effect. Watch especially for hepatic and renal impairment. Warn the patient about signs of pending toxicity, and tell him what to do if a toxic reaction occurs. Also, make sure to emphasize the importance of taking a drug exactly as prescribed. Warn the patient that serious problems could arise if he changes the dose or schedule or stops taking the drug without his prescriber's knowledge.

2

Drug therapy across the lifespan

Drug therapy is a fact of life for millions of people of all ages, and certain aspects of a patient's life, such as age, growth, and development, can affect drug therapy.

Drugs and pregnancy

Drug administration during pregnancy has been a source of serious medical concern and controversy since the thalidomide tragedy of the late 1950s, when thousands of malformed infants were born after their mothers were given this mild sedative–hypnotic while pregnant. To identify drugs that may cause such teratogenic effects, preclinical drug studies always include tests on pregnant laboratory animals. These studies may reveal gross teratogenicity but don't establish absolute safety. This is because different animal species react to drugs in different ways. Consequently, animal studies can't reveal all possible teratogenic effects in humans. For example, the preliminary studies on thalidomide gave no warning of teratogenic effects, and it was subsequently released for general use in Europe.

What about the placental barrier? Once thought to protect the fetus from drug effects, the placenta isn't much of a barrier at all. Almost every drug a pregnant woman takes crosses the placenta and enters the fetal circulation, except for drugs with exceptionally large molecular structure, such as heparin, the injectable anticoagulant. By this standard, heparin could be used in a pregnant woman without fear of harming the fetus, but even heparin carries a warning for cautious use during pregnancy. Conversely, just because a drug crosses the placenta doesn't necessarily mean it's harmful to the fetus. The relative risk to the fetus is expressed by the drug's pregnancy risk category.

Actually, only one factor—stage of fetal development—seems clearly related to greater risk during pregnancy. During the first and third trimesters of pregnancy, the fetus is especially vulnerable to damage from maternal use of drugs. During these times, give *all* drugs with extreme caution.

Organogenesis—when fetal organs differentiate—occurs in the first trimester. This is the most sensitive period for drug-induced fetal malformation. Withhold all drugs except those in category A or B during this time, unless this would jeopardize the mother's health. Strongly advise your patient to avoid *all* self-prescribed drugs during early pregnancy.

Fetal sensitivity to drugs is also of special concern during the last trimester. At birth, when separated from his mother, the neonate must rely on his own metabolism to eliminate any remaining drug. Because his detoxifying systems aren't fully developed, any residual drug may take a long time to be metabolized, and thus may induce prolonged toxic reactions. For this reason, discourage pregnant patients from taking drugs except when absolutely necessary during the last 3 months of pregnancy.

Of course, in many circumstances, pregnant women must continue to take certain drugs. For example, a woman with a seizure disorder that is well-controlled with an anticonvulsant should keep taking the drug during pregnancy. Similarly, a pregnant woman with a bacterial infection must receive antibiotics. In such cases, the potential risk to the fetus is outweighed by the mother's medical needs.

Complying with these general guidelines can prevent indiscriminate and harmful use of drugs in pregnancy:

- Before a drug is prescribed for a woman of childbearing age, ask the date of her last menstrual period and whether she may be pregnant. If a drug is a known teratogen (for example, isotretinoin), some manufacturers may recommend special precautions to ensure that the drug isn't given to a woman of childbearing age until pregnancy is ruled out and that contraceptives are used throughout the course of therapy.
- Caution a pregnant woman to avoid all drugs except those essential to maintain

her pregnancy or health—especially during the first and third trimesters.

- Topical drugs are subject to the same warning against use during pregnancy. Many topically applied drugs can be absorbed in large enough amounts to be harmful to the fetus.
- When a pregnant woman needs a drug, use the safest drug in the lowest possible dose to minimize harm to the fetus.
- Instruct a pregnant woman to check with her prescriber before taking any drug.

Drugs and breast-feeding

Most drugs a breast-feeding mother takes appear in breast milk. Drug levels in breast milk tend to be high when drug levels in maternal blood are high, especially right after each dose. Advise the mother to breast-feed *before* taking each drug dose, not *after.*

A mother who wants to breast-feed usually may continue to do so with her prescriber's advice. However, breast-feeding should be temporarily interrupted and replaced with bottle-feeding when the mother must take tetracycline, chloramphenicol, a sulfonamide (during the first 2 weeks postpartum), an oral anticoagulant, a drug that contains iodine, or an antineoplastic.

Caution the breast-feeding patient to protect her infant by not taking drugs indiscriminately. Instruct the mother to first check with her prescriber to be sure she's taking the safest drug at the lowest dose. Also instruct her to give her prescriber a list of all drugs and herbs she's currently taking.

Drug therapy in children

Providing drug therapy to infants, children, and adolescents is challenging. Physiologic differences between children and adults, including those in vital organ maturity and body composition, significantly influence a drug's effectiveness.

Physiologic changes affecting drug action

A child's absorption, distribution (including drug binding to plasma proteins), metabolism, and excretion processes undergo profound changes that affect drug dosage. To ensure optimal drug effect and minimal toxicity, consider these factors when giving drugs to a child.

Absorption

Drug absorption in children depends on the form of the drug, its physical properties, simultaneous ingestion of other drugs or food, physiologic changes, and concurrent disease.

The pH of neonatal gastric fluid is neutral or slightly acidic; it becomes more acidic as the infant matures, which affects drug absorption. For example, nafcillin and penicillin G are better absorbed in an infant than in an adult because of low gastric acidity.

Various infant formulas or milk products may increase gastric pH and impede absorption of acidic drugs. If possible, give a child oral drugs on an empty stomach.

Gastric emptying time and transit time through the small intestine—which takes longer in children than in adults—can affect absorption. Also, intestinal hypermotility (as occurs in patients with diarrhea) can diminish the drug's absorption.

A child's comparatively thin epidermis allows increased absorption of topical drugs.

Distribution

As with absorption, changes in body weight and physiology during childhood can significantly influence a drug's distribution and effects. In a premature infant, body fluid makes up about 85% of total body weight; in a full-term infant, it makes up 55% to 70%; in an adult, 50% to 55%. Extracellular fluid (mostly blood) constitutes 40% of a neonate's body weight, compared with 20% in an adult. Intracellular fluid remains fairly constant throughout life and has little effect on drug dosage.

Extracellular fluid volume influences a water-soluble drug's concentration and effect because most drugs travel through extracellular fluid to reach their receptors. Compared with adults, distribution area in children is proportionately greater because their fluid–to–solid body weight proportion is larger.

Because the proportion of fat to lean body mass increases with age, the distribution of fat-soluble drugs is more limited in children than in adults. As a result, a drug's fat or water solubility affects the dosage for a child.

Plasma protein binding

A decrease in albumin level or intermolecular attraction between drug and plasma protein causes many drugs to be less bound to plasma proteins in infants than in adults.

Strongly protein-bound drugs may displace endogenous compounds, such as bilirubin or free fatty acids. Displacement of bound bilirubin can increase unbound bilirubin, which can lead to increased risk of kernicterus at normal bilirubin levels. Conversely, an endogenous compound may displace a weakly bound drug.

Because only an unbound (free) drug has a pharmacologic effect, a change in ratio of a protein-bound to an unbound active drug can greatly influence its effect.

Several diseases and disorders, such as nephrotic syndrome and malnutrition, can decrease plasma protein and increase the level of an unbound drug, which can either intensify the drug's effect or produce toxicity.

Metabolism

A neonate's ability to metabolize a drug depends on the integrity of the hepatic enzyme system, intrauterine exposure to the drug, and the nature of the drug itself.

Certain metabolic mechanisms are underdeveloped in neonates. Glucuronidation is a metabolic process that renders most drugs more water soluble, facilitating renal excretion. This process isn't developed enough to permit full pediatric doses until the infant is age 1 month. The use of chloramphenicol in a neonate may cause gray baby syndrome because the infant's immature liver can't metabolize the drug and toxic levels accumulate in the blood. Reduce dosage in a neonate and periodically monitor his levels.

Conversely, intrauterine exposure to drugs may induce precocious development of hepatic enzyme mechanisms, increasing the infant's capacity to metabolize potentially harmful substances.

Older children can metabolize some drugs (theophylline, for example) more rapidly than adults. This ability may come from their increased hepatic metabolic activity. Doses larger than those recommended for adults may be required.

Also, more than one drug given to a child simultaneously may change the hepatic metabolism and initiate production of hepatic enzymes. Phenobarbital, for example, accelerates the metabolism of drugs taken with it and causes hepatic enzyme production.

Excretion

Renal excretion of a drug is the net result of glomerular filtration, active tubular secretion, and passive tubular reabsorption. Many drugs are excreted in the urine. The degree of renal development or presence of renal disease can greatly affect a child's dosage requirements because if a child can't excrete a drug renally, the drug may accumulate to toxic levels.

Physiologically, an infant's kidneys differ from an adult's because infants have a high resistance to blood flow and their kidneys receive a smaller proportion of cardiac output. Infants have incomplete glomerular and tubular development and short, incomplete loops of Henle. (A child's glomerular filtration rate (GFR) reaches an adult value between ages 2½ and 5 months; his tubular secretion rate may reach an adult value between ages 7 and 12 months.) Infants also are less able to concentrate urine or reabsorb certain filtered compounds. The proximal tubules in infants also are less able to secrete organic acids.

Children and adults have diurnal variations in urine pH that correlate with sleep patterns.

Special administration considerations

Biochemically, a drug displays the same mechanisms of action in all people. But the response to a drug can be affected by a child's age and size, as well as by the maturity of the target organ. To ensure optimal drug effect and minimal toxicity, consider the following factors when giving drugs to children.

Adjusting dosages for children

When calculating children's dosages, don't use formulas that just modify adult dosages. Base pediatric dosages on either body weight (mg/kg) or body surface area (mg/m^2). A child isn't a scaled-down version of an adult.

Reevaluate dosages at regular intervals to ensure needed adjustments as the child develops. Although body surface area provides a useful standard for adults and older children, use the body weight method instead in premature or full-term infants. Don't exceed the maximum adult dosage when calculating amounts per kilogram of body weight (except with certain drugs such as theophylline, if indicated).

Obtain an accurate maternal drug history, including prescription and nonprescription drugs, vitamins, herbs, or other health foods taken during pregnancy. Drugs passed into breast milk can have adverse effects on the breast-feeding infant. Before giving a drug to a breast-feeding mother, investigate its potential effects on the infant.

For example, a sulfonamide given to a breast-feeding mother for a UTI appears in breast milk and may cause kernicterus in an infant with low levels of unconjugated bilirubin. Also, high levels of isoniazid appear in the breast milk of a mother taking this drug. Because this drug is metabolized by the liver, the infant's immature hepatic enzyme mechanisms can't metabolize the drug, and he may develop CNS toxicity.

Giving oral drugs

Remember the following when giving oral drugs to a child:

If the patient is an infant, give drugs in liquid form, if possible. For accuracy, measure and give the preparation by oral syringe. It's very important to remove the syringe cap to keep the infant from aspirating it. Be sure to instruct parents to do the same. Never use a vial or cup. Lift the patient's head to prevent aspiration of the drug, and press down on his chin to prevent choking. You may also place the drug in a nipple and allow the infant to suck the contents.

If the patient is a toddler, explain how you're going to give him the drug. If possible, have the parents enlist the child's cooperation. Don't mix the drug with food or call it "candy," even if it has a pleasant taste. Let the child drink liquid drug from a calibrated medication cup rather than a spoon. It's easier and more accurate. If the preparation is available only in tablet form, crush and mix it with syrup. (First, verify with the pharmacist that the tablet can be crushed without compromising its effectiveness.)

If the patient is an older child who can swallow a tablet or capsule by himself, have him place the drug on the back of his tongue and swallow it with water or nonacidic fruit juice, because milk and milk products may interfere with drug absorption.

Giving I.V. infusions

For I.V. infusions, in infants, use a peripheral vein or a scalp vein in the temporal region. The scalp vein is safe because the needle isn't likely to dislodge. However, the head must be shaved around the site, and the needle and infiltrated fluids may cause temporary disfigurement. For these reasons, scalp veins aren't used as commonly today as they were in the past.

The arms and legs are the most accessible insertion sites, but because patients tend to move about, take these precautions:

- Protect the insertion site to keep the catheter or needle from being dislodged.
- Use a padded arm board to reduce the risk of dislodgment. Remove the arm board during range-of-motion exercises.
- Place the clamp out of the child's reach. If extension tubing is used to allow the child greater mobility, securely tape the connection.
- Explain in simple terms to the child why he must be restrained while asleep, to alleviate anxiety and maintain trust.

During an infusion, monitor flow rates and check the child's condition and insertion site at least every hour. Titrate the flow rate only while the patient is composed; crying and emotional upset can constrict blood vessels. Flow rate may vary if a pump isn't used. Flow should be adequate because some drugs (calcium, for example) can be irritating at low flow rates. Infants, small children, and children with compromised cardiopulmonary status are especially vulnerable to fluid overload with I.V. drug administration. To prevent this problem and help ensure that a limited amount of fluid is infused in a controlled manner, use a volume-control device in the I.V. tubing and an infusion pump or a syringe. Don't place more than 2 hours of I.V. fluid in the volume-control set at a time.

Giving I.M. injections

I.M. injections are preferred when a drug can't be given by other parenteral routes and rapid absorption is needed.

The vastus lateralis muscle is the preferred injection site in children younger than age 2. The ventrogluteal area or gluteus medius muscle can be used in older children. To select the correct needle size, consider the patient's age, muscle mass, nutritional status, and drug viscosity.

Record and rotate injection sites. Explain to the patient that the injection will hurt but that the drug will help him. Restrain him during the injection, if needed, and comfort him afterward.

Giving topical drugs and inhalants

When you give a child a topical drug or inhalant, consider the following:

Use eardrops warmed to room temperature. Cold drops can cause pain and vertigo. To give drops, turn the patient on his side, with the affected ear up. If he's younger than age 3, pull the pinna down and back; if age 3 or older, pull the pinna up and back.

Avoid using inhalants in young children because it's difficult to get them to cooperate. Before you try to give a drug to an older child through a metered-dose nebulizer, explain the inhaler to him. Then have him hold the nebulizer upside down and close his lips around the mouthpiece. Have him exhale and pinch his nostrils shut. When he starts to inhale, release one dose of the drug into his mouth. Tell the patient to continue inhaling until his lungs feel full; then he can breathe normally and unpinch his nostrils. Most inhaled drugs aren't useful if taken orally—if you doubt the patient's ability to use the inhalant correctly, don't use it. Such devices as spacers or assist devices may help. Check with a pharmacist, the prescriber, or a respiratory therapist.

Use topical corticosteroids cautiously because prolonged use in children may delay growth. When you apply topical corticosteroids to the diaper area of infants, don't cover the area with plastic or rubber pants, which act as an occlusive dressing and may enhance systemic absorption.

Giving parenteral nutrition

Give I.V. nutrition to patients who can't or won't take adequate food orally and to patients with hypermetabolic conditions who need supplementation. The latter group includes premature infants and children with burns or other major trauma, intractable diarrhea, malabsorption syndromes, GI abnormalities, emotional disorders (such as anorexia nervosa), and congenital abnormalities.

Before giving fat emulsions to infants and children, weigh the potential benefits against any possible risks. Fats—supplied as 10% or 20% emulsions—are given both peripherally and centrally. Their use is limited by the child's ability to metabolize them. For example, an infant or child with a diseased liver can't efficiently metabolize fats.

Some fats, however, must be supplied both to prevent essential fatty acid deficiency and to permit normal growth and development. A minimum of calories (2% to 4%) must be supplied as linoleic acid—an essential fatty acid found in lipids. In infants, fats are essential for normal neurologic development.

Nevertheless, fat solutions may decrease oxygen perfusion and may adversely affect children with pulmonary disease. This risk can be minimized by supplying only the minimum fat needed for essential fatty acid requirements and not the usual intake of 40% to 50% of the child's total calories.

Fatty acids can also displace bilirubin bound to albumin, causing a rise in free, unconjugated bilirubin and an increased risk of kernicterus. But fat solutions may interfere with some bilirubin assays and cause falsely elevated levels. To avoid this complication, draw a blood sample 4 hours after infusion of the lipid emulsion; or if the emulsion is introduced over 24 hours, centrifuge the blood sample before the assay is performed.

Drug therapy in elderly patients

If you're giving drugs to elderly patients, you'll need to understand the physiologic and pharmacokinetic changes that may affect drug dosage, cause common adverse reactions, or create compliance problems.

Physiologic changes affecting drug action

As a person ages, gradual physiologic changes occur. Some of these age-related changes may alter the therapeutic and toxic effects of drugs.

Body composition

Proportions of fat, lean tissue, and water in the body change with age. Total body mass and lean body mass tend to decrease, but the proportion of body fat tends to increase.

Body composition varies from person to person, and these changes in body composition affect the relationship between a drug's concentration and distribution in the body.

For example, a water-soluble drug such as gentamicin isn't distributed to fat. Because there's relatively less lean tissue in an elderly person, more drug remains in the blood.

Gastrointestinal function

In elderly patients, decreases in gastric acid secretion and GI motility slow the emptying of stomach contents and movement through the entire intestinal tract. Also, research suggests that elderly patients may have more difficulty absorbing drugs than younger patients. This is an especially significant problem with drugs that have a narrow therapeutic range, such as digoxin, in which any change in absorption can be crucial.

Hepatic function

The liver's ability to metabolize certain drugs decreases with age. This decrease is caused by diminished blood flow to the liver, which results from an age-related decrease in cardiac output, and from the lessened activity of certain liver enzymes. When an elderly patient takes a sleep medication such as flurazepam, for example, the liver's reduced ability to metabolize the drug can produce a hangover effect the next morning.

Decreased hepatic function may result in more intense drug effects caused by higher levels, longer-lasting drug effects because of prolonged levels, and a greater risk of drug toxicity.

Renal function

An elderly person's renal function is usually sufficient to eliminate excess body fluid and waste, but the ability to eliminate some drugs may be reduced by 50% or more.

Many drugs commonly used by elderly patients, such as digoxin, are excreted primarily through the kidneys. If the kidneys' ability to excrete the drug is decreased, high blood levels may result. Digoxin toxicity can be relatively common in elderly patients who don't receive a reduced digoxin dosage to accommodate decreased renal function.

Drug dosages can be modified to compensate for age-related decreases in renal function. Aided by results of laboratory tests, such as BUN and creatinine levels, adjust drug dosages so the patient receives therapeutic benefits without the risk of toxicity. Also, observe the patient for signs and symptoms of toxicity. A patient taking digoxin, for example, may experience anorexia, nausea, vomiting, or confusion.

Special administration considerations

Aging is usually accompanied by a decline in organ function that can affect drug distribution and clearance. This physiologic decline is likely to be worsened by a disease or a chronic disorder. Together, these factors can significantly increase the risk of adverse reactions and drug toxicity, as well as noncompliance.

Adverse reactions

Compared with younger people, elderly patients experience twice as many adverse drug reactions, mostly from greater drug use, poor compliance, and physiologic changes.

Signs and symptoms of adverse drug reactions—confusion, weakness, agitation, and lethargy—are often mistakenly attributed to senility or disease. If the adverse reaction isn't identified, the patient may continue to receive the drug. He may receive other, unnecessary drugs to treat complications caused by the original drug. This regimen can sometimes result in a pattern of inappropriate and excessive drug use.

Any drug can cause adverse reactions, but most of the serious reactions in the elderly are caused by relatively few drugs. Be particularly alert for toxicities resulting from diuretics, antihypertensives, digoxin, corticosteroids, anticoagulants, sleeping aids, and OTC drugs.

Diuretic toxicity

Because total body water content decreases with age, a normal dosage of a potassium-wasting diuretic, such as hydrochlorothiazide or furosemide, may result in fluid loss and even dehydration in an elderly patient.

These diuretics may deplete a patient's potassium level, making him feel weak, and they may raise blood uric acid and glucose levels, complicating gout and diabetes mellitus.

Antihypertensive toxicity

Many elderly patients experience lightheadedness or fainting when taking antihypertensives, partly in response to atherosclerosis and decreased elasticity of the blood vessels. Antihypertensives can lower blood pressure too rapidly, resulting in insufficient blood flow to the brain, which can cause dizziness, fainting, or even a stroke.

Consequently, dosages of antihypertensives must be carefully individualized. In elderly patients, aggressive treatment of high blood pressure may be harmful. Treatment goals should be reasonable. Reducing blood pressure to 135/90 mm Hg needs to be done more slowly in elderly patients.

Digoxin toxicity

As the body's renal function and rate of excretion decline, the digoxin level in the blood of an elderly patient may increase to the point of causing nausea, vomiting, diarrhea, and, most seriously, cardiac arrhythmias. Monitor the patient's digoxin level and observe him for early signs and symptoms of inotropic toxicity, such as appetite loss, confusion, or depression.

Corticosteroid toxicity

Elderly patients taking a corticosteroid may experience short-term effects, including fluid retention and psychological effects ranging from mild euphoria to acute psychotic reactions. Long-term toxic effects, such as osteoporosis, can be especially severe in elderly patients who have been taking prednisone or related steroidal compounds for months or even years. To prevent serious toxicity, carefully monitor patients on long-term regimens. Observe them for subtle changes in appearance, mood, and mobility; for impaired healing; and for fluid and electrolyte disturbances.

Anticoagulant effects

Elderly patients taking an anticoagulant have an increased risk of bleeding, especially when they take NSAIDs at the same time, which is common. They're also at increased risk of bleeding and bruising because they are more likely to fall. Observe the patient's INR carefully, and monitor him for bruising and other signs of bleeding.

Sleeping aid toxicity

Sedatives and sleeping aids such as flurazepam may cause excessive sedation or drowsiness. Keep in mind that consuming alcohol may increase depressant effects, even if the sleeping aid was taken the previous evening. Use these drugs sparingly in elderly patients.

Over-the-counter drug toxicity

Toxicity is minimal when aspirin, aspirin-containing analgesics, and other OTC NSAIDs (such as ibuprofen, ketoprofen, and naproxen) are used in moderation. But prolonged ingestion may cause GI irritation—even ulcers—and gradual blood loss resulting in severe anemia. Prescription NSAIDs may cause similar problems. Anemia from prolonged aspirin consumption can affect all age groups, but elderly patients may be less able to compensate because of their already reduced iron stores.

Laxatives may cause diarrhea in elderly patients, who are extremely sensitive to drugs such as bisacodyl. Long-term oral use of mineral oil as a lubricating laxative may result in lipid pneumonia from aspiration of small residual oil droplets in the patient's mouth.

Noncompliance

Poor compliance can be a problem with patients of any age. Many hospitalizations result from noncompliance with a medical regimen. In elderly patients, factors linked to aging, such as diminished visual acuity, hearing loss, forgetfulness, the need for multiple drug therapy, and socioeconomic factors, can combine to make compliance a special problem. About one-third of elderly patients fail to comply with their prescribed drug therapy. They may fail to take prescribed doses or to follow the correct schedule. They may take drugs prescribed for previous disorders, stop drugs prematurely, or indiscriminately use drugs that are to be taken as needed. Elderly patients may also have multiple prescriptions for the same drug and inadvertently take an overdose.

Review the patient's drug regimen with him. Make sure he understands the dose amount, the time and frequency of doses, and why he's taking the drug. Also, explain in detail if a drug is to be taken with food, water, or separate from other drugs.

Help the patient avoid drug therapy problems by suggesting that he use drug calendars, pill sorters, or other aids to help him comply. Refer him to the prescriber, a pharmacist, or social services if he needs further information or assistance with his drug therapy.

3
Safe drug administration

In the state where you practice nursing, a number of different health care professionals, including doctors, nurse practitioners, dentists, podiatrists, and optometrists, may be legally permitted to prescribe, dispense, and give drugs. Most often, however, doctors prescribe drugs, pharmacists dispense them, and nurses give them.

That means you're almost always on the front line when it comes to patients and their drugs. It also means you bear a major share of the responsibility for avoiding drug errors. Besides following your institution's administration policies, you can help prevent drug mistakes by reviewing the common errors outlined below and ways to prevent them.

Also included in this chapter is a section on important points to teach your patients so they may take their drugs safely at home.

Drug orders

Prescribing and filling drug orders must be done carefully to avoid potential problems.

Pharmacy computer systems

Error: The Institute for Safe Medication Practices (ISMP) performed a field test on 307 pharmacy computer systems; only four detected all of the unsafe orders. Many didn't detect potentially lethal orders, including doses that exceeded safe limits, drug ingredient duplications, and orders to give oral solutions I.V.
Best practice or prevention: Don't rely on the pharmacy computer system to detect all unsafe orders. Before you give a drug, understand the correct dosage, indications, and adverse effects. If necessary, check a current drug reference guide.

Confusing drug names

Error: According to the USP, insulin was the drug most often involved in medication errors in 2003. One type of error stems from name confusion. For instance, Lantus (insulin glargine [rDNA origin]) may easily be confused with Lente insulin. This mix-up could happen with either a verbal or written order.
Best practice or prevention: Be aware of the drugs your patient takes regularly, and question any deviations from his regular routine. As with any drug, take your time and read the label carefully.

Abbreviations

Error: Abbreviating drug names is risky. A cancer patient with anemia may receive epoetin alfa, commonly abbreviated EPO, to stimulate RBC production. In one case, when a cancer patient was admitted to a hospital, the doctor wrote, "May take own supply of EPO." But the patient wasn't anemic. Sensing that something was wrong, the pharmacist interviewed the patient, who confirmed that he was taking "EPO"—evening primrose oil—to lower his cholesterol level.
Best practice or prevention: Ask all prescribers to spell out drug names.

Unclear orders

Error: A patient was supposed to receive one dose of the antineoplastic lomustine to treat brain cancer. (Lomustine is typically given as a single oral dose once every 6 weeks.) The doctor's order read "Administer h.s." Because this was misinterpreted to mean every night, the patient received nine daily doses, developed severe thrombocytopenia and leukopenia, and died.
Best practice or prevention: If you're unfamiliar with a drug, check a drug reference before giving it. If a prescriber uses "h.s." but doesn't specify the frequency of administration, clarify the order. When documenting orders, note "h.s. nightly" or "h.s.—one dose today."

Misreading orders

Error: Two reports concerned incorrect use of the tricyclic antidepressant nortriptyline (Pamelor, Aventyl, or, in Australia, Allegron) when ordered for neuropathic pain syndromes. The cases involved

10-mg and 20-mg orders that were misread as 100 mg and 200 mg, respectively. One patient who received an incorrect dose required hospitalization; the other developed sedation and orthostatic hypotension after two doses, which led to recognition of the error.
Best practice or prevention: Nortriptyline and other tricyclic antidepressants aren't prescribed as frequently as they once were. To make sure you're familiar with recommended dosages, refer to a drug handbook and then ask a pharmacist, if necessary.

Misinterpretation of orders

Error: The ISMP reports that insulin orders may be especially prone to misinterpretation. In one case, an order was written as "add 10U of regular insulin to each TPN bag," and the pharmacist preparing the solution misinterpreted the dose as 100 units. In another case, a pharmacy technician entering orders misinterpreted a sliding scale when the insulin order used "u" for units, an error that could have caused a tenfold overdose if a nurse hadn't caught it. Yet another report involved a nurse who received a verbal order to resume an insulin drip but wrote "resume heparin drip." Fortunately, the pharmacist caught the error.
Best practice or prevention: Before you give a drug ordered in units, such as insulin or heparin, always check the prescriber's written order against the provided dose. Never abbreviate "units." If you must accept a verbal order, have another nurse listen in; then transcribe that order directly onto an order form and repeat it to ensure that you've transcribed it correctly.

Inadvertent overdose

Error: The inadvertent prescribing of harmful acetaminophen doses has become a disturbing trend. To relieve pain, prescribers may write orders for combined acetaminophen and opioid analgesic tablets (Lortab, Tylox, Darvocet-N) without realizing that the total acetaminophen dose could be toxic.

Consider this order: "Tylox, 1 to 2 tablets every 4 hours, as needed, for pain." By taking the higher dose, the patient would receive 1,000 mg of acetaminophen every 4 hours, exceeding the maximum recommended dose of 4 g/day.
Best practice or prevention: To prevent an acetaminophen overdose from combined analgesics, note the amount of acetaminophen in each drug. Beware of substitutions by the pharmacy because the amount of acetaminophen may vary.

Lipid-based drugs

Error: Serious drug errors, some fatal, have occurred because of confusion between certain lipid-based (liposomal) drugs and their conventional counterparts. The drugs involved include:

- lipid-based amphotericin B (Abelcet, Amphotec, AmBisome) and conventional amphotericin B for injection (available generically and as Amphocin and Fungizone)
- the pegylated liposomal form of doxorubicin (Doxil) and its conventional form, doxorubicin hydrochloride (Adriamycin, Rubex)
- a liposomal form of daunorubicin (DaunoXome, daunorubicin citrate liposomal) and conventional daunorubicin hydrochloride (Cerubidine).

Best practice or prevention: Lipid-based products have different dosages than their conventional counterparts. Check the original order and labels carefully to avoid confusion.

Drug preparation

When preparing to give a drug, be alert for potential problems.

Syringe tip caps and children

Error: A syringe tip cap poses a potential choking hazard to a small child: If you forget to remove the cap from an oral syringe before you give a drug, the cap could blow off into the child's mouth when you press the plunger. If a cap from an oral or a hypodermic syringe gets lost in the linens, the child may find it later and swallow or aspirate it.
Best practice or prevention: Remove and discard the cap in a secure sharps container before you give the drug; don't place it in a trash can where the child may find it later.

Teach parents about the potential danger of syringe tip caps. Tell them to store a capped syringe where children can't reach it and to remove the cap before giving the drug.

Inattentiveness

Error: When a hospital pharmacy received an order for Fludara (fludarabine), a pharmacy technician asked the pharmacist if Navelbine (vinorelbine) was the same as Fludara (both are antineoplastics). The preoccupied pharmacist said "yes." The technician prepared the Navelbine, but labeled it as Fludara. The pharmacist checked the preparation but didn't notice the error, and the patient received the wrong drug.

Best practice or prevention: To prevent errors of this type, the hospital posted tables of antineoplastics and their dosing guidelines in the pharmacy. As an added safeguard, the pharmacy now sends the empty drug vial or box top with the prepared solution for the nurse to double-check before infusing the drug.

Solution color changes

Error: In two cases, alert nurses noticed that antineoplastics prepared in the pharmacy didn't look the way they should.

In the first error, a 6-year-old child was to receive 12 mg of methotrexate intrathecally. In the pharmacy, a 1-g vial was mistakenly selected instead of a 20-mg vial, and the drug was reconstituted with 10 ml of normal saline solution. The vial containing 100 mg/ml was incorrectly labeled as containing 2 mg/ml, and 6 ml of the solution was drawn into a syringe. Although the syringe label indicated 12 mg of drug, the syringe actually contained 600 mg of drug.

When the nurse received the syringe and noted that the drug's color didn't appear right, she returned it to the pharmacy for verification. The pharmacist retrieved the vial used to prepare the dose and drew the remaining solution into another syringe. The solutions in both syringes matched, and no one noticed the vial's 1-g label. The pharmacist concluded that a manufacturing change caused the color difference.

The child received the 600-mg dose and experienced seizures 45 minutes later. A pharmacist responding to the emergency detected the error. The child received an antidote and recovered.

In the second error, a 20-year-old patient with leukemia received mitomycin instead of mitoxantrone. The nurse had questioned the drug's unusual bluish tint, but the pharmacist had assured her that the color difference was the result of a change in manufacturer. Fortunately, the patient didn't suffer any harm.

Best practice or prevention: If a familiar drug has an unfamiliar appearance, find out why. If the pharmacist cites a manufacturing change, ask him to double-check whether he has received verification from the manufacturer. Document the appearance discrepancy, your actions, and the pharmacist's response in the patient record.

Dropper confusion

Error: Ordering drugs such as liquid ferrous sulfate by the dropperful is a dangerous practice. One person might correctly consider the dropper full when the liquid meets the upper calibration mark; another might incorrectly fill the entire length of the dropper. Also, parents giving the drug at home may use a different dropper, which could significantly change the dose given.

Best practice or prevention: Dosing directions for liquid drugs should always be expressed as weight per volume, such as 15 mg/0.6 ml. Verify the correct dose and teach parents to use only the dropper provided. Show them the mark on the dropper that indicates a full dose and ask them to demonstrate the proper technique.

Incorrect allergy history

Error: After a patient was admitted to the hospital, a nurse faxed a list of the patient's allergies to the pharmacy. The pharmacist couldn't read it, so he accessed the files from the patient's previous admission. However, these records didn't reflect an allergy to the anti-infective cefazolin that the patient had recently developed.

A consulting doctor ordered cefazolin, and the pharmacy processed the order. The medication administration record (MAR) generated by the pharmacy's database didn't indicate the allergy, and the nurse didn't know about it either.

The patient received cefazolin and became hypotensive and unresponsive. The nurse immediately notified the doctor and gave the antihistamine diphenhydramine. The patient recovered and was discharged the next day.

Best practice or prevention: Obtain a new allergy history with each admission. If the patient's history must be faxed, name the drugs, note how many are included, and follow the facility's faxing safeguards. If the pharmacy also adheres to strict guidelines, the computer-generated MAR should be accurate.

Drug administration

According to the USP, the number of medication errors caused by administration problems declined almost 10% between 1999 and 2003. However, administration errors are still the most common type of medication error. When you give a drug, be careful to avoid the following potential problems.

Misidentifying patients

Error: Two common errors are inadvertently failing to check the patient's identification and confusing patients with similar names. Using a tactic that helps prevent wrongsite surgery—involving the patient in the identification process—can also help prevent these drug errors.

Best practice or prevention: Urge the patient to clearly state his full name, even without being asked, at admission and before accepting drugs, procedures, or treatments. Teach him to offer his identification bracelet for inspection when anyone arrives with drugs and to insist on having it replaced if it's removed.

Herbal remedies

Error: Surveys suggest that about one-third of Americans use herbs as medicine. Some people take them with conventional drugs; others use them as replacements. Herbs are available without a prescription. Because government quality assurance standards don't apply to herbs' manufacturing and labeling, their ingredients may be misrepresented or contaminated.

Research on the effects of herbs is limited. Because these products may contain a mixture of chemicals, their use carries risks.

Best practice or prevention: Ask the patient about his use of alternative therapies, including herbs, and record your findings in his medical record. Monitor the patient carefully and report unusual events. Ask the patient to keep a diary of all therapies he uses and to take the diary for review each time he visits a health care professional.

Calculation errors

Error: A physician assistant wrote the following order for a woman being admitted to the hospital for neck surgery: "methylprednisolone 10.6 g (30 mg/kg) over 1 hour IVPB before surgery" to minimize inflammation. The patient weighed 154 lb (70 kg), so the dose should have been 2.1 g, and not 10.6 g. Because neither the pharmacist nor the nurse independently checked the calculation, the patient received an overdose. She developed significant hyperglycemia and hypokalemia but recovered without injury.

Best practice or prevention: Writing the mg/kg or mg/m^2 dose and the calculated dose provides a safeguard against calculation errors. Whenever a prescriber provides the calculation, double-check it and document that the dose was verified.

Eyedrops for two or more

Error: Using one bottle of eyedrops to treat several patients may seem like a good way to prevent waste, control cost, and save time. Some facilities, for example, give shared eyedrops to multiple patients undergoing outpatient cataract surgery. But this practice has risks.

Eyedrops contain preservatives to prevent bacterial growth, but contaminants may remain on the bottle top's inner surfaces or outer grooves. The dropper can also become contaminated if it accidentally touches an infected eye. (Cross-infections have been reported.)

Giving the wrong drug or wrong concentration is more likely when containers are shared because patient names don't appear on the containers. A patient may receive the wrong drops because the nurse can't check the bottle label against the patient's identification.

Best practice or prevention: Just as sharing any drug is poor practice, eyedrops shouldn't be used for more than one patient. If unit doses aren't available for surgical patients, each patient should fill his prescriptions before admission and bring his drugs with him.

Trouble with liquids

Error: Liquid drugs may be more error-prone than solid drugs because of the calculations and dosage measurements needed. Here are a few examples: A 5-year-old boy who was receiving imipramine to treat his enuresis was given a fivefold overdose because of an incorrectly compounded suspension. A prescription of Augmentin was dispensed with the instruction to take 2½ tsp instead of 2½ ml. In another case, a mother who misunderstood the written directions gave her child 7 ml instead of 0.7 ml of a liquid drug.

Best practice or prevention: Don't assume that liquid drugs are less likely to cause harm than parenteral ones. Pediatric and geriatric patients often receive liquid drugs and may be especially sensitive to the effects of an inaccurate dose. If a unit-dose form isn't available, calculate carefully, and double-check your math and the drug label.

Labels and toxicity

Error: A container of 5% acetic acid, used to clean tracheostomy tubing, was left near nebulization equipment in the room of a 10-month-old infant. A respiratory therapist mistook the liquid for normal saline solution and used it to dilute albuterol for the child's nebulizer treatment. During treatment, the child experienced bronchospasm, hypercapnic dyspnea, tachypnea, and tachycardia.

Best practice or prevention: Leaving potentially dangerous chemicals near patients is extremely risky, especially when the container labels don't indicate toxicity. To prevent such problems, read the label on every drug you prepare and never give anything that isn't labeled.

Dosage equations

Error: A 13-month study at Albany (N.Y.) Medical Center examined 200 prescribing errors arising from the use of dosage equations. Almost 70% involved children, for whom dosage equations are commonly used. Mistakes in decimal point placement, mathematical calculation, or expression of the regimen accounted for more than 50% of the errors. Examples include prescribing the entire day's drug as a single dose instead of at intervals and giving an entire day's dose at each interval. Use of dosage equations invites drug errors.

Best practice or prevention: Alternatives to dosage equations include using preestablished ranges or tables, incorporating a calculator into a computer order entry system, and requiring both the calculated dose and dosage equation on orders to facilitate independent checks.

After you calculate a drug dosage, always have another nurse calculate it independently to double-check your results. If doubts or questions remain or if the calculations don't match, ask a pharmacist to calculate the dose before you give the drug.

Air bubbles in pump tubing

Error: After starting an I.V. drip to give insulin, 2 units/hour, to a 9-year-old patient, a nurse noted air bubbles in the tubing and pump chamber. To remove them and promote proper flow, she disconnected the tubing and increased the pump rate to 200 ml/hour. When the bubbles were cleared, she reconnected the tubing and restarted the infusion without resetting the rate. The child received about 50 units of insulin before the error was detected. Fortunately, the child wasn't harmed.

Best practice or prevention: To clear bubbles from I.V. tubing, never increase the pump's flow rate to flush the line. Instead, remove the tubing from the pump, disconnect it from the patient, and use the flow-control clamp to establish gravity flow. When the bubbles have been removed, return the tubing to the pump, restart the infusion, and recheck the flow rate.

Misplacing decimals

Error: A patient in the intensive care unit was to receive the opioid fentanyl, 12.5 to 25 mcg I.V. every 4 to 6 hours, p.r.n., for pain. Unit stock consisted of 5-ml ampules of fentanyl 0.05 mg/ml, so each ampule contained 0.25 mg (250 mcg). A nurse preparing a dose confused the volume needed when she converted from milligrams to micrograms and gave 5 ml, thinking it contained 25 mcg. The patient suffered respiratory arrest but was resuscitated.

Best practice or prevention: Numerous serious fentanyl errors have been reported, and a misplaced decimal point caused many of them. A safer alternative for intermittent dosing is I.V. morphine. Fentanyl doses are best prepared in the pharmacy rather than in the unit. If a fentanyl dose must be prepared, refer to dosing charts, follow the facility's protocols, and ask another nurse to check your calculations.

Incorrect administration route

Error: A nurse was caring for a patient who had a jejunostomy tube for oral drugs and a central I.V. line for hyperalimentation and I.V. drugs. At the bedside was a stock bottle of digoxin elixir. After checking the concentration, the nurse used a syringe to withdraw 2.5 ml of elixir for a 0.125-mg dose. She then mistakenly gave the elixir through the central line rather than the jejunostomy tube.

Using an incorrect route put the patient at risk for overdose and secondary infection from unsterile I.V. administration. Fortunately, he was receiving antibiotics for a preexisting infection and suffered no adverse reactions.

Best practice or prevention: This case emphasizes the need to ensure that the right route is being used to give any drug. When the patient has multiple lines, label the distal end of each line. Using a parenteral syringe to prepare oral liquid drugs increases the chance for error because the syringe tip fits easily into I.V. ports. To safely give an oral drug through a feeding tube, use a dose prepared by the pharmacy and a syringe with the appropriate tip.

Stress

Error: A nurse-anesthetist gave the sedative midazolam (Versed) to the wrong patient. When she discovered the error, she grabbed what she thought was a vial of the antidote flumazenil (Romazicon), withdrew 2.5 ml, and gave it. When the patient didn't respond, she realized she'd grabbed a vial of ondansetron (Zofran), an antiemetic, instead. Another practitioner assisted with proper I.V. administration of flumazenil, and the patient recovered without harm.

Best practice or prevention: Committing a serious error can cause enormous stress and cloud your judgment. If you're involved in a drug error, ask another professional to give the antidote.

Patient teaching

Patients being discharged from an acute care setting may be at a greater risk for adverse drug reactions arising from drug-drug interactions. Changes are frequently made to a patient's regular drug regimen before discharge, either by altering the dose or adding one or more new drugs. Adverse effects may go unnoticed by the practitioner or unreported when the patient is at home. Carefully review the patient's drugs upon discharge, inform him of any potential adverse drug effects to be aware of, and tell him to call the prescriber if adverse effects become bothersome.

The following general guidelines will help to ensure that the patient receives the maximum therapeutic benefit and avoids adverse reactions, accidental overdose, and harmful changes in effectiveness.

- Instruct the patient to learn the brand and generic names of all drugs he's taking and to inform his regular prescriber about their use. Before you give a patient a drug, ask him to report unusual reactions experienced in the past, allergies to foods and other substances, special medical problems, and drugs taken over the last few weeks, including OTC drugs or herbs.
- Advise the patient to always read the label before taking a drug, to take it exactly as prescribed, and never to share prescription drugs.

• Warn the patient not to change brands of a drug without consulting his prescriber, to avoid harmful changes in effectiveness. Certain generic preparations aren't equivalent in effect to brand-name preparations of the same drug.
• Tell the patient to check the expiration date before taking a drug.
• Instruct the patient to safely discard drugs that are outdated or no longer needed and to keep discarded drugs out of the reach of children and pets.
• Tell the patient to store each drug in its original container, at room temperature (unless directed otherwise), and in places that aren't accessible to children or exposed to sunlight. Discourage storage in the bathroom medicine cabinet, in the kitchen close to heat, or in the glove compartment or trunk of an automobile, where extremes of temperature and humidity will cause deterioration.
• Caution the patient about mixing different drugs in a single container, removing a drug from its original container, or removing the label. Relying on memory to identify a drug and specific directions for its use is dangerous.
• If the patient must remove pills from their original container to use a daily or weekly "medication planner" as a reminder, tell him to keep an index card with the planner that includes the drug's name, strength, dosage instructions, and physical description written on the card. This is particularly important when he's taking more than one prescription.
• Stress how important it is for the patient to tell the prescriber about adverse reactions he experiences during drug therapy.
• Advise the patient to have all prescriptions filled at the same pharmacy so that the pharmacist can identify and warn against potentially harmful drug interactions. Also, tell the patient to inform the pharmacist and prescriber about any OTC drugs or herbs he takes.
• Instruct the patient to call the prescriber, poison control center, or pharmacist immediately if he or someone else has taken an overdose. The National Poison Control Center phone number is 1-800-222-1222. Tell the patient to keep this and other emergency telephone numbers handy at all times.
• Advise the patient to inform medical personnel about use of drugs before undergoing surgery (including dental surgery).
• Tell the patient to have a sufficient supply of drugs when traveling. He should carry them with him in their original containers and not pack them in his luggage. Also, recommend that a patient who travels abroad should carry a letter from his prescriber authorizing the use of the drug, especially if the drug is a controlled substance.

4

Amebicides and antiprotozoals

atovaquone
chloroquine hydrochloride
(See Chapter 7, ANTIMALARIALS.)
chloroquine phosphate
(See Chapter 7, ANTIMALARIALS.)
metronidazole
metronidazole hydrochloride
nitazoxanide
pentamidine isethionate
tinidazole

atovaquone
Mepron

Pharmacologic class: ubiquinone analogue
Pregnancy risk category C

AVAILABLE FORMS
Suspension: 750 mg/5 ml

INDICATIONS & DOSAGES
➤ **Acute, mild to moderate *Pneumocystis jiroveci (carinii)* pneumonia in patients who can't tolerate co-trimoxazole**
Adults and adolescents ages 13 to 16: 750 mg P.O. b.i.d. with food for 21 days.
➤ **To prevent *P. jiroveci (carinii)* pneumonia in patients who are unable to tolerate co-trimoxazole**
Adults and adolescents ages 13 to 16: 1,500 mg (10 ml) P.O. daily with food.

ACTION
May interfere with electron transport in protozoal mitochondria, inhibiting enzymes needed to synthesize nucleic acids and adenosine triphosphate.

Route	Onset	Peak	Duration
P.O.	Unknown	Unknown	Unknown

Half-life: 2 to 3 days.

ADVERSE REACTIONS
CNS: *headache, insomnia, fever, pain,* asthenia, anxiety, dizziness.
CV: hypotension.
EENT: sinusitis, rhinitis.
GI: *abdominal pain, nausea, diarrhea, oral candidiasis, vomiting,* constipation, anorexia, dyspepsia, taste perversion.
Hematologic: ***neutropenia,*** anemia.
Metabolic: ***hypoglycemia,*** hyponatremia.
Respiratory: *cough.*
Skin: *rash, diaphoresis,* pruritus.

INTERACTIONS
Drug-drug. *Rifabutin, rifampin:* May decrease atovaquone's steady-state level. Avoid using together.

EFFECTS ON LAB TEST RESULTS
- May increase alkaline phosphatase, ALT, and AST levels. May decrease glucose, hemoglobin, and sodium levels.
- May decrease neutrophil count.

CONTRAINDICATIONS & CAUTIONS
- Contraindicated in patients hypersensitive to drug.
- Use cautiously in breast-feeding patients; it's unknown if drug appears in breast milk.
- Use cautiously with other highly protein-bound drugs; if used together, assess patient for toxicity.

NURSING CONSIDERATIONS
- ***Alert:*** Monitor patient closely during therapy because of risk of pulmonary infection.

PATIENT TEACHING
- Instruct patient to take drug with meals because food significantly enhances absorption.

Reactions may be *common,* uncommon, ***life-threatening,*** or COMMON AND LIFE-THREATENING.
Interaction may have a *rapid onset* or ***delayed onset.***

metronidazole
Apo-Metronidazole†, Flagyl, Flagyl 375, Flagyl ER, Metrogyl‡, Novo-Nidazol†, Trikacide†

metronidazole hydrochloride
Flagyl IV RTU, Novo-Nidazol†

Pharmacologic class: nitroimidazole
Pregnancy risk category B

AVAILABLE FORMS
Capsules: 375 mg
Injection: 500 mg/100 ml ready-to-use minibags
Powder for injection: 500-mg single-dose vials
Tablets: 200 mg‡, 250 mg, 400 mg‡, 500 mg
Tablets (extended-release [ER]): 750 mg

INDICATIONS & DOSAGES
➤**Amebic liver abscess**
Adults: 500 to 750 mg P.O. t.i.d. for 5 to 10 days; or 2.4 g P.O. once daily for 1 to 2 days. Or, 500 mg I.V. q 6 hours for 10 days if patient can't tolerate P.O. route.
Children: 30 to 50 mg/kg daily in 3 divided doses for 10 days. Maximum, 750 mg/dose.
➤**Intestinal amebiasis**
Adults: 750 mg P.O. t.i.d. for 5 to 10 days; then treat with a luminal amebicide, such as iodoquinol or paromomycin.
Children: 30 to 50 mg/kg daily in 3 divided doses for 10 days; then treat with a luminal amebicide, such as iodoquinol or paromomycin.
➤**Trichomoniasis**
Adults: 250 mg P.O. t.i.d. for 7 days, or 500 mg P.O. b.i.d. for 7 days, or 2 g P.O. in single dose (may give the 2-g dose in two 1-g doses, both on the same day); wait 4 to 6 weeks before repeating course.
Children: 5 mg/kg P.O. t.i.d. for 7 days.
➤**Refractory trichomoniasis**
Adults: 250 mg P.O. b.i.d. for 10 days. Or, 500 mg P.O. b.i.d. for 7 days.
➤**Bacterial infections caused by anaerobic microorganisms**
Adults: Loading dose is 15 mg/kg I.V. infused over 1 hour. Maintenance dose is 7.5 mg/kg I.V. or P.O. q 6 hours. Give first maintenance dose 6 hours after loading dose. Maximum dose shouldn't exceed 4 g daily.
➤**To prevent postoperative infection in contaminated or potentially contaminated colorectal surgery**
Adults: Infuse 15 mg/kg I.V. over 30 to 60 minutes and complete about 1 hour before surgery. Then, infuse 7.5 mg/kg I.V. over 30 to 60 minutes at 6 and 12 hours after first dose.
➤**Bacterial vaginosis**
Adults: 750 mg Flagyl ER P.O. daily for 7 days.
➤***Clostridium difficile*-associated diarrhea and colitis**♦
Adults: Usually 250 mg P.O. q.i.d. or 500 mg P.O. t.i.d. for 10 days. Or, 500 mg to 750 mg I.V. q 6 to 8 hours when P.O. route isn't practical.
Children: 30 to 50 mg/kg/day P.O. given in three to four equally divided doses for 7 to 10 days. Don't exceed adult dose.
➤**Pelvic inflammatory disease (PID)**♦
Adults: 500 mg I.V. q 8 hours with ofloxacin or with I.V. levofloxacin. For ambulatory patients, 500 mg P.O. b.i.d. with ofloxacin for 14 days.
➤**Bacterial vaginosis**♦
Nonpregnant women: 250 mg P.O. t.i.d. or 500 mg P.O. b.i.d. for 7 days. Or, 2 g P.O. as a single dose.
Pregnant women: 250 mg P.O. t.i.d. for 7 days or 2 g P.O. as a single dose.

I.V. ADMINISTRATION
- Flagyl IV ready-to-use (RTU) minibags need no preparation.
- Don't use aluminum needles or hubs to reconstitute the drug or to transfer reconstituted drug. Equipment that contains aluminum will turn the solution orange; the potency isn't affected.
- To reconstitute lyophilized vials, add 4.4 ml of sterile water for injection, bacteriostatic water for injection, sterile normal saline solution for injection, or bacteriostatic normal saline solution for injection. Reconstituted drug contains 100 mg/ml. Add contents of vial to 100 ml of D_5W, lactated Ringer injection, or normal saline solution to yield 5 mg/ml. Neutralize this highly acidic solution by carefully adding 5 mEq sodium bicarbon-

ate to each 500 mg; the carbon dioxide gas that forms may need to be vented.
- Infuse drug over at least 1 hour. Don't give by I.V. push.
- Don't refrigerate the neutralized diluted solution; precipitation may occur. Refrigerated Flagyl IV RTU may form crystals, which disappear after the solution warms to room temperature.

INCOMPATIBILITIES

Aluminum, amino acid 10%, amoxicillin sodium and clavulanate potassium, amphotericin B, aztreonam, ceftriaxone, dopamine, filgrastim, meropenem, other I.V. drugs, warfarin.

ACTION

Direct-acting trichomonacide and amebicide that works inside and outside the intestines. It's thought to enter the cells of microorganisms that contain nitroreductase, forming unstable compounds that bind to DNA and inhibit synthesis, causing cell death.

Route	Onset	Peak	Duration
P.O.	Unknown	2 hr	Unknown
I.V.	Immediate	1 hr	Unknown

Half-life: 6 to 8 hours.

ADVERSE REACTIONS

CNS: *headache, **seizures,*** fever, vertigo, ataxia, dizziness, syncope, incoordination, confusion, irritability, depression, weakness, insomnia, peripheral neuropathy.
CV: flattened T wave, edema, flushing, thrombophlebitis after I.V. infusion.
EENT: rhinitis, sinusitis, pharyngitis.
GI: *nausea,* abdominal cramping or pain, stomatitis, epigastric distress, vomiting, anorexia, diarrhea, constipation, proctitis, dry mouth, metallic taste.
GU: *vaginitis,* darkened urine, polyuria, dysuria, cystitis, dyspareunia, dryness of vagina and vulva, vaginal candidiasis, genital pruritus.
Hematologic: ***transient leukopenia, neutropenia.***
Musculoskeletal: transient joint pains.
Respiratory: upper respiratory tract infection.
Skin: rash.
Other: decreased libido, overgrowth of nonsusceptible organisms, especially *Candida.*

INTERACTIONS

Drug-drug. *Busulfan:* May increase busulfan toxicity. Avoid using together.
Cimetidine: May increase risk of metronidazole toxicity because of inhibited hepatic metabolism. Monitor patient.
Disulfiram: May cause acute psychosis and confusion. Avoid giving metronidazole within 2 weeks of disulfiram.
Lithium: May increase lithium level, which may cause toxicity. Monitor lithium level.
Phenobarbital, phenytoin: May decrease metronidazole effectiveness; may reduce total phenytoin clearance. Monitor patient.
Warfarin: May increase anticoagulant effects and risk of bleeding. Reduce warfarin as needed.
Drug-lifestyle. *Alcohol use:* May cause disulfiram-like reaction, including nausea, vomiting, headache, cramps, and flushing. Warn patient to avoid alcohol during and for 3 days after completing drug therapy.

EFFECTS ON LAB TEST RESULTS

- May decrease WBC and neutrophil counts.
- May falsely decrease triglyceride and aminotransferase levels.

CONTRAINDICATIONS & CAUTIONS

- Contraindicated in patients hypersensitive to drug or other nitroimidazole derivatives and in women in first trimester of pregnancy.
- ***Alert:*** If drug must be given to a pregnant woman for trichomoniasis, use the 7-day regimen, not the 2-g single-dose regimen. The 2-g dose produces a high level that's more likely to reach fetal circulation.
- Use cautiously in patients with history of blood dyscrasia, CNS disorder, or retinal or visual field changes.
- Use cautiously in patients who take hepatotoxic drugs or have hepatic disease or alcoholism.

NURSING CONSIDERATIONS

- Monitor liver function test results carefully in elderly patients.

- Give oral form with meals.
- Observe patient for edema, especially if he's receiving corticosteroids; Flagyl IV RTU may cause sodium retention.
- Record number and character of stools when drug is used to treat amebiasis. Give drug only after *Trichomonas vaginalis* infection is confirmed by wet smear or culture or *Entameba histolytica* is identified.
- Sexual partners of patients being treated for *T. vaginalis* infection, even if asymptomatic, must also be treated to avoid reinfection.

PATIENT TEACHING
- Instruct patient to take ER tablets from at least 1 hour before or 2 hours after meals but to take all other oral forms with food to minimize GI upset.
- Inform patient of need for sexual partners to be treated simultaneously to avoid reinfection.
- Instruct patient in proper hygiene.
- Tell patient to avoid alcohol and alcohol-containing drugs during and for at least 3 days after treatment course.
- Tell patient he may experience a metallic taste and have dark or red-brown urine.
- Tell patient to report to prescriber symptoms of candidal overgrowth.
- Tell patient to report to prescriber immediately any neurologic symptoms (seizures, peripheral neuropathy).

nitazoxanide
Alinia

Pharmacologic class: antiprotozoal
Pregnancy risk category B

AVAILABLE FORMS
Oral suspension: 100 mg/5 ml
Tablets: 500 mg

INDICATIONS & DOSAGES
➤ **Diarrhea caused by *Cryptosporidium parvum* or *Giardia lamblia***
Adults and children age 12 and older: 500 mg P.O. with food q 12 hours for 3 days.
Children ages 4 to 11: Give 10 ml (200 mg) P.O. with food q 12 hours for 3 days.
Children ages 1 to 3: Give 5 ml (100 mg) P.O. with food q 12 hours for 3 days.

ACTION
May interfere with an enzyme-dependent electron transfer reaction, essential for anaerobic energy metabolism.

Route	Onset	Peak	Duration
P.O.	Rapid	1–4 hr	Unknown

Half-life: Unknown.

ADVERSE REACTIONS
CNS: headache.
GI: abdominal pain, diarrhea, nausea, vomiting.

INTERACTIONS
Drug-drug. *Drugs that are highly protein-bound:* May compete for binding sites. Use together cautiously.

EFFECTS ON LAB TEST RESULTS
- May increase creatinine and glutamate pyruvate transaminase levels.

CONTRAINDICATIONS & CAUTIONS
- Contraindicated in patients hypersensitive to nitazoxanide.
- Use cautiously in patients with renal or hepatic dysfunction. Safety and effectiveness haven't been established in HIV-positive patients, other immunodeficient patients, or infants younger than age 1.

NURSING CONSIDERATIONS
- Give drug with food.
- ***Alert:*** A single tablet contains more of the drug than is recommended for pediatric doses and shouldn't be given to children age 11 or younger.
- Monitor glucose level in patients with diabetes who are taking the suspension.

PATIENT TEACHING
- Tell caregiver or patient to give drug with food.
- Instruct caregiver or patient to keep container tightly closed and to shake it well before each use.
- Advise caregiver or patient that drug may be stored at room temperature.
- Advise caregiver or patient to discard suspension after 7 days.
- Inform diabetic patient or his caregiver that suspension contains 1.48 g of sucrose per 5 ml.

pentamidine isethionate
NebuPent, Pentam 300

Pharmacologic class: diamidine derivative
Pregnancy risk category C

AVAILABLE FORMS
Aerosol, injection, powder for injection: 300-mg vial

INDICATIONS & DOSAGES
➤ ***Pneumocystis jiroveci (carinii)* pneumonia**
Adults and children age 4 months and older: 3 to 4 mg/kg I.V. or I.M. once daily for 14 to 21 days.
➤ **To prevent *P. jiroveci (carinii)* pneumonia in high-risk patients**
Adults and children capable of effectively using a nebulizer: 300 mg by inhalation using a Respirgard II nebulizer once q 4 weeks.
➤ **Visceral leishmaniasis caused by *Leishmania donovani*♦**
Adults and children: 2 to 4 mg/kg I.V. or I.M. once daily or once every other day for up to 15 doses.
➤ **Cutaneous leishmaniasis♦**
Adults and children: 2 mg/kg I.M. every other day for 7 doses or 3 mg/kg I.M. every other day for 4 doses.

I.V. ADMINISTRATION
- Reconstitute drug with 3 ml sterile water for injection.
- Dilute reconstituted drug in 50 to 250 ml D_5W.
- Infuse over at least 60 minutes.
- To minimize risk of hypotension, infuse drug slowly with patient lying down. Closely monitor blood pressure.

INCOMPATIBILITIES
Aldesleukin, cephalosporins, fluconazole, foscarnet, linezolid.

ACTION
May interfere with biosynthesis of DNA, RNA, phospholipids, and proteins in susceptible organisms.

Route	Onset	Peak	Duration
I.V.	Unknown	1 hr	Unknown
I.M., inhalation	Unknown	30 min	Unknown

Half-life: 9 to 13 hours for I.M., about 6½ hours for I.V. Unknown for inhalation.

ADVERSE REACTIONS
CNS: *dizziness, fatigue,* confusion, hallucinations, headache.
CV: *chest pain,* ***severe hypotension, ventricular tachycardia,*** edema.
EENT: *pharyngitis,* burning in throat (with inhaled form).
GI: *nausea, metallic taste, decreased appetite, vomiting,* ***pancreatitis,*** diarrhea, abdominal pain, anorexia.
GU: ***acute renal failure.***
Hematologic: ***leukopenia, thrombocytopenia,*** anemia.
Metabolic: ***hypoglycemia,*** hyperglycemia, hypocalcemia.
Musculoskeletal: myalgia.
Respiratory: *congestion, cough, shortness of breath,* **bronchospasm,** pneumothorax.
Skin: ***Stevens-Johnson syndrome,*** rash.
Other: *night sweats, chills, sterile abscess, pain, induration at injection site.*

INTERACTIONS
Drug-drug. *Aminoglycosides, amphotericin B, capreomycin, cisplatin, methoxyflurane, polymyxin B, vancomycin:* May increase risk of nephrotoxicity. Monitor renal function test results closely.
Antineoplastics: May cause additive bone marrow suppression. Use together cautiously; monitor hematologic study results.
Drugs that prolong the QT interval (antipsychotics; antiarrhythmics, such as amiodarone, disopyramide, procainamide, quinidine, and sotalol; fluoroquinolones; macrolides; tricyclic antidepressants): May cause additive effect. Use together cautiously; monitor patient for adverse cardiac effects.

EFFECTS ON LAB TEST RESULTS
- May increase BUN, creatinine, and potassium levels. May decrease hemoglobin level and hematocrit. May increase or decrease glucose level.

• May decrease WBC and platelet counts.

CONTRAINDICATIONS & CAUTIONS
• Contraindicated in patients with history of anaphylactic reaction to drug.
• Use cautiously in patients with hypertension, hypotension, hypoglycemia, hypocalcemia, leukopenia, thrombocytopenia, anemia, diabetes, pancreatitis, Stevens-Johnson syndrome, or hepatic or renal dysfunction.
• Use cautiously in breast-feeding women; it's unknown if drug appears in breast milk.

NURSING CONSIDERATIONS
• Give aerosol form only by Respirgard II nebulizer. Dosage recommendations are based on particle size and delivery rate of this device. To give aerosol, mix contents of 1 vial in 6 ml sterile water for injection. Don't use normal saline solution. Don't mix with other drugs.
• Don't use low-pressure (less than 20 pounds per square inch [psi]) compressors. The flow rate should be 5 to 7 L/minute from a 40- to 50-psi air or oxygen source.
• For I.M. use, reconstitute drug with 3 ml sterile water for a solution containing 100 mg/ml; give deep into muscle. Patient may have pain and induration at injection site. Rotate injection sites.
• ***Alert:*** Monitor glucose, calcium, creatinine, and BUN levels daily. After parenteral administration, glucose level may decrease initially; hypoglycemia may be severe in 5% to 10% of patients. After several months of therapy, this may be followed by hyperglycemia and type 1 diabetes mellitus, which may be permanent because of pancreatic cell damage.
• In patients with AIDS, drug may produce less severe adverse reactions than co-trimoxazole.

PATIENT TEACHING
• Instruct patient to use the aerosol device until the chamber is empty, which may take up to 45 minutes.
• Warn patient that I.M. injection is painful.
• Instruct patient to complete the full course, even if he's feeling better.

tinidazole
Tindamax

Pharmacologic class: antiprotozoal
Pregnancy risk category C

AVAILABLE FORMS
Tablets: 250 mg, 500 mg

INDICATIONS & DOSAGES
➤ **Trichomoniasis caused by *Trichomonas vaginalis***
Adults: 2 g P.O. as a single dose taken with food. Sexual partners should be treated at the same time with the same dose.
➤ **Giardiasis caused by *Giardia lamblia (G. duodenalis)***
Adults: 2 g P.O. as a single dose taken with food.
Children older than age 3: Give 50 mg/kg (up to 2 g) as a single dose taken with food.
➤ **Intestinal amebiasis caused by *Entamoeba histolytica***
Adults: 2 g P.O. daily for 3 days, taken with food.
Children older than age 3: Give 50 mg/kg (up to 2 g) P.O. daily for 3 days, taken with food.
➤ **Amebic liver abscess (amebiasis)**
Adults: 2 g P.O. daily for 3 to 5 days, taken with food.
Children older than age 3: Give 50 mg/kg (up to 2 g) P.O. daily for 3 to 5 days, taken with food.
Adjust-a-dose: For patients receiving hemodialysis, give an additional dose equal to one-half the recommended dose after the hemodialysis session.

ACTION
For *Trichomonas,* drug reduces the compound's nitro group into a free nitro radical. Mechanism of action against *Giardia* and *Entamoeba* is unknown.

Route	Onset	Peak	Duration
P.O.	Unknown	1½ hr	Unknown

Half-life: 12 to 14 hours.

ADVERSE REACTIONS

CNS: *seizures,* dizziness, fatigue, headache, malaise, peripheral neuropathy, weakness.
GI: anorexia, constipation, cramps, dyspepsia, metallic taste, nausea, vomiting.

INTERACTIONS

Drug-drug. *Cyclosporine, tacrolimus:* May increase cyclosporine or tacrolimus level. Monitor patient closely for toxicity, including headache, nausea, vomiting, nephrotoxicity, and electrolyte abnormalities.
Disulfiram: May increase abdominal cramping, nausea, vomiting, headaches, and flushing. Separate doses by 2 weeks.
Drugs that induce CYP-450, such as fosphenytoin, phenobarbital, phenytoin, and rifampin: May increase tinidazole elimination. Monitor patient.
Drugs that inhibit CYP-450, such as cimetidine and ketoconazole: May prolong tinidazole half-life and decrease clearance. Monitor patient.
Fluorouracil: May decrease fluorouracil clearance, increasing adverse effects without added benefit. Monitor patient for rash, nausea, vomiting, stomatitis, and leukopenia.
Fosphenytoin, phenytoin: May prolong phenytoin half-life and decrease clearance of I.V. drug. Monitor patient for toxicity.
Lithium: May increase lithium level. Monitor patient; monitor lithium and creatinine levels.
Oxytetracycline: May counteract tinidazole. Assess patient for lack of effect.
Warfarin and other oral anticoagulants: May increase anticoagulant effect. Anticoagulant dosage may need adjustment during and for up to 8 days after tinidazole therapy.
Drug-herb. *St. John's wort:* May increase or decrease drug level. Discourage use together.
Drug-lifestyle. *Use of alcohol and alcohol-containing products:* May increase abdominal cramping, nausea, vomiting, headaches, and flushing. Discourage use together and for 3 days after stopping drug.

EFFECTS ON LAB TEST RESULTS

- May increase AST, ALT, glucose, LDH, and triglyceride levels.
- May decrease WBC count.

CONTRAINDICATIONS & CAUTIONS

- Contraindicated in patients hypersensitive to drug, its component, or other nitroimidazole derivatives.
- Contraindicated in pregnant women during first trimester of pregnancy.
- Use cautiously in patients with CNS disorders and in those with blood dyscrasias or hepatic dysfunction.

NURSING CONSIDERATIONS

- If therapy exceeds 3 days, monitor children closely.
- For children who can't swallow pills, tablets may be crushed into a fine powder and mixed with artificial cherry syrup.
- Patient should take drug with food to minimize adverse GI effects.
- ***Alert:*** If abnormal neurologic signs, such as seizures or numbness of the arms or legs, occur, stop drug immediately.
- If candidiasis develops during therapy, the patient may need an antifungal.
- Women shouldn't breast-feed during therapy and for 3 days after the last dose.
- An elderly patient may have decreased liver or kidney function or other medical conditions and may be taking other drugs that may affect dosage.

PATIENT TEACHING

- Tell patient to take drug with food.
- ***Alert:*** Tell patient to report to prescriber seizures and numbness in arms or legs.
- Warn patient not to drink alcohol or use alcohol-containing products while taking drug and for 3 days afterward.
- Advise woman to immediately notify her prescriber if she becomes pregnant.
- Tell woman to stop breast-feeding during therapy and for 3 days after the last dose.
- If patient is being treated for a sexually transmitted infection, explain that his sexual partners should be treated at the same time.

5 Anthelmintics

mebendazole
pyrantel pamoate

mebendazole
Vermox

Pharmacologic class: benzimidazole
Pregnancy risk category C

AVAILABLE FORMS
Tablets (chewable): 100 mg

INDICATIONS & DOSAGES
➤ Pinworm
Adults and children older than age 2: 100 mg P.O. as a single dose; repeat if infestation persists 2 to 3 weeks later.
➤ Roundworm, whipworm, and hookworm
Adults and children older than age 2: 100 mg P.O. b.i.d. for 3 days; repeat if infestation persists 3 weeks later.
➤ Trichinosis ♦
Adults: 200 to 400 mg P.O. t.i.d. for 3 days; then 400 to 500 mg t.i.d. for 10 days.
➤ Capillariasis ♦
Adults and children: 200 mg P.O. b.i.d. for 20 days.
➤ Dracunculiasis ♦
Adults: 400 to 800 mg P.O. daily for 6 days.

ACTION
Selectively and irreversibly inhibits uptake of glucose and other nutrients by susceptible helminths.

Route	Onset	Peak	Duration
P.O.	Unknown	2–4 hr	Variable

Half-life: 3 to 9 hours.

ADVERSE REACTIONS
CNS: *seizures,* fever.
GI: transient abdominal pain and diarrhea in massive infestation and during expulsion of worms.
Skin: urticaria.

INTERACTIONS
Drug-drug. *Carbamazepine, hydantoin:* May decrease mebendazole level, which may decrease drug's effect. Monitor patient for drug effectiveness.
Cimetidine: May increase mebendazole level. Monitor patient for increased adverse effects.

EFFECTS ON LAB TEST RESULTS
None reported.

CONTRAINDICATIONS & CAUTIONS
- Contraindicated in patients hypersensitive to drug.
- Safe use in children younger than age 2 hasn't been established.

NURSING CONSIDERATIONS
- Tablets may be chewed, swallowed whole, or crushed and mixed with food.
- Give drug to all family members to decrease risk of spreading the infestation.
- No dietary restrictions, laxatives, or enemas are needed.

PATIENT TEACHING
- Teach patient about personal hygiene, especially good hand-washing technique. Advise him to refrain from preparing food for others.
- To avoid reinfestation, teach patient to wash perianal area daily, change undergarments and bedclothes daily, and wash hands and clean fingernails before meals and after bowel movements.

pyrantel pamoate
Antiminth ◇, Combantrin†, Pin-Rid ◇, Pin-X ◇, Reese's Pinworm ◇

Pharmacologic class: pyrimidine derivative
Pregnancy risk category C

AVAILABLE FORMS
Liquid: 50 mg/ml

Oral suspension: 50 mg/ml
Soft-gel capsules: 62.5 mg (as base)

INDICATIONS & DOSAGES

➤ **Roundworm and pinworm**
Adults and children age 2 and older: 11 mg/kg P.O. as a single dose. Maximum dose, 1 g. For pinworm, repeat dose in 2 weeks.

ACTION

Blocks neuromuscular action, paralyzing the worm, and causing its expulsion by normal peristalsis.

Route	Onset	Peak	Duration
P.O.	Variable	1–3 hr	Variable

Half-life: Unknown.

ADVERSE REACTIONS

CNS: headache, fever, dizziness, drowsiness, insomnia, weakness.
GI: anorexia, nausea, vomiting, gastralgia, abdominal cramps, diarrhea, tenesmus.
Skin: rash.

INTERACTIONS

Drug-drug. *Piperazine salts:* May antagonize drug effects. Avoid using together.

EFFECTS ON LAB TEST RESULTS

- May increase AST level.

CONTRAINDICATIONS & CAUTIONS

- Contraindicated in patients hypersensitive to drug.
- Use cautiously in patients with severe malnutrition, anemia, or hepatic dysfunction.

NURSING CONSIDERATIONS

- No dietary restrictions, laxatives, or enemas are needed.
- Give drug to all family members to decrease risk of spreading the infestation.

PATIENT TEACHING

- Inform patient that drug may be taken with food, milk, or fruit juices. Tell him to shake suspension well.
- Teach patient about personal hygiene, especially good hand-washing technique. To avoid reinfestation, teach patient to wash perianal area daily, to change undergarments and bedclothes daily, and to wash hands and clean fingernails before meals and after bowel movements.
- Advise patient not to prepare food for others.
- Tell patient to take entire dosage as prescribed.

6 Antifungals

amphotericin B cholesteryl sulfate complex
amphotericin B desoxycholate
amphotericin B lipid complex
amphotericin B liposomal
anidulafungin
caspofungin acetate
fluconazole
flucytosine
griseofulvin
itraconazole
ketoconazole
micafungin sodium
nystatin
posaconazole
terbinafine hydrochloride
voriconazole

SAFETY ALERT!

amphotericin B cholesteryl sulfate complex
Amphotec

Pharmacologic class: polyene antibiotic
Pregnancy risk category B

AVAILABLE FORMS
Injection: 50 mg/20 ml, 100 mg/50 ml

INDICATIONS & DOSAGES
➤ **Invasive aspergillosis in patients whose renal impairment or unacceptable toxicity precludes use of effective doses of amphotericin B deoxycholate or whose previous amphotericin B deoxycholate therapy has failed**
Adults and children: 3 to 4 mg/kg/day I.V. Dilute in D_5W and give by continuous infusion at 1 mg/kg/hour. Give a test dose before beginning new course of treatment; infuse 10 ml of final preparation containing 1.6 to 8.3 mg of drug over 15 to 30 minutes and monitor patient for next 30 minutes. May shorten infusion time to 2 hours or lengthen infusion time based on patient's tolerance.
➤ ***Candida*** **or** ***Cryptococcus*** **infections in patients who can't tolerate or who failed to respond to conventional amphotericin B ♦**
Adults: 3 to 6 mg/kg/day I.V. Dosages up to 7.5 mg/kg/day I.V. have been used for invasive fungal infections in bone marrow transplant patients.

I.V. ADMINISTRATION
- Don't give undiluted drug.
- Reconstitute 50-mg vial by rapidly adding 10 ml sterile water for injection; reconstitute 100-mg vial by rapidly adding 20 ml sterile water for injection. Shake vial gently.
- Don't use any diluent except sterile water for injection. Don't reconstitute lyophilized powder with saline or dextrose solution or mix reconstituted liquid with saline solution or electrolytes. A bacteriostatic product in the solution may cause drug to precipitate.
- Reconstituted drug should be clear or opalescent.
- Add reconstituted drug to D_5W to yield about 0.6 mg/ml.
- Don't use a filter (including an in-line filter), and don't freeze.
- If given through an existing I.V. line, flush line with D_5W before infusion.
- Infuse drug over at least 2 hours.
- Store unopened vials at room temperature; store reconstituted drug in refrigerator, where it's stable for 24 hours.
- Discard partially used vials.

INCOMPATIBILITIES
Bacteriostatic agents, electrolyte solutions, saline solutions. Don't mix with other drugs.

ACTION
Binds to sterols of fungal cell membranes, altering cell permeability and causing cell death.

Route	Onset	Peak	Duration
I.V.	Unknown	3 hr	Unknown

Half-life: Biphasic, with initial half-life of 24 hours and a second phase of about 15 days.

ADVERSE REACTIONS

CNS: *fever,* ***seizures,*** abnormal thinking, anxiety, agitation, confusion, depression, dizziness, hallucinations, headache, hypertonia, neuropathy, nervousness, paresthesia, psychosis, somnolence, speech disorder, stupor, asthenia, syncope.
CV: *tachycardia,* ***arrhythmias, bradycardia, cardiac arrest, heart failure, hemorrhage, shock, supraventricular tachycardia,*** atrial fibrillation, hypertension, hypotension, phlebitis, chest pain, orthostatic hypotension, vasodilation, edema.
EENT: amblyopia, deafness, epistaxis, eye hemorrhage, pharyngitis, tinnitus, rhinitis, sinusitis.
GI: *nausea, vomiting,* ***GI hemorrhage,*** abdominal pain, anorexia, diarrhea, dry mouth, gingivitis, glossitis, hematemesis, melena, mouth ulceration, oral candidiasis, stomatitis.
GU: ***renal failure,*** albuminuria, dysuria, glycosuria, hematuria, oliguria, urinary incontinence or urine retention.
Hematologic: ***leukopenia, thrombocytopenia,*** anemia, coagulation disorders, ecchymosis, hypochromic anemia, leukocytosis, petechiae.
Hepatic: *hyperbilirubinemia,* ***hepatic failure,*** jaundice.
Metabolic: *hypokalemia,* ***hypoglycemia, hyperkalemia,*** weight changes, acidosis, dehydration, hypocalcemia, hypoproteinemia, hyperglycemia, hypervolemia, hypophosphatemia, hyponatremia, hyperlipemia, hypernatremia, hypomagnesemia.
Musculoskeletal: arthralgia, myalgia, neck or back pain.
Respiratory: ***apnea,*** asthma, dyspnea, hemoptysis, hyperventilation, hypoxia, increased cough, lung or respiratory tract disorders, pleural effusion, pulmonary edema.
Skin: acne, alopecia, pruritus, rash, sweating, skin discoloration, nodules, ulcers, urticaria, pain or reaction at injection site.
Other: *chills,* ***anaphylaxis, sepsis,*** allergic reaction, peripheral or facial edema, infection, mucous membrane disorder.

INTERACTIONS

Drug-drug. *Antineoplastics:* May enhance renal toxicity, bronchospasm, and hypotension. Use together cautiously.
Cardiac glycosides: May enhance potassium excretion and increase digitalis toxicity. Monitor potassium level closely.
Corticosteroids: May enhance potassium depletion, which may increase risk of cardiac dysfunction. Monitor electrolyte levels.
Cyclosporine, tacrolimus: May increase creatinine level. Monitor renal function.
Flucytosine: May increase toxicity by amphotericin. Use together cautiously.
Imidazoles (clotrimazole, fluconazole, ketoconazole, miconazole): May antagonize effects of amphotericin. Monitor patient closely.
Leukocyte transfusions: May increase risk of pulmonary reactions, such as acute dyspnea, tachypnea, hypoxemia, hemoptysis, and interstitial infiltrates. Use together cautiously; separate doses as much as possible, and monitor pulmonary function.
Nephrotoxic drugs (such as aminoglycosides, pentamidine): May enhance renal toxicity. Monitor renal function closely.
Skeletal muscle relaxants: May enhance muscle relaxant effects because of amphotericin. Monitor potassium level closely.

EFFECTS ON LAB TEST RESULTS

- May increase alkaline phosphatase, ALT, AST, bilirubin, BUN, creatinine, GGT, and LDH levels. May decrease calcium, magnesium, phosphate, protein, and hemoglobin levels. May increase or decrease glucose, sodium, and potassium levels.
- May decrease platelet count and INR. May increase or decrease WBC count and PT.

CONTRAINDICATIONS & CAUTIONS

- Contraindicated in patients hypersensitive to drug or its components, unless the benefits outweigh the risks.
- It's unknown if drug appears in breast milk; if it does, breast-fed infants are at risk for serious adverse reactions. Patient should either stop breast-feeding or stop drug.

NURSING CONSIDERATIONS

- *Alert:* Dosages of different amphotericin B preparations will vary because the preparations aren't interchangeable. Confusing the preparations may cause permanent damage or death.
- *Alert:* Monitor vital signs every 30 minutes during initial therapy. Acute infusion-related reactions, including fever, chills, hypotension, nausea, and tachycardia, usually occur 1 to 3 hours after the I.V. infusion starts and are usually most severe after first dose, usually diminishing with each dose. If severe respiratory distress occurs, stop infusion immediately and don't restart.
- Reduce acute infusion-related reactions by pretreating with antihistamines, antipyretics, and corticosteroids; reducing infusion rate; and maintaining sodium balance.
- Hydrate patient before infusion to reduce risk of nephrotoxicity.
- Monitor intake and output; report changes in urine appearance or volume.
- Monitor renal and hepatic function test results, electrolyte levels (especially potassium, magnesium, and calcium), CBC, and PT.

PATIENT TEACHING

- Instruct patient to immediately report symptoms of hypersensitivity.
- Warn patient of possible discomfort at I.V. site.
- Advise patient of potential adverse reactions, such as fever, chills, nausea, and vomiting. Tell patient that these can be severe with first dose but usually subside with repeated doses.

SAFETY ALERT!

amphotericin B desoxycholate

Amphocin, Amphotericin B for Injection, Fungizone

Pharmacologic class: polyene antibiotic
Pregnancy risk category B

AVAILABLE FORMS

Powder for injection: 50 mg

INDICATIONS & DOSAGES

➤ **Systemic fungal infection (histoplasmosis, coccidioidomycosis, blastomycosis, cryptococcosis, disseminated candidiasis, aspergillosis, phycomycosis, zygomycosis) or meningitis**

Adults: Initially, test dose of 1 mg in 20 ml of D_5W infused I.V. over 20 to 30 minutes. If that dosage is tolerated, start daily dose at 0.25 to 0.3 mg/kg by slow I.V. infusion (0.1 mg/ml) over 2 to 6 hours. Daily dose is gradually increased to maximum of 1.5 mg/kg in patients with potentially fatal infections. If drug is stopped for 1 week or longer, resume with initial dose and increase gradually.

➤ **To prevent fungal infection in bone marrow transplant patients ♦**

Adults: 0.1 mg/kg/day as I.V. infusion.

I.V. ADMINISTRATION

- Reconstitute drug with 10 ml of sterile water.
- If solution contains precipitate or foreign matter, don't use.
- Drug seems to be compatible with limited amounts of heparin sodium, hydrocortisone sodium succinate, and methylprednisolone sodium succinate.
- Choose I.V. sites in distal veins. If veins become thrombosed, alternate administration sites.
- Use an infusion pump and in-line filter with mean pore diameter larger than 1 micron.
- After giving test dose, monitor patient's pulse, respiratory rate, temperature, and blood pressure for at least 4 hours.
- Rapid infusion may cause CV collapse.
- Monitor vital signs every 30 minutes; fever, shaking chills, and hypotension may appear 1 to 2 hours after start of infusion and should subside within 4 hours after stopping drug.
- Store the dry form at 36° to 46° F (2° to 8° C). Protect from light.
- Reconstituted solution is stable 1 week refrigerated or 24 hours at room temperature. It's stable 8 hours in room light.

INCOMPATIBILITIES

Amikacin, calcium chloride, chlorpromazine, cimetidine, diphenhydramine, edetate calcium disodium, gentamicin, kanamycin, lactated Ringer injection, melphalan, methyldopate, normal saline solution, paclitaxel, penicillin G potassium, penicillin G sodium, polymyxin B, potassium chloride, prochlorperazine mesylate, streptomycin, verapamil. To avoid precipitation, don't mix with solutions containing sodium chloride, other electrolytes, or bacteriostatic products such as benzyl alcohol. Give antibiotics separately; don't mix or piggyback them with amphotericin B.

ACTION

Binds to sterols of fungal cell membranes, altering cell permeability and causing cell death.

Route	Onset	Peak	Duration
I.V.	Immediate	Unknown	Unknown

Half-life: Adults and children older than age 9, 24 hours; children age 9 and younger, 18 hours.

ADVERSE REACTIONS

CNS: *headache, fever, malaise,* ***seizures,*** peripheral neuropathy, transient vertigo.
CV: ***arrhythmias, asystole,*** hypertension, hypotension, tachycardia, flushing, *phlebitis, thrombophlebitis.*
EENT: hearing loss, tinnitus, blurred vision, diplopia.
GI: *anorexia, nausea, vomiting, dyspepsia, diarrhea, epigastric pain, cramping,* ***hemorrhagic gastroenteritis,*** melena, steatorrhea.
GU: *abnormal renal function with azotemia, hyposthenuria, renal tubular acidosis, nephrocalcinosis,* ***permanent renal impairment,*** anuria, oliguria.
Hematologic: *normochromic anemia, normocytic anemia,* ***thrombocytopenia, leukopenia, agranulocytosis,*** eosinophilia, leukocytosis.
Hepatic: ***acute liver failure, hepatitis,*** jaundice.
Metabolic: *weight loss, hypokalemia,* ***hypoglycemia,*** hyperglycemia, hyperuricemia, hypomagnesemia.
Musculoskeletal: arthralgia, myalgia.
Respiratory: ***bronchospasm,*** dyspnea, tachypnea, wheezing.
Skin: *maculopapular rash, pain at injection site,* pruritus, tissue damage with extravasation.
Other: *chills, generalized pain,* ***anaphylactoid reaction.***

INTERACTIONS

Drug-drug. *Antineoplastics (such as mechlorethamine):* May cause renal toxicity, bronchospasm, and hypotension. Use together cautiously.
Cardiac glycosides: May increase risk of digitalis toxicity in potassium-depleted patients. Monitor digoxin level closely.
Corticosteroids: May increase potassium depletion. Monitor potassium level.
Flucytosine: May have synergistic effect; may cause increased toxicity of flucytosine. Monitor patient closely for toxicity.
Leukocyte transfusions: May increase risk of pulmonary reactions, such as acute dyspnea, tachypnea, hypoxemia, hemoptysis, and interstitial infiltrates. Use together cautiously; separate doses as much as possible and monitor pulmonary function if drugs are used together.
Nephrotoxic drugs such as antibiotics, pentamidine: May cause additive renal toxicity. Use together cautiously and monitor renal function studies.
Thiazides: May intensify depletion of electrolytes, especially potassium. Monitor patient for hypokalemia.
Drug-herb. *Gossypol:* May increase risk of renal toxicity. Discourage use together.

EFFECTS ON LAB TEST RESULTS

- May increase alkaline phosphatase, ALT, AST, bilirubin, BUN, creatinine, GGT, LDH, urine urea, and uric acid levels. May decrease hemoglobin, magnesium, and potassium levels. May increase or decrease glucose level.
- May decrease granulocyte and platelet counts. May increase or decrease eosinophil and WBC counts.

CONTRAINDICATIONS & CAUTIONS

- Contraindicated in patients hypersensitive to drug.
- Use cautiously in patients with impaired renal function.

NURSING CONSIDERATIONS

- Because of drug's dangerous adverse effects, it's used primarily to treat patients with progressive and potentially fatal fungal infections.

• Infusion-related reactions, including fever, shaking chills, hypotension, anorexia, nausea, vomiting, headache, dyspnea, and tachypnea, may occur 1 to 3 hours after starting infusion.
• ***Alert:*** Different amphotericin B preparations aren't interchangeable, so dosages will vary. Confusing the preparations may cause permanent damage or death.
• ***Alert:*** To reduce severe adverse effects, premedicate with antipyretics, antihistamines, antiemetics, or small doses of corticosteroids on an alternate-day schedule. For severe reactions, stop drug and notify prescriber.
• Infusion-related reactions occur most frequently with initial doses and usually lessen with subsequent doses.
• Monitor fluid intake and output; report change in urine appearance or volume. Monitor BUN and creatinine levels or creatinine clearance two or three times weekly. If BUN level exceeds 40 mg/100 ml or if creatinine level exceeds 3 mg/100 ml, prescriber may reduce or stop drug until renal function improves. Kidney damage may be reversible if drug is stopped at first sign of renal dysfunction.
• Hydrate patient before infusion to reduce risk of nephrotoxicity.
• Obtain liver function studies once or twice weekly. Drug may be stopped if alkaline phosphatase or bilirubin level increases. Monitor CBC weekly.
• Monitor potassium level closely and report signs of hypokalemia. Hypokalemia occurs commonly and can be life-threatening. Potassium supplementation may be needed.
• Check calcium and magnesium levels twice weekly.
• Drug may be ototoxic. Report evidence of hearing loss, tinnitus, vertigo, or unsteady gait.

PATIENT TEACHING

• Warn patient of possible discomfort at I.V. site and other potential adverse reactions. Instruct patient to report signs and symptoms of hypersensitivity immediately.
• Inform patient that therapy may take several months. Stress importance of compliance and follow-up.

SAFETY ALERT!

amphotericin B lipid complex
Abelcet

Pharmacologic class: polyene antibiotic
Pregnancy risk category B

AVAILABLE FORMS

Suspension for injection: 100 mg/20-ml vial

INDICATIONS & DOSAGES

➤ **Invasive fungal infections, including *Aspergillus* and *Candida* species, in patients refractory to or intolerant of conventional amphotericin B therapy**
Adults and children: 5 mg/kg daily I.V. as a single infusion given at rate of 2.5 mg/kg/hour.

I.V. ADMINISTRATION

• To prepare, shake vial gently until there's no yellow sediment. Using aseptic technique, withdraw calculated dose into one or more 20-ml syringes using an 18G needle. More than one vial will be needed.
• Attach a 5-micron filter needle to syringe and inject dose into I.V. bag of D_5W. Volume of D_5W should be sufficient to yield 1 mg/ml. One filter needle can be used for up to four vials of amphotericin B lipid complex.
• For children and patients with CV disease, dilute to 2 mg/ml.
• Don't use an in-line filter.
• If infusing through an existing I.V. line, flush first with D_5W.
• Use an infusion pump, and give by continuous infusion at 2.5 mg/kg/hour.
• If infusion time exceeds 2 hours, mix contents by shaking infusion bag every 2 hours.
• Monitor vital signs closely. Fever, shaking chills, and hypotension may appear within 2 hours of starting infusion. Slowing infusion rate may decrease risk of infusion-related reactions.
• If severe respiratory distress occurs, stop infusion, provide supportive therapy for anaphylaxis, and notify prescriber. Don't restart drug.

• Reconstituted drug is stable up to 48 hours if refrigerated (36° to 46° F [2° to 8° C]) and up to 6 hours at room temperature.
• Discard any unused drug because it contains no preservative.

INCOMPATIBILITIES

Electrolytes, other I.V. drugs, saline solutions.

ACTION

Binds to sterols of fungal cell membranes, altering cell permeability and causing cell death.

Route	Onset	Peak	Duration
I.V.	Unknown	Unknown	Unknown

Half-life: About 1 week.

ADVERSE REACTIONS

CNS: *fever,* headache, pain.
CV: ***cardiac arrest,*** chest pain, hypertension, hypotension.
GI: ***GI hemorrhage,*** abdominal pain, diarrhea, nausea, vomiting.
GU: ***renal failure.***
Hematologic: ***leukopenia, thrombocytopenia,*** anemia.
Hepatic: bilirubinemia.
Metabolic: hypokalemia.
Respiratory: ***respiratory failure,*** dyspnea, respiratory disorder.
Skin: rash.
Other: MULTIPLE ORGAN FAILURE, *chills, sepsis,* infection.

INTERACTIONS

Drug-drug. *Antineoplastics:* May increase risk of renal toxicity, bronchospasm, and hypotension. Use together cautiously.
Cardiac glycosides: May increase risk of digitalis toxicity from amphotericin B–induced hypokalemia. Monitor potassium level closely.
Clotrimazole, fluconazole, itraconazole, ketoconazole, miconazole: May counteract amphotericin B. Monitor patient closely.
Corticosteroids, corticotropin: May enhance hypokalemia, which could lead to cardiac toxicity. Monitor electrolyte levels and cardiac function.
Cyclosporine: May increase renal toxicity. Monitor renal function test results closely.
Flucytosine: May increase risk of flucytosine toxicity from increased cellular uptake or impaired renal excretion. Use together cautiously.
Leukocyte transfusions: May increase risk of pulmonary reactions, such as acute dyspnea, tachypnea, hypoxemia, hemoptysis, and interstitial infiltrates. Use together with caution; separate doses as much as possible, and monitor pulmonary function.
Nephrotoxic drugs (such as aminoglycosides, pentamidine): May increase risk of renal toxicity. Use together cautiously and monitor renal function closely.
Skeletal muscle relaxants: May enhance skeletal muscle relaxant effects of amphotericin B–induced hypokalemia. Monitor potassium level closely.
Zidovudine: May increase myelotoxicity and nephrotoxicity. Monitor renal and hematologic function.

EFFECTS ON LAB TEST RESULTS

• May increase alkaline phosphatase, ALT, AST, bilirubin, BUN, creatinine, GGT, and LDH levels. May decrease hemoglobin and potassium levels.
• May decrease platelet and WBC counts.

CONTRAINDICATIONS & CAUTIONS

• Contraindicated in patients hypersensitive to amphotericin B or its components.
• Use cautiously in patients with renal impairment. Adjust dosage based on patient's overall condition. Renal toxicity is more common at higher dosages.
• It's unknown if drug appears in breast milk. Encourage the patient to either stop breast-feeding or stop treatment.

NURSING CONSIDERATIONS

• ***Alert:*** Different amphotericin B preparations aren't interchangeable, so dosages will vary. Confusing the preparations may cause permanent damage or death.
• Premedicate patient with acetaminophen, antihistamines, or corticosteroids to prevent or lessen severity of infusion-related reactions such as fever, chills, nausea, and vomiting, which occur 1 to 2 hours after start of infusion.

• Hydrate before infusion to reduce risk of nephrotoxicity.
• Monitor creatinine and electrolyte levels (especially magnesium and potassium), liver function, and CBC during therapy.

PATIENT TEACHING
• Inform patient that he may develop fever, chills, nausea, and vomiting during infusion, but that they usually subside with subsequent doses.
• Instruct patient to report any redness or pain at infusion site.
• Teach patient to recognize and report to prescriber signs and symptoms of acute hypersensitivity such as respiratory distress.
• Warn patient that therapy may take several months.
• Tell patient to expect frequent laboratory testing to monitor kidney and liver function.

SAFETY ALERT!

amphotericin B liposomal
AmBisome

Pharmacologic class: polyene antibiotic
Pregnancy risk category B

AVAILABLE FORMS
Powder for injection: 50-mg vial

INDICATIONS & DOSAGES
➤ **Empirical therapy for presumed fungal infection in febrile, neutropenic patients**
Adults and children: 3 mg/kg I.V. infusion over 2 hours daily.
➤ **Systemic fungal infections caused by *Aspergillus* species, *Candida* species, or *Cryptococcus* species refractory to amphotericin B deoxycholate or in patients for whom renal impairment or unacceptable toxicity precludes use of amphotericin B deoxycholate**
Adults and children: 3 to 5 mg/kg I.V. infusion over 2 hours daily.
➤ **Visceral leishmaniasis in immunocompetent patients**
Adults and children: 3 mg/kg I.V. infusion over 2 hours daily on days 1 to 5, 14, and 21. A repeat course of therapy may be beneficial if initial treatment fails to clear parasites.
➤ **Visceral leishmaniasis in immunocompromised patients**
Adults and children: 4 mg/kg I.V. infusion over 2 hours daily on days 1 to 5, 10, 17, 24, 31, and 38. Refer patient for expert advice regarding further treatment if initial therapy fails or patient relapses.
➤ **Cryptococcal meningitis in patients with HIV-infection**
Adults and children: 6 mg/kg/day I.V. infusion over 2 hours. Reduce infusion time to 1 hour if treatment is well tolerated, and increase infusion time if discomfort occurs.

I.V. ADMINISTRATION
• Don't reconstitute with bacteriostatic water for injection, and don't allow bacteriostatic product in solution.
• Don't reconstitute with saline solution, add saline solution to reconstituted concentration, or mix with other drugs.
• Reconstitute each 50-mg vial with 12 ml of sterile water for injection to yield 4 mg/ml.
• After reconstitution, shake vial vigorously for 30 seconds or until particulate matter disperses.
• Dilute to 1 to 2 mg/ml by withdrawing calculated amount of reconstituted solution into a sterile syringe and injecting it through a 5-micron filter into D_5W. Use only 1 filter needle per vial. Concentrations of 0.2 to 0.5 mg/ml may provide sufficient volume of infusion for children.
• Flush existing I.V. line with D_5W before infusing drug. If this isn't possible, give drug through a separate line.
• Use a controlled infusion device and an in-line filter with a mean pore diameter of 1 micron or larger.
• Initially, infuse drug over at least 2 hours. If drug is tolerated well, reduce infusion time to 1 hour. If discomfort occurs, increase infusion time.
• Store unopened vial at 36° to 46° F (2° to 8° C). Store reconstituted drug for up to 24 hours at 36° to 46° F. Don't freeze.

INCOMPATIBILITIES

Other I.V. drugs, saline solutions.

ACTION

Binds to sterols of fungal cell membranes, altering cell permeability and causing cell death.

Route	Onset	Peak	Duration
I.V.	Unknown	Unknown	Unknown

Half-life: About 4 to 6 days.

ADVERSE REACTIONS

CNS: *fever, anxiety, confusion, headache, insomnia, asthenia, pain.*
CV: *chest pain, hypotension, tachycardia, hypertension, edema, flushing.*
EENT: *epistaxis, rhinitis.*
GI: *nausea, vomiting, abdominal pain, diarrhea,* ***GI hemorrhage.***
GU: *hematuria,* ***renal failure.***
Hepatic: *bilirubinemia,* ***hepatotoxicity.***
Metabolic: *hyperglycemia,* hypernatremia, *hypocalcemia, hypokalemia, hypomagnesemia.*
Musculoskeletal: *back pain.*
Respiratory: *increased cough, dyspnea,* hypoxia, *pleural effusion, lung disorder,* hyperventilation.
Skin: *pruritus, rash, sweating.*
Other: *chills, infection,* ***anaphylaxis, sepsis,*** *blood product infusion reaction.*

INTERACTIONS

Drug-drug. *Antineoplastics:* May enhance potential for renal toxicity, bronchospasm, and hypotension. Use together cautiously.
Cardiac glycosides: May increase risk of digitalis toxicity caused by amphotericin B–induced hypokalemia. Monitor potassium level closely.
clotrimazole, fluconazole, ketoconazole, miconazole: May induce fungal resistance to amphotericin B. Use together cautiously.
Corticosteroids, corticotropin: May increase potassium depletion, which could cause cardiac dysfunction. Monitor electrolyte levels and cardiac function.
Flucytosine: May increase flucytosine toxicity by increasing cellular reuptake or impairing renal excretion of flucytosine. Use together cautiously.
Leukocyte transfusions: May increase risk of pulmonary reactions, such as acute dyspnea, tachypnea, hypoxemia, hemoptysis, and interstitial infiltrates. Use together cautiously; separate doses as much as possible, and monitor pulmonary function.
Other nephrotoxic drugs, such as antibiotics and antineoplastics: May cause additive nephrotoxicity. Use together cautiously; monitor renal function closely.
Skeletal muscle relaxants: May enhance effects of skeletal muscle relaxants resulting from amphotericin B–induced hypokalemia. Monitor potassium level.

EFFECTS ON LAB TEST RESULTS

- May increase alkaline phosphatase, ALT, AST, bilirubin, BUN, creatinine, GGT, glucose, LDH, and sodium levels. May decrease calcium, magnesium, and potassium levels.

CONTRAINDICATIONS & CAUTIONS

- Contraindicated in patients hypersensitive to drug or its components.
- Use cautiously in patients with impaired renal function, in elderly patients, and in pregnant women.
- It's unknown if drug appears in breast milk. Because of risk of serious adverse reactions in breast-fed infants, encourage mothers to stop either breast-feeding or therapy, taking into account importance of drug.

NURSING CONSIDERATIONS

- Patients also receiving chemotherapy or bone marrow transplantation are at greater risk for additional adverse reactions, including seizures, arrhythmias, and thrombocytopenia.
- ***Alert:*** Different amphotericin B preparations aren't interchangeable, so dosages will vary. Confusing the preparations may cause permanent damage or death.
- Premedicate patient with antipyretics, antihistamines, antiemetics, or corticosteroids.
- Hydrate before infusion to reduce the risk of nephrotoxicity.
- Monitor BUN and creatinine and electrolyte levels (particularly magnesium and potassium), liver function, and CBC.

- Watch for signs and symptoms of hypokalemia (ECG changes, muscle weakness, cramping, drowsiness).
- Patients treated with this drug have a lower risk of chills, elevated BUN level, hypokalemia, hypertension, and vomiting than patients treated with conventional amphotericin B.
- Therapy may take several weeks or months.
- Observe patient closely for adverse reactions during infusion. If anaphylaxis occurs, stop infusion immediately, provide supportive therapy, and notify prescriber.

PATIENT TEACHING

- Teach patient signs and symptoms of hypersensitivity, and stress importance of reporting them immediately.
- Warn patient that therapy may take several months; teach personal hygiene and other measures to prevent spread and recurrence of lesions.
- Instruct patient to report any adverse reactions that occur while receiving drug.
- Tell patient to watch for and report signs and symptoms of low levels of potassium in the blood (muscle weakness, cramping, drowsiness).
- Advise patient that frequent laboratory testing will be needed.

✷ NEW DRUG

anidulafungin

Eraxis

Pharmacologic class: echinocandin
Pregnancy risk category C

AVAILABLE FORMS

Powder for injection: 50 mg/vial with companion diluent

INDICATIONS & DOSAGES

➤ **Candidemia and other *Candida* infections (intra-abdominal abscess, peritonitis)**

Adults: A single 200-mg loading dose given by I.V. infusion at no more than 1.1 mg/minute on day 1; then 100 mg daily for at least 14 days after last positive culture result.

➤ **Esophageal candidiasis**

Adults: A single 100-mg loading dose given by I.V. infusion at no more than 1.1 mg/minute on day 1; then 50 mg daily for at least 14 days and for at least 7 more days after symptoms resolve.

I.V. ADMINISTRATION

- Reconstitute each vial with 15 ml of supplied diluent.
- Further dilute with D_5W or normal saline solution to a final concentration of 0.5 mg/ml.
- For 50-mg dose, add to 85 ml for final infusion volume of 100 ml. For 100-mg dose, add to 170 ml for final infusion volume of 200 ml. For 200-mg dose, add to 340 ml for final infusion volume of 400 ml.
- Don't infuse at more than 1.1 mg/minute.
- Store at room temperature; don't freeze. Use reconstituted solution within 24 hours of preparation.

INCOMPATIBILITIES

Unknown. Only use supplied diluent to reconstitute and D_5W or normal saline solution to further dilute.

ACTION

Inhibits glucan synthase, which in turn inhibits formation of 1,3-β-D-glucan, an essential component of fungal cell walls.

Route	Onset	Peak	Duration
I.V.	< 24 hr	Unknown	Unknown

Half-life: 40 to 50 hours.

ADVERSE REACTIONS

CNS: headache.
CV: deep vein thrombosis, hypotension.
GI: abdominal pain, dyspepsia, nausea, vomiting.
Hematologic: ***leukopenia, neutropenia.***
Metabolic: hypokalemia.
Skin: flushing, pruritus, rash, urticaria.

INTERACTIONS

None reported.

EFFECTS ON LAB TEST RESULTS

- May increase AST, ALT, alkaline phosphatase, GGT, hepatic enzyme, amylase,

lipase, bilirubin, CK, creatinine, urea, calcium, glucose, potassium, and sodium levels. May decrease potassium and magnesium levels.
- May increase PT. May decrease neutrophil and WBC counts. May increase or decrease platelet count.

CONTRAINDICATIONS & CAUTIONS
- Contraindicated in patients hypersensitive to drug, other echinocandins, or any component of the drug.
- Use cautiously in patients with liver impairment and in pregnant or breast-feeding women.

NURSING CONSIDERATIONS
- Obtain specimens for culture and sensitivity tests and baseline laboratory tests before therapy.
- Use only the supplied diluent to reconstitute powder.
- To avoid histamine-mediated symptoms, such as rash, urticaria, flushing, itching, dyspnea, and hypotension, don't infuse faster than 1.1 mg/minute.
- Monitor patient closely for changes in liver function and blood cell counts during therapy.
- Notify prescriber about signs or symptoms of liver toxicity, such as dark urine, jaundice, abdominal pain, and fatigue.
- Patients with esophageal candidiasis who are HIV-positive may need suppressive antifungal therapy after drug to prevent relapse.
- Safety and effectiveness in children haven't been established.

PATIENT TEACHING
- Tell patient to call the nurse if he develops a rash, itching, trouble breathing, or other adverse effects during infusion.
- Explain that blood tests will be needed to monitor the drug's effects.

caspofungin acetate
Cancidas

Pharmacologic class: echinocandin
Pregnancy risk category C

AVAILABLE FORMS
Lyophilized powder for injection: 50-mg, 70-mg single-use vials

INDICATIONS & DOSAGES
➤ **Invasive aspergillosis in patients who are refractory to or intolerant of other therapies (amphotericin B, lipid forms of amphotericin B, or itraconazole); candidemia and *Candida*-caused intra-abdominal abscesses, peritonitis, and pleural space infections**
Adults: Single 70-mg I.V. loading dose on day 1, followed by 50 mg/day I.V. over about 1 hour. Base treatment duration on severity of patient's underlying disease, recovery from immunosuppression, and clinical response.
➤ **Empirical treatment of presumed fungal infections in febrile, neutropenic patients**
Adults: Single 70-mg I.V. loading dose on day 1, followed by 50 mg/day I.V. over 1 hour thereafter. Continue empirical therapy until neutropenia resolves. If fungal infection is confirmed, treat for a minimum of 14 days and continue therapy for at least 7 days after neutropenia and symptoms resolve. May increase daily dose to 70 mg if the 50-mg dose is well tolerated but clinical response is suboptimal.
➤ **Esophageal candidiasis**
Adults: 50 mg I.V. daily over 1 hour. After treatment, patients with HIV may require oral suppressive therapy to reduce risk of relapse.
Adjust-a-dose: For patients with Child-Pugh score 7 to 9, after initial 70-mg loading dose (when indicated), give 35 mg/day. Dosage adjustment in patients with Child-Pugh score of more than 9 is unknown.

I.V. ADMINISTRATION
- Let refrigerated vial warm to room temperature.

• For patients on fluid restriction, dilute the 35-mg and 50-mg doses in 100 ml normal saline solution. For other patients, dilute 35-mg, 50-mg, and 70-mg doses in 250 ml normal saline solution.
• Give drug by slow infusion over about 1 hour.
• Monitor site carefully for phlebitis.
• Use reconstituted vials within 1 hour or discard.
• The final product for infusion (solution in I.V. bag or bottle) can be stored at room temperature for 24 hours.

INCOMPATIBILITIES
Don't mix or infuse with other drugs or dextrose solutions.

ACTION
Inhibits synthesis of beta (1,3)-d-glucan in susceptible *Aspergillus* species. Drug is extensively distributed and has a prolonged half-life.

Route	Onset	Peak	Duration
I.V.	Unknown	Unknown	Unknown

Half-life: 9 to 11 hours.

ADVERSE REACTIONS
CNS: *paresthesia,* fever, headache.
CV: *tachycardia,* phlebitis, infused vein complications.
GI: *anorexia,* nausea, vomiting, diarrhea, abdominal pain.
GU: proteinuria, hematuria.
Hematologic: *anemia,* eosinophilia.
Metabolic: hypokalemia.
Musculoskeletal: *pain, myalgia.*
Respiratory: *tachypnea.*
Skin: histamine-mediated symptoms, including rash, facial swelling, pruritus, sensation of warmth.
Other: *chills, sweating.*

INTERACTIONS
Drug-drug. *Cyclosporine:* May increase caspofungin level. May increase risk of elevated ALT level, avoid using together unless benefit outweighs risk.
Inducers of drug clearance or mixed inducer-inhibitors (carbamazepine, dexamethasone, efavirenz, nelfinavir, nevirapine, phenytoin, rifampin): May reduce caspofungin level. May need to adjust dosage.
Tacrolimus: May reduce tacrolimus level. Monitor tacrolimus level; expect to adjust dosage.

EFFECTS ON LAB TEST RESULTS
• May increase alkaline phosphatase and liver enzyme levels. May decrease albumin, calcium, hemoglobin, potassium, and protein levels.
• May increase eosinophil count.

CONTRAINDICATIONS & CAUTIONS
• Contraindicated in patients hypersensitive to drug or its components.
• Safety and effectiveness in children younger than age 18 aren't known.
• It's unknown if drug appears in breast milk. Use cautiously in breast-feeding women.

NURSING CONSIDERATIONS
• Safety information is limited, but drug is well-tolerated for therapy lasting longer than 2 weeks.
• Observe patients for histamine-mediated reactions, including rash, facial swelling, pruritus, and a sensation of warmth.

PATIENT TEACHING
• Instruct patient to report signs and symptoms of phlebitis.
• Instruct patient to immediately report any signs of a hypersensitivity reaction.

fluconazole
Diflucan🖉

Pharmacologic class: bis-triazole derivative
Pregnancy risk category C

AVAILABLE FORMS
Injection: 200 mg/100 ml, 400 mg/200 ml
Powder for oral suspension: 10 mg/ml, 40 mg/ml
Tablets: 50 mg, 100 mg, 150 mg, 200 mg

INDICATIONS & DOSAGES
➤ **Oropharyngeal candidiasis**
Adults: 200 mg P.O. or I.V. on first day, then 100 mg once daily for at least 2 weeks.

Children: 6 mg/kg P.O. or I.V. on first day, then 3 mg/kg daily for 2 weeks.

➤ **Esophageal candidiasis**

Adults: 200 mg P.O. or I.V. on first day, then 100 mg once daily. Up to 400 mg daily has been used, depending on patient's condition and tolerance of treatment. Patients should receive drug for at least 3 weeks and for 2 weeks after symptoms resolve.

Children: 6 mg/kg P.O. or I.V. on first day, then 3 mg/kg daily for at least 3 weeks and for at least 2 weeks after symptoms resolve. Maximum daily dose 12 mg/kg.

➤ **Vulvovaginal candidiasis**

Adults: 150 mg P.O. for one dose only.

➤ **Systemic candidiasis**

Adults: 400 mg P.O. or I.V. on first day, then 200 mg once daily for at least 4 weeks and for 2 weeks after symptoms resolve. Doses up to 400 mg/day may be used.

Children: 6 to 12 mg/kg/day P.O. or I.V.

➤ **Cryptococcal meningitis**

Adults: 400 mg P.O. or I.V. on first day, then 200 mg once daily for 10 to 12 weeks after CSF culture result is negative. Doses up to 400 mg/day may be used.

Children: 12 mg/kg/day P.O. or I.V. on first day, then 6 mg/kg/day for 10 to 12 weeks after CSF culture result is negative.

➤ **To prevent candidiasis in bone marrow transplant**

Adults: 400 mg P.O. or I.V. once daily. Start treatment several days before anticipated agranulocytosis, and continue for 7 days after neutrophil count exceeds 1,000/mm^3.

➤ **To suppress relapse of cryptococcal meningitis in patients with AIDS**

Adults: 200 mg P.O. or I.V. daily.

Children: 3 to 6 mg/kg/day P.O. or I.V.

Adjust-a-dose: If creatinine clearance is less than 50 ml/minute and patient isn't receiving dialysis, reduce dosage by 50%. Patients receiving regular hemodialysis treatment should receive usual dose after each dialysis session.

I.V. ADMINISTRATION

- To ensure product sterility, don't remove protective wrap from I.V. bag until just before use.
- The plastic container may show some opacity from moisture absorbed during sterilization. This doesn't affect drug and diminishes over time.
- To prevent air embolism, don't connect in series with other infusions.
- Use an infusion pump.
- Give by continuous infusion at no more than 200 mg/hour.

INCOMPATIBILITIES

Amphotericin B, amphotericin B cholesteryl sulfate complex, ampicillin sodium, calcium gluconate, cefotaxime sodium, ceftazidime, ceftriaxone, cefuroxime sodium, chloramphenicol sodium succinate, clindamycin phosphate, co-trimoxazole, diazepam, digoxin, erythromycin lactobionate, furosemide, haloperidol lactate, hydroxyzine hydrochloride, imipenem and cilastatin sodium, pentamidine, piperacillin sodium, ticarcillin disodium, trimethoprim-sulfamethoxazole. Don't add other drugs to I.V. bag.

ACTION

Inhibits fungal cytochrome P-450 (responsible for fungal sterol synthesis); weakens fungal cell walls.

Route	Onset	Peak	Duration
P.O.	Unknown	1–2 hr	30 hr
I.V.	Immediate	Immediate	Unknown

Half-life: 20 to 50 hours.

ADVERSE REACTIONS

CNS: *headache,* dizziness.
GI: nausea, vomiting, abdominal pain, diarrhea, dyspepsia, taste perversion.
Hematologic: ***leukopenia, thrombocytopenia.***
Skin: rash.
Other: ***anaphylaxis.***

INTERACTIONS

Drug-drug. *Alprazolam, chlordiazepoxide, clonazepam, clorazepate, diazepam, estazolam, flurazepam, midazolam, quazepam, triazolam:* May increase and prolong levels of these drugs, CNS depression, and psychomotor impairment. Avoid using together.

Cimetidine: May decrease fluconazole level. Monitor patient's response to fluconazole.
Cyclosporine, phenytoin, theophylline: May increase levels of these drugs. Monitor cyclosporine, phenytoin, and theophylline levels.
HMG-CoA reductase inhibitors (atorvastatin, fluvastatin, lovastatin, pravastatin, simvastatin): May increase levels and adverse effects of these drugs. Avoid using together or reduce dosage of HMG-CoA reductase inhibitor.
Isoniazid, oral sulfonylureas, phenytoin, rifampin, valproic acid: May increase hepatic transaminase level. Monitor liver function test results closely.
Oral sulfonylureas (such as glipizide, glyburide, tolbutamide): May increase levels of these drugs. Monitor patient for enhanced hypoglycemic effect.
Rifampin: May enhance fluconazole metabolism. Monitor patient for lack of response to fluconazole.
Tacrolimus: May increase tacrolimus level and nephrotoxicity. Monitor patient carefully.
Warfarin: May increase risk of bleeding. Monitor PT and INR.
Zidovudine: May increase zidovudine activity. Monitor patient closely.

EFFECTS ON LAB TEST RESULTS
- May increase alkaline phosphatase, ALT, AST, bilirubin, and GGT levels.
- May decrease platelet and WBC counts.

CONTRAINDICATIONS & CAUTIONS
- Contraindicated in patients hypersensitive to drug and breast-feeding patients.
- Use cautiously in patients hypersensitive to other antifungal azole compounds.

NURSING CONSIDERATIONS
- Serious hepatotoxicity has occurred in patients with underlying medical conditions.
- If patient develops mild rash, monitor him closely. Stop drug if lesions progress.
- Likelihood of adverse reactions may be greater in HIV-infected patients.

PATIENT TEACHING
- Tell patient to take drug as directed, even after he feels better.
- Instruct patient to report adverse reactions promptly.

flucytosine (5-FC, 5-fluorocytosine)

Ancobon, Ancotil‡

Pharmacologic class: fluorinated pyrimidine
Pregnancy risk category C

AVAILABLE FORMS
Capsules: 250 mg, 500 mg

INDICATIONS & DOSAGES
➤ **Severe fungal infections from susceptible strains of *Candida* (including septicemia, endocarditis, and urinary tract or pulmonary infection), and of *Cryptococcus* (including meningitis and urinary tract or pulmonary infection)**
Adults: 50 to 150 mg/kg daily P.O. in four equally divided doses q 6 hours.

ACTION
Appears to penetrate fungal cells and cause defective protein synthesis.

Route	Onset	Peak	Duration
P.O.	Unknown	1–2 hr	Unknown

Half-life: 2½ to 6 hours.

ADVERSE REACTIONS
CNS: headache, vertigo, sedation, fatigue, weakness, confusion, hallucinations, psychosis, ataxia, hearing loss, paresthesia, parkinsonism, peripheral neuropathy.
CV: ***cardiac arrest,*** chest pain.
GI: ***hemorrhage,*** nausea, vomiting, diarrhea, abdominal pain, dry mouth, duodenal ulcer, ulcerative colitis, anorexia.
GU: ***renal failure,*** azotemia, crystalluria.
Hematologic: ***agranulocytosis, aplastic anemia, leukopenia, bone marrow suppression, thrombocytopenia,*** anemia, eosinophilia.
Hepatic: jaundice.
Metabolic: ***hypoglycemia,*** hypokalemia.
Respiratory: ***respiratory arrest,*** dyspnea.
Skin: rash, pruritus, urticaria, photosensitivity.

INTERACTIONS

Drug-drug. *Amphotericin B:* May cause synergistic effects, increasing risk of toxicity. Monitor patient for increased adverse reactions and toxicity.

EFFECTS ON LAB TEST RESULTS

- May increase alkaline phosphatase, ALT, AST, bilirubin, BUN, creatinine, and urine urea levels. May decrease glucose, hemoglobin, and potassium levels.
- May increase eosinophil count. May decrease granulocyte, platelet, and WBC counts.

CONTRAINDICATIONS & CAUTIONS

- Contraindicated in patients hypersensitive to drug.
- Use with extreme caution in patients with impaired hepatic or renal function or bone marrow suppression.

NURSING CONSIDERATIONS

- Monitor blood, liver, and renal function studies frequently during therapy; obtain susceptibility tests weekly to monitor drug resistance.
- Regularly perform drug level assays to maintain therapeutic level of 40 to 60 mcg/ml. Levels above 100 mcg/ml may be toxic.
- Monitor fluid intake and output; report marked changes.

PATIENT TEACHING

- Instruct patient to take a few capsules at a time over 15 minutes to reduce adverse GI reactions.
- Tell patient that drug may cause photosensitivity and to avoid prolonged exposure to sun or ultraviolet light, such as tanning beds, to use sunscreen, and to wear protective clothing.
- Tell patient that therapeutic response may take weeks or months.
- Advise patient to report adverse reactions promptly.

griseofulvin microsize

Grifulvin V

griseofulvin ultramicrosize

Gris-PEG

Pharmacologic class: penicillium antibiotic
Pregnancy risk category C

AVAILABLE FORMS

microsize
Tablets: 500 mg
Oral suspension: 125 mg/5 ml
ultramicrosize
Tablets (film-coated): 125 mg, 250 mg

INDICATIONS & DOSAGES

➤ ***Tinea corporis, t. capitis, t. barbae, t. cruris t. pedis,* or *t. unguium* infections**

Microsize
Adults: 500 mg P.O. daily. For more difficult fungal infections, such as tinea pedis or unguium, give 1 g P.O. daily.
Children: Approximately 5 mg per pound of body weight daily. For children who weigh 14 to 23 kg (30 to 50 lbs), acceptable range is 125 to 250 mg daily; children who weigh more than 23 kg, acceptable range is 250 to 500 mg daily.

Ultramicrosize
Adults: 375 mg P.O. daily. For more difficult fungal infections, such as tinea pedis or t. unguium, give 750 mg P.O. daily in divided doses.
Children older than age 2: Approximately 3.3 mg per pound of body weight daily. For children who weigh 16 to 27 kg (35 to 60 lbs), acceptable range is 125 to 187.5 mg daily; children who weigh more than 27 kg, acceptable range is 187.5 mg to 375 mg daily.

ACTION

Drug disrupts fungal cells' mitotic spindle, interfering with cell division; it also may inhibit DNA replication. Drug also enters keratin precursor cells, slowing fungal growth. Active against *Trichophyton, Microsporum,* and *Epidermophyton* species.

Route	Onset	Peak	Duration
P.O.	Unknown	4–8 hr	Unknown

Half-life: 9 to 24 hours.

ADVERSE REACTIONS
CNS: dizziness, fatigue, headache, impaired performance, insomnia, mental confusion, paresthesia of the hands and feet, psychotic symptoms.
EENT: oral thrush, transient decrease in hearing.
GI: ***bleeding,*** diarrhea, epigastric distress, flatulence, nausea, vomiting.
GU: menstrual irregularities, proteinuria.
Hematologic: ***granulocytopenia, leukopenia,*** porphyria.
Hepatic: ***hepatotoxicity.***
Skin: erythema multiforme-like reaction, photosensitivity, *rash, urticaria.*
Other: ***angioedema,*** hypersensitivity reactions, systemic lupus erythematosus.

INTERACTIONS
Drug-drug. *Barbiturates:* May impair griseofulvin absorption. Increase dosage as needed.
Cyclosporine, salicylates: May decrease levels of these drugs. Monitor patient for decreased drug effects.
Hormonal contraceptives: May decrease contraceptive efficacy. Suggest alternative method of contraception.
Warfarin: May decrease PT and INR. Adjust dosage if needed.
Drug-food. *High-fat meals:* May increase absorption. May be given together.
Drug-lifestyle. *Alcohol use:* May increase alcohol effect, producing tachycardia, diaphoresis, and flushing. Discourage alcohol use.

EFFECTS ON LAB TEST RESULTS
• May decrease WBC and granulocyte counts.

CONTRAINDICATIONS & CAUTIONS
• Contraindicated in patients hypersensitive to drug, women who intend to become pregnant during therapy, and patients with porphyria or hepatocellular failure.
• Use cautiously in penicillin-sensitive patients.

PATIENT TEACHING
• Tell patient to take drug with or after meals, preferably high-fat meals if allowed, to minimize GI distress.
• Encourage patient to maintain adequate nutritional intake.
• Stress importance of completing prescribed regimen, even if symptoms subside quickly, to prevent relapse.
• Tell patient to report adverse reactions immediately.
• Advise patient to avoid exposure to intense indoor light and sunlight to reduce the risk of photosensitivity reactions.
• Explain that drug may increase the effects of alcohol, and advise patient to avoid alcohol during therapy.

itraconazole
Sporanox

Pharmacologic class: synthetic triazole
Pregnancy risk category C

AVAILABLE FORMS
Capsules: 100 mg
Injection: 10 mg/ml
Oral solution: 10 mg/ml

INDICATIONS & DOSAGES
➤ **Pulmonary and extrapulmonary blastomycosis, nonmeningeal histoplasmosis**
Adults: 200 mg P.O. daily; increase as needed and tolerated by 100 mg to maximum of 400 mg daily. Give dosages exceeding 200 mg P.O. daily in two divided doses. Or, give 200 mg I.V. b.i.d. over 1 hour for 4 doses, followed by 200 mg I.V. daily for up to 14 days; then change to P.O. form. Continue treatment for at least 3 months. In life-threatening illness, give a loading dose of 200 mg P.O. t.i.d. for 3 days.
➤ **Aspergillosis**
Adults: 200 to 400 mg P.O. daily. Or, 200 mg I.V. b.i.d. over 1 hour for 4 doses, followed by 200 mg I.V. daily for up to 14 days; then change to P.O. form.

➤**Onychomycosis of the toenail (with or without fingernail involvement)**
Adults: 200 mg P.O. once daily for 12 consecutive weeks.
➤**Onychomycosis of the fingernail**
Adults: 200 mg P.O. b.i.d. for 1 week, followed by 3 weeks drug free. Repeat dosage.
➤**Oropharyngeal candidiasis**
Adults: 200 mg oral solution swished in mouth vigorously and swallowed daily, for 1 to 2 weeks.
➤**Oropharyngeal candidiasis in patients unresponsive to fluconazole tablets**
Adults: 100 mg oral solution swished in mouth vigorously and swallowed b.i.d., for 2 to 4 weeks.
➤**Esophageal candidiasis**
Adults: 100 to 200 mg oral solution swished in mouth vigorously and swallowed daily, for at least 3 weeks. Treatment should continue for 2 weeks after symptoms resolve.

I.V. ADMINISTRATION

- Use only components provided in the infusion kit. Don't substitute.
- Dilute contents of 250-mg ampule in the 50-ml bag of normal saline solution, then withdraw and discard 15 ml of solution before giving to patient. This provides 60 ml of a solution containing 3.33 mg/ml of drug.
- Give by I.V. infusion over 1 hour, using infusion set provided and a controlled infusion device.
- Don't mix with other drugs or give through same I.V. line as other drugs.
- Flush infusion set via the two-way stopcock with 15 to 20 ml of normal saline solution injection over 30 seconds to 15 minutes; then discard I.V. line.
- Store diluted injection at 36° to 46° F (2° to 8° C) or at 59° to 77° F (15° to 25° C) for up to 48 hours when protected from light.

INCOMPATIBILITIES

All other drugs and diluents excluding the one provided in the kit accompanying the drug.

ACTION

Interferes with fungal cell-wall synthesis by inhibiting ergosterol formation and increasing cell-wall permeability, leading to osmotic instability.

Route	Onset	Peak	Duration
P.O.	Unknown	3–4 hr	Unknown
I.V.	Unknown	Unknown	Unknown

Half-life: 1 to 8¼ hours.

ADVERSE REACTIONS

CNS: *headache,* fever, dizziness, somnolence, fatigue, malaise, asthenia, pain, tremor, abnormal dreams, anxiety, depression.
CV: ***heart failure,*** hypertension, edema, orthostatic hypotension.
EENT: rhinitis, sinusitis, pharyngitis.
GI: *nausea,* vomiting, diarrhea, abdominal pain, anorexia, dyspepsia, flatulence, increased appetite, constipation, gastritis, gastroenteritis, ulcerative stomatitis, gingivitis.
GU: albuminuria, impotence, cystitis, UTI.
Hematologic: ***neutropenia.***
Hepatic: ***hepatotoxicity, liver failure,*** impaired hepatic function.
Metabolic: hypokalemia, hypertriglyceridemia.
Musculoskeletal: myalgia.
Respiratory: ***pulmonary edema,*** upper respiratory tract infection.
Skin: rash, pruritus.
Other: decreased libido, injury, herpes zoster, ***hypersensitivity reactions (urticaria, angioedema, Stevens-Johnson syndrome).***

INTERACTIONS

Drug-drug. *Alprazolam, midazolam, triazolam:* May increase and prolong drug levels, CNS depression, and psychomotor impairment. Avoid using together.
Antacids, carbamazepine, H_2-receptor antagonists, isoniazid, phenobarbital, ***phenytoin,*** *rifabutin, rifampin:* May decrease itraconazole level. Avoid using together.
Chlordiazepoxide, clonazepam, clorazepate, diazepam, estazolam, flurazepam, quazepam: May increase and prolong drug levels, CNS depression, and psychomotor impairment. Avoid using together.

Reactions may be *common,* uncommon, ***life-threatening,*** or COMMON AND LIFE-THREATENING.
Interaction may have a *rapid onset* or ***delayed onset.***

Clarithromycin, erythromycin: May increase itraconazole levels. Monitor patient for signs of itraconazole toxicity.
Cyclosporine, **digoxin,** *tacrolimus:* May increase levels of these drugs. Monitor drug levels.
Dofetilide, pimozide, quinidine: May increase levels of these drugs by cytochrome P-450 metabolism, causing serious CV events, including torsades de pointes, QT interval prolongation, ventricular tachycardia, cardiac arrest, and sudden death. Avoid using together.
HMG-CoA reductase inhibitors (atorvastatin, fluvastatin, lovastatin, pravastatin, simvastatin): May increase levels and adverse effects of these drugs. Avoid using together, or reduce dose of HMG-CoA reductase inhibitor. Don't use itraconazole with lovastatin or simvastatin.
Indinavir, ritonavir, saquinavir: May increase levels of these drugs; indinavir and ritonavir may increase itraconazole levels. Monitor patient for toxicity.
Oral anticoagulants: May enhance anticoagulant effect. Monitor PT and INR.
Oral antidiabetics: May cause hypoglycemia, similar to effect of other antifungals. Monitor glucose level. Avoid using together.
Drug-food. *Grapefruit and orange juice:* May decrease drug level and therapeutic effect. Give with other liquids.

EFFECTS ON LAB TEST RESULTS

- May increase alkaline phosphatase, ALT, AST, bilirubin, triglyceride, and GGT levels. May decrease potassium level.

CONTRAINDICATIONS & CAUTIONS

- Contraindicated in patients hypersensitive to drug or those receiving alprazolam, triazolam, midazolam, pimozide, quinidine, dofetilide, lovastatin, or simvastatin; in those with ventricular dysfunction ora history of heart failure; and in those who are breast-feeding. If signs and symptoms of heart failure occur, stop itraconazole.
- Use cautiously in patients with hypochlorhydria; they may not absorb drug readily.
- Use cautiously in HIV-infected patients because hypochlorhydria can accompany HIV infection.
- Use cautiously in patients receiving other highly bound drugs.

NURSING CONSIDERATIONS

- ***Alert:*** Capsules and oral solution aren't interchangeable.
- Confirm the diagnosis of onychomycosis before starting therapy by sending nail specimens for testing.
- Perform baseline liver function tests and monitor results periodically. In patients with baseline hepatic impairment, give drug only if patient's condition is life threatening. If liver dysfunction occurs during therapy, notify prescriber immediately.

PATIENT TEACHING

- Teach patient to recognize and report signs and symptoms of liver disease (anorexia, dark urine, pale stools, unusual fatigue, and jaundice).
- Instruct patient not to use oral solution interchangeably with capsules.
- For the oral solution, tell patient to take 10 ml at a time.
- Advise patient to take solution without food and to take capsules with a full meal.
- Urge patient to list the other drugs he's taking for prescriber, to avoid drug interactions.
- Advise women of childbearing age that an effective form of contraception must be used during therapy and for two menstrual cycles after stopping therapy with capsules.

ketoconazole

Nizoral

Pharmacologic class: imidazole derivative
Pregnancy risk category C

AVAILABLE FORMS

Oral suspension: 100 mg/5 ml†
Tablets: 200 mg

INDICATIONS & DOSAGES

➤ **Systemic candidiasis, chronic mucocutaneous candidiasis, oral candidiasis, candiduria, coccidioidomycosis, blastomycosis, histoplasmosis, chromomycosis, and paracoccidioi-**

domycosis; severe cutaneous dermatophyte infections that are resistant to therapy with topical or oral griseofulvin
Adults and children who weigh more than 40 kg (88 lb): Initially, 200 mg P.O. daily in a single dose. Dosage may be increased to 400 mg once daily in patients who don't respond.
Children age 2 and older: 3.3 to 6.6 mg/kg P.O. daily in a single dose.
➤**Onychomycosis (caused by *Trichophyton* and *Candida* species); tinea versicolor; tinea pedis, tinea corporis, and tinea cruris**♦
Adults: 200 to 400 mg P.O. daily.
➤**Tinea capitis**♦
Adults: 3.3 to 6.6 mg/kg P.O. daily.

ACTION

Interferes with fungal cell-wall synthesis by inhibiting formation of ergosterol and increasing cell-wall permeability that makes the fungus susceptible to osmotic instability.

Route	Onset	Peak	Duration
P.O.	Unknown	1–2 hr	Unknown

Half-life: 8 hours.

ADVERSE REACTIONS

CNS: ***suicidal tendencies,*** fever, headache, nervousness, dizziness, somnolence, severe depression.
EENT: photophobia.
GI: *nausea, vomiting,* abdominal pain, diarrhea.
GU: impotence.
Hematologic: ***leukopenia, thrombocytopenia,*** hemolytic anemia.
Hepatic: ***fatal hepatotoxicity.***
Metabolic: hyperlipidemia.
Skin: pruritus.
Other: gynecomastia with tenderness, chills.

INTERACTIONS

Drug-drug. *Alprazolam, triazolam:* May increase and prolong levels of these drugs. May cause CNS depression and psychomotor impairment. Avoid using together.
Antacids, anticholinergics, H_2-receptor antagonists: May decrease absorption of ketoconazole. Wait at least 2 hours after ketoconazole dose before giving these drugs.
Chlordiazepoxide, clonazepam, clorazepate, diazepam, estazolam, flurazepam, midazolam, quazepam: May increase and prolong levels of these drugs. May cause CNS depression and psychomotor impairment. Avoid using together.
Cyclosporine, methylprednisolone, tacrolimus: May increase drug levels. Monitor drug levels, if appropriate.
Digoxin: May increase digoxin level. Monitor digoxin level.
Isoniazid, rifampin: May increase ketoconazole metabolism. Monitor patient for decreased antifungal effect.
HMG-CoA reductase inhibitors (atorvastatin, fluvastatin, lovastatin, pravastatin, simvastatin): May increase levels and adverse effects of these drugs. Avoid using together, or reduce dose of HMG-CoA reductase inhibitor.
Oral antidiabetics: May cause hypoglycemia. Monitor glucose level.
Paclitaxel: May inhibit metabolism. Use together cautiously.
Phenytoin: May alter the metabolism of one or both drugs. Monitor patient for adverse effects.
Rifampin, isoniazid: May decrease ketoconazole level. Avoid using together.
Theophylline: May decrease theophylline level. Monitor theophylline level.
Warfarin: May enhance effects of anticoagulant. Monitor INR, PT, and PTT and adjust dosage, as needed.
Drug-herb. *Yew:* May inhibit drug metabolism. Discourage use together.

EFFECTS ON LAB TEST RESULTS

- May increase lipid, alkaline phosphatase, ALT, and AST levels. May decrease hemoglobin level.
- May decrease platelet and WBC counts.

CONTRAINDICATIONS & CAUTIONS

- Contraindicated in patients hypersensitive to drug and in those taking alprazolam or oral triazolam.
- Use cautiously in patients with hepatic disease and in those taking other hepatotoxic drugs.

NURSING CONSIDERATIONS

- *Alert:* Because of risk of hepatotoxicity, drug shouldn't be used for less serious conditions, such as fungal infections of skin or nails.
- Monitor patient for signs and symptoms of hepatotoxicity, including elevated liver enzyme levels, nausea that doesn't subside, and unusual fatigue, jaundice, dark urine, or pale stool.
- Doses up to 800 mg/day can be used to treat fungal meningitis and intracerebral fungal lesions.
- *Alert:* Drug is a potent inhibitor of the cytochrome P-450 enzyme system. Giving this drug with drugs metabolized by the cytochrome P-450 3A4 enzyme system may lead to increased drug levels, which could increase or prolong therapeutic and adverse effects.

PATIENT TEACHING

- Instruct patient with achlorhydria to dissolve each tablet in 4 ml aqueous solution of 0.2 N hydrochloric acid, sip mixture through a glass or plastic straw, and then drink a glass of water because drug needs gastric acidity for dissolution and absorption.
- Instruct patient to wait at least 2 hours after dose before taking antacids.
- Make sure patient understands that treatment should continue until all tests indicate that active fungal infection has subsided. If drug is stopped too soon, infection will recur. Minimum treatment for candidiasis is 7 to 14 days; for other systemic fungal infections, 6 months; for resistant dermatophyte infections, at least 4 weeks.
- Reassure patient that nausea is common early in therapy but will subside. To minimize nausea, instruct patient to divide daily amount into 2 doses or take drug with meals.
- Review signs and symptoms of hepatotoxicity with patient; instruct him to stop drug and notify prescriber if they occur.
- Advise patient to discuss any new drugs or herbal supplements with prescriber.

micafungin sodium

Mycamine

Pharmacologic class: echinocandin
Pregnancy risk category C

AVAILABLE FORMS

Lyophilized powder for injection: 50 mg single-use vial

INDICATIONS & DOSAGES

➤ **Esophageal candidiasis**

Adults: 150 mg I.V. daily for 10 to 30 days.

➤ **To prevent candidal infection in hematopoietic stem cell transplant recipients**

Adults: 50 mg I.V. daily for 6 to 51 days.

I.V. ADMINISTRATION

- Use aseptic technique when preparing drug.
- Reconstitute each 50-mg vial with 5 ml of normal saline solution for injection or D_5W. To minimize foaming, dissolve powder by swirling the vial; don't shake it.
- Dilute dose in 100 ml of normal saline solution for injection.
- Flush line with normal saline solution for injection before infusing drug.
- Infuse drug over 1 hour.
- Reconstituted product and diluted infusion may be stored for up to 24 hours at room temperature.
- Protect diluted solution from light.

INCOMPATIBILITIES

Drug may precipitate when mixed with commonly used drugs.

ACTION

Inhibits synthesis of an essential component of fungal cell walls. Drug is active against *Candida albicans, C. glabrata, C. krusei, C. parapsilosis,* and *C. tropicalis.*

Route	Onset	Peak	Duration
I.V.	Unknown	Unknown	Unknown

Half-life: Unknown.

ADVERSE REACTIONS

CNS: headache.

GI: abdominal pain, diarrhea, nausea, vomiting.
Hematologic: ***leukopenia, neutropenia, thrombocytopenia,*** anemia.
Metabolic: hypocalcemia, hypokalemia, hypomagnesemia, hypophosphatemia.
Skin: infusion site inflammation, phlebitis, pruritus, rash.
Other: pyrexia, rigors.

INTERACTIONS

Drug-drug. *Nifedipine:* May increase nifedipine level. Monitor blood pressure, and decrease nifedipine dose if needed.
Sirolimus: May increase sirolimus level. Monitor patient for evidence of toxicity, and decrease sirolimus dose if needed.

EFFECTS ON LAB TEST RESULTS

- May increase alkaline phosphatase, ALT, AST, bilirubin, BUN, creatinine, and LDH levels. May decrease calcium, magnesium, phosphorus, potassium, and hemoglobin levels and hematocrit.
- May decrease neutrophil and platelet counts.

CONTRAINDICATIONS & CAUTIONS

- Contraindicated in patients hypersensitive to drug.
- Use cautiously in patients with severe hepatic disease.

NURSING CONSIDERATIONS

- Injection site reactions occur more often in patients receiving drug by peripheral I.V.
- To reduce the risk of histamine-mediated reactions, infuse drug over at least 1 hour.
- ***Alert:*** If patient develops signs of serious hypersensitivity reaction, including shock, stop infusion and notify prescriber.
- Monitor hepatic and renal function during therapy.
- Monitor patient for hemolysis and hemolytic anemia.
- Use drug in pregnant women only if clearly needed.
- It's unknown whether drug appears in breast milk. Use cautiously in breastfeeding women.

PATIENT TEACHING

- Advise patient to report pain or redness at infusion site.
- Tell patient he'll likely need laboratory tests to monitor his hematologic, renal, and hepatic function.

nystatin

Mycostatin*, Nadostine†, Nilstat, Nystex

Pharmacologic class: polyene macrolide
Pregnancy risk category C

AVAILABLE FORMS

Lozenges: 200,000 units
Oral suspension: 100,000 units/ml*
Powder: 50, 150, or 500 million units; 1, 2, or 5 billion units
Tablets: 500,000 units
Vaginal tablets: 100,000 units

INDICATIONS & DOSAGES

➤Intestinal candidiasis
Adults: 500,000 to 1 million units P.O. as tablets t.i.d.
➤Oral candidiasis (thrush)
Adults and children: 400,000 to 600,000 units P.O. as oral suspension q.i.d. or 200,000 to 400,000 units P.O. as lozenges 4 to 5 times daily for up to 14 days.
Infants: 200,000 units P.O. as oral suspension q.i.d.
Neonates and premature infants: 100,000 units P.O. oral suspension q.i.d.
➤Vaginal candidiasis
Adults: 100,000 units, as vaginal tablets, inserted high into vagina, daily at h.s. or b.i.d. for 14 days.

ACTION

Probably binds to sterols in fungal cell membrane, altering cell permeability and allowing leakage of intracellular components.

Route	Onset	Peak	Duration
P.O., topical	Unknown	Unknown	Unknown

Half-life: Unknown.

ADVERSE REACTIONS

GI: transient nausea, vomiting, diarrhea.
GU: irritation, sensitization, vulvovaginal burning (vaginal form).
Skin: rash.

INTERACTIONS
None significant.

EFFECTS ON LAB TEST RESULTS
None reported.

CONTRAINDICATIONS & CAUTIONS
- Contraindicated in patients hypersensitive to drug.

NURSING CONSIDERATIONS
- Drug isn't effective against systemic infections.
- Vaginal tablets can be used by pregnant patients up to 6 weeks before term to treat maternal infection that may cause oral candidiasis in neonates.
- To treat oral candidiasis, after the patient's mouth is clean of food debris, have him hold suspension in mouth for several minutes before swallowing. When treating infants, swab medication on oral mucosa. Prescriber may instruct immunosuppressed patients to suck on vaginal tablets (100,000 units) because this provides prolonged contact with oral mucosa.

PATIENT TEACHING
- Instruct patient not to chew or swallow lozenge but to allow it to dissolve slowly in mouth.
- Advise patient to continue taking drug for at least 2 days after signs and symptoms disappear. Consult prescriber for exact length of therapy.
- Instruct patient to continue therapy during menstruation.
- Explain that factors predisposing woman to vaginal infection include use of antibiotics, hormonal contraceptives, and corticosteroids; diabetes; reinfection by sexual partner; and tight-fitting pantyhose. Encourage woman to wear cotton underwear.
- Instruct women in careful hygiene for affected areas, including cleaning perineal area from front to back.
- Advise patient to report redness, swelling, or irritation.
- Tell patient, especially an older patient, that overusing mouthwash or wearing poorly fitting dentures may promote infection.

✱ NEW DRUG

posaconazole
Noxafil

Pharmacologic class: triazole antifungal
Pregnancy risk category C

AVAILABLE FORMS
Oral solution: 40 mg/ml

INDICATIONS & DOSAGES
➤ **Prevention of invasive *Aspergillus* and *Candida* infections in high-risk immunocompromised patients**
Adults and children age 13 and older: 200 mg (5 ml) P.O. t.i.d. with a full meal or a liquid nutritional supplement.

ACTION
Blocks the synthesis of ergosterol, a vital component of the fungal cell membrane.

Route	Onset	Peak	Duration
P.O.	Unknown	3–5 hr	Unknown

Half-life: 35 hours.

ADVERSE REACTIONS
CNS: *anxiety, dizziness, fatigue, fever, headache, insomnia, weakness.*
CV: *edema, hypertension, hypotension, tachycardia.*
EENT: *epistaxis, pharyngitis,* altered taste, blurred vision.
GI: *abdominal pain, constipation, diarrhea, dyspepsia, mucositis, nausea, vomiting.*
GU: *vaginal hemorrhage.*
Hematologic: *anemia, petechiae,* FEBRILE NEUTROPENIA, NEUTROPENIA, THROMBOCYTOPENIA.
Hepatic: *bilirubinemia.*
Metabolic: *anorexia, hyperglycemia, hypokalemia, hypomagnesemia,* hypocalcemia.
Musculoskeletal: *arthralgia, back pain, pain.*
Respiratory: *cough, dyspnea,* upper respiratory tract infection.
Other: *bacteremia, CMV infection, herpes simplex, rigors.*

INTERACTIONS

Drug-drug. *Cimetidine, phenytoin:* May decrease level and effectiveness of posaconazole. Avoid using together.
Calcium channel blockers, cyclosporine, HMG-CoA reductase inhibitors, midazolam, phenytoin, sirolimus, tacrolimus, vinca alkaloids: May increase levels of these drugs. Reduce dosages, increase monitoring of levels, and observe patient for adverse effects.
Rifabutin: May decrease level and effectiveness of posaconazole while increasing rifabutin level and risk of toxicity. Avoid using together. If unavoidable, monitor patient for uveitis, leukopenia, and other adverse effects.
Drug-food. *Food, liquid nutritional supplements:* May greatly enhance absorption of drug. Always give drug with liquid supplement or food.

EFFECTS ON LAB TEST RESULTS

- May increase AST, ALT, bilirubin, creatinine, alkaline phosphatase, and glucose levels. May decrease potassium, magnesium, and calcium levels.
- May decrease WBC, RBC, and platelet counts.

CONTRAINDICATIONS & CAUTIONS

- Contraindicated in patients hypersensitive to drug or its components and in patients taking astemizole, cisapride, ergot derivatives, pimozide, or quinidine.
- Use cautiously in patients hypersensitive to other azole antifungals, patients with potentially proarrhythmic conditions, and patients with hepatic or renal insufficiency.

NURSING CONSIDERATIONS

- Correct electrolyte imbalances, especially potassium, magnesium, and calcium imbalances, before therapy.
- Monitor patient for signs and symptoms of electrolyte imbalance including a slow, weak or irregular pulse; ECG change; nausea; neuromuscular irritability; and tetany.
- Obtain baseline liver function tests, including bilirubin level, before therapy and periodically during treatment. Notify prescriber if patient develops signs or symptoms of hepatic dysfunction.
- Give drug with a full meal or a liquid nutritional supplement.
- Monitor patient who has severe vomiting or diarrhea for breakthrough fungal infection.

PATIENT TEACHING

- If patient can't eat or take a liquid supplement, instruct him to notify prescriber. A different anti-infective may be needed, or monitoring may need to be increased.
- Tell patient to notify prescriber about an irregular heartbeat, fainting, or severe diarrhea or vomiting.
- Explain the signs and symptoms of liver dysfunction, including abdominal pain, yellowing skin or eyes, pale stools, and dark urine.
- Urge patient to contact the prescriber or pharmacist before taking other prescription or OTC drugs, and herbal or dietary supplements.
- Tell patient to shake the suspension well before taking it.
- Instruct patient to measure doses using the spoon provided with the drug. Household spoons vary in size and may yield an incorrect dose.
- Point out that the calibrated spoon has two markings, one for 2.5-ml and one for 5-ml. Make sure patient understands which mark to use for his prescribed dose.
- To ensure a full dose, tell patient to fill the spoon with water and drink it after taking a dose. Urge him to clean the spoon with water before putting it away.
- Tell patient to store oral solution at room temperature.

terbinafine hydrochloride

Lamisil

Pharmacologic class: synthetic allylamine derivative
Pregnancy risk category B

AVAILABLE FORMS

Tablets: 250 mg

INDICATIONS & DOSAGES

➤ **Fingernail onychomycosis caused by dermatophytes (tinea unguium)**
Adults: 250 mg P.O. once daily for 6 weeks.

➤ **Toenail onychomycosis caused by dermatophytes (tinea unguium)**
Adults: 250 mg P.O. once daily for 12 weeks.

ACTION
Inhibits squalene epoxidase, a key enzyme in sterol biosynthesis of fungi, leading to ergosterol deficiency and a corresponding accumulation of sterol within the fungal cell.

Route	Onset	Peak	Duration
P.O.	Unknown	2 hr	Unknown

Half-life: Unknown.

ADVERSE REACTIONS
CNS: *headache.*
EENT: visual disturbances.
GI: taste disturbances, diarrhea, dyspepsia, abdominal pain, nausea, flatulence.
Hematologic: ***neutropenia.***
Hepatic: hepatobiliary dysfunction, including cholestatic jaundice.
Skin: ***Stevens-Johnson syndrome, toxic epidermal necrolysis,*** rash, pruritus, urticaria.
Other: ***anaphylaxis,*** hypersensitivity reactions.

INTERACTIONS
Drug-drug. *Caffeine:* May decrease I.V. caffeine clearance. Use cautiously together.
Cimetidine: May decrease clearance of terbinafine by one-third. Avoid using together.
Cyclosporine: May increase cyclosporine clearance. Monitor cyclosporine level.

EFFECTS ON LAB TEST RESULTS
- May increase AST and ALT levels.
- May decrease neutrophil and lymphocyte counts.

CONTRAINDICATIONS & CAUTIONS
- Contraindicated in patients hypersensitive to drug, pregnant or breast-feeding women, those with liver disease, and those with creatinine clearance less than 50 ml/minute.

NURSING CONSIDERATIONS
- ***Alert:*** Rarely, patients with or without liver disease may suffer life-threatening liver failure.
- Obtain pretreatment transaminase levels for all patients taking drug. Tablets aren't recommended for patients with acute or chronic liver disease.
- Monitor CBC and hepatic enzyme levels in patients receiving drug for longer than 6 weeks. Stop drug if hepatobiliary dysfunction or cholestatic hepatitis develops.
- ***Look alike–sound alike:*** Don't confuse terbinafine with terbutaline or Lamisil with Lamictal.

PATIENT TEACHING
- Inform patient that successful treatment may take 10 weeks for toenail infections and 4 weeks for fingernail infections.
- Tell patient to report visual disturbances immediately; changes in the ocular lens and retina may occur. Patient should also immediately report persistent nausea, anorexia, fatigue, vomiting, right upper quadrant pain, jaundice, dark urine, or pale stools.

voriconazole
Vfend

Pharmacologic class: synthetic triazole
Pregnancy risk category D

AVAILABLE FORMS
Oral suspension: 40 mg/ml (after reconstitution)
Powder for injection: 200 mg
Tablets: 50 mg, 200 mg

INDICATIONS & DOSAGES
➤ **Esophageal candidiasis**
Adults who weigh 40 kg (88 lb) or more: 200 mg P.O. q 12 hours. Treat for a minimum of 14 days and for at least 7 days after symptoms resolve.
Adults who weigh less than 40 kg: 100 mg P.O. q 12 hours. Treat for a minimum of 14 days and for at least 7 days after symptoms resolve.
➤ **Invasive aspergillosis; serious infections caused by *Fusarium* species and *Scedosporium apiospermum* in**

patients intolerant of or refractory to other therapy
Adults: Initially, 6 mg/kg I.V. q 12 hours for 2 doses; then maintenance dose of 4 mg/kg I.V. q 12 hours. If patient can't tolerate 4 mg dose, decrease to 3 mg/kg. Switch to P.O. form as tolerated, using the maintenance dosages shown here.
Adults who weigh more than 40 kg: 200 mg P.O. q 12 hours. May increase to 300 mg P.O. q 12 hours, if needed. If unable to tolerate the 300 mg dose, reduce dose in 50-mg decrements to a minimum of 200 mg q 12 hours.
Adults who weigh less than 40 kg: 100 mg P.O. q 12 hours. May increase to 150 mg P.O. q 12 hours, if needed. If unable to tolerate the 150 mg dose, reduce dose to 100 mg q 12 hours.

➤ **Candidemia in nonneutropenic patients; *Candida* infections of the kidney, abdomen, bladder wall, or wounds and disseminated skin infections**
Adults: Initially, 6 mg/kg I.V. q 12 hours for 2 doses, then 3 to 4 mg/kg I.V. q 12 hours for maintenance, depending on severity of the infection. If patient can't tolerate 4 mg dose, decrease to 3 mg/kg. Switch to P.O. form as tolerated. For adults who weigh 40 kg or more, give 200 mg P.O. q 12 hours. May increase to 300 mg P.O. q 12 hours, if needed. If unable to tolerate the 300 mg dose, reduce dose in 50–mg decrements to a minimum of 200 mg q 12 hours. For adults who weigh less than 40 kg, give 100 mg P.O. q 12 hours. May increase to 150 mg P.O. q 12 hours, if needed. If unable to tolerate the 150 mg dose, reduce dose to 100 mg q 12 hours. Treat patients with candidemia for at least 14 days after symptoms resolve or after the last positive culture result, whichever is longer.
Adjust-a-dose: For patients in Child-Pugh classes A or B, decrease the maintenance dosage by 50%. In patients with a creatinine clearance of less than 50 ml/minute, use oral form instead of I.V. form to prevent accumulation of a component of the I.V. mixture. In patients also receiving phenytoin, increase maintenance dose of voriconazole to 5 mg/kg I.V. q 12 hours, or increase P.O. dose from 100 mg to 200 mg or from 200 mg to 400 mg.

I.V. ADMINISTRATION

- In patients with creatinine clearance less than 50 ml/minute, use cautiously.
- Reconstitute the powder with 19 ml of water for injection to obtain a volume of 20 ml of clear concentrate containing 10 mg/ml of drug. Discard the vial if a vacuum doesn't pull the diluent into the vial. Shake the vial until all the powder is dissolved. Use the reconstituted solution immediately.
- Further dilute the 10-mg/ml solution to 5 mg/ml or less. Follow the manufacturer's instructions for diluting.
- Infuse over 1 to 2 hours at 5 mg/ml or less and a maximum hourly rate of 3 mg/kg.

INCOMPATIBILITIES

Blood products, electrolyte supplements, 4.2% sodium bicarbonate infusion.

ACTION

Inhibits the cytochrome P-450–dependent synthesis of ergosterol, a vital component of fungal cell membranes.

Route	Onset	Peak	Duration
P.O., I.V.	Immediate	1–2 hr	12 hr

Half-life: Depends on dose.

ADVERSE REACTIONS

CNS: fever, headache, hallucinations, dizziness.
CV: tachycardia, hypertension, hypotension, vasodilatation.
EENT: *abnormal vision,* photophobia, chromatopsia, dry mouth.
GI: abdominal pain, nausea, vomiting, diarrhea.
Hepatic: cholestatic jaundice.
Metabolic: hypokalemia, hypomagnesemia.
Skin: rash, pruritus.
Other: chills, peripheral edema.

INTERACTIONS

Drug-drug. *Benzodiazepines, calcium channel blockers, methadone, omeprazole, sulfonylureas, vinca alkaloids:* May increase levels of these drugs. Adjust dosages of these drugs; monitor patient for adverse reactions.

Carbamazepine, long-acting barbiturates, rifabutin, rifampin, *ritonavir (high-dose therapy):* May decrease voriconazole level. Use together is contraindicated.
Cyclosporine, tacrolimus: May increase levels of these drugs. Adjust dosages; monitor levels.
Efavirenz: May significantly decrease voriconazole levels while significantly increasing efavirenz levels. Use together is contraindicated.
Ergot alkaloids (such as ergotamine), sirolimus: May increase levels of these drugs. Use together is contraindicated.
HIV protease inhibitors (amprenavir, nelfinavir, ritonavir, saquinavir), nonnucleoside reverse transcriptase inhibitors (delavirdine): May increase levels of both drugs. Monitor patient for adverse reactions and toxicity.
HMG-CoA reductase inhibitors (atorvastatin, fluvastatin, lovastatin, pravastatin, rosuvastatin, simvastatin): May increase levels and adverse effects, including rhabdomyolysis, of these drugs. Monitor patient closely and reduce dose of HMG-CoA reductase inhibitor as needed.
Oral contraceptives containing ethinyl estradiol and norethindrone: May increase levels and adverse effects of these drugs. Monitor patient closely.
Phenytoin: May decrease voriconazole level and increase phenytoin level. Increase voriconazole maintenance dose; monitor phenytoin level.
Pimozide, quinidine: May increase levels of these drugs, leading to torsades de pointes and prolonged QT interval. Use together is contraindicated.
Warfarin: May significantly increase PT. Monitor PT and other anticoagulant test results.
Drug-herb. *St. John's wort:* May increase drug level. Discourage use together.
Drug-lifestyle. *Sun exposure:* May cause photosensitivity. Advise patient to avoid excessive sunlight exposure.

EFFECTS ON LAB TEST RESULTS

- May increase alkaline phosphatase, AST, ALT, bilirubin, and creatinine levels. May decrease potassium and hemoglobin levels and hematocrit.
- May decrease platelet, WBC, and RBC counts.

CONTRAINDICATIONS & CAUTIONS

- Contraindicated in patients hypersensitive to drug or its components; in those with rare, hereditary galactose intolerance, Lapp lactase deficiency, or glucose-galactose malabsorption; and in those taking carbamazepine, efavirenz, an ergot alkaloid, a long-acting barbiturate, pimozide, quinidine, rifabutin, rifampin, ritonavir, or sirolimus.
- Use cautiously in patients hypersensitive to other azoles.

NURSING CONSIDERATIONS

- Infusion reactions, including flushing, fever, sweating, tachycardia, chest tightness, dyspnea, faintness, nausea, pruritus, and rash, may occur as soon as infusion starts. If reaction occurs, notify prescriber; infusion may need to be stopped.
- Monitor liver function test results at start of and during therapy. Monitor patients who develop abnormal liver function test results for more severe hepatic injury. If patient develops signs and symptoms of liver disease, drug may need to be stopped.
- Monitor renal function during treatment. For patients with creatinine clearance less than 50 ml/minute, give the oral form.
- If treatment lasts longer than 28 days, vision changes may occur.

PATIENT TEACHING

- Tell patient to take oral form at least 1 hour before or 1 hour after a meal.
- Tell patient taking the oral form to only use the dispenser provided with the medication pack.
- Advise patient not to mix oral suspension with other drugs or beverages.
- Tell patient to discard any unused portion of suspension after 14 days.
- Advise patient to avoid driving or operating machinery while taking drug, especially at night, because vision changes, including blurring and photophobia, may occur.
- Tell patient to avoid strong, direct sunlight during therapy.
- Advise patient to avoid becoming pregnant during therapy because of the risk of fetal harm.

7 Antimalarials

atovaquone and proguanil hydrochloride
chloroquine phosphate
doxycycline
(See Chapter 12, TETRACYCLINES.)
hydroxychloroquine sulfate
mefloquine hydrochloride
primaquine phosphate
pyrimethamine
pyrimethamine with sulfadoxine

atovaquone and proguanil hydrochloride

Malarone, Malarone Pediatric

Pharmacologic class: hydroxynaphthoquinone and biguanide derivative
Pregnancy risk category C

AVAILABLE FORMS

Tablets (pediatric-strength): 62.5 mg atovaquone and 25 mg proguanil hydrochloride
Tablets (adult-strength): 250 mg atovaquone and 100 mg proguanil hydrochloride

INDICATIONS & DOSAGES

➤To prevent *Plasmodium falciparum* malaria, including in areas where chloroquine resistance has been reported
Adults and children who weigh more than 40 kg (88 lb): 1 adult-strength tablet P.O. once daily with food or milk, beginning 1 or 2 days before entering a malaria-endemic area. Continue prophylactic treatment during stay and for 7 days after return.
Children who weigh 31 to 40 kg (68 to 88 lb): 3 pediatric-strength tablets P.O. once daily with food or milk, beginning 1 or 2 days before entering endemic area. Continue prophylactic treatment during stay and for 7 days after return.
Children who weigh 21 to 30 kg (46 to 66 lb): 2 pediatric-strength tablets P.O. once daily with food or milk, beginning 1 or 2 days before entering endemic area. Continue prophylactic treatment during stay and for 7 days after return.
Children who weigh 11 to 20 kg (24 to 44 lb): 1 pediatric-strength tablet P.O. daily with food or milk, beginning 1 or 2 days before entering endemic area. Continue prophylactic treatment during stay and for 7 days after return.

➤Acute, uncomplicated *P. falciparum* malaria
Adults and children who weigh more than 40 kg (88 lb): 4 adult-strength tablets P.O. once daily, with food or milk, for 3 consecutive days.
Children who weigh 31 to 40 kg (68 to 88 lb): 3 adult-strength tablets P.O. once daily, with food or milk, for 3 consecutive days.
Children who weigh 21 to 30 kg (46 to 66 lb): 2 adult-strength tablets P.O. once daily, with food or milk, for 3 consecutive days.
Children who weigh 11 to 20 kg (24 to 44 lb): 1 adult-strength tablet P.O. once daily, with food or milk, for 3 consecutive days.
Children who weigh 9 to 10 kg (20 to 22 lb): 3 pediatric-strength tablets P.O. once daily, with food or milk, for 3 consecutive days.
Children who weigh 5 to 8 kg (11 to 18 lb): 2 pediatric-strength tablets P.O. once daily, with food or milk, for 3 consecutive days.

ACTION

Thought to interfere with nucleic acid replication in the malarial parasite. Atovaquone selectively inhibits mitochondrial electron transport in the parasite. Cycloguanil, an active metabolite of proguanil hydrochloride, inhibits dihydrofolate reductase. Atovaquone and cycloguanil are active against the erythrocytic and exoerythrocytic stages of *Plasmodium* species.

Route	Onset	Peak	Duration
P.O.	Unknown	Unknown	Unknown

Half-life: atovaquone: 2 to 3 days in adults; proguanil: 12 to 21 hours in adults and children.

ADVERSE REACTIONS

CNS: *headache,* fever, asthenia, dizziness, dreams, insomnia.
GI: *abdominal pain, nausea, vomiting,* diarrhea, anorexia, dyspepsia, gastritis, oral ulcers.
Respiratory: cough.
Skin: pruritus.

INTERACTIONS

Drug-drug. *Metoclopramide:* May decrease atovaquone bioavailability. Use another antiemetic.
Rifampin, rifabutin: May decrease atovaquone level by about 50%. Avoid using together.
Tetracycline: May decrease atovaquone level by about 40%. Monitor patient with parasitemia closely.

EFFECTS ON LAB TEST RESULTS

- May increase alkaline phosphatase, ALT, and AST levels. May decrease hemoglobin level and hematocrit.
- May decrease WBC count.

CONTRAINDICATIONS & CAUTIONS

- Contraindicated in patients hypersensitive to atovaquone, proguanil hydrochloride, or any component of the drug.
- Use cautiously in patients with severe renal impairment and in those who are vomiting.
- Use cautiously in elderly patients because they have a greater frequency of decreased renal, hepatic, and cardiac function.
- It isn't known if atovaquone appears in breast milk, but proguanil does in small amounts. Use cautiously in breast-feeding women.
- Safety and effectiveness haven't been established for prevention in children who weigh less than 11 kg or for treatment in children who weigh less than 5 kg.

NURSING CONSIDERATIONS

- Persistent diarrhea or vomiting may decrease drug absorption. Patients with these symptoms may need a different antimalarial.
- Store tablets at controlled room temperature of 59° to 86° F (15° to 30° C).

PATIENT TEACHING

- Tell patient to take dose at the same time each day with food or milk.
- Tell parents, that if child has difficulty swallowing tablets, to crush and mix in condensed milk.
- Tell patient to repeat dose if he vomits within 1 hour.
- Advise patient to notify prescriber if he can't complete the course of therapy as prescribed.
- Instruct patient to supplement preventive malarial with use of protective clothing, bed nets, and insect repellents.

chloroquine phosphate

Aralen Phosphate, Chlorquin‡

Pharmacologic class: aminoquinoline
Pregnancy risk category C

AVAILABLE FORMS

Tablets: 250 mg (equivalent to 150 mg base), 500 mg (equivalent to 300 mg base)

INDICATIONS & DOSAGES

➤Acute malarial attacks caused by *Plasmodium vivax, P. malariae, P. ovale,* and susceptible strains of *P. falciparum*
Adults: Initially, 600 mg base P.O.; then 300 mg base at 6, 24, and 48 hours.
Children: Initially, 10 mg/kg base P.O.; then 5 mg/kg base at 6, 24, and 48 hours. Don't exceed adult dose.
➤To prevent malaria
Adults: 300 mg base P.O. once weekly on the same day each week, for 1 to 2 weeks before entering a malaria-endemic area and continued for 4 weeks after leaving the area. If treatment begins after exposure, give 600 mg base P.O. initially, in two divided doses 6 hours apart, followed by the usual dosing regimen.

Children: 5 mg/kg base P.O. once weekly on the same day each week, for 1 to 2 weeks before entering a malaria-endemic area and continued for 4 weeks after leaving the area. Don't exceed 300 mg. If treatment begins after exposure, give 10 mg/kg base P.O. initially, in two divided doses 6 hours apart, followed by the usual dosing regimen.

➤ **Extraintestinal amebiasis**

Adults: 600 mg base P.O. once daily for 2 days; then 300 mg base daily for 2 to 3 weeks. Treatment is usually combined with an intestinal amebicide.

Children: 10 mg/kg base P.O. once daily for 2 to 3 weeks. Maximum dose is 300 mg base daily.

ACTION

May bind to and alter the properties of DNA in susceptible parasites.

Route	Onset	Peak	Duration
P.O.	Unknown	1–3 hr	Unknown

Half-life: 1 to 2 months.

ADVERSE REACTIONS

CNS: ***seizures,*** mild and transient headache, psychic stimulation, dizziness, neuropathy.

CV: hypotension, ECG changes.

EENT: blurred vision, difficulty in focusing, reversible corneal changes, typically irreversible, sometimes progressive or delayed retinal changes such as narrowing of arterioles, macular lesions, pallor of optic disk, optic atrophy, patchy retinal pigmentation, typically leading to blindness, ototoxicity, nerve deafness, vertigo, tinnitus.

GI: anorexia, abdominal cramps, diarrhea, nausea, vomiting, stomatitis.

Hematologic: ***agranulocytosis, aplastic anemia, thrombocytopenia,*** hemolytic anemia.

Skin: pruritus, lichen planus eruptions, skin and mucosal pigmentary changes, pleomorphic skin eruptions.

INTERACTIONS

Drug-drug. *Aluminum salts (kaolin), magnesium:* May decrease GI absorption. Separate dose times.

Cimetidine: May decrease hepatic metabolism of chloroquine. Monitor patient for toxicity.

Drug-lifestyle. *Sun exposure:* May worsen drug-induced dermatoses. Advise patient to avoid excessive sun exposure.

EFFECTS ON LAB TEST RESULTS

- May decrease hemoglobin level.
- May decrease granulocyte and platelet counts.

CONTRAINDICATIONS & CAUTIONS

- Contraindicated in patients hypersensitive to drug and in those with retinal or visual field changes or porphyria.
- Use cautiously in patients with severe GI, neurologic, or blood disorders; hepatic disease or alcoholism; or G6PD deficiency or psoriasis.

NURSING CONSIDERATIONS

- ***Alert:*** Drug dosage may be discussed in "mg" or "mg base"; be aware of the difference.
- Ensure that baseline and periodic ophthalmic examinations are performed. Check periodically for ocular muscle weakness after long-term use.
- Make sure patient is tested with an audiometer before, during, and after therapy, especially if therapy is long-term.
- Monitor CBC and liver function studies periodically during long-term therapy. If a severe blood disorder—not caused by the disease—develops, drug may need to be stopped.
- ***Alert:*** Monitor patient for overdose, which can quickly lead to toxic symptoms: headache, drowsiness, visual disturbances, CV collapse, seizures, and then cardiopulmonary arrest. Children are extremely susceptible to toxicity; avoid long-term treatment.

PATIENT TEACHING

- To improve compliance when using drug for prevention, advise patient to take drug immediately before or after a meal on the same day each week.
- Instruct patient to avoid excessive sun exposure to prevent worsening of drug-induced dermatoses.
- Tell patient to report adverse reactions promptly, especially blurred vision, in-

creased sensitivity to light, tinnitus, hearing loss, or muscle weakness.
- Instruct patient to keep drug out of reach of children. Overdose may be fatal.

hydroxychloroquine sulfate
Plaquenil Sulfate

Pharmacologic class: aminoquinoline
Pregnancy risk category C

AVAILABLE FORMS
Tablets: 200 mg (equivalent to 155 mg base)

INDICATIONS & DOSAGES
➤ **Suppressive prevention of malaria attacks caused by *Plasmodium vivax, P. malariae, P. ovale,* and susceptible strains of *P. falciparum***
Adults: 310 mg base P.O. weekly on the same day each week, beginning 1 to 2 weeks before entering malaria-endemic area and continuing for 4 weeks after leaving area. If not started before exposure, double first dose to 620 mg base in two divided doses 6 hours apart.
Children: 5 mg/kg base P.O. weekly on the same day each week, beginning 1 to 2 weeks before entering malaria-endemic area and continuing for 4 weeks after leaving area. Don't exceed adult dose. If not started before exposure, double first dose to 10 mg/kg base in two divided doses, 6 hours apart.
➤ **Acute malarial attacks**
Adults: Initially, 620 mg base P.O., followed by 310 mg base 6 to 8 hours after first dose; then 310 mg base daily for 2 days.
Children: Initially, 10 mg/kg base P.O.; then 5 mg/kg base at 6, 24, and 48 hours after the first dose.
➤ **Lupus erythematosus**
Adults: 310 mg base P.O. daily or b.i.d., continued for several weeks or months, depending on response. For prolonged maintenance dose, 155 to 310 mg base daily.
➤ **Rheumatoid arthritis**
Adults: Initially, 310 to 465 mg base P.O. daily. When good response occurs, usually in 4 to 12 weeks, cut dosage in half.

ACTION
May bind to and alter the properties of DNA in susceptible organisms.

Route	Onset	Peak	Duration
P.O.	Unknown	2–4½ hr	Unknown

Half-life: 32 to 50 days.

ADVERSE REACTIONS
CNS: ***seizures,*** irritability, nightmares, ataxia, psychosis, vertigo, dizziness, hypoactive deep tendon reflexes, lassitude, headache.
CV: T-wave inversion or depression, widening of QRS complex.
EENT: blurred vision, difficulty in focusing, reversible corneal changes, typically irreversible nystagmus, sometimes progressive or delayed retinal changes such as narrowing of arterioles, macular lesions, pallor of optic disk, optic atrophy.
GI: anorexia, abdominal cramps, diarrhea, nausea, vomiting.
Hematologic: ***agranulocytosis, leukopenia, thrombocytopenia, hemolysis in patients with G6PD deficiency, aplastic anemia.***
Metabolic: weight loss.
Musculoskeletal: skeletal muscle weakness.
Skin: pruritus, lichen planus eruptions, skin and mucosal pigmentary changes, pleomorphic skin eruptions, worsened psoriasis, alopecia, bleaching of hair.

INTERACTIONS
Drug-drug. *Aluminum salts (kaolin), magnesium:* May decrease GI absorption. Separate dose times.
Cimetidine: May decrease hepatic metabolism of hydroxychloroquine. Monitor patient for toxicity.
Digoxin: May increase digoxin level. Monitor drug levels; monitor patient for toxicity.

EFFECTS ON LAB TEST RESULTS
- May decrease hemoglobin level.
- May decrease granulocyte, WBC, and platelet counts.

CONTRAINDICATIONS & CAUTIONS

- Contraindicated in patients hypersensitive to drug and in those with retinal or visual field changes or porphyria.
- Contraindicated for long-term therapy for children.
- Use with caution in patients with severe GI, neurologic, or blood disorders.
- Use with caution in patients with hepatic disease or alcoholism because drug concentrates in liver.
- Use with caution in those with G6PD deficiency or psoriasis because drug may worsen these conditions.

NURSING CONSIDERATIONS

- ***Alert:*** Drug dosage may be discussed in "mg" or "mg base;" be aware of the difference.
- Ensure that baseline and periodic ophthalmic examinations are performed. Check periodically for ocular muscle weakness after long-term use.
- Make sure patient is examined with an audiometer before, during, and after therapy, especially if therapy is long-term.
- Monitor CBC and liver function studies periodically during long-term therapy; if severe blood disorder—not caused by disease—develops, drug may need to be stopped.
- ***Alert:*** Monitor patient for possible overdose, which can quickly lead to toxic signs or symptoms: headache, drowsiness, visual disturbances, CV collapse, seizures, then cardiopulmonary arrest. Children are extremely susceptible to toxicity.

PATIENT TEACHING

- Advise patient taking drug for prevention to take drug immediately before or after a meal on the same day each week, to improve compliance.
- Instruct patient to report adverse reactions promptly.

mefloquine hydrochloride

Lariam

Pharmacologic class: quinidine derivative
Pregnancy risk category C

AVAILABLE FORMS

Tablets: 250 mg

INDICATIONS & DOSAGES

➤ Acute malaria infections caused by mefloquine-sensitive strains of *Plasmodium falciparum* or *P. vivax*

Adults: 1,250 mg (5 tablets) P.O. as a single dose with food and at least 8 ounces of water. Patients with *P. vivax* infections should receive further therapy with primaquine or other 8-aminoquinolines to avoid relapse after treatment of the initial infection.
Children: 20 to 25 mg/kg P.O. as a single dose with food and at least 8 ounces of water. Maximum dose 1,250 mg. Dosage may be divided into two doses given 6 to 8 hours apart to reduce the incidence and severity of adverse effects. Patients with *P. vivax* infections should receive further therapy with primaquine or other 8-aminoquinolines to avoid relapse after treatment of the initial infection.

➤ To prevent malaria

Adults and children weighing more than 45 kg (99 lb): 250 mg P.O. once weekly. Prevention therapy should start 1 week before entering endemic area and continue for 4 weeks after returning. If patient returns to an area without malaria after a prolonged stay in an endemic area, prevention therapy should end after three doses.
Children who weigh 31 to 45 kg (68 to 99 lb): 187.5 mg (¾ of a 250-mg tablet) P.O. once weekly.
Children who weigh 20 to 30 kg (44 to 66 lb): 125 mg (½ of a 250-mg tablet) P.O. once weekly.
Children who weigh 15 to 19 kg (33 to 42 lb): 62.5 mg (¼ of a 250-mg tablet) P.O. once weekly.
Children who weigh less than 15 kg (33 lb): 3 to 5 mg/kg P.O. once weekly.

ACTION

May be caused by drug's ability to form complexes with hemin and to raise intravesicular pH in parasite acid vesicles.

Route	Onset	Peak	Duration
P.O.	Unknown	7–24 hr	Unknown

Half-life: About 21 days.

ADVERSE REACTIONS

CNS: ***seizures, suicidal behavior,*** fever, dizziness, syncope, headache, psychotic changes, hallucinations, confusion, anxiety, fatigue, vertigo, depression, tremor, ataxia, mood changes, panic attacks.
CV: chest pain, edema.
EENT: tinnitus, visual disturbances.
GI: anorexia, vomiting, *nausea,* loose stools, diarrhea, abdominal discomfort or pain, dyspepsia.
Hematologic: ***leukopenia, thrombocytopenia.***
Musculoskeletal: myalgia.
Skin: rash.
Other: chills.

INTERACTIONS

Drug-drug. *Beta blockers, quinidine, quinine:* May cause ECG abnormalities and cardiac arrest. Avoid using together.
Carbamazepine, phenobarbital, phenytoin, valproic acid: May decrease drug levels and loss of seizure control at start of mefloquine therapy. Monitor anticonvulsant level.
Chloroquine, quinine: May increase risk of seizures and ECG abnormalities. Give mefloquine at least 12 hours after last dose.
Valproic acid: May decrease valproic acid level and loss of seizure control at start of mefloquine therapy. Monitor anticonvulsant level.

EFFECTS ON LAB TEST RESULTS

- May increase transaminase level. May decrease hematocrit.
- May decrease WBC and platelet counts.

CONTRAINDICATIONS & CAUTIONS

- Contraindicated in patients hypersensitive to mefloquine or related compounds.
- Contraindicated for prevention of malaria in patients with a history of seizures or an active or recent history of depression, generalized anxiety disorder, psychosis, schizophrenia, or other major psychiatric disorders.
- Use cautiously when treating patients with cardiac disease or seizure disorders.

NURSING CONSIDERATIONS

- Because giving quinine and mefloquine together poses a health risk, give mefloquine no sooner than 12 hours after the last dose of quinine or quinidine.
- Patients with *P. vivax* infections are at high risk for relapse because drug doesn't eliminate the hepatic-phase exoerythrocytic parasites. Give follow-up therapy with primaquine.
- Monitor liver function test results periodically.
- If overdose is suspected, induce vomiting or perform gastric lavage because of risk of cardiotoxicity. Mefloquine has produced cardiac reactions similar to quinidine and quinine.
- ***Alert:*** When drug is used for prevention, psychiatric symptoms (acute anxiety, depression, restlessness, confusion) that occur may precede onset of a more serious event. Replace drug with other therapy.

PATIENT TEACHING

- Advise patient taking drug for prevention to take dose immediately before or after a meal on the same day each week, to improve compliance.
- Tell patient not to take drug on an empty stomach and always to take it with at least 8 ounces of water.
- Advise patient to use caution when performing activities that require alertness and coordination because dizziness, disturbed sense of balance, and neuropsychiatric reactions may occur.
- Instruct patient taking drug for prevention to stop drug and notify prescriber if signs or symptoms of impending toxicity, such as anxiety, depression, confusion, or restlessness, occur.
- Advise patient undergoing long-term therapy to have periodic ophthalmic exams because drug may cause ocular lesions.
- Advise women of childbearing age to use reliable contraception during treatment.

primaquine phosphate

Pharmacologic class: aminoquinoline
Pregnancy risk category NR

AVAILABLE FORMS

Powder: 5 g, 25 g, 100 g, 500 g
Tablets: 26.3 mg (equivalent to 15 mg base)

INDICATIONS & DOSAGES

➤ **Relapsing *Plasmodium vivax* malaria, eliminating symptoms and infection completely; to prevent relapse**

Adults: 15 mg base P.O. daily for 14 days. Begin therapy during the last 2 weeks of, or after, a course of suppression with chloroquine or comparable drug.
Children: 0.3 mg/kg/day base P.O. for 14 days. Maximum 15 mg base/dose. Begin therapy during the last 2 weeks of, or after, a course of suppression with chloroquine or comparable drug.

ACTION

May bind to and alter the properties of DNA in susceptible parasites.

Route	Onset	Peak	Duration
P.O.	Unknown	1–3 hr	Unknown

Half-life: 4 to 10 hours.

ADVERSE REACTIONS

GI: nausea, vomiting, epigastric distress, abdominal cramps.
Hematologic: ***hemolytic anemia, leukopenia,*** methemoglobinemia.

INTERACTIONS

Drug-drug. *Aluminum salts, magnesium:* Decreases GI absorption. Separate dose times.

EFFECTS ON LAB TEST RESULTS

- May decrease hemoglobin level.
- May decrease RBC count. May increase or decrease WBC count.

CONTRAINDICATIONS & CAUTIONS

- Contraindicated in patients with systemic diseases in which agranulocytosis may develop, such as lupus erythematosus or rheumatoid arthritis, and in those taking a bone marrow suppressant, quinacrine, or hemolytic drugs.
- Use cautiously in patients with previous idiosyncratic reaction involving hemolytic anemia, methemoglobinemia, or leukopenia; in those with a family or personal history of favism; and in those with erythrocytic G6PD or nicotinamide-adenine-dinucleotide (NADH) methemoglobin reductase deficiency.

NURSING CONSIDERATIONS

- ***Alert:*** Drug dosage may be discussed in "mg" or "mg base;" be aware of the difference.
- Give drug with meals.
- Use drug with a fast-acting antimalarial such as chloroquine to reduce possibility of drug-resistant strains.
- Obtain frequent blood studies and urinalysis in light-skinned patients taking more than 30 mg base daily, dark-skinned patients taking more than 15 mg base daily, and patients with severe anemia or suspected sensitivity.
- Monitor patient for markedly darkened urine and for suddenly reduced hemoglobin level or erythrocyte or leukocyte count, which suggest impending hemolytic reactions. Stop drug immediately and notify prescriber.
- Safe use during pregnancy hasn't been established.

PATIENT TEACHING

- Instruct patient to take drug with meals to minimize stomach upset. If nausea, vomiting, or stomach pain persists, tell patient to notify prescriber.
- Tell patient to report to prescriber chills, fever, chest pain, and bluish skin discoloration; these signs and symptoms may suggest a hemolytic reaction.
- Tell patient to stop drug and notify prescriber immediately if urine darkens markedly.
- Stress importance of completing full course of therapy.

pyrimethamine
Daraprim
pyrimethamine with sulfadoxine
Fansidar

Pharmacologic class: folic acid antagonist
Pregnancy risk category C

AVAILABLE FORMS
pyrimethamine
Tablets: 25 mg
pyrimethamine with sulfadoxine
Tablets: 25 mg pyrimethamine and 500 mg sulfadoxine

INDICATIONS & DOSAGES
➤**To prevent and control transmission of malaria**
pyrimethamine
Adults and children age 10 and older: 25 mg P.O. weekly for 6 to 10 weeks or longer after leaving malaria-endemic areas.
Children ages 4 to 10: 12.5 mg P.O. weekly continued for 6 to 10 weeks or longer after leaving malaria-endemic areas.
Children younger than age 4: 6.25 mg P.O. weekly continued for 6 to 10 weeks or longer after leaving malaria-endemic areas.
pyrimethamine with sulfadoxine
Adults and children age 14 and older: 1 tablet weekly or 2 tablets q 2 weeks during exposure and for 4 to 6 weeks after exposure.
Children ages 9 to 14: Give ¾ tablet weekly, or 1½ tablets q 2 weeks during exposure and for 4 to 6 weeks after exposure.
Children ages 4 to 8: Give ½ tablet weekly or 1 tablet q 2 weeks during exposure and for 4 to 6 weeks after exposure.
Children younger than age 4: Give ¼ tablet weekly, or ½ tablet q 2 weeks during exposure and for 4 to 6 weeks after exposure.
➤**Acute attacks of malaria**
pyrimethamine
Adults: 50 mg P.O. daily for 2 days; then 25 mg once weekly for at least 10 weeks.
Children ages 4 to 10: 25 mg P.O. once daily for 2 days; then 12.5 mg once weekly for at least 10 weeks.
pyrimethamine with sulfadoxine
Adults and children age 14 and older: 3 tablets as a single dose, given on the last day of quinine therapy.
Children ages 9 to 14: Give 2 tablets as a single dose, given on the last day of quinine therapy.
Children ages 4 to 8: Give 1 tablet as a single dose, given on the last day of quinine therapy.
Children ages 1 to 3: Give ½ tablet as a single dose, given on the last day of quinine therapy.
Children ages 2 to 11 months: Give ¼ tablet as a single dose, given on the last day of quinine therapy.
➤**Toxoplasmosis**
pyrimethamine
Adults: Initially, 50 to 75 mg P.O. with 1 to 4 g sulfadiazine; continue for 1 to 3 weeks. After 3 weeks, reduce dosage by half and continue for 4 to 5 weeks.
Children: Initially, 1 mg/kg/day P.O. in two equally divided doses for 2 to 4 days; then 0.5 mg/kg daily for 4 weeks, along with 100 mg sulfadiazine/kg P.O. daily, divided q 6 hours. Don't exceed 100 mg.
➤**Primary prevention of toxoplasmosis in patients with HIV infection ♦**
Adults and adolescents: 50 mg P.O., once weekly, with leucovorin 25 mg P.O. once weekly and dapsone 50 mg P.O. daily; or 75 mg pyrimethamine with leucovorin 25 mg and dapsone 200 mg P.O., all once weekly.
➤**Secondary prevention of toxoplasmosis in patients with HIV infection ♦**
Adults and adolescents: 25 to 50 mg P.O., once daily, with leucovorin 10 to 25 mg P.O. once daily and either sulfadiazine 0.5 to 1 g P.O. q.i.d. or clindamycin 300 to 450 mg q 6 to 8 hours.

ACTION
Inhibits the enzyme dihydrofolate reductase, blocking the creation of folic acid, which is required for the reproduction of

the infecting organism. Sulfadoxine competitively inhibits use of PABA.

Route	Onset	Peak	Duration
P.O.	Unknown	1½–8 hr	2 wk

Half-life: 4 days.

ADVERSE REACTIONS

CNS: ***seizures,*** headache, peripheral neuritis, mental depression, ataxia, hallucinations, fatigue.
CV: ***arrhythmias,*** allergic myocarditis.
EENT: scleral irritation, periorbital edema.
GI: anorexia, vomiting, atrophic glossitis.
Hematologic: ***agranulocytosis, aplastic anemia, leukopenia, thrombocytopenia, pancytopenia,*** megaloblastic anemia.
Skin: ***Stevens-Johnson syndrome,*** generalized skin eruptions, urticaria, pruritus, photosensitivity.

INTERACTIONS

Drug-drug. *Co-trimoxazole, methotrexate, sulfonamides:* May increase risk of bone marrow suppression. Avoid using together.
Lorazepam: May increase risk of hepatotoxicity. Avoid using together.
PABA: May decrease action against toxoplasmosis. May need to adjust dosage.

EFFECTS ON LAB TEST RESULTS

- May decrease hemoglobin level.
- May decrease granulocyte, WBC, platelet, and RBC counts.

CONTRAINDICATIONS & CAUTIONS

- Pyrimethamine is contraindicated in patients hypersensitive to drug and in those with megaloblastic anemia from folic acid deficiency. Pyrimethamine with sulfadoxine is contraindicated in patients with porphyria.
- Repeated use of pyrimethamine with sulfadoxine is contraindicated in patients with severe renal insufficiency, marked parenchymal damage to the liver, blood dyscrasias, hypersensitivity to pyrimethamine or sulfonamides, or documented megaloblastic anemia from folic-acid deficiency.
- Contraindicated in infants younger than age 2 months and in pregnant (at term) and breast-feeding women.
- Use cautiously after treatment with chloroquine and in patients with impaired hepatic or renal function, severe allergy or bronchial asthma, G6PD deficiency, or seizure disorders (smaller doses may be needed).

NURSING CONSIDERATIONS

- Pyrimethamine alone isn't recommended for malaria. Use drug with faster-acting antimalarials, such as chloroquine, for 2 days to start transmission control and suppressive cure.
- For toxoplasmosis, obtain twice-weekly blood counts, including platelets, because usual dosages approach toxic levels. If signs of folic- or folinic-acid deficiency develop, reduce dosage or stop drug and give parenteral folinic acid (leucovorin) until blood counts return to normal.
- Adverse drug reactions related to sulfadiazine are similar to those related to sulfonamides.
- When used for toxoplasmosis in patients with AIDS, therapy may be lifelong.
- Use pyrimethamine with sulfadoxine only in areas where chloroquine-resistant malaria is prevalent and only if the traveler plans to stay longer than 3 weeks.

PATIENT TEACHING

- Instruct patient to take drug with meals.
- Inform patient with toxoplasmosis of importance of frequent laboratory studies and compliance with therapy. Tell patient he may need long-term therapy.
- Warn patient taking pyrimethamine with sulfadoxine to stop drug and notify prescriber at first sign of rash, sore throat, or glossitis.
- Tell patient to take first preventive dose 1 to 2 days before traveling.

8
Antituberculotics

cycloserine
ethambutol hydrochloride
isoniazid
rifabutin
rifampin
rifapentine
streptomycin sulfate
(See Chapter 9, AMINOGLYCOSIDES.)

cycloserine
Seromycin

Pharmacologic class: isoxazolidine derivative, d-alanine analogue
Pregnancy risk category C

AVAILABLE FORMS
Capsules: 250 mg

INDICATIONS & DOSAGES
➤ **Adjunctive treatment for pulmonary or extrapulmonary tuberculosis (TB)**
Adults: Initially, 250 mg P.O. q 12 hours for 2 weeks; then, if levels are below 25 to 30 mcg/ml and no toxicity has developed, increase dosage to 250 mg q 8 hours for 2 weeks. If optimum levels still aren't achieved and no toxicity has developed, then increase dosage to 250 mg q 6 hours. Maximum dosage is 1 g daily. If CNS toxicity occurs, stop drug for 1 week, then resume at 250 mg daily for 2 weeks. If no serious toxic effects occur, increase dosage by 250-mg increments q 10 days until level of 25 to 30 mcg/ml is obtained.
Children♦: 10 to 20 mg/kg/day P.O. in two divided doses. Maximum dosage is 1 g daily.
➤ **Acute UTIs**
Adults: 250 mg P.O. q 12 hours for 2 weeks.

ACTION
Inhibits cell-wall biosynthesis by interfering with the bacterial use of amino acids; may be bacteriostatic or bactericidal, depending on the drug level attained at the site of infection and the organism's susceptibility.

Route	Onset	Peak	Duration
P.O.	Unknown	4–8 hr	Unknown

Half-life: 10 hours.

ADVERSE REACTIONS
CNS: ***coma, seizures, suicidal behavior,*** drowsiness, somnolence, headache, tremor, dysarthria, vertigo, confusion, loss of memory, psychosis, hyperirritability, paresthesia, paresis, hyperreflexia.
CV: ***sudden heart failure.***
Other: hypersensitivity reactions (rash, photosensitivity).

INTERACTIONS
Drug-drug. *Ethionamide:* May increase neurotoxic adverse reactions. Monitor patient closely.
Isoniazid: May increase risk of CNS toxicity, causing dizziness or drowsiness. Monitor patient closely.
Drug-lifestyle. *Alcohol use:* May increase risk of CNS toxicity, causing seizures. Discourage use together.

EFFECTS ON LAB TEST RESULTS
- May increase transaminase levels.

CONTRAINDICATIONS & CAUTIONS
- Contraindicated in patients hypersensitive to drug, in those who use alcohol excessively, and in those with seizure disorders, depression, severe anxiety, psychosis, or severe renal insufficiency.
- Use cautiously in patients with impaired renal function; reduce dosage in these patients.

NURSING CONSIDERATIONS
- Obtain specimen for culture and sensitivity tests before therapy begins and then periodically to detect possible resistance.
- Drug is considered a second-line drug in TB treatment and should always be given with other antituberculotics to prevent the development of resistant organisms.

• Use to treat UTIs only when better alternatives are contraindicated and susceptibility to cycloserine is confirmed.
• Monitor level periodically, especially in patients receiving high dosages (more than 500 mg daily), because toxic reactions may occur with levels above 30 mcg/ml.
• Watch patient receiving dosages of more than 500 mg daily for signs and symptoms of CNS toxicity, such as seizures, anxiety, and tremor. Giving 200 to 300 mg pyridoxine daily may help prevent neurotoxic effects.
• Monitor results of hematologic tests and renal and liver function tests.
• Observe patient for psychotic symptoms, hallucinations, and suicidal behavior.
• Monitor patient for hypersensitivity reactions, such as allergic dermatitis.
• Give anticonvulsant, tranquilizer, or sedative to relieve adverse reactions.

PATIENT TEACHING

• Warn patient to avoid alcohol, which may cause serious neurologic reactions.
• Advise patient not to perform hazardous activities if drowsiness occurs.
• Tell patient to report adverse reactions promptly; dosage may need to be adjusted or other drugs prescribed to relieve adverse reactions.

ethambutol hydrochloride

Etibit†, Myambutol

Pharmacologic class: synthetic antituberculotic
Pregnancy risk category B

AVAILABLE FORMS

Tablets: 100 mg, 400 mg

INDICATIONS & DOSAGES

➤ **Adjunctive treatment for pulmonary tuberculosis**
Adults and children older than age 13: In patients who haven't received prior antitubercular therapy, 15 mg/kg P.O. daily as a single dose, combined with other antituberculotics. For retreatment, 25 mg/kg P.O. daily as a single dose for 60 days (or until bacteriologic smears and cultures become negative) with at least one other antituberculotic; then decrease to 15 mg/kg/day as a single dose.

ACTION

May inhibit synthesis of one or more metabolites of susceptible bacteria, changing cell metabolism during cell division; bacteriostatic.

Route	Onset	Peak	Duration
P.O.	Unknown	2–4 hr	Unknown

Half-life: About 3½ hours.

ADVERSE REACTIONS

CNS: headache, dizziness, fever, mental confusion, hallucinations, malaise, peripheral neuritis.
EENT: optic neuritis.
GI: anorexia, nausea, vomiting, abdominal pain, GI upset.
Hematologic: ***thrombocytopenia.***
Metabolic: hyperuricemia.
Musculoskeletal: joint pain.
Respiratory: bloody sputum.
Skin: ***toxic epidermal necrolysis,*** dermatitis, pruritus.
Other: ***anaphylactoid reactions,*** precipitation of acute gout.

INTERACTIONS

Drug-drug. *Aluminum salts:* May delay and reduce absorption of ethambutol. Separate doses by several hours.

EFFECTS ON LAB TEST RESULTS

• May increase ALT, AST, bilirubin, and uric acid levels. May decrease glucose level.
• May decrease platelet count.

CONTRAINDICATIONS & CAUTIONS

• Contraindicated in children younger than age 13, patients hypersensitive to drug, and patients with optic neuritis.
• Use cautiously in patients with impaired renal function, cataracts, recurrent eye inflammation, gout, or diabetic retinopathy.

NURSING CONSIDERATIONS

• Perform visual acuity and color discrimination tests before and during therapy.

• Ensure that any changes in vision don't result from an underlying condition.
• Obtain AST and ALT levels before therapy, and monitor these levels every 3 to 4 weeks.
• In patients with impaired renal function, base dosage on drug level.
• Always give drug with other antituberculotics to prevent development of resistant organisms.
• Monitor uric acid level; observe patient for signs and symptoms of gout.

PATIENT TEACHING

• Reassure patient that visual disturbances usually disappear several weeks to months after drug is stopped. Inflammation of the optic nerve is related to dosage and duration of treatment.
• Inform patient that drug is given with other antituberculotics.
• Stress importance of compliance with drug therapy.
• Advise patient to report adverse reactions to prescriber.

isoniazid (INH, isonicotinic acid hydrazide)

Isotamine†, Nydrazid, PMS-Isoniazid†

Pharmacologic class: isonicotinic acid hydrazine
Pregnancy risk category C

AVAILABLE FORMS

Injection: 100 mg/ml
Oral solution: 50 mg/5 ml
Tablets: 100 mg, 300 mg

INDICATIONS & DOSAGES

➤ **Actively growing tubercle bacilli**
Adults and children age 15 and older: 5 mg/kg daily P.O. or I.M. in a single dose, up to 300 mg/day, with other drugs, continued for 6 months to 2 years. For intermittent multiple-drug regimen, 15 mg/kg (up to 900 mg) P.O. or I.M. 1, 2, or 3 times weekly.
Infants and children: 10 to 15 mg/kg daily P.O. or I.M. in a single dose, up to 300 mg/day, continued long enough to prevent relapse. Give with at least one other antituberculotic. For intermittent multiple-drug regimen, 20 to 40 mg/kg (up to 900 mg) P.O. or I.M. 2 or 3 times weekly.
➤ **To prevent tubercle bacilli in those exposed to tuberculosis (TB) or those with positive skin test results whose chest X-rays and bacteriologic study results indicate nonprogressive TB**
Adults: 300 mg daily P.O. in a single dose, continued for 6 months to 1 year.
Infants and children: 10 mg/kg daily P.O. in a single dose, up to 300 mg/day, continued for up to 1 year.

ACTION

May inhibit cell-wall biosynthesis by interfering with lipid and DNA synthesis; bactericidal.

Route	Onset	Peak	Duration
P.O., I.M.	Unknown	1–2 hr	Unknown

Half-life: 1 to 4 hours.

ADVERSE REACTIONS

CNS: *peripheral neuropathy, **seizures, toxic encephalopathy,*** memory impairment, toxic psychosis.
EENT: optic neuritis and atrophy.
GI: nausea, vomiting, epigastric distress.
Hematologic: ***agranulocytosis, aplastic anemia, thrombocytopenia,*** hemolytic anemia, eosinophilia, sideroblastic anemia.
Hepatic: ***hepatitis,*** jaundice, bilirubinemia.
Metabolic: hyperglycemia, metabolic acidosis, hypocalcemia, hypophosphatemia.
Skin: irritation at injection site.
Other: rheumatic and lupuslike syndromes, hypersensitivity reactions, pyridoxine deficiency, gynecomastia.

INTERACTIONS

Drug-drug. *Antacids and laxatives containing aluminum:* May decrease isoniazid absorption. Give isoniazid at least 1 hour before antacid or laxative.
Benzodiazepines, such as diazepam, triazolam: May inhibit metabolic clearance of benzodiazepines that undergo oxidative metabolism, possibly increasing benzodiazepine activity. Monitor patient for adverse reactions.

Carbamazepine, phenytoin: May increase levels of these drugs. Monitor drug levels closely.
Cycloserine: May increase CNS adverse reactions. Use safety precautions.
Disulfiram: May cause neurologic symptoms, including changes in behavior and coordination. Avoid using together.
Enflurane: In rapid acetylators of isoniazid, may cause high-output renal failure because of nephrotoxic inorganic fluoride level. Monitor renal function.
Ketoconazole: May decrease ketoconazole level. Monitor patient for lack of efficacy.
Meperidine: May increase CNS adverse reactions and hypotension. Use safety precautions.
Oral anticoagulants: May enhance anticoagulant activity. Monitor PT and INR.
Phenytoin: May inhibit phenytoin metabolism and increase phenytoin level. Monitor patient for phenytoin toxicity.
Rifampin: May increase the risk of hepatoxicity. Monitor liver function tests closely.
Drug-food. *Foods containing tyramine (such as aged cheese, beer, and chocolate):* May cause hypertensive crisis. Tell patient to avoid such foods or eat in small quantities.
Drug-lifestyle. *Alcohol use:* May increase risk of drug-related hepatitis. Discourage use of alcohol.

EFFECTS ON LAB TEST RESULTS

- May increase transaminase, glucose, and bilirubin levels. May decrease calcium, phosphate, and hemoglobin levels.
- May increase eosinophil count. May decrease granulocyte and platelet counts.
- May alter result of urine glucose tests that use cupric sulfate method, such as Benedict reagent and Diastix.

CONTRAINDICATIONS & CAUTIONS

- Contraindicated in patients with acute hepatic disease or isoniazid-related liver damage.
- Use cautiously in elderly patients, in those with chronic non–isoniazid-related liver disease or chronic alcoholism, in those with seizure disorders (especially if taking phenytoin), and in those with severe renal impairment.

NURSING CONSIDERATIONS

- Always give drug with other antituberculotics to prevent development of resistant organisms.
- Drug's pharmacokinetics may vary among patients because drug is metabolized in the liver by genetically controlled acetylation. Fast acetylators metabolize drug up to five times as fast as slow acetylators. About 50% of blacks and whites are slow acetylators; more than 80% of Chinese, Japanese, and Inuits are fast acetylators.
- Peripheral neuropathy is more common in patients who are slow acetylators or who are malnourished, alcoholic, or diabetic.
- Monitor hepatic function closely for changes. Elevated liver function study results occur in about 15% of patients; most abnormalities are mild and transient, but some may persist throughout treatment.
- ***Alert:*** Severe and sometimes fatal hepatitis may develop, even after many months of treatment. Risk increases with age. Monitor liver study results closely.
- Give pyridoxine to prevent peripheral neuropathy, especially in malnourished patients.

PATIENT TEACHING

- Instruct patient to take drug exactly as prescribed; warn against stopping drug without prescriber's consent.
- Advise patient to take drug 1 hour before or 2 hours after meals.
- Tell patient to notify prescriber immediately if signs and symptoms of liver impairment occur, such as appetite loss, fatigue, malaise, yellow skin or eye discoloration, and dark urine.
- Advise patient to avoid alcoholic beverages while taking drug. Also tell him to avoid certain foods: fish, such as skipjack and tuna, and products containing tyramine, such as aged cheese, beer, and chocolate because drug has some MAO inhibitor activity.
- Encourage patient to comply fully with treatment, which may take months or years.

rifabutin
Mycobutin

Pharmacologic class: semisynthetic ansamycin
Pregnancy risk category B

AVAILABLE FORMS
Capsules: 150 mg

INDICATIONS & DOSAGES
➤ **To prevent disseminated *Mycobacterium avium* complex in patients with advanced HIV infection**
Adults: 300 mg P.O. daily as a single dose or divided b.i.d.

ACTION
Inhibits DNA-dependent RNA polymerase in susceptible bacteria, blocking bacterial protein synthesis.

Route	Onset	Peak	Duration
P.O.	Unknown	2–4 hr	Unknown

Half-life: About 2 days.

ADVERSE REACTIONS
CNS: headache, fever.
EENT: eye inflammation.
GI: dyspepsia, eructation, flatulence, diarrhea, nausea, vomiting, abdominal pain, anorexia, taste perversion.
GU: discolored urine.
Hematologic: ***neutropenia, leukopenia, thrombocytopenia,*** eosinophilia.
Musculoskeletal: myalgia.
Skin: *rash.*

INTERACTIONS
Drug-drug. *Benzodiazepines, beta blockers, buspirone,* ***corticosteroids, cyclosporine,*** *delavirdine, doxycycline, fluconazole, hydantoins, indinavir, itraconazole, ketoconazole, losartan, macrolides, methadone, morphine, nelfinavir, quinidine, quinine,* ***tacrolimus,*** *theophylline, tricyclic antidepressants, zolpidem:* May decrease effectiveness of these drugs. Monitor patient for drug effects.
Hormonal contraceptives: May decrease contraceptive effectiveness. Tell patient to use another form of birth control.
Indinavir: May increase rifabutin level. Decrease rifabutin dosage by 50%.
Ritonavir: May increase the risk of rifabutin hematologic toxicity. Using together is contraindicated.
Voriconazole: May decrease therapeutic effects of voriconazole while increasing the risk of rifabutin adverse effects. Using together is contraindicated.
Warfarin: May decrease effectiveness of warfarin. May require higher dosages of anticoagulants. Monitor PT and INR.
Drug-food. *High-fat foods:* May reduce rate but not extent of absorption. Discourage use together.

EFFECTS ON LAB TEST RESULTS
- May increase aminotransferase level.
- May decrease neutrophil, WBC, and platelet counts.

CONTRAINDICATIONS & CAUTIONS
- Contraindicated in patients hypersensitive to drug or other rifamycin derivatives, such as rifampin, and in patients with active tuberculosis, because single-drug therapy with rifabutin increases risk of inducing bacterial resistance to both rifabutin and rifampin.
- Use cautiously in patients with neutropenia and thrombocytopenia.

NURSING CONSIDERATIONS
- In patients with neutropenia or thrombocytopenia, obtain baseline hematologic studies and repeat periodically.
- Mix drug with soft foods such as applesauce for patients who have difficulty swallowing.
- ***Look alike–sound alike:*** Don't confuse rifabutin with rifampin or rifapentine.

PATIENT TEACHING
- Instruct patient to take drug for as long as prescribed, exactly as directed, even after feeling better.
- Tell patient experiencing GI adverse effects, such as nausea or vomiting, to divide total daily dose into 2 doses and to take with food.
- Tell patient that drug may cause brownish orange staining of urine, feces, sputum, saliva, tears, and skin. Tell him to avoid wearing soft contact lenses because they may be permanently stained.

• Instruct patient to report sensitivity to light, excessive tears, or eye pain immediately.
• Advise patient to report tingling and joint stiffness, swelling, or tenderness.

rifampin (rifampicin)

Rifadin, Rimactane, Rimycin‡, Rofact†

Pharmacologic class: semisynthetic rifamycin
Pregnancy risk category C

AVAILABLE FORMS

Capsules: 150 mg, 300 mg
Powder for injection: 600 mg

INDICATIONS & DOSAGES

➤ **Pulmonary tuberculosis, with other antituberculotics**
Adults: 10 mg/kg P.O. or I.V. daily in single dose. Give oral doses 1 hour before or 2 hours after meals with a full glass of water. Maximum daily dose is 600 mg.
Children age 5 and older: 10 to 20 mg/kg P.O. or I.V. daily in single dose. Give oral doses 1 hour before or 2 hours after meals with a full glass of water. Maximum daily dose is 600 mg. Give with other antituberculotics.
➤ **Meningococcal carriers**
Adults: 600 mg P.O. or I.V. q 12 hours for 2 days; or 600 mg P.O. or I.V. once daily for 4 days.
Children ages 1 month to 12 years: 10 mg/kg P.O. or I.V. q 12 hours for 2 days, not to exceed 600 mg/day; or 20 mg/kg once daily for 4 days.
Neonates: 5 mg/kg P.O. or I.V. q 12 hours for 2 days.
➤ ***Mycobacterium avium* complex ♦**
Adults: 600 mg P.O. or I.V. daily as part of a multiple-drug regimen.

I.V. ADMINISTRATION

• Reconstitute drug with 10 ml of sterile water for injection to yield 60 mg/ml.
• Add to 100 ml of D_5W and infuse over 30 minutes, or add to 500 ml of D_5W and infuse over 3 hours.
• When dextrose is contraindicated, dilute with normal saline solution for injection.
• Once prepared, dilutions in D_5W are stable for up to 4 hours and dilutions in normal saline solution are stable for up to 24 hours at room temperature.

INCOMPATIBILITIES

Diltiazem, minocycline, other IV solutions.

ACTION

Inhibits DNA-dependent RNA polymerase, which impairs RNA synthesis; bactericidal.

Route	Onset	Peak	Duration
P.O.	Unknown	2–4 hr	Unknown
I.V.	Unknown	Unknown	Unknown

Half-life: 1¼ to 5 hours.

ADVERSE REACTIONS

CNS: headache, fatigue, drowsiness, behavioral changes, dizziness, mental confusion, generalized numbness, ataxia.
CV: ***shock.***
EENT: visual disturbances, exudative conjunctivitis.
GI: ***pancreatitis, pseudomembranous colitis,*** epigastric distress, anorexia, nausea, vomiting, abdominal pain, diarrhea, flatulence, sore mouth and tongue.
GU: ***acute renal failure,*** hemoglobinuria, hematuria, menstrual disturbances.
Hematologic: ***thrombocytopenia, transient leukopenia,*** eosinophilia, hemolytic anemia.
Hepatic: ***hepatotoxicity.***
Metabolic: hyperuricemia.
Musculoskeletal: osteomalacia.
Respiratory: dyspnea, wheezing.
Skin: pruritus, urticaria, rash.
Other: flulike syndrome, discoloration of body fluids, porphyria exacerbation.

INTERACTIONS

Drug-drug. *Acetaminophen, amiodarone, analgesics, anticonvulsants, barbiturates, beta blockers, cardiac glycosides, chloramphenicol, clofibrate,* **corticosteroids, cyclosporine,** *dapsone, delavirdine, diazepam, digoxin, disopyramide, doxycycline, enalapril, fluoroquinolones, hormonal contraceptives, hydantoins, losartan, methadone, mexiletine, midazolam, nifedipine, ondansetron, opioids, progestins,*

propafenone, quinidine, ***ritonavir,*** *sulfonylureas,* ***tacrolimus,*** *theophylline, tocainide, triazolam, tricyclic antidepressants, verapamil, zidovudine, zolpidem:* May decrease effectiveness of these drugs. Monitor effectiveness.
Anticoagulants: May increase requirements for anticoagulant. Monitor PT and INR closely and adjust dosage of anticoagulants.
Halothane: May increase risk of hepatotoxicity. Monitor liver function test results.
Isoniazid: May increase risk of hepatotoxicity. Monitor liver function test results.
Ketoconazole, para-aminosalicylate sodium: May interfere with absorption of rifampin. Separate doses by 8 to 12 hours.
Macrolide antibiotics, protease inhibitors: May inhibit rifampin metabolism but increase metabolism of other drug. Monitor patient for effects.
Probenecid: May increase rifampin levels. Use together cautiously.
Voriconazole: May decrease voriconazole's therapeutic effects while increasing the risk of rifampin adverse effects. Using together is contraindicated.
Drug-lifestyle. *Alcohol use:* May increase risk of hepatotoxicity. Discourage use together.

EFFECTS ON LAB TEST RESULTS

- May increase ALT, AST, alkaline phosphatase, bilirubin, and uric acid levels. May decrease hemoglobin level.
- May increase eosinophil counts. May decrease platelet and WBC counts.
- May alter standard folate and vitamin B_{12} assay results.

CONTRAINDICATIONS & CAUTIONS

- Contraindicated in patients hypersensitive to rifampin or related drugs.
- Use cautiously in patients with liver disease.

NURSING CONSIDERATIONS

- Give drug with at least one other antituberculotic.
- For best absorption, give capsules 1 hour before or 2 hours after meals.
- Monitor hepatic function, hematopoietic studies, and uric acid levels. Drug's systemic effects may asymptomatically raise liver function test results and uric acid level.
- Watch for and report to prescriber signs and symptoms of hepatic impairment.
- Drug may cause hemorrhage in neonates of mothers taking drug.
- ***Look alike–sound alike:*** Don't confuse rifampin with rifabutin or rifapentine.

PATIENT TEACHING

- Instruct patient who can't tolerate capsules on an empty stomach to take drug with meals and a full glass of water.
- Warn patient that he may feel drowsy and that drug can turn body fluids red-orange and permanently stain contact lenses.
- Advise a woman using hormonal contraceptive to consider another form of birth control.
- Advise patient to contact prescriber if he experiences fever, loss of appetite, malaise, nausea, vomiting, dark urine, or yellow discoloration of the eyes or skin.
- Advise patient to avoid alcohol during drug therapy.

rifapentine

Priftin

Pharmacologic class: synthetic rifamycin
Pregnancy risk category C

AVAILABLE FORMS

Tablets (film-coated): 150 mg

INDICATIONS & DOSAGES

➤ **Pulmonary tuberculosis (TB), with at least one other antituberculotic to which the isolate is susceptible**

Adults: During intensive phase of short-course therapy, 600 mg P.O. twice weekly for 2 months, with an interval between doses of at least 3 days (72 hours). During continuation phase of short-course therapy, 600 mg P.O. once weekly for 4 months, combined with isoniazid or another drug to which the isolate is susceptible.

ACTION

Inhibits DNA-dependent RNA polymerase in susceptible strains of *Mycobacte-*

rium tuberculosis. Demonstrates bactericidal activity against the organism both intracellularly and extracellularly.

Route	Onset	Peak	Duration
P.O.	Unknown	5–6 hr	Unknown

Half-life: 13 hours.

ADVERSE REACTIONS

CNS: headache, dizziness, pain.
CV: hypertension.
GI: anorexia, nausea, vomiting, dyspepsia, diarrhea.
GU: pyuria, proteinuria, hematuria, urinary casts.
Hematologic: ***leukopenia, neutropenia,*** lymphopenia, anemia, thrombocytosis.
Metabolic: *hyperuricemia.*
Musculoskeletal: arthralgia.
Respiratory: hemoptysis.
Skin: rash, pruritus, acne, maculopapular rash.

INTERACTIONS

Drug-drug. *Antiarrhythmics (disopyramide, mexiletine, quinidine, tocainide), antibiotics (chloramphenicol, clarithromycin, dapsone, doxycycline, fluoroquinolones), anticonvulsants (phenytoin), antifungals (fluconazole, itraconazole, ketoconazole), barbiturates, benzodiazepines (diazepam), beta blockers, calcium channel blockers (diltiazem, nifedipine, verapamil), cardiac glycosides, clofibrate,* ***corticosteroids,*** *haloperidol, HIV protease inhibitors (indinavir, nelfinavir, ritonavir, saquinavir), hormonal contraceptives,* ***immunosuppressants (cyclosporine, tacrolimus),*** *levothyroxine, opioid analgesics (methadone), oral anticoagulants (warfarin), oral hypoglycemics (sulfonylureas), progestins, quinine, reverse transcriptase inhibitors (delavirdine, zidovudine), sildenafil, theophylline, tricyclic antidepressants (amitriptyline, nortriptyline):* May decrease activity of these drugs because of cytochrome P-450 enzyme metabolism. May need to adjust dosage.
Ritonavir: May decrease ritonavir levels. Carefully monitor patient's response.

EFFECTS ON LAB TEST RESULTS

- May increase uric acid, ALT, and AST levels. May decrease hemoglobin level.
- May increase platelet count. May decrease neutrophil and WBC counts.
- May alter folate and vitamin B_{12} assay results.

CONTRAINDICATIONS & CAUTIONS

- Contraindicated in patients hypersensitive to rifamycins (rifapentine, rifampin, or rifabutin).
- Use drug cautiously and with frequent monitoring in patients with liver disease.

NURSING CONSIDERATIONS

- Rifamycin antibiotics may cause hepatotoxicity. Obtain baseline liver function test results before therapy.
- Give drug with pyridoxine (vitamin B_6) in malnourished patients; in those predisposed to neuropathy, such as alcoholics and diabetics; and in adolescents.
- ***Alert:*** Give drug with appropriate daily companion drugs. Compliance with all drug regimens, especially with daily companion drugs on the days when rifapentine isn't given, is crucial for early sputum conversion and protection from relapse of TB.
- If used during the last 2 weeks of pregnancy, drug may lead to postnatal hemorrhage in mother or infant. Monitor clotting parameters closely if drug is used at that time.
- ***Look alike–sound alike:*** Don't confuse rifapentine with rifabutin or rifampin.

PATIENT TEACHING

- Stress importance of strict compliance with this drug regimen and that of daily companion drugs, as well as needed follow-up visits and laboratory tests.
- Advise a woman to use nonhormonal birth control methods.
- Tell patient to take drug with food if nausea, vomiting, or GI upset occurs.
- Instruct patient to report to prescriber fever, appetite loss, malaise, nausea, vomiting, darkened urine, yellowish skin and eyes, joint pain or swelling, or excessive loose stools or diarrhea.
- Instruct patient to protect pills from excessive heat.
- Tell patient that drug may turn body fluids red-orange and permanently stain contact lenses.

9 Aminoglycosides

amikacin sulfate
gentamicin sulfate
neomycin sulfate
streptomycin sulfate
tobramycin sulfate

amikacin sulfate
Amikin

Pharmacologic class: aminoglycoside
Pregnancy risk category D

AVAILABLE FORMS
Injection: 50 mg/ml (pediatric), 250 mg/ml, 5 mg/ml (500 mg) in normal saline solution

INDICATIONS & DOSAGES
➤ **Serious infections caused by sensitive strains of *Pseudomonas aeruginosa, Escherichia coli, Proteus, Klebsiella,* or *Staphylococcus***
Adults and children: 15 mg/kg/day I.M. or I.V. infusion, in divided doses q 8 to 12 hours for 7 to 10 days.
Neonates: Initially, loading dose of 10 mg/kg I.V.; then 7.5 mg/kg q 12 hours for 7 to 10 days.
➤ **Uncomplicated UTI caused by organisms not susceptible to less toxic drugs**
Adults: 250 mg I.M. or I.V. b.i.d.
➤ **Active tuberculosis, with other antituberculotics ♦**
Adults and children age 15 and older: 15 mg/kg (up to 1 g) I.M. or I.V. once daily five to seven times per week for 2 to 4 months or until culture conversion. Then reduce dose to 15 mg/kg daily given two or three times weekly depending on other drugs in regimen. Patients older than age 59 may receive a reduced dose of 10 mg/kg (up to 750 mg) daily.
Children younger than age 15: 15 to 30 mg/kg (up to 1 g) I.M. or I.V. once daily or twice weekly.
➤ ***Mycobacterium avium* complex (MAC) infection ♦**
Adults: 15 mg/kg/day I.V. in divided doses q 8 to 12 hours as part of a multiple-drug regimen.
Adjust-a-dose: For adults with impaired renal function, initially, 7.5 mg/kg I.M. or I.V. Subsequent doses and frequency determined by amikacin levels and renal function studies. For adults receiving hemodialysis, give supplemental doses of 50% to 75% of initial loading dose at end of each dialysis session. Monitor drug levels and adjust dosage accordingly.

I.V. ADMINISTRATION
- For adults, dilute I.V. drug in 100 to 200 ml of D_5W or normal saline solution. For children, the amount of fluid will depend on the ordered dose.
- In adults and children, infuse over 30 to 60 minutes. In infants, infuse over 1 to 2 hours.
- After infusion, flush line with normal saline solution or D_5W.

INCOMPATIBILITIES
Allopurinol, aminophylline, amphotericin B, ampicillin, azithromycin, bacitracin, cefazolin, ceftazidime, chlorothiazide sodium, cisplatin, heparin sodium, hetastarch in 0.9% sodium chloride, oxacillin, phenytoin, propofol, thiopental, vancomycin, vitamin B complex with C.

ACTION
Inhibits protein synthesis by binding directly to the 30S ribosomal subunit; bactericidal.

Route	Onset	Peak	Duration
I.V.	Immediate	30 min	8–12 hr
I.M.	Unknown	1 hr	8–12 hr

Half-life: Adults: 2 to 3 hours. Patients with severe renal damage, 30 to 86 hours.

ADVERSE REACTIONS
CNS: ***neuromuscular blockade.***
EENT: *ototoxicity.*

GU: *azotemia,* ***nephrotoxicity,*** increase in urinary excretion of casts.
Musculoskeletal: arthralgia.
Respiratory: ***apnea.***

INTERACTIONS

Drug-drug. *Acyclovir, amphotericin B, cephalosporins, cidofovir, cisplatin, methoxyflurane, vancomycin, other aminoglycosides:* May increase nephrotoxicity. Use together cautiously, and monitor renal function test results.
Atracurium, pancuronium, rocuronium, vecuronium: May increase effects of nondepolarizing muscle relaxants, including prolonged respiratory depression. Use together only when necessary, and expect to reduce dosage of nondepolarizing muscle relaxant.
Dimenhydrinate: May mask ototoxicity symptoms. Monitor patient's hearing.
General anesthetics: May increase neuromuscular blockade. Monitor patient for increased effects.
Indomethacin: May increase trough and peak amikacin levels. Monitor amikacin level.
I.V. loop diuretics such as furosemide: May increase ototoxicity. Use together cautiously, and monitor patient's hearing.
Parenteral penicillins: May inactivate amikacin in vitro. Don't mix.

EFFECTS ON LAB TEST RESULTS

- May increase BUN, creatinine, nonprotein nitrogen, and urine urea levels.

CONTRAINDICATIONS & CAUTIONS

- Contraindicated in patients hypersensitive to drug or other aminoglycosides.
- Use cautiously in patients with impaired renal function or neuromuscular disorders, in neonates and infants, and in elderly patients.

NURSING CONSIDERATIONS

- Obtain specimen for culture and sensitivity tests before giving first dose. Therapy may begin while awaiting results.
- Evaluate patient's hearing before and during therapy if he will be receiving drug for longer than 2 weeks. Notify prescriber if patient has tinnitus, vertigo, or hearing loss.
- Weigh patient and review renal function studies before therapy begins.
- Correct dehydration before therapy because of increased risk of toxicity.
- Obtain blood for peak level 1 hour after I.M. injection and 30 minutes to 1 hour after I.V. infusion ends; for trough levels, draw blood just before next dose. Don't collect blood in a heparinized tube; heparin is incompatible with aminoglycosides.
- Peak drug levels more than 35 mcg/ml and trough levels more than 10 mcg/ml may be linked to a higher risk of toxicity.
- Monitor renal function: urine output, specific gravity, urinalysis, BUN and creatinine levels, and creatinine clearance. Report to prescriber evidence of declining renal function.
- Watch for signs and symptoms of superinfection (especially of upper respiratory tract), such as continued fever, chills, and increased pulse rate.
- Therapy usually continues for 7 to 10 days. If no response occurs after 3 to 5 days, stop therapy and obtain new specimens for culture and sensitivity testing.
- ***Look alike–sound alike:*** Don't confuse Amikin with Amicar. Don't confuse amikacin with anakinra.

PATIENT TEACHING

- Instruct patient to promptly report adverse reactions to prescriber.
- Encourage patient to maintain adequate fluid intake.

gentamicin sulfate

Cidomycin†, Garamycin

Pharmacologic class: aminoglycoside
Pregnancy risk category D

AVAILABLE FORMS

Injection: 40 mg/ml (adults), 10 mg/ml (children)
I.V. infusion (premixed): 40 mg, 60 mg, 70 mg, 80 mg, 90 mg, 100 mg, 120 mg, in normal saline solution

INDICATIONS & DOSAGES

➤ **Serious infections caused by sensitive strains of *Pseudomonas aeru-***

ginosa, Escherichia coli, Proteus, Klebsiella,* or *Staphylococcus
Adults: 3 mg/kg daily in 3 divided doses I.M. or I.V. infusion q 8 hours. For life-threatening infections, may give up to 5 mg/kg daily in 3 to 4 divided doses; reduce dosage to 3 mg/kg daily as soon as patient improves.
Children: 2 to 2.5 mg/kg q 8 hours I.M. or by I.V. infusion.
Neonates older than 1 week and infants: 2.5 mg/kg q 8 hours I.M. or by I.V. infusion.
Neonates younger than 1 week and preterm infants: 2.5 mg/kg q 12 hours I.M. or by I.V. infusion.

➤To prevent endocarditis before GI or GU procedure or surgery
Adults: 1.5 mg/kg I.M. or I.V. 30 minutes before procedure or surgery. Maximum dose is 80 mg. Give with ampicillin (vancomycin in penicillin-allergic patients).
Children: 2 mg/kg I.M. or I.V. 30 minutes before procedure or surgery. Maximum dose is 80 mg. Give with ampicillin (vancomycin in penicillin-allergic patients).
Adjust-a-dose: For adults with impaired renal function, doses and frequency are determined by drug level and renal function. To maintain therapeutic levels, adults should receive 1 to 1.7 mg/kg I.M. or by I.V. infusion after each dialysis session, and children should receive 2 to 2.5 mg/kg I.M. or by I.V. infusion after each dialysis session.

I.V. ADMINISTRATION
- For intermittent infusion, dilute with 50 to 200 ml of D_5W or normal saline solution for injection.
- Infuse over 30 minutes to 2 hours.
- After completing infusion, flush the line with normal saline solution or D_5W.

INCOMPATIBILITIES
Allopurinol, amphotericin B, ampicillin, azithromycin, cefazolin, cefepime, cefotaxime, ceftazidime, ceftriaxone sodium, cefuroxime, certain parenteral nutrition formulations, cytarabine, dopamine, fat emulsions, furosemide, heparin, hetastarch, idarubicin, indomethacin sodium trihydrate, nafcillin, propofol, ticarcillin, warfarin.

ACTION
Inhibits protein synthesis by binding directly to the 30S ribosomal subunit; bactericidal.

Route	Onset	Peak	Duration
I.V.	Immediate	30–90 min	Unknown
I.M.	Unknown	30–90 min	Unknown

Half-life: 2 to 3 hours.

ADVERSE REACTIONS
CNS: ***encephalopathy, seizures,*** fever, headache, lethargy, confusion, dizziness, numbness, peripheral neuropathy, vertigo, ataxia, tingling.
CV: hypotension.
EENT: *ototoxicity,* blurred vision, tinnitus.
GI: vomiting, nausea.
GU: ***nephrotoxicity,*** possible increase in urinary excretion of casts.
Hematologic: ***agranulocytosis, leukopenia, thrombocytopenia,*** anemia, eosinophilia.
Musculoskeletal: muscle twitching, myasthenia gravis–like syndrome.
Respiratory: ***apnea.***
Skin: rash, urticaria, pruritus, injection site pain.
Other: ***anaphylaxis.***

INTERACTIONS
Drug-drug. *Acyclovir, amphotericin B, cephalosporins, cidofovir, cisplatin, methoxyflurane, vancomycin, other aminoglycosides:* May increase ototoxicity and nephrotoxicity. Monitor hearing and renal function test results.
Atracurium, pancuronium, rocuronium, vecuronium: May increase effects of nondepolarizing muscle relaxants, including prolonged respiratory depression. Use together only when necessary, and expect to reduce dosage of nondepolarizing muscle relaxant.
Dimenhydrinate: May mask ototoxicity symptoms. Monitor patient's hearing.
General anesthetics: May increase neuromuscular blockade. Monitor patient closely.
Indomethacin: May increase peak and trough levels of gentamicin. Monitor gentamicin level.

I.V. loop diuretics (such as furosemide): May increase risk of ototoxicity. Monitor patient's hearing.
Parenteral penicillins (such as ampicillin and ticarcillin): May inactivate gentamicin in vitro. Don't mix together.

EFFECTS ON LAB TEST RESULTS

- May increase ALT, AST, bilirubin, BUN, creatinine, LDH, and nonprotein nitrogen levels. May decrease hemoglobin level.
- May increase eosinophil count. May decrease granulocyte, platelet, and WBC counts.

CONTRAINDICATIONS & CAUTIONS

- Contraindicated in patients hypersensitive to drug or other aminoglycosides.
- Use cautiously in neonates, infants, elderly patients, and patients with impaired renal function or neuromuscular disorders.

NURSING CONSIDERATIONS

- Obtain specimen for culture and sensitivity tests before giving. Begin therapy, awaiting results.
- Evaluate patient's hearing before and during therapy. Notify prescriber if patient complains of tinnitus, vertigo, or hearing loss.
- Weigh patient and review renal function studies before therapy begins.
- ***Alert:*** Use preservative-free form when intrathecal route is used adjunctively for serious CNS infections, such as meningitis and ventriculitis.
- Obtain blood for peak level 1 hour after I.M. injection or 30 minutes after I.V. infusion finishes; for trough levels, draw blood just before next dose. Don't collect blood in a heparinized tube; heparin is incompatible with aminoglycosides.
- Maintain peak levels at 4 to 12 mcg/ml and trough levels at 1 to 2 mcg/ml. The maximum peak level is usually 8 mcg/ml, except in patients with cystic fibrosis, who need increased lung penetration. Prolonged peak levels of 10 to 12 mcg/ml or prolonged trough levels greater than 2 mcg/ml may increase risk of toxicity.
- Monitor renal function: urine output, specific gravity, urinalysis, BUN and creatinine levels, and creatinine clearance. Report to prescriber evidence of declining renal function.
- Hemodialysis for 8 hours may remove up to 50% of drug from blood.
- Watch for signs and symptoms of superinfection (especially of upper respiratory tract), such as continued fever, chills, and increased pulse rate.
- Therapy usually continues for 7 to 10 days. If no response occurs in 3 to 5 days, stop therapy and obtain new specimens for culture and sensitivity testing.

PATIENT TEACHING

- Instruct patient to promptly report adverse reactions, such as dizziness, vertigo, unsteady gait, ringing in the ears, hearing loss, numbness, tingling, or muscle twitching.
- Encourage patient to drink plenty of fluids.
- Warn patient to avoid hazardous activities if adverse CNS reactions occur.

neomycin sulfate

Mycifradin†, Neo-fradin, Neosulf‡, Neo-Tabs

Pharmacologic class: aminoglycoside
Pregnancy risk category D

AVAILABLE FORMS

Oral solution: 125 mg/5 ml
Tablets: 500 mg

INDICATIONS & DOSAGES

➤ **Infectious diarrhea caused by enteropathogenic *Escherichia coli***
Adults: 50 mg/kg daily P.O. in 4 divided doses for 2 to 3 days; maximum of 3 g/day.
Children: 50 to 100 mg/kg daily P.O. in divided doses q 4 to 6 hours for 2 to 3 days.

➤ **To suppress intestinal bacteria before surgery**
Adults: After saline cathartic, 1 g P.O. q hour for 4 doses; then 1 g q 4 hours for the balance of the 24 hours. Or, 88 mg/kg in 6 equally divided doses q 4 hours. Or, 1 g neomycin with 1 g erythromycin base at 1 p.m., 2 p.m., and 11 p.m. on day before 8 a.m. surgery.
Children: After saline cathartic, 40 to 100 mg/kg daily P.O. in divided doses q

4 to 6 hours. Or, 88 mg/kg in 6 equally divided doses q 4 hours.

➤**Adjunctive treatment for hepatic coma**

Adults: 1 to 3 g P.O. q.i.d. for 5 to 6 days; or 200 ml of 1% solution or 100 ml of 2% solution as enema retained for 20 to 60 minutes q 6 hours. For patients with chronic hepatic insufficiency, 4 g/day indefinitely may be needed.

Children: 50 to 100 mg/kg/day P.O. in divided doses for 5 to 6 days.

ACTION

Inhibits protein synthesis by binding directly to the 30S ribosomal subunit; bactericidal.

Route	Onset	Peak	Duration
P.O.	Unknown	1–4 hr	8 hr

Half-life: 2 to 3 hours.

ADVERSE REACTIONS

EENT: *ototoxicity.*

GI: nausea, vomiting, diarrhea, malabsorption syndrome, *Clostridium difficile*–related colitis.

GU: ***nephrotoxicity,*** possible increase in urinary excretion of casts.

INTERACTIONS

Drug-drug. *Acyclovir, amphotericin B, cephalosporins, cidofovir, cisplatin, methoxyflurane, vancomycin, other aminoglycosides:* May increase nephrotoxicity. Monitor renal function test results.

Atracurium, pancuronium, rocuronium, vecuronium: May increase effects of nondepolarizing muscle relaxants, including prolonged respiratory depression. Use together only when necessary, and expect to reduce dosage of nondepolarizing muscle relaxants.

Digoxin: May decrease digoxin absorption. Monitor digoxin level.

I.V. loop diuretics (such as furosemide): May increase ototoxicity. Monitor patient's hearing.

Oral anticoagulants: May inhibit vitamin K–producing bacteria; may increase anticoagulant effect. Monitor PT and INR.

EFFECTS ON LAB TEST RESULTS

- May increase BUN, creatinine, and nonprotein nitrogen levels.

CONTRAINDICATIONS & CAUTIONS

- Contraindicated in patients hypersensitive to other aminoglycosides and in those with intestinal obstruction.
- Use cautiously in elderly patients and in those with impaired renal function, neuromuscular disorders, or ulcerative bowel lesions.

NURSING CONSIDERATIONS

- Monitor renal function: urine output, specific gravity, urinalysis, BUN and creatinine levels, and creatinine clearance. Report to prescriber evidence of declining renal function.
- Evaluate patient's hearing before and during prolonged therapy. Notify prescriber if patient has tinnitus, vertigo, or hearing loss. Deafness may start several weeks after drug is stopped.
- Watch for signs and symptoms of superinfection, such as fever, chills, and increased pulse rate.
- For adjunctive treatment for hepatic coma, decrease patient's dietary protein and assess neurologic status frequently during therapy.
- For preoperative disinfection, provide a low-residue diet and a cathartic immediately before therapy.
- The ototoxic and nephrotoxic properties of drug limit its usefulness.

PATIENT TEACHING

- Instruct patient to report adverse reactions promptly.
- Encourage patient to maintain adequate fluid intake.

streptomycin sulfate

Pharmacologic class: aminoglycoside
Pregnancy risk category D

AVAILABLE FORMS

Injection: 1-g/2.5-ml ampules

INDICATIONS & DOSAGES

➤ Streptococcal endocarditis
Adults: 1 g q 12 hours I.M. for 1 week; then 500 mg I.M. q 12 hours for 1 week, given with penicillin.
Adjust-a-dose: In patients older than age 60, give 500 mg I.M. q 12 hours for entire 2 weeks, with penicillin.

➤ Second-line treatment of tuberculosis (TB), given with other antituberculotics
Adults: 15 mg/kg (maximum of 1 g) I.M. daily, continued long enough to prevent relapse. For intermittent use, 25 to 30 mg/kg (maximum of 1.5 g) 2 to 3 times weekly.
Children: 20 to 40 mg/kg (maximum of 1 g) I.M. daily. Give with other antituberculotics, except capreomycin; continue until sputum test result becomes negative. For intermittent use, 25 to 30 mg/kg (maximum of 1.5 g) 2 to 3 times weekly.
Adults older than 59: 10 mg/kg I.M. daily.

➤ Enterococcal endocarditis
Adults: 1 g I.M. q 12 hours for 2 weeks; then 500 mg I.M. q 12 hours for 4 weeks, given with penicillin.

➤ Tularemia
Adults: 1 to 2 g I.M. daily in divided doses injected deep into upper outer quadrant of buttocks; continued for 7 to 14 days or until patient is afebrile for 5 to 7 days.

ACTION

Inhibits protein synthesis by binding directly to the 30S ribosomal subunit; bactericidal.

Route	Onset	Peak	Duration
I.M.	Unknown	1–2 hr	Unknown

Half-life: 2 to 3 hours.

ADVERSE REACTIONS

CNS: ***neuromuscular blockade,*** vertigo, facial paresthesia.
EENT: *ototoxicity.*
GI: vomiting, nausea.
GU: ***nephrotoxicity,*** increase in urinary excretion of casts.
Hematologic: ***leukopenia, thrombocytopenia, hemolytic anemia,*** eosinophilia.
Respiratory: ***apnea.***
Skin: exfoliative dermatitis.
Other: ***anaphylaxis,*** hypersensitivity reactions.

INTERACTIONS

Drug-drug. *Acyclovir, amphotericin B, cephalosporins, cidofovir, cisplatin, methoxyflurane, vancomycin, other aminoglycosides:* May increase nephrotoxicity. Monitor renal function test results.
Atracurium, pancuronium, rocuronium, vecuronium: May increase effects of nondepolarizing muscle relaxants, including prolonged respiratory depression. Use together only when necessary, and expect to reduce dosage of nondepolarizing muscle relaxant.
General anesthetics: May increase neuromuscular blockade. Monitor patient closely.
I.V. loop diuretics such as furosemide: May increase ototoxicity. Monitor patient's hearing.
Penicillins: May inactivate streptomycin, decreasing the therapeutic effects. Don't mix together.

EFFECTS ON LAB TEST RESULTS

- May increase BUN, creatinine, and nonprotein nitrogen levels. May decrease hemoglobin level.
- May increase eosinophil count. May decrease WBC and platelet counts.
- May cause false-positive reaction in copper sulfate tests for urine glucose, such as Benedict reagent and Diastix.

CONTRAINDICATIONS & CAUTIONS

- Contraindicated in patients hypersensitive to drug or other aminoglycosides.
- Use cautiously in elderly patients and in patients with impaired renal function or neuromuscular disorders.

NURSING CONSIDERATIONS

- Obtain specimen for culture and sensitivity tests before giving, except when treating TB. Begin therapy, awaiting results.
- Evaluate patient's hearing before therapy and for 6 months afterward. Notify prescriber if patient has hearing loss, feels fullness in ears, or hears roaring noises.
- To avoid irritation, protect hands when preparing drug.

• When giving I.M., inject deep into upper outer quadrant of buttocks or midlateral thigh. Rotate injection sites.
• In children, give I.M. injection in midlateral thigh, if possible, to minimize possibility of damaging sciatic nerve.
• Obtain blood for peak level 1 to 2 hours after I.M. injection; obtain blood for trough level just before next dose. Don't use a heparinized tube; heparin is incompatible with aminoglycosides.
• Drug has been given as I.V. infusion over 30 to 60 minutes without unusual adverse effects in patients who can't tolerate I.M. injections.
• Watch for signs and symptoms of superinfection, such as continued fever, chills, and increased pulse rate.
• Nephrotoxicity occurs less frequently with streptomycin than with other aminoglycosides.
• When drug is used as primary treatment of TB, stop therapy when sputum test result becomes negative.
• Total dose for TB shouldn't exceed 120 g over the course of therapy unless there are no other treatment options.

PATIENT TEACHING

• Instruct patient to report adverse reactions promptly.
• Encourage patient to maintain adequate fluid intake.
• Emphasize need for blood tests to monitor levels and determine effectiveness of therapy.

tobramycin sulfate

Nebcin, TOBI

Pharmacologic class: aminoglycoside
Pregnancy risk category D

AVAILABLE FORMS

Multidose vials (pediatric): 40 mg/ml, 10 mg/ml
Nebulizer solution (for inhalation): 300 mg/5 ml
Premixed parenteral injection for infusion: 60 mg or 80 mg in normal saline solution

INDICATIONS & DOSAGES

➤ **Serious infection by sensitive strains of *Escherichia coli, Proteus, Klebsiella, Enterobacter, Serratia, Morganella morganii, Staphylococcus aureus, Citrobacter, Pseudomonas,* or *Providencia***

Adults: 3 mg/kg/day I.M. or I.V. in divided doses. For life-threatening infections, give up to 5 mg/kg/day in divided doses q 6 to 8 hours; reduce to 3 mg/kg daily as soon as clinically indicated.
Children: 6 to 7.5 mg/kg/day I.M. or I.V., divided t.i.d. or q.i.d.
Neonates younger than age 1 week or premature infants: Up to 4 mg/kg/day I.V. or I.M. in 2 equal doses q 12 hours.
Adjust-a-dose: For patients with renal impairment, give loading dose of 1 mg/kg; then give decreased doses at 8-hour intervals or same dose at prolonged intervals. For patients with severe cystic fibrosis, initial dose is 10 mg/kg/day I.V. or I.M., divided q.i.d.

➤ **To manage cystic fibrosis patients with *Pseudomonas aeruginosa***

Adults and children age 6 and older: 300 mg via nebulizer q 12 hours for 28 days. Continue cycle of 28 days on drug and 28 days off.

I.V. ADMINISTRATION

• For adults, dilute in 50 to 100 ml of normal saline solution or D_5W; use a smaller volume for children.
• Infuse over 20 to 60 minutes.
• After infusion, flush line with normal saline solution or D_5W.

INCOMPATIBILITIES

Allopurinol; amphotericin B; azithromycin; beta lactam antibiotics; cefepime; clindamycin; dextrose 5% in Isolyte E, M, or P; heparin sodium; hetastarch; indomethacin; propofol; sargramostim; solutions containing alcohol.

ACTION

Generally bactericidal. Inhibits protein synthesis by binding directly to the 30S ribosomal subunit.

Route	Onset	Peak	Duration
I.V.	Immediate	30 min	8 hr
I.M.	Unknown	30–60 min	8 hr
Inhalation	Unknown	Unknown	Unknown

Half-life: 2 to 3 hours.

ADVERSE REACTIONS

CNS: ***seizures,*** headache, lethargy, confusion, disorientation, fever.
EENT: *ototoxicity, hoarseness, pharyngitis.*
GI: vomiting, nausea, diarrhea.
GU: ***nephrotoxicity,*** possible increase in urinary excretion of casts.
Hematologic: anemia, eosinophilia, ***leukopenia, thrombocytopenia, agranulocytosis.***
Metabolic: electrolyte imbalances.
Musculoskeletal: muscle twitching.
Respiratory: ***bronchospasm.***
Skin: rash, urticaria, pruritus.

INTERACTIONS

Drug-drug. *Acyclovir, amphotericin B, cephalosporins, cidofovir, cisplatin, methoxyflurane, vancomycin, other aminoglycosides:* May increase nephrotoxicity. Monitor renal function test results.
Atracurium, pancuronium, rocuronium, vecuronium: May increase effects of nondepolarizing muscle relaxants, including prolonged respiratory depression. Use together only when necessary, and expect to reduce dosage of nondepolarizing muscle relaxant.
Dimenhydrinate: May mask symptoms of ototoxicity. Monitor patient's hearing.
General anesthetics: May increase neuromuscular blockade. Monitor patient for increased clinical effects.
I.V. loop diuretics such as furosemide: May increase ototoxicity. Monitor patient's hearing.
Parenteral penicillins: May inactivate tobramycin in vitro. Don't mix together.

EFFECTS ON LAB TEST RESULTS

- May increase BUN, creatinine, nonprotein nitrogen, and urine urea levels. May decrease calcium, magnesium, and potassium levels.
- May increase eosinophil count. May decrease WBC, platelet, and granulocyte counts.

CONTRAINDICATIONS & CAUTIONS

- Contraindicated in patients hypersensitive to drug or other aminoglycosides.
- Use cautiously in patients with impaired renal function or neuromuscular disorders and in elderly patients.

NURSING CONSIDERATIONS

- Obtain specimen for culture and sensitivity tests before giving. Begin therapy, awaiting results.
- Weigh patient and review renal function studies before therapy.
- Evaluate patient's hearing before and during therapy. If patient complains of tinnitus, vertigo, or hearing loss, notify prescriber.
- Don't dilute or mix with dornase alpha in a nebulizer.
- Unrefrigerated drug, which is normally slightly yellow, may darken with age. This change doesn't indicate a change in product quality.
- Avoid exposing ampules to intense light.
- Give nebulizer solution over 10 to 15 minutes using handheld Pari LC Plus reusable nebulizer with DeVilbiss Pulmo-Aide compressor.
- Obtain blood for peak level 1 hour after I.M. injection or ½ hour after infusion stops; draw blood for trough level just before next dose. Don't collect blood in a heparinized tube because of incompatibility.
- ***Alert:*** Peak levels over 12 mcg/ml and trough levels over 2 mcg/ml may increase the risk of toxicity. Reserve higher peak levels for cystic fibrosis patients, who need a greater lung penetration.
- Monitor renal function: urine output, specific gravity, urinalysis, creatinine clearance, and BUN and creatinine levels. Notify prescriber about signs and symptoms of decreasing renal function.
- Watch for signs and symptoms of superinfection, such as continued fever, chills, and increased pulse rate.
- If no response occurs in 3 to 5 days, therapy may be stopped and new specimens obtained for culture and sensitivity testing.

• ***Look alike–sound alike:*** Don't confuse tobramycin with Trobicin.

PATIENT TEACHING

• Instruct patient to report adverse reactions promptly.
• Caution patient not to perform hazardous activities if adverse CNS reactions occur.
• Encourage patient to maintain adequate fluid intake.
• Teach patient how to use and maintain nebulizer.
• Tell patient using several inhaled therapies to use this drug last.
• Instruct patient not to use if the solution is cloudy or contains particles or if it has been stored at room temperature for longer than 28 days.

10

Penicillins

amoxicillin and clavulanate potassium
amoxicillin trihydrate
ampicillin
ampicillin sodium
ampicillin sodium and sulbactam sodium
ampicillin trihydrate
penicillin G benzathine
penicillin G potassium
penicillin G procaine
penicillin G sodium
penicillin V potassium
piperacillin sodium and tazobactam sodium
ticarcillin disodium and clavulanate potassium

amoxicillin and clavulanate potassium (amoxycillin and clavulanate potassium)

Augmentin, Augmentin ES-600, Augmentin XR, Clavulin†

Pharmacologic class: aminopenicillin and beta-lactamase inhibitor
Pregnancy risk category B

AVAILABLE FORMS

Oral suspension: 125 mg amoxicillin trihydrate and 31.25 mg clavulanic acid/5 ml (after reconstitution); 200 mg amoxicillin trihydrate and 28.5 mg clavulanic acid/ 5 ml (after reconstitution); 250 mg amoxicillin trihydrate and 62.5 mg clavulanic acid/5 ml (after reconstitution); 400 mg amoxicillin trihydrate and 57 mg clavulanic acid/5 ml (after reconstitution); 600 mg amoxicillin trihydrate and 42.9 mg clavulanic acid/5 ml after reconstitution
Tablets (chewable): 125 mg amoxicillin trihydrate, 31.25 mg clavulanic acid; 200 mg amoxicillin trihydrate, 28.5 mg clavulanic acid; 250 mg amoxicillin trihydrate, 62.5 mg clavulanic acid; 400 mg amoxicillin trihydrate, 57 mg clavulanic acid
Tablets (extended-release): 1,000 mg amoxicillin trihydrate, 62.5 mg clavulanic acid
Tablets (film-coated): 250 mg amoxicillin trihydrate, 125 mg clavulanic acid; 500 mg amoxicillin trihydrate, 125 mg clavulanic acid; 875 mg amoxicillin trihydrate, 125 mg clavulanic acid

INDICATIONS & DOSAGES

➤ **Recurrent or persistent acute otitis media caused by *Streptococcus pneumoniae, Haemophilus influenzae,* or *Moraxella catarrhalis* in patients exposed to antibiotics within the previous 3 months, who are 2 years old or younger or in daycare facilities**
Children age 3 months and older: 90 mg/ kg/day Augmentin ES-600 P.O., based on amoxicillin component, q 12 hours for 10 days.

➤ **Lower respiratory tract infections, otitis media, sinusitis, skin and skin-structure infections, and UTIs caused by susceptible strains of gram-positive and gram-negative organisms**
Adults and children who weigh 40 kg (88 lb) or more: 250 mg P.O., based on amoxicillin component, q 8 hours; or 500 mg q 12 hours. For more severe infections, 500 mg q 8 hours or 875 mg q 12 hours.
Children age 3 months and older and weighing less than 40 kg: 20 to 45 mg/kg P.O., based on amoxicillin component and severity of infection, daily in divided doses q 8 to 12 hours.
Children younger than age 3 months: 30 mg/kg/day P.O., based on amoxicillin component of the 125-mg/5-ml oral suspension, in divided doses q 12 hours.
Adjust-a-dose: Don't give the 875-mg tablet to patients with creatinine clearance less than 30 ml/minute. If clearance is 10 to 30 ml/minute, give 250 to 500 mg P.O. q 12 hours. If clearance is less than 10 ml/minute, give 250 to 500 mg P.O. q 24 hours. Give hemodialysis patients

250 to 500 mg P.O. q 24 hours with an additional dose both during and after dialysis.

➤**Community-acquired pneumonia or acute bacterial sinusitis caused by *H. influenzae, M. catarrhalis, H. parainfluenzae, Klebsiella pneumoniae,* methicillin-susceptible *Staphylococcus aureus,* or *S. pneumoniae* with reduced susceptibility to penicillin**

Adults and children age 16 and older: 2,000 mg/125 mg Augmentin XR tablets q 12 hours for 7 to 10 days for pneumonia; 10 days for sinusitis.

Adjust-a-dose: In patients with creatinine clearance less than 30 ml/minute and patients receiving hemodialysis, don't use Augmentin XR.

ACTION

Prevents bacterial cell-wall synthesis during replication. Increases amoxicillin effectiveness by inactivating beta-lactamases, which destroy amoxicillin.

Route	Onset	Peak	Duration
P.O.	Unknown	1–2½ hr	6–8 hr
P.O. (Augmentin ES-600)	Unknown	1–4 hr	Unknown
P.O. (Augmentin XR)	Unknown	1–6 hr	Unknown

Half-life: 1 to 1½ hours. For patients with severe renal impairment, 7½ hours for amoxicillin and 4½ hours for clavulanate.

ADVERSE REACTIONS

CNS: agitation, anxiety, insomnia, confusion, behavioral changes, dizziness.

GI: nausea, vomiting, *diarrhea,* indigestion, gastritis, stomatitis, glossitis, black hairy tongue, enterocolitis, ***pseudomembranous colitis,*** mucocutaneous candidiasis, abdominal pain.

GU: vaginitis, vaginal candidiasis.

Hematologic: anemia, ***thrombocytopenia, thrombocytopenic purpura,*** eosinophilia, ***leukopenia, agranulocytosis.***

Other: hypersensitivity reactions, ***(anaphylaxis,*** rash, urticaria, pruritus, ***angioedema),*** overgrowth of nonsusceptible organisms, serum sickness–like reaction.

INTERACTIONS

Drug-drug. *Allopurinol:* May increase risk of rash. Monitor patient for rash.

Hormonal contraceptives: May decrease hormonal contraceptive effectiveness. Advise use of additional form of contraception during penicillin therapy.

Probenecid: May increase levels of amoxicillin and other penicillins. Probenecid may be used for this purpose.

Drug-herb. *Khat:* May decrease antimicrobial effect of certain penicillins. Discourage khat chewing, or tell patient to take amoxicillin 2 hours after khat chewing.

EFFECTS ON LAB TEST RESULTS

- May increase eosinophil count.
- May falsely decrease aminoglycoside level. May alter results of urine glucose tests that use cupric sulfate, such as Benedict reagent and Clinitest.

CONTRAINDICATIONS & CAUTIONS

- Contraindicated in patients hypersensitive to drug or other penicillins and in those with a history of amoxicillin-related cholestatic jaundice or hepatic dysfunction.
- Augmentin XR is contraindicated in patients receiving hemodialysis and those with creatinine clearance less than 30 ml/minute.
- Use cautiously in patients with other drug allergies (especially to cephalosporins) because of possible cross-sensitivity and in those with mononucleosis because of high risk of maculopapular rash.
- Use cautiously in breast-feeding women; it's unknown if drug appears in breast milk.
- Use cautiously in hepatically impaired patients, and monitor the hepatic function of these patients.

NURSING CONSIDERATIONS

- Before giving drug, ask patient about allergic reactions to penicillin. However, a negative history of penicillin allergy is no guarantee against an allergic reaction.
- Obtain specimen for culture and sensitivity tests before giving first dose. Therapy may begin pending results.
- Give drug at least 1 hour before a bacteriostatic antibiotic.

• Each Augmentin XR tablet contains 29.3 mg (1.27 mEq) of sodium.
• Augmentin XR isn't indicated for treating infections caused by *S. pneumoniae* with penicillin minimum inhibitory concentration (commonly known as MIC) 4 mcg/ml or greater.
• If large doses are given or therapy is prolonged, bacterial or fungal superinfection may occur, especially in elderly, debilitated, or immunosuppressed patients.
• ***Alert:*** Don't interchange the oral suspensions because of varying clavulanic acid contents.
• Augmentin ES-600 is intended only for children ages 3 months to 12 years with persistent or recurrent acute otitis media.
• Avoid use of 250-mg tablet in children weighing less than 40 kg (88 lb). Use chewable form instead.
• ***Alert:*** Both 250- and 500-mg film-coated tablets contain the same amount of clavulanic acid (125 mg). Therefore, two 250-mg tablets aren't equivalent to one 500-mg tablet. Regular tablets aren't equivalent to Augmentin XR.
• This drug combination is particularly useful in clinical settings with a high prevalence of amoxicillin-resistant organisms.
• After reconstitution, refrigerate the oral suspension; discard after 10 days.
• ***Look alike–sound alike:*** Don't confuse amoxicillin with amoxapine.

PATIENT TEACHING
• Tell patient to take entire quantity of drug exactly as prescribed, even after feeling better.
• Instruct patient to take drug with food to prevent GI upset. If he's taking the oral suspension, tell him to keep drug refrigerated, to shake it well before taking it, and to discard remaining drug after 10 days.
• Tell patient to call prescriber if a rash occurs because rash is a sign of an allergic reaction.

amoxicillin trihydrate (amoxycillin trihydrate)

Alphamox‡, Amoxil, Apo-Amoxi†, Cilamox‡, DisperMox, Moxacin‡, Novamoxin†, Nu-Amoxi†, Trimox

Pharmacologic class: aminopenicillin
Pregnancy risk category B

AVAILABLE FORMS
Capsules: 250 mg, 500 mg
Oral suspension: 50 mg/ml (pediatric drops), 125 mg/5 ml, 200 mg/5 ml, 250 mg/5 ml, 400 mg/5 ml (after reconstitution)
Tablets (chewable): 125 mg, 200 mg, 250 mg, 400 mg
Tablets (film-coated): 500 mg, 875 mg
Tablets for oral suspension: 200 mg, 400 mg

INDICATIONS & DOSAGES
➤ Mild to moderate infections of the ear, nose, and throat; skin and skin structure; or genitourinary tract
Adults and children who weigh 40 kg (88 lb) or more: 500 mg P.O. q 12 hours or 250 mg P.O. q 8 hours.
Children older than age 3 months who weigh less than 40 kg: 25 mg/kg/day P.O. divided q 12 hours or 20 mg/kg/day P.O. divided q 8 hours.
Neonates and infants up to age 3 months: Up to 30 mg/kg/day P.O. divided q 12 hours.
➤ Mild to severe infections of the lower respiratory tract and severe infections of the ear, nose, and throat; skin and skin structure; or genitourinary tract
Adults and children who weigh 40 kg or more: 875 mg P.O. q 12 hours or 500 mg P.O. q 8 hours.
Children older than age 3 months weighing less than 40 kg: 45 mg/kg/day P.O. divided q 12 hours or 40 mg/kg/day P.O. divided q 8 hours.
➤ Uncomplicated gonorrhea
Adults and children who weigh more than 45 kg (99 lb): 3 g P.O. with 1 g probenecid given as a single dose.
Children age 2 and older who weigh less than 45 kg: 50 mg/kg to a maximum of

3 g P.O. with 25 mg/kg, to a maximum of 1 g of probenecid as a single dose. Don't give probenecid to children younger than age 2.

➤**To prevent endocarditis in patients having dental, oral, or respiratory tract procedures and in moderate-risk patients undergoing GI and GU procedures♦**

Adults: 2 g P.O. 1 hour before procedure.
Children: 50 mg/kg P.O. 1 hour before procedure.

➤**To prevent penicillin-susceptible anthrax after exposure♦**

Adults and children older than age 9: 500 mg P.O. t.i.d. for 60 days.
Children younger than age 9: 80 mg/kg daily P.O., divided b.i.d. or t.i.d. for 60 days.

ACTION

Inhibits cell-wall synthesis during bacterial multiplication.

Route	Onset	Peak	Duration
P.O.	Unknown	1–2 hr	6–8 hr

Half-life: 1 to 1½ hours (7½ hours in severe renal impairment).

ADVERSE REACTIONS

CNS: ***seizures,*** lethargy, hallucinations, anxiety, confusion, agitation, depression, dizziness, fatigue.
GI: *diarrhea, nausea,* ***pseudomembranous colitis,*** vomiting, glossitis, stomatitis, gastritis, enterocolitis, abdominal pain, black hairy tongue.
GU: interstitial nephritis, nephropathy, vaginitis.
Hematologic: ***agranulocytosis, leukopenia, thrombocytopenia, thrombocytopenic purpura,*** anemia, eosinophilia, hemolytic anemia.
Other: ***anaphylaxis,*** hypersensitivity reactions, overgrowth of nonsusceptible organisms.

INTERACTIONS

Drug-drug. *Allopurinol:* May increase risk of rash. Monitor patient for rash.
Hormonal contraceptives: May decrease contraceptive effectiveness. Advise use of additional form of contraception during penicillin therapy.
Probenecid: May increase levels of amoxicillin and other penicillins. Probenecid may be used for this purpose.
Drug-herb. *Khat:* May decrease antimicrobial effect of certain penicillins. Discourage herb use, or tell patient to take drug 2 hours after herb use.

EFFECTS ON LAB TEST RESULTS

- May decrease hemoglobin level.
- May increase eosinophil count. May decrease granulocyte, platelet, and WBC counts.
- May falsely decrease aminoglycoside level. May alter results of urine glucose tests that use cupric sulfate, such as Benedict reagent and Clinitest.

CONTRAINDICATIONS & CAUTIONS

- Contraindicated in patients hypersensitive to drug or other penicillins.
- Use cautiously in patients with other drug allergies (especially to cephalosporins) because of possible cross-sensitivity.
- Use cautiously in those with mononucleosis because of high risk of maculopapular rash.

NURSING CONSIDERATIONS

- Obtain specimen for culture and sensitivity tests before giving first dose. Therapy may begin pending results.
- Before giving, ask patient about allergic reactions to penicillin. A negative history of penicillin allergy is no guarantee against allergic reaction.
- If large doses are given or if therapy is prolonged, bacterial or fungal superinfection may occur, especially in elderly, debilitated, or immunosuppressed patients.
- Store Trimox oral suspension in refrigerator, if possible. It also may be stored at room temperature for up to 2 weeks. Make sure to check individual product labels for storage information.
- Amoxicillin usually causes fewer cases of diarrhea than ampicillin.
- ***Look alike–sound alike:*** Don't confuse amoxicillin with amoxapine.

PATIENT TEACHING

- Tell patient to take entire quantity of drug exactly as prescribed, even after he feels better.

• Instruct patient to take drug with or without food.
• Tell patient to notify prescriber if rash, fever, or chills develop. A rash is the most common allergic reaction, especially if allopurinol is also being taken.
• Tell parent to place drops directly on child's tongue for swallowing or add to formula, milk, fruit juice, water, ginger ale, or a cold drink for immediate and complete consumption.
• If child takes DisperMox, tell parent to mix 1 tablet in about 10 ml of water, to have the child drink the resulting solution, to rinse container with a small amount of water, and to have the child drink again to ensure the whole dose is taken. Parent should mix tablet only in water. Caution parent against allowing child to chew tablets, to swallow them whole, or to let them dissolve in mouth.

ampicillin
Apo-Ampi†, Novo Ampicillin†, Nu-Ampi†

ampicillin sodium
Ampicin†, Ampicyn‡, Penbritin†

ampicillin trihydrate
Penbritin†, Principen

Pharmacologic class: aminopenicillin
Pregnancy risk category B

AVAILABLE FORMS
Capsules: 250 mg, 500 mg
Injection: 250 mg, 500 mg, 1 g, 2 g
Oral suspension: 125 mg/5 ml, 250 mg/5 ml

INDICATIONS & DOSAGES
➤ Respiratory tract or skin and skin-structure infections
Adults and children who weigh 40 kg (88 lb) or more: 250 to 500 mg P.O. q 6 hours.
Children who weigh less than 40 kg: 25 to 50 mg/kg/day P.O. in equally divided doses q 6 hours. Pediatric dosages shouldn't exceed recommended adult dosages.

➤ GI infections or UTIs
Adults and children who weigh 40 kg (88 lb) or more: 500 mg P.O. q 6 hours. For severe infections, larger doses may be needed.
Children who weigh less than 40 kg: 50 to 100 mg/kg/day P.O. in equally divided doses q 6 hours.

➤ Bacterial meningitis or septicemia
Adults: 150 to 200 mg/kg/day I.V. in divided doses q 3 to 4 hours. May be given I.M. after 3 days of I.V. therapy. Maximum recommended daily dose is 14 g.
Children: 150 to 200 mg/kg I.V. daily in divided doses q 3 to 4 hours. Give I.V. for 3 days; then give I.M.

➤ Uncomplicated gonorrhea
Adults and children who weigh more than 45 kg (99 lb): 3.5 g P.O. with 1 g probenecid given as a single dose.

➤ To prevent endocarditis in patients having dental, GI, and GU procedures♦
Adults: 2 g I.M. or I.V. within 30 minutes before procedure. For high-risk patients, also give 1.5 mg/kg gentamicin 30 minutes before the procedure; 6 hours later, give 1 g ampicillin I.M. or I.V. or 1 g amoxicillin P.O.
Children: 50 mg/kg I.M. or I.V. within 30 minutes before procedure. For high-risk patients, also give 1.5 mg/kg gentamicin 30 minutes before the procedure; 6 hours later, give 25 mg/kg ampicillin I.M. or I.V. or 25 mg/kg amoxicillin P.O.
Adjust-a-dose: In patients with creatinine clearance of 10 to 50 ml/minute, use same dose but increase dosing interval to 6 to 12 hours; for those with a clearance less than 10 ml/minute, increase dosing interval to 12 to 24 hours.

I.V. ADMINISTRATION
• Give drug intermittently to prevent vein irritation. Change site every 48 hours.
• For direct injection, reconstitute with bacteriostatic water for injection. Use 5 ml for 250-mg or 500-mg vials, 7.4 ml for 1-g vials, and 14.8 ml for 2-g vials. Give drug over 10 to 15 minutes to avoid seizures. Don't exceed 100 mg/minute.
• For intermittent infusion, dilute in 50 to 100 ml of normal saline solution for injection. Give drug over 15 to 30 minutes.

• Use first dilution within 1 hour. Follow manufacturer's directions for stability data when drug is further diluted for I.V. infusion.

INCOMPATIBILITIES

Amikacin, amino acid solutions, chlorpromazine, dextran solutions, dextrose solutions, dopamine, erythromycin lactobionate, 10% fat emulsions, fructose, gentamicin, heparin sodium, hetastarch, hydrocortisone sodium succinate, hydromorphone, kanamycin, lidocaine, lincomycin, polymyxin B, prochlorperazine edisylate, sodium bicarbonate, streptomycin, tobramycin.

ACTION

Inhibits cell-wall synthesis during bacterial multiplication.

Route	Onset	Peak	Duration
P.O.	Unknown	2 hr	6–8 hr
I.V.	Immediate	Immediate	Unknown
I.M.	Unknown	1 hr	Unknown

Half-life: 1 to 1½ hours (10 to 24 hours in severe renal impairment.

ADVERSE REACTIONS

CNS: ***seizures,*** lethargy, hallucinations, anxiety, confusion, agitation, depression, dizziness, fatigue.
CV: vein irritation, thrombophlebitis.
GI: *diarrhea, nausea,* ***pseudomembranous colitis,*** vomiting, glossitis, stomatitis, gastritis, abdominal pain, enterocolitis, black hairy tongue.
GU: interstitial nephritis, nephropathy, vaginitis.
Hematologic: ***leukopenia, thrombocytopenia, thrombocytopenic purpura,*** anemia, eosinophilia, hemolytic anemia, ***agranulocytosis.***
Skin: pain at injection site.
Other: hypersensitivity reactions, overgrowth of nonsusceptible organisms.

INTERACTIONS

Drug-drug. *Allopurinol:* May increase risk of rash. Monitor patient for rash.
H_2 antagonists, proton pump inhibitors: May decrease ampicillin absorption and level. Separate administration times. Monitor patient for continued antibiotic effectiveness.
Hormonal contraceptives: May decrease hormonal contraceptive effectiveness. Advise use of another form of contraception during therapy.
Oral anticoagulants: May increase risk of bleeding. Monitor PT and INR.
Probenecid: May increase levels of ampicillin and other penicillins. Probenecid may be used for this purpose.

EFFECTS ON LAB TEST RESULTS

• May decrease hemoglobin level.
• May increase eosinophil count. May decrease granulocyte, platelet, and WBC counts.
• May falsely decrease aminoglycoside level. May alter results of urine glucose tests that use cupric sulfate, such as Benedict reagent and Clinitest.

CONTRAINDICATIONS & CAUTIONS

• Contraindicated in patients hypersensitive to drug or other penicillins.
• Use cautiously in patients with other drug allergies (especially to cephalosporins) because of possible cross-sensitivity, and in those with mononucleosis because of high risk of maculopapular rash.

NURSING CONSIDERATIONS

• Before giving drug, ask patient about allergic reactions to penicillin. A negative history of penicillin allergy is no guarantee against a future allergic reaction.
• Obtain specimen for culture and sensitivity tests before giving. Therapy may begin pending results.
• Give drug I.M. or I.V. only if infection is severe or if patient can't take oral dose.
• Give drug 1 to 2 hours before or 2 to 3 hours after meals. When given orally, drug may cause GI disturbances. Food may interfere with absorption.
• Monitor sodium level because each gram of ampicillin contains 2.9 mEq of sodium.
• If large doses are given or if therapy is prolonged, bacterial or fungal superinfection may occur, especially in elderly, debilitated, or immunosuppressed patients.
• Watch for signs and symptoms of hypersensitivity, such as erythematous maculopapular rash, urticaria, and anaphylaxis.

- In patients with impaired renal function, decrease dosage.
- In pediatric meningitis, drug may be given with parenteral chloramphenicol for 24 hours, pending cultures.
- To prevent bacterial endocarditis in patients at high risk, give drug with gentamicin.

PATIENT TEACHING

- Tell patient to take entire quantity of drug exactly as prescribed, even after he feels better.
- Instruct patient to take oral form on an empty stomach 1 hour before or 2 hours after meals.
- Inform patient to notify prescriber if rash, fever, or chills develop. A rash is the most common allergic reaction, especially if allopurinol also is being taken.
- Advise patient to report discomfort at I.V. injection site.

ampicillin sodium and sulbactam sodium

Unasyn

Pharmacologic class: aminopenicillin and beta-lactamase inhibitor
Pregnancy risk category B

AVAILABLE FORMS

Injection: Vials and piggyback vials containing 1.5 g (1 g ampicillin sodium with 0.5 g sulbactam sodium), 3 g (2 g ampicillin sodium with 1 g sulbactam sodium)

INDICATIONS & DOSAGES

➤ Intra-abdominal, gynecologic, and skin-structure infections caused by susceptible strains

Adults: 1.5 to 3 g I.M. or I.V. q 6 hours. Don't exceed 4 g/day of sulbactam.

Children age 1 or older (skin and skin-structure infections only): 300 mg/kg/day I.V. in divided doses q 6 hours for no longer than 14 days.

Adjust-a-dose: If creatinine clearance in adults is 15 to 29 ml/minute, give 1.5 to 3 g q 12 hours; if clearance is 5 to 14 ml/minute, give 1.5 to 3 g q 24 hours.

I.V. ADMINISTRATION

- Reconstitute powder with one of these diluents: normal saline solution, sterile water for injection, D_5W, lactated Ringer injection, 1/6 M sodium lactate, dextrose 5% in half-normal saline solution for injection, or 10% invert sugar.
- After reconstitution, let vials stand for a few minutes so foam can dissipate. Inspect solution for particles.
- Give drug at least 1 hour before giving a bacteriostatic antibiotic.
- For direct injection, give drug slowly over 10 to 15 minutes.
- For infusion, dilute in 50 to 100 ml of compatible diluent and infuse over 15 to 30 minutes.
- Change I.V. site every 48 hours.
- Stability varies with diluent, temperature, and concentration of solution.

INCOMPATIBILITIES

Amikacin, amino acid solutions, amiodarone, amphotericin B, chlorpromazine, ciprofloxacin, dextran solutions, dopamine, erythromycin lactobionate, 10% fat emulsions, fructose, gentamicin, heparin sodium, hetastarch, hydrocortisone sodium succinate, idarubicin, kanamycin, lidocaine, lincomycin, netilmicin, polymyxin B, nicardipine, ondansetron, prochlorperazine edisylate, sargramostim, sodium bicarbonate, streptomycin, tobramycin.

ACTION

Inhibits cell-wall synthesis during bacterial multiplication.

Route	Onset	Peak	Duration
I.V.	Immediate	15 min	Unknown
I.M.	Unknown	Unknown	Unknown

Half-life: 1 to 1½ hours (10 to 24 in severe renal impairment).

ADVERSE REACTIONS

CV: thrombophlebitis, vein irritation.
GI: *diarrhea, nausea,* ***pseudomembranous colitis,*** vomiting, glossitis, stomatitis, gastritis, black hairy tongue, enterocolitis.
Hematologic: ***agranulocytosis, leukopenia, thrombocytopenia, thrombocytopenic purpura,*** anemia, eosinophilia.

Skin: *pain at injection site.*
Other: hypersensitivity reactions, ***anaphylaxis,*** overgrowth of nonsusceptible organisms.

INTERACTIONS
Drug-drug. *Allopurinol:* May increase risk of rash. Monitor patient for rash.
Hormonal contraceptives: May decrease hormonal contraceptive effectiveness. Strongly advise use of another contraceptive during therapy.
Oral anticoagulants: May increase risk of bleeding. Monitor PT and INR.
Probenecid: May increase ampicillin level. Probenecid may be used for this purpose.

EFFECTS ON LAB TEST RESULTS
- May increase alkaline phosphatase, ALT, AST, bilirubin, BUN, CK, creatinine, GGT, and LDH levels. May decrease hemoglobin level. May transiently decrease conjugated estriol, conjugated estrone, estradiol, and estriol glucuronide levels in pregnant women.
- May increase eosinophil count. May decrease granulocyte, platelet, and WBC counts.
- May alter results of urine glucose tests that use cupric sulfate, such as Benedict reagent and Clinitest.

CONTRAINDICATIONS & CAUTIONS
- Contraindicated in patients hypersensitive to drug or other penicillins.
- Use cautiously in patients with other drug allergies (especially to cephalosporins) because of possible cross-sensitivity, and in those with mononucleosis because of high risk of maculopapular rash.

NURSING CONSIDERATIONS
- Before giving drug, ask patient about allergic reactions to penicillin although a negative history of penicillin allergy is no guarantee against future allergic reaction. Also, obtain specimen for culture and sensitivity tests. Therapy may begin pending results.
- Dosage is expressed as total drug. Each 1.5-g vial contains 1 g ampicillin sodium and 0.5 g sulbactam sodium.
- In patients with impaired renal function, decrease dosage.
- For I.M. injection, reconstitute with sterile water for injection or 0.5% or 2% lidocaine hydrochloride injection. Add 3.2 ml to a 1.5-g vial (or 6.4 ml to a 3-g vial) to yield a concentration of 375 mg/ml. Give deep into muscle.
- In children, don't use I.M. route.
- Monitor liver function test results during therapy, especially in patients with impaired liver function.
- If large doses are given or if therapy is prolonged, bacterial or fungal superinfection may occur, especially in elderly, debilitated, or immunosuppressed patients.

PATIENT TEACHING
- Tell patient to report rash, fever, or chills. A rash is the most common allergic reaction.
- Advise patient to report discomfort at I.V. insertion site.
- Warn patient that I.M. injection may cause pain at injection site.

penicillin G benzathine (benzathine benzylpenicillin)
Bicillin L-A, Permapen

Pharmacologic class: natural penicillin
Pregnancy risk category B

AVAILABLE FORMS
Injection: 600,000 units/ml; 1.2 million units/2 ml; 2.4 million units/4 ml

INDICATIONS & DOSAGES
➤ **Congenital syphilis**
Children younger than age 2: Give 50,000 units/kg I.M. as a single dose.
➤ **Group A streptococcal upper respiratory tract infections**
Adults: Give 1.2 million units I.M. as a single injection.
Children who weigh 27 kg (59.5 lb) or more: Give 900,000 units I.M. as a single injection.
Children who weigh less than 27 kg: Give 300,000 to 600,000 units I.M. as a single injection.

➤ **To prevent poststreptococcal rheumatic fever**
Adults and children: Give 1.2 million units I.M. once monthly or 600,000 units I.M. q 2 weeks.
➤ **Syphilis of less than 1 year duration**
Adults: Give 2.4 million units I.M. as a single dose.
Children: Give 50,000 units/kg I.M. as a single dose. Don't exceed adult dosage.
➤ **Syphilis of more than 1 year duration**
Adults: Give 2.4 million units I.M. weekly for 3 weeks.
Children: Give 50,000 units/kg I.M. weekly for 3 weeks.

ACTION
Inhibits cell-wall synthesis during bacterial multiplication.

Route	Onset	Peak	Duration
I.M.	Unknown	13–24 hr	1–4 wk

Half-life: 30 to 60 minutes.

ADVERSE REACTIONS
CNS: ***seizures,*** neuropathy, lethargy, hallucinations, anxiety, confusion, agitation, depression, dizziness, fatigue.
GI: ***pseudomembranous colitis,*** nausea, vomiting, enterocolitis.
GU: interstitial nephritis, nephropathy.
Hematologic: ***agranulocytosis, leukopenia, thrombocytopenia,*** eosinophilia, hemolytic anemia, anemia.
Skin: maculopapular rash, exfoliative dermatitis.
Other: ***anaphylaxis,*** hypersensitivity reactions, pain, sterile abscess at injection site.

INTERACTIONS
Drug-drug. *Aminoglycosides:* Physical and chemical incompatibility. Give separately.
Colestipol: May decrease penicillin G benzathine level. Give penicillin G benzathine 1 hour before or 4 hours after colestipol.
Hormonal contraceptives: May decrease hormonal contraceptive effectiveness. Advise use of additional form of contraception during therapy.
Probenecid: May increase penicillin level. Probenecid may be used for this purpose.
Tetracycline: May antagonize penicillin G benzathine effects. Avoid using together.

EFFECTS ON LAB TEST RESULTS
- May decrease hemoglobin level.
- May increase eosinophil count. May decrease platelet, WBC, and granulocyte counts. May cause positive Coombs' test results.
- May falsely decrease aminoglycoside level. May cause false-positive CSF protein test results. May alter urine glucose testing using cupric sulfate (Benedict reagent).

CONTRAINDICATIONS & CAUTIONS
- Contraindicated in patients hypersensitive to drug or other penicillins.
- Use cautiously in patients allergic to other drugs, especially to cephalosporins, because of possible cross-sensitivity.

NURSING CONSIDERATIONS
- Before giving drug, ask patient about allergic reactions to penicillin.
- ***Alert:*** Bicillin L-A is the only penicillin G benzathine product indicated for sexually transmitted infections. Don't substitute Bicillin C-R because it may not be effective.
- Obtain specimen for culture and sensitivity tests before giving first dose. Therapy may begin pending results.
- Shake well before injection.
- ***Alert:*** Inadvertent I.V. use may cause cardiac arrest and death. Never give I.V.
- Inject deep into upper outer quadrant of buttocks in adults and in midlateral thigh in infants and small children. Rotate injection sites. Avoid injection into or near major nerves or blood vessels to prevent permanent neurovascular damage.
- Give drug at least 1 hour before a bacteriostatic antibiotic.
- Drug's extremely slow absorption time makes allergic reactions difficult to treat.
- If large doses are given or if therapy is prolonged, bacterial or fungal superinfection may occur, especially in elderly, debilitated, or immunosuppressed patients.

• ***Look alike–sound alike:*** Don't confuse drug with Polycillin, penicillamine, or the various types of penicillin.

PATIENT TEACHING

• Tell patient to report adverse reactions promptly.
• Inform patient that fever and increased WBC count are the most common reactions.
• Warn patient that I.M. injection may be painful but that ice applied to the site may ease discomfort.

penicillin G potassium (benzylpenicillin potassium)

Pfizerpen

Pharmacologic class: natural penicillin
Pregnancy risk category B

AVAILABLE FORMS

Injection: 1 million units, 5 million units, 20 million units
Premixed injection: 1 million units/50 ml, 2 million units/50 ml, 3 million units/ 50 ml
Tablets: 500,000 units†

INDICATIONS & DOSAGES

➤ **Moderate to severe systemic infection**

Adults and children age 12 and older: Highly individualized; 1 to 30 million units I.M. or I.V. daily in divided doses q 2 to 6 hours or via continuous I.V. infusion.
Children younger than age 12: 25,000 to 400,000 units/kg I.M. or I.V. daily in divided doses q 4 to 6 hours.

➤ **Anthrax**

Adults: 5 to 20 million units I.V. daily in divided doses q 4 to 6 hours, for at least 14 days after symptoms diminish. Or, 80,000 units/kg in the first hour, followed by a maintenance dose of 320,000 units/ kg/day. The average adult dosage is 4 million units q 4 hours or 2 million units q 2 hours.
Children: 100,000 to 150,000 units/kg/ day I.V. in divided doses q 4 to 6 hours for at least 14 days after symptoms diminish.

Adjust-a-dose: If creatinine clearance is 10 to 50 ml/minute, give the usual dose q 8 to 12 hours. If clearance is less than 10 ml/minute, give 50% of usual dose q 8 to 10 hours or the usual dose q 12 to 18 hours. If patient is uremic and creatinine clearance is more than 10 ml/minute, give full loading dose; then give half the loading dose q 4 to 5 hours for additional doses.

I.V. ADMINISTRATION

• Reconstitute drug with sterile water for injection, D_5W, or normal saline solution for injection. Volume of diluent varies with manufacturer.
• For intermittent infusion, give drug over 1 to 2 hours.
• For continuous infusion, add reconstituted drug to 1 to 2 L of compatible solution. Determine how much fluid is needed and what the rate should be for a 24-hour period; then, add the drug to this fluid.

INCOMPATIBILITIES

Alcohol 5%, amikacin, aminoglycosides, aminophylline, amphotericin B sodium, chlorpromazine, dextran, dopamine, heparin sodium, hydroxyzine hydrochloride, lincomycin, metoclopramide, pentobarbital sodium, phenytoin sodium, prochlorperazine mesylate, promethazine hydrochloride, sodium bicarbonate, thiopental, vancomycin, vitamin B complex with C.

ACTION

Inhibits cell-wall synthesis during bacterial multiplication.

Route	Onset	Peak	Duration
I.V.	Immediate	Immediate	Unknown
I.M.	Unknown	15–30 min	Unknown

Half-life: 30 to 60 minutes.

ADVERSE REACTIONS

CNS: ***seizures,*** neuropathy, lethargy, hallucinations, anxiety, confusion, agitation, depression, dizziness, fatigue.
CV: thrombophlebitis.
GI: ***pseudomembranous colitis,*** nausea, vomiting, enterocolitis.
GU: interstitial nephritis, nephropathy.

Hematologic: ***agranulocytosis, leukopenia, thrombocytopenia,*** anemia, eosinophilia, hemolytic anemia.
Metabolic: ***severe potassium poisoning.***
Skin: maculopapular eruptions, exfoliative dermatitis, pain at injection site.
Other: ***anaphylaxis,*** hypersensitivity reactions, overgrowth of nonsusceptible organisms.

INTERACTIONS

Drug-drug. *Aminoglycosides:* Physically and chemically incompatible. Give separately.
Colestipol: May decrease penicillin G potassium level. Give penicillin G potassium 1 hour before or 4 hours after colestipol.
Hormonal contraceptives: May decrease hormonal contraceptive effectiveness. Advise use of additional form of contraception during therapy.
Oral anticoagulants: May increase risk of bleeding. Monitor PT and INR.
Potassium-sparing diuretics: May increase risk of hyperkalemia. Avoid using together.
Probenecid: May increase penicillin level. Probenecid may be used for this purpose.

EFFECTS ON LAB TEST RESULTS

- May increase potassium level. May decrease hemoglobin level.
- May increase eosinophil count. May decrease platelet, WBC, and granulocyte counts. May cause positive Coombs test result.
- May falsely decrease aminoglycoside levels. May cause false-positive CSF protein test result. May alter urine glucose testing using cupric sulfate (Benedict reagent).

CONTRAINDICATIONS & CAUTIONS

- Contraindicated in patients hypersensitive to drug or other penicillins.
- Use cautiously in patients with other drug allergies, especially to cephalosporins, because of possible cross-sensitivity.

NURSING CONSIDERATIONS

- Before giving drug, ask patient about allergic reactions to penicillin.
- Obtain specimen for culture and sensitivity tests before giving first dose. Therapy may begin pending results.
- For I.M. use, give deep into large muscle; injection may be extremely painful.
- Monitor renal function closely. Patients with poor renal function are predisposed to high levels.
- Monitor potassium and sodium levels closely in patients receiving more than 10 million units I.V. daily.
- Observe patient closely. With large doses and prolonged therapy, bacterial or fungal superinfection may occur, especially in elderly, debilitated, or immunosuppressed patients.
- ***Look alike–sound alike:*** Don't confuse drug with Polycillin, penicillamine, or the various types of penicillin.

PATIENT TEACHING

- Tell patient to notify prescriber if rash, fever, or chills develop. A rash is the most common allergic reaction.
- Warn patient that I.M. injection may be painful but that ice applied to the site may help alleviate discomfort.

penicillin G procaine (benzylpenicillin procaine)

Ayercillin†, Wycillin

Pharmacologic class: natural penicillin
Pregnancy risk category B

AVAILABLE FORMS

Injection: 600,000 units/ml; 1.2 million units/ml

INDICATIONS & DOSAGES

➤ **Moderate to severe systemic infection**
Adults: 600,000 to 1.2 million units I.M. daily for a minimum of 10 days.
Children older than age 1 month: 25,000 to 50,000 units/kg I.M. daily in a single dose.

➤ **Anthrax caused by *Bacillus anthracis,* including inhalation anthrax after exposure**
Adults: 1,200,000 units I.M. q 12 hours.
Children: 25,000 units/kg I.M.; not to exceed 1,200,000 units q 12 hours.

➤ **Cutaneous anthrax**
Adults: 600,000 to 1,000,000 units I.M. daily.

ACTION
Inhibits cell-wall synthesis during bacterial multiplication.

Route	Onset	Peak	Duration
I.M.	Unknown	1–4 hr	1–5 days

Half-life: 30 to 60 minutes.

ADVERSE REACTIONS
CNS: ***seizures,*** lethargy, hallucinations, anxiety, confusion, agitation, depression, dizziness, fatigue.
GI: ***pseudomembranous colitis,*** nausea, vomiting, enterocolitis.
GU: interstitial nephritis, nephropathy.
Hematologic: ***agranulocytosis, thrombocytopenia, hemolytic anemia, leukopenia,*** anemia, eosinophilia.
Musculoskeletal: arthralgia.
Other: ***anaphylaxis,*** hypersensitivity reactions, overgrowth of nonsusceptible organisms.

INTERACTIONS
Drug-drug. *Aminoglycosides:* Physically and chemically incompatible. Give separately.
Colestipol: May decrease penicillin G procaine level. Give penicillin G procaine 1 hour before or 4 hours after colestipol.
Hormonal contraceptives: May decrease hormonal contraceptive effectiveness. Advise use of additional form of contraception during therapy.
Probenecid: May increase penicillin level. Probenecid may be used for this purpose.

EFFECTS ON LAB TEST RESULTS
- May decrease hemoglobin level.
- May increase eosinophil count. May decrease platelet, WBC, and granulocyte counts.

CONTRAINDICATIONS & CAUTIONS
- Contraindicated in patients hypersensitive to drug or other penicillins.
- Use cautiously in patients with other drug allergies, especially to cephalosporins, because of possible cross-sensitivity. Some formulations contain sulfites, which may cause allergic reactions in sensitive people.

NURSING CONSIDERATIONS
- Before giving drug, ask patient about allergic reactions to penicillin.
- Obtain specimen for culture and sensitivity tests before giving first dose. Therapy may begin pending results.
- Give deep I.M. in upper outer quadrant of buttocks in adults; in midlateral thigh in small children. Rotate injection sites. Don't give subcutaneously. Don't massage injection site. Avoid injection near major nerves or blood vessels to prevent permanent neurovascular damage.
- ***Alert:*** Continue postexposure treatment for inhalation anthrax for 60 days. Prescriber should consider the risk-benefit ratio of continuing penicillin longer than 2 weeks, compared with switching to another drug.
- ***Alert:*** Inadvertent I.V. use may cause CNS toxicity and death. Never give I.V.
- Allergic reactions are hard to treat because of drug's slow absorption rate.
- Monitor renal and hematopoietic function periodically.
- If large doses are given or if therapy is prolonged, bacterial or fungal superinfection may occur, especially in elderly, debilitated, or immunosuppressed patients.
- Treatment duration depends on site and cause of infection.
- ***Look alike–sound alike:*** Don't confuse drug with Polycillin, penicillamine, or the various types of penicillin.

PATIENT TEACHING
- Tell patient to report adverse reactions promptly. A rash is the most common allergic reaction.
- Warn patient that I.M. injection may be painful but that ice applied to the site may help alleviate discomfort.

penicillin G sodium (benzylpenicillin sodium)

Crystapen†

Pharmacologic class: natural penicillin

Pregnancy risk category B

AVAILABLE FORMS

Injection: 5 million-unit vial

INDICATIONS & DOSAGES

➤ Moderate to severe systemic infection

Adults and children age 12 and older: 1.2 to 24 million units daily I.M. or I.V. in divided doses q 4 to 6 hours.

Children younger than age 12: 25,000 to 400,000 units/kg daily I.M. or I.V. in divided doses q 4 to 6 hours.

➤ Neurosyphilis

Adults: 18 to 24 million units I.V. daily in divided doses q 4 hours for 10 to 14 days.

Adjust-a-dose: If creatinine clearance is 10 to 50 ml/minute, give the usual dose q 8 to 12 hours. If clearance is less than 10 ml/minute, give 50% of usual dose q 8 to 10 hours or the usual dose q 12 to 18 hours. If patient is uremic and creatinine clearance is more than 10 ml/minute, give full loading dose; then give half the loading dose q 4 to 5 hours for additional doses.

I.V. ADMINISTRATION

- Reconstitute drug with sterile water for injection, normal saline solution for injection, or D_5W. Check manufacturer's instructions for volume of diluent necessary to produce desired drug level.
- Give by intermittent infusion: Dilute drug in 50 to 100 ml, and give over 30 minutes to 2 hours q 4 to 6 hours.
- In neonates and children, give divided doses over 15 to 30 minutes.

INCOMPATIBILITIES

Aminoglycosides, amphotericin B, bleomycin, chlorpromazine, cytarabine, fat emulsions 10%, heparin sodium, hydroxyzine hydrochloride, invert sugar 10%, lincomycin, methylprednisolone sodium succinate, potassium chloride, prochlorperazine mesylate, promethazine hydrochloride.

ACTION

Inhibits cell-wall synthesis during bacterial multiplication.

Route	Onset	Peak	Duration
I.V.	Immediate	Immediate	Unknown
I.M.	Unknown	15–30 min	Unknown

Half-life: 30 to 60 minutes.

ADVERSE REACTIONS

CNS: neuropathy, ***seizures,*** lethargy, hallucinations, anxiety, confusion, agitation, depression, dizziness, fatigue.
CV: ***heart failure,*** thrombophlebitis.
GI: nausea, vomiting, enterocolitis, ischemic colitis, ***pseudomembranous colitis.***
GU: nephropathy.
Hematologic: hemolytic anemia, ***leukopenia, thrombocytopenia, agranulocytosis,*** anemia, eosinophilia.
Musculoskeletal: arthralgia.
Other: hypersensitivity reactions, ***anaphylaxis,*** overgrowth of nonsusceptible organisms, pain at injection site, vein irritation.

INTERACTIONS

Drug-drug. *Aminoglycosides:* Physically and chemically incompatible. Give separately.
Colestipol: May decrease penicillin G sodium level. Give penicillin G sodium 1 hour before or 4 hours after colestipol.
Hormonal contraceptives: May decrease hormonal contraceptive effectiveness. Advise use of additional form of contraception during penicillin therapy.
Oral anticoagulants: May increase risk of bleeding. Monitor PT and INR.
Probenecid: May increase penicillin level. Probenecid may be used for this purpose.

EFFECTS ON LAB TEST RESULTS

- May decrease hemoglobin level.
- May cause positive Coombs test result. May increase eosinophil count. May decrease platelet, WBC, and granulocyte counts.
- May cause false-positive CSF protein test result. May falsely decrease aminoglycoside level. May alter urine glucose test-

ing using cupric sulfate (Benedict reagent).

CONTRAINDICATIONS & CAUTIONS
- Contraindicated in patients hypersensitive to drug or other penicillins and in those on sodium-restricted diets.
- Use cautiously in patients with other drug allergies, especially to cephalosporins, because of possible cross-sensitivity.

NURSING CONSIDERATIONS
- Before giving drug, ask patient about allergic reactions to penicillin.
- Obtain specimen for culture and sensitivity tests before giving first dose. Therapy may begin pending results.
- Observe patient closely. With large doses and prolonged therapy, bacterial or fungal superinfection may occur, especially in elderly, debilitated, or immunosuppressed patients.
- ***Look alike–sound alike:*** Don't confuse drug with Polycillin, penicillamine, or the various types of penicillin.

PATIENT TEACHING
- Tell patient to report adverse reactions promptly.
- Instruct patient to report discomfort at I.V. site.
- Warn patient receiving I.M. injection that the injection may be painful, but that ice applied to site may help alleviate discomfort.

penicillin V potassium (phenoxymethylpenicillin potassium)

Abbocillin VK‡, Apo-Pen VK†, Cilicaine VK‡, Nadopen-V 200†, Nadopen-V 400†, Novo-Pen-VK†, Nu-Pen-VK†, Pen-Vee†, PVF K†, Veetids

Pharmacologic class: natural penicillin
Pregnancy risk category B

AVAILABLE FORMS
Capsules: 250 mg‡
Oral suspension: 125 mg/5 ml, 250 mg/5 ml (after reconstitution)
Tablets: 250 mg, 500 mg
Tablets (film-coated): 250 mg, 500 mg

INDICATIONS & DOSAGES

➤ Mild to moderate systemic infections
Adults and children age 12 and older: 125 to 500 mg or P.O. q 6 hours.
Children younger than age 12: 15 to 62.5 mg/kg P.O. daily in divided doses q 6 to 8 hours.

➤ To prevent recurrent rheumatic fever
Adults and children: 250 mg P.O. b.i.d.

➤ Erythema chronica migrans in Lyme disease♦
Adults: 250 to 500 mg P.O. q.i.d. for 10 to 20 days.
Children younger than age 2: 50 mg/kg/day (up to 2 g/day) P.O. in four divided doses for 10 to 20 days.

➤ To prevent inhalation anthrax after possible exposure♦
Adults: 7.5 mg/kg P.O. q.i.d. Continue treatment until exposure is ruled out. If exposure is confirmed, anthrax vaccine may be indicated. Continue treatment for 60 days.
Children younger than age 9: 50 mg/kg P.O. daily given in four divided doses. Continue treatment until exposure is ruled out. If exposure is confirmed, anthrax vaccine may be indicated. Continue treatment for 60 days.

ACTION
Inhibits cell-wall synthesis during bacterial multiplication.

Route	Onset	Peak	Duration
P.O.	Unknown	30–60 min	Unknown

Half-life: 30 minutes.

ADVERSE REACTIONS
CNS: neuropathy.
GI: *epigastric distress, nausea,* vomiting, diarrhea, black hairy tongue.
GU: nephropathy.
Hematologic: ***leukopenia, thrombocytopenia,*** eosinophilia, hemolytic anemia.
Other: ***anaphylaxis,*** hypersensitivity reactions, overgrowth of nonsusceptible organisms.

INTERACTIONS

Drug-drug. *Hormonal contraceptives:* May decrease hormonal contraceptive effectiveness. Advise use of another form of contraception during therapy.
Probenecid: May increase penicillin level. Probenecid may be used for this purpose.

EFFECTS ON LAB TEST RESULTS

- May decrease hemoglobin level.
- May increase eosinophil count. May decrease platelet, WBC, and granulocyte counts.
- May alter results of turbidimetric test methods using sulfosalicylic acid, acetic acid, trichloroacetic acid, and nitric acid.

CONTRAINDICATIONS & CAUTIONS

- Contraindicated in patients hypersensitive to drug or other penicillins.
- Use cautiously in patients with GI disturbances and in those with other drug allergies, especially to cephalosporins, because of possible cross-sensitivity.

NURSING CONSIDERATIONS

- Before giving drug, ask patient about allergic reactions to penicillins.
- Obtain specimen for culture and sensitivity tests before giving first dose. Therapy may begin pending results.
- Periodically assess renal and hematopoietic function in patients receiving long-term therapy.
- If large doses are given or if therapy is prolonged, bacterial or fungal superinfection may occur, especially in elderly, debilitated, or immunosuppressed patients.
- Amoxicillin is the preferred drug to prevent endocarditis because GI absorption is better and drug levels are sustained longer. Penicillin V is considered an alternate drug.
- ***Look alike–sound alike:*** Don't confuse drug with Polycillin, penicillamine, or the various types of penicillin.

PATIENT TEACHING

- Instruct patient to take entire quantity of drug exactly as prescribed, even after he feels better.
- Tell patient to take drug with food if stomach upset occurs.
- Advise patient to notify prescriber if rash, fever, or chills develop. A rash is the most common allergic reaction.

piperacillin sodium and tazobactam sodium

Zosyn

Pharmacologic class: extended-spectrum penicillin, beta-lactamase inhibitor
Pregnancy risk category B

AVAILABLE FORMS

Powder for injection: 2 g piperacillin and 0.25 g tazobactam per vial, 3 g piperacillin and 0.375 g tazobactam per vial, 4 g piperacillin and 0.5 g tazobactam per vial

INDICATIONS & DOSAGES

➤ **Moderate to severe infections from piperacillin-resistant, piperacillin and tazobactam-susceptible, beta-lactamase–producing strains of microorganisms in appendicitis (complicated by rupture or abscess) and peritonitis caused by *Escherichia coli, Bacteroides fragilis, B. ovatus, B. thetaiotaomicron, B. vulgatus;* skin and skin-structure infections caused by *Staphylococcus aureus;* postpartum endometritis or pelvic inflammatory disease caused by *E. coli;* moderately severe community-acquired pneumonia caused by *Haemophilus influenzae***

Adults: 3.375 g (3 g piperacillin/0.375 g tazobactam) q 6 hours as a 30-minute I.V. infusion. Duration of treatment is usually 7 to 10 days.
Adjust-a-dose: If creatinine clearance is 20 to 40 ml/minute, give 2.25 g (2 g piperacillin/0.25 g tazobactam) q 6 hours; if less than 20 ml/minute, give 2.25 g (2 g piperacillin/0.25 g tazobactam) q 8 hours. In continuous ambulatory peritoneal dialysis (CAPD) patients, give 2.25 g (2 g piperacillin/0.25 g tazobactam) q 12 hours. In hemodialysis patients, give 2.25 g (2 g piperacillin/0.25 g tazobactam) q 12 hours with a supplemental dose of 0.75 g (0.67 g piperacillin/0.08 g tazobactam) after each dialysis period.

➤ **Moderate to severe nosocomial pneumonia caused by piperacillin-resistant, beta-lactamase–producing strains of *S. aureus* and by piperacillin and tazobactam-susceptible *Acinetobacter baumannii, H. influenzae, Klebsiella pneumoniae,* and *Pseudomonas aeruginosa***

Adults: 4.5 g (4 g piperacillin/0.5 g tazobactam) q 6 hours with aminoglycoside. Patients with *P. aeruginosa* should continue aminoglycoside treatment; if *P. aeruginosa* isn't isolated, aminoglycoside treatment may be stopped. Duration of treatment is usually 7 to 14 days.

Adjust-a-dose: If creatinine clearance is 20 to 40 ml/minute, give 3.375 g (3 g piperacillin/0.375 g tazobactam) q 6 hours; if less than 20 ml/minute, give 2.25 g (2 g piperacillin/0.25 g tazobactam) q 6 hours. In CAPD patients, give 2.25 g (2 g piperacillin/0.25 g tazobactam) q 8 hours. In hemodialysis patients, give 2.25 g (2 g piperacillin/0.25 g tazobactam) q 8 hours with a supplemental dose of 0.75 g (0.67 g piperacillin/0.08 g tazobactam) after each dialysis period.

I.V. ADMINISTRATION

- Reconstitute each gram with 5 ml of diluent, such as sterile or bacteriostatic water for injection, normal saline solution for injection, bacteriostatic normal saline solution for injection, D_5W, dextrose 5% in normal saline solution for injection, or dextran 6% in normal saline solution for injection.
- Shake until dissolved.
- Further dilute to 50 to 150 ml before infusion.
- Use drug immediately after reconstitution.
- Stop any primary infusion during administration, if possible.
- Infuse over at least 30 minutes.
- Discard unused drug after 24 hours if stored at room temperature or 48 hours if refrigerated.
- Change I.V. site every 48 hours.
- Diluted drug is stable in I.V. bags for 24 hours at room temperature or for 1 week refrigerated.

INCOMPATIBILITIES

Acyclovir sodium, aminoglycosides, amphotericin B, chlorpromazine, cisatracurium, cisplatin, dacarbazine, daunorubicin, dobutamine, doxorubicin, doxycycline hyclate, droperidol, famotidine, ganciclovir, gemcitabine, haloperidol lactate, hydroxyzine hydrochloride, idarubicin, lactated Ringer solution, minocycline, mitomycin, mitoxantrone, nalbuphine, prochlorperazine edisylate, promethazine hydrochloride, streptozocin, vancomycin.

ACTION

Inhibits cell-wall synthesis during bacterial multiplication.

Route	Onset	Peak	Duration
I.V.	Immediate	Immediate	Unknown

Half-life: About 1 hour.

ADVERSE REACTIONS

CNS: *headache, insomnia,* fever, ***seizures,*** agitation, dizziness, anxiety.
CV: hypertension, tachycardia, chest pain, edema.
EENT: rhinitis.
GI: *diarrhea, nausea, constipation,* ***pseudomembranous colitis,*** vomiting, dyspepsia, stool changes, abdominal pain.
GU: interstitial nephritis, candidiasis.
Hematologic: ***leukopenia, neutropenia, thrombocytopenia,*** anemia, eosinophilia.
Respiratory: dyspnea.
Skin: rash, pruritus.
Other: ***anaphylaxis,*** pain, inflammation, phlebitis at I.V. site, hypersensitivity reactions.

INTERACTIONS

Drug-drug. *Hormonal contraceptives:* May decrease contraceptive effectiveness. Advise use of another form of contraception during therapy.
Oral anticoagulants: May prolong effectiveness. Monitor PT and INR closely.
Probenecid: May increase piperacillin level. Probenecid may be used for this purpose.
Vecuronium: May prolong neuromuscular blockade. Monitor patient closely.

EFFECTS ON LAB TEST RESULTS

- May decrease hemoglobin level.
- May increase eosinophil count. May decrease neutrophil, platelet, and WBC counts.
- May cause false-positive result for urine glucose tests using copper reduction method, such as Clinitest.

CONTRAINDICATIONS & CAUTIONS

- Contraindicated in patients hypersensitive to drug or other penicillins.
- Use cautiously in patients with bleeding tendencies, uremia, hypokalemia, and allergies to other drugs, especially cephalosporins, because of possible cross-sensitivity.

NURSING CONSIDERATIONS

- Before giving drug, ask patient about allergic reactions to penicillins.
- Obtain specimen for culture and sensitivity tests before giving first dose. Therapy may begin pending results.
- Because peritoneal dialysis removes 6% of the piperacillin dose and 21% of the tazobactam dose, and hemodialysis removes 30% to 40% of a dose in 4 hours, additional doses may be needed after each dialysis period.
- If large doses are given or if therapy is prolonged, bacterial or fungal superinfection may occur, especially in elderly, debilitated, or immunosuppressed patients.
- Drug contains 2.35 mEq sodium/g of piperacillin. Monitor patient's sodium intake.
- Monitor hematologic and coagulation parameters.
- Patients with cystic fibrosis may have a higher rate of fever and rash. Monitor these patients closely.

PATIENT TEACHING

- Tell patient to report adverse reactions promptly.
- Tell patient to alert a health care professional about discomfort at the I.V. site.

ticarcillin disodium and clavulanate potassium

Timentin

Pharmacologic class: extended-spectrum penicillin, beta-lactamase inhibitor
Pregnancy risk category B

AVAILABLE FORMS

Injection: 3 g ticarcillin and 100 mg clavulanic acid in 3.1-g vials
Premixed: 3.1 g/100 ml

INDICATIONS & DOSAGES

➤ Gynecologic infection

Women who weigh 60 kg (132 lb) or more: For moderate infections, 200 mg/kg (ticarcillin component) I.V. daily in divided doses q 6 hours. For severe infections, 300 mg/kg (ticarcillin component) I.V. daily in divided doses q 4 hours.
Women who weigh less than 60 kg: 200 to 300 mg/kg (ticarcillin component) I.V. daily in divided doses q 4 to 6 hours.

➤ Lower respiratory tract, urinary tract, bone and joint, intra-abdominal, or skin and skin-structure infection and septicemia caused by beta-lactamase–producing strains of bacteria or by ticarcillin-susceptible organisms

Adults and children who weigh more than 60 kg (132 lb): 3.1 g (Timentin) by I.V. infusion q 4 to 6 hours.
Adults and children ages 3 months to 16 years who weigh less than 60 kg: 200 mg/kg (ticarcillin component) I.V. daily in divided doses q 6 hours. For severe infections, 300 mg/kg (ticarcillin component) I.V. daily in divided doses q 4 hours.
Adjust-a-dose: If creatinine clearance is 30 to 60 ml/minute, dosage is 2 g I.V. q 4 hours; if clearance is 10 to 29 ml/minute, 2 g I.V. q 8 hours; if clearance is less than 10 ml/minute, 2 g I.V. q 12 hours; if clearance is less than 10 ml/minute and patient has hepatic dysfunction, 2 g I.V. q 24 hours. For patients receiving peritoneal dialysis or hemodialysis, give a loading dose of 3.1 g I.V. and then maintenance doses of 3.1 g I.V. q 12 hours for patients receiving peritoneal dialysis or 2 g I.V. q 12 hours for patients receiving

hemodialysis. Supplement with 3.1 g after each hemodialysis session.

I.V. ADMINISTRATION

- Reconstitute drug with 13 ml of sterile water for injection or normal saline solution for injection. Further dilute to a maximum of 10 to 100 mg/ml (based on drug component).
- Infuse over 30 minutes.

INCOMPATIBILITIES

Aminoglycosides, amphotericin B, azithromycin, cisatracurium, other anti-infectives, sodium bicarbonate, topotecan, vancomycin.

ACTION

Inhibits cell-wall synthesis during bacterial multiplication.

Route	Onset	Peak	Duration
I.V.	Immediate	Immediate	Unknown

Half-life: 1 hour.

ADVERSE REACTIONS

CNS: ***seizures,*** neuromuscular excitability, headache, giddiness.
CV: phlebitis, vein irritation.
EENT: taste and smell disturbances.
GI: ***pseudomembranous colitis,*** nausea, diarrhea, stomatitis, vomiting, epigastric pain, flatulence.
Hematologic: ***leukopenia, neutropenia, thrombocytopenia,*** eosinophilia, hemolytic anemia, anemia.
Metabolic: hypokalemia, hypernatremia.
Skin: ***Stevens-Johnson syndrome,*** pain at injection site, rash, pruritus.
Other: ***anaphylaxis,*** hypersensitivity reactions, overgrowth of nonsusceptible organisms.

INTERACTIONS

Drug-drug. *Hormonal contraceptives:* May decrease contraceptive effectiveness. Advise use of another form of contraception during therapy.
Oral anticoagulants: May increase risk of bleeding. Monitor PT and INR.
Probenecid: May increase ticarcillin level. Probenecid may be used for this purpose.

EFFECTS ON LAB TEST RESULTS

- May increase ALT, AST, alkaline phosphatase, LDH, and sodium levels. May decrease potassium and hemoglobin levels.
- May increase eosinophil count. May decrease platelet, WBC, and granulocyte counts.
- May alter results of turbidimetric tests that use sulfosalicylic acid, trichloroacetic acid, acetic acid, or nitric acid.

CONTRAINDICATIONS & CAUTIONS

- Contraindicated in patients hypersensitive to drug or other penicillins.
- Use cautiously in patients with other drug allergies, especially to cephalosporins because of possible cross-sensitivity, and in those with impaired renal function, hemorrhagic conditions, hypokalemia, or sodium restriction. Drug contains 4.5 mEq sodium/g.

NURSING CONSIDERATIONS

- Before giving, ask patient about allergic reactions to penicillin, and obtain specimen for culture and sensitivity tests. Therapy may begin pending results.
- Give drug at least 1 hour before a bacteriostatic antibiotic.
- Check CBC and platelet counts frequently. Drug may cause thrombocytopenia.
- Monitor PT and INR in patients taking oral anticoagulants.
- Monitor potassium and sodium levels.
- If large doses are given or if therapy is prolonged, bacterial or fungal superinfection may occur, especially in elderly, debilitated, or immunosuppressed patients.

PATIENT TEACHING

- Tell patient to report adverse reactions promptly.
- Instruct patient to report discomfort at I.V. site.
- Advise patient to limit salt intake during drug therapy because of high sodium content.

11 Cephalosporins

cefaclor
cefadroxil
cefazolin sodium
cefdinir
cefditoren pivoxil
cefepime hydrochloride
cefoperazone sodium
cefotaxime sodium
cefoxitin sodium
cefpodoxime proxetil
cefprozil
ceftazidime
ceftizoxime sodium
ceftriaxone sodium
cefuroxime axetil
cefuroxime sodium
cephalexin monohydrate
loracarbef

cefaclor

Ceclor, Ceclor CD, Raniclor

Pharmacologic class: second-generation cephalosporin
Pregnancy risk category B

AVAILABLE FORMS

Capsules: 250 mg, 500 mg
Oral suspension: 125 mg/5 ml, 187 mg/5 ml, 250 mg/5 ml, 375 mg/5 ml
Tablets (chewable): 125 mg, 187 mg, 250 mg, 375 mg
Tablets (extended-release): 375 mg, 500 mg

INDICATIONS & DOSAGES

➤ Respiratory tract infections, UTIs, skin and soft-tissue infections, and otitis media caused by *Haemophilus influenzae, Streptococcus pneumoniae, S. pyogenes, Escherichia coli, Proteus mirabilis, Klebsiella* species, and staphylococci

Adults: 250 to 500 mg P.O. q 8 hours. For pharyngitis or otitis media, daily dose may be given in two equally divided doses q 12 hours. For extended-release forms in bronchitis, 500 mg P.O. q 12 hours for 7 days; for extended-release forms in pharyngitis or skin and skin-structure infections, 375 mg P.O. q 12 hours for 10 days and 7 to 10 days, respectively.
Children: 20 mg/kg daily P.O. in divided doses q 8 hours. For pharyngitis or otitis media, daily dose may be given in two equally divided doses q 12 hours. In more serious infections, 40 mg/kg daily is recommended, not to exceed 1 g daily.

ACTION

Second-generation cephalosporin that inhibits cell-wall synthesis, promoting osmotic instability; usually bactericidal.

Route	Onset	Peak	Duration
P.O.	Unknown	30–60 min	Unknown
P.O. (extended)	Unknown	1½–2½ hr	Unknown

Half-life: ½ to 1 hour.

ADVERSE REACTIONS

CNS: fever, dizziness, headache, somnolence, malaise.
GI: *diarrhea, nausea,* ***pseudomembranous colitis,*** vomiting, anorexia, dyspepsia, abdominal cramps, oral candidiasis.
GU: vaginal candidiasis, vaginitis.
Hematologic: ***thrombocytopenia, transient leukopenia,*** anemia, eosinophilia, lymphocytosis.
Skin: *maculopapular rash,* dermatitis, pruritus.
Other: ***anaphylaxis,*** hypersensitivity reactions, serum sickness.

INTERACTIONS

Drug-drug. *Aminoglycosides:* May increase risk of nephrotoxicity. Avoid using together.
Antacids: May decrease absorption of extended-release cefaclor if taken within 1 hour. Separate doses by 1 hour.
Anticoagulants: May increase anticoagulant effects. Monitor PT and INR.
Chloramphenicol: May cause antagonistic effect. Avoid using together.

Probenecid: May inhibit excretion and increase cefaclor level. Monitor patient for increased adverse reactions.

EFFECTS ON LAB TEST RESULTS

• May increase alkaline phosphatase, ALT, AST, bilirubin, GGT, and LDH levels. May decrease hemoglobin level.
• May increase eosinophil count. May decrease platelet and WBC counts.
• May falsely increase serum or urine creatinine level in tests using Jaffe reaction. May cause false-positive results of Coombs test and urine glucose tests that use cupric sulfate, such as Benedict reagent and Clinitest.

CONTRAINDICATIONS & CAUTIONS

• Contraindicated in patients hypersensitive to drug or other cephalosporins.
• Use cautiously in patients hypersensitive to penicillin because of the possibility of cross-sensitivity with other beta-lactam antibiotics.
• Use cautiously in breast-feeding women and in patients with a history of colitis or renal insufficiency.

NURSING CONSIDERATIONS

• Before administration, ask patient if he is allergic to penicillins or cephalosporins.
• Obtain specimen for culture and sensitivity tests before giving. Therapy may begin pending results.
• If large doses are given, therapy is prolonged, or patient is at high risk, monitor patient for signs and symptoms of superinfection.
• Store reconstituted suspension in refrigerator. Suspension is stable for 14 days if refrigerated. Shake well before use.
• ***Look alike–sound alike:*** Don't confuse drug with other cephalosporins that sound alike.

PATIENT TEACHING

• Tell patient to take entire amount of drug exactly as prescribed, even after he feels better.
• Tell patient that drug may be taken with meals. If suspension is used, instruct him to shake container well before measuring dose and to keep the drug refrigerated.
• Advise patient to notify prescriber if rash develops or signs and symptoms of superinfection appear.
• Inform patient not to crush, cut, or chew extended-release tablets.

cefadroxil

Duricef✐

Pharmacologic class: first-generation cephalosporin
Pregnancy risk category B

AVAILABLE FORMS

Capsules: 500 mg
Oral suspension: 125 mg/5 ml, 250 mg/5 ml, 500 mg/5 ml
Tablets: 1 g

INDICATIONS & DOSAGES

➤ **UTIs caused by *Escherichia coli, Proteus mirabilis,* and *Klebsiella* species; skin and soft-tissue infections caused by staphylococci and streptococci; pharyngitis or tonsillitis caused by group A beta-hemolytic streptococci**

Adults: 1 to 2 g P.O. daily, depending on infection being treated. Usually given once daily or in two divided doses.
Children: 30 mg/kg P.O. daily in two divided doses q 12 hours.
Adjust-a-dose: In patients with renal impairment, give first dose of 1 g. Reduce additional doses based on creatinine clearance. If clearance is 25 to 50 ml/minute, give 500 mg P.O. q 12 hours. If clearance is 10 to 25 ml/minute, give 500 mg P.O. q 24 hours; if clearance is less than 10 ml/minute, give 500 mg P.O. q 36 hours.

ACTION

First-generation cephalosporin that inhibits cell-wall synthesis, promoting osmotic instability; usually bactericidal.

Route	Onset	Peak	Duration
P.O.	Unknown	1–2 hr	Unknown

Half-life: About 1 to 2 hours.

ADVERSE REACTIONS

CNS: ***seizures,*** fever, dizziness, headache.
GI: *diarrhea, nausea,* ***pseudomembranous colitis,*** vomiting, glossitis, abdominal cramps, oral candidiasis.
GU: genital pruritus, candidiasis, vaginitis, renal dysfunction.
Hematologic: ***transient neutropenia, leukopenia, agranulocytosis, thrombocytopenia,*** anemia, eosinophilia.
Respiratory: dyspnea.
Skin: *maculopapular and erythematous rashes,* urticaria.
Other: ***anaphylaxis, angioedema,*** hypersensitivity reactions.

INTERACTIONS

Drug-drug. *Aminoglycosides:* May increase risk of nephrotoxicity. Avoid using together.
Probenecid: May inhibit excretion and increase cefadroxil level. Use together cautiously.

EFFECTS ON LAB TEST RESULTS

- May increase alkaline phosphatase, ALT, AST, bilirubin, GGT, and LDH levels. May decrease hemoglobin level.
- May increase eosinophil count. May decrease granulocyte, neutrophil, platelet, and WBC counts.
- May falsely increase serum or urine creatinine level in tests using Jaffe reaction. May cause false-positive results of Coombs test and urine glucose tests that use cupric sulfate, such as Benedict reagent and Clinitest.

CONTRAINDICATIONS & CAUTIONS

- Contraindicated in patients hypersensitive to drug or other cephalosporins.
- Use cautiously in patients with a history of sensitivity to penicillin and in breast-feeding women.
- Use cautiously in patients with impaired renal function; adjust dosage as needed.

NURSING CONSIDERATIONS

- Before administration, ask patient if he is allergic to penicillins or cephalosporins.
- Obtain specimen for culture and sensitivity tests before giving first dose. Therapy may begin while awaiting results.
- If creatinine clearance is less than 50 ml/minute, lengthen dosage interval so drug doesn't accumulate. Monitor renal function in patients with renal dysfunction.
- If large doses are given, therapy is prolonged, or patient is high risk, monitor patient for superinfection.
- ***Look alike–sound alike:*** Don't confuse drug with other cephalosporins that sound alike.

PATIENT TEACHING

- Instruct patient to take drug with food or milk to lessen GI discomfort.
- Tell patient to take entire amount of drug exactly as prescribed, even after he feels better.
- Advise patient to notify prescriber if rash develops or if signs and symptoms of superinfection appear, such as recurring fever, chills, and malaise.

cefazolin sodium

Ancef

Pharmacologic class: first-generation cephalosporin
Pregnancy risk category B

AVAILABLE FORMS

Infusion: 500 mg/50-ml bag, 1 g/50-ml bag
Injection (parenteral): 250 mg, 500 mg, 1 g

INDICATIONS & DOSAGES

➤ **Perioperative prevention in contaminated surgery**
Adults: 1 g I.M. or I.V. 30 to 60 minutes before surgery; then 0.5 to 1 g I.M. or I.V. q 6 to 8 hours for 24 hours. In operations lasting longer than 2 hours, give another 0.5- to 1-g dose I.M. or I.V. intraoperatively. Continue treatment for 3 to 5 days if life-threatening infection is likely.
➤ **Infections of respiratory, biliary, and GU tracts; skin, soft-tissue, bone, and joint infections; septicemia; endocarditis caused by *Escherichia coli, Enterobacteriaceae,* gonococci, *Haemophilus influenzae, Klebsiella* species, *Proteus mirabilis, Staphylococcus aureus, Streptococ-***

***cus pneumoniae,* and group A beta-hemolytic streptococci**
Adults: 250 mg to 500 mg I.M. or I.V. q 8 hours for mild infections or 500 mg to 1.5 g I.M. or I.V. q 6 to 8 hours for moderate to severe or life-threatening infections. Maximum 12 g/day in life-threatening situations.
Children older than age 1 month: 25 to 50 mg/kg/day I.M. or I.V. in three or four divided doses. In severe infections, dose may be increased to 100 mg/kg/day.
Adjust-a-dose: For patients with creatinine clearance of 35 to 54 ml/minute, give full dose q 8 hours; if clearance is 11 to 34 ml/minute, give 50% of usual dose q 12 hours; if clearance is below 10 ml/minute, give 50% of usual dose q 18 to 24 hours.

I.V. ADMINISTRATION

- Give commercially available frozen solutions in D_5W only by intermittent or continuous I.V. infusion.
- Reconstitute drug with sterile water, bacteriostatic water, or normal saline solution as follows: Add 2 ml to 500-mg vial or 2.5 ml to 1-g vial, yielding 225 mg/ml or 330 mg/ml, respectively.
- Shake well until dissolved.
- For direct injection, further dilute with 5 ml of sterile water for injection.
- Inject into a large vein or into the tubing of a free-flowing I.V. solution over 3 to 5 minutes.
- For intermittent infusion, add reconstituted drug to 50 to 100 ml of compatible solution or use premixed solution.
- If I.V. therapy lasts longer than 3 days, alternate injection sites. Use of small I.V. needles in larger available veins may be preferable.
- Reconstituted drug is stable 24 hours at room temperature or 96 hours refrigerated.

INCOMPATIBILITIES

Aminoglycosides, amiodarone, amobarbital, ascorbic acid injection, bleomycin, calcium gluconate, cimetidine, colistimethate, hydrocortisone, idarubicin, lidocaine, norepinephrine, oxytetracycline, pentobarbital sodium, polymyxin B, ranitidine, tetracycline, theophylline, vitamin B complex with C.

ACTION

First-generation cephalosporin that inhibits cell-wall synthesis, promoting osmotic instability; usually bactericidal.

Route	Onset	Peak	Duration
I.V.	Immediate	Immediate	Unknown
I.M.	Unknown	1–2 hr	Unknown

Half-life: About 1 to 2 hours.

ADVERSE REACTIONS

CNS: ***seizures,*** headache, confusion.
CV: *phlebitis, thrombophlebitis with I.V. injection.*
GI: *diarrhea,* ***pseudomembranous colitis,*** nausea, anorexia, vomiting, glossitis, dyspepsia, abdominal cramps, anal pruritus, oral candidiasis.
GU: genital pruritus, candidiasis, vaginitis.
Hematologic: ***neutropenia, leukopenia, thrombocytopenia,*** eosinophilia.
Skin: *maculopapular and erythematous rashes, urticaria, pruritus, pain, induration, sterile abscesses, tissue sloughing at injection site,* ***Stevens-Johnson syndrome.***
Other: ***anaphylaxis,*** hypersensitivity reactions, serum sickness, drug fever.

INTERACTIONS

Drug-drug. *Aminoglycosides:* May increase risk of nephrotoxicity. Avoid using together.
Anticoagulants: May increase anticoagulant effects. Monitor PT and INR.
Probenecid: May inhibit excretion and increase cefazolin level. Use together cautiously.

EFFECTS ON LAB TEST RESULTS

- May increase alkaline phosphatase, ALT, AST, bilirubin, GGT, and LDH levels.
- May increase eosinophil count. May decrease neutrophil, platelet, and WBC counts.
- May falsely increase serum or urine creatinine level in tests using Jaffe reaction. May cause false-positive results of Coombs test and urine glucose tests that use cupric sulfate, such as Benedict reagent and Clinitest.

CONTRAINDICATIONS & CAUTIONS

- Contraindicated in patients hypersensitive to drug or other cephalosporins.
- Use cautiously in patients hypersensitive to penicillin because of the possibility of cross-sensitivity with other beta-lactam antibiotics.
- Use cautiously in breast-feeding women and in patients with a history of colitis or renal insufficiency.

NURSING CONSIDERATIONS

- Before giving drug, ask patient if he is allergic to penicillins or cephalosporins.
- Obtain specimen for culture and sensitivity tests before giving first dose. Therapy may begin while awaiting results.
- If creatinine clearance falls below 55 ml/minute, adjust dosage.
- After reconstitution, inject drug I.M. without further dilution. This drug isn't as painful as other cephalosporins. Give injection deep into a large muscle, such as the gluteus maximus or the side of the thigh.
- If large doses are given, therapy is prolonged, or patient is at high risk, monitor patient for signs and symptoms of superinfection.
- ***Look alike–sound alike:*** Don't confuse drug with other cephalosporins that sound alike.

PATIENT TEACHING

- Instruct patient to report adverse reactions promptly.
- Tell patient to report discomfort at I.V. injection site.
- Advise patient to notify prescriber if a rash develops or if signs and symptoms of superinfection appear, such as recurring fever, chills, and malaise.

cefdinir
Omnicef

Pharmacologic class: third-generation cephalosporin
Pregnancy risk category B

AVAILABLE FORMS

Capsules: 300 mg
Suspension: 125 mg/5 ml, 250 mg/5 ml

INDICATIONS & DOSAGES

➤ **Mild to moderate infections caused by susceptible strains of microorganisms in community-acquired pneumonia, acute worsening of chronic bronchitis, acute maxillary sinusitis, acute bacterial otitis media, and uncomplicated skin and skin-structure infections**

Adults and children age 12 and older: 300 mg P.O. q 12 hours or 600 mg P.O. q 24 hours for 10 days. Give q 12 hours for pneumonia and skin infections.

Children ages 6 months to 12 years: 7 mg/kg P.O. q 12 hours or 14 mg/kg P.O. q 24 hours, for 10 days, up to maximum dose of 600 mg daily. Give q 12 hours for skin infections.

➤ **Pharyngitis, tonsillitis**

Adults and children age 12 and older: 300 mg P.O. q 12 hours for 5 to 10 days or 600 mg P.O. q 24 hours for 10 days.

Children ages 6 months to 12 years: 7 mg/kg P.O. q 12 hours for 5 to 10 days; or 14 mg/kg P.O. q 24 hours, for 10 days.

Adjust-a-dose: If creatinine clearance is less than 30 ml/minute, reduce dosage to 300 mg P.O. once daily for adults and 7 mg/kg up to 300 mg P.O. once daily for children. In patients receiving long-term hemodialysis, give 300 mg or 7 mg/kg P.O. at end of each dialysis session and then every other day.

ACTION

Third-generation cephalosporin that inhibits cell-wall synthesis, promoting osmotic instability; usually bactericidal. Some microorganisms resistant to penicillins and cephalosporins are susceptible to cefdinir. Active against a broad range of gram-positive and gram-negative aerobic microorganisms.

Route	Onset	Peak	Duration
P.O.	Unknown	2–4 hr	Unknown

Half-life: 1¾ hours.

ADVERSE REACTIONS

CNS: headache.
GI: *diarrhea,* ***pseudomembranous colitis,*** abdominal pain, nausea, vomiting.
GU: vaginal candidiasis, vaginitis, increased urine proteins, WBCs, and RBCs.

Skin: rash, cutaneous candidiasis.
Other: ***hypersensitivity reactions, anaphylaxis.***

INTERACTIONS

Drug-drug. *Aminoglycosides:* May increase risk of nephrotoxicity. Avoid using together.
Antacids containing aluminum and magnesium, iron supplements, multivitamins containing iron: May decrease cefdinir rate of absorption and bioavailability. Give such preparations 2 hours before or after cefdinir.
Probenecid: May inhibit renal excretion of cefdinir. Monitor patient for adverse reactions.

EFFECTS ON LAB TEST RESULTS

- May increase alkaline phosphatase, GGT, and LDH levels. May decrease bicarbonate levels.
- May increase eosinophil, lymphocyte, and platelet counts.
- May falsely increase serum or urine creatinine level in tests using Jaffe reaction. May cause false-positive results of Coombs test and urine glucose tests that use cupric sulfate, such as Benedict reagent and Clinitest.

CONTRAINDICATIONS & CAUTIONS

- Contraindicated in patients hypersensitive to drug or other cephalosporins.
- Use cautiously in patients hypersensitive to penicillin because of the possibility of cross-sensitivity with other beta-lactam antibiotics.
- Use cautiously in patients with history of colitis or renal insufficiency.

NURSING CONSIDERATIONS

- Before administration, ask patient if he is allergic to penicillins or cephalosporins.
- Prolonged drug treatment may result in emergence and overgrowth of resistant organisms. Monitor patient for signs and symptoms of superinfection.
- Pseudomembranous colitis has been reported with cefdinir and should be considered in patients with diarrhea after antibiotic therapy and in those with history of colitis.
- ***Look alike–sound alike:*** Don't confuse drug with other cephalosporins that sound alike.

PATIENT TEACHING

- Instruct patient to take antacids and iron supplements 2 hours before or after a dose of cefdinir.
- Inform diabetic patient that each teaspoon of suspension contains 2.86 g of sucrose.
- Tell patient that drug may be taken without regard to meals.
- Tell patient to take drug as prescribed, even after he feels better.
- Advise patient to report severe diarrhea or diarrhea with abdominal pain.
- Tell patient to report adverse reactions or signs and symptoms of superinfection promptly.

cefditoren pivoxil

Spectracef

Pharmacologic class: third-generation cephalosporin
Pregnancy risk category B

AVAILABLE FORMS

Tablets: 200 mg

INDICATIONS & DOSAGES

➤ **Acute bacterial worsening of chronic bronchitis or community-acquired pneumonia caused by *Haemophilus influenzae, H. parainfluenzae, Streptococcus pneumoniae,* or *Moraxella catarrhalis***
Adults and adolescents age 12 and older: 400 mg P.O. b.i.d. with meals for 10 days (chronic bronchitis) or 14 days (community-acquired pneumonia).
➤ **Pharyngitis or tonsillitis caused by *Streptococcus pyogenes;* uncomplicated skin and skin-structure infections caused by *S. pyogenes* or *Staphylococcus aureus***
Adults and adolescents age 12 and older: 200 mg P.O. b.i.d. with meals for 10 days.
Adjust-a-dose: For patients with creatinine clearance of 30 to 49 ml/minute, don't exceed 200 mg b.i.d. For patients with clearance less than 30 ml/minute, give 200 mg daily.

ACTION
Adheres to bacterial penicillin-binding proteins, inhibiting cell-wall synthesis. Active against many gram-positive and gram-negative organisms.

Route	Onset	Peak	Duration
P.O.	Unknown	1½–3 hr	Unknown

Half-life: 1¼ to 2 hours.

ADVERSE REACTIONS
CNS: headache.
GI: *diarrhea,* abdominal pain, dyspepsia, nausea, vomiting.
GU: vaginal candidiasis, hematuria.
Metabolic: hyperglycemia.

INTERACTIONS
Drug-drug. *H_2-receptor antagonists, magnesium, and aluminum antacids:* May decrease cefditoren absorption. Avoid using together.
Probenecid: May increase cefditoren level. Avoid using together.
Drug-food. *Moderate- or high-fat meal:* May increase drug bioavailability. Advise patient to take drug with meals.

EFFECTS ON LAB TEST RESULTS
- May decrease glucose and hemoglobin level and hematocrit.
- May increase WBC count in urine.
- May cause a false-positive direct Coombs test result and a false-positive reaction for urine glucose in copper reduction tests (using Benedict or Fehling solution or Clinitest tablets).

CONTRAINDICATIONS & CAUTIONS
- Contraindicated in patients hypersensitive to drug or other cephalosporins.
- Contraindicated in patients with carnitine deficiency or inborn errors of metabolism that may result in significant carnitine deficiency.
- Because tablets contain sodium caseinate, a milk protein, don't give drug to patients hypersensitive to milk protein (not lactose intolerance).
- Use cautiously in breast-feeding women because cephalosporins appear in breast milk, and safe use hasn't been established.
- Use cautiously in patients with impaired renal function or penicillin allergy.

NURSING CONSIDERATIONS
- Before administration, ask patient if he is allergic to penicillins or cephalosporins.
- Obtain specimen for culture and sensitivity tests before giving. Therapy may begin pending results.
- Give drug with a fatty meal to increase its bioavailability.
- If patient develops diarrhea, keep in mind that this drug may cause pseudomembranous colitis.
- Don't use this drug if patient needs prolonged treatment.
- Monitor patient for overgrowth of resistant organisms.
- Patients with renal or hepatic impairment, in poor nutritional state, receiving a protracted course of antibiotics, or previously stabilized on anticoagulants may be at risk for decreased prothrombin activity. Monitor PT in these patients.

PATIENT TEACHING
- Instruct patient to take drug exactly as prescribed.
- Tell patient to take drug with food to increase its absorption.
- Caution patient not to take drug with an H_2-receptor antagonist or an antacid because either may reduce cefditoren absorption.
- Instruct patient not to stop drug before completing course and to call prescriber immediately if he experiences any unpleasant adverse reactions.
- Instruct patient to contact prescriber if signs and symptoms of infection don't improve after several days of therapy.
- Inform patient of potential adverse reactions.
- Urge patient not to miss any doses. However, if he does, tell him to take the missed dose as soon as possible unless it's within 4 hours of the next scheduled dose. In that case, tell him to skip the missed dose and go back to the regular dosing schedule. Tell him not to double the dose.

cefepime hydrochloride
Maxipime

Pharmacologic class: fourth-generation cephalosporin
Pregnancy risk category B

AVAILABLE FORMS
Injection: 500-mg vial, 1-g/100-ml piggyback bottle, 1-g ADD-Vantage vial, 1-g vial, 2-g/100-ml piggyback bottle, 2-g ADD-Vantage vial, 2-g vial

INDICATIONS & DOSAGES
➤ **Mild to moderate UTI caused by *Escherichia coli, Klebsiella pneumoniae,* or *Proteus mirabilis,* including concurrent bacteremia with these microorganisms**
Adults and children age 12 and older: 0.5 to 1 g I.M. or I.V. Infuse over 30 minutes q 12 hours for 7 to 10 days. Use I.M. only for *E. coli* infection.
➤ **Severe UTI, including pyelonephritis, caused by *E. coli* or *K. pneumoniae***
Adults and children age 12 and older: 2 g I.V. Infuse over 30 minutes q 12 hours for 10 days.
➤ **Moderate to severe pneumonia caused by *Streptococcus pneumoniae, Pseudomonas aeruginosa, K. pneumoniae,* or *Enterobacter* species (sp.)**
Adults and children age 12 and older: 1 to 2 g I.V. Infuse over 30 minutes q 12 hours for 10 days.
➤ **Moderate to severe skin infection, uncomplicated skin infection, and skin-structure infection caused by *Streptococcus pyogenes* or methicillin-susceptible strains of *Staphylococcus aureus***
Adults and children age 12 and older: 2 g I.V. Infuse over 30 minutes q 12 hours for 10 days.
➤ **Complicated intra-abdominal infection caused by *E. coli,* viridans group streptococci, *P. aeruginosa, K. pneumoniae, Enterobacter* sp., or *Bacteroides fragilis***
Adults: 2 g I.V. Infuse over 30 minutes q 12 hours for 7 to 10 days. Give with metronidazole.
➤ **Empiric therapy for febrile neutropenia**
Adults: 2 g I.V. q 8 hours for 7 days or until neutropenia resolves.
➤ **Uncomplicated and complicated UTI (including pyelonephritis), uncomplicated skin and skin-structure infection, pneumonia, empiric therapy for febrile neutropenic children**
Children ages 2 months to 16 years, who weigh up to 40 kg (88 lb): 50 mg/kg/dose I.V. Infuse over 30 minutes q 12 hours, or q 8 hours for febrile neutropenia, for 7 to 10 days. Don't exceed 2 g/dose.
Adjust-a-dose: Adjust dosage based on creatinine clearance, as shown in the table on page 106. For patients receiving hemodialysis, about 68% of drug is removed after a 3-hour dialysis session. Give a repeat dose, equivalent to the first dose, at the completion of dialysis. For patients receiving continuous ambulatory peritoneal dialysis, give normal dose q 48 hours.

I.V. ADMINISTRATION
- Follow manufacturer's guidelines closely when reconstituting drug. They vary with concentration of drug ordered and how drug is packaged (piggyback vial, ADD-Vantage vial, or regular vial).
- The type of diluent varies with the product used. Use only solutions recommended by the manufacturer.
- Give intermittent I.V. infusion with a Y-type administration and compatible solutions.
- Stop the main I.V. fluid while infusing.
- Infuse over about 30 minutes.

INCOMPATIBILITIES
Aminophylline, amphotericin B, amphotericin B cholesteryl sulfate complex, ciprofloxacin, gentamicin, metronidazole, tobramycin, vancomycin.

ACTION
Fourth-generation cephalosporin that inhibits bacterial cell-wall synthesis, promotes osmotic instability, and destroys bacteria.

Route	Onset	Peak	Duration
I.V., I.M.	30 min	1–2 hr	Unknown

Half-life: Adults: 2 to 2½ hours. Children: 1½ to 2 hours.

Dosage adjustments for renal impairment

Creatinine clearance (ml/min)	If normal dosage would be 500 mg q 12 hr	1 g q 12 hr	2 g q 12 hr	2 g q 8 hr
30–60	500 mg q 24 hr	1 g q 24 hr	2 g q 24 hr	2 g q 12 hr
11–29	500 mg q 24 hr	500 mg q 24 hr	1 g q 24 hr	2 g q 24 hr
< 11	250 mg q 24 hr	250 mg q 24 hr	500 mg q 24 hr	1 g q 24 hr

ADVERSE REACTIONS

CNS: fever, headache.
CV: phlebitis.
GI: colitis, diarrhea, nausea, vomiting, oral candidiasis.
GU: vaginitis.
Skin: rash, pruritus, urticaria.
Other: ***anaphylaxis,*** pain, inflammation, hypersensitivity reactions.

INTERACTIONS

Drug-drug. *Aminoglycosides:* May increase risk of nephrotoxicity. Monitor renal function closely.
Potent diuretics: May increase risk of nephrotoxicity. Monitor renal function closely.
Probenecid: May inhibit renal excretion of cefepime. Monitor patient for adverse reactions.

EFFECTS ON LAB TEST RESULTS

- May increase ALT and AST levels. May decrease phosphorus level.
- May increase eosinophil count. May alter PT and PTT.
- May falsely increase serum or urine creatinine level in tests using Jaffe reaction. May cause false-positive results of Coombs test and urine glucose tests that use cupric sulfate, such as Benedict reagent and Clinitest.

CONTRAINDICATIONS & CAUTIONS

- Contraindicated in patients hypersensitive to drug, cephalosporins, beta-lactam antibiotics, or penicillins.
- Use cautiously in patients hypersensitive to penicillin because of possibility of cross-sensitivity with other beta-lactam antibiotics.
- Use cautiously in breast-feeding women and in patients with history of colitis or renal insufficiency.

NURSING CONSIDERATIONS

- Before giving drug, ask patient if he is allergic to penicillins or cephalosporins.
- Obtain culture and sensitivity tests before giving. Therapy may begin pending results.
- Adjust dosage in patients with impaired renal function. If dosage isn't adjusted, serious adverse reactions, including encephalopathy, myoclonus, seizures, and renal failure may occur.
- For I.M. administration, reconstitute drug using sterile water for injection, normal saline solution for injection, D_5W injection, 0.5% or 1% lidocaine hydrochloride, or bacteriostatic water for injection with parabens or benzyl alcohol. Follow manufacturer's guidelines for quantity of diluent to use.
- Inspect solution for particulate matter before use. The powder and its solutions tend to darken, depending on storage conditions. If stored as recommended, potency isn't adversely affected.
- Monitor patient for superinfection. Drug may cause overgrowth of nonsusceptible bacteria or fungi.
- Drug may reduce PT activity. Patients at risk include those with renal or hepatic impairment or poor nutrition and those receiving prolonged therapy. Monitor PT and INR in these patients. Give vitamin K, as indicated.
- ***Look alike–sound alike:*** Don't confuse drug with other cephalosporins that sound alike.

PATIENT TEACHING

- Warn patient receiving drug I.M. that pain may occur at injection site.
- Advise patient to notify prescriber if a rash develops or if signs and symptoms of superinfection appear, such as recurring fever, chills, and malaise

- Instruct patient to report adverse reactions promptly.

cefoperazone sodium
Cefobid

Pharmacologic class: third-generation cephalosporin
Pregnancy risk category B

AVAILABLE FORMS
Infusion: 1 g, 2 g piggyback; 1 g, 2 g premixed
Injection: 1-g, 2-g vials

INDICATIONS & DOSAGES
➤ **Serious respiratory tract infection; intra-abdominal, gynecologic, and skin infection; bacteremia; septicemia caused by susceptible microorganisms (*Streptococcus pneumoniae* and *S. pyogenes; Staphylococcus aureus* [penicillinase- and non–penicillinase-producing] and *S. epidermidis;* enterococci; *Escherichia coli; Haemophilus influenzae; Enterobacter, Citrobacter, Klebsiella,* and *Proteus* species (sp.); some *Pseudomonas* sp., including *P. aeruginosa;* and *Bacteroides fragilis*)**
Adults: 1 to 2 g q12 hours I.M. or I.V. In severe infections or in infections caused by less-sensitive organisms, total daily dose or frequency may be increased to 16 g/day.
Adjust-a-dose: For patients with hepatic or biliary obstruction, don't exceed total dose of 4 g daily. For patients with hepatic and substantial renal impairment, don't exceed total dose of 2 g daily. Hemodialysis reduces drug's half-life; schedule dose to follow a dialysis session.

I.V. ADMINISTRATION
- Reconstitute drug in 1- or 2-g vial with at least 2.8 ml of compatible I.V. solution; manufacturer recommends using 5 ml/g.
- For direct injection, give over 3 to 5 minutes into a large vein or into tubing of a free-flowing I.V. solution.
- For intermittent infusion, add reconstituted drug to 20 to 40 ml of a compatible I.V. solution and infuse over 15 to 30 minutes.

INCOMPATIBILITIES
Amifostine, aminoglycosides, diltiazem, filgrastim, hetastarch, labetalol hydrochloride, meperidine hydrochloride, ondansetron hydrochloride, pentamidine isethionate, perphenazine, promethazine hydrochloride, sargramostim, vinorelbine tartrate.

ACTION
Third-generation cephalosporin that inhibits cell-wall synthesis, promoting osmotic instability; usually bactericidal.

Route	Onset	Peak	Duration
I.V.	Immediate	Immediate	Unknown
I.M.	Unknown	1–2 hr	Unknown

Half-life: About 1½ to 2½ hours.

ADVERSE REACTIONS
CNS: fever.
CV: *phlebitis, thrombophlebitis.*
GI: *diarrhea,* ***pseudomembranous colitis,*** nausea, vomiting.
Hematologic: ***transient neutropenia,*** eosinophilia, anemia, hypoprothrombinemia, bleeding.
Skin: *maculopapular and erythematous rashes, urticaria, pain, induration, sterile abscesses, temperature elevation, tissue sloughing at I.M. injection site.*
Other: ***anaphylaxis,*** hypersensitivity reactions, serum sickness.

INTERACTIONS
Drug-drug. *Aminoglycosides:* May increase risk of nephrotoxicity. Monitor renal function.
Anticoagulants: May increase anticoagulant effects. Monitor PT and INR.
Probenecid: May inhibit excretion and increase cefoperazone level. Use together cautiously.
Drug-lifestyle. *Alcohol use:* May cause a disulfiram-like reaction. Warn patient not to drink alcohol for several days after stopping drug.

EFFECTS ON LAB TEST RESULTS
- May increase alkaline phosphatase, ALT, AST, bilirubin, GGT, and LDH levels. May decrease hemoglobin level.
- May increase INR and eosinophil count. May decrease neutrophil count. May increase or decrease PT.

• May falsely increase serum or urine creatinine level in tests using Jaffe reaction. May cause false-positive results of Coombs test and urine glucose tests that use cupric sulfate, such as Benedict reagent and Clinitest.

CONTRAINDICATIONS & CAUTIONS
• Contraindicated in patients hypersensitive to drug or other cephalosporins.
• Use cautiously in patients hypersensitive to penicillin because of possibility of cross-sensitivity with other beta-lactam antibiotics.
• Use cautiously in breast-feeding women and in patients with history of colitis or renal insufficiency.
• Give doses of 4 g/day cautiously to patients with hepatic disease or biliary obstruction. Higher dosages require monitoring of drug level.

NURSING CONSIDERATIONS
• Before giving drug, ask patient if he is allergic to penicillins or cephalosporins.
• Periodically monitor liver and renal function and compare to baseline.
• Obtain specimen for culture and sensitivity tests before giving first dose. Therapy may begin while awaiting results.
• To prepare 1-g vial for I.M. injection, dissolve drug with 2 ml of sterile water for injection; then add 0.6 ml of 2% lidocaine hydrochloride for final concentration of 333 mg/ml. Or, dissolve drug with 2.6 ml of sterile water for injection; then add 1 ml of 2% lidocaine hydrochloride for final concentration of 250 mg/ml.
• To prepare 2-g vial for I.M. injection, dissolve drug with 3.8 ml of sterile water for injection; then add 1.2 ml of 2% lidocaine hydrochloride for final concentration of 333 mg/ml. Or, dissolve drug with 5.4 ml of sterile water for injection; then add 1.8 ml of 2% lidocaine hydrochloride for final concentration of 250 mg/ml.
• For I.M. administration, inject deep into a large muscle, such as the gluteus maximus or the side of the thigh.
• If large doses are given, therapy is prolonged, or patient is at high risk, monitor him for signs or symptoms of superinfection.
• Monitor PT and INR regularly. Bleeding disorder may occur; vitamin K promptly reverses it.
• ***Look alike–sound alike:*** Don't confuse drug with other cephalosporins that sound alike.

PATIENT TEACHING
• Tell patient to report adverse reactions and signs and symptoms of superinfection promptly.
• Instruct patient to report discomfort at I.V. insertion site.

cefotaxime sodium
Claforan

Pharmacologic class: third-generation cephalosporin
Pregnancy risk category B

AVAILABLE FORMS
Infusion: 1-g, 2-g premixed package
Injection: 500-mg, 1-g, 2-g vials

INDICATIONS & DOSAGES
➤ **Perioperative prevention in contaminated surgery**
Adults: 1 g I.M. or I.V. 30 to 90 minutes before surgery. In patients undergoing bowel surgery, provide preoperative mechanical bowel cleansing and give a nonabsorbable anti-infective, such as neomycin. In patients undergoing cesarean delivery, give 1 g I.M. or I.V. as soon as the umbilical cord is clamped; then 1 g I.M. or I.V. 6 and 12 hours later.
➤ **Uncomplicated gonorrhea caused by penicillinase-producing strains or non–penicillinase-producing strains of *Neisseria gonorrhoeae***
Adults and adolescents: 500 mg I.M. as a single dose.
➤ **Rectal gonorrhea**
Men: 1 g I.M. as a single dose.
Women: 500 mg I.M. as a single dose.
➤ **Serious infection of the lower respiratory and urinary tract, CNS, skin, bone, and joints; gynecologic and intra-abdominal infection; bacteremia; septicemia caused by susceptible microorganisms, such as streptococci (including *Streptococcus pneumoniae* and *S. pyogenes*,**

Staphylococcus aureus* [penicillinase- and non–penicillinase-producing] and *S. epidermidis*), *Escherichia coli, Klebsiella, Haemophilus influenzae, Serratia marcescens,* and species of *Pseudomonas* (including *P. aeruginosa*), *Enterobacter, Proteus,* and *Peptostreptococcus
Adults and children who weigh 50 kg (110 lb) or more: 1 to 2 g I.V. or I.M. q 6 to 8 hours. Up to 12 g daily can be given for life-threatening infections.
Children ages 1 month to 12 years who weigh less than 50 kg: 50 to 180 mg/kg/day I.M. or I.V. in four to six divided doses.
Neonates ages 1 to 4 weeks: 50 mg/kg I.V. q 8 hours.
Neonates to age 1 week: 50 mg/kg I.V. q 12 hours.
Adjust-a-dose: For patients with creatinine clearance less than 20 ml/minute, give half usual dose at usual interval.

I.V. ADMINISTRATION
- For direct injection, reconstitute drug in 500-mg, 1-g, or 2-g vials with 10 ml of sterile water for injection. Solutions containing 1 g/14 ml are isotonic.
- Inject drug over 3 to 5 minutes into a large vein or into the tubing of a free-flowing I.V. solution.
- For infusion, reconstitute drug in infusion vials with 50 to 100 ml of D_5W or normal saline solution.
- Interrupt flow of primary I.V. solution, and infuse this drug over 20 to 30 minutes.

INCOMPATIBILITIES
Allopurinol, aminoglycosides, aminophylline, azithromycin, doxapram, filgrastim, fluconazole, hetastarch, pentamidine isethionate, sodium bicarbonate injection, vancomycin.

ACTION
Third-generation cephalosporin that inhibits cell-wall synthesis, promoting osmotic instability; usually bactericidal.

Route	Onset	Peak	Duration
I.V.	Immediate	Immediate	Unknown
I.M.	Unknown	30 min	Unknown

Half-life: 1 to 2 hours.

ADVERSE REACTIONS
CNS: fever, headache, dizziness.
CV: *phlebitis, thrombophlebitis.*
GI: *diarrhea,* ***pseudomembranous colitis,*** nausea, vomiting.
GU: vaginitis, candidiasis, interstitial nephritis.
Hematologic: ***agranulocytosis, thrombocytopenia, transient neutropenia,*** eosinophilia, hemolytic anemia.
Skin: *maculopapular and erythematous rashes, urticaria, pain, induration, sterile abscesses, temperature elevation, tissue sloughing at I.M. injection site.*
Other: ***anaphylaxis,*** hypersensitivity reactions, serum sickness.

INTERACTIONS
Drug-drug. *Aminoglycosides:* May increase risk of nephrotoxicity. Monitor patient's renal function tests.
Probenecid: May inhibit excretion and increase cefotaxime. Use together cautiously.

EFFECTS ON LAB TEST RESULTS
- May increase alkaline phosphatase, ALT, AST, bilirubin, GGT, and LDH levels. May decrease hemoglobin level.
- May increase eosinophil count. May decrease granulocyte, neutrophil, and platelet counts.
- May cause positive Coombs test results.

CONTRAINDICATIONS & CAUTIONS
- Contraindicated in patients hypersensitive to drug or other cephalosporins.
- Use cautiously in patients hypersensitive to penicillin because of possibility of cross-sensitivity with other beta-lactam antibiotics.
- Use cautiously in breast-feeding women and in patients with history of colitis or renal insufficiency.

NURSING CONSIDERATIONS
- Before giving drug, ask patient if he is allergic to penicillins or cephalosporins.
- Obtain specimen for culture and sensitivity tests before giving. Therapy may begin pending results.
- For I.M. use, inject deep into a large muscle, such as the gluteus maximus or the side of the thigh.

- For I.M. doses of 2 g, divide the dose and give at different sites.
- If large doses are given, therapy is prolonged, or patient is at high risk, monitor patient for superinfection.
- ***Look alike–sound alike:*** Don't confuse drug with other cephalosporins that sound alike.

PATIENT TEACHING

- Tell patient to report adverse reactions and signs and symptoms of superinfection promptly.
- Instruct patient to report discomfort at I.V. insertion site.

cefoxitin sodium

Mefoxin

Pharmacologic class: second-generation cephalosporin
Pregnancy risk category B

AVAILABLE FORMS

Infusion: 1 g, 2 g in 50-ml or 100-ml container
Injection: 1 g, 2 g

INDICATIONS & DOSAGES

➤ **Serious infection of the respiratory and GU tracts; skin, soft-tissue, bone, or joint infection; bloodstream or intra-abdominal infection caused by susceptible organisms (such as *Escherichia coli* and other coliform bacteria, penicillinase- and non–penicillinase-producing *Staphylococcus aureus, S. epidermidis,* streptococci, *Klebsiella, Haemophilus influenzae,* and *Bacteroides,* including *B. fragilis*)**

Adults: 1 to 2 g I.V. or I.M. q 6 to 8 hours for uncomplicated infections. Up to 12 g daily in life-threatening infections.
Children older than age 3 months: 80 to 160 mg/kg daily I.V. or I.M., given in four to six equally divided doses. Maximum daily dose is 12 g.

➤ **Uncomplicated gonorrhea**

Adults: 2 g I.M. with 1 g probenecid P.O. as a single dose. Give probenecid within 30 minutes before cefoxitin dose.

➤ **Perioperative prevention**

Adults: 2 g I.M. or I.V. 30 to 60 minutes before surgery; then 2 g I.M. or I.V. q 6 hours for up to 24 hours. For transurethral prostatectomy, give 1 g I.M. or I.V. before surgery; then continue giving 1 g q 8 hours for up to 5 days.
Children age 3 months and older: 30 to 40 mg/kg I.M. or I.V. 30 to 60 minutes before surgery; then 30 to 40 mg/kg q 6 hours for up to 24 hours.
Adjust-a-dose: For patients with creatinine clearance of 30 to 50 ml/minute, give 1 to 2 g q 8 to 12 hours; if clearance is 10 to 29 ml/minute, give 1 to 2 g q 12 to 24 hours; if clearance is 5 to 9 ml/minute, give 0.5 to 1 g q 12 to 24 hours; and if clearance is less than 5 ml/minute, give 0.5 to 1 g q 24 to 48 hours. For patients receiving hemodialysis, give a loading dose of 1 to 2 g after each hemodialysis session; then give the maintenance dose based on creatinine level.

I.V. ADMINISTRATION

- Reconstitute 1 g with at least 10 ml of sterile water for injection and 2 g with 10 to 20 ml of sterile water for injection. Solutions of D_5W and normal saline solution for injection also may be used.
- For direct injection, give drug over 3 to 5 minutes into a large vein or into the tubing of a free-flowing I.V. solution.
- For intermittent infusion, add reconstituted drug to 50 or 100 ml of D_5W or normal saline solution for injection.
- Interrupt flow of primary solution during infusion.
- Assess site often to detect evidence of thrombophlebitis.

INCOMPATIBILITIES

Aminoglycosides, filgrastim, hetastarch, pentamidine isethionate, ranitidine.

ACTION

Second-generation cephalosporin that inhibits cell-wall synthesis, promoting osmotic instability; usually bactericidal.

Route	Onset	Peak	Duration
I.V.	Immediate	Immediate	Unknown
I.M.	Unknown	20–30 min	Unknown

Half-life: About ½ to 1 hours.

ADVERSE REACTIONS

CNS: fever.
CV: *phlebitis, thrombophlebitis,* hypotension.
GI: *diarrhea,* ***pseudomembranous colitis,*** nausea, vomiting.
GU: ***acute renal failure.***
Hematologic: ***thrombocytopenia, transient neutropenia,*** eosinophilia, hemolytic anemia, anemia.
Respiratory: dyspnea.
Skin: *maculopapular and erythematous rashes, urticaria, pain, induration, sterile abscesses, tissue sloughing at injection site,* exfoliative dermatitis.
Other: ***anaphylaxis,*** hypersensitivity reactions, serum sickness.

INTERACTIONS

Drug-drug. *Aminoglycosides:* May increase risk of nephrotoxicity. Monitor patient's renal function tests.
Probenecid: May inhibit excretion and increase cefoxitin level. Probenecid may be used for this effect.

EFFECTS ON LAB TEST RESULTS

- May increase alkaline phosphatase, ALT, AST, bilirubin, and LDH levels. May decrease hemoglobin level.
- May increase eosinophil count. May decrease neutrophil and platelet counts.
- May falsely increase serum or urine creatinine level in tests using Jaffe reaction. May cause false-positive results of Coombs test and urine glucose tests that use cupric sulfate, such as Benedict reagent and Clinitest.

CONTRAINDICATIONS & CAUTIONS

- Contraindicated in patients hypersensitive to drug or other cephalosporins.
- Use cautiously in patients hypersensitive to penicillin because of possibility of cross-sensitivity with other beta-lactam antibiotics.
- Use cautiously in breast-feeding women and in patients with history of colitis or renal insufficiency.

NURSING CONSIDERATIONS

- Before giving drug, ask patient if he is allergic to penicillins or cephalosporins.
- Obtain specimen for culture and sensitivity tests before giving. Start therapy, awaiting results.
- ***Alert:*** The premixed frozen product is for I.V. use only.
- For I.M. use, reconstitute each 1 g of drug with 2 ml of sterile water for injection or 0.5% or 1% lidocaine hydrochloride (without epinephrine) to minimize pain. Inject deep into a large muscle, such as the gluteus maximus or the lateral aspect of the thigh.
- After reconstitution, drug may be stored for 24 hours at room temperature or 1 week under refrigeration.
- If large doses are given, therapy is prolonged, or patient is at high risk, monitor patient for signs and symptoms of superinfection.
- ***Look alike–sound alike:*** Don't confuse drug with other cephalosporins that sound alike.

PATIENT TEACHING

- Tell patient to report adverse reactions and signs and symptoms of superinfection promptly.
- Instruct patient to report discomfort at I.V. site.
- Advise patient to notify prescriber about loose stools or diarrhea.

cefpodoxime proxetil

Vantin

Pharmacologic class: third-generation cephalosporin
Pregnancy risk category B

AVAILABLE FORMS

Oral suspension: 50 mg/5 ml or 100 mg/5 ml in 50, 75, or 100-ml bottles
Tablets (film-coated): 100 mg, 200 mg

INDICATIONS & DOSAGES

➤ Acute, community-acquired pneumonia caused by strains of *Haemophilus influenzae* or *Streptococcus pneumoniae*
Adults and children age 12 and older: 200 mg P.O. q 12 hours for 14 days.
➤ Acute bacterial worsening of chronic bronchitis caused by *S. pneumoniae* or *H. influenzae* (strains

that don't produce beta-lactamase only), or *Moraxella catarrhalis*
Adults and children age 12 and older: 200 mg P.O. q 12 hours for 10 days.

➤ **Uncomplicated gonorrhea in men and women; rectal gonococcal infections in women**
Adults and children age 12 and older: 200 mg P.O. as a single dose. Follow with doxycycline 100 mg P.O. b.i.d. for 7 days.

➤ **Uncomplicated skin and skin-structure infections caused by *Staphylococcus aureus* or *S. pyogenes***
Adults and children age 12 and older: 400 mg P.O. q 12 hours for 7 to 14 days.

➤ **Acute otitis media caused by *S. pneumoniae* (penicillin-susceptible strains only), *S. pyogenes, H. influenzae,* or *M. catarrhalis***
Children age 2 months to 12 years: 5 mg/kg P.O. q 12 hours for 5 days. Don't exceed 200 mg per dose.

➤ **Pharyngitis or tonsillitis caused by *S. pyogenes***
Adults: 100 mg P.O. q 12 hours for 5 to 10 days.
Children ages 2 months to 12 years: 5 mg/kg P.O. q 12 hours for 5 to 10 days. Don't exceed 100 mg per dose.

➤ **Uncomplicated UTIs caused by *Escherichia coli, Klebsiella pneumoniae, Proteus mirabilis,* or *Staphylococcus saprophyticus***
Adults: 100 mg P.O. q 12 hours for 7 days.

➤ **Mild to moderate acute maxillary sinusitis caused by *H. influenzae, S. pneumoniae,* or *M. catarrhalis***
Adults and adolescents age 12 and older: 200 mg P.O. q 12 hours for 10 days.
Children ages 2 months to 12 years: 5 mg/kg P.O. q 12 hours for 10 days; maximum is 200 mg/dose.
Adjust-a-dose: For patients with creatinine clearance less than 30 ml/minute, increase dosage interval to q 24 hours. Give to dialysis patients three times weekly after dialysis.

ACTION
Third-generation cephalosporin that inhibits cell-wall synthesis, promoting osmotic instability; usually bactericidal.

Route	Onset	Peak	Duration
P.O.	Unknown	2–3 hr	Unknown

Half-life: 2 to 3 hours.

ADVERSE REACTIONS
CNS: headache.
GI: *diarrhea,* ***pseudomembranous colitis,*** nausea, vomiting, abdominal pain.
GU: vaginal fungal infections.
Skin: rash.
Other: ***anaphylaxis,*** hypersensitivity reactions.

INTERACTIONS
Drug-drug. *Aminoglycosides:* May increase risk of nephrotoxicity. Monitor renal function tests closely.
Antacids, H_2-receptor antagonists: May decrease absorption of cefpodoxime. Avoid using together.
Probenecid: May decrease excretion of cefpodoxime. Monitor patient for toxicity.
Drug-food. *Any food:* May increase absorption. Give tablets with food to enhance absorption. Oral suspension may be given without regard to food.

EFFECTS ON LAB TEST RESULTS
- May falsely increase serum or urine creatinine level in tests using Jaffe reaction. May cause false-positive results of Coombs test and urine glucose tests that use cupric sulfate, such as Benedict reagent and Clinitest.

CONTRAINDICATIONS & CAUTIONS
- Contraindicated in patients hypersensitive to drug or other cephalosporins.
- Use cautiously in patients with a history of penicillin hypersensitivity because of risk of cross-sensitivity.
- Use cautiously in patients receiving nephrotoxic drugs because other cephalosporins have been shown to have nephrotoxic potential.
- Use cautiously in breast-feeding women because drug appears in breast milk.

NURSING CONSIDERATIONS
- Before administration, ask patient if he is allergic to penicillins or cephalosporins.

- Monitor renal function and compare with baseline.
- Obtain specimen for culture and sensitivity tests before giving first dose. Start therapy, awaiting results.
- Give drug with food to enhance absorption. Shake suspension well before using.
- Store suspension in the refrigerator (36° to 46° F [2° to 8° C]). Discard unused portion after 14 days.
- Monitor patient for superinfection. Drug may cause overgrowth of nonsusceptible bacteria or fungi.
- ***Look alike–sound alike:*** Don't confuse drug with other cephalosporins that sound alike.

PATIENT TEACHING

- Tell patient to take drug as prescribed, even after he feels better.
- Instruct patient to take drug with food. If patient is using suspension, tell him to shake container before measuring dose and to keep container refrigerated.
- Tell patient to call prescriber if rash or signs and symptoms of superinfection occur.
- Instruct patient to notify prescriber about loose stools or diarrhea.

cefprozil

Cefzil✐

Pharmacologic class: second-generation cephalosporin
Pregnancy risk category B

AVAILABLE FORMS

Oral suspension: 125 mg/5 ml, 250 mg/5 ml
Tablets: 250 mg, 500 mg

INDICATIONS & DOSAGES

➤ **Pharyngitis or tonsillitis caused by *Streptococcus pyogenes***
Adults and children age 13 and older: 500 mg P.O. daily for at least 10 days.
➤ **Otitis media caused by *Streptococcus pneumoniae, Haemophilus influenzae,* and *Moraxella catarrhalis***
Infants and children ages 6 months to 12 years: 15 mg/kg P.O. q 12 hours for 10 days.
➤ **Secondary bacterial infections of acute bronchitis and acute bacterial worsening of chronic bronchitis caused by *S. pneumoniae, H. influenzae,* and *M. catarrhalis***
Adults and children age 13 and older: 500 mg P.O. q 12 hours for 10 days.
➤ **Uncomplicated skin and skin-structure infections caused by *Staphylococcus aureus* and *S. pyogenes***
Adults and children age 13 and older: 250 or 500 mg P.O. q 12 hours or 500 mg daily for 10 days.
➤ **Acute sinusitis caused by *S. pneumoniae, H. influenzae* (beta-lactamase–positive and –negative strains), and *M. catarrhalis* (including strains that produce beta-lactamase)**
Adults and children age 13 and older: 250 mg P.O. q 12 hours for 10 days; for moderate to severe infection, 500 mg P.O. q 12 hours for 10 days.
Children ages 6 months to 12 years: 7.5 mg/kg P.O. q 12 hours for 10 days; for moderate to severe infections, 15 mg/kg P.O. q 12 hours for 10 days.
Adjust-a-dose: If creatinine clearance is less than 30 ml/minute, give 50% of standard dose at standard intervals. If patient is receiving dialysis, give dose after hemodialysis is completed; drug is removed by hemodialysis.

ACTION

Second-generation cephalosporin that inhibits cell-wall synthesis, promoting osmotic instability; usually bactericidal.

Route	Onset	Peak	Duration
P.O.	Unknown	1½ hr	Unknown

Half-life: 1¼ hours in patients with normal renal function; 2 hours in patients with impaired hepatic function; and 5¼ to 6 hours in patients with end-stage renal disease.

ADVERSE REACTIONS

CNS: dizziness, hyperactivity, headache, nervousness, insomnia, confusion, somnolence.
GI: diarrhea, nausea, vomiting, abdominal pain.
GU: genital pruritus, vaginitis.
Hematologic: eosinophilia.
Skin: rash, urticaria, diaper rash.

Other: ***anaphylaxis,*** superinfection, hypersensitivity reactions, serum sickness.

INTERACTIONS

Drug-drug. *Aminoglycosides:* May increase risk of nephrotoxicity. Monitor renal function tests closely.
Probenecid: May inhibit excretion and increase cefprozil level. Use together cautiously.

EFFECTS ON LAB TEST RESULTS

- May increase alkaline phosphatase, ALT, AST, bilirubin, BUN, creatinine, and LDH levels.
- May increase eosinophil count. May decrease leukocyte, platelet, and WBC counts.
- May falsely increase serum or urine creatinine level in tests using Jaffe reaction. May cause false-positive results of Coombs test and urine glucose tests that use cupric sulfate, such as Benedict reagent and Clinitest.

CONTRAINDICATIONS & CAUTIONS

- Contraindicated in patients hypersensitive to drug or other cephalosporins.
- Use cautiously in patients hypersensitive to penicillin because of possibility of cross-sensitivity with other beta-lactam antibiotics.
- Use cautiously in breast-feeding women and in patients with history of colitis and renal insufficiency.

NURSING CONSIDERATIONS

- Before administration, ask patient if he is allergic to penicillins or cephalosporins.
- Monitor renal function and liver function test results.
- Obtain specimen for culture and sensitivity tests before giving first dose. Start therapy, awaiting results.
- Monitor patient for superinfection. May cause overgrowth of nonsusceptible bacteria or fungi.
- ***Look alike–sound alike:*** Don't confuse drug with other cephalosporins that sound alike.

PATIENT TEACHING

- Advise patient to take drug as prescribed, even after he feels better.
- Tell patient to shake suspension well before measuring dose.
- Inform patient or parent that oral suspension is bubble gum–flavored to improve palatability and promote compliance in children. Tell him to refrigerate reconstituted suspension and to discard unused drug after 14 days.
- Instruct patient to notify prescriber if rash or signs and symptoms of superinfection occur.

ceftazidime

Ceptaz, Fortaz, Tazicef

Pharmacologic class: third-generation cephalosporin
Pregnancy risk category B

AVAILABLE FORMS

Infusion: 1 g, 2 g in 50-ml and 100-ml vials (premixed)
Injection (with arginine): 500 mg, 1 g, 2 g
Injection (with sodium carbonate): 500 mg, 1 g, 2 g

INDICATIONS & DOSAGES

➤ **Serious UTI and lower respiratory tract infection; skin, gynecologic, intra-abdominal, and CNS infection; bacteremia; and septicemia caused by susceptible microorganisms, such as streptococci (including *Streptococcus pneumoniae* and *S. pyogenes*), penicillinase- and non–penicillinase-producing *Staphylococcus aureus, Escherichia coli, Klebsiella, Proteus, Enterobacter, Haemophilus influenzae, Pseudomonas,* and some strains of *Bacteroides***

Adults and children age 12 and older: 1 to 2 g I.V. or I.M. q 8 to 12 hours; up to 6 g daily in life-threatening infections.
Children ages 1 month to 12 years: 30 to 50 mg/kg I.V. q 8 hours. Maximum dose is 6 g/day. Use sodium carbonate formulation.
Neonates up to age 4 weeks: 30 mg/kg I.V. q 12 hours. Use sodium carbonate formulation.

➤ **Uncomplicated UTI**

Adults: 250 mg I.V. or I.M. q 12 hours.

➤ **Complicated UTI**

Adults and children age 12 and older: 500 mg to 1 g I.V. or I.M. q 8 to 12 hours.

Adjust-a-dose: If creatinine clearance is 31 to 50 ml/minute, give 1 g q 12 hours; if clearance is 16 to 30 ml/minute, give 1 g q 24 hours; if clearance is 6 to 15 ml/minute, give 500 mg q 24 hours; if clearance is less than 5 ml/minute, give 500 mg q 48 hours. Ceftazidime is removed by hemodialysis; give a supplemental dose of drug after each dialysis session.

I.V. ADMINISTRATION

- Each brand of drug includes specific instructions for reconstitution. Read and follow them carefully.
- To reconstitute solution that contains sodium carbonate, add 5 ml sterile water for injection to a 500-mg vial, or add 10 ml to a 1-g or 2-g vial. Shake well to dissolve drug. Because carbon dioxide is released during dissolution, positive pressure will develop in vial.
- To reconstitute solution that contains arginine, use 10 ml of sterile water for injection. This product won't release gas bubbles.
- Infuse drug over 15 to 30 minutes.

INCOMPATIBILITIES

Aminoglycosides, aminophylline, amiodarone, amphotericin B cholesteryl sulfate complex, azithromycin, clarithromycin, fluconazole, idarubicin, midazolam, pentamidine isethionate, ranitidine hydrochloride, sargramostim, sodium bicarbonate solutions, vancomycin.

ACTION

Third-generation cephalosporin that inhibits cell-wall synthesis, promoting osmotic instability; usually bactericidal.

Route	Onset	Peak	Duration
I.V.	Immediate	Immediate	Unknown
I.M.	Unknown	1 hr	Unknown

Half-life: 1½ to 2 hours.

ADVERSE REACTIONS

CNS: ***seizures,*** headache, dizziness, paresthesia.
CV: *phlebitis, thrombophlebitis.*
GI: ***pseudomembranous colitis,*** nausea, vomiting, diarrhea, abdominal cramps.
GU: vaginitis, candidiasis.
Hematologic: ***agranulocytosis, leukopenia, thrombocytopenia,*** eosinophilia, thrombocytosis, hemolytic anemia.
Skin: *maculopapular and erythematous rashes, urticaria, pain, induration, sterile abscesses, tissue sloughing at injection site.*
Other: ***anaphylaxis,*** hypersensitivity reactions, serum sickness.

INTERACTIONS

Drug-drug. *Aminoglycosides:* May cause additive or synergistic effect against some strains of *Pseudomonas aeruginosa* and *Enterobacteriaceae;* may increase risk of nephrotoxicity. Monitor patient for effects and monitor renal function.
Chloramphenicol: May cause antagonistic effect. Avoid using together.

EFFECTS ON LAB TEST RESULTS

- May increase alkaline phosphatase, ALT, AST, bilirubin, and LDH levels. May decrease hemoglobin level.
- May increase eosinophil count. May decrease granulocyte and WBC counts. May increase or decrease platelet count.
- May falsely increase serum or urine creatinine level in tests using Jaffe reaction. May cause false-positive results of Coombs test and urine glucose tests that use cupric sulfate, such as Benedict reagent and Clinitest.

CONTRAINDICATIONS & CAUTIONS

- Contraindicated in patients hypersensitive to drug or other cephalosporins.
- Use cautiously in patients hypersensitive to penicillin because of possibility of cross-sensitivity with other beta-lactam antibiotics.
- Use cautiously in breast-feeding women and in patients with history of colitis or renal insufficiency.

NURSING CONSIDERATIONS

- Before administration, ask patient if he is allergic to penicillins or cephalosporins.
- Obtain specimen for culture and sensitivity tests before giving first dose. Therapy may begin while awaiting results.
- For I.M. use, inject deep into a large muscle, such as the gluteus maximus or the side of the thigh.

• If large doses are given, therapy is prolonged, or patient is at high risk, monitor patient for signs and symptoms of superinfection.
• ***Alert:*** Drug contains either sodium carbonate (Fortaz or Tazicef) or arginine (Ceptaz) to facilitate dissolution of drug. Safety and effectiveness of solutions containing arginine in children younger than age 12 haven't been established.
• ***Look alike–sound alike:*** Don't confuse drug with other cephalosporins that sound alike.

PATIENT TEACHING
• Tell patient to report adverse reactions or signs and symptoms of superinfection promptly.
• Instruct patient to report discomfort at I.V. insertion site.
• Advise patient to notify prescriber about loose stools or diarrhea.

ceftizoxime sodium
Cefizox

Pharmacologic class: third-generation cephalosporin
Pregnancy risk category B

AVAILABLE FORMS
Infusion: 1 g, 2 g in 100-ml vials or in 50 ml containers
Injection: 500 mg, 1 g, 2 g

INDICATIONS & DOSAGES
➤ **Serious UTI, lower respiratory tract infection, gynecologic infection, bacteremia, septicemia, meningitis, intra-abdominal infection, bone or joint infection, and skin infection caused by susceptible microorganisms, such as streptococci (including *Streptococcus pneumoniae* and *S. pyogenes*), *Staphylococcus aureus, S. epidermidis, Escherichia coli, Haemophilus influenzae,* and *Klebsiella, Enterobacter, Proteus, Peptostreptococcus,* and some *Pseudomonas* species**
Adults: 1 to 2 g I.V. or I.M. q 8 to 12 hours. For life-threatening infections, give up to 2 g q 4 hours.
Children older than age 6 months: 50 mg/kg I.V. q 6 to 8 hours. For serious infections, up to 200 mg/kg/day in divided doses may be used. Don't exceed 12 g/day.
➤ **Uncomplicated gonorrhea**
Adults: 1 g I.M. as a single dose.
Adjust-a-dose: If creatinine clearance is 50 to 79 ml/minute, give 500 mg to 1.5 g q 8 hours; if clearance is 5 to 49 ml/minute, give 250 mg to 1 g q 12 hours; if clearance is less than 5 ml/minute or patient undergoes hemodialysis, give 500 mg to 1 g q 48 hours, or 250 to 500 mg q 24 hours.

I.V. ADMINISTRATION
• To reconstitute powder, add 5 ml of sterile water to a 500-mg vial, 10 ml to a 1-g vial, or 20 ml to a 2-g vial.
• Reconstitute drug in piggyback vials with 50 to 100 ml of normal saline solution or D_5W. Shake well.
• For direct injection, give drug over 3 to 5 minutes or slowly into I.V. tubing of free-flowing compatible solution.
• For infusion, give drug over 15 to 30 minutes.

INCOMPATIBILITIES
Aminoglycosides, cisatracurium besylate, filgrastim. Possibly promethazine hydrochloride and vancomycin hydrochloride.

ACTION
Third-generation cephalosporin that inhibits cell-wall synthesis, promoting osmotic instability; usually bactericidal.

Route	Onset	Peak	Duration
I.V.	Immediate	Immediate	Unknown
I.M.	Unknown	30–90 min	Unknown

Half-life: 1½ to 2 hours.

ADVERSE REACTIONS
CNS: fever.
CV: *phlebitis, thrombophlebitis.*
GI: *diarrhea,* ***pseudomembranous colitis,*** nausea, anorexia, vomiting.
GU: vaginitis.
Hematologic: ***thrombocytopenia, thrombocytosis, transient neutropenia,*** eosinophilia, hemolytic anemia, anemia.
Respiratory: dyspnea.

Skin: *maculopapular and erythematous rashes, urticaria, pain, induration, sterile abscesses, tissue sloughing at injection site.*
Other: ***anaphylaxis,*** hypersensitivity reactions, serum sickness.

INTERACTIONS
Drug-drug. *Aminoglycosides:* May increase nephrotoxicity. Monitor renal function.
Probenecid: May inhibit excretion and increase ceftizoxime level. Use probenecid for this effect.

EFFECTS ON LAB TEST RESULTS
- May increase alkaline phosphatase, ALT, AST, bilirubin, BUN, creatinine, GGT, and LDH levels. May decrease albumin, hemoglobin, and protein levels.
- May decrease PT and granulocyte, neutrophil, platelet, RBC, and WBC counts.
- May falsely increase serum or urine creatinine level in tests using Jaffe reaction. May cause false-positive results of Coombs test and urine glucose tests that use cupric sulfate, such as Benedict reagent and Clinitest.

CONTRAINDICATIONS & CAUTIONS
- Contraindicated in patients hypersensitive to drug or other cephalosporins.
- Use cautiously in patients hypersensitive to penicillin because of possibility of cross-sensitivity with other beta-lactam antibiotics.
- Use cautiously in breast-feeding women and in patients with history of colitis or renal insufficiency.

NURSING CONSIDERATIONS
- Before giving drug, ask patient if he is allergic to penicillins or cephalosporins.
- Obtain specimen for culture and sensitivity tests before giving first dose. Start therapy, awaiting results.
- For I.M. use, mix 1.5 ml of diluent per 500 mg of drug. Inject deep into a large muscle, such as the gluteus maximus or the side of the thigh. Divide doses of more than 2 gand give at two separate sites.
- If large doses are given, therapy is prolonged, or patient is at high risk, monitor patient for signs or symptoms of superinfection.
- ***Look alike–sound alike:*** Don't confuse drug with other cephalosporins that sound alike.

PATIENT TEACHING
- Tell patient to report adverse reactions and signs and symptoms of superinfection promptly.
- Instruct patient to report discomfort at I.V. site.
- Tell patient to notify prescriber about loose stools or diarrhea.

ceftriaxone sodium
Rocephin

Pharmacologic class: third-generation cephalosporin
Pregnancy risk category B

AVAILABLE FORMS
Infusion: 1 g, 2 g piggyback; 1 g, 2 g/ 50 ml premixed
Injection: 250 mg, 500 mg, 1 g, 2 g

INDICATIONS & DOSAGES
➤ **Uncomplicated gonococcal vulvovaginitis**
Adults: 125 mg I.M. as a single dose, plus azithromycin 1 g P.O. as a single dose or doxycycline 100 mg P.O. b.i.d. for 7 days.
➤ **UTI; lower respiratory tract, gynecologic, bone or joint, intra-abdominal, skin, or skin structure infection; septicemia**
Adults and children older than age 12: 1 to 2 g I.M. or I.V. daily or in equally divided doses q 12 hours. Total daily dose shouldn't exceed 4 g.
Children age 12 and younger: 50 to 75 mg/kg I.M. or I.V., not to exceed 2 g/ day, given in divided doses q 12 hours.
➤ **Meningitis**
Adults and children: Initially, 100 mg/kg I.M. or I.V. Don't exceed 4 g; then 100 mg/kg I.M. or I.V., given once daily or in divided doses q 12 hours, not to exceed 4 g, for 7 to 14 days.
➤ **Perioperative prevention**
Adults: 1 g I.V. as a single dose 30 minutes to 2 hours before surgery.
➤ **Acute bacterial otitis media**
Children: 50 mg/kg I.M. as a single dose. Don't exceed 1 g.

➤Neurologic complications, carditis, and arthritis from penicillin G–refractory Lyme disease ♦
Adults: 2 g I.V. daily for 14 to 28 days.

I.V. ADMINISTRATION

- Reconstitute drug with sterile water for injection, normal saline solution for injection, D_5W, or a combination of normal saline solution and dextrose injection and other compatible solutions.
- Add 2.4 ml of diluent to the 250-mg vial, 4.8 ml to the 500-mg vial, 9.6 ml to the 1-g vial, and 19.2 ml to the 2-g vial. All reconstituted solutions average 100 mg/ml.
- For intermittent infusion, dilute further to achieve desired concentration.
- Diluted I.V. preparation is stable 24 hours at room temperature or 10 days if refrigerated.

INCOMPATIBILITIES

Aminoglycosides, aminophylline, amphotericin B cholesteryl sulfate complex, azithromycin, clindamycin phosphate, filgrastim, fluconazole, gentamicin, labetalol, lidocaine hydrochloride, linezolid, metronidazole, pentamidine isethionate, theophylline, vancomycin, vinorelbine tartrate.

ACTION

Third-generation cephalosporin that inhibits cell-wall synthesis, promoting osmotic instability; usually bactericidal.

Route	Onset	Peak	Duration
I.V.	Immediate	Immediate	Unknown
I.M.	Unknown	1½–4 hr	Unknown

Half-life: 5½ to 11 hours.

ADVERSE REACTIONS

CNS: fever, headache, dizziness.
CV: phlebitis.
GI: ***pseudomembranous colitis,*** diarrhea.
GU: genital pruritus, candidiasis.
Hematologic: eosinophilia, thrombocytosis, ***leukopenia.***
Skin: pain, induration, tenderness at injection site, *rash,* pruritus.
Other: hypersensitivity reactions, serum sickness, ***anaphylaxis,*** chills.

INTERACTIONS

Drug-drug. *Aminoglycosides:* May cause synergistic effect against some strains of *P. aeruginosa* and *Enterobacteriaceae* species. Monitor patient.
Probenecid: High doses (1 g or 2 g daily) may enhance hepatic clearance of ceftriaxone and shorten its half-life. Avoid using together.

EFFECTS ON LAB TEST RESULTS

- May increase alkaline phosphatase, ALT, AST, bilirubin, BUN, and LDH levels.
- May increase eosinophil and platelet counts. May decrease WBC count.
- May falsely increase serum or urine creatinine level in tests using Jaffe reaction. May cause false-positive results of Coombs test and urine glucose tests that use cupric sulfate, such as Benedict reagent and Clinitest.

CONTRAINDICATIONS & CAUTIONS

- Contraindicated in patients hypersensitive to drug or other cephalosporins.
- Use cautiously in patients hypersensitive to penicillin because of possibility of cross-sensitivity with other beta-lactam antibiotics.
- Use cautiously in breast-feeding women and in patients with history of colitis and renal insufficiency.

NURSING CONSIDERATIONS

- Before giving drug, ask patient if he is allergic to penicillins or cephalosporins.
- Obtain specimen for culture and sensitivity tests before giving first dose. Therapy may begin before results.
- An I.M. kit containing 1% lidocaine as a diluent is available from the manufacturer.
- For I.M. use, inject deep into a large muscle, such as the gluteus maximus or the lateral aspect of the thigh.
- If large doses are given, therapy is prolonged, or patient is at high risk, monitor patient for signs and symptoms of superinfection.
- Monitor PT and INR in patients with impaired vitamin K synthesis or low vitamin K stores. Vitamin K therapy may be needed.
- Drug is commonly used in home antibiotic programs for outpatient treatment of

serious infections such as osteomyelitis and community-acquired pneumonia.
• ***Look alike–sound alike:*** Don't confuse drug with other cephalosporins that sound alike.

PATIENT TEACHING
• Tell patient to report adverse reactions promptly.
• Instruct patient to report discomfort at I.V. insertion site.
• Teach patient and family receiving home care how to prepare and give drug.
• If home care patient is diabetic and is testing his urine for glucose, tell him drug may affect results of cupric sulfate tests; he should use an enzymatic test instead.
• Tell patient to notify prescriber about loose stools or diarrhea.

cefuroxime axetil
Ceftin

cefuroxime sodium
Zinacef

Pharmacologic class: second-generation cephalosporin
Pregnancy risk category B

AVAILABLE FORMS
cefuroxime axetil
Suspension: 125 mg/5 ml, 250 mg/5 ml
Tablets: 125 mg, 250 mg, 500 mg
cefuroxime sodium
Infusion: 750 mg, 1.5 g premixed, frozen solution
Injection: 750 mg, 1.5 g

INDICATIONS & DOSAGES
➤ **Serious lower respiratory tract infection, UTI, skin or skin-structure infections, bone or joint infection, septicemia, meningitis, and gonorrhea**
Adults and children age 13 and older: 750 mg to 1.5 g cefuroxime sodium I.V. or I.M. q 8 hours for 5 to 10 days. For life-threatening infections and infections caused by less susceptible organisms, 1.5 g I.V. or I.M. q 6 hours; for bacterial meningitis, up to 3 g I.V. q 8 hours.
Children age 3 months to 12 years: 50 to 100 mg/kg/day cefuroxime sodium I.V. or I.M. in equally divided doses q 6 to 8 hours. Use higher dosage of 100 mg/kg/day, not to exceed maximum adult dosage, for more severe or serious infections. For bacterial meningitis, 200 to 240 mg/kg cefuroxime sodium I.V. in divided doses q 6 to 8 hours.
➤ **Perioperative prevention**
Adults: 1.5 g I.V. 30 to 60 minutes before surgery; in lengthy operations, 750 mg I.V. or I.M. q 8 hours. For open-heart surgery, 1.5 g I.V. at induction of anesthesia and then q 12 hours for a total dose of 6 g.
➤ **Bacterial exacerbations of chronic bronchitis or secondary bacterial infection of acute bronchitis**
Adults: 250 or 500 mg P.O. b.i.d. for 10 days (chronic bronchitis) or 5 to 10 days (acute bronchitis).
➤ **Acute bacterial maxillary sinusitis**
Adults and children age 13 and older: 250 mg P.O. b.i.d. for 10 days.
Children ages 3 months to 12 years: 30 mg/kg/day oral suspension divided b.i.d. for 10 days.
➤ **Pharyngitis and tonsillitis**
Adults and children age 13 and older: 250 mg P.O. b.i.d. for 10 days.
Children ages 3 months to 12 years: 125 mg P.O. b.i.d. for 10 days. For children who can't swallow tablets whole, give 20 mg/kg daily of oral suspension divided b.i.d. for 10 days. Maximum daily dose for suspension is 500 mg.
➤ **Otitis media**
Children ages 3 months to 12 years: 250 mg P.O. b.i.d. for 10 days. For children who can't swallow tablets whole, give 30 mg/kg/day of oral suspension divided b.i.d. for 10 days. Maximum daily dose for suspension is 1,000 mg.
➤ **Uncomplicated skin and skin structure infection**
Adults and children age 13 and older: 250 or 500 mg P.O. b.i.d. for 10 days.
➤ **Uncomplicated UTI**
Adults: 125 or 250 mg P.O. b.i.d. for 7 to 10 days.
➤ **Uncomplicated gonorrhea**
Adults: 1.5 g I.M. with 1 g probenecid P.O. for one dose. Or, 1 g P.O. as a single dose.
➤ **Early Lyme disease**
Adults and children age 13 and older: 500 mg P.O. b.i.d. for 20 days.

➤**Impetigo**
Children ages 3 months to 12 years: 30 mg/kg/day of oral suspension divided b.i.d. for 10 days. Maximum daily dose, 1,000 mg.
Adjust-a-dose: In adults with creatinine clearance of 10 to 20 ml/minute, give 750 mg I.V. or I.M. q 12 hours; if clearance is less than 10 ml/min, give 750 mg I.V. or I.M. q 24 hours.

I.V. ADMINISTRATION
- Reconstitute each 750-mg vial with 8 ml and each 1.5-g vial with 16 ml of sterile water for injection.
- Withdraw entire contents of vial for a dose.
- For direct injection, inject over 3 to 5 minutes into a large vein or into the tubing of a free-flowing I.V. solution.
- For intermittent infusion, add reconstituted drug to 100 ml D_5W, normal saline solution for injection, or other compatible I.V. solution.
- Infuse over 15 to 60 minutes.

INCOMPATIBILITIES
Aminoglycosides, azithromycin, ciprofloxacin, cisatracurium, clarithromycin, cyclophosphamide, doxapram, filgrastim, fluconazole, gentamicin, midazolam, ranitidine, sodium bicarbonate injection, vancomycin, vinorelbine tartrate.

ACTION
Second-generation cephalosporin that inhibits cell-wall synthesis, promoting osmotic instability; usually bactericidal.

Route	Onset	Peak	Duration
P.O.	Unknown	15–60 min	Unknown
I.V.	Immediate	Immediate	Unknown
I.M.	Unknown	2 hr	Unknown

Half-life: 1 to 2 hours.

ADVERSE REACTIONS
CV: *phlebitis, thrombophlebitis.*
GI: *diarrhea, **pseudomembranous colitis,*** nausea, anorexia, vomiting.
Hematologic: *hemolytic anemia, **thrombocytopenia, transient neutropenia,*** eosinophilia.
Skin: *maculopapular and erythematous rashes, urticaria, pain, induration, sterile abscesses, temperature elevation, tissue sloughing at I.M. injection site.*
Other: ***anaphylaxis,*** hypersensitivity reactions, serum sickness.

INTERACTIONS
Drug-drug. *Aminoglycosides:* May cause synergistic activity against some organisms; may increase nephrotoxicity. Monitor patient's renal function closely.
Loop diuretics: May increase risk of adverse renal reactions. Monitor renal function test results closely.
Probenecid: May inhibit excretion and increase cefuroxime level. Probenecid may be used for this effect.
Drug-food. *Any food:* May increase absorption. Give drug with food.

EFFECTS ON LAB TEST RESULTS
- May increase alkaline phosphatase, ALT, AST, bilirubin, and LDH levels. May decrease hemoglobin level and hematocrit.
- May increase PT and INR and eosinophil count. May decrease neutrophil and platelet counts.
- May falsely increase serum or urine creatinine level in tests using Jaffe reaction. May cause false-positive results of Coombs test and urine glucose tests that use cupric sulfate, such as Benedict reagent and Clinitest.

CONTRAINDICATIONS & CAUTIONS
- Contraindicated in patients hypersensitive to drug or other cephalosporins.
- Use cautiously in patients hypersensitive to penicillin because of possibility of cross-sensitivity with other beta-lactam antibiotics.
- Use cautiously in breast-feeding women and in patients with history of colitis or renal insufficiency.

NURSING CONSIDERATIONS
- Before giving drug, ask patient if he is allergic to penicillins or cephalosporins.
- Obtain specimen for culture and sensitivity tests before giving first dose. Therapy may begin while awaiting results.
- For I.M. use, inject deep into a large muscle, such as the gluteus maximus or the side of the thigh.
- Absorption of oral drug is enhanced by food.

• Tablets may be crushed, if absolutely necessary, for patients who can't swallow tablets. Tablets may be dissolved in small amounts of apple, orange, or grape juice or chocolate milk. However, the drug has a bitter taste that is difficult to mask, even with food.
• ***Alert:*** Tablets and suspension aren't bioequivalent and can't be substituted milligram-for-milligram.
• Monitor patient for signs and symptoms of superinfection.
• ***Look alike–sound alike:*** Don't confuse drug with other cephalosporins that sound alike.

PATIENT TEACHING
• Tell patient to take drug as prescribed, even after he feels better.
• Instruct patient to take oral form with food.
• If patient has difficulty swallowing tablets, show him how to dissolve or crush tablets but warn him that the bitter taste is hard to mask, even with food.
• Tell parent to shake suspension well before measuring dose. Suspension may be stored at room temperature or refrigerated, but must be discarded after 10 days.
• Instruct patient to notify prescriber about rash, loose stools, diarrhea, or evidence of superinfection.
• Advise patient receiving drug I.V. to report discomfort at I.V. insertion site.

cephalexin monohydrate

Apo-Cephalex†, Biocef, Keflex, Novo-Lexin†, Nu-Cephalex†

Pharmacologic class: first-generation cephalosporin
Pregnancy risk category B

AVAILABLE FORMS
Capsules: 250 mg, 500 mg
Oral suspension: 125 mg/5 ml, 250 mg/5 ml
Tablets: 250 mg, 500 mg

INDICATIONS & DOSAGES
➤ **Respiratory tract, GI tract, skin, soft-tissue, bone, and joint infections and otitis media caused by *Escherichia coli* and other coliform bacteria, group A beta-hemolytic streptococci, *Klebsiella* species, *Proteus mirabilis, Streptococcus pneumoniae,* and staphylococci**
Adults: 250 mg to 1 g P.O. q 6 hours or 500 mg q 12 hours. Maximum 4 g daily.
Children: 25 to 50 mg/kg/day P.O. in two to four equally divided doses. In severe infections, dose can be doubled.
Adjust-a-dose: For adults with impaired renal function, initial dose is the same. Then, for those with creatinine clearance of 11 to 40 ml/minute, give 500 mg P.O. q 8 to 12 hours; for clearance of 5 to 10 ml/minute, give 250 mg P.O. q 12 hours; and for clearance of less than 5 ml/minute, give 250 mg P.O. q 12 to 24 hours.

ACTION
First-generation cephalosporin that inhibits cell-wall synthesis, promoting osmotic instability; usually bactericidal.

Route	Onset	Peak	Duration
P.O.	Unknown	1 hr	Unknown

Half-life: 30 minutes to 1 hour.

ADVERSE REACTIONS
CNS: dizziness, headache, fatigue, agitation, confusion, hallucinations.
GI: *anorexia, diarrhea, nausea,* ***pseudomembranous colitis,*** vomiting, gastritis, glossitis, dyspepsia, abdominal pain, anal pruritus, tenesmus, oral candidiasis.
GU: genital pruritus, candidiasis, vaginitis, interstitial nephritis.
Hematologic: ***neutropenia, thrombocytopenia,*** eosinophilia, anemia.
Musculoskeletal: arthritis, arthralgia, joint pain.
Skin: *maculopapular and erythematous rashes, urticaria.*
Other: ***anaphylaxis,*** hypersensitivity reactions, serum sickness.

INTERACTIONS
Drug-drug. *Aminoglycosides:* May increase risk of nephrotoxicity. Avoid using together.
Probenecid: May increase cephalosporin level. Use probenecid for this effect.

EFFECTS ON LAB TEST RESULTS

- May increase alkaline phosphatase, ALT, AST, bilirubin, and LDH levels. May decrease hemoglobin level.
- May increase eosinophil count. May decrease neutrophil and platelet counts.
- May falsely increase serum or urine creatinine level in tests using Jaffe reaction. May cause false-positive results of Coombs test and urine glucose tests that use cupric sulfate, such as Benedict reagent and Clinitest.

CONTRAINDICATIONS & CAUTIONS

- Contraindicated in patients hypersensitive to cephalosporins.
- Use cautiously in patients hypersensitive to penicillin because of possibility of cross-sensitivity with other beta-lactam antibiotics.
- Use cautiously in breast-feeding women and in patients with history of colitis or renal insufficiency.

NURSING CONSIDERATIONS

- Ask patient about past reaction to cephalosporin or penicillin therapy and obtain specimen for culture and sensitivity tests before giving. Start therapy, awaiting results.
- To prepare oral suspension: Add required amount of water to powder in two portions. Shake well after each addition. After mixing, store in refrigerator. Mixture will remain stable for 14 days. Keep tightly closed and shake well before using.
- If large doses are given or if therapy is prolonged, monitor patient for superinfection, especially if patient is high risk.
- Treat group A beta-hemolytic streptococcal infections for a minimum of 10 days.
- ***Look alike–sound alike:*** Don't confuse drug with other cephalosporins that sound alike.

PATIENT TEACHING

- Tell patient to take drug exactly as prescribed, even after he feels better.
- Instruct patient to take drug with food or milk to lessen GI discomfort. If patient is taking suspension form, instruct him to shake container well before measuring dose and to store in refrigerator.
- Tell patient to notify prescriber if rash or signs and symptoms of superinfection develop.

loracarbef

Lorabid

Pharmacologic class: second-generation carbacephem
Pregnancy risk category B

AVAILABLE FORMS

Capsules: 200 mg, 400 mg
Powder for oral suspension: 100 mg/5 ml, 200 mg/5 ml in 50-ml, 75-ml, and 100-ml bottles

INDICATIONS & DOSAGES

➤Secondary bacterial infections of acute bronchitis
Adults: 200 to 400 mg P.O. q 12 hours for 7 days.

➤Acute bacterial worsening of chronic bronchitis
Adults: 400 mg P.O. q 12 hours for 7 days.

➤Pneumonia
Adults: 400 mg P.O. q 12 hours for 14 days.

➤Pharyngitis, sinusitis, tonsillitis
Adults: 200 to 400 mg P.O. q 12 hours for 10 days.
Children ages 6 months to 12 years: 15 mg/kg P.O. daily in divided doses q 12 hours for 10 days.

➤Acute otitis media
Children ages 6 months to 12 years: 30 mg/kg oral suspension P.O. daily in divided doses q 12 hours for 10 days.

➤Uncomplicated skin and skin-structure infections
Adults: 200 mg P.O. q 12 hours for 7 days.

➤Impetigo
Children ages 6 months to 12 years: 15 mg/kg P.O. daily in divided doses q 12 hours for 7 days.

➤Uncomplicated cystitis
Adults: 200 mg P.O. daily for 7 days.

➤Uncomplicated pyelonephritis
Adults: 400 mg P.O. q 12 hours for 14 days.
Adjust-a-dose: For patients with creatinine clearance of 10 to 49 ml/minute, give half usual dose at usual interval; if clearance is less than 10 ml/minute, give usual

dose q 3 to 5 days. Hemodialysis patients require an additional dose after dialysis.

ACTION

Synthetic beta-lactam antibiotic of the carbacephem class that inhibits cell-wall synthesis, promoting osmotic instability; usually bactericidal.

Route	Onset	Peak	Duration
P.O.	Unknown	30–60 min	Unknown

Half-life: About 1 hour.

ADVERSE REACTIONS

CNS: headache, somnolence, nervousness, insomnia, dizziness.
CV: vasodilation.
GI: ***pseudomembranous colitis,*** diarrhea, nausea, vomiting, abdominal pain, anorexia.
GU: vaginal candidiasis.
Hematologic: ***transient thrombocytopenia, leukopenia, pancytopenia, neutropenia,*** eosinophilia.
Skin: ***erythema multiforme,*** rash, urticaria, pruritus.
Other: ***anaphylaxis,*** hypersensitivity reactions.

INTERACTIONS

Drug-drug. *Probenecid:* May decrease excretion of loracarbef, causing increased drug levels. Monitor patient for toxicity.
Drug-food. *Any food:* May decrease absorption. Have patient take drug on empty stomach at least 1 hour before or 2 hours after a meal.

EFFECTS ON LAB TEST RESULTS

- May increase alkaline phosphatase, ALT, AST, BUN, and creatinine levels.
- May increase eosinophil count and PT and INR. May decrease neutrophil, platelet, RBC, and WBC counts.

CONTRAINDICATIONS & CAUTIONS

- Contraindicated in patients hypersensitive to drug or other cephalosporins.
- Use cautiously in patients hypersensitive to penicillin because of possibility of cross-sensitivity with other beta-lactam antibiotics.
- Use cautiously in breast-feeding women and in patients with history of colitis or renal insufficiency.
- Safety and effectiveness of drug haven't been established in infants younger than age 6 months.

NURSING CONSIDERATIONS

- Before administration, ask patient if he is allergic to penicillins or cephalosporins.
- Obtain specimen for culture and sensitivity tests before giving. Start therapy, awaiting results.
- To reconstitute powder for oral suspension, add 30 ml of water in two portions to the 50-ml bottle, 45 ml of water in two portions to the 75-ml bottle, or 60 ml of water in two portions to the 100-ml bottle; shake after each addition.
- After reconstitution, store oral suspension for 14 days at 59° to 86° F (15° to 30° C).
- Monitor patient for superinfection. Drug may cause overgrowth of nonsusceptible bacteria or fungi.
- Monitor renal function.
- For otitis media, the more rapidly absorbed oral suspension produces higher peak drug levels than do capsules.
- ***Look alike–sound alike:*** Don't confuse Lorabid with Lortab.

PATIENT TEACHING

- Instruct patient to take drug prescribed, even after he feels better.
- Tell patient to take drug on an empty stomach, at least 1 hour before or 2 hours after meals. Tell him to shake container of suspension well before measuring dose.
- Advise patient to discard unused portion after 14 days.
- Instruct patient to notify prescriber if rash or signs and symptoms of superinfection appear.
- Instruct patient to notify prescriber if loose stools or diarrhea occur.

12

Tetracyclines

doxycycline calcium
doxycycline hyclate
doxycycline hydrochloride
doxycycline monohydrate
minocycline hydrochloride
tetracycline hydrochloride
tigecycline

doxycycline calcium
Vibramycin

doxycycline hyclate
Apo-Doxy†, Doryx, Doxy 100, Doxy 200, Doxycin†, Doxytec†, Novo-Doxylin†, Nu-Doxycycline†, Periostat, Vibramycin, Vibra-Tabs

doxycycline hydrochloride‡
Doryx‡, Doxsig‡, Doxylin‡, Doxy Tablets‡, Vibramycin‡, Vibra-Tabs 50‡

doxycycline monohydrate
Adoxa, Monodox, Vibramycin

Pharmacologic class: tetracycline
Pregnancy risk category D

AVAILABLE FORMS
doxycycline calcium
Syrup: 50 mg/5 ml
doxycycline hyclate
Capsules: 50 mg, 100 mg
Capsules (coated pellets): 75 mg, 100 mg
Injection: 100 mg, 200 mg
Tablets: 20 mg, 100 mg
doxycycline hydrochloride‡
Capsules: 50 mg‡, 100 mg‡
Tablets: 50 mg‡, 100 mg‡
doxycycline monohydrate
Capsules: 50 mg, 100 mg
Oral suspension: 25 mg/5 ml
Tablets: 50 mg, 75 mg, 100 mg

INDICATIONS & DOSAGES
➤ **Infections caused by susceptible gram-positive and gram-negative organisms (including *Haemophilus ducreyi, Yersinia pestis,* and *Campylobacter fetus*), *Rickettsiae* species, *Mycoplasma pneumoniae, Chlamydia trachomatis*, and *Borrelia burgdorferi* (Lyme disease); psittacosis; granuloma inguinale**
Adults and children older than age 8 who weigh at least 45 kg (99 lb): 100 mg P.O. q 12 hours on first day; then 100 mg P.O. daily as a single dose or divided b.i.d. Or, 200 mg I.V. on first day in one or two infusions; then 100 to 200 mg I.V. daily. Daily doses of 200 mg I.V. can be given as a single dose or divided b.i.d.
Children older than age 8 who weigh less than 45 kg: 4.4 mg/kg P.O. or I.V. daily, in divided doses q 12 hours on first day; then 2.2 to 4.4 mg/kg daily given as a single dose or divided b.i.d.

Give I.V. infusion slowly (minimum 1 hour). Infusion must be completed within 12 hours (within 6 hours in lactated Ringer solution or dextrose 5% in lactated Ringer solution).

➤ **Gonorrhea in patients allergic to penicillin**
Adults: 100 mg P.O. b.i.d. for 7 days. Use for 10 days for epididymitis.

➤ **Syphilis in patients allergic to penicillin (except Adoxa, Doryx, Monodox)**
Adults: 100 mg P.O. b.i.d. for 14 days (early). If more than 1 year duration, 100 mg P.O. daily for 4 weeks.

➤ **Primary or secondary syphilis in patients allergic to penicillin (Adoxa, Doryx, Monodox only)**
Adults: 300 mg P.O. daily in divided doses for at least 10 days.

➤ **Uncomplicated urethral, endocervical, or rectal infections caused by *C. trachomatis* or *Ureaplasma urealyticum***
Adults: 100 mg P.O. b.i.d. for at least 7 days. In those with epididymitis, treat for 10 days.

➤ **To prevent malaria**
Adults: 100 mg P.O. daily beginning 1 to 2 days before travel to endemic area and continued for 4 weeks after travel.

Children older than age 8: 2 mg/kg P.O. once daily beginning 1 to 2 days before travel to endemic area and continued for 4 weeks after travel. Don't exceed daily dose of 100 mg.

➤ **Pelvic inflammatory disease ♦**
Adults: 100 mg I.V. or P.O. q 12 hours with 2 g cefoxitin I.V. q 6 hours. May stop parenteral doxycycline and cefoxitin after 24 hours and continue with 100 mg doxycycline P.O. q 12 hours for 14 days total.

➤ **Adjunct to other antibiotics for inhalation, GI, and oropharyngeal anthrax**
Adults: 100 mg q 12 hours I.V. initially until susceptibility test results are known. Switch to 100 mg P.O. b.i.d. when appropriate. Treat for 60 days total.
Children older than age 8 who weigh more than 45 kg (99 lb): 100 mg q 12 hours I.V.; then switch to 100 mg P.O. b.i.d. when appropriate. Treat for 60 days total.
Children older than age 8 who weigh 45 kg or less: 2.2 mg/kg q 12 hours I.V.; then switch to 2.2 mg/kg P.O. b.i.d. when appropriate. Treat for 60 days total.
Children age 8 and younger: 2.2 mg/kg q 12 hours I.V.; then switch to 2.2 mg/kg P.O. b.i.d. when appropriate. Treat for 60 days total.

➤ **Cutaneous anthrax**
Adults: 100 mg P.O. q 12 hours for 60 days.
Children older than age 8 who weigh more than 45 kg (99 lb): 100 mg P.O. q 12 hours for 60 days.
Children older than age 8 who weigh 45 kg or less: 2.2 mg/kg q 12 hours P.O. for 60 days.
Children age 8 and younger: 2.2 mg/kg P.O. q 12 hours for 60 days.

➤ **Adjunct to scaling and root planing to improve attachment and reduce pocket depth in periodontitis**
Adults: 20 mg P.O. Periostat b.i.d., more than 1 hour before or 2 hours after the morning and evening meals and after scaling and root planing. Effective for 9 months.

➤ **Adjunctive treatment for severe acne**
Adults: 200 mg Adoxa P.O. on the first day of treatment (100 mg given q 12 hours or 50 mg q 6 hours), followed by a maintenance dose of 100 mg/day in single or divided doses.

➤ **To prevent traveler's diarrhea caused by *Escherichia coli* ♦**
Adults: 100 mg P.O. daily.

I.V. ADMINISTRATION

- Reconstitute powder for injection with sterile water for injection. Use 10 ml in 100-mg vial and 20 ml in 200-mg vial. Further dilute solution to a concentration of 0.1 mg/ml to 1 mg/ml; don't infuse solution that contains more than 1 mg/ml.
- Don't expose drug to light or heat. Protect it from sunlight during infusion.
- Infusion time varies with dose but usually ranges from 1 to 4 hours. Infusion must be completed within 12 hours.
- Monitor infusion site for evidence of thrombophlebitis.
- Reconstituted injectable solution is stable 72 hours if refrigerated and protected from light.

INCOMPATIBILITIES

Allopurinol; drugs that are unstable in acidic solutions, such as barbiturates; erythromycin lactobionate; heparin; meropenem; nafcillin; penicillin G potassium; piperacillin with tazobactam; riboflavin; and sulfonamides.

ACTION

May exert bacteriostatic effect by binding to the 30S and possibly 50S ribosomal subunits of microorganisms and inhibiting protein synthesis. May also alter the cytoplasmic membrane of susceptible microorganisms.

Route	Onset	Peak	Duration
P.O.	Unknown	1½–4 hr	Unknown
I.V.	Immediate	Unknown	Unknown

Half-life: About 1 day after multiple dosing.

ADVERSE REACTIONS

CNS: ***intracranial hypertension.***
CV: pericarditis, thrombophlebitis.
GI: *diarrhea, epigastric distress, nausea,* anorexia, glossitis, dysphagia, vomiting, oral candidiasis, enterocolitis, anogenital inflammation.
Hematologic: ***neutropenia, thrombocytopenia,*** eosinophilia, hemolytic anemia.

Musculoskeletal: bone growth retardation in children younger than age 8.
Skin: *maculopapular and erythematous rashes, photosensitivity, increased pigmentation, urticaria.*
Other: ***anaphylaxis,*** hypersensitivity reactions, superinfection, permanent discoloration of teeth, enamel defects.

INTERACTIONS

Drug-drug. *Antacids and laxatives containing aluminum, magnesium, or calcium, antidiarrheals:* May decrease antibiotic absorption. Give antibiotic 1 hour before or 2 hours after these drugs.
Carbamazepine, phenobarbital, rifamycins: May decrease antibiotic effect. Avoid using together.
Ferrous sulfate and other iron products, zinc: May decrease antibiotic absorption. Give drug 2 hours before or 3 hours after iron.
Hormonal contraceptives: May decrease contraceptive effectiveness and increase risk of breakthrough bleeding. Advise use of a nonhormonal contraceptive.
Methoxyflurane: May cause nephrotoxicity with tetracyclines. Avoid using together.
Oral anticoagulants: May increase anticoagulant effect. Monitor PT and INR, and adjust dosage.
Penicillins: May interfere with bactericidal action of penicillins. Avoid using together.
Drug-lifestyle. *Alcohol use:* May decrease drug's effect. Discourage use together.
Sun exposure: May cause photosensitivity reactions. Advise patient to avoid excessive sunlight exposure.

EFFECTS ON LAB TEST RESULTS

- May increase BUN and liver enzyme levels. May decrease hemoglobin level.
- May increase eosinophil count. May decrease platelet, neutrophil, and WBC counts.
- May falsely elevate fluorometric tests for urine catecholamines. May cause false-negative results in urine glucose tests using glucose oxidase reagent (Diastix or Chemstrip uG). Parenteral form may cause false-positive Clinitest results.

CONTRAINDICATIONS & CAUTIONS

- Contraindicated in patients hypersensitive to drug or other tetracyclines.
- Use cautiously in patients with impaired renal or hepatic function.
- In a fetus in the last half of gestation or a child younger than age 8, drug may cause permanent discoloration of teeth, enamel defects, and bone growth retardation.

NURSING CONSIDERATIONS

- Obtain specimen for culture and sensitivity tests before giving. Therapy may begin awaiting test results.
- ***Alert:*** Check expiration date. Outdated or deteriorated tetracyclines may cause reversible nephrotoxicity (Fanconi syndrome).
- If patient receives large doses or therapy is prolonged, or if patient is at high risk, monitor patient for signs and symptoms of superinfection.
- Cutaneous anthrax with signs of systemic involvement, extensive edema, or lesions on the head or neck requires I.V. therapy and a multidrug approach.
- Ciprofloxacin and doxycycline are first-line therapies for anthrax. If anthrax patient also has meningitis, ciprofloxacin is preferred because of better distribution to the CNS.
- In pregnant women and immunocompromised patients, use the usual dosage schedule for anthrax. In pregnant women, adverse effects on fetal teeth and bones are dose-limited, so drug may be used for 7 to 14 days before the third trimester.
- Check patient's tongue for signs of fungal infection. Stress good oral hygiene.
- Photosensitivity reactions may occur within a few minutes to several hours after exposure and may last after therapy ends.
- ***Look alike–sound alike:*** Don't confuse doxycycline, doxylamine, and dicyclomine.

PATIENT TEACHING

- Tell patient to take entire amount of drug exactly as prescribed, even after he feels better.
- Instruct patient to report adverse reactions promptly. If drug is being given I.V., tell him to report discomfort at I.V. site.

• Advise patient to take oral form of drug with food or milk if stomach upset occurs.
• Advise patient to increase fluid intake and not to take oral tablets or capsules within 1 hour of bedtime because of possible esophageal irritation or ulceration.
• Advise parent giving drug to a child that tablets may be crushed and mixed with low-fat milk, chocolate milk, chocolate pudding, or apple juice mixed equally with sugar. Tell parent to store mixtures in refrigerator (except apple juice mixture, which can be stored at room temperature) and to discard after 24 hours.
• Warn patient to avoid direct sunlight and ultraviolet light, wear protective clothing, and use sunscreen.
• Tell patient to report signs and symptoms of superinfection to prescriber.

minocycline hydrochloride

Akamin‡, Alti-Minocycline†, Apo-Minocycline†, Dynacin, Minocin, Minomycin‡, Novo-Minocycline†, PMS-Minocycline†

Pharmacologic class: tetracycline
Pregnancy risk category D

AVAILABLE FORMS

Capsules: 50 mg, 75 mg, 100 mg
Capsules (pellet-filled): 50 mg, 100 mg
Oral suspension: 50 mg/ml
Tablets: 50 mg, 75 mg, 100 mg

INDICATIONS & DOSAGES

➤ **Infections caused by susceptible gram-negative and gram-positive organisms (including *Haemophilus ducreyi, Yersinia pestis,* and *Campylobacter fetus*), *Rickettsiae* species, *Mycoplasma pneumoniae,* and *Chlamydia trachomatis;* psittacosis; granuloma inguinale**
Adults: 200 mg P.O. initially; then 100 mg P.O. q 12 hours. May use 100 or 200 mg P.O. initially; then 50 mg q.i.d.
Children older than age 8: Initially, 4 mg/kg P.O.; then, 2 mg/kg q 12 hours.
➤ **Gonorrhea in patients allergic to penicillin**
Adults: Initially, 200 mg P.O.; then 100 mg q 12 hours for at least 4 days. Obtain samples for follow-up cultures within 2 to 3 days after treatment.
➤ **Syphilis in patients allergic to penicillin**
Adults: Initially, 200 mg P.O.; then 100 mg q 12 hours for 10 to 15 days.
➤ **Meningococcal carrier state**
Adults: 100 mg P.O. q 12 hours for 5 days.
➤ **Uncomplicated urethral, endocervical, or rectal infection caused by *C. trachomatis* or *Ureaplasma urealyticum***
Adults: 100 mg P.O. q 12 hours for at least 7 days.
➤ **Uncomplicated gonococcal urethritis**
Men: 100 mg P.O. q 12 hours for 5 days.

ACTION

May be bacteriostatic by binding to microorganism's ribosomal subunits, inhibiting protein synthesis; may also alter the cytoplasmic membrane of susceptible microorganisms.

Route	Onset	Peak	Duration
P.O.	Unknown	1–4 hr	Unknown

Half-life: 11 to 26 hours.

ADVERSE REACTIONS

CNS: ***intracranial hypertension,*** headache, light-headedness, dizziness, vertigo.
CV: *thrombophlebitis,* pericarditis.
GI: *anorexia, diarrhea, nausea,* dysphagia, glossitis, epigastric distress, oral candidiasis, vomiting.
Hematologic: ***neutropenia, thrombocytopenia,*** eosinophilia, hemolytic anemia.
Musculoskeletal: bone growth retardation in children younger than age 8.
Skin: *increased pigmentation, maculopapular and erythematous rashes, photosensitivity, urticaria.*
Other: ***anaphylaxis,*** enamel defects, hypersensitivity reactions, permanent discoloration of teeth, superinfection.

INTERACTIONS

Drug-drug. *Antacids (including sodium bicarbonate) and laxatives containing aluminum, magnesium, or calcium, antidiarrheals:* May decrease antibiotic absorption. Give antibiotic 1 hour before or 2 hours after these drugs.

Ferrous sulfate and other iron products, zinc: May decrease antibiotic absorption. Give drug 2 hours before or 3 hours after iron.
Hormonal contraceptives: May decrease contraceptive effectiveness and increase risk of breakthrough bleeding. Advise patient to use nonhormonal contraceptive.
Methoxyflurane: May cause nephrotoxicity when given with tetracyclines. Avoid using together.
Oral anticoagulants: May increase anticoagulant effect. Monitor PT and INR, and adjust dosage.
Penicillins: May disrupt bactericidal action of penicillins. Avoid using together.
Drug-lifestyle. *Sun exposure:* May cause photosensitivity reactions. Advise patient to avoid excessive sunlight exposure.

EFFECTS ON LAB TEST RESULTS

- May increase BUN and liver enzyme levels. May decrease hemoglobin level.
- May increase eosinophil count. May decrease platelet and neutrophil counts.
- May falsely elevate fluorometric test results for urine catecholamines. Parenteral form may cause false-positive results of copper sulfate test (Clinitest). May cause false-negative results in urine glucose tests using glucose oxidase reagent (Diastix or Chemstrip uG).

CONTRAINDICATIONS & CAUTIONS

- Contraindicated in patients hypersensitive to drug or other tetracyclines.
- Use cautiously in patients with impaired renal or hepatic function. Use of these drugs during last half of pregnancy and in children younger than age 8 may cause permanent discoloration of teeth, enamel defects, and bone growth retardation.

NURSING CONSIDERATIONS

- Monitor renal and liver function test results.
- Obtain specimen for culture and sensitivity tests before first dose. Therapy may begin awaiting test results.
- ***Alert:*** Check expiration date. Outdated or deteriorated tetracyclines may cause reversible nephrotoxicity (Fanconi syndrome).
- Don't expose drug to light or heat. Keep cap tightly closed.
- If large doses are given, therapy is prolonged, or patient is at high risk, monitor patient for signs and symptoms of superinfection.
- Check patient's tongue for signs of candidal infection. Stress good oral hygiene.
- Drug may discolor teeth in older children and young adults, more commonly when used as long-term treatment. Watch for brown pigmentation, and notify prescriber if it occurs.
- Photosensitivity reactions may occur within a few minutes to several hours after exposure. Photosensitivity lasts after therapy ends.
- ***Look alike–sound alike:*** Don't confuse Minocin with niacin or Mithracin.

PATIENT TEACHING

- Tell patient to take entire amount of drug exactly as prescribed, even after he feels better.
- Instruct patient to take drug with a full glass of water. Drug may be taken with food. Tell patient not to take within 1 hour of bedtime, to avoid esophageal irritation or ulceration.
- Warn patient to avoid driving or other hazardous tasks because of possible adverse CNS effects.
- Caution patient to avoid direct sunlight and ultraviolet light, wear protective clothing, and use sunscreen.

tetracycline hydrochloride

Achromycin, Apo-Tetra†, Novo-Tetra†, Nu-Tetra†, Sumycin, Tetrex‡

Pharmacologic class: tetracycline
Pregnancy risk category D

AVAILABLE FORMS

Capsules: 250 mg, 500 mg
Oral suspension: 125 mg/5 ml

INDICATIONS & DOSAGES

➤ **Infections caused by susceptible gram-negative and -positive organisms, including *Haemophilus ducreyi, Yersinia pestis, Campylobacter fetus, Rickettsiae* species, *Mycoplasma pneumoniae,* and *Chlamydia***

***trachomatis;* psittacosis; granuloma inguinale**
Adults: 1 g to 2 g/day P.O. divided b.i.d. or q.i.d depending on the severity of infection.
Children older than age 8: 25 to 50 mg/kg P.O. daily, in divided doses q 6 hours.
➤ **Uncomplicated urethral, endocervical, or rectal infections caused by *C. trachomatis***
Adults: 500 mg P.O. q.i.d. for at least 7 days, 10 days for epididymitis, and for at least 14 days for lymphogranuloma venereum.
➤ **Brucellosis**
Adults: 500 mg P.O. q 6 hours for 3 weeks with 1 g of streptomycin I.M. q 12 hours for first week; once daily for second week.
➤ **Gonorrhea in patients allergic to penicillin**
Adults: Initially, 1.5 g P.O.; then 500 mg P.O. q 6 hours for total dose of 9 g. For epididymitis, 500 mg P.O. q 6 hours for 7 days.
➤ **Syphilis in patients allergic to penicillin ♦**
Adults and adolescents: 500 mg P.O. q.i.d. for 14 days. If infection has lasted 1 year or longer, treat for 28 days.
➤ **Acne**
Adults and adolescents: Initially, 250 mg P.O. q 6 hours; then 125 to 500 mg daily or every other day.
➤ ***Helicobacter pylori* infection**
Adults: 500 mg P.O. q 6 hours for 10 to 14 days with other drugs, such as metronidazole, bismuth subsalicylate, amoxicillin, or omeprazole.
➤ **Cholera**
Adults: 500 mg P.O. q 6 hours for 48 to 72 hours.
➤ **Malaria caused by *Plasmodium falciparum***
Adults: 250 to 500 mg P.O. daily for 7 days with quinine sulfate 650 mg P.O. q 8 hours for 3 to 7 days.
➤ **To prevent infection in rape victims**
Adults: 500 mg P.O. q.i.d. for 7 days.

ACTION
May exert bacteriostatic effect by binding to the 30S and possibly 50S ribosomal subunits of microorganisms, thus inhibiting protein synthesis. May also alter the cytoplasmic membrane of susceptible microorganisms.

Route	Onset	Peak	Duration
P.O.	Unknown	1–4 hr	Unknown

Half-life: 6 to 11 hours.

ADVERSE REACTIONS
CNS: ***intracranial hypertension,*** dizziness, headache.
CV: pericarditis.
EENT: sore throat.
GI: *diarrhea, epigastric distress, nausea,* anorexia, dysphagia, enterocolitis, esophagitis, glossitis, oral candidiasis, stomatitis, vomiting.
GU: inflammatory lesions in anogenital region.
Hematologic: ***neutropenia, thrombocytopenia,*** eosinophilia.
Musculoskeletal: *bone growth retardation in children younger than age 8.*
Skin: *candidal superinfection, increased pigmentation, maculopapular and erythematous rash, photosensitivity, urticaria.*
Other: enamel defects, hypersensitivity reactions, permanent discoloration of teeth.

INTERACTIONS
Drug-drug. *Antacids and laxatives containing aluminum, magnesium, or calcium,* *antidiarrheals containing kaolin, pectin, or bismuth subsalicylate:* May decrease antibiotic absorption. Give antibiotic 1 hour before or 2 hours after these drugs.
Digoxin: May increase digoxin absorption. Monitor digoxin levels and monitor patient for signs of toxicity.
Ferrous sulfate and other iron products, zinc: May decrease antibiotic absorption. Give tetracycline 2 hours before or 3 hours after these products.
Hormonal contraceptives: May decrease contraceptive effectiveness and increase risk of breakthrough bleeding. Advise patient to use nonhormonal contraceptive.
Methoxyflurane: May cause severe nephrotoxicity. Avoid using together.
Oral anticoagulants: May increase anticoagulant effects. Monitor PT and INR, and adjust anticoagulant dosage.
Penicillins: May interfere with bactericidal action of penicillins. Avoid using together.

Drug-food. ***Dairy products:*** May decrease antibiotic absorption. Give antibiotic 1 hour before or 2 hours after eating or drinking dairy products.
Drug-lifestyle. *Sun exposure:* May cause photosensitivity reactions. Advise patient to avoid excessive sunlight exposure.

EFFECTS ON LAB TEST RESULTS
- May increase BUN and liver enzyme levels.
- May increase eosinophil count. May decrease platelet and neutrophil counts.
- May falsely elevate fluorometric test results for urine catecholamines. May cause false-negative results in urine glucose tests using glucose oxidase reagent (Diastix or Chemstrip uG).

CONTRAINDICATIONS & CAUTIONS
- Contraindicated in patients hypersensitive to drug or other tetracyclines.
- Use cautiously in patients with renal or hepatic impairment. Avoid using or use cautiously during last half of pregnancy and in children younger than age 8 because drug may cause permanent discoloration of teeth, enamel defects, and bone growth retardation.

NURSING CONSIDERATIONS
- Obtain specimen for culture and sensitivity tests before giving first dose. Therapy may begin awaiting test results.
- ***Alert:*** Check expiration date. Outdated or deteriorated tetracyclines have been linked to reversible nephrotoxicity (Fanconi syndrome).
- Don't expose drug to light or heat.
- If large doses are given, therapy is prolonged, or patient is at high risk, monitor patient for signs and symptoms of superinfection.
- In patients with renal or hepatic impairment, monitor renal and liver function test results if drug is used.
- Check patient's tongue for signs of candidal infection. Stress good oral hygiene.
- Drug isn't indicated for treatment of neurosyphilis.
- Photosensitivity reactions may occur within a few minutes to several hours after sun exposure. Photosensitivity lasts after therapy ends.

PATIENT TEACHING
- Tell patient to take drug exactly as prescribed, even after he feels better, and to take entire amount prescribed.
- Explain that effectiveness is reduced when drug is taken with milk or other dairy products, antacids, or iron products. For best drug absorption, tell patient to take each dose with a full glass of water on an empty stomach, at least 1 hour before or 2 hours after meals. Also tell him to take it at least 1 hour before bedtime to prevent esophageal irritation or ulceration.
- Warn patient to avoid direct sunlight and ultraviolet light, wear protective clothing, and use sunscreen.
- Advise patient to promptly report adverse reactions to prescriber.

tigecycline
Tygacil

Pharmacologic class: glycylcycline antibacterial
Pregnancy risk category D

AVAILABLE FORMS
Lyophilized powder: 50-mg vial

INDICATIONS & DOSAGES
➤ **Complicated skin or skin structure infection; complicated intra-abdominal infection**
Adults: Initially 100 mg I.V.; then 50 mg q 12 hours for 5 to 14 days. Infuse drug over 30 to 60 minutes.
Adjust-a-dose: For patients with severe hepatic impairment, give initial dose of 100 mg I.V. and then 25 mg I.V. q 12 hours.

I.V. ADMINISTRATION
- Reconstitute powder with 5.3 ml of normal saline solution or D_5W to yield 10 mg/ml. Gently swirl the vial until the powder dissolves.
- Immediately withdraw the dose from the vial and add it to 100 ml of normal saline solution or D_5W. The maximum concentration is 1 mg/ml.
- Inspect the solution for particulates and discoloration (green or black) before giv-

ing. Reconstituted solution should be yellow or orange.
- Immediately dilute reconstituted drug.
- Use a dedicated I.V. line or a Y-site, and flush the line with normal saline or D_5W before and after infusion.
- Infuse the drug over 30 to 60 minutes.
- Store unopened vials at room temperature in the original package. Store diluted solution at room temperature for up to 6 hours, or refrigerate for up to 24 hours.

INCOMPATIBILITIES
Amphotericin B, chlorpromazine, methylprednisolone, and voriconazole.

ACTION
Inhibits protein translation in bacteria by binding to the 30S ribosomal unit.

Route	Onset	Peak	Duration
I.V.	Unknown	Unknown	Unknown

Half-life: 27 to 42 hours.

ADVERSE REACTIONS
CNS: asthenia, dizziness, fever, headache, insomnia, pain.
CV: hypertension, hypotension, peripheral edema.
GI: *diarrhea, nausea, vomiting,* abdominal pain, constipation, dyspepsia.
Hematologic: ***thrombocytopenia,*** anemia, leukocytosis.
Metabolic: hyperglycemia, hypokalemia, hypoproteinemia.
Musculoskeletal: back pain.
Respiratory: cough, dyspnea.
Skin: local reaction, phlebitis, pruritus, rash, sweating.
Other: ***sepsis,*** abnormal healing, abscess, allergic reaction, infection.

INTERACTIONS
Drug-drug. *Hormonal contraceptives:* May decrease contraceptive's effectiveness. Advise patient to use nonhormonal form of contraception during treatment.
Warfarin: May increase risk of bleeding. Monitor INR.

EFFECTS ON LAB TEST RESULTS
- May increase alkaline phosphatase, amylase, bilirubin, BUN, creatinine, LDH, and AST and ALT levels. May decrease potassium, protein, calcium, sodium, and hemoglobin levels and hematocrit. May increase or decrease glucose levels.
- May increase WBC count and INR. May prolong APTT and PT. May decrease platelet count.

CONTRAINDICATIONS & CAUTIONS
- Contraindicated in patients hypersensitive to drug.
- Use cautiously in patients with severe hepatic impairment and in those hypersensitive to tetracycline antibiotics. Also use cautiously as monotherapy in patients with complicated intra-abdominal infections caused by intestinal perforation.

NURSING CONSIDERATIONS
- Assess patient for tetracycline allergy before therapy.
- Obtain specimen for culture and sensitivity tests before first dose. Therapy may begin pending results.
- If patient develops diarrhea, monitor him closely for pseudomembranous colitis.
- If patient has abdominal infection caused by intestinal perforation, monitor for sepsis.
- Monitor for symptoms of dangerous toxicities of tetracyclines, such as photosensitivity, pseudotumor cerebri, pancreatitis, and antianabolic action (increased BUN level, azotemia, acidosis, and hypophosphatemia).

PATIENT TEACHING
- Tell patient that drug is used to treat only bacterial infections, not viral.
- Advise patient to take the full course of treatment, even if he feels better after a few days of therapy.
- Tell patient to report burning or pain at the I.V. site.
- Tell woman of childbearing age to avoid becoming pregnant during treatment. Urge those who use hormonal contraception to also use barrier contraception during treatment.
- Advise woman to notify her health care provider if pregnancy is suspected or confirmed.

13

Sulfonamides

co-trimoxazole
sulfadiazine
sulfisoxazole
sulfisoxazole acetyl

co-trimoxazole (sulfamethoxazole and trimethoprim)

Apo-Sulfatrim†, Apo-Sulfatrim DS†, Bactrim*, Bactrim DS, Bactrim IV, Cotrim, Cotrim D.S, Cotrim Pediatric*, Novo-Trimel†, Novo-Trimel DS†, Nu-Cotrimox†, Resprim‡, Roubac†, Septra*, Septra DS, Septra IV, Septrin‡, Sulfatrim, Sulfatrim Pediatric

Pharmacologic class: sulfonamide and folate antagonist
Pregnancy risk category C

AVAILABLE FORMS

Injection: trimethoprim 16 mg/ml and sulfamethoxazole 80 mg/ml in 5-ml, 10-ml, 20-ml, and 30-ml vials
Oral suspension: trimethoprim 40 mg and sulfamethoxazole 200 mg/5 ml*
Tablets (double-strength): trimethoprim 160 mg and sulfamethoxazole 800 mg
Tablets (single-strength): trimethoprim 80 mg and sulfamethoxazole 400 mg

INDICATIONS & DOSAGES

➤ **Shigellosis or UTIs caused by susceptible strains of *Escherichia coli, Proteus* (indole positive or negative), *Klebsiella,* or *Enterobacter* species**
Adults: 160 mg trimethoprim/800 mg sulfamethoxazole P.O. q 12 hours for 10 to 14 days in UTIs and for 5 days in shigellosis. If indicated, give I.V.: 8 to 10 mg/kg/day, based on trimethoprim component, divided b.i.d. to q.i.d. q 6, 8, or 12 hours for 5 days for shigellosis or up to 14 days for severe UTIs. Maximum daily dose is 960 mg trimethoprim (as co-trimoxazole).
Children age 2 months and older: 8 mg/kg/day, based on trimethoprim component P.O., in two divided doses q 12 hours for 10 days for UTIs and 5 days for shigellosis. If indicated, give I.V.: 8 to 10 mg/kg/day based on trimethoprim component, in two to four divided doses q 6, 8, or 12 hours. Don't exceed adult dose.

➤ **Otitis media in patients with penicillin allergy or penicillin-resistant infection**
Children age 2 months and older: 8 mg/kg/day, based on trimethoprim component P.O., in two divided doses q 12 hours for 10 to 14 days.

➤ **Chronic bronchitis, upper respiratory tract infections**
Adults: 160 mg trimethoprim and 800 mg sulfamethoxazole P.O. q 12 hours for 10 to 14 days.

➤ **Traveler's diarrhea**
Adults: 160 mg trimethoprim and 800 mg sulfamethoxazole P.O. b.i.d. for 3 to 5 days. Some patients may only need up to 2 days of therapy.

➤ **To prevent *Pneumocystis jiroveci (carinii)* pneumonia**
Adults: 160 mg of trimethoprim and 800 mg sulfamethoxazole P.O. daily; or 80 mg trimethoprim/400 mg sulfamethoxazole P.O. three times weekly.
Children age 2 months and older: 150 mg/m^2 trimethoprim and 750 mg/m^2 sulfamethoxazole P.O. daily in two divided doses on 3 consecutive days each week.

➤ ***P. jiroveci (carinii)* pneumonia**
Adults and children older than age 2 months: 15 to 20 mg/kg/day based on trimethoprim I.V. or P.O. in three or four divided doses for 14 to 21 days.
Adjust-a-dose: For patients with creatinine clearance of 15 to 30 ml/minute, reduce daily dose by 50%. Don't give to those with creatinine clearance less than 15 ml/minute.

I.V. ADMINISTRATION

- Don't give by rapid infusion or bolus injection.
- Dilute each 5 ml of concentrate in 75 to 125 ml of D_5W. Don't mix with other drugs or solutions.
- Infuse slowly over 60 to 90 minutes.

- Don't refrigerate; use within 6 hours if diluted in 125 ml and within 2 hours if diluted in 75 ml.
- Discard solution if it's cloudy or crystallized.

INCOMPATIBILITIES

Cisatracurium, fluconazole, foscarnet, linezolid, midazolam, verapamil, vinorelbine.

ACTION

Sulfamethoxazole inhibits formation of dihydrofolic acid from PABA; trimethoprim inhibits dihydrofolate reductase formation. Both decrease bacterial folic acid synthesis and are bactericidal.

Route	Onset	Peak	Duration
P.O.	Unknown	1–4 hr	Unknown
I.V.	Immediate	1–1½ hr	Unknown

Half-life: Trimethoprim, 8 to 11 hours; sulfamethoxazole, 10 to 13 hours.

ADVERSE REACTIONS

CNS: ***seizures,*** apathy, aseptic meningitis, ataxia, depression, fatigue, hallucinations, headache, insomnia, nervousness, tinnitus, vertigo.
CV: thrombophlebitis.
GI: ***pancreatitis, pseudomembranous colitis,*** *diarrhea, nausea, vomiting,* abdominal pain, anorexia, stomatitis.
GU: ***toxic nephrosis with oliguria and anuria,*** crystalluria, hematuria, interstitial nephritis.
Hematologic: ***agranulocytosis, aplastic anemia, leukopenia, thrombocytopenia,*** hemolytic anemia, megaloblastic anemia.
Hepatic: ***hepatic necrosis,*** jaundice.
Musculoskeletal: arthralgia, muscle weakness, myalgia.
Respiratory: pulmonary infiltrates.
Skin: *generalized skin eruption,* ***erythema multiforme, Stevens-Johnson syndrome, toxic epidermal necrolysis,*** exfoliative dermatitis, photosensitivity, pruritus, urticaria.
Other: ***anaphylaxis,*** drug fever, hypersensitivity reactions, serum sickness.

INTERACTIONS

Drug-drug. *Cyclosporine:* May decrease cyclosporine level and increase nephrotoxicity risk. Avoid using together.
Dofetilide: May increase dofetilide level and effects. May increase risk of prolonged QT-interval syndrome and fatal ventricular arrhythmias. Avoid using together.
Hormonal contraceptives: May decrease contraceptive effectiveness and increase risk of breakthrough bleeding. Advise patient to use a nonhormonal contraceptive.
Methotrexate: May increase methotrexate level. Monitor methotrexate level.
Oral antidiabetics: May increase hypoglycemic effect. Monitor glucose level.
Phenytoin: May inhibit hepatic metabolism of phenytoin. Monitor phenytoin level.
Warfarin: May increase anticoagulant effect. Monitor patient for bleeding; monitor PT and INR.
Drug-herb. *Dong quai, St. John's wort:* May cause photosensitivity reactions. Advise patient to avoid excessive sunlight exposure.
Drug-lifestyle. *Sun exposure:* May cause photosensitivity reactions. Advise patient to avoid excessive sunlight exposure.

EFFECTS ON LAB TEST RESULTS

- May increase aminotransferase, bilirubin, BUN, and creatinine levels. May decrease hemoglobin level.
- May decrease granulocyte, platelet, and WBC counts.

CONTRAINDICATIONS & CAUTIONS

- Contraindicated in patients hypersensitive to trimethoprim or sulfonamides.
- Contraindicated in those with creatinine clearance less than 15 ml/minute, porphyria, or megaloblastic anemia from folate deficiency.
- Contraindicated in pregnant women at term, breast-feeding women, and infants younger than age 2 months.
- Use cautiously and in reduced dosages in patients with creatinine clearance of 15 to 30 ml/minute, severe allergy or bronchial asthma, G6PD deficiency, or blood dyscrasia.

NURSING CONSIDERATIONS

- Before giving drug, ask patient if he is allergic to sulfa drugs.
- Obtain specimen for culture and sensitivity tests before giving. Start therapy, awaiting results.
- ***Alert:*** Double-check dosage, which may be written as trimethoprim component.
- ***Alert:*** "DS" product means "double strength."
- Never give drug I.M.
- Monitor renal and liver function test results.
- Promptly report rash, sore throat, fever, cough, mouth sores, or iris lesions—early signs and symptoms of erythema multiforme, which may progress to life-threatening Stevens-Johnson syndrome. These symptoms may also represent early signs of blood dyscrasias.
- Watch for signs and symptoms of superinfection, such as fever, chills, and increased pulse.
- ***Alert:*** Adverse reactions—especially hypersensitivity reactions, rash, and fever—occur much more frequently in patients with AIDS.

PATIENT TEACHING

- Tell patient to take drug as prescribed, even if he feels better.
- Encourage patient to drink plenty of fluids.
- Tell patient to report adverse reactions promptly.
- Instruct patient receiving drug I.V. to report discomfort at I.V. insertion site.
- Advise patient to avoid prolonged sun exposure, wear protective clothing, and use sunscreen.
- Instruct patient to take oral form with 8 ounces (240 ml) of water on an empty stomach.

sulfadiazine

Coptin†

Pharmacologic class: sulfonamide
Pregnancy risk category C

AVAILABLE FORMS

Tablets: 500 mg

INDICATIONS & DOSAGES

➤Asymptomatic meningococcal carrier

Adults: 1 g P.O. q 12 hours for 2 days.
Children ages 1 to 12: 500 mg P.O. q 12 hours for 2 days.
Children ages 2 to 12 months: 500 mg P.O. daily for 2 days.

➤To prevent rheumatic fever, as an alternative to penicillin

Children who weigh more than 30 kg (66 lb): 1 g P.O. daily.
Children who weigh less than 30 kg: 500 mg P.O. daily.

➤Adjunctive treatment for toxoplasmosis

Adults: Initial loading dose, 2 to 4 g P.O.; then a maintenance dose, 2 to 4 g P.O. daily in three to six divided doses. Maximum, 6 g daily. Usually given with pyrimethamine.
Children: Initial loading dose, 75 mg/kg or 2 g/m^2 P.O.; then maintenance dose, 150 mg/kg/day (4 g/m^2/day) P.O. in four to six divided doses. Maximum, 6 g daily. Usually given with pyrimethamine.

➤Nocardiosis

Adults: 4 to 8 g P.O. daily given in divided doses for at least 6 weeks.

ACTION

Inhibits formation of dihydrofolic acid from PABA, decreasing bacterial folic acid synthesis; bacteriostatic.

Route	Onset	Peak	Duration
P.O.	Unknown	4–6 hr	Unknown

Half-life: Adults, 17 hours; children, 24 hours.

ADVERSE REACTIONS

CNS: ***seizures,*** depression, hallucinations, headache.
GI: *diarrhea, nausea, vomiting,* abdominal pain, anorexia, stomatitis.
GU: ***toxic nephrosis with oliguria and anuria,*** crystalluria, hematuria.
Hematologic: ***agranulocytosis, aplastic anemia, leukopenia, thrombocytopenia,*** hemolytic anemia, megaloblastic anemia.
Hepatic: jaundice.
Skin: *generalized skin eruption,* ***erythema multiforme, Stevens-Johnson syndrome, toxic epidermal necrolysis,*** exfoliative

dermatitis, photosensitivity, pruritus, urticaria.
Other: ***anaphylaxis,*** drug fever, hypersensitivity reactions, serum sickness.

INTERACTIONS

Drug-drug. *Cyclosporine:* May decrease cyclosporine level. Monitor cyclosporine level.
Drugs containing PABA: May inhibit antibacterial action. Avoid using together.
Hormonal contraceptives: May decrease contraceptive effectiveness and increase risk of breakthrough bleeding. Advise patient to use a nonhormonal contraceptive.
Methotrexate: May increase methotrexate level. Monitor methotrexate level.
Oral antidiabetics: May increase hypoglycemic effect. Monitor glucose level.
Phenytoin: May increase phenytoin level. Monitor phenytoin level.
Warfarin: May increase anticoagulant effect. Monitor patient for bleeding; monitor PT and INR.
Drug-herb. *Dong quai, St. John's wort:* May cause photosensitivity reaction. Advise patient to avoid excessive sunlight exposure.
Drug-lifestyle. *Sun exposure:* May cause photosensitivity reaction. Advise patient to avoid excessive sunlight exposure.

EFFECTS ON LAB TEST RESULTS

- May increase bilirubin, BUN, creatinine, and transaminase levels. May decrease hemoglobin level.
- May increase eosinophil count. May decrease PT and fibrinogen, granulocyte, platelet, and WBC counts.
- May alter results of urine glucose tests that use cupric sulfate (Benedict reagent or Chemstrip uG).

CONTRAINDICATIONS & CAUTIONS

- Contraindicated in patients hypersensitive to sulfonamides, those with porphyria, infants younger than age 2 months (except in congenital toxoplasmosis), pregnant women at term, and breast-feeding women.
- Use cautiously and in reduced doses in patients with impaired hepatic or renal function, bronchial asthma, history of multiple allergies, G6PD deficiency, and blood dyscrasia.

NURSING CONSIDERATIONS

- Before giving drug, ask patient if he is allergic to sulfa drugs.
- Give drug on schedule to maintain constant level.
- Monitor patient for signs and symptoms of blood dyscrasia (purpura, ecchymoses, sore throat, fever, and pallor) and report to prescriber immediately.
- Promptly report rash, sore throat, fever, cough, mouth sores, or iris lesions—early signs and symptoms of erythema multiforme, which may progress to fatal Stevens-Johnson syndrome.
- Monitor urine cultures, CBCs, and urinalyses before and during therapy.
- Monitor renal and liver function test results.
- Watch for signs and symptoms of superinfection, such as fever, chills, and increased pulse.
- Folic or folinic acid may be used during rest periods in toxoplasmosis therapy to reverse hematopoietic depression or anemia caused by pyrimethamine and sulfadiazine.
- Monitor fluid intake and output. Maintain intake between 3,000 and 4,000 ml daily for adults to produce output of 1,500 ml daily. If fluid intake isn't adequate to prevent crystalluria, sodium bicarbonate may be given to alkalinize urine. Monitor urine pH daily.
- ***Look alike–sound alike:*** Don't confuse sulfadiazine with sulfasalazine. Don't confuse sulfonamide drugs.

PATIENT TEACHING

- Tell patient to take drug as prescribed, even if he feels better.
- Urge patient to drink a glass of water with each dose, plus plenty of water each day to prevent urine crystals.
- Instruct patient to report adverse reactions promptly.
- Warn patient to avoid prolonged exposure to sunlight, wear protective clothing, and use sunscreen.

sulfisoxazole (sulfafurazole, sulphafurazole)

Novo-Soxazole†

sulfisoxazole acetyl

Gantrisin

Pharmacologic class: sulfonamide
Pregnancy risk category C

AVAILABLE FORMS

sulfisoxazole
Tablets: 500 mg
sulfisoxazole acetyl
Liquid: 500 mg/5 ml*

INDICATIONS & DOSAGES

➤UTI, systemic infection
Adults: Initially, 2 to 4 g P.O.; then 4 to 8 g daily divided in four to six doses.
Children older than age 2 months: Initially, 75 mg/kg P.O. daily or 2 g/m^2 P.O.; then 150 mg/kg or 4 g/m^2 P.O. daily in divided doses q 6 hours. Don't exceed total daily dose of 6 g.
Adjust-a-dose: If creatinine clearance is 10 to 50 ml/minute, give normal dose q 8 to 12 hours. If clearance is less than 10 ml/minute, give normal dose q 12 to 24 hours.

ACTION

Inhibits formation of dihydrofolic acid from PABA, decreasing bacterial folic acid synthesis; bacteriostatic.

Route	Onset	Peak	Duration
P.O.	Unknown	1–4 hr	Unknown

Half-life: 4½ to 8 hours.

ADVERSE REACTIONS

CNS: ***seizures,*** depression, dizziness, hallucinations, headache, syncope.
CV: cyanosis, palpitations, tachycardia.
GI: *diarrhea, nausea, vomiting,* ***pseudomembranous colitis,*** abdominal pain, anorexia, stomatitis.
GU: ***acute renal failure, toxic nephrosis with oliguria and anuria,*** crystalluria, hematuria.
Hematologic: ***agranulocytosis, aplastic anemia, leukopenia, thrombocytopenia,*** hemolytic anemia, megaloblastic anemia.
Hepatic: ***hepatitis,*** jaundice.
Skin: *generalized skin eruption,* ***erythema multiforme, toxic epidermal necrolysis,*** exfoliative dermatitis, photosensitivity, pruritus, urticaria.
Other: ***anaphylaxis,*** drug fever, hypersensitivity reactions, serum sickness.

INTERACTIONS

Drug-drug. *Hormonal contraceptives:* May decrease contraceptive effectiveness and increase risk of breakthrough bleeding. Advise patient to use a nonhormonal contraceptive.
Methotrexate: May increase methotrexate level. Monitor methotrexate level.
Oral antidiabetics: May increase hypoglycemic effect. Monitor glucose level.
Warfarin: May increase anticoagulant effect. Monitor patient for bleeding; monitor PT and INR.
Drug-herb. *Dong quai, St. John's wort:* May cause photosensitivity reactions. Advise patient to avoid excessive sunlight exposure.
Drug-lifestyle. *Sun exposure:* May cause photosensitivity reactions. Advise patient to avoid excessive sunlight exposure.

EFFECTS ON LAB TEST RESULTS

- May increase aminotransferase, bilirubin, BUN, and creatinine levels. May decrease hemoglobin level.
- May increase eosinophil count. May decrease PT and fibrinogen, granulocyte, platelet, and WBC counts.
- May alter results of urine glucose tests that use cupric sulfate (Benedict reagent or Chemstrip uG).

CONTRAINDICATIONS & CAUTIONS

- Contraindicated in patients hypersensitive to sulfonamides, infants younger than age 2 months (except in congenital toxoplasmosis), pregnant women at term, and breast-feeding women.
- Use cautiously in patients with impaired hepatic or renal function, severe allergy, bronchial asthma, and G6PD deficiency.

NURSING CONSIDERATIONS

- Before giving drug, ask patient if he is allergic to sulfa drugs.

- Obtain specimen for culture and sensitivity tests before giving first dose. Start therapy, awaiting results.
- Monitor urine cultures, CBC, PT, INR, and urinalyses before and during therapy.
- Monitor renal and liver function test results.
- Report moderate to severe diarrhea to prescriber.
- Watch for signs and symptoms of superinfection, such as fever, chills, and increased pulse.
- Monitor fluid intake and output. Maintain intake between 3,000 and 4,000 ml daily for adults to produce output of 1,500 ml daily. If fluid intake isn't adequate to prevent crystalluria, sodium bicarbonate may be given to alkalinize urine. Monitor urine pH daily.
- ***Look alike–sound alike:*** Don't confuse sulfisoxazole with sulfasalazine. Don't confuse the combination products with sulfisoxazole alone.

PATIENT TEACHING

- Tell patient to take drug as prescribed, even if he feels better.
- Instruct patient to drink a glass of water with each dose, plus plenty of water each day to prevent urine crystals.
- Advise patient to report rash, sore throat, fever, pallor, or yellowed skin or eyes immediately.
- Warn patient to avoid prolonged exposure to sunlight, wear protective clothing, and use sunscreen.

14
Fluoroquinolones

ciprofloxacin
gemifloxacin mesylate
levofloxacin
moxifloxacin hydrochloride
norfloxacin
ofloxacin

ciprofloxacin
Cipro✐, Cipro I.V., Cipro XR, Ciproxin‡, Proquin XR

Pharmacologic class: fluoroquinolone
Pregnancy risk category C

AVAILABLE FORMS
Infusion (premixed): 200 mg in 100 ml D_5W, 400 mg in 200 ml D_5W
Injection: 200 mg, 400 mg
Suspension (oral): 5 g/100 ml (5%), 10 g/100 ml (10%)
Tablets (extended-release, film-coated): 500 mg, 1,000 mg
Tablets (film-coated): 100 mg, 250 mg, 500 mg, 750 mg

INDICATIONS & DOSAGES
➤ **Complicated intra-abdominal infection**
Adults: 500 mg P.O. or 400 mg I.V. q 12 hours for 7 to 14 days. Give with metronidazole.
➤ **Severe or complicated bone or joint infection, severe respiratory tract infection, severe skin or skin-structure infection**
Adults: 750 mg P.O. q 12 hours or 400 mg I.V. q 8 hours.
➤ **Severe or complicated UTI; mild to moderate bone or joint infection; mild to moderate respiratory infection; mild to moderate skin or skin-structure infection; infectious diarrhea; typhoid fever**
Adults: 500 mg P.O. or 400 mg I.V. q 12 hours. Or, 1,000 mg extended-release tablets P.O. q 24 hours.
➤ **Complicated UTI or pyelonephritis**
Children age 1 to 17: 6 to 10 mg/kg I.V. q 8 hours for 10 to 21 days. Maximum I.V. dose, 400 mg. Or, 10 to 20 mg/kg P.O. q 12 hours. Maximum P.O. dose, 750 mg. Don't exceed maximum dose, even in patients who weigh more than 51 kg (112 lbs).
➤ **Nosocomial pneumonia**
Adults: 400 mg I.V. q 8 hours for 10 to 14 days.
➤ **Mild to moderate UTI**
Adults: 250 mg P.O. or 200 mg I.V. q 12 hours for 7 to 14 days.
➤ **Uncomplicated UTI**
Adults: 500 mg extended-release tablet P.O. once daily for 3 days.
➤ **Chronic bacterial prostatitis**
Adults: 500 mg P.O. q 12 hours or 400 mg I.V. q 12 hours for 28 days.
➤ **Acute uncomplicated cystitis**
Adults: 100 mg or 250 mg P.O. q 12 hours for 3 days.
➤ **Mild to moderate acute sinusitis**
Adults: 500 mg P.O. or 400 mg I.V. q 12 hours for 10 days.
➤ **Empirical therapy in febrile neutropenic patients**
Adults: 400 mg I.V. q 8 hours used with piperacillin 50 mg/kg I.V. q 4 hours (not to exceed 24 g/day).
➤ **Inhalation anthrax (postexposure)**
Adults: 400 mg I.V. q 12 hours initially until susceptibility test results are known; then 500 mg P.O. b.i.d. Give drug with one or two additional antimicrobials. Switch to oral therapy when appropriate. Treat for 60 days (I.V. and P.O. combined).
Children: 10 mg/kg I.V. q 12 hours; then 15 mg/kg P.O. q 12 hours. Don't exceed 800 mg/day I.V. or 1,000 mg/day P.O. Give drug with one or two additional antimicrobials. Switch to oral therapy when appropriate. Treat for 60 days (I.V. and P.O. combined).
➤ **Cutaneous anthrax**♦
Adults: 500 mg P.O. b.i.d. for 60 days.

Children: 10 to 15 mg/kg q 12 hours. Don't exceed 1,000 mg/day. Treat for 60 days.

Adjust-a-dose: For patients with a creatinine clearance of 30 to 50 ml/minute, give 250 to 500 mg P.O. q 12 hours or the usual I.V. dose; if clearance is 5 to 29 ml/minute, give 250 to 500 mg P.O. q 18 hours or 200 to 400 mg I.V. q 18 to 24 hours. If patient is receiving hemodialysis, give 250 to 500 mg P.O. q 24 hours after dialysis.

I.V. ADMINISTRATION

- Dilute drug to 1 to 2 mg/ml using D_5W or normal saline solution for injection.
- If giving drug through a Y-type set, stop the other I.V. solution while infusing.
- Infuse over 1 hour into a large vein to minimize discomfort and vein irritation.

INCOMPATIBILITIES

Aminophylline, ampicillin-sulbactam, azithromycin, cefepime, clindamycin phosphate, dexamethasone sodium phosphate, furosemide, heparin sodium, methylprednisolone sodium succinate, phenytoin sodium.

ACTION

Inhibits bacterial DNA synthesis, mainly by blocking DNA gyrase; bactericidal.

Route	Onset	Peak	Duration
P.O.	Unknown	30–120 min	Unknown
P.O. (extended-release)	Unknown	1–4 hr	Unknown
I.V.	Unknown	Immediate	Unknown

Half-life: 4 hours; Cipro XR, 6 hours in adults with normal renal function.

ADVERSE REACTIONS

CNS: ***seizures,*** confusion, depression, dizziness, drowsiness, fatigue, hallucinations, headache, insomnia, lightheadedness, paresthesia, restlessness, tremor.
CV: chest pain, edema, thrombophlebitis.
GI: ***pseudomembranous colitis,*** *diarrhea, nausea,* abdominal pain or discomfort, constipation, dyspepsia, flatulence, oral candidiasis, vomiting.
GU: crystalluria, interstitial nephritis.
Hematologic: ***leukopenia, neutropenia, thrombocytopenia,*** eosinophilia.
Musculoskeletal: aching, arthralgia, arthropathy, joint inflammation, joint or back pain, joint stiffness, neck pain, tendon rupture.
Skin: *rash,* ***Stevens-Johnson syndrome, toxic epidermal necrolysis,*** burning, erythema, exfoliative dermatitis, photosensitivity, pruritus.
Other: hypersensitivity reactions.

INTERACTIONS

Drug-drug. *Aluminum hydroxide, aluminum-magnesium hydroxide, calcium carbonate, didanosine (chewable tablets, buffered tablets, or pediatric powder for oral solution), magnesium hydroxide, products containing zinc:* May decrease ciprofloxacin absorption and effects. Give ciprofloxacin 2 hours before or 6 hours after these drugs.
Cyclosporine: May increase risk for cyclosporine toxicity. Monitor cyclosporine level.
Iron salts: May decrease absorption of ciprofloxacin, reducing anti-infective response. Give at least 2 hours apart.
NSAIDs: May increase risk of CNS stimulation. Monitor patient closely.
Probenecid: May elevate level of ciprofloxacin. Monitor patient for toxicity.
Sucralfate: May decrease ciprofloxacin absorption, reducing anti-infective response. If use together can't be avoided, give at least 6 hours apart.
Theophylline: May increase theophylline level and prolong theophylline half-life. Monitor level of theophylline and watch for adverse effects.
Tizanidine: Increases tizanidine levels, causing low blood pressure, somnolence, dizziness and slowed psychomotor skills. Avoid use together.
Warfarin: May increase anticoagulant effects. Monitor PT and INR closely.
Drug-herb. *Dong quai, St. John's wort:* May cause photosensitivity. Advise patient to avoid excessive sunlight exposure.
Yerba maté: May decrease clearance of herb's methylxanthines and cause toxicity. Discourage use together.
Drug-food. *Caffeine:* May increase effect of caffeine. Monitor patient closely.

Dairy products, other foods: May delay peak drug levels. Advise patient to take drug on an empty stomach.
Orange juice fortified with calcium: May decrease GI absorption of drug, reducing its effects. Advise patient to avoid use together.
Drug-lifestyle. *Sun exposure:* May cause photosensitivity reactions. Advise patient to avoid excessive sunlight exposure.

EFFECTS ON LAB TEST RESULTS

- May increase alkaline phosphatase, ALT, AST, bilirubin, BUN, creatinine, LDH, and GGT levels.
- May increase eosinophil count. May decrease WBC, neutrophil, and platelet counts.

CONTRAINDICATIONS & CAUTIONS

- Contraindicated in patients sensitive to fluoroquinolones.
- Use cautiously in patients with CNS disorders, such as severe cerebral arteriosclerosis or seizure disorders, and in those at risk for seizures. Drug may cause CNS stimulation.
- Drug is associated with increased risk of adverse reactions involving joints, tendons, and surrounding tissues in children younger than age 18.

NURSING CONSIDERATIONS

- Obtain specimen for culture and sensitivity tests before giving first dose. Begin therapy, awaiting results.
- Some drugs require waiting up to 6 hours after giving this drug to avoid decreasing its effects. Food doesn't affect absorption but may delay peak levels.
- Monitor patient's intake and output and observe patient for signs of crystalluria.
- Tendon rupture may occur in patients receiving quinolones. If pain or inflammation occurs or if patient ruptures a tendon, stop drug.
- Long-term therapy may result in overgrowth of organisms resistant to drug.
- Cutaneous anthrax patients with signs of systemic involvement, extensive edema, or lesions on the head or neck need I.V. therapy and a multidrug approach.
- Additional antimicrobials for anthrax multidrug regimens can include rifampin, vancomycin, penicillin, ampicillin, chloramphenicol, imipenem, clindamycin, and clarithromycin.
- Steroids may be used as adjunctive therapy for anthrax patients with severe edema and for meningitis.
- Follow current CDC recommendations for anthrax.
- Pregnant women and immunocompromised patients should receive the usual doses and regimens for anthrax.

PATIENT TEACHING

- Tell patient to take drug as prescribed, even after he feels better.
- Advise patient to drink plenty of fluids to reduce risk of urine crystals.
- Advise patient not to crush, split, or chew the extended-release tablets.
- Warn patient to avoid hazardous tasks that require alertness, such as driving, until effects of drug are known.
- Instruct patient to avoid caffeine while taking drug because of potential for increased caffeine effects.
- Advise patient that hypersensitivity reactions may occur even after first dose. If a rash or other allergic reaction occurs, tell him to stop drug immediately and notify prescriber.
- Tell patient that tendon rupture can occur with drug and to notify prescriber if he experiences pain or inflammation.
- Tell patient to avoid excessive sunlight or artificial ultraviolet light during therapy.
- Because drug appears in breast milk, advise woman to stop breast-feeding during treatment or to consider treatment with another drug.

---

gemifloxacin mesylate
Factive

Pharmacologic class: fluoroquinolone
Pregnancy risk category C

AVAILABLE FORMS

Tablets: 320 mg

INDICATIONS & DOSAGES

➤ **Acute bacterial worsening of chronic bronchitis caused by *Strep-***

tococcus pneumoniae, Haemophilus influenzae, H. parainfluenzae,* or *Moraxella catarrhalis
Adults: 320 mg P.O. once daily for 5 days.

➤ **Mild to moderate community-acquired pneumonia caused by *S. pneumoniae* (including multidrug-resistant strains), *H. influenzae, M. catarrhalis, Mycoplasma pneumoniae, Chlamydia pneumoniae,* or *Klebsiella pneumoniae***
Adults: 320 mg P.O. once daily for 7 days.
Adjust-a-dose: If creatinine clearance is 40 ml/minute or less, or if patient receives routine hemodialysis or continuous ambulatory peritoneal dialysis, reduce dosage to 160 mg P.O. once daily.

ACTION

Prevents cell growth by inhibiting DNA gyrase and topoisomerase IV, which interferes with DNA synthesis.

Route	Onset	Peak	Duration
P.O.	Unknown	½–2 hr	Unknown

Half-life: 4 to 12 hours.

ADVERSE REACTIONS

CNS: headache.
GI: diarrhea, nausea.
Musculoskeletal: ruptured tendons.
Skin: rash.
Other: hypersensitivity reactions.

INTERACTIONS

Drug-drug. *Antacids (magnesium or aluminum), didanosine (chewable tablets, buffered tablets, or pediatric powder for oral solution), ferrous sulfate, multivitamins containing metal cations (such as zinc):* May decrease gemifloxacin level. Give these drugs at least 3 hours before or 2 hours after gemifloxacin.
Antiarrhythmics of class IA (procainamide, quinidine) or class III (amiodarone, sotalol): May increase risk of prolonged QTc interval. Avoid using together.
Antipsychotics, erythromycin, tricyclic antidepressants: May increase risk of prolonged QTc interval. Use together cautiously.
Probenecid: May increase gemifloxacin level. May use with probenecid for this reason.
Sucralfate: May decrease gemifloxacin level. Use together cautiously.
Warfarin: May increase anticoagulation effect. Monitor PT and INR.
Drug-lifestyle. *Sun exposure:* May increase risk of photosensitivity. Advise patient to avoid excessive sunlight exposure.

EFFECTS ON LAB TEST RESULTS

- May increase alkaline phosphatase, ALT, AST, bilirubin, BUN, CK, creatinine, GGT, and potassium levels. May decrease albumin, protein, and sodium levels. May increase or decrease calcium and hemoglobin levels and hematocrit.
- May increase or decrease neutrophil, platelet, and RBC counts.

CONTRAINDICATIONS & CAUTIONS

- Contraindicated in patients hypersensitive to fluoroquinolones, gemifloxacin, or their components.
- Contraindicated in patients with a history of prolonged QTc interval, those with uncorrected electrolyte disorders (such as hypokalemia or hypomagnesemia), and those taking a drug that could prolong the QTc interval.
- Use cautiously in patients with a proarrhythmic condition (such as bradycardia or acute myocardial ischemia), epilepsy, or a predisposition to seizures.
- Safety and effectiveness haven't been established for children younger than age 18.

NURSING CONSIDERATIONS

- Use drug only for infections caused by susceptible bacteria.
- ***Alert:*** Don't exceed recommended dosage because of increased risk of prolonging the QTc interval.
- Mild to moderate maculopapular rash may appear, usually 8 to 10 days after therapy starts. It's more likely in women younger than age 40, especially those taking hormone therapy. Stop drug if rash appears.
- ***Alert:*** Serious, occasionally fatal, hypersensitivity reactions may occur. Stop drug immediately if hypersensitivity reaction occurs.
- Fluoroquinolones may cause tendon rupture, arthropathy, or osteochondrosis; stop drug if patient reports pain or inflammation or ruptures a tendon.

- Stop drug if patient has a photosensitivity reaction.
- Fluoroquinolones may cause CNS effects, such as tremors and anxiety. Monitor patient carefully.
- Serious diarrhea may reflect pseudomembranous colitis; drug may need to be stopped.
- Keep patient adequately hydrated to avoid concentration of urine.

PATIENT TEACHING

- Urge patient to finish full course of treatment, even if symptoms improve.
- Tell patient that drug may be taken with or without food, but that it shouldn't be taken within 3 hours after or 2 hours before an antacid.
- Tell patient to stop drug and seek medical care if evidence of hypersensitivity reaction develops.
- Instruct patient to drink fluids liberally during treatment.
- Warn patient against taking OTC drugs or dietary supplements without consulting his prescriber.
- Tell patient to avoid excessive exposure to sunlight or ultraviolet light.
- Urge patient to report pain, inflammation, or rupture of tendons.
- Warn patient to avoid driving or other hazardous activities until effects of drug are known.

levofloxacin

Levaquin

Pharmacologic class: fluoroquinolone
Pregnancy risk category C

AVAILABLE FORMS

Infusion (premixed): 250 mg in 50 ml D_5W, 500 mg in 100 ml D_5W, 750 mg in 150 ml D_5W
Oral solution: 25 mg/ml
Single-use vials: 500 mg, 750 mg
Tablets: 250 mg, 500 mg, 750 mg

INDICATIONS & DOSAGES

➤**Acute bacterial sinusitis caused by susceptible strains of *Streptococcus pneumoniae, Moraxella catarrhalis,* or *Haemophilus influenzae***
Adults: 500 mg P.O. or I.V. infusion over 60 minutes q 24 hours for 10 to 14 days or 750 mg P.O. q 24 hours for 5 days.

➤**Mild to moderate skin and skin-structure infections caused by *Staphylococcus aureus* or *S. pyogenes***
Adults: 500 mg P.O. or I.V. infusion over 60 minutes q 24 hours for 7 to 10 days.

➤**Acute bacterial worsening of chronic bronchitis caused by *S. aureus, S. pneumoniae, M. catarrhalis, H. influenzae,* or *H. parainfluenzae***
Adults: 500 mg P.O. or I.V. infusion over 60 minutes q 24 hours for 7 days.

➤**Community-acquired pneumonia from *S. pneumoniae* (resistant to two or more of the following antibiotics: penicillin, second-generation cephalosporins, macrolides, trimethoprim-sulfamethoxazole, tetracyclines), *S. aureus, M. catarrhalis, H. influenzae, H. parainfluenzae, Klebsiella pneumoniae, Chlamydia pneumoniae, Legionella pneumophila,* or *Mycoplasma pneumoniae***
Adults: 500 mg P.O. or I.V. infusion over 60 minutes q 24 hours for 7 to 14 days.

➤**To prevent inhalation anthrax after confirmed or suspected exposure to *Bacillus anthracis***
Adults: 500 mg I.V. infusion or P.O. q 24 hours for 60 days.

➤**Chronic bacterial prostatitis caused by *Escherichia coli, Enterococcus faecalis,* or *Staphylococcus epidermidis***
Adults: 500 mg P.O. or I.V. over 60 minutes q 24 hours for 28 days.
Adjust-a-dose: In patients with a creatinine clearance of 20 to 49 ml/minute, give first dose of 500 mg and then 250 mg daily. If clearance is 10 to 19 ml/minute, give first dose of 500 mg and then 250 mg q 48 hours. For patients receiving dialysis or chronic ambulatory peritoneal dialysis, give first dose of 500 mg and then 250 mg q 48 hours. For patients using the 5-day regimen for acute bacterial sinusitis, use the adjust-a-dose schedule for nosocomial pneumonia.

➤**Community-acquired pneumonia from *S. pneumoniae* (excluding multidrug-resistant strains), *H. in-***

fluenzae, H. parainfluenzae, M. pneumoniae,* and *C. pneumoniae
Adults: 750 mg P.O. or I.V. over 90 minutes q 24 hours for 5 days.
➤**Complicated skin and skin-structure infections caused by methicillin-sensitive *S. aureus, E. faecalis, S. pyogenes,* or *Proteus mirabilis***
Adults: 750 mg P.O. or I.V. infusion over 90 minutes q 24 hours for 7 to 14 days.
➤**Nosocomial pneumonia caused by methicillin-susceptible *S. aureus, Pseudomonas aeruginosa, Serratia marcescens, E. coli, K. pneumoniae, H. influenzae,* or *S. pneumoniae***
Adults: 750 mg P.O. or I.V. infusion over 90 minutes q 24 hours for 7 to 14 days.
Adjust-a-dose: If creatinine clearance is 20 to 49 ml/minute, give 750 mg initially and then 750 mg q 48 hours; if clearance is 10 to 19 ml/minute, or patient is receiving hemodialysis or chronic ambulatory peritoneal dialysis, give 750 mg initially and then 500 mg q 48 hours.
➤**Mild to moderate UTI caused by *E. faecalis, Enterobacter cloacae, E. coli, K. pneumoniae, P. mirabilis,* or *P. aeruginosa;* mild to moderate acute pyelonephritis caused by *E. coli***
Adults: 250 mg P.O. or I.V. over 60 minutes q 24 hours for 10 days.
Adjust-a-dose: If creatinine clearance is 10 to 19 ml/minute, increase dosage interval to q 48 hours.
➤**Mild to moderate uncomplicated UTI caused by *E. coli, K. pneumoniae,* or *S. saprophyticus***
Adults: 250 mg P.O. daily for 3 days.
➤**Traveler's diarrhea ♦**
Adults: 500 mg P.O. daily for up to 3 days.
➤**To prevent traveler's diarrhea ♦**
Adults: 500 mg P.O. once daily during period of risk, for up to 3 weeks.
➤**Uncomplicated cervical, urethral, or rectal gonorrhea ♦**
Adults: 250 mg P.O. as a single dose with 1 g azithromycin as a single dose. Or, if chlamydia is ruled out, 100 mg doxycycline P.O. b.i.d. for 7 days.
➤**Disseminated gonococcal infection ♦**
Adults: 250 mg I.V. once daily and continued for 24 to 48 hours after patient starts to improve. Therapy may be switched to 500 mg P.O. daily to complete at least 1 week of therapy.
➤**Nongonococcal urethritis; chlamydia ♦**
Adults: 500 mg P.O. once daily for 7 days.
➤**Acute pelvic inflammatory disease ♦**
Adults: 500 mg I.V. once daily with or without metronidazole 500 mg q 8 hours. Stop parenteral therapy 24 hours after patient improves; then begin doxycycline 100 mg P.O. b.i.d. to complete 14 days of treatment. Or, 500 mg P.O. once daily for 14 days with or without metronidazole 500 mg b.i.d. for 14 days.

I.V. ADMINISTRATION

- Give this form only by infusion.
- Dilute drug in single-use vials, according to manufacturer's instructions, with D_5W or normal saline solution for injection to a final concentration of 5 mg/ml.
- Infuse doses of 500 mg or less over 60 minutes and doses of 750 mg over 90 minutes.
- Reconstituted solution should be clear, slightly yellow, and free of particulate matter.
- Reconstituted drug is stable for 72 hours at room temperature, for 14 days when refrigerated in plastic containers, and for 6 months when frozen.
- Thaw at room temperature or in refrigerator.

INCOMPATIBILITIES

Acyclovir sodium, alprostadil, azithromycin, furosemide, heparin sodium, indomethacin sodium trihydrate, insulin, mannitol 20%, nitroglycerin, propofol, sodium bicarbonate, sodium nitroprusside. The manufacturer recommends not mixing or infusing other drugs with levofloxacin.

ACTION

Inhibits bacterial DNA gyrase and prevents DNA replication, transcription, repair, and recombination in susceptible bacteria.

Route	Onset	Peak	Duration
P.O., I.V.	Unknown	1–2 hr	Unknown

Half-life: About 6 to 8 hours.

ADVERSE REACTIONS

CNS: ***encephalopathy, seizures,*** dizziness, headache, insomnia, pain, paresthesia.
CV: chest pain, palpitations, vasodilation.
GI: ***pseudomembranous colitis,*** abdominal pain, constipation, diarrhea, dyspepsia, flatulence, nausea, vomiting.
GU: vaginitis.
Hematologic: ***lymphopenia,*** eosinophilia, hemolytic anemia.
Metabolic: ***hypoglycemia.***
Musculoskeletal: back pain, tendon rupture.
Respiratory: allergic pneumonitis.
Skin: ***erythema multiforme, Stevens-Johnson syndrome,*** photosensitivity, pruritus, rash.
Other: ***anaphylaxis, multisystem organ failure,*** hypersensitivity reactions.

INTERACTIONS

Drug-drug. *Aluminum hydroxide, aluminum–magnesium hydroxide, calcium carbonate, didanosine, magnesium hydroxide, products containing zinc, sucralfate:* May interfere with GI absorption of levofloxacin. Give levofloxacin 2 hours before or 6 hours after these products.
Antidiabetics: May alter glucose level. Monitor glucose level closely.
Iron salts: May decrease absorption of levofloxacin, reducing anti-infective response. Separate doses by at least 2 hours.
NSAIDs: May increase CNS stimulation. Monitor patient for seizure activity.
Theophylline: May decrease clearance of theophylline. Monitor theophylline level.
Warfarin and derivatives: May increase effect of oral anticoagulant. Monitor PT and INR.
Drug-herb. *Dong quai, St. John's wort:* May cause photosensitivity reactions. Advise patient to avoid excessive sunlight exposure.
Drug-lifestyle. *Sun exposure:* May cause photosensitivity reactions. Advise patient to avoid excessive sunlight exposure.

EFFECTS ON LAB TEST RESULTS

- May decrease glucose and hemoglobin levels.
- May increase eosinophil count. May decrease WBC count.
- May produce false-positive opiate assay results.

CONTRAINDICATIONS & CAUTIONS

- Contraindicated in patients hypersensitive to drug, its components, or other fluoroquinolones.
- Use cautiously in patients with history of seizure disorders or other CNS diseases, such as cerebral arteriosclerosis.
- Use cautiously and with dosage adjustment in patients with renal impairment.
- Safety and effectiveness of drug in children younger than age 18 and in pregnant and breast-feeding women haven't been established.

NURSING CONSIDERATIONS

- If patient experiences symptoms of excessive CNS stimulation (restlessness, tremor, confusion, hallucinations), stop drug and notify prescriber. Begin seizure precautions.
- Patients with acute hypersensitivity reactions may need treatment with epinephrine, oxygen, I.V. fluids, antihistamines, corticosteroids, pressor amines, and airway management.
- Most antibacterials can cause pseudomembranous colitis. If diarrhea occurs, notify prescriber; drug may be stopped.
- Drug may cause an abnormal ECG.
- Obtain specimen for culture and sensitivity tests before therapy and as needed to determine if bacterial resistance has occurred.
- ***Alert:*** If *P. aeruginosa* is a confirmed or suspected pathogen, use with a beta-lactam.
- Monitor glucose level and renal, hepatic, and hematopoietic blood studies.

PATIENT TEACHING

- Tell patient to take drug as prescribed, even if signs and symptoms disappear.
- Advise patient to take drug with plenty of fluids and to space antacids, sucralfate, and products containing iron or zinc.
- Tell patient to take oral solution 1 hour before or 2 hours after eating.
- Warn patient to avoid hazardous tasks until adverse effects of drug are known.
- Advise patient to avoid excessive sunlight, use sunscreen, and wear protective clothing when outdoors.

- Instruct patient to stop drug and notify prescriber if rash or other signs or symptoms of hypersensitivity develop.
- Tell patient that tendon rupture may occur with drug and to notify prescriber if he experiences pain or inflammation.
- Instruct diabetic patient to monitor glucose level and notify prescriber about low-glucose reaction.
- Instruct patient to notify prescriber of loose stools or diarrhea.

moxifloxacin hydrochloride

Avelox, Avelox I.V.

Pharmacologic class: fluoroquinolone
Pregnancy risk category C

AVAILABLE FORMS

Injection: 400 mg/250 ml
Tablets (film-coated): 400 mg

INDICATIONS & DOSAGES

➤**Acute bacterial sinusitis caused by *Streptococcus pneumoniae, Haemophilus influenzae,* or *Moraxella catarrhalis***
Adults: 400 mg P.O. or I.V. q 24 hours for 10 days.

➤**Complicated skin and skin structure infections caused by methicillin-susceptible *Staphylococcus aureus, Escherichia coli, Klebsiella pneumoniae,* or *Enterobacter cloacae***
Adults: 400 mg P.O. or I.V. q 24 hours for 7 to 21 days.

➤**Complicated intra-abdominal infection caused by *E. coli, Bacteroides fragilis, Streptococcus anginosis, Streptococcus constellatus, Enterococcus faecalis, Proteus mirabilis, Clostridium perfringens, Bacteroides thetaiotaomicron,* or *Peptostreptococcus species***
Adults: 400 mg P.O. or I.V. every 24 hours for 5 to 14 days. Start with the I.V. form; switch to P.O. when appropriate.

➤**Community-acquired pneumonia from multidrug-resistant *S. pneumoniae* (resistance to two or more of the following antibiotics: penicillin, second-generation cephalosporins, macrolides, trimethoprim-sulfamethoxazole, tetracyclines), *S. aureus, M. catarrhalis, H. influenzae, H. parainfluenzae, K. pneumoniae, Chlamydia pneumoniae, Legionella pneumophila,* or *Mycoplasma pneumoniae***
Adults: 400 mg P.O. or I.V. q 24 hours for 7 to 14 days.

➤**Acute bacterial worsening of chronic bronchitis caused by *S. pneumoniae, H. influenzae, H. parainfluenzae, K. pneumoniae, S. aureus,* or *M. catarrhalis***
Adults: 400 mg P.O. or I.V. q 24 hours for 5 days.

➤**Uncomplicated skin-structure or skin infection caused by *S. aureus* or *S. pyogenes***
Adults: 400 mg P.O. or I.V. q 24 hours for 7 days.

I.V. ADMINISTRATION

- Don't use if particulate matter is visible.
- Flush I.V. line with a compatible solution such as D_5W, normal saline, or Ringer lactate solution before and after use.
- Give only by infusion over 1 hour. Avoid rapid or bolus infusion.

INCOMPATIBILITIES

Other I.V. drugs.

ACTION

Interferes with action of enzymes needed for bacterial replication. Inhibits topoisomerases I (DNA gyrase) and IV, impairing bacterial DNA replication, transcription, repair, and recombination.

Route	Onset	Peak	Duration
P.O., I.V.	Unknown	1–3 hr	Unknown

Half-life: About 12 hours.

ADVERSE REACTIONS

CNS: dizziness, headache, asthenia, pain, malaise, insomnia, nervousness, anxiety, confusion, somnolence, tremor, vertigo, paresthesia.
CV: ***prolonged QT interval,*** chest pain, hypertension, palpitations, peripheral edema, tachycardia.
GI: ***pseudomembranous colitis,*** abdominal pain, anorexia, constipation, diarrhea,

dyspepsia, dry mouth, flatulence, GI disorder, glossitis, nausea, oral candidiasis, stomatitis, taste perversion, vomiting.
GU: vaginal candidiasis, vaginitis.
Hematologic: ***leukopenia, thrombocytopenia, thrombocytosis,*** eosinophilia.
Hepatic: abnormal liver function, cholestatic jaundice.
Musculoskeletal: arthralgia, back pain, leg pain, myalgia, tendon rupture.
Respiratory: dyspnea.
Skin: injection site reaction, pruritus, rash (maculopapular, purpuric, pustular), sweating.
Other: allergic reaction, candidiasis.

INTERACTIONS

Drug-drug. *Aluminum hydroxide, aluminum-magnesium hydroxide, calcium carbonate, didanosine, magnesium hydroxide, multivitamins, products containing zinc:* May interfere with GI absorption of moxifloxacin. Give moxifloxacin 4 hours before or 8 hours after these products.
Class IA antiarrhythmics (such as procainamide, quinidine), class III antiarrhythmics (such as amiodarone, sotalol): May increase risk of cardiac arrhythmias. Avoid using together.
Drugs that prolong QT interval, such as antipsychotics, erythromycin, tricyclic antidepressants: May have additive effect. Avoid using together.
NSAIDs: May increase risk of CNS stimulation and seizures. Avoid using together.
Sucralfate: May decrease absorption of moxifloxacin, reducing anti-infective response. If use together can't be avoided, give at least 6 hours apart.
Warfarin: May increase anticoagulant effects. Monitor PT and INR closely.
Drug-lifestyle. *Sun exposure:* May cause photosensitivity reactions. Advise patient to avoid excessive sunlight exposure.

EFFECTS ON LAB TEST RESULTS

- May increase GGT, amylase, and LDH levels. May decrease hemoglobin level.
- May increase eosinophil count. May decrease PT and WBC count. May increase or decrease platelet count.

CONTRAINDICATIONS & CAUTIONS

- Contraindicated in patients hypersensitive to drug or other fluoroquinolones and in those with prolonged QT interval or uncorrected hypokalemia.
- Use cautiously in patients with ongoing proarrhythmic conditions, such as clinically significant bradycardia or acute myocardial ischemia.
- Use cautiously in patients who may have CNS disorders and in those with other risk factors that may lower the seizure threshold or predispose them to seizures.
- Safety and effectiveness in children, adolescents younger than age 18, and pregnant or breast-feeding women haven't been established.

NURSING CONSIDERATIONS

- Drug may be given without regard to meals. Give at same time each day.
- ***Alert:*** Monitor patient for adverse CNS effects, including seizures, dizziness, confusion, tremors, hallucinations, depression, and suicidal thoughts. If these occur, stop drug and notify prescriber.
- Monitor patient for hypersensitivity reactions, including anaphylaxis.
- If diarrhea develops during therapy, send stool specimen for *Clostridium difficile* test.
- Rupture of the Achilles and other tendons is linked to fluoroquinolone use. If pain, inflammation, or tendon rupture occurs, stop drug and notify prescriber.
- Store drug at controlled room temperature.

PATIENT TEACHING

- Instruct patient to take drug once daily, at the same time each day, without regard to meals.
- Tell patient to finish entire course of therapy, even if symptoms are relieved.
- Advise patient to drink plenty of fluids.
- Tell patient to space antacids, sucralfate, multivitamins, and products containing aluminum, magnesium, iron, and zinc to avoid decreasing drug's therapeutic effects.
- Instruct patient to contact prescriber and stop drug if he experiences allergic reaction, rash, heart palpitations, fainting, or persistent diarrhea.

• Direct patient to contact prescriber, stop drug, rest, and refrain from exercise if he experiences pain, inflammation, or tendon rupture.
• Warn patient that drug may cause dizziness and light-headedness. Tell patient to avoid hazardous activities, such as driving or operating machinery, until effects of drug are known.
• Instruct patient to avoid excessive sunlight exposure and ultraviolet light and to report photosensitivity reactions to prescriber.

norfloxacin
Noroxin

Pharmacologic class: fluoroquinolone
Pregnancy risk category C

AVAILABLE FORMS
Tablets (film-coated): 400 mg

INDICATIONS & DOSAGES
➤ **Complicated or uncomplicated UTI from susceptible strains of *Enterococcus faecalis, Escherichia coli, E. cloacae, Klebsiella pneumoniae, Enterobacter aerogenes, Proteus mirabilis, P. vulgaris, Pseudomonas aeruginosa, Citrobacter freundii, Staphylococcus agalactiae, S. aureus, S. epidermidis, S. saprophyticus,* or *Serratia marcescens***
Adults: 400 mg P.O. q 12 hours for 7 to 10 days (uncomplicated infection). Or, 400 mg P.O. q 12 hours for 10 to 21 days (complicated infection).
➤ **Prostatitis**
Adults: 400 mg P.O. q 12 hours for 28 days.
➤ **Cystitis caused by *E. coli, K. pneumoniae,* or *P. mirabilis***
Adults: 400 mg P.O. q 12 hours for 3 days.
Adjust-a-dose: If creatinine clearance is 30 ml/minute or less, give 400 mg once daily for above indications.
➤ **Acute, uncomplicated urethral and cervical gonorrhea**
Adults: 800 mg P.O. as a single dose, then doxycycline therapy to treat any coexisting chlamydial infection.

ACTION
Inhibits bacterial DNA synthesis, mainly by blocking DNA gyrase; bactericidal.

Route	Onset	Peak	Duration
P.O.	Unknown	15–120 min	Unknown

Half-life: 3 to 4 hours.

ADVERSE REACTIONS
CNS: ***seizures,*** depression, dizziness, fatigue, fever, headache, insomnia, somnolence.
GI: ***pseudomembranous colitis,*** abdominal pain, anorexia, constipation, dry mouth, diarrhea, flatulence, heartburn, nausea, vomiting.
GU: crystalluria.
Hematologic: ***leukopenia, neutropenia, thrombocytopenia,*** eosinophilia.
Musculoskeletal: back pain.
Skin: hyperhidrosis, photosensitivity, rash.
Other: ***anaphylaxis,*** hypersensitivity reactions.

INTERACTIONS
Drug-drug. *Aluminum hydroxide, calcium carbonate, aluminum–magnesium hydroxide, magnesium hydroxide:* May decrease norfloxacin level. Give antacid at least 6 hours before or 2 hours after norfloxacin.
Iron salts: May decrease absorption of norfloxacin, reducing anti-infective response. Give at least 2 hours apart.
Cyclosporine: May increase cyclosporine level. Monitor cyclosporine level.
Nitrofurantoin: May antagonize norfloxacin effect. Monitor patient closely.
Oral anticoagulants: May increase anticoagulant effect. Monitor PT and INR.
Probenecid: May increase norfloxacin level by decreasing its excretion. May give probenecid for this reason, but monitor high-risk patient for toxicity.
Sucralfate: May decrease absorption of norfloxacin, reducing anti-infective response. If use together can't be avoided, give at least 6 hours apart.
Theophylline: May impair theophylline metabolism, increasing drug level and risk of toxicity. Monitor patient closely.
Drug-herb. *Dong quai, St. John's wort:* May cause photosensitivity reactions. Ad-

vise patient to avoid excessive sunlight exposure.

EFFECTS ON LAB TEST RESULTS
- May increase BUN, creatinine, ALT, AST, and alkaline phosphatase levels. May decrease hematocrit.
- May increase eosinophil count. May decrease neutrophil count.

CONTRAINDICATIONS & CAUTIONS
- Contraindicated in patients hypersensitive to drug or other fluoroquinolones.
- Use cautiously in patients with conditions such as cerebral arteriosclerosis who may be predisposed to seizure disorders.
- Use cautiously and monitor renal function in those with renal impairment.
- Safety in children younger than age 18 hasn't been established.

NURSING CONSIDERATIONS
- Obtain specimen for culture and sensitivity testing before starting therapy.
- Tendon rupture may occur in patients receiving quinolones. Stop drug if pain or inflammation occurs or tendon ruptures.
- Monitor patient for adverse CNS effects, including dizziness, headache, seizures, or depression. Stop drug and notify prescriber if these effects occur.
- Monitor patient for hypersensitivity reactions. Stop drug and initiate supportive therapy as indicated.
- ***Look alike–sound alike:*** Don't confuse Noroxin with Neurontin or Floxin.

PATIENT TEACHING
- Tell patient to take drug as prescribed, even after he feels better.
- Advise patient to take drug 1 hour before or 2 hours after meals because food may hinder absorption.
- Advise patient to appropriately space iron products and antacids when taking norfloxacin.
- Warn patient not to exceed the recommended dosages and to drink several glasses of water throughout the day to maintain hydration and adequate urine output.
- Warn patient to avoid hazardous tasks that require alertness until effects of drug are known.
- Instruct patient to avoid exposure to sunlight, wear protective clothing, and use sunscreen while outdoors.
- Tell patient to report pain, inflammation, or tendon rupture, and to refrain from exercise until diagnosis of rupture or tendinitis is excluded.

ofloxacin

Floxin

Pharmacologic class: fluoroquinolone
Pregnancy risk category C

AVAILABLE FORMS
Tablets: 200 mg, 300 mg, 400 mg

INDICATIONS & DOSAGES

➤ **Acute bacterial worsening of chronic bronchitis, uncomplicated skin and skin-structure infections, and community-acquired pneumonia**
Adults: 400 mg P.O. q 12 hours for 10 days.

➤ **Sexually transmitted infections, such as acute uncomplicated urethral and cervical gonorrhea, nongonococcal urethritis and cervicitis, and mixed infections of urethra and cervix**
Adults: For acute uncomplicated gonorrhea, 400 mg P.O. once as a single dose; for cervicitis and urethritis, 300 mg P.O. q 12 hours for 7 days.

➤ **Cystitis from *Escherichia coli, Klebsiella pneumoniae,* or other organisms**
Adults: 200 mg P.O. q 12 hours for 3 days (*E. coli* or *K. pneumoniae*), 200 mg P.O. q 12 hours for 7 days (other organisms).

➤ **Complicated UTI**
Adults: 200 mg P.O. q 12 hours for 10 days.

➤ **Prostatitis**
Adults: 300 mg P.O. q 12 hours for 6 weeks.

➤ **Pelvic inflammatory disease**
Adults: 400 mg P.O. q 12 hours with metronidazole for 10 to 14 days.

➤ **To prevent inhalation anthrax ♦**
Adults: 400 mg P.O. b.i.d. Continue therapy for 60 days if no vaccine is available.

If vaccine is available, continue for 28 to 45 days and until three doses of the vaccine have been given.

➤ **Traveler's diarrhea**

Adults: 300 mg P.O. b.i.d. for 3 days.

Adjust-a-dose: For patients with creatinine clearance less than 20 ml/minute, give first dose as recommended; then give subsequent doses at 50% of recommended dose q 24 hours. For patients with hepatic impairment, don't exceed 400 mg/day.

ACTION

Interferes with DNA gyrase, which is needed for synthesis of bacterial DNA. Spectrum of action includes many gram-positive and gram-negative aerobic bacteria, including *Enterobacteriaceae* and *Pseudomonas aeruginosa.*

Route	Onset	Peak	Duration
P.O.	Unknown	15–120 min	Unknown

Half-life: 4 to 7½ hours.

ADVERSE REACTIONS

CNS: ***seizures,*** dizziness, drowsiness, fatigue, fever, headache, insomnia, lethargy, malaise, nervousness, sleep disorders, visual disturbances.
CV: chest pain, phlebitis.
GI: *nausea,* ***pseudomembranous colitis,*** abdominal pain or discomfort, anorexia, constipation, diarrhea, dry mouth, dysgeusia, flatulence, vomiting.
GU: genital pruritus, glucosuria, hematuria, proteinuria, vaginal discharge, vaginitis.
Hematologic: ***leukopenia, neutropenia,*** anemia, eosinophilia, leukocytosis.
Metabolic: ***hypoglycemia,*** hyperglycemia.
Musculoskeletal: body pain, tendon rupture.
Skin: photosensitivity, pruritus, rash.
Other: ***anaphylactoid reaction,*** hypersensitivity reactions.

INTERACTIONS

Drug-drug. *Aluminum hydroxide, calcium carbonate, aluminum–magnesium hydroxide, magnesium hydroxide:* May decrease effects of ofloxacin. Give antacid at least 6 hours before or 2 hours after ofloxacin.
Antidiabetics: May affect glucose level, causing hypoglycemia or hyperglycemia. Monitor patient closely.
Didanosine (chewable or buffered tablets or pediatric powder for oral solution): May interfere with GI absorption of ofloxacin. Separate doses by 2 hours.
Iron salts: May decrease absorption of ofloxacin, reducing anti-infective response. Separate doses by at least 2 hours.
Sucralfate: May decrease absorption of ofloxacin, reducing anti-infective response. If use together can't be avoided, separate doses by at least 6 hours.
Theophylline: May increase theophylline level. Monitor patient closely and adjust theophylline dosage as needed.
Warfarin: May prolong PT and INR. Monitor PT and INR.
Drug-lifestyle. *Sun exposure:* May cause photosensitivity reactions. Advise patient to avoid excessive sunlight exposure.

EFFECTS ON LAB TEST RESULTS

- May increase BUN, creatinine, and liver enzyme levels. May decrease hemoglobin level and hematocrit. May increase or decrease glucose level.
- May increase erythrocyte sedimentation rate and eosinophil count. May decrease neutrophil count. May increase or decrease WBC count.
- May produce false-positive opiate assay results.

CONTRAINDICATIONS & CAUTIONS

- Contraindicated in patients hypersensitive to drug or other fluoroquinolones.
- Use cautiously in pregnant patients and in those with seizure disorders, CNS diseases such as cerebral arteriosclerosis, hepatic disorders, or renal impairment.
- Ofloxacin appears in breast milk in levels similar to those found in plasma. Safety hasn't been established in breast-feeding women.
- Safety and efficacy in children younger than age 18 haven't been established.

NURSING CONSIDERATIONS

- ***Alert:*** Patients treated for gonorrhea should be tested for syphilis. Drug isn't effective against syphilis, and treating

gonorrhea may mask or delay syphilis symptoms.
- Periodically assess organ system functions during prolonged therapy.
- Monitor patient for overgrowth of nonsusceptible organisms.
- Monitor renal and hepatic studies and CBC in prolonged therapy.
- Monitor patient for adverse CNS effects, including dizziness, headache, seizures, or depression. Stop drug and notify prescriber if these effects occur.
- Monitor patient for hypersensitivity reactions. Stop drug and initiate supportive therapy, as indicated.

PATIENT TEACHING
- Tell patient to drink plenty of fluids during drug therapy and to finish the entire prescription even if he starts feeling better.
- Tell patient drug may be taken without regard to meals, but he shouldn't take antacids and vitamins at the same time as ofloxacin.
- Warn patient that dizziness and lightheadedness may occur. Advise caution when driving or operating hazardous machinery until effects of drug are known.
- Warn patient that hypersensitivity reactions may follow first dose; he should stop drug at first sign of rash or other allergic reaction and call prescriber immediately.
- Advise patient to avoid prolonged exposure to direct sunlight and to use a sunscreen when outdoors.

15

Antivirals

abacavir sulfate
acyclovir
acyclovir sodium
adefovir dipivoxil
amantadine hydrochloride
(See Chapter 33 ANTIPARKINSONIANS.)
amprenavir
atazanavir sulfate
cidofovir
darunavir ethanolate
delavirdine mesylate
didanosine
efavirenz
emtricitabine
enfuvirtide
entecavir
famciclovir
fosamprenavir calcium
foscarnet sodium
ganciclovir
indinavir sulfate
lamivudine
lopinavir and ritonavir
nelfinavir mesylate
nevirapine
oseltamivir phosphate
ribavirin
ritonavir
saquinavir mesylate
stavudine
tenofovir disoproxil fumarate
tipranavir
valacyclovir hydrochloride
valganciclovir
zanamivir
zidovudine

abacavir sulfate

Ziagen

Pharmacologic class: nucleoside reverse transcriptase inhibitor
Pregnancy risk category C

AVAILABLE FORMS

Oral solution: 20 mg/ml
Tablets: 300 mg

INDICATIONS & DOSAGES

➤ HIV-1 infection

Adults: 300 mg P.O. b.i.d. with other antiretrovirals.
Children ages 3 months to 16 years: 8 mg/kg P.O. b.i.d., up to maximum of 300 mg P.O. b.i.d., with other antiretrovirals.

ACTION

Converted intracellularly to the active metabolite carbovir triphosphate, which inhibits activity of HIV-1 reverse transcriptase, terminating viral DNA growth.

Route	Onset	Peak	Duration
P.O.	Unknown	Unknown	Unknown

Half-life: 1 to 2 hours.

ADVERSE REACTIONS

CNS: fever, headache, insomnia and sleep disorders.
GI: *anorexia, diarrhea, nausea, vomiting.*
Skin: rash.
Other: ***hypersensitivity reaction.***

INTERACTIONS

Drug-lifestyle. *Alcohol use:* May decrease elimination of drug, increasing overall exposure. Monitor alcohol consumption. Discourage use together.

EFFECTS ON LAB TEST RESULTS

- May increase GGT, glucose, and triglyceride levels.

CONTRAINDICATIONS & CAUTIONS

- Contraindicated in patients hypersensitive to drug or its components.
- Use cautiously when giving drug to patients at risk for liver disease. Lactic acidosis and severe hepatomegaly with steatosis, including fatal cases, have been reported with the use of nucleoside analogues alone or in combination, including abacavir and other antiretrovirals. Stop treatment with drug if events occur.
- Use cautiously in pregnant women because the effects are unknown. Use dur-

ing pregnancy only if the potential benefits outweigh the risk. Register pregnant women with the Antiretroviral Pregnancy Registry at 1-800-258-4263.

NURSING CONSIDERATIONS

- Women are more likely than men to experience lactic acidosis and severe hepatomegaly with steatosis. Obesity and prolonged nucleoside exposure may be risk factors.
- ***Alert:*** Drug can cause fatal hypersensitivity reactions; if patient develops signs or symptoms of hypersensitivity (such as fever, rash, fatigue, nausea, vomiting, diarrhea, or abdominal pain), stop drug and notify prescriber immediately.
- ***Alert:*** Don't restart drug after a hypersensitivity reaction because severe signs and symptoms will recur within hours and may include life-threatening hypotension and death. To facilitate reporting of hypersensitivity reactions, register patients with the Abacavir Hypersensitivity Reaction Registry at 1-800-270-0425.
- Always give drug with other antiretrovirals, never alone.
- Because of a high rate of early virologic resistance, triple antiretroviral therapy with abacavir, lamivudine, and tenofovir shouldn't be used as new treatment regimen for naïve or pretreated patients. Monitor patients currently controlled with this combination and those who use this combination in addition to other antiretrovirals, and consider modification of therapy.
- Drug may mildly elevate glucose level.
- ***Look alike–sound alike:*** Don't confuse abacavir with amprenavir.

PATIENT TEACHING

- Inform patient that drug can cause a life-threatening hypersensitivity reaction. Warn patient who develops signs or symptoms of hypersensitivity (such as fever, rash, severe tiredness, achiness, a generally ill feeling, nausea, vomiting, diarrhea, or stomach pain) to stop taking drug and notify prescriber immediately.
- Include information leaflet about drug with each new prescription and refill. Patient also should receive, and be instructed to carry, a warning card summarizing signs and symptoms of hypersensitivity reaction.
- Inform patient that this drug doesn't cure HIV infection. Tell patient that drug doesn't reduce the risk of transmission of HIV to others through sexual contact or blood contamination and that its long-term effects are unknown.
- Tell patient to take drug exactly as prescribed.
- Inform patient that drug can be taken with or without food.

---

acyclovir
Acihexal‡, Acyclo-V‡, Avirax†, Lovir‡, Zovirax

acyclovir sodium
Aciclovir‡, Acihexal‡, Avirax†, Zovirax🖉

Pharmacologic class: synthetic purine nucleoside
Pregnancy risk category B

AVAILABLE FORMS

Capsules: 200 mg
Injection: 500 mg/vial, 1 g/vial
Suspension: 200 mg/5 ml
Tablets: 400 mg, 800 mg

INDICATIONS & DOSAGES

➤ **First and recurrent episodes of mucocutaneous herpes simplex virus (HSV-1 and HSV-2) infections in immunocompromised patients; severe first episodes of genital herpes in patients who aren't immunocompromised**
Adults and children age 12 and older: 5 mg/kg given I.V. over 1 hour q 8 hours for 7 days. Give for 5 to 7 days for severe first episode of genital herpes.
Children younger than age 12: 10 mg/kg given I.V. over 1 hour q 8 hours for 7 days.

➤ **First genital herpes episode**
Adults: 200 mg P.O. q 4 hours while awake, five times daily; or 400 mg P.O. q 8 hours. Continue for 7 to 10 days.

➤ **Intermittent therapy for recurrent genital herpes**
Adults: 200 mg P.O. q 4 hours while awake, five times daily. Continue for

5 days. Begin therapy at first sign of recurrence.

➤ **Long-term suppressive therapy for recurrent genital herpes**
Adults: 400 mg P.O. b.i.d. for up to 12 months. Or, 200 mg P.O. three to five times daily for up to 12 months.

➤ **Varicella (chickenpox) infections in immunocompromised patients**
Adults and children age 12 and older: 10 mg/kg I.V. over 1 hour q 8 hours for 7 days. Dosage for obese patients is 10 mg/kg based on ideal body weight q 8 hours for 7 days. Don't exceed maximum dosage equivalent of 20 mg/kg q 8 hours.
Children younger than age 12: 20 mg/kg I.V. over 1 hour q 8 hours for 7 days.

➤ **Varicella infection in immunocompetent patients**
Adults and children who weigh more than 40 kg (88 lb): 800 mg P.O. q.i.d. for 5 days.
Children age 2 and older, who weigh less than 40 kg: 20 mg/kg (maximum 800 mg/dose) P.O. q.i.d. for 5 days. Start therapy as soon as symptoms appear.

➤ **Acute herpes zoster infection in immunocompetent patients**
Adults and children age 12 and older: 800 mg P.O. q 4 hours five times daily for 7 to 10 days.

➤ **Herpes simplex encephalitis**
Adults and children age 12 and older: 10 mg/kg I.V. over 1 hour q 8 hours for 10 days.
Children ages 3 months to 12 years: 20 mg/kg I.V. over 1 hour q 8 hours for 10 days.

➤ **Neonatal herpes simplex virus infection**
Neonates to 3 months old: 10 mg/kg I.V. over 1 hour q 8 hours for 10 days.

Adjust-a-dose: For patients receiving the I.V. form, if creatinine clearance is 25 to 50 ml/minute, give 100% of dose q 12 hours; if clearance is 10 to 24 ml/minute, give 100% of dose q 24 hours; if clearance is less than 10 ml/minute, give 50% of dose q 24 hours.

For patients receiving the P.O. form, if normal dose is 200 mg q 4 hours five times daily and creatinine clearance is less than 10 ml/minute, give 200 mg P.O. q 12 hours. If normal dose is 400 mg q 12 hours and clearance is less than 10 ml/minute, give 200 mg q 12 hours. If normal dose is 800 mg q 4 hours five times daily and clearance is 10 to 25 ml/minute, give 800 mg q 8 hours; if clearance is less than 10 ml/minute, give 800 mg q 12 hours.

I.V. ADMINISTRATION

- Solutions concentrated at 7 mg/ml or more may cause a higher risk of phlebitis.
- Encourage fluid intake because patient must be adequately hydrated during infusion.
- Bolus injection, dehydration (decreased urine output), renal disease, and use with other nephrotoxic drugs increase the risk of renal toxicity. Don't give by bolus injection.
- Give I.V. infusion over at least 1 hour to prevent renal tubular damage.
- Monitor intake and output, especially during the first 2 hours after administration.

INCOMPATIBILITIES

Amifostine, aztreonam, biological or colloidal solutions, cefepime, cisatracurium besylate, diltiazem hydrochloride, dobutamine hydrochloride, dopamine hydrochloride, fludarabine phosphate, foscarnet sodium, gemcitabine hydrochloride, idarubicin hydrochloride, levofloxacin, meperidine hydrochloride, meropenem, morphine sulfate, ondansetron hydrochloride, parabens, piperacillin sodium and tazobactam sodium, sargramostim, tacrolimus, vinorelbine tartrate.

ACTION

Interferes with DNA synthesis and inhibits viral multiplication.

Route	Onset	Peak	Duration
P.O.	Unknown	2½ hr	Unknown
I.V.	Immediate	Immediate	Unknown

Half-life: 2 to 3½ hours with normal renal function; up to 19 hours with renal impairment.

ADVERSE REACTIONS

CNS: *headache, malaise,* ***encephalopathic changes (including lethargy, ob-***

tundation, tremor, confusion, hallucinations, agitation, seizures, coma).
GI: *nausea, vomiting,* diarrhea.
GU: ***acute renal failure,*** hematuria.
Hematologic: ***leukopenia, thrombocytopenia,*** thrombocytosis.
Skin: *inflammation or phlebitis at injection site,* itching, rash, urticaria.

INTERACTIONS
Drug-drug. *Interferon:* May have synergistic effect. Monitor patient closely.
Probenecid: May increase acyclovir level. Monitor patient for possible toxicity.
Zidovudine: May cause drowsiness or lethargy. Use together cautiously.

EFFECTS ON LAB TEST RESULTS
- May increase BUN and creatinine levels.
- May decrease WBC count. May increase or decrease platelet count.

CONTRAINDICATIONS & CAUTIONS
- Contraindicated in patients hypersensitive to drug.
- Use cautiously in patients with neurologic problems, renal disease, or dehydration, and in those receiving other nephrotoxic drugs.
- Adequate studies haven't been done in pregnant women; use only if potential benefits outweigh risks to fetus.

NURSING CONSIDERATIONS
- ***Alert:*** Don't give I.M. or subcutaneously.
- In patients with renal disease or dehydration and in those taking other nephrotoxic drugs, monitor renal function.
- Encephalopathic changes are more likely to occur in patients with neurologic disorders and in those who have had neurologic reactions to cytotoxic drugs.
- ***Look alike–sound alike:*** Don't confuse acyclovir sodium (Zovirax) with acetazolamide sodium (Diamox) vials, which may look alike.
- ***Look alike–sound alike:*** Don't confuse Zovirax with Zyvox.

PATIENT TEACHING
- Tell patient to take drug as prescribed, even after he feels better.
- Tell patient drug is effective in managing herpes infection but doesn't eliminate or cure it. Warn patient that drug won't prevent spread of infection to others.
- Tell patient to avoid sexual contact while visible lesions are present.
- Teach patient about early signs and symptoms of herpes infection (such as tingling, itching, or pain). Tell him to notify prescriber and get a prescription for drug before the infection fully develops. Early treatment is most effective.

adefovir dipivoxil
Hepsera

Pharmacologic class: acyclic nucleotide analog
Pregnancy risk category C

AVAILABLE FORMS
Tablets: 10 mg

INDICATIONS & DOSAGES
➤ **Chronic hepatitis B infection**
Adults: 10 mg P.O. once daily.
Adjust-a-dose: In patients with creatinine clearance of 20 to 49 ml/minute, give 10 mg P.O. q 48 hours. In patients with clearance of 10 to 19 ml/minute, give 10 mg P.O. q 72 hours. In patients receiving hemodialysis, give 10 mg P.O. q 7 days, after dialysis session.

ACTION
An acyclic nucleotide analogue that inhibits hepatitis B virus reverse transcription via viral DNA chain termination.

Route	Onset	Peak	Duration
P.O.	Unknown	1–4 hr	Unknown

Half-life: Unknown.

ADVERSE REACTIONS
CNS: *asthenia,* fever, headache.
EENT: pharyngitis, sinusitis.
GI: abdominal pain, diarrhea, dyspepsia, flatulence, nausea, vomiting.
GU: ***renal failure, renal insufficiency,*** *hematuria,* glycosuria.
Hepatic: ***hepatic failure, hepatomegaly with steatosis.***
Metabolic: ***lactic acidosis.***
Respiratory: cough.
Skin: pruritus, rash.

INTERACTIONS
Drug-drug. *Ibuprofen:* May increase adefovir bioavailability. Monitor patient for adverse effects.
Nephrotoxic drugs (aminoglycosides, cyclosporine, NSAIDs, tacrolimus, vancomycin): May increase risk of nephrotoxicity. Use together cautiously.

EFFECTS ON LAB TEST RESULTS
- May increase ALT, amylase, AST, CK, creatinine, and lactate levels.

CONTRAINDICATIONS & CAUTIONS
- Contraindicated in patients hypersensitive to any component of the drug.
- Use cautiously in patients with renal dysfunction, in those receiving nephrotoxic drugs, and in those with known risk factors for hepatic disease.
- In elderly patients, use cautiously because they're more likely to have decreased renal and cardiac function.
- For pregnant women, call the Antiretroviral Pregnancy Registry at 1-800-258-4263 to monitor fetal outcome.
- Safety and effectiveness in children haven't been established.

NURSING CONSIDERATIONS
- Monitor renal function, especially in patients with renal dysfunction or those taking nephrotoxic drugs.
- ***Alert:*** Patients may develop lactic acidosis and severe hepatomegaly with steatosis during treatment. Women, obese patients, and those taking antiretrovirals are at higher risk.
- Monitor hepatic function. Notify prescriber if patient develops signs or symptoms of lactic acidosis and severe hepatomegaly with steatosis. Stop drug, if needed.
- Stopping adefovir may cause severe worsening of hepatitis. Monitor hepatic function closely in patients who stop anti-hepatitis B therapy.
- The ideal length of treatment hasn't been established.
- Offer patients HIV antibody testing; drug may promote resistance to antiretrovirals in patients with unrecognized or untreated HIV infection.

PATIENT TEACHING
- Inform the patient that drug may be taken without regard to meals.
- Tell patient to immediately report weakness, muscle pain, trouble breathing, stomach pain with nausea and vomiting, dizziness, light-headedness, fast or irregular heartbeat, and feeling cold, especially in arms and legs.
- Warn patient not to stop taking this drug unless directed because it could cause hepatitis to become worse.
- Instruct woman to tell her prescriber if she becomes pregnant or is breast-feeding. It's unknown if drug appears in breast milk. Use cautiously in breast-feeding women.

amprenavir
Agenerase

Pharmacologic class: protease inhibitor
Pregnancy risk category C

AVAILABLE FORMS
Capsules: 50 mg
Oral solution: 15 mg/ml

INDICATIONS & DOSAGES
➤ **HIV-1 infection (with other antiretrovirals)**
Adults and children ages 13 to 16 who weigh 50 kg (110 lb) or more: 1,200 mg (twenty-four 50-mg capsules) P.O. b.i.d. or 1,400 mg oral solution b.i.d. with other antiretrovirals.
Children ages 4 to 12, or ages 13 to 16 who weigh less than 50 kg (110 lb): For capsules, give 20 mg/kg P.O. b.i.d. or 15 mg/kg P.O. t.i.d., to maximum daily dose of 2,400 mg with other antiretrovirals.

For oral solution, give 22.5 mg/kg (1.5 ml/kg) P.O. b.i.d. or 17 mg/kg (1.1 ml/kg) P.O. t.i.d., to maximum daily dose of 2,800 mg with other antiretrovirals.

Adjust-a-dose: For patients with a Child-Pugh score of 5 to 8, reduce dose for capsules to 450 mg P.O. b.i.d. or oral solution to 513 mg b.i.d. For patients with a Child-Pugh score of 9 to 12, reduce dose for capsules to 300 mg P.O. b.i.d. or, for oral solution, 342 mg b.i.d.

ACTION

Inhibits HIV-1 protease by binding to the active site of HIV-1 protease, which causes immature noninfectious viral particles to form.

Route	Onset	Peak	Duration
P.O.	Unknown	1–2 hr	Unknown

Half-life: 7 to 10½ hours.

ADVERSE REACTIONS

CNS: *oral and perioral paresthesia,* depression or mood disorders.
GI: *diarrhea or loose stools, nausea, vomiting,* abdominal pain or discomfort, taste disorders.
Metabolic: *hyperglycemia, hypertriglyceridemia,* hypercholesterolemia.
Skin: *rash,* ***Stevens-Johnson syndrome.***

INTERACTIONS

Drug-drug. *Antacids:* May decrease amprenavir absorption. Separate doses by at least 1 hour.
Antiarrhythmics such as amiodarone, lidocaine (systemic), quinidine, anticoagulants such as warfarin, tricyclic antidepressants: May alter levels of these drugs. Monitor patient closely.
Dihydroergotamine, midazolam, ***rifampin,*** *triazolam:* May be life-threatening. Avoid using together.
Efavirenz: May decrease amprenavir exposure. May need to increase dose.
Ethinyl estradiol and norethindrone: May cause loss of virologic response and resistance to amprenavir. Avoid use together.
HMG-CoA reductase inhibitors, such as atorvastatin, lovastatin, simvastatin: May increase levels of these drugs; may increase risk of myopathy, including rhabdomyolysis. Avoid using together.
Indinavir, nelfinavir, ritonavir: May increase amprenavir level. Monitor patient closely for adverse reactions.
Ketoconazole: May increase levels of both drugs. Monitor patient closely for adverse reactions.
Macrolides: May increase amprenavir level. Don't adjust dosage.
Methadone: May decrease amprenavir level. Consider alternative antiretroviral or pain therapy. May need to increase methadone dosage if used together.
Phosphodiesterase (PDE) 5 inhibitors (sildenafil, tadalafil, vardenafil): May increase levels of these drugs, increasing the risk of adverse effects including hypotension, visual changes, and priapism. Reduce dosage and extend dosing interval of PDE 5 inhibitor.
Psychotherapeutic drugs: May increase CNS effects. Monitor patient closely.
Rifabutin: May decrease amprenavir exposure. May increase rifabutin level by 200%. May need to decrease rifabutin dose to 150 mg daily or 300 mg two to three times a week.
Saquinavir: May decrease amprenavir exposure. Monitor patient closely.
Drug-herb. ***St. John's wort*** **:** May decrease drug level. Discourage use together.
Drug-food. *Grapefruit juice:* May affect drug level. Monitor patient closely.
High-fat meals: May decrease drug absorption. Advise patient to avoid taking drug with a high-fat meal.

EFFECTS ON LAB TEST RESULTS

- May increase cholesterol, glucose, and triglyceride levels.

CONTRAINDICATIONS & CAUTIONS

- Contraindicated in patients hypersensitive to drug or its components. Contraindicated in infants, children younger than age 4, pregnant women, patients with liver or kidney failure, and patients treated with disulfiram (Antabuse) or metronidazole (Flagyl).
- Use cautiously in patients with moderate or severe hepatic impairment, diabetes mellitus, a known sulfonamide allergy, or hemophilia A or B.
- Use during pregnancy only if the potential benefits outweigh the risks.

NURSING CONSIDERATIONS

- ***Alert:*** Drug can cause severe or life-threatening rash, including Stevens-Johnson syndrome. Stop therapy if patient develops a severe or life-threatening rash or a moderate rash accompanied by systemic signs and symptoms.

- *Alert:* Because this drug may interact with many drugs, obtain patient's complete drug history. Ask patient to show you the drugs he's taking.
- Oral solution should only be used when the capsules or other protease inhibitor forms aren't possible.
- Monitor patient for adverse reactions. A patient taking a protease inhibitor may experience a redistribution of body fat, including central obesity, dorsocervical fat enlargement (buffalo hump), peripheral wasting, breast enlargement, and cushingoid appearance.
- Drug provides high daily doses of vitamin E, which may worsen coagulopathy caused by vitamin K deficiency.
- Protease inhibitors may cause spontaneous bleeding in some patients with hemophilia A or B. In some patients, additional factor VIII may be needed.
- Capsules aren't interchangeable with oral solution, milligram for milligram.
- *Look alike–sound alike:* Don't confuse amprenavir with abacavir.

PATIENT TEACHING

- Advise patient that drug doesn't cure HIV infection; patient may continue to develop opportunistic infections and other complications from the disease. Also, tell patient that drug doesn't reduce risk of HIV transmission through sexual contact.
- Tell patient that although drug can be taken without regard to food, he shouldn't take it with a high-fat meal because of decreased drug absorption.
- Tell patient to report adverse reactions, especially rash.
- Advise patient to take drug daily, as prescribed, with other antiretrovirals. Tell him not to stop or alter dosage without prescriber's approval.
- Inform patient not to take an antacid within 1 hour of amprenavir to prevent a decrease in amprenavir absorption.
- Advise patient receiving sildenafil, vardenafil, or tadalafil of increased adverse reactions. Caution against taking more than is recommended by prescriber.
- If a dose is missed by more than 4 hours, advise patient to wait and take the next dose at the regularly scheduled time. If a dose is missed by less than 4 hours, advise him to take the dose as soon as possible and then take the next dose at the regularly scheduled time. If a dose is skipped, patient shouldn't double the dose.
- Advise woman to notify prescriber if she becomes pregnant during therapy.
- Advise patient not to take supplemental vitamin E because drug contains a significant amount of the vitamin.

atazanavir sulfate
Reyataz✐

Pharmacologic class: protease inhibitor
Pregnancy risk category B

AVAILABLE FORMS

Capsules: 100 mg, 150 mg, 200 mg, 300 mg

INDICATIONS & DOSAGES

➤ **HIV-1 infection, with other antiretrovirals**

Adults: Give antiretroviral-experienced patients 300 mg (as one 300-mg capsule or two 150-mg capsules) once daily, plus 100 mg ritonavir once daily with food. Give antiretroviral-naive patients 400 mg (as two 200-mg capsules) once daily with food. When drug is given with efavirenz in antiretroviral-naive patients, give atazanavir 300 mg, ritonavir 100 mg, and efavirenz 600 mg as a single daily dose with food. Dosage recommendations for efavirenz and atazanavir in treatment-experienced patients haven't been established.

Adjust-a-dose: In patients with Child-Pugh class B hepatic insufficiency who haven't experienced prior virologic failure, reduce dosage to 300 mg P.O. once daily.

ACTION

Inhibits viral maturation in HIV-1–infected cells, resulting in the formation of immature noninfectious viral particles.

Route	Onset	Peak	Duration
P.O.	Unknown	2½ hr	Unknown

Half-life: About 7 hours.

ADVERSE REACTIONS

CNS: *headache,* depression, dizziness, fatigue, fever, insomnia, pain, peripheral neurologic symptoms.
EENT: scleral yellowing.
GI: *abdominal pain, diarrhea, nausea,* vomiting.
Hepatic: jaundice, hyperbilirubinemia.
Metabolic: lipodystrophy.
Musculoskeletal: arthralgia, back pain.
Respiratory: increased cough.
Skin: *rash.*

INTERACTIONS

Drug-drug. *Amiodarone, lidocaine (systemic), quinidine, tricyclic antidepressants:* May increase levels of these drugs. Monitor drug levels.
Antacids, buffered drugs, didanosine: May decrease atazanavir level. Give atazanavir 2 hours before or 1 hour after these drugs.
Atorvastatin: May increase atorvastatin levels, increasing the risk of myopathy and rhabdomyolysis. Use together cautiously.
Clarithromycin: May increase clarithromycin level and prolong QTc interval while reducing active metabolite. Avoid using together, except to treat *Mycobacterium avium* complex infection. Decrease clarithromycin by 50% when using together.
Cyclosporine, sirolimus, tacrolimus: May increase immunosuppressant level. Monitor immunosuppressant level.
Diltiazem, felodipine, nicardipine, nifedipine, verapamil: May increase calcium channel blocker level. Use together cautiously, with close ECG monitoring. Adjust calcium channel blocker dosage as needed. Decrease diltiazem dose by 50%.
Efavirenz: May alter atazanavir level. Reduce atazanavir dosage.
Ergot derivatives, pimozide: May cause serious or life-threatening reactions. Avoid using together.
Ethinyl estradiol and norethindrone: May increase ethinyl estradiol and norethindrone levels. Use cautiously together; give the lowest effective dose of hormonal contraceptive.
H_2-receptor antagonists: May decrease atazanavir level, reducing therapeutic effect. Separate doses by at least 12 hours.
Indinavir: May increase risk of indirect (unconjugated) hyperbilirubinemia. Avoid using together.
Irinotecan: May interfere with irinotecan metabolism and increase irinotecan toxicity. Avoid using together.
Lovastatin, simvastatin: May cause myopathy and rhabdomyolysis. Avoid using together.
Midazolam, triazolam: May cause prolonged or increased sedation or respiratory depression. Avoid using together.
Proton-pump inhibitors, *rifampin:* May significantly reduce atazanavir level. Avoid using together.
Rifabutin: May increase rifabutin level. Reduce rifabutin dose up to 75%.
Ritonavir: May increase atazanavir level. Decrease atazanavir dose to 300 mg.
Saquinavir (soft-gelatin capsules): May increase saquinavir level. Avoid using together.
Sildenafil, tadalafil, vardenafil: May increase levels of these drugs, causing hypotension, visual changes, and priapism. Tell patient to use together cautiously and reduce sildenafil dose to 25 mg every 48 hours, tadalafil dose to 10 mg every 72 hours, and vardenafil dose to 2.5 mg every 72 hours.
Tenofovir: May decrease atazanavir level, causing resistance. Give both drugs with ritonavir.
Warfarin: May increase warfarin level, which may cause life-threatening bleeding. Monitor INR.
Drug-herb. ***St. John's wort:*** May decrease drug level, reducing therapeutic effect and causing drug resistance. Discourage use together.
Drug-food. *Any food:* May increase bioavailability of drug. Tell patient to take drug with food.

EFFECTS ON LAB TEST RESULTS

- May increase ALT, amylase, AST, bilirubin, and lipase levels. May decrease hemoglobin level.
- May decrease neutrophil count.

CONTRAINDICATIONS & CAUTIONS

- Contraindicated in patients hypersensitive to drug or its ingredients.
- Contraindicated in patients taking drugs cleared mainly by CYP3A4 or drugs that

can cause serious or life-threatening reactions at high levels (dihydroergotamine, ergonovine, ergotamine, midazolam, methylergonovine, pimozide, triazolam).
- Don't use in patients with Child-Pugh class C hepatic insufficiency.
- Use cautiously in patients with conduction system disease or hepatic impairment.
- Use cautiously in elderly patients because of the increased likelihood of other disease, additional drug therapy, and decreased hepatic, renal, or cardiac function.

NURSING CONSIDERATIONS
- ***Alert:*** Drug may prolong the PR interval.
- Monitor the patient for hyperglycemia and new-onset diabetes or worsened diabetes. Insulin and oral hypoglycemic dosages may need adjustment.
- Monitor a patient with hepatitis B or C for elevated liver enzymes or hepatic decompensation.
- Watch for life-threatening lactic acidosis syndrome and symptomatic hyperlactatemia, especially in women and obese patients.
- If the patient has hemophilia, watch for bleeding.
- Most patients have an asymptomatic increase in indirect bilirubin, possibly with yellowed skin or sclerae. This hyperbilirubinemia will resolve when therapy stops.
- Although cross resistance occurs among protease inhibitors, resistance to drug doesn't preclude use of other protease inhibitors.
- Give drug to a pregnant woman only if the potential benefit justifies the risk to the fetus.
- Register pregnant women for monitoring of maternal-fetal outcomes by calling the Antiretroviral Pregnancy Registry at 1-800-258-4263.

PATIENT TEACHING
- Urge patient to take drug with food every day and to take other antiretrovirals as prescribed.
- Explain that drug doesn't cure HIV infection and that the patient may develop opportunistic infections and other complications of HIV disease.
- Caution the patient that drug doesn't reduce the risk of transmitting the HIV virus to others.
- Tell patient that drug may cause altered or increased body fat, central obesity, buffalo hump, peripheral wasting, facial wasting, breast enlargement, and a cushingoid appearance.
- Tell patient to report yellowed skin or eyes, dizziness, or light-headedness.
- Caution patient not to take other prescription, OTC, or herbal medicines without first consulting his prescriber.

cidofovir
Vistide

Pharmacologic class: nucleotide analogue
Pregnancy risk category C

AVAILABLE FORMS
Injection: 75 mg/ml in 5-ml vial

INDICATIONS & DOSAGES
➤ CMV retinitis in patients with AIDS
Adults: Initially, 5 mg/kg I.V. infused over 1 hour once weekly for 2 consecutive weeks; then maintenance dose of 5 mg/kg I.V. infused over 1 hour once q 2 weeks. Give probenecid and prehydration with normal saline solution I.V. simultaneously to reduce risk of nephrotoxicity.
Adjust-a-dose: For patients with creatinine level of 0.3 to 0.4 mg/dl above baseline, reduce dosage to 3 mg/kg at same rate and frequency. If creatinine level reaches 0.5 mg/dl or more above baseline, stop drug.

I.V. ADMINISTRATION
- Drug has mutagenic effects; prepare it in a class II laminar flow biological safety cabinet and wear surgical gloves and a closed-front surgical gown with knit cuffs.
- If drug contacts skin, wash and flush thoroughly with water.
- Place excess drug and all materials used to prepare and give it in a leak-proof, puncture-proof container.
- Let drug reach room temperature before use.

- Using a syringe, withdraw prescribed dose and add to an I.V. bag containing 100 ml of normal saline solution.
- Infuse over 1 hour using an infusion pump.
- Because of the risk of nephrotoxicity, don't exceed recommended dosages or frequency or rate of infusion.
- Discard any partially used vials.
- Give within 24 hours of preparing. Admixture may be refrigerated at 36° to 46° F (2° to 8° C) for up to 24 hours.

INCOMPATIBILITIES

Don't add other drugs or supplements to admixture. Compatibility with Ringer, lactated Ringer, and bacteriostatic solutions hasn't been evaluated.

ACTION

A nucleotide analogue that suppresses CMV replication by selective inhibition of viral DNA synthesis.

Route	Onset	Peak	Duration
I.V.	Unknown	Unknown	Unknown

Half-life: Unknown.

ADVERSE REACTIONS

CNS: *asthenia, fever, headache,* ***seizures,*** abnormal gait, amnesia, anxiety, confusion, depression, dizziness, hallucinations, insomnia, neuropathy, paresthesia, somnolence, malaise.
CV: hypotension, orthostatic hypotension, pallor, syncope, tachycardia, vasodilation.
EENT: *ocular hypotony,* abnormal vision, amblyopia, conjunctivitis, eye disorders, iritis, pharyngitis, retinal detachment, rhinitis, sinusitis, uveitis.
GI: *abdominal pain, anorexia, diarrhea, nausea, vomiting,* aphthous stomatitis, colitis, constipation, dry mouth, dyspepsia, dysphagia, flatulence, gastritis, melena, mouth ulcers, oral candidiasis, rectal disorders, stomatitis, taste perversion, tongue discoloration.
GU: *proteinuria,* ***nephrotoxicity,*** glycosuria, hematuria, urinary incontinence, UTI.
Hematologic: *anemia,* ***neutropenia, thrombocytopenia.***
Hepatic: hepatomegaly.
Metabolic: fluid imbalance, hyperglycemia, hyperlipemia, hypocalcemia, hypokalemia, weight loss.
Musculoskeletal: arthralgia, myalgia, myasthenia, pain in back, chest, or neck.
Respiratory: *dyspnea,* asthma, bronchitis, coughing, hiccups, increased sputum, lung disorders, pneumonia.
Skin: *alopecia, rash,* acne, dry skin, pruritus, skin discoloration, sweating, urticaria.
Other: *chills, infections,* ***sarcoma, sepsis,*** allergic reactions, facial edema, herpes simplex.

INTERACTIONS

Drug-drug. *Nephrotoxic drugs (such as aminoglycosides, amphotericin B, foscarnet, I.V. pentamidine):* May increase nephrotoxicity. Avoid using together.

EFFECTS ON LAB TEST RESULTS

- May increase alkaline phosphatase, ALT, AST, BUN, creatinine, and LDH levels. May decrease bicarbonate and hemoglobin levels.
- May decrease neutrophil and platelet counts.

CONTRAINDICATIONS & CAUTIONS

- Contraindicated in patients hypersensitive to drug, probenecid, and other sulfa drugs.
- Contraindicated in patients receiving other drugs with nephrotoxic potential (stop such drugs at least 7 days before starting cidofovir therapy) and in those with creatinine level exceeding 1.5 mg/dl, creatinine clearance of 55 ml/minute or less, or urine protein level of 100 mg/dl or more (equivalent to 2+ proteinuria or more).
- Use within 1 month of placement of a ganciclovir ocular implant may cause profound hypotony.
- Safety and effectiveness in children haven't been established.
- Use cautiously in patients with renal impairment. Monitor renal function tests and patient's fluid balance.

NURSING CONSIDERATIONS

- Drug is indicated for CMV retinitis only in patients with AIDS. Safety and efficacy of drug haven't been established for

treating other CMV infections, congenital or neonatal CMV disease, or CMV disease in patients not infected with HIV.
- Give 1 liter normal saline solution I.V. over 1- to 2-hour period, immediately before drug.
- Give probenecid with cidofovir.
- Monitor creatinine and urine protein levels and WBC counts with differential before each dose.
- Drug may cause Fanconi syndrome and decreased bicarbonate level with renal tubular damage. Monitor patient closely.
- Drug may cause granulocytopenia.
- Stop zidovudine therapy or reduce dosage by 50% on the days when cidofovir is given; probenecid reduces metabolic clearance of zidovudine.

PATIENT TEACHING
- Inform patient that drug doesn't cure CMV retinitis and that regular ophthalmologic examinations are needed.
- Alert patient taking zidovudine that he'll need to obtain dosage guidelines on days cidofovir is given.
- Tell patient that close monitoring of kidney function will be needed and that abnormalities may require a change in therapy.
- Stress importance of completing a full course of probenecid with each cidofovir dose. Tell patient to take probenecid after a meal to decrease nausea.
- Patients with AIDS should use effective contraception, especially during and for 1 month after treatment.
- Advise men to practice barrier contraception during and for 3 months after treatment.

✷ NEW DRUG

darunavir ethanolate
Prezista

Pharmacologic class: protease inhibitor
Pregnancy risk category B

AVAILABLE FORMS
Tablets: 300 mg

INDICATIONS & DOSAGES
➤With ritonavir and other antiretrovirals, for HIV infection in antiretroviral treatment–experienced patients
Adults: 600 mg P.O. b.i.d., given with 100 mg ritonavir P.O. b.i.d. and food.

ACTION
Binds to the protease-active site and selectively inhibits enzyme activity. This inhibition prevents cleavage of viral polyproteins, resulting in the formation of immature, noninfectious viral particles.

Route	Onset	Peak	Duration
P.O.	Unknown	2½–4 hr	Unknown

Half-life: About 15 hours when combined with ritonavir.

ADVERSE REACTIONS
CNS: *headache,* altered mood, anxiety, asthenia, confusion, disorientation, fatigue, hypoesthesia, irritability, memory impairment, nightmares, paresthesia, peripheral neuropathy, somnolence, transient ischemic attack, vertigo.
CV: ***MI,*** hypertension, tachycardia.
EENT: nasopharyngitis.
GI: *diarrhea, nausea,* abdominal distension, abdominal pain, anorexia, constipation, dry mouth, dyspepsia, flatulence, polydipsia, vomiting.
GU: ***acute renal failure,*** renal insufficiency, nephrolithiasis, polyuria.
Hematologic: LEUKOPENIA, ***neutropenia, thrombocytopenia.***
Metabolic: decreased appetite, diabetes mellitus, hypercholesterolemia, hyperlipidemia, hypernatremia, hyperuricemia, hyponatremia, obesity.
Musculoskeletal: arthralgia, myalgia, osteopenia, osteoporosis, pain in extremity.
Respiratory: cough, dyspnea, hiccups.
Skin: ***erythema multiforme, Stevens-Johnson syndrome,*** allergic dermatitis, alopecia, dermatitis medicamentosa, eczema, folliculitis, increased sweating, inflammation, lipoatrophy, maculopapular rash, night sweats, toxic skin eruption.
Other: fat redistribution, gynecomastia, hyperthermia, peripheral edema, pyrexia, rigors.

INTERACTIONS

Drug-drug. *Amiodarone, bepridil, cyclosporine, felodipine, fluticasone, lidocaine, nicardipine, nifedipine, quinidine, rifabutin, sildenafil, sirolimus, tacrolimus, tadalafil, trazodone, vardenafil:* May increase levels of these drugs, increasing the risk of adverse reactions. Use caution, and monitor patient carefully.
Astemizole, cisapride, ergot derivatives, midazolam, pimozide, terfenadine, triazolam: May cause life-threatening reactions. Using together is contraindicated.
Atorvastatin, pravastatin: May increase levels of these drugs. Start at the lowest possible dose, and monitor patient carefully.
Clarithromycin: May increase clarithromycin level. Reduce clarithromycin dose in patients with renal impairment.
CYP3A inducers (carbamazepine, dexamethasone, phenobarbital, phenytoin, rifabutin, rifampin), efavirenz, lopinavir, saquinavir: May increase darunavir clearance and decrease darunavir level. Avoid use together.
Ethinyl estradiol, norethindrone: May decrease estrogen level. Recommend alternative or additional contraception.
Itraconazole, ketoconazole: May increase levels of these drugs and darunavir. Don't exceed 200 mg of itraconazole or ketoconazole daily.
Lovastatin, simvastatin: May increase risk of myopathy, including rhabdomyolysis. Use caution.
Methadone: May decrease methadone level. Monitor patient for opioid abstinence syndrome, and consider increasing methadone dosage.
Rifabutin: May decrease darunavir level. If used together, give rifabutin as 150 mg every other day.
SSRIs (paroxetine, sertraline): May decrease levels of these drugs. Adjust dosage carefully based on antidepressant response.
Trazodone: May increase trazodone level and risk of toxicity. Decrease trazodone dosage.
Warfarin: May decrease warfarin level. Monitor patient carefully.
Drug-herb. *St. John's wort:* May decrease drug level significantly. Discourage use together.
Drug-food. *Food:* Increases drug absorption, which is needed for adequate therapeutic effect. Always give with food.

EFFECTS ON LAB TEST RESULTS

- May increase AST, ALT, GGT, alkaline phosphatase, bilirubin, pancreatic amylase, pancreatic lipase, cholesterol, triglyceride, and uric acid levels. May decrease albumin, bicarbonate, and calcium levels. May increase or decrease sodium and glucose levels.
- May decrease WBC, neutrophil, lymphocyte, and platelet counts.

CONTRAINDICATIONS & CAUTIONS

- Contraindicated in patients hypersensitive to any component of drug and patient taking drugs metabolized by CYP3A (astemizole, dihydroergotamine, ergonovine, ergotamine, methylergonovine, midazolam, pimozide, terfenadine, triazolam).
- Use cautiously in patients with liver or renal impairment, diabetes mellitus, hemophilia, known sulfonamide allergy, or a history of opportunistic infections.

PATIENT TEACHING

- Explain that many drugs interact with darunavir; advise patient to report all drugs he takes, including OTC products.
- ***Alert:*** Instruct patient to take darunavir and ritonavir at the same time every day, with food.
- Tell patient that drug doesn't cure HIV infection or AIDS and doesn't reduce the risk of passing HIV to others.
- Explain that opportunistic infections and other complications of HIV infection may still develop.
- If patient misses a dose by more than 6 hours, tell him to wait and take the next dose at the regularly scheduled time. If he remembers within 6 hours, tell him to take the missed dose immediately.

delavirdine mesylate

Rescriptor

Pharmacologic class: nonnucleoside reverse transcriptase inhibitor
Pregnancy risk category C

AVAILABLE FORMS

Tablets: 100 mg, 200 mg

INDICATIONS & DOSAGES

➤ HIV-1 infection when therapy is warranted

Adults: 400 mg P.O. t.i.d. with other appropriate antiretrovirals.

ACTION

A nonnucleoside reverse transcriptase inhibitor of HIV-1. Drug binds directly to reverse transcriptase and blocks RNA- and DNA-dependent DNA polymerase activities.

Route	Onset	Peak	Duration
P.O.	Unknown	1 hr	Unknown

Half-life: 5¼ hours.

ADVERSE REACTIONS

CNS: *asthenia, fatigue, headache,* depression, fever, insomnia, pain.
EENT: pharyngitis, sinusitis.
GI: *nausea,* abdominal cramps, diarrhea, distention or pain, vomiting.
GU: epididymitis, hematuria, hemospermia, impotence, metrorrhagia, nocturia, polyuria, proteinuria, renal calculi, renal pain, vaginal candidiasis.
Respiratory: bronchitis, cough, upper respiratory tract infection.
Skin: *rash.*
Other: flulike syndrome.

INTERACTIONS

Drug-drug. *Amphetamines, nonsedating antihistamines, benzodiazepines, calcium channel blockers, clarithromycin, dapsone, ergot alkaloid preparations, indinavir, quinidine, rifabutin, sedative-hypnotics, warfarin:* May increase or prolong therapeutic and adverse effects of these drugs. Avoid using together, or, if use together is unavoidable, reduce doses of indinavir and clarithromycin.
Antacids: May reduce absorption of delavirdine. Separate doses by at least 1 hour.
Carbamazepine, phenobarbital, phenytoin: May decrease delavirdine level. Use together cautiously.
Clarithromycin, fluoxetine, ketoconazole: May cause a 50% increase in delavirdine bioavailability. Monitor patient and reduce dose of clarithromycin.
Didanosine: May decrease absorption of both drugs by 20%. Separate doses by at least 1 hour.
H_2-receptor antagonists: May increase gastric pH and reduce absorption of delavirdine. Long-term use together isn't recommended.
HMG-CoA reductase inhibitors, such as atorvastatin, lovastatin, simvastatin: May increase levels of these drugs, which increases risk of myopathy, including rhabdomyolysis. Avoid using together.
Rifabutin, rifampin: May decrease delavirdine level. May increase rifabutin level by 100%. Avoid using together.
Saquinavir: May increase bioavailability of saquinavir fivefold. Monitor AST and ALT levels frequently when used together.
Sildenafil: May increase sildenafil level and may increase sildenafil adverse events, including hypotension, visual changes, and priapism. Tell patient not to exceed 25 mg of sildenafil in 48 hours.
Drug-herb. *St. John's wort:* May decrease drug level. Discourage use together.

EFFECTS ON LAB TEST RESULTS

- May increase alkaline phosphatase, ALT, amylase, AST, CK, creatinine, GGT, and lipase levels. May decrease glucose and hemoglobin levels and hematocrit.
- May increase eosinophil count, PT, and PTT. May decrease granulocyte, neutrophil, platelet, RBC, and WBC counts.

CONTRAINDICATIONS & CAUTIONS

- Contraindicated in patients hypersensitive to drug or its components.
- Use cautiously in patients with impaired hepatic function.

NURSING CONSIDERATIONS

- Because drug's effects in patients with hepatic or renal impairment haven't been

studied, monitor renal and liver function test results carefully.
- Drug-induced diffuse, maculopapular, erythematous, pruritic rash occurs most commonly on upper body and arms of patients with lower CD4 cell counts, usually within first 3 weeks of treatment. Dosage adjustment doesn't seem to affect rash. Treat symptoms with diphenhydramine, hydroxyzine, or topical corticosteroids.
- Drug doesn't reduce risk of transmission of HIV-1.
- Because resistance develops rapidly when used as monotherapy, always use drug with appropriate antiretrovirals.
- Monitor patient's fluid balance and weight.

PATIENT TEACHING
- Tell patient to stop drug and call prescriber if severe rash or such symptoms as fever, fatigue, headache, nausea, abdominal pain, or cough occur.
- Inform patient that drug doesn't cure HIV-1 infection and that he may continue to acquire illnesses including opportunistic infections related to HIV-1 infection. Therapy hasn't been shown to reduce the risk or frequency of such illnesses. Drug hasn't been shown to reduce transmission of HIV.
- Advise patient to remain under medical supervision when taking drug because the long-term effects aren't known.
- Tell patient to take drug as prescribed and not to alter doses without prescriber's approval. If a dose is missed, tell patient to take the next dose as soon as possible; he shouldn't double the next dose.
- Inform patient that drug may be dispersed in water before ingestion. Add tablets to at least 5 ounces (148 ml) of water, allow to stand for a few minutes, and stir until a uniform dispersion occurs. Tell patient to drink dispersion promptly, rinse glass, and swallow the rinse to ensure that entire dose is consumed.
- Tell patient that drug may be taken without regard to food.
- Instruct patient with absence of hydrochloric acid in the stomach to take drug with an acidic beverage, such as orange or cranberry juice.
- Instruct patient to take drug and antacids at least 1 hour apart.
- Advise patient to report use of other prescription or nonprescription drugs, including herbal remedies.
- Advise patient taking sildenafil about an increased risk of sildenafil-related adverse events, including low blood pressure, visual changes, and painful penile erection. Tell him to promptly report any symptoms to his prescriber. Tell patient not to exceed 25 mg of sildenafil in a 48-hour period.

didanosine (ddI)
Videx, Videx EC

Pharmacologic class: nucleoside reverse transcriptase inhibitor
Pregnancy risk category B

AVAILABLE FORMS
Delayed-release capsules: 125 mg, 200 mg, 250 mg, 400 mg
Powder for oral solution (buffered): 100 mg/packet, 250 mg/packet
Powder for oral solution (pediatric): 2 g/4-ounce glass bottle, 4 g/8-ounce glass bottle
Tablets (buffered, chewable): 25 mg, 50 mg, 100 mg, 200 mg

INDICATIONS & DOSAGES
➤ **HIV infection when antiretroviral therapy is warranted**
Adults who weigh 60 kg (132 lb) or more: 200 mg tablets P.O. q 12 hours or 400 mg P.O. once daily; or 250 mg buffered powder P.O. q 12 hours; or 400 mg capsule P.O. daily.
Adults who weigh less than 60 kg: 125 mg tablets P.O. q 12 hours or 250 mg P.O. once daily; or 167 mg buffered powder P.O. q 12 hours; or 250 mg capsule P.O. daily.
Children: 120 mg/m^2 P.O. q 12 hours; Videx EC hasn't been studied in children.
Adjust-a-dose: For dialysis patients, give 25% of usual Videx dose once daily. For patient who weighs 60 kg or more, give 125 mg of Videx EC once daily. Don't use in patients who weigh less than 60 kg. If creatinine clearance is less than 10 ml/

minute, don't give a supplemental dose after hemodialysis for either drug.

In adults who weigh 60 kg or more with creatinine clearance of 30 to 59 ml/minute, give 100-mg tablet b.i.d., 200-mg tablet or 200-mg capsule once daily, or 100-mg buffered powder b.i.d. If clearance is 10 to 29 ml/minute, give 150-mg tablet, 125-mg capsule, or 167-mg buffered powder once daily. If clearance is less than 10 ml/minute, give 100-mg tablet, 125-mg capsule, or 100-mg buffered powder once daily.

In adults who weigh less than 60 kg and have a clearance of 30 to 59 ml/minute, give 75-mg tablet b.i.d., 150-mg tablet or 125-mg capsule once daily, or 100-mg buffered powder b.i.d. If clearance is 10 to 29 ml/minute, give 100-mg tablet, 125-mg capsule, or 100-mg buffered powder once daily. For clearance less than 10 ml/minute, give 75-mg tablet or 100-mg buffered powder once daily; capsule not indicated for these patients.

ACTION

Inhibits the enzyme HIV-RNA–dependent DNA polymerase (reverse transcriptase) and terminates DNA chain growth.

Route	Onset	Peak	Duration
P.O.	Unknown	30–60 min	Unknown

Half-life: 48 minutes.

ADVERSE REACTIONS

CNS: *dizziness, fever, headache, peripheral neuropathy,* ***seizures,*** abnormal thinking, anxiety, asthenia, confusion, depression, insomnia, nervousness, pain, twitching.
CV: ***heart failure,*** hypertension, edema.
EENT: optic neuritis, retinal changes.
GI: *abdominal pain, diarrhea, nausea, vomiting,* ***pancreatitis,*** anorexia, dry mouth.
Hematologic: ***leukopenia, thrombocytopenia,*** anemia, granulocytosis.
Hepatic: ***hepatic failure.***
Metabolic: hyperuricemia.
Musculoskeletal: myopathy.
Respiratory: dyspnea, pneumonia.
Skin: alopecia, pruritus, rash.
Other: *chills,* ***sarcoma,*** allergic reactions, infection.

INTERACTIONS

Drug-drug. *Amprenavir, delavirdine, indinavir, nelfinavir, ritonavir, saquinavir:* May alter pharmacokinetics of didanosine or these drugs. Separate dosage times.
Antacids containing magnesium or aluminum hydroxides: May enhance adverse effects of the antacid component (including diarrhea or constipation) when given with didanosine tablets or pediatric suspension. Avoid using together.
Co-trimoxazole, pentamidine, other drugs linked to pancreatitis: May increase risk of pancreatic toxicity. Use together cautiously; consider temporarily stopping didanosine during administration of these drugs.
Dapsone, drugs that require gastric acid for adequate absorption, ketoconazole: May decrease absorption from buffering action. Give these drugs 2 hours before didanosine.
Fluoroquinolones, tetracyclines: May decrease absorption from buffering products in didanosine tablets or antacids in pediatric suspension. Separate dosage times by at least 2 hours.
Itraconazole: May decrease itraconazole level. Avoid using together.
Tenofovir: May increase didanosine levels and risk of life-threatening adverse effects including lactic acidosis and pancreatitis. Use cautiously with close monitoring.
Drug-herb. *St. John's wort:* May decrease drug level, decreasing therapeutic effects. Discourage use together.
Drug-food. *Any food:* May decrease rate of absorption. Advise patient to take drug on an empty stomach at least 30 minutes before a meal.

EFFECTS ON LAB TEST RESULTS

- May increase alkaline phosphatase, ALT, AST, bilirubin, and uric acid levels. May decrease hemoglobin level.
- May decrease granulocyte, platelet, and WBC counts.

CONTRAINDICATIONS & CAUTIONS

- Contraindicated in patients hypersensitive to drug or its components.
- Use cautiously in patients with history of pancreatitis; deaths have occurred. Also use cautiously in patients with peripheral

neuropathy, renal or hepatic impairment, or hyperuricemia. Monitor liver and renal function tests.

NURSING CONSIDERATIONS

- Give all forms of drug on an empty stomach, at least 30 minutes before or 2 hours after eating; giving drug with meals can decrease absorption by 50%.
- To give single-dose packets containing buffered powder for oral solution, pour contents into 4 ounces (120 ml) of water. Don't use fruit juice or other acidic beverages. Stir for 2 or 3 minutes until the powder dissolves completely. Give immediately.
- The powder for oral solution may cause diarrhea. Switch to the tablet form if diarrhea is a problem.
- ***Alert:*** The pediatric powder for oral solution must be prepared by a pharmacist before dispensing. It must be constituted with purified USP water and then diluted with an antacid (Mylanta Double Strength Liquid, Extra Strength Maalox Plus Suspension, or Maalox TC Suspension) to a final concentration of 10 mg/ml. The admixture is stable for 30 days at 36° to 46° F (2° to 8° C). Shake the solution well before measuring dose.
- Because of a high rate of early virologic failure and emergence of resistance, using tenofovir with didanosine and lamivudine isn't recommended as a new treatment regimen for therapy-naïve or -experienced patients with HIV infection. Patients on this regimen should be considered for treatment modification.
- ***Look alike–sound alike:*** Don't confuse drug with other antiretrovirals that use abbreviations for identification.

PATIENT TEACHING

- Instruct patient to take drug on an empty stomach, 30 minutes before or 2 hours after eating.
- Because the tablets contain buffers that raise stomach pH to levels that prevent degradation of the active drug, instruct patient to chew tablets thoroughly before swallowing and to drink at least 1 ounce (30 ml) of water with each dose. Teach patient how to prepare and take crushed tablets or buffered powder.
- Inform patient that drug doesn't cure HIV infection, that opportunistic infections and other complications of HIV infection may continue to occur, and that transmission of HIV to others through sexual contact or blood contamination is still possible.
- To reduce the risk of GI adverse effects from excess antacid, advise patient to take no more than 4 buffered tablets at a time.
- Inform patient on a sodium-restricted diet that each 2-tablet dose contains 529 mg of sodium and that each single packet of buffered powder for oral solution contains 1.38 g of sodium.
- Tell patient to report symptoms of inflammation of the pancreas, such as abdominal pain, nausea, vomiting, diarrhea, or symptoms of peripheral neuropathy.

efavirenz

Sustiva

Pharmacologic class: nonnucleoside reverse transcriptase inhibitor
Pregnancy risk category D

AVAILABLE FORMS

Capsules: 50 mg, 100 mg, 200 mg
Tablets: 600 mg

INDICATIONS & DOSAGES

➤ **HIV-1 infection, with a protease inhibitor or nucleoside analogue reverse transcriptase inhibitors**

Adults and children age 3 and older who weigh 40 kg (88 lb) or more: 600 mg (three 200-mg capsules or one 600-mg tablet) P.O. once daily on an empty stomach, preferably h.s.

Children age 3 and older who weigh 33 to less than 40 kg (72 to less than 88 lb): 400 mg P.O. once daily on an empty stomach, preferably h.s.

Children age 3 and older who weigh 25 to less than 33 kg (55 to less than 72 lb): 350 mg P.O. once daily on an empty stomach, preferably h.s.

Children age 3 and older who weigh 20 to less than 25 kg (44 to less than 55 lb): 300 mg P.O. once daily on an empty stomach, preferably h.s.

Children age 3 and older who weigh 15 to less than 20 kg (33 to less than 44 lb):

250 mg P.O. once daily on an empty stomach, preferably h.s.
Children age 3 and older who weigh 10 to less than 15 kg (22 to less than 33 lb): 200 mg P.O. once daily on an empty stomach, preferably h.s.

ACTION
A nonnucleoside reverse transcriptase inhibitor that inhibits the transcription of HIV-1 RNA to DNA, a critical step in the viral replication process.

Route	Onset	Peak	Duration
P.O.	Unknown	3–5 hr	Unknown

Half-life: 40 to 76 hours.

ADVERSE REACTIONS
CNS: *dizziness,* abnormal dreams or thinking, agitation, amnesia, confusion, depersonalization, depression, euphoria, fever, fatigue, hallucinations, headache, hypoesthesia, impaired concentration, insomnia, somnolence, nervousness.
GI: *diarrhea, nausea,* abdominal pain, anorexia, dyspepsia, flatulence, vomiting.
GU: hematuria, renal calculi.
Skin: *rash,* ***erythema multiforme, Stevens-Johnson syndrome, toxic epidermal necrolysis,*** increased sweating, pruritus.

INTERACTIONS
Drug-drug. *Amprenavir, clarithromycin, indinavir, lopinavir:* May decrease levels of these drugs. Consider alternative therapy or dosage adjustment.
Drugs that induce the cytochrome P-450 enzyme system (such as phenobarbital, rifampin): May increase clearance of efavirenz, resulting in lower drug level. Avoid using together.
Ergot derivatives, midazolam, triazolam: May inhibit metabolism of these drugs and cause serious or life-threatening adverse events (such as arrhythmias, prolonged sedation, or respiratory depression). Avoid using together.
Estrogens, ritonavir: May increase drug levels. Monitor patient.
Hormonal contraceptives: May increase ethinyl estradiol level. Advise use of a reliable method of barrier contraception in addition to use of hormonal contraceptives.
Psychoactive drugs: May cause additive CNS effects. Avoid using together.
Rifabutin: May decrease rifabutin level. Increase rifabutin dosage to 450 to 600 mg once daily or 600 mg two to three times a week.
Ritonavir: May increase levels of both drugs. Monitor patient and liver function closely.
Saquinavir: May decrease saquinavir level and efavirenz exposure to the body. Don't use with saquinavir as sole protease inhibitor.
Voriconazole: Efavirenz significantly decreases voriconazole levels while efavirenz levels significantly increase. Avoid using together.
Warfarin: May increase or decrease level and effects of warfarin. Monitor INR.
Drug-herb. *St. John's wort:* May decrease drug level. Discourage use together.
Drug-food. *High-fat meals:* May increase absorption of drug. Instruct patient to maintain a proper low-fat diet.
Drug-lifestyle. *Alcohol use:* May enhance CNS effects. Discourage use together.

EFFECTS ON LAB TEST RESULTS
- May increase ALT, AST, and cholesterol levels.
- May cause false-positive urine cannabinoid test results.

CONTRAINDICATIONS & CAUTIONS
- Contraindicated in patients hypersensitive to drug or its components.
- Use cautiously in patients with hepatic impairment and in those receiving hepatotoxic drugs. Monitor liver function test results in patients with history of hepatitis B or C and in those taking ritonavir.

NURSING CONSIDERATIONS
- Monitor cholesterol level.
- ***Alert:*** Drug shouldn't be used as monotherapy or added on as a single drug to a regimen failing because of viral resistance.
- Using drug with ritonavir may increase liver enzyme levels and adverse effects (such as dizziness, nausea, paresthesia).
- Give drug at bedtime to decrease CNS adverse effects.

• Pregnancy must be ruled out before starting therapy in women of childbearing age.
• Children may be more prone to adverse reactions, especially diarrhea, nausea, vomiting, and rash.

PATIENT TEACHING
• Instruct patient to take drug with water, preferably at bedtime and on an empty stomach.
• Inform patient about need for scheduled blood tests to monitor liver function and cholesterol level.
• Tell patient to use a barrier contraceptive with a hormonal contraceptive and to notify prescriber immediately if pregnancy is suspected; drug is a known risk to the fetus.
• Inform patient that drug doesn't cure HIV infection, that opportunistic infections and other complications of HIV infection may continue to occur, and that transmission of HIV to others through sexual contact or blood contamination is still possible.
• Instruct patient to take drug at the same time daily and always with other antiretrovirals.
• Tell patient to take drug exactly as prescribed and not to stop it without medical approval. Also instruct patient to report adverse reactions.
• Inform patient that rash is the most common adverse effect. Tell patient to report rash immediately because it may be serious in rare cases.
• Advise patient to report use of other drugs.
• Advise patient that dizziness, difficulty sleeping or concentrating, drowsiness, or unusual dreams may occur during the first few days of therapy. Reassure him that these symptoms typically resolve after 2 to 4 weeks and may be less problematic if drug is taken at bedtime.
• Tell patient to avoid alcohol, driving, or operating machinery until the drug's effects are known.

emtricitabine
Emtriva

Pharmacologic class: nucleoside reverse transcriptase inhibitor
Pregnancy risk category B

AVAILABLE FORMS
Capsules: 200 mg
Oral solution: 10 mg/ml

INDICATIONS & DOSAGES
➤ HIV-1 infection, with other antiretrovirals
Adults: One 200-mg capsule or 240 mg (24 ml) oral solution P.O. once daily.
Children age 3 months to 18 years: For children who weigh more than 33 kg (73 lb) and can swallow intact capsules, give one 200-mg capsule P.O. once daily. Otherwise, give 6 mg/kg, up to a maximum dose of 240 mg (24 ml) oral solution once daily.
Adjust-a-dose: In adults with creatinine clearance of 30 to 49 ml/minute, give one 200-mg capsule q 48 hours or 120 mg oral solution q 24 hours; if clearance is 15 to 29 ml/minute, give one 200-mg capsule q 72 hours or 80 mg oral solution q 24 hours; if clearance is less than 15 ml/minute or patient is receiving dialysis, give one 200-mg capsule q 96 hours or 60 mg oral solution q 24 hours. Give dose after dialysis session. In children with renal insufficiency, a dose reduction and increased dosing interval should be considered.

ACTION
Inhibits replication of HIV by blocking viral DNA synthesis. Also inhibits reverse transcriptase by acting as an alternative for the enzyme's substrate, deoxycytidine triphosphate.

Route	Onset	Peak	Duration
P.O.	Unknown	1–2 hr	Unknown

Half-life: About 10 hours.

ADVERSE REACTIONS
CNS: *abnormal dreams, asthenia, dizziness, headache, insomnia,* depressive dis-

orders, neuritis, paresthesia, peripheral neuropathy.
EENT: *rhinitis.*
GI: *abdominal pain, diarrhea, nausea,* dyspepsia, vomiting.
Hepatic: ***hepatotoxicity.***
Musculoskeletal: arthralgia, myalgia.
Respiratory: *increased cough.*
Skin: *allergic skin reaction, discoloration, maculopapular rash, pruritus, urticarial and purpuric lesions, vesiculobullous rash.*

INTERACTIONS
None reported.

EFFECTS ON LAB TEST RESULTS
- May increase ALT, amylase, AST, bilirubin, CK, lipase, serum glucose, and triglyceride levels.
- May decrease neutrophil count.

CONTRAINDICATIONS & CAUTIONS
- Contraindicated in patients hypersensitive to drug or its ingredients.
- Don't use drug for treating chronic hepatitis B virus (HBV); safety and efficacy haven't been established in patients infected with both HBV and HIV.
- Use cautiously in elderly patients because of the increased likelihood of concurrent disease or drug therapy, and decreased hepatic, renal, or cardiac function.
- Use cautiously in patients with impaired renal function.

NURSING CONSIDERATIONS
- Test all patients for HBV before starting drug.
- Hepatitis B may worsen after emtricitabine therapy stops. Patients with both HIV and HBV need close clinical and laboratory follow-up for several months or longer after stopping drug.
- Like other antiretrovirals, emtricitabine may cause changes or increases in body fat, including central obesity, buffalo hump, peripheral wasting, facial wasting, breast enlargement, and a cushingoid appearance.
- ***Alert:*** Notify prescriber immediately if lactic acidosis or pronounced hepatotoxicity occurs.
- Use drug only if clearly needed in pregnant women.

PATIENT TEACHING
- Remind patient that anti-HIV medicine must be taken for life.
- Inform patient that drug doesn't cure HIV infection, that opportunistic infections and other complications of HIV infection may continue to occur, and that transmission of HIV to others through sexual contact or blood contamination is still possible.
- Explain possible adverse reactions, including lactic acidosis, hepatotoxicity, and changes or increases in body fat.
- Tell woman to notify prescriber immediately if she is or could be pregnant.
- Inform patient the drug may be taken with or without food.
- Tell patient to refrigerate oral solution but if stored at room temperature, to use within 3 months.

enfuvirtide
Fuzeon

Pharmacologic class: fusion inhibitor
Pregnancy risk category B

AVAILABLE FORMS
Powder for injection: 108-mg single-use vials (90 mg/ml after reconstitution)

INDICATIONS & DOSAGES
➤ **To help control HIV-1 infection, with other antiretrovirals, in patients who have continued HIV-1 replication despite antiretroviral therapy**
Adults: 90 mg subcutaneously b.i.d., injected into the upper arm, anterior thigh, or abdomen.
Children ages 6 to 16: 2 mg/kg subcutaneously b.i.d.; maximum 90 mg per dose.

ACTION
Interferes with entry of HIV-1 into cells by inhibiting fusion of HIV-1 to cell membranes.

Route	Onset	Peak	Duration
SubQ	Unknown	4–8 hr	Unknown

Half-life: 4 hours.

ADVERSE REACTIONS

CNS: *fatigue, insomnia,* anxiety, asthenia, depression, peripheral neuropathy.
EENT: conjunctivitis, sinusitis, taste disturbance.
GI: *diarrhea, nausea,* ***pancreatitis,*** abdominal pain, constipation.
Metabolic: anorexia, weight decrease.
Musculoskeletal: myalgia.
Respiratory: ***bacterial pneumonia,*** cough.
Skin: *injection site reactions,* pruritus, skin papilloma.
Other: herpes simplex, influenza, influenza-like illness, lymphadenopathy.

INTERACTIONS

None reported.

EFFECTS ON LAB TEST RESULTS

- May increase ALT, amylase, AST, CK, GGT, lipase, and triglyceride, levels. May decrease hemoglobin level.
- May decrease eosinophil count.

CONTRAINDICATIONS & CAUTIONS

- Contraindicated in patients hypersensitive to drug and in those not infected with HIV.
- Use in pregnant women only if clearly needed. Pregnant women can be registered in the Antiretroviral Pregnancy Registry by calling 1-800-258-4263.
- Safety and effectiveness haven't been established in children younger than age 6.

NURSING CONSIDERATIONS

- For subcutaneous administration, reconstitute vial with 1.1 ml sterile water for injection. Tap vial for 10 seconds and then gently roll to prevent foaming. Let drug stand for up to 45 minutes to ensure reconstitution. Or, gently roll vial between hands until product is completely dissolved. Then draw up correct dose and inject drug.
- If you won't be using drug immediately after reconstitution, refrigerate in original vial and use within 24 hours. Don't inject drug until it's at room temperature.
- Store unreconstituted vials at room temperature.
- Vial is for single use; discard unused portion.
- Rotate injection sites. Don't inject into the same site for 2 consecutive doses, and don't inject into moles, scar tissue, bruises, or the navel.
- Injection site reactions (pain, discomfort, induration, erythema, pruritus, nodules, cysts, ecchymosis) are common and may require analgesics or rest.
- ***Alert:*** Monitor patient closely for evidence of bacterial pneumonia. Patients at high risk include those with a low initial CD4 count or high initial viral load, those who use I.V. drugs or smoke, and those with history of lung disease.
- Hypersensitivity may occur with the first dose or later doses. If symptoms occur, stop drug.

PATIENT TEACHING

- Teach patient how to prepare and give drug and how to safely dispose of used needles and syringes.
- Tell patient to rotate injection sites and to watch for cellulitis or local infection.
- Urge patient to immediately report evidence of pneumonia, such as cough with fever, rapid breathing, or shortness of breath.
- Tell patient to stop taking drug and seek medical attention if evidence of hypersensitivity develops, such as rash, fever, nausea, vomiting, chills, rigors, and hypotension.
- Teach patient that drug doesn't cure HIV infection and that it must be taken with other antiretrovirals.
- Tell patient to inform prescriber if she's pregnant, plans to become pregnant, or is breast-feeding while taking this drug. Because HIV could be transmitted to the infant, HIV-infected mothers shouldn't breast-feed.
- Tell patient that drug may effect his ability to drive or operate machinery.

---

entecavir

Baraclude

Pharmacologic class: guanosine nucleoside analogue
Pregnancy risk category C

AVAILABLE FORMS

Oral solution: 0.05 mg/ml
Tablets: 0.5 mg, 1 mg

INDICATIONS & DOSAGES

➤ **Chronic hepatitis B virus (HBV) infection in patients with active viral replication and either persistently increased aminotransferase levels or histologically active disease**

Adults and adolescents age 16 and older who have had no previous nucleoside treatment: 0.5 mg P.O. once daily at least 2 hours before or after a meal.

Adjust-a-dose: If creatinine clearance is 30 to 49 ml/minute, give 0.25 mg P.O. once daily. If clearance is 10 to 30 ml/minute, give 0.15 mg P.O. once daily. If clearance is less than 10 ml/minute or patient is undergoing hemodialysis or continuous ambulatory peritoneal dialysis, give 0.05 mg P.O. once daily.

Adults and adolescents age 16 and older who have a history of viremia and are taking lamivudine or have resistance mutations: 1 mg P.O. once daily at least 2 hours before or after a meal.

If creatinine clearance is 30 to 49 ml/minute, give 0.5 mg P.O. once daily. If clearance is 10 to 30 ml/minute, give 0.3 mg P.O. once daily. If clearance is less than 10 ml/minute or patient is undergoing hemodialysis or continuous ambulatory peritoneal dialysis, give 0.1 mg P.O. once daily.

ACTION

Inhibits HBV polymerase and reduces viral DNA levels.

Route	Onset	Peak	Duration
P.O.	Unknown	½–1½ hr	Unknown

Half-life: About 5 or 6 days.

ADVERSE REACTIONS

CNS: dizziness, fatigue, headache.
GI: diarrhea, dyspepsia, nausea.
GU: glycosuria, hematuria.

INTERACTIONS

Drug-drug. *Cyclosporine, tacrolimus:* May further decrease renal function. Monitor renal function carefully.

Drugs that reduce renal function or compete for active tubular secretion: May increase level of either drug. Monitor renal function, and watch for adverse effects.

Drug-food. *All foods:* Delays absorption and decreases drug level. Give drug at least 2 hours before or after a meal.

EFFECTS ON LAB TEST RESULTS

- May increase ALT, amylase, AST, blood glucose, creatinine, lipase, and total bilirubin levels.
- May decrease platelet count.

CONTRAINDICATIONS & CAUTIONS

- Contraindicated in patients hypersensitive to drug or its components.
- Use cautiously in patients with renal impairment and in patients who have had a liver transplant.

NURSING CONSIDERATIONS

- ***Alert:*** Drug may cause life-threatening lactic acidosis and severe hepatomegaly with steatosis.
- ***Alert:*** HBV infection may worsen severely after therapy stops.
- Monitor hepatic function for several months in patients who stop therapy. If appropriate, start therapy for HBV infection.
- Use cautiously in pregnant women only if maternal benefit outweighs fetal risk. For monitoring of fetal outcome data, call the pregnancy registry at 1-800-258-4263.
- It's unknown if drug appears in breast milk. Avoid use in breast-feeding women.
- In elderly patients, adjust dosage for age-related decrease in renal function.

PATIENT TEACHING

- Tell patient that drug should be taken on an empty stomach at least 2 hours before or after a meal.
- Caution against mixing or diluting oral solution with any other substance. Teach proper use of dosing spoon.
- Tell patient to report to prescriber any new adverse effects from this drug and any new drugs he's taking.
- Explain that drug doesn't reduce the risk of HBV transmission to others.
- Teach patient the signs and symptoms of lactic acidosis, such as muscle pain, weakness, dyspnea, GI distress, cold hands and feet, dizziness, or fast or irregular heartbeat.

• Teach patient the signs and symptoms of hepatotoxicity, such as jaundice, dark urine, light-colored stool, loss of appetite, nausea, and lower stomach pain.
• Warn patient not to stop drug abruptly.

famciclovir

Famvir

Pharmacologic class: synthetic acyclic guanine derivative
Pregnancy risk category B

AVAILABLE FORMS

Tablets: 125 mg, 250 mg, 500 mg

INDICATIONS & DOSAGES

➤ **Acute herpes zoster infection (shingles)**
Adults: 500 mg P.O. q 8 hours for 7 days.
Adjust-a-dose: For patients with creatinine clearance of 40 to 59 ml/minute, give 500 mg P.O. q 12 hours; if clearance is 20 to 39 ml/minute, give 500 mg P.O. q 24 hours; if clearance is less than 20 ml/minute, give 250 mg P.O. q 24 hours. For hemodialysis patients, give 250 mg P.O. after each hemodialysis session.

➤ **Recurrent genital herpes**
Adults: 1,000 mg P.O. b.i.d. for a single day. Begin therapy at the first sign or symptom.
Adjust-a-dose: For patients with creatinine clearance of 40 to 59 ml/minute, give 500 mg q 12 hours for one day; for clearance of 20 to 39 ml/minute, give 500 mg P.O. as a single dose; if clearance is less than 20 ml/minute, give 250 mg as a single dose. For hemodialysis patient, give 250 mg single dose following dialysis session.

➤ **Suppression of recurrent genital herpes**
Adults: 250 mg P.O. b.i.d. for up to 1 year.
Adjust-a-dose: For patients with creatinine clearance of 20 to 39 ml/minute, give 125 mg P.O. q 12 hours; if clearance is less than 20 ml/minute, give 125 mg P.O. q 24 hours. For hemodialysis patients, give 125 mg P.O. after each hemodialysis session.

➤ **Recurrent mucocutaneous herpes simplex infections in HIV-infected patients**
Adults: 500 mg P.O. b.i.d. for 7 days.
Adjust-a-dose: For patients with creatinine clearance of 20 to 39 ml/minute, give 500 mg P.O. q 24 hours; if clearance is less than 20 ml/minute, give 250 mg P.O. q 24 hours. For hemodialysis patients, give 250 mg P.O. after each hemodialysis session.

✷ ***NEW INDICATION:*** **Recurrent herpes labialis (cold sores)**
Adults: 1,500 mg P.O. for one dose. Give at the first sign or symptom of cold sore.
Adjust-a-dose: For patients with creatinine clearance of 40 to 59 ml/minute, give 750 mg as a single dose; for clearance of 20 to 39 ml/minute, give 500 mg P.O. as a single dose; if clearance is less than 20 ml/minute, give 250 mg as a single dose. For hemodialysis patient, give 250 mg single dose following dialysis session.

ACTION

A guanosine nucleoside that is converted to penciclovir, which enters viral cells and inhibits DNA polymerase and viral DNA synthesis.

Route	Onset	Peak	Duration
P.O.	Unknown	1 hr	Unknown

Half-life: 2 to 3 hours.

ADVERSE REACTIONS

CNS: *headache,* fatigue, fever, dizziness, paresthesia, somnolence.
EENT: pharyngitis, sinusitis.
GI: *nausea,* abdominal pain, anorexia, constipation, diarrhea, vomiting.
Musculoskeletal: arthralgia, back pain.
Skin: pruritus.
Other: zoster-related signs, symptoms, and complications.

INTERACTIONS

Drug-drug. *Probenecid:* May increase level of penciclovir, the active metabolite of famciclovir. Monitor patient for increased adverse reactions.

EFFECTS ON LAB TEST RESULTS

None reported.

CONTRAINDICATIONS & CAUTIONS

- Contraindicated in patients hypersensitive to drug.
- Use cautiously in patients with renal or hepatic impairment.

NURSING CONSIDERATIONS

- Drug may be taken without regard to meals.
- In patients with renal or hepatic impairment, adjust dosage as needed.
- Monitor renal and liver function tests in these patients.

PATIENT TEACHING

- Inform patient that drug doesn't cure genital herpes but can decrease the length and severity of symptoms.
- Teach patient how to avoid spreading infection to others.
- Urge patient to recognize the early signs and symptoms of herpes infection, such as tingling, itching, and pain, and to report them. Therapy is more effective if started within 48 hours of rash onset.

fosamprenavir calcium

Lexiva

Pharmacologic class: protease inhibitor
Pregnancy risk category C

AVAILABLE FORMS

Tablets: 700 mg

INDICATIONS & DOSAGES

➤ HIV infection, with other antiretrovirals

Adults: In patients not previously treated, 1,400 mg P.O. b.i.d. (without ritonavir). Or, 1,400 mg P.O. once daily and ritonavir 200 mg P.O. once daily. Or, 700 mg P.O. b.i.d. and ritonavir 100 mg P.O. b.i.d. In patients previously treated with a protease inhibitor, 700 mg P.O. b.i.d. plus ritonavir 100 mg P.O. b.i.d.

Adjust-a-dose: If the patient receives efavirenz, fosamprenavir, and ritonavir once daily, give an additional 100 mg/day of ritonavir (300 mg total). If the patient has mild or moderate hepatic impairment and takes fosamprenavir without ritonavir, reduce the dosage to 700 mg P.O. b.i.d.

ACTION

Converts rapidly to amprenavir, which binds to the active site of HIV-1 protease and forms immature noninfectious viral particles.

Route	Onset	Peak	Duration
P.O.	Unknown	1½–4 hr	Unknown

Half-life: 7¼ hours.

ADVERSE REACTIONS

CNS: *depression, fatigue, headache, oral paresthesia.*
GI: *abdominal pain, diarrhea, nausea, vomiting.*
Metabolic: hyperglycemia.
Skin: *rash,* pruritus.

INTERACTIONS

Drug-drug. *Amitriptyline, cyclosporine, imipramine, rapamycin, tacrolimus:* May increase levels of these drugs. Monitor drug levels.
Antiarrhythmics (amiodarone, systemic lidocaine, quinidine): May increase antiarrhythmic level. Use together cautiously and monitor antiarrhythmic levels.
Atorvastatin: May increase atorvastatin level. Give 20 mg/day or less of atorvastatin and monitor patient carefully. Or, consider other HMG-CoA reductase inhibitors, such as fluvastatin, pravastatin, or rosuvastatin.
Benzodiazepines (alprazolam, clorazepate, diazepam, flurazepam): May increase benzodiazepine level. Decrease benzodiazepine dosage as needed.
Bepridil: May increase bepridil level, possibly leading to arrhythmias. Use together cautiously.
Calcium channel blockers (amlodipine, diltiazem, felodipine, isradipine, nifedipine, nicardipine, nimodipine, nisoldipine, verapamil): May increase calcium channel blocker level. Use together cautiously.
Carbamazepine, dexamethasone, H_2-receptor antagonists, phenobarbital, phenytoin, proton-pump inhibitors: May decrease amprenavir level. Use together cautiously.
Delavirdine: May cause loss of virologic response and resistance to delavirdine. Avoid using together.

Dihydroergotamine, ergonovine, ergotamine, flecainide, methylergonovine, midazolam, pimozide, propafenone, triazolam: May cause serious adverse reactions. Avoid using together.
Efavirenz, nevirapine, saquinavir: May decrease amprenavir level. Appropriate combination doses haven't been established.
Efavirenz with ritonavir: May decrease amprenavir level. Increase ritonavir by 100 mg/day (300 mg total) when giving efavirenz, fosamprenavir, and ritonavir once daily. No change needed in ritonavir when giving efavirenz, fosamprenavir, and ritonavir twice daily.
Ethinyl estradiol and norethindrone: May increase ethinyl estradiol and norethindrone levels. Recommend nonhormonal contraception.
Indinavir, nelfinavir: May increase amprenavir level. Appropriate combination doses haven't been established.
Ketoconazole, itraconazole: May increase ketoconazole and itraconazole levels. Reduce ketoconazole or itraconazole dosage as needed if patient receives more than 400 mg/day. (More than 200 mg/day isn't recommended.).
Lopinavir with ritonavir: May decrease amprenavir and lopinavir levels. Appropriate combination doses haven't been established.
Lovastatin, simvastatin: May increase risk of myopathy, including rhabdomyolysis. Avoid using together.
Methadone: May decrease methadone level. Increase methadone dosage as needed.
Rifabutin: May increase rifabutin level. Obtain CBC weekly to watch for neutropenia, and decrease rifabutin dosage by at least half. If patient receives ritonavir, decrease dosage by at least 75% from the usual 300 mg/day. (Maximum, 150 mg every other day or three times weekly.).
Rifampin: May decrease amprenavir level and drug effect. Avoid using together.
Sildenafil, vardenafil: May increase sildenafil and vardenafil levels. Recommend cautious use of sildenafil at 25 mg every 48 hours or vardenafil at no more than 2.5 mg every 24 hours. If patient receives ritonavir, advise no more than 2.5 mg vardenafil every 72 hours, and tell patient to report adverse events.
Warfarin: May alter warfarin level. Monitor INR.
Drug-herb. *St. John's wort:* May cause loss of virologic response and resistance to drug or its class of protease inhibitors. Discourage use together.

EFFECTS ON LAB TEST RESULTS

- May increase ALT, AST, glucose, lipase, and triglyceride levels.
- May decrease neutrophil count.

CONTRAINDICATIONS & CAUTIONS

- Contraindicated in patients hypersensitive to drug or its components.
- Contraindicated with dihydroergotamine, ergonovine, ergotamine, flecainide, methylergonovine, midazolam, pimozide, propafenone, and triazolam.
- Avoid use in patients with severe hepatic impairment.
- Use cautiously in patients allergic to sulfonamides and those with mild to moderate hepatic impairment.
- Use in pregnant woman only when benefit to mother justifies risk to fetus.
- Tell woman not to breast-feed during therapy.

NURSING CONSIDERATIONS

- Patients with hepatitis B or C or marked increase in transaminases before treatment may have increased risk of transaminase elevation. Monitor patient closely during treatment.
- Monitor triglyceride, lipase, ALT, AST, and glucose levels before starting therapy and periodically throughout treatment.
- Ask patient if he's allergic to sulfa drugs.
- Monitor patient with hemophilia for spontaneous bleeding.
- During first treatment, monitor patient for opportunistic infections, such as mycobacterium avium complex, CMV, *Pneumocystis jiroveci (carinii)* pneumonia, and tuberculosis.
- Assess patient for redistribution or accumulation of body fat, as in central obesity, dorsocervical fat enlargement (buffalo hump), peripheral wasting, facial wasting, breast enlargement, and a cushingoid appearance.

PATIENT TEACHING

- Tell patient that drug doesn't reduce the risk of transmitting HIV to others.
- Inform patient that the drug may reduce the risk of progression to AIDS.
- Explain that fosamprenavir must be used with other antiretrovirals.
- Tell patient not to alter the dose or stop taking drug without consulting prescriber.
- Drug interacts with many other drugs; urge patient to tell prescriber about any prescription, OTC, or herbal medicines he's taking (especially St. John's wort).
- Explain that body fat may redistribute or accumulate.

foscarnet sodium (phosphonoformic acid)

Foscavir

Pharmacologic class: pyrophosphate analogue
Pregnancy risk category C

AVAILABLE FORMS

Injection: 24 mg/ml in 250- and 500-ml bottles

INDICATIONS & DOSAGES

➤ CMV retinitis in patients with AIDS

Adults: Initially, for induction, 60 mg/kg I.V. q 8 hours or 90 mg/kg I.V. q 12 hours for 2 to 3 weeks, depending on patient response. Follow with a maintenance infusion of 90 to 120 mg/kg daily.

➤ Acyclovir-resistant herpes simplex virus infections

Adults: 40 mg/kg I.V. over 1 hour q 8 to 12 hours for 2 to 3 weeks or until healed.

Adjust-a-dose: Adjust dosage when creatinine clearance is less than 1.4 ml/minute/kg. If clearance falls below 0.4 ml/minute/kg, stop drug. Consult manufacturer's package insert for specific dosage adjustments.

I.V. ADMINISTRATION

- To minimize renal toxicity, make sure patient is adequately hydrated before and during infusion.
- Don't exceed the recommended dosage, rate, or frequency of infusion. Doses must be individualized according to patient's renal function.
- Drug may be infused via a central or peripheral vein with enough blood flow for rapid distribution and dilution. If infusing into a central vein, don't dilute the commercially available form (24 mg/ml). If infusing into a peripheral vein, dilute to 12 mg/ml with D_5W or normal saline solution to decrease risk of local irritation. Use an infusion pump.
- Give induction treatment over 1 hour and maintenance infusions over 2 hours.

INCOMPATIBILITIES

Acyclovir, amphotericin B, co-trimoxazole, dextrose 30%, diazepam, digoxin, diphenhydramine, dobutamine, droperidol, ganciclovir, haloperidol, lactated Ringer solution, leucovorin, lorazepam, midazolam, pentamidine, phenytoin, prochlorperazine, promethazine, solutions containing calcium (such as total parenteral nutrition), trimetrexate, vancomycin.

ACTION

Inhibits all known herpes viruses in vitro by blocking the pyrophosphate-binding site on DNA polymerases and reverse transcriptases.

Route	Onset	Peak	Duration
I.V.	Unknown	Immediate	Unknown

Half-life: 3 hours.

ADVERSE REACTIONS

CNS: *asthenia, dizziness, fatigue, fever, headache, hypoesthesia, malaise, neuropathy, paresthesia,* ***seizures,*** abnormal coordination, agitation, aggression, amnesia, anxiety, aphasia, ataxia, cerebrovascular disorder, confusion, dementia, depression, EEG abnormalities, generalized spasms, hallucinations, insomnia, meningitis, nervousness, pain, sensory disturbances, somnolence, stupor, tremor.
CV: *ECG abnormalities, first-degree AV block, flushing, hypertension, hypotension, palpitations, sinus tachycardia,* chest pain, edema.
EENT: conjunctivitis, eye pain, pharyngitis, rhinitis, sinusitis, visual disturbances.
GI: *abdominal pain, anorexia, diarrhea, nausea, vomiting,* ***pancreatitis,*** constipa-

tion, dysphagia, dry mouth, dyspepsia, flatulence, melena, rectal hemorrhage, taste perversion, ulcerative stomatitis.
GU: ***acute renal failure,*** *abnormal renal function,* albuminuria, candidiasis, dysuria, polyuria, urethral disorder, urinary retention, UTI.
Hematologic: *anemia,* ***bone marrow suppression, granulocytopenia, leukopenia, thrombocytopenia,*** thrombocytosis.
Hepatic: abnormal hepatic function.
Metabolic: *hyperphosphatemia, hypocalcemia, hypokalemia, hypomagnesemia, hypophosphatemia, hyponatremia.*
Musculoskeletal: arthralgia, back pain, leg cramps, myalgia.
Respiratory: ***bronchospasm,*** *cough, dyspnea,* hemoptysis, pneumonitis, pneumothorax, pulmonary infiltration, respiratory insufficiency, stridor.
Skin: *diaphoresis, rash,* erythematous rash, facial edema, pruritus, seborrhea, skin ulceration, skin discoloration.
Other: ***sarcoma, sepsis,*** abscess, bacterial or fungal infections, flulike symptoms, inflammation and pain at infusion site, lymphadenopathy, lymphoma-like disorder, rigors.

INTERACTIONS

Drug-drug. *Nephrotoxic drugs (such as aminoglycosides, amphotericin B):* May increase risk of nephrotoxicity. Avoid using together.
Pentamidine: May increase risk of nephrotoxicity; severe hypocalcemia also has been reported. Monitor renal function tests and electrolytes.
Zidovudine: May increase risk or severity of anemia. Monitor blood counts.

EFFECTS ON LAB TEST RESULTS

- May increase alkaline phosphatase, ALT, AST, bilirubin, creatinine, and phosphate levels. May decrease calcium, hemoglobin, magnesium, phosphate, potassium, and sodium levels.
- May increase platelet count. May decrease granulocyte, platelet, and WBC counts.

CONTRAINDICATIONS & CAUTIONS

- Contraindicated in patients hypersensitive to drug.
- In patients with abnormal renal function, use cautiously and reduce dosage. Drug is nephrotoxic and can worsen renal impairment. Some degree of nephrotoxicity occurs in most patients.

NURSING CONSIDERATIONS

- ***Alert:*** Because drug is highly toxic, which is probably dose-related, always use the lowest effective maintenance dose.
- Monitor creatinine clearance frequently during therapy because of drug's adverse effects on renal function. Obtain a baseline 24-hour creatinine clearance. Monitor level two to three times weekly during induction and at least once every 1 to 2 weeks during maintenance.
- Drug can alter electrolyte levels; monitor levels using a schedule similar to that established for creatinine clearance. Assess patient for tetany and seizures caused by abnormal electrolyte levels.
- Monitor patient's hemoglobin level and hematocrit. Anemia occurs in about a third of patients and may be severe enough to require transfusions.
- Drug may cause a dose-related transient decrease in ionized calcium, which may not always show up in patient's lab values.

PATIENT TEACHING

- Explain the importance of adequate hydration throughout therapy.
- Advise patient to report tingling around the mouth, numbness in the arms and legs, and pins-and-needles sensations.
- Tell patient to alert nurse about discomfort at I.V. insertion site.

ganciclovir

Cytovene

Pharmacologic class: synthetic purine nucleoside analogue of guanine
Pregnancy risk category C

AVAILABLE FORMS

Capsules: 250 mg, 500 mg
Injection: 500 mg/vial

INDICATIONS & DOSAGES

➤ **CMV retinitis in immunocompromised patients, including those with AIDS and normal renal function**

Adults and children older than age 3 months: Induction treatment is 5 mg/kg I.V. q 12 hours for 14 to 21 days. Don't use capsules for induction. Maintenance treatment is 5 mg/kg I.V. daily or 6 mg/kg I.V. daily five times weekly. Or, for maintenance therapy, give 1,000 mg P.O. t.i.d. with food or 500 mg P.O. q 3 hours while awake (six times daily).

➤ **To prevent CMV disease in patients with advanced HIV infection and normal renal function**

Adults: 1,000 mg P.O. t.i.d. with food.

➤ **To prevent CMV disease in transplant recipients with normal renal function**

Adults: 5 mg/kg I.V. (given at a constant rate over 1 hour) q 12 hours for 7 to 14 days; then 5 mg/kg daily or 6 mg/kg daily five times weekly. Duration of therapy depends on degree of immunosuppression.

Adjust-a-dose: Adjust dosage in patients with renal impairment according to the table. If patient is receiving hemodialysis, give dose shortly after session is complete. First I.V. dosage is 1.25 mg/kg three times weekly; maintenance I.V. dosage is 0.625 mg/kg three times weekly; and P.O. dosage is 500 mg three times weekly.

Initial I.V. therapy

Creatinine clearance (ml/min)	Dose (mg/kg)	Interval
50–69	2.5	12 hr
25–49	2.5	24 hr
10–24	1.25	24 hr
< 10	1.25	3 times weekly

Maintenance I.V. therapy

Creatinine clearance (ml/min)	Dose (mg/kg)	Interval
50–69	2.5	24 hr
25–49	1.25	24 hr
10–24	0.625	24 hr
< 10	0.625	3 times weekly

P.O. therapy

Creatinine clearance (ml/min)	Dose (mg)	Interval
50–69	1,500	24 hr
	500	8 hr
25–49	1,000	24 hr
	500	12 hr
10–24	500	24 hr
< 10	500	3 times weekly

I.V. ADMINISTRATION

- To reconstitute, add 10 ml sterile water for injection to 500-mg vial. Shake vial well to dissolve drug.
- Further dilute in 50 to 250 ml (usually 100 ml) of compatible I.V. solution.
- If fluids are being restricted, dilute to no more than 10 mg/ml.
- Don't give as bolus.
- Use an infusion pump.
- Infuse over at least 1 hour.
- Infusing drug too rapidly has toxic effects.

INCOMPATIBILITIES

Aldesleukin, amifostine, aztreonam, cefepime, cytarabine, doxorubicin hydrochloride, fludarabine, foscarnet, ondansetron, other I.V. drugs, paraben (bacteriostatic agent), piperacillin sodium with tazobactam, sargramostim, vinorelbine.

ACTION

Inhibits binding of deoxyguanosine triphosphate to DNA polymerase, resulting in inhibition of DNA synthesis.

Route	Onset	Peak	Duration
P.O.	Unknown	2–3 hr	Unknown
I.V.	Unknown	Immediate	Unknown

Half-life: About 3 hours.

ADVERSE REACTIONS

CNS: *fever,* ***coma, seizures,*** abnormal thinking, agitation, altered dreams, amnesia, anxiety, asthenia, ataxia, confusion, dizziness, headache, somnolence, tremor, neuropathy, paresthesia.

EENT: retinal detachment in CMV retinitis patients.
GI: *abdominal pain, anorexia, diarrhea, nausea, vomiting,* dry mouth, dyspepsia, flatulence.
Hematologic: *anemia,* ***agranulocytosis, leukopenia, thrombocytopenia.***
Respiratory: pneumonia.
Skin: *rash, sweating,* inflammation, pruritus, pain and phlebitis at injection site.
Other: ***sepsis,*** chills, infection.

INTERACTIONS

Drug-drug. *Amphotericin B, cyclosporine, other nephrotoxic drugs:* May increase risk of nephrotoxicity. Monitor renal function.
Imipenem and cilastatin: May increase seizure activity. Use together only if potential benefits outweigh risks.
Cytotoxic drugs: May increase toxic effects, especially hematologic effects and stomatitis. Monitor patient closely.
Immunosuppressants (such as azathioprine, corticosteroids, cyclosporine): May enhance immune and bone marrow suppression. Use together cautiously.
Probenecid: May increase ganciclovir level. Monitor patient closely.
Zidovudine: May increase risk of agranulocytosis. Use together cautiously; monitor hematologic function closely.

EFFECTS ON LAB TEST RESULTS

- May increase alkaline phosphatase, ALT, AST, creatinine, and GGT levels. May decrease hemoglobin level.
- May decrease granulocyte, neutrophil, platelet, and WBC counts.

CONTRAINDICATIONS & CAUTIONS

- Contraindicated in patients hypersensitive to drug or acyclovir and in those with an absolute neutrophil count below 500/mm^3 or a platelet count below 25,000/mm^3.
- Use cautiously and reduce dosage in patients with renal dysfunction. Monitor renal function tests.

NURSING CONSIDERATIONS

- Use caution when preparing solution, which is alkaline.
- ***Alert:*** Don't give subcutaneously or I.M.
- Because of the frequency of agranulocytosis and thrombocytopenia, obtain neutrophil and platelet counts every 2 days during twice-daily doses and at least weekly thereafter.

PATIENT TEACHING

- Explain importance of drinking plenty of fluids during therapy.
- Instruct patient to report adverse reactions promptly.
- Tell patient to report discomfort at I.V. insertion site.
- Advise patient that drug causes birth defects. Instruct women to use effective birth control; men should use barrier contraception during and for at least 90 days after therapy.

indinavir sulfate

Crixivan

Pharmacologic class: protease inhibitor
Pregnancy risk category C

AVAILABLE FORMS

Capsules: 100 mg, 200 mg, 333 mg, 400 mg

INDICATIONS & DOSAGES

➤ **HIV infection, with other antiretrovirals, when antiretrovirals are warranted**

Adults: 800 mg P.O. q 8 hours.
Adjust-a-dose: For patients with mild to moderate hepatic insufficiency from cirrhosis, reduce dosage to 600 mg P.O. q 8 hours.

ACTION

Inhibits HIV protease by binding to the protease-active site and inhibiting activity of the enzyme, preventing cleavage of the viral polyproteins and forming immature noninfectious viral particles.

Route	Onset	Peak	Duration
P.O.	Unknown	< 1 hr	Unknown

Half-life: 2 hours.

ADVERSE REACTIONS

CNS: asthenia, dizziness, fatigue, headache, insomnia, malaise, somnolence.
CV: chest pain, palpitations.
EENT: blurred vision, eye pain or swelling.
GI: *nausea,* abdominal pain, acid regurgitation, anorexia, diarrhea, dry mouth, taste perversion, vomiting.
GU: hematuria, nephrolithiasis.
Hematologic: ***neutropenia, thrombocytopenia,*** anemia.
Metabolic: *hyperbilirubinemia,* hyperglycemia.
Musculoskeletal: back pain.
Other: flank pain.

INTERACTIONS

Drug-drug. *Amprenavir, saquinavir:* May increase levels of these drugs. Dosage adjustments not needed.
Carbamazepine: May decrease indinavir exposure to the body. Consider an alternative drug.
Clarithromycin: May alter clarithromycin level. Dosage adjustments not needed.
Delavirdine, itraconazole, ketoconazole: May increase indinavir level. Consider reducing indinavir to 600 mg q 8 hours.
Didanosine: May alter absorption of indinavir. Separate doses by 1 hour and give on an empty stomach.
Efavirenz, nevirapine: May decrease indinavir level. Increase indinavir to 1,000 mg q 8 hours.
HMG-CoA reductase inhibitors: May increase levels of these drugs and increase risk of myopathy and rhabdomyolysis. Avoid using together.
Lopinavir and ritonavir combination: May increase indinavir level. Adjust indinavir dosage to 600 mg b.i.d.
Midazolam, triazolam: May inhibit metabolism of these drugs, which may cause serious or life-threatening events, such as arrhythmias or prolonged sedation. Avoid using together.
Nelfinavir: May increase indinavir level by 50% and nelfinavir by 80%. May need to adjust dosage to indinavir 1,200 mg b.i.d. and nelfinavir 1,250 mg b.i.d. Monitor patient closely.
Proton-pump inhibitors (lansoprazole, omeprazole, pantoprazole, rabeprazole): May reduce the antiviral activity of indinavir. Avoid use together.
Rifabutin: May increase rifabutin level and decrease indinavir level. Give indinavir 1,000 mg q 8 hours and decrease the rifabutin dose to either 150 mg daily or 300 mg two to three times a week.
Rifampin: May decrease indinavir level. Avoid using together.
Rifapentine: May decrease indinavir level. Use with extreme caution, if at all.
Ritonavir: May increase indinavir level twofold to fivefold. Adjust dosage to indinavir 400 mg b.i.d. and ritonavir 400 mg b.i.d., or indinavir 800 mg b.i.d. and ritonavir 100 to 200 mg b.i.d.
Sildenafil, tadalafil, vardenafil: May increase levels of these drugs and increase adverse effects (hypotension, visual changes, and priapism). Tell patient not to exceed prescribed dosage.
Drug-herb. ***St. John's wort:*** May reduce drug level by more than half. Discourage use together.
Drug-food. *Grapefruit and grapefruit juice:* May decrease drug level and therapeutic effect. Discourage use together.

EFFECTS ON LAB TEST RESULTS

- May increase ALT, AST, bilirubin, amylase, hemoglobin, and glucose levels.
- May decrease neutrophil and platelet counts.

CONTRAINDICATIONS & CAUTIONS

- Contraindicated in patients hypersensitive to drug or its components.
- Use cautiously in patients with hepatic insufficiency from cirrhosis.
- Safety and effectiveness in children haven't been established.

NURSING CONSIDERATIONS

- Drug must be taken at 8-hour intervals.
- Drug may cause nephrolithiasis. If signs and symptoms of nephrolithiasis occur, prescriber may stop drug for 1 to 3 days during acute phases.
- To prevent nephrolithiasis, patient should maintain adequate hydration (at least 48 ounces or 1.5 L of fluids q 24 hours while taking indinavir).

PATIENT TEACHING

- Tell patient that drug doesn't cure HIV infection and that he may continue to develop opportunistic infections and other complications of HIV infection. Drug hasn't been shown to reduce the risk of HIV transmission.
- Advise patient to use barrier protection during sexual intercourse.
- Caution patient not to adjust dosage or stop therapy without first consulting prescriber.
- Advise patient that if a dose is missed, he should take the next dose at the regularly scheduled time and shouldn't double the dose.
- Instruct patient to take drug on an empty stomach with water 1 hour before or 2 hours after a meal. Or, he may take it with other liquids (such as skim milk, juice, coffee, or tea) or a light meal. Inform patient that a meal high in fat, calories, and protein reduces absorption of drug.
- Instruct patient to store capsules in the original container and to keep desiccant in the bottle; capsules are sensitive to moisture.
- Tell patient to drink at least 48 ounces (1.5 L) of fluid daily.
- Advise woman to avoid breast-feeding because drug may appear in breast milk. Also, to prevent transmitting virus to infant, advise an HIV-positive woman not to breast-feed.

lamivudine

Epivir, Epivir-HBV

Pharmacologic class: nucleoside reverse transcriptase inhibitor
Pregnancy risk category C

AVAILABLE FORMS

Epivir
Oral solution: 10 mg/ml
Tablets: 150 mg, 300 mg
Epivir-HBV
Oral solution: 5 mg/ml
Tablets: 100 mg

INDICATIONS & DOSAGES

➤ **HIV infection, with other antiretrovirals**
Adults and children older than age 16: 300 mg Epivir P.O. once daily or 150 mg P.O. b.i.d.
Children ages 3 months to 16 years: 4 mg/kg Epivir P.O. b.i.d. Maximum dose is 150 mg b.i.d.
Neonates age 30 days and younger♦: 2 mg/kg Epivir P.O. b.i.d.
Adjust-a-dose: For patients with creatinine clearance of 30 to 49 ml/minute, give 150 mg Epivir P.O. daily. If clearance is 15 to 29 ml/minute, give 150 mg P.O. on day 1 and then 100 mg daily; if it's 5 to 14 ml/minute, give 150 mg on day 1 and then 50 mg daily; if it's less than 5 ml/minute, give 50 mg on day 1 and then 25 mg daily.

➤ **Chronic hepatitis B with evidence of hepatitis B virus (HBV) replication and active liver inflammation**
Adults: 100 mg Epivir-HBV P.O. once daily.
Children ages 2 to 17: 3 mg/kg Epivir-HBV P.O. once daily, up to a maximum dose of 100 mg daily. Optimum duration of treatment isn't known; safety and effectiveness of treatment beyond 1 year haven't been established.
Adjust-a-dose: For adult patients with creatinine clearance of 30 to 49 ml/minute, give first dose of 100 mg Epivir-HBV; then give 50 mg P.O. once daily. If clearance is 15 to 29 ml/minute, give first dose of 100 mg; then give 25 mg P.O. once daily. If clearance is 5 to 14 ml/minute, give first dose of 35 mg; then give 15 mg P.O. once daily. If clearance is less than 5 ml/minute, give first dose of 35 mg; then give 10 mg P.O. once daily.

ACTION

A synthetic nucleoside analogue that inhibits HIV and HBV reverse transcription via viral DNA chain termination. RNA- and DNA-dependent DNA polymerase activities.

Route	Onset	Peak	Duration
P.O.	Unknown	1–3 hr	Unknown

Half-life: 5 to 7 hours.

ADVERSE REACTIONS

Adverse reactions pertain to the combination therapy of lamivudine and zidovudine.

CNS: *dizziness, fatigue, fever, headache, insomnia and other sleep disorders, malaise, neuropathy,* depressive disorders.
EENT: *nasal symptoms.*
GI: *anorexia, diarrhea, nausea, vomiting,* ***pancreatitis,*** abdominal cramps, abdominal pain, dyspepsia.
Hematologic: ***neutropenia, thrombocytopenia,*** anemia.
Hepatic: ***hepatotoxicity.***
Metabolic: ***lactic acidosis.***
Musculoskeletal: *musculoskeletal pain,* arthralgia, myalgia.
Respiratory: *cough.*
Skin: rash.
Other: *chills.*

INTERACTIONS

Drug-drug. *Trimethoprim and sulfamethoxazole:* May increase lamivudine level because of decreased clearance of drug. Monitor patient for toxicity.
Zalcitabine: May inhibit activation of both drugs. Avoid using together.
Zidovudine: May increase zidovudine level. Monitor patient closely for adverse reactions.

EFFECTS ON LAB TEST RESULTS

- May increase ALT and bilirubin levels. May decrease hemoglobin level.
- May decrease neutrophil and platelet counts.

CONTRAINDICATIONS & CAUTIONS

- Contraindicated in patients hypersensitive to drug.
- Use cautiously in patients with renal impairment.
- ***Alert:*** Use drug cautiously, if at all, in children with history of pancreatitis or other significant risk factors for development of pancreatitis.
- The Antiretroviral Pregnancy Registry monitors maternal-fetal outcomes of pregnant women exposed to lamivudine. To register a pregnant woman, call the Antiretroviral Pregnancy Registry at 1-800-258-4263.

NURSING CONSIDERATIONS

- ***Alert:*** Stop treatment immediately and notify prescriber if signs, symptoms, or laboratory abnormalities suggest pancreatitis. Monitor amylase level.
- ***Alert:*** Lactic acidosis and hepatotoxicity have been reported. Notify prescriber if signs of lactic acidosis or hepatotoxicity occurs.
- Hepatitis may recur in some patients with chronic HBV when they stop taking drug.
- Safety and effectiveness of Epivir-HBV for longer than 1 year haven't been established; optimum duration of treatment isn't known. Test patients for HIV before starting treatment and during therapy because form and dosage of lamivudine in Epivir-HBV aren't appropriate for those infected with both HBV and HIV. If lamivudine is given to patients with HBV and HIV, use the higher dosage indicated for HIV therapy as part of an appropriate combination regimen.
- Because of a high rate of early virologic resistance, don't use triple antiretroviral therapy with abacavir or didanosine, lamivudine, and tenofovir as new treatment for never-treated or pretreated patients. Monitor patients currently taking this therapy and those who take it with other antiretrovirals, and consider a different therapy.
- Monitor patient's CBC, platelet count, and renal and liver function studies. Report abnormalities.

PATIENT TEACHING

- Inform patient that long-term effects of drug aren't known.
- Stress importance of taking drug exactly as prescribed.
- Inform patient that drug doesn't cure HIV infection, that opportunistic infections and other complications of HIV infection may still occur, and that transmission of HIV to others through sexual contact or blood contamination is still possible.
- Teach parents or guardians the signs and symptoms of pancreatitis. Advise them to report signs and symptoms immediately.

lopinavir and ritonavir

Kaletra

Pharmacologic class: protease inhibitor
Pregnancy risk category C

AVAILABLE FORMS

Tablets: lopinavir 200 mg and ritonavir 50 mg
Solution: lopinavir 400 mg and ritonavir 100 mg/5 ml (80 mg and 20 mg/ml)

INDICATIONS & DOSAGES

➤ HIV infection, with other antiretrovirals in treatment-naive adults
Adults: 800 mg lopinavir and 200 mg ritonavir (4 tablets or 10 ml) P.O. once daily or divided evenly b.i.d.

➤ HIV infection, with other antiretrovirals in treatment-experienced patients
Adults and children older than age 12: 400 mg lopinavir and 100 mg ritonavir (2 tablets or 5 ml) P.O. b.i.d.
Children ages 6 months to 12 years, who weigh 15 to 40 kg (33 to 88 lb): 10 mg/kg (lopinavir content) P.O. b.i.d. with food up to a maximum of 400 mg lopinavir and 100 mg ritonavir.
Children ages 6 months to 12 years, who weigh 7 to 15 kg (15 to 33 lb): 12 mg/kg (lopinavir content) P.O. b.i.d. with food.
Adjust-a-dose: In treatment-experienced patients older than age 12 also taking efavirenz, nevirapine, fosamprenavir without ritonavir, or nelfinavir, consider dosage of 600 mg lopinavir and 150 mg ritonavir (3 tablets) P.O. b.i.d. For patients using oral solution and also taking efavirenz, nevirapine, amprenavir, or nelfinavir, 533 mg lopinavir and 133 mg ritonavir (6.5 ml) b.i.d. with food is recommended.

In treatment-experienced children age 6 months to 12 years who also take amprenavir, efavirenz, or nevirapine and who weigh 7 to 15 kg, give 13 mg/kg (lopinavir content) P.O. b.i.d. with food. For those who weigh 15 to 45 kg, give 11 mg/kg (lopinavir content) P.O. b.i.d. with food up to a maximum dose of 533 mg lopinavir, and 133 mg ritonavir b.i.d. in children who weigh more than 45 kg.

ACTION

Lopinavir is an HIV protease inhibitor, which produces immature, noninfectious viral particles. Ritonavir, also an HIV protease inhibitor, inhibits the metabolism of lopinavir, thereby increasing lopinavir level.

Route	Onset	Peak	Duration
P.O.	Unknown	4 hr	5–6 hr

Half-life: About 6 hours.

ADVERSE REACTIONS

CNS: ***encephalopathy,*** abnormal dreams, abnormal thinking, agitation, amnesia, anxiety, asthenia, ataxia, confusion, depression, dizziness, dyskinesia, emotional lability, fever, headache, hypertonia, insomnia, malaise, nervousness, neuropathy, pain, paresthesia, peripheral neuritis, somnolence, tremors.
CV: chest pain, deep vein thrombosis, edema, hypertension, palpitations, thrombophlebitis, vasculitis.
EENT: abnormal vision, eye disorder, otitis media, sinusitis, tinnitus.
GI: ***hemorrhagic colitis, pancreatitis,*** *diarrhea, nausea,* abdominal pain, abnormal stools, anorexia, cholecystitis, constipation, dry mouth, dyspepsia, dysphagia, enterocolitis, eructation, esophagitis, fecal incontinence, flatulence, gastritis, gastroenteritis, GI disorder, increased appetite, inflammation of the salivary glands, stomatitis, taste perversion, ulcerative stomatitis, vomiting.
GU: abnormal ejaculation, hypogonadism, renal calculus, urine abnormality.
Hematologic: ***leukopenia, neutropenia, thrombocytopenia in children,*** anemia.
Hepatic: hyperbilirubinemia in children.
Metabolic: Cushing's syndrome, dehydration, decreased glucose tolerance, hyperglycemia, hyperuricemia, hyponatremia in children, hypothyroidism, lactic acidosis, weight loss.
Musculoskeletal: arthralgia, arthrosis, back pain, myalgia.
Respiratory: bronchitis, dyspnea, lung edema.

Skin: acne, alopecia, benign skin neoplasm, dry skin, exfoliative dermatitis, furunculosis, nail disorder, pruritus, rash, skin discoloration, sweating.
Other: chills, decreased libido, facial edema, flu syndrome, gynecomastia, lymphadenopathy, peripheral edema, viral infection.

INTERACTIONS

Drug-drug. *Amiodarone, bepridil, lidocaine, quinidine:* May increase antiarrhythmic level. Use together cautiously. Monitor levels of these drugs, if possible.
Amprenavir , efavirenz, nelfinavir, nevirapine: May decrease lopinavir level. Consider increasing Kaletra dose. Don't use a once-daily Kaletra regimen with these drugs.
Antiarrhythmics (flecainide, propafenone), pimozide: May increase risk of cardiac arrhythmias. Avoid using together.
Atorvastatin: May increase level of this drug. Use lowest possible dose and monitor patient carefully.
Atovaquone, methadone: May decrease levels of these drugs. Consider increasing doses of these drugs.
Carbamazepine, dexamethasone, phenobarbital, phenytoin: May decrease lopinavir level. Use together cautiously.
Clarithromycin: May increase clarithromycin level in patients with renal impairment. Adjust clarithromycin dosage.
Cyclosporine, rapamycin, tacrolimus: May increase levels of these drugs. Monitor therapeutic levels.
Delavirdine: May increase lopinavir level. Avoid using together.
Didanosine: May decrease absorption of didanosine because Kaletra is taken with food. Give didanosine 1 hour before or 2 hours after Kaletra.
Dihydroergotamine, ergonovine, ergotamine, methylergonovine: May increase risk of ergot toxicity characterized by peripheral vasospasm and ischemia. Avoid using together.
Disulfiram, metronidazole: May cause disulfiram-like reaction. Avoid using together.
Felodipine, nicardipine, nifedipine: May increase levels of these drugs. Use together cautiously.
Hormonal contraceptives (ethinyl estradiol): May decrease effectiveness of contraceptives. Recommend nonhormonal contraceptives.
Indinavir, saquinavir: May increase levels of these drugs. Avoid using together.
Itraconazole, ketoconazole: May increase levels of these drugs. Don't give more than 200 mg/day of these drugs.
Lovastatin, simvastatin: May increase risk of adverse reactions, such as myopathy, rhabdomyolysis. Avoid using together.
Midazolam, triazolam: May cause prolonged or increased sedation or respiratory depression. Avoid using together.
Rifabutin: May increase rifabutin level. Decrease rifabutin dose by 75%. Monitor patient for adverse effects.
Rifampin: May decrease effectiveness of Kaletra. Avoid using together.
Sildenafil, tadalafil, vardenafil: May increase level of these drugs and adverse effects, such as hypotension and prolonged erection. Warn patient not to take more than 25 mg of sildenafil in 48 hours, more than 10 mg of tadalafil in 72 hours, or more than 2.5 mg vardenafil in 72 hours.
Warfarin: May affect warfarin level. Monitor PT and INR.
Drug-herb. *St. John's wort:* Loss of virologic response and possible resistance to drug. Discourage use together.
Drug-food. *Any food:* May increase absorption of oral solution. Tell patient to take with food.

EFFECTS ON LAB TEST RESULTS

- May increase amylase, cholesterol, and triglyceride levels. May decrease hemoglobin level and hematocrit.
- May decrease RBC, WBC, neutrophil, and platelet counts.

CONTRAINDICATIONS & CAUTIONS

- Contraindicated in patients hypersensitive to drug or any of its components.
- Use cautiously in patients with a history of pancreatitis or with hepatic impairment, hepatitis B or C, marked elevations in liver enzyme levels, or hemophilia.
- Use cautiously in elderly patients.
- The Antiretroviral Pregnancy Registry monitors maternal-fetal outcomes of pregnant women taking Kaletra. Health care

providers are encouraged to enroll women by calling 1-800-258-4263.

NURSING CONSIDERATIONS

- ***Alert:*** Many drug interactions are possible. Review all drugs patient is taking.
- Refrigerated drug remains stable until expiration date on package. If stored at room temperature, use drug within 2 months.
- Monitor patient for signs of fat redistribution, including central obesity, buffalo hump, peripheral wasting, breast enlargement, and cushingoid appearance.
- Monitor total cholesterol and triglycerides before starting therapy and periodically thereafter.
- Monitor patient for signs and symptoms of pancreatitis (nausea, vomiting, abdominal pain, or increased lipase and amylase values).
- Monitor patient for signs and symptoms of bleeding (hypotension, rapid heart rate).
- ***Look alike–sound alike:*** Don't confuse Kaletra with Keppra.

PATIENT TEACHING

- Tell patient to take oral solution with food. Tablets may be taken without regard to food.
- ***Alert:*** Tablets must be swallowed whole; don't crush or divide, and tell patient not to chew.
- Tell patient also taking didanosine to take it 1 hour before or 2 hours after lopinavir-ritonavir combination.
- Advise patient to report side effects to prescriber.
- Tell patient to immediately report severe nausea, vomiting, or abdominal pain.
- Inform patient that drug doesn't cure HIV infection, that opportunistic infections and other complications of HIV infection may still occur, and that transmission of HIV to others through sexual contact or blood contamination remains possible.
- Advise patient taking an erectile dysfunction drug of an increased risk of adverse effects, including low blood pressure, visual changes, and painful erections, and to promptly report any symptoms to his prescriber. Tell him not to take more often than directed.
- Warn patient to tell prescriber about any other prescription or nonprescription medicine that he's taking, including herbal supplements.

nelfinavir mesylate
Viracept

Pharmacologic class: protease inhibitor
Pregnancy risk category B

AVAILABLE FORMS

Powder: 50 mg/g powder in 144-g bottle
Tablets: 250 mg, 625 mg

INDICATIONS & DOSAGES

➤ **HIV infection, when antiretroviral therapy is warranted**
Adults: 1,250 mg b.i.d. or 750 mg P.O. t.i.d. with meals or light snack.
Children ages 2 to 13: 45 to 55 mg/kg P.O. b.i.d. or 25 to 35 mg/kg P.O. t.i.d. with meals or light snack; don't exceed 750 mg t.i.d.

➤ **To prevent infection after occupational exposure to HIV♦**
Adults: 750 mg P.O. t.i.d. with two other antiretrovirals (zidovudine and lamivudine, lamivudine and stavudine, or didanosine and stavudine) for 4 weeks.

ACTION

An HIV-1 protease inhibitor, which prevents cleavage of the viral polyprotein, resulting in the production of immature, noninfectious virus.

Route	Onset	Peak	Duration
P.O.	Unknown	2–4 hr	Unknown

Half-life: 3½ to 5 hours.

ADVERSE REACTIONS

CNS: ***seizures, suicidal ideation.***
GI: *diarrhea,* ***pancreatitis,*** flatulence, nausea.
Hematologic: ***leukopenia, thrombocytopenia.***
Hepatic: ***hepatitis.***
Metabolic: ***hypoglycemia,*** dehydration, diabetes mellitus, hyperlipidemia, hyperuricemia.
Skin: rash.

Other: redistribution or accumulation of body fat.

INTERACTIONS

Drug-drug. *Amiodarone, ergot derivatives, lovastatin, midazolam, pimozide, quinidine, simvastatin, triazolam:* May increase levels of these drugs, causing increased risk of life-threatening adverse events. Avoid using together.
Atorvastatin: May increase atorvastatin level. Use lowest possible dose or consider using pravastatin or fluvastatin instead.
Azithromycin: May increase azithromycin level. Monitor patient for liver impairment.
Carbamazepine, phenobarbital: May reduce the effectiveness of nelfinavir. Use together cautiously.
Cyclosporine, sirolimus, tacrolimus: May increase levels of these immunosuppressants. Use cautiously together.
Delavirdine, HIV protease inhibitors (indinavir, saquinavir): May increase levels of protease inhibitors. Use together cautiously.
Didanosine: May decrease didanosine absorption. Take nelfinavir with food at least 2 hours before or 1 hour after didanosine.
Ethinyl estradiol: May decrease contraceptive level and effectiveness. Advise patient to use alternative contraceptive measures during therapy.
Methadone, phenytoin: May decrease levels of these drugs. Adjust dosage of these drugs accordingly.
Rifabutin: May increase rifabutin level and decrease nelfinavir level. Reduce dosage of rifabutin to half the usual dose and increase nelfinavir to 1,250 mg b.i.d.
Sildenafil: May increase adverse effects of sildenafil. Caution patient not to exceed 25 mg of sildenafil in a 48-hour period.
Drug-herb. ***St. John's wort:*** May decrease drug level. Discourage use together.

EFFECTS ON LAB TEST RESULTS

- May increase ALT, AST, alkaline phosphatase, bilirubin, GGT, amylase, CK, and lipid levels. May decrease hemoglobin level. May increase or decrease glucose level.
- May decrease WBC and platelet counts.

CONTRAINDICATIONS & CAUTIONS

- Contraindicated in patients hypersensitive to drug or its components. Drug is also contraindicated in patients receiving amiodarone, ergot derivatives, lovastatin, midazolam, pimozide, quinidine, simvastatin, or triazolam.
- Use cautiously in patients with hepatic dysfunction or hemophilia types A or B. Monitor liver function test results.
- It's not known if drug appears in breast milk. Because safety hasn't been established, advise HIV-infected women not to breast-feed, to avoid transmitting virus to the infant.

NURSING CONSIDERATIONS

- Drug dosage is the same whether used alone or with other antiretrovirals.
- Give oral powder to children unable to take tablets. May mix oral powder with small amount of water, milk, formula, soy formula, soy milk, or dietary supplements. Patient should consume entire amount.
- Don't reconstitute with water in the original container.
- Use reconstituted powder within 6 hours.
- Mixing with acidic foods or juice isn't recommended because of bitter taste.
- ***Look alike–sound alike:*** Don't confuse nelfinavir with nevirapine.

PATIENT TEACHING

- Advise patient to take drug with food.
- Inform patient that drug doesn't cure HIV infection.
- Tell patient that long-term effects of drug are unknown and that there are no data stating that nelfinavir reduces risk of HIV transmission.
- Advise patient to take drug daily as prescribed and not to alter dose or stop drug without medical approval.
- If patient misses a dose, tell him to take it as soon as possible and then return to his normal schedule. Advise patient not to double the dose.
- Tell patient that diarrhea is the most common adverse effect and that it can be controlled with loperamide, if needed.
- Instruct patient taking hormonal contraceptives to use alternative or additional

contraceptive measures while taking nelfinavir.
- Advise patient taking sildenafil about an increased risk of sildenafil-related adverse events, including low blood pressure, visual changes, and painful erections. Tell him to promptly report any symptoms. Tell him not to exceed 25 mg of sildenafil in a 48-hour period.
- Warn patient with phenylketonuria that powder contains 11.2 mg phenylalanine per gram.
- Advise patient to report use of other prescribed or OTC drugs because of possible drug interactions.

nevirapine

Viramune

Pharmacologic class: nonnucleoside reverse transcriptase inhibitor
Pregnancy risk category C

AVAILABLE FORMS

Oral suspension: 50 mg/5 ml
Tablets: 200 mg

INDICATIONS & DOSAGES

➤ Adjunct treatment in HIV-infected adults who have experienced clinical or immunologic deterioration

Adults: 200 mg P.O. daily for the first 14 days; then 200 mg P.O. b.i.d. Used with nucleoside analogue antiretrovirals.

➤ Adjunct treatment in HIV-infected children

Children age 8 and older: 4 mg/kg P.O. once daily for first 14 days; then 4 mg/kg P.O. b.i.d. thereafter. Maximum daily dose is 400 mg.
Children ages 2 months to 8 years: 4 mg/kg P.O. once daily for first 14 days; then 7 mg/kg P.O. b.i.d. thereafter. Maximum daily dose is 400 mg.

ACTION

A nonnucleoside reverse transcriptase inhibitor that binds directly to reverse transcriptase and blocks RNA-dependent and DNA-dependent DNA polymerase activities by disrupting the enzyme's catalytic site.

Route	Onset	Peak	Duration
P.O.	Unknown	4 hr	Unknown

Half-life: 25 to 30 hours.

ADVERSE REACTIONS

CNS: *fever,* headache, paresthesia.
GI: *nausea,* abdominal pain, diarrhea, ulcerative stomatitis.
Hematologic: ***neutropenia.***
Hepatic: ***hepatitis.***
Musculoskeletal: myalgia.
Skin: *blistering, rash,* ***Stevens-Johnson syndrome.***

INTERACTIONS

Drug-drug. *Drugs extensively metabolized by cytochrome P-450 3A:* May lower levels of these drugs. Dosage adjustment of these drugs may be needed.
Ketoconazole: May decrease ketoconazole level. Avoid using together.
Protease inhibitors or hormonal contraceptives: May decrease levels of these drugs. Use together cautiously.
Rifabutin, rifampin: Dosage adjustment may be needed. Monitor patient closely.
Drug-herb. *St. John's wort:* May decrease drug level. Discourage use together.

EFFECTS ON LAB TEST RESULTS

- May increase ALT, AST, GGT, and bilirubin levels. May decrease hemoglobin level.
- May decrease neutrophil count.

CONTRAINDICATIONS & CAUTIONS

- Contraindicated in patients hypersensitive to drug.
- For patients with severe hepatic impairment from drug accumulation, don't give.
- In patients with impaired renal and hepatic function, use cautiously; pharmacokinetics haven't been evaluated in these patients.
- Drug appears in breast milk. Don't use drug in breast-feeding women.

NURSING CONSIDERATIONS

- Perform laboratory tests, including renal function tests, before therapy and regularly throughout.
- Use drug with at least one other antiretroviral.

• *Alert:* Severe, life-threatening hepatotoxicity, including fulminant and cholestatic hepatitis, hepatic necrosis, and hepatic failure, may occur in all patients, including those receiving drug for post-exposure prophylaxis, an unapproved use.
• Increased AST or ALT levels or coinfection with hepatitis B or C at the start of therapy suggest a greater risk of hepatic adverse events.
• In some cases, early signs or symptoms of hepatitis will be present and patient will progress to hepatic failure. These events are often linked with rash and fever. Women and patients with higher CD4+ cell counts are at increased risk of these hepatic events. Women with CD4+ cell counts greater than 250/mm^3, including pregnant women receiving long-term treatment for HIV infection, are at considerably higher risk of these events.
• Monitor patient for signs and symptoms of hepatitis including rash. Closely monitor liver function tests at baseline and during the first 18 weeks of treatment; then monitor frequently thereafter.
• Perform liver function tests immediately if hepatitis or hypersensitivity reactions are suspected.
• *Alert:* Monitor patient for blistering, oral lesions, conjunctivitis, muscle or joint aches, or general malaise. Especially look for a severe rash or rash accompanied by fever. Report these signs and symptoms to prescriber. Patients who experience a rash during the first 14 days of therapy shouldn't have the dosage increased until the rash has resolved. Most rashes occur within the first 6 weeks of therapy.
• *Alert:* If hepatitis occurs, permanently stop drug and don't restart after recovery. In some cases, hepatic injury progresses anyway.
• Patients who have stopped therapy for more than 7 days should restart therapy as if receiving drug for the first time.
• Antiretroviral therapy may be changed if disease progresses while patient is receiving this drug.
• *Look alike–sound alike:* Don't confuse nevirapine with nelfinavir.

PATIENT TEACHING

• Inform patient that drug doesn't cure HIV and that illnesses from advanced HIV infection still may occur. Explain that drug doesn't reduce risk of HIV transmission.
• Instruct patient to report rash immediately and to stop drug until told to resume.
• Tell patient with signs or symptoms of hepatitis (such as fatigue, malaise, anorexia, nausea, jaundice, liver tenderness or hepatomegaly, with or without initially abnormal transaminase levels) to stop drug and seek medical evaluation immediately.
• Stress importance of taking drug exactly as prescribed. If a dose is missed, tell patient to take the next dose as soon as possible and not to double next dose.
• Tell patient not to use other drugs unless approved by prescriber.
• Advise woman of childbearing age that hormonal contraceptives and other hormonal methods of birth control shouldn't be used with this drug.

oseltamivir phosphate
Tamiflu

Pharmacologic class: selective neuraminidase inhibitor
Pregnancy risk category C

AVAILABLE FORMS

Capsules: 75 mg
Oral suspension: 12 mg/ml after reconstitution

INDICATIONS & DOSAGES

➤ Uncomplicated, acute illness caused by influenza infection in patients who have had symptoms for 2 days or less
Adults and adolescents age 13 and older: 75 mg P.O. b.i.d. for 5 days.
Children age 1 and older who weigh more than 40 kg (88 lb): 75 mg oral suspension P.O. b.i.d. for 5 days.
Children age 1 and older who weigh 23 to 40 kg (51 to 88 lb): 60 mg oral suspension P.O. b.i.d. for 5 days.
Children age 1 and older who weigh 15 to 23 kg (33 to 51 lb): 45 mg oral suspension P.O. b.i.d. for 5 days.
Children age 1 and older who weigh 15 kg (33 lb) or less: 30 mg oral suspension P.O. b.i.d. for 5 days.

Adjust-a-dose: For adults and adolescents with creatinine clearance of 10 to 30 ml/minute, reduce dosage to 75 mg P.O. once daily for 5 days.

➤ **To prevent influenza after close contact with infected person within 2 days of exposure**

Adults and adolescents age 13 and older: 75 mg P.O. once daily for at least 10 days.

Children age 1 and older who weigh more than 40 kg (88 lb): 75 mg oral suspension P.O. once daily for 10 days.

Children age 1 and older who weigh 23 to 40 kg (51 to 88 lb): 60 mg oral suspension P.O. once daily for 10 days.

Children age 1 and older who weigh 15 to 23 kg (33 to 51 lb): 45 mg oral suspension P.O. once daily for 10 days.

Children age 1 and older who weigh 15 kg (33 lb) or less: 30 mg oral suspension P.O. once daily for 10 days.

Adjust-a-dose: For adults and adolescents with creatinine clearance of 10 to 30 ml/minute, reduce dosage to 75 mg P.O. (as capsule) every other day or 30 mg oral suspension once daily.

➤ **To prevent influenza during a community outbreak**

Adults and adolescents age 13 and older: 75 mg P.O. once daily for up to 6 weeks.

ACTION

Inhibits influenza A and B virus enzyme neuraminidase, which is thought to play a role in viral particle aggregation and release from the host cell and appears to interfere with viral replication.

Route	Onset	Peak	Duration
P.O.	Unknown	Unknown	Unknown

Half-life: 1 to 10 hours.

ADVERSE REACTIONS

CNS: dizziness, fatigue, headache, insomnia, vertigo.
GI: abdominal pain, diarrhea, nausea, vomiting.
Respiratory: bronchitis, cough.

INTERACTIONS

None significant.

EFFECTS ON LAB TEST RESULTS

None reported.

CONTRAINDICATIONS & CAUTIONS

- Contraindicated in patients hypersensitive to drug or its components.
- Use cautiously in patients with chronic cardiac or respiratory diseases, or any medical condition that may require imminent hospitalization. Also use cautiously in patients with renal failure.
- It's unknown if drug or its metabolite appears in breast milk. Use only if benefits to patient outweigh risks to infant.

NURSING CONSIDERATIONS

- Drug must be given within 2 days of onset of symptoms.
- Safety and effectiveness of repeated treatment courses haven't been established.
- Drug may be given with meals to decrease GI adverse effects.
- Store at controlled room temperature (59° F to 86° F [15° C to 30° C]).

PATIENT TEACHING

- Instruct patient to begin treatment as soon as possible after appearance of flu symptoms.
- Inform patient that drug may be taken with or without meals. If nausea or vomiting occurs, he can take drug with food or milk.
- Tell patient that, if a dose is missed, he should take it as soon as possible. However, if next dose is due within 2 hours, tell him to skip the missed dose and take the next dose on schedule.
- Advise patient to complete the full course of treatment, even if symptoms resolve.
- Alert patient that drug isn't a replacement for the annual influenza vaccination. Patients for whom vaccine is indicated should continue to receive the vaccine each fall.

ribavirin

Copegus, Rebetol, Ribaspheres, Virazole

Pharmacologic class: synthetic nucleoside
Pregnancy risk category X

AVAILABLE FORMS

Capsules: 200 mg
Oral solution: 40 mg/ml

Powder to be reconstituted for inhalation: 6 g in 100-ml glass vial
Tablets: 200 mg

INDICATIONS & DOSAGES

➤**Hospitalized infants and young children infected by respiratory syncytial virus (RSV)**
Infants and young children: Solution in concentration of 20 mg/ml delivered via the Viratek Small Particle Aerosol Generator (SPAG-2) and mechanical ventilator or oxygen hood, face mask, or oxygen tent at a rate of about 12.5 L of mist/minute. Treatment is given for 12 to 18 hours/day for at least 3 days, and no longer than 7 days.

➤**Chronic hepatitis C**
Adults who weigh more than 75 kg (165 lb): 1,000 mg Rebetol P.O. divided b.i.d. (600 in morning, 600 mg in evening) with interferon alfa-2b, 3 million units subcutaneously three times weekly. Or, 1,200 mg Copegus with 180 mcg of Pegasys (peginterferon alfa-2a).
Adults who weigh 75 kg or less: 1,000 mg Rebetol P.O. daily in divided dose (400 mg in morning, 600 mg in evening) with interferon alfa-2b 3 million units subcutaneously three times weekly. Or, 1,000 mg Copegus with 180 mcg of Pegasys.
Children age 3 and older who weigh 50 to 61 kg (110 to 134 lb): 400 mg P.O. (Rebetol) q morning and 400 mg P.O. q evening with interferon alfa-2b, 3 million units/m^2 subcutaneously three times weekly.
Children age 3 and older who weigh 37 to 49 kg (81 to 108 lb): 200 mg P.O. (Rebetol) q morning and 400 mg P.O. q evening with interferon alfa-2b, 3 million units/m^2 subcutaneously three times weekly.
Children age 3 and older who weigh 25 to 36 kg (55 to 79 lb): 200 mg P.O. (Rebetol) q morning and 200 mg P.O. q evening with interferon alfa-2b, 3 million units/m^2 subcutaneously three times weekly.

➤**Chronic hepatitis C (regardless of genotype) in HIV-infected patients who haven't previously been treated with interferon**
Adults: 800 mg (Copegus) P.O. daily given in two divided doses with peginterferon alfa-2a (Pegasys) 180 mcg subcutaneously weekly for 48 weeks.
Adjust-a-dose: In patient with no cardiac history and hemoglobin level less than 10 g/dl, reduce dosage to 600 mg daily (200 mg in a.m., 400 mg in p.m.) for adults and 7.5 mg/kg daily for children. If hemoglobin level is less than 8.5 g/dl, stop drug. In patient with cardiac history and whose hemoglobin level falls 2 g/dl or more during any 4–week period, reduce dosage to 600 mg daily (200 mg in a.m., 400 mg in p.m.) for adults and 7.5 mg/kg daily for children. If hemoglobin level is less than 12 g/dl after 4 weeks of reduced dosage, stop drug.

ACTION

Inhibits viral activity by an unknown mechanism, possibly by inhibiting RNA and DNA synthesis by depleting intracellular nucleotide pools.

Route	Onset	Peak	Duration
Inhalation	Unknown	Unknown	Unknown
P.O.	Unknown	2 hr	Unknown

Half-life: First phase, 9¼ hours; second phase, 40 hours.

ADVERSE REACTIONS

CV: ***bradycardia, cardiac arrest,*** hypotension.
EENT: conjunctivitis, rash or erythema of eyelids.
Hematologic: anemia, reticulocytosis.
Respiratory: ***apnea, bronchospasm,*** bacterial pneumonia, pneumothorax, pulmonary edema, worsening respiratory state.

INTERACTIONS

Drug-drug. *Acetaminophen, antacids that contain magnesium, aluminum, or simethicone, aspirin, cimetidine:* May affect drug level. Monitor patient.
Didanosine: May increase toxicity. Avoid using together.
Stavudine, zidovudine: May decrease antiretroviral activity. Use together cautiously.

EFFECTS ON LAB TEST RESULTS

- May increase ALT, AST, and bilirubin levels. May decrease hemoglobin level.
- May increase reticulocyte count.

CONTRAINDICATIONS & CAUTIONS

- Aerosol form contraindicated in patients hypersensitive to drug, and women who are or may become pregnant during exposure to aerosolized ribavirin.
- Oral form is contraindicated in patients hypersensitive to drug, pregnant women, men whose partners are pregnant or may become pregnant within 6 months, patients with thalassemia major or sickle cell anemia, patients with a history of significant or unstable cardiac disease, and patients whose creatinine clearance is less than 50 ml/min.
- Use cautiously in elderly patients and patients with hepatic or renal insufficiency.

NURSING CONSIDERATIONS

Aerosol form

- Give by the Viratek SPAG-2 only. Don't use any other aerosol-generating device.
- Use sterile USP water for injection, not bacteriostatic water. Water used to reconstitute this drug must not contain any antimicrobial product.
- Discard solutions placed in the SPAG-2 unit at least every 24 hours before adding newly reconstituted solution.
- ***Alert:*** The long-term and cumulative effects to health care personnel exposed to this form aren't known. Eye irritation and headache may occur. Advise pregnant women to be avoid unnecessary exposure.
- ***Alert:*** Monitor ventilator function frequently. Drug may precipitate in ventilator, causing equipment to malfunction with serious consequences.
- Store reconstituted solutions at room temperature for 24 hours.
- This form is indicated only for severe lower respiratory tract infection caused by RSV. Although you should begin treatment awaiting test results, an RSV infection must be documented eventually.
- Most infants and children with RSV infection don't require treatment with antivirals because the disease is commonly mild and self-limiting. Premature infants or those with cardiopulmonary disease experience RSV in its severest form and benefit most from treatment with ribavirin aerosol.

Oral form

- Don't start therapy until a negative pregnancy test is confirmed in patient or partner of patient; they should take a pregnancy test every month during therapy and for 6 months afterward.
- Women or female partner of patient should use two reliable forms of contraception before and during treatment and for 6 months afterward.
- Report pregnancies that occur during treatment by calling 800-727-7064 for capsules and 800-593-2214 for tablets.
- Monitor hematologic status, liver function, and thyroid-stimulating hormone level at baseline and throughout therapy.
- Ribavirin alone is ineffective for treating chronic hepatitis C.
- ***Alert:*** Monitor patient for suicidal ideation, severe depression, hemolytic anemia, bone marrow suppression, autoimmune and infective disorders, pulmonary dysfunction, pancreatitis, and diabetes.
- Stop drug if pulmonary infiltrates or severe pulmonary impairment occur.

PATIENT TEACHING

- Inform parents of need for drug, and answer any questions.
- Encourage parents to immediately report any subtle change in child.
- Inform patient that oral form may be taken without regard to meals but should be taken in a consistent manner.

---

ritonavir
Norvir

Pharmacologic class: protease inhibitor
Pregnancy risk category B

AVAILABLE FORMS

Capsules: 100 mg
Oral solution: 80 mg/ml

INDICATIONS & DOSAGES

➤ **HIV infection, with other antiretrovirals, when antiretrovirals are warranted**
Adults: 600 mg P.O. b.i.d. with meals. To reduce adverse GI effects, begin with 300 mg P.O. b.i.d. and increase by 100 mg b.i.d. at 2- to 3-day intervals.

Children older than age 1 month: 350 to 400 mg/m² P.O. b.i.d.; don't exceed 600 mg P.O. b.i.d. Initially, start with 250 mg/m² b.i.d. and increase by 50 mg/m² P.O. q 12 hours at 2- to 3-day intervals. If children can't reach b.i.d. doses of 400 mg/m² because of adverse effects, consider alternate therapy.

ACTION

An HIV protease inhibitor with activity against HIV-1 and HIV-2 proteases. HIV protease is an enzyme required for the proteolytic cleavage of viral polyprotein precursors into the individual functional proteins in infectious HIV. Ritonavir binds to the protease-active site and inhibits activity of the enzyme, preventing cleavage of the viral polyproteins and resulting in the formation of immature, noninfectious viral particles.

Route	Onset	Peak	Duration
P.O.	Unknown	2–4 hr	Unknown

Half-life: Unknown.

ADVERSE REACTIONS

CNS: *asthenia,* ***generalized tonic-clonic seizure,*** anxiety, circumoral paresthesia, confusion, depression, dizziness, fever, headache, malaise, insomnia, pain, paresthesia, peripheral paresthesia, somnolence, thinking abnormality, malaise.
CV: syncope, vasodilation.
EENT: pharyngitis.
GI: *diarrhea, nausea, taste perversion, vomiting,* ***pancreatitis, pseudomembranous colitis,*** abdominal pain, anorexia, constipation, dyspepsia, flatulence.
Hematologic: ***leukopenia, thrombocytopenia.***
Hepatic: ***hepatitis.***
Metabolic: ***diabetes mellitus,*** weight loss.
Musculoskeletal: arthralgia, myalgia.
Skin: rash, sweating.
Other: ***hypersensitivity reactions,*** fat redistribution or accumulation.

INTERACTIONS

Drug-drug. *Alfuzosin, amiodarone, cisapride, ergot derivatives, flecainide, midazolam, propafenone, quinidine, triazolam, voriconazole:* May cause life-threatening adverse reactions. Use together is contraindicated.
Atovaquone, divalproex, lamotrigine, phenytoin, warfarin: May decrease levels of these drugs. Use together cautiously and monitor drug levels closely.
Beta blockers, disopyramide, fluoxetine, mexiletine, nefazodone: May increase levels of these drugs, causing cardiac and neurologic events. Use together with caution.
Bupropion, buspirone, calcium channel blockers , carbamazepine, clonazepam, clorazepate, cyclosporine, desipramine, dexamethasone, diazepam, ***digoxin,*** *dronabinol, estazolam, ethosuximide, flurazepam, lidocaine, methamphetamine, metoprolol, perphenazine, prednisone, propoxyphene, quinine, risperidone, sirolimus, SSRIs, tacrolimus, tricyclic antidepressants, thioridazine, timolol, tramadol, zolpidem:* May increase levels of these drugs. Use cautiously together and consider decreasing the dosage of these drugs by almost 50%. Monitor therapeutic levels.
Clarithromycin: May increase clarithromycin level. If creatinine clearance is 30 to 60 ml/minute, reduce clarithromycin dose by 50%. If creatinine clearance is less than 30 ml/minute, reduce clarithromycin dose by 75%.
Clozapine, piroxicam: May increase levels and toxicity of these drugs. Avoid use together.
Delavirdine: May increase ritonavir level. Adjusted dose recommendations aren't established. Use cautiously.
Didanosine: May decrease didanosine absorption. Separate doses by 2½ hours.
Disulfiram, metronidazole: May increase risk of disulfiram-like reactions because ritonavir formulations contain alcohol. Monitor patient.
Ethinyl estradiol: May decrease ethinyl estradiol level. Use an alternative or additional method of birth control.
Fluticasone: May significantly increase fluticasone exposure, significantly decreasing cortisol concentrations and causing systemic corticosteroid effects (including Cushing syndrome). Don't use together, if possible.
HMG-CoA reductase inhibitors: May cause large increase in statin levels, result-

ing in myopathy. Avoid use with lovastatin and simvastatin. Use cautiously with atorvastatin. Consider using fluvastatin or pravastatin.
Indinavir: May increase indinavir levels. Use together cautiously.
Ketoconazole, itraconazole: May increase levels of these drugs. Don't exceed 200 mg per day of these drugs.
Meperidine: May decrease levels of meperidine and its metabolite. Dosage increases and long-term use together aren't recommended because of CNS effects. Use cautiously together.
Methadone: May decrease methadone levels. Consider increasing methadone dosage.
PDE5 inhibitors (sildenafil, tadalafil, vardenafil): May increase levels of PDE5 inhibitor, causing hypotension, syncope, visual changes, or prolonged erection. Use together cautiously and increase monitoring for adverse reactions. Tell patient not to exceed 25 mg of sildenafil in a 48-hour period, 10 mg of tadalafil in a 72-hour period, or 2.5 mg of vardenafil in a 72-hour period.
Rifabutin: May increase rifabutin levels. Monitor patient and reduce rifabutin daily dosage by at least 75% of usual dose.
Rifampin, rifapentine: May decrease ritonavir levels. Consider using rifabutin.
Saquinavir: May increase saquinavir plasma levels. Adjust dose by taking saquinavir 400 mg b.i.d. and ritonavir 400 mg b.i.d.
Theophylline: May decrease theophylline levels. Increase dose based on blood levels.
Trazodone: May increase trazodone level causing nausea, dizziness, hypotension and syncope. Avoid use together. If unavoidable, use cautiously and lower trazodone dose.
Drug-herb. ***St. John's wort:*** May substantially reduce drug levels. Discourage use together.
Drug-food. *Any food:* May increase absorption. Advise patient to take drug with food.
Drug-lifestyle. *Smoking:* May decrease drug levels. Discourage smoking.

EFFECTS ON LAB TEST RESULTS

- May increase ALT, AST, GGT, glucose, triglyceride, lipid, CK, and uric acid levels. May decrease hemoglobin level and hematocrit.
- May decrease WBC, RBC, platelet, and neutrophil counts.

CONTRAINDICATIONS & CAUTIONS

- Contraindicated in patients hypersensitive to drug or its components and in those taking alfuzosin, amiodarone, cisapride, flecainide, piroxicam, propafenone, quinidine, ergot derivatives, lovastatin, simvastatin, midazolam, triazolam, or voriconazole.
- Use cautiously in patients with hepatic insufficiency.
- Safety and effectiveness in children younger than 1 month haven't been established.
- It's unknown if ritonavir appears in breast milk. Use cautiously in breast-feeding women.

NURSING CONSIDERATIONS

- Patients beginning regimens with ritonavir and nucleosides may improve GI tolerance by starting ritonavir alone and then adding nucleosides before completing 2 weeks of ritonavir.
- ***Look alike–sound alike:*** Don't confuse Norvir with Norvasc.

PATIENT TEACHING

- Inform patient that drug doesn't cure HIV infection. He may continue to develop opportunistic infections and other complications of HIV infection. Drug hasn't been shown to reduce the risk of transmitting HIV to others through sexual contact or blood contamination.
- Caution patient to take drug as prescribed and not to adjust dosage or stop therapy without first consulting prescriber.
- Tell patient that taste of oral solution may be improved by mixing it with chocolate milk, Ensure, or Advera within 1 hour of the scheduled dose.
- Instruct patient to take drug with a meal to improve absorption.
- Tell patient that if a dose is missed, he should take the next dose as soon as possible. If a dose is skipped, he shouldn't double the next dose.

• Advise patients taking a PDE5 inhibitor for erectile dysfunction to promptly report hypotension, dizziness, visual changes, and prolonged erection to their prescriber. Caution against exceeding the recommended reduced dosage.
• Advise patient to report use of other drugs, including OTC drugs; this drug interacts with many drugs.

saquinavir mesylate
Invirase

Pharmacologic class: protease inhibitor
Pregnancy risk category B

AVAILABLE FORMS
Capsules (hard gelatin): 200 mg
Tablets (film-coated): 500 mg

INDICATIONS & DOSAGES
➤**Adjunct treatment of advanced HIV infection in selected patients**
Adults and adolescents age 16 and older: 1,000 mg P.O. b.i.d. given at the same time with 100 mg ritonavir P.O. b.i.d.

ACTION
Inhibits the activity of HIV protease and prevents the cleavage of HIV polyproteins, which are essential for HIV maturation.

Route	Onset	Peak	Duration
P.O.	Unknown	Unknown	Unknown

Half-life: 1 to 2 hours.

ADVERSE REACTIONS
CNS: anxiety, asthenia, depression, dizziness, headache, insomnia, numbness, paresthesia.
CV: chest pain.
GI: *diarrhea, nausea,* ***pancreatitis,*** altered taste, abdominal pain, constipation, dyspepsia, flatulence, ulcerated buccal mucosa, vomiting.
Hematologic: ***pancytopenia, thrombocytopenia.***
Musculoskeletal: musculoskeletal pain.
Respiratory: bronchitis, cough.
Skin: rash.

INTERACTIONS
Drug-drug. *Amprenavir:* May decrease amprenavir level. Use together cautiously.
Carbamazepine, phenobarbital, phenytoin: May decrease saquinavir level. Avoid using together.
Delavirdine: May increase saquinavir level. Use cautiously and monitor hepatic enzymes. Decrease dose when used together.
Dexamethasone: May decrease saquinavir level. Avoid using together.
Efavirenz: May decrease levels of both drugs. Avoid using together.
HMG-CoA reductase inhibitors: May increase levels of these drugs, which increases risk of myopathy, including rhabdomyolysis. Avoid using together.
Indinavir, lopinavir and ritonavir combination, nelfinavir, ritonavir: May increase saquinavir level. Use together cautiously.
Macrolide antibiotics, such as clarithromycin: May increase levels of both drugs. Use together cautiously.
Nevirapine: May decrease saquinavir level. Monitor patient.
PDE5 inhibitors (sildenafil, tadalafil, vardenafil): May increase levels of these drugs. Reduce dose and frequency of PDE5 inhibitor and monitor patient closely for adverse reactions.
Rifabutin, rifampin: May decrease saquinavir level. Use with rifabutin cautiously. Don't use with rifampin.
Drug-herb. *Garlic supplements,* ***St. John's wort:*** May substantially reduce drug level, causing loss of therapeutic effects. Discourage use together.
Drug-food. *Any food:* May increase drug absorption. Advise patient to take drug with food.
Grapefruit juice: May increase drug level. Tell patient to take with liquid other than grapefruit juice.

EFFECTS ON LAB TEST RESULTS
• May decrease WBC, RBC, and platelet counts.

CONTRAINDICATIONS & CAUTIONS
• Contraindicated in patients hypersensitive to drug or its components.
• Safety of drug hasn't been established in pregnant or breast-feeding women or in children younger than age 16.

NURSING CONSIDERATIONS

- Evaluate CBC, platelets, electrolytes, uric acid, liver enzymes, and bilirubin before therapy begins and at appropriate intervals throughout therapy.
- If serious toxicity occurs during treatment, stop drug until cause is identified or toxicity resolves. Drug may be resumed without dosage modifications.
- Monitor patient's hydration if adverse GI reactions occur.

PATIENT TEACHING

- Advise patient to take drug with food or within 2 hours of a full meal to increase drug absorption.
- Instruct patient to avoid missing any doses, to decrease the risk of developing HIV resistance.
- Inform patient that drug doesn't cure HIV infection, that opportunistic infections and other complications of HIV infection may continue to occur, and that transmission of HIV to others through sexual contact or blood contamination is still possible.
- Advise patient to keep an updated list of the drugs he's taking and to contact his healthcare provider before using any prescription or OTC drug because of the many interactions.

stavudine (2, 3 didehydro-3-deoxythymidine, d4T)

Zerit, Zerit XR

Pharmacologic class: nucleoside reverse transcriptase inhibitor
Pregnancy risk category C

AVAILABLE FORMS

Capsules: 15 mg, 20 mg, 30 mg, 40 mg
Capsules (extended-release): 37.5 mg, 50 mg, 75 mg, 100 mg
Oral solution: 1 mg/ml

INDICATIONS & DOSAGES

➤ **HIV-infection, with other antiretrovirals**

Adults who weigh 60 kg (132 lb) or more: 40 mg P.O. regular-release q 12 hours or 100 mg P.O. extended-release once daily.
Adults who weigh 30 kg (66 lb) to 60 kg: 30 mg P.O. regular-release q 12 hours or 75 mg P.O. extended-release once daily.
Children who weigh 60 kg or more: 40 mg P.O. regular-release q 12 hours.
Children who weigh 30 kg to 60 kg: 30 mg P.O. regular-release q 12 hours.
Neonates 14 days and older and children who weigh less than 30 kg: 1 mg/kg P.O. regular-release q 12 hours.
Neonates age 13 days and younger: 0.5 mg/kg P.O. regular-release q 12 hours.

Adjust-a-dose: For patients experiencing peripheral neuropathy, withdraw temporarily; then resume therapy at 50% recommended dose. Consider stopping therapy if neuropathy recurs. For patients with creatinine clearance 26 to 50 ml/minute, adjust dosage to 20 mg (if weight exceeds 60 kg) or 15 mg (if weight is less than 60 kg) P.O. q 12 hours; if clearance is 10 to 25 ml/minute, 20 mg (if weight exceeds 60 kg) or 15 mg (if weight is less than 60 kg) P.O. q 24 hours. Don't use extended-release form in patients with creatinine clearance of 50 ml/minute or less.

ACTION

A thymidine nucleoside analogue that prevents replication of retroviruses, including HIV, by inhibiting the enzyme reverse transcriptase and causing termination of DNA chain growth.

Route	Onset	Peak	Duration
P.O.	Unknown	1 hr	Unknown

Half-life: 1 to 2 hours.

ADVERSE REACTIONS

CNS: *asthenia, fever,* anxiety, depression, dizziness, headache, insomnia, malaise, nervousness, peripheral neuropathy.
CV: chest pain.
EENT: conjunctivitis.
GI: *abdominal pain, anorexia, diarrhea, nausea, vomiting,* ***pancreatitis,*** constipation, dyspepsia.
Hematologic: ***neutropenia, thrombocytopenia,*** anemia.
Hepatic: ***hepatotoxicity, severe hepatomegaly with steatosis.***
Metabolic: ***lactic acidosis,*** weight loss.

Musculoskeletal: *arthralgia, back pain, myalgia.*
Respiratory: *dyspnea.*
Skin: *diaphoresis, pruritus, rash,* maculopapular rash.
Other: *chills.*

INTERACTIONS

Drug-drug. *Methadone:* May decrease stavudine absorption and level. Separate dosage times and monitor patient for clinical effect if drugs must be used together.
Zidovudine: May inhibit phosphorylation of stavudine. Avoid using together.

EFFECTS ON LAB TEST RESULTS

- May increase ALT and AST levels. May decrease hemoglobin level.
- May decrease neutrophil and platelet counts.

CONTRAINDICATIONS & CAUTIONS

- Contraindicated in patients hypersensitive to drug.
- Use cautiously in patients with renal impairment or history of peripheral neuropathy. Adjust dosage for creatinine clearance of less than 50 ml/minute; adjust dosage or stop drug in patients with peripheral neuropathy.
- Use cautiously in pregnant women; fatal lactic acidosis may occur in pregnant women who receive stavudine and didanosine with other antiretrovirals.
- In children, safety and effectiveness of extended-release form haven't been established.

NURSING CONSIDERATIONS

- Monitor patient for signs and symptoms of pancreatitis, especially if he takes stavudine with didanosine or hydroxyurea. If patient has pancreatitis, reinstate drug cautiously.
- Monitor liver function test results.
- ***Alert:*** Motor weakness, mimicking the clinical presentation of Guillain-Barré syndrome (including respiratory failure) in HIV patients taking stavudine with other antiretrovirals may occur, especially in patients with lactic acidosis. Monitor patient for factors of lactic acidosis, including generalized fatigue, GI problems, tachypnea, or dyspnea. Symptoms may continue or worsen when drug is stopped. Patients with these symptoms should promptly interrupt antiretroviral therapy and rapidly receive a full medical workup. Consider permanently stopping drug.
- ***Alert:*** Peripheral neuropathy appears to be the major dose-limiting adverse effect; it may or may not resolve after drug is stopped.
- Monitor CBC results and creatinine.

PATIENT TEACHING

- Tell patient that drug may be taken without regard to meals.
- Warn patient not to take other drugs for HIV or AIDS unless prescriber has approved them.
- Inform patient that drug doesn't cure HIV infection, that opportunistic infections and other complications of HIV infection may still occur, and that transmission of HIV to others through sexual contact or blood contamination is still possible.
- Teach patient signs and symptoms of peripheral neuropathy (pain, burning, aching, weakness, or pins and needles in the limbs) and tell him to report these immediately.
- Tell patient to report symptoms of lactic acidosis, including fatigue, GI problems, dyspnea, or tachypnea.
- Tell patient to report symptoms of pancreatitis, including abdominal pain, nausea, vomiting, weight loss, or fatty stools.
- Tell patient to monitor weight patterns and report weight loss or gain.
- Explain to patient who has difficulty swallowing that extended-release capsules can be opened and contents mixed with 2 tablespoons of yogurt or applesauce. Caution patient not to chew or crush the beads while swallowing.

tenofovir disoproxil fumarate

Viread✐

Pharmacologic class: nucleotide reverse transcriptase inhibitor
Pregnancy risk category B

AVAILABLE FORMS

Tablets: 300 mg as the fumarate salt (equivalent to 245 mg of tenofovir disoproxil)

INDICATIONS & DOSAGES

➤ **HIV-1 infection, with other antiretrovirals**

Adults: 300 mg P.O. once daily without regard to food.

Adjust-a-dose: For patients with creatinine clearance of 30 to 49 ml/minute, 300 mg P.O. q 48 hours. For a clearance of 10 to 29 ml/minute, 300 mg P.O. twice weekly. For patients receiving hemodialysis, 300 mg P.O. q 7 days or after a total of about 12 hours of hemodialysis. Give dose after session. There are no recommendations for patients with a creatinine clearance of less than 10 ml/minute not receiving hemodialysis.

ACTION

Hydrolyzed to produce tenofovir, a nucleoside analogue of adenosine monophosphate that yields tenofovir diphosphate. Tenofovir diphosphate inhibits HIV replication.

Route	Onset	Peak	Duration
P.O.	Unknown	1–2 hr	Unknown

Half-life: Unknown.

ADVERSE REACTIONS

CNS: asthenia, headache.
GI: *nausea,* abdominal pain, anorexia, diarrhea, flatulence, vomiting.
GU: glycosuria.
Hematologic: ***neutropenia.***
Metabolic: hyperglycemia.

INTERACTIONS

Drug-drug. *Atazanavir:* May decrease atazanavir levels, causing resistance. Give both drugs with ritonavir.

Didanosine (buffered form): May increase didanosine bioavailability. Monitor patient for didanosine-related adverse effects, such as bone marrow suppression, GI distress, and peripheral neuropathy. Give tenofovir 2 hours before or 1 hour after didanosine.

Drugs that reduce renal function or compete for renal tubular secretion (acyclovir, cidofovir, ganciclovir, valacyclovir, valganciclovir): May increase levels of tenofovir or other renally eliminated drugs. Monitor patient for adverse effects.

EFFECTS ON LAB TEST RESULTS

- May increase amylase, AST, ALT, CK, serum and urine glucose, creatinine, phosphaturia, and triglyceride levels.
- May decrease neutrophil count.

CONTRAINDICATIONS & CAUTIONS

- Contraindicated in patients hypersensitive to any component of the drug.
- Use very cautiously in patients with risk factors for liver disease or with hepatic impairment.
- Because of a high rate of early virologic failure and emergence of resistance, combination therapy with tenofovir, didanosine, and lamivudine isn't recommended as a new regimen for therapy-naive or -experienced patients with HIV infection. Consider changing therapies in these patients.
- Because the effects of drug on pregnant women aren't known, use during pregnancy only if benefits clearly outweigh risks.

NURSING CONSIDERATIONS

- ***Alert:*** Drug may cause lactic acidosis and fatal hepatomegaly with steatosis. These effects may occur without elevated transaminase levels. Risk factors include long-term antiretroviral use, obesity, and being female. Monitor all patients closely.
- Drug may cause body fat to accumulate and be redistributed, resulting in central obesity, peripheral wasting, and buffalo hump. Monitor patient for changes in body fat.
- Drug may be linked to osteomalacia and decreased bone mineral density and increased creatinine and phosphaturia levels. Monitor patient carefully during long-term treatment.
- Drug may lead to decreased HIV RNA level and CD4+ cell counts.
- In elderly patients, use drug cautiously because they may be taking other drugs and may have a higher risk of decreased renal function.
- Because of a high rate of early virologic resistance, triple antiretroviral therapy with abacavir, lamivudine, and tenofovir shouldn't be used as new regimen for naive or pretreated patient. Monitor patients currently controlled with this regimen and those who use this regimen with

other antiretrovirals, and consider a different therapy.

PATIENT TEACHING

- Instruct patient to take drug with a meal to enhance bioavailability.
- Inform patient that drug doesn't cure HIV infection, that opportunistic infections and other complications of HIV infection may still occur, and that transmission of HIV to others through sexual contact or blood contamination is still possible.
- If patient takes tenofovir and didanosine (buffered form), instruct him to take tenofovir 2 hours before or 1 hour after didanosine.
- Tell patient to report adverse effects, including nausea, vomiting, diarrhea, flatulence, and headache.

tipranavir

Aptivus

Pharmacologic class: protease inhibitor
Pregnancy risk category C

AVAILABLE FORMS

Capsules: 250 mg

INDICATIONS & DOSAGES

➤ **HIV-1 in patients with viral replication who are highly treatment experienced or have HIV-1 strains resistant to multiple protease inhibitors**

Adults: 500 mg P.O. twice daily with 200 mg of ritonavir twice daily. Give with food.

ACTION

Inhibits virus-specific processing of polyproteins in HIV-1 infected cells, preventing formation of mature virions.

Route	Onset	Peak	Duration
P.O.	Unknown	3 hr	Unknown

Half-life: 5 to 6 hours.

ADVERSE REACTIONS

CNS: asthenia, depression, dizziness, fatigue, headache, insomnia, malaise, peripheral neuropathy, pyrexia, sleep disorder, somnolence.
GI: *diarrhea, **pancreatitis,*** abdominal distention, abdominal pain, dyspepsia, flatulence, GERD, nausea, vomiting.
GU: renal insufficiency.
Hematologic: ***neutropenia, thrombocytopenia,*** anemia.
Hepatic: ***hepatic failure,*** hepatitis.
Metabolic: anorexia, decreased appetite, dehydration, diabetes mellitus, facial wasting, hyperglycemia, weight loss.
Musculoskeletal: muscle cramps, myalgia.
Respiratory: bronchitis, cough, dyspnea.
Skin: *rash,* acquired lipodystrophy, exanthem, lipoatrophy, lipohypertrophy, pruritus.
Other: flulike illness, hypersensitivity, reactivation of herpes simplex and varicella zoster.

INTERACTIONS

Drug-drug. *Amiodarone, bepridil, flecainide, propafenone, quinidine:* May increase levels of these drugs and risk of life-threatening arrhythmias. Avoid use together.
Astemizole, cisapride, pimozide, terfenadine: May cause life-threatening arrhythmias. Avoid use together.
Atorvastatin: May increase levels of both drugs. Start with lowest dose of atorvastatin, and monitor patient closely or consider other drugs.
Clarithromycin: May increase levels of both drugs. If patient's creatinine clearance is 30 to 60 ml/minute, decrease clarithromycin dose by 50%. If patient's creatinine clearance is less than 30 ml/minute, decrease clarithromycin dose by 75%.
Cyclosporine, sirolimus, tacrolimus: May cause unpredictable interaction. Monitor drug levels closely until they've stabilized.
Desipramine: May increase desipramine level. Decrease dose and monitor desipramine level.
Dihydroergotamine, ergonovine, ergotamine, methylergonovine: May cause acute ergot toxicity, including peripheral vasospasm and ischemia of extremities. Avoid use together.

Diltiazem, felodipine, nicardipine, nisoldipine, verapamil: May cause unpredictable interaction. Use together cautiously, and monitor patient closely.
Disulfiram, metronidazole: May cause disulfiram-like reaction. Use together cautiously.
Estrogen-based hormone therapy: May decrease estrogen level, and rash may occur. Monitor patient carefully. Advise using nonhormonal contraception.
Fluoxetine, paroxetine, sertraline: May increase levels of these drugs. Adjust dosages as needed.
Glimepiride, glipizide, glyburide, pioglitazone, repaglinide, tolbutamide: May affect glucose levels. Monitor glucose level carefully.
Lovastatin, simvastatin: May increase risk of myopathy and rhabdomyolysis. Avoid use together.
Meperidine: May increase normeperidine metabolite. Avoid use together.
Methadone: May decrease methadone level by 50%. Consider increased methadone dose.
Midazolam, triazolam: May cause prolonged or increased sedation or respiratory depression. Avoid use together.
Rifampin: May lead to loss of virologic response and resistance to tipranavir and other protease inhibitors. Avoid use together.
Rifabutin: May increase rifabutin level. Decrease rifabutin dose by 75%.
Sildenafil, tadalafil, vardenafil: May increase levels of these drugs. Use together cautiously. Tell patient not to exceed 25 mg sildenafil in 48 hours, 10 mg tadalafil every 72 hours, or 2.5 mg vardenafil every 72 hours.
Warfarin: May cause unpredictable reaction. Check INR often.
Drug-herb. *St. John's wort:* May lead to loss of virologic response and resistance to this drug and other antiretrovirals. Warn patient to avoid use together.

EFFECTS ON LAB TEST RESULTS

- May increase total cholesterol, triglyceride, blood glucose, amylase, lipase, ALT, and AST levels.
- May decrease WBC count.

CONTRAINDICATIONS & CAUTIONS

- Contraindicated in patients hypersensitive to any ingredients of the product, patients with moderate (Child-Pugh class B) and severe (Child-Pugh class C) hepatic insufficiency, and patients taking drugs that depend on CYP3A for clearance, such as amiodarone, astemizole, bepridil, cisapride, dihydroergotamine, ergonovine, ergotamine, flecainide, methylergonovine, midazolam, pimozide, propafenone, quinidine, terfenadine, and triazolam.
- Use cautiously in patients with sulfonamide allergy, diabetes, liver disease, hepatitis B or C, or hemophilia A or B.

PATIENT TEACHING

- Explain that drug doesn't cure HIV infection and doesn't reduce the risk of transmitting the virus to others.
- ***Alert:*** Many drugs may interfere with this drug. Urge patient to tell prescriber about all prescription drugs, OTC drugs, and herbal products he takes.
- Tell patient that drug is effective only when taken with ritonavir and other antiretrovirals.
- Instruct patient to take drug with food.
- Urge patient to stop drug and contact prescriber if he has evidence of hepatitis, such as fatigue, malaise, anorexia, nausea, jaundice, bilirubinemia, acholic stools, or liver tenderness.
- If woman uses hormonal contraceptives, advise use of barrier contraception.
- Tell patient that redistribution or accumulation of body fat may occur.
- Advise woman that breast-feeding isn't recommended during therapy.

valacyclovir hydrochloride

Valtrex

Pharmacologic class: synthetic purine nucleoside
Pregnancy risk category B

AVAILABLE FORMS

Tablets: 500 mg, 1,000 mg

INDICATIONS & DOSAGES

➤ **Herpes zoster infection (shingles)**
Adults: 1 g P.O. t.i.d. for 7 days.

Adjust-a-dose: For patients with creatinine clearance of 30 to 49 ml/minute, give 1 g P.O. q 12 hours; if clearance is 10 to 29 ml/minute, give 1 g P.O. q 24 hours; if clearance is less than 10 ml/minute, give 500 mg P.O. q 24 hours.

➤ **First episode of genital herpes**
Adults: 1 g P.O. b.i.d. for 10 days.
Adjust-a-dose: For patients with creatinine clearance of 10 to 29 ml/minute, give 1 g P.O. q 24 hours; if clearance is less than 10 ml/minute, give 500 mg P.O. q 24 hours.

➤ **Recurrent genital herpes in immunocompetent patients**
Adults: 500 mg P.O. b.i.d. for 3 days, given at the first sign or symptom of an episode.
Adjust-a-dose: For patients with creatinine clearance of 29 ml/minute or less, give 500 mg P.O. q 24 hours.

➤ **Long-term suppression of recurrent genital herpes**
Adults: 1 g P.O. once daily. In patients with a history of nine or fewer recurrences per year, use alternative dose of 500 mg once daily.
Adjust-a-dose: For patients with creatinine clearance of 29 ml/minute or less, 500 mg P.O. q 24 hours (q 48 hours if patient has nine or fewer occurrences per year).

➤ **Cold sores (herpes labialis)**
Adults: 2 g P.O. q 12 hours for two doses.
Adjust-a-dose: For patients with creatinine clearance of 30 to 49 ml/minute, give 1 g q 12 hours for two doses; if clearance is 10 to 29 ml/minute, give 500 mg q 12 hours for two doses; if clearance is less than 10 ml/minute, give 500 mg as a single dose.

➤ **Long-term suppression of recurrent genital herpes in HIV-infected patients with CD4 cell count of 100 cells/mm³ or more**
Adults: 500 mg P.O. b.i.d. Safety and effectiveness of therapy beyond 6 months haven't been established.
Adjust-a-dose: For patients with creatinine clearance of 29 ml/minute or less, give 500 mg P.O. q 24 hours.

➤ **To reduce transmission of genital herpes in patients with history of nine or fewer occurrences per year**
Adults: 500 mg P.O. daily.

ACTION
Rapidly converts to acyclovir, which in turn becomes incorporated into viral DNA, thereby terminating growth of the DNA chain; inhibits viral DNA polymerase, causing inhibition of viral replication.

Route	Onset	Peak	Duration
P.O.	30 min	Unknown	Unknown

Half-life: 2½ to 3¼ hours.

ADVERSE REACTIONS
CNS: *headache,* depression, dizziness.
GI: *nausea,* abdominal pain, diarrhea, vomiting.
GU: dysmenorrhea.
Musculoskeletal: arthralgia.

INTERACTIONS
Drug-drug. *Cimetidine, probenecid:* May reduce rate but not extent of conversion of valacyclovir to acyclovir and may decrease renal clearance of acyclovir, thus increasing acyclovir level. Monitor patient for acyclovir toxicity.

EFFECTS ON LAB TEST RESULTS
- May increase alkaline phosphatase, ALT, AST, and creatinine levels. May decrease hemoglobin level.
- May decrease platelet and WBC counts.

CONTRAINDICATIONS & CAUTIONS
- Contraindicated in patients hypersensitive to or intolerant of valacyclovir, acyclovir, or components of the formulation.
- ***Alert:*** Drug isn't recommended for use in patients with HIV infection or in bone marrow or renal transplant recipients because thrombotic thrombocytopenic purpura and hemolytic uremic syndrome may occur in these patients at doses of 8 g/day.
- Use cautiously in elderly patients, those with renal impairment, and those receiving other nephrotoxic drugs. Monitor renal function test results.
- Consider use of drug during pregnancy only if the benefits outweigh the risks.
- If patient is breast-feeding, drug may need to be stopped.
- Safety and effectiveness in prepubertal children haven't been established.

NURSING CONSIDERATIONS

• ***Look alike–sound alike:*** Don't confuse valacyclovir (Valtrex) with valganciclovir (Valcyte).
• Although there are no reports of overdose, precipitation of acyclovir in renal tubules may occur when solubility (2.5 mg/ml) is exceeded in the intratubular fluid. With acute renal failure and anuria, the patient may benefit from hemodialysis until renal function is restored.

PATIENT TEACHING

• Inform patient that drug may be taken without regard to meals.
• Teach patient the signs and symptoms of herpes infection (rash, tingling, itching, and pain), and advise him to notify prescriber immediately if they occur. Treatment should begin as soon as possible after symptoms appear, preferably within 48 hours of the onset of zoster rash.
• Tell patient that drug isn't a cure for herpes but may decrease the length and severity of symptoms.

valganciclovir
Valcyte

Pharmacologic class: synthetic nucleoside
Pregnancy risk category C

AVAILABLE FORMS

Tablets: 450 mg

INDICATIONS & DOSAGES

➤ To prevent CMV disease in heart, kidney, and kidney-pancreas transplantation in patients at high risk (donor CMV seropositive or recipient CMV seronegative)
Adults: 900 mg P.O. once daily with food starting within 10 days of transplantation until 100 days after transplantation.
➤ Active CMV retinitis in patients with AIDS
Adults: 900 mg P.O. b.i.d. with food for 21 days; maintenance dose is 900 mg P.O. daily with food.
➤ Inactive CMV retinitis
Adults: 900 mg P.O. daily with food.
Adjust-a-dose: For patients with creatinine clearance of 40 to 59 ml/minute, induction dosage is 450 mg b.i.d.; maintenance dosage is 450 mg daily. If clearance is 25 to 39 ml/minute, induction dosage is 450 mg daily; maintenance dosage is 450 mg q 2 days. If clearance is 10 to 24 ml/minute, induction dosage is 450 mg q 2 days; maintenance dosage is 450 mg twice weekly.

ACTION

Drug is converted to the active drug ganciclovir, which inhibits replication of CMV.

Route	Onset	Peak	Duration
P.O.	Unknown	1–3 hr	Unknown

Half-life: 4 hours.

ADVERSE REACTIONS

CNS: *headache, insomnia, pyrexia,* ***seizures,*** agitation, confusion, hallucinations, paresthesia, peripheral neuropathy, psychosis.
EENT: *retinal detachment.*
GI: *abdominal pain, diarrhea, nausea, vomiting.*
Hematologic: **NEUTROPENIA,** *anemia,* ***aplastic anemia, bone marrow depression, pancytopenia, thrombocytopenia.***
Other: ***sepsis,*** catheter-related infection, hypersensitivity reactions, local or systemic infections.

INTERACTIONS

Drug-drug. *Didanosine:* May increase absorption of didanosine. Monitor patient closely for didanosine toxicity.
Immunosuppressants, zidovudine: May enhance neutropenia, anemia, thrombocytopenia, and bone marrow depression. Monitor CBC results.
Mycophenolate mofetil: May increase levels of both drugs in renally impaired patients. Use together cautiously.
Probenecid: May decrease renal clearance of ganciclovir. Monitor patient for ganciclovir toxicity.
Drug-food. *Any food:* May increase drug absorption. Give drug with food.

EFFECTS ON LAB TEST RESULTS

• May decrease hemoglobin level and hematocrit.

• May decrease neutrophil, platelet, RBC, and WBC counts.

CONTRAINDICATIONS & CAUTIONS

• Contraindicated in patients hypersensitive to valganciclovir or ganciclovir. Don't use in patients receiving hemodialysis.
• Drug isn't indicated for use in liver transplant patients.
• The safety and effectiveness of drug for the prevention of CMV disease in other solid organ transplant patients, such as lung transplant patients, haven't been established.
• Use cautiously in patients with cytopenias and in those who have received immunosuppressants or radiation.

NURSING CONSIDERATIONS

• Adhere to dosing guidelines for valganciclovir because ganciclovir and valganciclovir aren't interchangeable and overdose may occur.
• Toxicities include severe leukopenia, neutropenia, anemia, pancytopenia, bone marrow depression, aplastic anemia, and thrombocytopenia. Don't use if patient's absolute neutrophil count is less than 500/mm^3, platelet count is less than 25,000/mm^3, or hemoglobin level is less than 8 g/dl.
• Monitor CBC, platelet counts, and creatinine level or creatinine clearance values frequently during treatment.
• Cytopenia may occur at any time during treatment and increase with continued use. Counts usually recover 3 to 7 days after stopping drug.
• No drug interaction studies have been conducted, but, because drug is converted to ganciclovir, assume that drug interactions will be similar.
• Drug may cause temporary or permanent inhibition of spermatogenesis.
• ***Look alike–sound alike:*** Don't confuse valganciclovir hydrochloride (Valcyte) with valacyclovir (Valtrex).

PATIENT TEACHING

• Tell patient to take drug with food.
• Tell patient to follow dosage instructions precisely. Ganciclovir capsules and valganciclovir tablets aren't interchangeable.
• Advise patient that blood tests are needed during treatment. Doses may need to be adjusted based on blood counts.
• Tell woman of childbearing age to use contraception during treatment. Inform man that he should use barrier contraception during and for 90 days after treatment.
• Advise patient that ganciclovir is a carcinogen.
• Tell patient that CNS effects (seizures, ataxia, dizziness) can occur and to use care in driving or operating machinery.
• Advise patient that this drug isn't a cure for CMV retinitis and that the condition may recur. Tell patient to see an ophthalmologist at least every 4 to 6 weeks during treatment.

---

zanamivir

Relenza

Pharmacologic class: selective neuraminidase inhibitor
Pregnancy risk category C

AVAILABLE FORMS

Powder for inhalation: 5 mg/blister

INDICATIONS & DOSAGES

➤ **Uncomplicated acute illness caused by influenza virus A and B in patients who have had symptoms for no longer than 2 days**

Adults and children age 7 and older: 2 oral inhalations (one 5-mg blister per inhalation for total dose of 10 mg) b.i.d. using the dry-powder inhalation device for 5 days. Give two doses on first day of treatment, allowing at least 2 hours to elapse between doses. Give subsequent doses about 12 hours apart (in the morning and evening) at about the same time each day.

➤ **Prevention of influenza in a household setting**

Adults and children age 5 and older: 2 oral inhalations (one 5-mg blister per inhalation for total dose of 10 mg) once daily for 10 days.

➤**Prevention of influenza in a community setting**
Adults and adolescents: 2 oral inhalations (one 5-mg blister per inhalation for total dose of 10 mg) once daily for 28 days.

ACTION
Likely exerts its antiviral action by inhibiting neuraminidase on the surface of the influenza virus, altering virus particle aggregation and release.

Route	Onset	Peak	Duration
Inhalation	Unknown	1–2 hr	Unknown

Half-life: 2½ to 5¼ hours.

ADVERSE REACTIONS
CNS: dizziness, headache.
EENT: ear, nose, and throat infections, nasal signs and symptoms, sinusitis.
GI: diarrhea, nausea, vomiting.
Respiratory: ***bronchospasm,*** bronchitis, cough.
Skin: serious rash.
Other: ***anaphylaxis.***

INTERACTIONS
None significant.

EFFECTS ON LAB TEST RESULTS
- May increase CK and liver enzyme levels.
- May decrease lymphocyte and neutrophil counts.

CONTRAINDICATIONS & CAUTIONS
- Contraindicated in patients hypersensitive to drug or its components.
- Not recommended for patients with severe or decompensated COPD, asthma, or other underlying respiratory disease.

NURSING CONSIDERATIONS
- For a patient with underlying respiratory disease, have a fast-acting bronchodilator readily available and carefully monitor respiratory status. Patients using an inhaled bronchodilator for asthma simultaneously with this drug should use the bronchodilator first.
- Start drug within 48 hours of symptoms or as prevention after household contact, within 36 hours, or community outbreak, within 5 days.
- Drug doesn't replace annual influenza vaccine.
- Monitor patient for bronchospasm and decline in lung function. Stop drug in such situations.

PATIENT TEACHING
- Tell patient to carefully read the instructions for the dry-powder inhalation device.
- Teach parents how to give the drug to a child and to properly supervise use.
- Advise patient to keep the dry-powder inhaler level when loading and inhaling drug. Tell him to always check inside the mouthpiece of the dry-powder inhaler before each use to make sure it's free of foreign objects.
- Tell patient to exhale fully before putting the mouthpiece in his mouth; then, keeping the dry-powder inhaler level, to close his lips around the mouthpiece and inhale steadily and deeply. Advise patient to hold his breath for a few seconds after inhaling to help drug stay in the lungs.
- Instruct patient simultaneously using a bronchodilator with this drug, to use the bronchodilator first. Tell patient to have a fast-acting bronchodilator readily available in case of wheezing.
- ***Alert:*** Advise all patients to immediately report worsening of respiratory symptoms, wheezing, shortness of breath and bronchospasm.
- Advise patient that it's important to finish the entire treatment course.
- Tell patient that drug doesn't reduce the risk of transmitting the influenza virus to others.

zidovudine (azidothymidine, AZT)
Apo-Zidovudine†, Novo-AZT†, Retrovir✐

Pharmacologic class: nucleoside reverse transcriptase inhibitor
Pregnancy risk category C

AVAILABLE FORMS
Capsules: 100 mg
Injection: 10 mg/ml
Syrup: 50 mg/5 ml
Tablets: 300 mg

INDICATIONS & DOSAGES

➤ **HIV infection, with other antiretrovirals**

Adults: 600 mg daily P.O. in divided doses, with other antiretrovirals. If patient is unable to tolerate oral drug, give 1 mg/kg I.V. over 1 hour five to six times daily.

Children ages 6 weeks to 12 years: 160 mg/m^2 q 8 hours (480 mg/m^2/day up to a maximum of 200 mg q 8 hours) with other antiretrovirals. Some prescribers recommend 120 mg/m^2 I.V. q 6 hours, or 20 mg/m^2/hour continuous I.V. infusion.

➤ **To prevent maternal-fetal transmission of HIV**

Pregnant women at more than 14 weeks' gestation: 100 mg P.O. five times daily until the start of labor. Then, 2 mg/kg I.V. over 1 hour followed by a continuous I.V. infusion of 1 mg/kg/hour until the umbilical cord is clamped.

Neonates: 2 mg/kg P.O. q 6 hours starting within 12 hours after birth and continuing until 6 weeks old. Or, give 1.5 mg/kg via I.V. infusion over 30 minutes q 6 hours.

Adjust-a-dose: In patients with significant anemia (hemoglobin level less than 7.5 g/dl or more than 25% below baseline) or significant neutropenia (granulocyte count less than 750 cells/mm^3 or more than 50% below baseline), interrupt therapy until evidence proves marrow has recovered. In patients receiving hemodialysis or peritoneal dialysis, give 100 mg P.O. or 1 mg/kg I.V. q 6 to 8 hours. For patients with mild to moderate hepatic dysfunction or liver cirrhosis, daily dose may need to be reduced.

I.V. ADMINISTRATION

- Give by this route only until oral drug can be tolerated.
- Remove the calculated dose from the vial; add to D_5W to achieve a concentration no greater than 4 mg/ml.
- Infuse drug over 1 hour at a constant rate. Avoid rapid infusion or bolus injection.
- Protect undiluted vials from light.
- Give diluted solution within 8 hours if stored at room temperature or 24 hours if refrigerated.

INCOMPATIBILITIES

Biological or colloidal solutions, such as blood products or protein-containing solutions; meropenem.

ACTION

Nucleoside reverse transcriptase inhibitor that inhibits replication of HIV by blocking DNA synthesis.

Route	Onset	Peak	Duration
P.O., I.V.	Unknown	30–90 min	Unknown

Half-life: 1 hour.

ADVERSE REACTIONS

CNS: *asthenia, dizziness, fever, headache, malaise,* ***seizures,*** insomnia, paresthesia, somnolence.
GI: *anorexia, nausea, vomiting,* ***pancreatitis,*** abdominal pain, constipation, diarrhea, dyspepsia, taste perversion.
Hematologic: ***agranulocytosis, severe bone marrow suppression, thrombocytopenia,*** anemia.
Hepatic: *hepatomegaly.*
Metabolic: lactic acidosis.
Musculoskeletal: myalgia.
Respiratory: *cough,* wheezing.
Skin: *rash,* diaphoresis.

INTERACTIONS

Drug-drug. *Acetaminophen:* May decrease bioavailability of zidovudine. Adjust zidovudine dosage, as needed.
Atovaquone, fluconazole, methadone, probenecid, trimethoprim, valproic acid: May increase bioavailability of zidovudine. May need to adjust dosage.
Doxorubicin, ribavirin, stavudine: May have antagonistic effects. Avoid using together.
Ganciclovir, interferon alfa, other bone marrow suppressive or cytotoxic drugs: May increase hematologic toxicity of zidovudine. Use together cautiously.
Phenytoin: May alter phenytoin level and decrease zidovudine clearance by 30%. Monitor patient closely.

EFFECTS ON LAB TEST RESULTS

- May increase ALT, AST, alkaline phosphatase, and LDH levels. May decrease hemoglobin level.

• May decrease granulocyte and platelet counts.

CONTRAINDICATIONS & CAUTIONS
• Contraindicated in patients hypersensitive to drug.
• Use cautiously and with close monitoring in patients with advanced symptomatic HIV infection and in those with severe bone marrow depression.
• Use cautiously in patients with hepatomegaly, hepatitis, or other risk factors for liver disease and in those with renal insufficiency. Monitor renal and liver function tests.

NURSING CONSIDERATIONS
• ***Alert:*** Although rare, lactic acidosis without hypoxemia may occur. Notify prescriber if patient develops unexplained tachypnea, dyspnea, or a decrease in bicarbonate level. Therapy may need to be suspended until lactic acidosis is ruled out.
• Monitor blood studies every 2 weeks to detect anemia or agranulocytosis. Patients may need reduced dosage or temporary stop to therapy.
• Drug may temporarily decrease morbidity and mortality in certain patients with AIDS.
• ***Look alike–sound alike:*** Don't confuse Retrovir with ritonavir.

PATIENT TEACHING
• Tell patient to take drug exactly as directed and not to share it with others.
• Instruct patient to take drug on an empty stomach. To avoid esophageal irritation, tell patient to take drug while sitting upright and with adequate fluids.
• Remind patient to comply with the dosage schedule. Suggest ways to avoid missing doses, perhaps by using an alarm clock.
• Advise patient that blood transfusions may be needed during therapy because of drug-related anemia.
• Tell patient that dosages vary among patients and not to change his dosing instructions unless directed to do so by his prescriber.
• Tell patient that his gums may bleed. Recommend good mouth care with a soft toothbrush.
• Warn patient not to take other drugs for AIDS unless prescriber has approved them.
• Advise pregnant, HIV-infected patient that drug therapy only reduces the risk of HIV transmission to her newborn. Long-term risks to infants are unknown.
• Advise patient that monotherapy isn't recommended and to discuss any questions with prescriber.
• Advise health care worker considering prophylactic use after occupational exposure (such as needlestick injury) that drug's safety and effectiveness haven't been established.
• Tell patient not to keep capsules in the kitchen, bathroom, or other places that may be damp or hot. Heat and moisture may cause the drug to break down and affect the intended results.

16

Macrolides

azithromycin
clarithromycin
erythromycin base
erythromycin estolate
erythromycin ethylsuccinate
erythromycin lactobionate
erythromycin stearate

azithromycin

Zithromax✐, Zmax

Pharmacologic class: macrolide
Pregnancy risk category B

AVAILABLE FORMS

Injection: 500 mg
Oral suspension (extended-release): 2 g
Powder for oral suspension: 100 mg/5 ml, 200 mg/5 ml; 1,000 mg/packet
Tablets: 250 mg, 500 mg, 600 mg

INDICATIONS & DOSAGES

➤ **Acute bacterial worsening of COPD caused by *Haemophilus influenzae, Moraxella catarrhalis,* or *Streptococcus pneumoniae;* uncomplicated skin and skin-structure infections caused by *Staphylococcus aureus, Streptococcus pyogenes,* or *S. agalactiae;* second-line therapy for pharyngitis or tonsillitis caused by *Staphylococcus pyogenes***
Adults and adolescents age 16 and older: Initially, 500 mg P.O. as a single dose on day 1, followed by 250 mg daily on days 2 through 5. Or, for worsening COPD, 500 mg P.O. daily for 3 days.

➤ **Community-acquired pneumonia from *Chlamydia pneumoniae, H. influenzae, Mycoplasma pneumoniae,* or *S. pneumoniae;* or caused by *Legionella pneumophila, M. catarrhalis,* or *S. aureus***
Adults and adolescents age 16 and older: For mild infections, give 500 mg P.O. as a single dose on day 1; then 250 mg P.O. daily on days 2 through 5. For more severe infections or those caused by *S. aureus,* give 500 mg I.V. as a single daily dose for 2 days; then 500 mg P.O. as a single daily dose to complete a 7- to 10-day course of therapy. Switch from I.V. to P.O. therapy based on patient's response.

➤ **Community-acquired pneumonia from *C. pneumoniae, H. influenzae, M. pneumoniae, S. pneumoniae***
Children 6 months and older: 10 mg/kg P.O. (maximum of 500 mg) as a single dose on day 1, followed by 5 mg/kg (maximum of 250 mg) daily on days 2 through 5.

➤ **Single dose treatment for mild to moderate acute bacterial sinusitis from *H. influenzae, M. catarrhalis,* or *S. pneumoniae;* or community-acquired pneumonia caused by *C. pneumoniae, H. influenzae, M. pneumoniae,* or *S. pneumoniae***
Adults: 2 g Zmax P.O. as a single dose taken 1 hour before or 2 hours after a meal.

➤ **Chancroid**
Adults: 1 g P.O. as a single dose.
Infants and children♦: 20 mg/kg (maximum of 1 g) P.O. as a single dose.

➤ **Nongonococcal urethritis or cervicitis caused by *C. trachomatis***
Adults and adolescents age 16 and older: 1 g P.O. as a single dose.

➤ **To prevent disseminated *Mycobacterium avium* complex in patients with advanced HIV infection**♦
Adults and adolescents: 1.2 g P.O. once weekly alone or with rifabutin.
Infants and children: 20 mg/kg P.O. (maximum of 1.2 g) weekly or 5 mg/kg (maximum of 250 mg) can be given P.O. daily. Children age 6 and older may also receive 300 mg rifabutin P.O. daily.

➤ ***M. avium* complex in patients with advanced HIV infection**
Adults: 600 mg P.O. daily with 15 mg/kg daily ethambutol.

➤ **Urethritis and cervicitis caused by *Neisseria gonorrhoeae***
Adults: 2 g P.O. as a single dose.

➤ **Pelvic inflammatory disease caused by *C. trachomatis, N. gonor-***

***rhoeae,* or *M. hominis* in patients who need initial I.V. therapy**
Adults and adolescents age 16 and older: 500 mg I.V. as a single daily dose for 1 to 2 days; then 250 mg P.O. daily to complete a 7-day course of therapy. Switch from I.V. to P.O. therapy, based on patient's response.

➤**Otitis media**
Children older than age 6 months: 30 mg/kg P.O. as a single dose; or, 10 mg/kg P.O. once daily for 3 days; or, 10 mg/kg P.O. on day 1 and then 5 mg/kg once daily on days 2 to 5.

➤**Pharyngitis, tonsillitis**
Children age 2 and older: 12 mg/kg (maximum 500 mg) P.O. daily for 5 days.

➤**To prevent bacterial endocarditis in penicillin-allergic adults at moderate to high risk**♦
Adults: 500 mg P.O. 1 hour before procedure.
Children: 15 mg/kg P.O. 1 hour before procedure. Don't exceed adult dose.

➤**Chlamydial infections; uncomplicated gonococcal infections of the cervix, urethra, rectum, and pharynx; to prevent such infections after sexual assault**♦
Adults: 1 g P.O. as a single dose, with other drugs, as recommended by the Centers for Disease Control.

I.V. ADMINISTRATION

- Reconstitute drug in 500-mg vial with 4.8 ml of sterile water for injection to yield 100 mg/ml.
- Shake well until all drug is dissolved.
- Further dilute in 250 or 500 ml normal saline solution, half-normal saline solution, D_5W, or lactated Ringer solution to yield a final concentration of 1 or 2 mg/ml, respectively.
- Infuse a 500-mg dose of azithromycin I.V. over 1 hour or longer. Never give it as a bolus or I.M. injection.

INCOMPATIBILITIES

Amikacin sulfate, aztreonam, cefotaxime, ceftazidime, ceftriaxone sodium, cefuroxime, ciprofloxacin, clindamycin phosphate, famotidine, fentanyl citrate, furosemide, gentamicin sulfate, imipenem and cilastatin sodium, ketorolac tromethamine, levofloxacin, morphine sulfate, ondansetron hydrochloride, piperacillin and tazobactam sodium, potassium chloride, ticarcillin disodium and clavulanate potassium, tobramycin sulfate.

ACTION

Binds to the 50S subunit of bacterial ribosomes, blocking protein synthesis; bacteriostatic or bactericidal, depending on concentration.

Route	Onset	Peak	Duration
P.O.	Unknown	2–5 hr	Unknown
I.V.	Unknown	Unknown	Unknown

Half-life: About 3 days.

ADVERSE REACTIONS

CNS: dizziness, fatigue, headache, somnolence, vertigo.
CV: chest pain, palpitations.
GI: *abdominal pain, diarrhea, nausea, vomiting,* ***pseudomembranous colitis,*** dyspepsia, flatulence, melena.
GU: candidiasis, nephritis, vaginitis.
Hepatic: cholestatic jaundice.
Skin: photosensitivity, rash.
Other: ***angioedema.***

INTERACTIONS

Drug-drug. *Antacids containing aluminum and magnesium:* May lower peak azithromycin level (immediate-release form). Separate doses by at least 2 hours.
Carbamazepine, cyclosporine, digoxin, phenytoin, theophylline: May increase levels of these drugs. Monitor drug levels.
Ergotamine: May cause acute ergotamine toxicity. Monitor patient closely.
Nelfinavir: May increase azithromycin level. Monitor for liver enzyme abnormalities and hearing impairment.
Pimozide: May prolong QT interval and cause ventricular tachycardia. Monitor patient closely.
Triazolam: May decrease triazolam clearance. Monitor patient closely.
Warfarin: May increase INR. Monitor INR carefully.
Drug-food. *Any food:* May decrease absorption of multidose oral suspension form. Advise patient to take drug on empty stomach.

Drug-lifestyle. *Sun exposure:* May cause photosensitivity reactions. Advise patient to avoid excessive sunlight exposure.

EFFECTS ON LAB TEST RESULTS
None reported.

CONTRAINDICATIONS & CAUTIONS
- Contraindicated in patients hypersensitive to erythromycin or other macrolide or ketolide antibiotics.
- Use cautiously in patients with impaired hepatic function.

NURSING CONSIDERATIONS
- Obtain specimen for culture and sensitivity tests before giving first dose. Therapy may begin pending results.
- Give Zmax 1 hour before or 2 hours after a meal. Tablets and single-dose packets for oral suspension can be taken with or without food. Don't give with antacids.
- Monitor patient for superinfection. Drug may cause overgrowth of nonsusceptible bacteria or fungi.
- Reconstitute suspension with 2 ounces (60 ml) water. After taking, patient should rinse glass with additional 2 ounces water and drink it to ensure he has taken entire dose. Packets aren't for children.
- If patient vomits within 60 minutes of taking Zmax, notify prescriber; additional or different therapy may be needed.

PATIENT TEACHING
- Tell patient to take drug as prescribed, even after he feels better.
- Advise patient to avoid excessive sunlight and to wear protective clothing and use sunscreen when outside.
- Tell patient to report adverse reactions promptly.

clarithromycin
Biaxin✐, Biaxin XL✐

Pharmacologic class: macrolide
Pregnancy risk category C

AVAILABLE FORMS
Suspension: 125 mg/5 ml, 250 mg/5 ml
Tablets (extended-release [ER]): 500 mg
Tablets (film-coated): 250 mg, 500 mg

INDICATIONS & DOSAGES
➤ **Pharyngitis or tonsillitis caused by *Streptococcus pyogenes***
Adults: 250 mg P.O. q 12 hours for 10 days.
Children: 15 mg/kg/day P.O. divided q 12 hours for 10 days.
➤ **Acute maxillary sinusitis caused by *S. pneumoniae, Haemophilus influenzae,* or *Moraxella catarrhalis***
Adults: 500 mg P.O. q 12 hours for 14 days or two 500-mg extended-release tablets P.O. daily for 14 days.
Children: 15 mg/kg/day P.O. divided q 12 hours for 10 days.
➤ **Acute worsening of chronic bronchitis caused by *M. catarrhalis, S. pneumoniae;* community-acquired pneumonia caused by *H. influenzae, S. pneumoniae, Mycoplasma pneumoniae,* or *Chlamydia pneumoniae***
Adults: 250 mg P.O. q 12 hours for 7 days (*H. influenzae*) or 7 to 14 days (others).
➤ **Acute worsening of chronic bronchitis caused by *H. influenzae* or *H. parainfluenzae***
Adults: 500 mg P.O. q 12 hours for 7 days *H. parainfluenzae* or 7 to 14 days *H. influenzae.*
➤ **Acute worsening of chronic bronchitis caused by *M. catarrhalis, S. pneumoniae, H. parainfluenzae,* or *H. influenzae***
Adults: Two 500-mg P.O. extended-release tablets daily for 7 days.
➤ **Mild to moderate community-acquired pneumonia, caused by *H. influenzae, H. parainfluenzae, M. catarrhalis, S. pneumoniae, C. pneumoniae,* or *M. pneumoniae***
Adults: Two 500-mg P.O. extended-release tablets daily for 7 days.
➤ **Community-acquired pneumonia caused by *S. pneumoniae, C. pneumoniae,* and *M. pneumoniae***
Children: 15 mg/kg/day P.O. divided q 12 hours for 10 days.
➤ **Uncomplicated skin and skin-structure infections from *Staphylococcus aureus* or *S. pyogenes***
Adults: 250 mg P.O. q 12 hours for 7 to 14 days.
Children: 15 mg/kg/day P.O. divided q 12 hours for 10 days.

➤**Acute otitis media caused by *H. influenzae, M. catarrhalis,* or *S. pneumoniae***
Children: 15 mg/kg/day P.O. divided q 12 hours for 10 days.
➤**To prevent and treat disseminated infection caused by *Mycobacterium avium* complex**
Adults: 500 mg P.O. b.i.d.
Children: 7.5 mg/kg P.O. b.i.d., up to 500 mg b.i.d.
➤***Helicobacter pylori,* to reduce risk of duodenal ulcer recurrence**
Adults: 500 mg clarithromycin with 30 mg lansoprazole and 1 g amoxicillin, all given q 12 hours for 10 to 14 days. Or, 500 mg clarithromycin with 20 mg omeprazole and 1 g amoxicillin, all given q 12 hours for 10 days. Or, 500 mg clarithromycin b.i.d., 20 mg rabeprazole b.i.d., and 1 g amoxicillin b.i.d., all for 7 days. Or, two-drug regimen with 500 mg clarithromycin q 8 hours and 40 mg omeprazole once daily for 14 days. Continue omeprazole for 14 additional days.
Adjust-a-dose: In patients with creatinine clearance less than 30 ml/minute, cut dose in half or double frequency interval.

ACTION

Binds to the 50S subunit of bacterial ribosomes, blocking protein synthesis; bacteriostatic or bactericidal, depending on concentration.

Route	Onset	Peak	Duration
P.O.	Unknown	2–4 hr	Unknown
P.O. (extended)	Unknown	5–6 hr	Unknown

Half-life: 5 to 7 hours.

ADVERSE REACTIONS

CNS: headache.
GI: ***pseudomembranous colitis,*** diarrhea, nausea, taste perversion, abdominal pain or discomfort, vomiting (in children).
Hematologic: ***leukopenia,*** coagulation abnormalities.
Skin: rash (in children).

INTERACTIONS

Drug-drug. *Alprazolam, midazolam, triazolam:* May decrease clearance of these drugs, causing adverse reactions. Use together cautiously.
Carbamazepine, phenytoin: May inhibit metabolism of these drugs, increasing levels and risk of toxicity. Avoid using together.
Cyclosporine: May increase cyclosporine levels. Monitor cyclosporine level.
Digoxin: May increase digoxin level. Monitor patient for digoxin toxicity.
Dihydroergotamine, ergotamine: May cause acute ergot toxicity. Avoid using together.
Fluconazole: May increase clarithromycin level. Monitor patient closely.
HMG-CoA reductase inhibitors: May increase levels of these drugs; may rarely cause rhabdomyolysis. Use together cautiously.
Other drugs that prolong the QTc interval (amiodarone, antipsychotics, disopyramide, fluoroquinolones, procainamide, quinidine, sotalol, tricyclic antidepressants): May have additive effects. Monitor ECG for QTc interval prolongation. Avoid using together if possible.
Pimozide: May cause torsades de pointes. Use together is contraindicated.
Rifamycin: May decrease therapeutic effects of macrolide while increasing adverse effects of rifamycin. Monitor patient.
Ritonavir: May increase level of clarithromycin. May need to reduce clarithromycin dosage in renally impaired patients.
Sildenafil: May prolong absorption of sildenafil. May need to reduce sildenafil dosage.
Theophylline: May increase theophylline level. Monitor drug level.
Warfarin: May increase PT and INR. Monitor PT and INR carefully.
Zidovudine: May alter zidovudine level. Monitor patient closely.
Drug-food. ***Grapefruit juice:*** May inhibit metabolism, increasing adverse effects. Don't take with grapefruit juice.

EFFECTS ON LAB TEST RESULTS

- May increase alkaline phosphatase, ALT, AST, bilirubin, BUN, creatinine, GGT, and LDH levels.
- May increase PT and INR. May decrease neutrophil, thrombocyte, and WBC counts.

CONTRAINDICATIONS & CAUTIONS
- Contraindicated in patients hypersensitive to clarithromycin, erythromycin, or other macrolides and in those receiving pimozide or other drugs that prolong QT interval or cause cardiac arrhythmias.
- Use cautiously in patients with hepatic or renal impairment.

NURSING CONSIDERATIONS
- ***Alert:*** The safety and effectiveness of the ER form haven't been established for treating other infections for which the original form has been approved.
- Obtain specimen for culture and sensitivity tests before giving. Begin therapy awaiting results.
- Monitor patient for superinfection.
- Giving clarithromycin with a drug metabolized by CYP3A may increase drug levels and prolong therapeutic and adverse effects.

PATIENT TEACHING
- Tell patient to take drug as prescribed, even after he feels better.
- Advise patient to report persistent adverse reactions.
- Inform patient that drug may be taken with or without food.
- Tell patient not to refrigerate the suspension form, but to discard unused portion after 14 days.

erythromycin base
Apo-Erythro Base†, E-Base, E-Mycin🖉, Erybid†, Eryc🖉, Ery-Tab🖉, Erythromycin Base Filmtab, Erythromycin Delayed-Release, PCE Dispertab

erythromycin estolate

erythromycin ethylsuccinate
Apo-Erythro-ES†, E.E.S., E.E.S. Granules, EryPed, EryPed 200, EryPed 400

erythromycin lactobionate
Erythrocin Lactobionate

erythromycin stearate
Apo-Erythro-S†, Erythrocin Stearate

Pharmacologic class: macrolide
Pregnancy risk category B

AVAILABLE FORMS

erythromycin base
Capsules (delayed-release): 250 mg
Tablets (enteric-coated): 250 mg, 333 mg, 500 mg
Tablets (filmtabs): 250 mg, 500 mg
erythromycin estolate
Oral suspension: 125 mg/5 ml, 250 mg/5 ml
erythromycin ethylsuccinate
Oral suspension: 100 mg/2.5 ml, 200 mg/5 ml, 400 mg/5 ml (after reconstitution)
Tablets: 400 mg
Powder for oral suspension: 200 mg/5 ml, 400 mg/5 ml
erythromycin lactobionate
Injection: 500-mg, 1-g vials
erythromycin stearate
Tablets (film-coated): 250 mg, 500 mg

INDICATIONS & DOSAGES

➤ Acute pelvic inflammatory disease caused by *Neisseria gonorrhoeae*
Adults: 500 mg I.V. q 6 hours for 3 days; then 250 mg P.O. q 6 hours or 333 mg P.O. q 8 hours for 7 days.

➤ Intestinal amebiasis caused by *Entamoeba histolytica*
Adults: 250 mg P.O. q.i.d. or 333 mg P.O. q 8 hours, or 500 mg delayed-release tablets P.O. q 12 hours for 10 to 14 days.
Children: 30 to 50 mg/kg P.O. daily, in divided doses, for 10 to 14 days.

➤ Erythrasma
Adults: 250 mg P.O. q 6 hours for 14 days.

➤ To prevent rheumatic fever
Adults: 250 mg base, estolate, or stearate P.O. b.i.d.; or, 400 mg ethylsuccinate P.O. b.i.d.

➤ Mild to moderately severe respiratory tract, skin, or soft-tissue infection
Adults: 250 to 500 mg base, estolate, or stearate P.O. q 6 hours; or 400 to 800 mg ethylsuccinate P.O. q 6 hours; or 15 to 20 mg/kg I.V. daily, as continuous infusion or in divided doses q 6 hours for

10 days (3 weeks for *Mycoplasma*species infection).
Children: 30 to 50 mg/kg P.O. daily, in divided doses q 6 hours; or 15 to 20 mg/kg I.V. daily, in divided doses q 4 to 6 hours for 10 days (3 weeks for *Mycoplasma* species infection).

➤***Listeria monocytogenes* infection**
Adults: 250 mg P.O. q 6 hours or 500 mg P.O. q 12 hours.

➤**Nongonococcal urethritis caused by *Ureaplasma urealyticum***
Adults: 500 mg P.O. q 6 hours or 666 mg P.O. q 8 hours for at least 7 days.

➤**Syphilis in patients allergic to penicillin**
Adults: 500 mg P.O. q.i.d. for 2 weeks.

➤**Legionnaires' disease**
Adults: 1 to 4 g P.O. daily in divided doses for 10 to 14 days alone or with rifampin. I.V. route may be used initially in severe cases.

➤**Uncomplicated urethral, endocervical, or rectal infection caused by *Chlamydia trachomatis,* when tetracyclines are contraindicated**
Adults: 500 mg base P.O. q.i.d. for at least 7 days, or 666 mg P.O. q 8 hours for at least 7 days, or 250 mg P.O. q.i.d. for 14 days if patient can't tolerate higher doses.

➤**Urogenital *C. trachomatis* infection during pregnancy**
Adults: 500 mg base, estolate, or stearate P.O. q.i.d. for at least 7 days or 250 mg base, estolate, or stearate or 400 mg ethylsuccinate P.O. q.i.d. for at least 14 days.

➤**Conjunctivitis caused by *C. trachomatis* in neonates**
Neonates: 50 mg/kg base, estolate, or stearate P.O. daily in four divided doses for 14 days.

➤**Pneumonia in infants caused by *C. trachomatis***
Infants: 50 mg/kg/day base, estolate, or stearate P.O. in 4 divided doses for 21 days, or 15 to 20 mg/kg/day lactobionate I.V. as a continuous infusion or in four divided doses.

➤**Chancroid caused by *Haemophilus ducreyi*♦**
Adults: 500 mg base P.O. q.i.d. for 7 days.

➤**Diarrhea caused by *Campylobacter jejuni* enteritis or enterocolitis**
Adults: 500 mg base P.O. q.i.d. for 7 days.

I.V. ADMINISTRATION

- Reconstitute drug according to manufacturer's directions.
- Dilute each 250 mg in at least 100 ml of normal saline solution.
- Infuse over 1 hour.

INCOMPATIBILITIES

Ascorbic acid injection, colistimethate, dextrose 2.5% in half-strength Ringer lactate, dextrose 5% in lactated Ringer solution, dextrose 5% in normal saline solution, dextrose 5% in Normosol-M, dextrose 10% in water, D_5W, furosemide, heparin sodium, linezolid, metoclopramide, Normosol-R, Ringer injection, vitamin B complex with C.

ACTION

Inhibits bacterial protein synthesis by binding to the 50S subunit of the ribosome. Bacteriostatic or bactericidal, depending on concentration.

Route	Onset	Peak	Duration
P.O.	Unknown	1½ hr	Unknown
I.V.	Immediate	1½ hr	Unknown

Half-life: 1½ hours.

ADVERSE REACTIONS

CNS: fever.
CV: *vein irritation or thrombophlebitis after I.V. injection,* ***ventricular arrhythmias.***
EENT: hearing loss (with high I.V. doses).
GI: *abdominal pain and cramping, diarrhea, nausea, vomiting.*
Hepatic: cholestatic jaundice (with erythromycin estolate).
Skin: eczema, rash, urticaria.
Other: ***anaphylaxis,*** overgrowth of nonsusceptible bacteria or fungi.

INTERACTIONS

Drug-drug. *Carbamazepine:* May inhibit metabolism of carbamazepine, increasing blood level and risk of toxicity. Avoid using together.
Clindamycin, lincomycin: May be antagonistic. Avoid using together.
Cyclosporine: May increase cyclosporine level. Monitor drug level.
Digoxin: May increase digoxin level. Monitor patient for digoxin toxicity.

Dihydroergotamine, ergotamine: May cause acute ergot toxicity. Avoid using together.
Disopyramide: May increase disopyramide level, which may cause arrhythmias and prolonged QT intervals. Monitor ECG.
Midazolam, triazolam: May increase effects of these drugs. Monitor patient closely.
Oral anticoagulants: May increase anticoagulant effect. Monitor PT and INR closely.
Fluoroquinolones, *other drugs that prolong the QTc interval (amiodarone, antipsychotics, procainamide, quinidine, sotalol, tricyclic antidepressants):* May have additive effects. Monitor ECG for QTc interval prolongation. Avoid using together, if possible.
Rifamycins (rifabutin, rifampin, rifapentine): May decrease therapeutic effects of erythromycin while increasing adverse effects of rifamycin. Monitor patient.
Strong CYP3A inhibitors (such as diltiazem, verapamil, troleandomycin): May increase the risk of sudden death from cardiac causes. Don't use together.
Theophylline: May decrease erythromycin level and increase theophylline toxicity. Use together cautiously.
Drug-herb. *Pill-bearing spurge:* May inhibit CYP3A enzymes, affecting drug metabolism. Urge caution.
Drug-food. *Food, grapefruit juice:* Food can delay absorption; grapefruit juice may inhibit drug's metabolism. Don't give within 2 hours of a meal; caution patient to avoid grapefruit juice during therapy.

EFFECTS ON LAB TEST RESULTS

- May increase alkaline phosphatase, ALT, AST, and bilirubin levels.
- May interfere with fluorometric determination of urine catecholamines and with colorimetric assays.

CONTRAINDICATIONS & CAUTIONS

- Contraindicated in those hypersensitive to drug or other macrolides.
- Erythromycin estolate is contraindicated in patients with hepatic disease.
- Use erythromycin salts cautiously in patients with impaired hepatic function.
- Erythromycin estolate isn't recommended during pregnancy because of the risk of adverse effects for the mother and fetus.
- Drug appears in breast milk. Use cautiously in breast-feeding women.
- Don't use drug to treat neurosyphilis.

NURSING CONSIDERATIONS

- Obtain urine specimen for culture and sensitivity tests before giving. Begin therapy awaiting results.
- When giving suspension, note the concentration.
- Monitor patient for superinfection. Drug may cause overgrowth of nonsusceptible bacteria or fungi.
- Monitor hepatic function. Erythromycin estolate may cause serious hepatotoxicity in adults. Other salts cause less serious hepatotoxicity.
- Ototoxicity may occur, especially in patients with renal or hepatic insufficiency and in those receiving high doses of drug.
- Coated tablets or encapsulated pellets cause less GI upset, so they may be better tolerated by patients who have trouble tolerating drug.

PATIENT TEACHING

- Tell patient to take drug as prescribed, even after he feels better.
- Instruct patient to take oral form of drug with full glass of water within 2 hours of meals for best absorption.
- Drug may be taken with food if GI upset occurs. Tell patient not to take drug with fruit juice or to swallow the chewable tablets whole.
- Instruct patient to report adverse reactions, especially nausea, abdominal pain, vomiting, and fever.

17

Miscellaneous anti-infectives

aztreonam
chloramphenicol sodium succinate
clindamycin hydrochloride
clindamycin palmitate hydrochloride
clindamycin phosphate
daptomycin
ertapenem sodium
imipenem and cilastatin sodium
linezolid
meropenem
nitrofurantoin
quinupristin and dalfopristin
telithromycin
vancomycin hydrochloride

aztreonam

Azactam

Pharmacologic class: monobactam
Pregnancy risk category B

AVAILABLE FORMS

Injection: 500-mg vials, 1-g vials, 2-g vials

INDICATIONS & DOSAGES

➤**UTI; septicemia; infections of lower respiratory tract, skin, and skin structures; intra-abdominal infections, surgical infections, and gynecologic infections caused by susceptible *Escherichia coli, Klebsiella pneumoniae, Proteus mirabilis, Pseudomonas aeruginosa, Enterobacter cloacae, K. oxytoca, Citrobacter* species, and *Serratia marcescens;* respiratory infections caused by *Haemophilus influenzae***

Adults: 500 mg to 2 g I.V. or I.M. q 8 to 12 hours. For severe systemic or life-threatening infections, 2 g q 6 to 8 hours. Maximum dose is 8 g daily.

Children ages 9 months to 15 years: 30 mg/kg q 6 to 8 hours I.V. Maximum dose is 120 mg/kg/day.

Neonates age 1 to 4 weeks who weigh more than 2 kg (4.4 lbs)♦: 30 mg/kg I.V. q 6 hours.

Neonates age 1 to 4 weeks who weigh 2 kg or less♦: 30 mg/kg I.V. q 8 hours.

Neonates younger than 7 days who weigh more than 2 kg♦: 30 mg/kg I.V. q 8 hours.

Neonates younger than 7 days who weigh 2 kg or less♦: 30 mg/kg I.V. q 12 hours.

Adjust-a-dose: For adults with a creatinine clearance of 10 to 30 ml/minute, give 1 to 2 g; then give 50% of the usual dose at usual interval. If clearance is less than 10 ml/minute, give 500 mg to 2 g; then give 25% of the usual dose at usual interval. For serious infections, add 12½% of the initial dose to maintenance doses after each hemodialysis session. For adults with alcoholic cirrhosis, decrease dose by 20% to 25%.

I.V. ADMINISTRATION

- For direct injection, reconstitute with 6 to 10 ml of sterile water for injection and immediately shake vial vigorously.
- To give a bolus, inject drug over 3 to 5 minutes, directly into a vein or I.V. tubing.
- For infusion, reconstitute with a compatible I.V. solution to yield 20 mg/ml or less.
- Give infusions over 20 minutes to 1 hour.
- Give thawed solutions only by I.V. infusion.

INCOMPATIBILITIES

Acyclovir, amphotericin B, ampicillin sodium, azithromycin, cephradine, chlorpromazine, daunorubicin, ganciclovir, lorazepam, metronidazole, mitomycin, mitoxantrone, nafcillin, prochlorperazine, streptozocin, vancomycin.

ACTION

Inhibits bacterial cell-wall synthesis, ultimately causing cell-wall destruction; bactericidal.

Route	Onset	Peak	Duration
I.V.	Unknown	Immediate	Unknown
I.M.	Unknown	< 1 hr	Unknown

Half-life: 2 hours.

ADVERSE REACTIONS

CNS: ***seizures,*** confusion, headache, insomnia.
CV: hypotension, thrombophlebitis.
GI: ***pseudomembranous colitis,*** diarrhea, nausea, vomiting.
Hematologic: ***neutropenia, pancytopenia, thrombocytopenia,*** anemia, leukocytosis, thrombocytosis.
Skin: discomfort and swelling at I.M. injection site, rash.
Other: hypersensitivity reactions.

INTERACTIONS

Drug-drug. *Aminoglycosides:* May have synergistic nephrotoxic effects. Monitor renal function.
Cefoxitin, imipenem: May have antagonistic effect. Avoid using together.
Probenecid: May increase aztreonam level. Avoid using together.

EFFECTS ON LAB TEST RESULTS

- May increase ALT, AST, BUN, creatinine, and LDH levels. May decrease hemoglobin level.
- May increase PT, PTT, and INR. May decrease neutrophil and RBC counts. May increase or decrease platelet and WBC counts.
- May cause false-positive Coombs' test result. May alter urine glucose determinations using cupric sulfate (Clinitest or Benedict reagent).

CONTRAINDICATIONS & CAUTIONS

- Contraindicated in patients hypersensitive to drug or any of its components.
- Use cautiously in elderly patients and in those with impaired renal or hepatic function. Dosage adjustment may be needed. Monitor renal function tests.

NURSING CONSIDERATIONS

- Obtain specimen for culture and sensitivity tests before giving first dose. Begin therapy awaiting results.
- To prepare I.M. injection, add at least 3 ml of one of the following solutions per gram of aztreonam: sterile water for injection, bacteriostatic water for injection, normal saline solution, or bacteriostatic normal saline solution.
- Give I.M. injections deep into a large muscle, such as the upper outer quadrant of the gluteus maximus or the side of the thigh. Give doses more than 1 g by I.V. route.
- ***Alert:*** Don't give I.M. injection to children.
- Observe patient for signs and symptoms of superinfection.
- ***Alert:*** Because drug is ineffective against gram-positive and anaerobic organisms, combine it with other antibiotics for immediate treatment of life-threatening illnesses.
- ***Alert:*** Patients allergic to penicillins or cephalosporins may not be allergic to this drug. Monitor closely those who have had an immediate hypersensitivity reaction to these antibiotics, especially to ceftazidime.

PATIENT TEACHING

- Warn patient receiving I.M. drug that pain and swelling may occur at injection site.
- Tell patient to report discomfort at I.V. insertion site.
- Instruct patient to report adverse reactions and signs and symptoms of superinfection promptly.

chloramphenicol sodium succinate

Chloromycetin Sodium Succinate, Pentamycetin†

Pharmacologic class: dichloroacetic acid derivative
Pregnancy risk category C

AVAILABLE FORMS

Injection: 1-g vial

INDICATIONS & DOSAGES

➤ ***Haemophilus influenzae*** **meningitis, acute** ***Salmonella typhi*** **infection, and meningitis, bacteremia, or other severe infections caused by sensitive** ***Salmonella*** **species, rickettsia,**

lymphogranuloma, psittacosis, or various sensitive gram-negative organisms
Adults: 50 to 100 mg/kg I.V. daily, divided q 6 hours. Maximum dose is 100 mg/kg daily.
Full-term infants older than age 2 weeks with normal metabolic processes: Up to 50 mg/kg I.V. daily, divided q 6 hours. May use up to 100 mg/kg/day in four divided doses for meningitis.
Premature infants, neonates age 2 weeks and younger, and children and infants with immature metabolic processes: 25 mg/kg I.V. once daily.

I.V. ADMINISTRATION
- Reconstitute 1-g vial of powder for injection with 10 ml of sterile water for injection to yield 100 mg/ml.
- Give slowly over at least 1 minute.
- Check injection site daily for phlebitis and irritation.
- Solution is stable for 30 days at room temperature, but you should refrigerate it.
- Don't use cloudy solution.

INCOMPATIBILITIES
Chlorpromazine, fluconazole, glycopyrrolate, hydroxyzine, metoclopramide, polymyxin B sulfate, prochlorperazine, promethazine, vancomycin.

ACTION
Inhibits bacterial protein synthesis by binding to the 50S subunit of the ribosome; bacteriostatic.

Route	Onset	Peak	Duration
I.V.	Unknown	1–3 hr	Unknown

Half-life: 1½ to 4½ hours.

ADVERSE REACTIONS
CNS: confusion, delirium, headache, mild depression, peripheral neuropathy with prolonged therapy.
EENT: decreased visual acuity, optic neuritis in patients with cystic fibrosis.
GI: diarrhea, enterocolitis, glossitis, nausea, vomiting, stomatitis.
Hematologic: ***aplastic anemia, granulocytopenia, hypoplastic anemia, thrombocytopenia.***
Hepatic: jaundice.
Other: ***anaphylaxis, gray syndrome in neonates,*** hypersensitivity reactions.

INTERACTIONS
Drug-drug. *Anticoagulants, barbiturates, hydantoins, iron salts, sulfonylureas:* May increase levels of these drugs. Monitor patient for toxicity.
Penicillins: May have synergistic or antagonistic effects. Monitor patient for change in effectiveness.
Rifampin: May reduce chloramphenicol level. Monitor patient for changes in effectiveness.
Vitamin B_{12}: May decrease response of vitamin B_{12} in patients with pernicious anemia. Monitor patient closely.

EFFECTS ON LAB TEST RESULTS
- May decrease hemoglobin level.
- May decrease granulocyte and platelet counts.
- May falsely elevate urine PABA levels if given during a bentiromide test for pancreatic function. May cause false-positive results in urine glucose tests that use cupric sulfate (Clinitest).

CONTRAINDICATIONS & CAUTIONS
- Contraindicated in patients hypersensitive to drug.
- Use cautiously in patients with impaired hepatic or renal function, acute intermittent porphyria, and G6PD deficiency.
- Use cautiously in those taking other drugs that cause bone marrow suppression or blood disorders.
- ***Alert:*** Use cautiously in premature infants and newborns because potentially fatal gray syndrome may occur. Symptoms include abdominal distention, gray cyanosis, vasomotor collapse, respiratory distress, and death within a few hours of symptom onset.

NURSING CONSIDERATIONS
- Obtain specimen for culture and sensitivity tests before giving first dose. Begin therapy awaiting results.
- Obtain drug level measurement; maintain peak level of 10 to 20 mcg/ml and trough level of 5 to 10 mcg/ml.
- Monitor CBC, iron level, and platelet and reticulocyte counts before and every 2 days during therapy. Stop drug and no-

tify prescriber immediately if anemia, reticulocytopenia, leukopenia, or thrombocytopenia develops.
- Monitor patient for signs and symptoms of superinfection.

PATIENT TEACHING
- Instruct patient to notify prescriber if adverse reactions occur, especially nausea, vomiting, diarrhea, fever, confusion, sore throat, or mouth sores.
- Tell patient receiving drug I.V. to report discomfort at I.V. insertion site.
- Instruct patient to report signs and symptoms of superinfection.

clindamycin hydrochloride
Cleocin HCl, Dalacin C†‡

clindamycin palmitate hydrochloride
Cleocin Pediatric, Dalacin C Flavored Granules†

clindamycin phosphate
Cleocin Phosphate, Dalacin C Phosphate Sterile Solution†‡

Pharmacologic class: lincomycin derivative
Pregnancy risk category B

AVAILABLE FORMS
clindamycin hydrochloride
Capsules: 75 mg, 150 mg, 300 mg
clindamycin palmitate hydrochloride
Granules for oral solution: 75 mg/5 ml
clindamycin phosphate
Injectable infusion (in D_5W): 300 mg (50 ml), 600 mg (50 ml), 900 mg (50 ml)
Injection: 150-mg base/ml, 300-mg base/2 ml, 600-mg base/4 ml, 900-mg base/6 ml

INDICATIONS & DOSAGES
➤ Infections caused by sensitive staphylococci, streptococci, pneumococci, *Bacteroides, Fusobacterium, Clostridium perfringens* and other sensitive aerobic and anaerobic organisms
Adults: 150 to 450 mg P.O. q 6 hours; or 300 to 600 mg I.M. or I.V. q 6, 8, or 12 hours.
Children older than age 1 month: 8 to 20 mg/kg P.O. daily, in divided doses q 6 to 8 hours; or 15 to 40 mg/kg I.M. or I.V. daily, in divided doses q 6 or 8 hours.
➤ Pelvic inflammatory disease
Adults and adolescents: 900 mg I.V. q 8 hours, with gentamicin. Continue at least 48 hours after symptoms improve; then switch to oral clindamycin 450 mg q.i.d. for total of 10 to 14 days or doxycycline 100 mg P.O. q 12 hours for total of 10 to 14 days.
➤ *Pneumocystis jiroveci (carinii)* pneumonia ♦
Adults: 600 mg I.V. q 6 hours or 900 mg I.V. q 8 hours, with primaquine.
➤ CNS toxoplasmosis in AIDS patients, as alternative to sulfonamides with pyrimethamine ♦
Adults: 1,200 to 2,400 mg/day in divided doses.

I.V. ADMINISTRATION
- Never give undiluted as a bolus.
- For infusion, dilute each 300 mg in 50 ml solution and give over 10 to 60 minutes at no more than 30 mg/minute.
- Check site daily for phlebitis and irritation.

INCOMPATIBILITIES
Allopurinol, aminophylline, ampicillin, azithromycin, barbiturates, calcium gluconate, ceftriaxone, ciprofloxacin hydrochloride, doxapram, filgrastim, fluconazole, gentamicin sulfate with cefazolin sodium, idarubicin, magnesium sulfate, phenytoin sodium, ranitidine, rubber closures such as those on I.V. tubing, tobramycin sulfate.

ACTION
Inhibits bacterial protein synthesis by binding to the 50S subunit of the ribosome.

Route	Onset	Peak	Duration
P.O.	Unknown	45–60 min	Unknown
I.V.	Immediate	Immediate	Unknown
I.M.	Unknown	3 hr	Unknown

Half-life: 2½ to 3 hours.

ADVERSE REACTIONS

CV: thrombophlebitis.
GI: *nausea,* ***pseudomembranous colitis,*** abdominal pain, diarrhea, vomiting.
Hematologic: ***thrombocytopenia, transient leukopenia,*** eosinophilia.
Hepatic: jaundice.
Skin: maculopapular rash, urticaria.
Other: ***anaphylaxis.***

INTERACTIONS

Drug-drug. *Erythromycin:* May block access of clindamycin to its site of action. Avoid using together.
Kaolin: May decrease absorption of oral clindamycin. Separate dosage times.
Neuromuscular blockers: May increase neuromuscular blockade. Monitor patient closely.
Drug-food. *Diet foods with sodium cyclamate:* May decrease drug level. Discourage patient from eating of these foods.

EFFECTS ON LAB TEST RESULTS

- May increase alkaline phosphatase, AST, and bilirubin levels.
- May increase eosinophil count. May decrease platelet and WBC counts.

CONTRAINDICATIONS & CAUTIONS

- Contraindicated in patients hypersensitive to drug or lincomycin.
- Use cautiously in neonates and patients with renal or hepatic disease, asthma, history of GI disease, or significant allergies.

NURSING CONSIDERATIONS

- Obtain specimen for culture and sensitivity tests before giving first dose. Therapy may begin pending results.
- For I.M. administration, inject deep into muscle. Rotate sites. Don't exceed 600 mg per injection.
- I.M. injection may raise CK level in response to muscle irritation.
- Don't refrigerate reconstituted oral solution because it will thicken. Drug is stable for 2 weeks at room temperature.
- Monitor renal, hepatic, and hematopoietic functions during prolonged therapy.
- Observe patient for signs and symptoms of superinfection.
- ***Alert:*** Don't give opioid antidiarrheals to treat drug-induced diarrhea; they may prolong and worsen this condition.
- Drug doesn't penetrate blood-brain barrier.

PATIENT TEACHING

- Advise patient to take capsule form with a full glass of water to prevent esophageal irritation.
- Warn patient that I.M. injection may be painful.
- Tell patient to report discomfort at I.V. insertion site.
- Instruct patient to notify prescriber of adverse reactions (especially diarrhea). Warn him not to treat such diarrhea himself because drug may cause life-threatening colitis.

daptomycin
Cubicin

Pharmacologic class: cyclic lipopeptide
Pregnancy risk category B

AVAILABLE FORMS

Powder for injection: 250-mg vial, 500-mg vial

INDICATIONS & DOSAGES

✱***NEW INDICATION:*** **Bacteremia caused by *Staphylococcus aureus* (including right-sided endocarditis caused by methicillin-susceptible and methicillin-resistant strains)**
Adults: 6 mg/kg I.V. over 30 minutes q 24 hours for at least 2 to 6 weeks based on patient response.
➤ **Complicated skin or skin-structure infection (SSSI) caused by susceptible strains of *S. aureus* (including methicillin-resistant strains), *Streptococcus pyogenes, Streptococcus agalactiae, Streptococcus dysgalactiae,* and *Enterococcus faecalis* (vancomycin-susceptible strains only)**
Adults: 4 mg/kg I.V. over 30 minutes q 24 hours for 7 to 14 days.
Adjust-a-dose: In patients with SSSI with creatinine clearance less than 30 ml/minute, including those receiving hemodi-

alysis or continuous ambulatory peritoneal dialysis, give 4 mg/kg I.V. q 48 hours. For bacteremic patients with a clearance less than 30 ml/minute, give 6 mg/kg I.V. q 48 hours. When possible, give drug after hemodialysis.

I.V. ADMINISTRATION

- Reconstitute 250-mg vial with 5 ml and 500-mg vial with 10 ml of normal saline solution.
- Further dilute with normal saline solution.
- Infuse over 30 minutes.
- Refrigerate vials at 36° to 46° F (2° to 8° C).
- Vials are for single use; discard excess.
- Reconstituted and diluted solutions are stable 12 hours at room temperature or 48 hours at 36° to 46° F (2° to 8° C).

INCOMPATIBILITIES

Dextrose-containing solutions and other I.V. drugs. If an I.V. line is used for several drugs, flush the line with normal saline solution or lactated Ringer injection between drugs.

ACTION

Binds to and depolarizes bacterial membranes to inhibit protein, DNA, and RNA synthesis, thus causing bacterial cell death.

Route	Onset	Peak	Duration
I.V.	Rapid	< 1 hr	Unknown

Half-life: About 8 hours.

ADVERSE REACTIONS

CNS: anxiety, confusion, dizziness, fever, headache, insomnia.
CV: ***cardiac failure,*** chest pain, edema, hypertension, hypotension.
EENT: sore throat.
GI: ***pseudomembranous colitis,*** abdominal pain, constipation, decreased appetite, diarrhea, nausea, vomiting.
GU: ***renal failure,*** urinary tract infection.
Hematologic: anemia.
Metabolic: ***hypoglycemia,*** hyperglycemia, hypokalemia.
Musculoskeletal: limb and back pain, myopathy.
Respiratory: cough, dyspnea.
Skin: cellulitis, injection site reactions, pruritus, rash.
Other: fungal infections.

INTERACTIONS

Drug-drug. *HMG-CoA reductase inhibitors:* May increase risk of myopathy. Consider stopping these drugs while giving daptomycin.
Tobramycin: May affect levels of both drugs. Use together cautiously.
Warfarin: May alter anticoagulant activity. Monitor PT and INR for the first several days of daptomycin therapy.

EFFECTS ON LAB TEST RESULTS

- May increase alkaline phosphatase and CK levels. May decrease potassium and hemoglobin levels and hematocrit. May increase or decrease glucose level.
- May increase liver function test values.

CONTRAINDICATIONS & CAUTIONS

- Contraindicated in patients hypersensitive to drug.
- Use cautiously in patients with renal insufficiency and those who are older than age 65, pregnant, or breast-feeding.
- Safety and effectiveness haven't been established in patients younger than age 18.

NURSING CONSIDERATIONS

- Obtain specimen for culture and sensitivity tests before giving first dose.
- Monitor CBC and renal and liver function tests periodically.
- ***Alert:*** Because drug may increase the risk of myopathy, monitor CK level weekly. If CK level rises, monitor it more often. In patients with myopathy and CK level over 1,000 units/L or more than 10 times the upper limit of normal, stop drug. Consider stopping all other drugs linked with myopathy (such as HMG-CoA reductase inhibitors) during therapy.
- Monitor patient for superinfection because drug may cause overgrowth of nonsusceptible organisms.
- Watch for evidence of pseudomembranous colitis and treat accordingly.

PATIENT TEACHING

- Advise patient to immediately report muscle weakness and infusion site irritation.

• Tell patient to report severe diarrhea, rash, and infection.
• Inform patient about possible adverse reactions.

ertapenem sodium
Invanz

Pharmacologic class: carbapenem
Pregnancy risk category B

AVAILABLE FORMS
Injection: 1 g

INDICATIONS & DOSAGES
➤ **Complicated intra-abdominal infection caused by *Escherichia coli, Clostridium clostridiiforme, Eubacterium lentum, Peptostreptococcus* species, *Bacteroides fragilis, B. distasonis, B. ovatus, B. thetaiotaomicron,* or *B. uniformis***
Adults and children age 13 and older: 1 g I.V. or I.M. once daily for 5 to 14 days.
Infants and children ages 3 months to 13 years: 15 mg/kg I.V. or I.M. q 12 hours for 5 to 14 days. Don't exceed 1 g daily.
➤ **Complicated skin or skin-structure infection including diabetic foot infections without osteomyelitis caused by *Staphylococcus aureus* (methicillin-susceptible strains), *Streptococcus agalactiae, S. pyogenes, Escherichia coli, Klebsiella pneumoniae, Proteus mirabilis, Bacteroides fragilis, Peptostreptococcus* species, *Porphyromonas asaccharolytica,* or *Prevotella bivia***
Adults and children age 13 and older: 1 g I.V. or I.M. once daily for 7 to 14 days. Diabetic foot infections may need up to 28 days of treatment.
Infants and children ages 3 months to 13 years: 15 mg/kg I.V. or I.M. q 12 hours for 7 to 14 days. Don't exceed 1 g daily.
➤ **Community-acquired pneumonia from *S. pneumoniae* (penicillin-susceptible strains), *Haemophilus influenzae* (beta-lactamase–negative strains), or *Moraxella catarrhalis;* complicated UTI including pyelonephritis caused by *E. coli* or *K. pneumoniae***
Adults and children age 13 and older: 1 g I.V. or I.M. once daily for 10 to 14 days. If patient improves after at least 3 days of treatment, use appropriate oral therapy to complete the full course of therapy.
Infants and children ages 3 months to 13 years: 15 mg/kg I.V. or I.M. q 12 hours for 10 to 14 days. Don't exceed 1 g daily. If patient improves after at least 3 days of treatment, use appropriate oral therapy to complete the full course of therapy.
➤ **Acute pelvic infection, including postpartum endomyometritis, septic abortion, and postsurgical gynecologic infections caused by *S. agalactiae, E. coli, B. fragilis, P. asaccharolytica, Peptostreptococcus* species, or *P. bivia***
Adults and children age 13 and older: 1 g I.V. or I.M. once daily for 3 to 10 days.
Infants and children ages 3 months to 13 years: 15 mg/kg I.V. or I.M. q 12 hours for 3 to 10 days. Don't exceed 1 g daily.
Adjust-a-dose: In adult patients with creatinine clearance of 30 ml/minute or less, give 500 mg/day. In hemodialysis patients receiving daily 500-mg dose less than 6 hours before hemodialysis, give supplementary 150-mg dose afterward. In hemodialysis patients receiving dose 6 hours or more before hemodialysis, no supplementary dose is needed.

I.V. ADMINISTRATION
• Reconstitute 1-g vial with 10 ml of sterile water for injection, normal saline solution for injection, or bacteriostatic water for injection.
• Shake well to dissolve, and then immediately transfer contents to 50 ml of normal saline solution.
• Infuse over 30 minutes.
• Complete the infusion within 6 hours of reconstitution or refrigerate for up to 24 hours. Infuse within 4 hours once removed from refrigeration. Don't freeze.

INCOMPATIBILITIES
Diluents containing dextrose (alpha-D-glucose), other I.V. drugs.

ACTION
Inhibits cell-wall synthesis through penicillin-binding proteins.

Route	Onset	Peak	Duration
I.V.	Immediate	30 min	24 hr
I.M.	Unknown	2 hr	24 hr

Half-life: 4 hours.

ADVERSE REACTIONS
CNS: altered mental status, anxiety, asthenia, dizziness, fatigue, fever, headache, insomnia.
CV: chest pain, edema, hypertension, hypotension, infused vein complication, phlebitis, swelling, tachycardia, thrombophlebitis.
EENT: pharyngitis.
GI: *diarrhea,* abdominal pain, acid regurgitation, constipation, dyspepsia, nausea, oral candidiasis, vomiting.
GU: renal dysfunction, vaginitis.
Hematologic: ***leukopenia, neutropenia, thrombocytopenia,*** anemia, coagulation abnormalities, eosinophilia, thrombocytosis.
Hepatic: jaundice.
Metabolic: ***hyperkalemia,*** hyperglycemia.
Musculoskeletal: leg pain.
Respiratory: cough, dyspnea, rales, respiratory distress, rhonchi.
Skin: erythema, extravasation, infusion site pain and redness, pruritus, rash.
Other: hypersensitivity reactions.

INTERACTIONS
Drug-drug. *Probenecid:* May reduce renal clearance and may increase half-life. Don't give together with probenecid to extend half-life.

EFFECTS ON LAB TEST RESULTS
- May increase albumin, ALT, alkaline phosphatase, AST, bilirubin, creatinine, glucose, and potassium levels. May decrease hemoglobin level and hematocrit.
- May increase eosinophil count, PT, and urinary RBC or WBC counts. May decrease segmented neutrophil and WBC counts. May increase or decrease platelet count.

CONTRAINDICATIONS & CAUTIONS
- Contraindicated in patients hypersensitive to any component of the drug or to other drugs in the same class and in patients who have had anaphylactic reactions to beta-lactams. I.M. use is contraindicated in patients hypersensitive to local anesthetics of the amide type (because of drug's diluent, lidocaine hydrochloride).
- Use cautiously in patients with CNS disorders, compromised renal function, or both, as seizures may occur in these patients.

NURSING CONSIDERATIONS
- Check for previous penicillin, cephalosporin, or other beta-lactam hypersensitivity before giving first dose.
- If giving dose I.M., check for hypersensitivity to local amide-type anesthetics.
- Obtain specimens for culture and sensitivity testing before giving. Begin therapy awaiting results.
- To give I.M., reconstitute 1-g vial with 3.2 ml of 1% lidocaine hydrochloride injection (without epinephrine). Shake vial thoroughly to form solution. Immediately withdraw the contents of the vial and give by deep I.M. injection into a large muscle, such as the gluteal muscles or lateral part of the thigh. Use the reconstituted I.M. solution within 1 hour after preparation. Don't give reconstituted solution I.V.
- If patient has diarrhea during therapy, notify prescriber and collect stool specimen for culture to rule out pseudomembranous colitis.
- Vomiting occurs more frequently in children than adults. Monitor children closely for signs and symptoms of dehydration and electrolyte imbalance.
- If allergic reaction occurs, stop drug immediately.
- Anaphylactic reactions require immediate emergency treatment with epinephrine, oxygen, I.V. steroids, and airway management.
- Anticonvulsants may continue in patients with seizure disorders. If focal tremors, myoclonus, or seizures occur, notify prescriber. Drug may need to be decreased or stopped.

• Monitor renal, hepatic, and hematopoietic function during prolonged therapy.
• Methicillin-resistant staphylococci and *Enterococcus* species are resistant to drug.
• ***Look alike–sound alike:*** Don't confuse Invanz with Avinza.

PATIENT TEACHING

• Tell patient about adverse reactions.
• Tell patient to alert nurse if discomfort occurs at injection site.

imipenem and cilastatin sodium

Primaxin I.M., Primaxin I.V.

Pharmacologic class: carbapenem, beta-lactam
Pregnancy risk category C

AVAILABLE FORMS

Powder for injection: 250 mg, 500 mg, 750 mg

INDICATIONS & DOSAGES

➤ **Serious lower respiratory tract, bone, intra-abdominal, gynecologic, joint, skin, and soft-tissue infections; UTIs; endocarditis; and bacterial septicemia, caused by *Acinetobacter, Enterococcus, Staphylococcus, Streptococcus, Escherichia coli, Haemophilus, Klebsiella, Morganella, Proteus, Enterobacter, Pseudomonas aeruginosa,* and *Bacteroides,* including *B. fragilis***

Adults who weigh more than 70 kg (154 lb): 250 mg to 1 g by I.V. infusion q 6 to 8 hours. Maximum daily dose is 50 mg/kg/day or 4 g/day, whichever is less. Or, 500 to 750 mg I.M. q 12 hours. Maximum I.M. daily dose is 1,500 mg.
Children age 3 months and older (except for CNS infections): 15 to 25 mg/kg I.V. q 6 hours. Maximum daily dose is 2 to 4 g.
Infants ages 4 weeks to 3 months who weigh 1.5 kg (3.3 lb) or more (except for CNS infections): 25 mg/kg I.V. q 6 hours.
Neonates ages 1 to 4 weeks who weigh 1.5 kg or more (except for CNS infections): 25 mg/kg I.V. q 8 hours.
Neonates younger than age 1 week who weigh 1.5 kg or more (except for CNS infections): 25 mg/kg I.V. q 12 hours.

Adjust-a-dose: If creatinine clearance is less than 70 ml/minute, adjust dosage and monitor renal function test results. Consult manufacturer's package insert for specific dosage adjustments.

I.V. ADMINISTRATION

• Reconstitute piggyback units with 100 ml of compatible I.V. solution to provide solution containing 2.5 to 5 mg/ml.
• When reconstituting powder, shake until the solution is clear. Solutions may be colorless to yellow; variations of color within this range don't affect drug's potency.
• After reconstitution, solution is stable for 4 hours at room temperature and for 24 hours when refrigerated.
• Don't give by direct I.V. bolus injection.
• For adults, give each 250- or 500-mg dose by I.V. infusion over 20 to 30 minutes. Infuse each 750-mg to 1-g dose over 40 to 60 minutes.
• For children, infuse doses of 500 mg or less over 15 to 30 minutes. Infuse doses greater than 500 mg over 40 to 60 minutes. If nausea occurs, the infusion may be slowed.

INCOMPATIBILITIES

Allopurinol, antibiotics, amiodarone, amphotericin B cholesterol complex, azithromycin, dextrose 5% in lactated Ringer injection, etoposide, fluconazole, gemcitabine, lorazepam, meperidine, midazolam, milrinone, sargramostim, sodium bicarbonate.

ACTION

Inhibits bacterial cell-wall synthesis; enzymatic breakdown of drug in the kidneys causes adequate antibacterial levels of drug in the urine.

Route	Onset	Peak	Duration
I.V.	Immediate	Immediate	Unknown
I.M.	Unknown	1–2 hr	Unknown

Half-life: 1 hour after I.V. dose; 2 to 3 hours after I.M. dose.

ADVERSE REACTIONS

CNS: ***seizures,*** dizziness, fever, somnolence.
CV: hypotension, thrombophlebitis.

GI: ***pseudomembranous colitis,*** diarrhea, nausea, vomiting.
Hematologic: ***leukopenia, thrombocytopenia,*** eosinophilia.
Skin: injection site pain, pruritus, rash, urticaria.
Other: ***anaphylaxis,*** hypersensitivity reactions.

INTERACTIONS

Drug-drug. *Beta-lactam antibiotics:* May have antagonistic effect. Avoid using together.
Ganciclovir: May cause seizures. Avoid using together.
Probenecid: May increase cilastatin level. May be used together for this effect.

EFFECTS ON LAB TEST RESULTS

- May increase BUN, creatinine, ALT, AST, alkaline phosphatase, bilirubin, and LDH levels.
- May increase eosinophil count. May decrease WBC and platelet counts.
- May interfere with glucose determination by Benedict solution or Clinitest.

CONTRAINDICATIONS & CAUTIONS

- Contraindicated in patients hypersensitive to drug, in those with a history of hypersensitivity to local anesthetics of the amide type, and in those with severe shock or heart block.
- Use cautiously in patients allergic to penicillins or cephalosporins because drug has similar properties.
- Use cautiously in patients with history of seizure disorders, especially if they also have compromised renal function.
- Use cautiously in children younger than age 3 months.

NURSING CONSIDERATIONS

- ***Alert:*** Don't use for CNS infections in children because drug increases the risk of seizures.
- Obtain specimen culture and sensitivity tests before giving first dose. Begin therapy awaiting results.
- ***Alert:*** Don't give I.M. solution by I.V. route.
- ***Alert:*** If seizures develop and persist despite anticonvulsant therapy, stop drug and notify prescriber.
- Monitor patient for bacterial or fungal superinfections and resistant infections during and after therapy.

PATIENT TEACHING

- Instruct patient to report adverse reactions promptly.
- Tell patient to report discomfort at I.V. insertion site.
- Urge patient to notify prescriber about loose stools or diarrhea.

linezolid

Zyvox

Pharmacologic class: oxazolidinone
Pregnancy risk category C

AVAILABLE FORMS

Injection: 2 mg/ml
Powder for oral suspension: 100 mg/5 ml when reconstituted
Tablets: 400 mg, 600 mg

INDICATIONS & DOSAGES

➤ **Vancomycin-resistant *Enterococcus faecium* infections, including those with concurrent bacteremia**
Adults and children age 12 and older: 600 mg I.V. or P.O. q 12 hours for 14 to 28 days.
Neonates age 7 days or older and infants and children through age 11: 10 mg/kg I.V. or P.O. q 8 hours for 14 to 28 days.
Neonates younger than age 7 days: 10 mg/kg I.V. or P.O. q 12 hours for 14 to 28 days. Increase to 10 mg/kg q 8 hours when patient is 7 days old. Consider this dosage increase if neonate has inadequate response.
➤ **Hospital-acquired pneumonia caused by *Staphylococcus aureus* (methicillin-susceptible [MSSA] and methicillin-resistant [MRSA] strains) or *Streptococcus pneumoniae* (including multidrug-resistant strains [MDRSP]); complicated skin and skin-structure infections, including diabetic foot infections without osteomyelitis caused by *S. aureus* (MSSA and MRSA), *S. pyogenes, or S. agalactiae;* community-acquired pneumonia caused by *S. pneumoniae* (including MDRSP), including**

those with concurrent bacteremia, or *S. aureus* (MSSA only)
Adults and children age 12 and older: 600 mg I.V. or P.O. q 12 hours for 10 to 14 days.
Neonates 7 days or older, infants and children through 11 years: 10 mg/kg I.V. or P.O. q 8 hours for 10 to 14 days.
Neonates younger than age 7 days: 10 mg/kg I.V. or P.O. q 12 hours for 10 to 14 days. Increase to 10 mg/kg q 8 hours when patient is 7 days old. Consider this dosage increase if neonate has inadequate response.

➤ **Uncomplicated skin and skin-structure infections caused by *S. aureus* (MSSA only) or *S. pyogenes***
Adults: 400 mg P.O. q 12 hours for 10 to 14 days.
Children ages 12 to 18: 600 mg P.O. q 12 hours for 10 to 14 days.
Children ages 5 to 11: 10 mg/kg P.O. q 12 hours for 10 to 14 days.
Neonates age 7 days or older and infants and children younger than age 5: 10 mg/kg P.O. q 8 hours for 10 to 14 days.
Neonates younger than age 7 days: 10 mg/kg P.O. q 12 hours for 10 to 14 days. Increase to 10 mg/kg q 8 hours when patient is 7 days old. Consider this dosage increase if neonate has inadequate response.

I.V. ADMINISTRATION

- Inspect solution for particulate matter and leaks.
- Drug is compatible with D_5W injection, normal saline solution for injection, and lactated Ringer injection.
- Don't inject additives into infusion bag. Give other I.V. drugs separately or via a separate I.V. line to avoid incompatibilities. If single I.V. line is used, flush line before and after infusion with a compatible solution.
- Infuse over 30 minutes to 2 hours. Don't infuse drug in a series connection.
- Store drug at room temperature in its protective overwrap. Solution may turn yellow over time, but this doesn't affect drug's potency.

INCOMPATIBILITIES

Amphotericin B, ceftriaxone sodium, chlorpromazine hydrochloride, diazepam, erythromycin lactobionate, pentamidine isethionate, phenytoin sodium, trimethoprim-sulfamethoxazole.

ACTION

Prevents bacterial protein synthesis by interfering with DNA translation in the ribosomes. Also prevents formation of a functional 70S ribosomal subunit by binding to a site on the bacterial 50S ribosomal subunit.

Route	Onset	Peak	Duration
P.O.	Unknown	1 hr	Unknown
I.V.	Unknown	30 min	Unknown

Half-life: 6¼ hours.

ADVERSE REACTIONS

CNS: *headache,* dizziness, fever, insomnia.
GI: *diarrhea, nausea,* ***pseudomembranous colitis,*** altered taste, constipation, oral candidiasis, tongue discoloration, vomiting.
GU: vaginal candidiasis.
Hematologic: ***leukopenia, myelosuppression, neutropenia, thrombocytopenia,*** anemia.
Skin: rash.
Other: fungal infection.

INTERACTIONS

Drug-drug. *Adrenergic drugs (such as dopamine, epinephrine, pseudoephedrine):* May cause hypertension. Monitor blood pressure and heart rate; start continuous infusions of dopamine and epinephrine at lower doses and titrate to response.
Serotoninergic drugs: May cause serotonin syndrome, including confusion, delirium, restlessness, tremors, blushing, diaphoresis, and hyperpyrexia. Notify prescriber immediately of signs and symptoms of serotonin syndrome.
Drug-food. *Foods and beverages high in tyramine (such as aged cheeses, air-dried meats, red wines, sauerkraut, soy sauce, tap beers):* May increase blood pressure. Provide a list of foods containing tyramine and advise patient that tyramine content of meals shouldn't exceed 100 mg.

EFFECTS ON LAB TEST RESULTS

- May increase ALT, AST, bilirubin, alkaline phosphatase, creatinine, amylase, lipase, and BUN levels. May decrease hemoglobin level.
- May decrease WBC, neutrophil, and platelet counts.

CONTRAINDICATIONS & CAUTIONS

- Contraindicated in patients hypersensitive to drug or its components.

NURSING CONSIDERATIONS

- Obtain specimen for culture and sensitivity tests before therapy. Use sensitivity results to guide subsequent therapy.
- No dosage adjustment is needed when switching from I.V. to P.O. forms.
- Reconstitute oral suspension according to manufacturer's instructions. Store reconstituted suspension at room temperature and use within 21 days.
- ***Look alike–sound alike:*** Don't confuse Zyvox with Zovirax. Both come in a 400-mg strength.
- ***Alert:*** Drug may cause thrombocytopenia. In patients at increased risk for bleeding, those with existing thrombocytopenia, those taking other drugs that may cause thrombocytopenia, and those receiving this drug for longer than 14 days, monitor platelet count.
- ***Alert:*** Drug may lead to myelosuppression. Monitor CBC weekly.
- ***Alert:*** Pseudomembranous colitis or superinfection may occur. Consider these diagnoses and take appropriate measures in patients with persistent diarrhea or secondary infections.
- Inappropriate use of antibiotics may lead to development of resistant organisms; carefully consider other drugs before starting therapy, especially in outpatient setting.

PATIENT TEACHING

- Tell patient that tablets and oral suspension may be taken with or without meals.
- Stress importance of completing entire course of therapy, even if patient feels better.
- Tell patient to alert prescriber if he has high blood pressure, is taking cough or cold preparations, or is being treated with SSRIs or other antidepressants.
- Advise patient to avoid large quantities of tyramine-containing foods (such as aged cheeses, soy sauce, tap beers, red wine) during therapy.
- Inform patient with phenylketonuria that each 5 ml of oral suspension contains 20 mg of phenylalanine. Tablets and injection don't contain phenylalanine.

meropenem

Merrem IV

Pharmacologic class: carbapenem
Pregnancy risk category B

AVAILABLE FORMS

Powder for injection: 500 mg, 1 g

INDICATIONS & DOSAGES

➤ **Complicated skin and skin structure infections from *Staphylococcus aureus* (beta-lactamase or non–beta-lactamase producing, methicillin-susceptible isolates only), *Streptococcus pyogenes, S. agalactiae*, viridans group streptococci, *Enterococcus faecalis* (excluding vancomycin-resistant isolates), *Pseudomonas aeruginosa, Escherichia coli, Proteus mirabilis, Bacteroides fragilis,* and *Peptostreptococcus* species**

Adults and children who weigh more than 50 kg (110 lb): 500 mg I.V. q 8 hours over 15 to 30 minutes as I.V. infusion.

Children ages 3 months and older who weigh 50 kg or less: 10 mg/kg I.V. q 8 hours over 15 to 30 minutes as I.V. infusion or over 3 to 5 minutes as I.V. bolus injection (5 to 20 ml); maximum dose is 500 mg I.V. q 8 hours.

➤ **Complicated appendicitis and peritonitis from viridans group streptococci, *E. coli, Klebsiella pneumoniae, Pseudomonas aeruginosa, B. fragilis, B. thetaiotaomicron,* and *Peptostreptococcus* species**

Adults and children who weigh more than 50 kg: 1 g I.V. q 8 hours over 15 to 30 minutes as I.V. infusion or over 3 to 5 minutes as I.V. bolus injection (5 to 20 ml).

Children ages 3 months and older, who weigh 50 kg or less: 20 mg/kg I.V. q

8 hours over 15 to 30 minutes as I.V. infusion or over 3 to 5 minutes as I.V. bolus injection (5 to 20 ml); maximum dose is 1 g I.V. q 8 hours.
Adjust-a-dose: For adults with creatinine clearance of 26 to 50 ml/minute, give usual dose q 12 hours. If clearance is 10 to 25 ml/minute, give half usual dose q 12 hours; if clearance is less than 10 ml/minute, give half usual dose q 24 hours.

➤ **Bacterial meningitis from *S. pneumoniae, Haemophilus influenzae,* and *Neisseria meningitidis***
Children who weigh more than 50 kg: 2 g I.V. q 8 hours.
Children ages 3 months and older, who weigh 50 kg or less: 40 mg/kg I.V. q 8 hours; maximum dose, 2 g I.V. q 8 hours.

I.V. ADMINISTRATION
- Use freshly prepared solutions of drug immediately whenever possible. Stability of drug varies with form of drug used (injection vial, infusion vial, or ADD-Vantage container).
- For bolus, add 10 ml of sterile water for injection to 500 mg/20-ml vial or 20 ml to 1 g/30-ml vial. Shake to dissolve, and let stand until clear.
- For infusion, an infusion vial (500 mg/100 ml or 1 g/100 ml) may be directly reconstituted with a compatible infusion fluid. Or, an injection vial may be reconstituted and the resulting solution added to an I.V. container and further diluted with an appropriate infusion fluid. Don't use ADD-Vantage vials for this purpose.
- For ADD-Vantage vials, constitute only with half-normal saline solution for injection, normal saline solution for injection, or D_5W in 50-, 100-, or 250-ml Abbott ADD-Vantage flexible diluent containers. Follow manufacturer's guidelines closely when using ADD-Vantage vials.

INCOMPATIBILITIES
Other I.V. drugs.

ACTION
Inhibits cell-wall synthesis in bacteria. Readily penetrates cell wall of most gram-positive and -negative bacteria to reach penicillin-binding protein targets.

Route	Onset	Peak	Duration
I.V.	Unknown	1 hr	Unknown

Half-life: 1 hour.

ADVERSE REACTIONS
CNS: ***seizures,*** headache, pain.
CV: phlebitis, thrombophlebitis.
GI: ***pseudomembranous colitis,*** constipation, diarrhea, glossitis, nausea, oral candidiasis, vomiting.
GU: RBCs in urine.
Hematologic: anemia.
Respiratory: ***apnea,*** dyspnea.
Skin: injection site inflammation, pruritus, rash.
Other: ***anaphylaxis,*** hypersensitivity reactions, inflammation.

INTERACTIONS
Drug-drug. *Probenecid:* May decrease renal excretion of meropenem; probenecid competes with meropenem for active tubular secretion, which significantly increases elimination half-life of meropenem and extent of systemic exposure. Avoid using together.

EFFECTS ON LAB TEST RESULTS
- May increase ALT, AST, bilirubin, alkaline phosphatase, LDH, creatinine, and BUN levels. May decrease hemoglobin level and hematocrit.
- May increase eosinophil count. May decrease WBC count. May increase or decrease PT, PTT, and INR, and platelet count.

CONTRAINDICATIONS & CAUTIONS
- Contraindicated in patients hypersensitive to components of drug or other drugs in same class and in patients who have had anaphylactic reactions to beta-lactams.
- Use cautiously in elderly patients and in those with a history of seizure disorders or impaired renal function.
- Safety and effectiveness of drug haven't been established for infants younger than age 3 months.
- Use drug cautiously in breast-feeding women; it's unknown if drug appears in breast milk.

NURSING CONSIDERATIONS

- Obtain specimen for culture and sensitivity tests before giving. Begin therapy awaiting test results.
- ***Alert:*** Serious hypersensitivity reactions may occur in patients receiving beta-lactams. Before therapy begins, determine if patient has had previous hypersensitivity reactions to penicillins, cephalosporins, beta-lactams, or other allergens. If an allergic reaction occurs, stop drug and notify prescriber. Serious anaphylactic reactions require emergency treatment.
- In patients with CNS disorders, bacterial meningitis, and compromised renal function, drug may cause seizures and other CNS adverse reactions.
- If seizures occur during therapy, stop infusion and notify prescriber. Dosage adjustment may be needed.
- Monitor patient for signs and symptoms of superinfection. Drug may cause overgrowth of nonsusceptible bacteria or fungi.
- Periodic assessment of organ system functions, including renal, hepatic, and hematopoietic function, is recommended during prolonged therapy.
- Monitor patient's fluid balance and weight carefully.

PATIENT TEACHING

- Advise woman not to breast-feed during therapy.
- Instruct patient to report adverse reactions or signs and symptoms of superinfection.
- Advise patient to report loose stools to prescriber.

nitrofurantoin macrocrystals

Macrobid✐, Macrodantin

nitrofurantoin microcrystals

Apo-Nitrofurantoin†, Furadantin, Novo-Furantoin†

Pharmacologic class: nitrofuran
Pregnancy risk category B

AVAILABLE FORMS

nitrofurantoin macrocrystals
Capsules: 25 mg, 50 mg, 100 mg
nitrofurantoin microcrystals
Oral suspension: 25 mg/5 ml

INDICATIONS & DOSAGES

➤ **UTIs caused by susceptible *Escherichia coli, Staphylococcus aureus, enterococci;* or certain strains of *Klebsiella* and *Enterobacter* species**
Adults and children older than age 12: 50 to 100 mg P.O. q.i.d. with meals and h.s. Or, 100 mg Macrobid P.O. q 12 hours for 7 days.
Children ages 1 month to 12 years: 5 to 7 mg/kg P.O. daily, divided q.i.d.

➤ **Long-term suppression therapy**
Adults: 50 to 100 mg P.O. daily h.s.
Children: 1 mg/kg P.O. daily in a single dose h.s. or divided into two doses given q 12 hours.

ACTION

May interfere with bacterial enzyme systems and bacterial cell-wall formation.

Route	Onset	Peak	Duration
P.O.	Unknown	Unknown	Unknown

Half-life: 15 minutes to 1 hour.

ADVERSE REACTIONS

CNS: *ascending polyneuropathy with high doses or renal impairment,* dizziness, drowsiness, headache, peripheral neuropathy.
GI: *anorexia, diarrhea, nausea, vomiting,* abdominal pain.
GU: overgrowth of nonsusceptible organisms in urinary tract.
Hematologic: ***agranulocytosis, hemolysis in patients with G6PD deficiency, thrombocytopenia.***
Hepatic: ***hepatic necrosis, hepatitis.***
Metabolic: ***hypoglycemia.***
Respiratory: ***asthmatic attacks, pulmonary sensitivity reactions.***
Skin: ***Stevens-Johnson syndrome,*** exfoliative dermatitis, maculopapular, erythematous, or eczematous eruption, pruritus, transient alopecia, urticaria.
Other: ***anaphylaxis,*** drug fever, hypersensitivity reactions.

INTERACTIONS

Drug-drug. *Antacids containing magnesium:* May decrease nitrofurantoin absorption. Separate dosage times by 1 hour.
Probenecid, sulfinpyrazone: May inhibit excretion of nitrofurantoin, increasing

drug levels and risk of toxicity. The resulting decreased urinary levels could lessen antibacterial effects. Avoid using together.
Drug-food. *Any food:* May increase absorption. Advise patient to take drug with food or milk.

EFFECTS ON LAB TEST RESULTS

- May increase bilirubin and alkaline phosphatase levels. May decrease glucose level.
- May decrease granulocyte and platelet counts.
- May cause false-positive results in urine glucose tests using cupric sulfate (such as Benedict reagent, Fehling solution, or Chemstrip uG).

CONTRAINDICATIONS & CAUTIONS

- Contraindicated in infants age 1 month and younger and in patients with anuria, oliguria, or creatinine clearance less than 60 ml/minute. Also contraindicated in pregnant patients at 38 to 42 weeks' gestation and during labor and delivery.
- Use cautiously in patients with renal impairment, asthma, anemia, diabetes mellitus, electrolyte abnormalities, vitamin B deficiency, debilitating disease, and G6PD deficiency.

NURSING CONSIDERATIONS

- Obtain urine specimen for culture and sensitivity tests before giving. Repeat as needed. Begin therapy awaiting results.
- Give drug with food or milk to minimize GI distress and improve absorption.
- Drug may cause an asthma attack in patients with a history of asthma.
- Monitor fluid intake and output carefully. May turn urine brown or dark yellow.
- Monitor CBC and pulmonary status regularly.
- ***Alert:*** Monitor patient for signs and symptoms of superinfection. Use of nitrofurantoin may result in growth of nonsusceptible organisms, especially *Pseudomonas* species.
- Monitor patient for pulmonary sensitivity reactions, including cough, chest pain, fever, chills, dyspnea, and pulmonary infiltration with consolidation or effusions.
- ***Alert:*** Hypersensitivity may develop when drug is used for long-term therapy.
- Some patients may experience fewer adverse GI effects with nitrofurantoin macrocrystals.
- Dual-release capsules (25 mg nitrofurantoin macrocrystals combined with 75 mg nitrofurantoin monohydrate) enable patients to take drug only twice daily.
- Continue treatment for 3 days after sterile urine specimens have been obtained.
- Store drug in amber container. Don't store in metals other than stainless steel or aluminum to avoid precipitation.

PATIENT TEACHING

- Instruct patient to take drug for as long as prescribed, exactly as directed, even after he feels better.
- Tell patient to take drug with food or milk to minimize stomach upset.
- Instruct patient to report adverse reactions, especially peripheral neuropathy, which can become severe or irreversible.
- Alert patient that drug may turn urine dark yellow or brown.
- Warn patient not to store drug in metals other than stainless steel or aluminum.

quinupristin and dalfopristin
Synercid

Pharmacologic class: streptogramin
Pregnancy risk category B

AVAILABLE FORMS

Injection: 500 mg/10 ml (150 mg quinupristin and 350 mg dalfopristin)

INDICATIONS & DOSAGES

➤ **Serious or life-threatening infections with vancomycin-resistant *Enterococcus faecium* bacteremia**
Adults and adolescents age 16 and older: 7.5 mg/kg I.V. over 1 hour q 8 hours. Length of treatment depends on site and severity of infection.

➤ **Complicated skin and skin-structure infections caused by methicillin-susceptible *Staphylococcus aureus* or *Streptococcus pyogenes***
Adults and adolescents age 16 and older: 7.5 mg/kg I.V. over 1 hour q 12 hours for at least 7 days.

I.V. ADMINISTRATION

- Reconstitute powder for injection by adding 5 ml of either sterile water for injection or D_5W and gently swirling vial by manual rotation to ensure dissolution; avoid shaking to limit foaming. Reconstituted solutions must be further diluted within 30 minutes.
- Add appropriate dose of reconstituted solution to 250 ml of D_5W, according to patient's weight, to yield no more than 2 mg/ml. This diluted solution is stable for 5 hours at room temperature or 54 hours if refrigerated.
- Flush line with D_5W before and after each dose.
- Fluid-restricted patients with a central venous catheter may receive dose in 100 ml of D_5W. This concentration isn't recommended for peripheral venous administration.
- If moderate to severe peripheral venous irritation occurs, consider increasing infusion volume to 500 or 750 ml, changing injection site, or infusing by a central venous catheter.
- Give all doses by I.V. infusion over 1 hour. An infusion pump or device may be used to control infusion rate.

INCOMPATIBILITIES

Saline and heparin solutions.

ACTION

The two antibiotics work synergistically to inhibit or destroy susceptible bacteria through combined inhibition of protein synthesis in bacterial cells. Without the ability to manufacture new proteins, the bacterial cells are inactivated or die.

Route	Onset	Peak	Duration
I.V.	Unknown	Unknown	Unknown

Half-life: Quinupristin, 1 hour; dalfopristin, ¾ hours.

ADVERSE REACTIONS

CNS: headache.
CV: thrombophlebitis.
GI: diarrhea, nausea, vomiting.
Musculoskeletal: arthralgia, myalgia.
Skin: *edema at infusion site, inflammation, infusion site reaction, pain,* pruritus, rash.

INTERACTIONS

Drug-drug. *Cyclosporine:* May lower metabolism; may increase drug level. Monitor cyclosporine level.
Drugs metabolized by CYP3A4, such as carbamazepine, delavirdine, diazepam, diltiazem, disopyramide, docetaxel, indinavir, lidocaine, lovastatin, methylprednisolone, midazolam, nevirapine, nifedipine, paclitaxel, ritonavir, tacrolimus, verapamil, vinblastine: May increase levels of these drugs, which could increase both their therapeutic effects and adverse reactions. Use together cautiously.
Drugs metabolized by CYP3A4 that may prolong the QTc interval, such as quinidine: May decrease metabolism of these drugs, prolonging QTc interval. Avoid using together.

EFFECTS ON LAB TEST RESULTS

- May increase AST, ALT, and bilirubin levels.

CONTRAINDICATIONS & CAUTIONS

- Contraindicated in patients hypersensitive to drug or other streptogramin antibiotics.

NURSING CONSIDERATIONS

- Drug isn't active against *Enterococcus faecalis*. Blood cultures are needed to avoid misidentifying *E. faecalis* as *E. faecium*.
- Because drug may cause mild to life-threatening pseudomembranous colitis, consider this diagnosis in patient who develops diarrhea during or after therapy.
- Adverse reactions, such as arthralgia and myalgia, may be reduced by decreasing dosage interval to every 12 hours.
- Because overgrowth of nonsusceptible organisms may occur, monitor patient closely for signs and symptoms of superinfection.
- Monitor liver function test results during therapy.

PATIENT TEACHING

- Advise patient to immediately report irritation at I.V. site, pain in joints or muscles, and diarrhea.
- Tell patient about importance of reporting persistent or worsening signs and

symptoms of infection, such as pain or redness.

telithromycin
Ketek

Pharmacologic class: ketolide
Pregnancy risk category C

AVAILABLE FORMS
Tablets: 300 mg, 400 mg

INDICATIONS & DOSAGES
➤ **Mild to moderate community-acquired pneumonia caused by *S. pneumoniae* (including multi–drug-resistant isolates), *H. influenzae*, *M. catarrhalis*, *Chlamydophila pneumoniae*, or *Mycoplasma pneumoniae***
Adults: 800 mg P.O. once daily for 7 to 10 days.
Adjust-a-dose: In patients with creatinine clearance less than 30 ml/minute, including those on dialysis, give 600 mg P.O. once daily. On dialysis days, give after session. In patients with clearance less than 30 ml/minute and hepatic impairment, give 400 mg once daily.

ACTION
Inhibits bacterial protein synthesis.

Route	Onset	Peak	Duration
P.O.	Unknown	1 hr	Unknown

Half-life: 10 hours.

ADVERSE REACTIONS
CNS: dizziness, headache.
EENT: blurred vision, difficulty focusing, diplopia.
GI: *diarrhea,* loose stools, nausea, taste disturbance, vomiting.

INTERACTIONS
Drug-drug. *Atorvastatin, lovastatin, simvastatin:* May increase levels of these drugs, increasing the risk of myopathy. Avoid using together.
Benzodiazepines (midazolam): May increase benzodiazepine level. Monitor patient closely and adjust benzodiazepine dosage.
CYP3A4 inhibitors (itraconazole, ketoconazole): May increase telithromycin level. Monitor patient closely.
CYP3A4 inducers (carbamazepine, phenobarbital, phenytoin): May decrease telithromycin level. Avoid using together.
Digoxin: May increase digoxin level. Monitor digoxin level.
Drugs metabolized by the cytochrome P-450 system (carbamazepine, cyclosporine, hexobarbital, phenytoin, sirolimus, tacrolimus): May increase levels of these drugs, increasing or prolonging their effects. Use together cautiously.
Ergot alkaloid derivatives such as ergotamine: May increase the risk of ergot toxicity, characterized by severe peripheral vasospasm and dysesthesia. Avoid using together.
Metoprolol: May increase metoprolol level. Use together cautiously.
Oral anticoagulants: May increase anticoagulant effect. Monitor PT and INR.
Pimozide: May increase pimozide level. Avoid using together.
Rifamycins: May significantly decrease telithromycin level. Avoid using together.
Sotalol: May decrease sotalol level. Monitor patient for lack of effect.
Theophylline: May increase theophylline level and cause nausea and vomiting. Separate doses by 1 hour.

EFFECTS ON LAB TEST RESULTS
- May increase AST and ALT levels.
- May increase platelet count.

CONTRAINDICATIONS & CAUTIONS
- Contraindicated in patients hypersensitive to telithromycin or any macrolide antibiotic. Also contraindicated in patients taking cisapride or pimozide.
- Avoid use in those with congenitally prolonged QTc interval; those with ongoing proarrhythmic conditions, such as uncorrected hypokalemia, hypomagnesemia, or bradycardia; or those taking class IA antiarrhythmics, such as quinidine or procainamide, or class III antiarrhythmics such as dofetilide.
- Not for patients with myasthenia gravis because drug may worsen symptoms and increase the risk of acute respiratory failure.

• Use cautiously in patients with a history of drug-induced hepatitis or jaundice and in breast-feeding women.

NURSING CONSIDERATIONS

• Visual disturbances may occur, particularly in women and patients younger than age 40. Adverse visual effects occur most often after the first or second dose, last several hours, and sometimes return with later doses.
• Monitor patient for signs or symptoms of liver problems, including jaundice, pale stools, darkened urine, and abdominal pain.
• Patients with diarrhea may have pseudomembranous colitis.
• This drug may prolong the QTc interval. Rarely, an irregular heartbeat may cause the patient to faint.

PATIENT TEACHING

• Tell patient to take entire amount of drug exactly as directed, even if he feels better.
• Tell patient that drug can be taken with or without food.
• Explain that this drug may cause visual disturbances. Caution patient to avoid hazardous activities.
• Tell patient to report diarrhea or any episodes of fainting that occur while taking this drug.
• Advise patient to immediately report signs of liver problems to prescriber.

vancomycin hydrochloride

Vancocin, Vancoled

Pharmacologic class: glycopeptide
Pregnancy risk category C; B for capsules only

AVAILABLE FORMS

Capsules: 125 mg, 250 mg
Powder for injection: 500-mg vials, 1-g vials
Powder for oral solution: 1-g bottles, 10-g bottles

INDICATIONS & DOSAGES

➤ **Serious or severe infections when other antibiotics are ineffective or contraindicated, including those caused by methicillin-resistant *Staphylococcus aureus, S. epidermidis,* or diphtheroid organisms**
Adults: 500 mg I.V. q 6 hours or 1 g I.V. q 12 hours.
Children: 10 mg/kg I.V. q 6 hours.
Neonates and young infants: 15 mg/kg I.V. loading dose; then 10 mg/kg I.V. q 12 hours if child is younger than age 1 week or 10 mg/kg I.V. q 8 hours if age is older than 1 week but younger than 1 month.
Elderly patients: 15 mg/kg I.V. loading dose. Subsequent doses are based on renal function and drug levels.

➤ **Antibiotic-related pseudomembranous *Clostridium difficile* and *S. enterocolitis***
Adults: 125 to 500 mg P.O. q 6 hours for 7 to 10 days.
Children: 40 mg/kg P.O. daily, in divided doses q 6 hours for 7 to 10 days. Maximum daily dose is 2 g.

➤ **Endocarditis prophylaxis for dental procedures**
Adults: 1 g I.V. slowly over 1 to 2 hours, completing infusion 30 minutes before procedure.
Children: 20 mg/kg I.V. over 1 to 2 hours, completing infusion 30 minutes before procedure.
Adjust-a-dose: In renal insufficiency, adjust dosage based on degree of renal impairment, drug level, severity of infection, and susceptibility of causative organism. Initially, give 15 mg/kg, and adjust subsequent doses, p.r.n. One possible schedule is as follows: If creatinine level is less than 1.5 mg/dl, give 1 g q 12 hours. If creatinine level is 1.5 to 5 mg/dl, give 1 g q 3 to 6 days. If creatinine level is greater than 5 mg/dl, give 1 g q 10 to 14 days. Or, if glomerular filtration rate (GFR) is 10 to 50 ml/minute, give usual dose q 3 to 10 days, and if GFR is less than 10 ml/minute, give usual dose q 10 days.

➤ **Bacterial endocarditis from methicillin-resistant or methicillin-susceptible staphylococci in patients with native cardiac valves**
Adults: 30 mg/kg I.V. daily given in 2 divided doses for 4 to 6 weeks. Doses over 2 g require monitoring of drug level.

I.V. ADMINISTRATION
- This form is ineffective for pseudomembranous (*Clostridium difficile*) diarrhea.
- Reconstitute 500-mg vial with 10 ml or 1-g vial with 20 ml sterile water for injection to provide a solution containing 50 mg/ml.
- For infusion, further dilute 500 mg in 100 ml or 1 g in 200 ml normal saline solution for injection or D_5W, and infuse over 60 minutes; if dose is greater than 1 g, infuse over 90 minutes.
- Check site daily for phlebitis and irritation. Severe irritation and necrosis can result from extravasation.
- Refrigerate solution after reconstitution and use within 14 days.

INCOMPATIBILITIES
Albumin, alkaline solutions, aminophylline, amobarbital, amphotericin B, aztreonam, cephalosporins, chloramphenicol, chlorothiazide, corticosteroids, dexamethasone sodium phosphate, foscarnet, gatifloxacin, heavy metals, heparin, hydrocortisone, idarubicin, methotrexate, nafcillin, omeprazole, penicillin G potassium, pentobarbital, phenobarbital, phenytoin, piperacillin, piperacillin sodium and tazobactam sodium, sargramostim, sodium bicarbonate, ticarcillin disodium, ticarcillin disodium and clavulanate potassium, vitamin B complex with C, warfarin.

ACTION
Hinders bacterial cell-wall synthesis, damaging the bacterial plasma membrane and making the cell more vulnerable to osmotic pressure. Also interferes with RNA synthesis.

Route	Onset	Peak	Duration
P.O.	Unknown	Unknown	Unknown
I.V.	Immediate	Immediate	Unknown

Half-life: 6 hours.

ADVERSE REACTIONS
CNS: fever, pain.
CV: hypotension, thrombophlebitis at injection site.
EENT: ototoxicity, tinnitus.
GI: ***pseudomembranous colitis,*** nausea.
GU: ***nephrotoxicity.***
Hematologic: ***leukopenia, neutropenia,*** eosinophilia.
Respiratory: dyspnea, wheezing.
Skin: red-man syndrome (with rapid I.V. infusion).
Other: ***anaphylaxis,*** chills, superinfection.

INTERACTIONS
Drug-drug. *Aminoglycosides, amphotericin B, cisplatin, pentamidine:* May increase risk of nephrotoxicity and ototoxicity. Monitor renal function and hearing function tests.
Nondepolarizing muscle relaxants: May enhance neuromuscular blockade. Monitor patient closely.

EFFECTS ON LAB TEST RESULTS
- May increase BUN and creatinine levels.
- May increase eosinophil counts. May decrease neutrophil and WBC counts.

CONTRAINDICATIONS & CAUTIONS
- Contraindicated in patients hypersensitive to drug.

NURSING CONSIDERATIONS
- Use cautiously in patients receiving other neurotoxic, nephrotoxic, or ototoxic drugs; in patients older than age 60; and in those with impaired hepatic or renal function, hearing loss, or allergies to other antibiotics. Patients with renal dysfunction need dosage adjustment. Monitor blood levels to adjust I.V. dosage. Normal therapeutic levels of vancomycin are peak, 30 to 40 mg/L (drawn 1 hour after infusion ends), and trough, 5 to 10 mg/L (drawn just before next dose is given).
- Obtain specimen for culture and sensitivity tests before giving. Because of the emergence of vancomycin-resistant enterococci, reserve use of drug for treatment of serious infections caused by gram-positive bacteria resistant to beta-lactam anti-infectives.
- Obtain hearing evaluation and renal function studies before therapy.
- Monitor patient's fluid balance and watch for oliguria and cloudy urine.
- Monitor patient carefully for red-man syndrome, which can occur if drug is infused too rapidly. Signs and symptoms in-

clude maculopapular rash on face, neck, trunk, and limbs and pruritus and hypotension caused by histamine release. If wheezing, urticaria, or pain and muscle spasm of the chest and back occur, stop infusion and notify prescriber.

- Don't give drug I.M.
- ***Alert:*** Oral form is ineffective for systemic infections.
- Oral solution is stable for 2 weeks if refrigerated.
- Monitor renal function (BUN, creatinine and creatinine clearance levels, urinalysis, and urine output) during therapy.
- Monitor patient for signs and symptoms of superinfection.
- Have patient's hearing evaluated during prolonged therapy.
- For staphylococcal endocarditis, give for at least 4 weeks.

PATIENT TEACHING

- Tell patient to take entire amount of drug exactly as directed, even after he feels better.
- Instruct patient receiving drug I.V. to report discomfort at I.V. insertion site.
- Tell patient to report ringing in ears.
- Tell patient to report adverse reactions to prescriber immediately.

18

Inotropics

digoxin
inamrinone lactate
milrinone lactate

SAFETY ALERT!

digoxin

Digitek, Digoxin, Lanoxicaps, Lanoxin*

Pharmacologic class: cardiac glycoside
Pregnancy risk category C

AVAILABLE FORMS

Capsules: 0.05 mg, 0.1 mg, 0.2 mg
Elixir: 0.05 mg/ml (pediatric)
Injection: 0.05 mg/ml†, 0.1 mg/ml (pediatric), 0.25 mg/ml
Tablets: 0.125 mg, 0.25 mg

INDICATIONS & DOSAGES

➤ **Heart failure, paroxysmal supraventricular tachycardia, atrial fibrillation and flutter**

Capsules

Adults: For rapid digitalization, give 0.4 to 0.6 mg P.O. initially, followed by 0.1 to 0.3 mg q 6 to 8 hours, as needed and tolerated, for 24 hours. For slow digitalization, give 0.05 to 0.35 mg daily in two divided doses for 7 to 22 days, p.r.n., until therapeutic levels are reached. Maintenance dose is 0.05 to 0.35 mg daily in one or two divided doses.

Children: Digitalizing dose is based on child's age and is given in three or more divided doses over the first 24 hours. First dose is 50% of the total dose; subsequent doses are given q 6 to 8 hours as needed and tolerated.

Children age 10 and older: For rapid digitalization, give 8 to 12 mcg/kg P.O. over 24 hours, divided as described previously. Maintenance dose is 25% to 35% of total digitalizing dose, given daily as a single dose.

Children ages 5 to 10: For rapid digitalization, give 15 to 30 mcg/kg P.O. over 24 hours, divided as described previously. Maintenance dose is 25% to 35% of total digitalizing dose, divided and given in two or three equal portions daily.

Children ages 2 to 5: For rapid digitalization, give 25 to 35 mcg/kg P.O. over 24 hours, divided as described previously. Maintenance dose is 25% to 35% of total digitalizing dose, divided and given in two or three equal portions daily.

Elixir, tablets

Adults: For rapid digitalization, give 0.75 to 1.25 mg P.O. over 24 hours in two or more divided doses q 6 to 8 hours. For slow digitalization, give 0.125 to 0.5 mg daily for 5 to 7 days. Maintenance dose is 0.125 to 0.5 mg daily.

Children age 10 and older: 10 to 15 mcg/kg P.O. over 24 hours in two or more divided doses q 6 to 8 hours. Maintenance dose is 25% to 35% of total digitalizing dose.

Children ages 5 to 10: 20 to 35 mcg/kg P.O. over 24 hours in two or more divided doses q 6 to 8 hours. Maintenance dose is 25% to 35% of total digitalizing dose.

Children ages 2 to 5: 30 to 40 mcg/kg P.O. over 24 hours in two or more divided doses q 6 to 8 hours. Maintenance dose is 25% to 35% of total digitalizing dose.

Infants ages 1 month to 2 years: 35 to 60 mcg/kg P.O. over 24 hours in two or more divided doses q 6 to 8 hours. Maintenance dose is 25% to 35% of total digitalizing dose.

Neonates: 25 to 35 mcg/kg P.O. over 24 hours in two or more divided doses q 6 to 8 hours. Maintenance dose is 25% to 35% of total digitalizing dose.

Premature infants: 20 to 30 mcg/kg P.O. over 24 hours in two or more divided doses q 6 to 8 hours. Maintenance dose is 20% to 30% of total digitalizing dose.

Injection

Adults: For rapid digitalization, give 0.4 to 0.6 mg I.V. initially, followed by 0.1 to 0.3 mg I.V. q 6 to 8 hours, as needed and tolerated, for 24 hours. For slow digitalization, give appropriate daily maintenance dose for 7 to 22 days p.r.n. until therapeutic levels are reached. Maintenance dose

is 0.125 to 0.5 mg I.V. daily in one or two divided doses.
Children: Digitalizing dose is based on child's age; give in three or more divided doses over the first 24 hours. First dose is 50% of total dose; subsequent doses are given q 6 to 8 hours as needed and tolerated.
Children age 10 and older: For rapid digitalization, give 8 to 12 mcg/kg I.V. over 24 hours, divided as described previously. Maintenance dose is 25% to 35% of total digitalizing dose, given daily as a single dose.
Children ages 5 to 10: For rapid digitalization, give 15 to 30 mcg/kg I.V. over 24 hours, divided as described previously. Maintenance dose is 25% to 35% of total digitalizing dose, divided and given in two or three equal portions daily.
Children ages 2 to 5: For rapid digitalization, give 25 to 35 mcg/kg I.V. over 24 hours, divided as described previously. Maintenance dose is 25% to 35% of total digitalizing dose, divided and given in two or three equal portions daily.
Infants ages 1 month to 2 years: For rapid digitalization, give 30 to 50 mcg/kg I.V. over 24 hours, divided as described previously. Maintenance dose is 25% to 35% of total digitalizing dose, divided and given in two or three equal portions daily.
Neonates: For rapid digitalization, give 20 to 30 mcg/kg I.V. over 24 hours, divided as described previously. Maintenance dose is 25% to 35% of the total digitalizing dose, divided and given in two or three equal portions daily.
Premature infants: For rapid digitalization, give 15 to 25 mcg/kg I.V. over 24 hours, divided as described previously. Maintenance dose is 20% to 30% of the total digitalizing dose, divided and given in two or three equal portions daily.
Adjust-a-dose: For patients with impaired renal function, give smaller loading and maintenance doses.

I.V. ADMINISTRATION

- Dilute fourfold with D_5W, normal saline solution, or sterile water for injection to reduce the chance of precipitation.
- Infuse drug slowly over at least 5 minutes.
- Protect solution from light.

INCOMPATIBILITIES

Amiodarone, amphotericin B cholesteryl sulfate complex, dobutamine, doxapram, fluconazole, foscarnet, propofol, remifentanil. Mixing with other drugs isn't recommended.

ACTION

Inhibits sodium-potassium–activated adenosine triphosphatase, promoting movement of calcium from extracellular to intracellular cytoplasm and strengthening myocardial contraction. Also acts on CNS to enhance vagal tone, slowing conduction through the SA and AV nodes.

Route	Onset	Peak	Duration
P.O.	30–120 min	2–6 hr	3–4 days
I.V.	5–30 min	1–4 hr	3–4 days

Half-life: 30 to 40 hours.

ADVERSE REACTIONS

CNS: *agitation, fatigue, generalized muscle weakness, hallucinations,* dizziness, headache, malaise, paresthesia, stupor, vertigo.
CV: ***arrhythmias, heart block.***
EENT: blurred vision, diplopia, light flashes, photophobia, yellow-green halos around visual images.
GI: *anorexia, nausea,* diarrhea, vomiting.

INTERACTIONS

Drug-drug. *Amiloride:* May decrease digoxin effect and increase digoxin excretion. Monitor patient for altered digoxin effect.
Amiodarone, *diltiazem, indomethacin, nifedipine,* ***quinidine, verapamil:*** May increase digoxin level. Monitor patient for toxicity.
Amphotericin B, carbenicillin, corticosteroids, ***diuretics (such as chlorthalidone, loop diuretics, metolazone, thiazides),*** *ticarcillin:* May cause hypokalemia, predisposing patient to digitalis toxicity. Monitor potassium level.
Antacids, kaolin-pectin: May decrease absorption of oral digoxin. Separate doses as much as possible.
Antibiotics (azole antifungals, macrolides, telithromycin, tetracyclines), propafenone, ritonavir: May increase risk of toxicity. Monitor patient for toxicity.

Anticholinergics: May increase digoxin absorption of oral digoxin tablets. Monitor drug level and observe for toxicity.
Beta-blockers, calcium channel blockers: May have additive effects on AV node conduction causing advanced or complete heart block. Use cautiously.
Cholestyramine, colestipol, metoclopramide: May decrease absorption of oral digoxin. Monitor patient for decreased digoxin level and effect. Give digoxin 1½ hours before or 2 hours after other drugs.
Parenteral calcium, thiazides: May cause hypercalcemia and hypomagnesemia, predisposing patient to digitalis toxicity. Monitor calcium and magnesium levels.
Drug-herb. *Betel palm, fumitory, goldenseal, hawthorn, lily of the valley, motherwort, rue, shepherd's purse:* May increase cardiac effects. Discourage use together.
Gossypol, horsetail, licorice, oleander, Siberian ginseng, squill: May increase toxicity. Monitor patient closely.
Plantain, St. John's wort: May decrease effectiveness of drug. Discourage use together.

EFFECTS ON LAB TEST RESULTS

- May prolong PR interval or depress ST segment.

CONTRAINDICATIONS & CAUTIONS

- Contraindicated in patients hypersensitive to drug and in those with digitalis-induced toxicity, ventricular fibrillation, or ventricular tachycardia unless caused by heart failure.
- Don't use in patients with Wolff-Parkinson-White syndrome unless the conduction accessory pathway has been pharmacologically or surgically disabled.
- Use with extreme caution in elderly patients and in those with acute MI, incomplete AV block, sinus bradycardia, PVCs, chronic constrictive pericarditis, hypertrophic cardiomyopathy, renal insufficiency, severe pulmonary disease, or hypothyroidism.

NURSING CONSIDERATIONS

- Drug-induced arrhythmias may increase the severity of heart failure and hypotension.
- In children, cardiac arrhythmias, including sinus bradycardia, are usually early signs of toxicity.
- Patients with hypothyroidism are extremely sensitive to cardiac glycosides and may need lower doses.
- Before giving loading dose, obtain baseline data (heart rate and rhythm, blood pressure, and electrolytes) and ask patient about use of cardiac glycosides within the previous 2 to 3 weeks.
- Loading dose is usually divided over the first 24 hours with approximately half the loading dose given in the first dose.
- Before giving drug, take apical-radial pulse for 1 minute. Record and notify prescriber of significant changes (sudden increase or decrease in pulse rate, pulse deficit, irregular beats and, particularly, regularization of a previously irregular rhythm). If these occur, check blood pressure and obtain a 12-lead ECG.
- Toxic effects on the heart may be life-threatening and require immediate attention.
- Absorption of digoxin from liquid-filled capsules is superior to absorption from tablets or elixir. Expect dosage reduction of 20% to 25% when changing from tablets or elixir to liquid-filled capsules or parenteral therapy.
- Monitor digoxin level. Therapeutic level ranges from 0.8 to 2 ng/ml. Obtain blood for digoxin level at least 6 to 8 hours after last oral dose, preferably just before next scheduled dose.
- ***Alert:*** Excessively slow pulse rate (60 beats/minute or less) may be a sign of digitalis toxicity. Withhold drug and notify prescriber.
- Monitor potassium level carefully. Take corrective action before hypokalemia occurs. Hyperkalemia may result from digoxin toxicity.
- Reduce drug dose for 1 or 2 days before elective cardioversion. Adjust dosage after cardioversion.
- ***Look alike–sound alike:*** Don't confuse digoxin with doxepin.

PATIENT TEACHING

- Teach patient and a responsible family member about drug action, dosage regimen, how to take pulse, reportable signs, and follow-up care.

• Tell patient to report pulse less than 60 beats/minute or more than 110 beats/minute, or skipped beats or other rhythm changes.
• Instruct patient to report adverse reactions promptly. Nausea, vomiting, diarrhea, appetite loss, and visual disturbances may be indicators of toxicity.
• Encourage patient to eat potassium-rich foods.
• Tell patient not to substitute one brand for another.
• Advise patient to avoid the use of herbal drugs or to consult his prescriber before taking one.

SAFETY ALERT!

inamrinone lactate

Pharmacologic class: bipyridine phosphodiesterase inhibitor
Pregnancy risk category C

AVAILABLE FORMS

Injection: 5 mg/ml in 20-ml ampules

INDICATIONS & DOSAGES

➤ **Short-term management of heart failure**
Adults: Initially, 0.75 mg/kg I.V. bolus over 2 to 3 minutes. Then begin maintenance infusion of 5 to 10 mcg/kg/minute. May give additional bolus of 0.75 mg/kg after 30 minutes. Don't exceed total daily dose of 10 mg/kg.

I.V. ADMINISTRATION

• Give drug with an infusion pump. Use drug as supplied, or dilute in half-normal saline solution or normal saline solution to a concentration of 1 to 3 mg/ml. Use diluted solution within 24 hours.
• Don't dilute with solutions containing dextrose because a slow chemical reaction occurs over 24 hours. Inamrinone can be injected into free-flowing dextrose infusions through a Y-connector or directly into tubing.
• Monitor blood pressure and heart rate throughout the infusion. If patient's blood pressure falls, slow or stop infusion and notify prescriber.

INCOMPATIBILITIES

Bicarbonate, dextrose-containing solutions such as D_5W, furosemide, glucose, procainamide, sodium bicarbonate, torsemide.

ACTION

Produces inotropic action by increasing cellular levels of cAMP. Produces vasodilation through a direct relaxant effect on vascular smooth muscle.

Route	Onset	Peak	Duration
I.V.	2–5 min	10 min	30–120 min

Half-life: About 4 hours.

ADVERSE REACTIONS

CNS: fever.
CV: ***arrhythmias,*** chest pain, hypotension.
GI: abdominal pain, anorexia, nausea, vomiting.
Hematologic: ***thrombocytopenia.***
Hepatic: ***hepatotoxicity.***
Metabolic: hypokalemia.
Skin: burning at injection site.
Other: hypersensitivity reactions.

INTERACTIONS

Drug-drug. *Cardiac glycosides:* May increase inotropic effect, which is a beneficial drug interaction. Monitor patient.
Disopyramide: May cause excessive hypotension. Monitor blood pressure.

EFFECTS ON LAB TEST RESULTS

• May increase liver enzyme level. May decrease potassium level.
• May increase sedimentation rate. May decrease platelet count.

CONTRAINDICATIONS & CAUTIONS

• Contraindicated in patients hypersensitive to inamrinone or bisulfites.
• Contraindicated in patients with severe aortic or pulmonic valvular disease in place of surgery or during acute phase of MI.
• Use cautiously in patients with hypertrophic cardiomyopathy.
• Safety and effectiveness haven't been established in children, although drug has been used in preterm infants for heart failure.

NURSING CONSIDERATIONS

- Drug is prescribed primarily for patients who haven't responded to cardiac glycosides, diuretics, and vasodilators.
- Dosage depends on clinical response, including assessment of pulmonary wedge pressure and cardiac output, as well as lessening of dyspnea, orthopnea, and fatigue.
- In patients with atrial fibrillation and flutter, drug may be added to cardiac glycoside therapy because it slightly enhances AV conduction and increases ventricular response rate.
- Correct hypokalemia before or during therapy.
- Monitor platelet count. If it falls below 150,000/mm^3, decrease dosage.
- Monitor patient for hypersensitivity reactions, such as pericarditis, ascites, myositis, vasculitis, and pleuritis.
- Monitor intake and output and daily weight.
- Patients with end-stage cardiac disease may receive home treatment while awaiting heart transplantation.
- ***Look alike–sound alike:*** Because of confusion with amiodarone, the generic name "amrinone" was changed to "inamrinone."

PATIENT TEACHING

- Warn patient that burning may occur at injection site.
- Instruct home care patient and family about drug administration; tell them to report adverse reactions promptly.

SAFETY ALERT!

milrinone lactate

Primacor

Pharmacologic class: bipyridine phosphodiesterase inhibitor
Pregnancy risk category C

AVAILABLE FORMS

Injection: 1 mg/ml
Injection (premixed): 200 mcg/ml in D_5W

INDICATIONS & DOSAGES

➤ **Short-term treatment of acutely decompensated heart failure**

Adults: Give first loading dose of 50 mcg/kg I.V. slowly over 10 minutes; then give continuous I.V. infusion of 0.375 to 0.75 mcg/kg/minute. Titrate infusion dose based on clinical and hemodynamic responses. Don't exceed 1.13 mg/kg/day.

Adjust-a-dose: If creatinine clearance is 50 ml/minute, infusion rate is 0.43 mcg/kg/minute; if 40 ml/minute, infusion rate is 0.38 mcg/kg/minute; if 30 ml/minute, infusion rate is 0.33 mcg/kg/minute; if 20 ml/minute, infusion rate is 0.28 mcg/kg/minute; if 10 ml/minute, infusion rate is 0.23 mcg/kg/minute; and if 5 ml/minute, infusion rate is 0.2 mcg/kg/minute. Don't exceed 1.13 mg/kg/day.

I.V. ADMINISTRATION

- Give loading dose undiluted as a direct injection over 10 minutes.
- Prepare I.V. infusion solution using half-normal saline solution, normal saline solution, or D_5W. Prepare the 100-mcg/ml solution by adding 180 ml of diluent per 20-mg (20-ml) vial, the 150-mcg/ml solution by adding 113 ml of diluent per 20-mg (20-ml) vial, and the 200-mcg/ml solution by adding 80 ml of diluent per 20-mg (20-ml) vial.

INCOMPATIBILITIES

Bumetanide, furosemide, imipenem and cilastatin sodium, procainamide, torsemide

ACTION

Produces inotropic action by increasing cellular levels of cAMP and vasodilation by relaxing vascular smooth muscle.

Route	Onset	Peak	Duration
I.V.	5–15 min	1–2 hr	3–6 hr

Half-life: 2½ to 3¾ hours.

ADVERSE REACTIONS

CNS: headache.
CV: VENTRICULAR ARRHYTHMIAS, *ventricular ectopic activity,* ***sustained ventricular tachycardia, ventricular fibrilla-***

tion, hypotension, nonsustained ventricular tachycardia.

INTERACTIONS
None significant.

EFFECTS ON LAB TEST RESULTS
- May cause abnormal liver function tests.

CONTRAINDICATIONS & CAUTIONS
- Contraindicated in patients hypersensitive to drug.
- Contraindicated for use in patients with severe aortic or pulmonic valvular disease in place of surgery and during acute phase of MI.
- Use cautiously in patients with atrial flutter or fibrillation because drug slightly shortens AV node conduction time and may increase ventricular response rate.

NURSING CONSIDERATIONS
- Give digoxin before therapy. Drug is typically given with digoxin and diuretics.
- Improved cardiac output may increase urine output. Reduce diuretic dosage when heart failure improves. Potassium loss may cause digitalis toxicity.
- Monitor fluid and electrolyte status, blood pressure, heart rate, and renal function during therapy. Excessive decrease in blood pressure requires stopping or slowing rate of infusion.
- Correct hypoxemia.

PATIENT TEACHING
- Instruct patient to report adverse reactions to prescriber promptly, especially angina.
- Tell patient that drug may cause headache, which can be treated with analgesics.
- Tell patient to report discomfort at I.V. insertion site.

19

Antiarrhythmics

adenosine

Adenocard

Pharmacologic class: nucleoside
Pregnancy risk category C

AVAILABLE FORMS

Injection: 3 mg/ml in 2-ml, 4-ml, and 5-ml vials and syringes

INDICATIONS & DOSAGES

➤To convert paroxysmal supraventricular tachycardia (PSVT) to sinus rhythm

Adults and children who weigh 50 kg (110 lb) or more: 6 mg I.V. by rapid bolus injection over 1 to 2 seconds. If PSVT isn't eliminated in 1 to 2 minutes, give 12 mg by rapid I.V. push and repeat, if needed.

Children who weigh less than 50 kg: Initially, 0.05 to 0.1 mg/kg I.V. by rapid bolus injection followed by a saline flush. If PSVT isn't eliminated in 1 to 2 minutes, give additional bolus injections, increasing the amount given by 0.05- to 0.1-mg/kg increments, followed by a saline flush. Continue, p.r.n., until conversion or a maximum single dose of 0.3 mg/kg is given.

I.V. ADMINISTRATION

- Don't give single doses exceeding 12 mg.
- In adults, avoid giving drug through a central line because more prolonged asystole may occur.
- Give by rapid I.V. injection to ensure drug action.
- Give directly into a vein, if possible. When giving through an I.V. line, use the port closest to the patient.
- Flush immediately and rapidly with normal saline solution to ensure that drug quickly reaches the systemic circulation.

INCOMPATIBILITIES

Other I.V. drugs.

ACTION

A naturally occurring nucleoside that acts on the AV node to slow conduction and inhibit reentry pathways. Also useful in treating PSVTs, including those with accessory bypass tracts (Wolff-Parkinson-White syndrome).

Route	Onset	Peak	Duration
I.V.	Immediate	Immediate	Unknown

Half-life: Less than 10 seconds.

ADVERSE REACTIONS

CNS: dizziness, light-headedness, numbness, tingling in arms, headache.
CV: *facial flushing.*
GI: nausea.
Respiratory: *dyspnea, shortness of breath,* chest pressure.

INTERACTIONS

Drug-drug. *Carbamazepine:* May cause high-level heart block. Use together cautiously.
Digoxin, verapamil: May cause ventricular fibrillation. Monitor ECG closely.
Dipyridamole: May increase adenosine's effects. Adenosine dose may need to be reduced. Use together cautiously.
Methylxanthines (caffeine, theophylline): May decrease adenosine's effects. Adenosine dose may need to be increased or patients may not respond to adenosine therapy.
Drug-herb. *Guarana:* May decrease patient's response to drug. Monitor patient.

EFFECTS ON LAB TEST RESULTS

None reported.

CONTRAINDICATIONS & CAUTIONS

- Contraindicated in patients hypersensitive to drug.
- Contraindicated in those with second- or third-degree heart block or sinus node disease (such as sick sinus syndrome and symptomatic bradycardia), except those with a pacemaker.
- Use cautiously in patients with asthma, emphysema, or bronchitis because bronchoconstriction may occur.

NURSING CONSIDERATIONS

- ***Alert:*** By decreasing conduction through the AV node, drug may produce first-, second-, or third-degree heart block. Patients who develop high-level heart block after a single dose shouldn't receive additional doses.
- ***Alert:*** New arrhythmias, including heart block and transient asystole, may develop; monitor cardiac rhythm and treat as indicated.
- If solution is cold, crystals may form; gently warm solution to room temperature. Don't use solutions that aren't clear.
- Drug lacks preservatives. Discard unused portion.

PATIENT TEACHING

- Instruct patient to report adverse reactions promptly.
- Tell patient to report discomfort at I.V. site.
- Inform patient that he may experience flushing or chest pain lasting 1 to 2 minutes.

SAFETY ALERT!

amiodarone hydrochloride

Aratac‡, Cordarone✎, Cordarone X‡, Pacerone

Pharmacologic class: benzofuran derivative
Pregnancy risk category D

AVAILABLE FORMS

Injection: 50 mg/ml in 3-ml ampules, vials
Tablets: 100 mg‡, 200 mg, 400 mg

INDICATIONS & DOSAGES

➤ **Life-threatening recurrent ventricular fibrillation or recurrent hemodynamically unstable ventricular tachycardia unresponsive to adequate doses of other antiarrhythmics or when alternative drugs can't be tolerated**

Adults: Give loading dose of 800 to 1,600 mg P.O. daily divided b.i.d. for 1 to 3 weeks until first therapeutic response occurs; then 600 to 800 mg P.O. daily for 1 month, followed by maintenance dose 200 to 600 mg P.O. daily.

Or, give loading dose of 150 mg I.V. over 10 minutes (15 mg/minute); then 360 mg I.V. over next 6 hours (1 mg/minute), followed by 540 mg I.V. over next 18 hours (0.5 mg/minute). After first 24 hours, continue with maintenance I.V. infusion of 720 mg/24 hours (0.5 mg/minute).

I.V. ADMINISTRATION

- Give drug I.V. only if continuous ECG and electrophysiologic monitoring are available.
- Mix first dose of 150 mg in 100 ml of D_5W solution.
- If infusion will last 2 hours or longer, mix solution in glass or polyolefin bottles.

- If concentration is 2 mg/ml or more, give drug through a central line. If possible, use a dedicated line.
- Use an in-line filter.
- Continuously monitor patient's cardiac status. If hypotension occurs, reduce infusion rate.
- Cordarone I.V. leaches out plasticizers such as DEHP from I.V. tubing, which can adversely affect male reproductive tract development in fetuses, infants, and toddlers.

INCOMPATIBILITIES

Aminophylline, ampicillin sodium and sulbactam sodium, bivalirudin, cefazolin sodium, ceftazidime, digoxin, furosemide, heparin sodium, imipenem and cilastatin sodium, magnesium sulfate, normal saline solution, piperacillin sodium, piperacillin and tazobactam sodium, quinidine gluconate, sodium bicarbonate, sodium nitroprusside, sodium phosphates.

ACTION

Effects result from blockade of potassium chloride leading to a prolongation of action potential duration.

Route	Onset	Peak	Duration
P.O.	Variable	3–7 hr	Variable
I.V.	Unknown	Unknown	Variable

Half-life: 25 to 110 days (usually 40 to 50 days).

ADVERSE REACTIONS

CNS: *fatigue, malaise, tremor,* peripheral neuropathy, ataxia, paresthesia, insomnia, sleep disturbances, headache.
CV: *hypotension,* ***bradycardia, arrhythmias, heart failure, heart block, sinus arrest,*** edema.
EENT: *asymptomatic corneal microdeposits, visual disturbances,* optic neuropathy or neuritis resulting in visual impairment, abnormal smell.
GI: *nausea, vomiting,* abnormal taste, anorexia, constipation, abdominal pain.
Hematologic: ***coagulation abnormalities.***
Hepatic: ***hepatic failure,*** hepatic dysfunction.
Metabolic: *hypothyroidism,* hyperthyroidism.
Respiratory: ***acute respiratory distress syndrome,*** **SEVERE PULMONARY TOXICITY.**
Skin: *photosensitivity,* solar dermatitis, blue-gray skin.

INTERACTIONS

Drug-drug. *Antiarrhythmics:* May reduce hepatic or renal clearance of certain antiarrhythmics, especially flecainide, procainamide, and quinidine. Use of amiodarone with other antiarrhythmics, especially mexiletine, propafenone, disopyramide, and procainamide, may induce torsades de pointes. Avoid using together.
Antihypertensives: May increase hypotensive effect. Use together cautiously.
Azole antifungals, disopyramide, pimozide: May increase the risk of arrhythmias, including torsades de pointes. Avoid using together.
Beta blockers, calcium channel blockers: May increase cardiac depressant effects; may increase slowing of SA node and AV conduction. Use together cautiously.
Cimetidine: May increase amiodarone level. Use together cautiously.
Cyclosporine: May increase cyclosporine level, resulting in an increase in the serum creatinine level and renal toxicity. Monitor cyclosporine levels and renal function tests.
Digoxin: May increase digoxin level 70% to 100%. Monitor digoxin level closely and reduce digoxin dosage by half or stop drug completely when starting amiodarone therapy.
Fentanyl: May cause hypotension, bradycardia, and decreased cardiac output. Monitor patient closely.
Fluoroquinolones: May increase risk of arrhythmias, including torsades de pointes. Avoid using together.
Macrolide antibiotics (azithromycin, clarithromycin, erythromycin, telithromycin): May cause additive or prolongation of the QT interval. Use with caution. Avoid use with telithromycin.
Methotrexate: May impair methotrexate metabolism, causing toxicity. Use together cautiously.
Phenytoin: May decrease phenytoin metabolism and amiodarone level. Monitor phenytoin level and adjust dosages of drugs if needed.

Protease inhibitors (amprenavir, atazanavir, indinavir, lopinavir and ritonavir, nelfinavir, ritonavir, and saquinavir): May increase the risk of amiodarone toxicity. Use of ritonavir or nelfinavir with amiodarone is contraindicated. Use other protease inhibitors cautiously.
Quinidine: May increase quinidine level, causing life-threatening cardiac arrhythmias. Avoid using together, or monitor quinidine level closely if use together can't be avoided. Adjust quinidine dosage as needed.
Rifamycins: May decrease amiodarone level. Monitor patient closely.
Theophylline: May increase theophylline level and cause toxicity. Monitor theophylline level.
Warfarin: May increase anticoagulant response with the potential for serious or fatal bleeding. Decrease warfarin dosage 33% to 50% when starting amiodarone. Monitor patient closely.
Drug-herb. *Pennyroyal:* May change rate of formation of toxic metabolites of pennyroyal. Discourage use together.
St. John's wort: May decrease amiodarone levels. Discourage use together.
Drug-food. *Grapefruit juice:* May inhibit CYP3A4 metabolism of drug in the intestinal mucosa, causing increased levels and risk of toxicity. Discourage use together.
Drug-lifestyle. *Sun exposure:* May cause photosensitivity reaction. Advise patient to avoid excessive sunlight exposure and to take precautions while in the sun.

EFFECTS ON LAB TEST RESULTS

- May increase alkaline phosphatase, ALT, AST, GGT, and T_4 levels. May decrease T_3 level.
- May increase PT and INR.

CONTRAINDICATIONS & CAUTIONS

- Contraindicated in patients hypersensitive to drug or to iodine.
- Contraindicated in those with cardiogenic shock, second- or third-degree AV block, severe SA node disease resulting in bradycardia unless an artificial pacemaker is present, and in those for whom bradycardia has caused syncope.
- Use cautiously in patients receiving other antiarrhythmics.
- Use cautiously in patients with pulmonary, hepatic, or thyroid disease.

NURSING CONSIDERATIONS

- Be aware of the high risk of adverse reactions.
- Obtain baseline pulmonary, liver, and thyroid function test results and baseline chest X-ray.
- Give loading doses in a hospital setting and with continuous ECG monitoring because of the slow onset of antiarrhythmic effect and the risk of life-threatening arrhythmias.
- Divide oral loading dose into two or three equal doses and give with meals to decrease GI intolerance. Give maintenance dose once daily or divide into two doses, with meals to decrease GI intolerance.
- ***Alert:*** Drug may pose life-threatening management problems in patients at risk for sudden death. Use only in patients with life-threatening, recurrent ventricular arrhythmias unresponsive to or intolerant of other antiarrhythmics or alternative drugs. Amiodarone can cause fatal toxicities, including hepatic and pulmonary toxicity.
- ***Alert:*** Drug is highly toxic. Watch carefully for pulmonary toxicity. Risk increases in patients receiving doses over 400 mg/day.
- Watch for evidence of pneumonitis, exertional dyspnea, nonproductive cough, and pleuritic chest pain. Monitor pulmonary function tests and chest X-ray.
- Monitor liver and thyroid function test results and electrolyte, particularly potassium and magnesium, levels.
- Monitor PT and INR if patient takes warfarin and digoxin level if he takes digoxin.
- Instill methylcellulose ophthalmic solution during amiodarone therapy to minimize corneal microdeposits. About 1 to 4 months after starting amiodarone, most patients develop corneal microdeposits, although 10% or less have vision disturbances. Regular ophthalmic examinations are advised.

- Monitor blood pressure and heart rate and rhythm frequently. Perform continuous ECG monitoring when starting or changing dosage. Notify prescriber of significant change in assessment results.
- Life-threatening gasping syndrome may occur in neonates given I.V. solutions containing benzyl alcohol.
- ***Look alike–sound alike:*** Don't confuse amiodarone with amiloride.

PATIENT TEACHING

- Advise patient to wear sunscreen or protective clothing to prevent sensitivity reaction to the sun. Monitor patient for skin burning or tingling, followed by redness and blistering. Exposed skin may turn blue-gray.
- Tell patient to take oral drug with food if GI reactions occur.
- Inform patient that adverse effects of drug are more common at high doses and become more frequent with treatment lasting longer than 6 months, but are generally reversible when drug is stopped. Resolution of adverse reactions may take up to 4 months.

SAFETY ALERT!

atropine sulfate

Sal-Tropine

Pharmacologic class: anticholinergic, belladonna alkaloid
Pregnancy risk category C

AVAILABLE FORMS

Injection: 0.05 mg/ml, 0.1 mg/ml, 0.3 mg/ml, 0.4 mg/ml, 0.5 mg/ml, 0.8 mg/ml, 1 mg/ml
Prefilled auto-injectors: 0.25 mg, 0.5 mg, 1 mg, 2 mg
Tablets: 0.4 mg

INDICATIONS & DOSAGES

➤ **Symptomatic bradycardia, bradyarrhythmia (junctional or escape rhythm)**
Adults: Usually 0.5 to 1 mg I.V. push, repeated q 3 to 5 minutes to maximum of 2 mg p.r.n.
Children and adolescents: 0.02 mg/kg I.V., with minimum dose of 0.1 mg and maximum single dose of 0.5 mg in children or 1 mg in adolescents. May repeat dose at 5-minute intervals to a maximum total dose of 1 mg in children or 2 mg in adolescents.

➤ **Antidote for anticholinesterase-insecticide poisoning**
Adults: Initially, 1 to 2 mg I.V.; may repeat with 2 mg I.M. or I.V. q 5 to 60 minutes until muscarinic signs and symptoms disappear or signs of atropine toxicity appear. Severe poisoning may require up to 6 mg hourly.
Children: 0.05 mg/kg I.V. or I.M. repeated q 10 to 30 minutes until muscarinic signs and symptoms disappear (may be repeated if they reappear) or until atropine toxicity occurs.

➤ **Preoperatively to diminish secretions and block cardiac vagal reflexes**
Adults and children who weigh 20 kg (44 lb) or more: 0.4 to 0.6 mg I.V., I.M. or subcutaneously 30 to 60 minutes before anesthesia.
Children who weigh less than 20 kg: 0.01 mg/kg I.V., I.M. or subcutaneously up to maximum dose of 0.4 mg 30 to 60 minutes before anesthesia. May repeat q. 4 to 6 hours p.r.n.
Infants who weigh more than 5 kg (11 lb): 0.03 mg/kg q 4 to 6 hours p.r.n.
Infants who weigh 5 kg or less: 0.04 mg/kg q 4 to 6 hours p.r.n.

➤ **Adjunct treatment of peptic ulcer disease; functional GI disorders such as irritable bowel syndrome**
Adults: 0.4 to 0.6 mg P.O. q 4 to 6 hours.

I.V. ADMINISTRATION

- Give into a large vein or into I.V. tubing over at least 1 minute.
- Slow delivery may cause slowing of the heart rate.

INCOMPATIBILITIES

Alkalies, bromides, iodides, isoproterenol, methohexital, norepinephrine, pentobarbital sodium, sodium bicarbonate.

ACTION

An anticholinergic that inhibits acetylcholine at the parasympathetic neuroeffector junction, blocking vagal effects on the SA and AV nodes, enhancing conduction through the AV node and increasing the heart rate.

Route	Onset	Peak	Duration
P.O.	30–120 min	1–2 hr	4 hr
I.V.	Immediate	2–4 min	4 hr
I.M.	5–40 min	20–60 min	4 hr
SubQ	Unknown	Unknown	Unknown

Half-life: Initial, 2 hours; second phase, 12½ hours.

ADVERSE REACTIONS

CNS: *headache, restlessness, insomnia, dizziness,* ataxia, disorientation, hallucinations, delirium, excitement, agitation, confusion.
CV: ***bradycardia,*** palpitations, tachycardia.
EENT: *blurred vision, mydriasis,* photophobia, cycloplegia, increased intraocular pressure.
GI: *dry mouth, constipation,* thirst, nausea, vomiting.
GU: urine retention, impotence.
Other: ***anaphylaxis.***

INTERACTIONS

Drug-drug. *Antacids:* May decrease absorption of oral anticholinergics. Separate doses by at least 1 hour.
Anticholinergics, drugs with anticholinergic effects (amantadine, antiarrhythmics, antiparkinsonians, glutethimide, meperidine, phenothiazines, tricyclic antidepressants): May increase anticholinergic effects. Use together cautiously.
Ketoconazole, levodopa: May decrease absorption of these drugs. Separate doses by at least 2 hours, and monitor patient for clinical effect.
Potassium chloride wax-matrix tablets: May increase risk of mucosal lesions. Use together cautiously.
Drug-herb. *Jaborandi tree, pill-bearing spurge:* May decrease effectiveness of drug. Discourage use together.
Jimsonweed: May adversely affect CV function. Discourage use together.
Squaw vine: Tannic acid may decrease metabolic breakdown of drug. Monitor patient.

EFFECTS ON LAB TEST RESULTS

None reported.

CONTRAINDICATIONS & CAUTIONS

- Contraindicated in patients hypersensitive to drug.
- Contraindicated in those with acute angle-closure glaucoma, obstructive uropathy, obstructive disease of GI tract, paralytic ileus, toxic megacolon, intestinal atony, unstable CV status in acute hemorrhage, tachycardia, myocardial ischemia, asthma, or myasthenia gravis.
- Use cautiously in patients with Down syndrome because they may be more sensitive to drug.

NURSING CONSIDERATIONS

- Many adverse reactions (such as dry mouth and constipation) vary with the dose.
- In adults, avoid doses less than 0.5 mg because of the risk of paradoxical bradycardia.
- ***Alert:*** Watch for tachycardia in cardiac patients because it may lead to ventricular fibrillation.
- Monitor fluid intake and urine output. Drug causes urine retention and urinary hesitancy.

PATIENT TEACHING

- Teach patient receiving oral form of drug how to handle distressing anticholinergic effects.
- Instruct patient to report serious or persistent adverse reactions promptly.
- Tell patient about potential for sensitivity of the eyes to the sun and suggest use of sunglasses.

disopyramide
Rythmodan†‡

disopyramide phosphate
Norpace, Norpace CR, Rythmodan-LA†

Pharmacologic class: pyridine derivative
Pregnancy risk category C

AVAILABLE FORMS

disopyramide
Capsules: 100 mg†, 150 mg†
disopyramide phosphate
Capsules: 100 mg, 150 mg

Capsules (controlled-release): 100 mg, 150 mg
Tablets (sustained-release): 250 mg†

INDICATIONS & DOSAGES

➤Ventricular tachycardia and life-threatening ventricular arrhythmias
Adults who weigh more than 50 kg (110 lb): 150 mg P.O. q 6 hours with regular-release formulation or 300 mg q 12 hours with extended-release preparations.
Adults who weigh 50 kg or less: 100 mg P.O. q 6 hours with regular-release formulation or 200 mg P.O. q 12 hours with extended-release preparations.
Children ages 12 to 18: 6 to 15 mg/kg P.O. daily, divided into four doses (q 6 hours).
Children ages 4 to 12: 10 to 15 mg/kg P.O. daily, divided into four doses (q 6 hours).
Children ages 1 to 4: 10 to 20 mg/kg P.O. daily, divided into four doses (q 6 hours).
Children younger than age 1: 10 to 30 mg/kg P.O. daily, divided into four doses (q 6 hours).
Adjust-a-dose: If creatinine clearance is 30 to 40 ml/minute, give 100 mg q 8 hours; if clearance is 15 to 30 ml/minute, give 100 mg q 12 hours; if clearance is less than 15 ml/minute, give 100 mg q 24 hours. All dosages are for immediate-release form. Don't use extended-release capsules in patients with a creatinine clearance less than or equal to 40 ml/minute.

ACTION

A class IA antiarrhythmic that depresses phase 0, prolongs the action potential, and has membrane-stabilizing effects.

Route	Onset	Peak	Duration
P.O.	½–3½ hr	2–2½ hr	1½–8½ hr

Half-life: 7 hours.

ADVERSE REACTIONS

CNS: ***agitation,*** dizziness, depression, fatigue, headache, nervousness, acute psychosis, syncope.
CV: ***hypotension, heart failure, heart block, arrhythmias,*** edema, shortness of breath, chest pain.
EENT: blurred vision, dry eyes or nose.
GI: *dry mouth, constipation,* nausea, vomiting, anorexia, bloating, gas, weight gain, abdominal pain, diarrhea.
GU: *urinary hesitancy,* urine retention, urinary frequency, urinary urgency, impotence.
Hepatic: cholestatic jaundice.
Musculoskeletal: muscle weakness, aches, pain.
Skin: rash, pruritus, dermatosis.

INTERACTIONS

Drug-drug. *Antiarrhythmics:* May increase QRS complex or QT interval, which may lead to other arrhythmias. Monitor ECG closely.
Macrolides and related antibiotics (azithromycin, clarithromycin, erythromycin, telithromycin): May prolong the QT interval. Use with caution. Avoid use with telithromycin.
Phenytoin: May increase metabolism of disopyramide. Watch for decreased antiarrhythmic effect.
Quinidine: May increase disopyramide levels and decrease quinidine levels. Monitor patient closely.
Quinolones: May cause life-threatening arrhythmias, including torsades de pointes. Avoid using together.
Rifampin: May decrease disopyramide level. Monitor patient for lack of effect.
Thioridazine: May cause life-threatening arrhythmias, including torsades de pointes. Avoid using together.
Verapamil: May cause additive effects and impairment of left ventricular function. Don't give disopyramide 48 hours before starting verapamil or 24 hours after verapamil is stopped.
Drug-herb. *Jimsonweed:* May adversely affect CV function. Discourage use together.

EFFECTS ON LAB TEST RESULTS

None reported.

CONTRAINDICATIONS & CAUTIONS

- Contraindicated in patients hypersensitive to drug.
- Contraindicated with sparfloxacin, thioridazine, or ziprasidone because of increased risk of life-threatening arrhythmias.

• Contraindicated in those with sick sinus syndrome, cardiogenic shock, congenital QT interval prolongation, or second- or third-degree heart block in the absence of an artificial pacemaker.
• Use cautiously, or avoid if possible, in patients with heart failure.
• Use cautiously in patients with underlying conduction abnormalities, urinary tract diseases (especially prostatic hyperplasia), hepatic or renal impairment, myasthenia gravis, or acute angle-closure glaucoma.

NURSING CONSIDERATIONS
• Correct electrolyte abnormalities before starting therapy.
• Digitalize patients with atrial fibrillation or flutter before starting disopyramide because of the risk of enhancing AV conduction.
• Check apical pulse before giving drug. Notify prescriber if pulse rate is slower than 60 beats/minute or faster than 120 beats/minute.
• Don't use sustained- or controlled-release preparations to control ventricular arrhythmias when therapeutic drug level must be rapidly attained, in patients with cardiomyopathy or possible cardiac decompensation, or in those with severe renal impairment.
• ***Alert:*** Don't open the extended-release capsules.
• For use in young children, pharmacist may prepare disopyramide suspension using 100-mg capsules and cherry syrup. Pharmacist should dispense suspension in amber glass bottles. Protect suspension from light.
• Watch for recurrence of arrhythmias and check for adverse reactions; notify prescriber if any occur.
• Stop drug if heart block develops, if QRS complex widens by more than 25%, or if QT interval lengthens by more than 25% above baseline.
• ***Look alike–sound alike:*** Don't confuse disopyramide with desipramine or dipyridamole.

PATIENT TEACHING
• Teach patient importance of taking drug on time and exactly as prescribed.
• If transferring patient from immediate-release to sustained-release capsules, advise him to take the first sustained-release capsule 6 hours after taking the last immediate-release capsule.
• Tell patient not to crush or chew sustained-release capsules or tablets.
• If not contraindicated, advise patient to chew gum or hard candy to relieve dry mouth and to increase fiber and fluid intake to relieve constipation.

dofetilide
Tikosyn

Pharmacologic class: antiarrhythmic
Pregnancy risk category C

AVAILABLE FORMS
Capsules: 125 mcg, 250 mcg, 500 mcg

INDICATIONS & DOSAGES
➤ **To maintain normal sinus rhythm in patients with symptomatic atrial fibrillation or atrial flutter lasting longer than 1 week who have been converted to normal sinus rhythm; to convert atrial fibrillation and atrial flutter to normal sinus rhythm**
Adults: Individualized dosage based on creatinine clearance and baseline QTc interval (or QT interval if heart rate is below 60 beats/minute), determined before first dose; usually 500 mcg P.O. b.i.d. for patients with creatinine clearance greater than 60 ml/minute.
Adjust-a-dose: If creatinine clearance is 40 to 60 ml/minute, starting dose is 250 mcg P.O. b.i.d.; if clearance is 20 to 39 ml/minute, starting dose is 125 mcg P.O. b.i.d. Don't use drug at all if clearance is less than 20 ml/minute.

Determine QTc interval 2 to 3 hours after first dose. If QTc interval has increased by more than 15% above baseline or if it's more than 500 msec (550 msec in patients with ventricular conduction abnormalities), adjust dosage as follows: If starting dose based on creatinine clearance was 500 mcg P.O. b.i.d., give 250 mcg P.O. b.i.d. If starting dose based on clearance was 250 mcg b.i.d., give 125 mcg b.i.d. If starting dose based on clearance was 125 mcg b.i.d., give 125 mcg once a day.

Determine QTc interval 2 to 3 hours after each subsequent dose while patient is in hospital. If at any time after second dose the QTc interval exceeds 500 msec (550 msec in patients with ventricular conduction abnormalities), stop drug.

ACTION

Class III antiarrhythmic; prolongs repolarization without affecting conduction velocity. Drug doesn't affect sodium channels, alpha-adrenergic receptors, or beta-adrenergic receptors.

Route	Onset	Peak	Duration
P.O.	Unknown	2–3 hr	Unknown

Half-life: 10 hours.

ADVERSE REACTIONS

CNS: *headache,* ***stroke,*** dizziness, insomnia, anxiety, migraine, cerebral ischemia, asthenia, paresthesia, syncope.
CV: *chest pain,* ***ventricular fibrillation, ventricular tachycardia, torsades de pointes, AV block, heart block, bradycardia, cardiac arrest, MI,*** bundle-branch block, angina, atrial fibrillation, hypertension, palpitations, edema.
GI: nausea, diarrhea, abdominal pain.
GU: UTI.
Hepatic: liver damage.
Musculoskeletal: back pain, arthralgia, facial paralysis.
Respiratory: respiratory tract infection, dyspnea, increased cough.
Skin: rash, sweating.
Other: ***angioedema,*** flu syndrome, peripheral edema.

INTERACTIONS

Drug-drug. *Antiarrhythmics (classes I and III):* May increase dofetilide level. Withhold other antiarrhythmics for at least three plasma half-lives before giving dofetilide.
Drugs secreted by renal tubular cationic transport (amiloride, metformin, triamterene): May increase dofetilide level. Use together cautiously; monitor patient for adverse effects.
Drugs that prolong QT interval: May increase risk of QT interval prolongation. Avoid using together.
Inhibitors of CYP3A4 (amiodarone), ***azole antifungals,*** *cannabinoids, diltiazem,* ***macrolides,*** *nefazodone, norfloxacin, protease inhibitors, quinine, SSRIs, zafirlukast:* May decrease metabolism and increase dofetilide level. Use together cautiously.
Inhibitors of renal cationic secretion (cimetidine, ketoconazole, megestrol, prochlorperazine, trimethoprim with or without sulfamethoxazole), verapamil: May increase dofetilide level. Use together is contraindicated.
Potassium-depleting diuretics: May increase risk of hypokalemia or hypomagnesemia. Monitor potassium and magnesium levels.
Thiazide diuretics: May cause hypokalemia and arrhythmias. Use together is contraindicated.
Drug-food. *Grapefruit juice:* May decrease hepatic metabolism and increase drug level. Discourage use together.

EFFECTS ON LAB TEST RESULTS

None reported.

CONTRAINDICATIONS & CAUTIONS

- Contraindicated in patients hypersensitive to drug, in those with congenital or acquired long QT interval syndromes or with baseline QTc interval greater than 440 msec (500 msec in patients with ventricular conduction abnormalities), and in those with creatinine clearance less than 20 ml/minute.
- Contraindicated for use with verapamil and with cation transport system inhibitors (cimetidine, ketoconazole, megestrol, prochlorperazine, trimethoprim with or without sulfamethoxazole).
- Use cautiously in patients with severe hepatic impairment.

NURSING CONSIDERATIONS

- Provide continuous ECG monitoring for at least 3 days.
- Don't discharge patient within 12 hours of conversion to normal sinus rhythm.
- Monitor patient for prolonged diarrhea, sweating, and vomiting. Report these signs to prescriber because electrolyte im-

balance may increase potential for arrhythmia development.
- Monitor renal function and QTc interval every 3 months.
- Use of potassium-depleting diuretics may cause hypokalemia and hypomagnesemia, increasing the risk of torsades de pointes. Give dofetilide after potassium level reaches and stays in normal range.
- If patient doesn't convert to normal sinus rhythm within 24 hours of starting dofetilide, consider electrical conversion.
- Before starting dofetilide, stop previous antiarrhythmics while carefully monitoring patient for a minimum of three plasma half-lives. Don't give drug after amiodarone therapy until amiodarone level falls below 0.3 mcg/ml or until amiodarone has been stopped for at least 3 months.
- If dofetilide must be stopped to allow dosing with interacting drugs, allow at least 2 days before starting other drug therapy.

PATIENT TEACHING
- Tell patient to report any change in OTC or prescription drug use, or supplement or herb use.
- Inform patient that drug can be taken without regard to meals or antacid administration.
- Tell patient to immediately report excessive or prolonged diarrhea, sweating, vomiting, or loss of appetite or thirst.
- Advise patient not to take drug with grapefruit juice.
- Advise patient to use antacids, such as Zantac 75 mg, Pepcid, Prilosec, Axid, or Prevacid instead of Tagamet HB if needed for ulcers or heartburn.
- Instruct patient to tell prescriber if she becomes pregnant.
- Advise patient not to breast-feed while taking dofetilide because drug appears in breast milk.
- If a dose is missed, tell patient not to double a dose but to skip that dose and take the next regularly scheduled dose.

SAFETY ALERT!

esmolol hydrochloride
Brevibloc

Pharmacologic class: beta blocker
Pregnancy risk category C

AVAILABLE FORMS
Injection: 10 mg/ml in 10-ml vials, 20 mg/ml in 5-ml vials, 250 mg/ml in 10-ml ampules
Premixed bags in sodium chloride: 10 mg/ml in 250-ml bags; 20 mg/ml in 100-ml bags

INDICATIONS & DOSAGES
➤ Supraventricular tachycardia; postoperative tachycardia or hypertension; noncompensatory sinus tachycardias
Adults: 500 mcg/kg/minute as loading dose by I.V. infusion over 1 minute; then 4-minute maintenance infusion of 50 mcg/kg/minute. If adequate response doesn't occur within 5 minutes, repeat loading dose and follow with maintenance infusion of 100 mcg/kg/minute for 4 minutes. Repeat loading dose and increase maintenance infusion by increments of 50 mcg/kg/minute. Maximum maintenance infusion for tachycardia is 200 mcg/kg/minute.
➤ Intraoperative tachycardia or hypertension
Adults: For intraoperative treatment of tachycardia or hypertension, 80 mg (about 1 mg/kg) I.V. bolus over 30 seconds; then 150 mcg/kg/minute I.V. infusion, if needed. Titrate infusion rate, p.r.n., to maximum of 300 mcg/kg/minute.
➤ Unstable angina, non–ST-segment elevation MI ♦
Adults: Initially, 0.1 mg/kg/minute I.V.; increase by increments of 0.05 mg/kg/minute q 10 to 15 minutes, as tolerated. Maximum dose is 0.3 mg/kg/minute. Initial I.V. loading dose of 0.5 mg/kg may be given slowly over 2 to 5 minutes for a faster onset.

I.V. ADMINISTRATION
- Don't dilute 10-mg/ml single-dose, ready-to-use vials.

- Before infusion, dilute 250-mg/ml injection concentrate to maximum of 10 mg/ml. Remove and discard 20 ml from 500-ml bag of D_5W, lactated Ringer's solution, or half-normal or normal saline solution, and add two ampules of esmolol (final level 10 mg/ml) to the bag.
- Give with an infusion-control device rather than by I.V. push.
- If concentration exceeds 10 mg/ml, give drug through a central line.
- Don't use for longer than 48 hours. Watch infusion site carefully for signs of extravasation; if they occur, stop infusion immediately and call prescriber.

INCOMPATIBILITIES
Amphotericin B cholesteryl sulfate complex, diazepam, furosemide, procainamide, sodium bicarbonate 5%, thiopental sodium, warfarin sodium.

ACTION
A class II antiarrhythmic and ultra–short-acting selective beta blocker that decreases heart rate, contractility, and blood pressure.

Route	Onset	Peak	Duration
I.V.	Immediate	30 min	30 min after infusion

Half-life: About 9 minutes.

ADVERSE REACTIONS
CNS: anxiety, depression, dizziness, somnolence, headache, agitation, fatigue, confusion.
CV: **HYPOTENSION,** peripheral ischemia.
GI: nausea, vomiting.
Skin: inflammation or induration at infusion site.

INTERACTIONS
Drug-drug. *Digoxin:* May increase digoxin level by 10% to 20%. Monitor digoxin level.
Morphine: May increase esmolol level. Adjust esmolol dosage carefully.
Prazosin: May increase risk of orthostatic hypotension. Help patient to stand slowly until effects are known.
Reserpine, other catecholamine-depleting drugs: May increase bradycardia and hypotension. Adjust esmolol dosage carefully.
Succinylcholine: May prolong neuromuscular blockade. Monitor patient closely.
Verapamil: May increase the effects of both drugs. Monitor cardiac function closely and decrease dosages as necessary.

EFFECTS ON LAB TEST RESULTS
None reported.

CONTRAINDICATIONS & CAUTIONS
- Contraindicated in patients with sinus bradycardia, second- or third-degree heart block, cardiogenic shock, or overt heart failure.
- Use cautiously if patient has renal impairment, diabetes, or bronchospasm.

NURSING CONSIDERATIONS
- Dosage for postoperative treatment of tachycardia and hypertension is same as for supraventricular tachycardia.
- ***Alert:*** Monitor ECG and blood pressure continuously during infusion. Nearly half of patients will develop hypotension. Diaphoresis and dizziness may accompany hypotension. Monitor patient closely, especially if he had low blood pressure before treatment.
- Hypotension can usually be reversed within 30 minutes by decreasing the dose or, if needed, by stopping the infusion. Notify prescriber if this becomes necessary.
- If a local reaction develops at the infusion site, change to another site. Avoid using butterfly needles.
- When patient's heart rate becomes stable, replace drug with longer acting antiarrhythmics, such as propranolol, digoxin, or verapamil. Reduce infusion rate by half, 30 minutes after the first dose of the new drug. Monitor patient response and, if heart rate is controlled for 1 hour after administration of the second dose of the replacement drug, stop esmolol infusion.

PATIENT TEACHING
- Instruct patient to report adverse reactions promptly.
- Tell patient to report discomfort at I.V. site.

flecainide acetate
Tambocor

Pharmacologic class: benzamide derivative
Pregnancy risk category C

AVAILABLE FORMS
Injection: 10 mg/ml‡
Tablets: 50 mg, 100 mg, 150 mg

INDICATIONS & DOSAGES
➤ **Paroxysmal supraventricular tachycardia, including AV nodal reentrant tachycardia and AV reentrant tachycardia or paroxysmal atrial fibrillation or flutter in patients without structural heart disease; life-threatening ventricular arrhythmias such as sustained ventricular tachycardia**
Adults: For paroxysmal supraventricular tachycardia, 50 mg P.O. q 12 hours. Increase in increments of 50 mg b.i.d. q 4 days. Maximum dose is 300 mg/day. For life-threatening ventricular arrhythmias, 100 mg P.O. q 12 hours. Increase in increments of 50 mg b.i.d. q 4 days until desired effect occurs. Maximum dose for most patients is 400 mg/day. Or, where available for emergency treatment,‡ 2 mg/kg I.V. push over not less than 10 minutes to maximum dose of 150 mg; or dilute dose and give as an infusion over 10 to 30 minutes.
Adjust-a-dose: If creatinine clearance is 35 ml/minute or less, first dose is 100 mg P.O. once daily or 50 mg P.O. b.i.d.

I.V. ADMINISTRATION
- Give with I.V. lidocaine for first several days.
- Because of drug's long half-life, full therapeutic effect may take 3 to 5 days.
- For I.V. push, give over at least 10 minutes.
- For infusion, mix only with D_5W.

INCOMPATIBILITIES
Alkaline solutions, solutions containing chloride.

ACTION
A class IC antiarrhythmic that decreases excitability, conduction velocity, and automaticity by slowing atrial, AV node, His-Purkinje system, and intraventricular conduction; prolongs refractory periods in these tissues.

Route	Onset	Peak	Duration
P.O.	Unknown	2–3 hr	Unknown
I.V.	Immediate	Immediate	Unknown

Half-life: 12 to 27 hours.

ADVERSE REACTIONS
CNS: *dizziness, headache, lightheadedness, syncope,* fatigue, fever, tremor, anxiety, insomnia, depression, malaise, paresthesia, ataxia, vertigo, asthenia.
CV: ***new or worsened arrhythmias, heart failure, cardiac arrest,*** chest pain, palpitations, edema, flushing.
EENT: *blurred vision and other visual disturbances,* eye pain, eye irritation.
GI: nausea, constipation, abdominal pain, dyspepsia, vomiting, diarrhea, anorexia.
Respiratory: *dyspnea.*
Skin: rash.

INTERACTIONS
Drug-drug. *Amiodarone, cimetidine:* May increase level of flecainide. Watch for toxicity. Reduce usual flecainide dose by 30% to 50% several days after amiodarone is started.
Digoxin: May increase digoxin level by 15% to 25%. Monitor digoxin level.
Disopyramide, verapamil: May increase negative inotropic properties. Avoid using together.
Propranolol, other beta blockers: May increase flecainide and propranolol levels by 20% to 30%. Watch for propranolol and flecainide toxicity.
Ritonavir: May significantly increase flecainide levels and toxicity. Use together is contraindicated.
Urine-acidifying and urine-alkalinizing drugs: May cause extremes of urine pH, which may alter flecainide excretion. Monitor patient for flecainide toxicity or decreased effectiveness.
Drug-lifestyle. *Smoking:* May decrease flecainide level. Monitor patient closely.

EFFECTS ON LAB TEST RESULTS

None reported.

CONTRAINDICATIONS & CAUTIONS

- Contraindicated in patients hypersensitive to drug and in those with second- or third-degree AV block or right bundle-branch block with a left hemiblock (in the absence of an artificial pacemaker), recent MI, or cardiogenic shock, and in patients taking ritonavir.
- Use cautiously in patients with heart failure, cardiomyopathy, severe renal or hepatic disease, prolonged QT interval, sick sinus syndrome, or blood dyscrasia.

NURSING CONSIDERATIONS

- When used to prevent ventricular arrhythmias, reserve drug for patients with documented life-threatening arrhythmias.
- Check that pacing threshold was determined 1 week before and after starting therapy in a patient with a pacemaker; flecainide can alter endocardial pacing thresholds.
- Correct hypokalemia or hyperkalemia before giving flecainide because these electrolyte disturbances may alter drug's effect.
- Monitor ECG rhythm for proarrhythmic effects.
- Most patients can be adequately maintained on an every-12-hours dosing schedule, but some need to receive flecainide every 8 hours.
- Adjust dosage only once every 3 to 4 days.
- Monitor flecainide level, especially if patient has renal or heart failure. Therapeutic flecainide levels range from 0.2 to 1 mcg/ml. Risk of adverse effects increases when trough blood level exceeds 1 mcg/ml.

PATIENT TEACHING

- Stress importance of taking drug exactly as prescribed.
- Instruct patient to report adverse reactions promptly and to limit fluid and sodium intake to minimize fluid retention.
- Tell patient receiving drug I.V. to report discomfort at insertion site.

ibutilide fumarate

Corvert

Pharmacologic class: methanesulfonanilide derivative
Pregnancy risk category C

AVAILABLE FORMS

Injection: 0.1 mg/ml in 10-ml vials

INDICATIONS & DOSAGES

➤Rapid conversion of recent onset atrial fibrillation or atrial flutter to sinus rhythm

Adults who weigh 60 kg (132 lb) or more: 1 mg I.V. infusion over 10 minutes. May repeat dose if arrhythmia doesn't respond 10 minutes after completing first dose.
Adults who weigh less than 60 kg: 0.01 mg/kg I.V. infusion over 10 minutes. May repeat dose if arrhythmia doesn't respond 10 minutes after completing first dose.

I.V. ADMINISTRATION

- Give drug undiluted or diluted in 50 ml of diluent, and add to normal saline solution for injection or D_5W before infusion. Add contents of 10-ml vial (0.1 mg/ml) to 50-ml infusion bag to form admixture of about 0.017 mg/ml ibutilide. Use drug with polyvinyl chloride plastic bags or polyolefin bags.
- Give drug over 10 minutes.
- Stop infusion if arrhythmia is terminated or patient develops ventricular tachycardia or marked prolongation of QT or QTc interval. If arrhythmia doesn't respond 10 minutes after infusion ends, may repeat dose.
- Admixtures with approved diluents are stable for 24 hours at room temperature; 48 hours if refrigerated.
- Don't infuse parenteral products that contain particulate matter or are discolored.

INCOMPATIBILITIES

None reported.

ACTION

Prolongs action potential in isolated cardiac myocyte and increases atrial and ventricular refractoriness: namely, class III electrophysiologic effects.

Route	Onset	Peak	Duration
I.V.	Unknown	Unknown	Unknown

Half-life: Averages about 6 hours.

ADVERSE REACTIONS

CNS: headache.
CV: ***sustained polymorphic ventricular tachycardia, AV block, bradycardia, heart failure,*** ventricular extrasystoles, nonsustained ventricular tachycardia, hypotension, bundle-branch block, hypertension, prolonged QT interval, palpitations, tachycardia.
GI: nausea.

INTERACTIONS

Drug-drug. *Class IA antiarrhythmics (disopyramide, procainamide, quinidine), other class III drugs (amiodarone, sotalol):* May increase potential for prolonged refractoriness. Don't give these drugs for at least five half-lives before and 4 hours after ibutilide dose.
Digoxin: Supraventricular arrhythmias may mask cardiotoxicity from excessive digoxin level. Use with caution in patients who may have an increased digoxin therapeutic range.
H_1-receptor antagonist antihistamines, phenothiazines, tetracyclic antidepressants, tricyclic antidepressants, other drugs that prolong QT interval: May increase risk for proarrhythmia. Monitor patient closely.

EFFECTS ON LAB TEST RESULTS

None reported.

CONTRAINDICATIONS & CAUTIONS

- Contraindicated in patients hypersensitive to drug or its components.
- Contraindicated in patients with history of polymorphic ventricular tachycardia. Use not recommended in breast-feeding women.
- Use cautiously in patients with hepatic or renal dysfunction.
- Safety and effectiveness of drug haven't been established in children.

NURSING CONSIDERATIONS

- Only skilled personnel should give drug. Cardiac monitor, intracardiac pacing, cardioverter or defibrillator, and drugs to treat sustained ventricular tachycardia must be available.
- Before therapy, correct hypokalemia and hypomagnesemia to reduce risk of proarrhythmia. Patients with atrial fibrillation lasting longer than 2 to 3 days must be adequately anticoagulated, generally over at least 2 weeks.
- Monitor ECG continuously during administration and for at least 4 hours afterward or until QTc interval returns to baseline; drug can induce or worsen ventricular arrhythmias. Longer monitoring is required if ECG shows arrhythmia or patient has hepatic insufficiency.
- Don't give class IA or other class III antiarrhythmics with infusion or for 4 hours afterward.

PATIENT TEACHING

- Tell patient to report adverse reactions promptly.
- Instruct patient to alert nurse of discomfort at injection site.

SAFETY ALERT!

lidocaine hydrochloride (lignocaine hydrochloride)

LidoPen Auto-Injector, Xylocaine, Xylocard†‡

Pharmacologic class: amide derivative
Pregnancy risk category B

AVAILABLE FORMS

Infusion (premixed): 0.2% (2 mg/ml), 0.4% (4 mg/ml), 0.8% (8 mg/ml)
Injection (for direct I.V. use): 1% (10 mg/ml), 2% (20 mg/ml)
Injection (for I.V. admixtures): 4% (40 mg/ml), 10% (100 mg/ml), 20% (200 mg/ml)
Injection (for I.M. use): 300 mg/3 ml automatic injection device

INDICATIONS & DOSAGES

➤Ventricular arrhythmias caused by MI, cardiac manipulation, or cardiac glycosides

Adults: 50 to 100 mg (1 to 1.5 mg/kg) by I.V. bolus at 25 to 50 mg/minute. Bolus dose is repeated q 3 to 5 minutes until arrhythmias subside or adverse reactions develop. Don't exceed 300-mg total bolus during a 1-hour period. Simultaneously, constant infusion of 20 to 50 mcg/kg/minute (1 to 4 mg/minute) is begun. If single bolus has been given, smaller bolus dose may be repeated 15 to 20 minutes after start of infusion to maintain therapeutic level. Or, 200 to 300 mg I.M.; then second I.M. dose 60 to 90 minutes later, if needed.
Children: 1 mg/kg by I.V. or intraosseous bolus. If no response, start infusion of 20 to 50 mcg/kg/minute. Give an additional bolus dose of 0.5 to 1 mg/kg if delay of greater than 15 minutes between initial bolus and starting the infusion. Bolus doses shouldn't exceed 3 to 5 mg/kg.
Elderly patients: Reduce dosage and rate of infusion by 50%.
Adjust-a-dose: For patients with heart failure, with renal or liver disease, or who weigh less than 50 kg (110 lb), reduce dosage.

I.V. ADMINISTRATION

- Injections (additive syringes and single-use vials) containing 40, 100, or 200 mg/ml are for the preparation of I.V. infusion solutions only and must be diluted before use.
- Prepare I.V. infusion by adding 1 g (using 25 ml of 4% or 5 ml of 20% injection) to 1 L of D_5W injection to provide a solution containing 1 mg/ml.
- Use a more concentrated solution of up to 8 mg/ml if patient is fluid restricted.
- Patients receiving infusions must be on a cardiac monitor and must be attended at all times. Use an infusion control device for giving infusion precisely. Don't exceed 4 mg/minute; faster rate greatly increases risk of toxicity.
- Avoid giving injections containing preservatives.

INCOMPATIBILITIES

Amphotericin, ampicillin, cefazolin, ceftriaxone, fentanyl citrate (higher pH brands), methohexital sodium, phenytoin sodium, sodium bicarbonate, thiopental sodium.

ACTION

A class IB antiarrhythmic that decreases the depolarization, automaticity, and excitability in the ventricles during the diastolic phase by direct action on the tissues, especially the Purkinje network.

Route	Onset	Peak	Duration
I.V.	Immediate	Immediate	10–20 min
I.M.	5–15 min	10 min	2 hr

Half-life: 1½ to 2 hours (may be prolonged in patients with heart failure or hepatic disease).

ADVERSE REACTIONS

CNS: *confusion, tremor, stupor, restlessness, light-headedness,* ***seizures,*** lethargy, somnolence, anxiety, hallucinations, nervousness, paresthesia, muscle twitching.
CV: *hypotension,* **bradycardia, new or** ***worsened arrhythmias, cardiac arrest.***
EENT: *tinnitus, blurred or double vision.*
GI: vomiting.
Respiratory: ***respiratory depression and arrest.***
Skin: soreness at injection site.
Other: ***anaphylaxis,*** sensation of cold.

INTERACTIONS

Drug-drug. *Atenolol, metoprolol, nadolol, pindolol, propranolol:* May reduce hepatic metabolism of lidocaine, increasing the risk of toxicity. Give bolus doses of lidocaine at a slower rate, and monitor lidocaine level closely.
Cimetidine: May decrease clearance of lidocaine increasing the risk of toxicity. Consider using a different H_2 receptor antagonist if possible. Monitor lidocaine level closely.
Ergot-type oxytocic drugs: May cause severe, persistent hypertension or stroke. Avoid using together.
Mexiletine: May increase pharmacologic effects. Avoid using together.
Phenytoin, procainamide, propranolol, quinidine: May increase cardiac depressant effects. Monitor patient closely.
Succinylcholine: May prolong neuromuscular blockade. Monitor patient closely.

Drug-herb. *Pareira:* May increase the effects of neuromuscular blockade. Discourage use together.
Drug-lifestyle. *Smoking:* May increase metabolism of lidocaine. Monitor patient closely.

EFFECTS ON LAB TEST RESULTS
- May increase CPK levels with I.M. use.

CONTRAINDICATIONS & CAUTIONS
- Contraindicated in patients hypersensitive to the amide-type local anesthetics.
- Contraindicated in those with Adams-Stokes syndrome, Wolff-Parkinson-White syndrome, and severe degrees of SA, AV, or intraventricular block in the absence of an artificial pacemaker.
- Use cautiously and at reduced dosages in patients with complete or second-degree heart block or sinus bradycardia, in elderly patients, in those with heart failure or renal or hepatic disease, and in those who weigh less than 50 kg (110 lb).

NURSING CONSIDERATIONS
- Give I.M. injections in the deltoid muscle only.
- Monitor isoenzymes when using I.M. drug for suspected MI. A patient who has received I.M. lidocaine will show a sevenfold increase in CK level. Such an increase originates in the skeletal muscle, not the heart.
- Monitor drug level. Therapeutic levels are 2 to 5 mcg/ml.
- ***Alert:*** Monitor patient for toxicity. In many severely ill patients, seizures may be the first sign of toxicity, but severe reactions are usually preceded by somnolence, confusion, tremors, and paresthesia. If signs of toxicity occur, stop drug at once and notify prescriber. Continuing could lead to seizures and coma. Give oxygen through a nasal cannula if not contraindicated. Keep oxygen and cardiopulmonary resuscitation equipment available.
- Monitor patient's response, especially blood pressure and electrolytes, BUN, and creatinine levels. Notify prescriber promptly if abnormalities develop.
- If arrhythmias worsen or ECG changes (for example, QRS complex widens or PR interval substantially prolongs), stop infusion and notify prescriber.

PATIENT TEACHING
- For I.M. form, tell patient that drug may cause soreness at injection site. Tell him to report discomfort at the site.
- Tell patient to report adverse reactions promptly because toxicity can occur.

mexiletine hydrochloride
Mexitil

Pharmacologic class: lidocaine analogue
Pregnancy risk category C

AVAILABLE FORMS
Capsules: 50 mg‡, 100 mg†, 150 mg, 200 mg, 250 mg

INDICATIONS & DOSAGES
➤ Life-threatening ventricular arrhythmias, including ventricular tachycardia and PVCs
Adults: Initially, 200 mg P.O. q 8 hours. If satisfactory control isn't obtained at this dosage, increase dosage by 50 to 100 mg q 2 to 3 days up to maximum of 400 mg q 8 hours. If rapid control of ventricular rate is desired, give a loading dose of 400 mg P.O., followed by 200 mg 8 hours later. Patients controlled on 300 mg or less q 8 hours can receive the total daily dose in evenly divided doses q 12 hours.

ACTION
A class IB antiarrhythmic; blocks the fast sodium channel in cardiac tissues without involving the autonomic nervous system. Reduces rate of rise, amplitude, and duration of action potential, and automaticity and effective refractory period in the Purkinje fibers.

Route	Onset	Peak	Duration
P.O.	30–120 min	2–3 hr	Unknown

Half-life: 10 to 12 hours.

ADVERSE REACTIONS
CNS: *tremor, dizziness, light-headedness, incoordination, nervousness,* confusion, changes in sleep habits, paresthesia, weakness, fatigue, speech difficulties, depression, headache.

CV: NEW OR WORSENED ARRHYTHMIAS, palpitations, chest pain, nonspecific edema, angina.
EENT: blurred vision, diplopia, tinnitus.
GI: *nausea, vomiting, upper GI distress, heartburn,* diarrhea, constipation, dry mouth, changes in appetite, abdominal pain.
Skin: rash.

INTERACTIONS

Drug-drug. *Antacids, atropine, narcotics:* May slow mexiletine absorption. Monitor patient for effectiveness.
Cimetidine: May alter mexiletine level. Monitor patient.
Fluvoxamine: May decrease mexiletine clearance. Monitor patient for adverse effects and toxicity.
Methylxanthines (such as caffeine, theophylline): May reduce methylxanthine clearance, which may cause toxicity. Monitor drug level.
Metoclopramide: May speed up mexiletine absorption. Monitor patient for toxicity.
Phenobarbital, phenytoin, rifampin, urine acidifiers: May decrease mexiletine level. Monitor patient for effectiveness.
Urine alkalinizers: May increase mexiletine level. Monitor patient for adverse reactions.

EFFECTS ON LAB TEST RESULTS

- May increase AST level.

CONTRAINDICATIONS & CAUTIONS

- Contraindicated in patients with cardiogenic shock or second- or third-degree AV block in the absence of an artificial pacemaker.
- Use cautiously in patients with first-degree heart block, a ventricular pacemaker, sinus node dysfunction, intraventricular conduction disturbances, hypotension, severe heart failure, liver disease, or seizure disorder.

NURSING CONSIDERATIONS

- When changing from lidocaine to mexiletine, stop the lidocaine infusion when the first mexiletine dose is given. But keep the infusion line open until the arrhythmia is satisfactorily controlled.
- When switching to mexiletine from another oral class 1A antiarrhythmic, begin with a 200-mg dose 6 to 12 hours after the last dose of quinidine or disopyramide or 3 to 6 hours after the last dose of procainamide.
- Give oral dose with meals or antacids to lessen GI distress.
- If patient may be a good candidate for every-12-hours therapy, notify prescriber. Twice-daily dosage enhances compliance.
- Monitor therapeutic drug level, which may range from 0.5 to 2 mcg/ml.
- An early sign of mexiletine toxicity is tremor, usually a fine tremor of the hands, progressing to dizziness and then to ataxia and nystagmus as drug level in the blood increases. Watch for and ask patients about these symptoms.
- Monitor blood pressure and heart rate and rhythm frequently. Notify prescriber of significant change.

PATIENT TEACHING

- Tell patient to take drug exactly as prescribed and to take with food or antacids if GI reactions occur.
- Instruct patient to report adverse reactions promptly.
- Advise patient to notify prescriber if he develops jaundice, fever, or general tiredness; these symptoms may indicate liver damage.

moricizine hydrochloride
Ethmozine

Pharmacologic class: sodium channel blocker
Pregnancy risk category B

AVAILABLE FORMS

Tablets: 200 mg, 250 mg, 300 mg

INDICATIONS & DOSAGES

➤ **Life-threatening ventricular arrhythmias**
Adults: Individualized dosage is based on patient response and tolerance. Begin therapy in the hospital. Most patients respond to 600 to 900 mg P.O. daily in divided doses q 8 hours. Increase daily dose by 150 mg q 3 days until desired effect occurs.

Adjust-a-dose: For patients with hepatic or renal impairment, begin therapy with 600 mg or less P.O. daily.

ACTION
A class I antiarrhythmic; reduces fast inward current carried by sodium ions across myocardial cell membranes. Drug has potent local anesthetic activity and membrane-stabilizing effect.

Route	Onset	Peak	Duration
P.O.	Unknown	30–120 min	10–24 hr

Half-life: 1½ to 3½ hours.

ADVERSE REACTIONS
CNS: *dizziness,* headache, fatigue, hyperesthesia, anxiety, asthenia, depression, nervousness, paresthesia, sleep disorders.
CV: *ECG abnormalities including conduction defects, sinus pause, junctional rhythm and AV block,* ***heart failure, cardiac death, PVCs, supraventricular arrhythmias, ventricular tachycardia,*** palpitations, thrombophlebitis, chest pain, hypotension, hypertension, vasodilation, cerebrovascular events.
EENT: blurred vision.
GI: nausea, vomiting, abdominal pain, dyspepsia, diarrhea, dry mouth.
GU: urine retention, urinary frequency, dysuria.
Musculoskeletal: musculoskeletal pain.
Respiratory: dyspnea.
Skin: rash, diaphoresis.
Other: drug-induced fever.

INTERACTIONS
Drug-drug. *Cimetidine:* May increase level and decrease clearance of moricizine. Begin moricizine at no more than 600 mg daily, and monitor drug level and therapeutic effect closely.
Digoxin, propranolol: May increase PR interval prolongation. Monitor patient closely.
Diltiazem: May increase moricizine level and decrease diltiazem level. Monitor patient for adverse effects and expected therapeutic effect.
Theophylline: May increase clearance and reduces level of theophylline. Monitor drug level and therapeutic response; adjust theophylline dosage, as needed.

EFFECTS ON LAB TEST RESULTS
- May increase liver function test results.

CONTRAINDICATIONS & CAUTIONS
- Contraindicated in patients hypersensitive to drug, cardiogenic shock, or second- or third-degree AV block or right bundle-branch block with left hemiblock (bifascicular block), unless an artificial pacemaker is present.
- Use with caution in patients with sick sinus syndrome because drug may cause sinus bradycardia or sinus arrest.
- Use with caution in patients with coronary artery disease and left ventricular dysfunction because these patients may be at risk for sudden death when treated with the drug.
- Use with caution in patients with hepatic or renal dysfunction and in breast-feeding patients.

NURSING CONSIDERATIONS
- Monitor patients with heart failure carefully for worsening of heart failure.
- When substituting moricizine for another antiarrhythmic, withdraw previous drug for one to two of the drug's half-lives before starting moricizine. During withdrawal and adjustment to moricizine, hospitalize patients who developed life-threatening arrhythmias after withdrawal of previous antiarrhythmic. Guidelines for when to start moricizine therapy are as follows: disopyramide, 6 to 12 hours after last dose; flecainide, 12 to 24 hours after last dose; mexiletine, 8 to 12 hours after last dose; procainamide, 3 to 6 hours after last dose; propafenone, 8 to 12 hours after last dose; and quinidine, 6 to 12 hours after last dose.
- Determine electrolyte status and correct imbalances before therapy, as prescribed. Hypokalemia, hyperkalemia, and hypomagnesemia may alter drug's effects.
- Because drug appears in breast milk, the decision to stop breast-feeding or stop taking the drug depends on importance of drug to the mother.
- ***Look alike–sound alike:*** Don't confuse Ethmozine with Erythrocin.

PATIENT TEACHING
- Inform patient that he'll need to be hospitalized for start of therapy.

- Instruct patient to take drug exactly as prescribed and not to abruptly stop use.
- Tell patient to avoid hazardous activities if adverse CNS reactions or blurred vision occurs.
- Instruct patient to report persistent or serious adverse reactions promptly.

procainamide hydrochloride
Procanbid, Pronestyl, Pronestyl Filmlok, Pronestyl-SR Filmlok

Pharmacologic class: procaine derivative
Pregnancy risk category C

AVAILABLE FORMS
Capsules: 250 mg, 375 mg, 500 mg
Injection: 100 mg/ml, 500 mg/ml
Tablets: 250 mg, 375 mg, 500 mg
Tablets (extended-release): 250 mg, 500 mg, 750 mg, 1,000 mg

INDICATIONS & DOSAGES
➤ Symptomatic PVCs, life-threatening ventricular tachycardia

For oral therapy, start at 50 mg/kg/day of P.O. of conventional tablets or capsules in divided doses q 3 hours until therapeutic level is reached. For maintenance, substitute extended-release form to deliver the total daily dose divided q 6 hours or extended-release form (Procanbid) at a dose of 50 mg/kg P.O. in two divided doses q 12 hours.
Adults: 100 mg q 5 minutes by slow I.V. push, no faster than 25 to 50 mg/minute, until arrhythmias disappear, adverse effects develop, or 500 mg has been given. Usual effective loading dose is 500 to 600 mg. Or, give a loading dose of 500 to 600 mg I.V. infusion over 25 to 30 minutes. Maximum total dose is 1 g. When arrhythmias disappear, give continuous infusion of 2 to 6 mg/minute. If arrhythmias recur, repeat bolus as above and increase infusion rate.

For I.M. administration, give 50 mg/kg divided q 3 to 6 hours; if arrhythmias occur during surgery, give 100 to 500 mg I.M.
Children♦: Dosage not established. Recommendations include 2 to 5 mg/kg I.V., not exceeding 100 mg, repeated p.r.n. at 5- to 10-minute intervals, not exceeding 15 mg/kg in 24 hours or 500 mg in 30 minutes. Or, 15 mg/kg infused over 30 to 60 minutes; then maintenance infusion of 0.02 to 0.08 mg/kg/minute.

➤ To convert atrial fibrillation or paroxysmal atrial tachycardia♦
Adults: 1.25 g P.O. of conventional tablets or capsules. If arrhythmias persist after 1 hour, give additional 750 mg. If no change occurs, give 500 mg to 1 g P.O. q 2 hours until arrhythmias disappear or adverse effects occur. Maintenance dose is 1 g extended-release q 6 hours.
Children: 15 to 50 mg/kg/day P.O. divided q 3 to 6 hours. Maximum dose 4 g daily. Or, 20 to 30 mg/kg/day I.M. Or, loading dose of 3 to 6 mg/kg I.V. over 5 minutes, up to 100 mg/dose; then maintenance dose 20 to 80 mcg/kg/minute as continuous I.V. infusion. Maximum daily dose is 2 g.

➤ To maintain normal sinus rhythm after conversion of atrial flutter♦
Adults: 0.5 to 1 g P.O. of conventional tablets or capsules q 4 to 6 hours.

➤ Malignant hyperthermia♦
Adults: 200 to 900 mg I.V., followed by maintenance infusion.
Adjust-a-dose: For patients with renal or hepatic dysfunction, decrease dose or increase dosing interval, as needed.

I.V. ADMINISTRATION
- Vials for I.V. injection contain 1 g of drug: 100 mg/ml (10 ml) or 500 mg/ml (2 ml).
- Dilute with compatible I.V. solution, such as D_5W injection, and give with the patient supine at a rate not exceeding 25 to 50 mg/minute. Keep patient supine during I.V. administration.
- Attend patient receiving infusion at all times. Use an infusion-control device to give infusion precisely.
- Monitor blood pressure and ECG continuously during I.V. administration. Watch for prolonged QTc intervals and QRS complexes, heart block, or increased arrhythmias. If such reactions occur, withhold drug, obtain rhythm strip, and notify prescriber immediately. If drug is given too rapidly, hypotension can occur. Watch closely for adverse reactions during infusion, and notify prescriber if they occur.

INCOMPATIBILITIES
Bretylium, esmolol, ethacrynate, milrinone, phenytoin sodium.

ACTION
A class IA antiarrhythmic that decreases excitability, conduction velocity, automaticity, and membrane responsiveness with prolonged refractory period. Larger than usual doses may induce AV block.

Route	Onset	Peak	Duration
P.O.	Unknown	90–120 min	Unknown
I.V.	Immediate	Immediate	Unknown
I.M.	10–30 min	15–60 min	Unknown

Half-life: About 2½ to 4¾ hours.

ADVERSE REACTIONS
CNS: *fever, **seizures,*** hallucinations, psychosis, giddiness, confusion, depression, dizziness.
CV: *hypotension, **bradycardia, AV block, ventricular fibrillation, ventricular asystole.***
GI: abdominal pain, nausea, vomiting, anorexia, diarrhea, bitter taste.
Skin: *maculopapular rash, urticaria, pruritus, flushing, angioneurotic edema.*
Other: *lupuslike syndrome.*

INTERACTIONS
Drug-drug. *Amiodarone:* May increase procainamide level and toxicity and have additive effects on QTc interval and QRS complex. Avoid using together.
Anticholinergics: May increase antivagal effects. Monitor patient closely.
Anticholinesterases: May decrease effect of anticholinesterases. Anticholinesterase dosage may need to be increased.
Beta blockers, ranitidine, trimethoprim: May increase procainamide level. Watch for toxicity.
Cimetidine: May increase procainamide level. Avoid using together if possible. Monitor procainamide level closely and adjust the dosage as necessary.
Macrolides and related antibiotics (azithromycin, clarithromycin, erythromycin, telithromycin): May prolong the QT interval. Use with caution. Avoid use with telithromycin.
Neuromuscular blockers: May increase skeletal muscle relaxant effect. Monitor patient closely.
Quinidine, disopyramide: May enhance antiarrhythmic and hypotensive effects. Avoid using together.
Quinolones: Life-threatening arrhythmias, including torsades de pointes, can occur. Avoid using together; sparfloxacin is contraindicated.
Thioridazine, ziprasidone: May prolong QTc interval. Avoid using together.
Drug-herb. *Jimsonweed:* May adversely affect CV function. Discourage use together.
Licorice: May prolong QTc interval. Urge caution.
Drug-lifestyle. *Alcohol use:* May reduce drug level. Discourage use together.

EFFECTS ON LAB TEST RESULTS
- May increase ALT, AST, alkaline phosphatase, LDH, and bilirubin levels.
- May cause positive antinuclear antibody (ANA) titers and positive direct antiglobulin (Coombs) tests.

CONTRAINDICATIONS & CAUTIONS
- Contraindicated in patients hypersensitive to this drug and related drugs.
- Contraindicated in those with complete, second- or third-degree heart block in the absence of an artificial pacemaker. Also contraindicated in those with myasthenia gravis, systemic lupus erythematosus, or atypical ventricular tachycardia (torsades de pointes).
- Use with extreme caution in patients with ventricular tachycardia during coronary occlusion.
- Use cautiously in patients with heart failure or other conduction disturbances, such as bundle-branch heart block, sinus bradycardia, or digitalis intoxication; in those with hepatic or renal insufficiency; and in those with blood dyscrasias or bone marrow suppression.
- Digitalize patients with atrial flutter or fibrillation before therapy with procainamide to prevent ventricular rate acceleration in patient.

NURSING CONSIDERATIONS
- Monitor level of drug and its active metabolite NAPA. To suppress ventricular

arrhythmias, therapeutic levels of procainamide are 4 to 8 mcg/ml; therapeutic levels of NAPA are 10 to 30 mcg/ml.
- Monitor QTc interval closely. Dosage reduction may be needed if QTc interval is prolonged more than 50% from baseline.
- Hypokalemia predisposes patient to arrhythmias. Monitor electrolytes, especially potassium level.
- Elderly patients may be more likely to develop hypotension. Monitor blood pressure carefully.
- Monitor CBC frequently during first 3 months of therapy.
- Positive ANA titer is common in about 60% of patients who don't have symptoms of lupuslike syndrome. This response seems to be related to prolonged use, not dosage. May progress to systemic lupus erythematosus if drug isn't stopped.
- ***Alert:*** Don't crush the extended-release tablets.
- The Filmlok formulation may contain tartrazine.
- ***Look alike–sound alike:*** Don't confuse Procanbid with probenecid.

PATIENT TEACHING
- Stress importance of taking drug exactly as prescribed. This may require use of an alarm clock for nighttime doses.
- Instruct patient to report fever, rash, muscle pain, diarrhea, bleeding, bruises, or pleuritic chest pain.
- Tell patient not to crush or break extended-release tablets.
- Reassure patient who is taking extended-release form that a wax-matrix "ghost" from the tablet may be passed in stools. Drug is completely absorbed before this occurs.

propafenone hydrochloride
Rythmol, Rythmol SR

Pharmacologic class: sodium channel antagonist
Pregnancy risk category C

AVAILABLE FORMS
Capsules (extended-release): 225 mg, 325 mg, 425 mg
Tablets (immediate-release): 150 mg, 225 mg, 300 mg

INDICATIONS & DOSAGES
➤ To suppress life-threatening ventricular arrhythmias such as sustained ventricular tachycardia (SVT); to prevent life-threatening paroxysmal SVT and paroxysmal atrial fibrillation or flutter
Adults: Initially, 150 mg immediate-release tablet P.O. q 8 hours. May increase dosage q 3 or 4 days to 225 mg q 8 hours. If needed, increase dosage to 300 mg q 8 hours. Maximum daily dose, 900 mg.
➤ To prolong time until recurrence of symptomatic atrial fibrillation
Adults: Initially, 225 mg extended-release capsule P.O. q 12 hours. May increase dose after 5 days to 325 mg P.O. q 12 hours. Mayincrease dose to 425 mg q 12 hours.
Adjust-a-dose: For patients with hepatic impairment, reduce initial dose of immediate-release tablets by 70% to 80%.

ACTION
Class IC antiarrhythmic that reduces inward sodium current in cardiac cells, prolongs refractory period in AV node, and decreases excitability, conduction velocity, and automaticity in cardiac tissue.

Route	Onset	Peak	Duration
P.O. (immediate-release)	Unknown	3½ hr	Unknown
P.O. (extended-release)	Unknown	3–8 hr	Unknown

Half-life: 2 to 32 hours.

ADVERSE REACTIONS
CNS: *dizziness,* anxiety, ataxia, drowsiness, fatigue, headache, insomnia, syncope, tremor, weakness.
CV: ***heart failure, bradycardia, arrhythmias, ventricular tachycardia, premature ventricular contractions, ventricular fibrillation,*** atrial fibrillation, bundle-branch block, angina, chest pain, edema, first-degree AV block, hypotension, increased QRS complex, intraventricular conduction delay, palpitations.
EENT: blurred vision.

GI: *nausea, vomiting,* abdominal pain or cramps, constipation, diarrhea, dyspepsia, anorexia, flatulence, dry mouth, unusual taste.
Musculoskeletal: arthralgia.
Respiratory: dyspnea.
Skin: rash, diaphoresis.

INTERACTIONS

Drug-drug. *Antiarrhythmics:* May increase risk of prolonged QTc interval. Monitor patient closely.
Beta blockers (metoprolol, propranolol): May decrease metabolism of these drugs. Adjust dosage of beta blocker as needed.
Cimetidine: May increase propafenone levels. Monitor patient for adverse effects and toxicity.
Cyclosporine, ***digoxin:*** May increase levels of these drugs, causing toxicity. Monitor patient closely; dosage adjustment may be necessary.
Desipramine: May decrease desipramine metabolism. Monitor patient closely.
Lidocaine: May decrease lidocaine metabolism. Monitor patient for increased CNS adverse effects and lidocaine toxicity.
Local anesthetics: May increase risk of CNS toxicity. Monitor patient closely.
Mexiletine: May decrease mexiletine metabolism, increasing level and adverse reactions. Monitor mexiletine level and patient closely.
Phenobarbital, rifampin: May increase propafenone clearance. Watch for decreased antiarrhythmic effect.
Quinidine: May decrease propafenone metabolism; may be useful in certain patients refractory to propafenone and quinidine monotherapy. Monitor patient closely.
Ritonavir: May increase propafenone level, causing life-threatening arrhythmias. Avoid using together.
Theophylline: May decrease theophylline metabolism. Monitor theophylline level and ECG closely.
Warfarin: May increase warfarin level. Monitor PT and INR closely, and adjust warfarin dose as needed.

EFFECTS ON LAB TEST RESULTS

- May increase alkaline phosphatase, ALT, and AST levels.
- May cause positive ANA titers.

CONTRAINDICATIONS & CAUTIONS

- Contraindicated in patients hypersensitive to drug and in those with severe or uncontrolled heart failure; cardiogenic shock; SA, AV, or intraventricular disorders of impulse conduction without a pacemaker; bradycardia; marked hypotension; bronchospastic disorders; or electrolyte imbalances.
- Use cautiously in patients with a history of heart failure because drug may weaken the contraction of the heart.
- Use cautiously in patients taking other cardiac depressants and in those with hepatic or renal impairment.
- Avoid using in patients with myasthenia gravis.

NURSING CONSIDERATIONS

- To minimize adverse GI reactions, give drug with food.
- ***Alert:*** Perform continuous cardiac monitoring at start of therapy and during dosage adjustments. If PR interval or QRS complex increases by more than 25%, reduce dosage.
- If using with digoxin, frequently monitor ECG and digoxin level.
- Pacing and sensing thresholds of artificial pacemakers may change; monitor pacemaker function.
- Agranulocytosis may develop during the first 2 to 3 months of therapy. If patient has an unexplained fever, monitor leukocyte count.

PATIENT TEACHING

- Stress importance of taking drug exactly as prescribed.
- Tell patient not to double the dose if he misses one, but to take the next dose at the usual time.
- Tell patient to report adverse reactions promptly, including fever, sore throat, chills, and other signs and symptoms of infection.
- Instruct patient to notify prescriber if prolonged diarrhea, sweating, vomiting, or loss of appetite or thirst occurs; these may cause an electrolyte imbalance.
- Tell patient not to crush, chew, or open the extended-release capsules.

quinidine gluconate
Quinaglute Dura-Tabs, Quinate†

quinidine sulfate
Apo-Quinidine†, Novoquinidin†, Quinidex Extentabs

Pharmacologic class: cinchona alkaloid
Pregnancy risk category C

AVAILABLE FORMS
quinidine gluconate (62% quinidine base)
Injection: 80 mg/ml
Tablets (extended-release): 324 mg, 325 mg†
quinidine sulfate (83% quinidine base)
Injection: 200 mg/ml†
Tablets: 200 mg, 300 mg
Tablets (extended-release): 300 mg

INDICATIONS & DOSAGES
➤Atrial flutter or fibrillation
Adults: 300 to 400 mg quinidine sulfate or equivalent base P.O. q 6 hours. Or, 200 mg P.O. q 2 to 3 hours for five to eight doses, increased daily until sinus rhythm is restored or toxic effects develop. Maximum, 3 to 4 g daily.
Children♦: 30 mg/kg or 900 mg/m^2 P.O. (sulfate) or I.V. or I.M. (gluconate) daily in five divided doses.
➤Paroxysmal supraventricular tachycardia
Adults: 400 to 600 mg P.O. gluconate q 2 to 3 hours until toxic adverse reactions develop or arrhythmia subsides.
Children♦: 30 mg/kg or 900 mg/m^2 P.O. (sulfate) or I.V. or I.M. (gluconate) daily in five divided doses.
➤Premature atrial and ventricular contractions, paroxysmal AV junctional rhythm, paroxysmal atrial tachycardia, paroxysmal ventricular tachycardia, maintenance after cardioversion of atrial fibrillation or flutter
Adults: Test dose is 200 mg P.O. or I.M. Quinidine sulfate or equivalent base 200 to 400 mg P.O. q 4 to 6 hours or 600 mg quinidine sulfate extended-release q 8 to 12 hours; or quinidine gluconate 800 mg (10 ml of commercially available solution) added to 40 ml of D_5W, infused I.V. at 0.25 mg/kg/minute.
Children♦: 30 mg/kg or 900 mg/m^2 P.O. (sulfate) or I.V. or I.M. (gluconate) daily in five divided doses.
➤Severe *Plasmodium falciparum* malaria
Adults: 10 mg/kg gluconate I.V. diluted in 250 ml normal saline solution and infused over 1 to 2 hours; then begin a continuous infusion of 0.02 mg/kg/minute for at least 24 hours, and until parasitemia is reduced to less than 1% and oral therapy can be started. Or, give a loading dose of 24 mg/kg of quinidine gluconate I.V. diluted in 250 ml of normal saline and infused over 4 hours; then 4 hours later, give maintenance dose of 12 mg/kg of quinidine gluconate given by I.V. infusion over 4 hours at 8-hour intervals until three maintenance doses have been given and parasitemia is reduced to less than 1% and oral quinidine sulfate can be initiated.
Children♦: 10 mg/kg gluconate I.V. over 1 to 2 hours; then continuous infusion of 0.02 mg/kg/minute.
Adjust-a-dose: In patients with hepatic impairment or heart failure, reduce dosage.

I.V. ADMINISTRATION
- For quinidine gluconate infusion to treat atrial fibrillation or flutter in adults, dilute 800 mg (10 ml of injection) with 40 ml D_5W and infuse at up to 0.25 mg/kg/minute.
- For quinidine gluconate infusion to treat malaria, dilute in 5 ml/kg (usually 250 ml) normal saline solution and infuse over 1 to 2 hours, followed by a continuous maintenance infusion.
- During infusion, continuously monitor patient's blood pressure and ECG.
- Adjust rate so that the arrhythmia is corrected without disturbing the normal mechanism of the heartbeat.

INCOMPATIBILITIES
Alkalies, amiodarone, atracurium besylate, furosemide, heparin sodium, iodides.

ACTION
A class IA antiarrhythmic with direct and indirect (anticholinergic) effects on cardiac tissue. Decreases automaticity, con-

duction velocity, and membrane responsiveness; prolongs effective refractory period; and reduces vagal tone.

Route	Onset	Peak	Duration
P.O.	1–3 hr	1–6 hr	6–8 hr
I.V.	Immediate	Immediate	Unknown
I.M.	Unknown	30–90 min	Unknown

Half-life: 5 to 12 hours.

ADVERSE REACTIONS

CNS: *vertigo, fever, headache, lightheadedness,* ataxia, confusion, depression, dementia.
CV: *ECG changes, tachycardia,* ***PVCs, ventricular tachycardia, atypical ventricular tachycardia, complete AV block, aggravated heart failure,*** hypotension.
EENT: *tinnitus,* blurred vision, diplopia, photophobia.
GI: *diarrhea, nausea, vomiting,* anorexia, excessive salivation, abdominal pain.
Hematologic: ***thrombocytopenia, agranulocytosis,*** hemolytic anemia.
Hepatic: ***hepatotoxicity.***
Respiratory: ***acute asthmatic attack, respiratory arrest.***
Skin: rash, petechial hemorrhage of buccal mucosa, pruritus, urticaria, photosensitivity.
Other: *cinchonism,* ***angioedema,*** lupus erythematosus.

INTERACTIONS

Drug-drug. *antacids, sodium bicarbonate:* May increase quinidine level. Monitor patient for increased effect.
Amiloride: May increase the risk of arrhythmias. If use together can't be avoided, monitor ECG closely.
Amiodarone: May increase quinidine level, producing life-threatening cardiac arrhythmias. Monitor quinidine level closely if use together can't be avoided. Adjust quinidine as needed.
Azole antifungals: May increase the risk of cardiovascular events. Use together is contraindicated.
Barbiturates, phenytoin, rifampin: May decrease quinidine level. Monitor patient for decreased effect.
Cimetidine: May increase quinidine level. Monitor patient for increased arrhythmias.
Digoxin: May increase digoxin level after starting quinidine therapy. Monitor digoxin level.
Drugs that prolong the QT interval (antipsychotics, disopyramide, procainamide, tricyclic antidepressants, sotalol): May have additive effect with quinidine and cause life-threatening cardiac arrhythmias. Avoid using together when possible.
Fluvoxamine, nefazodone, tricyclic antidepressants: May increase antidepressant level, thus increasing its effect. Monitor patient for adverse reactions.
Macrolides and related antibiotics (azithromycin, clarithromycin, erythromycin, telithromycin): May cause additive effects or prolongation of the QT interval. Use with caution. Avoid use with telithromycin.
Neuromuscular blockers: May potentiate effects of these drugs. Avoid use of quinidine immediately after surgery.
Nifedipine: May decrease quinidine level. May need to adjust dosage.
Other antiarrhythmics (such as lidocaine, procainamide, propranolol): May increase risk of toxicity. Use together cautiously.
Protease inhibitors (nelfinavir, ritonavir): May significantly increase quinidine levels and toxicity. Use together is contraindicated.
Quinolones: Life-threatening arrhythmias, including torsades de pointes, can occur. Avoid use together.
Verapamil: May decrease quinidine clearance and cause hypotension, bradycardia, AV block, or pulmonary edema. Monitor blood pressure and heart rate.
Warfarin: May increase anticoagulant effect. Monitor patient closely.
Drug-herb. *Jimsonweed:* May adversely affect CV function. Discourage use together.
Licorice: May have additive effect and prolong QT interval. Urge caution.
Drug-food. *Grapefruit:* May delay absorption and onset of action of drug. Discourage use together.

EFFECTS ON LAB TEST RESULTS

- May decrease hemoglobin level.
- May decrease platelet and granulocyte counts.

CONTRAINDICATIONS & CAUTIONS

- Contraindicated in patients with idiosyncrasy or hypersensitivity to quinidine or related cinchona derivatives.
- Contraindicated in those with myasthenia gravis, intraventricular conduction defects, digitalis toxicity when AV conduction is grossly impaired, abnormal rhythms caused by escape mechanisms, complete AV block, history of drug-induced torsades de pointes, and history of prolonged QT interval syndrome.
- Contraindicated in patients who developed thrombocytopenia after exposure to quinidine or quinine.
- Use cautiously in patients with asthma, muscle weakness, or infection accompanied by fever because hypersensitivity reactions to drug may be masked.
- Use cautiously in patients with hepatic or renal impairment because systemic accumulation may occur.

NURSING CONSIDERATIONS

- Check apical pulse rate and blood pressure before therapy. If extremes in pulse rate are detected, withhold drug and notify prescriber at once.
- ***Alert:*** For atrial fibrillation or flutter, give quinidine only after AV node has been blocked with a beta blocker, digoxin, or a calcium channel blocker to avoid increasing AV conduction.
- Anticoagulant therapy is commonly advised before quinidine therapy in long-standing atrial fibrillation because restoration of normal sinus rhythm may result in thromboembolism caused by dislodgment of thrombi from atrial wall.
- Monitor patient for atypical ventricular tachycardia, such as torsades de pointes and ECG changes, particularly widening of QRS complex, widened QT and PR intervals.
- ***Alert:*** When changing route of administration or oral salt form, prescriber should alter dosage to compensate for variations in quinidine base content.
- Never use discolored (brownish) quinidine solution.
- Quinidine gluconate I.M. is no longer recommended for arrhythmias because of erratic absorption.
- ***Alert:*** Hospitalize patients with severe malaria in an intensive care setting, with continuous monitoring. Decrease infusion rate if quinidine level exceeds 6 mcg/ml, uncorrected QT interval exceeds 0.6 seconds, or QRS complex widening exceeds 25% of baseline.
- Monitor liver function test results during first 4 to 8 weeks of therapy.
- Monitor quinidine level. Therapeutic levels for antiarrhythmic effects are 4 to 8 mcg/ml.
- Monitor patient response carefully. If adverse GI reactions occur, especially diarrhea, notify prescriber. Check quinidine level, which is increasingly toxic when greater than 10 mcg/ml. GI symptoms may be decreased by giving drug with meals or aluminum hydroxide antacids.
- Store drug away from heat and direct light.
- ***Look alike–sound alike:*** Don't confuse quinidine with quinine or clonidine.

PATIENT TEACHING

- Stress importance of taking drug exactly as prescribed and taking it with food if adverse GI reactions occur.
- ***Alert:*** Instruct patient not to crush or chew extended-release tablets. If necessary, they may be broken in half to adjust quinidine dose.
- Tell patient to avoid grapefruit juice because it may delay drug absorption and inhibit drug metabolism.
- Advise patient to report persistent or serious adverse reactions promptly, especially signs and symptoms of quinidine toxicity (ringing in the ears, visual disturbances, dizziness, headache, nausea).

sotalol hydrochloride

Betapace, Betapace AF, Sotacor†‡

Pharmacologic class: nonselective beta blocker
Pregnancy risk category B

AVAILABLE FORMS

Betapace
Tablets: 80 mg, 120 mg, 160 mg, 240 mg
Betapace AF
Tablets: 80 mg, 120 mg, 160 mg

INDICATIONS & DOSAGES

➤ **Documented, life-threatening ventricular arrhythmias**

Adults: Initially, 80 mg Betapace P.O. b.i.d. Increase dosage q 3 days as needed and tolerated. Most patients respond to 160 to 320 mg/day, although some patients with refractory arrhythmias need up to 640 mg/day.

Adjust-a-dose: If creatinine clearance is 30 to 60 ml/minute, increase dosage interval to q 24 hours; if clearance is 10 to 29 ml/minute, increase interval to q 36 to 48 hours; and if clearance is less than 10 ml/minute, individualize dosage.

➤ **To maintain normal sinus rhythm or to delay recurrence of atrial fibrillation or atrial flutter in patients with symptomatic atrial fibrillation or flutter who are currently in sinus rhythm**

Adults: 80 mg Betapace AF P.O. b.i.d. Increase dosage p.r.n. to 120 mg P.O. b.i.d. after 3 days if the QTc interval is less than 500 msec. Maximum dose is 160 mg P.O. b.i.d.

Adjust-a-dose: If creatinine clearance is 40 to 60 ml/minute, increase dosage interval to q 24 hours. If clearance is less than 40 ml/minute, Betapace AF is contraindicated.

ACTION

A nonselective beta blocker that depresses sinus heart rate, slows AV conduction, decreases cardiac output, and lowers systolic and diastolic blood pressure. Drug also has class III antiarrhythmic action potential's duration and prolongation.

Route	Onset	Peak	Duration
P.O.	Unknown	2½–4 hr	Unknown

Half-life: 12 hours.

ADVERSE REACTIONS

CNS: *asthenia, headache, dizziness, weakness, fatigue, light-headedness,* sleep problems.

CV: *chest pain, palpitations,* ***bradycardia, arrhythmias, heart failure, AV block, proarrhythmic events (including polymorphic ventricular tachycardia, PVCs, ventricular fibrillation),*** edema, ECG abnormalities, hypotension.

GI: *nausea, vomiting,* diarrhea, dyspepsia.

Metabolic: hyperglycemia.

Respiratory: *dyspnea,* ***bronchospasm.***

INTERACTIONS

Drug-drug. *Antiarrhythmics:* May increase drug effects. Avoid using together.

Antihypertensives, catecholamine-depleting drugs (such as guanethidine, reserpine): May increase hypotensive effects or cause marked bradycardia. Monitor blood pressure and pulse closely.

Calcium channel blockers: May increase myocardial depression. Avoid using together.

Clonidine: May enhance rebound effect after withdrawal of clonidine. Stop sotalol several days before withdrawing clonidine.

Drugs that prolong the QT interval (Class I and III antiarrhythmics, bepridil, phenothiazines, tricyclics): May cause excessive QT prolongation. Monitor QT interval.

General anesthetics: May increase myocardial depression. Monitor patient closely.

Insulin, oral antidiabetics: May cause hyperglycemia and may mask signs and symptoms of hypoglycemia. Adjust dosage accordingly.

Macrolides and related antibiotics (azithromycin, clarithromycin, erythromycin, telithromycin): May cause additive effects or prolong the QT interval. Use with caution. Avoid use with telithromycin.

Prazosin: May increase the risk of orthostatic hypotension. Assist patient to stand slowly until effects are known.

Quinolones: May cause life-threatening arrhythmias, including torsades de pointes. Avoid using together.

Drug-food. *Any food:* May decrease absorption by 20%. Advise patient to take on empty stomach.

EFFECTS ON LAB TEST RESULTS

- May increase glucose level.
- May cause false-positive catecholamine level.

CONTRAINDICATIONS & CAUTIONS

- Contraindicated in patients hypersensitive to drug.

• Contraindicated in those with severe sinus node dysfunction, sinus bradycardia, second- and third-degree AV block unless patient has a pacemaker, congenital or acquired long QT-interval syndrome, cardiogenic shock, uncontrolled heart failure, and bronchial asthma.
• Use cautiously in patients with renal impairment or diabetes mellitus (beta blockers may mask signs and symptoms of hypoglycemia).

NURSING CONSIDERATIONS
• Because proarrhythmic events may occur at start of therapy and during dosage adjustments, hospitalize patient for a minimum of 3 days. Facilities and personnel should be available for cardiac rhythm monitoring and interpretation of ECG.
• The baseline QTc interval must be less than or equal to 450 msec before starting Betapace AF.
• Assess patient for new or worsened symptoms of heart failure.
• Although patients receiving I.V. lidocaine may start sotalol therapy without ill effect, withdraw other antiarrhythmics before therapy begins. Sotalol therapy typically is delayed until two or three half-lives of the withdrawn drug have elapsed. After withdrawing amiodarone, give sotalol only after QT interval normalizes.
• Adjust dosage slowly, allowing 3 days between dosage increments for adequate monitoring of QT intervals and for drug levels to reach a steady-state level.
• ***Alert:*** Don't substitute Betapace for Betapace AF.
• Monitor electrolytes regularly, especially if patient is receiving diuretics. Electrolyte imbalances, such as hypokalemia or hypomagnesemia, may enhance QT-interval prolongation and increase the risk of serious arrhythmias such as torsades de pointes.
• ***Look alike–sound alike:*** Don't confuse sotalol with Stadol.

PATIENT TEACHING
• Explain to patient that he will need to be hospitalized for initiation of drug therapy.
• Stress need to take drug as prescribed, even when he is feeling well. Caution patient against stopping drug suddenly.
• Caution patient against using nonprescription drugs and decongestants while taking drug.
• Because food and antacids can interfere with absorption, tell patient to take drug on an empty stomach, 1 hour before or 2 hours after meals or antacids.

20
Antianginals

amlodipine besylate
diltiazem hydrochloride
isosorbide dinitrate
isosorbide mononitrate
nadolol
nicardipine hydrochloride
nifedipine
nitroglycerin
propranolol hydrochloride
ranolazine
verapamil hydrochloride

amlodipine besylate
Norvasc✐

Pharmacologic class: calcium channel blocker
Pregnancy risk category C

AVAILABLE FORMS
Tablets: 2.5 mg, 5 mg, 10 mg

INDICATIONS & DOSAGES
➤ Chronic stable angina, vasospastic angina (Prinzmetal or variant angina)
Adults: Initially, 5 to 10 mg P.O. daily. Most patients need 10 mg daily.
Elderly patients: Initially, 5 mg P.O. daily.
Adjust-a-dose: For patients who are small or frail or have hepatic insufficiency, initially, 5 mg P.O. daily.
➤ Hypertension
Adults: Initially, 2.5 to 5 mg P.O. daily. Dosage adjusted according to patient response and tolerance. Maximum daily dose is 10 mg.
Elderly patients: Initially, 2.5 mg P.O. daily.
Adjust-a-dose: For patients who are small or frail, are taking other antihypertensives, or have hepatic insufficiency, initially, 2.5 mg P.O. daily.

ACTION
Inhibits calcium ion influx across cardiac and smooth-muscle cells, dilates coronary arteries and arterioles, and decreases blood pressure and myocardial oxygen demand.

Route	Onset	Peak	Duration
P.O.	Unknown	6–12 hr	24 hr

Half-life: 30 to 50 hours.

ADVERSE REACTIONS
CNS: headache, somnolence, fatigue, dizziness, light-headedness, paresthesia.
CV: *edema,* flushing, palpitations.
GI: nausea, abdominal pain.
GU: sexual difficulties.
Musculoskeletal: muscle pain.
Respiratory: dyspnea.
Skin: rash, pruritus.

INTERACTIONS
None reported.

EFFECTS ON LAB TEST RESULTS
None reported.

CONTRAINDICATIONS & CAUTIONS
- Contraindicated in patients hypersensitive to drug.
- Use cautiously in patients receiving other peripheral vasodilators, especially those with severe aortic stenosis, and in those with heart failure. Because drug is metabolized by the liver, use cautiously and in reduced dosage in patients with severe hepatic disease.

NURSING CONSIDERATIONS
- ***Alert:*** Monitor patient carefully. Some patients, especially those with severe obstructive coronary artery disease, have developed increased frequency, duration, or severity of angina or acute MI after initiation of calcium channel blocker therapy or at time of dosage increase.
- Monitor blood pressure frequently during initiation of therapy. Because drug-induced vasodilation has a gradual onset, acute hypotension is rare.

- Notify prescriber if signs of heart failure occur, such as swelling of hands and feet or shortness of breath.
- ***Alert:*** Abrupt withdrawal of drug may increase frequency and duration of chest pain. Taper dose gradually under medical supervision.
- ***Look alike–sound alike:*** Don't confuse amlodipine with amiloride.

PATIENT TEACHING

- Caution patient to continue taking drug, even when feeling better.
- Tell patient S.L. nitroglycerin may be taken as needed when angina symptoms are acute. If patient continues nitrate therapy during adjustment of amlodipine dosage, urge continued compliance.

diltiazem hydrochloride

Apo-Diltiaz†, Cardizem✐, Cardizem CD✐, Cardizem LA✐, Cartia XT, Dilacor XR, Diltia XT, Dilt-XR, Taztia XT, Tiazac

Pharmacologic class: calcium channel blocker
Pregnancy risk category C

AVAILABLE FORMS

Capsules (extended-release): 120 mg, 180 mg, 240 mg, 300 mg, 360 mg, 420 mg
Injection: 5 mg/ml in 5-, 10-, 25-ml vials
Powder for injection: 25 mg
Tablets: 30 mg, 60 mg, 90 mg, 120 mg

INDICATIONS & DOSAGES

➤ **To manage Prinzmetal or variant angina or chronic stable angina pectoris**
Adults: 30 mg P.O. q.i.d. before meals and at bedtime. Increase dose gradually to maximum of 360 mg/day divided into three to four doses, as indicated. Or, give 120 or 180 mg extended-release capsule P.O. once daily. Adjust over a 7- to 14-day period as needed and tolerated up to a maximum dose of 360 mg/day (Cardizem LA), 480 mg/day (Cardizem CD, Cartia XT, Dilacor XR, Dilacor XT), or 540 mg/day (Tiazac).

➤ **Hypertension**
Adults: 180 to 240 mg extended-release capsule P.O. once daily. Adjust dosage based on patient response to a maximum dose of 480 mg/day. Or, 120 to 240 mg P.O. (Cardizem LA) once daily. Dosage can be adjusted about every 2 weeks to a maximum of 540 mg daily.

➤ **Atrial fibrillation or flutter; paroxysmal supraventricular tachycardia**
Adults: 0.25 mg/kg I.V. as a bolus injection over 2 minutes. Repeat after 15 minutes if response isn't adequate with a dose of 0.35 mg/kg I.V. over 2 minutes. Follow bolus with continuous I.V. infusion at 5 to 15 mg/hour (for up to 24 hours).

I.V. ADMINISTRATION

- For 100-mg Cardizem Monovials, reconstitute according to manufacturer's directions.
- For direct injection, you need not dilute the 5 mg/ml injection.
- For continuous infusion, add 25 ml of drug to 100 ml solution, 50 ml of drug to 250 ml solution, or 50 ml of drug to 500 ml solutionof 5 mg/ml injection to yield 1 mg/ml, 0.83 mg/ml, or 0.45 mg/ml, respectively. Compatible solutions include normal saline solution, D_5W, or 5% dextrose and half-normal saline solution.
- For direct injection or continuous infusion; give slowly while monitoring ECG and blood pressure continuously.
- Don't infuse for longer than 24 hours.

INCOMPATIBILITIES

Acetazolamide, acyclovir, aminophylline, ampicillin, ampicillin sodium and sulbactam sodium, cefoperazone, diazepam, furosemide, heparin, hydrocortisone, insulin, methylprednisolone, nafcillin, phenytoin, rifampin, sodium bicarbonate, thiopental.

ACTION

A calcium channel blocker that inhibits calcium ion influx across cardiac and smooth-muscle cells, decreasing myocardial contractility and oxygen demand. Also dilates coronary arteries and arterioles.

Route	Onset	Peak	Duration
P.O.	30–60 min	2–3 hr	6–8 hr
P.O. (extended-release)	2–3 hr	10–14 hr	12–24 hr
P.O. (Cardizem LA)	3–4 hr	11–18 hr	6–9 hr
I.V.	< 3 min	2–7 min	1–10 hr

Half-life: 3 to 9 hours.

ADVERSE REACTIONS

CNS: *headache,* dizziness, asthenia, somnolence.
CV: *edema,* ***arrhythmias, AV block, bradycardia, heart failure,*** flushing, hypotension, conduction abnormalities, abnormal ECG.
GI: nausea, constipation, abdominal discomfort.
Hepatic: ***acute hepatic injury.***
Skin: rash.

INTERACTIONS

Drug-drug. *Anesthetics:* May increase effects of anesthetics. Monitor patient.
Carbamazepine: May increase level of carbamazepine. Monitor carbamazepine level, and watch for signs and symptoms of toxicity.
Cimetidine: May inhibit diltiazem metabolism, increasing additive AV node conduction slowing. Monitor patient for toxicity.
Cyclosporine: May increase cyclosporine level, possibly by decreasing its metabolism, leading to increased risk of cyclosporine toxicity. Monitor cyclosporine level with each dosage change.
Diazepam, midazolam, triazolam: May increase CNS depression and prolonged effects of these drugs. Use lower dose of these benzodiazepines.
Digoxin: May increase digoxin level. Monitor patient for digoxin toxicity.
Furosemide: May form a precipitate when mixed with diltiazem injection. Give through separate I.V. lines.
Lithium: May reduce lithium levels, causing loss of mania control, and neurotoxic and psychotic symptoms. Monitor patient for signs of neurotoxicity.
Propranolol, other beta blockers: May precipitate heart failure or prolong conduction time. Use together cautiously.
Sirolimus, tacrolimus: May increase level of these drugs. Monitor drug level and patient for toxicity.
Theophylline: May enhance action of theophylline, causing intoxication. Monitor theophylline levels.

EFFECTS ON LAB TEST RESULTS

None reported.

CONTRAINDICATIONS & CAUTIONS

- Contraindicated in patients hypersensitive to drug and in those with sick sinus syndrome or second- or third-degree AV block in the absence of an artificial pacemaker, cardiogenic shock, ventricular tachycardia, systolic blood pressure below 90 mm Hg, acute MI, or pulmonary congestion (documented by X-ray).
- I.V. form is contraindicated in patients who have atrial fibrillation or flutter with an accessory bypass tract, as in Wolff-Parkinson-White syndrome or short PR interval syndrome.
- Use cautiously in elderly patients and in those with heart failure or impaired hepatic or renal function.

NURSING CONSIDERATIONS

- Patients controlled on drug alone or with other drugs may be switched to Cardizem LA tablets once a day at the nearest equivalent total daily dose.
- Monitor blood pressure and heart rate when starting therapy and during dosage adjustments.
- Maximal antihypertensive effect may not be seen for 14 days.
- If systolic blood pressure is below 90 mm Hg or heart rate is below 60 beats/minute, withhold dose and notify prescriber.

PATIENT TEACHING

- Instruct patient to take drug as prescribed, even when feeling better.
- Advise patient to avoid hazardous activities during start of therapy.
- If nitrate therapy is prescribed during dosage adjustment, stress patient compliance. Tell patient that S.L. nitroglycerin

may be taken with drug, as needed, when angina symptoms are acute.
• ***Alert:*** Tell patient to swallow extended-release capsules whole, and not to open, crush, or chew them.

isosorbide dinitrate
Apo-ISDN†, Cedocard SR†, Dilatrate-SR, Isordil, Isordil Titradose

isosorbide mononitrate
Imdur, ISMO, Monoket

Pharmacologic class: nitrate
Pregnancy risk category C; B for mononitrate

AVAILABLE FORMS
isosorbide dinitrate
Capsules (sustained-release): 40 mg
Tablets: 5 mg, 10 mg, 20 mg, 30 mg, 40 mg
Tablets (S.L.): 2.5 mg, 5 mg,
Tablets (sustained-release): 40 mg
isosorbide mononitrate
Tablets: 10 mg, 20 mg
Tablets (extended-release): 30 mg, 60 mg, 120 mg

INDICATIONS & DOSAGES
➤ **Acute anginal attacks (S.L. isosorbide dinitrate only); to prevent situations that may cause anginal attacks**
Adults: 2.5 to 5 mg S.L. tablets for prompt relief of angina, repeated q 5 to 10 minutes (maximum of three doses for each 30-minute period). For prevention, 2.5 to 10 mg q 2 to 3 hours. Or, 5 to 40 mg isosorbide dinitrate P.O. b.i.d. or t.i.d. for prevention only (use smallest effective dose). Or, 30 to 60 mg Imdur P.O. once daily on arising; increase to 120 mg once daily after several days, if needed. Or, 20 mg ISMO or Monoket b.i.d. with the two doses given 7 hours apart.

ACTION
Thought to reduce cardiac oxygen demand by decreasing preload and afterload. Drug also may increase blood flow through the collateral coronary vessels.

Route	Onset	Peak	Duration
P.O.	15–40 min	Unknown	4–8 hr
P.O. (extended-release)	½–4 hr	Unknown	6–12 hr
P.O. (S.L.)	2–5 min	Unknown	1–4 hr

Half-life: dinitrate P.O., 5 to 6 hours; S.L., 2 hours; mononitrate, about 5 hours.

ADVERSE REACTIONS
CNS: *headache,* dizziness, weakness.
CV: *orthostatic hypotension, tachycardia, palpitations, ankle edema, flushing,* fainting.
EENT: S.L. burning.
GI: nausea, vomiting.
Skin: cutaneous vasodilation, rash.

INTERACTIONS
Drug-drug. *Antihypertensives:* May increase hypotensive effects. Monitor patient closely during initial therapy.
Sildenafil, tadalafil, vardenafil: May cause severe hypotension. Use of nitrates in any form with these drugs is contraindicated.
Drug-lifestyle. *Alcohol use:* May increase hypotension. Discourage use together.

EFFECTS ON LAB TEST RESULTS
• May cause falsely reduced value in cholesterol tests using the Zlatkis-Zak color reaction.

CONTRAINDICATIONS & CAUTIONS
• Contraindicated in patients with hypersensitivity or idiosyncrasy to nitrates and in those with severe hypotension, angle-closure glaucoma, increased intracranial pressure, shock, or acute MI with low left ventricular filling pressure.
• Use cautiously in patients with blood volume depletion (such as from diuretic therapy) or mild hypotension.

NURSING CONSIDERATIONS
• To prevent tolerance, a nitrate-free interval of 10 to 14 hours per day is recommended. The regimen for isosorbide mononitrate (1 tablet on awakening with the second dose in 7 hours, or 1 extended-release tablet daily) is intended to minimize nitrate tolerance by providing a substantial nitrate-free interval.

• Monitor blood pressure and intensity and duration of drug response.
• Drug may cause headaches, especially at beginning of therapy. Dosage may be reduced temporarily, but tolerance usually develops. Treat headache with aspirin or acetaminophen.
• Methemoglobinemia has been seen with nitrates. Symptoms are those of impaired oxygen delivery despite adequate cardiac output and adequate arterial partial pressure of oxygen.
• ***Look alike–sound alike:*** Don't confuse Isordil with Isuprel or Inderal.

PATIENT TEACHING
• Caution patient to take drug regularly, as prescribed, and to keep it accessible at all times.
• ***Alert:*** Advise patient that stopping drug abruptly may cause spasm of the coronary arteries with increased angina symptoms and potential risk of heart attack.
• Tell patient to take S.L. tablet at first sign of attack. He should wet tablet with saliva and place under his tongue until absorbed; he should sit down and rest. Dose may be repeated every 10 to 15 minutes for a maximum of three doses. If drug doesn't provide relief, tell patient to seek medical help promptly.
• Advise patient who complains of tingling sensation with S.L. drug to try holding tablet in cheek.
• Warn patient not to confuse S.L. with P.O. form.
• Advise patient taking P.O. form of isosorbide dinitrate to take oral tablet on an empty stomach either 30 minutes before or 1 to 2 hours after meals and to swallow oral tablets whole.
• Tell patient to minimize dizziness upon standing up by changing to upright position slowly. Advise him to go up and down stairs carefully and to lie down at first sign of dizziness.
• Caution patient to avoid alcohol because it may worsen low blood pressure effects.
• Advise patient that use of sildenafil, tadalafil, or vardenafil with any nitrate may cause severe low blood pressure. Patient should talk to his prescriber before using these drugs together.
• Instruct patient to store drug in a cool place, in a tightly closed container, and away from light.

nadolol
Corgard

Pharmacologic class: nonselective beta blocker
Pregnancy risk category C

AVAILABLE FORMS
Tablets: 20 mg, 40 mg, 80 mg, 120 mg, 160 mg

INDICATIONS & DOSAGES
➤Angina pectoris
Adults: 40 mg P.O. once daily. Increase in 40- to 80-mg increments at 3- to 7-day intervals until optimal response occurs. Usual maintenance dose is 40 to 80 mg once daily; up to 240 mg once daily may be needed.
➤Hypertension
Adults: 40 mg P.O. once daily. Increase in 40- to 80-mg increments until optimal response occurs. Usual maintenance dose is 40 to 80 mg once daily. Doses of 320 mg may be needed.
Adjust-a-dose: If creatinine clearance is 31 to 50 ml/minute, change dosing interval to q 24 to 36 hours; if clearance is 10 to 30 ml/minute, q 24 to 48 hours; and if clearance is less than 10 ml/minute, q 40 to 60 hours.

ACTION
A nonselective beta blocker that reduces cardiac oxygen demand by blocking catecholamine-induced increases in heart rate, blood pressure, and force of myocardial contraction. Depresses renin secretion.

Route	Onset	Peak	Duration
P.O.	Unknown	2–4 hr	Unknown

Half-life: About 10 to 24 hours.

ADVERSE REACTIONS
CNS: fatigue, dizziness, fever.
CV: BRADYCARDIA, HEART FAILURE, *hypotension,* peripheral vascular disease, rhythm and conduction disturbances.

GI: nausea, vomiting, diarrhea, abdominal pain, constipation, anorexia.
Respiratory: *increased airway resistance.*
Skin: rash.

INTERACTIONS

Drug-drug. *Antihypertensives:* May increase antihypertensive effect. Monitor blood pressure closely.
Cardiac glycosides: May cause excessive bradycardia and additive effects on AV conduction. Use together cautiously.
Epinephrine: May decrease the patient response to epinephrine for treatment of an allergic reaction. Monitor patient closely for decreased clinical effect.
General anesthetics: May increase hypotensive effects. Consider stopping nadolol before surgery.
Insulin: May mask symptoms of hypoglycemia, as a result of beta blockade (such as tachycardia). Use with caution in patients with diabetes.
I.V. lidocaine: May reduce hepatic metabolism of lidocaine, increasing the risk of toxicity. Give bolus doses of lidocaine at a slower rate and monitor lidocaine level closely.
NSAIDs: May decrease antihypertensive effect. Monitor blood pressure and adjust dosage.
Oral antidiabetics: May alter dosage requirements in previously stabilized diabetic patients. Monitor glucose closely.
Phenothiazines: May increase hypotensive effects. Monitor blood pressure.
Prazosin: May increase risk of orthostatic hypotension in the early phases of use together. Assist patient to stand slowly until effects are known.
Reserpine: May increase hypotension or bradycardia. Monitor patient for adverse effects, such as dizziness, syncope, and postural hypotension.
Verapamil: May increase effects of both drugs. Monitor cardiac function closely and decrease dosages as necessary.

EFFECTS ON LAB TEST RESULTS

None reported.

CONTRAINDICATIONS & CAUTIONS

- Contraindicated in patients with bronchial asthma, sinus bradycardia and greater than first-degree heart block, cardiogenic shock, and overt heart failure.
- Use cautiously in patients with heart failure, chronic bronchitis, emphysema, or renal or hepatic impairment and in patients undergoing major surgery involving general anesthesia.
- Use cautiously in diabetic patients because beta blockers may mask certain signs and symptoms of hypoglycemia.

NURSING CONSIDERATIONS

- Check apical pulse before giving drug. If slower than 60 beats/minute, withhold drug and call prescriber.
- Monitor blood pressure frequently. If patient develops severe hypotension, give a vasopressor, as prescribed.
- ***Alert:*** Abrupt stoppage can worsen angina and cause an MI. Reduce dosage gradually over 1 to 2 weeks.
- Drug masks signs and symptoms of shock and hyperthyroidism.

PATIENT TEACHING

- Explain importance of taking drug as prescribed, even when patient is feeling well.
- Teach patient how to check pulse rate and tell him to check it before each dose. If pulse rate is below 60 beats/minute, tell patient to notify prescriber.
- Warn patient not to stop drug suddenly.

nicardipine hydrochloride

Cardene, Cardene I.V, Cardene SR

Pharmacologic class: calcium channel blocker
Pregnancy risk category C

AVAILABLE FORMS

Capsules: 20 mg, 30 mg
Capsules (sustained-release): 30 mg, 45 mg, 60 mg
Injection: 2.5 mg/ml

INDICATIONS & DOSAGES

➤ **Chronic stable angina (used alone or with other antianginals)**
Adults: Initially, 20 mg immediate-release capsule P.O. t.i.d. Adjust dosage based

on patient response q 3 days. Usual range, 20 to 40 mg t.i.d.

➤ **Hypertension**

Adults: Initially, 20 mg immediate-release capsule P.O. t.i.d.; range, 20 to 40 mg t.i.d. Or, 30 mg sustained-release capsule b.i.d.; range, 30 to 60 mg b.i.d. Increase dosage based on patient response. Or, for patient who can't take oral form, 5 mg/hour (50 ml/hour) I.V. infusion initially; then, increase by 2.5 mg/hour (25 ml/hour) q 15 minutes to maximum of 15 mg/hour (150 ml/hour).

I.V. ADMINISTRATION

- Dilute to a concentration of 0.1 mg/ml with D_5W, dextrose 5% in normal saline solution or half-normal saline solution, and normal saline solution or half-normal saline solution.
- Give by slow infusion.
- Closely monitor blood pressure during and after completion of infusion.
- If hypotension or tachycardia occurs, titrate infusion rate.
- Change peripheral infusion site every 12 hours to minimize risk of venous irritation.
- When switching to oral form, give first dose of t.i.d. regimen 1 hour before stopping infusion. If also using a different oral drug, start it when infusion ends.
- If solution is kept at room temperature, use within 24 hours.

INCOMPATIBILITIES

Ampicillin sodium, ampicillin and sulbactam sodium, cefoperazone, ceftazidime, furosemide, heparin sodium, lactated Ringer's solution, sodium bicarbonate, thiopental.

ACTION

A calcium channel blocker that inhibits calcium ion influx across cardiac and smooth muscle cells but is more selective to vascular smooth muscle than cardiac muscle. Also dilates coronary arteries and arterioles.

Route	Onset	Peak	Duration
P.O. (immediate-release)	20 min	1–2 hr	Unknown
P.O. (sustained-release)	20 min	1–4 hr	12 hr
I.V.	Immediate	Immediate	Unknown

Half-life: 2 to 4 hours.

ADVERSE REACTIONS

CNS: *headache,* dizziness, light-headedness, asthenia.
CV: *peripheral edema, palpitations, flushing,* angina, tachycardia.
GI: nausea, abdominal discomfort, dry mouth.
Skin: rash.

INTERACTIONS

Drug-drug. *Antihypertensives:* May increase antihypertensive effect. Monitor blood pressure closely.
Cimetidine: May decrease metabolism of calcium channel blockers. Monitor patient for increased pharmacologic effect.
Cyclosporine: May increase plasma level of cyclosporine. Monitor patient for toxicity.

EFFECTS ON LAB TEST RESULTS

None reported.

CONTRAINDICATIONS & CAUTIONS

- Contraindicated in patients hypersensitive to drug and in those with advanced aortic stenosis.
- Use cautiously in patients with hypotension, heart failure, or impaired hepatic and renal function.

NURSING CONSIDERATIONS

- Measure blood pressure frequently during initial therapy. Maximal response occurs about 1 hour after giving the immediate-release form and 2 to 4 hours after giving the sustained-release form. Check for orthostatic hypotension. Because large swings in blood pressure may occur based on drug level, assess antihypertensive effect 8 hours after dosing.
- Extended-release form is preferred because of improved compliance, fewer fluc-

tuations in blood pressure, and less risk of death than with shorter-acting drugs.
• ***Look alike–sound alike:*** Don't confuse Cardene with Cardura or codeine.

PATIENT TEACHING
• Tell patient to take oral form exactly as prescribed.
• Advise patient to report chest pain immediately. Some patients may experience increased frequency, severity, or duration of chest pain at beginning of therapy or during dosage adjustments.
• Inform patient to get up from a sitting or lying position slowly to avoid dizziness caused by a decrease in blood pressure.

nifedipine
Adalat CC, Apo-Nifed†, Nifedical XL, Novo-Nifedin†, Nu-Nifedin†, Procardia XL

Pharmacologic class: calcium channel blocker
Pregnancy risk category C

AVAILABLE FORMS
Capsules: 10 mg, 20 mg
Tablets (extended-release): 30 mg, 60 mg, 90 mg

INDICATIONS & DOSAGES
➤ Vasospastic angina (Prinzmetal or variant angina), classic chronic stable angina pectoris
Adults: Initially, 10 mg short-acting capsule P.O. t.i.d. Usual effective dosage range is 10 to 20 mg t.i.d. Some patients may require up to 30 mg q.i.d. Maximum daily dose is 180 mg. Adjust dosage over 7 to 14 days to evaluate response. Or, 30 to 60 mg (extended-release tablets, except Adalat CC) P.O. once daily. Maximum daily dose is 120 mg. Adjust dosage over 7 to 14 days to evaluate response.
➤ Hypertension
Adults: 30 or 60 mg P.O. extended-release tablet once daily. Adjusted over 7 to 14 days. Doses larger than 90 mg (Adalat CC) and 120 mg (Procardia XL) aren't recommended.

ACTION
Thought to inhibit calcium ion influx across cardiac and smooth muscle cells, decreasing contractility and oxygen demand. Also may dilate coronary arteries and arterioles.

Route	Onset	Peak	Duration
P.O.	20 min	30–60 min	4–8 hr
P.O. (extended)	20 min	6 hr	24 hr

Half-life: 2 to 5 hours.

ADVERSE REACTIONS
CNS: *dizziness, light-headedness, headache, weakness,* somnolence, syncope, nervousness.
CV: *flushing, peripheral edema,* ***heart failure, MI,*** hypotension, palpitations.
EENT: nasal congestion.
GI: *nausea,* diarrhea, constipation, abdominal discomfort.
Musculoskeletal: muscle cramps.
Respiratory: dyspnea, pulmonary edema, cough.
Skin: rash, pruritus.

INTERACTIONS
Drug-drug. *Antiretrovirals, verapamil, cimetidine:* May decrease nifedipine metabolism. Monitor blood pressure closely and adjust nifedipine dosage as needed.
Azole antifungals, erythromycin, quinupristin and dalfopristin: May increase the effects of nifedipine. Monitor blood pressure closely and decrease nifedipine dosage as needed.
Digoxin: May cause elevated digoxin level. Monitor digoxin level.
Diltiazem: May increase the effects of nifedipine. Monitor patient closely.
Fentanyl: May cause severe hypotension. Monitor blood pressure.
Phenytoin: May reduce phenytoin metabolism. Monitor phenytoin level.
Propranolol, other beta blockers: May cause hypotension and heart failure. Use together cautiously.
Quinidine: May decrease levels and effects of quinidine while increasing effects of nifedipine. Monitor heart rate and adjust nifedipine dose as needed.
Rifamycins: May decrease nifedipine levels. Monitor patient.

Tacrolimus: May increase tacrolimus levels and risk for toxicity. Decrease tacrolimus dose as needed.
Drug-herb. *Ginkgo:* May increase effects of drug. Discourage use together.
Ginseng: May increase drug levels with possible toxicity. Discourage use together.
Melatonin, St. John's wort: May interfere with antihypertensive effect. Discourage use together.
Drug-food. *Grapefruit juice:* May increase bioavailability of drug. Discourage use together.

EFFECTS ON LAB TEST RESULTS

- May increase ALT, AST, alkaline phosphatase, and LDH levels.

CONTRAINDICATIONS & CAUTIONS

- Contraindicated in patients hypersensitive to drug.
- Use cautiously in patients with heart failure or hypotension and in elderly patients. Use extended-release tablets cautiously in patients with severe GI narrowing.

NURSING CONSIDERATIONS

- Don't give immediate-release capsules within 1 week of acute MI or in acute coronary syndrome.
- ***Alert:*** Don't use capsules S.L. to rapidly reduce severe high blood pressure because the result may be fatal.
- Monitor blood pressure regularly, especially in patients who take beta blockers or antihypertensives.
- Watch for symptoms of heart failure.
- ***Look alike–sound alike:*** Don't confuse nifedipine with nimodipine or nicardipine.

PATIENT TEACHING

- If patient is kept on nitrate therapy while nifedipine dosage is being adjusted, urge continued compliance. Patient may take S.L. nitroglycerin, as needed, for acute chest pain.
- Tell patient that chest pain may worsen briefly as therapy starts or dosage increases.
- Instruct patient to swallow extended-release tablets without breaking, crushing, or chewing them.
- Advise patient to avoid taking drug with grapefruit juice.
- Reassure patient taking the extended-release tablet that the wax mold may be passed in the stools. Assure him that drug has already been completely absorbed.
- Tell patient to protect capsules from direct light and moisture and to store at room temperature.

SAFETY ALERT!

nitroglycerin (glyceryl trinitrate)

Anginine‡, Deponit, Minitran, Nitradisc‡, Nitrek, Nitro-Bid, Nitro-Bid IV, Nitrodisc, Nitro-Dur, Nitrogard, Nitroglyn, Nitrolingual, Nitrong, NitroQuick, Nitrostat✐, NitroTab, Nitro-Time, NTS, Transderm-Nitro, Transiderm-Nitro‡, Tridil

Pharmacologic class: nitrate
Pregnancy risk category C

AVAILABLE FORMS

Aerosol (translingual): 0.4 mg/metered spray
Capsules (sustained-release): 2.5 mg, 6.5 mg, 9 mg,
Injection: 5 mg/ml; 100 mcg/ml, 200 mcg/ml, 400 mcg/ml
Tablets (S.L.): 0.3 mg (1/200 grain), 0.4 mg (1/150 grain), 0.6 mg (1/100 grain)
Tablets (sustained-release): 2.6 mg, 6.5 mg, 9 mg, 13 mg
Topical: 2% ointment
Transdermal: 0.1 mg/hour, 0.2 mg/hour, 0.3 mg/hour, 0.4 mg/hour, 0.6 mg/hour, 0.8 mg/hour release rate

INDICATIONS & DOSAGES

➤To prevent chronic anginal attacks

Adults: 2.5 or 2.6 mg sustained-release capsule or tablet q 8 to 12 hours. Increase to an effective dose in 2.5- or 2.6-mg increments b.i.d. to q.i.d. Or, use 2% ointment: Start dosage with ½-inch ointment, increasing by ½-inch increments until desired results are achieved. Range of dosage with ointment is ½ to 5 inches. Usual dose is 1 to 2 inches q 6 to 8 hours. Or, transdermal disc or pad (Nitrodisc, Nitro-

Dur, or Transderm-Nitro) 0.2 to 0.4 mg/hour once daily.

➤ **Acute angina pectoris; to prevent or minimize anginal attacks before stressful events**
Adults: 1 S.L. tablet (1/400 grain, 1/200 grain, 1/150 grain, 1/100 grain) dissolved under the tongue or in the buccal pouch as soon as angina begins. Repeat q 5 minutes, if needed, for 15 minutes. Or, one or two sprays Nitrolingual into mouth, preferably onto or under the tongue. Repeat q 3 to 5 minutes, if needed, to a maximum of three doses within a 15-minute period. Or, 1 to 3 mg transmucosally q 3 to 5 hours while awake.

➤ **Hypertension from surgery, heart failure after MI, angina pectoris in acute situations, to produce controlled hypotension during surgery (by I.V. infusion)**
Adults: Initially, infuse at 5 mcg/minute, increasing p.r.n. by 5 mcg/minute q 3 to 5 minutes until response occurs. If a 20-mcg/minute rate doesn't produce a response, increase dosage by as much as 20 mcg/minute q 3 to 5 minutes. Up to 100 mcg/minute may be needed.

I.V. ADMINISTRATION

- Dilute with D_5W or normal saline solution for injection. Concentration shouldn't exceed 400 mcg/ml.
- Always give with an infusion control device and titrate to desired response.
- Regular polyvinyl chloride tubing can bind up to 80% of drug, making it necessary to infuse higher dosages. A special nonabsorbent polyvinyl chloride tubing is available from the manufacturer. Always mix in glass bottles and avoid using a filter.
- Use the same type of infusion set when changing lines.
- When changing the concentration of infusion, flush the administration set with 15 to 20 ml of the new concentration before use. This will clear the line of the old drug solution.

INCOMPATIBILITIES

Alteplase, bretylium, hydralazine, levofloxacin, phenytoin sodium.

ACTION

A nitrate that reduces cardiac oxygen demand by decreasing left ventricular end-diastolic pressure (preload) and, to a lesser extent, systemic vascular resistance (afterload). Also increases blood flow through the collateral coronary vessels.

Route	Onset	Peak	Duration
P.O.	20–45 min	Unknown	3–8 hr
I.V.	Immediate	Immediate	3–5 min
Topical	30 min	Unknown	2–12 hr
Transdermal	30 min	Unknown	24 hr
S.L.	1–3 min	Unknown	30–60 min
Buccal	3 min	Unknown	3–5 hr
Translingual	2–4 min	Unknown	30–60 min

Half-life: About 1 to 4 minutes.

ADVERSE REACTIONS

CNS: *headache, dizziness,* weakness.
CV: *orthostatic hypotension, tachycardia, flushing, palpitations,* fainting.
EENT: S.L. burning.
GI: nausea, vomiting.
Skin: cutaneous vasodilation, contact dermatitis, rash.
Other: hypersensitivity reactions.

INTERACTIONS

Drug-drug. *Alteplase:* May decrease tissue plasminogen activator-antigen level. Avoid using together; if unavoidable, use lowest effective dose of nitroglycerin.
Antihypertensives: May increase hypotensive effect. Monitor blood pressure closely.
Heparin: I.V. nitroglycerin may interfere with anticoagulant effect of heparin. Monitor PTT.
Sildenafil, tadalafil, vardenafil: May cause severe hypotension. Use of nitrates in any form with these drugs is contraindicated.
Drug-lifestyle. *Alcohol use:* May increase hypotension. Discourage use together.

EFFECTS ON LAB TEST RESULTS

- May falsely decrease values in cholesterol determination tests using the Zlatkis-Zak color reaction.

CONTRAINDICATIONS & CAUTIONS

- Contraindicated in patients with early MI (oral and sublingual), severe anemia, increased intracranial pressure, angle-closure glaucoma, orthostatic hypotension, allergy to adhesives (transdermal), or hypersensitivity to nitrates. I.V. nitroglycerin is contraindicated in patients hypersensitive to I.V. form, with cardiac tamponade, restrictive cardiomyopathy, or constrictive pericarditis.
- Use cautiously in patients with hypotension or volume depletion.

NURSING CONSIDERATIONS

- Closely monitor vital signs during infusion, particularly blood pressure, especially in a patient with an MI. Excessive hypotension may worsen the MI.
- To apply ointment, measure the prescribed amount on the application paper; then place the paper on any nonhairy area. Don't rub in. Cover with plastic film to aid absorption and to protect clothing. Remove all excess ointment from previous site before applying the next dose. Avoid getting ointment on fingers.
- Transdermal dosage forms can be applied to any nonhairy part of the skin except distal parts of the arms or legs. (Absorption won't be maximal at distal sites.) Patch may cause contact dermatitis.
- Remove transdermal patch before defibrillation. Because of the aluminum backing on the patch, the electric current may cause arcing that can damage the paddles and burn the patient.
- When stopping transdermal treatment of angina, gradually reduce the dosage and frequency of application over 4 to 6 weeks.
- Monitor blood pressure and intensity and duration of drug response.
- Drug may cause headaches, especially at beginning of therapy. Dosage may be reduced temporarily, but tolerance usually develops. Treat headache with aspirin or acetaminophen.
- Tolerance to drug can be minimized with a 10- to 12-hour nitrate-free interval. To achieve this, remove the transdermal system in the early evening and apply a new system the next morning or omit the last daily dose of a buccal, sustained-release, or ointment form. Check with the prescriber for alterations in dosage regimen if tolerance is suspected.
- ***Look alike–sound alike:*** Don't confuse Nitro-Bid with Nicobid or nitroglycerin with nitroprusside.

PATIENT TEACHING

- Caution patient to take nitroglycerin regularly, as prescribed, and to have it accessible at all times.
- ***Alert:*** Advise patient that stopping drug abruptly causes spasm of the coronary arteries.
- Teach patient how to give the prescribed form of nitroglycerin.
- Tell patient to take S.L. tablet at first sign of attack. Patient should wet the tablet with saliva and place under the tongue until absorbed; he should sit down and rest. Dose may be repeated every 5 minutes for a maximum of three doses. If drug doesn't provide relief, he should obtain medical help promptly.
- Advise patient who complains of a tingling sensation with S.L. drug to try holding tablet in cheek.
- Tell patient to take oral tablets on an empty stomach either 30 minutes before or 1 to 2 hours after meals, to swallow oral tablets whole, and not to chew tablets.
- Remind patient using translingual aerosol form that he shouldn't inhale the spray, but should release it onto or under the tongue. Tell him to wait about 10 seconds or so before swallowing.
- Tell patient to place the buccal tablet between the lip and gum above the incisors or between the cheek and gum. Tablets shouldn't be swallowed or chewed.
- Tell patient to take an additional dose before anticipated stress or at bedtime if chest pain occurs at night.
- Urge patient using skin patches to dispose of them carefully because enough medication remains after normal use to be hazardous to children and pets.
- Advise patient to avoid alcohol.
- To minimize dizziness when standing up, tell patient to rise slowly. Advise him to go up and down stairs carefully and to lie down at the first sign of dizziness.
- Advise patient that use of sildenafil, tadalafil, or vardenafil with any nitrate may cause severe low blood pressure. The pa-

tient should talk to his prescriber before considering use of these drugs together.
• Tell patient to store drug in cool, dark place in a tightly closed container. Tell him to remove cotton from container because it absorbs drug.
• Tell patient to store S.L. tablets in original container or other container specifically approved for this use and to carry the container in a jacket pocket or purse, not in a pocket close to the body.

SAFETY ALERT!

propranolol hydrochloride
Apo-Propranolol†, Deralin‡, Inderal, Inderal LA, InnoPran XL, Novopranol†, pms Propranolol†

Pharmacologic class: beta blocker
Pregnancy risk category C

AVAILABLE FORMS
Capsules (extended-release): 60 mg, 80 mg, 120 mg, 160 mg
Injection: 1 mg/ml
Oral solution: 4 mg/ml, 8 mg/ml, 80 mg/ml (concentrate)
Tablets: 10 mg, 20 mg, 40 mg, 60 mg, 80 mg, 90 mg

INDICATIONS & DOSAGES
➤ **Angina pectoris**
Adults: Total daily doses of 80 to 320 mg P.O. when given b.i.d., t.i.d., or q.i.d. Or, one 80-mg extended-release capsule daily. Dosage increased at 3- to 7-day intervals.
➤ **To decrease risk of death after MI**
Adults: 180 to 240 mg P.O. daily in divided doses beginning 5 to 21 days after MI has occurred. Usually given t.i.d. or q.i.d.
➤ **Supraventricular, ventricular, and atrial arrhythmias; tachyarrhythmias caused by excessive catecholamine action during anesthesia, hyperthyroidism, or pheochromocytoma**
Adults: 1 to 3 mg by slow I.V. push, not to exceed 1 mg/minute. After 3 mg have been given, another dose may be given in 2 minutes; subsequent doses, no sooner than q 4 hours. Usual maintenance dose is 10 to 30 mg P.O. t.i.d. or q.i.d.
➤ **Hypertension**
Adults: Initially, 80 mg P.O. daily in two divided doses or extended-release form once daily. Increase at 3- to 7-day intervals to maximum daily dose of 640 mg. Usual maintenance dose is 120 to 240 mg daily or 120 to 160 mg daily as extended-release. For InnoPran XL, dose is 80 mg P.O. once daily at bedtime. Give consistently with or without food. Adjust to maximum of 120 mg daily if needed. Full effects are seen in about 2 to 3 weeks.
Children: 0.5 mg/kg (conventional tablets) P.O. b.i.d. Increase q 3 to 5 days to a maximum dose of 16 mg/kg daily. Usual dose is 2 to 4 mg/kg daily in two equally divided doses.
➤ **To prevent frequent, severe, uncontrollable, or disabling migraine or vascular headache**
Adults: Initially, 80 mg P.O. daily in divided doses or 1 extended-release capsule daily. Usual maintenance dose is 160 to 240 mg daily, t.i.d. or q.i.d.
➤ **Essential tremor**
Adults: 40 mg (tablets or oral solution) P.O. b.i.d. Usual maintenance dose is 120 to 320 mg daily in three divided doses.
➤ **Hypertrophic subaortic stenosis**
Adults: 20 to 40 mg P.O. t.i.d. or q.i.d.; or 80 to 160 mg extended-release capsules once daily.
➤ **Adjunct therapy in pheochromocytoma**
Adults: 60 mg P.O. daily in divided doses with an alpha blocker 3 days before surgery.

I.V. ADMINISTRATION
• For direct injection, give into a large vessel or into the tubing of a free-flowing, compatible I.V. solution; don't give by continuous I.V. infusion.
• Drug is compatible with D_5W, half-normal saline solution, normal saline solution, and lactated Ringer's solution.
• Infusion rate shouldn't exceed 1 mg/minute.
• Double-check dose and route. I.V. doses are much smaller than oral doses.
• Monitor blood pressure, ECG, central venous pressure, and heart rate and

rhythm frequently, especially during I.V. administration. If patient develops severe hypotension, notify prescriber; a vasopressor may be prescribed.
• For overdose, give I.V. isoproterenol, I.V. atropine, or glucagon; refractory cases may require a pacemaker.

INCOMPATIBILITIES

Amphotericin B, diazoxide.

ACTION

A nonselective beta blocker that reduces cardiac oxygen demand by blocking catecholamine-induced increases in heart rate, blood pressure, and force of myocardial contraction. Depresses renin secretion and prevents vasodilation of cerebral arteries.

Route	Onset	Peak	Duration
P.O.	30 min	60–90 min	12 hr
P.O. (extended)	Unknown	6–14 hr	24 hr
I.V.	Immediate	1 min	5 min

Half-life: About 4 hours; 8 hours for InnoPran XL.

ADVERSE REACTIONS

CNS: *fatigue, lethargy,* fever, vivid dreams, hallucinations, mental depression, light-headedness, dizziness, insomnia.
CV: *hypotension,* ***bradycardia, heart failure, intensification of AV block,*** intermittent claudication.
GI: abdominal cramping, constipation, diarrhea, nausea, vomiting.
Hematologic: ***agranulocytosis.***
Respiratory: ***bronchospasm.***
Skin: rash.

INTERACTIONS

Drug-drug. *Aminophylline:* May antagonize beta-blocking effects of propranolol. Use together cautiously.
Cardiac glycosides: May reduce the positive inotrope effect of the glycoside. Monitor patient for clinical effect.
Cimetidine: May inhibit metabolism of propranolol. Watch for increased beta-blocking effect.
Diltiazem, verapamil: May cause hypotension, bradycardia, and increased depressant effect on myocardium. Use together cautiously.
Epinephrine: May cause severe vasoconstriction. Monitor blood pressure and observe patient carefully.
Glucagon, isoproterenol: May antagonize propranolol effect. May be used therapeutically and in emergencies.
Haloperidol: May cause cardiac arrest. Avoid using together.
Insulin, oral antidiabetics: May alter requirements for these drugs in previously stabilized diabetics. Monitor patient for hypoglycemia.
Phenothiazines (chlorpromazine, thioridazine): May increase risk of serious adverse reactions of either drug. Use with thioridazine is contraindicated. If chlorpromazine must be used, monitor patient's pulse and blood pressure; decrease propranolol dose as needed.
Propafenone: May increase propranolol level. Monitor cardiac function, and adjust propranolol dose as needed.
Drug-herb. *Betel palm:* May decrease temperature-elevating effects and enhanced CNS effects. Discourage use together.
Ma huang: May decrease antihypertensive effects. Discourage use together.
Drug-lifestyle. *Cocaine use:* May increase angina-inducing potential of cocaine. Inform patient of this interaction.

EFFECTS ON LAB TEST RESULTS

• May increase BUN, transaminase, alkaline phosphatase, and LDH levels.
• May decrease granulocyte count.
• May alter thyroid function tests, increasing T_4 and reverse T_3 and decreasing T_3.

CONTRAINDICATIONS & CAUTIONS

• Contraindicated in patients with bronchial asthma, sinus bradycardia and heart block greater than first-degree, cardiogenic shock, and overt and decompensated heart failure (unless failure is secondary to a tachyarrhythmia that can be treated with propranolol).
• Use cautiously in patients with hepatic or renal impairment, nonallergic bronchospastic diseases, or hepatic disease and in those taking other antihypertensives.

• Because drug blocks some symptoms of hypoglycemia, use cautiously in patients who have diabetes mellitus.
• In patients with thyrotoxicosis, use drug cautiously because it may mask the signs and symptoms.
• Elderly patients may experience enhanced adverse reactions and may need dosage adjustment.

NURSING CONSIDERATIONS

• Always check patient's apical pulse before giving drug. If extremes in pulse rates occur, withhold drug and notify prescriber immediately.
• Give drug consistently with meals. Food may increase absorption of propranolol.
• Drug masks common signs and symptoms of shock and hypoglycemia.
• ***Alert:*** Don't stop drug before surgery for pheochromocytoma. Before any surgical procedure, tell anesthesiologist that patient is receiving propranolol.
• Compliance may be improved by giving drug twice daily or as extended-release capsules. Check with prescriber.
• ***Look alike–sound alike:*** Don't confuse propranolol with Pravachol. Don't confuse Inderal with Inderide, Isordil, Adderall, or Imuran.

PATIENT TEACHING

• Caution patient to continue taking this drug as prescribed, even when he's feeling well.
• Instruct patient to take drug with food.
• ***Alert:*** Tell patient not to stop drug suddenly because this can worsen chest pain and trigger a heart attack.

✱ NEW DRUG

ranolazine
Ranexa

Pharmacologic class: CV drug
Pregnancy risk category C

AVAILABLE FORMS

Tablets (extended-release): 500 mg

INDICATIONS & DOSAGES

➤ **Chronic angina, given with amlodipine, beta blockers, or nitrates, in patients who haven't achieved an adequate response with other antianginals**
Adults: Initially, 500 mg P.O. b.i.d. Increase, if needed, to maximum of 1,000 mg b.i.d.

ACTION

May result from increased efficiency of myocardial oxygen use when myocardial metabolism is shifted away from fatty acid oxidation toward glucose oxidation. Antianginal and anti-ischemic properties don't decrease heart rate or blood pressure and don't increase myocardial work.

Route	Onset	Peak	Duration
P.O.	Rapid	2–5 hr	Unknown

Half-life: 7 hours.

ADVERSE REACTIONS

CNS: dizziness, headache.
CV: palpitations, peripheral edema, syncope.
EENT: tinnitus, vertigo.
GI: abdominal pain, constipation, dry mouth, nausea, vomiting.
Respiratory: dyspnea.

INTERACTIONS

Drug-drug. *Antipsychotics or tricyclic antidepressants metabolized by CYP2D6:* May increase levels of these drugs. Dosage reduction may be needed.
Cyclosporine, paroxetine, ritonavir: May increase ranolazine level. Use cautiously together, and monitor patient for increased adverse effects.
Digoxin: May increase digoxin level. Monitor digoxin level periodically; digoxin dosage may need to be reduced .
Diltiazem, HIV protease inhibitors, macrolide antibiotics (azithromycin, erythromycin), verapamil: May increase ranolazine level and prolong QT interval. Avoid use together.
Drugs that prolong the QT interval (antiarrhythmics such as dofetilide, quinidine, and sotalol), antipsychotics, such as Thorazine and ziprasidone: May increase the risk of prolonged QT interval. Avoid use together.
Potent CYP3A inhibitors such as ketoconazole: May increase ranolazine level. Use together is contraindicated.

Simvastatin: May increase simvastatin level. Monitor patient for adverse effects, and decrease simvastatin dosage as needed.
Drug-food. *Grapefruit:* May increase drug level and prolong QT interval. Avoid use together.

EFFECTS ON LAB TEST RESULTS
- May increase creatinine and BUN levels. May decrease hemoglobin level and hematocrit.
- May decrease eosinophil count.

CONTRAINDICATIONS & CAUTIONS
- Contraindicated in patients taking QT interval-prolonging drugs or CYP3A inhibitors (including diltiazem), and in patients with ventricular tachycardia, hepatic impairment, or a prolonged QT interval.
- Use cautiously in patients with renal impairment.

NURSING CONSIDERATIONS
- ***Alert:*** Drug prolongs the QT interval according to the dose. If drug is given with other drugs that prolong the QTc interval, torsades de pointes or sudden death may occur. Don't exceed maximum dosage.
- Monitor ECG for prolonged QT interval and measure the QTc interval regularly.
- If patient has renal insufficiency, monitor blood pressure closely.
- Drug may be taken without regard to meals.
- Don't crush or cut tablets.

PATIENT TEACHING
- Educate patient about this drug's potential to affect the heart's rhythm. Advise patient to immediately report palpitations or fainting.
- Urge patient to tell prescriber about all other prescription or OTC drugs or herbal supplements he takes.
- Tell patient that he should keep taking other drugs prescribed for angina.
- Tell patient that drug may be taken with or without food.
- Advise patient to avoid grapefruit juice while taking this drug.
- ***Alert:*** Warn patient that tablets must be swallowed whole and not crushed, broken, or chewed.
- Explain that drug won't stop a sudden anginal attack; advise him to keep other treatments, such as sublingual nitroglycerin, readily available.
- Tell patient to avoid activities that require mental alertness until effects of the drug are known.

verapamil hydrochloride

Anpec‡, Anpec SR‡, Apo-Verap†, Calan✐, Calan SR, Cordilox‡, Cordilox SR‡, Covera-HS, Isoptin‡, Isoptin SR✐, Novo-Veramil†, Nu-Verap†, Veracaps SR‡, Verahexal‡, Verelan✐, Verelan PM

Pharmacologic class: calcium channel blocker
Pregnancy risk category C

AVAILABLE FORMS
Capsules (extended-release): 100 mg, 120 mg, 180 mg, 200 mg, 240 mg, 300 mg
Capsules (sustained-release): 120 mg, 160 mg‡, 180 mg, 240 mg, 360 mg
Injection: 2.5 mg/ml
Tablets: 40 mg, 80 mg, 120 mg, 160 mg‡
Tablets (extended-release): 120 mg, 180 mg, 240 mg
Tablets (sustained-release): 120 mg, 180 mg, 240 mg

INDICATIONS & DOSAGES
➤ **Vasospastic angina (Prinzmetal's or variant angina); classic chronic, stable angina pectoris; chronic atrial fibrillation**
Adults: Starting dose is 80 to 120 mg P.O. t.i.d. Increase dosage at daily or weekly intervals, p.r.n. Some patients may require up to 480 mg daily.
➤ **To prevent paroxysmal supraventricular tachycardia**
Adults: 80 to 120 mg P.O. t.i.d. or q.i.d.
➤ **Supraventricular arrhythmias**
Adults: 0.075 to 0.15 mg/kg (5 to 10 mg) by I.V. push over 2 minutes with ECG and blood pressure monitoring. Repeat dose

of 0.15 mg/kg (10 mg) in 30 minutes if no response occurs.
Children ages 1 to 15: 0.1 to 0.3 mg/kg as I.V. bolus over 2 minutes; not to exceed 5 mg. Repeat dose in 30 minutes if response is inadequate.
Children younger than age 1: 0.1 to 0.2 mg/kg as I.V. bolus over 2 minutes with continuous ECG monitoring. Repeat dose in 30 minutes if no response occurs.

➤ **Digitalized patients with chronic atrial fibrillation or flutter**
Adults: 240 to 320 mg P.O. daily, divided t.i.d. or q.i.d.

➤ **Hypertension**
Adults: 240 mg extended-release tablet P.O. once daily in the morning. If response isn't adequate, give an additional 120 mg in the evening or 240 mg q 12 hours, or an 80-mg immediate-release tablet t.i.d. If using Verelan PM, 200 mg P.O. daily at bedtime. May increase to 300 mg at bedtime if response is inadequate. Maximum dose is 400 mg. If using Covera-HS, 180 mg P.O. daily at bedtime. May increase to 240 mg daily if response is inadequate. Subsequent dosage adjustments may be made in 120-mg increments up to a maximum of 420 mg at bedtime.

I.V. ADMINISTRATION
- This form is contraindicated in patients receiving I.V. beta blockers and in those with ventricular tachycardia.
- Directly inject into a vein or into the tubing of a free-flowing, compatible solution, such as D_5W, half-normal saline solution, normal saline solution, Ringer's solution, or lactated Ringer's solution.
- Give doses over at least 2 minutes (3 minutes in elderly patients) to minimize the risk of adverse reactions.
- Monitor ECG and blood pressure continuously.

INCOMPATIBILITIES
Albumin, aminophylline, amphotericin B, ampicillin sodium, co-trimoxazole, dobutamine, hydralazine, nafcillin, oxacillin, propofol, sodium bicarbonate, solutions with a pH greater than 6.

ACTION
Not clearly defined. A calcium channel blocker that inhibits calcium ion influx across cardiac and smooth-muscle cells, thus decreasing myocardial contractility and oxygen demand; it also dilates coronary arteries and arterioles.

Route	Onset	Peak	Duration
P.O.	30 min	1–2 hr	8–10 hr
P.O. (extended)	30 min	5–9 hr	24 hr
I.V.	Immediate	1–5 min	1–6 hr

Half-life: 6 to 12 hours.

ADVERSE REACTIONS
CNS: dizziness, headache, asthenia, fatigue, sleep disturbances.
CV: *transient hypotension,* ***heart failure, bradycardia, AV block, ventricular asystole, ventricular fibrillation,*** peripheral edema, pulmonary edema.
GI: *constipation,* nausea, diarrhea, dyspepsia.
Respiratory: dyspnea, pharyngitis, rhinitis, sinusitis, upper respiratory infection.
Skin: rash.

INTERACTIONS
Drug-drug. *Acebutolol, atenolol, betaxolol, carteolol,* ***digoxin,*** *esmolol, metoprolol, nadolol, penbutolol, pindolol, propranolol, timolol:* May increase effects of both drugs. Monitor cardiac function closely and decrease doses as needed.
Amiodarone: May cause bradycardia and decrease cardiac output. Monitor patient closely.
Antihypertensives, quinidine: May cause hypotension. Monitor blood pressure.
Carbamazepine: May increase levels of carbamazepine. Monitor patient for toxicity and adjust dosage p.r.n.
Cyclosporine: May increase cyclosporine level. Monitor cyclosporine level.
Disopyramide, flecainide: May cause heart failure. Avoid using together.
Dofetilide: May increase dofetilide level. Avoid using together.
Lithium: May decrease or increase lithium level. Monitor lithium level.
Phenytoin: May decrease effects of verapamil. Monitor patient closely and adjust dose p.r.n.

Rifampin: May decrease oral bioavailability of verapamil. Monitor patient for lack of effect.
Neuromuscular blocking drugs: May potentiate the activity of these drugs. Monitor neuromuscular function and adjust dosages of either drug as needed.
Sirolimus, tacrolimus: May increase levels of these drugs. Monitor drug levels closely and adjust dosage p.r.n.
Drug-herb. *Black catechu:* May cause additive effects. Discourage use together.
St. John's wort: May decrease drug level and effect. Discourage use together.
Yerba maté: May decrease clearance of herb's methylxanthines and cause toxicity. Urge caution.
Drug-food. *Grapefruit juice:* May increase drug level. Discourage use together.
Drug-lifestyle. *Alcohol use:* May enhance the effects of alcohol. Discourage use together.

EFFECTS ON LAB TEST RESULTS

- May increase ALT, AST, alkaline phosphatase, and bilirubin levels.

CONTRAINDICATIONS & CAUTIONS

- Contraindicated in patients hypersensitive to drug and in those with severe left ventricular dysfunction, cardiogenic shock, second- or third-degree AV block or sick sinus syndrome except in presence of functioning pacemaker, atrial flutter or fibrillation and accessory bypass tract syndrome, severe heart failure (unless secondary to therapy), and severe hypotension.
- I.V. form is contraindicated in patients receiving I.V. beta blockers and in those with ventricular tachycardia.
- Use cautiously in elderly patients and in those with increased intracranial pressure or hepatic or renal disease.

NURSING CONSIDERATIONS

- Pellet-filled capsules may be given by carefully opening the capsule and sprinkling the pellets on a spoonful of applesauce. This should be swallowed immediately without chewing, followed by a glass of cool water to ensure all the pellets are swallowed.
- Patients with severely compromised cardiac function or those receiving beta blockers should receive lower doses of this drug. Monitor these patients closely.
- For supraventricular tachycardia, have the patient perform vagal maneuvers after receiving drug.
- Monitor blood pressure at the start of therapy and during dosage adjustments. Assist patient with walking because dizziness may occur.
- If signs and symptoms of heart failure occur, such as swelling of hands and feet and shortness of breath, notify prescriber.
- Monitor liver function test results during prolonged treatment.
- ***Look alike–sound alike:*** Don't confuse Verelan with Vivarin, Voltaren, or Virilon.

PATIENT TEACHING

- Instruct patient to take oral form of drug exactly as prescribed.
- Tell patient that long-acting forms shouldn't be crushed or chewed.
- Caution patient against abruptly stopping drug.
- If patient continues nitrate therapy during oral verapamil dosage adjustment, urge continued compliance. S.L. nitroglycerin may be taken, as needed, for acute chest pain.
- Encourage patient to increase fluid and fiber intake to combat constipation. Give a stool softener.
- Drug significantly inhibits alcohol elimination. Advise patient to avoid or severely limit alcohol use.
- Inform patient taking Covera-HS that the outer shell of the drug may be excreted in feces.

21 Antihypertensives

amlodipine besylate
(See Chapter 20, ANTIANGINALS.)
atenolol
benazepril hydrochloride
candesartan cilexetil
captopril
carvedilol
clonidine
clonidine hydrochloride
diltiazem hydrochloride
(See Chapter 20, ANTIANGINALS.)
doxazosin mesylate
enalaprilat
enalapril maleate
eplerenone
eprosartan mesylate
felodipine
fosinopril sodium
guanfacine hydrochloride
hydralazine hydrochloride
irbesartan
labetalol hydrochloride
lisinopril
losartan potassium
methyldopa
methyldopate hydrochloride
metoprolol succinate
metoprolol tartrate
minoxidil
nadolol
(See Chapter 20, ANTIANGINALS.)
nicardipine hydrochloride
(See Chapter 20, ANTIANGINALS.)
nifedipine
(See Chapter 20, ANTIANGINALS.)
nisoldipine
nitroprusside sodium
olmesartan medoxomil
perindopril erbumine
phentolamine mesylate
prazosin hydrochloride
propranolol hydrochloride
(See Chapter 20, ANTIANGINALS.)
quinapril hydrochloride
ramipril
telmisartan
terazosin hydrochloride
trandolapril
valsartan
verapamil hydrochloride
(See Chapter 20, ANTIANGINALS.)

SAFETY ALERT!

atenolol

Anselol‡, Apo-Atenolol†, Noten‡, Tenormin, Tensig‡

Pharmacologic class: beta blocker
Pregnancy risk category D

AVAILABLE FORMS

Injection: 5 mg/10 ml
Tablets: 25 mg, 50 mg, 100 mg

INDICATIONS & DOSAGES

➤ Hypertension
Adults: Initially, 50 mg P.O. daily alone or in combination with a diuretic as a single dose, increased to 100 mg once daily after 7 to 14 days. Dosages of more than 100 mg daily are unlikely to produce further benefit.

➤ Angina pectoris
Adults: 50 mg P.O. once daily, increased p.r.n. to 100 mg daily after 7 days for optimal effect. Maximum, 200 mg daily.

➤ Acute MI
Adults: 5 mg I.V. over 5 minutes; then another 5 mg after 10 minutes. After another 10 minutes, if patient tolerates the full 10-mg I.V. dose, give 50 mg P.O.; then give another 50 mg P.O. in 12 hours. Subsequently, give 100 mg P.O. daily (as a single dose or 50 mg b.i.d.) for at least 6 to 9 days or until discharged.

➤ Migraine prophylaxis ♦
Adults: 100 mg P.O. daily.

➤ Unstable angina, non–ST-segment elevation MI in patients at high risk for ischemic events ♦
Adults: Initially, 5 mg I.V. over 2 to 5 minutes, repeat q 5 minutes to maximum of 10 mg. Initiate oral therapy 1 to 2 hours after last I.V. dose at 50 to 100 mg P.O. daily. Maintenance dose, 50 to 200 mg daily.

Adjust-a-dose: If creatinine clearance is 15 to 35 ml/minute, maximum dose is 50 mg daily; if clearance is below 15 ml/minute, maximum dose is 25 mg daily. Hemodialysis patients need 25 to 50 mg after each dialysis session.

I.V. ADMINISTRATION

- May mix with D_5W, normal saline solution, or dextrose and saline solution.
- Give by slow I.V. injection, not exceeding 1 mg/minute.
- Solution is stable for 48 hours after mixing.

INCOMPATIBILITIES

Other I.V. drugs.

ACTION

A beta blocker that selectively blocks $beta_1$ beta-adrenergic receptors, decreases cardiac output and cardiac oxygen consumption, and depresses renin secretion.

Route	Onset	Peak	Duration
P.O.	1 hr	2–4 hr	24 hr
I.V.	5 min	5 min	12 hr

Half-life: 6 to 7 hours.

ADVERSE REACTIONS

CNS: *dizziness, fatigue,* lethargy, vertigo, drowsiness, fever.
CV: *hypotension,* ***bradycardia, heart failure,*** intermittent claudication.
GI: nausea, diarrhea.
Musculoskeletal: leg pain.
Respiratory: ***bronchospasm,*** dyspnea.
Skin: rash.

INTERACTIONS

Drug-drug. *Amiodarone:* May increase risk of bradycardia, AV block, and myocardial depression. Monitor ECG and vital signs.
Antihypertensives: May increase hypotensive effect. Use together cautiously.
Calcium channel blockers, hydralazine, methyldopa: May cause additive hypotensive effects. Adjust dosage as needed.
Cardiac glycosides, diltiazem, verapamil: May cause excessive bradycardia and increased depressant effect on myocardium. Use together cautiously.
Clonidine: May exacerbate rebound hypertension if clonidine is withdrawn. Atenolol should be withdrawn before clonidine by several days or added several days after clonidine is stopped.
Dolasetron: May decrease clearance of dolasetron and increase risk of toxicity. Monitor patient for toxicity.
Insulin, oral antidiabetics: May alter dosage requirements in previously stabilized diabetic patient. Observe patient carefully.
I.V. lidocaine: May reduce hepatic metabolism of lidocaine, increasing risk of toxicity. Give bolus doses of lidocaine at a slower rate and monitor lidocaine level closely.
NSAIDs: May decrease antihypertensive effects. Monitor blood pressure.
Prazosin: May increase the risk of orthostatic hypotension in the early phases of use together. Help patient stand slowly until effects are known.
Reserpine: May cause hypotension or marked bradycardia. Use together cautiously.

EFFECTS ON LAB TEST RESULTS

- May increase alkaline phosphatase, BUN, creatinine, glucose, LDH, potassium, transaminase, and uric acid levels. May decrease glucose level.
- May increase platelet count.

CONTRAINDICATIONS & CAUTIONS

- Contraindicated in patients with sinus bradycardia, heart block greater than first degree, overt cardiac failure, untreated pheochromocytoma, or cardiogenic shock.
- Use cautiously in patients at risk for heart failure and in those with bronchospastic disease, diabetes, hyperthyroidism, and impaired renal or hepatic function.

NURSING CONSIDERATIONS

- Check apical pulse before giving drug; if slower than 60 beats/minute, withhold drug and call prescriber.
- Monitor patient's blood pressure.
- Monitor hemodialysis patients closely because of hypotension risk.
- Beta blockers may mask tachycardia caused by hyperthyroidism. In patients with suspected thyrotoxicosis, withdraw beta blocker gradually to avoid thyroid storm.

- Drug may mask signs and symptoms of hypoglycemia in diabetic patients.
- Drug may cause changes in exercise tolerance and ECG.
- ***Alert:*** Withdraw drug gradually over 2 weeks to avoid serious adverse reactions.
- ***Look alike–sound alike:*** Don't confuse atenolol with timolol or albuterol.

PATIENT TEACHING

- Instruct patient to take drug exactly as prescribed, at the same time every day.
- Caution patient not to stop drug suddenly, but to notify prescriber if unpleasant adverse reactions occur.
- Teach patient how to take his pulse. Tell him to withhold drug and call prescriber if pulse rate is below 60 beats/minute.
- Tell woman of childbearing age to notify prescriber about planned, suspected, or known pregnancy. Drug will need to be stopped.
- Advise breast-feeding mother to contact prescriber; drug isn't recommended for breast-feeding women.

benazepril hydrochloride

Lotensin

Pharmacologic class: ACE inhibitor
Pregnancy risk category C; D in 2nd and 3rd trimesters

AVAILABLE FORMS

Tablets: 5 mg, 10 mg, 20 mg, 40 mg

INDICATIONS & DOSAGES

➤ **Hypertension**

Adults: For patients not receiving a diuretic, 10 mg P.O. daily initially. Adjust dosage as needed and tolerated; usually 20 to 40 mg daily in one or two divided doses. For patients receiving a diuretic, 5 mg P.O. daily initially.
Children age 6 and older: 0.2 mg/kg (up to 10 mg) P.O. daily. Adjust as needed up to 0.6 mg/kg (maximum 40 mg) P.O. daily.
Adjust-a-dose: If creatinine clearance is below 30 ml/minute, give 5 mg P.O. daily. Daily dose may be adjusted up to 40 mg.

ACTION

Inhibits ACE, preventing conversion of angiotensin I to angiotensin II, a potent vasoconstrictor. Less angiotensin II decreases peripheral arterial resistance, decreasing aldosterone secretion, which reduces sodium and water retention and lowers blood pressure. Drug also acts as antihypertensive in patients with low-renin hypertension.

Route	Onset	Peak	Duration
P.O.	1 hr	2–4 hr	24 hr

Half-life: benazepril, 0.6 hour; benazeprilat, 10 to 12 hours.

ADVERSE REACTIONS

CNS: headache, dizziness, drowsiness, fatigue, somnolence.
CV: symptomatic hypotension.
GI: nausea.
GU: impotence.
Metabolic: hyperkalemia.
Musculoskeletal: arthralgia, arthritis, myalgia.
Respiratory: dry, persistent, nonproductive cough.
Skin: increased diaphoresis.
Other: hypersensitivity reactions.

INTERACTIONS

Drug-drug. *Azathioprine:* May increase risk of anemia or leukopenia. Monitor hematologic study results if used together.
Diuretics, other antihypertensives: May cause excessive hypotension. Stop diuretic or lower dosage of benazepril, as needed.
Lithium: May increase lithium level and toxicity. Use together cautiously; monitor lithium level.
Nesiritide: May increase risk of hypotension. Monitor blood pressure.
NSAIDs: May decrease antihypertensive effects. Monitor blood pressure.
Potassium-sparing diuretics, potassium supplements: May cause hyperkalemia. Monitor patient closely.
Drug-herb. *Capsaicin:* May cause cough. Discourage use together.
Ma huang: May decrease antihypertensive effects. Discourage use together.
Drug-food. *Salt substitutes containing potassium:* May cause hyperkalemia. Monitor patient closely.

EFFECTS ON LAB TEST RESULTS
• May increase BUN, creatinine, and potassium levels.

CONTRAINDICATIONS & CAUTIONS
• Contraindicated in patients hypersensitive to ACE inhibitors.
• Use cautiously in patients with impaired hepatic or renal function.

NURSING CONSIDERATIONS
• Monitor patient for hypotension. Excessive hypotension can occur when drug is given with diuretics. If possible, diuretic therapy should be stopped 2 to 3 days before starting benazepril to decrease potential for excessive hypotensive response. If drug doesn't adequately control blood pressure, diuretic may be cautiously reinstituted.
• Ask pharmacist to make oral suspension for patients having difficulty swallowing tablets.
• Although ACE inhibitors reduce blood pressure in all races, they reduce it less in blacks taking the ACE inhibitor alone. Black patients should take drug with a thiazide diuretic for a more favorable response.
• Drug may increase risk of angioedema in black patients.
• Measure blood pressure when drug level is at peak (2 to 6 hours after administration) and at trough (just before a dose) to verify adequate blood pressure control.
• Assess renal and hepatic function before and periodically during therapy. Monitor potassium level.
• ***Look alike–sound alike:*** Don't confuse benazepril with Benadryl or Lotensin with Loniten or lovastatin.

PATIENT TEACHING
• Instruct patient to avoid salt substitutes because they may contain potassium, which can cause high potassium level in patients taking drug.
• Inform patient that light-headedness can occur, especially during first few days of therapy. Tell him to rise slowly to minimize this effect and to report dizziness to prescriber. If fainting occurs, he should stop drug and call prescriber immediately.
• Warn patient to use caution in hot weather and during exercise. Inadequate fluid intake, vomiting, diarrhea, and excessive perspiration can lead to light-headedness and fainting.
• Advise patient to report signs of infection, such as fever and sore throat. Tell him to call prescriber if he develops easy bruising or bleeding; swelling of tongue, lips, face, eyes, mucous membranes, or extremities; difficulty swallowing or breathing; or hoarseness.
• Tell woman of childbearing age to notify prescriber if she becomes pregnant. Drug will need to be stopped.

candesartan cilexetil
Atacand

Pharmacologic class: angiotensin II receptor antagonist
Pregnancy risk category C; D in 2nd and 3rd trimesters

AVAILABLE FORMS
Tablets: 4 mg, 8 mg, 16 mg, 32 mg

INDICATIONS & DOSAGES
➤**Hypertension (used alone or with other antihypertensives)**
Adults: Initially, 16 mg P.O. once daily when used alone; usual range is 8 to 32 mg P.O. daily as a single dose or divided b.i.d.
➤**Heart failure**
Adults: Initially, 4 mg P.O. once daily. Double the dose about every 2 weeks as tolerated, to a target dose of 32 mg once daily.
Adjust-a-dose: If patient takes a diuretic, consider a lower starting dose.

ACTION
Inhibits vasoconstrictive action of angiotensin II by blocking angiotensin II receptor on the surface of vascular smooth muscle and other tissue cells.

Route	Onset	Peak	Duration
P.O.	Unknown	3–4 hr	24 hr

Half-life: 9 hours.

ADVERSE REACTIONS
CNS: dizziness, fatigue, headache.
CV: chest pain, peripheral edema.

EENT: pharyngitis, rhinitis, sinusitis.
GI: abdominal pain, diarrhea, nausea, vomiting.
GU: albuminuria.
Musculoskeletal: arthralgia, back pain.
Respiratory: coughing, bronchitis, upper respiratory tract infection.

INTERACTIONS

Drug-drug. *Lithium:* May increase lithium concentration. Monitor lithium levels closely.
Potassium-sparing diuretics, potassium supplements: May cause hyperkalemia. Monitor patient closely.
Drug-herb. *Ma huang:* May decrease antihypertensive effects. Discourage use together.
Drug-food. *Salt substitutes containing potassium:* May cause hyperkalemia. Monitor patient closely.

EFFECTS ON LAB TEST RESULTS

- May increase potassium level, BUN, and serum creatinine.

CONTRAINDICATIONS & CAUTIONS

- Contraindicated in patients hypersensitive to drug or its components.
- Use cautiously in patients whose renal function depends on the renin-angiotensin-aldosterone system (such as patients with heart failure) because of risk of oliguria and progressive azotemia with acute renal failure or death.
- Avoid use in pregnant patients, especially in the second and third trimesters.
- Use cautiously in patients who are volume or salt depleted because they could develop symptoms of hypotension. Start therapy with a lower dosage range, and monitor blood pressure carefully.

NURSING CONSIDERATIONS

- ***Alert:*** Drugs, such as candesartan, that act directly on the renin-angiotensin system can cause fetal and neonatal illness and death when given to pregnant women. If pregnancy is suspected, notify prescriber immediately.
- If hypotension occurs after a dose of candesartan, place patient in the supine position and, if needed, give an I.V. infusion of normal saline solution.
- Most of drug's antihypertensive effect occurs within 2 weeks. Maximal effect may take 4 to 6 weeks. Diuretic may be added if blood pressure isn't controlled by drug alone.
- Carefully monitor elderly patients and those with renal disease for therapeutic response and adverse reactions.

PATIENT TEACHING

- Inform woman of childbearing age of the consequences of second and third trimester exposure to drug. Prescriber should be notified immediately if pregnancy is suspected.
- Advise breast-feeding woman of the risk of adverse effects on the infant and the need to stop either breast-feeding or drug.
- Instruct patient to store drug at room temperature and to keep container tightly sealed.
- Inform patient to report adverse reactions without delay.
- Tell patient that drug may be taken without regard to meals.

captopril

Acenorm‡, Capoten✐, Enzace‡, Novo-Captoril†

Pharmacologic class: ACE inhibitor
Pregnancy risk category C; D in 2nd and 3rd trimesters

AVAILABLE FORMS

Tablets: 12.5 mg, 25 mg, 50 mg, 100 mg

INDICATIONS & DOSAGES

➤ **Hypertension**
Adults: Initially, 25 mg P.O. b.i.d. or t.i.d. If dosage doesn't control blood pressure satisfactorily in 1 or 2 weeks, increase it to 50 mg b.i.d. or t.i.d. If that dosage doesn't control blood pressure satisfactorily after another 1 or 2 weeks, expect to add a diuretic. If patient needs further blood pressure reduction, dosage may be raised to 150 mg t.i.d. while continuing diuretic. Maximum daily dose is 450 mg.
➤ **Diabetic nephropathy**
Adults: 25 mg P.O. t.i.d.
➤ **Heart failure**
Adults: Initially, 25 mg P.O. t.i.d. Patients with normal or low blood pressure who

have been vigorously treated with diuretics and who may be hyponatremic or hypovolemic may start with 6.25 or 12.5 mg P.O. t.i.d.; starting dosage may be adjusted over several days. Gradually increase dosage to 50 mg P.O. t.i.d.; once patient reaches this dosage, delay further dosage increases for at least 2 weeks. Maximum dosage is 450 mg daily.
Elderly patients: Initially, 6.25 mg P.O. b.i.d. Increase gradually p.r.n.

➤**Left ventricular dysfunction after acute MI**
Adults: Start therapy as early as 3 days after MI with 6.25 mg P.O. for one dose, followed by 12.5 mg P.O. t.i.d. Increase over several days to 25 mg P.O. t.i.d.; then increase to 50 mg P.O. t.i.d. over several weeks.

ACTION

Inhibits ACE, preventing conversion of angiotensin I to angiotensin II, a potent vasoconstrictor. Less angiotensin II decreases peripheral arterial resistance, decreasing aldosterone secretion, which reduces sodium and water retention and lowers blood pressure.

Route	Onset	Peak	Duration
P.O.	15–60 min	60–90 min	6–12 hr

Half-life: Less than 2 hours.

ADVERSE REACTIONS

CNS: dizziness, fainting, headache, malaise, fatigue, fever.
CV: tachycardia, hypotension, angina pectoris.
GI: abdominal pain, anorexia, constipation, diarrhea, dry mouth, dysgeusia, nausea, vomiting.
Hematologic: ***leukopenia, agranulocytosis, thrombocytopenia, pancytopenia,*** anemia.
Metabolic: hyperkalemia.
Respiratory: *dry, persistent, nonproductive cough,* dyspnea.
Skin: *urticarial rash, maculopapular rash,* pruritus, alopecia.
Other: ***angioedema.***

INTERACTIONS

Drug-drug. *Antacids:* May decrease captopril effect. Separate dosage times.
Digoxin: May increase digoxin level by 15% to 30%. Monitor digoxin level, and observe patient for signs of digoxin toxicity.
Diuretics, other antihypertensives: May cause excessive hypotension. May need to stop diuretic or reduce captopril dosage.
Insulin, oral antidiabetics: May cause hypoglycemia when captopril therapy is started. Monitor patient closely.
Lithium: May increase lithium level, and symptoms of toxicity possible. Monitor patient closely.
NSAIDs: May reduce antihypertensive effect. Monitor blood pressure.
Potassium-sparing diuretics, potassium supplements: May cause hyperkalemia. Avoid using together unless hypokalemia is confirmed.
Drug-herb. *Black catechu:* May cause additional hypotensive effect. Discourage use together.
Capsaicin: May worsen cough. Discourage use together.
Drug-food. *Salt substitutes containing potassium:* May cause hyperkalemia. Monitor patient closely.

EFFECTS ON LAB TEST RESULTS

- May increase alkaline phosphatase, bilirubin, and potassium levels. May decrease hemoglobin level and hematocrit.
- May decrease granulocyte, platelet, RBC, and WBC counts.
- May cause false-positive urine acetone test results.

CONTRAINDICATIONS & CAUTIONS

- Contraindicated in patients hypersensitive to drug or other ACE inhibitors.
- Use cautiously in patients with impaired renal function or serious autoimmune disease, especially systemic lupus erythematosus, and in those who have been exposed to other drugs that affect WBC counts or immune response.

NURSING CONSIDERATIONS

- Monitor patient's blood pressure and pulse rate frequently.
- ***Alert:*** Elderly patients may be more sensitive to drug's hypotensive effects.
- Assess patient for signs of angioedema.

- Drug causes the most frequent occurrence of cough, compared with other ACE inhibitors.
- In patients with impaired renal function or collagen vascular disease, monitor WBC and differential counts before starting treatment, every 2 weeks for the first 3 months of therapy, and periodically thereafter.
- ***Look alike–sound alike:*** Don't confuse captopril with Capitrol.

PATIENT TEACHING

- Instruct patient to take drug 1 hour before meals; food in the GI tract may reduce absorption.
- Inform patient that light-headedness is possible, especially during first few days of therapy. Tell him to rise slowly to minimize this effect and to report occurrence to prescriber. If fainting occurs, he should stop drug and call prescriber immediately.
- Tell patient to use caution in hot weather and during exercise. Lack of fluids, vomiting, diarrhea, and excessive perspiration can lead to light-headedness and syncope.
- Advise patient to report signs and symptoms of infection, such as fever and sore throat.
- Tell women to notify prescriber if pregnancy occurs. Drug will need to be stopped.
- Urge patient to promptly report swelling of the face, lips, or mouth; or difficulty breathing.

carvedilol
Coreg

Pharmacologic class: alpha-nonselective beta blocker
Pregnancy risk category C

AVAILABLE FORMS

Tablets: 3.125 mg, 6.25 mg, 12.5 mg, 25 mg

INDICATIONS & DOSAGES

➤ **Hypertension**

Adults: Dosage highly individualized. Initially, 6.25 mg P.O. b.i.d. Measure standing blood pressure 1 hour after first dose. If tolerated, continue dosage for 7 to 14 days. May increase to 12.5 mg P.O. b.i.d. for 7 to 14 days, following same blood pressure monitoring protocol as before. Maximum dose is 25 mg P.O. b.i.d. as tolerated.

➤ **Left ventricular dysfunction after MI**

Adults: Dosage individualized. Start therapy after patient is hemodynamically stable and fluid retention has been minimized. Initially, 6.25 mg P.O. b.i.d. Increase after 3 to 10 days to 12.5 mg b.i.d., then again to a target dose of 25 mg b.i.d. Or start with 3.25 mg b.i.d., or adjust dosage slower if indicated.

➤ **Mild to severe heart failure**

Adults: Dosage highly individualized. Initially, 3.125 mg P.O. b.i.d. for 2 weeks; if tolerated, may increase to 6.25 mg P.O. b.i.d. Dosage may be doubled q 2 weeks as tolerated. Maximum dose for patients who weigh less than 85 kg (187 lb) is 25 mg P.O. b.i.d.; for those weighing more than 85 kg, dose is 50 mg P.O. b.i.d.

Adjust-a-dose: In patient with pulse rate below 55 beats/minute, use reduced dosage.

➤ **Angina pectoris** ♦

Adults: 25 to 50 mg P.O. b.i.d.

➤ **Idiopathic cardiomyopathy** ♦

Adults: 6.25 to 25 mg P.O. b.i.d.

ACTION

Nonselective beta blocker with alpha-blocking activity.

Route	Onset	Peak	Duration
P.O.	Unknown	1–2 hr	7–10 hr

Half-life: 7 to 10 hours.

ADVERSE REACTIONS

CNS: *asthenia, dizziness, fatigue,* ***stroke,*** pain, headache, malaise, fever, hypesthesia, paresthesia, vertigo, somnolence, depression, insomnia.
CV: *hypotension, postural hypertension,* ***AV block, bradycardia,*** edema, syncope, angina pectoris, peripheral edema, hypovolemia, fluid overload, hypertension, palpitations, peripheral vascular disorder, chest pain.
EENT: sinusitis, abnormal vision, blurred vision, pharyngitis, rhinitis.

GI: *diarrhea,* vomiting, nausea, melena, periodontitis, abdominal pain, dyspepsia.
GU: impotence, abnormal renal function, albuminuria, hematuria, UTI.
Hematologic: ***thrombocytopenia,*** purpura, anemia.
Metabolic: *hyperglycemia, weight gain,* ***hyperkalemia, hypoglycemia,*** weight loss, hypercholesterolemia, hyperuricemia, hyponatremia, glycosuria, hypervolemia, diabetes mellitus, gout, hypertriglyceridemia.
Musculoskeletal: arthralgia, back pain, muscle cramps, hypotonia, arthritis.
Respiratory: *upper respiratory tract infection,* ***lung edema,*** bronchitis, cough, rales, dyspnea.
Other: *hypersensitivity reactions,* infection, flulike syndrome, viral infection, injury.

INTERACTIONS

Drug-drug. *Amiodarone:* May increase risk of bradycardia, AV block, and myocardial depression. Monitor patient's ECG and vital signs.
Catecholamine-depleting drugs such as MAO inhibitors, reserpine: May cause bradycardia or severe hypotension. Monitor patient closely.
Cimetidine: May increase bioavailability of carvedilol. Monitor vital signs closely.
Clonidine: May increase blood pressure– and heart rate–lowering effects. Monitor vital signs closely.
Cyclosporine: May increase cyclosporine level. Monitor cyclosporine level.
Digoxin: May increase digoxin level by about 15% when given together. Monitor digoxin level.
Diltiazem, verapamil: May cause isolated conduction disturbances. Monitor patient's heart rhythm and blood pressure.
Fluoxetine, paroxetine, propafenone, quinidine: May increase level of carvedilol. Monitor patient for hypotension and dizziness.
Insulin, oral antidiabetics: May enhance hypoglycemic properties. Monitor glucose level.
NSAIDs: May decrease antihypertensive effects. Monitor blood pressure.
Rifampin: May reduce carvedilol level by 70%. Monitor vital signs closely.
Drug-herb. *Ma huang:* May decrease antihypertensive effects. Discourage use together.
Drug-food. *Any food:* May delay rate of absorption of carvedilol with no change in bioavailability. Advise patient to take drug with food to minimize orthostatic effects.

EFFECTS ON LAB TEST RESULTS

- May increase alkaline phosphatase, ALT, AST, BUN, cholesterol, creatinine, GGT, nonprotein nitrogen, potassium, triglyceride, sodium, and uric acid levels. May increase or decrease glucose level.
- May decrease PT and platelet count.

CONTRAINDICATIONS & CAUTIONS

- Contraindicated in patients hypersensitive to drug and in those with New York Heart Association class IV decompensated cardiac failure requiring I.V. inotropic therapy.
- Contraindicated in those with bronchial asthma or related bronchospastic conditions, second- or third-degree AV block, sick sinus syndrome (unless a permanent pacemaker is in place), cardiogenic shock, severe bradycardia, or symptomatic hepatic impairment.
- Use cautiously in hypertensive patients with left-sided heart failure, perioperative patients who receive anesthetics that depress myocardial function (such as cyclopropane and trichloroethylene), and diabetic patients receiving insulin or oral antidiabetics, and in those subject to spontaneous hypoglycemia.
- Use with caution in patients with thyroid disease (may mask hyperthyroidism; withdrawal may precipitate thyroid storm or exacerbation of hyperthyroidism), pheochromocytoma, Prinzmetal or variant angina, bronchospastic disease (in those who can't tolerate other antihypertensives), or peripheral vascular disease (may precipitate or aggravate symptoms of arterial insufficiency).
- Use cautiously in breast-feeding women.
- Safety and effectiveness in children younger than age 18 haven't been established.

NURSING CONSIDERATIONS

- ***Alert:*** Patients who have a history of severe anaphylactic reaction to several allergens may be more reactive to repeated challenge (accidental, diagnostic, or therapeutic). They may be unresponsive to dosages of epinephrine typically used to treat allergic reactions.

- Mild hepatocellular injury may occur during therapy. At first sign of hepatic dysfunction, perform tests for hepatic injury or jaundice; if present, stop drug.
- If drug must be stopped, do so gradually over 1 to 2 weeks.
- Monitor patient with heart failure for worsened condition, renal dysfunction, or fluid retention; diuretics may need to be increased.
- Monitor diabetic patient closely; drug may mask signs of hypoglycemia, or hyperglycemia may be worsened.
- Observe patient for dizziness or lightheadedness for 1 hour after giving each new dose.
- Monitor elderly patients carefully; drug levels are about 50% higher in elderly patients than in younger patients.

PATIENT TEACHING

- Tell patient not to interrupt or stop drug without medical approval.
- Inform patient that improvement of heart failure symptoms might take several weeks of drug therapy.
- Advise patient with heart failure to call prescriber if weight gain or shortness of breath occurs.
- Inform patient that he may experience low blood pressure when standing. If dizziness or fainting occurs (rare), advise him to sit or lie down and to notify prescriber if symptoms persist.
- Caution patient against performing hazardous tasks during start of therapy.
- Advise diabetic patient to promptly report changes in glucose level.
- Inform patient who wears contact lenses that his eyes may feel dry.

clonidine
Catapres-TTS

clonidine hydrochloride
Catapres, Dixarit†‡, Duraclon

Pharmacologic class: centrally acting alpha agonist
Pregnancy risk category C

AVAILABLE FORMS

clonidine
Transdermal: TTS-1 (releases 0.1 mg/24 hours), TTS-2 (releases 0.2 mg/24 hours), TTS-3 (releases 0.3 mg/24 hours)

clonidine hydrochloride
Injection for epidural use: 100 mcg/ml
Injection for epidural use, concentrate: 500 mcg/ml
Tablets: 0.025 mg†‡, 0.1 mg, 0.2 mg, 0.3 mg

INDICATIONS & DOSAGES

➤ **Essential and renal hypertension**
Adults and children age 12 and older: Initially, 0.1 mg P.O. b.i.d.; then increased by 0.1 to 0.2 mg daily on a weekly basis. Usual range is 0.2 to 0.6 mg daily in divided doses; infrequently, dosages as high as 2.4 mg daily are used.

Or, apply transdermal patch to nonhairy area of intact skin on upper arm or torso once q 7 days, starting with 0.1-mg system and adjusted with another 0.1-mg or larger system.

➤ **Severe cancer pain that is unresponsive to epidural or spinal opiate analgesia or other more conventional methods of analgesia**
Adults: Initially, 30 mcg/hour by continuous epidural infusion. Experience with rates greater than 40 mcg/hour is limited.
Children: Initially, 0.5 mcg/kg/hour by epidural infusion. Dosage should be cautiously adjusted, based on response.

➤ **Pheochromocytoma diagnosis ♦**
Adults: 0.3 mg P.O. for a single dose.

➤ **Migraine prophylaxis ♦**
Adults: 0.025 mg P.O. two to four times daily or up to 0.15 mg P.O. daily in divided doses.

➤**Dysmenorrhea** ♦
Adults: 0.025 mg P.O. b.i.d. for 14 days before and during menses.
➤**Vasomotor symptoms of menopause** ♦
Adults: 0.025 to 0.2 mg P.O. b.i.d. or 0.1-mg/24-hour patch applied once q 7 days.
➤**Opiate dependence** ♦
Adults: Initially, 0.005 or 0.006 mg/kg test dose, followed by 0.017 mg/kg P.O. daily in three or four divided doses for 10 days. Or, initially, 0.1 mg P.O. three or four times daily, with dosage adjusted by 0.1 to 0.2 mg daily. Dosage range is 0.3 to 1.2 mg P.O. daily. Stop drug gradually. Follow protocols.
➤**Alcohol dependence** ♦
Adults: 0.5 mg P.O. b.i.d. to t.i.d.
➤**Smoking cessation** ♦
Adults: Initially, 0.1 mg P.O. b.i.d., beginning on or shortly before the day of smoking cessation. Increase dosage q 7 days by 0.1 mg daily, if needed. Or, 0.1-mg/24-hour transdermal patch applied q 7 days. Therapy should begin on or shortly before the day of smoking cessation. Increase dosage by 0.1 mg/24 hours at weekly intervals, if needed.
➤**Attention deficit hyperactivity disorder** ♦
Children: Initially, 0.05 mg P.O. at bedtime. May increase dosage cautiously over 2 to 4 weeks. Maintenance dosage is 0.05 to 0.4 mg P.O. daily.

ACTION

Unknown. Thought to stimulate $alpha_2$ receptors and inhibit the central vasomotor centers, decreasing sympathetic outflow to the heart, kidneys, and peripheral vasculature, and lowering peripheral vascular resistance, blood pressure, and heart rate.

Route	Onset	Peak	Duration
P.O.	30–60 min	2–4 hr	12–24 hr
Transdermal	2–3 days	2–3 days	7–8 days
Epidural	Unknown	30–60 min	Unknown

Half-life: 6 to 20 hours.

ADVERSE REACTIONS

CNS: *drowsiness, dizziness, sedation, weakness,* fatigue, malaise, agitation, depression.
CV: ***bradycardia, severe rebound hypertension,*** orthostatic hypotension.
GI: *constipation, dry mouth,* nausea, vomiting, anorexia.
GU: urine retention, impotence.
Metabolic: weight gain.
Skin: *pruritus, dermatitis with transdermal patch,* rash.
Other: loss of libido.

INTERACTIONS

Drug-drug. *Amitriptyline, amoxapine, clomipramine, desipramine, doxepin, imipramine, nortriptyline, protriptyline, trimipramine:* May cause loss of blood pressure control with life-threatening elevations in blood pressure. Avoid using together.
CNS depressants: May increase CNS depression. Use together cautiously.
Digoxin, verapamil: May cause AV block and severe hypotension. Monitor BP and ECG.
Diuretics, other antihypertensives: May increase hypotensive effect. Monitor patient closely.
Beta blockers : May cause life-threatening hypertension. Closely monitor blood pressure.
Levodopa: May reduce effectiveness of levodopa. Monitor patient.
MAO inhibitors, prazosin: May decrease antihypertensive effect. Use together cautiously.
Propranolol, other beta blockers: May cause paradoxical hypertensive response. Monitor patient carefully.
Drug-herb. *Capsicum, ma huang:* May reduce antihypertensive effectiveness. Discourage use together.

EFFECTS ON LAB TEST RESULTS

• May decrease urinary excretion of vanillylmandelic acid and catecholamines. May cause a weakly positive Coombs' test result.

CONTRAINDICATIONS & CAUTIONS

• Contraindicated in patients hypersensitive to drug.

• Transdermal form is contraindicated in patients hypersensitive to any component of the adhesive layer of transdermal system.
• Epidural form is contraindicated in patients receiving anticoagulant therapy, in those with bleeding diathesis, in those with an injection site infection, and in those who are hemodynamically unstable or have severe CV disease.
• Use cautiously in patients with severe coronary insufficiency, conduction disturbances, recent MI, cerebrovascular disease, chronic renal failure, or impaired liver function.

NURSING CONSIDERATIONS
• Drug may be given to lower blood pressure rapidly in some hypertensive emergencies.
• Monitor blood pressure and pulse rate frequently. Dosage is usually adjusted to patient's blood pressure and tolerance.
• Elderly patients may be more sensitive than younger ones to drug's hypotensive effects.
• Observe patient for tolerance to drug's therapeutic effects, which may require increased dosage.
• Noticeable antihypertensive effects of transdermal clonidine may take 2 to 3 days. Oral antihypertensive therapy may have to be continued in the interim.
• ***Alert:*** Remove transdermal patch before defibrillation to prevent arcing.
• Stop drug gradually by reducing dosage over 2 to 4 days to avoid rapid rise in blood pressure, agitation, headache, and tremor. When stopping therapy in patients receiving both clonidine and a beta blocker, gradually withdraw the beta blocker several days before gradually stopping clonidine to minimize adverse reactions.
• Don't stop drug before surgery.
• ***Look alike–sound alike:*** Don't confuse clonidine with quinidine or clomiphene; or Catapres with Cetapred or Combipres.
• ***Alert:*** The injection form is for epidural use only.
• The injection form concentrate containing 500 mcg/ml must be diluted before use in normal saline injection to yield 100 mcg/ml.
• When drug is given epidurally, carefully monitor infusion pump, and inspect catheter tubing for obstruction or dislodgment.

PATIENT TEACHING
• Advise patient that stopping drug abruptly may cause severe rebound high blood pressure. Tell him dosage must be reduced gradually over 2 to 4 days as instructed by prescriber.
• Tell patient to take the last dose immediately before bedtime.
• Reassure patient that the transdermal patch usually remains attached despite showering and other routine daily activities. Instruct him on the use of the adhesive overlay to provide additional skin adherence, if needed. Also tell him to place patch at a different site each week.
• Caution patient that drug may cause drowsiness but that this adverse effect usually diminishes over 4 to 6 weeks.
• Inform patient that dizziness upon standing can be minimized by rising slowly from a sitting or lying position and avoiding sudden position changes.

doxazosin mesylate
Cardura✍, Carduran‡

Pharmacologic class: alpha blocker
Pregnancy risk category C

AVAILABLE FORMS
Tablets: 1 mg, 2 mg, 4 mg, 8 mg

INDICATIONS & DOSAGES
➤ **Essential hypertension**
Adults: Initially, 1 mg P.O. daily; determine effect on standing and supine blood pressure at 2 to 6 hours and 24 hours after dose. May increase at 2-week intervals to 2 mg and, thereafter, 4 mg and 8 mg once daily, if needed. Maximum daily dose is 16 mg, but doses over 4 mg daily increase the risk of adverse reactions.
➤ **BPH**
Adults: Initially, 1 mg P.O. once daily in the morning or evening; may increase at 1- or 2-week intervals to 2 mg and, thereafter, 4 mg and 8 mg once daily, if needed.

ACTION

An alpha blocker that acts on the peripheral vasculature to reduce peripheral vascular resistance and produce vasodilation. Drug also decreases smooth muscle tone in the prostate and bladder neck.

Route	Onset	Peak	Duration
P.O.	1–2 hr	2–3 hr	24 hr

Half-life: 19 to 22 hours.

ADVERSE REACTIONS

CNS: *dizziness, asthenia, headache,* vertigo, somnolence, drowsiness, pain.
CV: *orthostatic hypotension,* ***arrhythmias,*** hypotension, edema, palpitations, tachycardia.
EENT: rhinitis, pharyngitis, abnormal vision.
GI: nausea, vomiting, diarrhea, constipation.
Hematologic: ***leukopenia, neutropenia.***
Musculoskeletal: arthralgia, myalgia.
Respiratory: dyspnea.
Skin: rash, pruritus.

INTERACTIONS

Drug-drug. *Midodrine:* May decrease the effectiveness of midodrine. Monitor patient for therapeutic effect.
Drug-herb. *Butcher's broom:* May decrease effect of doxazosin. Discourage use together.
Ma huang: May decrease antihypertensive effects. Discourage use together.

EFFECTS ON LAB TEST RESULTS

- May decrease WBC and neutrophil counts.

CONTRAINDICATIONS & CAUTIONS

- Contraindicated in patients hypersensitive to drug and quinazoline derivatives (including prazosin and terazosin).
- Use cautiously in patients with impaired hepatic function.

NURSING CONSIDERATIONS

- Monitor blood pressure closely.
- If syncope occurs, place patient in a recumbent position and treat supportively. A transient hypotensive response isn't considered a contraindication to continued therapy.
- ***Look alike–sound alike:*** Don't confuse doxazosin with doxapram, doxorubicin, or doxepin. Don't confuse Cardura with Coumadin, K-Dur, Cardene, or Cordarone.

PATIENT TEACHING

- Instruct patient to take drug exactly as prescribed.
- ***Alert:*** Advise patient that he is susceptible to a first-dose effect (marked low blood pressure on standing up with dizziness or fainting). This is most common after first dose but also can occur during dosage adjustment or interruption of therapy.
- Advise patient to avoid driving and other hazardous activities until drug's effects are known.

enalaprilat

enalapril maleate

Amprace‡, Renitec‡, Vasotec✎

Pharmacologic class: ACE inhibitor
Pregnancy risk category C; D in 2nd and 3rd trimesters

AVAILABLE FORMS

enalaprilat
Injection: 1.25 mg/ml
enalapril maleate
Tablets: 2.5 mg, 5 mg, 10 mg, 20 mg

INDICATIONS & DOSAGES

➤ Hypertension

Adults: In patients not taking diuretics, initially, 5 mg P.O. once daily; then adjusted based on response. Usual dosage range is 10 to 40 mg daily as a single dose or two divided doses. Or, 1.25 mg I.V. infusion over 5 minutes q 6 hours.
Children ages 1 month to 16 years: 0.08 mg/kg (up to 5 mg) P.O. once daily; dosage should be adjusted as needed up to 0.58 mg/kg (maximum 40 mg). Don't use if creatinine clearance is less than 30 ml/minute.
Adjust-a-dose: If patient is taking diuretics or creatinine clearance is 30 ml/minute or less, initially, 2.5 mg P.O. once daily. Or, 0.625 mg I.V. over 5 minutes, and re-

peat in 1 hour, if needed; then 1.25 mg I.V. q 6 hours.

➤**To convert from I.V. therapy to oral therapy**
Adults: Initially, 2.5 mg P.O. once daily; if patient was receiving 0.625 mg I.V. q 6 hours, then 2.5 mg P.O. once daily. Adjust dosage based on response.

➤**To convert from oral therapy to I.V. therapy**
Adults: 1.25 mg I.V. over 5 minutes q 6 hours. Higher dosages aren't more effective.
Adjust-a-dose: If creatinine level is more than 1.6 mg/dl or sodium level below 130 mEq/L, initially, 2.5 mg P.O. daily and adjust slowly.

➤**To manage symptomatic heart failure**
Adults: Initially, 2.5 mg P.O. daily or b.i.d., increased gradually over several weeks. Maintenance is 5 to 20 mg daily in two divided doses. Maximum daily dose is 40 mg in two divided doses.

➤**Asymptomatic left ventricular dysfunction**
Adults: Initially, 2.5 mg P.O. b.i.d. Increase as tolerated to target daily dose of 20 mg P.O. in divided doses.

I.V. ADMINISTRATION
- Compatible solutions include D_5W, normal saline solution for injection, dextrose 5% in lactated Ringer's injection, dextrose 5% in normal saline solution for injection, and Isolyte E.
- Inject drug slowly over at least 5 minutes, or dilute in 50 ml of a compatible solution and infuse over 15 minutes.

INCOMPATIBILITIES
Amphotericin B, cefepime hydrochloride, phenytoin sodium.

ACTION
May inhibit ACE, preventing conversion of angiotensin I to angiotensin II, a potent vasoconstrictor. Less angiotensin II decreases peripheral arterial resistance, decreasing aldosterone secretion, reducing sodium and water retention, and lowering blood pressure.

Route	Onset	Peak	Duration
P.O.	1 hr	4–6 hr	24 hr
I.V.	15 min	1–4 hr	6 hr

Half-life: 12 hours.

ADVERSE REACTIONS
CNS: *asthenia,* headache, dizziness, fatigue, vertigo, syncope.
CV: hypotension, chest pain, angina pectoris.
GI: diarrhea, nausea, abdominal pain, vomiting.
GU: decreased renal function (in patients with bilateral renal artery stenosis or heart failure).
Hematologic: bone marrow depression.
Respiratory: *dry, persistent, tickling, nonproductive cough,* dyspnea.
Skin: rash.
Other: ***angioedema.***

INTERACTIONS
Drug-drug. *Azathioprine:* May increase risk of anemia or leukopenia. Monitor hematologic studies if used together.
Diuretics: May excessively reduce blood pressure. Use together cautiously.
Insulin, oral antidiabetics: May cause hypoglycemia, especially at start of enalapril therapy. Monitor patient closely.
Lithium: May cause lithium toxicity. Monitor lithium level.
NSAIDs: May reduce antihypertensive effect. Monitor blood pressure.
Potassium-sparing diuretics, potassium supplements: May cause hyperkalemia. Avoid using together unless hypokalemia is confirmed.
Drug-herb. *Capsaicin:* May cause cough. Discourage use together.
Ma huang: May decrease antihypertensive effects. Discourage use together.
Drug-food. *Salt substitutes containing potassium:* May cause hyperkalemia. Monitor patient closely.

EFFECTS ON LAB TEST RESULTS
- May increase bilirubin, BUN, creatinine, and potassium levels. May decrease sodium and hemoglobin levels and hematocrit.
- May increase liver function test values.

CONTRAINDICATIONS & CAUTIONS

- Contraindicated in patients hypersensitive to drug and in those with a history of angioedema related to previous treatment with an ACE inhibitor.
- Use cautiously in renally impaired patients or those with aortic stenosis or hypertrophic cardiomyopathy.

NURSING CONSIDERATIONS

- Closely monitor blood pressure response to drug.
- ***Look alike–sound alike:*** Similar packaging and labeling of enalaprilat injection and pancuronium, a neuromuscular-blocking drug, could result in a fatal medication error. Check all labels carefully.
- Monitor CBC with differential counts before and during therapy.
- Diabetic patients, those with impaired renal function or heart failure, and those receiving drugs that can increase potassium level may develop hyperkalemia. Monitor potassium intake and potassium level.
- Ask pharmacist to make an oral suspension for patient who has difficulty swallowing.
- ***Look alike–sound alike:*** Don't confuse enalapril with Anafranil or Eldepryl.

PATIENT TEACHING

- Instruct patient to report breathing difficulty or swelling of face, eyes, lips, or tongue. Swelling of the face and throat (including swelling of the larynx) may occur, especially after first dose.
- Advise patient to report signs of infection, such as fever and sore throat.
- Inform patient that light-headedness can occur, especially during first few days of therapy. Tell him to rise slowly to minimize this effect and to notify prescriber if symptoms develop. If he faints, he should stop taking drug and call prescriber immediately.
- Tell patient to use caution in hot weather and during exercise. Inadequate fluid intake, vomiting, diarrhea, and excessive perspiration can lead to light-headedness and fainting.
- Advise patient to avoid salt substitutes; these products may contain potassium, which can cause high potassium levels in patients taking this drug.
- Tell woman of childbearing age to notify prescriber if pregnancy occurs. Drug will need to be stopped.

eplerenone

Inspra

Pharmacologic class: selective aldosterone receptor antagonist
Pregnancy risk category B

AVAILABLE FORMS

Tablets: 25 mg, 50 mg

INDICATIONS & DOSAGES

➤ Hypertension

Adults: 50 mg P.O. once daily. If response is inadequate after 4 weeks, increase dosage to 50 mg P.O. b.i.d. Maximum daily dose, 100 mg.

Adjust-a-dose: In patients taking weak CYP3A4 inhibitors (erythromycin, fluconazole, saquinavir, verapamil), reduce eplerenone starting dose to 25 mg P.O. once daily.

➤ Heart failure after an MI

Adults: Initially, 25 mg P.O. once daily. Increase within 4 weeks, as tolerated and according to potassium level, to 50 mg P.O. once daily.

Adjust-a-dose: If potassium level is less than 5 mEq/L, increase dosage from 25 mg every other day to 25 mg daily; or increase dosage from 25 mg daily to 50 mg daily. If potassium level is 5 to 5.4 mEq/L, don't adjust dosage. If potassium level is 5.5 to 5.9 mEq/L, decrease dosage from 50 mg daily to 25 mg daily; or decrease dosage from 25 mg daily to 25 mg every other day; or if dosage was 25 mg every other day, withhold drug. If potassium level is greater than 6 mEq/L, withhold drug. May restart drug at 25 mg every other day when potassium level is less than 5.5 mEq/L. In patients taking weak CYP3A4 inhibitors (erythromycin, fluconazole, saquinavir, verapamil), reduce eplerenone starting dose to 25 mg P.O. once daily.

ACTION

Binds to mineralocorticoid receptors and blocks aldosterone, which increases blood pressure through induction of sodium reabsorption and possibly other mechanisms.

Route	Onset	Peak	Duration
P.O.	Unknown	90 min	Unknown

Half-life: 4 to 6 hours.

ADVERSE REACTIONS

CNS: dizziness, fatigue.
GI: diarrhea, abdominal pain.
GU: albuminuria, abnormal vaginal bleeding.
Metabolic: ***hyperkalemia.***
Respiratory: cough.
Other: flulike syndrome, gynecomastia.

INTERACTIONS

Drug-drug. *ACE inhibitors, angiotensin II receptor antagonists:* May increase risk of hyperkalemia. Use together cautiously.
Azole antifungals (itraconazole, ketoconazole), macrolides (clarithromycin), nefazodone, protease inhibitors (nelfinavir, ritonavir): Inhibits the CYP3A4 metabolism of eplerenone. Use together is contraindicated.
Lithium: May increase risk of lithium toxicity. Monitor lithium level.
NSAIDs: May reduce the antihypertensive effect and cause severe hyperkalemia in patients with impaired renal function. Monitor blood pressure and potassium level.
Potassium supplements, potassium-sparing diuretics (amiloride, spironolactone, triamterene): May increase risk of hyperkalemia and sometimes-fatal arrhythmias. Use together is contraindicated.
Weak CYP3A4 inhibitors (erythromycin, fluconazole, saquinavir, verapamil): May increase eplerenone level. Reduce eplerenone starting dose to 25 mg P.O. once daily.
Drug-herb. *St. John's wort:* May decrease eplerenone level over time. Discourage use together.

EFFECTS ON LAB TEST RESULTS

- May increase ALT, BUN, cholesterol, creatinine, GGT, potassium, triglyceride, and uric acid levels. May decrease sodium level.

CONTRAINDICATIONS & CAUTIONS

- When used for hypertension, contraindicated in patients with type 2 diabetes with microalbuminuria, creatinine level greater than 2 mg/dl in men or greater than 1.8 mg/dl in women, or creatinine clearance less than 50 ml/minute and in patients taking potassium supplements or potassium-sparing diuretics (amiloride, spironolactone, or triamterene).
- Contraindicated in patients with potassium level greater than 5.5 mEq/ml or creatinine clearance 30 ml/minute or less and in patients taking strong CYP3A4 inhibitors, such as ketoconazole, clarithromycin, ritonavir, nelfinavir, nefazodone, or itraconazole.
- Use cautiously in patient with mild to moderate hepatic impairment.
- Use in pregnant woman only if the potential benefits justify the potential risk to the fetus. Use cautiously in breast-feeding women; it's unknown if drug appears in breast milk.

NURSING CONSIDERATIONS

- Drug may be used alone or with other antihypertensives.
- Full therapeutic effect of the drug occurs in 4 weeks.
- In patients with heart failure, measure potassium level at baseline, within the first week, at 1 month after starting therapy, and periodically thereafter.
- Monitor patient for signs and symptoms of hyperkalemia.

PATIENT TEACHING

- Inform patient that drug may be taken with or without food.
- Advise patient to avoid potassium supplements and salt substitutes during treatment.
- Tell patient to report adverse reactions.

eprosartan mesylate

Teveten

Pharmacologic class: angiotensin II receptor antagonist
Pregnancy risk category C; D in 2nd and 3rd trimesters

AVAILABLE FORMS

Tablets: 400 mg, 600 mg

INDICATIONS & DOSAGES

➤ **Hypertension (alone or with other antihypertensives)**
Adults: Initially, 600 mg P.O. daily. Dosage ranges from 400 to 800 mg daily, given as single daily dose or two divided doses.

ACTION

An angiotensin II receptor antagonist that reduces blood pressure by blocking the vasoconstrictor and aldosterone-secreting effects of angiotensin II. Drug selectively blocks the binding of angiotensin II to its receptor sites found in many tissues, such as vascular smooth muscle and the adrenal gland.

Route	Onset	Peak	Duration
P.O.	1–2 hr	1–3 hr	24 hr

Half-life: 5 to 9 hours.

ADVERSE REACTIONS

CNS: depression, fatigue, headache, dizziness.
CV: chest pain, dependent edema.
EENT: pharyngitis, rhinitis, sinusitis.
GI: abdominal pain, dyspepsia, diarrhea.
GU: UTI.
Hematologic: ***neutropenia.***
Musculoskeletal: arthralgia, myalgia.
Respiratory: cough, upper respiratory tract infection, bronchitis.
Other: injury, viral infection.

INTERACTIONS

Drug-drug. *NSAIDs:* May decrease antihypertensive effects. Monitor blood pressure.
Drug-herb. *Ma huang:* May decrease antihypertensive effects. Discourage use together.

EFFECTS ON LAB TEST RESULTS

- May increase BUN and triglyceride levels.

CONTRAINDICATIONS & CAUTIONS

- Contraindicated in patients hypersensitive to eprosartan or its components.
- Use cautiously in patients with renal artery stenosis; in patients with an activated renin-angiotensin system, such as volume- or salt-depleted patients; and in patients whose renal function may depend on the renin-angiotensin-aldosterone system, such as those with severe heart failure.
- Safety and effectiveness in children haven't been established.

NURSING CONSIDERATIONS

- Correct hypovolemia and hyponatremia before starting therapy to reduce risk of symptomatic hypotension.
- Monitor blood pressure closely for 2 hours at start of treatment. If hypotension occurs, place patient in a supine position and, if needed, give an I.V. infusion of normal saline solution.
- A transient episode of hypotension isn't a contraindication to continued treatment. Drug may be restarted once patient's blood pressure has stabilized.
- Drug may be used alone or with other antihypertensives, such as diuretics and calcium channel blockers. Maximal blood pressure response may take 2 or 3 weeks.
- Monitor patient for facial or lip swelling because angioedema has occurred with other angiotensin II antagonists.
- Closely observe infants exposed to eprosartan in utero for hypotension, oliguria, and hyperkalemia.

PATIENT TEACHING

- Advise woman of childbearing age to use a reliable form of contraception and to notify her prescriber immediately if pregnancy is suspected. Treatment may need to be stopped under medical supervision.
- Advise patient to report facial or lip swelling and signs and symptoms of infection, such as fever and sore throat.

• Tell patient to notify prescriber before taking OTC medication to treat a dry cough.
• Inform patient that drug may be taken without regard to meals.
• Advise breast-feeding woman to either stop therapy or stop breast-feeding because of potential for adverse reactions in infant.

felodipine
Agon SR‡, Plendil, Plendil ER‡, Renedil†

Pharmacologic class: calcium channel blocker
Pregnancy risk category C

AVAILABLE FORMS
Tablets (extended-release): 2.5 mg, 5 mg, 10 mg

INDICATIONS & DOSAGES
➤Hypertension
Adults: Initially, 5 mg P.O. daily. Adjust dosage based on patient response, usually at intervals not less than 2 weeks. Usual dose is 2.5 to 10 mg daily; maximum dosage is 10 mg daily.
Elderly patients: 2.5 mg P.O. daily; adjust dosage as for adults. Maximum dosage is 10 mg daily.
Adjust-a-dose: For patients with impaired hepatic function, 2.5 mg P.O. daily; adjust dosage as for adults. Maximum daily dose is 10 mg.

ACTION
Unknown. A dihydropyridine-derivative calcium channel blocker that prevents entry of calcium ions into vascular smooth muscle and cardiac cells; shows some selectivity for smooth muscle compared with cardiac muscle.

Route	Onset	Peak	Duration
P.O.	2–5 hr	2½–5 hr	24 hr

Half-life: 11 to 16 hours.

ADVERSE REACTIONS
CNS: *headache,* dizziness, paresthesia, asthenia.
CV: *peripheral edema,* chest pain, palpitations, flushing.
EENT: rhinorrhea, pharyngitis.
GI: abdominal pain, nausea, constipation, diarrhea.
Musculoskeletal: muscle cramps, back pain.
Respiratory: upper respiratory tract infection, cough.
Skin: rash.

INTERACTIONS
Drug-drug. *Anticonvulsants:* May decrease felodipine level. Avoid using together.
CYP3A4 inhibitors such as azole antifungals, cimetidine, erythromycin: May decrease clearance of felodipine. Reduce doses of felodipine; monitor patient for toxicity.
Metoprolol: May alter pharmacokinetics of metoprolol. Monitor patient for adverse reactions.
NSAIDs: May decrease antihypertensive effects. Monitor blood pressure.
Tacrolimus: May increase tacrolimus level. Monitor patient closely.
Theophylline: May slightly decrease theophylline level. Monitor patient response closely.
Drug-herb. *Ma huang:* May decrease antihypertensive effects. Discourage use together.
Drug-food. *Grapefruit, lime:* May increase drug level and adverse effects. Discourage use together.

EFFECTS ON LAB TEST RESULTS
None reported.

CONTRAINDICATIONS & CAUTIONS
• Contraindicated in patients hypersensitive to drug.
• Use cautiously in patients with heart failure, particularly those receiving beta blockers, and in patients with impaired hepatic function.

NURSING CONSIDERATIONS
• Monitor blood pressure for response.
• Monitor patient for peripheral edema, which appears to be both dose- and age-related. It's more common in patients taking higher doses, especially those older than age 60.

• ***Look alike–sound alike:*** Don't confuse Plendil with pindolol.

PATIENT TEACHING
• Tell patient to swallow tablets whole and not to crush or chew them.
• Tell patient to take drug without food or with a light meal.
• Advise patient not to take drug with grapefruit juice.
• Advise patient to continue taking drug even when he feels better, to watch his diet, and to check with prescriber or pharmacist before taking other drugs, including OTC drugs, nutritional supplements, or herbal remedies.
• Advise patient to observe good oral hygiene and to see a dentist regularly; use of drug may cause mild gum problems.

fosinopril sodium
Monopril✐

Pharmacologic class: ACE inhibitor
Pregnancy risk category C; D in 2nd and 3rd trimesters

AVAILABLE FORMS
Tablets: 10 mg, 20 mg, 40 mg

INDICATIONS & DOSAGES
➤ **Hypertension**
Adults: Initially, 10 mg P.O. daily; adjust dosage based on blood pressure response at peak and trough levels. Usual dosage is 20 to 40 mg daily; maximum is 80 mg daily. Dosage may be divided.
➤ **Heart failure**
Adults: Initially, 10 mg P.O. once daily. Increase dosage over several weeks to a maximum of 40 mg P.O. daily, if needed.
Adjust-a-dose: For patients with moderate to severe renal failure or vigorous diuresis, start with 5 mg P.O. once daily.

ACTION
May inhibit ACE, preventing conversion of angiotensin I to angiotensin II, a potent vasoconstrictor. Less angiotensin II decreases peripheral arterial resistance, thus decreasing aldosterone secretion, which reduces sodium and water retention and lowers blood pressure.

Route	Onset	Peak	Duration
P.O.	1 hr	3 hr	24 hr

Half-life: 11½ hours.

ADVERSE REACTIONS
CNS: *dizziness, **stroke,*** headache, fatigue, syncope, paresthesia, sleep disturbance.
CV: ***MI,*** chest pain, angina pectoris, rhythm disturbances, palpitations, hypotension, orthostatic hypotension.
EENT: tinnitus, sinusitis.
GI: ***pancreatitis,*** nausea, vomiting, diarrhea, dry mouth, abdominal distention, abdominal pain, constipation.
GU: sexual dysfunction, renal insufficiency.
Hepatic: ***hepatitis.***
Metabolic: ***hyperkalemia.***
Musculoskeletal: arthralgia, musculoskeletal pain, myalgia.
Respiratory: *dry, persistent, tickling, nonproductive cough, **bronchospasm.***
Skin: urticaria, rash, photosensitivity reactions, pruritus.
Other: ***angioedema,*** decreased libido, gout.

INTERACTIONS
Drug-drug. *Antacids:* May impair absorption. Separate dosage times by at least 2 hours.
Azathioprine: May increase risk of anemia or leukopenia. Monitor hematologic studies if used together.
Diuretics, other antihypertensives: May cause excessive hypotension. Stop diuretic or lower fosinopril dosage.
Lithium: May increase lithium level and lithium toxicity. Monitor lithium level.
Nesiritide: May increase hypotensive effects. Monitor blood pressure.
NSAIDs: May decrease antihypertensive effects. Monitor blood pressure.
Potassium-sparing diuretics, potassium supplements: May cause risk of hyperkalemia. Monitor patient closely.
Drug-herb. *Capsaicin:* May cause cough. Discourage use together.
Ma huang: May decrease antihypertensive effects. Discourage use together.
Drug-food. *Salt substitutes containing potassium:* May cause hyperkalemia. Discourage use together.

EFFECTS ON LAB TEST RESULTS

- May increase BUN, creatinine, potassium, and hemoglobin levels and hematocrit.
- May increase liver function test values.
- May cause falsely low digoxin level with the Digi-Tab radioimmunoassay kit for digoxin.

CONTRAINDICATIONS & CAUTIONS

- Contraindicated in patients hypersensitive to drug or other ACE inhibitors and in breast-feeding women.
- Use cautiously in patients with impaired renal or hepatic function.

NURSING CONSIDERATIONS

- Monitor blood pressure for drug effect.
- Although ACE inhibitors reduce blood pressure in all races, they reduce it less in blacks taking the ACE inhibitor alone. Black patients should take drug with a thiazide diuretic for a more favorable response.
- ACE inhibitors appear to cause a higher risk of angioedema in black patients.
- Monitor potassium intake and potassium level. Diabetic patients, those with impaired renal function, and those receiving drugs that can increase potassium level may develop hyperkalemia.
- Other ACE inhibitors may cause agranulocytosis and neutropenia. Monitor CBC with differential counts before therapy and periodically thereafter.
- Assess renal and hepatic function before and periodically throughout therapy.
- ***Look alike–sound alike:*** Don't confuse fosinopril with lisinopril. Don't confuse Monopril with Monurol.

PATIENT TEACHING

- Tell patient to avoid salt substitutes; these products may contain potassium, which can cause high potassium level in patients taking drug.
- Instruct patient to contact prescriber if light-headedness or fainting occurs.
- Advise patient to report evidence of infection, such as fever and sore throat.
- Instruct patient to call prescriber if he develops easy bruising or bleeding; swelling of tongue, lips, face, eyes, mucous membranes, arms, or legs; difficulty swallowing or breathing; and hoarseness.
- Urge patient to use caution in hot weather and during exercise. Inadequate fluid intake, vomiting, diarrhea, and excessive perspiration can lead to light-headedness and fainting.
- Tell woman of childbearing age to notify prescriber if pregnancy occurs. Drug will need to be stopped.

guanfacine hydrochloride

Tenex

Pharmacologic class: centrally acting antiadrenergic
Pregnancy risk category B

AVAILABLE FORMS

Tablets: 1 mg, 2 mg

INDICATIONS & DOSAGES

➤Hypertension

Adults: Initially, 1 mg P.O. once daily at bedtime. If response isn't adequate after 3 to 4 weeks, increase dosage to 2 mg daily. Dosage may be further increased to 3 mg P.O. after an additional 3 to 4 weeks.

➤To relieve symptoms of heroin withdrawal ♦

Adults: 0.03 mg to 1.5 mg P.O. once daily.

➤Migraine ♦

Adults: 1 mg P.O. once daily for 12 weeks.

ACTION

Centrally acting $alpha_2$-adrenoreceptor agonist. Reduces sympathetic outflow from the vasomotor center to the heart and blood vessels, resulting in a decrease in peripheral vascular resistance and a reduction in heart rate.

Route	Onset	Peak	Duration
P.O.	Unknown	1–4 hr	24 hr

Half-life: About 17 hours.

ADVERSE REACTIONS

CNS: *dizziness, somnolence,* fatigue, headache, insomnia, asthenia.
CV: ***bradycardia.***
GI: *constipation, dry mouth,* diarrhea, nausea.
GU: impotence.
Skin: dermatitis, pruritus.

INTERACTIONS

Drug-drug. *CNS depressants:* May increase sedation. Use together cautiously.
Tricyclic antidepressants: May inhibit antihypertensive effects. Monitor blood pressure.
Drug-lifestyle. *Alcohol:* May increase sedation. Discourage alcohol use.

EFFECTS ON LAB TEST RESULTS

None reported.

CONTRAINDICATIONS & CAUTIONS

- Contraindicated in patients hypersensitive to drug.
- Use cautiously in patients with severe coronary insufficiency, recent MI, cerebrovascular disease, or chronic renal or hepatic insufficiency.

NURSING CONSIDERATIONS

- Monitor blood pressure frequently.
- Risk and severity of adverse reactions increase with higher dosages.
- Drug may be used alone or with a diuretic.
- Rebound hypertension may occur and, if it occurs, will be noticeable within 2 to 4 days after therapy ends.
- ***Look alike–sound alike:*** Don't confuse guanfacine with guanidine, guaifenesin, or guanabenz. Don't confuse Tenex with Xanax, Entex, or Ten-K.

PATIENT TEACHING

- Tell patient not to stop therapy abruptly. Rebound high blood pressure may occur but is less common than that which occurs with similar drugs.
- Advise patient to avoid activities that require alertness before drug's effects on him are known; drowsiness may occur.
- Warn patient that he may have a lower tolerance to alcohol and other CNS depressants during therapy.

hydralazine hydrochloride

Alphapress‡, Apresoline, Novo-Hylazin†, Supres†

Pharmacologic class: peripheral dilator
Pregnancy risk category C

AVAILABLE FORMS

Injection: 20 mg/ml in 1-ml vial
Tablets: 10 mg, 25 mg, 50 mg, 100 mg

INDICATIONS & DOSAGES

➤ Hypertension

Adults: Initially, 10 mg P.O. q.i.d.; gradually increase over 2 weeks to 50 mg q.i.d., based on patient tolerance and response. Once stabilized, maintenance dosage can be divided b.i.d. Recommended range is 12.5 to 50 mg b.i.d.
Children: Initially, 0.75 mg/kg daily P.O. divided into four doses; gradually increased over 3 to 4 weeks to maximum of 7.5 mg/kg or 200 mg daily. Maximum first P.O. dose is 25 mg.

Or, 0.1 to 0.2 mg/kg I.V. q 4 to 6 hours, p.r.n. Maximum first parenteral dose is 20 mg.

➤ Hypertensive crisis

Adults: 10 to 20 mg I.V. slowly or 10 to 50 mg I.M.; repeat p.r.n. Switch to oral form as soon as possible.

➤ Preeclampsia, eclampsia

Adults: Initially, 5 to 10 mg I.V., followed by 5- to 10-mg I.V. doses (range 5 to 20 mg) q 20 to 30 minutes, p.r.n; or, 0.5 to 10 mg/hour I.V. infusion.

➤ Heart failure ♦

Adults: Initially, 50 to 75 mg P.O. daily. Maintenance doses range from 200 to 600 mg P.O. daily in divided doses q 6 to 12 hours.

I.V. ADMINISTRATION

- Give drug slowly and repeat as needed, generally q 4 to 6 hours. Hydralazine changes color in most infusion solutions; these color changes don't indicate loss of potency.
- Drug is compatible with normal saline, Ringer's, lactated Ringer's, and several other common I.V. solutions.

• Oral therapy should replace parenteral therapy as soon as possible.

INCOMPATIBILITIES
Aminophylline, ampicillin sodium, chlorothiazide, dextrose 10% in lactated Ringer's solution, dextrose 10% in normal saline solution, D_5W, diazoxide, doxapram, edetate calcium disodium, ethacrynate, fructose 10% in normal saline solution, fructose 10% in water, furosemide, hydrocortisone sodium succinate, mephentermine, metaraminol bitartrate, methohexital, nitroglycerin, phenobarbital sodium, verapamil.

ACTION
Unknown. A direct-acting peripheral vasodilator that relaxes arteriolar smooth muscle.

Route	Onset	Peak	Duration
P.O.	20–30 min	1–2 hr	2–4 hr
I.V.	5–20 min	10–80 min	2–6 hr
I.M.	10–30 min	1 hr	2–6 hr

Half-life: 3 to 7 hours.

ADVERSE REACTIONS
CNS: *headache,* peripheral neuritis, dizziness.
CV: *angina pectoris, palpitations, tachycardia,* orthostatic hypotension, edema, flushing.
EENT: nasal congestion.
GI: *nausea, vomiting, diarrhea, anorexia,* constipation.
Hematologic: ***neutropenia, leukopenia, agranulocytopenia, agranulocytosis, thrombocytopenia with or without purpura.***
Skin: rash.
Other: *lupuslike syndrome.*

INTERACTIONS
Drug-drug. *Diazoxide, MAO inhibitors:* May cause severe hypotension. Use together cautiously.
Diuretics, other hypotensive drugs: May cause excessive hypotension. Dosage adjustment may be needed.
Indomethacin: May decrease effects of hydralazine. Monitor blood pressure.
Metoprolol, propranolol: May increase levels and effects of these beta blockers. Monitor patient closely. May need to adjust dosage of either drug.

EFFECTS ON LAB TEST RESULTS
• May decrease hemoglobin level.
• May decrease neutrophil, WBC, granulocyte, platelet, and RBC counts.
• May cause positive ANA titers.

CONTRAINDICATIONS & CAUTIONS
• Contraindicated in patients hypersensitive to drug.
• Contraindicated in those with coronary artery disease or mitral valvular rheumatic heart disease.
• Use cautiously in patients with suspected cardiac disease, stroke, or severe renal impairment and in those taking other antihypertensives.

NURSING CONSIDERATIONS
• Monitor patient's blood pressure, pulse rate, and body weight frequently. Drug may be given with diuretics and beta blockers to decrease sodium retention and tachycardia and to prevent angina attacks.
• Elderly patients may be more sensitive to drug's hypotensive effects.
• Monitor CBC, lupus erythematosus cell preparation, and antinuclear antibody titer determination before therapy and periodically during long-term therapy.
• ***Alert:*** Monitor patient closely for signs and symptoms of lupuslike syndrome (sore throat, fever, muscle and joint aches, rash), and notify prescriber immediately if they develop.
• Improve patient compliance by giving drug b.i.d. Check with prescriber.
• ***Look alike–sound alike:*** Don't confuse hydralazine with hydroxyzine or Apresoline with Apresazide.
• Apresoline may contain tartrazine.

PATIENT TEACHING
• Instruct patient to take oral form with meals to increase absorption.
• Inform patient that low blood pressure and dizziness upon standing can be minimized by rising slowly and avoiding sudden position changes.
• Tell woman of childbearing age to notify prescriber if she suspects pregnancy. Drug will need to be stopped.

• Tell patient to notify prescriber of unexplained prolonged general tiredness or fever, muscle or joint aching, or chest pain.

irbesartan

Avapro

Pharmacologic class: angiotensin II receptor antagonist
Pregnancy risk category C; D in 2nd and 3rd trimesters

AVAILABLE FORMS

Tablets: 75 mg, 150 mg, 300 mg

INDICATIONS & DOSAGES

➤ Hypertension

Adults and children age 13 and older: Initially, 150 mg P.O. daily, increased to maximum of 300 mg daily, if needed.
Children ages 6 to 12: Initially, 75 mg P.O. once daily, increased to maximum of 150 mg daily, if needed.
Adjust-a-dose: For volume- and sodium-depleted patients, initially, 75 mg P.O. daily.

➤ Nephropathy in patients with type 2 diabetes

Adults: 300 mg P.O. once daily.

ACTION

Produces antihypertensive effect by competitive antagonist activity at the angiotensin II receptor.

Route	Onset	Peak	Duration
P.O.	Unknown	½–2 hr	24 hr

Half-life: 11 to 15 hours.

ADVERSE REACTIONS

CNS: fatigue, anxiety, dizziness, headache.
CV: chest pain, edema, tachycardia.
EENT: pharyngitis, rhinitis, sinus abnormality.
GI: diarrhea, dyspepsia, abdominal pain, nausea, vomiting.
GU: UTI.
Musculoskeletal: musculoskeletal trauma or pain.
Respiratory: upper respiratory tract infection, cough.
Skin: rash.

INTERACTIONS

None reported.

EFFECTS ON LAB TEST RESULTS

None reported.

CONTRAINDICATIONS & CAUTIONS

• Contraindicated in patients hypersensitive to drug or its components.
• Use cautiously in patients with impaired renal function, heart failure, and renal artery stenosis and in breast-feeding women.
• Use during pregnancy can cause injury and death to the developing fetus. When pregnancy is detected, stop drug as soon as possible.

NURSING CONSIDERATIONS

• Drug may be given with a diuretic or other antihypertensive, if needed, for control of hypertension.
• Symptomatic hypotension may occur in volume- or sodium-depleted patients (vigorous diuretic use or dialysis). Correct the cause of volume depletion before administration or before a lower dose is used.
• If hypotension occurs, place patient in a supine position and give an I.V. infusion of normal saline solution, if needed. Once blood pressure has stabilized after a transient hypotensive episode, drug may be continued.
• Dizziness and orthostatic hypotension may occur more frequently in patients with type 2 diabetes and renal disease.

PATIENT TEACHING

• Warn woman of childbearing age of consequences of drug exposure to fetus. Tell her to call prescriber immediately if pregnancy is suspected.
• Tell patient that drug may be taken once daily without regard to food.

SAFETY ALERT!

labetalol hydrochloride
Normodyne, Presolol‡, Trandate

Pharmacologic class: alpha and beta blocker
Pregnancy risk category C

AVAILABLE FORMS
Injection: 5 mg/ml in 20- and 40-ml multiple-dose vials and 4- and 8-ml prefilled syringes
Tablets: 100 mg, 200 mg, 300 mg

INDICATIONS & DOSAGES
➤ **Hypertension**
Adults: 100 mg P.O. b.i.d. with or without a diuretic. If needed, dosage is increased to 200 mg b.i.d. after 2 days. Further increases may be made q 2 to 3 days until optimal response is reached. Usual maintenance dosage is 200 to 400 mg b.i.d.

➤ **Severe hypertension, hypertensive emergencies**
Adults: 200 mg diluted in 160 ml of D_5W, infused at 2 mg/minute until satisfactory response is obtained; then infusion is stopped. May be repeated q 6 to 12 hours.

Or, give by repeated I.V. injection: initially, 20 mg I.V. slowly over 2 minutes. Repeat injections of 40 to 80 mg q 10 minutes until maximum dose of 300 mg is reached, p.r.n.

I.V. ADMINISTRATION
- Drug may be given by slow, direct I.V. injection over 2 minutes at 10-minute intervals.
- For I.V. infusion, prepare by diluting with D_5W or normal saline solutions; for example, 200 mg of drug to 160 ml D_5W to yield 1 mg/ml.
- Give labetalol infusion with an infusion control device.
- Monitor blood pressure closely every 5 minutes for 30 minutes; then every 30 minutes for 2 hours. Then monitor it hourly for 6 hours.
- Patient should remain supine for 3 hours after infusion. When given I.V. for hypertensive emergencies, drug produces a rapid, predictable fall in blood pressure within 5 to 10 minutes.
- Store at room temperature. Protect from light.

INCOMPATIBILITIES
Alkali solutions, amphotericin B, cefoperazone, ceftriaxone, furosemide, heparin, nafcillin, sodium bicarbonate, thiopental, warfarin.

ACTION
May be related to reduced peripheral vascular resistance, as a result of alpha and beta blockade.

Route	Onset	Peak	Duration
P.O.	20 min	2–4 hr	8–12 hr
I.V.	2–5 min	5 min	2–4 hr

Half-life: About 5½ hours after I.V. use; 6 to 8 hours after P.O. use.

ADVERSE REACTIONS
CNS: *dizziness,* vivid dreams, fatigue, headache, paresthesia, transient scalp tingling, syncope.
CV: *orthostatic hypotension,* ***ventricular arrhythmias.***
EENT: nasal congestion.
GI: nausea, vomiting.
GU: sexual dysfunction, urine retention.
Respiratory: ***bronchospasm,*** dyspnea.
Skin: rash.

INTERACTIONS
Drug-drug. *Beta agonists:* May blunt bronchodilator effect of these drugs in patients with bronchospasm. May need to increase dosages of these drugs.
Cimetidine: May enhance labetalol's effect. Use together cautiously.
Halothane: May increase hypotensive effect. Monitor blood pressure closely.
Insulin, oral antidiabetics: May alter dosage requirements in previously stabilized diabetic patient. Monitor patient closely.
Nitroglycerin: May blunt reflex tachycardia produced by nitroglycerin but not the hypotension. Monitor BP if used together.
NSAIDs: May decrease antihypertensive effects. Monitor blood pressure.
Tricyclic antidepressants: May increase incidence of tremor. Monitor patient for tremor.

Drug-herb. *Ma huang:* May decrease antihypertensive effects. Discourage use together.

EFFECTS ON LAB TEST RESULTS
- May increase transaminase and urea levels.
- May cause a false-positive increase of urine free and total catecholamine levels when measured by a nonspecific trihydroxyindole fluorometric method.
- May cause false-positive test for amphetamines when screening urine for drugs.

CONTRAINDICATIONS & CAUTIONS
- Contraindicated in patients hypersensitive to drug and in those with bronchial asthma, overt cardiac failure, greater than first-degree heart block, cardiogenic shock, severe bradycardia, and other conditions that may cause severe and prolonged hypotension.
- Use cautiously in patients with heart failure, hepatic failure, chronic bronchitis, emphysema, peripheral vascular disease, and pheochromocytoma.

NURSING CONSIDERATIONS
- Monitor blood pressure frequently. Drug masks common signs and symptoms of shock.
- If dizziness occurs, give dose at bedtime or in smaller doses t.i.d.
- When switching from I.V. to P.O. form, begin P.O. regimen at 200 mg after blood pressure begins to rise; repeat dose with 200 to 400 mg in 6 to 12 hours. Adjust dosage according to blood pressure response.
- In diabetic patients, monitor glucose level closely because beta blockers may mask certain signs and symptoms of hypoglycemia.
- ***Look alike–sound alike:*** Don't confuse Trandate with Trental or Tridrate.

PATIENT TEACHING
- ***Alert:*** Tell patient that stopping drug abruptly can worsen chest pain and trigger a heart attack.
- Advise patient that dizziness is the most troublesome adverse reaction and tends to occur in the early stages of treatment, in patients taking diuretics, and with higher dosages. Inform patient that dizziness can be minimized by rising slowly and avoiding sudden position changes.
- Warn patient that occasional, harmless scalp tingling may occur, especially when therapy begins.

lisinopril

Prinivil✐, Zestril✐

Pharmacologic class: ACE inhibitor
Pregnancy risk category C; D in 2nd and 3rd trimesters

AVAILABLE FORMS
Tablets: 2.5 mg, 5 mg, 10 mg, 20 mg, 30 mg, 40 mg

INDICATIONS & DOSAGES

➤ Hypertension
Adults: Initially, 10 mg P.O. daily for patients not taking a diuretic. Most patients are well controlled on 20 to 40 mg daily as a single dose. For patients taking a diuretic, initially, 5 mg P.O. daily.
Children age 6 and older: Initially, 0.07 mg/kg (up to 5 mg) P.O. once daily. Increase dosage based on patient response and tolerance. Maximum dose, 0.61 mg/kg (don't exceed 40 mg). Don't use in children with a creatinine clearance less than 30 ml/minute.
Adjust-a-dose: In adults, if creatinine clearance is 10 to 30 ml/minute, give 5 mg P.O. daily; if clearance is less than 10 ml/minute, give 2.5 mg P.O. daily.

➤ Adjunct treatment (with diuretics and cardiac glycosides) for heart failure
Adults: Initially, 5 mg P.O. daily; increased p.r.n. to maximum of 20 mg P.O. daily.
Adjust-a-dose: If sodium level is less than 130 mEq/L or creatinine clearance less than 30 ml/minute, start treatment at 2.5 mg daily.

➤ Hemodynamically stable patients within 24 hours of acute MI to improve survival
Adults: Initially, 5 mg P.O.; then 5 mg after 24 hours, 10 mg after 48 hours, followed by 10 mg once daily for 6 weeks.
Adjust-a-dose: For patients with systolic blood pressure 120 mm Hg or less when treatment is started or during first 3 days

after an infarct, decrease dosage to 2.5 mg P.O. If systolic blood pressure drops to 100 mm Hg or less, reduce daily maintenance dose of 5 mg to 2.5 mg, if needed. If prolonged systolic blood pressure stays under 90 mm Hg for longer than 1 hour, withdraw drug.

➤ **Hypertension in children**
Children ages 6 to 16: Initially, 0.07 mg/kg P.O. once daily (up to 5 mg total). Adjust dosage according to blood pressure response. Doses above 0.61 mg/kg (or above 40 mg) haven't been studied in children.

ACTION

Unknown. Thought to result primarily from ACE, resulting in decreased production of angiotensin II, and suppression of the renin-angiotensin-aldosterone system.

Route	Onset	Peak	Duration
P.O.	1 hr	7 hr	24 hr

Half-life: 12 hours.

ADVERSE REACTIONS

CNS: *dizziness,* headache, fatigue, paresthesia.
CV: *orthostatic hypotension,* hypotension, chest pain.
EENT: *nasal congestion.*
GI: *diarrhea,* nausea, dyspepsia.
GU: impaired renal function, impotence.
Metabolic: ***hyperkalemia.***
Respiratory: dyspnea, dry, persistent, tickling, nonproductive cough.
Skin: rash.

INTERACTIONS

Drug-drug. *Allopurinol:* May cause hypersensitivity reaction. Use together cautiously.
Azathioprine: May increase risk of anemia or leukopenia. Monitor hematologic studies if used together.
Diuretics, thiazide diuretics: May cause excessive hypotension with diuretics. Monitor blood pressure closely.
Indomethacin, NSAIDs: May reduce hypotensive effects of drug. Adjust dose as needed.
Insulin, oral antidiabetics: May cause hypoglycemia, especially at start of lisinopril therapy. Monitor glucose level.
Lithium: May cause lithium toxicity. Monitor lithium levels.
Phenothiazines: May increase hypotensive effects. Monitor BP closely.
Potassium-sparing diuretics, potassium supplements: May cause hyperkalemia. Monitor laboratory values.
Tizanidine: May cause severe hypotension. Monitor patient.
Drug-herb. *Capsaicin:* May cause ACE inhibitor-induced cough. Discourage use together.
Ma huang: May decrease antihypertensive effects. Discourage use together.
Drug-food. *Potassium-containing salt substitutes:* May cause hyperkalemia. Monitor laboratory values.

EFFECTS ON LAB TEST RESULTS

- May increase BUN, creatinine, potassium, and bilirubin levels.
- May increase liver function test values.

CONTRAINDICATIONS & CAUTIONS

- Contraindicated in patients hypersensitive to ACE inhibitors and in those with a history of angioedema related to previous treatment with ACE inhibitor.
- Use cautiously in patients with impaired renal function; adjust dosage.
- Use cautiously in patients at risk for hyperkalemia and in those with aortic stenosis or hypertrophic cardiomyopathy.

NURSING CONSIDERATIONS

- When using drug in acute MI, give patient the appropriate and standard recommended treatment, such as thrombolytics, aspirin, and beta blockers.
- The safety and efficacy of lisinopril on blood pressure in pediatric patients younger than age 6 or in pediatric patients with glomerular filtration rate less than 30 ml/minute hasn't been established.
- Although ACE inhibitors reduce blood pressure in all races, they reduce it less in blacks taking the ACE inhibitor alone. Black patients should take drug with a thiazide diuretic for a more favorable response.
- ACE inhibitors appear to increase risk of angioedema in black patients.
- Monitor blood pressure frequently. If drug doesn't adequately control blood pressure, diuretics may be added.

• Monitor WBC with differential counts before therapy, every 2 weeks for first 3 months of therapy, and periodically thereafter.
• ***Look alike–sound alike:*** Don't confuse lisinopril with fosinopril or Lioresal. Don't confuse Zestril with Zostrix, Zetia, Zebeta, or Zyrtec. Don't confuse Prinivil with Proventil or Prilosec.

PATIENT TEACHING

• ***Alert:*** Rarely, facial and throat swelling (including swelling of the larynx) may occur, especially after first dose. Advise patient to report signs or symptoms of breathing problems or swelling of face, eyes, lips, or tongue.
• Inform patient that light-headedness can occur, especially during first few days of therapy. Tell him to rise slowly to minimize this effect and to report symptoms to prescriber. If he faints, advise patient to stop taking drug and call prescriber immediately.
• If unpleasant adverse reactions occur, tell patient not to stop drug suddenly but to notify prescriber.
• Advise patient to report signs and symptoms of infection, such as fever and sore throat.
• Tell woman of childbearing age to notify prescriber if pregnancy occurs. Drug will need to be stopped.
• Instruct patient not to use salt substitutes that contain potassium without first consulting prescriber.

losartan potassium
Cozaar✎

Pharmacologic class: angiotensin II receptor antagonist
Pregnancy risk category C; D in 2nd and 3rd trimesters

AVAILABLE FORMS

Tablets: 25 mg, 50 mg, 100 mg

INDICATIONS & DOSAGES

➤ **Hypertension**

Adults: Initially, 25 to 50 mg P.O. daily. Maximum daily dose is 100 mg in one or two divided doses.
Children age 6 and older: 0.7 mg/kg (up to 50 mg) P.O. daily, adjust as needed up to 1.4 mg/kg/day (maximum 100 mg).
Adjust-a-dose: For adults who are hepatically impaired or intravascularly volume depleted (such as those taking diuretics), initially, 25 mg.

➤ **Nephropathy in type 2 diabetic patients**

Adults: 50 mg P.O. once daily. Increase dosage to 100 mg once daily based on BP response.

➤ **To reduce risk of stroke in patients with hypertension and left ventricular hypertrophy**

Adults: Initially, 50 mg P.O. once daily. Adjust dosage based on BP response, adding hydrochlorothiazide 12.5 mg once daily, increasing losartan to 100 mg daily, or both. If further adjustments are required, may increase the daily dosage of hydrochlorothiazide to 25 mg.

ACTION

Inhibits vasoconstrictive and aldosterone-secreting action of angiotensin II by blocking angiotensin II receptor on the surface of vascular smooth muscle and other tissue cells.

Route	Onset	Peak	Duration
P.O.	Unknown	1 hr	Unknown

Half-life: 2 hours.

ADVERSE REACTIONS

Patients with hypertension or left ventricular hypertrophy
CNS: dizziness, asthenia, fatigue, headache, insomnia.
CV: edema, chest pain.
EENT: nasal congestion, sinusitis, pharyngitis, sinus disorder.
GI: abdominal pain, nausea, diarrhea, dyspepsia.
Musculoskeletal: muscle cramps, myalgia, back or leg pain.
Respiratory: cough, upper respiratory infection.
Other: ***angioedema.***
Patients with nephropathy
CNS: *asthenia, fatigue,* fever, hypesthesia.
CV: *chest pain,* hypotension, orthostatic hypotension.

EENT: sinusitis, cataract.
GI: *diarrhea,* dyspepsia, gastritis.
GU: *UTI.*
Hematologic: *anemia.*
Metabolic: ***hyperkalemia, hypoglycemia,*** weight gain.
Musculoskeletal: *back pain,* leg or knee pain, muscle weakness.
Respiratory: *cough, bronchitis.*
Skin: cellulitis.
Other: *flulike syndrome,* ***diabetic vascular disease, angioedema,*** infection, trauma, diabetic neuropathy.

INTERACTIONS

Drug-drug. *Lithium:* May increase lithium level. Monitor lithium level and patient for toxicity.
NSAIDs: May decrease antihypertensive effects. Monitor blood pressure.
Potassium-sparing diuretics, potassium supplements: May cause hyperkalemia. Monitor patient closely.
Drug-herb. *Ma huang:* May decrease antihypertensive effects. Discourage use together.
Drug-food. *Salt substitutes containing potassium:* May cause hyperkalemia. Monitor patient closely.

EFFECTS ON LAB TEST RESULTS

None reported.

CONTRAINDICATIONS & CAUTIONS

- Contraindicated in patients hypersensitive to drug. Breast-feeding isn't recommended during losartan therapy.
- Use cautiously in patients with impaired renal or hepatic function.
- Drugs that act directly on the renin-angiotensin system (such as losartan) can cause fetal and neonatal morbidity and death when given to women in the second or third trimester of pregnancy. These problems haven't been detected when exposure was limited to the first trimester. If pregnancy is suspected, notify prescriber because drug should be stopped.

NURSING CONSIDERATIONS

- Drug can be used alone or with other antihypertensives.
- If antihypertensive effect is inadequate using once-daily doses, a twice-daily regimen using the same or increased total daily dose may give a more satisfactory response.
- Monitor patient's BP closely to evaluate effectiveness of therapy. When used alone, drug has less of an effect on blood pressure in black patients than in patients of other races.
- Monitor patients who are also taking diuretics for symptomatic hypotension.
- Regularly assess the patient's renal function (via creatinine and BUN levels).
- Patients with severe heart failure whose renal function depends on the angiotensin-aldosterone system may develop acute renal failure during therapy. Closely monitor patient, especially during first few weeks of therapy.
- ***Look alike–sound alike:*** Don't confuse Cozaar with Zocor.

PATIENT TEACHING

- Tell patient to avoid salt substitutes; these products may contain potassium, which can cause high potassium level in patients taking losartan.
- Inform woman of childbearing age about consequences of second and third trimester exposure to drug. Prescriber should be notified immediately if pregnancy is suspected.
- Advise patient to immediately report swelling of face, eyes, lips, or tongue or any breathing difficulty.

SAFETY ALERT!

methyldopa

Aldopren‡, Apo-Methyldopa†, Dopamet†, Hydopa‡, Novo-Medopa†, Nu-Medopa†

methyldopate hydrochloride

Pharmacologic class: centrally acting antiadrenergic
Pregnancy risk category B for P.O.; C for I.V.

AVAILABLE FORMS

methyldopa
Tablets: 250 mg, 500 mg
methyldopate hydrochloride
Injection: 50 mg/ml

INDICATIONS & DOSAGES

➤ **Hypertension, hypertensive crisis**
Adults: Initially, 250 mg P.O. b.i.d. to t.i.d. in first 48 hours. Increase if needed q 2 days. May give entire daily dose in evening or at bedtime. Adjust dosages if other antihypertensives are added to or deleted from therapy. Maintenance dosage is 500 mg to 2 g daily in two to four divided doses. Maximum recommended daily dose is 3 g. Or, 250 to 500 mg I.V. q 6 hours. Maximum dosage is 1 g q 6 hours. Switch to oral antihypertensives as soon as possible.
Children: Initially, 10 mg/kg P.O. daily in two to four divided doses; or, 20 to 40 mg/kg I.V. daily in four divided doses. Increase dose daily until desired response occurs. Maximum daily dose is 65 mg/kg or 3 g, whichever is less.

I.V. ADMINISTRATION

- Dilute appropriate dose in 100 ml D_5W. Infuse slowly over 30 to 60 minutes.

INCOMPATIBILITIES

Amphotericin B; drugs with poor solubility in acidic media, such as barbiturates and sulfonamides; methohexital; some total parenteral nutrition solutions.

ACTION

May inhibit the central vasomotor centers, decreasing sympathetic outflow to the heart, kidneys, and peripheral vasculature.

Route	Onset	Peak	Duration
P.O.	4–6 hr	Unknown	12–48 hr
I.V.	4–6 hr	Unknown	10–16 hr

Half-life: About 2 hours.

ADVERSE REACTIONS

CNS: *decreased mental acuity, sedation, headache,* weakness, dizziness, paresthesia, parkinsonism, involuntary choreoathetoid movements, psychic disturbances, depression, nightmares.
CV: *orthostatic hypotension, edema,* ***bradycardia, myocarditis,*** aggravated angina.
EENT: *nasal congestion.*
GI: *dry mouth,* ***pancreatitis,*** nausea, vomiting, diarrhea, constipation.
GU: galactorrhea.
Hematologic: ***thrombocytopenia, leukopenia, bone marrow depression,*** hemolytic anemia.
Hepatic: ***hepatic necrosis, hepatitis.***
Musculoskeletal: arthralgia.
Skin: rash.
Other: drug-induced fever, gynecomastia.

INTERACTIONS

Drug-drug. *Amphetamines, nonselective beta blockers, norepinephrine, phenothiazines, tricyclic antidepressants:* May cause hypertensive effects. Monitor patient closely.
Anesthetics: May need lower doses of anesthetics. Use together cautiously.
Barbiturates: May decrease actions of methyldopa. Monitor patient closely.
Ferrous sulfate: May decrease bioavailability of methyldopa. Separate doses.
Haloperidol: May increase antipsychotic effects of haloperidol or cause psychosis. Use together cautiously.
Levodopa: May increase hypotensive effects, which may increase adverse CNS reactions. Monitor patient closely.
Lithium: May increase lithium level. Watch for increased lithium level and signs and symptoms of toxicity.
MAO inhibitors: May cause excessive sympathetic stimulation. Avoid using together.
Tolbutamide: May impair metabolism of tolbutamide. Monitor patient for hypoglycemic effect.
Drug-herb. *Capsicum:* May reduce antihypertensive effect. Discourage use together.

EFFECTS ON LAB TEST RESULTS

- May increase creatinine level. May decrease hemoglobin level and hematocrit.
- May increase liver function test values. May decrease platelet and WBC counts.
- May falsely increase urine catecholamine level, interfering with the diagnosis of pheochromocytoma.
- May interfere with urinary uric acid testing, serum creatinine testing, and AST testing.
- May cause positive Coombs test.

CONTRAINDICATIONS & CAUTIONS
- Contraindicated in patients hypersensitive to drug and in those with active hepatic disease (such as acute hepatitis) or active cirrhosis.
- Contraindicated in those whose previous methyldopa therapy caused liver problems and in those taking MAO inhibitors.
- Use cautiously in patients with history of impaired hepatic function or sulfite sensitivity and in breast-feeding women.

NURSING CONSIDERATIONS
- Monitor patient's blood pressure regularly. Elderly patients are more likely to experience hypotension and sedation.
- Occasionally, tolerance may occur, usually between the second and third months of therapy. Adding a diuretic or adjusting dosage may be needed. If patient's response changes significantly, notify prescriber.
- After dialysis, monitor patient for hypertension and notify prescriber, if needed. Patient may need an extra dose of drug.
- Monitor CBC with differential counts before therapy and periodically thereafter.
- Patients who need blood transfusions should have direct and indirect Coombs tests to prevent crossmatching problems.
- Monitor patient's Coombs test results. In patients who have received drug for several months, positive reaction to direct Coombs test indicates hemolytic anemia.
- Report involuntary choreoathetoid movements. Drug may be stopped.
- ***Look alike–sound alike:*** Don't confuse Aldomet with Anzemet.

PATIENT TEACHING
- Tell patient not to suddenly stop taking drug, but to notify prescriber if unpleasant adverse reactions occur.
- Instruct patient to report signs and symptoms of infection.
- Tell patient to check his weight daily and to notify prescriber if he gains more than 5 lb. Sodium and water retention may occur, but can be relieved with diuretics.
- Warn patient that, particularly at the start of therapy, drug may impair ability to perform tasks that require mental alertness. A once-daily dose at bedtime minimizes daytime drowsiness.
- Inform patient that low blood pressure and dizziness upon rising can be minimized by rising slowly and avoiding sudden position changes and that dry mouth can be relieved by chewing gum or sucking on hard candy or ice chips.
- Tell patient that urine may turn dark if left sitting in toilet bowl or if toilet bowl has been treated with bleach.

metoprolol succinate
Toprol-XL

metoprolol tartrate
Apo-Metoprolol†, Apo-Metoprolol (Type L)†, Betaloc†‡, Betaloc Durules†, Lopresor†, Lopresor SR†, Lopressor, Minax‡, Novo-Metoprol†, Nu-Metop†

Pharmacologic class: beta blocker
Pregnancy risk category C

AVAILABLE FORMS
metoprolol succinate
Tablets (extended-release): 25 mg, 50 mg, 100 mg, 200 mg
metoprolol tartrate
Injection: 1 mg/ml in 5-ml ampules
Tablets: 50 mg, 100 mg
Tablets (extended-release): 100 mg†, 200 mg†

INDICATIONS & DOSAGES
➤ **Hypertension**
Adults: Initially, 50 mg P.O. b.i.d. or 100 mg P.O. once daily; then up to 100 to 450 mg daily in two or three divided doses. Or, 50 to 100 mg of extended-release tablets (tartrate equivalent) once daily. Adjust dosage as needed and tolerated at intervals of not less than 1 week to maximum of 400 mg daily.
➤ **Early intervention in acute MI**
Adults: 5 mg metoprolol tartrate I.V. bolus q 2 minutes for three doses. Then, 15 minutes after the last I.V. dose, give 25 to 50 mg P.O. q 6 hours for 48 hours. Maintenance dosage is 100 mg P.O. b.i.d.
➤ **Angina pectoris**
Adults: Initially, 100 mg P.O. daily as a single dose or in two equally divided doses; increased at weekly intervals until an adequate response or a pronounced de-

crease in heart rate is seen. Effects of daily dose beyond 400 mg aren't known. Or, give 100 mg of extended-release tablets (tartrate equivalent) once daily. Adjust dosage as needed and tolerated at intervals of not less than 1 week to maximum of 400 mg daily.

➤ **Stable symptomatic heart failure (New York Heart Association class II) resulting from ischemia, hypertension, or cardiomyopathy**

Adults: 25 mg Toprol-XL P.O. once daily for 2 weeks. Double the dose q 2 weeks, as tolerated, to a maximum of 200 mg daily.

Adjust-a-dose: In patients with more severe heart failure, start with 12.5 mg Toprol-XL P.O. once daily for 2 weeks.

I.V. ADMINISTRATION

- Give drug undiluted by direct injection.
- Although best avoided, drug can be mixed with meperidine hydrochloride or morphine sulfate or given with an alteplase infusion at a Y-site connection.
- Store drug at room temperature and protect from light. Discard solution if it's discolored or contains particles.

INCOMPATIBILITIES

Amphotericin B.

ACTION

Unknown. A selective beta blocker that selectively blocks $beta_1$ receptors; decreases cardiac output, peripheral resistance, and cardiac oxygen consumption; and depresses renin secretion.

Route	Onset	Peak	Duration
P.O.	15 min	1 hr	6–12 hr
P.O. (extended-release)	15 min	6–12 hr	24 hr
I.V.	5 min	20 min	5–8 hr

Half-life: 3 to 7 hours.

ADVERSE REACTIONS

CNS: *fatigue, dizziness,* depression.
CV: *hypotension,* ***bradycardia, heart failure, AV block,*** edema.
GI: nausea, diarrhea.
Respiratory: dyspnea.
Skin: rash.

INTERACTIONS

Drug-drug. *Amobarbital, butabarbital, butalbital, pentobarbital, phenobarbital, primidone, secobarbital:* May reduce metoprolol effect. May need to increase metoprolol dose.
Cardiac glycosides, diltiazem: May cause excessive bradycardia and increased depressant effect on myocardium. Use together cautiously.
Catecholamine-depleting drugs such as MAO inhibitors, reserpine: May have additive effect. Monitor patient for hypotension and bradycardia.
Chlorpromazine: May decrease hepatic clearance. Watch for greater beta-blocking effect.
Cimetidine: May increase metoprolol effects. Give another H_2 agonist or decrease dose of metoprolol.
Fluoxetine, paroxetine, propafenone, quinidine: May increase metoprolol level. Monitor vital signs.
Hydralazine: May increase levels and effects of both drugs. Monitor patient closely. May need to adjust dosage.
Indomethacin, NSAIDs: May decrease antihypertensive effect. Monitor blood pressure and adjust dosage.
Insulin, oral antidiabetics: May alter dosage requirements in previously stabilized diabetic patients. Monitor patient closely.
I.V. lidocaine: May reduce hepatic metabolism of lidocaine, increasing risk of toxicity. Give bolus doses of lidocaine at a slower rate, and monitor lidocaine level closely.
Prazosin: May increase risk of orthostatic hypotension in the early phases of use together. Assist patient to stand slowly until effects are known.
Rifampin: May increase metoprolol metabolism. Watch for decreased effect.
Terbutaline: May antagonize bronchodilatory effects of terbutaline. Monitor patient.
Verapamil: May increase effects of both drugs. Monitor cardiac function closely, and decrease dosages as needed.
Drug-herb. *Ma huang:* May decrease antihypertensive effects. Discourage use together.
Drug-food. *Food:* May increase absorption. Encourage patient to take drug with food.

EFFECTS ON LAB TEST RESULTS

- May increase transaminase, alkaline phosphatase, LDH, and uric acid levels.

CONTRAINDICATIONS & CAUTIONS

- Contraindicated in patients hypersensitive to drug or other beta blockers.
- Contraindicated in patients with sinus bradycardia, greater than first-degree heart block, cardiogenic shock, or overt cardiac failure when used to treat hypertension or angina. When used to treat MI, drug is contraindicated in patients with heart rate less than 45 beats/minute, greater than first-degree heart block, PR interval of 0.24 second or longer with first-degree heart block, systolic blood pressure less than 100 mm Hg, or moderate to severe cardiac failure.
- Use cautiously in patients with heart failure, diabetes, or respiratory or hepatic disease.

NURSING CONSIDERATIONS

- Always check patient's apical pulse rate before giving drug. If it's slower than 60 beats/minute, withhold drug and call prescriber immediately.
- In diabetic patients, monitor glucose level closely because drug masks common signs and symptoms of hypoglycemia.
- Monitor blood pressure frequently; drug masks common signs and symptoms of shock.
- Beta blockers may mask tachycardia caused by hyperthyroidism. In patients with suspected thyrotoxicosis, taper off beta blocker to avoid thyroid storm.
- When stopping therapy, taper dose over 1 to 2 weeks.
- Beta selectivity is lost at higher doses. Watch for peripheral side effects.
- ***Look alike–sound alike:*** Don't confuse metoprolol with metaproterenol or metolazone. Don't confuse Toprol-XL with Topamax, Tegretol, or Tegretol-XR.

PATIENT TEACHING

- Instruct patient to take drug exactly as prescribed and with meals.
- Caution patient to avoid driving and other tasks requiring mental alertness until response to therapy has been established.
- Advise patient to inform dentist or prescriber about use of this drug before procedures or surgery.
- Tell patient to alert prescriber if shortness of breath occurs.
- Instruct patient not to stop drug suddenly but to notify prescriber about unpleasant adverse reactions. Inform him that drug must be withdrawn gradually over 1 or 2 weeks.
- Inform patient that use isn't advisable in breast-feeding women.

minoxidil

Loniten

Pharmacologic class: peripheral vasodilator

Pregnancy risk category C

AVAILABLE FORMS

Tablets: 2.5 mg, 10 mg

INDICATIONS & DOSAGES

➤ Severe hypertension

Adults and children older than age 12: Initially, 2.5 to 5 mg P.O. as a single dose. Effective dosage range is usually 10 to 40 mg daily. Maximum dose is 100 mg daily.

Children younger than age 12: 0.2 mg/kg P.O. (maximum 5 mg) as a single daily dose. Effective dosage range is usually 0.25 to 1 mg/kg daily. Maximum dose is 50 mg daily.

ACTION

Unknown. Predominantly produces direct arteriolar vasodilation.

Route	Onset	Peak	Duration
P.O.	30 min	2–3 hr	2–5 days

Half-life: Average is 4¼ hours.

ADVERSE REACTIONS

CV: *edema, tachycardia, pericardial effusion and tamponade, ECG changes,* ***heart failure,*** rebound hypertension.
GI: nausea, vomiting.
Metabolic: weight gain.
Skin: ***Stevens-Johnson syndrome,*** rash.
Other: *hypertrichosis,* breast tenderness.

INTERACTIONS
Drug-drug. *Antihypertensives:* May cause severe orthostatic hypotension. Advise patient to stand up slowly.
NSAIDs: May decrease antihypertensive effects. Monitor blood pressure.
Drug-herb. *Ma huang:* May decrease antihypertensive effects. Discourage use together.

EFFECTS ON LAB TEST RESULTS
- May increase alkaline phosphatase, BUN, and creatinine levels. May decrease hemoglobin level and hematocrit.

CONTRAINDICATIONS & CAUTIONS
- Contraindicated in patients hypersensitive to drug and in those with pheochromocytoma. Also contraindicated in patients with acute MI or dissecting aortic aneurysm.
- Use cautiously in patients with impaired renal function and after recent MI (within past month).

NURSING CONSIDERATIONS
- Closely monitor blood pressure and pulse rate at beginning of therapy and periodically thereafter.
- Elderly patients may be more sensitive to drug's hypotensive effects.
- Initially, assess CBC, electrolytes, alkaline phosphatase, renal function, ECG, chest X-ray, and echocardiogram. Repeat tests that are abnormal at 1- to 3-month intervals and every 6 to 12 months when stabilized.
- Drug is removed by hemodialysis. Be sure to give dose after dialysis.
- Administer with a thiazide or loop diuretic to prevent fluid retention and heart failure.
- Monitor fluid intake and urine output. Check for weight gain and edema.
- Monitor patient for elongated, thickened, and enhanced pigmentation of fine body hair.
- Minoxidil may elevate antinuclear antibody titers.
- ***Look alike–sound alike:*** Don't confuse Loniten with Lotensin.

PATIENT TEACHING
- Make sure patient receives and reads manufacturer's package insert that describes the drug and its adverse reactions. Also provide an oral explanation.
- Tell patient not to suddenly stop taking drug but to notify prescriber if unpleasant adverse effects occur.
- Make sure patient understands importance of compliance with total treatment regimen. Drug is usually prescribed with a beta blocker to control rapid heart rate and a diuretic to counteract fluid retention.
- Teach patient how to take his own pulse and to notify prescriber of increases of more than 20 beats/minute.
- Tell patient to weigh himself at least weekly and to report weight gain of more than 5 lb.
- About 8 of 10 patients experience elongation, thickening, and enhanced pigmentation of fine body hair within 3 to 6 weeks of beginning treatment. Shaving or using a depilatory can control unwanted hair. Assure patient that extra hair disappears within 1 to 6 months of stopping minoxidil. Advise patient not to stop drug without prescriber's approval.
- Advise woman of childbearing age to discuss drug therapy with prescriber if considering pregnancy or currently breast-feeding.

nisoldipine
Sular

Pharmacologic class: calcium channel blocker
Pregnancy risk category C

AVAILABLE FORMS
Tablets (extended-release): 10 mg, 20 mg, 30 mg, 40 mg

INDICATIONS & DOSAGES
➤ **Hypertension**
Adults: Initially, 20 mg P.O. once daily; increased by 10 mg/week or at longer intervals, p.r.n. Usual maintenance dose is 20 to 40 mg daily. Doses of more than 60 mg daily aren't recommended.
Patients older than age 65: Initially, 10 mg P.O. once daily; adjust dosage as for other adults.

Adjust-a-dose: For patients with impaired liver function, initially, 10 mg P.O. once daily; dosage is adjusted as for adults.

ACTION

Prevents calcium ions from entering vascular smooth muscle cells, causing dilation of arterioles, which decreases peripheral vascular resistance.

Route	Onset	Peak	Duration
P.O.	Unknown	6–12 hr	24 hr

Half-life: 7 to 12 hours.

ADVERSE REACTIONS

CNS: *headache,* dizziness.
CV: *peripheral edema,* vasodilation, palpitations, chest pain.
EENT: sinusitis, pharyngitis.
GI: nausea.
Skin: rash.

INTERACTIONS

Drug-drug. *Cimetidine:* May increase bioavailability and peak nisoldipine level. Monitor blood pressure closely.
CYP3A4 inducers such as phenytoin: May decrease nisoldipine level. Avoid using together; consider alternative antihypertensive therapy.
Quinidine: May decrease bioavailability of nisoldipine. Adjust dosage accordingly.
Drug-herb. *Ma huang:* May decrease antihypertensive effects. Discourage use together.
Peppermint oil: May decrease drug effect. Discourage use together.
Drug-food. *Grapefruit, grapefruit juice:* May increase drug level, increasing adverse reactions. Discourage use together.
High-fat foods: May increase peak drug level. Discourage use together.

EFFECTS ON LAB TEST RESULTS

None reported.

CONTRAINDICATIONS & CAUTIONS

- Contraindicated in patients hypersensitive to dihydropyridine calcium channel blockers.
- Contraindicated in breast-feeding women.
- Use cautiously in patients with heart failure or compromised ventricular function, particularly those receiving beta blockers and those with severe hepatic dysfunction.

NURSING CONSIDERATIONS

- Monitor patient carefully. Some patients, especially those with severe obstructive coronary artery disease, have developed increased frequency, duration, or severity of angina or even acute MI after starting calcium channel blocker therapy or at time of dosage increase.
- Monitor blood pressure regularly, especially when starting therapy and during dosage adjustment.

PATIENT TEACHING

- Tell patient to take drug as prescribed, even if he feels better.
- Advise patient to swallow tablet whole and not to chew, divide, or crush it.
- Remind patient not to take drug with a high-fat meal or with grapefruit juice. Both may increase drug level in the body beyond intended amount.

SAFETY ALERT!

nitroprusside sodium

Nipride†, Nitropress

Pharmacologic class: vasodilator
Pregnancy risk category C

AVAILABLE FORMS

Injection: 50 mg/vial in 2- and 5-ml vials

INDICATIONS & DOSAGES

➤ **To lower blood pressure quickly in hypertensive emergencies, to produce controlled hypotension during anesthesia, to reduce preload and afterload in cardiac pump failure or cardiogenic shock (may be used with or without dopamine)**
Adults and children: Begin infusion at 0.25 to 0.3 mcg/kg/minute I.V. and gradually titrate q few minutes to a maximum infusion rate of 10 mcg/kg/minute.
Adjust-a-dose: Patients also taking other antihypertensives are extremely sensitive to nitroprusside. Titrate dosage accordingly. Use with caution in patients

with renal failure; reduce dosage as much as possible.

I.V. ADMINISTRATION

- Prepare solution by dissolving 50 mg in 2 to 3 ml of D_5W injection or according to manufacturer's instructions. Further dilute concentration in 250, 500, or 1,000 ml of D_5W to provide solutions with 200, 100, or 50 mcg/ml, respectively. Reconstitute ADD-Vantage vials labeled as containing 50 mg of drug according to manufacturer's directions.
- Because drug is sensitive to light, wrap solution in foil or other opaque material; it's not necessary to wrap the tubing. Fresh solution should have a faint brownish tint. Discard if highly discolored after 24 hours.
- Use an infusion pump. Drug is best given via piggyback through a peripheral line with no other drug. Don't titrate rate of main I.V. line while drug is being infused. Even a small bolus can cause severe hypotension.
- Check blood pressure every 5 minutes at start of infusion and every 15 minutes thereafter.
- If severe hypotension occurs, stop infusion—effects of drug quickly reverse. Notify prescriber.
- If possible, start an arterial pressure line. Regulate drug flow to desired blood pressure response.

INCOMPATIBILITIES

Amiodarone, atracurium besylate, bacteriostatic water for injection, levofloxacin. Don't mix with other I.V. drugs or preservatives.

ACTION

Relaxes arteriolar and venous smooth muscle.

Route	Onset	Peak	Duration
I.V.	Immediate	1–2 min	10 min

Half-life: 2 minutes.

ADVERSE REACTIONS

CNS: *headache, dizziness,* ***increased intracranial pressure,*** loss of consciousness, apprehension, restlessness.
CV: ***bradycardia,*** hypotension, tachycardia, palpitations, ECG changes, flushing.
GI: *nausea, abdominal pain,* ileus.
Hematologic: ***methemoglobinemia.***
Metabolic: acidosis, hypothyroidism.
Musculoskeletal: *muscle twitching.*
Skin: *diaphoresis,* pink color, rash.
Other: ***thiocyanate toxicity, cyanide toxicity,*** venous streaking, irritation at infusion site.

INTERACTIONS

Drug-drug. *Antihypertensives:* May cause sensitivity to nitroprusside. Adjust dosage.
Ganglionic-blocking drugs, general anesthetics, negative inotropic drugs, other antihypertensives: May cause additive effects. Monitor blood pressure closely.
Sildenafil, vardenafil: May increase hypotensive effects. Monitor blood pressure.

EFFECTS ON LAB TEST RESULTS

- May increase creatinine level.
- May decrease RBC and WBC counts.

CONTRAINDICATIONS & CAUTIONS

- Contraindicated in patients hypersensitive to drug.
- Contraindicated in those with compensatory hypertension (such as in arteriovenous shunt or coarctation of the aorta), inadequate cerebral circulation, acute heart failure with reduced peripheral vascular resistance, congenital optic atrophy, or tobacco-induced amblyopia.
- Use with extreme caution in patients with increased intracranial pressure.
- Use cautiously in patients with hypothyroidism, hepatic or renal disease, hyponatremia, or low vitamin B level.

NURSING CONSIDERATIONS

- Obtain baseline vital signs before giving drug; find out parameters prescriber wants to achieve.
- Keep patient in the supine position when starting therapy or titrating drug.
- ***Alert:*** Giving excessive doses of 500 mcg/kg delivered faster than 2 mcg/kg/minute or using maximum infusion rate of 10 mcg/kg/minute for more than 10 minutes can cause cyanide toxicity. If patient is at risk, check thiocyanate level every 72 hours. Level higher than

100 mcg/ml may be toxic. If profound hypotension, metabolic acidosis, dyspnea, headache, loss of consciousness, ataxia, or vomiting occurs, stop drug immediately and notify prescriber.
• ***Look alike–sound alike:*** Don't confuse nitroprusside with nitroglycerin.

PATIENT TEACHING
• Instruct patient to report adverse reactions promptly.
• Tell patient to alert nurse if discomfort occurs at I.V. insertion site.

olmesartan medoxomil
Benicar

Pharmacologic class: angiotensin II receptor antagonist
Pregnancy risk category C; D in 2nd and 3rd trimesters

AVAILABLE FORMS
Tablets: 5 mg, 20 mg, 40 mg

INDICATIONS & DOSAGES
➤ Hypertension
Adults: 20 mg P.O. once daily if patient has no volume depletion. May increase dosage to 40 mg P.O. once daily if blood pressure isn't reduced after 2 weeks of therapy.
Adjust-a-dose: In patients with possible depletion of intravascular volume (those with impaired renal function who are taking diuretics), consider using lower starting dose.

ACTION
Blocks vasoconstrictor and aldosterone-secreting effects of angiotensin II by selectively blocking the binding of angiotensin II to the angiotensin I, or AT_1, receptor in the vascular smooth muscle.

Route	Onset	Peak	Duration
P.O.	Rapid	1–2 hr	24 hr

Half-life: 13 hours.

ADVERSE REACTIONS
CNS: headache.
EENT: pharyngitis, rhinitis, sinusitis.
GI: diarrhea.
GU: hematuria.
Metabolic: hyperglycemia, hypertriglyceridemia.
Musculoskeletal: back pain.
Respiratory: bronchitis, upper respiratory tract infection.
Other: flulike symptoms, accidental injury.

INTERACTIONS
Drug-herb. *Ma huang:* May decrease antihypertensive effects. Discourage use together.

EFFECTS ON LAB TEST RESULTS
• May increase glucose, triglyceride, uric acid, liver enzyme, bilirubin, and CK levels. May decrease hemoglobin level and hematocrit.

CONTRAINDICATIONS & CAUTIONS
• Contraindicated in patients hypersensitive to the drug or any of its components and in patients who are pregnant.
• Use cautiously in patients who are volume- or sodium-depleted, those whose renal function depends on the renin-angiotensin-aldosterone system (such as patients with severe heart failure), and those with unilateral and bilateral renal artery stenosis.
• It's unknown if drug appears in breast milk. Patient should stop either breast-feeding or drug.
• Safety and efficacy in children haven't been established.

NURSING CONSIDERATIONS
• Symptomatic hypotension may occur in patients who are volume- or salt-depleted, especially those being treated with high doses of a diuretic. If hypotension occurs, place patient supine and treat supportively. Treatment may continue once blood pressure is stabilized.
• If blood pressure isn't adequately controlled, a diuretic or other antihypertensive drugs also may be prescribed.
• Overdose may cause hypotension and tachycardia, along with bradycardia from parasympathetic (vagal) stimulation. Treatment should be supportive.
• Closely monitor patients with heart failure for oliguria, azotemia, and acute renal failure.

• Monitor BUN and creatinine level in patients with unilateral or bilateral renal artery stenosis.
• Drugs that act on the renin-angiotensin system may cause fetal and neonatal complications and death when given to pregnant women after the first trimester. If patient taking drug becomes pregnant, stop drug immediately.

PATIENT TEACHING
• Tell patient to take drug exactly as prescribed and not to stop taking it. even if he feels better.
• Tell patient that drug may be taken without regard to meals.
• Tell patient to report to health care provider any adverse reactions promptly, especially light-headedness and fainting.
• Advise woman of childbearing age to immediately report pregnancy to health care provider.
• Inform diabetic patients that glucose readings may rise and that the dosage of their diabetes drugs may need adjustment.
• Warn patients that inadequate fluid intake, excessive perspiration, diarrhea, or vomiting may lead to an excessive drop in blood pressure, light-headedness, and possibly fainting.
• Instruct patients that other antihypertensives can have additive effects. Patient should inform his prescriber of all medications he's taking, including OTC drugs.

perindopril erbumine
Aceon

Pharmacologic class: ACE inhibitor
Pregnancy risk category C; D in 2nd and 3rd trimesters

AVAILABLE FORMS
Tablets: 2 mg, 4 mg, 8 mg

INDICATIONS & DOSAGES
➤ **To reduce the risk of CV death or nonfatal MI in patients with stable CAD**
Adults age 70 or younger: 4 mg P.O. once daily for 2 weeks; then, increase as tolerated to 8 mg once daily.
Elderly adults older than age 70: Initially, 2 mg P.O. once daily for the first week; then, 4 mg once daily for the second week and 8 mg once daily after that, if tolerated.
➤ **Essential hypertension**
Adults: Initially, 4 mg P.O. once daily. Increase dosage until blood pressure is controlled or to maximum of 16 mg/day; usual maintenance dosage is 4 to 8 mg once daily; may be given in two divided doses.
Patients older than age 65: Initially, 4 mg P.O. daily as one dose or in two divided doses. Dosage may be increased by more than 8 mg/day only under close medical supervision.
Adjust-a-dose: For renally insufficient patients with creatinine clearance 30 ml/minute or greater, initially 2 mg P.O. daily. Maximum daily maintenance dose is 8 mg. In patients taking diuretics, initially 2 to 4 mg P.O. daily as single dose or in two divided doses, with close medical supervision for several hours and until blood pressure has stabilized. Adjust dosage based on patient's blood pressure response.

ACTION
ACE inhibitors prevent the conversion of angiotensin I to angiotensin II, a potent vasoconstrictor. Less angiotensin II decreases peripheral arterial resistance, decreasing aldosterone secretion, which reduces sodium and water retention and lowers blood pressure.

Route	Onset	Peak	Duration
P.O.	Unknown	1 hr	Unknown

Half-life: About 1 hour for perindopril; mean half-life, 3 to 10 hours, and terminal elimination half-life, 30 to 120 hours for perindoprilat.

ADVERSE REACTIONS
CNS: *headache,* dizziness, asthenia, sleep disorder, paresthesia, depression, somnolence, nervousness, fever.
CV: palpitations, edema, chest pain, hypotension, abnormal ECG.
EENT: rhinitis, sinusitis, ear infection, pharyngitis, tinnitus.
GI: dyspepsia, diarrhea, abdominal pain, nausea, vomiting, flatulence.
GU: proteinuria, UTI, male sexual dysfunction, menstrual disorder.
Metabolic: ***hyperkalemia.***

Musculoskeletal: back pain, hypertonia, neck pain, joint pain, myalgia, arthritis, arm or leg pain.
Respiratory: *cough,* upper respiratory tract infection.
Skin: rash.
Other: viral infection, injury, seasonal allergy.

INTERACTIONS

Drug-drug. *Diuretics:* May increase hypotensive effect. Monitor patient closely.
Lithium: May increase lithium level and risk of lithium toxicity. Use together cautiously; monitor lithium level.
NSAIDs: May decrease antihypertensive effects. Monitor blood pressure.
Potassium-sparing diuretics (amiloride, spironolactone, triamterene), potassium supplements, other drugs capable of increasing potassium level (cyclosporine, heparin, indomethacin): May increase hyperkalemic effect. Use together cautiously; monitor potassium level frequently.
Drug-herb. *Capsaicin:* May cause cough. Discourage use together.
Drug-food. *Salt substitutes containing potassium:* May cause hyperkalemia. Discourage use together.

EFFECTS ON LAB TEST RESULTS

- May increase ALT, alkaline phosphatase, uric acid, cholesterol, and creatinine. May increase potassium level.

CONTRAINDICATIONS & CAUTIONS

- Contraindicated in patients hypersensitive to drug or other ACE inhibitors and in those with a history of angioedema caused by ACE inhibitor use.
- Use cautiously in patients with a history of angioedema unrelated to ACE inhibitor use.
- Use cautiously in patients with renal impairment, heart failure, ischemic heart disease, cerebrovascular disease, or renal artery stenosis and in those with collagen vascular disease, such as systemic lupus erythematosus or scleroderma.

NURSING CONSIDERATIONS

- When used alone in black patients, drug affects blood pressure less than in other patients. Monitor blood pressure closely.
- Patients with a history of angioedema unrelated to ACE inhibitor use may be at increased risk for angioedema during therapy. Black patients are at a higher risk for angioedema regardless of prior ACE inhibitor use.
- ***Alert:*** If angioedema occurs, stop drug and observe patient until swelling disappears. Antihistamines may relieve swelling of the face and lips. Swelling of the tongue, glottis, or throat may cause life-threatening airway obstruction. Give prompt treatment such as epinephrine.
- Monitor CBC with differential for agranulocytosis and neutropenia before therapy, especially in renally impaired patients with lupus or scleroderma.
- Monitor patient for hypotension when starting therapy and when adjusting dosage. If severe hypotension occurs, place patient in supine position and treat symptomatically.
- Severe hypotension can occur when drug is given with diuretics. If possible, stop diuretic 2 to 3 days before starting this drug. If impossible, use lower doses of either drug.
- In patient who is volume- or sodium-depleted from prolonged diuretic therapy, dietary sodium restriction, dialysis, diarrhea, or vomiting, correct fluid and sodium deficits before starting drug.
- Monitor renal function before and periodically throughout therapy.
- Monitor potassium level closely.

PATIENT TEACHING

- Inform patient that throat and facial swelling, including swelling of the throat, can occur during therapy, especially with the first dose. Advise patient to stop taking drug and immediately report any signs or symptoms of swelling of face, extremities, eyes, lips, or tongue; hoarseness; or difficulty in swallowing or breathing.
- Advise patient to report promptly any sign or symptom of infection (sore throat, fever) or jaundice (yellowing of eyes or skin).
- Advise patient to avoid salt substitutes containing potassium unless instructed otherwise by prescriber.
- Caution patient that light-headedness may occur, especially during first few days of therapy. Advise patient to report light-

headedness and, if fainting occurs, to stop drug and consult prescriber promptly.
• Caution patient that inadequate fluid intake or excessive perspiration, diarrhea, or vomiting can lead to an excessive drop in blood pressure.
• Advise woman of childbearing age of the consequences of second- and third-trimester exposure to drug. Advise her to notify prescriber immediately if she suspects pregnancy.

phentolamine mesylate

Regitine, Rogitine†

Pharmacologic class: alpha blocker
Pregnancy risk category C

AVAILABLE FORMS

Injection: 5 mg/ml, 10 mg/ml†

INDICATIONS & DOSAGES

➤ **To aid in diagnosis of pheochromocytoma, to control or prevent hypertension before or during pheochromocytomectomy**
Adults: I.V. or I.M. diagnostic dose is 5 mg with close monitoring of blood pressure. Give 5 mg I.V. or I.M 1 to 2 hours before surgical removal of tumor. During surgery, patient may need an additional 5 mg I.V.
Children: I.V. diagnostic dose is 1 mg, and I.M. diagnostic dose is 3 mg with close monitoring of blood pressure. Give 1 mg I.V. or I.M 1 to 2 hours before surgical removal of tumor. During surgery, patient may need an additional 1 mg I.V.
➤ **To prevent dermal necrosis from norepinephrine extravasation**
Adults: Add 10 mg of phentolamine to each liter of solution containing norepinephrine; the pressor effect of norepinephrine is unaffected.
➤ **Dermal necrosis and sloughing after I.V. extravasation of norepinephrine or dopamine**
Adults: Infiltrate area with 5 to 10 mg phentolamine in 10 to 15 ml of normal saline solution. Must be done within 12 hours of extravasation.
Children: Inject 0.1 to 0.2 mg/kg up to a maximum of 10 mg in the extravasation area.

I.V. ADMINISTRATION

• Reconstitute drug by adding 1 ml of sterile water for injection to vial containing 5 mg of drug; resulting solution contains 5 mg/ml of drug.
• Delay injection until effect of venipuncture on blood pressure has passed, then inject drug rapidly.
• For pheochromocytoma diagnosis, inject drug rapidly. Test result is positive if severe hypotension develops.

INCOMPATIBILITIES

None reported.

ACTION

An alpha blocker that competitively blocks the effects of catecholamines on alpha-adrenergic receptors.

Route	Onset	Peak	Duration
I.V.	Immediate	< 2 min	15–30 min
I.M.	Unknown	< 20 min	30–45 min

Half-life: 19 minutes after I.V. administration.

ADVERSE REACTIONS

CNS: *dizziness, weakness, flushing,* ***cerebrovascular occlusion,*** cerebrovascular spasm.
CV: *hypotension, tachycardia,* ***shock, arrhythmias, MI.***
EENT: *nasal congestion.*
GI: *diarrhea, nausea, vomiting.*

INTERACTIONS

Drug-drug. *Ephedrine, epinephrine:* May cause excessive hypotension. Don't use together.

EFFECTS ON LAB TEST RESULTS

None reported.

CONTRAINDICATIONS & CAUTIONS

• Contraindicated in patients with hypersensitivity to drug and in those with angina, coronary artery disease, or MI or history of MI.
• Use cautiously in patients with gastritis or peptic ulcer.

NURSING CONSIDERATIONS

• When drug is given as a diagnostic test for pheochromocytoma, take patient's blood pressure first; monitor blood pressure frequently during administration.

- ***Alert:*** Don't give epinephrine to treat phentolamine-induced hypotension because it may cause additional fall in blood pressure ("epinephrine reversal"). Use norepinephrine instead.
- ***Look alike–sound alike:*** Don't confuse phentolamine with phentermine.

PATIENT TEACHING

- Explain use and administration of drug.
- Tell patient to report adverse reactions promptly.

prazosin hydrochloride
Minipress

Pharmacologic class: alpha blocker
Pregnancy risk category C

AVAILABLE FORMS

Capsules: 1 mg, 2 mg, 5 mg

INDICATIONS & DOSAGES

➤ **Mild to moderate hypertension**
Adults: Test dose is 1 mg P.O. at bedtime to prevent first-dose syncope (severe syncope with loss of consciousness). First dosage is 1 mg P.O. b.i.d. or t.i.d. Dosage may be increased slowly. Maximum daily dose is 20 mg. Maintenance dosage is 6 to 15 mg daily in three divided doses. Some patients need larger dosages (up to 40 mg daily).

If other antihypertensives or diuretics are added to therapy, decrease prazosin dosage to 1 to 2 mg t.i.d. and readjust to maintenance dosage.

➤ **Benign prostatic hyperplasia ♦**
Adults: 2 mg P.O. b.i.d. Dose range is 1 to 9 mg P.O. daily.

ACTION

Unknown. Thought to act by blocking alpha-adrenergic receptors.

Route	Onset	Peak	Duration
P.O.	30–90 min	2–4 hr	7–10 hr

Half-life: 2 to 4 hours.

ADVERSE REACTIONS

CNS: *dizziness, first-dose syncope,* headache, drowsiness, nervousness, paresthesia, weakness, depression, fever.
CV: orthostatic hypotension, palpitations, edema.
EENT: blurred vision, tinnitus, conjunctivitis, epistaxis, nasal congestion.
GI: vomiting, diarrhea, abdominal cramps, nausea.
GU: priapism, impotence, urinary frequency, incontinence.
Musculoskeletal: arthralgia, myalgia.
Respiratory: dyspnea.
Skin: pruritus.

INTERACTIONS

Drug-drug. *Acebutolol, atenolol, betaxolol, carteolol, esmolol, metoprolol, nadolol, pindolol, propranolol, sotalol, timolol:* May increase the risk of orthostatic hypotension in the early phases of use together. Help patient stand slowly until effects are known.
Diuretics: May increase frequency of syncope with loss of consciousness. Advise patient to sit or lie down if dizziness occurs.
Verapamil: May increase prazosin level. Monitor patient closely.
Drug-herb. *Butcher's broom:* May reduce effect. Discourage use together.
Ma huang: May decrease antihypertensive effects. Discourage use together.

EFFECTS ON LAB TEST RESULTS

- May increase BUN and uric acid levels. May increase levels of the urinary metabolite of norepinephrine and vanillylmandelic acid.
- May increase liver function test values.
- May alter results of screening tests for pheochromocytoma.
- May cause positive antinuclear antibody titer.

CONTRAINDICATIONS & CAUTIONS

- Contraindicated in patients hypersensitive to drug or other alpha blockers.
- Use cautiously in patients receiving other antihypertensives.

NURSING CONSIDERATIONS

- Monitor patient's blood pressure and pulse rate frequently.

- Elderly patients may be more sensitive to drug's hypotensive effects.
- Compliance might be improved with twice-daily dosing. Discuss this dosing change with prescriber if compliance problems are suspected.
- ***Alert:*** If first dose is more than 1 mg, first-dose syncope may occur.

PATIENT TEACHING

- Warn patient that dizziness may occur with first dose. If he experiences dizziness, tell him to sit or lie down. Reassure him that this effect disappears with continued dosing.
- Caution patient to avoid driving or performing hazardous tasks for the first 24 hours after starting this drug or increasing the dose.
- Tell patient not to suddenly stop taking drug, but to notify prescriber if unpleasant adverse reactions occur.
- Advise patient to minimize low blood pressure and dizziness upon standing by rising slowly and avoiding sudden position changes. Dry mouth can be relieved by chewing gum or sucking on hard candy or ice chips.

quinapril hydrochloride

Accupril✐, Asig‡

Pharmacologic class: ACE inhibitor
Pregnancy risk category C; D in 2nd and 3rd trimesters

AVAILABLE FORMS

Tablets: 5 mg, 10 mg, 20 mg, 40 mg

INDICATIONS & DOSAGES

➤ **Hypertension**

Adults: Initially, 10 to 20 mg P.O. daily. Dosage may be adjusted based on patient response at intervals of about 2 weeks. Most patients are controlled at 20, 40, or 80 mg daily as a single dose or in two divided doses. If patient is taking a diuretic, start therapy with 5 mg daily.
Elderly patients: For patients older than age 65, start therapy at 10 mg P.O. daily.
Adjust-a-dose: For adults with creatinine clearance over 60 ml/minute, initially, 10 mg maximum daily; for clearance of 30 to 60 ml/minute, 5 mg; for clearance of 10 to 30 ml/minute, 2.5 mg.

➤ **Heart failure**

Adults: If patient is taking a diuretic, give 5 mg P.O. b.i.d. initially. If patient isn't taking a diuretic, give 10 to 20 mg P.O. b.i.d. Dosage may be increased at weekly intervals. Usual effective dose is 20 to 40 mg daily in two equally divided doses.
Adjust-a-dose: For patients with creatinine clearance over 30 ml/minute, first dose is 5 mg daily; if clearance is 10 to 30 ml/minute, 2.5 mg.

ACTION

Unknown. Thought to inhibit ACE, preventing conversion of angiotensin I to angiotensin II, a potent vasoconstrictor. Less angiotensin II decreases peripheral arterial resistance, decreasing aldosterone secretion, which reduces sodium and water retention and lowers blood pressure.

Route	Onset	Peak	Duration
P.O.	1 hr	2–6 hr	24 hr

Half-life: Elimination half-life, 2 hours; terminal half-life, 25 hours.

ADVERSE REACTIONS

CNS: somnolence, vertigo, nervousness, headache, dizziness, fatigue, depression.
CV: ***hypertensive crisis,*** palpitations, tachycardia, angina pectoris, orthostatic hypotension, rhythm disturbances.
GI: ***hemorrhage,*** dry mouth, abdominal pain, constipation, vomiting, nausea, diarrhea.
Metabolic: ***hyperkalemia.***
Respiratory: dry, persistent, tickling, nonproductive cough.
Skin: pruritus, photosensitivity reactions, diaphoresis.

INTERACTIONS

Drug-drug. *Diuretics, other antihypertensives:* May cause excessive hypotension. Stop diuretic or reduce dose of quinapril, as needed.
Lithium: May increase lithium level and lithium toxicity. Monitor lithium level.
NSAIDs: May decrease antihypertensive effects. Monitor blood pressure.

Potassium-sparing diuretics, potassium supplements: May cause hyperkalemia. Monitor patient closely.
Tetracycline: May decrease absorption if taken with quinapril. Avoid using together.
Drug-herb. *Capsaicin:* May cause cough. Discourage use together.
Ma huang: May decrease antihypertensive effects. Discourage use together.
Drug-food. *Salt substitutes containing potassium:* May cause hyperkalemia. Discourage use together.

EFFECTS ON LAB TEST RESULTS

- May increase potassium, BUN, and creatinine levels.
- May increase liver function test values.

CONTRAINDICATIONS & CAUTIONS

- Contraindicated in patients hypersensitive to ACE inhibitors and in those with a history of angioedema related to treatment with an ACE inhibitor.
- Use cautiously in patients with impaired renal function.

NURSING CONSIDERATIONS

- Assess renal and hepatic function before and periodically throughout therapy.
- Monitor blood pressure for effectiveness of therapy.
- Monitor potassium level. Risk factors for the development of hyperkalemia include renal insufficiency, diabetes, and concomitant use of drugs that raise potassium level.
- Although ACE inhibitors reduce blood pressure in all races, they reduce it less in blacks taking the ACE inhibitor alone. Black patients should take drug with a thiazide diuretic for a more favorable response.
- ACE inhibitors appear to increase risk of angioedema in black patients.
- Other ACE inhibitors have caused agranulocytosis and neutropenia. Monitor CBC with differential counts before therapy and periodically thereafter.

PATIENT TEACHING

- Advise patient to report signs of infection, such as fever and sore throat.
- ***Alert:*** Facial and throat swelling (including swelling of the larynx) may occur, especially after first dose. Advise patient to report signs or symptoms of breathing difficulty or swelling of face, eyes, lips, or tongue.
- Light-headedness can occur, especially during first few days of therapy. Tell patient to rise slowly to minimize effect and to report signs and symptoms to prescriber. If he faints, patient should stop taking drug and call prescriber immediately.
- Inform patient that inadequate fluid intake, vomiting, diarrhea, and excessive perspiration can lead to light-headedness and fainting. Tell him to use caution in hot weather and during exercise.
- Tell patient to avoid salt substitutes. These products may contain potassium, which can cause high potassium level in patients taking quinapril.
- Advise woman of childbearing age to notify prescriber if pregnancy occurs. Drug will need to be stopped.

ramipril

Altace, Ramace‡, Tritace‡

Pharmacologic class: ACE inhibitor
Pregnancy risk category C; D in 2nd and 3rd trimesters

AVAILABLE FORMS

Capsules: 1.25 mg, 2.5 mg, 5 mg, 10 mg

INDICATIONS & DOSAGES

➤Hypertension
Adults: Initially, 2.5 mg P.O. once daily for patients not taking a diuretic, and 1.25 mg P.O. once daily for patients taking a diuretic. Increase dosage, if needed, based on patient response. Maintenance dose is 2.5 to 20 mg daily as a single dose or in divided doses.
Adjust-a-dose: For patients with creatinine clearance less than 40 ml/minute, give 1.25 mg P.O. daily. Adjust dosage gradually based on response. Maximum daily dose is 5 mg.

➤Heart failure after an MI
Adults: Initially, 2.5 mg P.O. b.i.d. If hypotension occurs; decrease dosage to 1.25 mg P.O. b.i.d. Adjust as tolerated to target dosage of 5 mg P.O. twice daily.
Adjust-a-dose: For patients with creatinine clearance less than 40 ml/minute,

give 1.25 mg P.O. daily. Adjust dosage gradually based on response. Maximum dosage is 2.5 mg b.i.d.

➤ **To reduce risk of MI, stroke, and death from CV causes**

Adults age 55 and older: 2.5 mg P.O. once daily for 1 week, then 5 mg P.O. once daily for 3 weeks. Increase as tolerated to a maintenance dose of 10 mg P.O. once daily.

Adjust-a-dose: In patients who are hypertensive or who have recently had an MI, daily dose may be divided.

ACTION

Unknown. Thought to inhibit ACE, preventing conversion of angiotensin I to angiotensin II, a potent vasoconstrictor. Less angiotensin II decreases peripheral arterial resistance, decreasing aldosterone secretion, which reduces sodium and water retention and lowers blood pressure.

Route	Onset	Peak	Duration
P.O.	1–2 hr	1–3 hr	24 hr

Half-life: 13 to 17 hours.

ADVERSE REACTIONS

CNS: headache, dizziness, fatigue, asthenia, malaise, light-headedness, anxiety, amnesia, depression, insomnia, nervousness, neuralgia, neuropathy, paresthesia, somnolence, tremor, vertigo, syncope.
CV: *hypotension,* ***heart failure, MI,*** postural hypotension, angina pectoris, chest pain, palpitations, edema.
EENT: epistaxis, tinnitus.
GI: nausea, vomiting, abdominal pain, anorexia, constipation, diarrhea, dyspepsia, dry mouth, gastroenteritis.
GU: impotence.
Metabolic: ***hyperkalemia,*** hyperglycemia, weight gain.
Musculoskeletal: arthralgia, arthritis, myalgia.
Respiratory: dyspnea, dry, persistent, tickling, nonproductive cough.
Skin: rash, dermatitis, pruritus, photosensitivity reactions, increased diaphoresis.
Other: hypersensitivity reactions.

INTERACTIONS

Drug-drug. *Diuretics:* May cause excessive hypotension, especially at start of therapy. Stop diuretic at least 3 days before therapy begins, increase sodium intake, or reduce starting dose of ramipril.
Insulin, oral antidiabetics: May cause hypoglycemia, especially at start of ramipril therapy. Monitor glucose level closely.
Lithium: May increase lithium level. Use together cautiously and monitor lithium level.
Nesiritide: May increase hypotensive effects. Monitor blood pressure.
NSAIDs: May decrease antihypertensive effects. Monitor blood pressure.
Potassium-sparing diuretics, potassium supplements: May cause hyperkalemia; ramipril attenuates potassium loss. Monitor potassium level closely.
Drug-herb. *Capsaicin:* May cause cough. Discourage use together.
Ma huang: May decrease antihypertensive effects. Discourage use together.
Drug-food. *Salt substitutes containing potassium:* May cause hyperkalemia; ramipril attenuates potassium loss. Discourage use of salt substitutes during therapy.

EFFECTS ON LAB TEST RESULTS

- May increase BUN, creatinine, bilirubin, liver enzymes, glucose, and potassium levels. May decrease hemoglobin level and hematocrit.
- May decrease RBC and platelet counts.

CONTRAINDICATIONS & CAUTIONS

- Contraindicated in patients hypersensitive to ACE inhibitors and in those with a history of angioedema related to treatment with an ACE inhibitor.
- Use cautiously in patients with renal impairment.

NURSING CONSIDERATIONS

- Monitor blood pressure regularly for drug effectiveness.
- Closely assess renal function in patients during first few weeks of therapy. Regular assessment of renal function is advisable. Patients with severe heart failure whose renal function depends on the renin-angiotensin-aldosterone system have experienced acute renal failure during ACE inhibitor therapy. Hypertensive patients with renal artery stenosis also

may show signs of worsening renal function during first few days of therapy.
- Although ACE inhibitors reduce blood pressure in all races, they reduce it less in blacks taking the ACE inhibitor alone. Black patients should take drug with a thiazide diuretic for a more favorable response.
- ACE inhibitors appear to increase risk of angioedema in black patients.
- Monitor CBC with differential counts before therapy and periodically thereafter.
- Drug may reduce hemoglobin and WBC, RBC, and platelet counts, especially in patients with impaired renal function or collagen vascular diseases (systemic lupus erythematosus or scleroderma).
- Monitor potassium level. Risk factors for the development of hyperkalemia include renal insufficiency, diabetes, and concomitant use of drugs that raise potassium level.

PATIENT TEACHING
- Tell patient to notify prescriber if any adverse reactions occur. Dosage adjustment or discontinuation of drug may be needed.
- ***Alert:*** Rarely, swelling of the face and throat (including swelling of the larynx) may occur, especially after first dose. Advise patient to report signs or symptoms of breathing difficulty or swelling of face, eyes, lips, or tongue.
- Inform patient that light-headedness can occur, especially during the first few days of therapy. Tell him to rise slowly to minimize this effect and to report signs and symptoms to prescriber. If he faints, patient should stop taking drug and call prescriber immediately.
- Tell patient that if he has difficulty swallowing capsules, he can open drug and sprinkle contents on a small amount of applesauce.
- Advise patient to report signs and symptoms of infection, such as fever and sore throat.
- Tell patient to avoid salt substitutes. These products may contain potassium, which can cause high potassium level in patients taking ramipril.
- Tell woman of childbearing age to notify prescriber if pregnancy occurs. Drug will need to be stopped.

telmisartan
Micardis

Pharmacologic class: angiotensin II receptor antagonist
Pregnancy risk category C; D in 2nd and 3rd trimesters

AVAILABLE FORMS
Tablets: 20 mg, 40 mg, 80 mg

INDICATIONS & DOSAGES
➤ **Hypertension (used alone or with other antihypertensives)**
Adults: 40 mg P.O. daily. Blood pressure response is dose-related over a range of 20 to 80 mg daily.

ACTION
Blocks vasoconstricting and aldosterone-secreting effects of angiotensin II by selectively blocking the binding of angiotensin II to the angiotensin I, or AT_1, receptor in many tissues, such as vascular smooth muscle and the adrenal gland.

Route	Onset	Peak	Duration
P.O.	Unknown	30–60 min	24 hr

Half-life: 24 hours.

ADVERSE REACTIONS
CNS: dizziness, pain, fatigue, headache.
CV: chest pain, hypertension, peripheral edema.
EENT: pharyngitis, sinusitis.
GI: *nausea,* abdominal pain, diarrhea, dyspepsia.
GU: UTI.
Musculoskeletal: back pain, myalgia.
Respiratory: cough, upper respiratory tract infection.
Other: flulike symptoms.

INTERACTIONS
Drug-drug. *Digoxin:* May increase digoxin level. Monitor digoxin level closely.
Warfarin: May decrease warfarin level. Monitor INR.
Drug-herb. *Ma huang:* May decrease antihypertensive effects. Discourage use together.

Drug-food. *Salt substitutes containing potassium:* May cause hyperkalemia. Discourage use together.

EFFECTS ON LAB TEST RESULTS
- May increase liver enzyme levels.

CONTRAINDICATIONS & CAUTIONS
- Contraindicated in patients hypersensitive to drug or its components.
- Use cautiously in patients with biliary obstruction disorders or renal and hepatic insufficiency and in those with an activated renin-angiotensin system, such as volume- or salt-depleted patients (for example, those being treated with high doses of diuretics).
- Drug may cause fetal and neonatal death when given to pregnant women after the first trimester. If pregnancy is suspected, notify prescriber to stop drug.

NURSING CONSIDERATIONS
- Monitor patient for hypotension after starting drug. Place patient supine if hypotension occurs, and give I.V. normal saline, if needed.
- Most of the antihypertensive effect occurs within 2 weeks. Maximal blood pressure reduction is usually reached after 4 weeks. Diuretic may be added if blood pressure isn't controlled by drug alone.
- ***Alert:*** In patients whose renal function may depend on the activity of the renin-angiotensin-aldosterone system (such as those with severe heart failure), drug may cause oliguria or progressive azotemia and (rarely) acute renal failure or death.
- Drug isn't removed by hemodialysis. Patients undergoing dialysis may develop orthostatic hypotension. Closely monitor blood pressure.

PATIENT TEACHING
- Instruct patient to report suspected pregnancy to prescriber immediately.
- Inform woman of childbearing age of the consequences of second and third trimester exposure to drug.
- Advise breast-feeding woman about risk of adverse drug effects in infants and the need to stop either drug or breast-feeding.
- Tell patient that if he feels dizzy or has low blood pressure on standing, he should lie down, rise slowly from a lying to standing position, and climb stairs slowly.
- Tell patient that drug may be taken without regard to meals.
- Tell patient not to remove drug from blister-sealed packet until immediately before use.

terazosin hydrochloride
Hytrin✐

Pharmacologic class: alpha blocker
Pregnancy risk category C

AVAILABLE FORMS
Capsules: 1 mg, 2 mg, 5 mg, 10 mg
Tablets: 1 mg, 2 mg, 5 mg, 10 mg

INDICATIONS & DOSAGES
➤ **Hypertension**
Adults: Initially, 1 mg P.O. at bedtime. Dosage may be increased gradually based on response. Usual dosage range is 1 to 5 mg daily. Maximum recommended dose is 20 mg daily.
➤ **Symptomatic BPH**
Adults: Initially, 1 mg P.O. at bedtime. Dosage may be increased in a stepwise fashion to 2, 5, or 10 mg once daily to achieve optimal response. Most patients need 10 mg daily for optimal response.

ACTION
Improves urine flow in patients with BPH by blocking alpha-adrenergic receptors in the bladder neck and prostate, relieving urethral pressure.

Reduces peripheral vascular resistance and blood pressure via arterial and venous dilation.

Route	Onset	Peak	Duration
P.O.	15 min	2–3 hr	24 hr

Half-life: About 12 hours.

ADVERSE REACTIONS
CNS: *headache, dizziness,* asthenia, first-dose syncope, nervousness, paresthesia, somnolence.
CV: *peripheral edema,* palpitations, orthostatic hypotension, tachycardia, atrial fibrillation.

EENT: *nasal congestion,* sinusitis, blurred vision.
GI: nausea.
GU: impotence, priapism.
Hematologic: ***thrombocytopenia.***
Musculoskeletal: back pain, muscle pain.
Respiratory: dyspnea.

INTERACTIONS

Drug-drug. *Antihypertensives:* May cause excessive hypotension. Use together cautiously.
Drug-herb. *Butcher's broom:* May decrease drug effect. Discourage use together.
Ma huang: May decrease antihypertensive effects. Discourage use together.

EFFECTS ON LAB TEST RESULTS

- May decrease total protein and albumin levels. May decrease hemoglobin level and hematocrit.
- May decrease WBC and platelet counts.

CONTRAINDICATIONS & CAUTIONS

- Contraindicated in patients hypersensitive to drug.

NURSING CONSIDERATIONS

- Monitor blood pressure frequently.
- ***Alert:*** If terazosin is stopped for several days, readjust dosage using first dosing regimen (1 mg P.O. at bedtime).

PATIENT TEACHING

- Tell patient not to stop drug suddenly, but to notify prescriber if adverse reactions occur.
- Warn patient to avoid hazardous activities that require mental alertness, such as driving or operating heavy machinery, for 12 hours after first dose.
- Tell patient that light-headedness can occur, especially during the first few days of therapy. Advise him to rise slowly to minimize this effect and to report signs and symptoms to prescriber.

trandolapril
Mavik

Pharmacologic class: ACE inhibitor
Pregnancy risk category C; D in 2nd and 3rd trimesters

AVAILABLE FORMS

Tablets: 1 mg, 2 mg, 4 mg

INDICATIONS & DOSAGES

➤ Hypertension

Adults: For patients not taking a diuretic, initially 2 mg P.O. for a black patient and 1 mg P.O. for all other races, once daily. If control isn't adequate, increase dosage at intervals of at least 1 week. Maintenance doses for most patients range from 2 to 4 mg daily. Some patients taking once-daily doses of 4 mg may need b.i.d. doses. For patients also taking a diuretic, initially, 0.5 mg P.O. once daily. Subsequent dosage adjustment is based on blood pressure response.

➤ Heart failure or ventricular dysfunction after MI

Adults: Initially, 1 mg P.O. daily, adjusted to 4 mg P.O. daily. If patient can't tolerate 4 mg, continue at highest tolerated dose.
Adjust-a-dose: If creatinine clearance is below 30 ml/minute, first dose is 0.5 mg daily.

ACTION

Thought to inhibit ACE, reducing angiotensin II formation, which decreases peripheral arterial resistance, decreases aldosterone secretion, reduces sodium and water retention, and lowers blood pressure. Drug is converted in the liver to the prodrug, trandolaprilat.

Route	Onset	Peak	Duration
P.O.	4 hr	1–10 hr	24 hr

Half-life: 5 to 10 hours; longer in patients with renal impairment.

ADVERSE REACTIONS

CNS: *dizziness,* headache, fatigue, drowsiness, insomnia, paresthesia, vertigo, anxiety.

CV: *hypotension, **bradycardia,*** chest pain, first-degree AV block, edema, flushing, palpitations.
EENT: epistaxis, throat irritation.
GI: ***pancreatitis,*** diarrhea, dyspepsia, abdominal distention, abdominal pain or cramps, constipation, vomiting.
GU: urinary frequency, impotence.
Hematologic: ***neutropenia, leukopenia.***
Metabolic: ***hyperkalemia,*** hyponatremia.
Respiratory: *persistent, nonproductive cough,* dyspnea, upper respiratory tract infection.
Skin: rash, pruritus, pemphigus.
Other: decreased libido.

INTERACTIONS

Drug-drug. *Azathioprine:* May increase risk of anemia or leukopenia. Monitor hematologic studies.
Diuretics: May cause excessive hypotension. Stop diuretic or reduce first dosage of trandolapril.
Lithium: May increase lithium level and lithium toxicity. Avoid using together; monitor lithium level.
NSAIDs: May decrease antihypertensive effects. Monitor blood pressure.
Potassium-sparing diuretics, potassium supplements: May cause hyperkalemia. Monitor potassium level closely.
Drug-herb. *Capsaicin:* May cause cough. Discourage use together.
Ma huang: May decrease antihypertensive effects. Discourage use together.
Drug-food. *Salt substitutes containing potassium:* May cause hyperkalemia. Discourage use of salt substitutes.

EFFECTS ON LAB TEST RESULTS

- May increase BUN, creatinine, potassium, and liver enzyme levels. May decrease sodium level.
- May decrease neutrophil and WBC counts.

CONTRAINDICATIONS & CAUTIONS

- Contraindicated in patients hypersensitive to drug and in those with a history of angioedema related to previous treatment with an ACE inhibitor. Also contraindicated in pregnant patients.
- Use cautiously in patients with impaired renal function, heart failure, or renal artery stenosis.
- Safety and effectiveness of drug in children haven't been established.
- Don't use drug in breast-feeding women.

NURSING CONSIDERATIONS

- Monitor potassium level closely.
- Watch for hypotension. Excessive hypotension can occur when drug is given with diuretics. If possible, stop diuretic therapy 2 to 3 days before starting trandolapril to decrease potential for excessive hypotension response. If drug doesn't adequately control blood pressure, diuretic therapy may be started again cautiously.
- Assess patient's renal function before and periodically throughout therapy.
- Other ACE inhibitors have caused agranulocytosis and neutropenia. Monitor CBC with differential before therapy, especially in patients with collagen vascular disease and impaired renal function.
- Although drug reduces blood pressure in patients of all races, drug reduces pressure less in blacks taking this drug alone. Blacks should take drug with a thiazide diuretic for a more favorable response.
- ***Alert:*** Angioedema involving the tongue, glottis, or larynx may be fatal because of airway obstruction. Give appropriate therapy, including epinephrine 1:1,000 (0.3 to 0.5 ml) subcutaneously; have resuscitation equipment for maintaining a patent airway readily available. The risk of angioedema is higher in blacks.
- If patient develops jaundice, stop drug under prescriber's advice because, although rare, ACE inhibitors have been linked to a syndrome of cholestatic jaundice, fulminant hepatic necrosis, and death.

PATIENT TEACHING

- Instruct patient to report yellowing of skin or eyes.
- Advise patient to report fever and sore throat (signs of infection), easy bruising or bleeding; swelling of the tongue, lips, face, eyes, mucous membranes, or extremities; difficulty swallowing or breathing; hoarseness; and nonproductive, persistent cough.
- Tell patient to avoid salt substitutes during drug therapy. These products may

contain potassium, which can cause high potassium level in patients taking drug.
- Tell patient that light-headedness can occur, especially during first few days of therapy. Advise him to rise slowly to minimize this effect and to report it immediately.
- Advise patient to use caution in hot weather and during exercise. Inadequate fluid intake, vomiting, diarrhea, and excessive perspiration can lead to light-headedness and fainting.
- Tell woman of childbearing age to report suspected pregnancy immediately. Drug will need to be stopped.
- Advise patient planning to undergo surgery or receive anesthesia to inform prescriber that he is taking this drug.

valsartan

Diovan

Pharmacologic class: angiotensin II receptor antagonist
Pregnancy risk category C; D in 2nd and 3rd trimesters

AVAILABLE FORMS

Tablets: 40 mg, 80 mg, 160 mg, 320 mg

INDICATIONS & DOSAGES

➤ Hypertension (used alone or with other antihypertensives)
Adults: Initially, 80 mg P.O. once daily. Expect to see a reduction in blood pressure in 2 to 4 weeks. If additional antihypertensive effect is needed, dose may be increased to 160 or 320 mg daily, or a diuretic may be added. (Addition of a diuretic has a greater effect than dosage increases beyond 80 mg.) Usual dosage range is 80 to 320 mg daily.

➤ New York Heart Association class II to IV heart failure
Adults: Initially, 40 mg P.O. b.i.d.; increase as tolerated to 80 mg b.i.d., and then to target dose of 160 mg b.i.d.

➤ To reduce CV death in stable post-MI patients with left-ventricular failure or dysfunction
Adults: 20 mg P.O. b.i.d. Initial dose may be given as soon as 12 hours after MI. Increase dose to 40 mg b.i.d. within 7 days. Increase subsequent doses, as tolerated, to target dose of 160 mg b.i.d.

ACTION

Blocks the binding of angiotensin II to receptor sites in vascular smooth muscle and the adrenal gland, which inhibits the pressor effects of the renin-angiotensin-aldosterone system.

Route	Onset	Peak	Duration
P.O.	2 hr	2–4 hr	24 hr

Half-life: 6 hours.

ADVERSE REACTIONS

CNS: *dizziness,* headache, insomnia, fatigue, vertigo.
CV: edema, hypotension, orthostatic hypotension, syncope.
EENT: rhinitis, sinusitis, pharyngitis, blurred vision.
GI: abdominal pain, diarrhea, nausea, dyspepsia.
GU: renal impairment.
Hematologic: ***neutropenia.***
Metabolic: hyperkalemia.
Musculoskeletal: arthralgia, back pain.
Respiratory: upper respiratory tract infection, cough.
Other: ***angioedema,*** viral infection.

INTERACTIONS

Drug-drug. *Lithium:* May increase lithium level. Monitor lithium level and patient for toxicity.
Potassium supplements, potassium-sparing diuretics, other angiotensin II blockers: May increase potassium level. May also increase creatinine level in heart failure patients. Avoid using together.
Drug-herb. *Ma huang:* May decrease antihypertensive effects. Discourage use together.
Drug-food. *Salt substitutes containing potassium:* May increase potassium level. May also increase creatinine level in heart failure patients. Avoid using together.

EFFECTS ON LAB TEST RESULTS

- May increase potassium, BUN, and creatinine levels.
- May decrease neutrophil count.

CONTRAINDICATIONS & CAUTIONS

- Contraindicated in patients hypersensitive to drug.
- Use cautiously in patients with renal or hepatic disease.
- For pregnant woman in the second or third trimester, drug can cause fetal or neonatal death. Breast-feeding women shouldn't take drug.
- Safety and effectiveness of drug in children haven't been established.

NURSING CONSIDERATIONS

- Watch for hypotension. Excessive hypotension can occur when drug is given with high doses of diuretics.
- Correct volume and sodium depletions before starting drug.

PATIENT TEACHING

- Tell woman of childbearing age to notify prescriber if pregnancy occurs. Drug will need to be stopped.
- Advise patient that drug may be taken without regard to food.

22

Antilipemics

atorvastatin calcium
cholestyramine
colesevelam hydrochloride
ezetimibe
fenofibrate
fluvastatin sodium
gemfibrozil
lovastatin
niacin
(See Chapter 89, VITAMINS AND MINERALS)
omega-3–acid ethyl esters
pravastatin sodium
rosuvastatin calcium
simvastatin

atorvastatin calcium
Lipitor

Pharmacologic class: HMG-CoA reductase inhibitor
Pregnancy risk category X

AVAILABLE FORMS
Tablets: 10 mg, 20 mg, 40 mg, 80 mg

INDICATIONS & DOSAGES
➤ **Adjunct to diet to reduce LDL, total cholesterol, apolipoprotein B, and triglyceride levels and to increase HDL levels in patients with primary hypercholesterolemia (heterozygous familial and nonfamilial) and mixed dyslipidemia (Fredrickson types IIa and IIb); adjunct to diet to reduce triglyceride level (Fredrickson type IV); primary dysbetalipoproteinemia (Fredrickson type III) in patients who don't respond adequately to diet**
Adults: Initially, 10 or 20 mg P.O. once daily. Patient who requires a reduction of more than 45% in LDL level may be started at 40 mg once daily. Increase dose, p.r.n., to maximum of 80 mg daily as single dose. Dosage based on lipid levels drawn within 2 to 4 weeks of starting therapy and after dosage adjustment.
➤ **Alone or as an adjunct to lipid-lowering treatments, such as LDL apheresis, to reduce total and LDL cholesterol in patients with homozygous familial hypercholesterolemia**
Adults: 10 to 80 mg P.O. once daily.
➤ **Heterozygous familial hypercholesterolemia**
Children ages 10 to 17 (girls should be 1 year postmenarche): Initially, 10 mg P.O. once daily. Adjustment intervals should be at least 4 weeks. Maximum daily dose is 20 mg.
➤ **To reduce the risk of MI, stroke, angina, or revascularization procedures in patients with multiple risk factors for CAD but who don't yet have the disease**
Adults: 10 mg P.O. daily.

ACTION
Inhibits HMG-CoA reductase, an early (and rate-limiting) step in cholesterol biosynthesis.

Route	Onset	Peak	Duration
P.O.	Unknown	1–2 hr	Unknown

Half-life: 14 hours.

ADVERSE REACTIONS
CNS: *headache,* asthenia, insomnia.
CV: peripheral edema.
EENT: pharyngitis, rhinitis, sinusitis.
GI: abdominal pain, constipation, diarrhea, dyspepsia, flatulence, nausea.
GU: UTI.
Musculoskeletal: ***rhabdomyolysis,*** arthritis, arthralgia, myalgia.
Respiratory: bronchitis.
Skin: rash.
Other: allergic reactions, flulike syndrome, infection.

INTERACTIONS
Drug-drug. *Antacids, cholestyramine, colestipol:* May decrease atorvastatin level. Monitor patient.
Cyclosporine, diltiazem, *fibric acid derivatives,* ***macrolides (azithromycin, clarithro-***

mycin, erythromycin, telithromycin), nefazodone, *niacin, protease inhibitors,* ***verapamil:*** May decrease metabolism of HMG-CoA reductase inhibitors, increasing toxicity. Monitor patient for adverse effects and report unexplained muscle pain.
Digoxin: May increase digoxin level. Monitor digoxin level and patient for evidence of toxicity.
Fluconazole, itraconazole, ketoconazole, voriconazole: May increase atorvastatin level and adverse effects. Avoid using together; or if unavoidable, reduce dose of atorvastatin.
Hormonal contraceptives: May increase hormone levels. Consider increased hormone levels when selecting a hormonal contraceptive.
Drug-herb. *Eucalyptus, jin bu huan, kava:* May increase risk of hepatotoxicity. Discourage use together.
Red yeast rice: May increase risk of adverse reactions because herb contains compounds similar to those in drug. Discourage use together.
Drug-food. *Grapefruit juice:* May increase drug levels, increasing risk of adverse reactions. Discourage use together.

EFFECTS ON LAB TEST RESULTS
- May increase ALT, AST, and CPK levels.

CONTRAINDICATIONS & CAUTIONS
- Contraindicated in patients hypersensitive to drug and in those with active liver disease or unexplained persistent elevations of transaminase levels.
- Contraindicated in pregnant and breast-feeding women and in women of child-bearing age.
- Use cautiously in patients with history of liver disease or heavy alcohol use.
- Withhold or stop drug in patients at risk for renal failure caused by rhabdomyolysis resulting from trauma; in serious, acute conditions that suggest myopathy; and in major surgery, severe acute infection, hypotension, uncontrolled seizures, or severe metabolic, endocrine, or electrolyte disorders.
- Limit use in children to those older than age 9 with homozygous familial hypercholesterolemia.

NURSING CONSIDERATIONS
- Use only after diet and other nondrug therapies prove ineffective. Patient should follow a standard low-cholesterol diet before and during therapy.
- Before treatment, assess patient for underlying causes for hypercholesterolemia and obtain a baseline lipid profile. Obtain periodic liver function test results and lipid levels before starting treatment and at 6 and 12 weeks after initiation, or after an increase in dosage and periodically thereafter.
- Drug may be given as a single dose at any time of day, with or without food.
- Watch for signs of myositis.
- ***Look alike–sound alike:*** Don't confuse Lipitor with Levatol.

PATIENT TEACHING
- Teach patient about proper dietary management, weight control, and exercise. Explain their importance in controlling high fat levels.
- Warn patient to avoid alcohol.
- Tell patient to inform prescriber of adverse reactions, such as muscle pain, malaise, and fever.
- Advise patient that drug can be taken at any time of day, without regard to meals.
- ***Alert:*** Tell woman to stop drug and notify prescriber immediately if she is or may be pregnant or if she's breast-feeding.

cholestyramine
LoCHOLEST, LoCHOLEST Light, Prevalite, Questran, Questran Light, Questran Lite‡

Pharmacologic class: bile acid sequestrant
Pregnancy risk category C

AVAILABLE FORMS
Powder: 378-g cans, 9-g single-dose packets. Each scoop of powder or single-dose packet contains 4 g of cholestyramine resin.

INDICATIONS & DOSAGES
➤ **Primary hyperlipidemia or pruritus caused by partial bile obstruction, adjunct for reduction of in-**

creased cholesterol level in patients with primary hypercholesterolemia
Adults: 4 g once or twice daily. Maintenance dose is 8 to 16 g daily divided into two doses. Maximum daily dose is 24 g.
Children: 240 mg/kg daily in two to three divided doses, not to exceed 8 g/day.

ACTION
Binds bile acids in the intestinal tract, impeding their absorption and causing their elimination in feces. In response to this bile acid depletion, LDL cholesterol levels decrease as the liver uses LDL cholesterol to replenish reduced bile acid stores.

Route	Onset	Peak	Duration
P.O.	Unknown	Unknown	2–4 wk

Half-life: Unknown.

ADVERSE REACTIONS
CNS: *dizziness, headache, vertigo,* anxiety, fatigue, insomnia, syncope, tinnitus.
GI: *abdominal discomfort, constipation, fecal impaction, nausea,* anorexia, diarrhea, flatulence, GI bleeding, hemorrhoids, steatorrhea, vomiting.
GU: dysuria, hematuria.
Hematologic: anemia, bleeding tendencies, ecchymoses.
Metabolic: hyperchloremic acidosis.
Musculoskeletal: backache, muscle and joint pains, osteoporosis.
Skin: *rash,* irritation of skin, tongue, and perianal area.
Other: *vitamin A, D, E, and K deficiencies from decreased absorption.*

INTERACTIONS
Drug-drug. *Acetaminophen, beta blockers, cardiac glycosides, corticosteroids, estrogens, fat-soluble vitamins (A, D, E, and K), iron preparations, niacin, penicillin G, phenobarbital, progestins, tetracycline, thiazide diuretics, thyroid hormones, warfarin and other coumarin derivatives:* May decrease absorption of these drugs. Give other drugs 1 hour before or 4 to 6 hours after cholestyramine.

EFFECTS ON LAB TEST RESULTS
- May increase alkaline phosphatase level. May decrease hemoglobin level and hematocrit.
- May increase PT.
- May cause abnormal results in cholecystography that uses iopanoic acid because iopanoic acid is also bound by cholestyramine.

CONTRAINDICATIONS & CAUTIONS
- Contraindicated in patients hypersensitive to bile-acid sequestering resins and in those with complete biliary obstruction.
- Use cautiously in patients predisposed to constipation and in those with conditions aggravated by constipation, such as severe, symptomatic coronary artery disease.

NURSING CONSIDERATIONS
- Monitor cholesterol and triglyceride levels regularly during therapy.
- Monitor levels of cardiac glycosides in patients receiving cardiac glycosides and cholestyramine together. If cholestyramine therapy is stopped, adjust dosage of cardiac glycosides to avoid toxicity.
- Monitor bowel habits. Encourage a diet high in fiber and fluids. If severe constipation develops, decrease dosage, add a stool softener, or stop drug.
- Watch for hyperchloremic acidosis with long-term use or very high doses.
- Long-term use may lead to deficiencies of vitamins A, D, E, and K, and folic acid.
- For patients with phenylketonuria, light form contains 28.1 mg of phenylalanine per 6.4-g dose.
- ***Look alike–sound alike:*** Don't confuse Questran with Quarzan.

PATIENT TEACHING
- ***Alert:*** Tell patient never to take drug in its dry form because it may irritate the esophagus or cause severe constipation.
- Tell patient to prepare drug in a large glass containing water, milk, or juice (especially pulpy fruit juice). Tell him to sprinkle powder on the surface of the beverage, let the mixture stand for a few minutes, and then stir thoroughly. Discourage mixing with carbonated beverages because of excessive foaming. After drinking preparation, patient should swirl a small additional amount of liquid in the same glass and then drink again to make sure he has taken the entire dose.

• Tell patient to avoid sipping or holding the suspension in the mouth because drug may damage tooth surfaces. Advise patient to maintain good oral hygiene.
• Advise patient to take at mealtime, if possible.
• Advise patient to take all other drugs at least 1 hour before or 4 to 6 hours after cholestyramine to avoid blocking their absorption.
• Teach patient about proper dietary management of fats. When appropriate, recommend weight control, exercise, and smoking cessation programs.
• Tell patient that drug may deplete body stores of vitamins A, D, E, and K, and folic acid. Patient should discuss need for supplements with prescriber.

colesevelam hydrochloride
WelChol

Pharmacologic class: bile acid sequestrant
Pregnancy risk category B

AVAILABLE FORMS
Tablets: 625 mg

INDICATIONS & DOSAGES
➤ **Adjunct to diet and exercise, either alone or with an HMG-CoA reductase inhibitor, to reduce elevated LDL cholesterol in patients with primary hypercholesterolemia (Fredrickson type IIa)**
Adults: 3 tablets (1,875 mg) P.O. b.i.d. with meals and liquid, or 6 tablets (3,750 mg) once daily with a meal and liquid. Maximum dosage is 7 tablets (4,375 mg) daily.

ACTION
Binds bile acids in the intestinal tract, impeding their absorption and causing their elimination in feces. In response to this bile acid depletion, LDL cholesterol levels decrease as the liver uses LDL cholesterol to replenish reduced bile acid stores.

Route	Onset	Peak	Duration
P.O.	Unknown	2 wk	Unknown

Half-life: Unknown.

ADVERSE REACTIONS
CNS: *headache,* asthenia, pain.
EENT: pharyngitis, rhinitis, sinusitis.
GI: *constipation, flatulence,* abdominal pain, diarrhea, dyspepsia, nausea.
Musculoskeletal: back pain, myalgia.
Respiratory: increased cough.
Other: *infection,* accidental injury, flulike syndrome.

INTERACTIONS
None reported.

EFFECTS ON LAB TEST RESULTS
None reported.

CONTRAINDICATIONS & CAUTIONS
• Contraindicated in patients hypersensitive to drug or any of its components and in patients with bowel obstruction.
• Use cautiously in patients susceptible to vitamin K or fat-soluble vitamin deficiencies and in patients with swallowing disorders, severe GI motility disorders, or major GI tract surgery.
• Use cautiously in patients with triglyceride levels greater than 300 mg/dl.

NURSING CONSIDERATIONS
• Before starting drug, assess patient for underlying causes of hypercholesterolemia, such as poorly controlled diabetes, hypothyroidism, nephrotic syndrome, dysproteinemias, obstructive liver disease, other drug therapy, and alcoholism.
• Give drug with a meal and a liquid.
• Store tablets at room temperature and protect them from moisture.
• Monitor patient's bowel habits. If severe constipation develops, decrease dosage, add a stool softener, or stop drug.
• Monitor the effects of patient's other drugs to identify drug interactions.
• Monitor total and LDL cholesterol and triglyceride levels periodically during therapy.
• Use only when clearly needed in breast-feeding women because it's not known if drug appears in breast milk.

PATIENT TEACHING
• Instruct patient to take drug with a meal and a liquid.
• Teach patient to monitor bowel habits. Encourage a diet high in fiber and fluids.

Instruct patient to notify prescriber promptly if severe constipation develops.
• Encourage patient to follow prescribed diet, exercise, and monitoring of cholesterol and triglyceride levels.
• Tell patient to notify prescriber if she is pregnant or breast-feeding.

ezetimibe
Zetia

Pharmacologic class: selective cholesterol absorption inhibitor
Pregnancy risk category C

AVAILABLE FORMS
Tablets: 10 mg

INDICATIONS & DOSAGES
➤ **Adjunct to diet and exercise to reduce total-cholesterol (C) , LDL-C, and apolipoprotein B (Apo B) levels in patients with primary hypercholesterolemia, alone or combined with HMG-CoA reductase inhibitors (statins) or bile acid sequestrants; adjunct to other lipid-lowering drugs (combined with atorvastatin or simvastatin) in patients with homozygous familial hypercholesterolemia; adjunct to diet in patients with homozygous sitosterolemia to reduce sitosterol and campesterol levels; adjunct to fenofibrate and diet to reduce total-C, LDL-C, Apo B, and non-HDL-C levels in patients with mixed hyperlipidemia**
Adults and children age 10 and older: 10 mg P.O. daily.

ACTION
Inhibits absorption of cholesterol by the small intestine, unlike other drugs used for cholesterol reduction; causes reduced hepatic cholesterol stores and increased cholesterol clearance from the blood.

Route	Onset	Peak	Duration
P.O.	Unknown	4–12 hr	Unknown

Half-life: 22 hours.

ADVERSE REACTIONS
CNS: dizziness, fatigue, headache.
CV: chest pain.
EENT: pharyngitis, sinusitis.
GI: abdominal pain, diarrhea.
Musculoskeletal: arthralgia, back pain, myalgia.
Respiratory: *upper respiratory tract infection,* cough.
Other: viral infection.

INTERACTIONS
Drug-drug. *Bile acid sequestrant (cholestyramine):* May decrease ezetimibe level. Give ezetimibe at least 2 hours before or 4 hours after cholestyramine.
Cyclosporine, fenofibrate, gemfibrozil: May increase ezetimibe level. Monitor patient for adverse reactions.
Fibrates: May increase excretion of cholesterol into the gallbladder bile. Avoid using together.

EFFECTS ON LAB TEST RESULTS
• May increase liver function test values.

CONTRAINDICATIONS & CAUTIONS
• Contraindicated in patients allergic to any component of the drug.
• Contraindicated with HMG-CoA reductase inhibitor in pregnant or breast-feeding women and in patients with active hepatic disease or unexplained increased transaminase level.
• Use cautiously in elderly patients.

NURSING CONSIDERATIONS
• Before starting treatment, assess patient for underlying causes of dyslipidemia.
• Obtain baseline triglyceride and total, LDL, and HDL cholesterol levels.
• Using drug with an HMG-CoA reductase inhibitor significantly decreases total and LDL cholesterol, apolipoprotein B, and triglyceride levels and (except with pravastatin) increases HDL cholesterol level more than use of an HMG-CoA reductase inhibitor alone. Check liver function test values when therapy starts and thereafter according to the HMG-CoA reductase inhibitor manufacturer's recommendations.
• Patient should maintain a cholesterol-lowering diet during treatment.

PATIENT TEACHING

- Emphasize importance of following a cholesterol-lowering diet during drug therapy.
- Tell patient he may take drug without regard to meals.
- Advise patient to notify prescriber of unexplained muscle pain, weakness, or tenderness.
- Urge patient to tell his prescriber about any herbal or dietary supplements he's taking.
- Advise patient to visit his prescriber for routine follow-ups and blood tests.
- Tell woman to notify prescriber if she becomes pregnant.

fenofibrate

Antara, Lipofen, Lofibra, TriCor, Triglide

Pharmacologic class: fibric acid derivative
Pregnancy risk category C

AVAILABLE FORMS

Capsules (micronized): 43 mg, 50 mg, 67 mg, 87 mg, 100 mg, 130 mg, 134 mg, 150 mg, 200 mg
Tablets: 48 mg, 50 mg, 54 mg, 145 mg, 160 mg

INDICATIONS & DOSAGES

➤ **Hypertriglyceridemia (Fredrickson types IV and V hyperlipidemia) in patients who don't respond adequately to diet alone**
Adults: For Antara, initial dose is 43 to 130 mg P.O. daily. Maximum dose, 130 mg daily. For Lipofen, initial dose is 50 to 150 mg daily. Maximum dose, 150 mg daily. For Lofibra capsules, initial dose is 67 to 200 mg daily. Maximum dose, 200 mg daily. For Lofibra tablets, initial dose is 54 to 160 mg daily. Maximum dose, 160 mg daily. For TriCor, initial dose is 48 to 145 mg daily. Maximum dose, 145 mg daily. For Triglide, initial dose is 50 to 160 mg daily. Maximum dose, 160 mg daily. For all forms, adjust dose based on patient response and repeat lipid determinations q 4 to 8 weeks.
➤ **Primary hypercholesterolemia or mixed dyslipidemia (Fredrickson types IIa and IIb) in patients who don't respond adequately to diet alone**
Adults: For Antara, initial dose is 130 mg P.O. daily. For Lipofen, initial dose is 150 mg daily. For Lofibra, initial dose is 200 mg (capsules) or 160 mg (tablets) daily. For TriCor, initial dose is 145 mg daily. For Triglide, initial dose is 160 mg daily. May reduce dose if lipid levels fall significantly below the target range.
Adjust-a-dose: If creatinine clearance is less than 50 ml/minute or in elderly patients, initially 43 mg daily for Antara, 50 mg daily for Lipofen, 67 mg daily for Lofibra capsules or 54 mg daily for Lofibra tablets, 48 mg daily for TriCor, or 50 mg daily for Triglide. Increase only after evaluating effects on renal function and triglyceride level at this dose.

ACTION

May lower triglyceride levels by inhibiting triglyceride synthesis with less very–low-density lipoproteins released into circulation. Drug may also stimulate breakdown of triglyceride-rich protein.

Route	Onset	Peak	Duration
P.O.	Unknown	6–8 hr	Unknown

Half-life: 20 hours.

ADVERSE REACTIONS

CNS: *dizziness, headache,* asthenia, fatigue, insomnia, localized pain, paresthesia.
CV: ***arrhythmias.***
EENT: blurred vision, conjunctivitis, earache, eye discomfort, eye floaters, rhinitis, sinusitis.
GI: abdominal pain, constipation, diarrhea, dyspepsia, eructation, flatulence, increased appetite, nausea, vomiting.
GU: polyuria, vaginitis.
Musculoskeletal: arthralgia.
Respiratory: cough.
Skin: pruritus, rash.
Other: *infection,* decreased libido, flulike syndrome, hypersensitivity reactions.

INTERACTIONS

Drug-drug. *Bile-acid sequestrants:* May bind and inhibit absorption of fenofibrate.

Give drug 1 hour before or 4 to 6 hours after bile-acid sequestrants.
Coumarin-type anticoagulants: May potentiate anticoagulant effect, prolonging PT and INR. Monitor PT and INR closely. May need to reduce anticoagulant dosage.
Cyclosporine, immunosuppressants, nephrotoxic drugs: May induce renal dysfunction that may affect fenofibrate elimination. Use together cautiously.
HMG-CoA reductase inhibitors: May increase risk of adverse musculoskeletal effects. Avoid using together, unless potential benefit outweighs risk.
Drug-food. *Any food:* May increase capsule absorption. Advise patient to take capsule with meals.
Drug-lifestyle. *Alcohol use:* May increase triglyceride levels. Discourage use together.

EFFECTS ON LAB TEST RESULTS
- May increase ALT, AST, BUN, CPK, and creatinine levels. May decrease uric acid and hemoglobin levels and hematocrit.
- May decrease WBC count.

CONTRAINDICATIONS & CAUTIONS
- Contraindicated in patients hypersensitive to drug and in those with gallbladder disease, hepatic dysfunction, primary biliary cirrhosis, severe renal dysfunction, or unexplained persistent liver function abnormalities.
- Use cautiously in patients with a history of pancreatitis.

NURSING CONSIDERATIONS
- Obtain baseline lipid levels and liver function test results before therapy, and monitor liver function periodically during therapy. Stop drug if enzyme levels persist above three times normal.
- Watch for signs and symptoms of pancreatitis, myositis, rhabdomyolysis, cholelithiasis, and renal failure. Monitor patient for muscle pain, tenderness, or weakness, especially with malaise or fever.
- If an adequate response isn't obtained after 2 months of treatment with maximum daily dose, stop therapy.
- Drug lowers uric acid level by increasing uric acid excretion in patients with or without hyperuricemia.
- Beta blockers, estrogens, and thiazide diuretics may increase triglyceride levels; evaluate need for continued use of these drugs.
- Hemoglobin level, hematocrit, and WBC count may decrease when therapy starts but will stabilize with long-term administration.

PATIENT TEACHING
- Inform patient that drug therapy doesn't reduce need for following a triglyceride-lowering diet.
- Advise patient to promptly report unexplained muscle weakness, pain, or tenderness, especially with malaise or fever.
- Inform patient to take capsules with meals for best drug absorption.
- Advise patient to continue weight control measures, including diet and exercise, and to limit alcohol before therapy.
- Instruct patient who is also taking a bile-acid resin to take fenofibrate 1 hour before or 4 to 6 hours after resin.
- Advise patient about risk of tumor growth.
- Tell breast-feeding woman to either stop breast-feeding or stop taking drug.

fluvastatin sodium
Lescol✐, Lescol XL

Pharmacologic class: HMG-CoA reductase inhibitor
Pregnancy risk category X

AVAILABLE FORMS
Capsules: 20 mg, 40 mg
Tablets (extended-release): 80 mg

INDICATIONS & DOSAGES
➤ **To reduce LDL and total cholesterol levels in patients with primary hypercholesterolemia (types IIa and IIb); to slow progression of coronary atherosclerosis in patients with coronary artery disease; elevated triglyceride and apolipoprotein B levels in patients with primary hypercholesterolemia and mixed dyslipidemia whose response to die-**

tary restriction and other nonpharmacologic measures has been inadequate
Adults: Initially, 20 to 40 mg P.O. at bedtime, increasing if needed to maximum of 80 mg daily in divided doses or 80 mg Lescol XL P.O. at bedtime.
➤ **To reduce the risk of undergoing coronary revascularization procedures**
Adults: In patients who must reduce LDL cholesterol level by at least 25%, initially, 40 mg P.O. once daily or b.i.d.; or one 80-mg extended-release tablet as a single dose in the evening. In patients who must reduce LDL cholesterol level by less than 25%, initially, 20 mg P.O. daily. Dosages range from 20 to 80 mg daily.

ACTION

Inhibits HMG-CoA reductase, an early (and rate-limiting) step in the synthetic pathway of cholesterol.

Route	Onset	Peak	Duration
P.O.	Unknown	1 hr	Unknown

Half-life: Less than 1 hour.

ADVERSE REACTIONS

CNS: dizziness, fatigue, headache, insomnia.
EENT: pharyngitis, rhinitis, sinusitis.
GI: abdominal pain, constipation, diarrhea, dyspepsia, flatulence, nausea, vomiting.
Hematologic: ***leukopenia, thrombocytopenia,*** hemolytic anemia.
Musculoskeletal: ***rhabdomyolysis,*** arthralgia, back pain, myalgia.
Respiratory: *upper respiratory tract infection,* bronchitis, cough.
Other: hypersensitivity reactions.

INTERACTIONS

Drug-drug. *Cholestyramine, colestipol:* May bind with fluvastatin in the GI tract and decrease absorption. Separate doses by at least 4 hours.
Cimetidine, omeprazole, ranitidine: May decrease fluvastatin metabolism. Monitor patient for enhanced effects.
Cyclosporine and other immunosuppressants, erythromycin, gemfibrozil, niacin: May increase risk of polymyositis and rhabdomyolysis. Avoid using together.
Digoxin: May alter digoxin pharmacokinetics. Monitor digoxin level carefully.
Fluconazole, itraconazole, ketoconazole: May increase fluvastatin level and adverse effects. Avoid using together, or, if they must be given together, reduce dose of fluvastatin.
Glyburide: May increase levels of both drugs. Monitor patient closely.
Phenytoin: May increase phenytoin levels. Monitor phenytoin levels.
Rifampin: May enhance fluvastatin metabolism and decrease levels. Monitor patient for lack of effect.
Warfarin: May increase anticoagulant effect with bleeding. Monitor patient.
Drug-herb. *Eucalyptus, jin bu huan, kava:* May increase risk of hepatotoxicity. Discourage use together.
Red yeast rice: May increase risk of adverse reactions because herb contains compounds similar to those in drug. Discourage use together.
Drug-lifestyle. *Alcohol use:* May increase risk of hepatotoxicity. Discourage use together.

EFFECTS ON LAB TEST RESULTS

- May increase ALT, AST, and CK levels. May decrease hemoglobin level and hematocrit.
- May decrease platelet and WBC counts.

CONTRAINDICATIONS & CAUTIONS

- Contraindicated in patients hypersensitive to drug and in those with active liver disease or unexplained persistent elevations of transaminase levels; also contraindicated in pregnant and breast-feeding women and in women of childbearing age.
- Use cautiously in patients with severe renal impairment and history of liver disease or heavy alcohol use.

NURSING CONSIDERATIONS

- Use only after diet and other nondrug therapies prove ineffective. Patient should follow a standard low-cholesterol diet during therapy.
- Test liver function at start of therapy, at 12 weeks after start of therapy, 12 weeks after an increase in dose, and then periodically. Stop drug if there is a persistent in-

crease in ALT or AST levels of at least three times the upper limit of normal.
- Watch for signs of myositis.
- ***Look alike–sound alike:*** Don't confuse fluvastatin with fluoxetine.

PATIENT TEACHING
- Tell patient that drug may be taken without regard to meals, but it will work better if it's taken in the evening.
- Advise the patient who is also taking a bile-acid resin such as cholestyramine to take fluvastatin at bedtime, at least 4 hours after taking the resin.
- Teach patient about proper dietary management, weight control, and exercise. Explain their importance in controlling elevated cholesterol and triglyceride levels.
- Warn patient to avoid alcohol.
- Tell patient to notify prescriber of adverse reactions, especially muscle aches and pains.
- Advise patient that it may take up to 4 weeks for the drug to be completely effective.
- ***Alert:*** Tell woman of childbearing age to stop drug and notify prescriber immediately if she is or may be pregnant or if she's breast-feeding.

gemfibrozil
Apo-Gemfibrozil†, Lopid✐

Pharmacologic class: fibric acid derivative
Pregnancy risk category C

AVAILABLE FORMS
Tablets: 600 mg

INDICATIONS & DOSAGES
➤ **Types IV and V hyperlipidemia unresponsive to diet and other drugs; to reduce risk of coronary heart disease in patients with type IIb hyperlipidemia who can't tolerate or who are refractory to treatment with bile-acid sequestrants or niacin**
Adults: 1,200 mg P.O. daily in two divided doses, 30 minutes before morning and evening meals.

ACTION
Inhibits peripheral lipolysis and reduces triglyceride synthesis in the liver; lowers triglyceride levels and increases HDL cholesterol levels.

Route	Onset	Peak	Duration
P.O.	2–5 days	4 wk	Unknown

Half-life: 1¼ hours.

ADVERSE REACTIONS
CNS: fatigue, headache, vertigo.
CV: atrial fibrillation.
GI: *abdominal and epigastric pain, dyspepsia,* acute appendicitis, constipation, diarrhea, nausea, vomiting.
Hematologic: ***leukopenia, thrombocytopenia,*** anemia, eosinophilia.
Hepatic: bile duct obstruction.
Metabolic: hypokalemia.
Skin: dermatitis, eczema, pruritus, rash.

INTERACTIONS
Drug-drug. *Cyclosporine:* May decrease cyclosporine levels. Monitor cyclosporine levels and adjust dose as needed.
Glyburide: May increase hypoglycemic effects. Monitor glucose level, and watch for signs of hypoglycemia.
HMG-CoA reductase inhibitors: May cause myopathy with rhabdomyolysis. Avoid using together.
Oral anticoagulants: May enhance effects of oral anticoagulants. Monitor patient closely.
Repaglinide: May increase repaglinide level. Avoid using together if possible. If already taking both drugs, monitor glucose levels and adjust repaglinide dosage.

EFFECTS ON LAB TEST RESULTS
- May increase ALT, AST, and CK levels. May decrease potassium and hemoglobin levels and hematocrit.
- May decrease eosinophil, WBC, and platelet counts.

CONTRAINDICATIONS & CAUTIONS
- Contraindicated in patients hypersensitive to drug and in those with hepatic or severe renal dysfunction (including primary biliary cirrhosis) or gallbladder disease.

NURSING CONSIDERATIONS

- Check CBC and test liver function periodically during the first 12 months of therapy.
- If drug has no benefits after 3 months of therapy, stop drug.
- Patient shouldn't take drug together with repaglinide or itraconazole.

PATIENT TEACHING

- Instruct patient to take drug 30 minutes before breakfast and dinner.
- Teach patient about proper dietary management of cholesterol and triglycerides. When appropriate, recommend weight control, exercise, and smoking cessation programs.
- Because of possible dizziness and blurred vision, advise patient to avoid driving and other hazardous activities until effects of drug are known.
- Tell patient to observe bowel movements and to report evidence of excess fat in feces or other signs of bile duct obstruction.

lovastatin (mevinolin)

Altoprev, Mevacor🖉

Pharmacologic class: HMG-CoA reductase inhibitor
Pregnancy risk category X

AVAILABLE FORMS

Tablets: 10 mg, 20 mg, 40 mg
Tablets (extended-release): 10 mg, 20 mg, 40 mg, 60 mg

INDICATIONS & DOSAGES

➤ To prevent and treat coronary heart disease; hyperlipidemia
Adults: Initially, 20 mg P.O. once daily with evening meal. Recommended range is 10 to 80 mg as a single dose or in two divided doses; maximum daily recommended dose is 80 mg.

Or, 20 to 60 mg extended-release tablets P.O. at bedtime. Starting dose of 10 mg can be used for patients requiring smaller reductions; usual dosage range is 10 to 60 mg daily.

➤ Heterozygous familial hypercholesterolemia in adolescents
Adolescents ages 10 to 17: 10 to 40 mg daily P.O. with evening meal. Patients requiring reductions in LDL cholesterol level of 20% or more should start with 20 mg daily.
Adjust-a-dose: For patients also taking cyclosporine, give 10 mg P.O. daily, not to exceed 20 mg daily. Avoid use of lovastatin with fibrates or niacin; if combined with either, the dosage of lovastatin shouldn't exceed 20 mg daily. For patients also taking amiodarone or verapamil, the dosage of lovastatin shouldn't exceed 40 mg daily. For patients with creatinine clearance less than 30 ml/minute, carefully consider dosage increase greater than 20 mg daily and implement cautiously if necessary.

ACTION

Inhibits HMG-CoA reductase, an early (and rate-limiting) step in cholesterol biosynthesis.

Route	Onset	Peak	Duration
P.O.	Unknown	2 hr	Unknown
P.O. (extended-release)	Unknown	14 hr	Unknown

Half-life: 3 hours.

ADVERSE REACTIONS

CNS: *headache,* dizziness, insomnia, peripheral neuropathy.
CV: chest pain.
EENT: blurred vision.
GI: abdominal pain or cramps, constipation, diarrhea, dyspepsia, flatulence, heartburn, nausea, vomiting.
Musculoskeletal: muscle cramps, myalgia, myositis, ***rhabdomyolysis.***
Skin: alopecia, rash, pruritus.

INTERACTIONS

Drug-drug. *Amiodarone,* ***verapamil:*** May cause myopathy and rhabdomyolysis. Don't exceed 40 mg lovastatin daily.
Azole antifungals, ***protease inhibitors:*** May cause myopathy and rhabdomyolysis. Avoid using together.
Cyclosporine, *danazol, gemfibrozil or other fibrates, niacin:* May cause myopa-

thy and rhabdomyolysis. Don't exceed 20 mg lovastatin daily.
Diltiazem, macrolides (azithromycin, clarithromycin, erythromycin, telithromycin), nefazodone: May decrease metabolism of HMG-CoA reductase inhibitor, increasing toxicity. Monitor patient for adverse effects and report unexplained muscle pain.
Oral anticoagulants: May increase oral anticoagulant effect. Monitor patient closely.
Drug-herb. *Eucalyptus, jin bu huan, kava:* May increase risk of hepatotoxicity. Discourage use together.
Pectin: May decrease drug effect. Discourage use together.
Red yeast rice: May increase risk of adverse reactions because herb contains compounds similar to those in drug. Discourage use together.
Drug-food. *Grapefruit juice:* May increase drug level, increasing risk of adverse effects. Discourage use together.
Drug-lifestyle. *Alcohol use:* May increase risk of hepatotoxicity. Discourage use together.

EFFECTS ON LAB TEST RESULTS

- May increase ALT, AST, and CK levels.

CONTRAINDICATIONS & CAUTIONS

- Contraindicated in patients hypersensitive to drug and in those with active liver disease or unexplained persistently increased transaminase level.
- Contraindicated in pregnant and breast-feeding women and in women of childbearing age.
- Use cautiously in patients who consume substantial quantities of alcohol or have a history of liver disease.

NURSING CONSIDERATIONS

- Use only after diet and other nondrug therapies prove ineffective. Have patient follow a standard low-cholesterol diet during therapy.
- Obtain liver function test results at the start of therapy, at 6 and 12 weeks after the start of therapy, and when increasing dose; then monitor results periodically.
- Heterozygous familial hypercholesterolemia can be diagnosed in adolescent boys and in girls who are at least 1 year postmenarche and are 10 to 17 years old; if after an adequate trial of diet therapy LDL cholesterol level remains over 189 mg/dl or LDL cholesterol over 160 mg/dl and patient has a positive family history of premature CV disease or two or more other CV disease risk factors.
- ***Look alike–sound alike:*** Don't confuse lovastatin with Lotensin, Leustatin, or Livostin. Don't confuse Mevacor with Mivacron.

PATIENT TEACHING

- Instruct patient to take drug with the evening meal, which improves absorption and cholesterol biosynthesis.
- Teach patient about proper dietary management of cholesterol and triglycerides. When appropriate, recommend weight control, exercise, and smoking cessation programs.
- Advise patient to have periodic eye examinations; related compounds cause cataracts.
- Instruct patient to store tablets at room temperature in a light-resistant container.
- Advise patient to promptly report unexplained muscle pain, tenderness, or weakness, particularly when accompanied by malaise or fever.
- ***Alert:*** Tell woman to stop drug and notify prescriber immediately if she is or may be pregnant or if she's breast-feeding.
- ***Alert:*** Advise patient not to crush or chew extended-release tablets.

omega-3–acid ethyl esters
Omacor

Pharmacologic class: ethyl ester
Pregnancy risk category C

AVAILABLE FORMS

Capsules: 1 g

INDICATIONS & DOSAGES

➤ **Adjunct to diet to reduce triglyceride levels 500 mg/dl or higher**
Adults: 4 g P.O. once daily or divided as 2 g b.i.d.

ACTION

May reduce hepatic formation of triglycerides because two components of drug are poor substrates for the necessary enzymes. These components also block formation of other fatty acids.

Route	Onset	Peak	Duration
P.O.	Unknown	Unknown	Unknown

Half-life: Unknown.

ADVERSE REACTIONS
CNS: pain.
CV: angina pectoris.
GI: altered taste, belching, dyspepsia.
Musculoskeletal: back pain.
Skin: rash.
Other: flulike syndrome, infection.

INTERACTIONS
Drug-drug. *Anticoagulants:* May prolong bleeding time. Monitor patient.

EFFECTS ON LAB TEST RESULTS
• May increase ALT and LDL cholesterol levels.

CONTRAINDICATIONS & CAUTIONS
• Contraindicated in patients hypersensitive to drug or its components.
• Use cautiously in patients sensitive to fish.

NURSING CONSIDERATIONS
• Assess patient for conditions that contribute to increased triglycerides, such as diabetes and hypothyroidism, before treatment.
• Evaluate patient's current drug regimen for any drugs known to sharply increase triglyceride levels, including estrogen therapy, thiazide diuretics, and beta blockers. Stopping these drugs, if appropriate, may negate the need for drug.
• Start therapy only after diet and lifestyle modifications have proven unsuccessful.
• Obtain baseline triglyceride levels to confirm that they're consistently abnormal before therapy; then recheck periodically during treatment. If patient has an inadequate response after 2 months, stop drug.
• Monitor LDL level to make sure it doesn't increase excessively during treatment.
• ***Look alike–sound alike:*** Don't confuse Omacor with Amicar.

PATIENT TEACHING
• Explain that taking drug doesn't reduce the importance of following the recommended diet and exercise plan.
• Remind patient of the need for follow-up blood work to evaluate progress.
• Advise patient to notify prescriber about bothersome side effects.
• Tell patient to report planned or suspected pregnancy.

pravastatin sodium (eptastatin)
Pravachol✐

Pharmacologic class: HMG-CoA reductase inhibitor
Pregnancy risk category X

AVAILABLE FORMS
Tablets: 10 mg, 20 mg, 40 mg, 80 mg

INDICATIONS & DOSAGES
➤ **Primary and secondary prevention of coronary events; hyperlipidemia**
Adults: Initially, 40 mg P.O. once daily at the same time each day, with or without food. Adjust dosage q 4 weeks, based on patient tolerance and response; maximum daily dose is 80 mg.
➤ **Heterozygous familial hypercholesterolemia**
Adolescents ages 14 to 18: 40 mg P.O. once daily.
Children ages 8 to 13: 20 mg P.O. once daily.
Adjust-a-dose: In patients with renal or hepatic dysfunction, start with 10 mg P.O. daily. In patients taking immunosuppressants, begin with 10 mg P.O. at bedtime and adjust to higher dosages with caution. Most patients treated with the combination of immunosuppressants and pravastatin receive up to 20 mg pravastatin daily.

ACTION
Inhibits HMG-CoA reductase, an early (and rate-limiting) step in cholesterol biosynthesis.

Route	Onset	Peak	Duration
P.O.	Unknown	60–90 min	Unknown

Half-life: 1¼ to 2¼ hours.

ADVERSE REACTIONS

CNS: dizziness, fatigue, headache.
CV: chest pain.
EENT: rhinitis.
GI: *nausea,* abdominal pain, constipation, diarrhea, flatulence, heartburn, vomiting.
GU: ***renal failure caused by myoglobinuria,*** urinary abnormality.
Musculoskeletal: *localized muscle pain,* ***rhabdomyolysis,*** myalgia, myopathy, myositis.
Respiratory: common cold, cough.
Skin: rash.
Other: flulike symptoms, influenza.

INTERACTIONS

Drug-drug. *Cholestyramine, colestipol:* May decrease pravastatin level. Give pravastatin 1 hour before or 4 hours after these drugs.
Cyclosporine: May decrease metabolism of HMG-CoA reductase inhibitor, increasing toxicity. Monitor patient for adverse effects and report unexplained muscle pain.
Erythromycin, fibric acid derivatives (such as clofibrate, gemfibrozil), immunosuppressants , high doses (1 g or more daily) of niacin (nicotinic acid): May cause rhabdomyolysis. Avoid using together; if unavoidable, monitor patient closely.
Fluconazole, itraconazole, ketoconazole: May increase pravastatin level and adverse effects. Avoid using together; if unavoidable, reduce dose of pravastatin.
Gemfibrozil: May decrease protein-binding and urinary clearance of pravastatin. Avoid using together.
Hepatotoxic drugs: May increase risk of hepatotoxicity. Avoid using together.
Drug-herb. *Eucalyptus, jin bu huan, kava:* May increase the risk of hepatotoxicity. Discourage use together.
Red yeast rice: May increase risk of adverse reactions because herb contains compounds similar to those in drug. Discourage use together.
Drug-lifestyle. *Alcohol use:* May increase risk of hepatotoxicity. Discourage use together.

EFFECTS ON LAB TEST RESULTS

- May increase ALT, AST, CK, alkaline phosphatase, and bilirubin levels.
- May alter thyroid function test values.

CONTRAINDICATIONS & CAUTIONS

- Contraindicated in patients hypersensitive to drug and in those with active liver disease or conditions that cause unexplained, persistent elevations of transaminase levels.
- Contraindicated in pregnant and breast-feeding women and in women of childbearing age.
- Safety and efficacy in children younger than age 8 haven't been established.
- Use cautiously in patients who consume large quantities of alcohol or have history of liver disease.

NURSING CONSIDERATIONS

- Use only after diet and other nondrug therapies prove ineffective. Patients should follow a standard low-cholesterol diet during therapy.
- Use in children with heterozygous familial hypercholesterolemia if LDL cholesterol level is at least 190 mg/dl, or if LDL cholesterol is at least 160 mg/dl and patient has either a positive family history of premature CV disease or two or more other CV disease risk factors.
- Obtain liver function test results at start of therapy and then periodically. A liver biopsy may be performed if elevated liver enzyme levels persist.
- ***Look alike–sound alike:*** Don't confuse Pravachol with Prevacid or propranolol.

PATIENT TEACHING

- Tell patient to take the prescribed dose in the evening, preferably at bedtime.
- Advise patient who is also taking a bile-acid resin such as cholestyramine to take pravastatin at least 1 hour before or 4 hours after taking resin.
- Tell patient to notify prescriber of adverse reactions, particularly muscle aches and pains.
- Teach patient about proper dietary management of cholesterol and triglycerides. When appropriate, recommend weight control, exercise, and smoking cessation programs.
- Inform patient that it will take up to 4 weeks to achieve full therapeutic effect.
- ***Alert:*** Tell woman of childbearing age to stop drug and notify prescriber immedi-

ately if she is or may be pregnant or if she's breast-feeding.

rosuvastatin calcium
Crestor

Pharmacologic class: HMG-CoA reductase inhibitor
Pregnancy risk category X

AVAILABLE FORMS
Tablets: 5 mg, 10 mg, 20 mg, 40 mg

INDICATIONS & DOSAGES
➤ **Adjunct to diet to reduce LDL cholesterol, total cholesterol, apolipoprotein B, non-HDL cholesterol, and triglyceride (TG) levels and to increase HDL cholesterol level in patients with primary hypercholesterolemia (heterozygous familial and nonfamilial) and mixed dyslipidemia (Fredrickson types IIa and IIb); adjunct to diet to treat elevated TG level (Fredrickson type IV)**
Adults: Initially, 10 mg P.O. once daily; 5 mg P.O. once daily in patients needing less-aggressive LDL cholesterol level reduction or those predisposed to myopathy. For aggressive lipid lowering, initially, 20 mg P.O. once daily. Increase p.r.n. to maximum of 40 mg P.O. daily. Dosage may be increased every 2 to 4 weeks, based on lipid levels.
➤ **Adjunct to lipid-lowering therapies; to reduce LDL cholesterol, apolipoprotein B, and total cholesterol levels in homozygous familial hypercholesterolemia**
Adults: Initially, 20 mg P.O. once daily. Maximum, 40 mg once daily.
Adjust-a-dose: If creatinine clearance is less than 30 ml/minute, initially, 5 mg once daily; don't exceed 10 mg once daily. For patient's requiring less-aggressive treatment, those at risk for myopathy, Asian patients, and patients also taking cyclosporine, initial dose is 5 mg.

ACTION
Inhibits HMG-CoA reductase, increases LDL receptors on liver cells, and inhibits hepatic synthesis of very–low-density lipoprotein.

Route	Onset	Peak	Duration
P.O.	Unknown	3–5 hr	Unknown

Half-life: About 19 hours.

ADVERSE REACTIONS
CNS: anxiety, asthenia, depression, dizziness, headache, insomnia, neuralgia, paresthesia, vertigo.
CV: angina pectoris, chest pain, hypertension, palpitations, peripheral edema, vasodilation.
EENT: pharyngitis, rhinitis, sinusitis.
GI: abdominal pain, constipation, diarrhea, dyspepsia, flatulence, gastritis, gastroenteritis, nausea, periodontal abscess, vomiting.
GU: UTI.
Hematologic: anemia, ecchymosis.
Metabolic: diabetes mellitus.
Musculoskeletal: arthralgia, arthritis, back pain, hypertonia, myalgia, neck pain, pain, pathologic fracture, pelvic pain.
Respiratory: asthma, bronchitis, dyspnea, increased cough, pneumonia.
Skin: pruritus, rash.
Other: accidental injury, flulike syndrome, infection.

INTERACTIONS
Drug-drug. *Antacids:* May decrease rosuvastatin level. Give antacids at least 2 hours after rosuvastatin.
Cimetidine, ketoconazole, spironolactone: May decrease level or effect of endogenous steroid hormones. Use together cautiously.
Cyclosporine: May increase rosuvastatin level and risk of myopathy or rhabdomyolysis. Don't exceed 5 mg of rosuvastatin daily. Watch for evidence of toxicity.
Gemfibrozil: May increase rosuvastatin level and risk of myopathy or rhabdomyolysis. Don't exceed 10 mg of rosuvastatin once daily. Watch for evidence of toxicity.
Hormonal contraceptives: May increase ethinyl estradiol and norgestrel levels. Watch for adverse effects.
Warfarin: May increase INR and risk of bleeding. Monitor INR, and watch for evidence of increased bleeding.
Drug-lifestyle. *Alcohol use:* May increase risk of hepatotoxicity. Discourage use together.

EFFECTS ON LAB TEST RESULTS

- May increase CK, transaminase, glucose, glutamyl transpeptidase, alkaline phosphatase, and bilirubin levels. May decrease hemoglobin level and hematocrit.
- May cause thyroid function abnormalities, dipstick-positive proteinuria, and microscopic hematuria.

CONTRAINDICATIONS & CAUTIONS

- Contraindicated in patients hypersensitive to rosuvastatin or its components, pregnant patients, patients with active liver disease, and those with unexplained persistently increased transaminases.
- Use cautiously in patients who drink substantial amounts of alcohol or have a history of liver disease and in those at increased risk for myopathies, such as those with renal impairment, advanced age, or hypothyroidism.
- Use cautiously in Asian patients because they have a greater risk of elevated drug levels.

NURSING CONSIDERATIONS

- Before therapy starts, assess patient for underlying causes of hypercholesterolemia, including poorly controlled diabetes, hypothyroidism, nephrotic syndrome, dyslipoproteinemias, obstructive liver disease, drug interaction, and alcoholism.
- Before therapy starts, advise patient to control hypercholesterolemia with diet, exercise, and weight reduction.
- Test liver function before therapy starts, 12 weeks afterward, 12 weeks after any increase in dosage, and twice a year routinely. If AST or ALT level persists at more than three times the upper limit of normal, decrease dose or stop drug.
- ***Alert:*** Rarely, rhabdomyolysis with acute renal failure has developed in patients taking drugs in this class, including rosuvastatin.
- Patients who are 65 or older, have hypothyroidism, or have renal insufficiency may be at a greater risk for developing myopathy while receiving a statin.
- Notify prescriber if CK level becomes markedly elevated or myopathy is suspected, or if routine urinalysis shows persistent proteinuria and patient is taking 40 mg daily.
- Withhold drug temporarily if patient becomes predisposed to myopathy or rhabdomyolysis because of sepsis, hypotension, major surgery, trauma, uncontrolled seizures, or severe metabolic, endocrine, or electrolyte disorders.

PATIENT TEACHING

- Instruct patient to take drug exactly as prescribed.
- Teach patient about diet, exercise, and weight control.
- Tell patient to immediately report unexplained muscle pain, tenderness, or weakness, especially if accompanied by malaise or fever.
- Instruct patient to take drug at least 2 hours before taking antacids containing aluminum or magnesium.

simvastatin (synvinolin)

Lipex‡, Zocor

Pharmacologic class: HMG-CoA reductase inhibitor
Pregnancy risk category X

AVAILABLE FORMS

Tablets: 5 mg, 10 mg, 20 mg, 40 mg, 80 mg

INDICATIONS & DOSAGES

➤To reduce risk of death from CV disease and CV events in patients at high-risk for coronary events

Adults: Initially, 20 to 40 mg P.O. daily in evening. In patients at high risk for a coronary heart disease event due to existing coronary heart disease, diabetes, peripheral vascular disease, or history of stroke, the recommended initial dose is 40 mg P.O. daily. Adjust dosage every 4 weeks based on patient tolerance and response. Maximum, 80 mg daily.

➤To reduce total and LDL cholesterol levels in patients with homozygous familial hypercholesterolemia

Adults: 40 mg daily in evening; or, 80 mg daily in three divided doses of 20 mg in morning, 20 mg in afternoon, and 40 mg in evening.

➤ **Heterozygous familial hypercholesterolemia**
Children ages 10 to 17: 10 mg P.O. once daily in the evening. Maximum, 40 mg daily.
Adjust-a-dose: For patients taking cyclosporine, begin with 5 mg P.O. simvastatin daily; don't exceed 10 mg P.O. simvastatin daily. In patients taking fibrates or niacin, maximum is 10 mg P.O. simvastatin daily. In patients taking amiodarone or verapamil, maximum is 20 mg P.O. simvastatin daily. In patients with severe renal insufficiency, start with 5 mg P.O. daily.

ACTION

Inhibits HMG-CoA reductase, an early (and rate-limiting) step in cholesterol biosynthesis.

Route	Onset	Peak	Duration
P.O.	Unknown	1–2 hr	Unknown

Half-life: 3 hours.

ADVERSE REACTIONS

CNS: asthenia, headache.
GI: abdominal pain, constipation, diarrhea, dyspepsia, flatulence, *nausea, vomiting.*
Musculoskeletal: myalgia.
Respiratory: upper respiratory tract infection.

INTERACTIONS

Drug-drug. *Amiodarone,* ***verapamil:*** May increase risk of myopathy and rhabdomyolysis. Don't exceed 20 mg simvastatin daily.
Cyclosporine, *fibrates, niacin:* May increase risk of myopathy and rhabdomyolysis. Avoid using together; if unavoidable, monitor patient closely and don't exceed 10 mg simvastatin daily.
Digoxin: May slightly increase digoxin level. Closely monitor digoxin levels at the start of simvastatin therapy.
Diltiazem, macrolides (azithromycin, clarithromycin, erythromycin, telithromycin), nefazodone: May decrease metabolism of HMG-CoA reductase inhibitor, increasing toxicity. Monitor patient for adverse effects and report unexplained muscle pain.
Fluconazole, itraconazole, ketoconazole: May increase simvastatin level and adverse effects. Avoid using together, or, if it can't be avoided, reduce dose of simvastatin.
Hepatotoxic drugs: May increase risk for hepatotoxicity. Avoid using together.
Protease inhibitors (amprenavir, atazanavir, indinavir, lopinavir and ritonavir, nelfinavir, ritonavir, saquinavir): May inhibit metabolism of simvastatin and increase the risk of adverse effects, including rhabdomyolysis. Avoid using together.
Warfarin: May slightly enhance anticoagulant effect. Monitor PT and INR when therapy starts or dose is adjusted.
Drug-herb. *Eucalyptus, jin bu huan, kava:* May increase risk of hepatotoxicity. Discourage use together.
Red yeast rice: May increase risk of adverse events or toxicity because it contains similar components to those in drugs. Discourage use together.
Drug-food. *Grapefruit juice:* May increase drug levels, increasing risk of adverse effects including myopathy and rhabdomyolysis. Discourage use together.
Drug-lifestyle. *Alcohol use:* May increase risk of hepatotoxicity. Discourage use together.

EFFECTS ON LAB TEST RESULTS

- May increase ALT, AST, and CK levels.

CONTRAINDICATIONS & CAUTIONS

- Contraindicated in patients hypersensitive to drug and in those with active liver disease or conditions that cause unexplained persistent elevations of transaminase levels.
- Contraindicated in pregnant and breastfeeding women and in women of childbearing age.
- Use cautiously in patients who consume large amounts of alcohol or have a history of liver disease.

NURSING CONSIDERATIONS

- Use drug only after diet and other nondrug therapies prove ineffective. Patient should follow a standard low-cholesterol diet during therapy.
- Obtain liver function test results at start of therapy and then periodically. A liver

biopsy may be performed if enzyme elevations persist.

- 40 mg daily significantly reduces risk of death from coronary heart disease, nonfatal MIs, stroke, and revascularization procedures.
- ***Look alike–sound alike:*** Don't confuse Zocor with Cozaar.

PATIENT TEACHING

- Instruct patient to take drug with the evening meal because this enhances absorption and increases cholesterol biosynthesis.
- Teach patient about proper dietary management of cholesterol and triglycerides. When appropriate, recommend weight control, exercise, and smoking cessation programs.
- Tell patient to inform prescriber if adverse reactions occur, particularly muscle aches and pains.
- ***Alert:*** Tell woman to stop drug and notify prescriber immediately if she is or may be pregnant or if she's breast-feeding.

23

Miscellaneous cardiovascular drugs

abciximab
alprostadil
bosentan
cilostazol
clopidogrel bisulfate
dipyridamole
eptifibatide
iloprost
midodrine hydrochloride
nesiritide
pentoxifylline
sildenafil citrate
ticlopidine hydrochloride
tirofiban hydrochloride
treprostinil sodium

abciximab

ReoPro

Pharmacologic class: antiplatelet aggregator
Pregnancy risk category C

AVAILABLE FORMS

Injection: 2 mg/ml

INDICATIONS & DOSAGES

➤ **Adjunct to percutaneous coronary intervention (PCI) to prevent acute cardiac ischemic complications**

Adults: 0.25 mg/kg as an I.V. bolus given 10 to 60 minutes before start of PCI; then, a continuous I.V. infusion of 0.125 mcg/kg/minute to maximum 10 mcg/minute for 12 hours.

➤ **Unstable angina not responding to conventional medical therapy in patients scheduled for PCI within 24 hours**

Adults: 0.25 mg/kg as an I.V. bolus; then an 18- to 24-hour infusion of 10 mcg/minute concluding 1 hour after PCI.

I.V. ADMINISTRATION

- Inspect solution for particulate matter before administration. If opaque particles are visible, discard solution and obtain new vial.
- For bolus, withdraw needed amount of drug through a low–protein-binding 0.2- or 5-micron syringe filter.
- Give bolus 10 to 60 minutes before procedure.
- For continuous infusion, filter drug either by withdrawing needed amount of drug through a low–protein-binding 0.2- or 5-micron syringe filter into a syringe or by infusing with a continuous infusion set equipped with a low-protein-binding 0.2 or 0.22–micron in-line filter. Use normal saline solution or D_5W.
- Infuse at 0.125 mcg/kg/minute (maximum, 10 mcg/minute) for 12 hours via a continuous infusion pump.
- Discard unused portion after 12-hour infusion.

INCOMPATIBILITIES

None reported. Give drug in a separate I.V. line. Don't add other drugs to infusion solution.

ACTION

Binds to the glycoprotein IIb/IIIa (GPIIb/IIIa) receptor of human platelets and inhibits platelet aggregation.

Route	Onset	Peak	Duration
I.V.	Immediate	Immediate	48 hr

Half-life: 10 to 30 minutes.

ADVERSE REACTIONS

CNS: confusion, headache, hyperesthesia, hypoesthesia, pain.
CV: *hypotension,* ***bradycardia,*** peripheral edema.
EENT: abnormal vision.
GI: *nausea,* abdominal pain, vomiting.
Hematologic: ***bleeding, thrombocytopenia,*** anemia, leukocytosis.
Respiratory: pleural effusion, pleurisy, pneumonia.

INTERACTIONS

Drug-drug. *Antiplatelet drugs, dipyridamole, heparin, NSAIDs, other anticoagulants, thrombolytics, ticlopidine:* May increase risk of bleeding. Monitor patient closely.

EFFECTS ON LAB TEST RESULTS
- May decrease hemoglobin level.
- May increase WBC count. May decrease platelet count.

CONTRAINDICATIONS & CAUTIONS
- Contraindicated in patients hypersensitive to drug, its ingredients, or murine proteins.
- Contraindicated in those with active internal bleeding, significant GI or GU bleeding within 6 weeks, stroke within past 2 years, or significant residual neurologic deficit, bleeding diathesis, thrombocytopenia (platelet count lower than 100,000/mm^3), major surgery or trauma within 6 weeks, intracranial neoplasm, intracranial arteriovenous malformation, intracranial aneurysm, severe uncontrolled hypertension, or history of vasculitis.
- Contraindicated when oral anticoagulants have been given within past 7 days unless PT is 1.2 times control or less, or when I.V. dextran is used before or during PCI.
- Use with caution in patients at increased risk for bleeding, including those who weigh less than 165 lb (75 kg) or who are older than age 65, those who have a history of GI disease, and those who are receiving thrombolytics. Conditions that increase patient's risk of bleeding include PCI within 12 hours of onset of symptoms for acute MI, prolonged PCI (lasting longer than 70 minutes), or failed PCI. Heparin use may also increase the risk of bleeding.

NURSING CONSIDERATIONS
- The risk of bleeding is reduced by using low-dose, weight-adjusted heparin, early sheath removal, and careful maintenance of access site immobility.
- Drug is intended for use with aspirin and heparin; review and monitor other drugs patient is taking.
- ***Alert:*** Keep epinephrine, dopamine, theophylline, antihistamines, and corticosteroids readily available in case of anaphylaxis.
- Monitor patient closely for bleeding at the arterial access site used for cardiac catheterization and internal bleeding involving the GI or GU tract or retroperitoneal sites.
- Institute bleeding precautions. Keep patient on bed rest for 6 to 8 hours after sheath removal or end of drug infusion, whichever is later. Minimize arterial and venous punctures, I.M. injections, urinary catheters, nasogastric tubes, automatic blood pressure cuffs, and nasotracheal intubation; avoid, if possible.
- During infusion, remove sheath only after heparin has been stopped and its effects largely reversed.
- Before treatment, obtain platelet count, PT, ACT, and activated PTT.
- Monitor platelet count closely. Obtain levels 2 to 4 hours after bolus dose, and 24 hours after bolus dose or before discharge, whichever is first.
- Anticipate stopping drug and giving platelets for severe bleeding or thrombocytopenia.
- ***Look alike–sound alike:*** Don't confuse abciximab with infliximab.

PATIENT TEACHING
- Explain use and administration of drug to patient and family.
- Instruct patient to report adverse reactions immediately.

SAFETY ALERT!

alprostadil
Prostin VR Pediatric

Pharmacologic class: prostaglandin
Pregnancy risk category NR

AVAILABLE FORMS
Injection: 500 mcg/ml

INDICATIONS & DOSAGES
➤ **Palliative therapy for temporary maintenance of patency of ductus arteriosus until surgery can be performed**

Neonates: 0.05 to 0.1 mcg/kg/minute by I.V. infusion. When therapeutic response is achieved, reduce infusion rate to lowest dose that will maintain response. Maximum dose is 0.4 mcg/kg/minute. Or, give drug through umbilical artery catheter placed at ductal opening.

I.V. ADMINISTRATION

- Dilute drug before giving. Prepare fresh solution daily; discard solution after 24 hours.
- For infusion, dilute 1 ml of concentrate labeled as containing 500 mcg in normal saline solution or D_5W injection to yield a solution containing 2 to 20 mcg/ml.
- When using a device with a volumetric infusion chamber, add appropriate volume of diluent to the chamber; then add 1 ml of alprostadil concentrate.
- During dilution, avoid direct contact between concentrate and wall of plastic volumetric infusion chamber because solution may become hazy. If this occurs, discard solution.
- Don't use diluents that contain benzyl alcohol. Fatal toxic syndrome may occur.
- Drug isn't recommended for direct injection or intermittent infusion. Give by continuous infusion using an infusion pump. Infuse through a large peripheral or central vein or through an umbilical artery catheter placed at the level of the ductus arteriosus. If flushing from peripheral vasodilation occurs, reposition catheter.
- Reduce infusion rate if patient develops fever or significant hypotension.

INCOMPATIBILITIES

None reported.

ACTION

A prostaglandin derivative that relaxes the smooth muscle of the ductus arteriosus.

Route	Onset	Peak	Duration
I.V.	20 min	1–2 hr	Length of infusion

Half-life: About 5 to 10 minutes.

ADVERSE REACTIONS

CNS: *fever,* ***seizures.***
CV: *flushing,* ***bradycardia, cardiac arrest,*** edema, hypotension, tachycardia.
GI: diarrhea.
Hematologic: ***DIC.***
Metabolic: hypokalemia.
Respiratory: **APNEA.**
Other: ***sepsis.***

INTERACTIONS

None significant.

EFFECTS ON LAB TEST RESULTS

- May decrease potassium level.

CONTRAINDICATIONS & CAUTIONS

- Contraindicated in neonates before making differential diagnosis between respiratory distress syndrome and cyanotic heart disease and in those with respiratory distress syndrome.
- Use cautiously in neonates with bleeding tendencies because drug inhibits platelet aggregation.

NURSING CONSIDERATIONS

- Keep respiratory support available.
- In infants with restricted pulmonary blood flow, measure drug's effectiveness by monitoring blood oxygenation. In infants with restricted systemic blood flow, measure drug's effectiveness by monitoring systemic blood pressure and blood pH.
- Monitor arterial pressure by umbilical artery catheter, auscultation, or Doppler transducer. If arterial pressure falls significantly, slow infusion rate.
- Carefully monitor neonates receiving drug at recommended doses for longer than 120 hours for gastric outlet obstruction and antral hyperplasia.
- ***Alert:*** Apnea is most often seen in neonates weighing less than 2 kg (4.5 lb) at birth and usually appears during the first hour of drug infusion. CV and CNS adverse reactions occur more often in infants weighing less than 2 kg and in those receiving infusions for longer than 48 hours.
- ***Alert:*** Apnea and bradycardia may reflect drug overdose; if either occurs, stop infusion immediately.
- ***Look alike–sound alike:*** Don't confuse alprostadil with alprazolam.

PATIENT TEACHING

- Inform parents of the need for drug, and explain its use.
- Encourage parents to ask questions and express concerns.

bosentan

Tracleer

Pharmacologic class: endothelin receptor antagonist
Pregnancy risk category X

AVAILABLE FORMS

Tablets: 62.5 mg, 125 mg

INDICATIONS & DOSAGES

➤**Pulmonary arterial hypertension in patients with World Health Organization class III or IV symptoms, to improve exercise ability and decrease rate of clinical worsening**
Adults: 62.5 mg P.O. b.i.d. in the morning and evening for 4 weeks. Increase to maintenance dosage of 125 mg P.O. b.i.d. in the morning and evening.
Adjust-a-dose: For patients who develop ALT and AST abnormalities, the dose may need to be decreased or the therapy stopped until ALT and AST levels return to normal. If therapy is resumed, begin with initial dose. Test levels within 3 days; then give using the following table. If liver function abnormalities are accompanied by symptoms of liver injury or if bilirubin level is at least twice the upper limit of normal (ULN), stop treatment and don't restart. In patients who weigh less than 40 kg (88 lb), the initial and maintenance dosage is 62.5 mg b.i.d.

ALT and AST levels	Treatment and monitoring recommendations
> 3 and < 5 times upper limit of normal (ULN)	Confirm with repeat test; if confirmed, reduce dose or interrupt treatment and retest q 2 wk. Once ALT and AST levels return to pretreatment levels, continue or reintroduce treatment at starting dose.
> 5 and < 8 times ULN	Confirm with repeat test; if confirmed, stop treatment and retest at least q 2 wk. Once levels return to pretreatment levels, consider reintroduction of treatment.
> 8 times ULN	Stop treatment; don't consider restarting drug.

ACTION

Specific and competitive antagonist for endothelin-1 (ET-1). ET-1 levels are elevated in patients with pulmonary arterial hypertension, suggesting a pathogenic role for ET-1 in this disease.

Route	Onset	Peak	Duration
P.O.	Unknown	3–5 hr	Unknown

Half-life: About 5 hours.

ADVERSE REACTIONS

CNS: *headache,* fatigue.
CV: edema, flushing, hypotension, palpitations.
EENT: *nasopharyngitis.*
GI: dyspepsia.
Hematologic: *anemia.*
Hepatic: HEPATOTOXICITY.
Skin: pruritus.
Other: leg edema.

INTERACTIONS

Drug-drug. ***Cyclosporine A:*** May increase bosentan level and decrease cyclosporine level. Use together is contraindicated.
Glyburide: May increase risk of elevated liver function test values and decrease levels of both drugs. Use together is contraindicated.
Hormonal contraceptives: May cause contraceptive failure. Advise use of an additional method of birth control.
Ketoconazole: May increase bosentan effect. Watch for adverse effects.
Simvastatin, other statins: May decrease levels of these drugs. Monitor cholesterol levels to assess need to adjust statin dose.
Tacrolimus: May increase bosentan levels. Use together cautiously.

EFFECTS ON LAB TEST RESULTS

- May increase liver aminotransferase level. May decrease hemoglobin level and hematocrit.

CONTRAINDICATIONS & CAUTIONS

- Contraindicated in patients hypersensitive to drug, in pregnant patients, and in those taking cyclosporine A or glyburide.
- Generally avoid using in patients with moderate to severe liver impairment or in

those with elevated aminotransferase levels greater than three times the ULN.
• Use cautiously in patients with mild liver impairment.
• Drug may harm fetus. Be sure woman isn't pregnant before starting treatment.
• Because it's unknown whether drug appears in breast milk, drug isn't recommended for breast-feeding women.
• Safety and effectiveness in children haven't been established.

NURSING CONSIDERATIONS
• Use of this drug can cause serious liver injury. AST and ALT level elevations may be dose dependent and reversible, so measure these levels before treatment and monthly thereafter, adjusting dosage accordingly. If elevations are accompanied by symptoms of liver injury (nausea, vomiting, fever, abdominal pain, jaundice, or unusual lethargy or fatigue) or if bilirubin level increases by greater than twice the ULN, notify prescriber immediately.
• Fluid retention and heart failure may occur. Patient may require diuretics, fluid management, or hospitalization for decompensating heart failure.
• Monitor hemoglobin level after 1 and 3 months of therapy; then every 3 months.
• Gradually reduce dose before stopping drug.

PATIENT TEACHING
• Advise patient to take doses in the morning and evening, with or without food.
• Warn patient to avoid becoming pregnant while taking this drug. Hormonal contraceptives, including oral, implantable, and injectable methods, may not be effective when used with this drug. Advise patient to use a backup method of contraception. A monthly pregnancy test must be performed.
• Advise patient to have liver function tests and blood counts performed regularly.

cilostazol
Pletal

Pharmacologic class: quinolone phosphodiesterase inhibitor
Pregnancy risk category C

AVAILABLE FORMS
Tablets: 50 mg, 100 mg

INDICATIONS & DOSAGES
➤ **To reduce symptoms of intermittent claudication**
Adults: 100 mg P.O. b.i.d., at least 30 minutes before or 2 hours after breakfast and dinner.
Adjust-a-dose: Decrease dose to 50 mg P.O. b.i.d. when giving with drugs that may interact to cause an increase in cilostazol level.

ACTION
A quinolinone derivative thought to inhibit the enzyme phosphodiesterase III, thus inhibiting platelet aggregation and causing vasodilation.

Route	Onset	Peak	Duration
P.O.	Unknown	2–4 hr	Unknown

Half-life: 11 to 13 hours.

ADVERSE REACTIONS
CNS: *dizziness, headache,* vertigo.
CV: *palpitations,* peripheral edema, tachycardia.
EENT: *pharyngitis, rhinitis.*
GI: *abnormal stools, diarrhea,* abdominal pain, dyspepsia, flatulence, nausea.
Musculoskeletal: back pain, myalgia.
Respiratory: increased cough.
Other: *infection,* bleeding.

INTERACTIONS
Drug-drug. *Diltiazem:* May increase cilostazol level. Reduce cilostazol dosage to 50 mg b.i.d.
Erythromycin, other macrolides: May increase level of cilostazol and its metabolites. Reduce cilostazol dosage to 50 mg b.i.d.
Omeprazole: May increase level of cilostazol metabolite. Reduce cilostazol dosage to 50 mg b.i.d.

Strong inhibitors of CYP3A4 (such as fluconazole, fluoxetine, fluvoxamine, itraconazole, ketoconazole, miconazole, nefazodone, sertraline): May increase level of cilostazol and its metabolites. Reduce cilostazol dosage to 50 mg b.i.d.
Drug-food. *Grapefruit juice:* May increase drug level. Discourage use together.
Drug-lifestyle. *Smoking:* May decrease drug exposure. Discourage smoking.

EFFECTS ON LAB TEST RESULTS
None reported.

CONTRAINDICATIONS & CAUTIONS
- Contraindicated in patients hypersensitive to drug or its components and in those with heart failure of any severity.
- Contraindicated in patients with hemostatic disorders or active bleeding, such as bleeding peptic ulcer and intracranial bleeding.
- Use cautiously in patients with severe underlying heart disease; also use cautiously with other drugs having antiplatelet activity.

NURSING CONSIDERATIONS
- Give drug at least 30 minutes before or 2 hours after breakfast and dinner.
- Beneficial effects may not be seen for up to 12 weeks after therapy starts.
- ***Alert:*** Cilostazol and similar drugs that inhibit the enzyme phosphodiesterase decrease the likelihood of survival in patients with class III and IV heart failure.
- ***Alert:*** CV risk is unknown in patients who use drug on long-term basis and in those with severe underlying heart disease.
- Dosage can be reduced or stopped without such rebound effects as platelet hyperaggregation.
- Drug may reduce triglyceride levels and increase HDL cholesterol level.

PATIENT TEACHING
- Instruct patient to take drug on an empty stomach, at least 30 minutes before or 2 hours after breakfast and dinner.
- Tell patient that beneficial effect of drug on cramping pain isn't likely to be noticed for 2 to 4 weeks and that it may take as long as 12 weeks.
- Advise patient to avoid drinking grapefruit juice during drug therapy.
- Inform patient that CV risk is unknown in patients who use drug on a long-term basis and in those with severe underlying heart disease.
- Tell patient that drug may cause dizziness. Caution patient not to drive or perform other activities that require alertness until response to drug is known.

clopidogrel bisulfate
Plavix

Pharmacologic class: inhibitor of adenosine diphosphate (ADP)-induced platelet aggregation
Pregnancy risk category B

AVAILABLE FORMS
Tablets: 75 mg

INDICATIONS & DOSAGES
➤ **To reduce thrombotic events in patients with atherosclerosis documented by recent stroke, MI, or peripheral arterial disease**
Adults: 75 mg P.O. daily.
➤ **To reduce thrombotic events in patients with acute coronary syndrome (unstable angina and non–Q-wave MI), including those receiving drugs and those having percutaneous coronary intervention (with or without stent) or coronary artery bypass graft (CABG)**
Adults: Initially, a single 300-mg P.O. loading dose; then 75 mg P.O. once daily. Start and continue aspirin (75 to 325 mg once daily) with clopidogrel.
✱ ***NEW INDICATION:*** **ST-segment elevation acute MI**
Adults: 75 mg P.O. once daily, with aspirin, with or without thrombolytics. An 300-mg loading dose is optional.

ACTION
Inhibits the binding of adenosine diphosphate (ADP) to its platelet receptor, impeding ADP-mediated activation and subsequent platelet aggregation, and irre-

versibly modifies the platelet ADP receptor.

Route	Onset	Peak	Duration
P.O.	2 hr	Unknown	5 days

Half-life: 8 hours.

ADVERSE REACTIONS

CNS: depression, dizziness, fatigue, headache, pain.
CV: edema, hypertension.
EENT: epistaxis, rhinitis.
GI: ***hemorrhage,*** abdominal pain, constipation, diarrhea, dyspepsia, gastritis, ulcers.
GU: UTI.
Hematologic: purpura.
Musculoskeletal: arthralgia.
Respiratory: bronchitis, coughing, dyspnea, upper respiratory tract infection.
Skin: *rash,* pruritus.
Other: flulike syndrome.

INTERACTIONS

Drug-drug. *Aspirin, NSAIDs:* May increase risk of GI bleeding. Monitor patient.
Heparin, warfarin: Safety hasn't been established. Use together cautiously.
Salicylates: May increase the risk of serious bleeding in patients with TIA or ischemic stroke. Avoid using together.
Drug-herb. *Red clover:* May increase risk of bleeding. Discourage use together.

EFFECTS ON LAB TEST RESULTS

- May decrease platelet count.

CONTRAINDICATIONS & CAUTIONS

- Contraindicated in patients hypersensitive to drug or its components and in those with pathologic bleeding (such as peptic ulcer or intracranial hemorrhage).
- Use cautiously in patients at risk for increased bleeding from trauma, surgery, or other pathologic conditions and in those with renal or hepatic impairment.

NURSING CONSIDERATIONS

- Platelet aggregation won't return to normal for at least 5 days after drug has been stopped.
- ***Alert:*** Drug may cause fatal thrombotic thrombocytopenic purpura (thrombocytopenia, hemolytic anemia, neurologic findings, renal dysfunction, and fever) that requires urgent treatment, including plasmapheresis.
- ***Look alike–sound alike:*** Don't confuse Plavix with Paxil.

PATIENT TEACHING

- Advise patient it may take longer than usual to stop bleeding. Tell him to refrain from activities in which trauma and bleeding may occur, and encourage him to wear a seatbelt when in a car.
- Instruct patient to notify prescriber if unusual bleeding or bruising occurs.
- Tell patient to inform all health care providers, including dentists, before undergoing procedures or starting new drug therapy, that he is taking drug.
- Inform patient that drug may be taken without regard to meals.

dipyridamole

Apo-Dipyridamole FC†, Novo-Dipiradol†, Persantin SR‡, Persantine

Pharmacologic class: pyrimidine analogue
Pregnancy risk category B

AVAILABLE FORMS

Injection: 5 mg/ml in 2- and 10-ml vials
Tablets: 25 mg, 50 mg, 75 mg

INDICATIONS & DOSAGES

➤ **To inhibit platelet adhesion in prosthetic heart valves (given together with warfarin)**
Adults: 75 to 100 mg P.O. q.i.d.
➤ **Alternative to exercise in evaluation of coronary artery disease during thallium myocardial perfusion scintigraphy**
Adults: 0.57 mg/kg as an I.V. infusion at a constant rate over 4 minutes (0.142 mg/kg/minute).

I.V. ADMINISTRATION

- For use as a diagnostic drug, dilute in half-normal or normal saline solution or D_5W in at least a 1:2 ratio for a total volume of 20 to 50 ml.

• Inject thallium-201 within 5 minutes after completing the 4-minute dipyridamole infusion.

INCOMPATIBILITIES
None reported.

ACTION
May involve drug's ability to increase adenosine, which is a coronary vasodilator and platelet aggregation inhibitor.

Route	Onset	Peak	Duration
P.O.	Unknown	75 min	Unknown
I.V.	Unknown	2 min	Unknown

Half-life: 1 to 12 hours.

ADVERSE REACTIONS
CNS: *dizziness, headache,* syncope.
CV: *angina pectoris, chest pain,* ***ECG abnormalities,*** blood pressure lability, flushing, hypertension, hypotension.
GI: *nausea,* abdominal distress, diarrhea, vomiting.

INTERACTIONS
Drug-drug. *Adenosine:* May increase levels and cardiac effects of adenosine. Adjust adenosine dose as needed.
Cholinesterase inhibitors: May counteract anticholinesterase effects and aggravate myasthenia gravis. Monitor patient.
Heparin: May increase risk of bleeding. Monitor patient closely.
Theophylline: May prevent coronary vasodilation by I.V. dipyridamole, causing a false-negative thallium-imaging result. Avoid using together.

EFFECTS ON LAB TEST RESULTS
• May increase liver enzyme levels.

CONTRAINDICATIONS & CAUTIONS
• Contraindicated in patients hypersensitive to drug.
• Use cautiously in patients with hypotension and those with severe coronary artery disease.

NURSING CONSIDERATIONS
• If GI distress develops, give drug 1 hour before meals or with meals.
• Observe for adverse reactions, especially with large doses. Monitor blood pressure.
• Observe for signs and symptoms of bleeding; note prolonged bleeding time (especially with large doses or long-term therapy).
• The value of drug as part of an antithrombotic regimen is controversial; its use may not provide significantly better results than aspirin alone.
• ***Look alike–sound alike:*** Don't confuse dipyridamole with disopyramide. Don't confuse Persantine with Periactin.
• Persantine may contain tartrazine.

PATIENT TEACHING
• Instruct patient to take drug exactly as prescribed.
• Tell patient to report adverse reactions promptly.
• Tell patient receiving drug I.V. to report discomfort at insertion site.

eptifibatide
Integrilin

Pharmacologic class: glycoprotein IIb/IIIa (GPIIb/IIIa) inhibitor
Pregnancy risk category B

AVAILABLE FORMS
Injection: 10-ml (2 mg/ml), 100-ml (0.75 mg/ml and 2 mg/ml) vials

INDICATIONS & DOSAGES
➤ **Acute coronary syndrome (unstable angina or non–ST-segment elevation MI) in patients receiving drug therapy and in those having a percutaneous coronary intervention (PCI)**
Adults: 180 mcg/kg I.V. bolus as soon as possible after diagnosis, followed by a continuous I.V. infusion at a rate of 2 mcg/kg/minute until hospital discharge or start of coronary artery bypass graft (CABG) surgery, for up to 72 hours. If patient is having a PCI, continue infusion until hospital discharge or for 18 to 24 hours after the procedure, whichever comes first, for up to 96 hours. Patients who weigh more than 121 kg (266 lb) should receive a bo-

lus not to exceed 22.6 mg, followed by a maximum infusion rate of 15 mg/hour.
Adjust-a-dose: If creatinine clearance is less than 50 ml/minute or creatinine level is greater than 2 mg/dl, give 180 mcg/kg I.V. bolus as soon as possible after diagnosis, followed by a continuous I.V. infusion at 1 mcg/kg/minute. Patients with this creatinine clearance who weigh more than 121 kg should receive a bolus not to exceed 22.6 mg, followed by a maximum infusion rate of 7.5 mg/hour.

➤ **PCI**

Adults: 180 mcg/kg I.V. bolus given just before the procedure, immediately followed by an infusion of 2 mcg/kg/minute and a second I.V. bolus of 180 mcg/kg given 10 minutes after the first bolus. Continue infusion until hospital discharge or for 18 to 24 hours, whichever comes first; the minimum duration of infusion is 12 hours. Patients weighing more than 121 kg should receive a bolus not to exceed 22.6 mg, followed by a maximum infusion rate of 15 mg/hour.
Adjust-a-dose: If creatinine clearance is less than 50 ml/minute or creatinine level is greater than 2 mg/dl, give 180 mcg/kg I.V. bolus just before the procedure, immediately followed by a continuous I.V. infusion at 1 mcg/kg/minute and a second bolus of 180 mcg/kg given 10 minutes after the first bolus. Patients with this creatinine clearance who weigh more than 121 kg should receive a bolus not to exceed 22.6 mg, followed by a maximum infusion rate of 7.5 mg/hour.

I.V. ADMINISTRATION

- Inspect solution for particles before use; if they appear, drug may not be sterile. Discard it.
- Protect drug from light before giving.
- Drug may be given in same line with normal saline solution, D_5W, alteplase, atropine, dobutamine, heparin, lidocaine, meperidine, metoprolol, midazolam, morphine, nitroglycerin, or verapamil. Main infusion may also contain up to 60 mEq/L of potassium chloride.
- For I.V. push, withdraw bolus dose from 10-ml vial into a syringe and give over 1 or 2 minutes.
- For infusion, give undiluted drug directly from 100-ml vial using an infusion pump.
- If patient needs thrombolytics, stop infusion.
- Refrigerate vials at 36° to 46° F (2° to 8° C). Store vials at room temperature for no longer than 2 months; afterward, discard them.

INCOMPATIBILITIES

Furosemide.

ACTION

Reversibly binds to the GP IIb/IIIa receptor on human platelets and inhibits platelet aggregation.

Route	Onset	Peak	Duration
I.V.	Immediate	Immediate	4–6 hr

Half-life: 2½ hours.

ADVERSE REACTIONS

CV: hypotension.
GU: hematuria.
Hematologic: *bleeding,* ***thrombocytopenia.***
Other: bleeding at femoral artery access site.

INTERACTIONS

Drug-drug. *Clopidogrel, dipyridamole, NSAIDs, oral anticoagulants (warfarin), thrombolytics, ticlopidine:* May increase risk of bleeding. Monitor patient closely.
Other inhibitors of platelet receptor IIb/IIIa: May cause serious bleeding. Avoid using together.

EFFECTS ON LAB TEST RESULTS

- May decrease platelet count.

CONTRAINDICATIONS & CAUTIONS

- Contraindicated in patients hypersensitive to drug or its ingredients and in those with history of bleeding diathesis or evidence of active abnormal bleeding within previous 30 days; severe hypertension (systolic blood pressure higher than 200 mm Hg or diastolic blood pressure higher than 110 mm Hg) not adequately controlled with antihypertensives; major surgery within previous 6 weeks; history of stroke within 30 days or history of

hemorrhagic stroke; current or planned use of another parenteral GP IIb/IIIa inhibitor; or platelet count less than 100,000/mm^3.
• Contraindicated in patients with creatinine level 4 mg/dl or higher and in patients dependent on renal dialysis.
• Use cautiously in patients at increased risk for bleeding, in those with platelet count less than 150,000/mm^3, in those with hemorrhagic retinopathy, and in those weighing more than 143 kg (315 lb).

NURSING CONSIDERATIONS

• Drug is intended for use with heparin and aspirin.
• At least 4 hours before hospital discharge, stop this drug and heparin and achieve sheath hemostasis by standard compressive techniques.
• Remove sheath during infusion only after heparin has been stopped and its effects largely reversed.
• If patient is to have a CABG, stop infusion before surgery.
• Minimize use of arterial and venous punctures, I.M. injections, urinary catheters, and nasotracheal and nasogastric tubes.
• When obtaining I.V. access, avoid use of noncompressible sites (such as subclavian or jugular veins).
• Monitor patient for bleeding.
• ***Alert:*** If patient's platelet count is less than 100,000/mm^3, stop this drug and heparin.
• Perform baseline laboratory tests before start of drug therapy; also determine hemoglobin level, hematocrit, PT, INR, APTT, platelet count, and creatinine level.

PATIENT TEACHING

• Explain that drug is a blood thinner used to prevent chest pain and heart attack.
• Explain that benefits of drug far outweigh risk of serious bleeding.
• Tell patient to report to prescriber chest discomfort or other adverse effects immediately.

iloprost

Ventavis

Pharmacologic class: prostacyclin analog
Pregnancy risk category C

AVAILABLE FORMS

Inhalation solution: 10 mcg/ml in 1- and 2-ml single-dose ampules

INDICATIONS & DOSAGES

➤Pulmonary arterial hypertension in patients with NYHA Class III or IV symptoms
Adults: Initially, 2.5 mcg inhaled using the I-neb or the Prodose Adaptive Aerosol Delivery (AAD) systems. As tolerated, increase to 5 mcg inhaled six to nine times daily while patient is awake, p.r.n., but to no more than q 2 hours. Maximum, 5 mcg nine times daily.

ACTION

Lowers pulmonary arterial pressure by dilating systemic and pulmonary arterial beds. Drug also affects platelet aggregation, although effect in pulmonary hypertension treatment isn't known.

Route	Onset	Peak	Duration
Inhalation	Unknown	Unknown	30-60 min

Half-life: 20 to 30 minutes.

ADVERSE REACTIONS

CNS: *headache,* insomnia, syncope.
CV: *hypotension, vasodilation,* ***chest pain, heart failure, supraventricular tachycardia,*** palpitations, peripheral edema.
GI: *nausea,* tongue pain, vomiting.
GU: ***renal failure.***
Musculoskeletal: *trismus,* back pain, muscle cramps.
Respiratory: *cough,* dyspnea, hemoptysis, pneumonia.
Other: *flulike syndrome.*

INTERACTIONS

Drug-drug. *Antihypertensives, vasodilators:* May increase effects of these drugs. Monitor patient's blood pressure.
Anticoagulants: May increase risk of bleeding. Monitor patient closely.

EFFECTS ON LAB TEST RESULTS
- May increase alkaline phosphatase and GGT levels.

CONTRAINDICATIONS & CAUTIONS
- No contraindications known. Avoid using in patients whose systolic blood pressure is less than 85 mm Hg.
- Use cautiously in elderly patients, patients with hepatic or renal impairment, and patients with COPD, severe asthma, or acute pulmonary infection.

NURSING CONSIDERATIONS
- Keep drug away from skin and eyes.
- The 2-ml ampule must be used with the Prodose AAD System and may be used with the I-neb AAD System. The 1-ml ampule must be used only with the I-neb AAD System.
- Take care not to inhale drug while providing treatment.
- Monitor patient's vital signs carefully at start of treatment.
- Watch for syncope.
- If patient develops evidence of pulmonary edema, stop treatment immediately.

PATIENT TEACHING
- Advise patient to take drug exactly as prescribed and using Prodose AAD or I-neb AAD.
- Urge patient to follow manufacturer instructions for preparing and inhaling drug.
- Advise patient to keep a backup Prodose AAD or I-neb AAD in case the original malfunctions.
- Tell patient to keep drug away from skin and eyes and to rinse the area immediately if contact occurs.
- Caution patient not to ingest drug solution.
- Inform patient that drug may cause dizziness and fainting. Urge him to stand up slowly from a sitting or lying position and to report to prescriber worsening of symptoms.
- Tell patient to take drug before physical exertion but no more than every 2 hours.
- Tell patient not to expose others, especially pregnant women and infants, to drug.
- Teach patient how to clean equipment and safely dispose of used ampules after each treatment. Caution patient not to save or use leftover solution.

midodrine hydrochloride
ProAmatine

Pharmacologic class: synthetic sympathomimetic amine
Pregnancy risk category C

AVAILABLE FORMS
Tablets: 2.5 mg, 5 mg, 10 mg

INDICATIONS & DOSAGES
➤ **Symptomatic orthostatic hypotension unresponsive to standard clinical care**
Adults: 10 mg P.O. t.i.d. The patient takes the first dose upon arising in the morning, the second dose at noon, and the third dose in late afternoon but no later than 6 p.m. or 4 hours before bedtime.
Adjust-a-dose: For patients with renal impairment, initially, 2.5 mg.

ACTION
Forms an active metabolite, desglymidodrine, which is an $alpha_1$ agonist. It increases blood pressure by activating alpha-adrenergic receptors in arteriolar and venous vasculature.

Route	Onset	Peak	Duration
P.O.	Unknown	1–2 hr	Unknown

Half-life: 3 to 4 hours.

ADVERSE REACTIONS
CNS: *paresthesia,* anxiety, confusion, headache.
CV: *vasodilation,* ***supine and sitting hypertension.***
GI: abdominal pain, dry mouth.
GU: *dysuria,* frequency and urgency, urine retention.
Skin: *piloerection, pruritus,* rash.
Other: chills, pain.

INTERACTIONS
Drug-drug. *Alpha agonists:* May enhance vasopressor effects. Monitor blood pressure closely.
Alpha blockers: May antagonize drug effects. Avoid using together.

Beta blockers, cardiac glycosides: May cause or worsen bradycardia, AV block, or arrhythmias. Avoid using together.
Fludrocortisone: May increase risk of supine hypertension and lead to increased intraocular pressure and worsened glaucoma. Monitor patient closely.

EFFECTS ON LAB TEST RESULTS
None reported.

CONTRAINDICATIONS & CAUTIONS
- Contraindicated in patients with severe organic heart disease, persistent and excessive supine hypertension, acute renal disease, urine retention, pheochromocytoma, or thyrotoxicosis.
- Use cautiously in patients with history of urine retention, visual problems, diabetes, or renal or hepatic impairment, and in breast-feeding women.
- Safety and effectiveness of drug in children haven't been established.

NURSING CONSIDERATIONS
- Drug should be used in pregnancy only if benefit justifies risk to fetus.
- Perform renal and hepatic tests before and during drug therapy.
- Monitor supine and sitting blood pressures closely, and notify prescriber if supine blood pressure increases excessively.
- Monitor patient for signs and symptoms of bradycardia, such as slowed pulse, syncope or dizziness, especially after giving the drug.
- Drug should be taken during the day when patient can be upright and performing activities of daily living. Space doses at least 3 hours apart. Midodrine shouldn't be given after the evening meal or within 4 hours of bedtime, to reduce risk of supine hypertension during sleep.
- Drug should be continued only if symptoms improve during initial therapy.
- ***Look alike–sound alike:*** Don't confuse ProAmatine with protamine.

PATIENT TEACHING
- Instruct patient to separate doses by 3 to 4 hours; tell him to take last dose of the day 4 hours before bedtime.
- Instruct patient to stop drug and immediately notify prescriber about signs and symptoms of supine hypertension (cardiac awareness, pounding in ears, headache, blurred vision).
- Tell patient to consult prescriber before taking OTC drugs.

SAFETY ALERT!

nesiritide
Natrecor

Pharmacologic class: human B-type natriuretic peptide
Pregnancy risk category C

AVAILABLE FORMS
Injection: Single-dose vials of 1.5 mg sterile, lyophilized powder

INDICATIONS & DOSAGES
➤ **Acutely decompensated heart failure in patients with dyspnea at rest or with minimal activity**
Adults: 2 mcg/kg by I.V. bolus over 60 seconds, followed by continuous infusion of 0.01 mcg/kg/minute.
Adjust-a-dose: If hypotension develops during administration, reduce dosage or stop drug. Restart drug at dosage reduced by 30% with no bolus doses.

I.V. ADMINISTRATION
- Reconstitute one 1.5-mg vial with 5 ml of diluent (such as D_5W, normal saline solution, 5% dextrose and 0.2% saline solution injection, or 5% dextrose and half-normal saline solution) from a prefilled 250-ml I.V. bag.
- Gently rock (don't shake) vial until solution becomes clear and colorless.
- Withdraw contents of vial and add back to the 250-ml I.V. bag to yield 6 mcg/ml. Invert the bag several times to ensure complete mixing, and use the solution within 24 hours.
- Use the formulas below to calculate bolus volume (2 mcg/kg) and infusion flow rate (0.01 mcg/kg/minute):

$$\underset{(ml)}{\text{Bolus volume}} = 0.33 \times \underset{(kg)}{\text{patient weight}}$$

$$\underset{(ml/hr)}{\text{Infusion flow rate}} = 0.1 \times \underset{(kg)}{\text{patient weight}}$$

- Before giving bolus dose, prime the I.V. tubing. Withdraw the bolus and give over 60 seconds through an I.V. port in the tubing.
- Immediately after giving bolus, infuse drug at 0.1 ml/kg/hr to deliver 0.01 mcg/kg/minute.
- Store drug at 68° to 77° F (20° to 25° C).

INCOMPATIBILITIES
Bumetanide, enalaprilat, ethacrynate sodium, furosemide, heparin, hydralazine, insulin, sodium metabisulfite.

ACTION
A human B-type natriuretic peptide that increases cGMP level, relaxes smooth muscle, and dilates veins and arteries. Reduces pulmonary capillary wedge pressure and systemic arterial pressure in patients with heart failure.

Route	Onset	Peak	Duration
I.V.	15 min	1 hr	3 hr

Half-life: 18 minutes.

ADVERSE REACTIONS
CNS: anxiety, confusion, dizziness, fever, headache, insomnia, paresthesia, somnolence, tremor.
CV: *hypotension,* ***bradycardia, ventricular tachycardia,*** angina, atrial fibrillation, AV node conduction abnormalities, ventricular extrasystoles.
GI: abdominal pain, nausea, vomiting.
Hematologic: anemia.
Musculoskeletal: back pain, leg cramps.
Respiratory: ***apnea,*** cough.
Skin: injection site reactions, rash, pruritus, sweating.

INTERACTIONS
Drug-drug. *ACE inhibitors:* May increase hypotension symptoms. Monitor blood pressure closely.

EFFECTS ON LAB TEST RESULTS
- May increase creatinine level more than 0.5 mg/dl above baseline. May decrease hemoglobin level and hematocrit.

CONTRAINDICATIONS & CAUTIONS
- Contraindicated in patients hypersensitive to drug or its components.
- Contraindicated in patients with cardiogenic shock, systolic blood pressure below 90 mm Hg, low cardiac filling pressures, conditions in which cardiac output depends on venous return, or conditions that make vasodilators inappropriate, such as valvular stenosis, restrictive or obstructive cardiomyopathy, constrictive pericarditis, and pericardial tamponade.

NURSING CONSIDERATIONS
- Don't start drug at higher-than-recommended dosage because this may cause hypotension and may increase creatinine level.
- ***Alert:*** This drug may cause hypotension. Monitor patient's blood pressure closely, particularly if he also takes an ACE inhibitor.
- ***Alert:*** Drug binds to heparin, including the heparin lining of a coated catheter, decreasing the amount of nesiritide delivered. Don't give nesiritide through a central heparin-coated catheter.
- Drug may affect renal function. In patients with severe heart failure whose renal function depends on the renin-angiotensin-aldosterone system, treatment may lead to azotemia.
- Results of giving this drug for longer than 48 hours are unknown.

PATIENT TEACHING
- Tell patient to report discomfort at I.V. site.
- Urge patient to report to prescriber symptoms of hypotension, such as dizziness, light-headedness, blurred vision, or sweating.
- Tell patient to report to prescriber other adverse effects promptly.

pentoxifylline
Trental✐

Pharmacologic class: xanthine derivative
Pregnancy risk category C

AVAILABLE FORMS
Tablets (extended-release): 400 mg

INDICATIONS & DOSAGES

➤Intermittent claudication from chronic occlusive vascular disease
Adults: 400 mg P.O. t.i.d. with meals. May decrease to 400 mg b.i.d. if GI and CNS adverse effects occur.

ACTION

Unknown. Improves capillary blood flow, probably by increasing RBC flexibility and lowering blood viscosity.

Route	Onset	Peak	Duration
P.O.	Unknown	1 hr	Unknown

Half-life: About 30 to 45 minutes.

ADVERSE REACTIONS

CNS: dizziness, headache.
GI: dyspepsia, nausea, vomiting.

INTERACTIONS

Drug-drug. *Anticoagulants:* May increase anticoagulant effect. Monitor PT.
Antihypertensives: May increase hypotensive effect. May need to adjust dosage.
Theophylline: May increase theophylline level. Monitor patient closely.
Drug-lifestyle. *Smoking:* May cause vasoconstriction. Advise patient to avoid smoking.

EFFECTS ON LAB TEST RESULTS

None reported.

CONTRAINDICATIONS & CAUTIONS

- Contraindicated in patients intolerant to this drug or to methylxanthines, such as caffeine, theophylline, and theobromine, and in those with recent cerebral or retinal hemorrhage.

NURSING CONSIDERATIONS

- Drug is useful in patients who aren't good surgical candidates.
- Elderly patients may be more sensitive to drug's effects.
- ***Look alike–sound alike:*** Don't confuse Trental with Trandate.

PATIENT TEACHING

- Advise patient to take drug with meals to minimize GI upset.
- Instruct patient to swallow tablet whole, without breaking, crushing, or chewing.
- Tell patient to report GI or CNS adverse reactions; prescriber may reduce dosage.
- Urge patient not to stop drug during the first 8 weeks of therapy unless directed by prescriber.

sildenafil citrate

Revatio

Pharmacologic class: cyclic guanosine monophosphate (c-GMP)-specific phosphodiesterase type-5, or PDE5, inhibitor
Pregnancy risk category B

AVAILABLE FORMS

Tablets: 20 mg

INDICATIONS & DOSAGES

➤To improve exercise ability in patients with World Health Organization group I pulmonary arterial hypertension (PAH)
Adults: 20 mg P.O. t.i.d., 4 to 6 hours apart.

ACTION

Increases c-GMP level by preventing its breakdown by phosphodiesterase, prolonging smooth muscle relaxation of the pulmonary vasculature, which leads to vasodilation.

Route	Onset	Peak	Duration
P.O.	15–30 min	30–120 min	4 hr

Half-life: 4 hours.

ADVERSE REACTIONS

CNS: *headache,* dizziness, fever.
CV: *flushing,* hypotension.
EENT: blurred vision, burning, epistaxis, impaired color discrimination, photophobia, rhinitis, sinusitis.
GI: *dyspepsia,* diarrhea, gastritis.
Musculoskeletal: myalgia.
Skin: erythema.

INTERACTIONS

Drug-drug. *Alpha blockers:* May cause symptomatic hypotension. Use together cautiously.

Amlodipine: May further reduce blood pressure. Monitor blood pressure closely.
Bosentan: May decrease sildenafil level. Monitor patient.
Cytochrome P-450 inducers, rifampin: May reduce sildenafil level. Monitor effect.
Hepatic isoenzyme inhibitors (such as cimetidine, erythromycin, itraconazole, ketoconazole): May increase sildenafil level. Avoid using together.
Isosorbide, nitroglycerin: May cause severe hypotension. Use of nitrates in any form is contraindicated during therapy.
Protease inhibitors (ritonavir): May significantly increase sildenafil level. Don't use together.
Vitamin K antagonists: May increase risk of bleeding (primarily epistaxis). Monitor patient.
Drug-food. *Grapefruit:* May increase drug level, while delaying absorption. Advise patient to avoid using together.

EFFECTS ON LAB TEST RESULTS
None reported.

CONTRAINDICATIONS & CAUTIONS
- Contraindicated in patients hypersensitive to drug or its components and in those taking organic nitrates.
- Don't use in patients with pulmonary veno-occlusive disease.
- Use cautiously in patients with resting hypotension, severe left ventricular outflow obstruction, autonomic dysfunction, and volume depletion.
- Use cautiously in elderly patients; in patients with hepatic or severe renal impairment, retinitis pigmentosa, bleeding disorders, or active peptic ulcer disease; in those who have suffered an MI, stroke, or life-threatening arrhythmia in last 6 months; in those with history of coronary artery disease causing unstable angina or of uncontrolled high or low blood pressure; in those with deformation of the penis or with conditions that may cause priapism (such as sickle cell anemia, multiple myeloma, or leukemia); and in those taking bosentan.

NURSING CONSIDERATIONS
- The serious CV events linked to this drug's use in erectile dysfunction mainly involve patients with underlying CV disease who are at increased risk for cardiac effects related to sexual activity.
- Patients with PAH caused by connective tissue disease are more prone to epistaxis during therapy than those with primary pulmonary hypertension.
- ***Alert:*** Don't substitute Viagra for Revatio because there isn't an equivalent dose.
- It's unknown if drug appears in breast milk. Use cautiously in breast-feeding women.
- Safety and effectiveness in children haven't been established.

PATIENT TEACHING
- Warn patient that drug should never be used with nitrates.
- Advise patient to rise slowly from lying down.
- Inform patient that drug can be taken with or without food.
- Warn patient that discrimination between colors, such as blue and green, may become impaired during therapy; warn him to avoid hazardous activities that rely on color discrimination.
- Instruct patient to notify prescriber of visual changes, dizziness, or fainting.
- Caution patient to take drug only as prescribed.

ticlopidine hydrochloride
Ticlid🖉

Pharmacologic class: platelet aggregation inhibitor
Pregnancy risk category B

AVAILABLE FORMS
Tablets: 250 mg

INDICATIONS & DOSAGES
➤To reduce risk of thrombotic stroke in patients who have had a stroke or stroke precursors
Adults: 250 mg P.O. b.i.d. with meals.
➤Adjunct to aspirin to prevent subacute stent thrombosis in patients having coronary stent placement
Adults: 250 mg P.O. b.i.d., combined with antiplatelet doses of aspirin. Start therapy after stent placement and continue for 30 days.

ACTION

Unknown. An antiplatelet that probably blocks adenosine diphosphate-induced platelet-to-fibrinogen and platelet-to-platelet binding.

Route	Onset	Peak	Duration
P.O.	Unknown	2 hr	Unknown

Half-life: 1½ hours after single dose; 4 to 5 days after multiple doses.

ADVERSE REACTIONS

CNS: ***intracranial bleeding,*** dizziness, peripheral neuropathy.
CV: vasculitis.
EENT: conjunctival hemorrhage.
GI: *diarrhea,* abdominal pain, anorexia, bleeding, dyspepsia, flatulence, nausea, vomiting.
GU: dark urine, hematuria.
Hematologic: ***agranulocytosis, aplastic anemia, immune thrombocytopenia, neutropenia, pancytopenia.***
Musculoskeletal: arthropathy, myositis.
Respiratory: *allergic pneumonitis.*
Skin: ***thrombocytopenic purpura,*** ecchymoses, maculopapular rash, pruritus, rash, urticaria.
Other: hypersensitivity reactions, postoperative bleeding.

INTERACTIONS

Drug-drug. *Antacids:* May decrease ticlopidine level. Separate doses by at least 2 hours.
Aspirin: May increase effect of aspirin on platelets. Use together cautiously.
Cimetidine: May decrease clearance of ticlopidine and increase risk of toxicity. Avoid using together.
Digoxin: May decrease digoxin level. Monitor digoxin level.
Phenytoin: May increase phenytoin level. Monitor patient closely.
Theophylline: May decrease theophylline clearance and risk of toxicity. Monitor patient closely and adjust theophylline dosage.
Drug-herb. *Red clover:* May cause bleeding. Discourage use together.

EFFECTS ON LAB TEST RESULTS

- May increase ALT, AST, alkaline phosphatase, cholesterol, and triglyceride levels.
- May decrease neutrophil, WBC, RBC, platelet, and granulocyte counts.

CONTRAINDICATIONS & CAUTIONS

- Contraindicated in patients hypersensitive to drug and in those with severe hepatic impairment, hematopoietic disorders, active pathologic bleeding from peptic ulceration, or active intracranial bleeding.
- Use cautiously and with close monitoring of CBC and WBC differentials, watching for signs and symptoms of neutropenia and agranulocytosis.

NURSING CONSIDERATIONS

- Because of life-threatening adverse reactions, use drug only in patients who are allergic to, can't tolerate, or have failed aspirin therapy.
- Obtain baseline liver function test results before therapy.
- Determine CBC and WBC differentials at second week of therapy and repeat every 2 weeks until end of third month.
- Monitor liver function test results and repeat if dysfunction is suspected.
- Thrombocytopenia has occurred rarely. Stop drug in patients with platelet count of 80,000/mm^3 or less. If needed, give methylprednisolone 20 mg I.V. to normalize bleeding time within 2 hours.
- When used preoperatively, drug may decrease risk of graft occlusion in patients receiving coronary artery bypass grafts and reduce severity of drop in platelet count in patients receiving extracorporeal hemoperfusion during open heart surgery.

PATIENT TEACHING

- Tell patient to take drug with meals.
- Warn patient to avoid aspirin and aspirin-containing products and to check with prescriber or pharmacist before taking OTC drugs.
- Explain that drug will prolong bleeding time and that patient should report unusual or prolonged bleeding. Advise patient to tell dentists and other health care providers that he takes ticlopidine.
- Stress importance of regular blood tests. Because neutropenia can result with in-

creased risk of infection, tell patient to immediately report signs and symptoms of infection, such as fever, chills, or sore throat.
- If drug is being substituted for a fibrinolytic or anticoagulant, tell patient to stop those drugs before starting ticlopidine therapy.
- Advise patient to stop drug 10 to 14 days before undergoing elective surgery.
- Tell patient to immediately report to prescriber yellow skin or sclera, severe or persistent diarrhea, rashes, bleeding under the skin, light-colored stools, or dark urine.

SAFETY ALERT!

tirofiban hydrochloride
Aggrastat

Pharmacologic class: glycoprotein (GP) IIb/IIIa receptor antagonist
Pregnancy risk category B

AVAILABLE FORMS
Injection: 25-ml and 50-ml vials (250 mcg/ml), 250-ml and 500-ml premixed vials (50 mcg/ml)

INDICATIONS & DOSAGES
➤ **Acute coronary syndrome, with heparin or aspirin, including patients who are to be managed medically and those undergoing percutaneous transluminal coronary angioplasty (PTCA) or atherectomy**
Adults: I.V. loading dose of 0.4 mcg/kg/minute for 30 minutes; then continuous I.V. infusion of 0.1 mcg/kg/minute. Continue infusion through angiography and for 12 to 24 hours after PTCA or atherectomy.
Adjust-a-dose: If creatinine clearance is less than 30 ml/minute, use a loading dose of 0.2 mcg/kg/minute for 30 minutes; then continuous infusion of 0.05 mcg/kg/minute. Continue infusion through angiography and for 12 to 24 hours after PTCA or atherectomy.

I.V. ADMINISTRATION
- Dilute injections of 250 mcg/ml to same strength as 500-ml premixed vials (50 mcg/ml) as follows: Withdraw and discard 100 ml from a 500-ml bag of sterile normal saline solution or D_5W and replace this volume with 100 ml of tirofiban injection (from four 25-ml vials or two 50-ml vials); or withdraw 50 ml from a 250-ml bag of sterile normal saline solution or D_5W and replace this volume with 50 ml of tirofiban injection (from two 25-ml vials or one 50-ml vial), to yield 50 mcg/ml.
- Inspect solution for particulate matter before giving, and check for leaks by squeezing the inner bag firmly. If bag leaks or particles are visible, discard solution.
- Avoid use of noncompressible sites (such as subclavian or jugular veins).
- Heparin and tirofiban may be given through the same I.V. catheter. Tirofiban may be given through the same I.V. line as dopamine, lidocaine, potassium chloride, and famotidine.
- Discard unused solution 24 hours after the start of infusion.
- Store drug at room temperature. Protect from light.

INCOMPATIBILITIES
Diazepam.

ACTION
Reversibly binds to the GP IIb/IIIa receptor on human platelets and inhibits platelet aggregation.

Route	Onset	Peak	Duration
I.V.	Immediate	Immediate	4–6 hr

Half-life: About 2 hours.

ADVERSE REACTIONS
CNS: dizziness, fever, headache.
CV: ***bradycardia, coronary artery dissection,*** edema, vasovagal reaction.
GI: *occult bleeding,* nausea.
Hematologic: *bleeding,* ***thrombocytopenia.***
Musculoskeletal: leg pain.
Skin: sweating.
Other: *bleeding at arterial access site,* pelvic pain.

INTERACTIONS
Drug-drug. *Anticoagulants such as warfarin, aspirin, clopidogrel, dipyridam-*

ole, heparin, NSAIDs, thrombolytics, ticlopidine: May increase risk of bleeding. Monitor patient closely.
Levothyroxine, omeprazole: May increase tirofiban renal clearance. Monitor patient.

EFFECTS ON LAB TEST RESULTS
- May decrease hemoglobin level and hematocrit.
- May decrease platelet count.

CONTRAINDICATIONS & CAUTIONS
- Contraindicated in patients hypersensitive to drug or its components.
- Contraindicated in those with active internal bleeding or history of bleeding diathesis within the previous 30 days and in those with history of intracranial hemorrhage, intracranial neoplasm, arteriovenous malformation, aneurysm, thrombocytopenia after previous exposure to drug, stroke within 30 days, or hemorrhagic stroke.
- Contraindicated in those with history, symptoms, or findings suggestive of aortic dissection; severe hypertension (systolic blood pressure higher than 180 mm Hg or diastolic blood pressure higher than 110 mm Hg); acute pericarditis; major surgical procedure or severe physical trauma within previous month; or concomitant use of another parenteral GP IIb/IIIa inhibitor.
- Use cautiously in patients with increased risk of bleeding, including those with hemorrhagic retinopathy or platelet count less than 150,000/mm^3.
- Safety and effectiveness of drug haven't been studied in patients younger than age 18.
- Elderly patients have a higher risk of bleeding complications.

NURSING CONSIDERATIONS
- Monitor hemoglobin level, hematocrit, and platelet count before starting therapy, 6 hours after loading dose, and at least daily during therapy. If thrombocytopenia occurs, notify prescriber.
- Give drug with aspirin and heparin.
- Monitor patient for bleeding.
- ***Alert:*** The most common adverse effect is bleeding at the arterial access site for cardiac catheterization.
- The risk of bleeding may decrease with early sheath removal and by keeping the access site immobile. The sheath may be removed during infusion, but only after heparin has been stopped and its effects largely reversed.
- Minimize use of arterial and venous punctures, I.M. injections, urinary catheters, and nasotracheal and nasogastric tubes.
- ***Look alike–sound alike:*** Don't confuse Aggrastat with argatroban.

PATIENT TEACHING
- Explain that drug is a blood thinner used to prevent chest pain and heart attack.
- Explain that risk of serious bleeding is far outweighed by the benefits of drug.
- Instruct patient to report chest discomfort or other adverse effects immediately.
- Tell patient that frequent blood sampling may be needed to evaluate therapy.

treprostinil sodium
Remodulin

Pharmacologic class: vasodilator
Pregnancy risk category B

AVAILABLE FORMS
Injection: 1 mg/ml, 2.5 mg/ml, 5 mg/ml, 10 mg/ml in 20-ml vials

INDICATIONS & DOSAGES
➤ **To reduce symptoms caused by exercise in patients with New York Heart Association class II to IV pulmonary arterial hypertension (PAH)**
Adults: Initially, 1.25 nanogram/kg/minute by continuous subcutaneous infusion. If patient doesn't tolerate initial dose, reduce infusion rate to 0.625 nanogram/kg/minute. Increase by 1.25 nanogram/kg/minute each week for the first 4 weeks and then by no more than 2.5 nanogram/kg/minute each week for the remaining duration of infusion. Maximum infusion rate is 40 nanogram/kg/minute. May be given I.V. through a central catheter if subcutaneous route isn't tolerated.
Adjust-a-dose: In patients with mild or moderate hepatic insufficiency, initially, 0.625 nanogram/kg ideal body weight per minute, and increase cautiously.

➤To decrease the rate of clinical deterioration in patients requiring transition from epoprostenol sodium (Flolan)
Adults: Start with 10% of the starting epoprostenol dose. Decrease epoprostenol dose in 20% increments and increase treprostinil in 20% increments, always maintaining a total dose of 110% of epoprostenol starting dose. Once epoprostenol is at 20% of starting dose and treprostinil is at 90%, decrease epoprostenol to 5% and increase treprostinil to 110%. Finally, stop epoprostenol and maintain treprostinil dose at 110% of epoprostenol starting dose plus an additional 5% to 10% p.r.n. Change rate based on individual patient response. Treat worsening of PAH symptoms with increases in treprostinil dose. Treat adverse effects associated with prostacyclin and prostacyclin analogs with decreases in epoprostenol dose.

I.V. ADMINISTRATION

- Give I.V. only if subcutaneous route isn't tolerated.
- Dilute with either sterile water for injection or normal saline solution.
- Inspect for particulate matter and discoloration before giving.
- Give by continuous infusion through a surgically placed indwelling central venous catheter, using an infusion pump designed for I.V. drug delivery.
- To avoid potential interruptions in drug delivery, make sure patient has immediate access to a backup infusion pump and infusion sets.
- Diluted drug is stable at room temperature for up to 48 hours.

INCOMPATIBILITIES

Other I.V. drugs.

ACTION

Directly vasodilates pulmonary and systemic arterial vascular beds and inhibits platelet aggregation.

Route	Onset	Peak	Duration
I.V.	Unknown	Unknown	Unknown
SubQ	Unknown	Unknown	Unknown

Half-life: 2 to 4 hours.

ADVERSE REACTIONS

CNS: dizziness, fatigue, *headache.*
CV: *vasodilation,* ***right ventricular heart failure,*** chest pain, edema, hypotension.
GI: *diarrhea, nausea.*
Musculoskeletal: *jaw pain.*
Respiratory: dyspnea.
Skin: *infusion site pain, infusion site reaction, rash,* pallor, pruritus.

INTERACTIONS

Drug-drug. *Antihypertensives, diuretics, vasodilators:* May exacerbate reduction in blood pressure. Monitor blood pressure.
Anticoagulants: May increase risk of bleeding. Monitor patient closely for bleeding.

EFFECTS ON LAB TEST RESULTS

None reported.

CONTRAINDICATIONS & CAUTIONS

- Contraindicated in patients hypersensitive to drug or structurally related compounds.
- Use cautiously in patients with hepatic or renal impairment and in elderly patients.

NURSING CONSIDERATIONS

- Assess the patient's ability to accept, place, and care for a subcutaneous catheter and to use an infusion pump.
- Preferred route is continuous subcutaneous infusion via a self-inserted subcutaneous catheter, using an infusion pump designed for subcutaneous drug delivery. The infusion pump should be small and lightweight; adjustable to about 0.002 ml/hour; have occlusion/no delivery, low-battery, programming-error, and motor-malfunction alarms; have delivery accuracy of ± 6% or better; and be positive-pressure driven. The reservoir should be made of polyvinyl chloride, polypropylene, or glass.
- During use, a single reservoir syringe can be given for up to 72 hours at 98.6° F (37° C).
- Don't use a single vial longer than 14 days after the initial introduction to the vial.
- Start treatment in setting where adequate monitoring and emergency care are available.

- Increase dose if patient doesn't improve or symptoms worsen, and decrease if drug effects become excessive or unacceptable infusion site symptoms develop.
- Avoid abrupt withdrawal or sudden large dose reductions because PAH symptoms may worsen.

PATIENT TEACHING

- Inform patient that he'll need to continue therapy for a prolonged period, possibly years.
- Tell patient that subsequent disease management may require I.V. therapy.
- Inform patient that many side effects, such as labored breathing, fatigue, and chest pain, may be related to the underlying disease.
- Tell patient that the most common local reactions are pain, redness, tissue hardening, and rash at the infusion site.
- Tell patient that a backup infusion pump must be available to avoid interruption in therapy.

24

Nonopioid analgesics and antipyretics

acetaminophen
aspirin
diflunisal

acetaminophen (APAP, paracetamol)

Abenol† ◊, Acephen, Aceta ◊, Acetaminophen ◊, Actamin ◊, Aminofen ◊, Apacet ◊, Apo-Acetaminophen† ◊, Atasol† ◊, Banesin ◊, Dapa ◊, Dymadon‡ ◊, Dymadon P‡ ◊, Exdol†, Feverall ◊, Genapap ◊, Genebs ◊, Liquiprin ◊, Neopap ◊, Oraphen-PD ◊, Panadol ◊, Panamax‡ ◊, Paralgin‡ ◊, Redutemp ◊, Robigesic† ◊, Rounox† ◊, Snaplets-FR ◊, St. Joseph Aspirin-Free Fever Reducer for Children ◊, Suppap ◊, Tapanol ◊, Tempra ◊, Tylenol ◊, Valorin ◊

Pharmacologic class: para-aminophenol derivative
Pregnancy risk category B

AVAILABLE FORMS

Caplets: 160 mg ◊, 500 mg ◊
Caplets (extended-release): 650 mg ◊
Capsules: 325 mg ◊, 500 mg ◊
Elixir: 80 mg/2.5 ml, 80 mg/5 ml, 120 mg/5 ml, 160 mg/5 ml* ◊, 325 mg/5 ml* ◊
Gelcaps: 500 mg ◊
Oral liquid: 160 mg/5 ml ◊, 500 mg/15 ml ◊
Oral solution: 48 mg/ml ◊, 100 mg/ml ◊
Oral suspension: 80 mg/0.8 ml ◊, 120 mg/5 ml‡, 160 mg/5 ml ◊
Oral syrup: 16 mg/ml ◊
Sprinkles: 80 mg/capsule ◊, 160 mg/capsule ◊
Suppositories: 80 mg ◊, 120 mg ◊, 125 mg ◊, 300 mg ◊, 325 mg ◊, 650 mg ◊
Tablets: 160 mg ◊, 325 mg ◊, 500 mg ◊, 650 mg ◊
Tablets (chewable): 80 mg ◊

INDICATIONS & DOSAGES

➤Mild pain or fever

P.O.

Adults: 325 to 650 mg P.O. q 4 to 6 hours; or 1 g P.O. t.i.d. or q.i.d., p.r.n. Or, two extended-release caplets P.O. q 8 hours. Maximum, 4 g daily. For long-term therapy, don't exceed 2.6 g daily unless prescribed and monitored closely by health care provider.
Children older than age 14: 650 mg P.O. q 4 to 6 hours, p.r.n.
Children ages 12 to 14: 640 mg P.O. q 4 to 6 hours, p.r.n.
Children age 11: 480 mg P.O. q 4 to 6 hours, p.r.n.
Children ages 9 to 10: 400 mg P.O. q 4 to 6 hours, p.r.n.
Children ages 6 to 8: 320 mg P.O. q 4 to 6 hours, p.r.n.
Children ages 4 to 5: 240 mg P.O. q 4 to 6 hours, p.r.n.
Children ages 2 to 3: 160 mg P.O. q 4 to 6 hours, p.r.n.
Children ages 12 to 23 months: 120 mg P.O. q 4 to 6 hours, p.r.n.
Children ages 4 to 11 months: 80 mg P.O. q 4 to 6 hours, p.r.n.
Children up to age 3 months: 40 mg P.O. q 4 to 6 hours, p.r.n. Or, 10 to 15 mg/kg/dose q 4 hours, p.r.n. Don't exceed five doses in 24 hours.

P.R.

Adults: 650 mg P.R. q 4 to 6 hours, p.r.n. Maximum, 4 g daily. For long-term therapy, don't exceed 2.6 g daily unless prescribed and monitored closely by health care provider.
Children ages 6 to 12: 325 mg P.R. q 4 to 6 hours, p.r.n.
Children ages 3 to 6: 120 to 125 mg P.R. q 4 to 6 hours, p.r.n.
Children ages 1 to 3: 80 mg P.R. q 4 to 6 hours, p.r.n.
Children ages 3 months to 11 months: 80 mg P.R. q 6 hours, p.r.n.

ACTION

Thought to produce analgesia by blocking pain impulses by inhibiting synthesis of prostaglandin in the CNS or of other substances that sensitize pain receptors to stimulation. The drug may relieve fever through central action in the hypothalamic heat-regulating center.

Route	Onset	Peak	Duration
P.O., P.R.	Unknown	½–2 hr	3–4 hr

Half-life: 1 to 4 hours.

ADVERSE REACTIONS

Hematologic: hemolytic anemia, ***leukopenia, neutropenia, pancytopenia.***
Hepatic: jaundice.
Metabolic: ***hypoglycemia.***
Skin: rash, urticaria.

INTERACTIONS

Drug-drug. *Barbiturates, carbamazepine, hydantoins, rifampin, sulfinpyrazone:* High doses or long-term use of these drugs may reduce therapeutic effects and enhance hepatotoxic effects of acetaminophen. Avoid using together.
Lamotrigine: May decrease lamotrigine level. Monitor patient for therapeutic effects.
Warfarin: May increase hypoprothrombinemic effects with long-term use with high doses of acetaminophen. Monitor INR closely.
Zidovudine: May decrease zidovudine effect. Monitor patient closely.
Drug-herb. *Watercress:* May inhibit oxidative metabolism of acetaminophen. Discourage use together.
Drug-food. *Caffeine:* May enhance analgesic effects of acetaminophen. Products may combine caffeine and acetaminophen for therapeutic advantage.
Drug-lifestyle. *Alcohol use:* May increase risk of hepatic damage. Discourage use together.

EFFECTS ON LAB TEST RESULTS

- May decrease glucose and hemoglobin levels and hematocrit.
- May decrease neutrophil, WBC, RBC, and platelet counts.
- May cause false-positive test result for urinary 5-hydroxyindoleacetic acid. May falsely decrease glucose level in home monitoring systems.

CONTRAINDICATIONS & CAUTIONS

- Contraindicated in patients hypersensitive to drug.
- Use cautiously in patients with long-term alcohol use because therapeutic doses cause hepatotoxicity in these patients.

NURSING CONSIDERATIONS

- ***Alert:*** Many OTC and prescription products contain acetaminophen; be aware of this when calculating total daily dose.
- Use liquid form for children and patients who have difficulty swallowing.
- In children, don't exceed five doses in 24 hours.

PATIENT TEACHING

- Tell parents to consult prescriber before giving drug to children younger than age 2.
- Advise parents that drug is only for short-term use; urge them to consult prescriber if giving to children for longer than 5 days or adults for longer than 10 days.
- ***Alert:*** Advise patient or caregiver that many OTC products contain acetaminophen and should be counted when calculating total daily dose.
- Tell patient not to use for marked fever (temperature higher than 103.1° F [39.5° C]), fever persisting longer than 3 days, or recurrent fever unless directed by prescriber.
- ***Alert:*** Warn patient that high doses or unsupervised long-term use can cause liver damage. Excessive alcohol use may increase the risk of liver damage. Caution long-term alcoholics to limit drug to 2 g/day or less.
- Tell breast-feeding woman that drug appears in breast milk in low levels (less than 1% of dose). Drug may be used safely if therapy is short-term and doesn't exceed recommended doses.

aspirin (acetylsalicylic acid)

Artria S.R ◇, ASA ◇, Aspergum ◇, Aspro‡, Bayer Aspirin ◇, Bex‡, Coryphen† ◇, Easprin ◇, Ecotrin ◇, Empirin ◇, Entrophen† ◇, Halfprin, Norwich Extra-Strength ◇, Novasen† ◇, Solprin‡, Vincent's Powders‡, ZORprin ◇

Pharmacologic class: salicylate
Pregnancy risk category D

AVAILABLE FORMS

Chewing gum: 227.5 mg ◇
Suppositories: 120 mg ◇, 200 mg ◇, 300 mg ◇, 600 mg ◇
Tablets: 325 mg ◇, 500 mg ◇
Tablets (chewable): 81 mg ◇
Tablets (controlled-release): 800 mg
Tablets (enteric-coated): 81 mg ◇, 165 mg ◇, 325 mg ◇, 500 mg ◇, 650 mg ◇, 975 mg
Tablets (extended-release): 650 mg ◇

INDICATIONS & DOSAGES

➤Rheumatoid arthritis, osteoarthritis, or other polyarthritic or inflammatory conditions
Adults: Initially, 2.4 to 3.6 g P.O. daily in divided doses. Maintenance dosage is 3.2 to 6 g P.O. daily in divided doses.

➤Juvenile rheumatoid arthritis
Children who weigh more than 25 kg (55 lb): 2.4 to 3.6 g P.O. daily in divided doses.
Children who weigh 25 kg or less: 60 to 130 mg/kg daily P.O. in divided doses. Increase by 10 mg/kg daily at no more than weekly intervals. Maintenance dosages usually range from 80 to 100 mg/kg daily; up to 130 mg/kg daily.

➤Mild pain or fever
Adults and children older than age 11: 325 to 650 mg P.O. or P.R. q 4 hours, p.r.n.
Children ages 2 to 11: 10 to 15 mg/kg/dose P.O. or P.R. q 4 hours up to 80 mg/kg daily.

➤To prevent thrombosis
Adults: 1.3 g P.O. daily, divided b.i.d. to q.i.d.

➤To reduce risk of MI in patients with previous MI or unstable angina
Adults: 75 to 325 mg P.O. daily.

➤Kawasaki syndrome (mucocutaneous lymph node syndrome)
Children: 80 to 100 mg/kg P.O. daily, divided q.i.d. with immune globulin I.V. After the fever subsides, reduce dosage to 3 to 5 mg/kg once daily. Aspirin therapy usually continues for 6 to 8 weeks.

➤Acute rheumatic fever
Adults: 5 to 8 g P.O. daily.
Children: 100 mg/kg daily P.O. for 2 weeks; then 75 mg/kg daily P.O. for 4 to 6 weeks.

➤To reduce risk of recurrent transient ischemic attacks and stroke or death in patients at risk
Adults: 50 to 325 mg P.O. daily.

➤Acute ischemic stroke
Adults: 160 to 325 mg P.O. daily, started within 48 hours of stroke onset and continued for up to 2 to 4 weeks.

➤Acute pericarditis after MI
Adults: 160 to 325 mg P.O. daily. Higher doses (650 mg P.O. q 4 to 6 hours) may be needed.

ACTION

Thought to produce analgesia by inhibiting prostaglandin and other substances that sensitize pain receptors. Drug may relieve fever by acting on the hypothalamic heat-regulating center and may exert its anti-inflammatory effect by inhibiting prostaglandin and other substances. In low doses, drug also appears to interfere with clotting by keeping a platelet-aggregating substance from forming.

Route	Onset	Peak	Duration
P.O. (buffered)	5–30 min	1–2 hr	1–4 hr
P.O. (enteric-coated)	5–30 min	Variable	1-4 hr
P.O. (extended-release)	5–30 min	1–4 hr	1–4 hr
P.O. (solution)	5–30 min	15–40 min	1–4 hr
P.O. (tablet)	5–30 min	25–40 min	1–4 hr
P.R.	Unknown	3–4 hr	Unknown

Half-life: 15 to 20 minutes.

ADVERSE REACTIONS

EENT: *tinnitus, hearing loss.*

GI: *nausea,* ***GI bleeding,*** dyspepsia, GI distress, occult bleeding.
Hematologic: *prolonged bleeding time,* ***leukopenia, thrombocytopenia.***
Hepatic: ***hepatitis.***
Skin: *rash,* bruising, urticaria.
Other: ***angioedema, Reye syndrome,*** hypersensitivity reactions.

INTERACTIONS

Drug-drug. *ACE inhibitors:* May decrease antihypertensive effects. Monitor blood pressure closely.
Ammonium chloride and other urine acidifiers: May increase levels of aspirin products. Watch for aspirin toxicity.
Antacids in high doses and other urine alkalinizers: May decrease levels of aspirin products. Watch for decreased aspirin effect.
Anticoagulants: May increase risk of bleeding. Use with extreme caution if must be used together.
Beta blockers: May decrease antihypertensive effect. Avoid long-term aspirin use if patient is taking antihypertensives.
Corticosteroids: May enhance salicylate elimination and decrease drug level. Watch for decreased aspirin effect.
Heparin: May increase risk of bleeding. Monitor coagulation studies and patient closely if used together.
Ibuprofen, other NSAIDs: May negate the anti-platelet effect of low-dose aspirin therapy. Patients using immediate-release aspirin (not enteric coated) should take ibuprofen at least 30 minutes after aspirin, or more than 8 hours before aspirin. Occasional use of ibuprofen is unlikely to have a negative impact.
Methotrexate: May increase risk of methotrexate toxicity. Avoid using together.
Nizatidine: May increase risk of salicylate toxicity in patients receiving high doses of aspirin. Monitor patient closely.
Oral antidiabetics: May increase hypoglycemic effect. Monitor patient closely.
Probenecid, sulfinpyrazone: May decrease uricosuric effect. Avoid using together.
Valproic acid: May increase valproic acid level. Avoid using together.
Drug-herb. *Dong quai, feverfew, ginkgo, horse chestnut, kelpware, red clover:* May increase risk of bleeding. Monitor patient closely for increased effects. Discourage use together.
White willow: May increase risk of adverse effects. Discourage use together.
Drug-food. *Caffeine:* May increase drug absorption . Watch for increased effects.
Drug-lifestyle. *Alcohol use:* May increase risk of GI bleeding. Discourage use together.

EFFECTS ON LAB TEST RESULTS

- May increase liver function test values. May decrease platelet and WBC counts.
- May falsely increase protein-bound iodine level. May interfere with urine glucose analysis with Diastix, Chemstrip uG, Clinitest, and Benedict solution; with urinary 5-hydroxyindoleacetic acid and vanillylmandelic acid tests; and with Gerhardt test for urine acetoacetic acid.

CONTRAINDICATIONS & CAUTIONS

- Contraindicated in patients hypersensitive to drug and in those with NSAID-induced sensitivity reactions, G6PD deficiency, or bleeding disorders, such as hemophilia, von Willebrand disease, or telangiectasia.
- Use cautiously in patients with GI lesions, impaired renal function, hypoprothrombinemia, vitamin K deficiency, thrombocytopenia, thrombotic thrombocytopenic purpura, or severe hepatic impairment.
- ***Alert:*** Oral and rectal OTC products containing aspirin and nonaspirin salicylates shouldn't be given to children or teenagers who have or are recovering from chickenpox or flulike symptoms because of the risk of Reye syndrome.

NURSING CONSIDERATIONS

- For inflammatory conditions, rheumatic fever, and thrombosis, give aspirin on a schedule rather than as needed.
- Because enteric-coated and sustained-release tablets are slowly absorbed, they aren't suitable for rapid relief of acute pain, fever, or inflammation. They cause less GI bleeding and may be better suited for long-term therapy, such as for arthritis.
- For patient with swallowing difficulties, crush non–enteric-coated aspirin and dissolve in soft food or liquid. Give liquid

immediately after mixing because drug will break down rapidly.
• For patients who can't tolerate oral drugs, ask prescriber about using aspirin rectal suppositories. Watch for rectal mucosal irritation or bleeding.
• Febrile, dehydrated children can develop toxicity rapidly.
• Monitor elderly patients closely because they may be more susceptible to aspirin's toxic effects.
• Monitor salicylate level. Therapeutic salicylate level for arthritis is 150 to 300 mcg/ml. Tinnitus may occur at levels above 200 mcg/ml, but this isn't a reliable indicator of toxicity, especially in very young patients and those older than age 60. With long-term therapy, severe toxic effects may occur with levels exceeding 400 mcg/ml.
• During prolonged therapy, assess hematocrit, hemoglobin level, PT, INR, and renal function periodically.
• Drug irreversibly inhibits platelet aggregation. Stop drug 5 to 7 days before elective surgery to allow time for production and release of new platelets.
• Monitor patient for hypersensitivity reactions, such as anaphylaxis and asthma.
• ***Look alike–sound alike:*** Don't confuse aspirin with Asendin or Afrin.

PATIENT TEACHING
• Tell patient who is allergic to tartrazine to avoid aspirin.
• Advise patient on a low-salt diet that 1 tablet of buffered aspirin contains 553 mg of sodium.
• Advise patient to take drug with food, milk, antacid, or large glass of water to reduce GI reactions.
• Tell patient not to crush or chew sustained-release or enteric-coated forms but to swallow them whole.
• Instruct patient to discard aspirin tablets that have a strong vinegar-like odor.
• Tell patient to consult prescriber if giving drug to children for longer than 5 days or adults for longer than 10 days.
• Advise patient receiving prolonged treatment with large doses of aspirin to watch for small, round, red pinprick spots, bleeding gums, and signs of GI bleeding, and to drink plenty of fluids. Encourage use of a soft-bristled toothbrush.
• Because of the many drug interactions with aspirin, warn patient taking prescription drugs to check with prescriber or pharmacist before taking aspirin or OTC products containing aspirin.
• Urge pregnant woman to avoid aspirin during last trimester of pregnancy unless specifically directed by prescriber.
• Drug is a leading cause of poisoning in children. Caution parents to keep drug out of reach of children. Encourage use of child-resistant containers.

diflunisal
Dolobid

Pharmacologic class: salicylate; NSAID
Pregnancy risk category C

AVAILABLE FORMS
Tablets: 250 mg, 500 mg

INDICATIONS & DOSAGES
➤ **Osteoarthritis, rheumatoid arthritis**
Adults: 500 to 1,000 mg P.O. daily in two divided doses, usually q 12 hours. Maximum, 1,500 mg daily.
Elderly patients: In patients older than age 65, one-half usual adult dosage.
➤ **Mild to moderate pain**
Adults: 1 g P.O., then 500 mg q 8 to 12 hours. A lower dosage of 500 mg P.O., then 250 mg q 8 to 12 hours may be appropriate.

ACTION
Unknown. Probably related to inhibition of prostaglandin synthesis.

Route	Onset	Peak	Duration
P.O.	1 hr	2–3 hr	8–12 hr

Half-life: 8 to 12 hours.

ADVERSE REACTIONS
CNS: dizziness, fatigue, headache, insomnia, somnolence.
EENT: tinnitus.
GI: constipation, diarrhea, dyspepsia, flatulence, GI pain, nausea, stomatitis, vomiting.

GU: ***interstitial nephritis,*** hematuria, renal impairment.
Skin: ***erythema multiforme, Stevens-Johnson syndrome,*** pruritus, rash, sweating.

INTERACTIONS

Drug-drug. *Acetaminophen, hydrochlorothiazide, indomethacin:* May substantially increase levels of these drugs, increasing risk of toxicity. Avoid using together.
Antacids, aspirin: May decrease diflunisal level. Monitor patient for reduced therapeutic effect.
Anticoagulants, thrombolytics: May enhance effects of these drugs. Use together cautiously.
Cyclosporine: May enhance the nephrotoxicity of cyclosporine. Avoid using together.
Methotrexate: May enhance the toxicity of methotrexate. Avoid using together.
Sulindac: May decrease level of sulindac's metabolite. Monitor patient for reduced effect.

EFFECTS ON LAB TEST RESULTS

- May falsely elevate salicylate level.

CONTRAINDICATIONS & CAUTIONS

- Contraindicated in patients hypersensitive to drug and in those for whom acute asthmatic attacks, urticaria, or rhinitis are precipitated by aspirin or other NSAIDs.
- Use cautiously in patients with GI bleeding, history of peptic ulcer disease, renal impairment, compromised cardiac function, hypertension, or other conditions predisposing patient to fluid retention.

NURSING CONSIDERATIONS

- ***Alert:*** The Centers for Disease Control and Prevention recommend not giving salicylates to children and teenagers with chickenpox or flulike illness because of the link to Reye's syndrome.

PATIENT TEACHING

- Advise patient to take with water, milk, or meals.
- Tell patient that tablets must be swallowed whole.
- Instruct patient to avoid aspirin or acetaminophen while using diflunisal.
- Inform breast-feeding woman that drug appears in breast milk and that she should stop either breast-feeding or taking drug.

25

Nonsteroidal anti-inflammatory drugs

celecoxib
diclofenac potassium
diclofenac sodium
etodolac
ibuprofen
indomethacin
indomethacin sodium trihydrate
ketoprofen
ketorolac tromethamine
meloxicam
nabumetone
naproxen
naproxen sodium
piroxicam
sulindac

celecoxib
Celebrex✐

Pharmacologic class:
cyclooxygenase-2 (COX-2) inhibitor
Pregnancy risk category C; D in 3rd trimester

AVAILABLE FORMS
Capsules: 100 mg, 200 mg

INDICATIONS & DOSAGES
➤ **To relieve signs and symptoms of osteoarthritis**
Adults: 200 mg P.O. daily as a single dose or divided equally b.i.d.
➤ **To relieve signs and symptoms of rheumatoid arthritis**
Adults: 100 to 200 mg P.O. b.i.d.
➤ **To relieve signs and symptoms of ankylosing spondylitis**
Adults: 200 mg P.O. once daily or divided b.i.d. If no response after 6 weeks, may increase dose to 400 mg daily. If no response after 6 more weeks, consider other treatment.
➤ **Adjunctive treatment for familial adenomatous polyposis to reduce the number of adenomatous colorectal polyps**
Adults: 400 mg P.O. b.i.d. with food, for up to 6 months.
Elderly patients: Start at lowest dosage.
➤ **Acute pain and primary dysmenorrhea**
Adults: 400 mg P.O., initially, followed by another 200-mg dose if needed. On subsequent days, 200 mg P.O. b.i.d., p.r.n.
Elderly patients: Start at lowest dosage.
Adjust-a-dose: For patients who weigh less than 50 kg (110 lb), start at lowest dosage. For patients with Child-Pugh class II hepatic impairment, start with reduced dosage.

ACTION
Thought to inhibit prostaglandin synthesis, impeding cyclooxygenase-2 (COX-2), to produce anti-inflammatory, analgesic, and antipyretic effects.

Route	Onset	Peak	Duration
P.O.	Unknown	3 hr	Unknown

Half-life: 11 hours.

ADVERSE REACTIONS
CNS: *headache,* dizziness, insomnia.
CV: hypertension, peripheral edema.
EENT: pharyngitis, rhinitis, sinusitis.
GI: abdominal pain, diarrhea, dyspepsia, flatulence, nausea.
Metabolic: hyperchloremia.
Musculoskeletal: back pain.
Respiratory: upper respiratory tract infection.
Skin: ***erythema multiforme, exfoliative dermatitis, Stevens-Johnson syndrome, toxic epidermal necrolysis,*** rash.
Other: accidental injury.

INTERACTIONS
Drug-drug. *ACE inhibitors:* May decrease antihypertensive effects. Monitor patient's blood pressure.
Antacids containing aluminum or magnesium: May decrease celecoxib level. Separate doses.
Aspirin: May increase risk of ulcers; low aspirin dosages can be used safely to reduce the risk of CV events. Monitor patient for signs and symptoms of GI bleeding.

Fluconazole: May increase celecoxib level. Reduce dosage of celecoxib to minimal effective dose.
Furosemide, thiazides: May reduce sodium excretion caused by diuretics, leading to sodium retention. Monitor patient for swelling and increased blood pressure.
Lithium: May increase lithium level. Monitor lithium level closely during treatment.
Warfarin: May increase PT and bleeding complications. Monitor PT and INR, and check for signs and symptoms of bleeding.
Drug-herb. *Dong quai, feverfew, garlic, ginger, horse chestnut, red clover:* May increase risk of bleeding. Discourage use together.
White willow: Herb and drug contain similar components. Discourage use together.
Drug-lifestyle. *Long-term alcohol use, smoking:* May cause GI irritation or bleeding. Check for signs and symptoms of bleeding.

EFFECTS ON LAB TEST RESULTS

- May increase ALT, AST, BUN, and chloride levels. May decrease phosphate level.

CONTRAINDICATIONS & CAUTIONS

- Contraindicated in patients hypersensitive to drug, sulfonamides, aspirin, or other NSAIDs.
- Contraindicated in those with severe hepatic impairment and in the treatment of perioperative pain after coronary artery bypass graft surgery.
- Avoid use in the third trimester of pregnancy.
- Use cautiously in patients with history of ulcers or GI bleeding, advanced renal disease, dehydration, anemia, symptomatic liver disease, hypertension, edema, heart failure, or asthma and in poor CYP2C9 metabolizers.
- Use cautiously in elderly or debilitated patients.

NURSING CONSIDERATIONS

- ***Alert:*** Patients allergic to or with a history of anaphylactic reactions to sulfonamides, aspirin, or other NSAIDs may be allergic to this drug.
- Patient with history of ulcers or GI bleeding is at higher risk for GI bleeding while taking NSAIDs such as celecoxib. Other risk factors for GI bleeding include treatment with corticosteroids or anticoagulants, longer duration of NSAID treatment, smoking, alcoholism, older age, and poor overall health.
- ***Alert:*** NSAIDs may increase the risk of serious thrombotic events, MI, or stroke. The risk may be greater with longer use or in patients with CV disease or risk factors for CV disease.
- Although drug may be used with low aspirin dosages, the combination may increase risk of GI bleeding.
- Watch for signs and symptoms of overt and occult bleeding.
- Drug can cause fluid retention; monitor patient with hypertension, edema, or heart failure.
- Assess patient for CV risk factors before therapy.
- Drug may be hepatotoxic; watch for signs and symptoms of liver toxicity.
- Before starting drug therapy, rehydrate dehydrated patient.
- Drug can be given without regard to meals, but food may decrease GI upset.
- ***Look alike–sound alike:*** Don't confuse Celebrex with Cerebyx or Celexa.

PATIENT TEACHING

- Tell patient to report history of allergic reactions to sulfonamides, aspirin, or other NSAIDs before therapy.
- Instruct patient to promptly report signs of GI bleeding such as blood in vomit, urine, or stool; or black, tarry stools.
- ***Alert:*** Advise patient to immediately report rash, unexplained weight gain, or swelling.
- Tell woman to notify prescriber if she becomes pregnant or is planning to become pregnant during drug therapy.
- Instruct patient to take drug with food if stomach upset occurs.
- Tell patient that drug may harm the liver. Advise patient to stop therapy and notify prescriber immediately if he experiences signs and symptoms of liver toxicity, including nausea, fatigue, lethargy, itching, yellowing of skin or eyes, right upper quadrant tenderness, and flulike syndrome.

• Inform patient that it may take several days before he feels consistent pain relief.
• Advise patient that using OTC NSAIDs with celecoxib may increase the risk of GI toxicity.

diclofenac potassium
Cataflam

diclofenac sodium
Fenac‡, Voltaren, Voltaren-XR, Voltaren Rapide†, Voltaren SR†

Pharmacologic class: NSAID
Pregnancy risk category B; D in 3rd trimester

AVAILABLE FORMS
diclofenac potassium
Tablets: 50 mg
diclofenac sodium
Suppositories: 50 mg†, 100 mg†
Tablets (delayed-release): 25 mg, 50 mg, 75 mg
Tablets (extended-release): 100 mg

INDICATIONS & DOSAGES
➤ Ankylosing spondylitis
Adults: 25 mg delayed-release diclofenac sodium P.O. q.i.d.; may add another 25-mg dose at bedtime.
➤ Osteoarthritis
Adults: 50 mg P.O. b.i.d. or t.i.d., or 75 mg P.O. b.i.d. diclofenac potassium or delayed-release diclofenac sodium only. Or, 100 mg P.O. daily or b.i.d. extended-release diclofenac sodium only.
➤ Rheumatoid arthritis
Adults: 50 mg P.O. t.i.d. or q.i.d., or 75 mg P.O. b.i.d. diclofenac potassium or delayed-release diclofenac sodium only. Or, 100 mg P.O. daily or b.i.d. extended-release diclofenac sodium only, or 50 to 100 mg diclofenac sodium P.R. h.s. as substitute for last P.O. dose of the day. Don't exceed 150 mg daily.
➤ Analgesia, primary dysmenorrhea
Adults: 50 mg diclofenac potassium P.O. t.i.d. For some patients, the first dose on the first day may be 100 mg, followed by 50 mg for the second and third doses; maximum dose for first day is 200 mg. Don't exceed 150 mg daily after the first day.

ACTION
May inhibit prostaglandin synthesis, to produce anti-inflammatory, analgesic, and antipyretic effects.

Route	Onset	Peak	Duration
P.O. (delayed-release)	30 min	2–3 hr	8 hr
P.O. (extended-release)	Unknown	5–6 hr	Unknown
P.O., P.R.	10 min	1 hr	8 hr

Half-life: 1 to 2 hours.

ADVERSE REACTIONS
CNS: ***aseptic meningitis,*** anxiety, depression, dizziness, drowsiness, headache, insomnia, irritability.
CV: ***heart failure,*** edema, fluid retention, hypertension.
EENT: ***laryngeal edema,*** blurred vision, epistaxis, eye pain, night blindness, reversible hearing loss, swelling of the lips and tongue, tinnitus.
GI: abdominal distention, abdominal pain or cramps, bleeding, constipation, diarrhea, flatulence, indigestion, melena, nausea, peptic ulceration, taste disorder, bloody diarrhea, appetite change, colitis.
GU: *nephrotic syndrome,* ***acute renal failure,*** fluid retention, interstitial nephritis, oliguria, papillary necrosis, proteinuria.
Hepatic: jaundice, ***hepatitis, hepatotoxicity.***
Metabolic: ***hypoglycemia,*** hyperglycemia.
Musculoskeletal: back, leg or joint pain.
Respiratory: asthma.
Skin: ***Stevens-Johnson syndrome,*** allergic purpura, alopecia, bullous eruption, dermatitis, eczema, photosensitivity reactions, pruritus, rash, urticaria.
Other: ***anaphylactoid reactions, anaphylaxis, angioedema.***

INTERACTIONS
Drug-drug. *Anticoagulants, including warfarin:* May cause bleeding. Monitor patient closely.

Aspirin: May decrease effectiveness of diclofenac and increase GI toxicity. Avoid using together.
Beta blockers: May decrease antihypertensive effects. Monitor patient closely.
Cyclosporine, digoxin, lithium, methotrexate: May reduce renal clearance of these drugs and increase risk of toxicity. Monitor patient closely.
Diuretics: May decrease effectiveness of diuretics. Avoid using together.
Insulin, oral antidiabetics: May alter requirements for antidiabetics. Monitor patient closely.
Potassium-sparing diuretics: May enhance retention and increase level of potassium. Monitor potassium level.
Drug-herb. *Dong quai, feverfew, garlic, ginger, horse chestnut, red clover:* May cause bleeding based on the known effects or components. Discourage use together.
White willow: Herb and drug contain similar components. Discourage use together.
Drug-lifestyle. *Sun exposure:* May cause photosensitivity reactions. Advise patient to avoid excessive sunlight exposure.

EFFECTS ON LAB TEST RESULTS

- May increase ALT, AST, bilirubin, BUN, and creatinine levels. May increase or decrease glucose level.

CONTRAINDICATIONS & CAUTIONS

- Contraindicated in patients hypersensitive to drug and in those with hepatic porphyria or history of asthma, urticaria, or other allergic reactions after taking aspirin or other NSAIDs.
- Avoid using during late pregnancy or while breast-feeding.
- Use cautiously in patients with history of peptic ulcer disease, hepatic dysfunction, cardiac disease, hypertension, fluid retention, or impaired renal function.

NURSING CONSIDERATIONS

- Because NSAIDs impair the synthesis of renal prostaglandins, they can decrease renal blood flow and lead to reversible renal impairment, especially in patients with renal or heart failure or liver dysfunction, in elderly patients, and in those taking diuretics. Monitor these patients closely.
- Liver function test values may increase during therapy. Monitor transaminase, especially ALT, levels periodically in patients undergoing long-term therapy. Make first transaminase measurement no later than 8 weeks after therapy begins.
- Because of their antipyretic and anti-inflammatory actions, NSAIDs may mask the signs and symptoms of infection.
- Serious GI toxicity, including peptic ulcers and bleeding, can occur in patient taking NSAIDs, despite lack of symptoms.
- ***Look alike–sound alike:*** Don't confuse diclofenac with Diflucan.

PATIENT TEACHING

- Tell patient to take drug with milk, meals, or antacids to minimize GI distress.
- Instruct patient not to crush, break, or chew enteric-coated tablets.
- Advise patient not to take this drug with any other diclofenac-containing products (such as Arthrotec).
- Teach patient signs and symptoms of GI bleeding, including blood in vomit, urine, or stool; coffee-ground vomit; and black, tarry stool. Tell him to notify prescriber immediately if any of these occurs.
- Teach patient the signs and symptoms of damage to the liver, including nausea, fatigue, lethargy, itching, yellowed skin or eyes, right upper quadrant tenderness, and flulike symptoms. Tell patient to contact prescriber immediately if these symptoms occur.
- Advise patient to avoid consuming alcohol or aspirin during drug therapy.
- Tell patient to wear sunscreen or protective clothing because drug may cause sensitivity to sunlight.
- Warn patient to avoid hazardous activities that require alertness until it is known whether the drug causes CNS symptoms.
- Tell pregnant woman to avoid use of drug during last trimester.
- Advise patient that use of OTC NSAIDs and diclofenac may increase the risk of GI toxicity.

etodolac

Lodine, Lodine XL

Pharmacologic class: NSAID
Pregnancy risk category C; D in 3rd trimester

AVAILABLE FORMS

Capsules: 200 mg, 300 mg
Tablets: 400 mg, 500 mg
Tablets (extended-release): 400 mg, 500 mg, 600 mg

INDICATIONS & DOSAGES

➤ **Acute pain**
Adults: 200 to 400 mg P.O. q 6 to 8 hours, p.r.n., not to exceed 1,200 mg daily. In patients who weigh 60 kg (132 lb) or less, don't exceed total daily dose of 20 mg/kg.
➤ **Short- and long-term management of osteoarthritis and rheumatoid arthritis**
Adults: 600 to 1,000 mg P.O. daily, divided into two or three doses. Maximum daily dose is 1,200 mg. For extended-release tablets, 400 to 1,000 mg P.O. daily. Maximum daily dose is 1,200 mg.

ACTION

Unknown. Produces anti-inflammatory, analgesic, and antipyretic effects, possibly by inhibiting prostaglandin synthesis.

Route	Onset	Peak	Duration
P.O.	30 min	1–2 hr	4–12 hr
P.O. (extended-release)	Unknown	3–12 hr	6–12 hr

Half-life: 7¼ hours.

ADVERSE REACTIONS

CNS: asthenia, malaise, dizziness, depression, drowsiness, nervousness, insomnia, syncope, fever.
CV: hypertension, ***heart failure,*** flushing, palpitations, edema, fluid retention.
EENT: blurred vision, tinnitus, photophobia.
GI: *dyspepsia,* flatulence, abdominal pain, diarrhea, nausea, constipation, gastritis, melena, vomiting, anorexia, ***peptic ulceration with or without GI bleeding or perforation,*** ulcerative stomatitis, thirst, dry mouth.
GU: dysuria, urinary frequency, ***renal failure.***
Hematologic: anemia, ***leukopenia,*** hemolytic anemia.
Hepatic: ***hepatitis.***
Metabolic: weight gain.
Respiratory: asthma.
Skin: pruritus, rash, cutaneous vasculitis, ***Stevens-Johnson syndrome.***
Other: chills.

INTERACTIONS

Drug-drug. *Antacids:* May decrease etodolac's peak level. Watch for decreased effect of etodolac.
Aspirin: May decrease protein-binding of etodolac without altering its clearance. May increase GI toxicity. Avoid using together.
Beta blockers, diuretics: May blunt effects of these drugs. Monitor patient closely.
Cyclosporine: May increase risk of nephrotoxicity. Avoid using together.
Digoxin, lithium, methotrexate: May impair elimination of these drugs, increasing risk of toxicity. Monitor drug levels.
Phenylbutazone: May increase etodolac level. Avoid using together.
Phenytoin: May increase phenytoin level. Monitor patient for toxicity.
Warfarin: May decrease the protein binding of warfarin but doesn't change its clearance. Although no dosage adjustment is needed, monitor INR closely and watch for bleeding.
Drug-herb. *Dong quai, feverfew, garlic, ginger, horse chestnut, red clover:* May increase risk of bleeding. Discourage use together.
White willow: Herb and drug contain similar components. Discourage use together.
Drug-lifestyle. *Alcohol use:* May increase risk of adverse effects. Discourage use together.
Sun exposure: May cause photosensitivity reactions. Advise patient to avoid excessive sunlight exposure.

EFFECTS ON LAB TEST RESULTS

- May decrease uric acid and hemoglobin levels and hematocrit.
- May decrease WBC count.

• May cause a false-positive test result for urine bilirubin, possibly from phenolic metabolites and ketone bodies.

CONTRAINDICATIONS & CAUTIONS

• Contraindicated in patients hypersensitive to drug and in those with history of aspirin- or NSAID-induced asthma, rhinitis, urticaria, or other allergic reactions.
• Use cautiously in patients with history of renal or hepatic impairment, preexisting asthma, or GI bleeding, ulceration, and perforation.

NURSING CONSIDERATIONS

• Because NSAIDs impair the synthesis of renal prostaglandins, they can decrease renal blood flow and lead to reversible renal impairment, especially in patients with renal or heart failure or liver dysfunction, in elderly patients, and in those taking diuretics. Monitor these patients closely.
• Serious GI toxicity, including peptic ulcers and bleeding, can occur in patient taking NSAIDs, despite lack of symptoms.
• ***Look alike–sound alike:*** Don't confuse Lodine with codeine, iodine, or Iopidine.

PATIENT TEACHING

• Tell patient to take drug with milk or meals to minimize GI discomfort.
• Teach patient signs and symptoms of GI bleeding, including blood in vomit, urine, or stool; coffee-ground vomit; and black, tarry stool. Tell him to notify prescriber immediately if any of these occurs.
• Advise patient to avoid consuming alcohol or aspirin while taking drug.
• Warn patient to avoid hazardous activities that require alertness until harmful CNS effects of drug are known.
• Teach patient signs and symptoms of liver damage, including nausea, fatigue, lethargy, itching, yellowed skin or eyes, right upper quadrant tenderness, and flu-like symptoms. Tell him to contact prescriber immediately if any of these symptoms occur.
• Advise patient to use a sunblock, wear protective clothing, and avoid prolonged exposure to sunlight because of possible sensitivity to sunlight.
• Tell pregnant woman to avoid use of drug during last trimester.
• Advise patient that use of OTC NSAIDs and etodolac may increase the risk of GI toxicity.

ibuprofen

ACT-3‡, Actiprofen‡, Advil ◊, Apo-Ibuprofen†, Bayer Select Ibuprofen Pain Relief Formula, Brufen‡, Children's Advil, Children's Motrin ◊, Excedrin IB ◊, Genpril ◊, Haltran ◊, Ibu-Tab ◊, Medipren ◊, Menadol, Midol IB, Motrin ◊ ✐, Novo-Profen†, Nuprin ◊, Nurofen‡, Nurofen Junior‡, Pamprin-IB, Rafen‡, Rufen, Saleto-200, Trendar ◊

Pharmacologic class: NSAID
Pregnancy risk category D in 3rd trimester

AVAILABLE FORMS

Capsules: 200 mg ◊
Oral drops: 40 mg/ml ◊
Oral suspension: 100 mg/2.5 ml ◊, 100 mg/5 ml ◊
Tablets: 100 mg, 200 mg ◊, 300 mg, 400 mg, 600 mg, 800 mg
Tablets (chewable): 50 mg ◊, 100 mg ◊

INDICATIONS & DOSAGES

➤ **Rheumatoid arthritis, osteoarthritis, arthritis**
Adults: 300 to 800 mg P.O. t.i.d. or q.i.d. Maximum daily dose is 3.2 g.
➤ **Mild to moderate pain, dysmenorrhea**
Adults: 400 mg P.O. q 4 to 6 hours, p.r.n.
➤ **Fever**
Adults: 200 to 400 mg P.O. q 4 to 6 hours, for no longer than 3 days. Maximum daily dose is 1.2 g.
Children ages 6 months to 12 years: If child's temperature is below 102.5° F (39.2° C), give 5 mg/kg P.O. q 6 to 8 hours. Treat higher temperatures with 10 mg/kg q 6 to 8 hours. Maximum daily dose is 40 mg/kg.
➤ **Juvenile arthritis**
Children: 30 to 40 mg/kg daily P.O. in three or four divided doses. Maximum daily dose is 50 mg/kg.

ACTION

May inhibit prostaglandin synthesis, to produce anti-inflammatory, analgesic, and antipyretic effects.

Route	Onset	Peak	Duration
P.O.	Variable	1–2 hr	4–6 hr

Half-life: 2 to 4 hours.

ADVERSE REACTIONS

CNS: ***aseptic meningitis,*** dizziness, headache, nervousness.
CV: edema, fluid retention, peripheral edema.
EENT: tinnitus.
GI: abdominal pain, bloating, constipation, decreased appetite, diarrhea, dyspepsia, epigastric distress, flatulence, GI fullness, heartburn, nausea, occult blood loss, peptic ulceration.
GU: ***acute renal failure,*** azotemia, cystitis, hematuria.
Hematologic: ***agranulocytosis, aplastic anemia, leukopenia, neutropenia, pancytopenia, thrombocytopenia,*** anemia, prolonged bleeding time.
Metabolic: ***hyperkalemia, hypoglycemia.***
Respiratory: ***bronchospasm.***
Skin: ***Stevens-Johnson syndrome,*** pruritus, rash, urticaria.

INTERACTIONS

Drug-drug. *Antihypertensives, furosemide, thiazide diuretics:* May decrease the effectiveness of diuretics or antihypertensives. Monitor patient closely.
Aspirin: May negate the antiplatelet effect of low-dose aspirin therapy. Advise patient on the appropriate spacing of doses.
Aspirin, corticosteroids: May cause adverse GI reactions. Avoid using together.
Bisphosphonates: May increase risk of gastric ulceration. Monitor patient for signs of gastric irritation or bleeding.
Cyclosporine: May increase nephrotoxicity of both drugs. Avoid using together.
Digoxin, lithium, oral anticoagulants: May increase levels or effects of these drugs. Monitor patient toxicity.
Methotrexate: May decrease methotrexate clearance and increases toxicity. Use together cautiously.
Drug-herb. *Dong quai, feverfew, garlic, ginger, ginkgo biloba, horse chestnut, red clover:* May increase risk of bleeding, based on the known effects of components. Discourage use together.
White willow: Herb and drug contain similar components. Discourage use together.
Drug-lifestyle. *Alcohol use:* May cause adverse GI reactions. Discourage use together.
Sun exposure: May cause photosensitivity reactions. Advise patient to avoid excessive sunlight exposure.

EFFECTS ON LAB TEST RESULTS

- May increase BUN, creatinine, ALT, AST, and potassium levels. May decrease glucose and hemoglobin levels and hematocrit.
- May decrease neutrophil, WBC, RBC, platelet, and granulocyte counts.

CONTRAINDICATIONS & CAUTIONS

- Contraindicated in patients hypersensitive to drug and in those with angioedema, syndrome of nasal polyps, or bronchospastic reaction to aspirin or other NSAIDs.
- Contraindicated in pregnant women.
- Use cautiously in patients with GI disorders, history of peptic ulcer disease, hepatic or renal disease, cardiac decompensation, hypertension, asthma, or intrinsic coagulation defects.

NURSING CONSIDERATIONS

- Check renal and hepatic function periodically in patients on long-term therapy. Stop drug if abnormalities occur and notify prescriber.
- Because of their antipyretic and anti-inflammatory actions, NSAIDs may mask signs and symptoms of infection.
- Blurred or diminished vision and changes in color vision may occur.
- It may take 1 or 2 weeks before full anti-inflammatory effects occur.
- Serious GI toxicity, including peptic ulcers and bleeding, can occur in patient taking NSAIDs, despite lack of symptoms.
- If patient consumes three or more alcoholic drinks per day, drug may cause stomach bleeding.

• ***Look alike–sound alike:*** Don't confuse Trendar with Trandate.

PATIENT TEACHING

• Tell patient to take with meals or milk to reduce adverse GI reactions.

• ***Alert:*** Drug is available OTC. Instruct patient not to exceed 1.2 g daily, not to give to children younger than age 12, and not to take for extended periods (longer than 3 days for fever or longer than 10 days for pain) without consulting prescriber.

• Tell patient that full therapeutic effect for arthritis may be delayed for 2 to 4 weeks. Although pain relief occurs at low dosage levels, inflammation doesn't improve at dosages less than 400 mg q.i.d.

• Caution patient that use with aspirin, alcohol, or corticosteroids may increase risk of GI adverse reactions.

• Teach patient to watch for and report to prescriber immediately signs and symptoms of GI bleeding, including blood in vomit, urine, or stool; coffee-ground vomit; and black, tarry stool.

• Tell patient to contact prescriber before using this drug if fluid intake hasn't been adequate or if fluids have been lost as a result of vomiting or diarrhea.

• Warn patient to avoid hazardous activities that require mental alertness until effects on CNS are known.

• Advise patient to wear sunscreen to avoid hypersensitivity to sunlight.

indomethacin

Apo-Indomethacin†, Arthrexin‡, Indocid†‡, Indocid SR†, Indocin, Indocin SR, Novo-Methacin†

indomethacin sodium trihydrate

Apo-Indomethacin†, Indocin I.V, Novo-Methacin†

Pharmacologic class: NSAID
Pregnancy risk category B; D in 3rd trimester

AVAILABLE FORMS

indomethacin
Capsules: 25 mg, 50 mg
Capsules (sustained-release): 75 mg
Oral suspension: 25 mg/5 ml
Suppositories: 50 mg
indomethacin sodium trihydrate
Injection: 1-mg vials

INDICATIONS & DOSAGES

➤ **Moderate to severe rheumatoid arthritis or osteoarthritis, ankylosing spondylitis**
Adults: 25 mg P.O. or P.R. b.i.d. or t.i.d. with food or antacids; increase daily dose by 25 or 50 mg q 7 days, up to 200 mg daily. Or, 75 mg sustained-release capsules P.O. to start, in morning or at bedtime, followed by 75 mg sustained-release capsules b.i.d. if needed.

➤ **Acute gouty arthritis**
Adults: 50 mg P.O. t.i.d. Reduce dose as soon as possible; then stop therapy. Don't use sustained-release form.

➤ **Acute painful shoulders (bursitis or tendinitis)**
Adults: 75 to 150 mg P.O. daily in divided doses t.i.d. or q.i.d. for 7 to 14 days.

➤ **To close a hemodynamically significant patent ductus arteriosus in premature neonates**
Neonates older than age 7 days: 0.2 mg/kg I.V.; then two doses of 0.25 mg/kg at 12- to 24-hour intervals.
Neonates ages 2 to 7 days: 0.2 mg/kg I.V.; then two doses of 0.2 mg/kg at 12- to 24-hour intervals.
Neonates younger than age 48 hours: 0.2 mg/kg I.V.; then two doses of 0.1 mg/kg at 12- to 24-hour intervals.

I.V. ADMINISTRATION

• Reconstitute powder for injection with sterile water or normal saline solution. For each 1-mg vial, add 1 or 2 ml of diluent for a solution containing 1 mg/ml or 0.5 mg/ml, respectively. Give over 20 to 30 minutes.

• Use only preservative-free sterile saline solution or sterile water to prepare. Never use diluents containing benzyl alcohol because it has been linked to toxicity in newborns.

• Because injection contains no preservatives, reconstitute drug immediately before use, and discard unused solution.

• If anuria or marked oliguria is evident, withhold administration of second or third scheduled I.V. dose and notify prescriber.

• Watch carefully for bleeding and for reduced urine output.

INCOMPATIBILITIES
Amino acid injection, calcium gluconate, cimetidine, dextrose injection, dobutamine, dopamine, gentamicin, levofloxacin, solutions with pH less than 6, tobramycin sulfate, tolazoline.

ACTION
May inhibit prostaglandin synthesis, to produce anti-inflammatory, analgesic, and antipyretic effects.

Route	Onset	Peak	Duration
P.O.	30 min	1–4 hr	4–6 hr
I.V.	Immediate	Immediate	4–6 hr
P.R.	Unknown	Unknown	4–6 hr

Half-life: 4¼ hours.

ADVERSE REACTIONS
P.O. and P.R.
CNS: *headache,* confusion, dizziness, depression, drowsiness, fatigue, peripheral neuropathy, psychic disturbances, somnolence, syncope, vertigo.
CV: edema, hypertension.
EENT: hearing loss, tinnitus.
GI: ***pancreatitis,*** abdominal pain, anorexia, constipation, diarrhea, dyspepsia, GI bleeding, nausea, peptic ulceration.
GU: hematuria.
Hematologic: iron-deficiency anemia.
Metabolic: ***hyperkalemia.***
Skin: ***Stevens-Johnson syndrome,*** pruritus, urticaria.
Other: hypersensitivity reactions.
I.V.
GU: hematuria, interstitial nephritis, proteinuria.

INTERACTIONS
Drug-drug. *Aminoglycosides, cyclosporine, methotrexate:* May enhance toxicity of these drugs. Avoid using together.
Anticoagulants: May cause bleeding. Monitor patient closely.
Antihypertensives: May decrease antihypertensive effect. Monitor patient closely.
Antihypertensives, furosemide, thiazide diuretics: May impair response to both drugs. Avoid using together, if possible.
Aspirin: May decrease level of indomethacin. Avoid using together.
Aspirin, corticosteroids: May increase risk of GI toxicity. Avoid using together.
Bisphosphonates: May increase risk of gastric ulceration. Monitor patient for symptoms of gastric irritation or GI bleeding.
Diflunisal, probenecid: May decrease indomethacin excretion. Watch for increased indomethacin adverse reactions.
Digoxin: May prolong half-life of digoxin. Use together cautiously.
Dipyridamole: May enhance fluid retention. Avoid using together.
Lithium: May increase lithium level. Monitor patient for toxicity.
Penicillamine: May increase bioavailability of penicillamine. Monitor patient closely.
Phenytoin: May increase phenytoin level. Monitor patient closely.
Triamterene: May cause nephrotoxicity. Avoid using together.
Drug-herb. *Dong quai, feverfew, garlic, ginger, horse chestnut, red clover:* May cause bleeding. Discourage use together.
Senna: May inhibit diarrheal effects. Discourage use together.
White willow: Herb and drug contain similar components. Discourage use together.
Drug-lifestyle. *Alcohol use:* May cause GI toxicity. Discourage use together.

EFFECTS ON LAB TEST RESULTS
• May increase potassium level. May decrease hemoglobin level and hematocrit.
• May increase liver function test values.

CONTRAINDICATIONS & CAUTIONS
• Contraindicated in patients hypersensitive to drug and in those with a history of aspirin- or NSAID-induced asthma, rhinitis, or urticaria.
• Contraindicated in pregnant or breast-feeding women and in neonates with untreated infection, active bleeding, coagulation defects or thrombocytopenia, congenital heart disease needing patency of the ductus arteriosus, necrotizing enterocolitis, or significant renal impairment. Suppositories are contraindicated in patients with history of proctitis or recent rectal bleeding.

- Contraindicated in pregnant women.
- Use cautiously in elderly patients, those with history of GI disease, and those with epilepsy, parkinsonism, hepatic or renal disease, CV disease, infection, and mental illness or depression.

NURSING CONSIDERATIONS

- Because of the high risk of adverse effects from long-term use, drug shouldn't be used routinely as an analgesic or antipyretic.
- Sustained-release capsules shouldn't be used for acute gouty arthritis.
- Give oral dose with food, milk, or antacid to decrease GI upset.
- If ductus arteriosus reopens, a second course of one to three doses may be given. If ineffective, surgery may be needed.
- Watch for bleeding in patients receiving anticoagulants, patients with coagulation defects, and neonates.
- Because NSAIDs impair synthesis of renal prostaglandins, they can decrease renal blood flow and lead to reversible renal impairment, especially in patients with renal failure, heart failure, or liver dysfunction; in elderly patients; and in those taking diuretics. Monitor these patients closely.
- Drug causes sodium retention; watch for weight gain (especially in elderly patients) and increased blood pressure in patients with hypertension.
- Monitor patient for rash and respiratory distress, which may indicate a hypersensitivity reaction.
- Because of their antipyretic and anti-inflammatory actions, NSAIDs may mask signs and symptoms of infection.
- Serious GI toxicity (including peptic ulcers and bleeding) can occur in patient taking NSAIDs, despite lack of symptoms.
- NSAIDs may cause increased risk of thrombotic events, MI, and stroke. Risk may be increased with duration of use and in patients with history of cardiovascular disease or risk factors of cardiovascular disease.
- Monitor patient on long-term oral therapy for toxicity by conducting regular eye examinations, hearing tests, CBCs, and kidney function tests.

PATIENT TEACHING

- Tell patient to take oral drug with food, milk, or antacid to prevent GI upset.
- Alert patient that using oral form with aspirin, alcohol, other NSAIDs, or corticosteroids may increase risk of adverse GI reactions.
- Teach patient signs and symptoms of GI bleeding, including blood in vomit, urine, or stool; coffee-ground vomit; and black, tarry stool. Tell him to notify prescriber immediately if any of these occurs.
- Tell patient to immediately report signs or symptoms of cardiac events, such as chest pain, shortness of breath, weakness, and slurred speech.
- Warn patient to avoid hazardous activities that require mental alertness until CNS effects are known.
- Tell patient to notify prescriber immediately if visual or hearing changes occur.

ketoprofen

Apo-Keto†, Apo-Keto-E†, Novo-Keto-EC†, Orudis, Orudis KT◊, Orudis SR†‡, Oruvail

Pharmacologic class: NSAID
Pregnancy risk category B; D in 3rd trimester

AVAILABLE FORMS

Capsules: 25 mg, 50 mg, 75 mg
Capsules (extended-release): 100 mg, 150 mg, 200 mg
Suppositories: 50 mg†, 100 mg†
Tablets: 12.5 mg◊
Tablets (enteric-coated): 50 mg†, 100 mg†
Tablets (extended-release): 200 mg†

INDICATIONS & DOSAGES

➤ **Rheumatoid arthritis, osteoarthritis**

Adults: 75 mg t.i.d. or 50 mg q.i.d., or 200 mg as an extended-release tablet once daily. Maximum dose is 300 mg daily, or 200 mg daily for extended-release capsules. Or, 50 or 100 mg P.R. b.i.d.; or one suppository h.s. (with oral ketoprofen during the day).
Adults older than age 75: 75 to 150 mg P.O. daily. Adjust dose according to patient's response and tolerance.

➤ **Mild to moderate pain, dysmenorrhea**
Adults: 25 to 50 mg P.O. q 6 to 8 hours, p.r.n. Maximum dose is 300 mg daily.
➤ **Minor aches and pain or fever**
Adults: 12.5 mg q 4 to 6 hours. Don't exceed 25 mg in 4 to 6 hours or 75 mg in 24 hours.
Adjust-a-dose: For elderly patients and those with impaired renal function, reduce first dose to between one-third and one-half normal first dose.

ACTION

Unknown. Produces anti-inflammatory, analgesic, and antipyretic effects, possibly by inhibiting prostaglandin synthesis.

Route	Onset	Peak	Duration
P.O. (extended-release)	2–3 hr	6–7 hr	Unknown
P.O., P.R.	1–2 hr	30–120 min	3–4 hr

Half-life: 2 to 5½ hours for extended-release forms.

ADVERSE REACTIONS

CNS: headache, dizziness, CNS excitation (which includes insomnia, nervousness, and dreams) or CNS depression (which includes somnolence and malaise).
CV: peripheral edema.
EENT: tinnitus, visual disturbances.
GI: *dyspepsia,* abdominal pain, anorexia, constipation, diarrhea, flatulence, nausea, stomatitis, peptic ulceration, vomiting.
GU: ***nephrotoxicity.***
Hematologic: prolonged bleeding time.
Respiratory: dyspnea.
Skin: photosensitivity reactions, rash.

INTERACTIONS

Drug-drug. *Aspirin, corticosteroids:* May increase risk of adverse GI reactions. Avoid using together.
Aspirin, probenecid: May increase ketoprofen level. Avoid using together.
Cyclosporine: May increase nephrotoxicity. Avoid using together.
Hydrochlorothiazide, other diuretics: May decrease diuretic effectiveness. Monitor patient for lack of effect.
Lithium, methotrexate, phenytoin: May increase levels of these drugs, leading to toxicity. Monitor patient closely.
Warfarin: May increase risk of bleeding. Monitor patient closely.
Drug-herb. *Dong quai, feverfew, garlic, ginger, horse chestnut, red clover:* May cause bleeding based on the known effects of components. Discourage use together.
White willow: Herb and drug contain similar components. Discourage use together.
Drug-lifestyle. *Alcohol use:* May cause GI toxicity. Discourage use together.
Sun exposure: May cause photosensitivity reactions. Advise patient to avoid excessive sunlight exposure.

EFFECTS ON LAB TEST RESULTS

- May increase creatinine, BUN, ALT, and AST levels.
- May increase bleeding time. May increase or decrease iron test results.
- May falsely increase bilirubin level.

CONTRAINDICATIONS & CAUTIONS

- Contraindicated in patients hypersensitive to drug and in those with history of aspirin- or NSAID-induced asthma, urticaria, or other allergic reactions.
- Avoid use during last trimester of pregnancy.
- Drug isn't recommended for children or breast-feeding women.
- Use cautiously in patients with history of peptic ulcer disease, renal dysfunction, hypertension, heart failure, or fluid retention.

NURSING CONSIDERATIONS

- Don't use sustained-release form for patients in acute pain.
- Because NSAIDs impair synthesis of renal prostaglandins, they can decrease renal blood flow and lead to reversible renal impairment, especially in patients with renal or heart failure or liver dysfunction, in elderly patients, and in those taking diuretics. Monitor these patients closely.
- Check renal and hepatic function every 6 months or as indicated.

• Drug decreases platelet adhesion and aggregation, and can prolong bleeding time about 3 to 4 minutes from baseline.
• NSAIDs may mask signs and symptoms of infection because of their antipyretic and anti-inflammatory actions.
• Serious GI toxicity, including peptic ulcers and bleeding, can occur in patient taking NSAIDs, despite lack of symptoms.

PATIENT TEACHING
• ***Alert:*** Drug is available without prescription. Instruct patient not to exceed 75 mg daily.
• Tell patient to take drug 30 minutes before or 2 hours after meals with a full glass of water. If adverse GI reactions occur, patient may take drug with milk or meals.
• Tell patient not to crush delayed-release or extended-release tablets.
• Tell patient that full therapeutic effect may be delayed for 2 to 4 weeks.
• Teach patient signs and symptoms of GI bleeding, including blood in vomit, urine, or stool; coffee-ground vomit; and black, tarry stool. Tell him to notify prescriber immediately if any of these occurs.
• Alert patient that using with aspirin, alcohol, other NSAIDs, or corticosteroids may increase risk of adverse GI reactions.
• Warn patient to avoid hazardous activities that require mental alertness until CNS effects are known.
• Because of possibility of sensitivity to the sun, advise patient to use a sunblock, wear protective clothing, and avoid prolonged exposure to sunlight.
• Instruct patient to report problems with vision or hearing immediately.
• Tell patient to protect drug from direct light and excessive heat and humidity.

ketorolac tromethamine
Toradol

Pharmacologic class: NSAID
Pregnancy risk category C; D in 3rd trimester

AVAILABLE FORMS
Injection: 15 mg/ml in 1- and 2-ml vials and 1-ml Tubex syringes, 30 mg/ml in 1- and 2-ml single dose vials, 1- and 2-ml Tubex syringes, and 10-ml multiple dose vials
Tablets: 10 mg

INDICATIONS & DOSAGES
➤ **Short-term management of moderately severe, acute pain for single-dose treatment**
Adults younger than age 65: Give 60 mg I.M. or 30 mg I.V.
Children ages 2 to 16: Give 1 mg/kg I.M. (maximum dose 30 mg) or 0.5 mg/kg I.V. (maximum dose 15 mg).
Adults age 65 and older: Give 30 mg I.M. or 15 mg I.V.
Adjust-a-dose: For renally impaired patients or those who weigh less than 50 kg (110 lb), give 30 mg I.M. or 15 mg I.V.
➤ **Short-term management of moderately severe, acute pain for multiple-dose treatment**
Adults younger than age 65: Give 30 mg I.M. or I.V. q 6 hours for maximum of 5 days. Maximum daily dose is 120 mg.
Adults age 65 and older: Give 15 mg I.M. or I.V. q 6 hours for maximum of 5 days. Maximum daily dose is 60 mg.
Adjust-a-dose: For renally impaired patients or those who weigh less than 50 kg, give 15 mg I.M. or I.V. q 6 hours. Maximum daily dose is 60 mg.
➤ **Short-term management of moderately severe, acute pain when switching from parenteral to oral administration (oral therapy is indicated only as continuation of parenterally given drug and should never be given without patient first having received parenteral therapy)**
Adults younger than age 65: 20 mg P.O. as single dose; then 10 mg P.O. q 4 to 6 hours for maximum of 5 days. Maximum daily dose is 40 mg.
Adults age 65 and older: Give 10 mg P.O. as single dose; then 10 mg P.O. q 4 to 6 hours for maximum of 5 days. Maximum daily dose is 40 mg.
Adjust-a-dose: For renally impaired patients or those who weigh less than 50 kg, give 10 mg P.O. as single dose; then 10 mg P.O. q 4 to 6 hours. Maximum daily dose is 40 mg.

I.V. ADMINISTRATION

- Dilute with normal saline solution, D_5W, 5% dextrose and normal saline solution, Ringer solution, lactated Ringer solution, or Plasma-Lyte A.
- Give injection over at least 15 seconds.
- Protect from light.

INCOMPATIBILITIES

Azithromycin; fenoldopam mesylate; haloperidol lactate; nalbuphine; solutions that result in a relatively low pH, such as hydroxyzine, meperidine, morphine sulfate, and prochlorperazine; thiethylperazine.

ACTION

May inhibit prostaglandin synthesis, to produce anti-inflammatory, analgesic, and antipyretic effects.

Route	Onset	Peak	Duration
P.O.	30–60 min	30–60 min	6–8 hr
I.V.	Immediate	1–3 min	6–8 hr
I.M.	10 min	30–60 min	6–8 hr

Half-life: 4 to 6 hours.

ADVERSE REACTIONS

CNS: *headache,* dizziness, drowsiness, sedation.
CV: ***arrhythmias,*** edema, hypertension, palpitations.
GI: *dyspepsia, GI pain, nausea,* constipation, diarrhea, flatulence, peptic ulceration, stomatitis, vomiting.
Hematologic: decreased platelet adhesion, prolonged bleeding time, purpura.
Skin: diaphoresis, pruritus, rash.
Other: pain at injection site.

INTERACTIONS

Drug-drug. *ACE inhibitors:* May cause renal impairment, particularly in volume-depleted patients. Avoid using together in volume-depleted patients.
Anticoagulants: May increase anticoagulant levels in the blood. Use together with extreme caution and monitor patient closely.
Antihypertensives, diuretics: May decrease effectiveness. Monitor patient closely.
Lithium: May increase lithium level. Monitor patient closely.
Methotrexate: May decrease methotrexate clearance and increased toxicity. Avoid using together.
Probenecid: May increase level and toxicity of ketorolac. Avoid using together.
Salicylates: May increase the risk of serious ketorolac adverse effects. Avoid using together.
Drug-herb. *Dong quai, feverfew, garlic, ginger, horse chestnut, red clover:* May cause bleeding. Discourage use together.
White willow: Herb and drug contain similar components. Discourage use together.

EFFECTS ON LAB TEST RESULTS

- May increase ALT and AST levels.
- May increase bleeding time.

CONTRAINDICATIONS & CAUTIONS

- Contraindicated in patients hypersensitive to drug and in those with active peptic ulcer disease, recent GI bleeding or perforation, advanced renal impairment, cerebrovascular bleeding, hemorrhagic diathesis, or incomplete hemostasis, and those at risk for renal impairment from volume depletion or at risk of bleeding.
- Contraindicated in children younger than age 2 and in patients with history of peptic ulcer disease or GI bleeding, past allergic reactions to aspirin or other NSAIDs, and during labor and delivery or breast-feeding.
- Contraindicated as prophylactic analgesic before major surgery or intraoperatively when hemostasis is critical; and in patients currently receiving aspirin, an NSAID, or probenecid.
- Use cautiously in patients who are elderly or have hepatic or renal impairment or cardiac decompensation.

NURSING CONSIDERATIONS

- Correct hypovolemia before giving.
- ***Alert:*** The maximum combined duration of parenteral and oral therapy is 5 days.
- When appropriate, give by deep I.M. injection. Patient may feel pain at injection site. Put pressure on site for 15 to 30 seconds after injection to minimize local effects.
- In children age 2 and older, use as a single dose only.

• Don't give drug epidurally or intrathecally because of alcohol content.
• Carefully observe patients with coagulopathies and those taking anticoagulants. Drug inhibits platelet aggregation and can prolong bleeding time. This effect disappears within 48 hours of stopping drug and doesn't alter platelet count, INR, PTT, or PT.
• NSAIDs may mask signs and symptoms of infection because of their antipyretic and anti-inflammatory actions.
• Serious GI toxicity, including peptic ulcers and bleeding, can occur in patient taking NSAIDs, despite lack of symptoms.
• ***Look alike–sound alike:*** Don't confuse Toradol with Tegretol or Foradil.

PATIENT TEACHING

• Warn patient receiving drug I.M. that pain may occur at injection site.
• Teach patient signs and symptoms of GI bleeding, including blood in vomit, urine, or stool; coffee-ground vomit; and black, tarry stool. Tell him to notify prescriber immediately if any of these occurs.
• Tell patient not to take drug for more than 5 days in a row.

meloxicam
Mobic

Pharmacologic class: NSAID
Pregnancy risk category C; D in 3rd trimester

AVAILABLE FORMS

Oral suspension: 7.5 mg/5 ml
Tablets: 7.5 mg, 15 mg

INDICATIONS & DOSAGES

➤ To relieve signs and symptoms of osteoarthritis or rheumatoid arthritis (RA)
Adults: 7.5 mg P.O. once daily. May increase p.r.n. to maximum dose of 15 mg daily.
➤ To relieve signs and symptoms of pauciarticular or polyarticular course juvenile RA
Children ages 2 to 17: 0.125 mg/kg P.O. once daily up to a maximum dose of 7.5 mg.

ACTION

May inhibit prostaglandin synthesis, to produce anti-inflammatory, analgesic, and antipyretic effects.

Route	Onset	Peak	Duration
P.O.	Unknown	4–5 hr	Unknown

Half-life: 15 to 20 hours.

ADVERSE REACTIONS

CNS: ***seizures,*** anxiety, confusion, depression, dizziness, fatigue, fever, headache, insomnia, malaise, nervousness, paresthesia, somnolence, syncope, tremor, vertigo.
CV: ***arrhythmias, heart failure, MI,*** angina pectoris, edema, hypertension, hypotension, palpitations, tachycardia.
EENT: abnormal vision, conjunctivitis, pharyngitis, taste perversion, tinnitus.
GI: ***hemorrhage, pancreatitis,*** abdominal pain, colitis, constipation, diarrhea, dyspepsia, dry mouth, duodenal ulcer, esophagitis, flatulence, gastric ulcer, gastritis, gastroesophageal reflux, increased appetite, nausea, vomiting.
GU: ***renal failure,*** albuminuria, hematuria, urinary frequency, UTI.
Hematologic: ***agranulocytosis, leukopenia, thrombocytopenia,*** anemia, purpura.
Hepatic: ***hepatitis, liver failure,*** jaundice.
Metabolic: dehydration, weight increase or decrease.
Musculoskeletal: arthralgia, back pain.
Respiratory: ***asthma, bronchospasm,*** coughing, dyspnea, upper respiratory tract infection.
Skin: ***erythema multiforme, exfoliative dermatitis, Stevens-Johnson syndrome, toxic epidermal necrolysis,*** alopecia, bullous eruption, photosensitivity reactions, pruritus, rash, sweating, urticaria.
Other: ***anaphylactoid reactions including shock, angioedema,*** accidental injury, allergic reaction, flulike symptoms.

INTERACTIONS

Drug-drug. *ACE inhibitors:* May decrease antihypertensive effects. Monitor blood pressure.
Aspirin: May cause adverse effects. Avoid using together.
Furosemide, thiazide diuretics: May reduce sodium excretion caused by diuretics, leading to sodium retention. Monitor

patient for edema and increased blood pressure.
Lithium: May increase lithium level. Monitor lithium level closely.
Methotrexate: May increase the toxicity of methotrexate. Use cautiously together.
Warfarin: May increase PT, INR, and risk of bleeding complications. Monitor PT and INR, and check for signs and symptoms of bleeding.
Drug-lifestyle. *Alcohol use:* May cause GI irritation and bleeding. Discourage use together.
Smoking: May cause GI irritation and bleeding. Discourage use together.

EFFECTS ON LAB TEST RESULTS

- May increase BUN, creatinine, ALT, AST, and bilirubin levels. May decrease hemoglobin level and hematocrit.
- May decrease WBC and platelet counts.

CONTRAINDICATIONS & CAUTIONS

- Contraindicated in patients hypersensitive to drug and in those who have experienced asthma, urticaria, or allergic reactions after taking aspirin or other NSAIDs.
- Contraindicated in perioperative pain following coronary artery bypass graft surgery.
- Avoid use late in pregnancy.
- Use with caution in patients with history of ulcers, GI bleeding, or asthma. Use cautiously in patients with dehydration, anemia, hepatic disease, renal disease, hypertension, fluid retention, heart failure, or asthma. Also use cautiously in elderly and debilitated patients because of increased risk of fatal GI bleeding.

NURSING CONSIDERATIONS

- ***Alert:*** Patients, including those hypersensitive to aspirin and other NSAIDs, may have allergic reactions to drug.
- ***Alert:*** NSAIDs may increase the risk of serious thrombotic events, MI, or stroke. The risk may be greater with longer use or in patients with CV disease or risk factors for CV disease.
- Rehydrate dehydrated patients before starting drug. Patient with a history of ulcers or GI bleeding is at higher risk for GI bleeding while taking NSAIDs. Other risk factors for GI bleeding include treatment with corticosteroids or anticoagulants, longer duration of NSAID treatment, smoking, alcoholism, older age, and poor overall health.
- Watch for signs and symptoms of overt and occult bleeding.
- NSAIDs can cause fluid retention; closely monitor patients who have hypertension, edema, or heart failure.
- Drug may be hepatotoxic. Watch for elevated ALT and AST levels. If signs and symptoms of liver disease develop, or if systemic signs and symptoms such as eosinophilia or rash occur, stop drug and call prescriber.
- Abdominal pain, vomiting, diarrhea, headache, and pyrexia may occur more frequently in children than in adults. Monitor children for these symptoms.
- Monitor hemoglobin level and hematocrit in patients on long-term therapy.
- The oral solution may be substituted for the tablets, milligram for milligram. Shake solution gently before use.

PATIENT TEACHING

- Tell patient to report history of allergic reactions to aspirin or other NSAIDs before starting therapy.
- Tell patient drug can be taken without regard to meals.
- Advise patient to report signs and symptoms of GI ulcers and bleeding, such as blood in vomit or stool, and black, tarry stools, and to contact prescriber if they occur.
- Instruct patient to report any skin rash, weight gain, or swelling.
- Advise patient to report warning signs of liver damage, such as nausea, fatigue, lethargy, itching, yellowed skin or eyes, right upper quadrant tenderness, and flu-like symptoms.
- Warn patient with history of asthma that drug may trigger an asthmatic attack. Tell him to stop drug and contact prescriber if he has an attack.
- Tell woman of childbearing age to notify prescriber if she becomes pregnant or is planning to become pregnant while taking drug.
- Inform patient that it may take several days to achieve consistent pain relief.
- Advise patient that use of OTC NSAIDs with meloxicam may increase the risk of GI toxicity.

nabumetone
Relafen

Pharmacologic class: NSAID
Pregnancy risk category C; D in 3rd trimester

AVAILABLE FORMS
Tablets: 500 mg, 750 mg

INDICATIONS & DOSAGES
➤ **Rheumatoid arthritis, osteoarthritis**
Adults: Initially, 1,000 mg P.O. daily as a single dose or in divided doses b.i.d. Maximum, 2,000 mg daily.

ACTION
Unknown. Produces anti-inflammatory, analgesic, and antipyretic effects, possibly by inhibiting prostaglandin synthesis.

Route	Onset	Peak	Duration
P.O.	Unknown	9–12 hr	Unknown

Half-life: About 24 hours.

ADVERSE REACTIONS
CNS: dizziness, fatigue, headache, insomnia, nervousness, somnolence.
CV: edema, vasculitis.
EENT: tinnitus.
GI: *abdominal pain, diarrhea, dyspepsia,* ***bleeding,*** anorexia, constipation, dry mouth, flatulence, gastritis, nausea, stomatitis, ulceration, vomiting.
Respiratory: dyspnea, pneumonitis.
Skin: increased diaphoresis, pruritus, rash.

INTERACTIONS
Drug-drug. *Diuretics:* May decrease diuretic effectiveness. Monitor patient closely.
Warfarin, other highly protein-bound drugs: May cause adverse effects from displacement of drugs by nabumetone. Use together cautiously.
Drug-herb. *Dong quai, feverfew, garlic, ginger, horse chestnut, red clover:* May cause bleeding. Discourage use together.
White willow: Herb and drug contain similar components. Discourage use together.
Drug-food. *Any food:* May increase absorption. Advise patient to take drug with food.
Drug-lifestyle. *Alcohol use:* May increase risk of additive GI toxicity. Discourage use together.

EFFECTS ON LAB TEST RESULTS
None reported.

CONTRAINDICATIONS & CAUTIONS
- Contraindicated in patients with hypersensitivity reactions and history of aspirin- or NSAID-induced asthma, urticaria, or other allergic-type reactions.
- Contraindicated in children and in pregnant women during third trimester of pregnancy.
- Use cautiously in patients with renal or hepatic impairment; heart failure, hypertension, or other conditions that may predispose patient to fluid retention; or a history of peptic ulcer disease.

NURSING CONSIDERATIONS
- Because NSAIDs impair synthesis of renal prostaglandins, they can decrease renal blood flow and lead to reversible renal impairment, especially in patients with renal or heart failure or liver dysfunction, in elderly patients, and in those taking diuretics. Monitor these patients closely.
- During long-term therapy, periodically monitor renal and liver function, CBC, and hematocrit; assess patients for signs and symptoms of GI bleeding.
- Serious GI toxicity, including peptic ulcers and bleeding, can occur in patients taking NSAIDs, despite lack of symptoms.

PATIENT TEACHING
- Instruct patient to take drug with food, milk, or antacids. Drug is absorbed more rapidly when taken with food or milk.
- Advise patient to limit alcohol intake because using drug with alcohol increases the risk of GI problems.
- Teach patient signs and symptoms of GI bleeding, including blood in vomit, urine, or stool; coffee-ground vomit; and black, tarry stool. Tell him to notify prescriber immediately if any of these occurs.

• Warn patient against hazardous activities that require mental alertness until CNS effects are known.
• Advise patient that use of OTC NSAIDs in combination with nabumetone may increase the risk of GI toxicity.

naproxen

Apo-Naproxen†, EC-Naprosyn, Naprosyn✐, Naprosyn-E†, Naprosyn-SR, Naxen†, Novo-Naprox†, Nu-Naprox†

naproxen sodium

Aleve ◇, Anaprox, Anaprox DS, Apo-Napro-Na† ◇, Naprelan, Naprogesic‡, Novo-Naprox Sodium†, Synflex†

Pharmacologic class: NSAID
Pregnancy risk category B; D in 3rd trimester

AVAILABLE FORMS

naproxen
Oral suspension: 125 mg/5 ml
Suppositories: 500 mg‡
Tablets: 250 mg, 375 mg, 500 mg
Tablets (delayed-release): 375 mg, 500 mg
Tablets (extended-release): 750 mg, 1,000 mg
naproxen sodium
Tablets (controlled-release): 412.5 mg, 550 mg
Tablets (film-coated): 220 mg ◇, 275 mg, 550 mg
Note: 275 mg of naproxen sodium contains 250 mg of naproxen.

INDICATIONS & DOSAGES

➤ **Rheumatoid arthritis, osteoarthritis, ankylosing spondylitis, pain, dysmenorrhea, tendinitis, bursitis**
Adults: 250 to 500 mg naproxen b.i.d.; maximum, 1.5 g daily for a limited time. Or, 375 to 500 mg delayed-release EC-Naprosyn b.i.d. Or, 750 to 1,000 mg controlled-release Naprelan daily. Or, 275 to 550 mg naproxen sodium b.i.d.
➤ **Juvenile arthritis**
Children: 10 mg/kg P.O. in two divided doses.
➤ **Acute gout**
Adults: 750 mg naproxen P.O.; then 250 mg q 8 hours until attack subsides. Or, 825 mg naproxen sodium; then 275 mg q 8 hours until attack subsides. Or, 1,000 to 1,500 mg daily controlled-release Naprelan on first day; then 1,000 mg daily until attack subsides.
➤ **Mild to moderate pain, primary dysmenorrhea**
Adults: 500 mg naproxen P.O.; then 250 mg q 6 to 8 hours up to 1.25 g daily. Or, 550 mg naproxen sodium; then 275 mg q 6 to 8 hours up to 1,375 mg daily. Or, 1,000 mg controlled-release Naprelan once daily. In patients older than age 65, don't exceed 400 mg daily.

ACTION

May inhibit prostaglandin synthesis to produce anti-inflammatory, analgesic, and antipyretic effects.

Route	Onset	Peak	Duration
P.O.	1 hr	2–4 hr	7 hr
P.R.	Unknown	Unknown	Unknown

Half-life: 10 to 20 hours.

ADVERSE REACTIONS

CNS: dizziness, drowsiness, headache, vertigo.
CV: edema, palpitations.
EENT: *tinnitus,* auditory disturbances, visual disturbances.
GI: abdominal pain, constipation, diarrhea, dyspepsia, epigastric pain, heartburn, nausea, occult blood loss, peptic ulceration, stomatitis, thirst.
Hematologic: ecchymoses, increased bleeding time.
Metabolic: ***hyperkalemia.***
Respiratory: dyspnea.
Skin: diaphoresis, pruritus, purpura, rash, urticaria.

INTERACTIONS

Drug-drug. *ACE inhibitors:* May cause renal impairment. Use together cautiously.
Antihypertensives, diuretics: May decrease effect of these drugs. Monitor patient closely.
Aspirin, corticosteroids: May cause adverse GI reactions. Avoid using together.

Lithium: May increase lithium level. Observe patient for toxicity and monitor level. Adjustment of lithium dosage may be required.
Methotrexate: May cause toxicity. Monitor patient closely.
Oral anticoagulants, other sulfonylureas, highly protein-bound drugs: May cause toxicity. Monitor patient closely.
Probenecid: May decrease elimination of naproxen. Monitor patient for toxicity.
Drug-herb. *Dong quai, feverfew, garlic, ginger, horse chestnut, red clover:* May cause bleeding, based on the known effects of components. Discourage use together.
White willow: Herb and drug contain similar components. Discourage use together.
Drug-lifestyle. *Alcohol use:* May cause adverse GI reactions. Discourage use together.

EFFECTS ON LAB TEST RESULTS

- May increase BUN, creatinine, ALT, AST, and potassium levels.
- May increase bleeding time.
- May interfere with urinary 5-hydroxyindoleacetic acid and 17-hydroxycorticosteroid determinations.

CONTRAINDICATIONS & CAUTIONS

- Contraindicated in patients hypersensitive to drug and in those with the syndrome of asthma, rhinitis, and nasal polyps.
- Patient should avoid drug during last trimester of pregnancy.
- Use cautiously in elderly patients and in patients with renal disease, CV disease, GI disorders, hepatic disease, or history of peptic ulcer disease.

NURSING CONSIDERATIONS

- Because NSAIDs impair synthesis of renal prostaglandins, they can decrease renal blood flow and lead to reversible renal impairment, especially in patients with renal failure, heart failure, or liver dysfunction; in elderly patients; and in those taking diuretics. Monitor these patients closely.
- Monitor CBC and renal and hepatic function every 4 to 6 months during long-term therapy.
- Serious GI toxicity, including peptic ulcers and bleeding, can occur in patient taking NSAIDs, despite lack of symptoms.
- Because of their antipyretic and anti-inflammatory actions, NSAIDs may mask signs and symptoms of infection.
- Drug may have a heart benefit, similar to aspirin, in preventing blood clotting.

PATIENT TEACHING

- ***Alert:*** Drug is available without prescription (naproxen sodium, 200 mg). Instruct patient not to take more than 600 mg in 24 hours. Dosage in patient older than age 65 shouldn't exceed 400 mg daily.
- Advise patient to take drug with food or milk to minimize GI upset. Tell him to drink a full glass of water or other liquid with each dose.
- Tell patient taking prescription doses for arthritis that full therapeutic effect may be delayed 2 to 4 weeks.
- Warn patient against taking naproxen and naproxen sodium at the same time.
- Teach patient signs and symptoms of GI bleeding, including blood in vomit, urine, or stool; coffee-ground vomit; and black, tarry stool. Tell him to notify prescriber immediately if any of these occur.
- Caution patient that use with aspirin, alcohol, other NSAIDs, or corticosteroids may increase risk of adverse GI reactions.
- Warn patient against hazardous activities that require mental alertness until CNS effects are known.

piroxicam

Apo-Piroxicam†, Feldene, Novo-Pirocam†, Pirox‡

Pharmacologic class: NSAID
Pregnancy risk category B ; D in 3rd trimester

AVAILABLE FORMS

Capsules: 10 mg, 20 mg

INDICATIONS & DOSAGES

➤ **Osteoarthritis, rheumatoid arthritis**
Adults: 20 mg P.O. daily. If desired, dose may be divided b.i.d.

ACTION
May inhibit prostaglandin synthesis, to produce anti-inflammatory, analgesic, and antipyretic effects.

Route	Onset	Peak	Duration
P.O.	1 hr	3–5 hr	48–72 hr

Half-life: 50 hours.

ADVERSE REACTIONS
CNS: *dizziness, headache,* drowsiness, somnolence, vertigo.
CV: peripheral edema.
EENT: auditory disturbances.
GI: ***severe GI bleeding,*** abdominal pain, anorexia, constipation, diarrhea, dyspepsia, epigastric distress, flatulence, heartburn, nausea, occult blood loss, peptic ulceration, stomatitis, vomiting.
GU: ***nephrotoxicity.***
Hematologic: ***agranulocytosis, leukopenia,*** anemia, eosinophilia, prolonged bleeding time.
Metabolic: ***hyperkalemia, hypoglycemia in diabetic patients.***
Skin: *pruritus, rash.*

INTERACTIONS
Drug-drug. *Antihypertensives, diuretics:* May decrease effects of these drugs. Avoid using together.
Aspirin, corticosteroids: May cause GI toxicity and may decrease level of piroxicam. Avoid using together.
Cyclosporine, methotrexate: May increase toxicity. Monitor patient closely.
Lithium: May increase lithium level. Monitor patient for toxicity.
Oral anticoagulants, other highly protein-bound drugs: May be toxic. Monitor patient closely.
Oral antidiabetics: May enhance antidiabetic effects. Monitor patient closely.
Ritonavir: May increase piroxicam level. Avoid using together.
Drug-herb. *Dong quai, feverfew, garlic, ginger, horse chestnut, red clover:* May cause bleeding. Discourage use together.
St. John's wort: May cause photosensitivity reaction. Advise patient to avoid excessive sunlight exposure.
White willow: Herb contains components similar to those of aspirin. Discourage use together.
Drug-lifestyle. *Alcohol use:* May cause GI toxicity and may decrease level of piroxicam. Discourage use together.
Sun exposure: May cause photosensitivity reaction. Advise patient to avoid excessive sunlight exposure.

EFFECTS ON LAB TEST RESULTS
- May increase BUN, creatinine, liver enzyme, and potassium levels. May decrease glucose and hemoglobin levels and hematocrit.
- May decrease WBC, granulocyte, and eosinophil counts.

CONTRAINDICATIONS & CAUTIONS
- Contraindicated in patients hypersensitive to drug and in those with bronchospasm or angioedema precipitated by aspirin or NSAIDs.
- Contraindicated in pregnant or breastfeeding patients.
- Use cautiously in elderly patients and in patients with GI disorders, history of renal or peptic ulcer disease, cardiac disease, hypertension, or conditions predisposing to fluid retention.

NURSING CONSIDERATIONS
- Because NSAIDs impair renal prostaglandin synthesis, they can decrease renal blood flow and lead to reversible renal impairment, especially in elderly patients, those taking diuretics, and those with renal failure, heart failure, or liver dysfunction. Monitor these patients closely.
- Check renal, hepatic, and auditory function and CBC periodically during prolonged therapy. Stop drug and notify prescriber if abnormalities occur.
- Serious GI toxicity, including peptic ulcers and bleeding, can occur in patient taking NSAIDs, despite lack of symptoms.
- NSAIDs may mask signs and symptoms of infection because of their antipyretic and anti-inflammatory actions.

PATIENT TEACHING
- Tell patient to take drug with milk, antacids, or meals if adverse GI reactions occur.
- Inform patient that full therapeutic effects may be delayed for 2 to 4 weeks.

• Teach patient signs and symptoms of GI bleeding, including blood in vomit, urine, or stool; coffee-ground vomit; and black, tarry stool. Tell him to notify prescriber immediately if any of these occur.
• Warn patient against hazardous activities that require mental alertness until CNS effects are known.
• Because drug causes adverse skin reactions more often than other drugs in its class, advise patient to use a sunblock, wear protective clothing, and avoid prolonged exposure to sunlight. Sensitivity to the sun is the most common reaction.
• Advise patient that use of OTC NSAIDs in combination with piroxicam may increase the risk of GI toxicity.

sulindac

Aclin‡, Apo-Sulin†, Clinoril, Novo-Sundac†, Saldac‡

Pharmacologic class: NSAID
Pregnancy risk category B; D in 3rd trimester

AVAILABLE FORMS

Tablets: 100 mg‡, 150 mg, 200 mg

INDICATIONS & DOSAGES

➤ **Osteoarthritis, rheumatoid arthritis, ankylosing spondylitis**
Adults: Initially, 150 mg P.O. b.i.d.; increase to 200 mg b.i.d., p.r.n. Maximum dose is 400 mg daily.

➤ **Acute subacromial bursitis or supraspinatus tendinitis, acute gouty arthritis**
Adults: 200 mg P.O. b.i.d. for 7 to 14 days. Reduce dosage as symptoms subside. Maximum dose is 400 mg daily.

ACTION

May inhibit prostaglandin synthesis, to produce anti-inflammatory, analgesic, and antipyretic effects.

Route	Onset	Peak	Duration
P.O.	Unknown	2–4 hr	Unknown

Half-life: Parent drug, 8 hours; active metabolite, about 16 hours.

ADVERSE REACTIONS

CNS: dizziness, headache, nervousness, psychosis.
CV: ***heart failure,*** edema, hypertension, palpitations.
EENT: tinnitus, transient visual disturbances.
GI: *epigastric distress,* anorexia, constipation, dyspepsia, flatulence, GI bleeding, nausea, occult blood loss, peptic ulceration.
GU: interstitial nephritis.
Hematologic: prolonged bleeding time.
Metabolic: ***hyperkalemia.***
Skin: pruritus, rash.
Other: ***anaphylaxis, angioedema,*** drug fever, hypersensitivity reactions.

INTERACTIONS

Drug-drug. *Anticoagulants:* May cause bleeding. Monitor PT and INR closely.
Aspirin: May decrease sulindac level and increase risk of GI adverse reactions. Avoid using together.
Cyclosporine: May increase nephrotoxicity of cyclosporine. Avoid using together.
Diflunisal, dimethyl sulfoxide: May hinder metabolism of sulindac to its metabolite, reducing its effectiveness. Avoid using together.
Methotrexate: May increase methotrexate toxicity. Avoid using together.
Probenecid: May increase levels of sulindac and its metabolite. Monitor patient for toxicity.
Sulfonamides, sulfonylureas, other highly protein-bound drugs: May cause these drugs to be displaced from protein-binding sites, increasing toxicity. Monitor patient closely.
Drug-herb. *Dong quai, feverfew, garlic, ginger, horse chestnut, red clover:* May cause bleeding, based on the known effects of components. Discourage use together.
White willow: Herb contains components similar to those of aspirin. Discourage use together.
Drug-lifestyle. *Alcohol use:* May increase risk of adverse GI reactions. Discourage use together.

EFFECTS ON LAB TEST RESULTS

• May increase BUN, creatinine, ALT, AST, and potassium levels.

CONTRAINDICATIONS & CAUTIONS

- Contraindicated in patients hypersensitive to drug and in those for whom aspirin or NSAIDs precipitate acute asthmatic attacks, urticaria, or rhinitis.
- Don't use drug in pregnant women.
- Use cautiously in patients with a history of ulcers and GI bleeding, renal dysfunction, compromised cardiac function, hypertension, or conditions predisposing to fluid retention.

NURSING CONSIDERATIONS

- Periodically monitor hepatic and renal function and CBC in patient receiving long-term therapy.
- Serious GI toxicity, including peptic ulcers and bleeding, can occur in patient taking NSAIDs, despite lack of symptoms.
- NSAIDs may mask signs and symptoms of infection.

PATIENT TEACHING

- Tell patient to take drug with food, milk, or antacids.
- Teach patient signs and symptoms of GI bleeding, including blood in vomit, urine, or stool; coffee-ground vomit; and black, tarry stool. Tell him to notify prescriber immediately if any of these occur.
- ***Alert:*** Tell patient to notify prescriber immediately if easy bruising or prolonged bleeding occurs.
- Advise patient to avoid hazardous activities that require mental alertness until CNS effects are known.
- Instruct patient to report edema and have blood pressure checked monthly.
- Advise patient to notify prescriber and have complete eye examination if visual disturbances occur.
- Advise patient that use of OTC NSAIDs in combination with sulindac may increase the risk of GI toxicity.

26
Opioid analgesics

buprenorphine hydrochloride
butorphanol tartrate
codeine phosphate
codeine sulfate
fentanyl citrate
fentanyl iontophoretic transdermal
fentanyl transdermal system
fentanyl transmucosal
hydromorphone hydrochloride
meperidine hydrochloride
methadone hydrochloride
morphine hydrochloride
morphine sulfate
nalbuphine hydrochloride
oxycodone hydrochloride
oxycodone pectinate
oxymorphone hydrochloride
pentazocine hydrochloride
pentazocine hydrochloride and naloxone hydrochloride
pentazocine lactate
propoxyphene hydrochloride
propoxyphene napsylate
tramadol hydrochloride

SAFETY ALERT!

buprenorphine hydrochloride
Buprenex, Subutex, Temgesic‡

Pharmacologic class: opioid agonist-antagonist, opioid partial agonist
Pregnancy risk category C
Controlled substance schedule III

AVAILABLE FORMS
Injection: 0.324 mg (equivalent to 0.3 mg base/ml)
Sublingual tablets: 2 mg, 8 mg (as base)

INDICATIONS & DOSAGES
➤ **Moderate to severe pain**
Adults and children age 13 and older: 0.3 mg I.M. or slow I.V. q 6 hours, p.r.n., or around the clock; repeat dose (up to 0.3 mg), p.r.n., 30 to 60 minutes after first dose.
Children ages 2 to 12: 2 to 6 mcg/kg I.M. or I.V. q 4 to 6 hours.
Elderly patients: Reduce dose by one-half.
Adjust-a-dose: In high-risk patients, such as debilitated patients, reduce dose by one-half.

➤ **Postoperative pain ♦**
Adults: 25 to 250 mcg/hr by continuous I.V. infusion. Or, 60 mcg by epidural administration in single doses, up to a mean total dose of 180 mcg over 48 hours.

➤ **Adjunct to surgical anesthesia with a local anesthetic ♦**
Adults: 0.3 mg by the epidural route.

➤ **Severe, chronic pain in terminally ill patients ♦**
Adults: 0.15 to 0.3 mg by the epidural route q 6 hours, up to a mean total daily dose of 0.86 mg (range 0.15 to 7.2 mg).

➤ **Adjunct to surgical anesthesia during circumcision ♦**
Children ages 9 months to 9 years: 3 mcg/kg I.M., followed by additional 3 mcg/kg doses postoperatively, p.r.n.

➤ **To reverse fentanyl-induced anesthesia and provide analgesia after surgery ♦**
Adults: 0.3 to 0.8 mg I.M. or I.V. 1 to 4 hours after induction of anesthesia and 30 minutes before surgery ends.

➤ **Opioid dependence**
Adults: 12 to 16 mg tablets S.L. as a single daily dose.

I.V. ADMINISTRATION
- When mixed in a 1:1 volume ratio, drug is compatible with atropine sulfate, diphenhydramine hydrochloride, droperidol, glycopyrrolate, haloperidol lactate, hydroxyzine hydrochloride, promethazine hydrochloride, scopolamine hydrochloride, D_5W, 5% dextrose and normal saline solution, sodium chloride solution, lactated Ringer solution, and normal saline solution injections.
- For direct injection, give drug slowly over at least 2 minutes into a vein or through tubing of a free-flowing, compatible I.V. solution.

INCOMPATIBILITIES
Diazepam, furosemide, lorazepam.

ACTION

Unknown. Binds with opiate receptors in the CNS, altering perception of and emotional response to pain.

Route	Onset	Peak	Duration
I.V.	Immediate	2 min	6 hr
I.M.	15 min	1 hr	6 hr
S.L.	Unknown	Unknown	Unknown

Half-life: 1 to 7 hours.

ADVERSE REACTIONS

CNS: *dizziness, sedation, vertigo,* ***increased intracranial pressure,*** asthenia (tablets only), confusion, depression, dreaming, euphoria, fatigue, headache, insomnia (tablets only), nervousness, pain (tablets only), paresthesia, psychosis, slurred speech, weakness.
CV: ***bradycardia,*** cyanosis, flushing, hypertension, hypotension, tachycardia, Wenckebach block.
EENT: blurred vision, conjunctivitis, diplopia, miosis, rhinitis (tablets only), tinnitus, visual abnormalities.
GI: *nausea,* abdominal pain (tablets only), constipation, diarrhea (tablets only), dry mouth, vomiting.
GU: urine retention.
Respiratory: ***respiratory depression,*** dyspnea, hypoventilation.
Skin: diaphoresis, injection site reactions, pruritus, sweating (tablets only).
Other: back pain (tablets only), chills, infection (tablets only), withdrawal syndrome.

INTERACTIONS

Drug-drug. *CNS depressants, MAO inhibitors:* May cause additive effects. Use together cautiously.
CYP3A4 inducers (carbamazepine, phenobarbital, phenytoin, rifampin): May increase clearance of buprenorphine. Monitor patient for clinical effects of drug.
CYP3A4 inhibitors (erythromycin, indinavir, ketoconazole, ritonavir, saquinavir): May decrease clearance of buprenorphine. Monitor patient for increased adverse effects.
Drug-lifestyle. *Alcohol use:* May cause additive effects. Discourage use together.

EFFECTS ON LAB TEST RESULTS

None reported.

CONTRAINDICATIONS & CAUTIONS

- Contraindicated in patients hypersensitive to drug.
- Use cautiously in elderly or debilitated patients; in those undergoing biliary tract surgery; and in those with head injury, intracranial lesions, and increased intracranial pressure; severe respiratory, liver, or kidney impairment; CNS depression or coma; thyroid irregularities; adrenal insufficiency; and prostatic hypertrophy, urethral stricture, acute alcoholism, delirium tremens, or kyphoscoliosis.

NURSING CONSIDERATIONS

- Reassess patient's level of pain 15 and 30 minutes after parenteral administration.
- Buprenorphine 0.3 mg is equal to 10 mg of morphine and 75 mg of meperidine in analgesic potency. It has longer duration of action than morphine or meperidine.
- ***Alert:*** Naloxone won't completely reverse the respiratory depression caused by buprenorphine overdose; an overdose may require mechanical ventilation. Larger-than-usual doses of naloxone (more than 0.4 mg) and doxapram also may be indicated.
- Treat accidental skin exposure by removing exposed clothing and rinsing skin with water.
- Drug may cause constipation. Assess bowel function and need for stool softeners or laxatives.
- ***Alert:*** Drug's opioid antagonist properties may cause withdrawal syndrome in opioid-dependent patients.
- If dependence occurs, withdrawal symptoms may appear up to 14 days after drug is stopped.
- ***Look alike–sound alike:*** Don't confuse Buprenex with Bumex or bupropion.

PATIENT TEACHING

- Caution ambulatory patient about getting out of bed or walking.
- When drug is used after surgery, encourage patient to turn, cough, and breathe deeply to prevent breathing problems.
- Tell patient to place all the tablets of the dose under his tongue until dissolved;

if this is uncomfortable, tell him to take at least two at the same time.

SAFETY ALERT!

butorphanol tartrate
Stadol, Stadol NS

Pharmacologic class: opioid agonist-antagonist, opioid partial agonist
Pregnancy risk category C
Controlled substance schedule IV

AVAILABLE FORMS
Injection: 1 mg/ml, 2 mg/ml
Nasal spray: 10 mg/ml

INDICATIONS & DOSAGES
➤Moderate to severe pain
Adults: 1 to 4 mg I.M. q 3 to 4 hours, p.r.n., or around the clock. Not to exceed 4 mg per dose. Or, 0.5 to 2 mg I.V. q 3 to 4 hours, p.r.n. or around the clock. Or, 1 mg by nasal spray q 3 to 4 hours (1 spray in one nostril); repeat in 60 to 90 minutes if pain relief is inadequate. For severe pain, 2 mg (1 spray in each nostril) q 3 to 4 hours.
Elderly patients: 1 mg I.M. or 0.5 mg I.V., wait 6 hours before repeating dose. For nasal use, 1 mg (1 spray in one nostril). May give another 1 mg in 1.5 to 2 hours. Wait 6 hours before repeating sequence.
Adjust-a-dose: For patients with renal or hepatic impairment, increase dosage interval to 6 to 8 hours.
➤Labor for patients at full term and in early labor
Adults: 1 or 2 mg I.V. or I.M.; repeat after 4 hours, p.r.n.
➤Preoperative anesthesia or preanesthesia
Adults: 2 mg I.M. 60 to 90 minutes before surgery.
➤Adjunct to balanced anesthesia
Adults: 2 mg I.V. shortly before induction, or 0.5 to 1 mg I.V. in increments during anesthesia.
Elderly patients: One-half usual dose at twice the interval for I.V. use.

I.V. ADMINISTRATION
- Compatible solutions include D_5W and normal saline solutions.
- Give by direct injection into a vein or into the tubing of a free-flowing I.V. solution.

INCOMPATIBILITIES
Dimenhydrinate, pentobarbital sodium.

ACTION
May bind with opiate receptors in the CNS, altering perception of and emotional response to pain.

Route	Onset	Peak	Duration
I.V.	1 min	4–5 min	2–4 hr
I.M.	10–30 min	30–60 min	3–4 hr
Nasal	15 min	1–2 hr	2½–5 hr

Half-life: About 2 to 9¼ hours.

ADVERSE REACTIONS
CNS: *dizziness, insomnia, somnolence,* ***increased intracranial pressure,*** anxiety, asthenia, confusion, euphoria, hallucinations, headache, lethargy, nervousness, paresthesia.
CV: flushing, hypotension, palpitations, vasodilation.
EENT: *nasal congestion,* blurred vision, tinnitus.
GI: *nausea, unpleasant taste, vomiting,* anorexia, constipation.
Respiratory: ***respiratory depression.***
Skin: clamminess, excessive diaphoresis, hives, rash.
Other: sensation of heat.

INTERACTIONS
Drug-drug. *CNS depressants:* May cause additive effects. Use together cautiously.
Drug-lifestyle. *Alcohol use:* May cause additive effects. Discourage use together.

EFFECTS ON LAB TEST RESULTS
None reported.

CONTRAINDICATIONS & CAUTIONS
- Contraindicated in patients hypersensitive to drug or to preservative, benzethonium chloride, and in those with opioid addiction; may cause withdrawal syndrome.
- Use cautiously in patients with head injury, increased intracranial pressure, acute MI, ventricular dysfunction, coronary in-

sufficiency, respiratory disease or depression, and renal or hepatic dysfunction.
• Use cautiously in patients who have recently received repeated doses of opioid analgesic.

NURSING CONSIDERATIONS

• Reassess patient's level of pain 15 and 30 minutes after administration.
• Don't give subcutaneously.
• Respiratory depression apparently doesn't increase with larger dosage.
• Drug may cause constipation. Assess bowel function and need for stool softener or laxatives.
• Psychological and physical addiction may occur.
• Periodically monitor postoperative vital signs and bladder function. Because drug decreases both rate and depth of respirations, monitor arterial oxygen saturation to help assess respiratory depression.
• Watch for nasal congestion with nasal spray use.
• ***Look alike–sound alike:*** Don't confuse Stadol with sotalol.

PATIENT TEACHING

• Caution ambulatory patient about getting out of bed or walking. Warn outpatient to avoid driving and other hazardous activities that require mental alertness until it is clear how the drug affects the CNS.
• Teach patient how to take and store nasal spray.
• Instruct patient to avoid alcohol during therapy.

SAFETY ALERT!

codeine phosphate
Paveral†

codeine sulfate

Pharmacologic class: opioid
Pregnancy risk category C
Controlled substance schedule II

AVAILABLE FORMS

codeine phosphate
Injection: 15 mg/ml, 30 mg/ml
Oral solution: 15 mg/5 ml, 10 mg/ml†
codeine sulfate
Tablets: 15 mg, 30 mg, 60 mg

INDICATIONS & DOSAGES

➤ Mild to moderate pain
Adults: 15 to 60 mg P.O. or 15 to 60 mg (phosphate) subcutaneously, I.M., or I.V. q 4 to 6 hours, p.r.n. Maximum daily dose is 360 mg.
Children older than age 1: 0.5 mg/kg P.O., subcutaneously, or I.M. q 4 to 6 hours, p.r.n. Don't give I.V. in children.
➤ Nonproductive cough
Adults: 10 to 20 mg P.O. q 4 to 6 hours. Maximum daily dose is 120 mg.
Children ages 6 to 12: 5 to 10 mg P.O. q 4 to 6 hours. Maximum daily dose is 60 mg.
Children ages 2 to 5: 2.5 to 5 mg P.O. q 4 to 6 hours. Maximum daily dose is 30 mg.

I.V. ADMINISTRATION

• Don't give discolored solution.
• Give drug by direct injection into a large vein. Give very slowly.

INCOMPATIBILITIES

Aminophylline, ammonium chloride, amobarbital, bromides, chlorothiazide, heparin, iodides, pentobarbital, phenobarbital, phenytoin, salts of heavy metals, sodium bicarbonate, sodium iodide, thiopental.

ACTION

May bind with opiate receptors in the CNS, altering perception of and emotional response to pain. Also suppresses the cough reflex by direct action on the cough center in the medulla.

Route	Onset	Peak	Duration
P.O.	30–45 min	1–2 hr	4–6 hr
I.V.	Immediate	Immediate	4–6 hr
I.M.	10–30 min	30–60 min	4–6 hr
SubQ	10–30 min	Unknown	4–6 hr

Half-life: 2½ to 4 hours.

ADVERSE REACTIONS

CNS: *clouded sensorium, sedation,* dizziness, euphoria, light-headedness, physical dependence.
CV: ***bradycardia,*** flushing, hypotension.
GI: *constipation,* dry mouth, ileus, nausea, vomiting.
GU: urine retention.
Respiratory: ***respiratory depression.***
Skin: *diaphoresis,* pruritus.

INTERACTIONS

Drug-drug. *CNS depressants, general anesthetics, hypnotics, MAO inhibitors, other opioid analgesics, sedatives, tranquilizers, tricyclic antidepressants:* May cause additive effects. Use together cautiously; monitor patient response.
Drug-lifestyle. *Alcohol use:* May cause additive effects. Discourage use together.

EFFECTS ON LAB TEST RESULTS

- May increase amylase and lipase levels.

CONTRAINDICATIONS & CAUTIONS

- Contraindicated in patients hypersensitive to drug.
- I.V. use contraindicated in children.
- Use cautiously in elderly or debilitated patients and in those with head injury, increased intracranial pressure, increased CSF pressure, hepatic or renal disease, hypothyroidism, Addison disease, acute alcoholism, seizures, severe CNS depression, bronchial asthma, COPD, respiratory depression, and shock.

NURSING CONSIDERATIONS

- Reassess patient's level of pain at least 15 and 30 minutes after use.
- Codeine and aspirin or acetaminophen are commonly prescribed together to provide enhanced pain relief.
- For full analgesic effect, give drug before patient has intense pain.
- Drug is an antitussive and shouldn't be used when cough is a valuable diagnostic sign or is beneficial (as after thoracic surgery).
- Monitor cough type and frequency.
- Monitor respiratory and circulatory status.
- Opiates may cause constipation. Assess bowel function and need for stool softeners or laxatives.
- Codeine may delay gastric emptying, increase biliary tract pressure from contraction of the sphincter of Oddi, and interfere with hepatobiliary imaging studies.
- ***Look alike–sound alike:*** Don't confuse codeine with Cardene, Lodine, or Cordran.

PATIENT TEACHING

- Advise patient that GI distress caused by taking drug P.O. can be eased by taking drug with milk or meals.
- Instruct patient to ask for or to take drug before pain is intense.
- Caution ambulatory patient about getting out of bed or walking. Warn outpatient to avoid driving and other hazardous activities that require mental alertness until drug's effects on the CNS are known.
- Advise patient to avoid alcohol during therapy.

SAFETY ALERT!

fentanyl citrate
Sublimaze

fentanyl iontophoretic transdermal
Ionsys

fentanyl transdermal system
Duragesic

fentanyl transmucosal
Actiq, Fentora

Pharmacologic class: opioid agonist
Pregnancy risk category C
Controlled substance schedule II

AVAILABLE FORMS

Injection: 50 mcg/ml
Transdermal system: Patches that release 12.5 mcg, 25 mcg, 50 mcg, 75 mcg, or 100 mcg of drug per hour
Transmucosal: 100 mcg, 200 mcg; 400 mcg; 600 mcg; 800 mcg; 1,200 mcg; 1,600 mcg
Iontophoretic transdermal: 40 mcg/dose

INDICATIONS & DOSAGES

➤ **Adjunct to general anesthetic**
Adults: For low-dose therapy, 2 mcg/kg I.V. For moderate-dose therapy, 2 to 20 mcg/kg I.V.; then 25 to 100 mcg I.V., p.r.n. For high-dose therapy, 20 to 50 mcg/kg I.V.; then 25 mcg to one-half initial loading dose I.V., p.r.n.
➤ **Adjunct to regional anesthesia**
Adults: 50 to 100 mcg I.M. or slowly I.V. over 1 to 2 minutes, p.r.n.

➤ **To induce and maintain anesthesia**
Children ages 2 to 12: 2 to 3 mcg/kg I.V.
➤ **Postoperative pain, restlessness, tachypnea, and emergence delirium**
Adults: 50 to 100 mcg I.M. q 1 to 2 hours, p.r.n.
➤ **Preoperative medication**
Adults: 50 to 100 mcg I.M. 30 to 60 minutes before surgery.
➤ **Short-term management of acute postoperative pain in patients requiring opioid analgesia during hospitalization**
Adults: First, use another form of opioid to make patient comfortable. Apply the Ionsys system to intact, nonirritated skin on the chest or upper outer arm. To activate a dose, instruct the patient to firmly press the system's dose-delivery button twice within 3 seconds. Each actuation of the system delivers 40 mcg of fentanyl. An audible beep indicates the start of delivery of each dose and a red light remains on throughout the 10-minute dosing period. A maximum of six 40 mcg doses can be delivered each hour. Each system operates for 80 doses or up to 24 hours. A maximum of three systems can be used sequentially, applied to a different skin site, for a total of 72 hours of pain management.
➤ **To manage persistent, moderate to severe chronic pain in opioid-tolerant patients who require around-the-clock opioid analgesics for an extended time**
Adults and children age 2 and older: When converting to Duragesic, base the first dose on the daily dose, potency, and characteristics of the current opioid therapy; the reliability of the relative potency estimates used to calculate the needed dose; the degree of opioid tolerance; and the patient's condition. Each patch may be worn for 72 hours, although some adult patients may need a patch to be applied q 48 hours during the first dosage period. May increase dose 3 days after the first dose, then q 6 days thereafter.
➤ **To manage breakthrough cancer pain in patients already receiving and tolerating an opioid**
Adults: 200 mcg Actiq initially; may give second dose 15 minutes after completing the first (30 minutes after first lozenge placed in mouth). Maximum dose is 2 lozenges per breakthrough episode. If several episodes of breakthrough pain requiring 2 lozenges occur, dose may be increased to the next available strength. Once a successful dosage has been reached, patient should limit use to no more than 4 lozenges daily.

Or, initially 100 mcg Fentora between the upper cheek and gum. May repeat same dose once per breakthrough episode after at least 30 minutes. Adjust in 100-mcg increments. Doses above 400 mcg can be increased by 200 mcg. Generally, dosage should be increased when patient requires more than one dose per breakthrough episode. Once a successful maintenance dose has been established, re-evaluate if patient experiences more than 4 breakthrough episodes per day.
➤ **Switching from Actiq to Fentora to manage breakthrough cancer pain in opioid-tolerant patients**
Adults: If current Actiq dose is 200 to 400 mcg, start with 100 mcg Fentora; if current Actiq dose is 600 to 800 mcg, use 200 mcg Fentora; if current Actiq dose is 1,200 to 1,600 mcg, use 400 mcg Fentora. Actiq and Fentora aren't bioequivalent.

I.V. ADMINISTRATION
- Only those trained to give I.V. anesthetics and manage adverse effects should give this form.
- Keep opioid antagonist (naloxone) and resuscitation equipment available.
- This form is often used with droperidol to produce neuroleptanalgesia.
- Inject slowly over 1 to 2 minutes.

INCOMPATIBILITIES
Azithromycin, fluorouracil, lidocaine, methohexital, pentobarbital sodium, phenytoin, thiopental.

ACTION
Unknown. Binds with opiate receptors in the CNS, altering perception of and emotional response to pain.

Route	Onset	Peak	Duration
I.V.	1–2 min	3–5 min	30–60 min
I.M.	7–15 min	20–30 min	1–2 hr
Transdermal	12–24 hr	1–3 days	Variable
Transmucosal	5–15 min	20–30 min	Unknown

Half-life: 3½ hours after parenteral use; 5 to 15 hours after transmucosal use; 18 hours after transdermal use.

ADVERSE REACTIONS

CNS: *asthenia, clouded sensorium, confusion, euphoria, sedation, somnolence,* ***seizures,*** anxiety, depression, dizziness, hallucinations, headache, nervousness.
CV: ***arrhythmias,*** chest pain, hypertension, hypotension.
GI: *constipation,* abdominal pain, anorexia, diarrhea, dyspepsia, dry mouth, ileus, nausea, vomiting.
GU: urine retention.
Musculoskeletal: skeletal muscle rigidity (dose-related).
Respiratory: ***apnea, hypoventilation, respiratory depression,*** dyspnea.
Skin: *diaphoresis, pruritus,* erythema at application site (transdermal).
Other: physical dependence.

INTERACTIONS

Drug-drug. *Amiodarone:* May cause hypotension, bradycardia, and decreased cardiac output. Monitor patient closely.
CNS depressants, general anesthetics, hypnotics, MAO inhibitors, other opioid analgesics, sedatives, tricyclic antidepressants: May cause additive effects. Use together cautiously. Reduce dosages of these drugs and reduce fentanyl dose by one-fourth to one-third.
CYP3A4 inducers (carbamazepine, phenytoin, rifampin): May decrease analgesic effects. Monitor patient for adequate pain relief.
Diazepam: May cause CV depression when given with high doses of fentanyl. Monitor patient closely.
Droperidol: May cause hypotension and decrease pulmonary arterial pressure. Use together cautiously.
Potent CYP3A4 inhibitors (clarithromycin, erythromycin, itraconazole, ketoconazole, nefazodone, nelfinavir, ritonavir, troleandomycin): May cause increased analgesia, CNS depression, and hypotensive effects. Monitor patient's respiratory status and vital signs.
Protease inhibitors: May increase fentanyl levels and adverse effects. Monitor patient closely for respiratory depression.
Drug-lifestyle. *Alcohol use:* May cause additive effects. Discourage use together.

EFFECTS ON LAB TEST RESULTS

- May increase amylase and lipase levels.

CONTRAINDICATIONS & CAUTIONS

- Contraindicated in patients intolerant to drug.
- Transdermal form is contraindicated in patients hypersensitive to adhesives, those who aren't opioid tolerant, those who need postoperative pain management, and those with acute, mild, or intermittent pain that can be managed with nonopioids. Don't use in patients with increased intracranial pressure, head injury, impaired consciousness, or coma.
- Actiq is contraindicated in children and in those who need acute or postoperative pain management.
- Use with caution in patients with brain tumors, COPD, decreased respiratory reserve, potentially compromised respirations, hepatic or renal disease, or cardiac bradyarrhythmias.
- Use with caution in elderly or debilitated patients.

NURSING CONSIDERATIONS

- For better analgesic effect, give drug before patient has intense pain.
- ***Alert:*** High doses can produce muscle rigidity, which can be reversed with neuromuscular blockers; however, patient must be artificially ventilated.
- Monitor circulatory and respiratory status and urinary function carefully. Drug may cause respiratory depression, hypotension, urine retention, nausea, vomiting, ileus, or altered level of consciousness, no matter how it's given.
- Periodically monitor postoperative vital signs and bladder function. Because drug decreases both rate and depth of respirations, monitoring of arterial oxygen saturation (SaO_2) may help assess respiratory depression. Immediately report respira-

tory rate below 12 breaths/minute, decreased respiratory volume, or decreased SaO_2.
• Drug may cause constipation. Assess bowel function and need for stool softeners or laxatives.

Transdermal form

• Dosage equivalent charts are available to calculate the fentanyl transdermal dose based on the daily morphine intake; for example, for every 90 mg of oral morphine or 15 mg of I.M. morphine per 24 hours, 25 mcg/hour of transdermal fentanyl is needed.
• ***Alert:*** Transdermal drug levels peak between 24 and 72 hours after initial application and dose increases. Monitor patients for life-threatening hypoventilation, especially during these times.
• Make dosage adjustments gradually in patient using the transdermal system. Reaching steady-state level of a new dosage may take up to 6 days; delay dosage adjustment until after at least two applications.
• Monitor patient who develops adverse reactions to the transdermal system for at least 12 hours after removal. Drug level drops gradually and may take as long as 17 hours to decline by 50%.
• Most patients experience good control of pain for 3 days while wearing the transdermal system, but a few may need a new application after 48 hours.
• Because the drug level rises for the first 24 hours after application, analgesic effect can't be evaluated on the first day. Make sure patient has adequate supplemental analgesic to prevent breakthrough pain.
• When reducing opioid therapy or switching to a different analgesic, withdraw the transdermal system gradually. Because the drug level drops gradually after removal, give half the equianalgesic dose of the new analgesic 12 to 18 hours after removal.
• ***Alert:*** Only the patient should activate the Ionsys transdermal system.

Transmucosal form

• ***Alert:*** Fentora and Actiq are used only to manage breakthrough cancer pain in patients who are already receiving and tolerating opioids.
• ***Alert:*** Fentora and Actiq aren't bioequivalent and can't be substituted on a mcg per mcg basis.
• Remove foil just before giving.
• Place tablet or lozenge between the cheek and gum and allow to dissolve over about 15 to 20 minutes. Actiq may be moved from one side to the other using the stick. Don't allow patient to bite, suck, or chew the tablets or lozenge. Discard Actiq stick in the trash after use or, if any drug matrix remains on the stick, place under hot running tap water until dissolved or place in child-resistant container provided, and discard as appropriate for schedule II drugs.
• ***Look alike–sound alike:*** Don't confuse fentanyl with alfentanil.

PATIENT TEACHING

• When drug is used for pain control, instruct patient to request drug before pain becomes intense.
• ***Alert:*** Inform family members only the patient should activate the Ionsys system for pain control to decrease the risk of fatal respiratory depression.
• When drug is used after surgery, encourage patient to turn, cough, and breathe deeply to prevent lung problems.
• Instruct patient to avoid hazardous activities until CNS effects subside.
• Tell home care patient to avoid drinking alcohol or taking other CNS-type drugs because additive effects can occur.
• Advise patient not to stop drug abruptly.
• Teach patient about proper application of transdermal patch. Tell patient to clip hair at application site, but not to use a razor, which may irritate skin. Wash area with clear water, if needed, but not with soaps, oils, lotions, alcohol, or other substances that may irritate skin or prevent adhesion. Dry area completely before application.
• Tell patient to remove transdermal system from package just before applying, hold in place for 30 seconds, and be sure the edges of patch stick to skin.
• ***Alert:*** Teach patient not to alter the transdermal patch (such as by cutting it) before applying.
• Advise parent or caregiver to place transdermal patch on the upper back for a child or a patient who's cognitively im-

paired, to reduce the chance the patch will be removed and placed in the mouth.
- Teach patient to dispose of the transdermal patch by folding it so the adhesive side adheres to itself and then flushing it down the toilet.
- Tell patient that, if another patch is needed after 48 to 72 hours, he should apply it to a different skin site.
- Tell patient that pain relief with the patch may not occur for several hours after the patch is applied. Oral, immediate release opioids may be needed for initial pain relief
- Inform patient that heat from fever or environment, such as from heating pads, electric blankets, heat lamps, hot tubs, or water beds, may increase transdermal delivery and cause toxicity requiring dosage adjustment. Instruct patient to notify prescriber if fever occurs or if he'll be spending time in a hot climate.
- ***Alert:*** Warn patient and patient's family that the amount of drug in one Actiq lozenge or Fentora tablet can be fatal to a child. Keep well secured and out of children's reach.

SAFETY ALERT!

hydromorphone hydrochloride (dihydromorphinone hydrochloride)

Dilaudid, Dilaudid-5, Dilaudid-HP

Pharmacologic class: opioid
Pregnancy risk category C
Controlled substance schedule II

AVAILABLE FORMS

Cough syrup: 1 mg/5 ml
Injection: 1 mg/ml, 2 mg/ml, 3 mg/ml, 4 mg/ml, 10 mg/ml
Liquid: 5 mg/5 ml
Lyophilized powder for injection: 10 mg/ml
Suppositories: 3 mg
Tablets: 1 mg, 2 mg, 3 mg, 4 mg, 8 mg

INDICATIONS & DOSAGES

➤ Moderate to severe pain

Adults: 2 to 4 mg P.O. q 4 to 6 hours, p.r.n. Or, 1 to 4 mg I.M., subcutaneously, or I.V. (slowly over at least 2 to 5 minutes) q 4 to 6 hours, p.r.n. Or, 3 mg P.R. suppository q 6 to 8 hours, p.r.n.

➤ Cough

Adults and children older than age 12: 1 mg cough syrup P.O. q 3 to 4 hours, p.r.n.
Children ages 6 to 12 years: 0.5 mg cough syrup P.O. q 3 to 4 hours, p.r.n.

I.V. ADMINISTRATION

- For infusion, drug may be mixed in D_5W, normal saline solution, dextrose 5% in normal saline solution, dextrose 5% in half-normal saline solution, or Ringer or lactated Ringer solutions.
- Give by direct injection over no less than 2 minutes.
- Respiratory depression and hypotension can occur. Give slowly, and monitor patient constantly. Keep resuscitation equipment available.

INCOMPATIBILITIES

Alkalies, amphotericin B cholesterol complex, ampicillin sodium, bromides, cefazolin, dexamethasone, diazepam, gallium nitrate, haloperidol, heparin sodium, iodides, minocycline, phenobarbital sodium, phenytoin sodium, prochlorperazine edisylate, sargramostim, sodium bicarbonate, sodium phosphate, thiopental.

ACTION

Unknown. Binds with opiate receptors in the CNS, altering perception of and emotional response to pain. Also suppresses the cough reflex by direct action on the cough center in the medulla.

Route	Onset	Peak	Duration
P.O.	15–30 min	30–60 min	4–5 hr
I.V.	10–15 min	15–30 min	2–3 hr
I.M.	15 min	30–60 min	4–5 hr
SubQ	15 min	30–90 min	4 hr
P.R.	Unknown	Unknown	4 hr

Half-life: 2½ to 4 hours.

ADVERSE REACTIONS

CNS: sedation, somnolence, clouded sensorium, dizziness, euphoria, lightheadedness.
CV: hypotension, flushing, ***bradycardia.***

EENT: blurred vision, diplopia, nystagmus.
GI: nausea, vomiting, *constipation,* ileus, dry mouth.
GU: urine retention.
Respiratory: ***respiratory depression, bronchospasm.***
Skin: diaphoresis, pruritus.
Other: induration with repeated subcutaneous injections, physical dependence.

INTERACTIONS

Drug-drug. *CNS depressants, general anesthetics, hypnotics, MAO inhibitors, other opioid analgesics, sedatives, tranquilizers, tricyclic antidepressants:* May cause additive effects. Use together with caution; reduce hydromorphone dose and monitor patient response.
Drug-lifestyle. *Alcohol use:* May cause additive effects. Advise patient to use together cautiously.

EFFECTS ON LAB TEST RESULTS

- May increase amylase and lipase levels.
- May interfere with hepatobiliary imaging studies because delayed gastric emptying and contraction of sphincter of Oddi may increase biliary tract pressure.

CONTRAINDICATIONS & CAUTIONS

- Contraindicated in patients hypersensitive to drug; in those with intracranial lesions that cause increased intracranial pressure; and in those with depressed ventilation, such as in status asthmaticus, COPD, cor pulmonale, emphysema, and kyphoscoliosis.
- Use with caution in elderly or debilitated patients and in those with hepatic or renal disease, hypothyroidism, Addison disease, prostatic hyperplasia, or urethral stricture.

NURSING CONSIDERATIONS

- Reassess patient's level of pain at least 15 and 30 minutes after administration.
- For better analgesic effect, give drug on a regular schedule, before patient has intense pain.
- Dilaudid-HP, a highly concentrated form (10 mg/ml), may be given in smaller volumes to prevent the discomfort of large-volume I.M. or subcutaneous injections. Check dosage carefully.
- Rotate injection sites to avoid induration with subcutaneous injection.
- Monitor respiratory and circulatory status and bowel function.
- Keep opioid antagonist (naloxone) available.
- Drug may worsen or mask gallbladder pain.
- Drug is a commonly abused opioid.
- ***Alert:*** Cough syrup may contain tartrazine.
- ***Look alike–sound alike:*** Don't confuse hydromorphone with morphine or oxymorphone or Dilaudid with Dilantin.

PATIENT TEACHING

- Instruct patient to request or take drug before pain becomes intense.
- Tell patient to store suppositories in refrigerator.
- Advise patient to take drug with food if GI upset occurs.
- When drug is used after surgery, encourage patient to turn, cough, and breathe deeply to avoid lung problems.
- Caution patient about getting out of bed or walking. Warn outpatient to avoid hazardous activities that require mental alertness until drug's CNS effects are known.
- Advise patient to avoid alcohol during therapy.

SAFETY ALERT!

meperidine hydrochloride (pethidine hydrochloride)

Demerol✐

Pharmacologic class: opioid
Pregnancy risk category B; D if used for prolonged periods or in high doses at term
Controlled substance schedule II

AVAILABLE FORMS

Injection: 10 mg/ml, 25 mg/ml, 50 mg/ml, 75 mg/ml, 100 mg/ml
Syrup: 50 mg/5 ml
Tablets: 50 mg, 100 mg

INDICATIONS & DOSAGES

➤ **Moderate to severe pain**
Adults: 50 to 150 mg P.O., I.M., or subcutaneously q 3 to 4 hours, p.r.n.

Children: 1.1 to 1.8 mg/kg P.O., I.M., or subcutaneously q 3 to 4 hours. Maximum, 100 mg q 4 hours, p.r.n.

➤ **Preoperative analgesia**
Adults: 50 to 100 mg I.M. or subcutaneously 30 to 90 minutes before surgery.
Children: 1 to 2.2 mg/kg I.M. or subcutaneously up to the adult dose 30 to 90 minutes before surgery.

➤ **Adjunct to anesthesia**
Adults: Repeated slow I.V. injections of fractional doses (10 mg/ml). Or, continuous I.V. infusion of a more dilute solution (1 mg/ml) titrated to patient's needs.

➤ **Obstetric analgesia**
Adults: 50 to 100 mg I.M. or subcutaneously when pain becomes regular; repeated at 1- to 3-hour intervals.

I.V. ADMINISTRATION

- Keep opioid antagonist (naloxone) available.
- Give drug slowly by direct injection.
- Drug may also be given by slow continuous infusion. Drug is compatible with most solutions, including D_5W, normal saline solution, and Ringer or lactated Ringer solutions.
- Protect from light and store at room temperature.

INCOMPATIBILITIES

Acyclovir, allopurinol, aminophylline, amobarbital, amphotericin B, cefepime, cefoperazone, doxorubicin liposomal, ephedrine, furosemide, heparin, hydrocortisone sodium succinate, idarubicin, imipenem and cilastatin sodium, methylprednisolone sodium succinate, morphine, pentobarbital, phenobarbital sodium, phenytoin, sodium bicarbonate, sodium iodide, thiopental.

ACTION

Unknown. Binds with opiate receptors in the CNS, altering perception of and emotional response to pain.

Route	Onset	Peak	Duration
P.O.	15 min	60–90 min	2–4 hr
I.V.	1 min	5–7 min	2–4 hr
I.M., SubQ	10–15 min	30–50 min	2–4 hr

Half-life: 2½ to 4 hours.

ADVERSE REACTIONS

CNS: *clouded sensorium, dizziness, euphoria, light-headedness, sedation, somnolence,* ***seizures,*** hallucinations, headache, paradoxical anxiety, physical dependence, syncope, tremor.
CV: ***bradycardia, cardiac arrest, shock,*** hypotension, tachycardia.
GI: biliary tract spasms, constipation, dry mouth, ileus, *nausea, vomiting.*
GU: urine retention.
Musculoskeletal: muscle twitching.
Respiratory: ***respiratory arrest, respiratory depression.***
Skin: *diaphoresis,* pruritus, urticaria.
Other: induration, local tissue irritation, pain at injection site, phlebitis after I.V. delivery.

INTERACTIONS

Drug-drug. *Aminophylline, barbiturates, heparin, methicillin, morphine sulfate, phenytoin, sodium bicarbonate, sulfonamides:* Incompatible when mixed in same I.V. container. Avoid using together.
Cimetidine: May increase respiratory and CNS depression. Monitor patient closely.
Chlorpromazine: May cause excessive sedation and hypotension. Avoid using together.
CNS depressants, general anesthetics, hypnotics, other opioid analgesics, phenothiazines, sedatives, tricyclic antidepressants: May cause respiratory depression, hypotension, profound sedation, or coma. Use together with caution; reduce meperidine dosage.
MAO inhibitors: May increase CNS excitation or depression that can be severe or fatal. Avoid using together.
Phenytoin: May decrease meperidine level. Watch for decreased analgesia.
Protease inhibitors: May increase respiratory and CNS depression. Avoid using together.
Ritonavir: May significantly increase level and toxic effects of meperidine. Avoid using together.
Drug-lifestyle. *Alcohol use:* May cause additive effects. Discourage use together.

EFFECTS ON LAB TEST RESULTS

- May increase amylase and lipase levels.

CONTRAINDICATIONS & CAUTIONS

- Contraindicated in patients hypersensitive to drug and in those who have received MAO inhibitors within past 14 days.
- Avoid use in patients with end-stage renal disease.
- Use with caution in elderly or debilitated patients and in those with increased intracranial pressure, head injury, asthma and other respiratory conditions, supraventricular tachycardias, seizures, acute abdominal conditions, hepatic or renal disease, hypothyroidism, Addison disease, urethral stricture, and prostatic hyperplasia.

NURSING CONSIDERATIONS

- In elderly patients or in those with renal dysfunction, active metabolite may accumulate, causing increased adverse CNS reactions.
- Drug may be used in some patients who are allergic to morphine.
- Reassess patient's level of pain at least 15 and 30 minutes after administration.
- Subcutaneous injection isn't recommended because it's very painful, but it may be suitable for occasional use. Monitor patient for pain at injection site, local tissue irritation, and induration after subcutaneous injection.
- ***Alert:*** Oral dose is less than half as effective as parenteral dose. Give I.M. if possible. When changing from parenteral to oral route, increase dosage.
- Syrup has local anesthetic effect. Give with full glass of water.
- Because drug toxicity frequently appears after several days of treatment, drug isn't recommended for treatment of chronic pain.
- In neonates exposed to drug during labor, monitor respirations. Have resuscitation equipment and naloxone available.
- Monitor respiratory and CV status carefully. Don't give if respirations are below 12 breaths/minute, if respiratory rate or depth is decreased, or if change in pupils is noted.
- If drug is stopped abruptly after long-term use, monitor patient for withdrawal symptoms.
- In postoperative patients, monitor bladder function.
- Monitor bowel function. Patient may need a laxative or stool softener.
- ***Look alike–sound alike:*** Don't confuse Demerol with Demulen.

PATIENT TEACHING

- Encourage postoperative patient to turn, cough, deep-breathe, and use an incentive spirometer to prevent lung problems.
- Caution ambulatory patient about getting out of bed or walking. Warn outpatient to avoid driving and other potentially hazardous activities that require mental alertness until drug's CNS effects are known.
- Advise patient to avoid alcohol during therapy.
- Caution patient that drug isn't intended for long-term use.

SAFETY ALERT!

methadone hydrochloride

Dolophine, Methadose, Physeptone‡

Pharmacologic class: opiate agonist
Pregnancy risk category C
Controlled substance schedule II

AVAILABLE FORMS

Dispersible tablets (for methadone maintenance therapy): 40 mg
Injection: 10 mg/ml
Oral solution: 5 mg/5 ml, 10 mg/5 ml, 10 mg/ml (concentrate)
Tablets: 5 mg, 10 mg

INDICATIONS & DOSAGES

➤ **Severe pain**
Adults: 2.5 to 10 mg P.O., I.M., or subcutaneously q 3 to 4 hours, p.r.n.

➤ **Severe chronic pain**
Adults: 5 to 20 mg P.O. q. 6 to 8 hours, p.r.n.

➤ **Opioid withdrawal syndrome**
Adults: 15 to 20 mg P.O. daily often suppresses withdrawal symptoms (highly individualized; some patients may require a higher dose). Maintenance dose is 20 to 120 mg P.O. daily. Dosage adjusted, p.r.n.

ACTION

Unknown. Binds with opiate receptors in the CNS, altering perception of and emotional response to pain.

Route	Onset	Peak	Duration
P.O.	30–60 min	90–120 min	4–6 hr
I.M., SubQ	10–20 min	1–2 hr	4–5 hr

Half-life: 15 to 25 hours.

ADVERSE REACTIONS

CNS: *clouded sensorium, dizziness, lightheadedness, sedation, somnolence, **seizures,*** agitation, choreic movements, euphoria, headache, insomnia, syncope.
CV: ***arrhythmias, bradycardia, cardiac arrest, shock,*** edema, hypotension, palpitations.
EENT: visual disturbances.
GI: *nausea, vomiting,* anorexia, biliary tract spasm, constipation, dry mouth, ileus.
GU: urine retention.
Respiratory: ***respiratory arrest, respiratory depression.***
Skin: diaphoresis, pruritus, urticaria.
Other: decreased libido, induration, pain at injection site, physical dependence, tissue irritation.

INTERACTIONS

Drug-drug. *Ammonium chloride, other urine acidifiers, phenytoin:* May reduce methadone effect. Watch for decreased pain control.
CNS depressants, general anesthetics, hypnotics, MAO inhibitors, sedatives, tranquilizers, tricyclic antidepressants: May cause respiratory depression, hypotension, profound sedation, or coma. Use together with caution. Monitor patient response.
Nonnucleoside reverse transcriptase inhibitors (delavirdine, efavirenz, nevirapine), protease inhibitors (lopinavir and ritonavir, nelfinavir, ritonavir), rifamycins: May increase methadone metabolism causing opiate withdrawal symptoms. Monitor patient and adjust dose as needed.
Protease inhibitors, cimetidine, fluvoxamine: May increase respiratory and CNS depression. Monitor patient closely.
Drug-lifestyle. *Alcohol use:* May cause additive effects. Discourage use together.

EFFECTS ON LAB TEST RESULTS

- May increase amylase level.

CONTRAINDICATIONS & CAUTIONS

- Contraindicated in patients hypersensitive to drug.
- Use with caution in elderly or debilitated patients and in those with acute abdominal conditions, severe hepatic or renal impairment, hypothyroidism, Addison disease, prostatic hyperplasia, urethral stricture, head injury, increased intracranial pressure, asthma, and other respiratory conditions.

NURSING CONSIDERATIONS

- Reassess patient's level of pain at least 15 and 30 minutes after parenteral administration and 30 minutes after oral administration.
- When used in opioid withdrawal syndrome, daily doses of more than 120 mg require special state and federal approval.
- Oral liquid form legally required in maintenance programs. Completely dissolve tablets in ½ cup of orange juice or powdered citrus drink.
- For parenteral use, I.M. injection is preferred. Rotate injection sites.
- Monitor patient for pain at injection site, tissue irritation, and induration after subcutaneous injection.
- Oral dose is one-half as potent as injected dose.
- An around-the-clock regimen is needed to manage severe, chronic pain.
- Patient treated for opioid withdrawal syndrome usually needs an additional analgesic if pain control is needed.
- Monitor patient closely because drug has cumulative effect; marked sedation can occur after repeated doses.
- Monitor circulatory and respiratory status and bladder and bowel function. Patient may need a stool softener or laxative.
- When used as an adjunct in the treatment of opioid addiction (maintenance), withdrawal is usually delayed and mild.
- ***Alert:*** High doses of methadone may cause or contribute to torsades de pointes and a prolonged QT interval.

PATIENT TEACHING

- Caution ambulatory patient about getting out of bed or walking. Warn outpatient to avoid hazardous activities that require mental alertness until drug's CNS effects are known.
- Instruct patient to increase fluid and fiber in diet, if not contraindicated, to combat constipation.
- Advise patient to avoid alcohol during therapy.

SAFETY ALERT!

morphine hydrochloride
Morphitec†, M.O.S†, M.O.S.-S.R†

morphine sulfate
Anamorph‡, Astramorph PF, Avinza, DepoDur, Duramorph, Epimorph†, Infumorph, Infumorph 500, Kadian, M-Eslon†, Morphine H.P†, MS Contin, MSIR, Oramorph SR, RMS Uniserts, Roxanol, Statex†

Pharmacologic class: opioid
Pregnancy risk category C
Controlled substance schedule II

AVAILABLE FORMS

morphine hydrochloride
Oral solution: 1 mg/ml†, 5 mg/ml†, 10 mg/ml†, 20 mg/ml†, 50 mg/ml†
Suppositories: 10 mg†, 20 mg†, 30 mg†
Syrup: 1 mg/ml*†, 5 mg/ml*†, 10 mg/ml*†, 20 mg/ml*†, 50 mg/ml*†
Tablets: 10 mg†, 20 mg†, 40 mg†, 60 mg†
Tablets (extended-release): 30 mg†, 60 mg†

morphine sulfate
Capsules: 15 mg, 30 mg
Capsules (extended-release beads): 30 mg, 60 mg, 90 mg, 120 mg
Capsules (extended-release pellets): 20 mg, 30 mg, 50 mg, 60 mg, 80 mg, 100 mg
Injection (with preservative): 0.5 mg/ml, 1 mg/ml, 2 mg/ml, 4 mg/ml, 5 mg/ml, 8 mg/ml, 10 mg/ml, 15 mg/ml, 25 mg/ml, 50 mg/ml
Injection (without preservative): 0.5 mg/ml, 1 mg/ml, 10 mg/ml, 15 mg/ml, 25 mg/ml
Oral solution: 10 mg/5 ml, 20 mg/5 ml, 20 mg/ml (concentrate), 100 mg/5 ml (concentrate)
Soluble tablets: 10 mg, 15 mg, 30 mg
Suppositories: 5 mg, 10 mg, 20 mg, 30 mg
Tablets: 15 mg, 30 mg
Tablets (extended-release): 15 mg, 30 mg, 60 mg, 100 mg, 200 mg

INDICATIONS & DOSAGES

➤ **Severe pain**

Adults: 5 to 20 mg subcutaneously or I.M. or 2.5 to 15 mg I.V. q 4 hours, p.r.n. Or, 5 to 30 mg P.O. or 10 to 20 mg P.R. q 4 hours, p.r.n.

For continuous I.V. infusion, give loading dose of 15 mg I.V.; then continuous infusion of 0.8 to 10 mg/hour.

For extended-release tablet, give 15 or 30 mg P.O,. q 8 to 12 hours.

For extended-release Kadian capsules used as a first opioid, give 20 mg P.O. q 12 hours or 40 mg P.O. once daily; increase conservatively in opioid-naive patients.

For epidural injection, give 5 mg by epidural catheter; then, if pain isn't relieved adequately in 1 hour, give supplementary doses of 1 to 2 mg at intervals sufficient to assess effectiveness. Maximum total epidural dose shouldn't exceed 10 mg/24 hours.

For intrathecal injection, a single dose of 0.2 to 1 mg may provide pain relief for 24 hours (only in the lumbar area). Don't repeat injections.

Children: 0.1 to 0.2 mg/kg subcutaneously or I.M. q 4 hours. Maximum single dose, 15 mg.

➤ **Moderate to severe pain requiring continuous, around-the-clock opioid**

Adults: Individualize dosage of Avinza. For patients with no tolerance to opioids, begin with 30 mg Avinza P.O. daily; adjust dosage by no more than 30 mg q 4 days. When converting from another oral morphine form, individualize the dosage schedule according to patient's schedule.

➤ **Single-dose, epidural extended pain relief after major surgery**

Adults: Inject 10 to 15 mg (maximum 20 mg) DepoDur via lumbar epidural administration before surgery or after clamping of umbilical cord during cesarean section. May be injected undiluted or may be diluted up to 5 ml total volume with preservative-free normal saline solution.

I.V. ADMINISTRATION

- For direct injection, dilute 2.5 to 15 mg in 4 or 5 ml of sterile water for injection and give slowly over 4 to 5 minutes.
- For continuous infusion, mix drug with D_5W to yield 0.1 to 1 mg/ml and give by a continuous infusion device.
- In adults with severe, chronic pain, maintenance I.V. infusion is 0.8 to 80 mg/hour; sometimes higher doses are needed.
- Don't mix DepoDur with other drugs. Once DepoDur is given, don't give any other drugs into epidural space for at least 48 hours. Don't use in-line filter during administration.
- Store DepoDur in refrigerator. Unopened vials can be stored at room temperature for up to 7 days. After drug is withdrawn from vial, it can be stored at room temperature for up to 4 hours before use.

INCOMPATIBILITIES

Aminophylline, amobarbital, cefepime, chlorothiazide, fluorouracil, haloperidol, heparin sodium, meperidine, pentobarbital, phenobarbital sodium, phenytoin sodium, prochlorperazine, promethazine hydrochloride, sodium bicarbonate, thiopental.

ACTION

Unknown. Binds with opiate receptors in the CNS, altering perception of and emotional response to pain.

Route	Onset	Peak	Duration
P.O.	1 hr	1–2 hr	4–12 hr
P.O. (morphine sulfate)	30 min	Unknown	24 hr
I.V.	5 min	20 min	4–5 hr
I.M.	10–30 min	30–60 min	4–5 hr
SubQ	10–30 min	50–90 min	4–5 hr
P.R.	20–60 min	20–60 min	4–5 hr
Epidural	15–60 min	15–60 min	24 hr
Intrathecal	15–60 min	30–60 min	24 hr

Half-life: 2 to 3 hours.

ADVERSE REACTIONS

CNS: *dizziness, euphoria, light-headedness, nightmares, sedation, somnolence,* ***seizures,*** depression, hallucinations, nervousness, physical dependence, syncope.
CV: ***bradycardia, cardiac arrest, shock,*** hypertension, hypotension, tachycardia.
GI: *constipation, nausea, vomiting,* anorexia, biliary tract spasms, dry mouth, ileus.
GU: urine retention.
Hematologic: ***thrombocytopenia.***
Respiratory: ***apnea, respiratory arrest, respiratory depression.***
Skin: diaphoresis, edema, pruritus and skin flushing.
Other: decreased libido.

INTERACTIONS

Drug-drug. *Cimetidine:* May increase respiratory and CNS depression when given with morphine sulfate. Monitor patient closely.
CNS depressants, general anesthetics, hypnotics, MAO inhibitors, other opioid analgesics, sedatives, tranquilizers, tricyclic antidepressants: May cause respiratory depression, hypotension, profound sedation, or coma. Use together with caution, reduce morphine dose, and monitor patient response.
Drug-lifestyle. *Alcohol use:* May cause the extended-release capsules' protective coating to fail, causing overdose. Warn patient to avoid alcohol.

EFFECTS ON LAB TEST RESULTS

- May increase amylase level. May decrease hemoglobin level (morphine sulfate).
- May decrease platelet count. May cause abnormal liver function test values (morphine sulfate).

CONTRAINDICATIONS & CAUTIONS

- Contraindicated in patients hypersensitive to drug and in those with conditions that would preclude administration of opioids by I.V. route (acute bronchial asthma or upper airway obstruction).
- Contraindicated in patients with GI obstruction.
- Use with caution in elderly or debilitated patients and in those with head

injury, increased intracranial pressure, seizures, chronic pulmonary disease, prostatic hyperplasia, severe hepatic or renal disease, acute abdominal conditions, hypothyroidism, Addison disease, and urethral stricture.
• Use with caution in patients with circulatory shock, biliary tract disease, CNS depression, toxic psychosis, acute alcoholism, delirium tremens, and seizure disorders.

NURSING CONSIDERATIONS
• Reassess patient's level of pain at least 15 and 30 minutes after giving parenterally and 30 minutes after giving orally.
• Keep opioid antagonist (naloxone) and resuscitation equipment available.
• Monitor circulatory, respiratory, bladder, and bowel functions carefully. Drug may cause respiratory depression, hypotension, urine retention, nausea, vomiting, ileus, or altered level of consciousness regardless of the route. If respirations drop below 12 breaths/minute, withhold dose and notify prescriber.
• Oral solutions of various concentrations and an intensified oral solution (20 mg/ml) are available. Carefully note the strength given.
• Oral capsules may be carefully opened and the entire contents poured into cool, soft foods, such as water, orange juice, applesauce, or pudding; patient should consume mixture immediately.
• For S.L. use, measure oral solution with tuberculin syringe. Give dose a few drops at a time to allow maximal S.L. absorption and minimize swallowing.
• Preservative-free preparations are available for epidural and intrathecal use.
• When drug is given epidurally, monitor patient closely for respiratory depression up to 24 hours after the injection. Check respiratory rate and depth every 30 to 60 minutes for 24 hours. Watch for pruritus and skin flushing.
• Morphine is drug of choice in relieving MI pain; may cause transient decrease in blood pressure.
• An around-the-clock regimen best manages severe, chronic pain.
• Morphine may worsen or mask gallbladder pain.
• Constipation is commonly severe with maintenance dose. Ensure that stool softener or other laxative is ordered.
• Give morphine sulfate without regard to food.
• Taper morphine sulfate therapy gradually when stopping therapy.
• Refrigeration of rectal suppository isn't needed.
• ***Look alike–sound alike:*** Don't confuse morphine with hydromorphone or Avinza with Invanz.

PATIENT TEACHING
• When drug is used after surgery, encourage patient to turn, cough, deep-breathe, and use incentive spirometer to prevent lung problems.
• Caution ambulatory patient about getting out of bed or walking. Warn outpatient to avoid driving and other potentially hazardous activities that require mental alertness until drug's adverse CNS effects are known.
• ***Alert:*** Drinking alcohol or taking drugs containing alcohol while taking extended-release capsules may cause the drug's protective coating to fail, releasing a potentially fatal dose of morphine. Warn patient to read labels on OTC drugs carefully and not to use alcohol in any form.
• Tell patient to swallow morphine sulfate whole or to open capsule and sprinkle beads or pellets on a small amount of applesauce immediately before taking.
• ***Alert:*** Warn patient not to crush, break, or chew extended-release form.

SAFETY ALERT!

nalbuphine hydrochloride
Nubain

Pharmacologic class: opioid agonist-antagonist, opioid partial agonist
Pregnancy risk category B

AVAILABLE FORMS
Injection: 10 mg/ml, 20 mg/ml

INDICATIONS & DOSAGES
➤ **Moderate to severe pain**
Adults: For a patient of about 70 kg (154 lb), 10 to 20 mg subcutaneously,

I.M., or I.V. q 3 to 6 hours, p.r.n. Maximum, 160 mg daily.

➤ **Adjunct to balanced anesthesia**

Adults: 0.3 mg/kg to 3.0 mg/kg I.V. over 10 to 15 minutes; then maintenance doses of 0.25 to 0.50 mg/kg in single I.V. dose, p.r.n.

Adjust-a-dose: In patients with renal or hepatic impairment, decrease dosage.

I.V. ADMINISTRATION

- Inject slowly over at least 2 to 3 minutes into a vein or into an I.V. line containing a compatible, free-flowing I.V. solution, such as D_5W, normal saline solution, or lactated Ringer solution.
- Respiratory depression can be reversed with naloxone. Keep resuscitation equipment available, particularly when giving I.V.

INCOMPATIBILITIES

Allopurinol, amphotericin B, cefepime, diazepam, docetaxel, ketorolac, methotrexate sodium, nafcillin, pentobarbital sodium, piperacillin and tazobactam sodium, promethazine, sargramostim, sodium bicarbonate, thiethylperazine.

ACTION

Unknown. Binds with opiate receptors in the CNS, altering perception of and emotional response to pain.

Route	Onset	Peak	Duration
I.V.	2–3 min	30 min	3–6 hr
I.M.	15 min	1 hr	3–6 hr
SubQ	15 min	Unknown	3–6 hr

Half-life: 5 hours.

ADVERSE REACTIONS

CNS: *dizziness, headache, sedation, vertigo,* confusion, crying, delusions, depression, euphoria, hallucinations, hostility, nervousness, restlessness, speech disorders, unusual dreams.
CV: ***bradycardia,*** hypertension, hypotension, tachycardia.
EENT: blurred vision, dry mouth.
GI: biliary tract spasms, constipation, cramps, dyspepsia, nausea, vomiting.
GU: urinary urgency.
Respiratory: ***respiratory depression,*** asthma, dyspnea, pulmonary edema.
Skin: burning, clamminess, diaphoresis, pruritus, urticaria.

INTERACTIONS

Drug-drug. *CNS depressants, general anesthetics, hypnotics, MAO inhibitors, sedatives, tranquilizers, tricyclic antidepressants:* May cause respiratory depression, hypertension, profound sedation, or coma. Use together with caution, and monitor patient response.
Opioid analgesics: May decrease analgesic effect. Avoid using together.
Drug-lifestyle. *Alcohol use:* May cause additive effects. Discourage use together.

EFFECTS ON LAB TEST RESULTS

None reported.

CONTRAINDICATIONS & CAUTIONS

- Contraindicated in patients hypersensitive to drug.
- Use cautiously in patients with history of drug abuse and in those with emotional instability, head injury, increased intracranial pressure, impaired ventilation, MI accompanied by nausea and vomiting, upcoming biliary surgery, and hepatic or renal disease.
- ***Alert:*** Certain commercial preparations contain sodium metabisulfite.

NURSING CONSIDERATIONS

- Reassess patient's level of pain at least 15 and 30 minutes after parenteral administration.
- Drug acts as an opioid antagonist and may cause withdrawal syndrome. For patients who have received long-term opioids, give 25% of the usual dose initially. Watch for signs of withdrawal.
- ***Alert:*** Drug causes respiratory depression, which at 10 mg is equal to respiratory depression produced by 10 mg of morphine.
- Monitor circulatory and respiratory status and bladder and bowel function. If respirations are shallow or rate is below 12 breaths/minute, withhold dose and notify prescriber.
- Constipation is often severe with maintenance therapy. Make sure stool softener or other laxative is ordered.
- Psychological and physical dependence may occur with prolonged use.

• *Look alike–sound alike:* Don't confuse Nubain with Navane.

PATIENT TEACHING

• Caution ambulatory patient about getting out of bed or walking. Warn outpatient to avoid driving and other hazardous activities that require mental alertness until drug's CNS effects are known.
• Teach patient how to manage troublesome adverse effects such as constipation.

SAFETY ALERT!

oxycodone hydrochloride
Endocodone, Endone‡, OxyContin, Oxydose, OxyFAST, OxyIR, Roxicodone, Roxicodone Intensol, Supeudol†

oxycodone pectinate
Proladone‡

Pharmacologic class: opioid
Pregnancy risk category B
Controlled substance schedule II

AVAILABLE FORMS
oxycodone hydrochloride
Capsules: 5 mg
Oral solution: 5 mg/5 ml, 20 mg/ml
Suppository: 10 mg*†, 20 mg*†
Tablets (immediate-release): 5 mg, 15 mg, 30 mg
Tablets (controlled-release): 10 mg, 20 mg, 40 mg, 80 mg
oxycodone pectinate
Suppositories: 30 mg‡

INDICATIONS & DOSAGES
➤ **Moderate to severe pain**
Adults: 5 mg P.O. q 6 hours. Or, one suppository P.R. three to four times daily, p.r.n. Patients not currently receiving opioids, who need a continuous, around-the-clock analgesic for an extended period of time, give 10 mg controlled-release tablets P.O. q 12 hours. May increase dose q 1 to 2 days p.r.n. The 80-mg formulation is for opioid-tolerant patients only.

ACTION
Unknown. Binds with opiate receptors in the CNS, altering perception of and emotional response to pain.

Route	Onset	Peak	Duration
P.O.	10–15 min	1 hr	3–6 hr
P.R.	Unknown	Unknown	Unknown

Half-life: 2 to 3 hours.

ADVERSE REACTIONS
CNS: clouded sensorium, dizziness, euphoria, light-headedness, physical dependence, sedation, somnolence.
CV: ***bradycardia,*** hypotension.
GI: *constipation, nausea, vomiting,* ileus.
GU: urine retention.
Respiratory: ***respiratory depression.***
Skin: diaphoresis, pruritus.

INTERACTIONS
Drug-drug. *Anticoagulants:* Oxycodone hydrochloride products containing aspirin may increase anticoagulant effect. Monitor clotting times. Use together cautiously.
CNS depressants, general anesthetics, hypnotics, MAO inhibitors, other opioid analgesics, sedatives, tranquilizers, tricyclic antidepressants: May cause additive effects. Use together with caution. Reduce oxycodone dose, and monitor patient response.
Drug-lifestyle. *Alcohol use:* May cause additive effects. Discourage use together.

EFFECTS ON LAB TEST RESULTS
• May increase amylase and lipase levels.

CONTRAINDICATIONS & CAUTIONS
• Contraindicated in patients hypersensitive to drug.
• Contraindicated in those suspected of having paralytic ileus.
• Use with caution in elderly and debilitated patients and in those with head injury, increased intracranial pressure, seizures, asthma, COPD, prostatic hyperplasia, severe hepatic or renal disease, acute abdominal conditions, urethral stricture, hypothyroidism, Addison disease, and arrhythmias.

NURSING CONSIDERATIONS
• Reassess patient's level of pain at least 15 and 30 minutes after administration.
• For full analgesic effect, give drug before patient has intense pain.

- To minimize GI upset, give drug after meals or with milk.
- Single-drug oxycodone solution or tablets are especially useful for patients who shouldn't take aspirin or acetaminophen.
- Monitor circulatory and respiratory status. Withhold dose and notify prescriber if respirations are shallow or if respiratory rate falls below 12 breaths/minute.
- Monitor patient's bladder and bowel patterns. Patient may need a laxative because drug has a constipating effect.
- Reserve the 80-mg controlled-release tablets for opioid-tolerant patients who are taking daily doses of 160 mg or more.
- Patients taking the controlled-release form around-the-clock may need to take the immediate-release form for pain exacerbation or for prevention of incident pain.
- For patients who are taking more than 60 mg daily, stop drug gradually to prevent withdrawal symptoms.
- OxyContin isn't intended for as-needed use or for immediate postoperative pain. Drug is indicated only for postoperative use if patient was receiving it before surgery or if pain is expected to persist for an extended time.
- ***Alert:*** OxyContin is potentially addictive and abused as much as morphine. Chewing, crushing, snorting, or injecting it can lead to overdose and death.

PATIENT TEACHING

- Instruct patient to take drug before pain is intense.
- Tell patient to take drug with milk or after eating.
- Tell patient to swallow extended-release tablets whole.
- Caution ambulatory patient about getting out of bed or walking. Warn outpatient to avoid driving and other hazardous activities that require mental alertness until drug's CNS effects are known.
- Advise patient to avoid alcohol use during therapy.
- Tell patient not to stop drug abruptly.

SAFETY ALERT!

oxymorphone hydrochloride

Numorphan, Opana, Opana ER

Pharmacologic class: opioid
Pregnancy risk category C; D if used for prolonged periods or high doses at term
Controlled substance schedule II

AVAILABLE FORMS

Injection: 1 mg/ml
Tablets: 5 mg, 10 mg
Tablets (extended-release [ER]): 5 mg, 10 mg, 20 mg, 40 mg

INDICATIONS & DOSAGES

➤ Moderate to severe pain

Adults: 1 to 1.5 mg I.M. or subcutaneously q 4 to 6 hours, p.r.n. Or, 0.5 mg I.V. q 4 to 6 hours, p.r.n. Or, in opioid-naïve patients, give 10 to 20 mg P.O. q 4 to 6 hours. If needed, begin dosing at 5 mg P.O. and adjust based on patient response.

➤ Moderate to severe pain in patients requiring continuous, around-the-clock opioid treatment for an extended period of time

Opioid naïve adults: Using ER form, give 5 mg P.O. q 12 hours. Increase 5 to 10 mg q 12 hours every 3 to 7 days as needed and tolerated. Patients taking Opana immediate-release tablets can be switched to Opana ER tablets by giving one-half the patient's total daily dose as Opana ER q 12 hours.

Adjust-a-dose: For patients with mild hepatic impairment or creatinine clearance less than 50 ml/minute, start with the lowest possible dose and slowly increase as tolerated.

➤ Analgesia during labor

Adults: 0.5 to 1 mg I.M.

I.V. ADMINISTRATION

- If necessary, dilute drug in normal saline solution.
- Give drug by direct I.V. injection.

INCOMPATIBILITIES

None reported.

ACTION

May bind with opiate receptors in the CNS, altering perception of and emotional response to pain.

Route	Onset	Peak	Duration
P.O.	Varies	Varies	Varies
I.V.	5–10 min	15–30 min	3–4 hr
I.M.	10–15 min	30–90 min	3–6 hr
SubQ	10–20 min	60–90 min	3–6 hr

Half-life: For parenteral, unknown. For ER tablets, 7 to 12 hours. For immediate-release tablets, 3 to 12 hours.

ADVERSE REACTIONS

CNS: *clouded sensorium, dizziness, euphoria, headache, sedation, somnolence,* ***seizures,*** dysphoria, light-headedness, hallucinations, physical dependence, restlessness.
CV: *hypotension,* ***bradycardia.***
EENT: blurred vision, diplopia, miosis.
GI: *constipation, nausea, vomiting,* ileus.
GU: *urine retention.*
Respiratory: ***respiratory depression.***
Skin: *increased sweating,* pruritus.

INTERACTIONS

Drug-drug. *Agonist or antagonist analgesics:* May reduce analgesic effect or precipitate withdraw symptoms. Don't use together.
Anticholinergics: May increase risk of urine retention or severe constipation, leading to paralytic ileus. Monitor patient for abdominal pain or distention.
CNS depressants, general anesthetics, MAO inhibitors, phenothiazines, sedative hypnotics, tricyclic antidepressants: May cause additive effects. Use together with caution and reduce opioid dosage.
Drug-lifestyle. *Alcohol use:* May cause additive effects. Discourage use together.

EFFECTS ON LAB TEST RESULTS

- May increase amylase and lipase levels.

CONTRAINDICATIONS & CAUTIONS

- Contraindicated in patients hypersensitive to drug and in those with acute asthma attacks, severe respiratory depression, upper airway obstruction, paralytic ileus, or those with moderate to severe hepatic impairment.
- Contraindicated in patients with pulmonary edema caused by a respiratory irritant.
- Use with caution in elderly or debilitated patients and in those with head injury, increased intracranial pressure, seizures, asthma, COPD, acute abdominal conditions, biliary tract disease (including pancreatitis), acute alcoholism, delirium tremens, prostatic hyperplasia, renal or mild hepatic impairment, urethral stricture, respiratory depression, hypothyroidism, Addison disease, and arrhythmias.

NURSING CONSIDERATIONS

- Keep opioid antagonist (naloxone) and resuscitation equipment available.
- Use of this drug may worsen gallbladder pain.
- Drug isn't for mild pain. For better effect, give drug before patient has intense pain.
- ER tablets aren't for p.r.n. use.
- Monitor CV and respiratory status. Withhold dose and notify prescriber if respirations decrease or rate is below 12 breaths/minute.
- Monitor bladder and bowel function. Patient may need a laxative.
- ***Look alike–sound alike:*** Don't confuse oxymorphone with oxymetholone or oxycodone, and don't confuse Numorphan with nalbuphine.

PATIENT TEACHING

- Instruct patient to ask for drug before pain is intense. Inform patient that ER tablets must be taken around-the-clock.
- When drug is used I.M. or I.V. after surgery, encourage patient to turn, cough, and deep-breathe and to use incentive spirometer to avoid lung problems.
- Caution ambulatory patient about getting out of bed or walking. Warn outpatient to avoid driving and other hazardous activities that require mental alertness until drug's CNS effects are known.
- ***Alert:*** Caution patient not to consume alcohol or take any prescription or OTC drug containing alcohol with oral form as this can lead to an overdose.
- ***Alert:*** Warn patient not to crush, break, chew, or dissolve ER tablets; doing so may lead to a fatal overdose.

• Instruct patient to keep tablets in a child-resistant container in a safe place. Accidental ingestion by a child can result in death.

SAFETY ALERT!

pentazocine hydrochloride
Fortral†‡, Talwin†

pentazocine hydrochloride and naloxone hydrochloride
Talwin NX

pentazocine lactate
Fortral‡, Talwin

Pharmacologic class: opioid agonist-antagonist, opioid partial agonist
Pregnancy risk category C
Controlled substance schedule IV

AVAILABLE FORMS
pentazocine hydrochloride
Tablets: 25 mg‡, 50 mg†‡
pentazocine hydrochloride and naloxone hydrochloride
Tablets: 50 mg pentazocine hydrochloride and 500 mcg naloxone hydrochloride
pentazocine lactate
Injection: 30 mg/ml

INDICATIONS & DOSAGES
➤ Moderate to severe pain
Adults: 50 to 100 mg P.O. q 3 to 4 hours, p.r.n. Maximum oral dose is 600 mg/day. Or, 30 mg I.M., I.V., or subcutaneously q 3 to 4 hours, p.r.n. Maximum parenteral dose is 360 mg/day. Single doses above 30 mg I.V. or 60 mg I.M. or subcutaneously aren't recommended.
➤ Labor
Adults: 30 mg I.M. as a single dose or 20 mg I.V. q 2 to 3 hours when contractions become regular for two to three doses.

I.V. ADMINISTRATION
• Give drug by direct I.V. injection slowly.
• Talwin NX, the oral form available in the United States, contains the opioid antagonist naloxone, which discourages illicit I.V. use.

INCOMPATIBILITIES
Alkaline solutions, aminophylline, amobarbital, glycopyrrolate, heparin sodium, nafcillin sodium, pentobarbital sodium, phenobarbital sodium, sodium bicarbonate.

ACTION
Unknown. Binds with opiate receptors in the CNS, altering perception of and emotional response to pain.

Route	Onset	Peak	Duration
P.O.	15–30 min	1–3 hr	2–3 hr
I.V.	2–3 min	15–30 min	2–3 hr
I.M., SubQ	15–20 min	30–60 min	2–3 hr

Half-life: 2 to 3 hours.

ADVERSE REACTIONS
CNS: *dizziness, euphoria, lightheadedness, sedation,* confusion, drowsiness, hallucinations, headache, psychotomimetic effects, visual disturbances.
CV: ***shock,*** circulatory depression, hypertension, hypotension.
EENT: dry mouth.
GI: *nausea, vomiting,* constipation.
GU: urine retention.
Respiratory: ***apnea, respiratory depression,*** dyspnea.
Skin: diaphoresis, induration, nodules, sclerosis at injection site, pruritus, sloughing.
Other: ***anaphylaxis,*** hypersensitivity reactions, physical and psychological dependence.

INTERACTIONS
Drug-drug. *CNS depressants:* May cause additive effects. Use together cautiously.
Fluoxetine: May cause additive effects resulting in serotonin syndrome. Use together cautiously.
Opioid analgesics: May decrease analgesic effect. Avoid using together.
Drug-lifestyle. *Alcohol use:* May cause additive effects. Discourage use together.
Smoking: May increase requirements for pentazocine. Monitor drug's effectiveness.

EFFECTS ON LAB TEST RESULTS

- May interfere with laboratory tests for urinary 17-hydroxycorticosteroids.

CONTRAINDICATIONS & CAUTIONS

- Contraindicated in patients hypersensitive to drug or its components and in children younger than age 12.
- Use cautiously in patients with hepatic or renal disease, acute MI, head injury, increased intracranial pressure, and respiratory depression.

NURSING CONSIDERATIONS

- Reassess patient's level of pain at least 15 and 30 minutes after parenteral administration and 30 minutes after oral administration.
- Drug may cause constipation. Assess bowel function and need for stool softeners or laxatives
- Have naloxone readily available. Respiratory depression can be reversed with naloxone.
- ***Alert:*** For subcutaneous or I.M. use, rotate injection sites to minimize tissue irritation. If possible, avoid giving subcutaneously.
- Drug has opioid antagonist properties. May cause withdrawal syndrome in opioid-dependent patients.
- Psychological and physical dependence may occur with prolonged use.

PATIENT TEACHING

- Instruct patient to ask for drug before pain is intense.
- Caution ambulatory patient about getting out of bed or walking. Warn outpatient to avoid driving and other hazardous activities that require mental alertness until drug's CNS effects are known.
- Advise patient to avoid alcohol during therapy.
- Instruct patient or family to report skin rash, disorientation, or confusion to prescriber.

SAFETY ALERT!

propoxyphene hydrochloride (dextropropoxyphene hydrochloride)

Darvon, Darvon Pulvules, 642†

propoxyphene napsylate (dextropropoxyphene napsylate)

Darvon N, Doloxene‡

Pharmacologic class: opioid
Pregnancy risk category C
Controlled substance schedule IV

AVAILABLE FORMS

propoxyphene hydrochloride
Capsules: 65 mg
propoxyphene napsylate
Oral suspension: 10 mg/ml
Tablets: 100 mg

INDICATIONS & DOSAGES

➤Mild to moderate pain
Adults: 65 mg propoxyphene hydrochloride P.O. q 4 hours, p.r.n. Maximum daily dose is 390 mg. Or, 100 mg propoxyphene napsylate P.O. q 4 hours, p.r.n. Maximum daily dose is 600 mg.
Adjust-a-dose: For patients with hepatic or renal dysfunction, reduce dosage. Consider increasing dosing interval in elderly patients.

ACTION

Unknown. Binds with opiate receptors in the CNS, altering perception of and emotional response to pain.

Route	Onset	Peak	Duration
P.O.	15–60 min	2–2½ hr	4–6 hr

Half-life: 6 to 12 hours.

ADVERSE REACTIONS

CNS: *dizziness, sedation,* euphoria, hallucinations, headache, light-headedness, psychological and physical dependence, weakness.
GI: *nausea, vomiting,* abdominal pain, constipation.
Respiratory: ***respiratory depression.***

INTERACTIONS

Drug-drug. *Carbamazepine:* May increase carbamazepine level. Monitor patient closely.
CNS depressants: May cause additive effects. Use together cautiously.
Tricyclic antidepressants (such as doxepin): May inhibit antidepressant metabolism. Monitor patient for toxicity.
Warfarin: May increase anticoagulant effect. Monitor PT and INR.
Drug-lifestyle. *Alcohol use:* May cause additive effects. Discourage use together.
Smoking: May increase metabolism of propoxyphene. Monitor patient closely.

EFFECTS ON LAB TEST RESULTS

- May alter liver function test values.

CONTRAINDICATIONS & CAUTIONS

- Contraindicated in patients hypersensitive to drug.
- Contraindicated in suicidal or addiction-prone patients.
- Use cautiously in patients with hepatic or renal disease, emotional instability, or history of drug or alcohol abuse.

NURSING CONSIDERATIONS

- Reassess patient's pain level at least 30 minutes after giving drug.
- Sixty-five mg propoxyphene hydrochloride equals 100 mg propoxyphene napsylate.
- Drug may cause constipation. Assess bowel function and need for stool softeners or laxatives.
- Drug is considered a mild opioid analgesic, but pain relief is equivalent to that provided by aspirin. Drug is used with aspirin or acetaminophen to maximize analgesia. Patient may become tolerant and physically dependent on drug.
- Smokers may need increased dosage because smoking may induce liver enzymes responsible for the metabolism of the drug, decreasing its effectiveness.

PATIENT TEACHING

- Advise patient to take drug with food or milk to minimize GI upset.
- Warn patient not to exceed recommended dosage. Respiratory depression, low blood pressure, profound sedation, coma, and death may result if used in excessive doses or with other CNS depressants. Advise patient to avoid alcohol or other CNS-type drugs when taking propoxyphene.
- Caution ambulatory patient about getting out of bed or walking. Warn outpatient to avoid driving and other hazardous activities that require mental alertness until drug's CNS effects are known.

tramadol hydrochloride

Ultram

Pharmacologic class: synthetic, centrally active analgesic
Pregnancy risk category C

AVAILABLE FORMS

Tablets: 50 mg

INDICATIONS & DOSAGES

➤ Moderate to moderately severe pain
Adults: Initially, 25 mg P.O. in the morning. Adjust by 25 mg q 3 days to 100 mg/day (25 mg q.i.d.). Thereafter, adjust by 50 mg q 3 days to reach 200 mg/day (50 mg q.i.d.). Thereafter, give 50 to 100 mg P.O. q 4 to 6 hours, p.r.n. Maximum, 400 mg daily.
Elderly patients: For patients older than age 75, maximum is 300 mg daily in divided doses.
Adjust-a-dose: If creatinine clearance is less than 30 ml/minute, increase dose interval to q 12 hours; maximum is 200 mg daily. For patients with cirrhosis, give 50 mg q 12 hours.

ACTION

Unknown. A centrally acting synthetic analgesic compound not chemically related to opioids. Thought to bind to opioid receptors and inhibit reuptake of norepinephrine and serotonin.

Route	Onset	Peak	Duration
P.O.	Unknown	2 hr	Unknown

Half-life: 6 to 7 hours.

ADVERSE REACTIONS

CNS: *dizziness, headache, somnolence, vertigo,* ***seizures,*** anxiety, asthenia, CNS

stimulation, confusion, coordination disturbance, euphoria, malaise, nervousness, sleep disorder.
CV: vasodilation.
EENT: visual disturbances.
GI: *constipation, nausea, vomiting,* abdominal pain, anorexia, diarrhea, dry mouth, dyspepsia, flatulence.
GU: menopausal symptoms, proteinuria, urinary frequency, urine retention.
Musculoskeletal: hypertonia.
Respiratory: ***respiratory depression.***
Skin: diaphoresis, pruritus, rash.

INTERACTIONS

Drug-drug. *Carbamazepine:* May increase tramadol metabolism. Patients receiving long-term carbamazepine therapy up to 800 mg daily may need up to twice the recommended tramadol dose.
CNS depressants: May cause additive effects. Use together cautiously; tramadol dosage may need to be reduced.
Cyclobenzaprine, MAO inhibitors, neuroleptics, other opioids, tricyclic antidepressants: May increase risk of seizures. Monitor patient closely.
Quinidine: May increase level of tramadol. Monitor patient closely.
SSRIs: May increase risk of serotonin syndrome. Use cautiously and monitor patient for adverse effects.

EFFECTS ON LAB TEST RESULTS

- May increase liver enzyme level. May decrease creatinine and hemoglobin levels.

CONTRAINDICATIONS & CAUTIONS

- Contraindicated in patients hypersensitive to drug or other opioids, in breast-feeding women, and in those with acute intoxication from alcohol, hypnotics, centrally acting analgesics, opioids, or psychotropic drugs. Serious hypersensitivity reactions can occur, usually after the first dose. Patients with history of anaphylactic reaction to codeine and other opioids may be at increased risk.
- Use cautiously in patients at risk for seizures or respiratory depression; in patients with increased intracranial pressure or head injury, acute abdominal conditions, or renal or hepatic impairment; or in patients with physical dependence on opioids.

NURSING CONSIDERATIONS

- Reassess patient's level of pain at least 30 minutes after administration.
- Monitor CV and respiratory status. Withhold dose and notify prescriber if respirations decrease or rate is below 12 breaths/minute.
- Monitor bowel and bladder function. Anticipate need for laxative.
- For better analgesic effect, give drug before onset of intense pain.
- Monitor patients at risk for seizures. Drug may reduce seizure threshold.
- In the case of an overdose, naloxone may also increase risk of seizures.
- Monitor patient for drug dependence. Drug can produce dependence similar to that of codeine or dextropropoxyphene and thus has potential for abuse.
- Withdrawal symptoms may occur if drug is stopped abruptly. Reduce dosage gradually.
- ***Look alike–sound alike:*** Don't confuse tramadol with trazodone or trandolapril.

PATIENT TEACHING

- Tell patient to take drug as prescribed and not to increase dose or dosage interval unless ordered by prescriber.
- Caution ambulatory patient to be careful when rising and walking. Warn outpatient to avoid driving and other potentially hazardous activities that require mental alertness until drug's CNS effects are known.
- Advise patient to check with prescriber before taking OTC drugs because drug interactions can occur.
- Warn patient not to stop the drug abruptly.

27 Sedative-hypnotics

chloral hydrate
dexmedetomidine hydrochloride
diazepam
(See Chapter 33, ANXIOLYTICS.)
estazolam
eszopiclone
flurazepam hydrochloride
pentobarbital
pentobarbital sodium
phenobarbital sodium
(See Chapter 28, ANTICONVULSANTS.)
ramelteon
temazepam
triazolam
zaleplon
zolpidem tartrate

SAFETY ALERT!

chloral hydrate

Aquachloral Supprettes, Novo-Chlorhydrate†, PMS-Chloral hydrate†, Somnote

Pharmacologic class: CNS depressant
Pregnancy risk category C
Controlled substance schedule IV

AVAILABLE FORMS

Capsules: 250 mg, 500 mg
Suppositories: 324 mg, 500 mg, 648 mg
Syrup: 250 mg/5 ml, 500 mg/5 ml

INDICATIONS & DOSAGES

➤ Sedation
Adults: 250 mg P.O. or P.R. t.i.d. after meals. Maximum single or daily dose is 2 g.
Children: 8 mg/kg P.O. t.i.d. Maximum dosage is 500 mg t.i.d.
➤ Insomnia
Adults: 500 mg to 1 g P.O. or P.R. 15 to 30 minutes before h.s. Maximum daily dose is 2 g.
Children: 50 mg/kg P.O. or P.R. 15 to 30 minutes before h.s. Maximum single dose is 1 g.
➤ Preoperatively to produce sedation and relieve anxiety
Adults: 500 mg to 1 g P.O. or P.R. 30 minutes before surgery.
➤ Premedication for EEG
Children: 20 to 25 mg/kg P.O. or P.R. up to 500 mg/single dose. May give divided doses.

ACTION

Unknown. Sedative effects may be caused by drug's main metabolite, trichloroethanol.

Route	Onset	Peak	Duration
P.O.	30 min	Unknown	4–8 hr
P.R.	Unknown	Unknown	4–8 hr

Half-life: 8 to 10 hours for trichloroethanol.

ADVERSE REACTIONS

CNS: drowsiness, nightmares, dizziness, ataxia, paradoxical excitement, hangover, somnolence, disorientation, delirium, light-headedness, hallucinations, confusion, somnambulism, vertigo, malaise, physical and psychological dependence.
GI: *nausea, vomiting, diarrhea,* flatulence.
Hematologic: eosinophilia, ***leukopenia.***
Other: hypersensitivity reactions.

INTERACTIONS

Drug-drug. *CNS depressants including opioid analgesics:* May cause excessive CNS depression or vasodilation reaction. Use together cautiously.
Furosemide I.V.: May cause sweating, flushes, variable blood pressure, nausea, and uneasiness. Use together cautiously or use a different hypnotic drug.
Oral anticoagulants: May increase risk of bleeding. Monitor patient closely.
Phenytoin: May decrease phenytoin level. Monitor patient closely.
Drug-lifestyle. *Alcohol use:* May react synergistically, increasing CNS depression, or, rarely, may produce a disulfiram-

like reaction. Strongly discourage alcohol use with these drugs.

EFFECTS ON LAB TEST RESULTS
• May increase eosinophil count. May decrease WBC count.
• May cause false-positive results in urine glucose tests that use cupric sulfate, such as Benedict reagent, and in phentolamine tests.

CONTRAINDICATIONS & CAUTIONS
• Contraindicated in patients hypersensitive to drug and in those with hepatic or renal impairment.
• Oral administration is contraindicated in patients with gastric disorders.
• Use with caution in patients with severe cardiac disease.
• Use cautiously in patients with mental depression, suicidal tendencies, or history of drug abuse.
• Some products may contain tartrazine; use cautiously in patients with aspirin sensitivity.

NURSING CONSIDERATIONS
• ***Alert:*** Note two strengths of oral liquid form. Double-check dose, especially when giving to children. Fatal overdoses have occurred.
• To minimize unpleasant taste and stomach irritation, dilute or give with liquid. Tell patient to take drug after meals.
• Take precautions to prevent hoarding or overdosing by patients who are depressed, suicidal, or drug dependent or who have history of drug abuse.
• Long-term use isn't recommended; drug loses its effectiveness in promoting sleep after 14 days of continued use. Long-term use may cause drug dependence, and patient may experience withdrawal symptoms if drug is suddenly stopped.
• Monitor BUN level; large doses may raise BUN level.
• Don't give drug for 48 hours before fluorometric test.

PATIENT TEACHING
• Instruct patient to take capsule with a full glass of water or juice and to swallow capsule whole.
• Tell patient to avoid alcohol during drug therapy.
• Caution patient to avoid performing activities that require mental alertness or physical coordination.
• Advise patient to store drug in dark container and to store suppositories in refrigerator.

SAFETY ALERT!

dexmedetomidine hydrochloride
Precedex

Pharmacologic class: selective alpha-$_2$ adrenergic agonist
Pregnancy risk category C

AVAILABLE FORMS
Injection: 100 mcg/ml in 2-ml vials and 2-ml ampules

INDICATIONS & DOSAGES
➤ **To sedate initially intubated and mechanically ventilated patients in intensive care unit**
Adults: Loading infusion of 1 mcg/kg I.V. over 10 minutes; then maintenance infusion of 0.2 to 0.7 mcg/kg/hour for up to 24 hours, titrated to achieve desired level of sedation.

I.V. ADMINISTRATION
• Dilute in normal saline solution. Withdraw 2 ml of drug and add to 48 ml of normal saline injection to total of 50 ml. Shake gently to mix well.
• Infusion is compatible with lactated Ringer solution, D_5W, normal saline solution in water, and 20% mannitol. It's also compatible with atracurium besylate, atropine sulfate, etomidate, fentanyl citrate, glycopyrrolate bromide, midazolam, morphine sulfate, pancuronium bromide, phenylephrine hydrochloride, plasma substitute, succinylcholine, thiopental sodium, and vecuronium bromide.
• Don't infuse drug for longer than 24 hours.

INCOMPATIBILITIES
Blood, plasma.

ACTION
Produces sedation by selective stimulation of alpha$_2$-adrenergic receptors.

Route	Onset	Peak	Duration
I.V.	Unknown	Unknown	Unknown

Half-life: About 2 hours.

ADVERSE REACTIONS
CNS: pain.
CV: *hypotension,* ***bradycardia, arrhythmias,*** *hypertension,* atrial fibrillation.
GI: *nausea,* vomiting, thirst.
GU: oliguria.
Hematologic: anemia, leukocytosis.
Respiratory: ***hypoxia,*** pleural effusion, ***pulmonary edema.***
Other: infection, rigors.

INTERACTIONS
Drug-drug. *Anesthetics, hypnotics, opioids, sedatives:* May enhance effects of dexmedetomidine. May need to reduce dexmedetomidine dose.

EFFECTS ON LAB TEST RESULTS
- May increase ALT, AST, and serum glutamic-oxaloacetic transaminase levels. May decrease hemoglobin level.
- May increase WBC count.

CONTRAINDICATIONS & CAUTIONS
- Contraindicated in patients hypersensitive to dexmedetomidine hydrochloride.
- Use cautiously in patients with advanced heart block or renal or hepatic impairment and in elderly patients.

NURSING CONSIDERATIONS
- Only health care professionals skilled in managing patients in the intensive care unit, where cardiac status can be continuously monitored, should give drug.
- ***Alert:*** Use controlled-infusion device at rate calculated for body weight.
- Determine renal and hepatic function before giving, and consider dosage adjustments in patients with renal or hepatic impairment and in elderly patients.
- Some patients receiving drug can awaken when stimulated. This alone shouldn't be considered evidence of lack of efficacy in absence of other signs and symptoms.
- Drug may be continuously infused in mechanically ventilated patients before, during, and after extubation. Drug doesn't need to be stopped before extubation.

PATIENT TEACHING
- Tell patient he will be sedated while drug is being given but that he may awaken when stimulated.
- Reassure patient that he will be closely monitored and attended while sedated.

SAFETY ALERT!

estazolam
ProSom

Pharmacologic class: benzodiazepine
Pregnancy risk category X
Controlled substance schedule IV

AVAILABLE FORMS
Tablets: 1 mg, 2 mg

INDICATIONS & DOSAGES
➤ Insomnia
Adults: 1 mg P.O. before bedtime. Some patients may need 2 mg.
Elderly patients: 1 mg P.O. before bedtime. Use higher doses with extreme care. Frail, elderly, or debilitated patients may take 0.5 mg, but this low dose may be only marginally effective.

ACTION
Thought to act on the limbic system and thalamus of CNS by binding to specific benzodiazepine receptors.

Route	Onset	Peak	Duration
P.O.	Unknown	1–3 hr	Unknown

Half-life: 10 to 24 hours.

ADVERSE REACTIONS
CNS: fatigue, dizziness, daytime drowsiness, *somnolence, asthenia,* hypokinesia, abnormal thinking.
GI: dyspepsia, abdominal pain.
Musculoskeletal: back pain, stiffness.
Respiratory: cold symptoms, pharyngitis.

INTERACTIONS

Drug-drug. *Cimetidine, disulfiram, hormonal contraceptives, isoniazid:* May impair metabolism and clearance of benzodiazepines and prolong their half-life. Watch for increased CNS depression.
CNS depressants, including antihistamines, opioid analgesics, other benzodiazepines: May increase CNS depression. Avoid using together.
Digoxin: May increase digoxin level, resulting in toxicity. Monitor patient closely.
Fluconazole, itraconazole, ketoconazole, miconazole: May increase drug level, CNS depression, and psychomotor impairment. Avoid using together.
Phenytoin: May increase phenytoin level, resulting in toxicity. Monitor patient closely.
Rifampin: May increase metabolism and clearance and decrease drug half-life of estazolam. Watch for decreased effectiveness.
Theophylline: May have antagonistic effect. Watch for decreased effectiveness of estazolam.
Drug-herb. *Calendula, hops, kava, lemon balm, passion flower, skullcap, valerian:* May enhance sedative effect of drug. Discourage use together.
Drug-lifestyle. *Alcohol use:* May cause additive CNS effects. Discourage use together.
Smoking: May increase metabolism and clearance. Advise patient to watch for signs of decreased effectiveness.

EFFECTS ON LAB TEST RESULTS
- May increase AST level.

CONTRAINDICATIONS & CAUTIONS
- Contraindicated in pregnant women and in those hypersensitive to drug.
- Use cautiously in patients with depression, suicidal tendencies, or hepatic, renal, or pulmonary disease.

NURSING CONSIDERATIONS
- Check liver and renal function and CBC before and periodically during long-term therapy.
- Take precautions to prevent depressed, suicidal, or drug-dependent patients or those with history of drug abuse from hoarding drug.
- Patients who receive prolonged treatment with benzodiazepines may experience withdrawal symptoms if drug is suddenly stopped (possibly after 6 weeks of continuous therapy).
- ***Look alike–sound alike:*** Don't confuse ProSom with Proscar, Prozac, or Psorcon E.

PATIENT TEACHING
- Advise patient to notify prescriber about planned, suspected, or known pregnancy during therapy.
- Tell patient not to increase dosage if he thinks that drug is no longer effective but instead to tell the prescriber.
- Caution patient to avoid performing activities that require mental alertness or physical coordination.
- Warn patient that drinking alcohol while taking drug or within 24 hours after taking drug can increase depressant effects.
- Warn patient not to abruptly stop use after taking drug for 1 month or longer.
- Tell breast-feeding patient to avoid using drug.

SAFETY ALERT!

eszopiclone
Lunesta✐

Pharmacologic class: pyrrolopyrazine derivative
Pregnancy risk category C
Controlled substance schedule IV

AVAILABLE FORMS
Tablets: 1 mg, 2 mg, 3 mg

INDICATIONS & DOSAGES
➤ **Insomnia**
Adults: 2 mg P.O. immediately before bedtime. Increase to 3 mg, p.r.n.
Elderly patients having trouble falling asleep: 1 mg P.O. immediately before bedtime. Increase to 2 mg, p.r.n.
Elderly patients having trouble staying asleep: 2 mg P.O. immediately before bedtime.
Adjust-a-dose: In patients with severe hepatic impairment, start with 1 mg P.O. In patients who also take a potent CYP3A4 inhibitor, start with 1 mg and increase to 2 mg, p.r.n.

ACTION
Probably interacts with GABA receptors at binding sites close or connected to benzodiazepine receptors.

Route	Onset	Peak	Duration
P.O.	Rapid	1 hr	Unknown

Half-life: 6 hours.

ADVERSE REACTIONS
CNS: abnormal dreams, anxiety, confusion, decreased libido, depression, dizziness, hallucinations, *headache,* nervousness, pain, *somnolence,* neuralgia.
EENT: *unpleasant taste.*
GI: diarrhea, dry mouth, dyspepsia, nausea, vomiting.
GU: UTI.
Respiratory: *respiratory tract infection.*
Skin: pruritus, rash.
Other: accidental injury, viral infection.

INTERACTIONS
Drug-drug. *CNS depressants:* May have additive CNS effects. Adjust dosage of either drug as needed.
CYP3A4 inhibitors (clarithromycin, itraconazole, ketoconazole, nefazodone, nelfinavir, ritonavir, troleandomycin): May decrease eszopiclone elimination, increasing the risk of toxicity. Use together cautiously.
Olanzapine: May impair cognitive function or memory. Use together cautiously.
Rifampicin: May decrease eszopiclone activity. Don't use together.
Drug-food. *High-fat meals:* May decrease drug absorption and effects. Discourage high-fat meals with or just before taking drug.
Drug-lifestyle. *Alcohol use:* May decrease psychomotor ability. Discourage use together.

EFFECTS ON LAB TEST RESULTS
None reported.

CONTRAINDICATIONS & CAUTIONS
- Use cautiously in patients with diseases or conditions that could affect metabolism or hemodynamic responses. Also use cautiously in patients with compromised respiratory function, severe hepatic impairment, or signs and symptoms of depression.

NURSING CONSIDERATIONS
- Evaluate patient for physical and psychiatric disorders before treatment.
- Use the lowest effective dose.
- ***Alert:*** Give drug immediately before patient goes to bed or after patient has gone to bed and has trouble falling asleep.
- Use only for short periods (for example, 7 to 10 days). If patient still has trouble sleeping, check for other psychological disorders.
- Monitor patient for changes in behavior, including those that suggest depression or suicidal thinking.

PATIENT TEACHING
- Urge patient to take drug immediately before going to bed because drug may cause dizziness or light-headedness.
- Caution patient not to take drug unless he can get a full night's sleep.
- Advise patient to avoid taking drug after a high-fat meal.
- Tell patient to avoid activities that require mental alertness until the drug's effects are known.
- Advise patient to avoid alcohol while taking drug.
- Urge patient to immediately report changes in behavior and thinking.
- Warn patient not to stop drug abruptly or change dose without consulting the prescriber.
- Inform patient that tolerance or dependence may develop if drug is taken for a prolonged period.

SAFETY ALERT!

flurazepam hydrochloride
Apo-Flurazepam†, Dalmane, Novo-Flupam†

Pharmacologic class: benzodiazepine
Pregnancy risk category X
Controlled substance schedule IV

AVAILABLE FORMS
Capsules: 15 mg, 30 mg

INDICATIONS & DOSAGES
➤ **Insomnia**
Adults: 15 to 30 mg P.O. at bedtime. May repeat dose once, p.r.n.

Elderly patients: 15 mg P.O. at bedtime initially, until response is determined.

ACTION
A benzodiazepine that is thought to act on the limbic system, thalamus, and hypothalamus of CNS to produce hypnotic effects.

Route	Onset	Peak	Duration
P.O.	15–45 min	30–60 min	7–8 hr

Half-life: 2 to 4 days.

ADVERSE REACTIONS
CNS: *daytime sedation, dizziness, drowsiness, disturbed coordination,* lethargy, confusion, physical or psychological dependence, *headache,* light-headedness, nervousness, hallucinations, staggering, ataxia, disorientation, ***coma.***
GI: nausea, vomiting, heartburn, diarrhea, abdominal pain.

INTERACTIONS
Drug-drug. *Cimetidine:* May increase sedation. Monitor patient carefully.
CNS depressants, including opioid analgesics: May cause excessive CNS depression. Use together cautiously.
Digoxin: May increase digoxin level, resulting in toxicity. Monitor patient closely.
Disulfiram, hormonal contraceptives, isoniazid: May decrease metabolism of benzodiazepines, leading to toxicity. Monitor patient closely.
Fluconazole, itraconazole, ketoconazole, miconazole: May increase and prolong drug level, CNS depression, and psychomotor impairment. Avoid using together.
Phenytoin: May increase phenytoin level. Watch for toxicity.
Rifampin: May enhance metabolism of benzodiazepines. Watch for decreased effectiveness of benzodiazepine.
Theophylline: May act as antagonist with flurazepam. Watch for decreased effectiveness of flurazepam.
Drug-herb. *Calendula, hops, kava, lemon balm, passion flower, skullcap, valerian:* May enhance sedative effect of drug. Discourage use together.
Drug-lifestyle. *Alcohol use:* May cause additive CNS effects. Discourage use together.
Smoking: May increase metabolism and clearance and decrease drug half-life. Advise patient to watch for signs of decreased effectiveness.

EFFECTS ON LAB TEST RESULTS
- May increase alkaline phosphatase, ALT, AST, and bilirubin levels.

CONTRAINDICATIONS & CAUTIONS
- Contraindicated in patients hypersensitive to drug and during pregnancy.
- Use cautiously in elderly patients and in those with impaired hepatic or renal function, chronic pulmonary insufficiency, mental depression, suicidal tendencies, or history of drug abuse.

NURSING CONSIDERATIONS
- Check hepatic and renal function and CBC before and periodically during long-term therapy.
- Minor changes in EEG patterns (usually low-voltage, fast activity) may occur during and after therapy.
- Assess mental status before starting. Elderly patients are more sensitive to drug's adverse CNS reactions.
- Take precautions to prevent hoarding or self-overdosing by depressed, suicidal, or drug-dependent patients and those with history of drug abuse.
- Patient may become physically and psychologically dependent with long-term use.
- ***Look alike–sound alike:*** Don't confuse Dalmane with Demulen.

PATIENT TEACHING
- Inform patient that drug is more effective on second, third, and fourth nights of treatment because drug builds up in the body.
- Warn patient not to abruptly stop drug after taking it for 1 month or longer.
- Tell patient to avoid alcohol use while taking drug.
- Caution patient to avoid performing activities that require mental alertness or physical coordination.
- Warn patient that prolonged use of this drug may produce psychological and physical dependence.
- Advise patient to warn prescriber about planned, suspected, or known pregnancy.

SAFETY ALERT!

pentobarbital
Nembutal*†

pentobarbital sodium
Nembutal Sodium*, Nova Rectal†, NovoPentobarb†

Pharmacologic class: barbiturate
Pregnancy risk category D
Controlled substance schedule II; III for suppositories

AVAILABLE FORMS
pentobarbital
Elixir: 18.2 mg/5 ml
pentobarbital sodium
Capsules: 50 mg, 100 mg
Injection: 50 mg/ml
Suppositories: 30 mg, 60 mg, 120 mg, 200 mg

INDICATIONS & DOSAGES
➤Sedation
Adults: 20 mg P.O. t.i.d. or q.i.d.
Children: 2 to 6 mg/kg P.O. daily in three divided doses. Maximum daily dose is 100 mg.
➤Insomnia
Adults: 100 to 200 mg P.O. h.s. Or, 150 to 200 mg deep I.M. Or, 100 mg I.V. initially, with further small doses up to total of 500 mg. Or, 120 or 200 mg P.R.
Children: 2 to 6 mg/kg or 125 mg/m^2 I.M. Maximum dose is 100 mg.
Children ages 12 to 14: 60 or 120 mg P.R.
Children ages 5 to 11: 60 mg P.R.
Children ages 1 to 4: 30 or 60 mg P.R.
Children ages 2 months to 1 year: 30 mg P.R.
➤Preoperative sedation
Adults: 150 to 200 mg I.M.
Children: 2 to 6 mg/kg P.O.. P.R., or I.M. Maximum dose is 100 mg.

I.V. ADMINISTRATION
- I.V. barbiturates may cause severe respiratory depression, laryngospasm, or hypotension. Reserve their use for emergencies, under close supervision, with resuscitation equipment nearby.
- To minimize deterioration, use injection solution within 30 minutes of opening container. Don't use cloudy solution.
- Don't mix in syringe or in solutions or lines with other drugs.
- Give slowly at no more than 50 mg/minute.
- Parenteral solution is alkaline. Local tissue reactions and injection site pain may occur. Monitor site for extravasation. Assess patency of site before and during administration.

INCOMPATIBILITIES
Other I.V. drugs or solutions.

ACTION
May interfere with transmission of impulses from the thalamus to the cortex of the brain and alter cerebellar function.

Route	Onset	Peak	Duration
P.O.	20 min	30–60 min	1–4 hr
I.V.	Immediate	Immediate	15 min
I.M.	10–25 min	Unknown	Unknown
P.R.	20 min	Unknown	1–4 hr

Half-life: 35 to 50 hours.

ADVERSE REACTIONS
CNS: *drowsiness, lethargy, hangover,* paradoxical excitement in elderly patients, somnolence, physical and psychological dependence.
GI: nausea, vomiting.
Hematologic: worsening porphyria.
Respiratory: ***respiratory depression.***
Skin: rash, urticaria, ***Stevens-Johnson syndrome.***
Other: ***angioedema.***

INTERACTIONS
Drug-drug. *CNS depressants including opioid analgesics:* May cause excessive CNS and respiratory depression. Use together cautiously.
Corticosteroids, doxycycline, estrogens and hormonal contraceptives, oral anticoagulants, theophylline, verapamil: May enhance metabolism of these drugs. Watch for decreased effect.
Griseofulvin: May decrease absorption of griseofulvin. Monitor effectiveness of griseofulvin.
MAO inhibitors, valproic acid: May inhibit metabolism of barbiturates; may prolong CNS depression. Reduce barbiturate dosage.

Metoprolol, propranolol: May reduce effects of these drugs. May need to increase beta-blocker dose.
Rifampin: May decrease barbiturate level. Watch for decreased effect of pentobarbital.
Drug-lifestyle. *Alcohol use:* May impair coordination, increase CNS effects, and cause death. Strongly discourage alcohol use with these drugs.

EFFECTS ON LAB TEST RESULTS
None reported.

CONTRAINDICATIONS & CAUTIONS
- Contraindicated in patients hypersensitive to barbiturates and in those with porphyria, bronchopneumonia, or other severe pulmonary insufficiency, and in severe liver or renal dysfunction.
- Use cautiously in elderly or debilitated patients and in patients with acute or chronic pain, mental depression, suicidal tendencies, history of drug abuse, or hepatic impairment.

NURSING CONSIDERATIONS
- Assess mental status before starting therapy and reduce doses in elderly patients; these patients may be more sensitive to drug's adverse CNS effects.
- ***Alert:*** Give deep I.M. injection with no more than 5 ml of drug at any one site. Superficial injection may cause pain, sterile abscess, and sloughing.
- To ensure accurate dosage, don't divide suppositories.
- Take precautions to prevent hoarding by patients who are depressed, suicidal, or drug-dependent or who have a history of drug abuse.
- Watch for signs of barbiturate toxicity: coma, pupillary constriction, cyanosis, clammy skin, and hypotension. Overdose can be fatal.
- Inspect patient's skin. Skin eruptions may precede fatal reactions. If skin reactions occur, stop drug and call prescriber. In some patients, high temperature, stomatitis, headache, or rhinitis may precede skin reactions.
- Drug has no analgesic effect and may cause restlessness or delirium in patients with pain.
- Long-term use for insomnia isn't recommended; drug loses its effectiveness in promoting sleep after 14 days of continuous use. Long-term high dosage may cause drug dependence, and patient may experience withdrawal symptoms if drug is suddenly stopped. Withdraw barbiturates gradually.
- EEG patterns show a change in low-voltage, fast activity; changes persist after therapy.
- ***Look alike–sound alike:*** Don't confuse pentobarbital with phenobarbital.
- ***Alert:*** Nembutal may contain tartrazine.

PATIENT TEACHING
- Inform patient that morning hangover is common after hypnotic dose, which suppresses REM sleep. Patient may experience increased dreaming after drug is stopped.
- Caution patient to avoid performing activities that require mental alertness or physical coordination.
- Tell patient to avoid alcohol use while taking drug.
- Because drug may decrease the effect of hormonal contraceptives, instruct patient to also use a barrier contraceptive.

SAFETY ALERT!

ramelteon
Rozerem

Pharmacologic class: melatonin receptor agonist
Pregnancy risk category C

AVAILABLE FORMS
Tablets: 8 mg

INDICATIONS & DOSAGES
➤ **Insomnia characterized by trouble falling asleep**
Adults: 8 mg P.O. within 30 minutes h.s. Don't give with or immediately after a high-fat meal.

ACTION
Acts on receptors believed to maintain the circadian rhythm underlying the normal sleep-wake cycle.

Route	Onset	Peak	Duration
P.O.	Rapid	½–1½ hr	Unknown

Half-life: Parent compound, 1 to 2½ hours; metabolite M-II, 2 to 5 hours.

ADVERSE REACTIONS

CNS: depression, dizziness, fatigue, headache, somnolence, worsened insomnia.
GI: diarrhea, impaired taste, nausea.
Musculoskeletal: arthralgia, myalgia .
Respiratory: upper respiratory tract infection.
Other: flulike symptoms.

INTERACTIONS

Drug-drug. *CNS depressants:* May cause excessive CNS depression. Use together cautiously.
Fluconazole (strong CYP2C9 inhibitor), ketoconazole (strong CYP3A4 inhibitor), weak CYP1A2 inhibitors: May increase ramelteon level. Use together cautiously.
Fluvoxamine (strong CYP1A2 inhibitor): May increase ramelteon level. Avoid using together .
Rifampin (strong CYP enzyme inducer): May decrease ramelteon level. Monitor patient for lack of effect.
Drug-food. *Food (especially high-fat meals):* May delay time to peak drug effect. Tell patient to take drug on an empty stomach.
Drug-lifestyle. *Alcohol use:* May cause excessive CNS depression. Discourage alcohol use.

EFFECTS ON LAB TEST RESULTS

- May increase prolactin level. May alter blood cortisol and testosterone levels.

CONTRAINDICATIONS & CAUTIONS

- Contraindicated in those hypersensitive to drug or its components. Don't use in patients taking fluvoxamine or in those with severe hepatic impairment, severe sleep apnea, or severe COPD.
- Use cautiously in patients with depression or moderate hepatic impairment.

NURSING CONSIDERATIONS

- Thoroughly evaluate the cause of insomnia before starting drug.
- Assess patient for behavioral or cognitive disorders.
- Drug doesn't cause physical dependence.

PATIENT TEACHING

- Instruct patient to take dose within 30 minutes of bedtime.
- Tell patient not to take drug with or after a heavy meal.
- Caution against performing activities that require mental alertness or physical coordination after taking drug.
- Caution patient to avoid alcohol while taking drug.
- Tell patient to consult prescriber if insomnia worsens or behavior changes.
- Urge woman to consult prescriber if menses stops, libido decreases, or galactorrhea or fertility problems develop.

SAFETY ALERT!

temazepam

Euhypnos 10‡, Euhypnos 20‡, Nomapam‡, Normison‡, Restoril✐, Temaze‡, Temtabs‡

Pharmacologic class: benzodiazepine
Pregnancy risk category X
Controlled substance schedule IV

AVAILABLE FORMS

Capsules: 7.5 mg, 10 mg‡, 15 mg, 20 mg‡, 30 mg

INDICATIONS & DOSAGES

➤Insomnia

Adults: 15 to 30 mg P.O. at bedtime.
Elderly or debilitated patients: 15 mg P.O. at bedtime until individualized response is determined.

ACTION

A benzodiazepine that probably acts on the limbic system, thalamus, and hypothalamus of the CNS to produce hypnotic effects.

Route	Onset	Peak	Duration
P.O.	Unknown	1–2 hr	3–18 hr

Half-life: 10 to 17 hours.

ADVERSE REACTIONS

CNS: drowsiness, dizziness, lethargy, disturbed coordination, daytime sedation, confusion, nightmares, vertigo, euphoria, weakness, headache, fatigue, nervousness, anxiety, depression, minor changes in EEG patterns (usually low-voltage fast activity).

EENT: blurred vision.
GI: diarrhea, nausea, dry mouth.
Other: physical and psychological dependence.

INTERACTIONS

Drug-drug. *CNS depressants:* May increase CNS depression. Use together cautiously.
Drug-herb. *Calendula, hops, kava, lemon balm, passion flower, skullcap, valerian:* May enhance sedative effect of drug. Discourage use together.
Drug-lifestyle. *Alcohol use:* May cause additive CNS effects. Discourage use together.

EFFECTS ON LAB TEST RESULTS

- May increase liver function test values.

CONTRAINDICATIONS & CAUTIONS

- Contraindicated in pregnant patients and those hypersensitive to drug or other benzodiazepines.
- Use cautiously in patients with chronic pulmonary insufficiency, impaired hepatic or renal function, severe or latent depression, suicidal tendencies, and history of drug abuse.

NURSING CONSIDERATIONS

- In elderly patients, assess mental status before starting therapy, and reduce doses; these patients may be more sensitive to drug's adverse CNS effects.
- Take precautions to prevent hoarding by patients who are depressed, suicidal, or drug-dependent or who have history of drug abuse.
- ***Look alike–sound alike:*** Don't confuse Restoril with Vistaril.

PATIENT TEACHING

- Tell patient to avoid alcohol during therapy.
- Caution patient to avoid performing activities that require mental alertness or physical coordination.
- Warn patient not to stop drug abruptly if taken for 1 month or longer.
- Tell patient that onset of drug's effects may take as long as 2 to 2¼ hours.

SAFETY ALERT!

triazolam
Apo-Triazo†, Halcion, Novo-Triolam†

Pharmacologic class: benzodiazepine
Pregnancy risk category X
Controlled substance schedule IV

AVAILABLE FORMS

Tablets: 0.125 mg, 0.25 mg

INDICATIONS & DOSAGES

➤ Insomnia
Adults: 0.125 to 0.5 mg P.O. at bedtime.
Elderly or debilitated patients: 0.125 mg P.O.at bedtime; increased, p.r.n., to 0.25 mg P.O. at bedtime.

ACTION

Unknown. A benzodiazepine that probably acts on the limbic system, thalamus, and hypothalamus of the CNS to produce hypnotic effects.

Route	Onset	Peak	Duration
P.O.	Unknown	1–2 hr	1½–5½ hr

Half-life: 1½ to 5½ hours.

ADVERSE REACTIONS

CNS: *drowsiness,* amnesia, ataxia, depression, dizziness, headache, lack of coordination, mental confusion, nervousness, physical or psychological dependence, rebound insomnia.
GI: nausea, vomiting.

INTERACTIONS

Drug-drug. *Cimetidine, erythromycin, fluoxetine, fluvoxamine, isoniazid, nefazodone, ranitidine:* May increase triazolam level. Avoid using with azole antifungals or nefazodone. Watch for increased sedation if used with other drugs.
CNS depressants: May cause excessive CNS depression. Use together cautiously.
Diltiazem: May increase CNS depression and prolonged effects of triazolam. Reduce triazolam dose.
Fluconazole, itraconazole, ketoconazole, miconazole: May increase and prolong

drug level, CNS depression, and psychomotor impairment. Avoid using together.
Drug-herb. *Calendula, hops, kava, lemon balm, passion flower, skullcap, valerian:* May enhance sedative effect of drug. Discourage use together.
Drug-food. *Grapefruit:* May delay onset and increase drug effects. Discourage use together.
Drug-lifestyle. *Alcohol use:* May cause additive CNS effects. Discourage use together.
Smoking: May increase metabolism and clearance of drug. Advise patient who smokes to watch for decreased effectiveness of drug.

EFFECTS ON LAB TEST RESULTS

- May increase liver function test values.

CONTRAINDICATIONS & CAUTIONS

- Contraindicated in pregnant patients and those hypersensitive to benzodiazepines.
- Use cautiously in patients with impaired hepatic or renal function, chronic pulmonary insufficiency, sleep apnea, mental depression, suicidal tendencies, or history of drug abuse.
- Use cautiously in breast-feeding women.

NURSING CONSIDERATIONS

- Assess mental status before starting therapy and reduce doses in elderly patients; these patients may be more sensitive to drug's adverse CNS effects.
- Monitor CBC, chemistry, and urinalysis.
- Take precautions to prevent hoarding or overdosing by patients who are depressed, suicidal, or drug-dependent or who have history of drug abuse.
- Minor changes in EEG patterns (usually low-voltage fast activity) may occur during and after therapy.
- ***Look alike–sound alike:*** Don't confuse Halcion with Haldol or halcinonide.

PATIENT TEACHING

- Warn patient not to take more than prescribed amount; overdose can occur at total daily dose of 2 mg (or four times highest recommended amount).
- Tell patient to avoid alcohol use while taking drug.
- Warn patient not to stop drug abruptly after taking for 2 weeks or longer.
- Caution patient to avoid performing activities that require mental alertness or physical coordination.
- Inform patient that drug doesn't tend to cause morning drowsiness.
- Tell patient that rebound insomnia may occur for 1 or 2 nights after stopping therapy.

SAFETY ALERT!

zaleplon
Sonata

Pharmacologic class: pyrazolopyrimidine
Pregnancy risk category C
Controlled substance schedule IV

AVAILABLE FORMS

Capsules: 5 mg, 10 mg

INDICATIONS & DOSAGES

➤Insomnia
Adults: 10 mg P.O. daily h.s.; may increase to 20 mg, p.r.n. Low-weight adults may respond to 5-mg dose. Limit use to 7 to 10 days. Reevaluate patient if drug is used for more than 2 to 3 weeks.
Elderly patients: Initially, 5 mg P.O. daily h.s.; doses of more than 10 mg aren't recommended.
Adjust-a-dose: For debilitated patients, initially, 5 mg P.O. daily h.s.; doses of more than 10 mg aren't recommended. For patients with mild to moderate hepatic impairment or those also taking cimetidine, 5 mg P.O. daily h.s.

ACTION

A hypnotic with chemical structure unrelated to benzodiazepines that interacts with the gamma-aminobutyric acid-benzodiazepine receptor complex in the CNS. Modulation of this complex is thought to be responsible for sedative, anxiolytic, muscle relaxant, and anticonvulsant effects of benzodiazepines.

Route	Onset	Peak	Duration
P.O.	1 hr	1 hr	3–4 hr

Half-life: 1 hour.

ADVERSE REACTIONS

CNS: *headache,* amnesia, anxiety, asthenia, depersonalization, depression, difficulty concentrating, dizziness, fever, hallucinations, hypertonia, hypesthesia, malaise, migraine, nervousness, paresthesia, somnolence, tremor, vertigo.
CV: chest pain, peripheral edema.
EENT: abnormal vision, conjunctivitis, ear discomfort, epistaxis, eye discomfort, hyperacusis, smell alteration.
GI: abdominal pain, anorexia, colitis, constipation, dry mouth, dyspepsia, nausea.
GU: dysmenorrhea.
Musculoskeletal: arthritis, back pain, myalgia.
Respiratory: bronchitis.
Skin: photosensitivity reactions, pruritus, rash.

INTERACTIONS

Drug-drug. *Carbamazepine, phenobarbital, phenytoin, rifampin, other CYP3A4 inducers:* May reduce zaleplon bioavailability and peak level by 80%. Consider using a different hypnotic.
Cimetidine: May increase zaleplon bioavailability and peak level by 85%. Use an initial zaleplon dose of 5 mg.
CNS depressants (imipramine, thioridazine): May cause additive CNS effects. Use together cautiously.
Drug-food. *High-fat foods, heavy meals:* May prolong absorption, delaying peak zaleplon level by about 2 hours; may delay sleep onset. Advise patient to avoid taking with meals.
Drug-lifestyle. *Alcohol use:* May increase CNS effects. Discourage use together.

EFFECTS ON LAB TEST RESULTS

None reported.

CONTRAINDICATIONS & CAUTIONS

- Contraindicated in patients with severe hepatic impairment.
- Use cautiously in elderly, depressed, or debilitated patients, in breast-feeding women, and in patients with compromised respiratory function.

NURSING CONSIDERATIONS

- Because drug works rapidly, give immediately before bedtime or after patient has gone to bed and has had difficulty falling asleep.
- Closely monitor patients who have compromised respiratory function caused by illness or who are elderly or debilitated because they are more sensitive to respiratory depression.
- Start treatment only after carefully evaluating patient because sleep disturbances may be a symptom of an underlying physical or psychiatric disorder.
- Adverse reactions are usually dose-related. Consult prescriber about dose reduction if adverse reactions occur.

PATIENT TEACHING

- Advise patient that drug works rapidly and should only be taken immediately before bedtime or after he has gone to bed and has had trouble falling asleep.
- Advise patient to take drug only if he will be able to sleep for at least 4 undisturbed hours.
- Caution patient that drowsiness, dizziness, light-headedness, and coordination problems occur most often within 1 hour after taking drug.
- Advise patient to avoid performing activities that require mental alertness until CNS adverse reactions are known.
- Advise patient to avoid alcohol use while taking drug and to notify prescriber before taking other prescription or OTC drugs.
- Tell patient not to take drug after a high-fat or heavy meal.
- Advise patient to report sleep problems that continue despite use of drug.
- Notify patient that dependence can occur and that drug is recommended for short-term use only.
- Warn patient not to abruptly stop drug because of the risk of withdrawal symptoms, including unpleasant feelings, stomach and muscle cramps, vomiting, sweating, shakiness, and seizures.
- Notify patient that insomnia may recur for a few nights after stopping drug, but should resolve on its own.
- Warn patient that drug may cause changes in behavior and thinking, including outgoing or aggressive behavior, loss of personal identity, confusion, strange behavior, agitation, hallucinations, worsening of depression, or suicidal thoughts.

Tell patient to notify prescriber immediately if these symptoms occur.

SAFETY ALERT!

zolpidem tartrate
Ambien, Ambien CR

Pharmacologic class: imidazopyridine
Pregnancy risk category C
Controlled substance schedule IV

AVAILABLE FORMS
Tablets: 5 mg, 10 mg
Tablets (extended-release): 6.25 mg, 12.5 mg

INDICATIONS & DOSAGES
➤ **Short-term management of insomnia**
Adults: 10 mg (immediate-release) or 12.5 mg (extended-release) P.O. immediately before bedtime.
Elderly patients: 5 mg (immediate-release) or 6.25 mg (extended-release) P.O. immediately before bedtime. Maximum daily dose is 10 mg (immediate-release) or 6.25 mg (extended-release).
Adjust-a-dose: For debilitated patients and those with hepatic insufficiency, 5 mg P.O. immediately before bedtime. Maximum daily dose (immediate-release) is 10 mg; maximum daily dose (extended-release) is 6.25 mg.

ACTION
Although drug interacts with one of three identified gamma-aminobutyric acid-benzodiazepine receptor complexes, it isn't a benzodiazepine. It exhibits hypnotic activity and minimal muscle relaxant and anticonvulsant properties.

Route	Onset	Peak	Duration
P.O.	Rapid	30–120 min	Unknown

Half-life: 2½ hours.

ADVERSE REACTIONS
CNS: *headache,* amnesia, change in dreams, daytime drowsiness, depression, dizziness, hangover, lethargy, lightheadedness, nervousness, sleep disorder.
CV: palpitations.
EENT: pharyngitis, sinusitis.
GI: abdominal pain, constipation, diarrhea, dry mouth, dyspepsia, nausea, vomiting.
Musculoskeletal: arthralgia, myalgia.
Skin: rash.
Other: back or chest pain, flulike syndrome, hypersensitivity reactions.

INTERACTIONS
Drug-drug. *CNS depressants:* May cause excessive CNS depression. Use together cautiously.
Rifampin: May decrease effects of zolpidem. Avoid using together, if possible. Consider alternative hypnotic.
Drug-lifestyle. *Alcohol use:* May cause excessive CNS depression. Discourage use together.

EFFECTS ON LAB TEST RESULTS
None reported.

CONTRAINDICATIONS & CAUTIONS
- No known contraindications.
- Use cautiously in patients with compromised respiratory status.

NURSING CONSIDERATIONS
- Use drug only for short-term management of insomnia, usually 7 to 10 days.
- Use the smallest effective dose in all patients.
- Take precautions to prevent hoarding by patients who are depressed, suicidal, or drug-dependent, or who have a history of drug abuse.
- ***Look alike–sound alike:*** Don't confuse Ambien with Amen.
- ***Alert:*** Don't crush or divide extended-release tablets.

PATIENT TEACHING
- For rapid sleep onset, instruct patient not to take drug with or immediately after meals.
- Instruct patient to take drug immediately before going to bed; onset of action is rapid.
- Tell patient to avoid alcohol use while taking drug.
- ***Alert:*** Tell patient not to crush, chew, or divide the extended-release tablets.
- Caution patient to avoid performing activities that require mental alertness or physical coordination during therapy.

28
Anticonvulsants

acetazolamide sodium
(See Chapter 60, DIURETICS.)
carbamazepine
clonazepam
clorazepate dipotassium
(See Chapter 30, ANXIOLYTICS.)
diazepam
(See Chapter 30, ANXIOLYTICS.)
divalproex sodium
fosphenytoin sodium
gabapentin
lamotrigine
levetiracetam
magnesium sulfate
oxcarbazepine
phenobarbital
phenobarbital sodium
phenytoin
phenytoin sodium
primidone
tiagabine hydrochloride
topiramate
valproate sodium
valproic acid
zonisamide

carbamazepine
Apo-Carbamazepine†, Carbatrol, Epitol, Equetro, Novo-Carbamaz†, Tegretol, Tegretol CR†, Tegretol-XR

Pharmacologic class: iminostilbene derivative
Pregnancy risk category D

AVAILABLE FORMS
Capsules (extended-release): 100 mg, 200 mg, 300 mg
Oral suspension: 100 mg/5 ml
Tablets: 200 mg
Tablets (chewable): 100 mg, 200 mg
Tablets (extended-release): 100 mg, 200 mg, 300 mg, 400 mg†

INDICATIONS & DOSAGES
➤ **Generalized tonic-clonic and complex partial seizures, mixed seizure patterns**
Adults and children older than age 12: Initially, 200 mg P.O. b.i.d. (conventional or extended-release tablets), or 100 mg P.O. q.i.d. of suspension with meals. May be increased weekly by 200 mg P.O. daily in divided doses at 12-hour intervals for extended-release tablets or 6- to 8-hour intervals for conventional tablets or suspension, adjusted to minimum effective level. Maximum, 1,000 mg daily in children ages 12 to 15, and 1,200 mg daily in patients older than age 15. Usual maintenance dosage is 800 to 1,200 mg daily.
Children ages 6 to 12: Initially, 100 mg P.O. b.i.d. (conventional or extended-release tablets) or 50 mg of suspension P.O. q.i.d. with meals, increased at weekly intervals by up to 100 mg P.O. divided in three to four doses daily (divided b.i.d. for extended-release form). Maximum, 1,000 mg daily. Usual maintenance dosage is 400 to 800 mg daily; or, 20 to 30 mg/kg in divided doses three to four times daily.
Children younger than age 6: 10 to 20 mg/kg in two to three divided doses (conventional tablets) or four divided doses (suspension). Maximum dosage is 35 mg/kg in 24 hours.
➤ **Acute manic and mixed episodes associated with bipolar I disorder**
Adults: Initially, 200 mg Equetro P.O. b.i.d. Increase by 200 mg daily to achieve therapeutic response. Doses higher than 1,600 mg daily haven't been studied.
➤ **Trigeminal neuralgia**
Adults: Initially, 100 mg P.O. b.i.d. (conventional or extended-release tablets) or 50 mg of suspension q.i.d. with meals, increased by 100 mg q 12 hours for tablets or 50 mg of suspension q.i.d. until pain is relieved. Maximum, 1,200 mg daily. Maintenance dosage is usually 200 to 400 mg P.O. b.i.d.
➤ **Restless legs syndrome ♦**
Adults: 100 to 300 mg P.O. at bedtime.

➤ **Nonneuritic pain syndromes (painful neuromas, phantom limb pain)** ♦
Adults: Initially, 100 mg P.O. b.i.d. Maintenance dose is 600 to 1,400 mg daily.

ACTION
Thought to stabilize neuronal membranes and limit seizure activity by either increasing efflux or decreasing influx of sodium ions across cell membranes in the motor cortex during generation of nerve impulses.

Route	Onset	Peak	Duration
P.O.	Unknown	1½–12 hr	Unknown
P.O. (extended-release)	Unknown	4–8 hr	Unknown

Half-life: 25 to 65 hours with single dose; 8 to 29 hours with long-term use.

ADVERSE REACTIONS
CNS: *ataxia, dizziness, drowsiness, vertigo,* ***worsening of seizures,*** confusion, fatigue, fever, headache, syncope.
CV: ***arrhythmias, AV block, heart failure,*** aggravation of coronary artery disease, hypertension, hypotension.
EENT: blurred vision, conjunctivitis, diplopia, dry pharynx, nystagmus.
GI: *nausea, vomiting,* abdominal pain, anorexia, diarrhea, dry mouth, glossitis, stomatitis.
GU: albuminuria, glycosuria, impotence, urinary frequency, urine retention.
Hematologic: ***agranulocytosis, aplastic anemia, thrombocytopenia,*** eosinophilia, leukocytosis.
Hepatic: ***hepatitis.***
Metabolic: hyponatremia, SIADH.
Respiratory: pulmonary hypersensitivity.
Skin: ***erythema multiforme, Stevens-Johnson syndrome,*** excessive diaphoresis, rash, urticaria.
Other: chills.

INTERACTIONS
Drug-drug. *Atracurium, cisatracurium, pancuronium, rocuronium, vecuronium:* May decrease the effects of nondepolarizing muscle relaxant, causing it to be less effective. May need to increase the dose of the nondepolarizing muscle relaxant.
Cimetidine, danazol, diltiazem, fluoxetine, fluvoxamine, isoniazid, macrolides, propoxyphene, valproic acid, verapamil: May increase carbamazepine level. Use together cautiously.
Clarithromycin, erythromycin, troleandomycin: May inhibit metabolism of carbamazepine, increasing carbamazepine level and risk of toxicity. Avoid using together.
Doxycycline, felbamate, haloperidol, hormonal contraceptives, phenytoin, theophylline, tiagabine, topiramate, valproate, warfarin: May decrease levels of these drugs. Watch for decreased effect.
Lamotrigine: May decrease lamotrigine level and increase carbamazepine level. Monitor patient for clinical effects and toxicity.
Lithium: May increase CNS toxicity of lithium. Avoid using together.
MAO inhibitors: May increase depressant and anticholinergic effects. Avoid using together.
Phenobarbital, phenytoin, primidone: May decrease carbamazepine level. Watch for decreased effect.
Nefazodone: May increase carbamazepine levels and toxicity while reducing nefazodone levels and therapeutic benefits. Use together is contraindicated.
Drug-herb. *Plantains (psyllium seed):* May inhibit GI absorption of drug. Discourage use together.

EFFECTS ON LAB TEST RESULTS
- May increase BUN level. May decrease hemoglobin level and hematocrit.
- May increase liver function test values and eosinophil and WBC counts. May decrease thyroid function test values and granulocyte and platelet counts.
- May cause false pregnancy test results.

CONTRAINDICATIONS & CAUTIONS
- Contraindicated in patients hypersensitive to this drug or tricyclic antidepressants and in those with a history of bone marrow suppression; also contraindicated in those who have taken an MAO inhibitor within 14 days.
- Use cautiously in patients with mixed seizure disorders because they may experience an increased risk of seizures. Also,

use with caution in patients with hepatic dysfunction.

NURSING CONSIDERATIONS

- Watch for worsening of seizures, especially in patients with mixed seizure disorders, including atypical absence seizures.
- Obtain baseline determinations of urinalysis, BUN and iron levels, liver function, CBC, and platelet and reticulocyte counts. Monitor these values periodically thereafter.
- Shake oral suspension well before measuring dose.
- Contents of extended-release capsules may be sprinkled over applesauce if patient has difficulty swallowing capsules. Capsules and tablets shouldn't be crushed or chewed, unless labeled as chewable form.
- When giving by nasogastric tube, mix dose with an equal volume of water, normal saline solution, or D_5W. Flush tube with 100 ml of diluent after giving dose.
- Never stop drug suddenly when treating seizures. Notify prescriber immediately if adverse reactions occur.
- Adverse reactions may be minimized by gradually increasing dosage.
- Therapeutic level is 4 to 12 mcg/ml. Monitor level and effects closely. Ask patient when last dose was taken to better evaluate drug level.
- When managing seizures, take appropriate precautions.
- ***Alert:*** Watch for signs of anorexia or subtle appetite changes, which may indicate excessive drug level.
- ***Look alike–sound alike:*** Don't confuse Tegretol or Tegretol-XR with Topamax, Toprol-XL, or Toradol. Don't confuse Carbatrol with carvedilol.

PATIENT TEACHING

- Instruct patient to take drug with food to minimize GI distress. Tell patient taking suspension form to shake container well before measuring dose.
- Tell patient not to crush or chew extended-release form and not to take broken or chipped tablets.
- Tell patient that Tegretol-XR tablet coating may appear in stool because it isn't absorbed.
- Advise patient to keep tablets in the original container and to keep the container tightly closed and away from moisture. Some formulations may harden when exposed to excessive moisture, so that less is available in the body, decreasing seizure control.
- Inform patient that when drug is used for trigeminal neuralgia, an attempt to decrease dosage or withdraw drug is usually made every 3 months.
- Advise patient to notify prescriber immediately if fever, sore throat, mouth ulcers, or easy bruising or bleeding occurs.
- Tell patient that drug may cause mild to moderate dizziness and drowsiness when first taken. Advise him to avoid hazardous activities until effects disappear, usually within 3 to 4 days.
- Advise patient that periodic eye examinations are recommended.
- Advise woman of risks to fetus if pregnancy occurs while taking carbamazepine.
- Advise woman that breast-feeding isn't recommended during therapy.

SAFETY ALERT!

clonazepam

Klonopin

Pharmacologic class: benzodiazepine
Pregnancy risk category D
Controlled substance schedule IV

AVAILABLE FORMS

Tablets: 0.5 mg, 1 mg, 2 mg

INDICATIONS & DOSAGES

➤ Lennox-Gastaut syndrome, atypical absence seizures, akinetic and myoclonic seizures

Adults: Initially, no more than 1.5 mg P.O. daily in three divided doses. May be increased by 0.5 to 1 mg q 3 days until seizures are controlled. If given in unequal doses, give largest dose at bedtime. Maximum recommended daily dose is 20 mg.
Children up to age 10 or 30 kg (66 lb): Initially, 0.01 to 0.03 mg/kg P.O. daily (not to exceed 0.05 mg/kg daily) in two or three divided doses. Increase by 0.25 to 0.5 mg q third day to maximum maintenance dose of 0.1 to 0.2 mg/kg daily, p.r.n.

➤ **Panic disorder**
Adults: Initially, 0.25 mg P.O. b.i.d.; increase to target dose of 1 mg daily after 3 days. Some patients may benefit from dosages up to maximum of 4 mg daily. To achieve 4 mg daily, increase dosage in increments of 0.125 to 0.25 mg b.i.d. q 3 days, as tolerated, until panic disorder is controlled. Taper drug with decrease of 0.125 mg b.i.d. q 3 days until drug is stopped.
➤ **Acute manic episodes of bipolar disorder** ♦
Adults: 0.75 to 16 mg daily P.O.
➤ **Adjunct treatment for schizophrenia** ♦
Adults: 0.5 to 2 mg daily P.O.
➤ **Periodic leg movements during sleep** ♦
Adults: 0.5 to 2 mg P.O. at bedtime.
➤ **Parkinsonian (hypokinetic) dysarthria** ♦
Adults: 0.25 to 0.5 mg daily P.O.
➤ **Multifocal tic disorders** ♦
Adults: 1.5 to 12 mg daily P.O.
➤ **Neuralgias (deafferentation pain syndromes)** ♦
Adults: 2 to 4 mg daily P.O.

ACTION
Unknown. Probably facilitates the effects of the inhibitory neurotransmitter GABA.

Route	Onset	Peak	Duration
P.O.	Unknown	1–2 hr	Unknown

Half-life: 18 to 50 hours.

ADVERSE REACTIONS
CNS: *drowsiness,* agitation, ataxia, behavioral disturbances, confusion, depression, slurred speech, tremor.
CV: palpitations.
EENT: abnormal eye movements, nystagmus.
GI: anorexia, change in appetite, constipation, diarrhea, gastritis, nausea, sore gums, vomiting.
GU: dysuria, enuresis, nocturia, urine retention.
Hematologic: ***leukopenia, thrombocytopenia,*** eosinophilia.
Respiratory: ***respiratory depression,*** chest congestion, shortness of breath.
Skin: rash.

INTERACTIONS
Drug-drug. *Carbamazepine, phenobarbital, phenytoin:* May lower clonazepam level. Monitor patient closely.
CNS depressants: May increase CNS depression. Avoid using together.
Fluconazole, itraconazole, ketoconazole, miconazole: May increase and prolong drug levels, CNS depression, and psychomotor impairment. Avoid using together.
Drug-lifestyle. *Alcohol use:* May cause additive CNS effects. Discourage use together.
Smoking: May increase clearance of clonazepam. Monitor patient for decreased drug effects.

EFFECTS ON LAB TEST RESULTS
- May increase liver function test values and eosinophil count. May decrease platelet and WBC counts.

CONTRAINDICATIONS & CAUTIONS
- Contraindicated in patients hypersensitive to benzodiazepines and in those with significant hepatic disease or acute angle-closure glaucoma.
- Use cautiously in patients with mixed-type seizures because drug may cause generalized tonic-clonic seizures.
- Use cautiously in children and in patients with chronic respiratory disease or open-angle glaucoma.

NURSING CONSIDERATIONS
- Watch for behavioral disturbances, especially in children.
- Don't stop drug abruptly because this may worsen seizures. Call prescriber at once if adverse reactions develop.
- Assess elderly patient's response closely. Elderly patients are more sensitive to drug's CNS effects.
- Monitor patient for oversedation.
- Monitor CBC and liver function tests.
- Withdrawal symptoms are similar to those of barbiturates.
- To reduce inconvenience of somnolence when drug is used for panic disorder, giving one dose at bedtime may be desirable.

PATIENT TEACHING
- Advise patient to avoid driving and other hazardous activities that require mental

alertness until drug's CNS effects are known.
- Instruct parent to monitor child's school performance because drug may interfere with attentiveness.
- Warn patient and parents not to stop drug abruptly because seizures may occur.
- Advise patient that drug isn't for use while pregnant or breast-feeding.

fosphenytoin sodium
Cerebyx

Pharmacologic class: hydantoin derivative
Pregnancy risk category D

AVAILABLE FORMS
Injection: 2 ml (150 mg fosphenytoin sodium equivalent to 100 mg phenytoin sodium), 10 ml (750 mg fosphenytoin sodium equivalent to 500 mg phenytoin sodium)

INDICATIONS & DOSAGES
➤ **Status epilepticus**
Adults: 15 to 20 mg phenytoin sodium equivalent (PE)/kg I.V. at 100 to 150 mg PE/minute as loading dose; then 4 to 6 mg PE/kg daily I.V. as maintenance dose.
➤ **To prevent and treat seizures during neurosurgery (nonemergent loading or maintenance dosage)**
Adults: Loading dose of 10 to 20 mg PE/kg I.M. or I.V. at infusion rate not exceeding 150 mg PE/minute. Maintenance dose is 4 to 6 mg PE/kg daily I.V. or I.M.
➤ **Short-term substitution for oral phenytoin therapy**
Adults: Same total daily dose equivalent as oral phenytoin sodium therapy given as a single daily dose I.M. or I.V. at infusion rate not exceeding 150 mg PE/minute. Some patients may need more frequent doses.
Elderly patients: Phenytoin clearance is decreased slightly in elderly patients; lower or less-frequent doses may be required.

I.V. ADMINISTRATION
- If rapid phenytoin loading is a main goal, this form is preferred.
- For status epilepticus, give I.V. rather than I.M. because therapeutic phenytoin level occurs more rapidly.
- For infusion, dilute in D_5W or normal saline solution for injection to yield 1.5 to 25 mg PE/ml.
- Don't give more than 150 mg PE/minute. For a 50-kg (110-lb) patient, infusion should take 5 to 7 minutes. (Infusion of identical molar dose of phenytoin takes at least 15 minutes because giving phenytoin I.V. at more than 50 mg/minute causes adverse CV effects.)
- Patients receiving 20 mg PE/kg at 150 mg PE/minute typically feel discomfort, usually in the groin. To reduce discomfort, slow or temporarily stop infusion.
- Monitor patient's ECG, blood pressure, and respirations continuously during maximal phenytoin level—about 10 to 20 minutes after end of fosphenytoin infusion. Severe CV complications are most common in elderly or gravely ill patients. If needed, decrease rate or stop infusion.

INCOMPATIBILITIES
Other I.V. drugs.

ACTION
A prodrug of phenytoin with the same anticonvulsant action. Stabilizes neuronal membranes and limits seizure activity by modulating voltage-dependent neuron channels, inhibiting calcium flux across neuronal membranes, and enhancing sodium-potassium ATPase activity.

Route	Onset	Peak	Duration
I.V.	Unknown	End of infusion	Unknown
I.M.	Unknown	30 min	Unknown

Half-life: 15 minutes.

ADVERSE REACTIONS
CNS: *ataxia, dizziness, somnolence, **brain edema, intracranial hypertension,*** agitation, asthenia, dysarthria, extrapyramidal syndrome, fever, headache, hypesthesia, incoordination, increased or decreased reflexes, nervousness, paresthesia, speech disorders, stupor, thinking abnormalities, tremor, vertigo.
CV: hypertension, hypotension, tachycardia, vasodilation.

EENT: *nystagmus,* amblyopia, deafness, diplopia, tinnitus.
GI: constipation, dry mouth, taste perversion, tongue disorder, vomiting.
Metabolic: hypokalemia.
Musculoskeletal: back pain, pelvic pain, myasthenia.
Respiratory: pneumonia.
Skin: *pruritus,* ecchymoses, injection site reaction and pain, rash.
Other: accidental injury, chills, facial edema, infection.

INTERACTIONS

Drug-drug. *Amiodarone, chloramphenicol, chlordiazepoxide, cimetidine, diazepam, disulfiram, estrogens, ethosuximide, fluoxetine, H_2 antagonists, halothane, isoniazid, methylphenidate, phenothiazines, phenylbutazone, salicylates, succinimides, sulfonamides, tolbutamide, trazodone:* May increase phenytoin level and effect. Use together cautiously.
Carbamazepine, reserpine: May decrease phenytoin level. Monitor patient.
Corticosteroids, doxycycline, estrogens, furosemide, hormonal contraceptives, quinidine, rifampin, theophylline, vitamin D, warfarin: May decrease effects of these drugs because of increased hepatic metabolism. Monitor patient closely.
Lithium: May increase lithium toxicity. Monitor patient's neurologic status closely. Marked neurologic symptoms have been reported despite normal lithium level.
Phenobarbital, valproate sodium, valproic acid: May increase or decrease phenytoin level. May increase or decrease levels of these drugs. Monitor patient.
Tricyclic antidepressants: May lower seizure threshold and require adjustments in phenytoin dosage. Use together cautiously.
Drug-lifestyle. *Alcohol use:* Acute intoxication may increase phenytoin level and effect. Discourage use together.
Long-term alcohol use: May decrease phenytoin level. Monitor patient.

EFFECTS ON LAB TEST RESULTS

- May increase alkaline phosphatase, GGT, and glucose levels. May decrease folate, potassium, and T_4 levels.
- May cause falsely low dexamethasone and metyrapone test results.

CONTRAINDICATIONS & CAUTIONS

- Contraindicated in patients hypersensitive to drug or its components, phenytoin, or other hydantoins.
- Contraindicated in those with sinus bradycardia, SA block, second- or third-degree AV block, or Adams-Stokes syndrome.
- Use cautiously in patients with porphyria and in those with history of hypersensitivity to similarly structured drugs, such as barbiturates, oxazolidinediones, and succinimide.

NURSING CONSIDERATIONS

- Most significant drug interactions are those commonly seen with phenytoin.
- ***Alert:*** Drug should always be prescribed and dispensed in phenytoin sodium equivalent units (PE). Don't make adjustments in the recommended doses when substituting fosphenytoin for phenytoin, and vice versa.
- In status epilepticus, phenytoin may be used instead of fosphenytoin as maintenance, using the appropriate dose.
- Phosphate load provided by fosphenytoin (0.0037 millimole phosphate/mg PE fosphenytoin) must be taken into consideration when treating patients who need phosphate restriction, such as those with severe renal impairment. Monitor laboratory values.
- If patient gets exfoliative, purpuric, or bullous rash or signs and symptoms of lupus erythematosus, Stevens-Johnson syndrome, or toxic epidermal necrolysis, stop drug and notify prescriber. If rash is mild (measles-like or scarlatiniform), therapy may resume after rash disappears. If rash recurs when therapy is resumed, further fosphenytoin or phenytoin administration is contraindicated. Document that patient is allergic to drug.
- Stop drug in patients with acute hepatotoxicity.
- I.M. administration generates systemic phenytoin levels similar enough to oral phenytoin sodium to allow essentially interchangeable use.
- After administration, phenytoin levels shouldn't be monitored until conversion to phenytoin is essentially complete—about 2 hours after the end of an I.V. infusion or 4 hours after I.M. administration.

• Interpret total phenytoin levels cautiously in patients with renal or hepatic disease or hypoalbuminemia caused by an increased fraction in unbound phenytoin. It may be more useful to monitor unbound phenytoin levels in these patients. When giving drug I.V., monitor patients with renal and hepatic disease because they are at increased risk for more frequent and severe adverse reactions.
• Monitor glucose level closely in diabetic patients; drug may cause hyperglycemia.
• Abrupt withdrawal of drug may precipitate status epilepticus.
• Store drug under refrigeration. Don't store at room temperature longer than 48 hours. Discard vials that develop particulate matter.
• ***Look alike–sound alike:*** Don't confuse Cerebyx with Cerezyme, Celexa, or Celebrex.

PATIENT TEACHING
• Warn patient that sensory disturbances may occur with I.V. administration.
• Instruct patient to report adverse reactions, especially rash, immediately.
• Warn patient not to stop drug abruptly or adjust dosage without discussing with prescriber.
• Advise woman of childbearing age to discuss drug therapy with prescriber if she's considering pregnancy.
• Advise woman of childbearing age that breast-feeding isn't recommended during therapy.

gabapentin
Neurontin🖉, Gabarone

Pharmacologic class: gamma-aminobutyric acid (GABA) structural analog
Pregnancy risk category C

AVAILABLE FORMS
Capsules: 100 mg, 300 mg, 400 mg
Oral solution: 250 mg/5 ml
Tablets: 100 mg, 300 mg, 400 mg, 600 mg, 800 mg

INDICATIONS & DOSAGES
➤ Adjunctive treatment of partial seizures with or without secondary generalization in patients with epilepsy
Adults and children older than 12: Initially, 300 mg P.O. t.i.d. Increase dosage as needed and tolerated to 1,800 mg daily in divided doses. Dosages up to 3,600 mg daily have been well tolerated.
➤ Adjunctive treatment to control partial seizures in children
Starting dosage, children ages 3 to 12: 10 to 15 mg/kg daily P.O. in three divided doses, adjusting over 3 days to reach effective dosage.
Effective dosage, children ages 5 to 12: 25 to 35 mg/kg daily P.O. in three divided doses.
Effective dosage, children ages 3 to 4: 40 mg/kg daily P.O. in three divided doses.
➤ Postherpetic neuralgia
Adults: 300 mg P.O. once daily on first day, 300 mg b.i.d. on day 2, and 300 mg t.i.d. on day 3. Adjust p.r.n. for pain to a maximum daily dose of 1,800 mg in three divided doses.
Adjust-a-dose: In patients age 12 and older with creatinine clearance 30 to 59 ml/minute, give 400 to 1,400 mg daily, divided into two doses. For clearance 15 to 29 ml/minute, give 200 to 700 mg daily in single dose. For clearance less than 15 ml/minute, give 100 to 300 mg daily, in single dose. Reduce daily dose in proportion to creatinine clearance (patients with a clearance of 7.5 ml/minute should receive one-half the daily dose of those with a clearance of 15 ml/minute). For patients receiving hemodialysis, maintenance dose is based on estimates of creatinine clearance. Give supplemental dose of 125 to 350 mg after each 4 hours of hemodialysis.
➤ Pain from diabetic neuropathy ♦
Adults: 3.6 g P.O. daily in divided doses.

ACTION
Unknown. Structurally related to GABA but doesn't interact with GABA receptors, isn't converted into GABA or GABA agonist, doesn't inhibit GABA reuptake, and doesn't prevent degradation.

Route	Onset	Peak	Duration
P.O.	Unknown	Unknown	Unknown

Half-life: 5 to 7 hours.

ADVERSE REACTIONS

CNS: *ataxia, dizziness, fatigue, somnolence,* abnormal thinking, amnesia, depression, dysarthria, incoordination, nervousness, nystagmus, tremor, twitching.
CV: peripheral edema, vasodilation.
EENT: amblyopia, diplopia, dry throat, pharyngitis, rhinitis.
GI: constipation, dry mouth, dyspepsia, increased appetite, nausea, vomiting.
GU: impotence.
Hematologic: ***leukopenia.***
Metabolic: weight gain.
Musculoskeletal: back pain, fractures, myalgia.
Respiratory: coughing.
Skin: abrasion, pruritus.
Other: dental abnormalities.

INTERACTIONS

Drug-drug. *Antacids:* May decrease absorption of gabapentin. Separate dosage times by at least 2 hours.
Hydrocodone: May increase gabapentin level and decrease hydrocodone level. Monitor patient for increased adverse effects or loss of clinical effect.

EFFECTS ON LAB TEST RESULTS

- May decrease WBC count.
- May cause false-positive results with the Ames-N-Multistix SG dipstick test for urine protein when drug is used with other antiepileptics.

CONTRAINDICATIONS & CAUTIONS

- Contraindicated in patients hypersensitive to drug.

NURSING CONSIDERATIONS

- Give first dose at bedtime to minimize drowsiness, dizziness, fatigue, and ataxia.
- If drug is to be stopped or another drug substituted, do so gradually over at least 1 week to minimize risk of seizures.
- ***Alert:*** Don't suddenly withdraw other anticonvulsants in patients starting gabapentin therapy.
- Routine monitoring of drug levels isn't necessary. Drug doesn't appear to alter levels of other anticonvulsants.
- ***Look alike–sound alike:*** Don't confuse Neurontin with Noroxin.

PATIENT TEACHING

- Advise patient that drug may be taken without regard to meals.
- Instruct patient to take first dose at bedtime to minimize adverse reactions.
- Tell patient with seizures the maximum time interval between doses shouldn't exceed 12 hours.
- Warn patient to avoid driving and operating heavy machinery until drug's CNS effects are known.
- Advise patient not to stop drug abruptly.
- Advise woman to discuss drug therapy with prescriber if she's considering pregnancy.
- Tell patient to keep oral solution refrigerated.

lamotrigine

Lamictal

Pharmacologic class: phenyltriazine
Pregnancy risk category C

AVAILABLE FORMS

Tablets: 25 mg, 100 mg, 150 mg, 200 mg
Tablets (chewable dispersible): 2 mg, 5 mg, 25 mg

INDICATIONS & DOSAGES

➤ **Adjunct treatment of partial seizures caused by epilepsy or generalized seizures of Lennox-Gastaut syndrome**

Adults and children older than age 12 taking other enzyme-inducing anticonvulsants with valproic acid: 25 mg P.O. every other day for 2 weeks; then 25 mg P.O. daily for 2 weeks. Continue to increase, p.r.n., by 25 to 50 mg daily q 1 to 2 weeks until an effective maintenance dosage of 100 to 400 mg daily given in one or two divided doses is reached. When added to valproic acid alone, the usual daily maintenance dose is 100 to 200 mg.
Adults and children older than age 12 taking other enzyme-inducing anticonvulsants but not valproic acid: 50 mg P.O. daily for 2 weeks; then 100 mg P.O. daily in two divided doses for 2 weeks. Increase, p.r.n., by 100 mg daily q 1 to 2 weeks. Usual maintenance dosage is 300 to 500 mg P.O. daily in two divided doses.

Children ages 2 to 12 weighing 6.7 to 40 kg (15 to 88 lb) taking other enzyme-inducing anticonvulsants with valproic acid: 0.15 mg/kg P.O. daily in one or two divided doses (rounded down to nearest whole tablet) for 2 weeks, followed by 0.3 mg/kg daily in one or two divided doses for another 2 weeks. Thereafter, usual maintenance dosage is 1 to 5 mg/kg daily (maximum, 200 mg daily in one to two divided doses).
Children ages 2 to 12 weighing 6.7 to 40 kg (15 to 88 lb) taking other enzyme-inducing anticonvulsants but not valproic acid: 0.6 mg/kg P.O. daily in two divided doses (rounded down to nearest whole tablet) for 2 weeks; then 1.2 mg/kg daily in two divided doses for another 2 weeks. Usual maintenance dosage is 5 to 15 mg/kg P.O. daily (maximum 400 mg daily in two divided doses).

➤ To convert patients from therapy with a hepatic enzyme–inducing anticonvulsant alone to lamotrigine therapy

Adults and children age 16 and older: Add lamotrigine 50 mg P.O. once daily to current drug regimen for 2 weeks, followed by 100 mg P.O. daily in two divided doses for 2 weeks. Then increase daily dosage by 100 mg q 1 to 2 weeks until maintenance dose of 500 mg daily in two divided doses is reached. The hepatic enzyme–inducing anticonvulsant can then be gradually reduced by 20% q week for 4 weeks.
Adjust-a-dose: For patients with severe renal impairment, use lower maintenance dosage.

➤ To convert patients with partial seizures from adjunctive therapy with valproate to therapy with lamotrigine alone

Adults and children age 16 and older: Add lamotrigine until 200 mg daily is achieved; then gradually decrease valproate to 500 mg daily by decrements of no more than 500 mg daily per week. Maintain these dosages for 1 week; then increase lamotrigine to 300 mg daily while decreasing valproate to 250 mg daily. Maintain these dosages for 1 week; then stop valproate completely while increasing lamotrigine by 100 mg daily q week until a dose of 500 mg daily is reached.

➤ Bipolar disorder

Adults: Initially, 25 mg P.O. once daily for 2 weeks; then 50 mg P.O. once daily for 2 weeks. Dosage may then be doubled at weekly intervals, to maintenance dosage of 200 mg daily.
Adults taking carbamazepine or other hepatic enzyme–inducing drugs without valproic acid: Initially, 50 mg P.O. once daily for 2 weeks; then 100 mg daily in two divided doses for 2 weeks. Dosage is then increased by 100 mg weekly to maintenance dosage of 400 mg daily, given in two divided doses.
Adults taking valproic acid: Initially, 25 mg P.O. every other day for 2 weeks; then 25 mg P.O. once daily for 2 weeks. Dosage may then be doubled at weekly intervals to maintenance dosage of 100 mg daily.

✷***NEW INDICATION:*** **Adjunctive therapy for primary generalized tonic-clonic seizures**

Adults and children age 12 and older also taking valproate: 25 mg P.O. every other day in weeks 1 and 2; then, 25 mg/day in weeks 3 and 4. Increase by 25 to 50 mg/day q 1 to 2 weeks to maintenance dose of 100 to 400 mg/day in 1 or 2 divided doses or 100 to 200 mg/day with valproate alone.
Adults and children age 12 and older taking carbamazepine, phenytoin, phenobarbital, or primidone but not valproate: 50 mg/day P.O. in weeks 1 and 2; then, 100 mg/day in 2 divided doses in weeks 3 and 4. Increase by 100 mg/day q 1 to 2 weeks to maintenance dose of 300 to 500 mg/day in 2 divided doses.
Adults and children age 12 and older taking antiepileptics other than carbamazepine, phenytoin, phenobarbital, primidone, and valproate: 25 mg/day P.O. in weeks 1 and 2; then, 50 mg/day in weeks 3 and 4. Increase by 50 mg/day q 1 to 2 weeks to maintenance dose of 225 to 375 mg/day in 2 divided doses.
Children ages 2 to 12 also taking valproate: 0.15 mg/kg/day P.O. in 1 to 2 divided doses in weeks 1 and 2; then, 0.3 mg/kg/day in 1 or 2 divided doses in weeks 3 and 4. Increase to maintenance dose of 1 to 5 mg/kg/day. Maximum, 200 mg/day or 1 to 3 mg/kg/day with valproate alone.

Children ages 2 to 12 taking carbamazepine, phenytoin, phenobarbital, or primidone but not valproate: 0.6 mg/kg/day P.O. in 2 divided doses in weeks 1 and 2; then, 1.2 mg/kg/day in 2 divided doses in weeks 3 and 4; then, maintenance dose of 5 to 15 mg/kg/day in 2 divided doses. Maximum, 400 mg/day.
Children ages 2 to 12 taking antiepileptics other than carbamazepine, phenytoin, phenobarbital, primidone, or valproate: 0.3 mg/kg/day P.O. in 1 or 2 divided doses in weeks 1 and 2; then, 0.6 mg/kg/day in 2 divided doses in weeks 3 and 4. Maintenance dose is 4.5 to 7.5 mg/kg/day in 2 divided doses. Maximum, 300 mg/day.

ACTION

Unknown. May inhibit release of glutamate and aspartate (excitatory neurotransmitters) in the brain via an action at voltage-sensitive sodium channels.

Route	Onset	Peak	Duration
P.O.	Unknown	1–5 hr	Unknown

Half-life: 14½ to 70¼ hours, depending on dosage schedule and use of other anticonvulsants.

ADVERSE REACTIONS

CNS: *ataxia, dizziness, headache, somnolence,* ***seizures,*** aggravated reaction, anxiety, concentration disturbance, decreased memory, depression, dysarthria, emotional lability, fever, incoordination, insomnia, irritability, malaise, mind racing, speech disorder, sleep disorder, tremor, vertigo.
CV: palpitations.
EENT: *blurred vision, diplopia, rhinitis,* nystagmus, pharyngitis, vision abnormality.
GI: *nausea, vomiting,* abdominal pain, anorexia, constipation, diarrhea, dry mouth, dyspepsia.
GU: amenorrhea, dysmenorrhea, vaginitis.
Musculoskeletal: muscle spasm, neck pain.
Respiratory: cough, dyspnea.
Skin: *rash,* ***Stevens-Johnson syndrome, toxic epidermal necrolysis,*** acne, alopecia, hot flashes, pruritus.
Other: chills, flulike syndrome, infection, tooth disorder.

INTERACTIONS

Drug-drug. *Acetaminophen:* May decrease therapeutic effects of lamotrigine. Monitor patient.
Carbamazepine: May decrease effects of lamotrigine while increasing toxicity of carbamazepine. Adjust doses and monitor patient.
Ethosuximide, oxcarbazepine, phenobarbital, phenytoin, primidone: May decrease lamotrigine level. Monitor patient closely.
Folate inhibitors, such as co-trimoxazole and methotrexate: May have additive effect because lamotrigine inhibits dihydrofolate reductase, an enzyme involved in folic acid synthesis. Monitor patient.
Oral contraceptives containing estrogen, rifampin: May decrease lamotrigine levels. Adjust dosage. By the end of the "pill-free" week, lamotrigine levels may double.
Valproic acid: May decrease clearance of lamotrigine, which increases lamotrigine level; also decreases valproic acid level. Monitor patient for toxicity.
Drug-lifestyle. *Sun exposure:* May cause photosensitivity reactions. Advise patient to avoid excessive sun exposure.

EFFECTS ON LAB TEST RESULTS

None reported.

CONTRAINDICATIONS & CAUTIONS

- Contraindicated in patients hypersensitive to drug or its components.
- Use cautiously in patients with renal, hepatic, or cardiac impairment.

NURSING CONSIDERATIONS

- Don't stop drug abruptly because this may increase seizure frequency. Instead, taper drug over at least 2 weeks.
- ***Alert:*** Stop drug at first sign of rash, unless rash is clearly not drug related.
- Reduce lamotrigine dose if drug is added to a multidrug regimen that includes valproic acid.
- Chewable dispersible tablets may be swallowed whole, chewed, or dispersed in water or diluted fruit juice. If tablets are chewed, give a small amount of water or diluted fruit juice to aid in swallowing.
- Evaluate patients for changes in seizure activity. Check adjunct anticonvulsant level.

• ***Look alike–sound alike:*** Don't confuse lamotrigine with lamivudine or Lamictal with Lamisil, Ludiomil, labetalol, or Lomotil.

PATIENT TEACHING

• Inform patient that drug may cause rash. Combination therapy of valproic acid and lamotrigine may cause a serious rash. Tell patient to report rash or signs or symptoms of hypersensitivity promptly because they may warrant stopping drug.
• Warn patient not to engage in hazardous activity until drug's CNS effects are known.
• Warn patient that the drug may trigger sensitivity to the sun and to take precautions until tolerance is determined.
• Warn patient not to stop drug abruptly.
• ***Alert:*** Advise woman of childbearing age to discuss drug therapy with prescriber if she's considering pregnancy. Babies exposed to drug during the first trimester have a greater risk of cleft lip or palate.
• Advise woman of childbearing age that breast-feeding isn't recommended during therapy.

levetiracetam

Keppra

Pharmacologic class: pyrrolidine derivative
Pregnancy risk category C

AVAILABLE FORMS

Injection: 500 mg/5 ml single-use vial
Oral solution: 100 mg/ml
Tablets: 250 mg, 500 mg, 750 mg

INDICATIONS & DOSAGES

➤ Adjunct for myoclonic seizures of juvenile myoclonic epilepsy

Adults and adolescents age 12 and older: Initially, 500 mg P.O. b.i.d. Increase by 1,000 mg/day q 2 weeks to daily dose of 3,000 mg.

➤ Adjunct for partial-onset seizures in patients with epilepsy

Adults and adolescents age 16 or older: Initially, 500 mg P.O. or I.V. b.i.d. Increase dosage by 500 mg b.i.d., p.r.n., for seizure control at 2-week intervals to maximum of 1,500 mg b.i.d.

Children ages 4 to 16: Initially, 10 mg/kg P.O. b.i.d. Increase dose by 10 mg/kg b.i.d. at 2-week intervals to recommended dose of 30 mg/kg b.i.d. If patient can't tolerate this dose, reduce it. For children who weigh 20 kg (44 lb) or less, use the oral solution.

Adjust-a-dose: For adults with creatinine clearance of 50 to 80 ml/minute, give 500 to 1,000 mg q 12 hours; if clearance is 30 to 50 ml/minute, give 250 to 750 mg q 12 hours; if clearance is less than 30 ml/minute, give 250 to 500 mg q 12 hours. For dialysis patients, give 500 to 1,000 mg q 24 hours. Give a 250- to 500-mg dose after dialysis.

I.V. ADMINISTRATION

• Dilute 500-mg, 1,000-mg, or 1,500-mg dose in 100 ml normal saline, D_5W, or lactated Ringer injection and infuse over 15 minutes.
• Drug is compatible with diazepam, lorazepam, and valproate sodium for 24 hours at a controlled room temperature.

INCOMPATIBILITIES

Unknown with other antiepileptics, besides diazepam, lorazepam, and valproate sodium.

ACTION

May act by inhibiting simultaneous neuronal firing that leads to seizure activity.

Route	Onset	Peak	Duration
P.O., I.V.	1 hr	1 hr	12 hr

Half-life: About 7 hours in patients with normal renal function.

ADVERSE REACTIONS

CNS: *asthenia, headache, somnolence,* amnesia, anxiety, ataxia, depression, dizziness, emotional lability, hostility, nervousness, paresthesia, vertigo.
EENT: diplopia, pharyngitis, rhinitis, sinusitis.
GI: anorexia.
Hematologic: ***leukopenia, neutropenia.***
Musculoskeletal: pain.
Respiratory: cough, infection.

INTERACTIONS

Drug-drug. *Antihistamines, benzodiazepines, opioids, other drugs that cause*

drowsiness, tricyclic antidepressants: May lead to severe sedation. Avoid using together.
Drug-lifestyle. *Alcohol use:* May lead to severe sedation. Discourage use together.

EFFECTS ON LAB TEST RESULTS

- May decrease hemoglobin level and hematocrit.
- May decrease WBC, RBC, and neutrophil counts. May alter liver function test results.

CONTRAINDICATIONS & CAUTIONS

- Contraindicated in patients hypersensitive to drug.
- Leukopenia and neutropenia have been reported with drug use. Use cautiously in immunocompromised patients, such as those with cancer or HIV infection.
- Patients with poor renal function need dosage adjustment.

NURSING CONSIDERATIONS

- Drug can be taken with or without food.
- Oral and I.V. forms are bioequivalent.
- Use drug only with other anticonvulsants; it's not recommended for monotherapy.
- Seizures can occur if drug is stopped abruptly. Tapering is recommended.
- Monitor patients closely for such adverse reactions as dizziness, which may lead to falls.
- ***Look alike–sound alike:*** Don't confuse Keppra with Kaletra.

PATIENT TEACHING

- Warn patient to use extra care when sitting up or standing up to avoid falling.
- Advise patient to call prescriber if adverse reactions occur and not to stop drug suddenly.
- Tell patient to take with other prescribed seizure drugs.
- For the oral solution, tell patient or parent to use a calibrated measuring device, not a household spoon.
- Warn patient that drug may cause dizziness and somnolence and that he should avoid driving, bike riding, or other hazardous activities until he knows how the drug will affect him.
- Inform patient that drug can be taken with or without food.

SAFETY ALERT!

magnesium sulfate

Pharmacologic class: mineral; electrolyte
Pregnancy risk category A

AVAILABLE FORMS

Injection: 4%, 8%, 10%, 12.5%, 25%, 50%
Injection solution: 1% in D_5W, 2% in D_5W

INDICATIONS & DOSAGES

➤ To prevent or control seizures in preeclampsia or eclampsia
Women: Initially, 4 g I.V. in 250 ml D_5W or normal saline and 4 to 5 g deep I.M. into each buttock; then 4 to 5 g deep I.M. into alternate buttock q 4 hours, p.r.n. Or, 4 g I.V. loading dose; then 1 to 3 g hourly as I.V. infusion. Total dose shouldn't exceed 30 or 40 g daily.
➤ Hypomagnesemia
Adults: For mild deficiency, 1 g I.M. q 6 hours for four doses; for severe deficiency, 5 g in 1,000 ml D_5W or normal saline solution infused over 3 hours.
➤ Seizures, hypertension, and encephalopathy with acute nephritis in children
Children: 20 to 40 mg/kg I.M. p.r.n to control seizures. Dilute the 50% concentration to a 20% solution and give 0.1 to 0.2 ml/kg of the 20% solution.
➤ To manage paroxysmal atrial tachycardia
Adults: 3 to 4 g I.V. over 30 seconds, with extreme caution.
➤ To manage life-threatening ventricular arrhythmias, such as sustained ventricular tachycardia or torsades de pointes ♦
Adults: 1 to 6 g I.V. over several minutes; then continuous I.V. infusion of 3 to 20 mg/minute for 5 to 48 hours. Base dosage and duration of therapy on patient response and magnesium level.
➤ To manage preterm labor ♦
Adults: 4 to 6 g I.V. over 20 minutes, followed by 2 to 4 g/hr I.V. infusion for 12 to 24 hours, as tolerated, after contractions have stopped.

I.V. ADMINISTRATION

- If necessary, dilute to maximum level of 20%. Infuse no faster than 150 mg/minute (1.5 ml/minute of a 10% solution or 0.75 ml/minute of a 20% solution). Drug is compatible with D_5W and normal saline solution.
- Maximum infusion rate is 150 mg/minute. Too-rapid infusion induces uncomfortable feeling of heat.
- Monitor vital signs every 15 minutes when giving drug I.V.

INCOMPATIBILITIES

Alkali carbonates and bicarbonates, amiodarone, amphotericin B, calcium gluconate, cefepime, ciprofloxacin, clindamycin, cyclosporine, dobutamine, heavy metals, I.V. fat emulsion 10%, polymyxin B, procaine, salicylates, sodium bicarbonate, soluble phosphates.

ACTION

May decrease acetylcholine released by nerve impulses, but its anticonvulsant mechanism is unknown.

Route	Onset	Peak	Duration
I.V.	1–2 min	Rapid	30 min
I.M.	1 hr	Unknown	3–4 hr

Half-life: Unknown.

ADVERSE REACTIONS

CNS: *depressed reflexes,* drowsiness, flaccid paralysis, hypothermia.
CV: *flushing, hypotension,* ***bradycardia, circulatory collapse,*** depressed cardiac function.
EENT: diplopia.
Metabolic: hypocalcemia.
Respiratory: ***respiratory paralysis.***
Skin: diaphoresis.

INTERACTIONS

Drug-drug. *Anesthetics, CNS depressants:* May cause additive CNS depression. Use together cautiously.
Cardiac glycosides: May worsen arrhythmias. Use together cautiously.
Neuromuscular blockers: May cause increased neuromuscular blockade. Use together cautiously.

EFFECTS ON LAB TEST RESULTS

- May increase magnesium level. May decrease calcium level.

CONTRAINDICATIONS & CAUTIONS

- Parenteral administration contraindicated in patients with heart block or myocardial damage.
- Contraindicated in patients with toxemia of pregnancy during 2 hours preceding delivery.
- Use cautiously in patients with impaired renal function.
- Use cautiously in pregnant women during labor.

NURSING CONSIDERATIONS

- If used to treat seizures, take appropriate seizure precautions.
- ***Alert:*** Watch for respiratory depression and signs and symptoms of heart block.
- Keep I.V. calcium gluconate available to reverse magnesium intoxication, but use cautiously in digitalized patients because of danger of arrhythmias.
- Check magnesium level after repeated doses. Disappearance of knee-jerk and patellar reflexes is sign of impending magnesium toxicity.
- Signs of hypermagnesemia begin to appear at levels of 4 mEq/L.
- Effective anticonvulsant level ranges from 2.5 to 7.5 mEq/L.
- Monitor fluid intake and output. Make sure urine output is 100 ml or more in 4-hour period before each dose.
- Observe neonates for signs of magnesium toxicity, including neuromuscular or respiratory depression, when giving I.V. form of drug to toxemic mothers within 24 hours before delivery.
- ***Look alike–sound alike:*** Don't confuse magnesium sulfate with manganese sulfate.

PATIENT TEACHING

- Inform patient of short-term need for drug, answer any questions, and address concerns.
- Review potential adverse reactions and instruct patient to promptly report any occurrences. Reassure patient that, although adverse reactions can occur, vital signs, reflexes, and drug level will be monitored frequently to ensure safety.

oxcarbazepine
Trileptal

Pharmacologic class: carboxamide derivative
Pregnancy risk category C

AVAILABLE FORMS
Oral suspension: 300 mg/5 ml (60 mg/ml)
Tablets (film-coated): 150 mg, 300 mg, 600 mg

INDICATIONS & DOSAGES
➤ **Adjunctive treatment of partial seizures in patients with epilepsy**
Adults: Initially, 300 mg P.O. b.i.d. Increase by a maximum of 600 mg daily (300 mg P.O. b.i.d.) at weekly intervals. Recommended daily dose is 1,200 mg P.O. divided b.i.d.
Children ages 4 to 16: Initially, 8 to 10 mg/kg daily P.O. divided b.i.d., not to exceed 600 mg daily. The target maintenance dose depends on patient's weight and should be divided b.i.d. If patient weighs between 20 and 29 kg (44 and 64 lb), target maintenance dose is 900 mg daily. If patient weighs between 29 and 39 kg (64 and 86 lb), target maintenance dose is 1,200 mg daily. If patient weighs more than 39 kg (86 lb), target maintenance dose is 1,800 mg daily. Target doses should be achieved over 2 weeks.
➤ **To change from multidrug to single-drug treatment of partial seizures in patients with epilepsy**
Adults: Initially, 300 mg P.O. b.i.d., while reducing dose of concomitant anticonvulsant. Increase oxcarbazepine by a maximum of 600 mg daily at weekly intervals over 2 to 4 weeks. Recommended daily dose is 2,400 mg P.O. divided b.i.d. Withdraw other anticonvulsant completely over 3 to 6 weeks.
Children ages 4 to 16: Initially, 8 to 10 mg/kg daily P.O. divided b.i.d., while reducing dose of concomitant anticonvulsant. Increase oxcarbazepine by a maximum of 10 mg/kg daily at weekly intervals. Withdraw other anticonvulsant completely over 3 to 6 weeks.
➤ **To start single-drug treatment of partial seizures in patients with epilepsy**
Adults: Initially, 300 mg P.O. b.i.d. Increase dosage by 300 mg daily q third day to a daily dose of 1,200 mg divided b.i.d.
Children ages 4 to 16: Initially, 8 to 10 mg/kg daily P.O. divided b.i.d., increasing the dosage by 5 mg/kg daily q third day to the recommended daily dose range shown in the table.

Weight (kg)	Dose (mg/day)
20	600–900
25	900–1,200
30	900–1,200
35	900–1,500
40	900–1,500
45	1,200–1,500
50	1,200–1,800
55	1,200–1,800
60	1,200–2,100
65	1,200–2,100
70	1,500–2,100

Adjust-a-dose: If creatinine clearance is less than 30 ml/minute, start therapy at 150 mg P.O. b.i.d. (one-half usual starting dose) and increase slowly to achieve desired response.

ACTION
Thought to prevent seizure spread in the brain by blocking voltage-sensitive sodium channels, and to produce anticonvulsant effects by increasing potassium conduction and modulating high-voltage activated calcium channels.

Route	Onset	Peak	Duration
P.O.	Unknown	Variable	Unknown

Half-life: About 2 hours for the drug; about 9 hours for the active metabolite. Children younger than age 8 have a 30% to 40% increase in clearance.

ADVERSE REACTIONS
CNS: *abnormal gait, ataxia, dizziness, fatigue, headache, somnolence, tremor, vertigo,* ***aggravated seizures,*** abnormal coordination, agitation, amnesia, anxiety, asthenia, confusion, emotional lability, feeling abnormal, fever, hypesthesia, im-

paired concentration, insomnia, nervousness, speech disorder.
CV: chest pain, edema, hypotension.
EENT: *abnormal vision, diplopia, nystagmus,* abnormal accommodation, ear pain, epistaxis, pharyngitis, rhinitis, sinusitis.
GI: *abdominal pain, nausea, vomiting,* ***rectal hemorrhage,*** anorexia, constipation, diarrhea, dry mouth, dyspepsia, gastritis, taste perversion, thirst.
GU: urinary frequency, UTI, vaginitis.
Metabolic: hyponatremia, weight increase.
Musculoskeletal: back pain, muscular weakness.
Respiratory: *upper respiratory tract infection,* bronchitis, chest infection, coughing.
Skin: acne, bruising, hot flushes, increased sweating, purpura, rash.
Other: allergic reaction, infection, lymphadenopathy, toothache.

INTERACTIONS

Drug-drug. *Carbamazepine, valproic acid, verapamil:* May decrease level of active metabolite of oxcarbazepine. Monitor patient and level closely.
Felodipine: May decrease felodipine level. Monitor patient closely.
Hormonal contraceptives: May decrease levels of ethinyl estradiol and levonorgestrel, reducing hormonal contraceptive effectiveness. Caution women of childbearing age to use alternative forms of contraception.
Phenobarbital: May decrease level of active metabolite of oxcarbazepine; may increase phenobarbital level. Monitor patient closely.
Phenytoin: May decrease level of active metabolite of oxcarbazepine; may increase phenytoin level in adults receiving high doses of oxcarbazepine. Monitor phenytoin level closely when starting therapy in these patients.
Drug-lifestyle. *Alcohol use:* May increase CNS depression. Discourage use together.

EFFECTS ON LAB TEST RESULTS

- May decrease sodium and thyroxine levels.

CONTRAINDICATIONS & CAUTIONS

- Contraindicated in patients hypersensitive to drug or its components.

NURSING CONSIDERATIONS

- ***Alert:*** Between 25% and 30% of patients with history of hypersensitivity reaction to carbamazepine may develop hypersensitivities to oxcarbazepine. Ask patient about carbamazepine hypersensitivity and stop drug immediately if signs or symptoms of hypersensitivity occur.
- Shake oral suspension well. Suspension can be mixed with water or swallowed directly from syringe.
- Oral suspension and tablets may be interchanged at equal doses.
- ***Alert:*** Withdraw drug gradually to minimize potential for increased seizure frequency.
- Watch for signs and symptoms of hyponatremia, including nausea, malaise, headache, lethargy, confusion, and decreased sensation.
- Monitor sodium level in patients receiving oxcarbazepine for maintenance treatment, especially patients receiving other therapies that may decrease sodium levels.
- Oxcarbazepine use has been linked to several nervous system-related adverse reactions, including psychomotor slowing, difficulty with concentration, speech or language problems, somnolence, fatigue, and coordination abnormalities, such as ataxia and gait disturbances.

PATIENT TEACHING

- Drug may be taken with or without food.
- Tell patient to contact prescriber before interrupting or stopping drug.
- Advise patient to report signs and symptoms of low sodium in the blood, such as nausea, malaise, headache, lethargy, and confusion.
- ***Alert:*** Multiorgan hypersensitivity reactions may occur. Tell patient to report fever and swollen lymph nodes to his prescriber.
- ***Alert:*** Serious skin reactions, including Stevens-Johnson syndrome and toxic epidermal necrosis, can occur. Advise patient to immediately report skin rashes to his prescriber.
- Caution patient to avoid driving and other potentially hazardous activities that require mental alertness until effects of drug are known.

• Instruct woman using oral contraceptives to use alternative form of contraception while taking drug.
• Tell patient to avoid alcohol while taking drug.
• Advise patient to inform prescriber if he has ever experienced hypersensitivity reaction to carbamazepine.

SAFETY ALERT!

phenobarbital (phenobarbitone)
Solfoton

phenobarbital sodium
Luminal Sodium

Pharmacologic class: barbiturate
Pregnancy risk category D
Controlled substance schedule IV

AVAILABLE FORMS
Elixir: 20 mg/5 ml*
Injection: 30 mg/ml, 60 mg/ml, 130 mg/ml
Tablets: 15 mg, 30 mg, 60 mg, 100 mg

INDICATIONS & DOSAGES
➤ Anticonvulsant, febrile seizures
Adults: 60 to 100 mg P.O. daily. For acute seizures, 200 to 320 mg I.M. or I.V., repeat in 6 hours as necessary.
Children: 3 to 6 mg/kg P.O. daily, usually divided q 12 hours. Drug can be given once daily, usually h.s. Or, 10 to 15 mg/kg daily I.V. or I.M.
➤ Status epilepticus
Adults: 200 to 600 mg I.V.
Children: 15 to 20 mg/kg I.V. over 10 to 15 minutes.
➤ Sedation
Adults: 30 to 120 mg P.O., I.V., or I.M daily in two or three divided doses. Maximum dose is 400 mg/24 hours.
Children: 8 to 32 mg P.O.
➤ Short-term treatment of insomnia
Adults: 100 to 200 mg P.O. or 100 to 320 mg I.M. or I.V. h.s.
➤ Preoperative sedation
Adults: 100 to 200 mg I.M. 60 to 90 minutes before surgery.
Children: 1 to 3 mg/kg I.V. or I.M. 60 to 90 minutes before surgery.

I.V. ADMINISTRATION
• I.V. use is reserved for emergency treatment. Give slowly under close supervision. Monitor respirations closely. Don't give more than 60 mg/minute. Have resuscitation equipment available.
• If solution contains precipitate, don't use.
• Dilute drug in half-normal or normal saline, D_5W, lactated Ringer, or Ringer solution.
• Inadvertent intra-arterial injection can cause spasm of the artery and severe pain and may lead to gangrene.
• Up to 30 minutes may be required for maximum effect; allow time for anticonvulsant effect to develop to avoid overdose.

INCOMPATIBILITIES
Acidic solutions, amphotericin B, chlorpromazine, dimenhydrinate, diphenhydramine, ephedrine, hydralazine, hydrocortisone sodium succinate, hydromorphone, insulin, kanamycin, levorphanol, meperidine, morphine, norepinephrine, pentazocine lactate, phenytoin, prochlorperazine mesylate, promethazine hydrochloride, ranitidine hydrochloride, streptomycin, vancomycin.

ACTION
As a barbiturate, may depress CNS and increase seizure threshold. As a sedative, may interfere with transmission of impulses from thalamus to cortex of brain.

Route	Onset	Peak	Duration
P.O.	1 hr	8–12 hr	10–12 hr
I.V.	5 min	30 min	4–10 hr
I.M.	> 5 min	> 30 min	4–10 hr

Half-life: 5 to 7 days.

ADVERSE REACTIONS
CNS: *drowsiness, lethargy, hangover,* paradoxical excitement in elderly patients, somnolence, changes in EEG patterns, physical and psychological dependence.
CV: ***bradycardia,*** hypotension, syncope.
GI: nausea, vomiting.
Hematologic: exacerbation of porphyria.
Respiratory: ***respiratory depression, apnea.***
Skin: rash, ***erythema multiforme, Stevens-Johnson syndrome,*** urticaria,

pain, swelling, thrombophlebitis, necrosis, nerve injury at injection site.
Other: injection site pain, ***angioedema.***

INTERACTIONS

Drug-drug. *Chloramphenicol, MAO inhibitors:* May potentiate barbiturate effect. Monitor patient for increased CNS and respiratory depression.
CNS depressants including opioid analgesics: Excessive CNS depression. Monitor patient closely.
Corticosteroids, doxycycline, estrogens and hormonal contraceptives, oral anticoagulants, tricyclic antidepressants: May enhance metabolism of these drugs. Watch for decreased effect.
Diazepam: May increase effects of both drugs. Use together cautiously.
Griseofulvin: May decrease absorption of griseofulvin. Monitor effectiveness of griseofulvin.
Mephobarbital, primidone: May cause excessive phenobarbital level. Monitor patient closely.
Metoprolol, propranolol: May reduce the effects of these drugs. Consider an increased beta-blocker dose.
Rifampin: May decrease barbiturate level. Watch for decreased effect.
Valproic acid: May increase phenobarbital level. Watch for toxicity.
Warfarin: May increase warfarin metabolism and decrease effect. Monitor patient for decreased warfarin effect.
Drug-herb. *Evening primrose oil:* May increase anticonvulsant dosage requirement. Discourage use together.
Drug-lifestyle. *Alcohol use:* May impair coordination, increase CNS effects, and lead to death. Strongly discourage use together.

EFFECTS ON LAB TEST RESULTS

- May decrease bilirubin level.
- May cause false-positive phentolamine test result.

CONTRAINDICATIONS & CAUTIONS

- Contraindicated in patients hypersensitive to barbiturates and in those with history of manifest or latent porphyria.
- Contraindicated in patients with hepatic or renal dysfunction, respiratory disease with dyspnea or obstruction, or nephritis.
- Use cautiously in patients with acute or chronic pain, depression, suicidal tendencies, history of drug abuse, fever, hyperthyroidism, diabetes mellitus, severe anemia, blood pressure alterations, CV disease, shock, or uremia, and in elderly or debilitated patients.

NURSING CONSIDERATIONS

- Give I.M. injection deeply into large muscles. Superficial injection may cause pain, sterile abscess, and tissue sloughing.
- ***Alert:*** Watch for signs of barbiturate toxicity: coma, cyanosis, asthmatic breathing, clammy skin, and hypotension. Overdose can be fatal.
- Therapeutic level is 15 to 40 mcg/ml.
- Elderly patients are more sensitive to drug's effects; drug may produce paradoxical excitement.
- Don't stop drug abruptly because this may worsen seizures. Call prescriber immediately if adverse reactions develop.
- First withdrawal symptoms occur within 8 to 12 hours and include anxiety, muscle twitching, tremor of hands and fingers, progressive weakness, dizziness, visual distortion, nausea, vomiting, insomnia, and orthostatic hypotension. Seizures and delirium may occur within 16 hours and last up to 5 days after abruptly stopping drug.
- Use for insomnia isn't recommended, and treatment shouldn't last longer than 14 days.
- Some products contain tartrazine; use cautiously in patients with aspirin sensitivity.
- EEG patterns show a change in low-voltage fast activity. Changes persist after therapy ends.
- Drug may decrease bilirubin level in neonates, patients with epilepsy, and those with congenital nonhemolytic, unconjugated hyperbilirubinemia.
- The physiologic effects of drug may impair the absorption of cyanocobalamin Co 57.
- ***Look alike–sound alike:*** Don't confuse phenobarbital with pentobarbital.

PATIENT TEACHING

- Ensure that patient is aware that drug is available in different milligram strengths and sizes. Advise him to check prescription and refills closely.

- Inform patient that full therapeutic effects aren't seen for 2 to 3 weeks, except when loading dose is used.
- Advise patient to avoid driving and other potentially hazardous activities that require mental alertness until drug's CNS effects are known.
- Warn patient and parents not to stop drug abruptly.
- Tell woman using hormonal contraceptives to consider a nonhormonal form because drug may decrease effectiveness.

phenytoin (diphenylhydantoin)

Dilantin 125, Dilantin Infatabs

phenytoin sodium (prompt)

Dilantin

phenytoin sodium (extended)

Dilantin Kapseals✐, Phenytek

Pharmacologic class: hydantoin derivative
Pregnancy risk category D

AVAILABLE FORMS

phenytoin
Oral suspension: 125 mg/5 ml
Tablets (chewable): 50 mg
phenytoin sodium (extended)
Capsules: 30 mg (27.6 mg base), 100 mg (92 mg base), 200 mg (184 mg base), 300 mg (276 mg base)
phenytoin sodium (prompt)
Capsules: 100 mg (92 mg base)
Injection: 50 mg/ml (46 mg base)

INDICATIONS & DOSAGES

➤ To control tonic-clonic (grand mal) and complex partial (temporal lobe) seizures
Adults: Highly individualized. Initially, 100 mg P.O. t.i.d., increasing by 100 mg P.O. q 2 to 4 weeks until desired response is obtained. Usual range is 300 to 600 mg daily. If patient is stabilized with extended-release capsules, once-daily dosing with 300-mg extended-release capsules is possible as an alternative.
Children: 5 mg/kg or 250 mg/m² P.O. divided b.i.d. or t.i.d. Usual dose range is 4 to 8 mg/kg daily. Maximum daily dose is 300 mg.

➤ For patient requiring a loading dose
Adults: Initially, 1 g P.O. daily divided into three doses and given at 2-hour intervals. Or, 10 to 15 mg/kg I.V. at a rate not exceeding 50 mg/minute. Normal maintenance dosage is started 24 hours after loading dose.
Children: 500 to 600 mg P.O. in divided doses, followed by maintenance dosage 24 hours after loading dose.

➤ To prevent and treat seizures occurring during neurosurgery
Adults: 100 to 200 mg I.M. q 4 hours during and after surgery.

➤ Status epilepticus
Adults: Loading dose of 10 to 15 mg/kg I.V. (1 to 1.5 g may be needed) at a rate not exceeding 50 mg/minute; then maintenance dosage of 100 mg P.O. or I.V. q 6 to 8 hours.
Children: Loading dose of 15 to 20 mg/kg I.V., at a rate not exceeding 1 to 3 mg/kg/minute; then highly individualized maintenance dosages.
Elderly patients: May need lower dosages.

I.V. ADMINISTRATION

- Clear tubing with normal saline solution. Use only clear solution for injection. A slight yellow color is acceptable.
- Mix with normal saline solution, if needed, and give as an infusion over 30 minutes to 1 hour, when possible.
- Infusion must begin within 1 hour after preparation and should run through an inline filter.
- Check patency of catheter before giving. Monitor site for extravasation because it can cause severe tissue damage.
- Give bolus slowly at 50 mg/minute.
- If possible, don't give by I.V. push into veins on back of hand to avoid purple glove syndrome. Inject into larger veins or central venous catheter, if available.
- Check vital signs, blood pressure, and ECG during I.V. administration.
- Discard 4 hours after preparation. Don't refrigerate.

INCOMPATIBILITIES

Amikacin, aminophylline, amphotericin B, bretylium, cephapirin, ciprofloxacin, D_5W, diltiazem, dobutamine, enalaprilat, fat emulsions, hydromorphone, insulin (regular), levorphanol, lidocaine, lincomycin, meperidine, morphine sulfate, nitroglycerin, norepinephrine, other I.V. drugs or infusion solutions, pentobarbital sodium, potassium chloride, procaine, propofol, streptomycin, sufentanil citrate, theophylline, vitamin B complex with C. If giving as an infusion, don't mix drug with D_5W because it will precipitate.

ACTION

May stabilize neuronal membranes and limit seizure activity either by increasing efflux or decreasing influx of sodium ions across cell membranes in the motor cortex during generation of nerve impulses.

Route	Onset	Peak	Duration
P.O.	Unknown	1½–12 hr	Unknown
P.O. (Phenytek)	Unknown	4–12 hr	Unknown
I.V.	Immediate	1–2 hr	Unknown
I.M.	Unknown	Unknown	Unknown

Half-life: Varies with dose and concentration changes.

ADVERSE REACTIONS

CNS: *ataxia, decreased coordination, mental confusion, slurred speech,* dizziness, headache, insomnia, nervousness, twitching.
CV: periarteritis nodosa.
EENT: *diplopia, nystagmus,* blurred vision.
GI: *gingival hyperplasia, nausea, vomiting,* constipation.
Hematologic: ***agranulocytosis, leukopenia, pancytopenia, thrombocytopenia,*** macrocythemia, megaloblastic anemia.
Hepatic: ***toxic hepatitis.***
Metabolic: hyperglycemia.
Musculoskeletal: osteomalacia.
Skin: ***Stevens-Johnson syndrome, toxic epidermal necrolysis,*** bullous or purpuric dermatitis, discoloration of skin if given by I.V. push in back of hand, exfoliative dermatitis, hypertrichosis, inflammation at injection site, lupus erythematosus, necrosis, pain, photosensitivity reactions, scarlatiniform or morbilliform rash.
Other: *hirsutism,* lymphadenopathy.

INTERACTIONS

Drug-drug. *Acetaminophen:* May decrease the therapeutic effects of acetaminophen and increase the incidence of hepatotoxicity. Monitor for toxicity.
Amiodarone, antihistamines, chloramphenicol, ***cimetidine,*** *cycloserine, diazepam,* ***fluconazole, isoniazid,*** *metronidazole, omeprazole, phenylbutazone, salicylates,* ***sulfonamides, ticlodipine,*** *valproate:* May increase phenytoin activity and toxicity. Monitor patient for toxicity and adjust dose as needed.
Atracurium, cisatracurium, pancuronium, rocuronium, vecuronium: May decrease the effects of nondepolarizing muscle relaxant. May need to increase the nondepolarizing muscle relaxant dose.
Barbiturates, carbamazepine, dexamethasone, diazoxide, folic acid, rifampin: May decrease phenytoin activity. Monitor phenytoin level.
Carbamazepine, cardiac glycosides, doxycycline, hormonal contraceptives, quinidine, theophylline, valproic acid: May decrease effects of these drugs. Monitor patient.
Cyclosporine: May decrease cyclosporine levels, risking organ rejection. Monitor cyclosporine levels closely and adjust dose as needed.
Disulfiram: May increase toxic effects of phenytoin. Monitor phenytoin level closely and adjust dose as needed.
Lithium: May increase toxicity of lithium, despite normal lithium levels. Monitor patient for adverse effects.
Warfarin: May increase effects of warfarin. Monitor patient for bleeding.
Drug-food. *Enteral tube feedings:* May interfere with absorption of oral drug. Stop enteral feedings for 2 hours before and 2 hours after drug use.
Drug-lifestyle. *Long-term alcohol use:* May decrease drug's activity. Strongly discourage patient from heavy alcohol use.

EFFECTS ON LAB TEST RESULTS

- May increase alkaline phosphatase, GGT, and glucose levels. May decrease

urinary 17-hydroxysteroid, 17-ketosteroid, and hemoglobin levels and hematocrit.
- May increase urine 6-hydroxycortisol excretion. May decrease dexamethasone suppression, metyrapone test results, and platelet, WBC, RBC, and granulocyte counts.
- May falsely reduce protein-bound iodine or free thyroxine level test results.

CONTRAINDICATIONS & CAUTIONS
- Contraindicated in patients hypersensitive to hydantoin and in those with sinus bradycardia, SA block, second- or third-degree AV block, or Adams-Stokes syndrome.
- Use cautiously in patients with hepatic dysfunction, hypotension, myocardial insufficiency, diabetes, or respiratory depression; in elderly or debilitated patients; and in those receiving other hydantoin derivatives.
- Elderly patients tend to metabolize drug slowly and may need reduced dosages.

NURSING CONSIDERATIONS
- Therapeutic dose usually increases during pregnancy.
- Don't give I.M. unless dosage adjustments are made; drug may precipitate at injection site, cause pain, and be absorbed erratically.
- Divided doses given with or after meals may decrease adverse GI reactions.
- If rash appears, stop drug. If rash is scarlatiniform or morbilliform, resume drug after rash clears. If rash reappears, stop therapy. If rash is exfoliative, purpuric, or bullous, don't resume drug.
- Don't stop drug suddenly because this may worsen seizures. Call prescriber immediately if adverse reactions develop.
- Monitor drug level. Therapeutic level is 10 to 20 mcg/ml.
- Allow at least 7 to 10 days to elapse between dosage changes.
- Monitor CBC and calcium level every 6 months, and periodically monitor hepatic function. If megaloblastic anemia is evident, prescriber may order folic acid and vitamin B_{12}.
- If using to treat seizures, take appropriate safety precautions.
- Mononucleosis may decrease level. Watch for increased seizures.
- Watch for gingival hyperplasia, especially in children.
- ***Alert:*** Doubling the dose doesn't double the level but may cause toxicity. Consult pharmacist for specific dosing recommendations.
- If seizure control is established with divided doses, once-daily dosing may be considered.
- ***Look alike–sound alike:*** Don't confuse phenytoin with mephenytoin or fosphenytoin or Dilantin with Dilaudid.

PATIENT TEACHING
- Tell patient to notify prescriber if skin rash develops.
- Advise patient to avoid driving and other potentially hazardous activities that require mental alertness until drug's CNS effects are known.
- Advise patient not to change brands or dosage forms once he's stabilized on therapy.
- Dilantin capsules are the only oral form that can be given once daily. Toxic levels may result if any other brand or form is given once daily. Dilantin tablets and oral suspension should never be taken once daily.
- Tell patient not to use capsules that are discolored.
- Advise patient to avoid alcohol.
- Warn patient and parents not to stop drug abruptly.
- Stress importance of good oral hygiene and regular dental examinations. Surgical removal of excess gum tissue may be needed periodically if dental hygiene is poor.
- Caution patient that drug may color urine pink, red, or reddish brown.

primidone
Apo-Primidone†, Mysoline, PMS Primidone†, Sertan†

Pharmacologic class: barbiturate analogue
Pregnancy risk category D

AVAILABLE FORMS
Tablets: 50 mg, 250 mg

INDICATIONS & DOSAGES

➤ **Tonic-clonic, complex partial, and simple partial seizures**

Adults and children age 8 and older: Initially, 100 to 125 mg P.O. h.s. on days 1 to 3; then 100 to 125 mg P.O. b.i.d. on days 4 to 6; then 100 to 125 mg P.O. t.i.d. on days 7 to 9, followed by maintenance dose of 250 mg P.O. t.i.d. Maintenance dose may be increased to 250 mg q.i.d., if needed. Dosage may be increased to maximum of 2 g daily in divided doses.
Children younger than age 8: Initially, 50 mg P.O. h.s. for 3 days; then 50 mg P.O. b.i.d. for days 4 to 6; then 100 mg P.O. b.i.d. for days 7 to 9, followed by maintenance dose of 125 to 250 mg P.O. t.i.d. or 10 to 25 mg/kg daily in divided doses.

➤ **Essential tremor ♦**

Adults: 750 mg P.O. daily.

ACTION

Unknown. Some activity may be caused by phenylethylmalonamide and phenobarbital, which are active metabolites.

Route	Onset	Peak	Duration
P.O.	Unknown	3–4 hr	Unknown

Half-life: 5 to 15 hours.

ADVERSE REACTIONS

CNS: *ataxia, drowsiness,* emotional disturbances, fatigue, hyperirritability, paranoid symptoms, vertigo.
EENT: *diplopia,* nystagmus.
GI: *nausea, vomiting,* anorexia.
GU: impotence, polyuria.
Hematologic: megaloblastic anemia, ***thrombocytopenia.***
Skin: morbilliform rash.

INTERACTIONS

Drug-drug. *Acetazolamide, succinimide:* May decrease primidone level. Monitor level.
Anticoagulants, felodipine: May decrease the effects of these drugs. Adjust doses as needed.
Carbamazepine: May increase carbamazepine level and decrease primidone and phenobarbital levels. Watch for toxicity.
CNS depressants: May cause additive CNS depression. Avoid using together.
Corticosteroids, doxycycline: May decrease the effects of these drugs. Avoid using together, if possible.
Hormonal contraceptives: May decrease the effectiveness of contraceptives. Recommend alternative birth control method.
Isoniazid: May increase primidone level. Monitor level.
Metoprolol, propranolol, ***other beta blockers:*** May reduce effects of these drugs. Consider increasing beta-blocker dose.
Phenytoin: May stimulate conversion of primidone to phenobarbital. Watch for increased phenobarbital effect.
Valproic acid: May increase primidone levels. Decrease primidone dose as needed.
Drug-lifestyle. *Alcohol use:* May impair coordination, increase CNS effects, and cause death. Strongly discourage alcohol use with this drug.

EFFECTS ON LAB TEST RESULTS

- May decrease hemoglobin level.
- May alter liver function test values. May decrease platelet count.

CONTRAINDICATIONS & CAUTIONS

- Contraindicated in patients hypersensitive to phenobarbital and in those with porphyria.

NURSING CONSIDERATIONS

- Don't withdraw drug suddenly because seizures may worsen. Notify prescriber immediately if adverse reactions develop.
- Therapeutic level of primidone is 5 to 12 mcg/ml. Therapeutic level of phenobarbital is 15 to 40 mcg/ml.
- Monitor CBC and routine blood chemistry every 6 months.
- Brand interchange isn't recommended because of documented bioequivalence problems for primidone products marketed by different manufacturers.
- ***Look alike–sound alike:*** Don't confuse primidone with prednisone or Prinivil.

PATIENT TEACHING

- Advise patient to avoid driving and other potentially hazardous activities that require mental alertness until drug's CNS effects are known.
- Warn patient and parents not to stop taking drug suddenly.

• Tell patient that full therapeutic response may take 2 weeks or longer.
• Advise woman of childbearing age to discuss drug therapy with prescriber if she's considering pregnancy.
• Caution woman of childbearing age that breast-feeding is contraindicated while taking this drug.

tiagabine hydrochloride
Gabitril

Pharmacologic class: gamma aminobutyric acid (GABA) enhancer
Pregnancy risk category C

AVAILABLE FORMS
Tablets: 4 mg, 12 mg, 16 mg

INDICATIONS & DOSAGES
➤ **Adjunctive treatment of partial seizures**
Adults: Initially, 4 mg P.O. once daily. Total daily dose may be increased by 4 to 8 mg at weekly intervals until clinical response or up to 56 mg daily. Give total daily dose in divided doses b.i.d. to q.i.d.
Children ages 12 to 18: Initially, 4 mg P.O. once daily. Total daily dose may be increased by 4 mg at beginning of week 2 and thereafter by 4 to 8 mg per week until clinical response or up to 32 mg daily. Give total daily dose in divided doses b.i.d. to q.i.d.
Adjust-a-dose: For patients with hepatic impairment, reduce first and maintenance doses or increase dosing intervals.

ACTION
Unknown. May act by facilitating the effects of the inhibitory neurotransmitter GABA. By binding to recognition sites linked to GABA uptake carrier, drug may make more GABA available.

Route	Onset	Peak	Duration
P.O.	Rapid	45 min	7–9 hr

Half-life: 7 to 9 hours.

ADVERSE REACTIONS
CNS: *asthenia, dizziness, nervousness, somnolence,* abnormal gait, agitation, ataxia, confusion, depression, difficulty with concentration and attention, difficulty with memory, emotional lability, hostility, insomnia, language problems, paresthesia, speech disorder, tremor.
CV: vasodilation.
EENT: nystagmus, pharyngitis.
GI: *nausea,* abdominal pain, diarrhea, increased appetite, mouth ulceration, vomiting.
Musculoskeletal: generalized weakness, myasthenia, pain.
Respiratory: increased cough.
Skin: pruritus, rash.

INTERACTIONS
Drug-drug. *Carbamazepine, phenobarbital, phenytoin:* May increase tiagabine clearance. Monitor patient closely.
CNS depressants: May enhance CNS effects. Use together cautiously.
Drug-lifestyle. *Alcohol use:* May enhance CNS effects. Discourage use together.

EFFECTS ON LAB TEST RESULTS
None reported.

CONTRAINDICATIONS & CAUTIONS
• Contraindicated in patients hypersensitive to drug or its components.
• ***Alert:*** Drug may cause new-onset seizures and status epilepticus in patients without a history of epilepsy. In these patients, stop drug and evaluate for underlying seizure disorder. Drug shouldn't be used for off-label uses.
• Use cautiously in breast-feeding women.

NURSING CONSIDERATIONS
• Withdraw drug gradually unless safety concerns require a more rapid withdrawal because sudden withdrawal may cause more frequent seizures.
• ***Alert:*** Use of anticonvulsants, including tiagabine, may cause status epilepticus and sudden unexpected death in patients with epilepsy.
• ***Look alike–sound alike:*** Don't confuse tiagabine with tizanidine; both have 4-mg starting doses.
• Patients who aren't receiving at least one enzyme-inducing anticonvulsant when starting tiagabine may need lower doses or slower dosage adjustment.
• Drug may cause moderately severe to incapacitating generalized weakness, which

resolves after dosage is reduced or drug stopped.

PATIENT TEACHING

- Advise patient to take drug only as prescribed.
- Tell patient to take drug with food.
- Warn patient that drug may cause dizziness, somnolence, and other signs and symptoms of CNS depression. Advise patient to avoid driving and other potentially hazardous activities that require mental alertness until drug's CNS effects are known.
- Tell woman of childbearing age to call prescriber if she becomes pregnant or plans to become pregnant during therapy.
- Instruct woman of childbearing age to notify prescriber if she's planning to breast-feed because drug may appear in breast milk.

topiramate

Topamax

Pharmacologic class: sulfamate-substituted monosaccharide
Pregnancy risk category C

AVAILABLE FORMS

Capsules, sprinkles: 15 mg, 25 mg
Tablets: 25 mg, 50 mg, 100 mg, 200 mg

INDICATIONS & DOSAGES

➤ **Initial monotherapy for partial-onset or primary generalized tonic-clonic seizures**

Adults and children age 10 or older: Recommended daily dose is 400 mg P.O. divided b.i.d. (morning and evening). To achieve this dosage, adjust as follows: first week, 25 mg P.O. b.i.d.; second week, 50 mg P.O. b.i.d.; third week, 75 mg P.O. b.i.d.; fourth week, 100 mg P.O. b.i.d.; fifth week, 150 mg P.O. b.i.d.; and sixth week, 200 mg P.O. b.i.d.

➤ **Adjunct treatment for partial-onset or primary generalized tonic-clonic seizures**

Adults: Initially, 25 to 50 mg P.O. daily; increase gradually by 25 to 50 mg/week until an effective daily dose is reached. Adjust to recommended daily dose of 200 to 400 mg P.O in two divided doses for adults with partial seizures or 400 mg P.O. in two divided doses for adults with primary generalized tonic-clonic seizures.

Children ages 2 to 16: Initially, 1 to 3 mg/kg daily given h.s. for 1 week. Increase at 1- or 2-week intervals by 1 to 3 mg/kg daily in two divided doses to achieve optimal response. Recommended daily dose is 5 to 9 mg/kg, in two divided doses.

➤ **Lennox-Gastaut syndrome**

Children ages 2 to 16: Initially, 1 to 3 mg/kg daily given h.s. for 1 week. Increase at 1- or 2-week intervals by 1 to 3 mg/kg daily in two divided doses to achieve optimal response. Recommended daily dose is 5 to 9 mg/kg, in two divided doses.

➤ **To prevent migraine headache**

Adults: Initially, 25 mg P.O. daily in evening for first week. Then, 25 mg P.O. b.i.d. in morning and evening for second week. For third week, 25 mg P.O. in morning and 50 mg P.O. in evening. For fourth week, 50 mg P.O. b.i.d. in morning and evening.

Adjust-a-dose: If creatinine clearance is less than 70 ml/minute, reduce dosage by 50%. For hemodialysis patients, supplemental doses may be needed to avoid rapid drops in drug level during prolonged dialysis treatment.

ACTION

Unknown. May block a sodium channel, potentiate the activity of GABA, and inhibit kainate's ability to activate an amino acid receptor.

Route	Onset	Peak	Duration
P.O.	Unknown	2 hr	Unknown

Half-life: 21 hours.

ADVERSE REACTIONS

CNS: *ataxia, confusion, difficulty with memory, dizziness, fatigue, nervousness, paresthesia, psychomotor slowing, somnolence, speech disorders, tremor,* ***generalized tonic-clonic seizures, suicide attempts,*** abnormal coordination, aggressive reaction, agitation, apathy, asthenia, depression, depersonalization, difficulty with concentration, attention, or language, emotional lability, euphoria, fever, hallu-

cination, hyperkinesia, hypertonia, hypoesthesia, hypokinesia, insomnia, malaise, mood problems, personality disorder, psychosis, stupor, vertigo.
CV: chest pain, edema, palpitations, vasodilation.
EENT: *abnormal vision, diplopia, nystagmus,* conjunctivitis, epistaxis, eye pain, hearing problems, pharyngitis, sinusitis, tinnitus.
GI: *anorexia, nausea,* abdominal pain, constipation, diarrhea, dry mouth, dyspepsia, flatulence, gastroenteritis, gingivitis, taste perversion, vomiting.
GU: amenorrhea, dysuria, dysmenorrhea, hematuria, impotence, intermenstrual bleeding, leukorrhea, menstrual disorder, menorrhagia, urinary frequency, renal calculi, urinary incontinence, UTI, vaginitis.
Hematologic: ***leukopenia,*** anemia.
Metabolic: *decreased weight,* increased weight.
Musculoskeletal: arthralgia, back or leg pain, muscle weakness, myalgia, rigors.
Respiratory: *upper respiratory tract infection,* bronchitis, coughing, dyspnea.
Skin: acne, alopecia, increased sweating, pruritus, rash.
Other: body odor, breast pain, decreased libido, flulike syndrome, hot flashes, lymphadenopathy.

INTERACTIONS

Drug-drug. *Carbamazepine:* May decrease topiramate level. Monitor patient.
Carbonic anhydrase inhibitors (acetazolamide, dichlorphenamide): May cause renal calculus formation. Avoid using together.
CNS depressants: May cause CNS depression and other adverse cognitive and neuropsychiatric events. Use together cautiously.
Hormonal contraceptives: May decrease efficacy. Report changes in menstrual patterns. Advise patient to use another contraceptive method.
Phenytoin: May decrease topiramate level and increase phenytoin level. Monitor levels.
Valproic acid: May decrease valproic acid and topiramate level. Monitor patient.
Drug-lifestyle. *Alcohol use:* May cause CNS depression and other adverse cognitive and neuropsychiatric events. Discourage use together.

EFFECTS ON LAB TEST RESULTS

- May increase liver enzyme levels. May decrease bicarbonate and hemoglobin levels and hematocrit.
- May decrease WBC count.

CONTRAINDICATIONS & CAUTIONS

- Contraindicated in patients hypersensitive to drug or its components.
- Use with caution in breast-feeding or pregnant women and in those with hepatic impairment.
- Use cautiously with other drugs that predispose patients to heat-related disorders, including other carbonic anhydrase inhibitors and anticholinergics.

NURSING CONSIDERATIONS

- If needed, withdraw anticonvulsant (including topiramate) gradually to minimize risk of increased seizure activity.
- Monitoring topiramate level isn't necessary.
- Drug may infrequently cause oligohidrosis and hyperthermia, mainly in children. Monitor patient closely, especially in hot weather.
- Topiramate may cause hyperchloremic, non-anion gap metabolic acidosis from renal bicarbonate loss. Factors that may predispose patients to acidosis, such as renal disease, severe respiratory disorders, status epilepticus, diarrhea, surgery, ketogenic diet, or drugs, may add to topiramate's bicarbonate-lowering effects.
- Measure baseline and periodic bicarbonate levels. If metabolic acidosis develops and persists, consider reducing the dose, gradually stopping the drug, or alkali treatment.
- Drug is rapidly cleared by dialysis. A prolonged period of dialysis may cause low drug level and seizures. A supplemental dose may be needed.
- Stop drug if patient experiences acute myopia and secondary angle-closure glaucoma.
- ***Look alike–sound alike:*** Don't confuse Topamax with Toprol-XL, Tegretol or Tegretol-XR.

PATIENT TEACHING

- Tell patient to drink plenty of fluids during therapy to minimize risk of forming kidney stones.
- Advise patient not to drive or operate hazardous machinery until CNS effects of drug are known. Drug can cause sleepiness, dizziness, confusion, and concentration problems.
- Tell woman of childbearing age that drug may decrease effectiveness of hormonal contraceptives. Advise woman using hormonal contraceptives to report change in menstrual patterns.
- Tell patient to avoid crushing or breaking tablets because of bitter taste.
- Inform patient that drug can be taken without regard to food.
- Tell patient that capsules may either be swallowed whole or carefully opened and contents sprinkled on a teaspoonful of soft food. Tell patient to swallow immediately without chewing.
- Tell patient to notify prescriber immediately if he experiences changes in vision.

---

valproate sodium

Depacon, Depakene, Epilim‡, Valpro‡

valproic acid

Depakene

divalproex sodium

Depakote✐, Depakote ER, Depakote Sprinkle✐, Epival†

Pharmacologic class: carboxylic acid derivative
Pregnancy risk category D

AVAILABLE FORMS

valproate sodium
Injection: 100 mg/ml
Syrup: 250 mg/5 ml
valproic acid
Capsules: 250 mg
Syrup: 200 mg/5 ml‡
Tablets (crushable): 100 mg‡
Tablets (enteric-coated): 200 mg‡, 500 mg‡
divalproex sodium
Capsules (sprinkle): 125 mg
Tablets (delayed-release): 125 mg, 250 mg, 500 mg
Tablets (extended-release): 250 mg, 500 mg

INDICATIONS & DOSAGES

➤ Simple and complex absence seizures, mixed seizure types (including absence seizures)
Adults and children: Initially, 15 mg/kg P.O. or I.V. daily; then increase by 5 to 10 mg/kg daily at weekly intervals up to maximum of 60 mg/kg daily. Don't use Depakote ER in children younger than age 10.

➤ Complex partial seizures
Adults and children age 10 and older: 10 to 15 mg/kg Depakote or Depakote ER P.O. or valproate sodium I.V. daily; then increase by 5 to 10 mg/kg daily at weekly intervals, up to 60 mg/kg daily.

➤ Mania
Adults: Initially, 750 mg Depakote daily P.O. in divided doses, or 25 mg/kg Depakote ER once daily. Adjust dosage based on patient's response; maximum dose for either form is 60 mg/kg daily.

➤ To prevent migraine headache
Adults: Initially, 250 mg delayed-release divalproex sodium P.O. b.i.d. Some patients may need up to 1,000 mg daily. Or, 500 mg Depakote ER P.O. daily for 1 week; then 1,000 mg P.O. daily.
Adjust-a-dose: For elderly patients, start at lower dosage. Increase dosage more slowly and with regular monitoring of fluid and nutritional intake, and watch for dehydration, somnolence, and other adverse reactions.

I.V. ADMINISTRATION

- I.V. use is indicated only in patients who can't take drug orally. Switch patient to oral form as soon as feasible; effects of I.V. use for longer than 14 days are unknown.
- Dilute valproate sodium injection with at least 50 ml of a compatible diluent. It's physically compatible and chemically stable in D_5W, normal saline, and lactated Ringer solution for 24 hours.
- Infuse drug over 60 minutes at no more than 20 mg/minute and at the same frequency as oral dosage.

• Monitor drug level, and adjust dosage as needed.

INCOMPATIBILITIES
None reported.

ACTION
Unknown. Probably facilitates the effects of the inhibitory neurotransmitter GABA.

Route	Onset	Peak	Duration
P.O.	Unknown	15 min–4 hr	Unknown
I.V.	Unknown	1 hr	Unknown

Half-life: 6 to 16 hours.

ADVERSE REACTIONS
CNS: *asthenia, dizziness, headache, insomnia, nervousness, somnolence, tremor,* abnormal thinking, amnesia, ataxia, depression, emotional upset, fever.
CV: chest pain, edema, hypertension, hypotension, tachycardia.
EENT: *blurred vision, diplopia,* nystagmus, pharyngitis, rhinitis, tinnitus.
GI: *abdominal pain, anorexia, diarrhea, dyspepsia, nausea, vomiting,* ***pancreatitis,*** constipation, increased appetite.
Hematologic: ***bone marrow suppression, hemorrhage, thrombocytopenia,*** bruising, petechiae.
Hepatic: ***hepatotoxicity.***
Metabolic: hyperammonemia, weight gain or loss.
Musculoskeletal: back and neck pain.
Respiratory: bronchitis, dyspnea.
Skin: *alopecia, flu syndrome, infection,* ***erythema multiforme, hypersensitivity reactions, Stevens-Johnson syndrome,*** rash, photosensitivity, pruritus.

INTERACTIONS
Drug-drug. *Aspirin, chlorpromazine, cimetidine, erythromycin, felbamate:* May cause valproic acid toxicity. Use together cautiously and monitor drug level.
Benzodiazepines, other CNS depressants: May cause excessive CNS depression. Avoid using together.
Carbamazepine: May cause carbamazepine CNS toxicity; may decrease valproic acid level and cause loss of seizure control. Use together cautiously, if at all. Monitor patient for seizure activity and toxicity during therapy and for at least 1 month after stopping either drug.
Lamotrigine: May increase lamotrigine level; may decrease valproate level. Monitor levels closely.
Phenobarbital: May increase phenobarbital level; may increase clearance of valproate. Monitor patient closely.
Phenytoin: May increase or decrease phenytoin level; may decrease valproate level. Monitor patient closely.
Rifampin: May decrease valproate level. Monitor level of valproate.
Warfarin: May displace warfarin from binding sites. Monitor PT and INR.
Zidovudine: May decrease zidovudine clearance. Avoid using together.
Drug-lifestyle. *Alcohol use:* May cause excessive CNS depression. Discourage use together.

EFFECTS ON LAB TEST RESULTS
• May increase ammonia, ALT, AST, and bilirubin levels.
• May increase eosinophil count and bleeding time. May decrease platelet, RBC, and WBC counts.
• May cause false-positive results for urine ketone levels.

CONTRAINDICATIONS & CAUTIONS
• Contraindicated in patients hypersensitive to drug and in those with hepatic disease or significant hepatic dysfunction, and in patients with a urea cycle disorder (UCD).
• Safety and efficacy of Depakote ER in children younger than age 10 haven't been established.

NURSING CONSIDERATIONS
• Obtain liver function test results, platelet count, and PT and INR before starting therapy, and monitor these values periodically.
• Don't give syrup to patients who need sodium restriction. Check with prescriber.
• Adverse reactions may not be caused by valproic acid alone because it's usually used with other anticonvulsants.
• When converting adults and children age 10 and older with seizures from Depakote to Depakote ER, make sure the extended-release dose is 8% to 20% higher than the regular dose taken previ-

ously. See manufacturer's package insert for more details.
• Divalproex sodium has a lower risk of adverse GI reactions.
• Never withdraw drug suddenly because sudden withdrawal may worsen seizures. Call prescriber at once if adverse reactions develop.
• ***Alert:*** Fatal hepatotoxicity may follow nonspecific symptoms, such as malaise, fever, and lethargy. If these symptoms occur during therapy, notify prescriber at once because patient who might be developing hepatic dysfunction must stop taking drug.
• Patients at high risk for hepatotoxicity include those with congenital metabolic disorders, mental retardation, or organic brain disease; those taking multiple anticonvulsants; and children younger than age 2.
• Notify prescriber if tremors occur; a dosage reduction may be needed.
• Monitor drug level. Therapeutic level is 50 to 100 mcg/ml.
• When converting patients from a brand-name drug to a generic drug, use caution because breakthrough seizures may occur.
• ***Alert:*** Sometimes fatal, hyperammonemic encephalopathy may occur when starting valproate therapy in patients with a UCD. Evaluate patients with UCD risk factors before starting valproate therapy. Patients who develop symptoms of unexplained hyperammonemic encephalopathy during valproate therapy should stop drug, undergo prompt appropriate treatment, and be evaluated for underlying UCD.
• ***Look alike–sound alike:*** Don't confuse Depakote with Depakote ER.

PATIENT TEACHING
• Tell patient to take drug with food or milk to reduce adverse GI effects.
• Advise patient not to chew capsules; irritation of mouth and throat may result.
• Tell patient that capsules may be either swallowed whole or carefully opened and contents sprinkled on a teaspoonful of soft food. Tell patient to swallow immediately without chewing.
• Tell patient and parents that syrup shouldn't be mixed with carbonated beverages; mixture may be irritating to mouth and throat.
• Tell patient and parents to keep drug out of children's reach.
• Warn patient and parents not to stop drug therapy abruptly.
• Advise patient to avoid driving and other potentially hazardous activities that require mental alertness until drug's CNS effects are known.
• Instruct patient or parents to call prescriber if malaise, weakness, lethargy, facial swelling, loss of appetite, or vomiting occurs.
• Tell woman to call prescriber if she becomes pregnant or plans to become pregnant during therapy.

zonisamide
Zonegran

Pharmacologic class: sulfonamide
Pregnancy risk category C

AVAILABLE FORMS
Capsules: 25 mg, 50 mg, 100 mg

INDICATIONS & DOSAGES
➤ **Adjunct therapy for partial seizures in adults with epilepsy**
Adults and children older than age 16: Initially, 100 mg P.O. as a single daily dose for 2 weeks. Then, dosage may be increased to 200 mg daily for at least 2 weeks. Dosage can be increased to 300 mg and 400 mg P.O. daily, with the dose stable for at least 2 weeks to achieve steady state at each level. Doses can be given once or twice daily, except for the daily dose of 100 mg at start of therapy. Maximum dose is 600 mg daily.

ACTION
May stabilize neuronal membranes and suppress neuronal hypersynchronization, which prevents seizures.

Route	Onset	Peak	Duration
P.O.	Unknown	2–6 hr	Unknown

Half-life: 63 hours.

ADVERSE REACTIONS
CNS: *dizziness, headache, somnolence,* ***seizures, status epilepticus,*** agitation or irritability, anxiety, asthenia, ataxia, confu-

sion, depression, difficulties in concentration or memory, difficulties in verbal expression, fatigue, hyperesthesia, incoordination, insomnia, mental slowing, nervousness, nystagmus, paresthesia, schizophrenic or schizophreniform behavior, speech disorders, tremor.
EENT: amblyopia, diplopia, pharyngitis, rhinitis, taste perversion, tinnitus.
GI: *anorexia,* abdominal pain, constipation, diarrhea, dry mouth, dyspepsia, nausea, vomiting.
GU: kidney stones.
Hematologic: ecchymoses.
Metabolic: weight loss.
Respiratory: cough.
Skin: pruritus, rash.
Other: accidental injury, flulike syndrome.

INTERACTIONS

Drug-drug. *Drugs that induce or inhibit CYP3A4:* Changes zonisamide level; phenytoin, carbamazepine, phenobarbital, and valproate increase zonisamide clearance. Monitor patient closely.

EFFECTS ON LAB TEST RESULTS

- May increase BUN and creatinine levels.

CONTRAINDICATIONS & CAUTIONS

- Contraindicated in patients hypersensitive to drug or to sulfonamides.
- Contraindicated in those with glomerular filtration rate less than 50 ml/minute.
- Use cautiously in patients with renal and hepatic dysfunction.
- Use cautiously with other drugs that predispose patients to heat-related disorders, including but not limited to carbonic anhydrase inhibitors and drugs with anticholinergic activity.
- Safety and effectiveness in children younger than age 16 haven't been established. Children are at increased risk for oligohidrosis and hyperthermia caused by zonisamide.

NURSING CONSIDERATIONS

- ***Alert:*** Rarely, patients receiving sulfonamides have died because of severe reactions such as Stevens-Johnson syndrome, fulminant hepatic necrosis, aplastic anemia, otherwise unexplained rashes, and agranulocytosis. If signs and symptoms of hypersensitivity or other serious reactions occur, stop drug immediately and notify prescriber.
- If patient develops acute renal failure or a significant sustained increase in creatinine or BUN level, stop drug and notify prescriber.
- Achieving steady-state levels may take 2 weeks.
- Monitor patient for signs and symptoms of hypersensitivity.
- Don't stop drug abruptly because this may cause increased seizures or status epilepticus; reduce dosage or stop drug gradually.
- Increase fluid intake and urine output to help prevent kidney stones, especially in patients with predisposing factors.
- Monitor renal function periodically.

PATIENT TEACHING

- Tell patient to take drug with or without food and not to bite or break capsule.
- Advise patient to call prescriber immediately if rash develops or seizures worsen.
- Tell patient to contact prescriber immediately if he develops sudden back or abdominal pain, pain when urinating, bloody or dark urine, fever, sore throat, mouth sores or easy bruising, decreased sweating, fever, depression, or speech or language problems.
- Tell patient to drink 6 to 8 glasses of water a day.
- Caution patient that this drug can cause drowsiness and not to drive or operate dangerous machinery until drug's effects are known.
- Advise patient not to stop taking drug without prescriber's approval.
- Instruct woman to call prescriber if she is pregnant or breast-feeding or plans to become pregnant or to breast-feed.
- Advise woman to use contraceptives while taking drug.

29
Antidepressants

amitriptyline hydrochloride
bupropion hydrochloride
citalopram hydrobromide
clomipramine hydrochloride
desipramine hydrochloride
doxepin hydrochloride
duloxetine hydrochloride
escitalopram oxalate
fluoxetine hydrochloride
fluvoxamine maleate
imipramine hydrochloride
imipramine pamoate
mirtazapine
nefazodone hydrochloride
nortriptyline hydrochloride
paroxetine hydrochloride
sertraline hydrochloride
trazodone hydrochloride
venlafaxine hydrochloride

amitriptyline hydrochloride
Apo-Amitriptyline†, Endep‡, Tryptanol‡

Pharmacologic class: tricyclic antidepressant
Pregnancy risk category C

AVAILABLE FORMS
amitriptyline hydrochloride
Injection: 10 mg/ml
Tablets: 10 mg, 25 mg, 50 mg, 75 mg, 100 mg, 150 mg

INDICATIONS & DOSAGES
➤ **Depression**
Adults: Initially, 50 to 100 mg P.O. at bedtime, increasing to 150 mg daily. Maximum, 300 mg daily, if needed. Maintenance, 50 to 100 mg daily. Or, 20 to 30 mg I.M. q.i.d.
Elderly patients and adolescents: 10 mg P.O. t.i.d. and 20 mg at bedtime daily.

ACTION
Unknown. A tricyclic antidepressant that increases the amount of norepinephrine, serotonin, or both in the CNS by blocking their reuptake by the presynaptic neurons.

Route	Onset	Peak	Duration
P.O., I.M.	Unknown	2–12 hr	Unknown

Half-life: Not established, varies widely.

ADVERSE REACTIONS
CNS: ***stroke, seizures, coma,*** ataxia, tremor, peripheral neuropathy, anxiety, insomnia, restlessness, drowsiness, dizziness, weakness, fatigue, headache, extrapyramidal reactions, hallucinations, delusions, disorientation.
CV: *orthostatic hypotension, tachycardia,* ***heart block, arrhythmias, MI,*** ECG changes, hypertension, edema.
EENT: blurred vision, tinnitus, mydriasis, increased intraocular pressure.
GI: *dry mouth,* nausea, vomiting, anorexia, epigastric pain, diarrhea, constipation, paralytic ileus.
GU: urine retention, altered libido, impotence.
Hematologic: ***agranulocytosis, thrombocytopenia, leukopenia,*** eosinophilia.
Metabolic: ***hypoglycemia,*** hyperglycemia.
Skin: rash, urticaria, photosensitivity reactions, diaphoresis.
Other: hypersensitivity reactions.

INTERACTIONS
Drug-drug. *Barbiturates, CNS depressants:* May enhance CNS depression. Avoid using together.
Cimetidine, ***fluoxetine, fluvoxamine,*** *hormonal contraceptives,* ***paroxetine, sertraline:*** May increase tricyclic antidepressant level. Monitor drug levels and patient for signs of toxicity.
Clonidine: May cause life-threatening hypertension. Avoid using together.
Epinephrine, norepinephrine: May increase hypertensive effect. Use together cautiously.
MAO inhibitors: May cause severe excitation, hyperpyrexia, or seizures, usually

with high doses. Avoid using within 14 days of MAO inhibitor therapy.
Quinolones: May increase the risk of life-threatening arrhythmias. Avoid using together.
Drug-herb. *Evening primrose:* May cause additive or synergistic effect, resulting in lower seizure threshold and increasing the risk of seizures. Discourage use together.
St. John's wort, SAM-e, yohimbe: May cause serotonin syndrome and decrease amitriptyline level. Discourage use together.
Drug-lifestyle. *Alcohol use:* May enhance CNS depression. Discourage use together.
Smoking: May lower drug level. Watch for lack of effect.
Sun exposure: May increase risk of photosensitivity reactions. Advise patient to avoid excessive sunlight exposure.

EFFECTS ON LAB TEST RESULTS

- May increase or decrease glucose level.
- May increase eosinophil count and liver function test values. May decrease granulocyte, platelet, and WBC counts.

CONTRAINDICATIONS & CAUTIONS

- Contraindicated in patients hypersensitive to drug and in those who have received an MAO inhibitor within the past 14 days.
- Contraindicated during acute recovery phase of MI.
- Use cautiously in patients with history of seizures, urine retention, angle-closure glaucoma, or increased intraocular pressure; in those with hyperthyroidism, CV disease, diabetes, or impaired liver function; and in those receiving thyroid drugs.
- Use cautiously in those receiving electroconvulsive therapy.

NURSING CONSIDERATIONS

- ***Alert:*** Parenteral form of drug is for I.M. administration only. Drug shouldn't be given I.V.
- ***Alert:*** Drug may increase the risk of suicidal thinking and behavior in children and adolescents with major depressive disorder or other psychiatric disorder. Don't use in children younger than age 12.
- Amitriptyline has strong anticholinergic effects and is one of the most sedating tricyclic antidepressants. Anticholinergic effects have rapid onset even though therapeutic effect is delayed for weeks.
- Elderly patients may have an increased sensitivity to anticholinergic effects of drug; sedating effects of drug may increase the risk of falls in this population.
- If signs or symptoms of psychosis occur or increase, expect prescriber to reduce dosage. Record mood changes. Monitor patient for suicidal tendencies and allow only minimum supply of drug.
- Because patients using tricyclic antidepressants may suffer hypertensive episodes during surgery, stop drug gradually several days before surgery.
- Monitor glucose level.
- Watch for nausea, headache, and malaise after abrupt withdrawal of long-term therapy; these symptoms don't indicate addiction.
- Don't withdraw drug abruptly.
- ***Look alike–sound alike:*** Don't confuse amitriptyline with nortriptyline or aminophylline.

PATIENT TEACHING

- Whenever possible, advise patient to take full dose at bedtime, but warn him of possible morning orthostatic hypotension.
- Tell patient to avoid alcohol during drug therapy.
- Advise patient to consult prescriber before taking other drugs.
- Warn patient to avoid activities that require alertness and good psychomotor coordination until CNS effects of drug are known. Drowsiness and dizziness usually subside after a few weeks.
- Inform patient that dry mouth may be relieved with sugarless hard candy or gum. Saliva substitutes may be useful.
- To prevent photosensitivity reactions, advise patient to use a sunblock, wear protective clothing, and avoid prolonged exposure to strong sunlight.
- Warn patient not to stop drug abruptly.
- Advise patient that it may take as long as 30 days to achieve full therapeutic effect.

bupropion hydrochloride
Wellbutrin✐, Wellbutrin SR✐, Wellbutrin XL, Zyban✐

Pharmacologic class: aminoketone
Pregnancy risk category B

AVAILABLE FORMS
Tablets (extended-release): 150 mg, 300 mg
Tablets (immediate-release): 75 mg, 100 mg
Tablets (sustained-release): 100 mg, 150 mg, 200 mg

INDICATIONS & DOSAGES
✱*NEW INDICATION:* **Seasonal affective disorder**
Adults: Start treatment in autumn, before depressive symptoms appear. Initially, 150 mg P.O. (Wellbutrin XL) once daily in the morning. After 1 week, increase to 300 mg once daily, if tolerated. Continue 300 mg daily during the autumn and winter and taper to 150 mg daily for 2 weeks before stopping the drug in the early spring.

➤ **Depression**
Adults: For immediate-release, initially, 100 mg Wellbutrin P.O. b.i.d.; increase after 3 days to 100 mg P.O. t.i.d., if needed. If patient doesn't improve after several weeks of therapy, increase dosage to 150 mg t.i.d. No single dose should exceed 150 mg. Allow at least 6 hours between doses. Maximum dose is 450 mg daily. For sustained-release, initially, 150 mg Wellbutrin P.O. q morning; increase to target dose of 150 mg P.O. b.i.d., as tolerated, as early as day 4 of dosing. Allow at least 8 hours between doses. Maximum dose is 400 mg daily. For extended-release, initially, 150 mg Wellbutrin P.O. q morning; increase to target dosage of 300 mg P.O. daily, as tolerated, as early as day 4 of dosing. Allow at least 24 hours between doses. Maximum is 450 mg daily.

➤ **Aid to smoking cessation treatment**
Adults: 150 mg Zyban P.O. daily for 3 days; increased to maximum of 300 mg daily in two divided doses at least 8 hours apart.

Adjust-a-dose: In patients with mild to moderate hepatic cirrhosis or renal impairment, reduce frequency and dose. In patients with severe hepatic cirrhosis, don't exceed 75 mg immediate-release P.O. daily, 100 mg sustained-release P.O. daily, 150 mg (sustained-release) P.O. every other day, or 150 mg extended-release P.O. every other day.

ACTION
Unknown. Drug doesn't inhibit MAO, but it weakly inhibits norepinephrine, dopamine, and serotonin reuptake. Noradrenergic or dopaminergic mechanisms, or both, may cause drug's effect.

Route	Onset	Peak	Duration
P.O. (immediate-release)	Unknown	2 hr	Unknown
P.O. (sustained-release)	Unknown	3 hr	Unknown
P.O. (extended-release)	Unknown	5 hr	Unknown

Half-life: 8 to 24 hours.

ADVERSE REACTIONS
CNS: *abnormal dreams, insomnia, headache, sedation, tremor, agitation, dizziness,* ***seizures, suicidal behavior,*** anxiety, confusion, delusions, euphoria, fever, hostility, impaired concentration, impaired sleep quality, akinesia, akathisia, fatigue, syncope.
CV: *tachycardia,* ***arrhythmias,*** hypertension, hypotension, palpitations, chest pain.
EENT: *blurred vision, rhinitis,* auditory disturbances, epistaxis, pharyngitis, sinusitis.
GI: *constipation, nausea, vomiting, anorexia, dry mouth,* taste disturbance, dyspepsia, diarrhea, abdominal pain.
GU: impotence, menstrual complaints, urinary frequency, urine retention.
Metabolic: increased appetite, *weight loss, weight gain.*
Musculoskeletal: arthritis, myalgia, arthralgia, muscle spasm or twitch.
Respiratory: upper respiratory complaints, increase in coughing.

Skin: *excessive sweating,* pruritus, rash, cutaneous temperature disturbance, urticaria.
Other: fever and chills, decreased libido, accidental injury.

INTERACTIONS

Drug-drug. *Amantadine, levodopa:* May increase risk of adverse reactions. If used together, give small first doses of bupropion and increase dosage gradually.
Antidepressants, antipsychotics, systemic corticosteroids, theophylline: May lower seizure threshold. Use cautiously together.
Beta blockers, class IC antiarrhythmics: May increase levels of these drugs and adverse reactions. Use a reduced dose if used with bupropion.
Carbamazepine, phenobarbital, phenytoin: May enhance metabolism of bupropion and decrease its effect. Monitor patient closely.
MAO inhibitors: May increase the risk of bupropion toxicity. Don't use drugs within 14 days of each other.
Nicotine replacement agents: May cause hypertension. Monitor blood pressure.
Ritonavir: May increase bupropion level. Monitor patient closely for adverse reactions.
Drug-lifestyle. *Alcohol use:* May alter seizure threshold. Discourage use together.
Sun exposure: May increase risk of photosensitivity reactions. Advise patient to avoid excessive sunlight exposure.

EFFECTS ON LAB TEST RESULTS

- May increase liver function test values.

CONTRAINDICATIONS & CAUTIONS

- Contraindicated in patients hypersensitive to drug, in those who have taken MAO inhibitors within previous 14 days, and in those with seizure disorders or history of bulimia or anorexia nervosa because of a higher risk of seizures.
- Don't use with other drugs containing bupropion.
- Contraindicated in patients abruptly stopping use of alcohol or sedatives (including benzodiazepines).
- Use cautiously in patients with recent history of MI, unstable heart disease, renal or hepatic impairment, a history of seizures, head trauma, or other predisposition to seizures, and in those being treated with drugs that lower seizure threshold.

NURSING CONSIDERATIONS

- Many patients experience a period of increased restlessness, including agitation, insomnia, and anxiety, especially at start of therapy.
- ***Alert:*** To minimize the risk of seizures, don't exceed maximum recommended dose.
- ***Alert:*** Patient with major depressive disorder may experience a worsening of depression and suicidal thoughts. Carefully monitor patient for worsening depression or suicidal thoughts, especially at the beginning of therapy and during dosage changes.
- ***Alert:*** Drug may increase the risk of suicidal thinking and behavior in children and adolescents with major depressive disorder or other psychiatric disorder.
- In switching patients from regular- or sustained-release tablets to extended-release tablets, give the same total daily dose (when possible) as the once-daily dosage provided.
- Closely monitor patient with history of bipolar disorder. Antidepressants can cause manic episodes during the depressed phase of bipolar disorder. This may be less likely to occur with bupropion than with other antidepressants.
- Begin smoking cessation treatment while patient is still smoking; about 1 week is needed to achieve steady-state drug levels.
- Stop smoking cessation treatment if patient hasn't progressed toward abstinence by week 7. Treatment usually lasts up to 12 weeks. Patient can stop taking drug without tapering off.
- ***Look alike–sound alike:*** Don't confuse bupropion with buspirone or Wellbutrin with Wellcovorin.

PATIENT TEACHING

- ***Alert:*** Explain that excessive use of alcohol, abrupt withdrawal from alcohol or other sedatives, and addiction to cocaine, opiates, or stimulants during therapy may increase risk of seizures. Seizure risk is also increased in those using OTC stimu-

lants, in anorectics, and in diabetic patients using oral antidiabetics or insulin.
- Advise patient to consult prescriber before taking other prescription or OTC drugs.
- Advise patient to avoid hazardous activities that require alertness and good psychomotor coordination until effects of drug are known.
- ***Alert:*** Advise patient that Zyban and Wellbutrin contain the same active ingredient and shouldn't be used together.
- Tell patient that it may take 4 weeks to reach full antidepressant effect.
- ***Alert:*** Advise patient to report mood swings or suicidal thoughts immediately.
- Tell patient not to chew, crush or divide tablets.
- Inform patient that tablets may have an odor.

citalopram hydrobromide
Celexa✎

Pharmacologic class: SSRI
Pregnancy risk category C

AVAILABLE FORMS
Solution: 10 mg/5 ml
Tablets: 10 mg, 20 mg, 40 mg
Tablets (orally disintegrating): 10 mg, 20 mg, 40 mg

INDICATIONS & DOSAGES
➤Depression
Adults: Initially, 20 mg P.O. once daily, increasing to 40 mg daily after no less than 1 week. Maximum recommended dose is 40 mg daily.
Elderly patients: 20 mg daily P.O. with adjustment to 40 mg daily only for unresponsive patients.
Adjust-a-dose: For patients with hepatic impairment, use 20 mg daily P.O. with adjustment to 40 mg daily only for unresponsive patients.

ACTION
An SSRI whose action is presumed to be linked to potentiation of serotonergic activity in the CNS resulting from inhibition of neuronal reuptake of serotonin.

Route	Onset	Peak	Duration
P.O.	Unknown	4 hr	Unknown

Half-life: 35 hours.

ADVERSE REACTIONS
CNS: *somnolence, insomnia,* ***suicide attempt,*** anxiety, agitation, dizziness, paresthesia, migraine, impaired concentration, amnesia, depression, apathy, tremor, confusion, fatigue, fever.
CV: tachycardia, orthostatic hypotension, hypotension.
EENT: rhinitis, sinusitis, abnormal accommodation.
GI: *dry mouth, nausea,* diarrhea, anorexia, dyspepsia, vomiting, abdominal pain, taste perversion, increased saliva, flatulence, increased appetite.
GU: dysmenorrhea, amenorrhea, ejaculation disorder, impotence, anorgasmia, polyuria.
Metabolic: decreased or increased weight.
Musculoskeletal: arthralgia, myalgia.
Respiratory: upper respiratory tract infection, coughing.
Skin: rash, pruritus.
Other: *increased sweating,* yawning, decreased libido.

INTERACTIONS
Drug-drug. *Amphetamines, buspirone, dextromethorphan, dihydroergotamine, meperidine, other SSRIs or selective serotonin-norepinephrine reuptake inhibitors (duloxetine, venlafaxine),* ***tramadol,*** *trazodone, tricyclic antidepressants, tryptophan:* May increase the risk of serotonin syndrome. Avoid other drugs that increase the availability of serotonin in the CNS; monitor patient closely if used together.
Carbamazepine: May increase citalopram clearance. Monitor patient for effects.
CNS drugs: May cause additive effects. Use together cautiously.
Drugs that inhibit cytochrome P-450 isoenzymes 3A4 and 2C19: May cause decreased clearance of citalopram. Monitor patient for increased adverse effects.
Imipramine, other tricyclic antidepressants: May increase level of imipramine metabolite desipramine by about 50%. Use together cautiously.

Lithium: May enhance serotonergic effect of citalopram. Use together cautiously, and monitor lithium level.
MAO inhibitors (phenelzine, selegiline, tranylcypromine): May cause serotonin syndrome. Avoid using within 14 days of MAO inhibitor therapy.
Sumatriptan: May cause weakness, hyperreflexia, and incoordination. Monitor patient closely.
Drug-herb. *St. John's wort:* May increase the risk of serotonin syndrome. Discourage use together.
Drug-lifestyle. *Alcohol use:* May increase CNS effects. Discourage use together.

EFFECTS ON LAB TEST RESULTS
None reported.

CONTRAINDICATIONS & CAUTIONS
- Contraindicated in patients hypersensitive to drug or its inactive components, within 14 days of MAO inhibitor therapy, and in patients taking pimozide.
- Use cautiously in patients with history of mania, seizures, suicidal thoughts, or hepatic or renal impairment.
- Use in third trimester of pregnancy may be linked to neonatal complications at birth. Consider the risk versus benefit of treatment during this time.
- Safety and effectiveness of drug haven't been established in children.

NURSING CONSIDERATIONS
- Although drug hasn't been shown to impair psychomotor performance, any psychoactive drug has the potential to impair judgment, thinking, or motor skills.
- The possibility of a suicide attempt is inherent in depression and may persist until significant remission occurs. Closely supervise high-risk patients at start of drug therapy. Reduce risk of overdose by limiting amount of drug available per refill.
- ***Alert:*** Drug may increase the risk of suicidal thinking and behavior in children and adolescents with major depressive disorder or other psychiatric disorders.
- At least 14 days should elapse between MAO inhibitor therapy and citalopram therapy.
- ***Look alike–sound alike:*** Don't confuse Celexa with Celebrex or Cerebyx.

PATIENT TEACHING
- Caution patient against use of MAO inhibitors while taking citalopram.
- Inform patient that, although improvement may take 1 to 4 weeks, he should continue therapy as prescribed.
- Advise patient not to stop drug abruptly.
- Tell patient that drug may be taken in the morning or evening without regard to meals. If drowsiness occurs, he should take drug in evening.
- Tell patient to allow orally disintegrating tablet to dissolve on his tongue then swallow, with or without water. Tell him not to cut, crush, or chew.
- Instruct patient to exercise caution when driving or operating hazardous machinery; drug may impair judgment, thinking, and motor skills.
- Advise patient to consult prescriber before taking other prescription or OTC drugs.
- Advise woman of childbearing age to consult prescriber before breast-feeding.
- Warn patient to avoid alcohol during drug therapy.
- Instruct woman of childbearing age to use contraceptives during drug therapy and to notify prescriber immediately if pregnancy is suspected.

clomipramine hydrochloride
Anafranil, Placil‡

Pharmacologic class: tricyclic antidepressant (TCA)
Pregnancy risk category C

AVAILABLE FORMS
Capsules: 25 mg, 50 mg, 75 mg

INDICATIONS & DOSAGES
➤ **Obsessive-compulsive disorder**
Adults: Initially, 25 mg P.O. daily with meals, gradually increased to 100 mg daily in divided doses during first 2 weeks. Thereafter, increase to maximum dose of 250 mg daily in divided doses with meals, p.r.n. After adjustment, give total daily dose at bedtime.
Children and adolescents: Initially, 25 mg P.O. daily with meals, gradually increased over first 2 weeks to daily maximum of 3 mg/kg or 100 mg P.O. in divided doses,

whichever is smaller. Maximum daily dose is 3 mg/kg or 200 mg, whichever is smaller; give at bedtime after adjustment. Reassess and adjust dosage periodically.

➤ **To manage panic disorder with or without agoraphobia**

Adults: 12.5 to 150 mg P.O. daily (maximum 200 mg).

➤ **Depression, chronic pain** ♦

Adults: 100 to 250 mg P.O. daily.

➤ **Cataplexy and related narcolepsy** ♦

Adults: 25 to 200 mg P.O. daily.

ACTION

Unknown. A TCA that inhibits reuptake of serotonin and norepinephrine at the presynaptic neuron.

Route	Onset	Peak	Duration
P.O.	Unknown	2–6 hr	Unknown

Half-life: Parent compound, 32 hours; active metabolite, 69 hours.

ADVERSE REACTIONS

CNS: *somnolence, tremor, dizziness, headache, insomnia, nervousness, myoclonus, fatigue,* ***seizures,*** EEG changes.
CV: orthostatic hypotension, palpitations, tachycardia.
EENT: *pharyngitis, rhinitis, visual changes.*
GI: *dry mouth, constipation, nausea, dyspepsia, increased appetite, anorexia, abdominal pain,* diarrhea.
GU: *urinary hesitancy,* UTI, *dysmenorrhea, ejaculation failure, impotence.*
Hematologic: purpura.
Metabolic: *weight gain.*
Musculoskeletal: *myalgia.*
Skin: *diaphoresis,* rash, pruritus, dry skin.
Other: *altered libido.*

INTERACTIONS

Drug-drug. *Barbiturates:* May decrease TCA level. Watch for decreased antidepressant effect.
Cimetidine, ***fluoxetine, fluvoxamine, paroxetine, sertraline:*** May increase TCA level. Monitor drug level and patient for signs of toxicity.
Clonidine: May cause life-threatening hypertension. Avoid using together.
CNS depressants: May enhance CNS depression. Avoid using together.
Epinephrine, norepinephrine: May increase hypertensive effect. Use together cautiously.
MAO inhibitors: May cause hyperpyretic crisis, seizures, coma, or death. Avoid using within 14 days of MAO inhibitor therapy.
Quinolones: May increase the risk of life-threatening arrhythmias. Avoid using together.
Drug-herb. *Evening primrose oil:* May cause additive or synergistic effect, resulting in lower seizure threshold and increasing the risk of seizure. Discourage use together.
St. John's wort, SAM-e, yohimbe: May cause serotonin syndrome. Discourage use together.
Drug-lifestyle. *Alcohol use:* May enhance CNS depression. Discourage use together.
Sun exposure: May increase risk of photosensitivity reactions. Advise patient to avoid excessive sunlight exposure.

EFFECTS ON LAB TEST RESULTS

None reported.

CONTRAINDICATIONS & CAUTIONS

- Contraindicated in patients hypersensitive to drug or other tricyclic antidepressants, in those who have taken MAO inhibitors within previous 14 days, and in patients in acute recovery period after MI.
- Use cautiously in patients with history of seizure disorders or with brain damage of varying cause; in patients receiving other seizure threshold–lowering drugs; in patients at risk for suicide; in patients with history of urine retention or angle-closure glaucoma, increased intraocular pressure, CV disease, impaired hepatic or renal function, or hyperthyroidism; in patients with tumors of the adrenal medulla; in patients receiving thyroid drug or electroconvulsive therapy; and in those undergoing elective surgery.

NURSING CONSIDERATIONS

- Monitor mood and watch for suicidal tendencies. Allow patient to have only the minimal amount of drug.
- ***Alert:*** Drug may increase risk of suicidal thinking and behavior in children

and adolescents with major depressive disorder or other psychiatric disorder.
- Don't withdraw drug abruptly.
- Because patients may suffer hypertensive episodes during surgery, stop drug gradually several days before surgery.
- Relieve dry mouth with sugarless candy or gum. Saliva substitutes may be needed.
- ***Look alike–sound alike:*** Don't confuse clomipramine with chlorpromazine or clomiphene, or Anafranil with enalapril, nafarelin, or alfentanil.

PATIENT TEACHING
- Warn patient to avoid hazardous activities requiring alertness and good coordination, especially during adjustment. Daytime sedation and dizziness may occur.
- Tell patient to avoid alcohol during drug therapy.
- Warn patient not to stop drug suddenly.
- Advise patient to use sunblock, wear protective clothing, and avoid prolonged exposure to strong sunlight to prevent oversensitivity to the sun.

desipramine hydrochloride
Apo-Desipramine†, Norpramin, Novo-Desipramine†

Pharmacologic class: tricyclic antidepressant (TCA)
Pregnancy risk category NR

AVAILABLE FORMS
Tablets: 10 mg, 25 mg, 50 mg, 75 mg, 100 mg, 150 mg

INDICATIONS & DOSAGES
➤ **Depression**
Adults: 100 to 200 mg P.O. daily in divided doses; increase to maximum of 300 mg daily. Or, give entire dose at bedtime.
Adolescents and elderly patients: 25 to 100 mg P.O. daily in divided doses; increase gradually to maximum of 150 mg daily, if needed.

ACTION
Unknown. A TCA that increases amount of norepinephrine, serotonin, or both in the CNS by blocking their reuptake by the presynaptic neurons.

Route	Onset	Peak	Duration
P.O.	Unknown	4–6 hr	Unknown

Half-life: Unknown.

ADVERSE REACTIONS
CNS: *drowsiness, dizziness,* ***seizures,*** excitation, tremor, weakness, confusion, anxiety, restlessness, agitation, headache, nervousness, EEG changes, extrapyramidal reactions.
CV: *tachycardia,* orthostatic hypotension, ECG changes, hypertension.
EENT: *blurred vision,* tinnitus, mydriasis.
GI: *dry mouth,* constipation, nausea, vomiting, anorexia, paralytic ileus.
GU: urine retention.
Metabolic: ***hypoglycemia,*** hyperglycemia.
Skin: rash, urticaria, photosensitivity reactions, diaphoresis.
Other: ***sudden death in children,*** hypersensitivity reactions.

INTERACTIONS
Drug-drug. *Barbiturates, CNS depressants:* May enhance CNS depression. Avoid using together.
Cimetidine, ***fluoxetine, fluvoxamine, paroxetine, sertraline:*** May increase desipramine level. Monitor drug levels and patient for signs of toxicity.
Clonidine: May cause life-threatening blood pressure elevations. Avoid using together.
Epinephrine, norepinephrine: May increase hypertensive effect. Use together cautiously.
MAO inhibitors: May cause severe excitation, hyperpyrexia, or seizures, usually with high doses. Avoid using within 14 days of MAO inhibitor therapy.
Quinolones: May increase the risk of life-threatening arrhythmias. Avoid using together.
Drug-herb. *Evening primrose oil:* May cause additive or synergistic effect, resulting in lower seizure threshold and increasing the risk of seizure. Discourage use together.
St. John's wort, SAM-e, yohimbe: May cause serotonin syndrome. Discourage use together.

Drug-lifestyle. *Alcohol use:* May enhance CNS depression. Discourage use together.
Smoking: May lower drug level. Monitor patient for lack of effect.
Sun exposure: May increase risk of photosensitivity reactions. Advise patient to avoid excessive sunlight exposure.

EFFECTS ON LAB TEST RESULTS
- May increase or decrease glucose level.
- May increase liver function test values.

CONTRAINDICATIONS & CAUTIONS
- Contraindicated in patients hypersensitive to drug and in those who have taken MAO inhibitors within previous 14 days.
- Contraindicated during acute recovery phase after MI.
- Use with extreme caution in patients with CV disease; in those with history of urine retention, glaucoma, seizure disorders, or thyroid disease; and in those taking thyroid drug.

NURSING CONSIDERATIONS
- Monitor patient for nausea, headache, and malaise after abrupt withdrawal of long-term therapy; these symptoms don't indicate addiction.
- Don't withdraw drug abruptly.
- Because patients may suffer hypertensive episodes during surgery, stop drug gradually several days before surgery.
- If signs or symptoms of psychosis occur or increase, notify prescriber. Record mood changes. Monitor patient for suicidal tendencies.
- ***Alert:*** Drug may increase the risk of suicidal thinking and behavior in children and adolescents with major depressive disorder or other psychiatric disorders.
- Because drug produces fewer anticholinergic effects than other TCAs, it's often prescribed for cardiac patients.
- Recommend sugarless hard candy or gum to relieve dry mouth. Saliva substitutes may be needed.
- ***Alert:*** Norpramin may contain tartrazine.
- ***Look alike–sound alike:*** Don't confuse desipramine with disopyramide or imipramine.

PATIENT TEACHING
- Advise patient to take full dose at bedtime to avoid daytime sedation; if insomnia occurs, tell him to take drug in the morning.
- Warn patient to avoid hazardous activities that require alertness and good coordination until effects of drug are known. Drowsiness and dizziness usually subside after a few weeks.
- Advise patient to call prescriber if fever and sore throat occur. Blood counts may need to be obtained.
- Tell patient to avoid alcohol during therapy because it may antagonize effects of drug.
- Tell patient to consult prescriber before taking other prescription or OTC drugs.
- Warn patient not to stop drug suddenly.
- To prevent sensitivity to the sun, advise patient to use sunblock, wear protective clothing, and avoid prolonged exposure to strong sunlight.

doxepin hydrochloride
Deptran‡, Novo-Doxepin†, Sinequan, Triadapin†

Pharmacologic class: tricyclic antidepressant (TCA)
Pregnancy risk category C

AVAILABLE FORMS
Capsules: 10 mg, 25 mg, 50 mg, 75 mg, 100 mg, 150 mg
Oral concentrate: 10 mg/ml

INDICATIONS & DOSAGES
➤ Depression; anxiety
Adults: Initially, 75 mg P.O. daily. Usual dosage range is 75 to 150 mg daily to maximum of 300 mg daily in divided doses. Or, entire maintenance dose may be given once daily with maximum dose of 150 mg.

ACTION
Unknown. Increases amount of norepinephrine, serotonin, or both in the CNS by blocking their reuptake by the presynaptic neurons.

Route	Onset	Peak	Duration
P.O.	Unknown	2 hr	Unknown

Half-life: 6 to 8 hours.

ADVERSE REACTIONS

CNS: *drowsiness, dizziness, **seizures,*** confusion, numbness, hallucinations, paresthesia, ataxia, weakness, headache, extrapyramidal reactions.
CV: *orthostatic hypotension, tachycardia,* ECG changes.
EENT: *blurred vision,* tinnitus.
GI: *dry mouth, constipation,* nausea, vomiting, anorexia.
GU: urine retention.
Metabolic: ***hypoglycemia,*** hyperglycemia.
Skin: *diaphoresis,* rash, urticaria, photosensitivity reactions.
Other: hypersensitivity reactions.

INTERACTIONS

Drug-drug. *Barbiturates, CNS depressants:* May enhance CNS depression. Avoid using together.
Cimetidine, ***fluoxetine, fluvoxamine, paroxetine, sertraline:*** May increase doxepin level. Monitor drug levels and patient for signs of toxicity.
Clonidine: May cause life-threatening hypertension. Avoid using together.
Epinephrine, norepinephrine: May increase hypertensive effect. Use together cautiously.
MAO inhibitors: May cause severe excitation, hyperpyrexia, or seizures, usually with high dosage. Avoid using within 14 days of MAO inhibitor therapy.
Quinolones: May increase the risk of life-threatening arrhythmias. Avoid using together.
Drug-herb. *Evening primrose oil:* May cause additive or synergistic effect, resulting in lower seizure threshold and increasing the risk of seizure. Discourage use together.
St. John's wort, SAM-e, yohimbe: May cause serotonin syndrome. Discourage use together.
Drug-lifestyle. *Alcohol use:* May enhance CNS depression. Discourage use together.
Sun exposure: May increase risk of photosensitivity reactions. Advise patient to avoid excessive sunlight exposure.

EFFECTS ON LAB TEST RESULTS

- May increase or decrease glucose level.
- May increase liver function test values.

CONTRAINDICATIONS & CAUTIONS

- Contraindicated in patients hypersensitive to drug and in those with glaucoma or tendency toward urine retention; also contraindicated in those who have received an MAO inhibitor within past 14 days and during acute recovery phase of an MI.

NURSING CONSIDERATIONS

- Don't withdraw drug abruptly.
- Monitor patient for nausea, headache, and malaise after abrupt withdrawal of long-term therapy; these symptoms don't indicate addiction.
- ***Alert:*** Because hypertensive episodes may occur during surgery in patients receiving drug, stop it gradually several days before surgery.
- If signs or symptoms of psychosis occur or increase, expect prescriber to reduce dosage. Record mood changes. Monitor patient for suicidal tendencies and allow only a minimum supply of drug.
- ***Alert:*** Drug may increase the risk of suicidal thinking and behavior in children and adolescents with major depressive disorder or other psychiatric disorders.
- Drug has strong anticholinergic effects and is one of the most sedating TCAs. Adverse anticholinergic effects can occur rapidly.
- Recommend use of sugarless hard candy or gum to relieve dry mouth.
- ***Look alike–sound alike:*** Don't confuse doxepin with doxazosin, digoxin, doxapram, or Doxidan; don't confuse Sinequan with saquinavir.

PATIENT TEACHING

- Tell patient to dilute oral concentrate with 4 ounces (120 ml) of water, milk, or juice (orange, grapefruit, tomato, prune, or pineapple, but not grape); preparation shouldn't be mixed with carbonated beverages.
- Tell patient to take full dose at bedtime whenever he can, but warn him of possible morning dizziness on standing up quickly.
- Advise patient to consult prescriber before taking other prescription or OTC drugs.
- Warn patient to avoid hazardous activities that require alertness and good psychomotor coordination until effects of

drug are known. Drowsiness and dizziness usually subside after a few weeks.
- Tell patient to avoid alcohol during drug therapy.
- Tell patient that maximal effect may not be evident for 2 to 3 weeks.
- Warn patient not to stop drug suddenly.
- To prevent sensitivity to the sun, advise patient to use sunblock, wear protective clothing, and avoid prolonged exposure to strong sunlight.

duloxetine hydrochloride

Cymbalta

Pharmacologic class: selective serotonin and norepinephrine reuptake inhibitor
Pregnancy risk category C

AVAILABLE FORMS

Capsules (delayed-release): 20 mg, 30 mg, 60 mg

INDICATIONS & DOSAGES

➤Major depressive disorder
Adults: Initially, 20 mg P.O. b.i.d.; then, 60 mg P.O. once daily or divided in two equal doses. Maximum, 60 mg daily.

➤Neuropathic pain related to diabetic peripheral neuropathy
Adults: 60 mg P.O. once daily.
Adjust-a-dose: In patients with impaired renal function, reduce starting dose and increase gradually.

ACTION

May inhibit serotonin and norepinephrine reuptake in the CNS.

Route	Onset	Peak	Duration
P.O.	Unknown	6 hr	Unknown

Half-life: 12 hours.

ADVERSE REACTIONS

CNS: *dizziness, fatigue, headache, insomnia, somnolence,* ***suicidal thoughts,*** fever, hypoesthesia, initial insomnia, irritability, lethargy, nervousness, nightmares, restlessness, sleep disorder, anxiety, asthenia, tremor.
CV: hot flushes, hypertension, increased heart rate.
EENT: blurred vision, nasopharyngitis, pharyngolaryngeal pain.
GI: *constipation, diarrhea, dry mouth, nausea,* dyspepsia, gastritis, vomiting.
GU: abnormal orgasm, abnormally increased frequency of urinating, delayed or dysfunctional ejaculation, dysuria, erectile dysfunction, urinary hesitation.
Metabolic: *decreased appetite,* ***hypoglycemia,*** increased appetite, weight gain or loss.
Musculoskeletal: muscle cramps, myalgia.
Respiratory: cough.
Skin: increased sweating, night sweats, pruritus, rash.
Other: decreased libido, rigors.

INTERACTIONS

Drug-drug. *Antiarrhythmics of type 1C (flecainide, propafenone), phenothiazines:* May increase levels of these drugs. Use together cautiously.
CNS drugs: May increase adverse effects. Use together cautiously.
CYP1A2 inhibitors (cimetidine, fluvoxamine, certain quinolones): May increase duloxetine level. Avoid using together.
CYP2D6 inhibitors (fluoxetine, paroxetine, quinidine): May increase duloxetine level. Use together cautiously.
Drugs that reduce gastric acidity: May cause premature breakdown of duloxetine's protective coating and early release of the drug. Monitor patient for effects.
MAO inhibitors: May cause hyperthermia, rigidity, myoclonus, autonomic instability, rapid fluctuations of vital signs, agitation, delirium, and coma. Avoid use within 2 weeks after MAO inhibitor therapy; wait at least 5 days after stopping duloxetine before starting MAO inhibitor.
Thioridazine: May prolong the QT interval and increase risk of serious ventricular arrhythmias and sudden death. Avoid using together.
Tricyclic antidepressants (amitriptyline, nortriptyline, imipramine): May increase levels of these drugs. Reduce tricyclic antidepressant dose, and monitor drug levels closely.
Triptans: May cause serotonin syndrome (restlessness, hallucinations, loss of coordination, fast heartbeat, rapid changes in blood pressure, increased body tempera-

ture, hyperreflexia,nausea, vomiting, and diarrhea). Use cautiously and with increased monitoring, especially when starting or increasing dosages.
Drug-lifestyle. *Alcohol use:* May increase risk of liver damage. Discourage use together.

EFFECTS ON LAB TEST RESULTS
• May increase alkaline phosphatase, ALT, AST, bilirubin, and CK levels.

CONTRAINDICATIONS & CAUTIONS
• Contraindicated in patients hypersensitive to drug or its ingredients, patients taking MAO inhibitors, patients with uncontrolled angle-closure glaucoma, and patients with a creatinine clearance less than 30 ml/minute. Drug isn't recommended for patients with hepatic dysfunction or end-stage renal disease.
• Use cautiously in patients with a history of mania or seizures, patients who drink substantial amounts of alcohol, patients with hypertension, patients with controlled angle-closure glaucoma, and those with conditions that slow gastric emptying.

NURSING CONSIDERATIONS
• Monitor patient for worsening of depression or suicidal behavior, especially when therapy starts or dosage changes.
• ***Alert:*** Drug may increase the risk of suicidal thinking and behavior in children and adolescents with major depressive disorder or other psychiatric disorder.
• Treatment of overdose is symptomatic. Don't induce emesis; gastric lavage or activated charcoal may be performed soon after ingestion or if patient is still symptomatic. Because drug undergoes extensive distribution, forced diuresis, dialysis, hemoperfusion, and exchange transfusion aren't useful. Contact a poison control center for information.
• If taken with tricyclic antidepressants, duloxetine metabolism will be prolonged, and patient will need extended monitoring.
• Periodically reassess patient to determine the need for continued therapy.
• Decrease dosage gradually, and watch for symptoms that may arise when drug is stopped, such as dizziness, nausea, headache, paresthesia, vomiting, irritability, and nightmares.
• If intolerable symptoms arise when decreasing or stopping drug, restart at previous dose and decrease even more gradually.
• Monitor blood pressure periodically during treatment.
• Use during the third trimester of pregnancy may cause neonatal complications including respiratory distress, cyanosis, apnea, seizures, vomiting, hypoglycemia, and hyperreflexia, which may require prolonged hospitalization, respiratory support, and tube feeding. Consider potential benefit of drug to the mother versus risks to the fetus.
• Older patients may be more sensitive to drug effects than younger adults.

PATIENT TEACHING
• ***Alert:*** Warn families or caregivers to report signs of worsening depression (such as agitation, irritability, insomnia, hostility, impulsivity) and signs of suicidal behavior to prescriber immediately.
• Tell patient to consult his prescriber or pharmacist if he plans to take other prescription or OTC drugs or an herbal or other dietary supplement.
• Instruct patient to swallow capsules whole and not to chew, crush, or open them because they have an enteric coating.
• Urge patient to avoid activities that are hazardous or require mental alertness until he knows how the drug affects him.
• Warn against drinking alcohol during therapy.
• If patient takes drug for depression, explain that it may take 1 to 4 weeks to notice an effect.

---

escitalopram oxalate
Lexapro

Pharmacologic class: SSRI
Pregnancy risk category C

AVAILABLE FORMS
Oral solution: 5 mg/5 ml
Tablets: 5 mg, 10 mg, 20 mg

INDICATIONS & DOSAGES

➤ **Treatment and maintenance therapy for patients with major depressive disorder; general anxiety disorder**

Adults: Initially, 10 mg P.O. once daily, increasing to 20 mg if needed after at least 1 week.

Adjust-a-dose: For elderly patients and those with hepatic impairment, 10 mg P.O. daily, initially and as maintenance dosages.

ACTION

Antidepressant action may be linked to increase of serotonergic activity in the CNS from inhibition of neuronal reuptake of serotonin. Drug is closely related to citalopram, which may be the active component.

Route	Onset	Peak	Duration
P.O.	Unknown	5 hr	Unknown

Half-life: 27 to 32 hours.

ADVERSE REACTIONS

CNS: ***suicidal behavior,*** fever, insomnia, dizziness, somnolence, paresthesia, lightheadedness, migraine, tremor, vertigo, abnormal dreams, irritability, impaired concentration, fatigue, lethargy.
CV: palpitations, hypertension, flushing, chest pain.
EENT: rhinitis, sinusitis, blurred vision, tinnitus, earache.
GI: *nausea,* diarrhea, constipation, indigestion, abdominal pain, vomiting, increased or decreased appetite, dry mouth, flatulence, heartburn, cramps, gastroesophageal reflux.
GU: ejaculation disorder, impotence, anorgasmia, menstrual cramps, UTI, urinary frequency.
Metabolic: weight gain or loss.
Musculoskeletal: arthralgia, myalgia, muscle cramps, pain in arms or legs.
Respiratory: bronchitis, cough.
Skin: rash, increased sweating.
Other: decreased libido, yawning, flulike symptoms.

INTERACTIONS

Drug-drug. *Aspirin, NSAIDs, other drugs known to affect coagulation:* May increase the risk of bleeding. Use together cautiously.
Carbamazepine: May increase escitalopram clearance. Monitor patient for expected antidepressant effect and adjust dose as needed.
Cimetidine: May increase escitalopram level. Monitor patient for increased adverse reactions to escitalopram.
Citalopram: May cause additive effects. Using together is contraindicated.
CNS drugs: May cause additive effects. Use together cautiously.
Desipramine, other drugs metabolized by CYP2D6: May increase levels of these drugs. Use together cautiously.
Lithium: May enhance serotonergic effect of escitalopram. Use together cautiously, and monitor lithium level.
MAO inhibitors: May cause fatal serotonin syndrome. Avoid using within 14 days of MAO inhibitor therapy.
Triptans: May increase serotonergic effects, leading to weakness, hyperreflexia, incoordination, rapid changes in blood pressure, nausea, and diarrhea. Use together cautiously, especially at the start of therapy or at dosage increases.
Tramadol: May cause serotonin syndrome. Monitor patient closely.
Drug-lifestyle. *Alcohol use:* May increase CNS effects. Discourage use together.

EFFECTS ON LAB TEST RESULTS

None reported.

CONTRAINDICATIONS & CAUTIONS

- Contraindicated in patients taking pimozide, MAO inhibitors, or within 14 days of MAO inhibitor therapy and in those hypersensitive to escitalopram, citalopram, or any of its inactive ingredients.
- Use cautiously in patients with a history of mania, seizure disorders, suicidal thoughts, or renal or hepatic impairment.
- Use cautiously in patients with diseases that produce altered metabolism or hemodynamic responses.
- Use with caution in elderly patients because they may have greater sensitivity to drug.
- Use in third trimester of pregnancy may cause complications at birth. Consider the risk versus benefit of treatment during this time.

• Drug appears in breast milk. Patient should either stop breast-feeding or stop taking drug.

NURSING CONSIDERATIONS

• Closely monitor patients at high risk of suicide.
• ***Alert:*** Drug may increase the risk of suicidal thinking and behavior in children and adolescents with major depressive disorder or other psychiatric disorder.
• ***Look alike–sound alike:*** Don't confuse escitalopram with estazolam.
• Evaluate patient for history of drug abuse and observe for signs of misuse or abuse.
• Periodically reassess patient to determine need for maintenance treatment and appropriate dosing.

PATIENT TEACHING

• Inform patient that symptoms should improve gradually over several weeks, rather than immediately.
• Tell patient that although improvement may occur within 1 to 4 weeks, he should continue drug as prescribed.
• ***Alert:*** Caution patient and patient's family to report signs of worsening depression (such as agitation, irritability, insomnia, hostility, impulsivity) and signs of suicidal behavior to prescriber immediately.
• Tell patient to use caution while driving or operating hazardous machinery because of drug's potential to impair judgment, thinking, and motor skills.
• Advise patient to consult health care provider before taking other prescription or OTC drugs.
• Tell patient that drug may be taken in the morning or evening without regard to meals.
• Encourage patient to avoid alcohol while taking drug.
• Tell woman to notify health care provider if she's pregnant or breast-feeding.

fluoxetine hydrochloride

Erocap‡, Lovan‡, Prozac, Prozac-20‡, Prozac Weekly, Sarafem, Zactin‡

Pharmacologic class: SSRI
Pregnancy risk category C

AVAILABLE FORMS

Capsules (delayed-release): 90 mg
Capsules (pulvules): 10 mg, 20 mg, 40 mg
Oral solution: 20 mg/5 ml
Tablets: 10 mg, 20 mg

INDICATIONS & DOSAGES

➤ **Depression, obsessive-compulsive disorder (OCD)**

Adults: Initially, 20 mg P.O. in the morning; increase dosage based on patient response. Maximum daily dose is 80 mg.
Children ages 7 to 17 (OCD): 10 mg P.O. daily. After 2 weeks, increase to 20 mg daily. Dosage is 20 to 60 mg daily.
Children ages 8 to 18 (depression): 10 mg P.O. once daily for 1 week; then increase to 20 mg daily.

➤ **Depression in elderly patients**

Adults age 65 and older: Initially, 20 mg P.O. daily in the morning. Increase dose based on response. Doses may be given b.i.d., morning and noon. Maximum daily dose is 80 mg. Consider using a lower dosage or less-frequent doses in these patients, especially those with systemic illness and those who are receiving drugs for other illnesses.

➤ **Maintenance therapy for depression in stabilized patients (not for newly diagnosed depression)**

Adults: 90 mg Prozac Weekly P.O. once weekly. Start once-weekly doses 7 days after the last daily dose of Prozac 20 mg.

➤ **Short-term and long-term treatment of bulimia nervosa**

Adults: 60 mg P.O. daily in the morning.

➤ **Short-term treatment of panic disorder with or without agoraphobia**

Adults: 10 mg P.O. once daily for 1 week; then increase dose as needed to 20 mg daily. Maximum daily dose is 60 mg.
Adjust-a-dose: For patients with renal or hepatic impairment, reduce dose or increase interval.

➤**Anorexia nervosa in weight-restored patients** ♦
Adults: 40 mg P.O. daily.
➤**Depression caused by bipolar disorder** ♦
Adults: 20 to 60 mg P.O. daily.
➤**Cataplexy** ♦
Adults: 20 mg P.O. once or twice daily with CNS stimulant therapy.
➤**Alcohol dependence** ♦
Adults: 60 mg P.O. daily.
➤**Premenstrual dysphoric disorder**
Adults: 20 mg Sarafem P.O. daily continuously (every day of the menstrual cycle) or intermittently (daily dose starting 14 days before the anticipated onset of menstruation through the first full day of menses and repeating with each new cycle). Maximum daily dose is 80 mg P.O.
Adjust-a-dose: For patients with renal or hepatic impairment and those taking several drugs at the same time, reduce dose or increase dosing interval.

ACTION
Thought to be linked to drug's inhibition of CNS neuronal uptake of serotonin.

Route	Onset	Peak	Duration
P.O.	Unknown	6–8 hr	Unknown

Half-life: Fluoxetine, 2 to 3 days; norfluoxetine, 7 to 9 days.

ADVERSE REACTIONS
CNS: *nervousness, somnolence, anxiety, insomnia, headache, drowsiness, tremor, dizziness, asthenia,* ***suicidal behavior,*** fatigue, fever.
CV: palpitations, hot flashes.
EENT: nasal congestion, pharyngitis, sinusitis.
GI: *nausea, diarrhea, dry mouth, anorexia,* dyspepsia, constipation, abdominal pain, vomiting, flatulence, increased appetite.
GU: sexual dysfunction.
Metabolic: weight loss.
Musculoskeletal: muscle pain.
Respiratory: upper respiratory tract infection, cough, respiratory distress.
Skin: rash, pruritus, diaphoresis.
Other: flulike syndrome.

INTERACTIONS
Drug-drug. *Amphetamines, buspirone, dextromethorphan, dihydroergotamine, lithium salts, meperidine, other SSRIs or selective serotonin-norepinephrine reuptake inhibitors (duloxetine, venlafaxine),* ***tramadol,*** *trazodone, tricyclic antidepressants, tryptophan:* May increase the risk of serotonin syndrome. Avoid combinations of drugs that increase the availability of serotonin in the CNS; monitor patient closely if used together.
Benzodiazepines, lithium, tricyclic antidepressants: May increase CNS effects. Monitor patient closely.
Beta blockers, carbamazepine, flecainide, vinblastine: May increase levels of these drugs. Monitor drug levels and monitor patient for adverse reactions.
Cyproheptadine: May reverse or decrease fluoxetine effect. Monitor patient closely.
Dextromethorphan: May cause unusual side effects, such as visual hallucinations. Advise use of cough suppressant that doesn't contain dextromethorphan while taking fluoxetine.
Highly protein-bound drugs: May increase level of fluoxetine or other highly protein-bound drugs. Monitor patient closely.
Insulin, oral antidiabetics: May alter glucose level and antidiabetic requirements. Adjust dosage.
MAO inhibitors (phenelzine, selegiline, tranylcypromine): May cause serotonin syndrome. Avoid using at the same time and for at least 5 weeks after stopping.
Phenytoin: May increase phenytoin level and risk of toxicity. Monitor phenytoin level and adjust dosage.
Triptans: May cause weakness, hyperreflexia, incoordination, rapid changes in blood pressure, nausea, and diarrhea. Monitor patient closely, especially at the start of treatment and when dosage increases.
Thioridazine: May increase thioridazine level, increasing risk of serious ventricular arrhythmias and sudden death. Avoid using at the same time and for at least 5 weeks after stopping.
Warfarin: May increase risk for bleeding. Monitor PT and INR.
Drug-herb. *St. John's wort:* May increase sedative and hypnotic effects; may cause

serotonin syndrome. Discourage use together.
Drug-lifestyle. *Alcohol use:* May increase CNS depression. Discourage use together.

EFFECTS ON LAB TEST RESULTS
None reported.

CONTRAINDICATIONS & CAUTIONS
- Contraindicated in patients hypersensitive to drug and in those taking MAO inhibitors within 14 days of starting therapy. MAO inhibitors shouldn't be started within 5 weeks of stopping fluoxetine. Avoid using thioridazine with fluoxetine or within 5 weeks after stopping fluoxetine.
- Use cautiously in patients at high risk for suicide and in those with history of diabetes mellitus, seizures, mania, or hepatic, renal, or CV disease.
- Use in third trimester of pregnancy may be associated with neonatal complications at birth. Consider the risk versus benefit of treatment during this time.

NURSING CONSIDERATIONS
- Use antihistamines or topical corticosteroids to treat rashes or pruritus.
- Watch for weight change during therapy, particularly in underweight or bulimic patients.
- Record mood changes. Watch for suicidal tendencies.
- ***Alert:*** Drug may increase the risk of suicidal thinking and behavior in children and adolescents with major depressive disorder or other psychiatric disorder.
- Drug has a long half-life; monitor patient for adverse effects for up to 2 weeks after drug is stopped.
- ***Look alike–sound alike:*** Don't confuse fluoxetine with fluvoxamine or fluvastatin. Don't confuse Prozac with Proscar, Prilosec, or ProSom.

PATIENT TEACHING
- Tell patient to avoid taking drug in the afternoon whenever possible because doing so commonly causes nervousness and insomnia.
- Drug may cause dizziness or drowsiness. Warn patient to avoid driving and other hazardous activities that require alertness and good psychomotor coordination until effects of drug are known.
- Tell patient to consult prescriber before taking other prescription or OTC drugs.
- Advise patient that full therapeutic effect may not be seen for 4 weeks or longer.

fluvoxamine maleate

Pharmacologic class: SSRI
Pregnancy risk category C

AVAILABLE FORMS
Tablets: 25 mg, 50 mg, 100 mg.

INDICATIONS & DOSAGES
➤ Obsessive-compulsive disorder (OCD)
Adults: Initially, 50 mg P.O. daily at bedtime; increase by 50 mg q 4 to 7 days. Maximum, 300 mg daily. Give total daily amounts above 100 mg in two divided doses.
Children ages 8 to 17: Initially, 25 mg P.O. daily at bedtime; increase by 25 mg q 4 to 7 days. Maximum, 200 mg daily for children ages 8 to 11 and 300 mg daily for children ages 11 to 17. Give total daily amounts over 50 mg in two divided doses.
Adjust-a-dose: In elderly patients and those with hepatic impairment, give lower first dose and adjust dose more slowly.

ACTION
Unknown. Selectively inhibits the presynaptic neuronal uptake of serotonin, which may improve OCD.

Route	Onset	Peak	Duration
P.O.	Unknown	3–8 hr	Unknown

Half-life: 17 hours.

ADVERSE REACTIONS
CNS: *agitation, headache, asthenia, somnolence, insomnia, nervousness, dizziness,* tremor, anxiety, hypertonia, depression, CNS stimulation.
CV: palpitations, vasodilation.
EENT: amblyopia.
GI: *nausea, diarrhea, constipation, dyspepsia, vomiting, dry mouth,* anorexia, flatulence, dysphagia, taste perversion.

GU: abnormal ejaculation, urinary frequency, impotence, anorgasmia, urine retention.
Respiratory: upper respiratory tract infection, dyspnea, yawning.
Skin: sweating.
Other: tooth disorder, flulike syndrome, chills, decreased libido.

INTERACTIONS

Drug-drug. *Benzodiazepines, theophylline, warfarin:* May reduce clearance of these drugs. Use together cautiously (except for diazepam, which shouldn't be used with fluvoxamine). Adjust dosage as needed.
Carbamazepine, clozapine, methadone, metoprolol, propranolol, theophylline, tricyclic antidepressants: May increase levels of these drugs. Use together cautiously, and monitor patient closely for adverse reactions. Dosage adjustments may be needed.
Diltiazem: May cause bradycardia. Monitor heart rate.
Lithium, tryptophan: May enhance effects of fluvoxamine. Use together cautiously.
MAO inhibitors (phenelzine, selegiline, tranylcypromine): May cause serotonin syndrome (CNS irritability, shivering, and altered consciousness). Avoid using within 2 weeks of MAO inhibitor.
Pimozide, thioridazine: May prolong QTc interval. Avoid using together.
Sumatriptan: May cause weakness, hyperreflexia, and incoordination. Monitor patient closely. May cause serotonin syndrome. Avoid using within 2 weeks of MAO inhibitor.
Tramadol: May cause serotonin syndrome. Monitor patient closely.
Drug-lifestyle. *Alcohol use:* May increase CNS effects. Discourage use together.
Smoking: May decrease drug's effectiveness. Urge patient to stop smoking.

EFFECTS ON LAB TEST RESULTS

None reported.

CONTRAINDICATIONS & CAUTIONS

- Contraindicated in patients hypersensitive to drug or to other phenyl piperazine antidepressants, in those receiving pimozide or thioridazine therapy, and within 2 weeks of MAO inhibitor.
- Use cautiously in patients with hepatic dysfunction, other conditions that may affect hemodynamic responses or metabolism, or history of mania or seizures.

NURSING CONSIDERATIONS

- Record mood changes. Monitor patient for suicidal tendencies.
- Don't use for the treatment of major depressive disorders in children younger than age 18 because of an increased risk of suicidal behavior.
- ***Alert:*** Combining an SSRI with a triptan may cause serotonin syndrome. Signs and symptoms may include restlessness, hallucinations, loss of coordination, fast heart beat, rapid changes in blood pressure, increased body temperature, hyperreflexia, nausea, vomiting, and diarrhea. Serotonin syndrome is more likely to occur when starting or increasing the dose of a triptan.
- ***Look alike–sound alike:*** Don't confuse fluvoxamine with fluoxetine.
- Patients shouldn't stop drug without first consulting prescriber; abruptly stopping drug may cause withdrawal syndrome, including headache, muscle ache, and flulike symptoms.

PATIENT TEACHING

- Warn patient to avoid hazardous activities until CNS effects of drug are known.
- Tell woman to notify prescriber about planned, suspected, or known pregnancy.
- Tell patient who develops a rash, hives, or a related allergic reaction to notify prescriber.
- Inform patient that several weeks of therapy may be needed to obtain full therapeutic effect. Once improvement occurs, advise patient not to stop drug until directed by prescriber.
- Suggest that patient keep a diary of changes in mood or behavior. Tell patient to report suicidal thoughts immediately.
- Advise patient to check with prescriber before taking OTC drugs; drug interactions can occur.
- Tell patient drug can be taken with or without food.

imipramine hydrochloride
Apo-Imipramine†, Impril†, Melipramine‡, Novopramine†, Tofranil

imipramine pamoate
Tofranil-PM

Pharmacologic class: tricyclic antidepressant (TCA)
Pregnancy risk category D

AVAILABLE FORMS
imipramine hydrochloride
Tablets: 10 mg, 25 mg, 50 mg
imipramine pamoate
Capsules: 75 mg, 100 mg, 125 mg, 150 mg

INDICATIONS & DOSAGES
➤ **Depression**
Adults: 75 to 100 mg P.O. daily in divided doses, increased by 25 to 50 mg. Maximum daily dose is 200 mg for outpatients and 300 mg for hospitalized patients. Give entire dose at bedtime.
Adolescents and elderly patients: Initially, 30 to 40 mg daily; maximum shouldn't exceed 100 mg daily.
➤ **Childhood enuresis**
Children age 5 and older: 25 mg P.O. 1 hour before bedtime. If patient doesn't improve within 1 week, increase dose to 50 mg if child is younger than age 12; increase dose to 75 mg for children age 12 and older. In either case, maximum daily dose is 2.5 mg/kg.

ACTION
Unknown. A TCA that increases norepinephrine, serotonin, or both in the CNS by blocking their reuptake by the presynaptic neurons.

Route	Onset	Peak	Duration
P.O.	Unknown	1–2 hr	Unknown

Half-life: 11 to 25 hours.

ADVERSE REACTIONS
CNS: *drowsiness, dizziness,* ***seizures, stroke,*** excitation, tremor, confusion, hallucinations, anxiety, ataxia, paresthesia, nervousness, EEG changes, extrapyramidal reactions.
CV: *orthostatic hypotension, tachycardia, ECG changes,* ***MI, arrhythmias, heart block,*** hypertension, precipitation of heart failure.
EENT: *blurred vision,* tinnitus, mydriasis.
GI: *dry mouth, constipation,* nausea, vomiting, anorexia, paralytic ileus, abdominal cramps.
GU: *urine retention.*
Metabolic: ***hypoglycemia,*** hyperglycemia.
Skin: rash, urticaria, photosensitivity reactions, pruritus, diaphoresis.
Other: hypersensitivity reactions.

INTERACTIONS
Drug-drug. *Barbiturates, CNS depressants:* May enhance CNS depression. Avoid using together.
Cimetidine, ***fluoxetine, fluvoxamine, paroxetine, sertraline:*** May increase imipramine level. Monitor drug levels and patient for signs of toxicity.
Clonidine: May cause life-threatening hypertension. Avoid using together.
Epinephrine, norepinephrine: May increase hypertensive effect. Use together cautiously.
MAO inhibitors: May cause hyperpyretic crisis, severe seizures, and death. Avoid using within 14 days of MAO inhibitor therapy.
Quinolones: May increase the risk of life-threatening arrhythmias. Avoid using together.
Drug-herb. *Evening primrose oil:* May cause additive or synergistic effect, lowering the seizure threshold and increasing the risk of seizure. Discourage use together.
St. John's wort, SAM-e, yohimbe: May cause serotonin syndrome. Discourage use together.
Drug-lifestyle. *Alcohol use:* May enhance CNS depression. Discourage use together.
Smoking: May lower level of drug. Monitor patient for lack of effect.
Sun exposure: May increase risk of photosensitivity reactions. Advise patient to avoid excessive sunlight exposure.

EFFECTS ON LAB TEST RESULTS
- May increase or decrease glucose level.
- May increase liver function test values.

CONTRAINDICATIONS & CAUTIONS
- Contraindicated in patients hypersensitive to drug and in those receiving MAO inhibitors; also contraindicated during acute recovery phase of MI.
- Use with extreme caution in patients at risk for suicide; in patients with history of urine retention, angle-closure glaucoma, or seizure disorders; in patients with increased intraocular pressure, CV disease, impaired hepatic function, hyperthyroidism, or impaired renal function; and in patients receiving thyroid drugs. Injectable form contains sulfites, which may cause allergic reactions in hypersensitive patients.

NURSING CONSIDERATIONS
- Monitor patient for nausea, headache, and malaise after abrupt withdrawal of long-term therapy; these symptoms don't indicate addiction.
- Don't withdraw drug abruptly.
- Because of hypertensive episodes during surgery in patients receiving TCAs, stop drug gradually several days before surgery.
- If signs or symptoms of psychosis occur or increase, expect prescriber to reduce dosage. Record mood changes. Monitor patient for suicidal tendencies, and allow only a minimum supply of drug.
- ***Alert:*** Drug may increase the risk of suicidal thinking and behavior in children and adolescents with major depressive disorder or other psychiatric disorder.
- To prevent relapse in children receiving drug for enuresis, withdraw drug gradually.
- Recommend sugarless hard candy or gum to relieve dry mouth. Saliva substitutes may be useful.
- ***Alert:*** Tofranil and Tofranil-PM may contain tartrazine.
- ***Look alike–sound alike:*** Don't confuse imipramine with desipramine.

PATIENT TEACHING
- Tell patient to take full dose at bedtime whenever possible, but warn him of possible morning dizziness upon standing up quickly.
- If child is an early-night bed wetter, tell parents it may be more effective to divide dose and give the first dose earlier in day.
- Tell patient to avoid alcohol while taking this drug.
- Advise patient to consult prescriber before taking other prescription or OTC drugs.
- Warn patient to avoid hazardous activities that require alertness and good coordination until effects of the drug are known. Drowsiness and dizziness usually subside after a few weeks.
- Warn patient not to stop drug suddenly.
- To prevent oversensitivity to the sun, advise patient to use sunblock, wear protective clothing, and avoid prolonged exposure to strong sunlight.

mirtazapine

Remeron, Remeron Soltab

Pharmacologic class: tetracyclic antidepressant
Pregnancy risk category C

AVAILABLE FORMS
Orally disintegrating tablets (ODTs): 15 mg, 30 mg, 45 mg
Tablets: 15 mg, 30 mg, 45 mg

INDICATIONS & DOSAGES
➤ **Depression**
Adults: Initially, 15 mg P.O. at bedtime. Maintenance dose is 15 to 45 mg daily. Adjust dosage at intervals of at least 1 week.

ACTION
Thought to enhance central noradrenergic and serotonergic activity.

Route	Onset	Peak	Duration
P.O.	Unknown	2 hr	Unknown

Half-life: About 20 to 40 hours.

ADVERSE REACTIONS
CNS: *somnolence,* ***suicidal behavior,*** dizziness, asthenia, abnormal dreams, abnormal thinking, tremors, confusion.

CV: edema, peripheral edema.
GI: *increased appetite, dry mouth, constipation,* nausea.
GU: urinary frequency.
Metabolic: *weight gain.*
Musculoskeletal: back pain, myalgia.
Respiratory: dyspnea.
Other: flulike syndrome.

INTERACTIONS
Drug-drug. *Diazepam, other CNS depressants:* May cause additive CNS effects. Avoid using together.
MAO inhibitors: May sometimes cause fatal reactions. Avoid using within 14 days of MAO inhibitor therapy.
Drug-lifestyle. *Alcohol use:* May cause additive CNS effects. Discourage use together.

EFFECTS ON LAB TEST RESULTS
• May increase ALT, cholesterol and triglyceride levels.

CONTRAINDICATIONS & CAUTIONS
• Contraindicated in patients hypersensitive to drug and within 14 days of MAO inhibitor (MAOI) therapy.
• Use cautiously in patients with CV or cerebrovascular disease, seizure disorders, suicidal thoughts, hepatic or renal impairment, or history of mania or hypomania.
• Use cautiously in patients with conditions that predispose them to hypotension, such as dehydration, hypovolemia, or antihypertensive therapy.
• Give drug cautiously to elderly patients; decreased clearance has occurred in this age group.

NURSING CONSIDERATIONS
• Don't use within 14 days of MAOI therapy.
• Record mood changes. Watch for suicidal tendencies.
• ***Alert:*** Drug may increase the risk of suicidal thinking and behavior in children and adolescents with major depressive disorder or other psychiatric disorder.
• Although agranulocytosis occurs rarely, stop drug and monitor patient closely if he develops a sore throat, fever, stomatitis, or other signs and symptoms of infection with a low WBC count.
• Lower dosages tend to be more sedating than higher dosages.

PATIENT TEACHING
• Caution patient not to perform hazardous activities if he gets too sleepy.
• Tell patient to report signs and symptoms of infection, such as fever, chills, sore throat, mucous membrane irritation, or flulike syndrome.
• Instruct patient not to use alcohol or other CNS depressants while taking drug.
• Stress importance of following prescriber's orders.
• Instruct patient not to take other drugs without prescriber's approval.
• Tell woman of childbearing age to report suspected pregnancy immediately and to notify prescriber if she is breastfeeding.
• Instruct patient to remove ODTs from blister pack and place immediately on tongue.
• Advise patient not to break or split tablet.

nefazodone hydrochloride

Pharmacologic class: phenylpiperazine
Pregnancy risk category C

AVAILABLE FORMS
Tablets: 50 mg, 100 mg, 150 mg, 250 mg

INDICATIONS & DOSAGES
➤ **Depression**
Adults: Initially, 200 mg daily P.O. in two divided doses. Dosage may be increased by 100 to 200 mg daily at intervals of at least 1 week, p.r.n. Usual dosage range is 300 to 600 mg daily.
Elderly patients: Initially, 100 mg daily P.O. in two divided doses.
Adjust-a-dose: For debilitated patients, initially, 100 mg daily P.O. in two divided doses.

ACTION
Thought to be linked to drug's inhibition of CNS neuronal uptake of serotonin ($5\text{-}HT_2$) and norepinephrine; it also occupies serotonin and $alpha_1$-adrenergic receptors in the CNS.

Route	Onset	Peak	Duration
P.O.	Unknown	1 hr	Unknown

Half-life: 2 to 4 hours.

ADVERSE REACTIONS

CNS: *headache, somnolence, dizziness, asthenia, insomnia, light-headedness, confusion,* ***suicidal behavior,*** fever, memory impairment, paresthesia, vasodilation, abnormal dreams, impaired concentration, ataxia, incoordination, psychomotor retardation, tremor, hypertonia.
CV: orthostatic hypotension, hypotension, peripheral edema.
EENT: blurred vision, abnormal vision, tinnitus, visual field defect, pharyngitis.
GI: *dry mouth, nausea, constipation,* taste perversion, dyspepsia, diarrhea, increased appetite, vomiting.
GU: urinary frequency, UTI, urine retention, vaginitis.
Hepatic: ***liver failure.***
Musculoskeletal: neck rigidity, arthralgia.
Respiratory: cough.
Skin: pruritus, rash.
Other: infection, flulike syndrome, chills, breast tenderness, thirst.

INTERACTIONS

Drug-drug. *Alprazolam, triazolam:* May potentiate effects of these drugs. Avoid using together; if use together is unavoidable, greatly reduce doses of alprazolam and triazolam.
CNS drugs: May alter CNS activity. Avoid using together.
Cyclosporine: May cause cyclosporine toxicity. Monitor cyclosporine level.
Digoxin: May increase digoxin level. Use together cautiously and monitor digoxin level.
Haloperidol: May increase haloperidol level. Monitor patient for increased adverse reactions.
HMG-CoA reductase inhibitors: May increase atorvastatin, lovastatin, and simvastatin levels. Monitor patient for increased adverse effects.
MAO inhibitors (MAOIs), such as phenelzine, selegiline, tranylcypromine: May cause serotonin syndrome. Avoid using within 14 days of MAOI therapy.
Other highly protein-bound drugs: May increase risk and severity of adverse reactions. Monitor patient closely.
Tramadol: May cause serotonin syndrome. Monitor patient closely.
Drug-herb. *St. John's wort:* May cause additive effects and serotonin syndrome. Discourage use together.
Drug-lifestyle. *Alcohol use:* May enhance CNS depression. Discourage use together.

EFFECTS ON LAB TEST RESULTS

- May decrease hemoglobin level and hematocrit.
- May increase liver function test values.

CONTRAINDICATIONS & CAUTIONS

- Contraindicated in patients hypersensitive to drug or other phenylpiperazine antidepressants; also contraindicated within 14 days of MAOI therapy.
- Contraindicated in patients with liver disease or who stopped using drug because of liver injury.
- Use cautiously in patients with CV or cerebrovascular disease that could be worsened by hypotension (such as history of MI, angina, or stroke) and conditions that would predispose patients to hypotension (such as dehydration, hypovolemia, and antihypertensive therapy).
- Use cautiously in patients with a history of mania.

NURSING CONSIDERATIONS

- ***Alert:*** Drug may cause hepatic failure. Don't start drug in patients with active liver disease or with elevated baseline transaminase level. Although preexisting hepatic disease doesn't increase the likelihood of developing hepatic failure, baseline abnormalities can complicate patient monitoring. Stop drug if clinical signs and symptoms of hepatic dysfunction appear, such as increased AST or ALT level exceeding three times the upper limit of normal. Don't restart therapy.
- Don't use within 14 days of MAOI therapy.
- ***Alert:*** Do a thorough risk-versus-benefit assessment before using drug to treat depression, taking into account the risk for

hepatic failure and emergence of suicidal thoughts and attempts.
- **Alert:** Drug may increase the risk of suicidal thinking and behavior in children and adolescents with major depressive disorder or other psychiatric disorders.

PATIENT TEACHING
- Warn patient not to engage in hazardous activity until effects of drug are known.
- **Alert:** Instruct men who experience prolonged or inappropriate erections to stop drug immediately and notify prescriber.
- Instruct woman of childbearing age to notify prescriber if she becomes pregnant or is planning pregnancy during therapy or if she's breast-feeding.
- **Alert:** Teach patient the signs and symptoms of liver problems, including yellowed skin or eyes, appetite loss, GI complaints, and malaise. Tell patient to report these adverse events to prescriber immediately.
- **Alert:** Inform family members to be particularly vigilant for suicidal tendencies during therapy.
- Tell patient to notify prescriber if rash, hives, or related allergic reactions occur.
- Instruct patient to avoid alcohol during therapy.
- Tell patient to notify prescriber before taking OTC drugs.
- Inform patient that several weeks of therapy may be needed to obtain full antidepressant effect. Once improvement occurs, advise him not to stop drug until directed by prescriber.

nortriptyline hydrochloride
Aventyl, Allegron‡, Pamelor*

Pharmacologic class: tricyclic antidepressant
Pregnancy risk category D

AVAILABLE FORMS
Capsules: 10 mg, 25 mg, 50 mg, 75 mg
Oral solution: 10 mg/5 ml*
Tablets: 10 mg‡, 25 mg‡

INDICATIONS & DOSAGES
➤ Depression
Adults: 25 mg P.O. t.i.d. or q.i.d., gradually increased to maximum of 150 mg daily. Give entire dose at bedtime. Monitor level when doses above 100 mg daily are given.
Adolescents and elderly patients: 30 to 50 mg daily given once or in divided doses.

ACTION
Unknown. Increases the amount of norepinephrine, serotonin, or both in the CNS by blocking reuptake by the presynaptic neurons.

Route	Onset	Peak	Duration
P.O.	Unknown	7–8½ hr	Unknown

Half-life: 18 to 24 hours.

ADVERSE REACTIONS
CNS: *drowsiness, dizziness,* ***seizures, stroke,*** tremor, weakness, confusion, headache, nervousness, EEG changes, extrapyramidal syndrome, insomnia, nightmares, hallucinations, paresthesia, ataxia, agitation.
CV: *tachycardia,* ***heart block, MI,*** ECG changes, hypertension, hypotension.
EENT: *blurred vision,* tinnitus, mydriasis.
GI: *constipation,* dry mouth, nausea, vomiting, anorexia, paralytic ileus.
GU: *urine retention.*
Hematologic: ***agranulocytosis, thrombocytopenia,*** bone marrow depression, eosinophilia.
Metabolic: ***hypoglycemia,*** hyperglycemia.
Skin: rash, urticaria, photosensitivity reactions, diaphoresis.
Other: hypersensitivity reactions.

INTERACTIONS
Drug-drug. *Barbiturates, CNS depressants:* May enhance CNS depression. Avoid using together.
Cimetidine, ***fluoxetine, fluvoxamine, paroxetine, sertraline:*** May increase nortriptyline level. Monitor drug levels and patient for signs of toxicity.
Clonidine: May cause life-threatening hypertension. Avoid using together.

Epinephrine, norepinephrine: May increase hypertensive effect. Use together cautiously.
MAO inhibitors (MAOIs): May cause severe excitation, hyperpyrexia, or seizures, usually with high doses. Avoid using within 14 days of MAOI therapy.
Quinolones: May increase the risk of life-threatening arrhythmias. Avoid using together.
Drug-herb. *Evening primrose oil:* May cause additive or synergistic effect, lowering seizure threshold and increasing the risk of seizure. Discourage use together.
St. John's wort, SAM-e, yohimbe: May cause serotonin syndrome and reduced drug level. Discourage use together.
Drug-lifestyle. *Alcohol use:* May enhance CNS depression. Discourage use together.
Smoking: May decrease drug level. Monitor patient for lack of effect.
Sun exposure: May increase risk of photosensitivity reactions. Advise patient to avoid excessive sunlight exposure.

EFFECTS ON LAB TEST RESULTS

- May increase or decrease glucose level.
- May increase eosinophil count and liver function test values. May decrease WBC, RBC, granulocyte, and platelet counts.

CONTRAINDICATIONS & CAUTIONS

- Contraindicated in patients hypersensitive to drug and during acute recovery phase of MI; also contraindicated within 14 days of MAO therapy.
- Use with extreme caution in patients with glaucoma, suicidal tendency, history of urine retention or seizures, CV disease, or hyperthyroidism and in those receiving thyroid drugs.

NURSING CONSIDERATIONS

- Monitor patient for nausea, headache, and malaise after abrupt withdrawal of long-term therapy; these symptoms don't indicate addiction.
- Because patients using tricyclic antidepressants may suffer hypertensive episodes during surgery, stop drug gradually several days before surgery.
- If signs or symptoms of psychosis occur or increase, expect to reduce dosage. Record mood changes. Monitor patient for suicidal tendencies and allow him only a minimum supply of drug.
- ***Alert:*** Drug may increase the risk of suicidal thinking and behavior in children and adolescents with major depressive disorder or other psychiatric disorder.
- ***Look alike–sound alike:*** Don't confuse nortriptyline with amitriptyline.

PATIENT TEACHING

- Advise patient to take full dose at bedtime whenever possible to reduce risk of dizziness upon standing quickly.
- Warn patient to avoid activities that require alertness and good coordination until effects of drug are known. Drowsiness and dizziness usually subside after a few weeks.
- Recommend use of sugarless hard candy or gum to relieve dry mouth. Saliva substitutes may be needed.
- Tell patient to consult prescriber before taking other prescription or OTC drugs.
- Warn patient not to stop drug suddenly.
- To prevent oversensitivity to the sun, advise patient to use sunblock, wear protective clothing, and avoid prolonged exposure to strong sunlight.

paroxetine hydrochloride

Aropax‡, Paxil, Paxil CR

Pharmacologic class: SSRI
Pregnancy risk category D

AVAILABLE FORMS

Suspension: 10 mg/5 ml
Tablets: 10 mg, 20 mg, 30 mg, 40 mg
Tablets (controlled-release): 12.5 mg, 25 mg, 37.5 mg

INDICATIONS & DOSAGES

➤ Depression

Adults: Initially, 20 mg P.O. daily, preferably in morning, as indicated. If patient doesn't improve, increase dose by 10 mg daily at intervals of at least 1 week to a maximum of 50 mg daily. If using controlled-release form, initially, 25 mg P.O. daily. Increase dose by 12.5 mg daily at weekly intervals to a maximum of 62.5 mg daily.
Elderly patients: Initially, 10 mg P.O. daily, preferably in morning, as indicated.

If patient doesn't improve, increase dose by 10 mg daily at weekly intervals, to a maximum of 40 mg daily. If using controlled-release form, start therapy at 12.5 mg P.O. daily. Don't exceed 50 mg daily.

➤ **Obsessive-compulsive disorder (OCD)**

Adults: Initially, 20 mg P.O. daily, preferably in morning. Increase dose by 10 mg daily at weekly intervals. Recommended daily dose is 40 mg. Maximum daily dose is 60 mg.

➤ **Panic disorder**

Adults: Initially, 10 mg P.O. daily. Increase dose by 10 mg at no less than weekly intervals to maximum of 60 mg daily. Or, 12.5 mg Paxil CR P.O. as a single daily dose, usually in the morning, with or without food; increase dose at intervals of at least 1 week by 12.5 mg daily, up to a maximum of 75 mg daily.

Adjust-a-dose: In elderly or debilitated patients and in those with severe renal or hepatic impairment, the first dose of Paxil CR is 12.5 mg daily; increase if indicated. Dosage shouldn't exceed 50 mg daily.

➤ **Social anxiety disorder**

Adults: Initially, 20 mg P.O. daily, preferably in morning. Dosage range is 20 to 60 mg daily. Adjust dosage to maintain patient on lowest effective dose. Or, 12.5 mg Paxil CR P.O. as a single daily dose, usually in the morning, with or without food. Increase dosage at weekly intervals in increments of 12.5 mg daily, up to a maximum of 37.5 mg daily.

➤ **Generalized anxiety disorder**

Adults: 20 mg P.O. daily initially, increasing by 10 mg per day weekly up to 50 mg daily.

Adjust-a-dose: For debilitated patients or those with renal or hepatic impairment taking immediate-release form, initially, 10 mg P.O. daily, preferably in morning. If patient doesn't respond after full antidepressant effect has occurred, increase dose by 10 mg per day at weekly intervals to a maximum of 40 mg daily. If using controlled-release form, start therapy at 12.5 mg daily. Don't exceed 50 mg daily.

➤ **Posttraumatic stress disorder**

Adults: Initially, 20 mg P.O. daily. Increase dose by 10 mg daily at intervals of at least 1 week. Maximum daily dose is 50 mg P.O.

➤ **Premenstrual dysphoric disorder (PMDD)**

Adults: Initially, 12.5 mg Paxil CR P.O. as a single daily dose, usually in the morning, with or without food, daily or during the luteal phase of the menstrual cycle. Dose changes should occur at intervals of at least 1 week. Maximum dose is 25 mg P.O. daily.

➤ **Premature ejaculation ♦**

Adults: 10 to 40 mg P.O. daily. Or, 20 mg P.O. p.r.n. 3 to 4 hours before planned intercourse.

➤ **Diabetic neuropathy ♦**

Adults: 40 mg P.O. daily.

ACTION

Thought to be linked to drug's inhibition of CNS neuronal uptake of serotonin.

Route	Onset	Peak	Duration
P.O.	Unknown	2–8 hr	Unknown
P.O. (controlled-release)	Unknown	6–10 hr	Unknown

Half-life: About 24 hours.

ADVERSE REACTIONS

CNS: *asthenia, dizziness, headache, insomnia, somnolence, tremor, nervousness,* ***suicidal behavior,*** anxiety, paresthesia, confusion, agitation.
CV: palpitations, vasodilation, orthostatic hypotension.
EENT: lump or tightness in throat.
GI: *dry mouth, nausea, constipation, diarrhea,* flatulence, vomiting, dyspepsia, dysgeusia, increased or decreased appetite, abdominal pain.
GU: *ejaculatory disturbances, sexual dysfunction,* urinary frequency, other urinary disorders.
Musculoskeletal: myopathy, myalgia, myasthenia.
Skin: *diaphoresis,* rash, pruritus.
Other: *decreased libido,* yawning.

INTERACTIONS

Drug-drug. *Amphetamines, buspirone, dextromethorphan, dihydroergotamine, lithium salts, meperidine, other SSRIs or selective serotonin-norepinephrine reuptake inhibitors (duloxetine, venlafax-*

*ine), **tramadol**, trazodone, tricyclic antidepressants, tryptophan:* May increase the risk of serotonin syndrome. Avoid combining drugs that increase the availability of serotonin in the CNS; monitor patient closely if used together.
Cimetidine: May decrease hepatic metabolism of paroxetine, leading to risk of adverse reactions. Dosage adjustments may be needed.
Digoxin: May decrease digoxin level. Use together cautiously.
MAO inhibitor (MAOI), such as phenelzine, selegiline, tranylcypromine: May cause serotonin syndrome. Avoid using within 14 days of MAOI therapy.
Phenobarbital, phenytoin: May alter pharmacokinetics of both drugs. Dosage adjustments may be needed.
Procyclidine: May increase procyclidine level. Watch for excessive anticholinergic effects.
Sumatriptan: May cause weakness, hyperreflexia, and incoordination. Monitor patient closely.
Theophylline: May decrease theophylline clearance. Monitor theophylline level.
Thioridazine: May prolong QTc interval and increase risk of serious ventricular arrhythmias, such as torsades de pointes, and sudden death. Avoid using together.
Tricyclic antidepressants: May inhibit tricyclic antidepressant metabolism. Dose of tricyclic antidepressant may need to be reduced. Monitor patient closely.
Triptans: May cause serotonin syndrome (restlessness, hallucinations, loss of coordination, fast heartbeat, rapid changes in blood pressure, increased body temperature, overactive reflexes, nausea, vomiting, and diarrhea). Use cautiously, especially at the start of therapy and at dosage increases.
Warfarin: May cause bleeding. Use together cautiously.
Drug-herb. *St. John's wort:* May increase sedative-hypnotic effects. Discourage use together.
Drug-lifestyle. *Alcohol use:* May alter psychomotor function. Discourage use together.

EFFECTS ON LAB TEST RESULTS

None reported.

CONTRAINDICATIONS & CAUTIONS

- Contraindicated in patients hypersensitive to drug, within 14 days of MAOI therapy, and in those taking thioridazine.
- Contraindicated in children and adolescents under age 18 for major depressive disorders.
- Use cautiously in patients with history of seizure disorders or mania and in those with other severe, systemic illness.
- Use cautiously in patients at risk for volume depletion and monitor them appropriately.
- Using drug in the first trimester may increase the risk of congenital fetal malformations; using drug in the third trimester may cause neonatal complications at birth. Consider the risk versus benefit of therapy.

NURSING CONSIDERATIONS

- Patients taking drug may be at increased risk for developing suicidal behavior, but this hasn't been definitively attributed to use of the drug.
- Patients taking Paxil CR for PMDD should be periodically reassessed to determine the need for continued treatment.
- If signs or symptoms of psychosis occur or increase, expect prescriber to reduce dosage. Record mood changes. Monitor patient for suicidal tendencies, and allow only a minimum supply of drug.
- ***Alert:*** Drug may increase the risk of suicidal thinking and behavior in children and adolescents with major depressive disorder or other psychiatric disorder.
- Monitor patient for complaints of sexual dysfunction. In men, they include anorgasmy, erectile difficulties, delayed ejaculation or orgasm, or impotence; in women, they include anorgasmy or difficulty with orgasm.
- ***Alert:*** Don't stop drug abruptly. Withdrawal or discontinuation syndrome may occur if drug is stopped abruptly. Symptoms include headache, myalgia, lethargy, and general flulike symptoms. Taper drug slowly over 1 to 2 weeks.
- ***Look alike–sound alike:*** Don't confuse paroxetine with paclitaxel, or Paxil with Doxil, paclitaxel, Plavix, or Taxol.

PATIENT TEACHING

- Tell patient that drug may be taken with or without food, usually in morning.
- Tell patient not to break, crush, or chew controlled-release tablets.
- Warn patient to avoid activities that require alertness and good coordination until effects of drug are known.
- Advise woman of childbearing age to contact prescriber if she becomes pregnant or plans to become pregnant during therapy or if she's currently breastfeeding.
- Tell patient to avoid alcohol and to consult prescriber before taking other prescription or OTC drugs or herbal medicines.
- Instruct patient not to stop taking drug abruptly.

sertraline hydrochloride
Zoloft

Pharmacologic class: SSRI
Pregnancy risk category C

AVAILABLE FORMS

Capsules†: 25 mg, 50 mg, 100 mg
Oral concentrate: 20 mg/ml
Tablets: 25 mg, 50 mg, 100 mg

INDICATIONS & DOSAGES

➤ **Depression**
Adults: 50 mg P.O. daily. Adjust dosage as needed and tolerated; dosage range is 50 to 200 mg daily.

➤ **Obsessive-compulsive disorder**
Adults: 50 mg P.O. once daily. If patient doesn't improve, increase dosage, up to 200 mg daily.
Children ages 6 to 17: Initially, 25 mg P.O. daily in children ages 6 to 12, or 50 mg P.O. daily in adolescents ages 13 to 17. Increase dosage, p.r.n., up to 200 mg daily at intervals of no less than 1 week.

➤ **Panic disorder**
Adults: Initially, 25 mg P.O. daily. After 1 week, increase dose to 50 mg P.O. daily. If patient doesn't improve, increase dose to maximum of 200 mg daily.

➤ **Posttraumatic stress disorder**
Adults: Initially, 25 mg P.O. once daily. Increase dosage to 50 mg P.O. once daily after 1 week. Increase at weekly intervals to a maximum of 200 mg daily. Maintain patient on lowest effective dose.

➤ **Premenstrual dysphoric disorder**
Adults: Initially, 50 mg daily P.O. either continuously or only during the luteal phase of the menstrual cycle. If patient doesn't respond, dose may be increased 50 mg per menstrual cycle, up to 150 mg daily for use throughout the menstrual cycle or 100 mg daily for luteal-phase doses. If a 100-mg daily dose has been established with luteal-phase dose, use a 50-mg daily adjustment for 3 days at the beginning of each luteal phase.

➤ **Social anxiety disorder**
Adults: Initially, 25 mg P.O. once daily. Increase dosage to 50 mg P.O. once daily after 1 week of therapy. Dose range is 50 to 200 mg daily. Adjust to the lowest effective dosage and periodically reassess patient to determine the need for long-term treatment.

➤ **Premature ejaculation ♦**
Adults: 25 to 50 mg P.O. daily or p.r.n.
Adjust-a-dose: For patients with hepatic disease, use lower or less-frequent doses.

ACTION

Thought to be linked to drug's inhibition of CNS neuronal uptake of serotonin.

Route	Onset	Peak	Duration
P.O.	Unknown	4–8 hr	Unknown

Half-life: 26 hours.

ADVERSE REACTIONS

CNS: *fatigue, headache, tremor, dizziness, insomnia, somnolence,* ***suicidal behavior,*** paresthesia, hypesthesia, nervousness, anxiety, agitation, hypertonia, twitching, confusion.
CV: palpitations, chest pain, hot flashes.
GI: *dry mouth, nausea, diarrhea, loose stools, dyspepsia,* vomiting, constipation, thirst, flatulence, anorexia, abdominal pain, increased appetite.
GU: *male sexual dysfunction.*
Musculoskeletal: myalgia.
Skin: rash, pruritus, diaphoresis.

INTERACTIONS

Drug-drug. *Amphetamines, buspirone, dextromethorphan, dihydroergota-*

mine, lithium salts, meperidine, other SSRIs or selective serotonin-norepinephrine reuptake inhibitors (duloxetine, venlafaxine), sumatriptan, **tramadol,** *trazodone, tricyclic antidepressants, tryptophan:* May increase the risk of serotonin syndrome. Avoid combinations of drugs that increase the availability of serotonin in the CNS; monitor patient closely if used together.
Benzodiazepines, tolbutamide: May decrease clearance of these drugs. Significance unknown; monitor patient for increased drug effects.
Cimetidine: May decrease clearance of sertraline. Monitor patient closely.
Disulfiram: Oral concentrate contains alcohol, which may react with drug. Avoid using together.
MAO inhibitors (MAOIs), such as phenelzine, selegiline, tranylcypromine: May cause serotonin syndrome. Avoid using within 14 days of MAOI therapy.
Pimozide: May increase pimozide level. Avoid using together.
Triptans: May cause serotonin syndrome (restlessness, hallucinations, loss of coordination, fast heartbeat, rapid changes in blood pressure, increased body temperature, hyperreflexia, nausea, vomiting, and diarrhea). Use cautiously, with close monitoring, especially at the start of treatment and during dosage adjustments.
Warfarin, other highly protein-bound drugs: May increase level of sertraline or other highly protein-bound drug. May increase PT, or INR may increase by 8%. Monitor patient closely; monitor PT and INR.
Drug-herb. *St. John's wort:* May cause additive effects and serotonin syndrome. Discourage use together.

EFFECTS ON LAB TEST RESULTS

- May increase ALT and AST levels.

CONTRAINDICATIONS & CAUTIONS

- Contraindicated in patients with a hypersensitivity to drug or its components. Contraindicated in patients taking pimozide or MAO inhibitors or within 14 days of MAOI therapy.
- Use cautiously in patients at risk for suicide and in those with seizure disorders, major affective disorder, or diseases or conditions that affect metabolism or hemodynamic responses.
- Use in third trimester of pregnancy may cause neonatal complications at birth. Consider the risk versus benefit of treatment during this time.

NURSING CONSIDERATIONS

- Give sertraline once daily, either in morning or evening, with or without food.
- Make dosage adjustments at intervals of no less than 1 week.
- Record mood changes. Monitor patient for suicidal tendencies and allow only a minimum supply of drug.
- ***Alert:*** Drug may increase the risk of suicidal thinking and behavior in children and adolescents with major depressive disorder or other psychiatric disorder.
- Don't use the oral concentrate dropper, which is made of rubber, in a patient with latex allergy.

PATIENT TEACHING

- Advise patient to use caution when performing hazardous tasks that require alertness.
- Tell patient to avoid alcohol and to consult prescriber before taking OTC drugs.
- Advise patient to mix the oral concentrate with 4 ounces (½ cup) of water, ginger ale, lemon or lime soda, lemonade, or orange juice only, and to take the dose right away.
- Instruct patient to avoid stopping drug abruptly.

trazodone hydrochloride

Pharmacologic class: triazolopyridine derivative
Pregnancy risk category C

AVAILABLE FORMS

Tablets: 50 mg, 100 mg, 150 mg, 300 mg

INDICATIONS & DOSAGES

➤ **Depression**
Adults: Initially, 150 mg P.O. daily in divided doses; then increased by 50 mg daily q 3 to 4 days, p.r.n. Dose ranges from 150 to 400 mg daily. Maximum, 600 mg daily for inpatients and 400 mg daily for outpatients.

ACTION

Unknown. Inhibits CNS neuronal uptake of serotonin; not a tricyclic derivative.

Route	Onset	Peak	Duration
P.O.	Unknown	1–2 hr	Unknown

Half-life: First phase, 3 to 6 hours; second phase, 5 to 9 hours.

ADVERSE REACTIONS

CNS: *drowsiness, dizziness,* nervousness, fatigue, confusion, tremor, weakness, hostility, anger, nightmares, vivid dreams, headache, insomnia, syncope.
CV: orthostatic hypotension, tachycardia, hypertension, shortness of breath, ECG changes.
EENT: blurred vision, tinnitus, nasal congestion.
GI: dry mouth, dysgeusia, constipation, nausea, vomiting, anorexia.
GU: urine retention, priapism possibly leading to impotence, hematuria.
Hematologic: anemia.
Skin: rash, urticaria, diaphoresis.
Other: decreased libido.

INTERACTIONS

Drug-drug. *Amphetamines, buspirone, dextromethorphan, dihydroergotamine, lithium salts, meperidine, SSRIs or selective serotonin-norepinephrine reuptake inhibitors (duloxetine, venlafaxine), sumatriptan, tramadol, tricyclic antidepressants, tryptophan:* May increase the risk of serotonin syndrome. Avoid combining drugs that increase the availability of serotonin in the CNS; monitor patient closely if used together.
Antihypertensives: May increase hypotensive effect of trazodone. Antihypertensive dosage may need to be decreased.
Clonidine, CNS depressants: May enhance CNS depression. Avoid using together.
CYP3A4 inducers (carbamazepine): May reduce trazodone level. Monitor patient closely; may need to increase trazodone dose.
CYP3A4 inhibitors (ketoconazole): May slow the clearance of trazodone and increase trazodone level. May cause nausea, hypotension, and fainting. Consider decreasing trazodone dose.
Digoxin, phenytoin: May increase levels of these drugs. Watch for toxicity.
MAO inhibitors: Effects unknown. Use together with extreme caution.
Protease inhibitors (amprenavir, atazanavir, fosamprenavir, indinavir, lopinavir and ritonavir, nelfinavir, ritonavir, saquinavir): May increase trazodone levels and adverse effects. Monitor patient and adjust trazodone dose, as needed.
Drug-herb. *Ginkgo biloba:* May cause sedation. Discourage use together.
St. John's wort: May cause serotonin syndrome. Discourage use together.
Drug-lifestyle. *Alcohol use:* May enhance CNS depression. Discourage use together.

EFFECTS ON LAB TEST RESULTS

- May increase ALT and AST levels. May decrease hemoglobin level.

CONTRAINDICATIONS & CAUTIONS

- Contraindicated in patients hypersensitive to drug.
- Use cautiously in patients with cardiac disease or in the initial recovery phase of MI and in patients at risk for suicide.

NURSING CONSIDERATIONS

- Give drug after meals or a light snack for optimal absorption and to decrease risk of dizziness.
- Record mood changes. Monitor patient for suicidal tendencies and allow only minimum supply of drug.
- ***Alert:*** Drug may increase the risk of suicidal thinking and behavior in children and adolescents with major depressive disorder or other psychiatric disorder.
- ***Look alike–sound alike:*** Don't confuse trazodone hydrochloride with tramadol hydrochloride.

PATIENT TEACHING

- ***Alert:*** Tell patient to report a persistent, painful erection (priapism) right away because he may need immediate intervention.
- Warn patient to avoid activities that require alertness and good coordination until effects of drug are known. Drowsiness and dizziness usually subside after first few weeks.

• Teach caregivers how to recognize signs and symptoms of suicidal tendency or suicidal thoughts.

venlafaxine hydrochloride
Effexor‡, Effexor, Effexor XR

Pharmacologic class: selective serotonin and norepinephrine reuptake inhibitor (SNRI)
Pregnancy risk category C

AVAILABLE FORMS
Capsules (extended-release): 37.5 mg, 75 mg, 150 mg
Tablets: 25 mg, 37.5 mg, 50 mg, 75 mg, 100 mg

INDICATIONS & DOSAGES
➤ Depression
Adults: Initially, 75 mg P.O. daily in two or three divided doses with food. Increase as tolerated and needed by 75 mg daily q 4 days. For moderately depressed outpatients, usual maximum is 225 mg daily; in certain severely depressed patients, dose may be as high as 375 mg daily. For extended-release capsules, 75 mg P.O. daily in a single dose. For some patients, it may be desirable to start at 37.5 mg P.O. daily for 4 to 7 days before increasing to 75 mg daily. Dosage may be increased by 75 mg daily q 4 days to maximum of 225 mg daily.
➤ Generalized anxiety disorder
Adults: Initially, 75 mg extended-release capsule P.O. daily in a single dose. For some patients, it may be desirable to start at 37.5 mg P.O. daily for 4 to 7 days before increasing to 75 mg daily. Dosage may be increased by 75 mg daily q 4 days to maximum of 225 mg daily.
➤ Panic disorder
Adults: Initially, 37.5 mg extended-release capsule P.O. daily for 1 week, then increase dose to 75 mg daily. If patient isn't responding, may increase dose by up to 75 mg/day in no less than weekly intervals, p.r.n., to a maximum dose of 225 mg daily.
➤ Social anxiety disorder
Adults: Initially, 75 mg extended-release capsule daily as a single dose. For some patients, it may be desirable to start at 37.5 mg P.O. daily for 4 to 7 days before increasing to 75 mg daily. Increase dosage p.r.n. by 75 mg daily q 4 days. Maximum dose is 225 mg daily.
Adjust-a-dose: For patients with renal impairment, reduce daily amount by 25%. For those undergoing hemodialysis, reduce daily amount by 50% and withhold dose until dialysis is completed. For patients with hepatic impairment, reduce daily amount by 50%.
➤ To prevent major depressive disorder relapse ♦
Adults: 100 to 200 mg daily P.O. regular-release tablets or 75 to 225 mg daily P.O. extended-release capsules.

ACTION
May increase the amount of norepinephrine, serotonin, or both in the CNS by blocking their reuptake by the presynaptic neurons.

Route	Onset	Peak	Duration
P.O.	Unknown	1–2 hr	Unknown

Half-life: 5 hours.

ADVERSE REACTIONS
CNS: *asthenia, headache, somnolence, dizziness, nervousness, insomnia,* ***suicidal behavior,*** anxiety, tremor, abnormal dreams, paresthesia, agitation.
CV: hypertension, tachycardia, vasodilation.
EENT: blurred vision.
GI: *nausea, constipation, dry mouth, anorexia,* vomiting, diarrhea, dyspepsia, flatulence.
GU: *abnormal ejaculation,* impotence, urinary frequency, impaired urination.
Metabolic: weight loss.
Skin: *diaphoresis,* rash.
Other: yawning, chills, infection.

INTERACTIONS
Drug-drug. *MAO inhibitor (MAOI), such as phenelzine, selegiline, tranylcypromine:* May cause serotonin syndrome. Avoid using within 14 days of MAOI therapy.
Tramadol: May cause serotonin syndrome. Monitor patient closely.
Triptans: May cause serotonin syndrome (restlessness, hallucinations, loss of coordination, fast heartbeat, rapid changes in

blood pressure, increased body temperature, hyperreflexia, nausea, vomiting, and diarrhea). Use cautiously and with increased monitoring at the start of therapy and with dose increase.
Drug-herb. *Yohimbe:* May cause additive stimulation. Urge caution.

EFFECTS ON LAB TEST RESULTS
None reported.

CONTRAINDICATIONS & CAUTIONS
- Contraindicated in patients hypersensitive to drug or within 14 days of MAOI therapy.
- Use cautiously in patients with renal impairment, diseases or conditions that could affect hemodynamic responses or metabolism, and in those with history of mania or seizures.
- Use in third trimester of pregnancy may be associated with neonatal complications at birth. Consider the risk versus benefit of treatment during this time.

NURSING CONSIDERATIONS
- ***Alert:*** Closely monitor patients being treated for depression for signs and symptoms of clinical worsening and suicidal ideation, especially at the beginning of therapy and with dosage adjustments. Symptoms may include agitation, insomnia, anxiety, aggressiveness, or panic attacks.
- ***Alert:*** Drug may increase the risk of suicidal thinking and behavior in children and adolescents with major depressive disorder or other psychiatric disorder.
- Carefully monitor blood pressure. Drug therapy may cause sustained, dose-dependent increases in blood pressure. Greatest increases (averaging about 7 mm Hg above baseline) occur in patients taking 375 mg daily.
- Monitor patient's weight, particularly underweight, depressed patients.

PATIENT TEACHING
- If medication is to be stopped, inform patient who has received drug for 6 weeks or longer that drug will be stopped gradually by tapering dosage over a 2-week period as instructed by prescriber. Patient shouldn't abruptly stop taking the drug.
- ***Alert:*** Warn family members to closely monitor patient for signs of worsening condition or suicidal ideation.
- Warn patient to avoid hazardous activities that require alertness and good coordination until effects of drug are known.
- Tell patient to avoid alcohol and to consult prescriber before taking other prescription or OTC drugs.
- Advise woman of childbearing age to contact prescriber if she becomes pregnant or intends to become pregnant during therapy or if she's breast-feeding.

30
Anxiolytics

alprazolam
buspirone hydrochloride
chlordiazepoxide hydrochloride
diazepam
doxepin hydrochloride
(See Chapter 29, ANTIDEPRESSANTS)
hydroxyzine hydrochloride
hydroxyzine pamoate
lorazepam
midazolam hydrochloride

SAFETY ALERT!

alprazolam
Apo-Alpraz†, Kalma‡, Niravam, Novo-Alprazol†, Nu-Alpraz†, Xanax🖉, Xanax XR

Pharmacologic class: benzodiazepine
Pregnancy risk category D
Controlled substance schedule IV

AVAILABLE FORMS
Oral solution: 1 mg/ml (concentrate)
Orally disintegrating tablets: 0.25 mg, 0.5 mg, 1 mg, 2 mg
Tablets: 0.25 mg, 0.5 mg, 1 mg, 2 mg
Tablets (extended-release): 0.5 mg, 1 mg, 2 mg, 3 mg

INDICATIONS & DOSAGES
➤ **Anxiety**
Adults: Usual first dose, 0.25 to 0.5 mg P.O. t.i.d. Maximum, 4 mg daily in divided doses.
Elderly patients: Usual first dose, 0.25 mg P.O. b.i.d. or t.i.d. Maximum, 4 mg daily in divided doses.
➤ **Panic disorders**
Adults: 0.5 mg P.O. t.i.d., increased at intervals of 3 to 4 days in increments of no more than 1 mg. Maximum, 10 mg daily in divided doses. If using extended-release tablets, start with 0.5 to 1 mg P.O. once daily. Increase by no more than 1 mg q 3 to 4 days. Maximum daily dose is 10 mg.
Adjust-a-dose: For debilitated patients or those with advanced hepatic disease, usual first dose is 0.25 mg P.O. b.i.d. or t.i.d. Maximum, 4 mg daily in divided doses.

ACTION
Unknown; a benzodiazepine that probably potentiates the effects of GABA, depresses the CNS, and suppresses the spread of seizure activity.

Route	Onset	Peak	Duration
P.O.	Unknown	1–2 hr	Unknown
P.O. (extended-release)	Unknown	Unknown	Unknown

Half-life: Immediate-release, 12 to 15 hours; extended-release, 11 to 16 hours.

ADVERSE REACTIONS
CNS: *insomnia, irritability, dizziness, headache, anxiety, confusion, drowsiness, light-headedness, sedation, somnolence, difficulty speaking, impaired coordination, memory impairment, fatigue, depression,* ***suicide,*** mental impairment, ataxia, paresthesia, dyskinesia, hypoesthesia, lethargy, decreased or increased libido, vertigo, malaise, tremor, nervousness, restlessness, agitation, nightmare, syncope, akathisia, mania.
CV: hot flushes, palpitation, chest pain, hypotension.
EENT: sore throat, allergic rhinitis, blurred vision, nasal congestion.
GI: *diarrhea, dry mouth, constipation,* nausea, increased or decreased appetite, anorexia, vomiting, dyspepsia, abdominal pain.
GU: dysmenorrhea, sexual dysfunction, premenstrual syndrome, difficulty urinating.
Metabolic: increased or decreased weight.
Musculoskeletal: arthralgia, myalgia, arm or leg pain, back pain, muscle rigidity, muscle cramps, muscle twitch.
Respiratory: upper respiratory tract infection, dyspnea, hyperventilation.
Skin: pruritus, increased sweating, dermatitis.
Other: influenza, injury, emergence of anxiety between doses, dependence.

INTERACTIONS

Drug-drug. *Anticonvulsants, antidepressants, antihistamines, barbiturates, benzodiazepines, general anesthetics, narcotics, phenothiazines:* May increase CNS depressant effects. Avoid using together.
Azole antifungals (including fluconazole, itraconazole, ketoconazole, miconazole): May increase and prolong alprazolam level, CNS depression, and psychomotor impairment. Avoid using together.
Carbamazepine, *propoxyphene:* May induce alprazolam metabolism and may reduce therapeutic effects. May need to increase dose.
Cimetidine, fluoxetine, fluvoxamine, hormonal contraceptives, nefazodone: May increase alprazolam level. Use cautiously together, and consider alprazolam dosage reduction.
Tricyclic antidepressants: May increase levels of these drugs. Monitor patient closely.
Drug-herb. *Kava, valerian root:* May increase sedation. Discourage use together.
St. John's wort: May decrease drug level. Discourage use together.
Drug-food. *Grapefruit juice:* May increase drug level. Discourage use together.
Drug-lifestyle. *Alcohol use:* May cause additive CNS effects. Discourage use together.
Smoking: May decrease effectiveness of drug. Monitor patient closely.

EFFECTS ON LAB TEST RESULTS

- May increase ALT and AST levels.

CONTRAINDICATIONS & CAUTIONS

- Contraindicated in patients hypersensitive to drug or other benzodiazepines and in those with acute angle-closure glaucoma.
- Use cautiously in patients with hepatic, renal, or pulmonary disease.

NURSING CONSIDERATIONS

- The optimum duration of therapy is unknown.
- ***Alert:*** Don't withdraw drug abruptly; withdrawal symptoms, including seizures, may occur. Abuse or addiction is possible.
- Monitor hepatic, renal, and hematopoietic function periodically in patients receiving repeated or prolonged therapy.
- ***Look alike–sound alike:*** Don't confuse alprazolam with alprostadil. Don't confuse Xanax with Zantac or Tenex.

PATIENT TEACHING

- Warn patient to avoid hazardous activities that require alertness and good coordination until effects of drug are known.
- Tell patient to avoid alcohol while taking drug.
- Advise patient that smoking may decrease drug's effectiveness.
- Warn patient not to stop drug abruptly because withdrawal symptoms or seizures may occur.
- Tell patient to swallow extended-release tablets whole.
- Tell patient using orally disintegrating tablet to remove it from bottle using dry hands and to immediately place it on his tongue where it will dissolve and can be swallowed with saliva.
- Tell patient taking half of a scored orally disintegrating tablet to discard the unused half.
- Advise patient to discard the cotton from the bottle of orally disintegrating tablets and keep it tightly sealed to prevent moisture from dissolving the tablets.

buspirone hydrochloride

BuSpar

Pharmacologic class: azaspirodecanedione derivative
Pregnancy risk category B

AVAILABLE FORMS

Tablets: 5 mg, 10 mg, 15 mg, 30 mg

INDICATIONS & DOSAGES

➤ Anxiety disorders
Adults: Initially, 7.5 mg P.O. b.i.d. Increase dosage by 5 mg daily at 2- to 3-day intervals. Usual maintenance dosage is 20 to 30 mg daily in divided doses. Don't exceed 60 mg daily.

ACTION
May inhibit neuronal firing and reduce serotonin turnover in cortical, amygdaloid, and septohippocampal tissue.

Route	Onset	Peak	Duration
P.O.	Unknown	40–90 min	Unknown

Half-life: 2 to 3 hours.

ADVERSE REACTIONS
CNS: *dizziness, drowsiness, headache,* nervousness, insomnia, light-headedness, fatigue, numbness.
CV: tachycardia, nonspecific chest pain.
EENT: blurred vision.
GI: dry mouth, nausea, diarrhea, abdominal distress.

INTERACTIONS
Drug-drug. ***Azole antifungals:*** May inhibit first-pass metabolism of buspirone. Monitor patient closely for adverse effects; adjust dosage as needed.
CNS depressants: May increase CNS depression. Use together cautiously.
Drugs metabolized by CYP3A4 (erythromycin, nefazodone): May increase buspirone level. Monitor patient; decrease buspirone dosage and adjust carefully.
MAO inhibitors: May elevate blood pressure. Avoid using together.
Drug-food. *Grapefruit juice:* May increase drug level, increasing adverse effects. Give with liquid other than grapefruit juice.
Drug-lifestyle. *Alcohol use:* May increase CNS depression. Discourage use together.

EFFECTS ON LAB TEST RESULTS
None reported.

CONTRAINDICATIONS & CAUTIONS
- Contraindicated in patients hypersensitive to drug and within 14 days of MAO inhibitor therapy.
- Drug isn't recommended for patients with severe hepatic or renal impairment.

NURSING CONSIDERATIONS
- Monitor patient closely for adverse CNS reactions. Drug is less sedating than other anxiolytics, but CNS effects may be unpredictable.
- ***Alert:*** Before starting therapy, don't stop a previous benzodiazepine regimen abruptly because a withdrawal reaction may occur.
- Drug shows no potential for abuse and isn't classified as a controlled substance.
- ***Look alike–sound alike:*** Don't confuse buspirone with bupropion.

PATIENT TEACHING
- Warn patient to avoid hazardous activities that require alertness and good coordination until effects of drug are known.
- Remind patient that drug effects may not be noticeable for several weeks.
- Warn patient not to abruptly stop a benzodiazepine because of risk of withdrawal symptoms.
- Tell patient to avoid alcohol during therapy.

SAFETY ALERT!

chlordiazepoxide hydrochloride
Apo-Chlordiazepoxide†, Librium, Novo-Poxide†

Pharmacologic class: benzodiazepine
Pregnancy risk category D
Controlled substance schedule IV

AVAILABLE FORMS
Capsules: 5 mg, 10 mg, 25 mg
Powder for injection: 100-mg ampule

INDICATIONS & DOSAGES
➤ Mild to moderate anxiety
Adults: 5 to 10 mg P.O. t.i.d. or q.i.d.
Children older than age 6: 5 mg P.O. b.i.d. to q.i.d. Maximum, 10 mg P.O. b.i.d. or t.i.d.
➤ Severe anxiety
Adults: 20 to 25 mg P.O. t.i.d. or q.i.d.
Elderly patients: 5 mg P.O. b.i.d. to q.i.d.
Adjust-a-dose: For debilitated patients, 5 mg P.O. b.i.d. to q.i.d.
➤ Withdrawal symptoms of acute alcoholism
Adults: 50 to 100 mg P.O., I.V., or I.M. Repeat in 2 to 4 hours, p.r.n. Maximum, 300 mg daily.

➤ Preoperative apprehension and anxiety
Adults: 5 to 10 mg P.O. t.i.d. or q.i.d. on day before surgery; or 50 to 100 mg I.M. 1 hour before surgery.

I.V. ADMINISTRATION
- Parenteral form isn't recommended for children younger than age 12.
- Make sure equipment and staff needed for emergency airway management are available. Monitor respirations every 5 to 15 minutes and before each I.V. dose.
- Keep powder refrigerated and away from light; mix just before use and discard remainder.
- Injectable form comes in two ampules—diluent and powdered drug. Read directions carefully.
- Don't give prepackaged diluent I.V. because air bubbles may form.
- Use 5 ml of normal saline solution or sterile water for injection as diluent for an ampule containing 100 mg of drug.
- Give over 1 minute.

INCOMPATIBILITIES
Other I.V. drugs.

ACTION
A benzodiazepine that may potentiate the effects of GABA, depress the CNS, and suppress the spread of seizure activity.

Route	Onset	Peak	Duration
P.O.	Unknown	½–4 hr	Unknown
I.V.	1–5 min	Unknown	15–60 min
I.M.	Unknown	Unknown	Unknown

Half-life: 5 to 30 hours.

ADVERSE REACTIONS
CNS: *drowsiness, lethargy,* ataxia, confusion, extrapyramidal reactions, minor changes in EEG patterns.
CV: edema.
GI: nausea, constipation.
GU: menstrual irregularities.
Hematologic: ***agranulocytosis.***
Hepatic: jaundice.
Skin: *swelling and pain at injection site,* skin eruptions.
Other: altered libido.

INTERACTIONS
Drug-drug. *Cimetidine:* May decrease chlordiazepoxide clearance and increase risk of adverse reactions. Monitor patient carefully.
CNS depressants: May increase CNS depression. Use together cautiously.
Digoxin: May increase digoxin level and risk of toxicity. Monitor patient and digoxin level closely.
Disulfiram: May decrease clearance and increase half-life of chlordiazepoxide. Monitor patient for enhanced effects. Consider dosage adjustment.
Fluconazole, itraconazole, ketoconazole, miconazole: May increase and prolong chlordiazepoxide levels, CNS depression, and psychomotor impairment. Avoid using together.
Levodopa: May decrease control of parkinsonian symptoms in patients with Parkinson disease. Use together cautiously.
Drug-herb. *Kava:* May increase sedation. Discourage use together.
Drug-lifestyle. *Alcohol use:* May cause additive CNS effects. Discourage use together.
Smoking: May decrease effectiveness of drug. Monitor patient closely.

EFFECTS ON LAB TEST RESULTS
- May increase liver function test values. May decrease granulocyte count.
- May cause a false-positive pregnancy test result. May alter urinary 17-ketosteroid (Zimmerman reaction), urine alkaloid (Frings thin-layer chromatography method), and urinary glucose determinations (with Chemstrip uG and Diastix).

CONTRAINDICATIONS & CAUTIONS
- Contraindicated in patients hypersensitive to drug and in pregnant women, especially in first trimester.
- Use cautiously in patients with mental depression, porphyria, or hepatic or renal disease.

NURSING CONSIDERATIONS
- ***Alert:*** 5-mg and 25-mg capsules may look similar in color through the packaging. Verify contents and read label carefully.

• For I.M. use, add 2 ml of diluent to powder and agitate gently until clear. Don't use the supplied diluent for I.V. use. Use immediately. I.M. form may be absorbed erratically.
• In patients receiving repeated or prolonged therapy, monitor hepatic, renal, and hematopoietic function periodically.
• ***Alert:*** Use of this drug may lead to abuse and addiction. Don't withdraw drug abruptly after long-term use because withdrawal symptoms may occur.

PATIENT TEACHING
• Warn patient to avoid hazardous activities that require alertness and coordination until effects of drug are known.
• Tell patient to avoid alcohol while taking drug.
• Notify patient that smoking may decrease drug's effectiveness.
• Warn patient not to abruptly stop the drug because withdrawal symptoms may occur.
• Warn woman to avoid use during pregnancy.

SAFETY ALERT!

diazepam

Antenex‡, Apo-Diazepam†, Diastat, Diazemuls†‡, Diazepam Intensol, Ducene‡, Novo-Dipam†, PMS-Diazepam†, Valium, Vivol†

Pharmacologic class: benzodiazepine
Pregnancy risk category D
Controlled substance schedule IV

AVAILABLE FORMS
Injection: 5 mg/ml
Oral solution: 5 mg/5 ml, 5 mg/ml
Rectal gel twin packs: 2.5 mg (pediatric), 5 mg (pediatric), 10 mg, 15 mg (adult), 20 mg (adult)
Tablets: 2 mg, 5 mg, 10 mg

INDICATIONS & DOSAGES
➤ **Anxiety**
Adults: Depending on severity, 2 to 10 mg P.O. b.i.d. to q.i.d. Or, 2 to 10 mg I.M. or I.V. q 3 to 4 hours, p.r.n.
Children age 6 months and older: 1 to 2.5 mg P.O. t.i.d. or q.i.d., increase gradually, as needed and tolerated.
Elderly patients: Initially, 2 to 2.5 mg once daily or b.i.d.; increase gradually.
➤ **Acute alcohol withdrawal**
Adults: 10 mg P.O. t.i.d. or q.i.d. first 24 hours; reduce to 5 mg P.O. t.i.d. or q.i.d., p.r.n. Or, initially, 10 mg I.V. or I.M. Then, 5 to 10 mg I.V. or I.M. q 3 to 4 hours, p.r.n.
➤ **Before endoscopic procedures**
Adults: Adjust I.V. dose to desired sedative response (up to 20 mg). Or, 5 to 10 mg I.M. 30 minutes before procedure.
➤ **Muscle spasm**
Adults: 2 to 10 mg P.O. b.i.d. to q.i.d. Or, 5 to 10 mg I.V. or I.M. initially; then 5 to 10 mg I.V. or I.M. q 3 to 4 hours, p.r.n. For tetanus, larger doses up to 20 mg q 2 to 8 hours may be needed.
Children age 5 and older: 5 to 10 mg I.V. or I.M. q 3 to 4 hours, p.r.n.
Children ages 1 month to 5 years: 1 to 2 mg I.V. or I.M. slowly, repeat q 3 to 4 hours, p.r.n.
➤ **Preoperative sedation**
Adults: 10 mg I.M. (preferred) or I.V. before surgery.
➤ **Cardioversion**
Adults: 5 to 15 mg I.V. within 5 to 10 minutes before procedure.
➤ **Adjunct treatment for seizure disorders**
Adults: 2 to 10 mg P.O. b.i.d. to q.i.d.
Children age 6 months and older: 1 to 2.5 mg P.O. t.i.d. or q.i.d. initially; increase as needed and as tolerated.
➤ **Status epilepticus, severe recurrent seizures**
Adults: 5 to 10 mg I.V. or I.M. initially. Use I.M. route only if I.V. access is unavailable. Repeat q 10 to 15 minutes, p.r.n., up to maximum dose of 30 mg. Repeat q 2 to 4 hours, if needed.
Children age 5 and older: 1 mg I.V. q 2 to 5 minutes up to maximum of 10 mg. Repeat q 2 to 4 hours, if needed.
Children ages 1 month to 5 years: 0.2 to 0.5 mg I.V. slowly q 2 to 5 minutes up to maximum of 5 mg. Repeat q 2 to 4 hours, if needed.
➤ **Patients on stable regimens of antiepileptic drugs who need diaze-**

pam intermittently to control bouts of increased seizure activity
Adults and children age 12 and older: 0.2 mg/kg P.R., rounding up to the nearest available dose form. A second dose may be given 4 to 12 hours later.
Children ages 6 to 11: 0.3 mg/kg P.R., rounding up to the nearest available dose form. A second dose may be given 4 to 12 hours later.
Children ages 2 to 5: 0.5 mg/kg P.R., rounding up to the nearest available dose form. A second dose may be given 4 to 12 hours later.
Adjust-a-dose: For elderly and debilitated patients, reduce dosage to decrease the likelihood of ataxia and oversedation.

I.V. ADMINISTRATION

- I.V. route is the more reliable parenteral route; I.M. route isn't recommended because absorption is variable and injection is painful.
- Keep emergency resuscitation equipment and oxygen at bedside.
- Avoid infusion sets or containers made from polyvinyl chloride.
- If possible, inject directly into a large vein. If not, inject slowly through infusion tubing as near to the insertion site as possible. Give at no more than 5 mg/minute. Watch closely for phlebitis at injection site.
- Monitor respirations every 5 to 15 minutes and before each dose.
- Don't store parenteral solution in plastic syringes.

INCOMPATIBILITIES

All other I.V. drugs, most I.V. solutions.

ACTION

A benzodiazepine that probably potentiates the effects of GABA, depresses the CNS, and suppresses the spread of seizure activity.

Route	Onset	Peak	Duration
P.O.	30 min	2 hr	20–80 hr
I.V.	1–5 min	1–5 min	15–60 min
I.M.	Unknown	2 hr	Unknown
P.R.	Unknown	90 min	Unknown

Half-life: About 1 to 12 days.

ADVERSE REACTIONS

CNS: *drowsiness,* dysarthria, slurred speech, tremor, transient amnesia, fatigue, ataxia, headache, insomnia, paradoxical anxiety, hallucinations, minor changes in EEG patterns.
CV: ***CV collapse, bradycardia,*** hypotension.
EENT: diplopia, blurred vision, nystagmus.
GI: nausea, constipation, diarrhea with rectal form.
GU: incontinence, urine retention.
Hematologic: ***neutropenia.***
Hepatic: jaundice.
Respiratory: ***respiratory depression, apnea.***
Skin: rash.
Other: *pain, phlebitis at injection site,* altered libido, physical or psychological dependence.

INTERACTIONS

Drug-drug. *Cimetidine, disulfiram, fluoxetine, fluvoxamine, hormonal contraceptives, isoniazid, metoprolol, propoxyphene, propranolol, valproic acid:* May decrease clearance of diazepam and increase risk of adverse effects. Monitor patient for excessive sedation and impaired psychomotor function.
CNS depressants: May increase CNS depression. Use together cautiously.
Digoxin: May increase digoxin level and risk of toxicity. Monitor patient and digoxin level closely.
Diltiazem: May increase CNS depression and prolong effects of diazepam. Reduce dose of diazepam.
Fluconazole, itraconazole, ketoconazole, miconazole: May increase and prolong diazepam level, CNS depression, and psychomotor impairment. Avoid using together.
Levodopa: May decrease levodopa effectiveness. Monitor patient.
Phenobarbital: May increase effects of both drugs. Use together cautiously.
Drug-herb. *Kava:* May increase sedation. Discourage use together.
Drug-lifestyle. *Alcohol use:* May cause additive CNS effects. Discourage use together.
Smoking: May decrease effectiveness of drug. Monitor patient closely.

EFFECTS ON LAB TEST RESULTS
- May increase liver function test values. May decrease neutrophil count.

CONTRAINDICATIONS & CAUTIONS
- Contraindicated in patients hypersensitive to drug or soy protein; in patients experiencing shock, coma, or acute alcohol intoxication (parenteral form); in pregnant women, especially in first trimester; and in children younger than age 6 months (oral form).
- Diastat rectal gel is contraindicated in patients with acute angle-closure glaucoma.
- Use cautiously in patients with liver or renal impairment, depression, or chronic open-angle glaucoma. Use cautiously in elderly and debilitated patients.

NURSING CONSIDERATIONS
- Use Diastat rectal gel to treat no more than five episodes per month and no more than one episode every 5 days because tolerance may develop.
- When using oral solution, dilute dose just before giving.
- ***Alert:*** Only caregivers who can distinguish the distinct cluster of seizures or events from the patient's ordinary seizure activity, who have been instructed and can give the treatment competently, who understand which seizures may or may not be treated with Diastat, and who can monitor the clinical response and recognize when immediate professional medical evaluation is needed should give Diastat rectal gel.
- Monitor periodic hepatic, renal, and hematopoietic function studies in patients receiving repeated or prolonged therapy.
- Monitor elderly patients for dizziness, ataxia, mental status changes. Patients are at an increased risk for falls.
- ***Alert:*** Use of this drug may lead to abuse and addiction. Don't withdraw drug abruptly after long-term use; withdrawal symptoms may occur.
- ***Look alike–sound alike:*** Don't confuse diazepam with diazoxide.

PATIENT TEACHING
- Warn patient to avoid activities that require alertness and good coordination until effects of drug are known.
- Tell patient to avoid alcohol while taking drug.
- Notify patient that smoking may decrease drug's effectiveness.
- Warn patient not to abruptly stop drug because withdrawal symptoms may occur.
- Warn woman to avoid use during pregnancy.
- Instruct patient's caregiver on the proper use of Diastat rectal gel.

---

hydroxyzine hydrochloride
Anx, Apo-Hydroxyzine†, Atarax*, Novo-Hydroxyzin†, PMS-Hydroxyzine†, Vistaril

hydroxyzine pamoate
Vistaril

Pharmacologic class: piperazine derivative
Pregnancy risk category NR

AVAILABLE FORMS
hydroxyzine hydrochloride
Capsules: 10 mg†, 25 mg†, 50 mg†
Injection: 25 mg/ml, 50 mg/ml
Syrup: 10 mg/5 ml
Tablets: 10 mg, 25 mg, 50 mg, 100 mg
hydroxyzine pamoate
Capsules: 25 mg, 50 mg, 100 mg
Oral suspension: 25 mg/5 ml

INDICATIONS & DOSAGES
➤ **Anxiety**
Adults: 50 to 100 mg P.O. q.i.d.
Children age 6 and older: 50 to 100 mg P.O. daily in divided doses.
Children younger than age 6: 50 mg P.O. daily in divided doses.
➤ **Preoperative and postoperative adjunctive therapy for sedation**
Adults: 25 to 100 mg I.M. or 50 to 100 mg P.O.
Children: 1.1 mg/kg I.M. or 0.6 mg/kg P.O.
➤ **Pruritus from allergies**
Adults: 25 mg P.O. t.i.d. or q.i.d.
Children age 6 and older: 50 to 100 mg P.O. daily in divided doses.
Children younger than age 6: 50 mg P.O. daily in divided doses.

➤ **Psychiatric and emotional emergencies, including acute alcoholism**
Adults: 50 to 100 mg I.M. q 4 to 6 hours, p.r.n.
➤ **Nausea and vomiting (excluding nausea and vomiting of pregnancy)**
Adults: 25 to 100 mg I.M.
Children: 1.1 mg/kg I.M.
➤ **Antepartum and postpartum adjunctive therapy**
Adults: 25 to 100 mg I.M.

ACTION
Suppresses activity in certain essential regions of the subcortical area of the CNS.

Route	Onset	Peak	Duration
P.O.	15–30 min	2 hr	4–6 hr
I.M.	Unknown	Unknown	4–6 hr

Half-life: 3 hours.

ADVERSE REACTIONS
CNS: *drowsiness,* involuntary motor activity.
GI: *dry mouth,* constipation.
Other: pain at I.M. injection site, hypersensitivity reactions.

INTERACTIONS
Drug-drug. *Anticholinergics:* May cause additive anticholinergic effects. Use together cautiously.
CNS depressants: May increase CNS depression. Use together cautiously; dosage adjustments may be needed.
Epinephrine: May inhibit and reverse vasopressor effect of epinephrine. Avoid using together.
Drug-lifestyle. *Alcohol use:* May increase CNS depression. Discourage use together.

EFFECTS ON LAB TEST RESULTS
- May cause false increase in urinary 17-hydroxycorticosteroid level. May cause false-negative skin allergen tests by reducing or inhibiting the cutaneous response to histamine.

CONTRAINDICATIONS & CAUTIONS
- Contraindicated in patients hypersensitive to drug, patients in early pregnancy, and breast-feeding women.

NURSING CONSIDERATIONS
- Parenteral form (hydroxyzine hydrochloride) is for I.M. use only, preferably by Z-track injection. Never give drug I.V. or subcutaneously.
- Aspirate I.M. injection carefully to prevent inadvertent I.V. injection. Inject deeply into a large muscle.
- If patient takes other CNS drugs, observe for oversedation.
- Elderly patients may be more sensitive to adverse anticholinergic effects; monitor these patients for dizziness, excessive sedation, confusion, hypotension, and syncope.
- ***Look alike–sound alike:*** Don't confuse hydroxyzine with hydroxyurea or hydralazine.

PATIENT TEACHING
- Warn patient to avoid hazardous activities that require alertness and good coordination until effects of drug are known.
- Tell patient to avoid alcohol while taking drug.
- Advise patient to use sugarless hard candy or gum to relieve dry mouth.
- Warn woman of childbearing age to avoid use during pregnancy and breast-feeding.

SAFETY ALERT!

lorazepam
Apo-Lorazepam†, Ativan, Lorazepam Intensol, Novo-Lorazem†, Nu-Loraz† ◊

Pharmacologic class: benzodiazepine
Pregnancy risk category D
Controlled substance schedule IV

AVAILABLE FORMS
Injection: 2 mg/ml, 4 mg/ml
Oral solution (concentrated): 2 mg/ml
Tablets: 0.5 mg, 1 mg, 2 mg

INDICATIONS & DOSAGES
➤ **Anxiety**
Adults: 2 to 6 mg P.O. daily in divided doses. Maximum, 10 mg daily.
Elderly patients: 1 to 2 mg P.O. daily in divided doses. Maximum, 10 mg daily.

➤ **Insomnia from anxiety**
Adults: 2 to 4 mg P.O. at bedtime.
➤ **Preoperative sedation**
Adults: 2 mg I.V. total or 0.044 mg/kg I.V., whichever is smaller. Larger doses up to 0.05 mg/kg I.V., to total of 4 mg, may be needed. Or, 0.05 mg/kg I.M. 2 hours before procedure. Total dose shouldn't exceed 4 mg.
➤ **Status epilepticus**
Adults: 4 mg I.V. If seizures continue or recur after 10 to 15 minutes; then, an additional 4-mg dose may be given. Drug may be given I.M. if I.V. access isn't available.
Children♦: 0.05 to 0.1 mg/kg I.V.
➤ **Nausea and vomiting caused by emetogenic cancer chemotherapy**♦
Adults: 2.5 mg P.O. the evening before and just after starting chemotherapy. Or, 1.5 mg/m^2 (usually up to a maximum dose of 3 mg) I.V. (over 5 minutes) 45 minutes before starting chemotherapy.

I.V. ADMINISTRATION

- Keep emergency resuscitation equipment and oxygen available.
- Dilute with an equal volume of sterile water for injection, normal saline solution for injection, or D_5W. Give slowly at no more than 2 mg/minute.
- Monitor respirations every 5 to 15 minutes and before each I.V. dose.
- Contains benzyl alcohol. Avoid use in neonates.
- Refrigerate intact vials and protect from light.

INCOMPATIBILITIES

Aldesleukin, aztreonam, buprenorphine, caffeine citrate, floxacillin, foscarnet, idarubicin, imipenem-cilastatin sodium, omeprazole, ondansetron hydrochloride, sargramostim, sufentanil citrate, thiopental.

ACTION

May potentiate the effects of GABA, depress the CNS, and suppress the spread of seizure activity.

Route	Onset	Peak	Duration
P.O.	1 hr	2 hr	12–24 hr
I.V.	5 min	60–90 min	6–8 hr
I.M.	15–30 min	60–90 min	6–8 hr

Half-life: 10 to 20 hours.

ADVERSE REACTIONS

CNS: *drowsiness, sedation,* amnesia, insomnia, agitation, dizziness, weakness, unsteadiness, disorientation, depression, headache.
CV: hypotension.
EENT: visual disturbances, nasal congestion.
GI: abdominal discomfort, nausea, change in appetite.

INTERACTIONS

Drug-drug. *CNS depressants:* May increase CNS depression. Use together cautiously.
Digoxin: May increase digoxin level and risk of toxicity. Monitor patient and digoxin level closely.
Drug-herb. *Kava:* May increase sedation. Discourage use together.
Drug-lifestyle. *Alcohol use:* May cause additive CNS effects. Discourage use together.
Smoking: May decrease drug's effectiveness. Monitor patient closely.

EFFECTS ON LAB TEST RESULTS

- May increase liver function test values.

CONTRAINDICATIONS & CAUTIONS

- Contraindicated in patients hypersensitive to drug, other benzodiazepines, or the vehicle used in parenteral dosage form; in patients with acute angle-closure glaucoma; and in pregnant women, especially in the first trimester.
- Use cautiously in patients with pulmonary, renal, or hepatic impairment.
- Use cautiously in elderly, acutely ill, or debilitated patients.

NURSING CONSIDERATIONS

- For I.M. use, inject deeply into a muscle. Don't dilute.
- Refrigerate parenteral form to prolong shelf life.

- Monitor hepatic, renal, and hematopoietic function periodically in patients receiving repeated or prolonged therapy.
- ***Alert:*** Use of this drug may lead to abuse and addiction. Don't stop drug abruptly after long-term use because withdrawal symptoms may occur.
- ***Look alike–sound alike:*** Don't confuse lorazepam with alprazolam.

PATIENT TEACHING

- When used before surgery, drug causes substantial preoperative amnesia. Patient teaching requires extra care to ensure adequate recall. Provide written materials or inform a family member, if possible.
- Warn patient to avoid hazardous activities that require alertness or good coordination until effects of drug are known.
- Tell patient to avoid alcohol while taking drug.
- Notify patient that smoking may decrease drug's effectiveness.
- Warn patient not to stop drug abruptly because withdrawal symptoms may occur.
- Advise woman to avoid becoming pregnant while taking drug.

SAFETY ALERT!

midazolam hydrochloride
Hypnovel‡

Pharmacologic class: benzodiazepine
Pregnancy risk category D
Controlled substance schedule IV

AVAILABLE FORMS

Injection: 1 mg/ml, 5 mg/ml
Syrup: 2 mg/ml

INDICATIONS & DOSAGES

➤ **Preoperative sedation (to induce sleepiness or drowsiness and relieve apprehension)**
Adults: 0.07 to 0.08 mg/kg I.M. about 1 hour before surgery.

➤ **Conscious sedation before short diagnostic or endoscopic procedures**
Adults younger than age 60: Initially, small dose not to exceed 2.5 mg I.V. given slowly; repeat in 2 minutes, if needed, in small increments of first dose over at least 2 minutes to achieve desired effect. Total dose of up to 5 mg may be used. Additional doses to maintain desired level of sedation may be given by slow titration in increments of 25% of dose used to first reach the sedative end point.
Patients age 60 or older and debilitated patients: 0.5 to 1.5 mg I.V. over at least 2 minutes. Incremental doses shouldn't exceed 1 mg. A total dose of up to 3.5 mg is usually sufficient.

➤ **To induce sleepiness and amnesia and to relieve apprehension before anesthesia or before and during procedures**
P.O.
Children ages 6 to 16 who are cooperative: 0.25 to 0.5 mg/kg P.O. as a single dose, up to 20 mg.
Infants and children ages 6 months to 5 years or less cooperative, older children: 0.25 to 1 mg/kg P.O. as a single dose, up to 20 mg.
I.V.
Children ages 12 to 16: Initially, no more than 2.5 mg I.V. given slowly; repeat in 2 minutes, if needed, in small increments of first dose over at least 2 minutes to achieve desired effect. Total dose of up to 10 mg may be used. Additional doses to maintain desired level of sedation may be given by slow titration in increments of 25% of dose used to first reach the sedative end point.
Children ages 6 to 12: 0.025 to 0.05 mg/kg I.V. over 2 to 3 minutes. Additional doses may be given in small increments after 2 to 3 minutes. Total dose of up to 0.4 mg/kg, not to exceed 10 mg, may be used.
Children ages 6 months to 5 years: 0.05 to 0.1 mg/kg I.V. over 2 to 3 minutes. Additional doses may be given in small increments after 2 to 3 minutes. Total dose of up to 0.6 mg/kg, not to exceed 6 mg, may be used.
I.M.
Children: 0.1 to 0.15 mg/kg I.M. Use up to 0.5 mg/kg in more anxious patients.
Adjust-a-dose: For obese children, base dose on ideal body weight; high-risk or debilitated children and children receiving other sedatives need lower doses.

➤ **To induce general anesthesia**
Adults older than age 55: 0.3 mg/kg I.V. over 20 to 30 seconds if patient hasn't re-

ceived premedication, or 0.2 mg/kg I.V. over 20 to 30 seconds if patient has received a sedative or opioid premedication. Additional increments of 25% of first dose may be needed to complete induction.
Adults younger than age 55: 0.3 to 0.35 mg/kg I.V. over 20 to 30 seconds if patient hasn't received premedication, or 0.25 mg/kg I.V. over 20 to 30 seconds if patient has received a sedative or opioid premedication. Additional increments of 25% of first dose may be needed to complete induction.
Adjust-a-dose: For debilitated patients, initially, 0.2 to 0.25 mg/kg. As little as 0.15 mg/kg may be needed.

➤ **As continuous infusion to sedate intubated patients in critical care unit**

Adults: Initially, 0.01 to 0.05 mg/kg may be given I.V. over several minutes, repeated at 10- to 15-minute intervals until adequate sedation is achieved. To maintain sedation, usual initial infusion rate is 0.02 to 0.1 mg/kg/hour. Higher loading dose or infusion rates may be needed in some patients. Use the lowest effective rate.
Children: Initially, 0.05 to 0.2 mg/kg may be given I.V. over 2 to 3 minutes or longer; then continuous infusion at rate of 0.06 to 0.12 mg/kg/hour. Increase or decrease infusion to maintain desired effect.
Neonates more than 32 weeks' gestational age: Initially, 0.06 mg/kg/hour. Adjust rate, p.r.n., using lowest possible rate.
Neonates less than 32 weeks' gestational age: Initially, 0.03 mg/kg/hour. Adjust rate, p.r.n., using lowest possible rate.

I.V. ADMINISTRATION

- Drug may be mixed in the same syringe with morphine sulfate, meperidine, atropine, or scopolamine.
- When mixing infusion, use 5-mg/ml vial and dilute to 0.5 mg/ml with D_5W or normal saline solution.
- Give slowly over at least 2 minutes, and wait at least 2 minutes when titrating doses to produce therapeutic effect.

INCOMPATIBILITIES

Albumin, amoxicillin sodium, amphotericin B, ampicillin sodium, bumetanide, butorphanol, ceftazidime, cefuroxime, clonidine, dexamethasone sodium phosphate, dimenhydrinate, dobutamine, foscarnet, fosphenytoin, furosemide, heparin sodium, hydrocortisone, imipenem-cilastatin sodium, lactated Ringer injection, methotrexate sodium, nafcillin, omeprazole sodium, pentobarbital sodium, perphenazine, prochlorperazine edisylate, ranitidine hydrochloride, sodium bicarbonate, thiopental, some total parenteral nutrition formulations, trimethoprim-sulfamethoxazole.

ACTION

May potentiate the effects of GABA, depress the CNS, and suppress the spread of seizure activity.

Route	Onset	Peak	Duration
P.O.	10–20 min	45–60 min	2–6 hr
I.V.	90 sec–5 min	Rapid	2–6 hr
I.M.	15 min	15–60 min	2–6 hr

Half-life: 2 to 6 hours.

ADVERSE REACTIONS

CNS: *oversedation, drowsiness,* amnesia, headache, involuntary movements, nystagmus, paradoxical behavior or excitement.
CV: variations in blood pressure and pulse rate.
GI: *nausea,* vomiting.
Respiratory: APNEA, *decreased respiratory rate, hiccups.*
Other: *pain at injection site.*

INTERACTIONS

Drug-drug. *CNS depressants:* May cause apnea. Use together cautiously. Adjust dosage of midazolam if used with opiates or other CNS depressants.
Diltiazem: May increase CNS depression and prolonged effects of midazolam. Use lower dose of midazolam.
Erythromycin: May alter metabolism of midazolam. Use together cautiously.
Fluconazole, itraconazole, ketoconazole, miconazole: May increase and prolong midazolam level, CNS depression, and psychomotor impairment. Avoid using together.
Hormonal contraceptives: May prolong half-life of midazolam. Use together cautiously.

Rifampin: May decrease midazolam level. Monitor for midazolam effectiveness.
Theophylline: May antagonize sedative effect of midazolam. Use together cautiously.
Verapamil: May increase midazolam level. Monitor patient closely.
Drug-herb. *St. John's wort:* May decrease drug level. Discourage use together.
Drug-food. *Grapefruit juice:* May increase bioavailability of oral drug. Discourage use together.
Drug-lifestyle. *Alcohol use:* May cause additive CNS effects. Discourage use together.

EFFECTS ON LAB TEST RESULTS

None reported.

CONTRAINDICATIONS & CAUTIONS

- Contraindicated in patients hypersensitive to drug and in those with acute angle-closure glaucoma, shock, coma, or acute alcohol intoxication.
- Use cautiously in patients with uncompensated acute illness and in elderly or debilitated patients.

NURSING CONSIDERATIONS

- ***Alert:*** Have oxygen and resuscitation equipment available in case of severe respiratory depression. Excessive amounts and rapid infusion have been linked to respiratory arrest. Continuously monitor patient, including children taking syrup form, for life-threatening respiratory depression.
- When injecting I.M., give deeply into a large muscle.
- Monitor blood pressure, heart rate and rhythm, respirations, airway integrity, and arterial oxygen saturation during procedure.

PATIENT TEACHING

- Because drug diminishes patient's recall of events around the time of surgery, provide written information, family member instructions, and follow-up contact.
- Warn patient to avoid hazardous activities that require alertness or good coordination until effects of drug are known.

31 Antipsychotics

aripiprazole
chlorpromazine hydrochloride
clozapine
fluphenazine decanoate
fluphenazine hydrochloride
haloperidol
haloperidol decanoate
haloperidol lactate
loxapine succinate
olanzapine
perphenazine
prochlorperazine
(See Chapter 48, ANTIEMETICS.)
quetiapine fumarate
risperidone
thioridazine hydrochloride
thiothixene
thiothixene hydrochloride
trifluoperazine hydrochloride
ziprasidone

aripiprazole

Abilify, Abilify Discmelt

Pharmacologic class: quinolone derivative
Pregnancy risk category C

AVAILABLE FORMS

Injection: 9.75 mg/1.3 ml (7.5 mg/ml) single-dose vial
Oral solution: 1 mg/ml
Orally disintegrating tablets (ODTs): 10 mg, 15 mg, 20 mg, 30 mg
Tablets: 2 mg, 5 mg, 10 mg, 15 mg, 20 mg, 30 mg

INDICATIONS & DOSAGES

➤ **Schizophrenia**

Adults: Initially, 10 to 15 mg P.O. daily; increase to maximum daily dose of 30 mg if needed, after at least 2 weeks.

Adjust-a-dose: When using with CYP3A4 inhibitors such as ketoconazole or CYP2D6 inhibitors, such as quinidine, fluoxetine, or paroxetine, give half the aripiprazole dose. When using with CYP3A4 inducers such as carbamazepine, double the aripiprazole dose. Return to original dosing after the other drugs are stopped.

➤ **Bipolar mania, including manic and mixed episodes**

Adults: Initially, 30 mg P.O. once daily. May reduce dose to 15 mg daily based on patient tolerance. Safety of doses greater than 30 mg daily and treatment lasting beyond 6 weeks hasn't been established.

✱ ***NEW INDICATION:*** **Agitation associated with schizophrenia or bipolar 1 disorder, mixed or manic**

Adults: 5.25 to 15 mg by deep I.M. injection. Recommended dose is 9.75 mg. May give a 2nd dose after 2 hours, if needed. Safety of giving more frequently than every 2 hours or a total daily dose more than 30 mg isn't known. Switch to oral form as soon as possible.

ACTION

Thought to exert partial agonist activity at D2 and serotonin 1A receptors and antagonist activity at serotonin 2A receptors.

Route	Onset	Peak	Duration
I.M.	Unknown	1–3 hr	Unknown
P.O.	Unknown	3–5 hr	Unknown

Half-life: About 75 hours in patients with normal metabolism; about 6 days in those who can't metabolize the drug through CYP2D6.

ADVERSE REACTIONS

CNS: *headache, anxiety, insomnia, lightheadedness, somnolence, akathisia,* ***increased suicide risk, neuroleptic malignant syndrome, seizures, suicidal thoughts,*** tremor, asthenia, depression, fatigue, dizziness, nervousness, hostility, manic behavior, confusion, abnormal gait, cogwheel rigidity, fever, tardive dyskinesia.

CV: peripheral edema, chest pain, hypertension, tachycardia, orthostatic hypotension, ***bradycardia.***

EENT: rhinitis, blurred vision, increased salivation, conjunctivitis, ear pain.

GI: *nausea, vomiting, constipation,* anorexia, dry mouth , dyspepsia, diarrhea, abdominal pain, esophageal dysmotility.
GU: urinary incontinence.
Hematologic: ecchymosis, anemia.
Metabolic: weight gain, weight loss, hyperglycemia, hypercholesterolemia.
Musculoskeletal: neck pain, neck stiffness, muscle cramps.
Respiratory: dyspnea, pneumonia, cough.
Skin: rash, dry skin, pruritus, sweating, ulcer.
Other: flulike syndrome.

INTERACTIONS

Drug-drug. *Antihypertensives:* May enhance antihypertensive effects. Monitor blood pressure.
Carbamazepine and other CYP3A4 inducers: May decrease levels and effectiveness of aripiprazole. Double the usual dose of aripiprazole, and monitor the patient closely.
Ketoconazole and other CYP3A4 inhibitors: May increase risk of serious toxic effects. Start treatment with one-half the usual dose of aripiprazole, and monitor patient closely.
Potential CYP2D6 inhibitors (fluoxetine, paroxetine, quinidine): May increase levels and toxicity of aripiprazole. Give half the usual dose of aripiprazole.
Drug-food. *Grapefruit juice:* May increase drug level. Tell patient not to take drug with grapefruit juice.
Drug-lifestyle. *Alcohol use:* May increase CNS effects. Discourage use together.

EFFECTS ON LAB TEST RESULTS

- May increase CK and glucose levels.

CONTRAINDICATIONS & CAUTIONS

- Contraindicated in patients hypersensitive to drug.
- Use cautiously in patients with CV disease, cerebrovascular disease, or conditions that could predispose the patient to hypotension, such as dehydration or hypovolemia.
- Use cautiously in patients with history of seizures or with conditions that lower the seizure threshold.
- Use cautiously in patients who engage in strenuous exercise, are exposed to extreme heat, take anticholinergics, or are susceptible to dehydration.
- Use cautiously in patients at risk for aspiration pneumonia, such as those with Alzheimer disease.
- Use cautiously in pregnant and breast-feeding women.

NURSING CONSIDERATIONS

- ***Alert:*** Neuroleptic malignant syndrome may occur. Monitor patient for hyperpyrexia, muscle rigidity, altered mental status, irregular pulse or blood pressure, tachycardia, diaphoresis, and cardiac dysrhythmias.
- If signs and symptoms of neuroleptic malignant syndrome occur, immediately stop drug and notify prescriber.
- Monitor patient for signs and symptoms of tardive dyskinesia. The elderly, especially elderly women, are at highest risk of developing this adverse effect.
- ***Alert:*** Fatal cerebrovascular adverse events (stroke, TIA) may occur in elderly patients with dementia. Drug isn't safe or effective in these patients.
- ***Alert:*** Hyperglycemia may occur. Monitor patient with diabetes regularly. Patient with risk factors for diabetes should undergo fasting blood glucose testing at baseline and periodically. Monitor all patients for symptoms of hyperglycemia including increased hunger, thirst, frequent urination, and weakness. Hyperglycemia may resolve when patient stops taking drug.
- ***Alert:*** Monitor patient for symptoms of metabolic syndrome (significant weight gain and increased BMI, hypertension, hyperglycemia, hypercholesterolemia, and hypertriglyceridemia).
- Treat patient with the smallest dose for the shortest time and periodically reevaluate for need for continuing.
- Give prescriptions only for small quantities of drug, to reduce risk of overdose.
- Substitute the oral solution on a milligram-by-milligram basis for the 5-, 10-, 15-, or 20-mg tablets, up to 25 mg. Give patients taking 30-mg tablets 25 mg of solution.
- Don't give I.V. or subcutaneously.

PATIENT TEACHING

- Tell patient to use caution while driving or operating hazardous machinery because psychoactive drugs may impair judgment, thinking, or motor skills.
- Tell patient that drug may be taken without regard to meals.
- Advise patients that grapefruit juice may interact with aripiprazole and to limit or avoid its use.
- Advise patient that gradual improvement in symptoms should occur over several weeks rather than immediately.
- Tell patients to avoid alcohol use while taking drug.
- Advise patients to limit strenuous activity while taking drug to avoid dehydration.
- Tell patient to keep ODT in blister package until ready to use. Using dry hands, he should carefully peel open the foil backing and place tablet on the tongue. Tell him not to split tablet.
- Tell patient to store oral solution in refrigerator and that the solution can be used for up to 6 months after opening.

---

chlorpromazine hydrochloride

Chlorpromanyl-20†, Chlorpromanyl-40†, Largactil†‡, Novo-Chlorpromazine†, Thorazine

Pharmacologic class: phenothiazine
Pregnancy risk category C

AVAILABLE FORMS

Capsules (extended-release): 200 mg, 300 mg
Injection: 25 mg/ml
Oral concentrate: 30 mg/ml, 100 mg/ml
Suppositories: 25 mg, 100 mg
Syrup: 10 mg/5 ml
Tablets: 10 mg, 25 mg, 50 mg, 100 mg, 200 mg

INDICATIONS & DOSAGES

➤ **Psychosis, mania**

Adults: For hospitalized patients with acute disease, 25 mg I.M.; may give an additional 25 to 50 mg I.M. in 1 hour if needed. Increase over several days to 400 mg q 4 to 6 hours. Switch to oral therapy as soon as possible. Or, 25 mg P.O. t.i.d. initially; then gradually increase to 400 mg daily in divided doses. For outpatients, 30 to 75 mg daily in two to four divided doses. Increase dosage by 20 to 50 mg twice weekly until symptoms are controlled.

Children age 6 months and older: 0.55 mg/kg P.O. q 4 to 6 hours or I.M. q 6 to 8 hours. Or, 1.1 mg/kg P.R. q 6 to 8 hours. Maximum I.M. dose in children younger than age 5 or who weigh less than 22.7 kg (50 lb) is 40 mg. Maximum I.M. dose in children ages 5 to 12 or who weigh 22.7 to 45.4 kg (50 to 100 lb) is 75 mg.

➤ **Nausea and vomiting**

Adults: 10 to 25 mg P.O. q 4 to 6 hours, p.r.n. Or, 50 to 100 mg P.R. q 6 to 8 hours, p.r.n. Or, 25 mg I.M. initially. If no hypotension occurs, 25 to 50 mg I.M. q 3 to 4 hours may be given, p.r.n., until vomiting stops.

Children age 6 months and older: 0.55 mg/kg P.O. q 4 to 6 hours or I.M. q 6 to 8 hours. Or, 1.1 mg/kg P.R. q 6 to 8 hours. Maximum I.M. dose in children younger than age 5 or who weigh less than 22.7 kg (50 lb) is 40 mg. Maximum I.M. dose in children ages 5 to 12 or who weigh 22.7 to 45.4 kg (50 to 100 lb) is 75 mg.

➤ **Acute intermittent porphyria, intractable hiccups**

Adults: 25 to 50 mg P.O. t.i.d. or q.i.d. If symptoms persist for 2 to 3 days, 25 to 50 mg I.M. For hiccups, if symptoms still persist, 25 to 50 mg diluted in 500 to 1,000 ml of normal saline solution and infused slowly with patient in supine position.

➤ **Tetanus**

Adults: 25 to 50 mg I.V. or I.M. t.i.d. or q.i.d.

Children age 6 months and older: 0.55 mg/kg I.M. or I.V. q 6 to 8 hours. Maximum parenteral dosage in children who weigh less than 22.7 kg (50 lb) is 40 mg daily; for children who weigh 22.7 to 45.4 kg (50 to 100 lb), 75 mg, except in severe cases. If giving I.V., dilute to 1 mg/ml with normal saline and give at a rate of 0.5 mg/minute.

➤ **Surgery**

Adults: Preoperatively, 25 to 50 mg P.O. 2 to 3 hours before surgery or 12.5 to 25 mg I.M. 1 to 2 hours before surgery;

during surgery, 12.5 mg I.M., repeated in 30 minutes, if needed, or fractional 2-mg doses I.V. at 2-minute intervals to maximum dose of 25 mg; postoperatively, 10 to 25 mg P.O. q 4 to 6 hours or 12.5 to 25 mg I.M., repeated in 1 hour, if needed.
Children age 6 months and older: Preoperatively, 0.55 mg/kg P.O. 2 to 3 hours before surgery or I.M. 1 to 2 hours before surgery. During surgery, 0.275 mg/kg I.M., repeated in 30 minutes if needed, or fractional 1-mg doses I.V. at 2-minute intervals to maximum of 0.275 mg/kg. May repeat fractional I.V. regimen in 30 minutes if needed. Postoperatively, 0.55 mg/kg P.O. or I.M. q 4 to 6 hours (oral dose) or 1 hour (I.M. dose), if needed and if hypotension doesn't occur.
Elderly patients: Lower dosages are sufficient; dosage increments should be more gradual than in adults.

I.V. ADMINISTRATION
- Drug is compatible with most common I.V. solutions, including D_5W, Ringer injection, lactated Ringer injection, and normal saline solution for injection.
- For direct injection, dilute with normal saline solution for injection and give into a large vein or through the tubing of a free-flowing I.V. solution.
- Don't exceed 1 mg/minute for adults or 0.5 mg/minute for children.
- For intermittent infusion, dilute with 50 or 100 ml of a compatible solution.
- Infuse over 30 minutes.

INCOMPATIBILITIES
Aminophylline, amphotericin B, ampicillin, chloramphenicol sodium succinate, chlorothiazide, cimetidine, dimenhydrinate, furosemide, heparin sodium, linezolid, melphalan, methohexital, paclitaxel, penicillin, pentobarbital, phenobarbital, solutions with a pH of 4 to 5, thiopental.

ACTION
A piperidine phenothiazine that may block postsynaptic dopamine receptors in the brain.

Route	Onset	Peak	Duration
P.O.	30–60 min	Unknown	4–6 hr
P.O. (extended)	30–60 min	Unknown	10–12 hr
I.V., I.M.	Unknown	Unknown	Unknown
P.R.	> 1 hr	Unknown	3–4 hr

Half-life: 20 to 24 hours.

ADVERSE REACTIONS
CNS: *extrapyramidal reactions, sedation, tardive dyskinesia, pseudoparkinsonism,* ***neuroleptic malignant syndrome, seizures,*** dizziness, drowsiness.
CV: *orthostatic hypotension,* tachycardia, quinidine-like ECG effects.
EENT: ocular changes, blurred vision, nasal congestion.
GI: *dry mouth, constipation,* nausea.
GU: *urine retention,* menstrual irregularities, inhibited ejaculation, priapism.
Hematologic: ***leukopenia, agranulocytosis, aplastic anemia, thrombocytopenia,*** eosinophilia, hemolytic anemia.
Hepatic: jaundice.
Skin: *mild photosensitivity reactions, pain at I.M. injection site,* allergic reactions, sterile abscess, skin pigmentation changes.
Other: gynecomastia, lactation, galactorrhea.

INTERACTIONS
Drug-drug. *Antacids:* May inhibit absorption of oral phenothiazines. Separate antacid and phenothiazine doses by at least 2 hours.
Anticholinergics such as tricyclic antidepressants, antiparkinsonians: May increase anticholinergic activity, aggravated parkinsonian symptoms. Use together cautiously.
Anticonvulsants: May lower seizure threshold. Monitor patient closely.
Barbiturates, lithium: May decrease phenothiazine effect. Monitor patient.
Centrally acting antihypertensives: May decrease antihypertensive effect. Monitor blood pressure.
CNS depressants: May increase CNS depression. Use together cautiously.
Electroconvulsive therapy, insulin: May cause severe reactions. Monitor patient closely.

Lithium: May increase neurologic effects. Monitor patient closely.
Meperidine: May cause excessive sedation and hypotension. Don't use together.
Propranolol: May increase levels of both propranolol and chlorpromazine. Monitor patient closely.
Warfarin: May decrease effect of oral anticoagulants. Monitor PT and INR.
Drug-herb. *St. John's wort:* May cause photosensitivity reactions. Advise patient to avoid excessive sunlight exposure.
Drug-lifestyle. *Alcohol use:* May increase CNS depression, particularly psychomotor skills. Strongly discourage alcohol use.
Sun exposure: May increase risk of photosensitivity reactions. Advise patient to avoid excessive sunlight exposure.

EFFECTS ON LAB TEST RESULTS

- May decrease hemoglobin level and hematocrit.
- May increase liver function test values and eosinophil count. May decrease granulocyte, platelet, and WBC counts.
- May cause false-positive results for urinary porphyrin, urobilinogen, amylase, and 5-hydroxyindoleacetic acid tests and for urine pregnancy tests that use human chorionic gonadotropin.

CONTRAINDICATIONS & CAUTIONS

- Contraindicated in patients hypersensitive to drug; in those with CNS depression, bone marrow suppression, or subcortical damage, and in those in coma.
- Use cautiously in elderly or debilitated patients and in patients with hepatic or renal disease, severe CV disease (may suddenly decrease blood pressure), respiratory disorders, hypocalcemia, glaucoma, or prostatic hyperplasia. Also use cautiously in those exposed to extreme heat or cold (including antipyretic therapy) or organophosphate insecticides.
- Use cautiously in acutely ill or dehydrated children.

NURSING CONSIDERATIONS

- Obtain baseline blood pressure measurements before therapy, and monitor regularly. Watch for orthostatic hypotension, especially with parenteral administration. Monitor blood pressure before and after I.M. administration; keep patient supine for 1 hour afterward and have him get up slowly.
- Wear gloves when preparing solutions and avoid contact with skin and clothing. Oral liquid and parenteral forms can cause contact dermatitis.
- Slight yellowing of injection or concentrate is common and doesn't affect potency. Discard markedly discolored solutions.
- Protect liquid concentrate from light. Dilute with fruit juice, milk, or semisolid food just before giving.
- Give deep I.M. only in upper outer quadrant of buttocks. Consider giving injection by Z-track method. Massage slowly afterward to prevent sterile abscess. Injection stings. Rotate injection sites.
- Monitor patient for tardive dyskinesia, which may occur after prolonged use. It may not appear until months or years later and may disappear spontaneously or persist for life, despite stopping drug.
- After abrupt withdrawal of long-term therapy, gastritis, nausea, vomiting, dizziness, or tremor may occur.
- ***Alert:*** Watch for evidence of neuroleptic malignant syndrome (extrapyramidal effects, hyperthermia, autonomic disturbance), which is rare but usually fatal. It may not be related to length of drug use or type of neuroleptic; more than 60% of affected patients are men.
- If jaundice, symptoms of blood dyscrasia (fever, sore throat, infection, cellulitis, weakness), or persistent extrapyramidal reactions (longer than a few hours) develop, or if such reactions occur in children or pregnant women, withhold dose and notify prescriber.
- Don't withdraw drug abruptly unless required by severe adverse reactions.
- ***Look alike–sound alike:*** Don't confuse chlorpromazine with clomipramine or with chlorpropamide, a hypoglycemic.

PATIENT TEACHING

- Warn patient to avoid activities that require alertness or good coordination until effects of drug are known. Drowsiness and dizziness usually subside after first few weeks.
- ***Alert:*** Advise patient not to crush, chew, or break extended-release capsule before swallowing.

- Tell patient to avoid alcohol while taking drug.
- Have patient report signs of urine retention or constipation.
- Tell patient to use sunblock and to wear protective clothing to avoid oversensitivity to the sun. This drug is more likely to cause sun sensitivity than other drugs in its class.
- Tell patient to relieve dry mouth with sugarless gum or hard candy.
- Advise patient receiving drug by any method other than by mouth to remain lying down for 1 hour afterward and to rise slowly.

SAFETY ALERT!

clozapine
Clozaril, FazaClo

Pharmacologic class: dibenzapine derivative

Pregnancy risk category B

AVAILABLE FORMS
Tablets: 25 mg, 100 mg, 200 mg
Tablets (orally disintegrating): 25 mg, 100 mg

INDICATIONS & DOSAGES
➤ **Schizophrenia in severely ill patients unresponsive to other therapies; to reduce risk of recurrent suicidal behavior in schizophrenia or schizoaffective disorders**

Adults: Initially, 12.5 mg P.O. once daily or b.i.d. If using the orally disintegrating tablet, cut in half and discard the unused half. Adjust dose upward by 25 to 50 mg daily (if tolerated) to 300 to 450 mg daily by end of 2 weeks. Individual dosage is based on response, patient tolerance, and adverse reactions. Subsequent dosage shouldn't be increased more than once or twice weekly and shouldn't exceed 50- to 100-mg increments. Many patients respond to dosages of 200 to 600 mg daily, but some may need as much as 900 mg daily. Don't exceed 900 mg daily.

ACTION
Unknown. Binds selectively to dopaminergic receptors in the CNS and may interfere with adrenergic, cholinergic, histaminergic, and serotonergic receptors.

Route	Onset	Peak	Duration
P.O.	Unknown	2½ hr	4–12 hr

Half-life: Appears proportional to dose and may range from 8 to 12 hours.

ADVERSE REACTIONS
CNS: *drowsiness, sedation, dizziness, vertigo, headache,* ***seizures,*** syncope, tremor, disturbed sleep or nightmares, restlessness, hypokinesia or akinesia, agitation, rigidity, akathisia, confusion, fatigue, insomnia, hyperkinesia, weakness, lethargy, ataxia, slurred speech, depression, myoclonus, anxiety, fever.
CV: *tachycardia,* ***cardiomyopathy, myocarditis, pulmonary embolism, cardiac arrest,*** hypotension, hypertension, chest pain, ECG changes, orthostatic hypotension.
EENT: visual disturbances.
GI: *constipation, excessive salivation,* dry mouth, nausea, vomiting, heartburn, diarrhea.
GU: urinary frequency or urgency, urine retention, incontinence, abnormal ejaculation.
Hematologic: ***leukopenia, agranulocytosis, granulocytopenia,*** eosinophilia.
Metabolic: *hyperglycemia,* weight gain, hypercholesterolemia, hypertriglyceridemia.
Musculoskeletal: muscle pain or spasm, muscle weakness.
Respiratory: ***respiratory arrest.***
Skin: rash, diaphoresis.

INTERACTIONS
Drug-drug. *Anticholinergics:* May potentiate anticholinergic effects of clozapine. Use together cautiously.
Antihypertensives: May potentiate hypotensive effects. Monitor blood pressure.
Benzodiazepines: May increase risk of sedation and CV and respiratory arrest. Use together cautiously.
Bone marrow suppressants: May increase bone marrow toxicity. Avoid using together.
Citalopram, *fluoroquinolones,* **fluoxetine, fluvoxamine,** *paroxetine,* **sertraline:** May

increase clozapine levels and toxicity. Adjust clozapine dose as needed.
Digoxin, other highly protein-bound drugs, warfarin: May increase levels of these drugs. Monitor patient closely for adverse reactions.
Phenytoin: May decrease clozapine level and cause breakthrough psychosis. Monitor patient for psychosis and adjust clozapine dosage.
Psychoactive drugs: May cause additive effects. Use together cautiously.
Ritonavir: May increase clozapine levels and toxicity. Avoid using together.
Drug-herb. *St. John's wort:* May decrease drug level. Discourage use together.
Drug-lifestyle. *Alcohol use:* May increase CNS depression. Discourage use together.
Smoking: May decrease drug level. Urge patient to quit smoking. Monitor patient for effectiveness and adjust dosage.

EFFECTS ON LAB TEST RESULTS

- May increase glucose, cholesterol, and triglyceride levels.
- May increase eosinophil count. May decrease granulocyte and WBC counts.

CONTRAINDICATIONS & CAUTIONS

- Contraindicated in patients with uncontrolled epilepsy, history of clozapine-induced agranulocytosis, WBC count below 3,500/mm^3, severe CNS depression or coma, paralytic ileus, and myelosuppressive disorders.
- Contraindicated in patients taking other drugs that suppress bone marrow function.
- Use cautiously in patients with prostatic hyperplasia or angle-closure glaucoma because drug has potent anticholinergic effects.

NURSING CONSIDERATIONS

- ***Alert:*** Drug carries significant risk of agranulocytosis. If possible, give patient at least two trials of standard antipsychotic before starting clozapine. Obtain baseline WBC and differential counts before clozapine therapy. Baseline WBC count must be at least 3,500/mm^3 and baseline ANC at least 2,000/mm^3. Monitor WBC and ANC values weekly for at least 4 weeks after stopping drug, regardless of how often you were monitoring when therapy stopped.
- During the first 6 months of therapy, monitor patient weekly and dispense no more than a 1-week supply of the drug. If acceptable WBC and ANC values [WBC 3,500/mm^3 or higher and ANC 2,000/mm^3 or higher] are maintained during the first 6 months of continuous therapy, reduce monitoring to every other week. After 6 months of every-other-week monitoring without interruption by leukopenia, reduce frequency of monitoring WBC and ANC to monthly.
- If WBC count drops below 3,500/mm^3 after therapy begins or if it drops substantially from baseline, monitor patient closely for signs and symptoms of infection. If WBC count is 3,000 to 3,500/mm^3 and granulocyte count is above 1,500/mm^3, perform WBC and differential count twice weekly. If WBC count drops to 2,000/mm^3 to 3,000/mm^3 or granulocyte count drops to 1,000/mm^3 to 1,500/mm^3, interrupt therapy and notify prescriber. Monitor WBC and differential daily until WBC exceeds 3,000/mm^3 and ANC exceeds 1,500/mm^3, and monitor patient for signs and symptoms of infection. Continue monitoring WBC and differential counts twice weekly until WBC count exceeds 3,500/mm^3 and ANC exceeds 2,000/mm^3. Then, restart therapy with weekly monitoring for 1 year before returning to the usual monitoring schedule of every 2 weeks for 6 months and then every 4 weeks.
- If WBC count drops below 2,000/mm^3 and granulocyte count drops below 1,000/mm^3, patient may need protective isolation. Bone marrow aspiration may be needed to assess bone marrow function. Future clozapine therapy is contraindicated in these patients.
- ***Alert:*** Drug increases the risk of fatal myocarditis, especially during, but not limited to, the first month of therapy. In patients in whom myocarditis is suspected (unexplained fatigue, dyspnea, tachypnea, chest pain, tachycardia, fever, palpitations, and other signs or symptoms of heart failure or ECG abnormalities, such as ST-T wave abnormalities or arrhythmias), stop therapy immediately and don't restart.
- ***Alert:*** Drug may cause hyperglycemia. Monitor patients with diabetes regularly.

In patients with risk factors for diabetes, obtain fasting blood glucose test results at baseline and periodically.

- ***Alert:*** Monitor patient for metabolic syndrome, which includes symptoms of significant weight gain and increased body mass index, hypertension, hyperglycemia, hypercholesterolemia, and hypertriglyceridemia.
- Monitor patient for signs and symptoms of cardiomyopathy.
- Seizures may occur, especially in patients receiving high doses.
- Some patients experience transient fever with temperature higher than 100.4° F (38° C), especially in the first 3 weeks of therapy. Monitor these patients closely.
- ***Alert:*** Drug isn't indicated for use in elderly patients with dementia-related psychoses because of an increased risk for death from CV disease or infection..
- After abrupt withdrawal of long-term therapy, abrupt recurrence of psychosis is possible.
- If therapy must be stopped, withdraw drug gradually over 1 or 2 weeks. If changes in patient's medical condition (including development of leukopenia) require that drug be stopped immediately, monitor patient closely for recurrence of psychosis.
- If therapy is reinstated in patients withdrawn from drug, follow usual guidelines for dosage increase. Reexposure of patient to drug may increase severity and risk of adverse reactions. If therapy was stopped because WBC counts were below $2,000/mm^3$ or granulocyte counts were below $1,000/mm^3$, don't restart.
- ***Look alike–sound alike:*** Don't confuse clozapine with clonidine, clofazimine, or Klonopin.
- Orally disintegrating tablets contain phenylalanine.

PATIENT TEACHING

- Tell patient about need for weekly blood tests to check for blood-cell deficiency. Advise him to report flulike symptoms, fever, sore throat, lethargy, malaise, or other signs of infection.
- Warn patient to avoid hazardous activities that require alertness and good coordination while taking drug.
- Tell patient to check with prescriber before taking alcohol or nonprescription drugs.
- Advise patient that smoking may decrease drug effectiveness.
- Tell patient to rise slowly to avoid dizziness.
- Tell patient to keep orally disintegrating tablets in the blister package until ready to take it.
- Inform patient that ice chips or sugarless candy or gum may help relieve dry mouth.

fluphenazine decanoate
Modecate†‡, Modecate Concentrate†, Prolixin Decanoate

fluphenazine hydrochloride
Apo-Fluphenazine†, Prolixin*, Prolixin Concentrate

Pharmacologic class: phenothiazine
Pregnancy risk category C

AVAILABLE FORMS

fluphenazine decanoate
Depot injection: 25 mg/ml
fluphenazine hydrochloride
Elixir: 2.5 mg/5 ml*
I.M. injection: 2.5 mg/ml
Oral concentrate: 5 mg/ml*
Tablets: 1 mg, 2.5 mg, 5 mg, 10 mg

INDICATIONS & DOSAGES

➤Psychotic disorders
Adults: Initially, 0.5 to 10 mg fluphenazine hydrochloride P.O. daily in divided doses q 6 to 8 hours; may increase cautiously to 20 mg. Maintenance dose is 1 to 5 mg P.O. daily. I.M. doses are one-third to one-half of P.O. doses. Usual I.M. dose is 1.25 mg. Give more than 10 mg daily with caution.

Or, 12.5 to 25 mg of fluphenazine decanoate I.M. or subcutaneously q 1 to 6 weeks; maintenance dose is 25 to 100 mg, p.r.n.
Elderly patients: 1 to 2.5 mg fluphenazine hydrochloride P.O daily.

ACTION

A piperazine phenothiazine that probably blocks postsynaptic dopamine receptors in the brain.

Route	Onset	Peak	Duration
P.O.	< 1 hr	30 min	6–8 hr
I.M. (decanoate)	24–72 hr	Unknown	1–6 wk
I.M. (hydro-chloride)	< 1 hr	90–120 min	6–8 hr
SubQ	Unknown	Unknown	Unknown

Half-life: Hydrochloride, 15 hours; decanoate, 7 to 10 days.

ADVERSE REACTIONS

CNS: *extrapyramidal reactions, tardive dyskinesia, pseudoparkinsonism,* ***seizures, neuroleptic malignant syndrome,*** sedation, EEG changes, drowsiness, dizziness.
CV: orthostatic hypotension, tachycardia, ECG changes.
EENT: *blurred vision,* ocular changes, nasal congestion.
GI: *dry mouth, constipation,* increased appetite.
GU: *urine retention,* dark urine, menstrual irregularities, inhibited ejaculation.
Hematologic: ***leukopenia, agranulocytosis, aplastic anemia, thrombocytopenia,*** eosinophilia, hemolytic anemia.
Hepatic: cholestatic jaundice.
Metabolic: weight gain.
Skin: *mild photosensitivity reactions,* allergic reactions.
Other: gynecomastia, galactorrhea.

INTERACTIONS

Drug-drug. *Antacids:* May inhibit absorption of oral phenothiazines. Separate antacid and phenothiazine doses by at least 2 hours.
Anticholinergics: May increase anticholinergic effects. Use together cautiously.
Barbiturates, lithium: May decrease phenothiazine effect and increase neurologic adverse effects. Monitor patient.
Centrally acting antihypertensives: May decrease antihypertensive effect. Monitor blood pressure.
CNS depressants: May increase CNS depression. Use together cautiously.
Drug-herb. *St. John's wort:* May increase risk of photosensitivity reactions. Advise patient to avoid excessive sunlight exposure.
Drug-lifestyle. *Alcohol use:* May increase CNS depression, especially that involving psychomotor skills. Strongly discourage alcohol use.
Sun exposure: May increase risk of photosensitivity reactions. Advise patient to avoid excessive sunlight exposure.

EFFECTS ON LAB TEST RESULTS

- May decrease hemoglobin level and hematocrit.
- May increase eosinophil count and liver function test values. May decrease granulocyte, platelet, and WBC counts.
- May cause false-positive results for amylase, 5-hydroxyindoleacetic acid, urinary porphyrin, and urobilinogen tests and for urine pregnancy tests that use human chorionic gonadotropin.

CONTRAINDICATIONS & CAUTIONS

- Contraindicated in patients hypersensitive to drug and in those with coma, CNS depression, bone marrow suppression or other blood dyscrasia, subcortical damage, or liver damage.
- Use cautiously in elderly or debilitated patients and in those with pheochromocytoma, severe CV disease (may cause sudden drop in blood pressure), peptic ulcer, respiratory disorder, hypocalcemia, seizure disorder (may lower seizure threshold), severe reactions to insulin or electroconvulsive therapy, mitral insufficiency, glaucoma, or prostatic hyperplasia.
- Use cautiously in those exposed to extreme heat or cold (including antipyretic therapy) or phosphorus insecticides.
- Use parenteral form cautiously in patients who have asthma or are allergic to sulfites.

NURSING CONSIDERATIONS

- Prolixin Concentrate and Permitil Concentrate are 10 times more concentrated than Prolixin elixir (5 mg/ml versus 0.5 mg/ml). Check dosage order carefully.
- Oral liquid and parenteral forms can cause contact dermatitis. Wear gloves when preparing solutions, and avoid contact with skin and clothing.

• Protect drug from light. Slight yellowing of injection or concentrate is common and doesn't affect potency. Discard markedly discolored solutions.
• Dilute liquid concentrate with water, fruit juice, milk, or semisolid food just before administration.
• For long-acting form (decanoate), which is an oil preparation, use a dry needle of at least 21G. Allow 24 to 96 hours for onset of action. Note and report to prescriber adverse reactions in patients taking this form.
• Monitor patient for tardive dyskinesia, which may occur after prolonged use. It may not appear until months or years later and may disappear spontaneously or persist for life, despite ending drug.
• ***Alert:*** Watch for signs and symptoms of neuroleptic malignant syndrome (extrapyramidal effects, hyperthermia, autonomic disturbance), which is rare but commonly fatal. It may not be related to length of drug use or type of neuroleptic; more than 60% of affected patients are men.
• Withhold dose and notify prescriber if patient—especially child or pregnant woman—develops signs or symptoms of blood dyscrasia (fever, sore throat, infection, cellulitis, weakness) or extrapyramidal reactions persisting longer than a few hours.
• Don't withdraw drug abruptly unless serious adverse reactions occur.
• Abrupt withdrawal of long-term therapy may cause gastritis, nausea, vomiting, dizziness, tremor, feeling of warmth or cold, diaphoresis, tachycardia, headache, or insomnia.
• ***Alert:*** Prolixin may contain tartrazine.

PATIENT TEACHING
• Warn patient to avoid activities that require alertness and good coordination until effects of drug are known. Drowsiness and dizziness usually subside after first few weeks.
• Warn patient to avoid alcohol while taking drug.
• Tell patient to relieve dry mouth with sugarless gum or hard candy.
• Have patient report signs of urine retention or constipation.
• Advise patient to use sunblock and wear protective clothing to avoid sensitivity to the sun.
• Tell patient that drug may discolor urine.

haloperidol
Apo-Haloperidol†, Haldol, Novo-Peridol†, Peridol†, Serenace‡

haloperidol decanoate
Haldol Decanoate, Haldol LA†

haloperidol lactate
Haldol, Haldol Concentrate, Haloperidol Intensol

Pharmacologic class: phenylbutylpiperadine derivative
Pregnancy risk category C

AVAILABLE FORMS
haloperidol
Tablets: 0.5 mg, 1 mg, 2 mg, 5 mg, 10 mg, 20 mg
haloperidol decanoate
Injection: 50 mg/ml, 100 mg/ml
haloperidol lactate
Injection: 5 mg/ml
Oral concentrate: 2 mg/ml

INDICATIONS & DOSAGES
➤ **Psychotic disorders**
Adults and children older than age 12: Dosage varies for each patient. Initially, 0.5 to 5 mg P.O. b.i.d. or t.i.d. Or, 2 to 5 mg I.M. lactate q 4 to 8 hours, although hourly administration may be needed until control is obtained. Maximum, 100 mg P.O. daily.
Children ages 3 to 12 who weigh 15 to 40 kg (33 to 88 lb): Initially, 0.5 mg P.O. daily divided b.i.d. or t.i.d. May increase dose by 0.5 mg at 5- to 7-day intervals, depending on therapeutic response and patient tolerance. Maintenance dose, 0.05 mg/kg to 0.15 mg/kg P.O. daily given in two to three divided doses. Severely disturbed children may need higher doses.
➤ **Chronic psychosis requiring prolonged therapy**
Adults: 50 to 100 mg I.M. decanoate q 4 weeks.

➤ **Nonpsychotic behavior disorders**
Children ages 3 to 12: 0.05 to 0.075 mg/kg P.O. daily, in two or three divided doses. Maximum, 6 mg daily.
➤ **Tourette syndrome**
Adults: 0.5 to 5 mg P.O. b.i.d., t.i.d., or p.r.n.
Children ages 3 to 12: 0.05 to 0.075 mg/kg P.O. daily, in two or three divided doses.
Elderly patients: 0.5 to 2 mg P.O. b.i.d. or t.i.d.; increase gradually, p.r.n.
Adjust-a-dose: For debilitated patients, initially, 0.5 to 2 mg P.O. b.i.d. or t.i.d.; increase gradually, p.r.n.
➤ **Delirium ♦**
Adults: 1 to 2 mg I.V. lactate q 2 to 4 hours. Severely agitated patients may require higher doses.
Elderly patients: 0.25 to 0.5 mg I.V. q 4 hours.

I.V. ADMINISTRATION

- Only the lactate form can be given I.V.
- Monitor patient receiving single doses higher than 50 mg or total daily doses greater than 500 mg closely for prolonged QTc interval and torsades de pointes.
- Store at controlled room temperature, and protect from light.

INCOMPATIBILITIES

Allopurinol, amphotericin B cholesteryl sulfate complex, benztropine, cefepime, diphenhydramine, fluconazole, foscarnet, heparin, hydromorphone, hydroxyzine, ketorolac, morphine, nitroprusside sodium, piperacillin and tazobactam sodium, sargramostim

ACTION

A butyrophenone that probably exerts antipsychotic effects by blocking postsynaptic dopamine receptors in the brain.

Route	Onset	Peak	Duration
P.O.	Unknown	3–6 hr	Unknown
I.V.	Unknown	Unknown	Unknown
I.M. (decanoate)	Unknown	3–9 days	Unknown
I.M. (lactate)	Unknown	10–20 min	Unknown

Half-life: P.O., 24 hours; I.M., 21 hours.

ADVERSE REACTIONS

CNS: *severe extrapyramidal reactions, tardive dyskinesia,* ***neuroleptic malignant syndrome, seizures,*** sedation, drowsiness, lethargy, headache, insomnia, confusion, vertigo.
CV: ***torsades de pointes with I.V. use*** , tachycardia, hypotension, hypertension, ECG changes.
EENT: blurred vision.
GI: dry mouth, anorexia, constipation, diarrhea, nausea, vomiting, dyspepsia.
GU: urine retention, menstrual irregularities, priapism.
Hematologic: ***leukopenia,*** leukocytosis.
Hepatic: jaundice.
Skin: rash, other skin reactions, diaphoresis.
Other: gynecomastia.

INTERACTIONS

Drug-drug. *Anticholinergics:* May increase anticholinergic effects and glaucoma. Use together cautiously.
Azole antifungals, buspirone, macrolides: May increase haloperidol level. Monitor patient for increased adverse reactions; haloperidol dose may need to be adjusted.
Carbamazepine: May decrease haloperidol level. Monitor patient.
CNS depressants: May increase CNS depression. Use together cautiously.
Lithium: May cause lethargy and confusion after high doses. Monitor patient.
Methyldopa: May cause dementia. Monitor patient closely.
Rifampin: May decrease haloperidol level. Monitor patient for clinical effect.
Drug-lifestyle. *Alcohol use:* May increase CNS depression. Discourage use together.

EFFECTS ON LAB TEST RESULTS

- May increase liver function test values. May increase or decrease WBC count.

CONTRAINDICATIONS & CAUTIONS

- Contraindicated in patients hypersensitive to drug and in those with parkinsonism, coma, or CNS depression.
- Use cautiously in elderly and debilitated patients; in patients with history of seizures or EEG abnormalities, severe CV disorders, allergies, glaucoma, or urine retention; and in those taking anticonvul-

sants, anticoagulants, antiparkinsonians, or lithium.

NURSING CONSIDERATIONS

- Protect drug from light. Slight yellowing of injection or concentrate is common and doesn't affect potency. Discard very discolored solutions.
- When switching from tablets to decanoate injection, give 10 to 15 times the oral dose once a month (maximum 100 mg).
- Dilute oral dose with water or a beverage, such as orange juice, apple juice, tomato juice, or cola, immediately before administration.
- ***Alert:*** Don't give decanoate form I.V.
- Monitor patient for tardive dyskinesia, which may occur after prolonged use. It may not appear until months or years later and may disappear spontaneously or persist for life, despite ending drug.
- ***Alert:*** Watch for signs and symptoms of neuroleptic malignant syndrome (extrapyramidal effects, hyperthermia, autonomic disturbance), which is rare but commonly fatal.
- Don't withdraw drug abruptly unless required by severe adverse reactions.
- ***Alert:*** Haldol may contain tartrazine.
- ***Look alike–sound alike:*** Don't confuse Haldol with Halcion or Halog.

PATIENT TEACHING

- Although drug is the least sedating of the antipsychotics, warn patient to avoid activities that require alertness and good coordination until effects of drug are known. Drowsiness and dizziness usually subside after a few weeks.
- Warn patient to avoid alcohol during therapy.
- Tell patient to relieve dry mouth with sugarless gum or hard candy.

---

loxapine succinate

Loxitane

Pharmacologic class: dibenzapine derivative

Pregnancy risk category NR

AVAILABLE FORMS

Capsules: 5 mg, 10 mg, 25 mg, 50 mg

INDICATIONS & DOSAGES

➤ Psychotic disorders

Adults: 10 mg P.O. b.i.d. to q.i.d., rapidly increasing to 60 to 100 mg P.O. daily for most patients; dosage varies.

Elderly patients: Initially, 5 mg P.O. b.i.d. Adjust dosage as needed and as tolerated.

ACTION

Unknown. A dibenzoxazepine that probably exerts antipsychotic effects by blocking postsynaptic dopamine receptors in the brain.

Route	Onset	Peak	Duration
P.O.	30 min	90 min–3 hr	12 hr

Half-life: 8 hours.

ADVERSE REACTIONS

CNS: *extrapyramidal reactions, sedation, tardive dyskinesia,* ***neuroleptic malignant syndrome, seizures,*** drowsiness, numbness, confusion, syncope, pseudoparkinsonism, EEG changes, dizziness.
CV: orthostatic hypotension, tachycardia, ECG changes, hypertension.
EENT: *blurred vision,* nasal congestion.
GI: *dry mouth, constipation,* nausea, vomiting, paralytic ileus.
GU: *urine retention,* menstrual irregularities.
Hematologic: ***leukopenia, agranulocytosis, thrombocytopenia.***
Hepatic: jaundice.
Metabolic: weight gain.
Skin: allergic reactions, rash, pruritus.
Other: gynecomastia, galactorrhea.

INTERACTIONS

Drug-drug. *Anticholinergics:* May increase anticholinergic effect. Use together cautiously.
CNS depressants: May increase CNS depression. Use together cautiously.
Epinephrine: May inhibit vasopressor effect of epinephrine. Avoid using together.
Drug-lifestyle. *Alcohol use:* May increase CNS depression. Discourage use together.

EFFECTS ON LAB TEST RESULTS

- May increase liver function test values. May decrease WBC, granulocyte, and platelet counts.

• May cause false-positive results for urinary porphyrin, urobilinogen, amylase, and 5-hydroxyindoleacetic acid tests and for urine pregnancy tests that use human chorionic gonadotropin.

CONTRAINDICATIONS & CAUTIONS
• Contraindicated in patients hypersensitive to dibenzapines, in those in a coma, and in those with severe CNS depression or drug-induced depressed states.
• Use with caution in patients with seizure disorder, CV disorder, glaucoma, or history of urine retention.

NURSING CONSIDERATIONS
• Obtain baseline blood pressure measurements before starting therapy and monitor pressure regularly.
• Monitor patient for tardive dyskinesia, which may occur after prolonged use. It may not appear until months or years later and may disappear spontaneously or persist for life, despite ending drug.
• ***Alert:*** Watch for evidence of neuroleptic malignant syndrome (extrapyramidal effects, hyperthermia, autonomic disturbance), a rare but deadly disorder.

PATIENT TEACHING
• Warn patient to avoid activities that require alertness and good coordination until effects of drug are known. Drowsiness and dizziness usually subside after first few weeks.
• Advise patient to report bruising, fever, or sore throat immediately.
• Tell patient to avoid alcohol while taking drug.
• Advise patient to get up slowly to avoid dizziness upon standing quickly.
• Tell patient to relieve dry mouth with sugarless gum or hard candy.
• Recommend periodic eye examinations.

olanzapine
Zyprexa, Zyprexa Zydis

Pharmacologic class: dibenzapine derivative
Pregnancy risk category C

AVAILABLE FORMS
Injection: 10 mg
Tablets: 2.5 mg, 5 mg, 7.5 mg, 10 mg, 15 mg, 20 mg
Tablets (orally disintegrating): 5 mg, 10 mg, 15 mg, 20 mg

INDICATIONS & DOSAGES
➤ **Schizophrenia**
Adults: Initially, 5 to 10 mg P.O. once daily with the goal to be at 10 mg daily within several days of starting therapy. Adjust dose in 5-mg increments at intervals of 1 week or more. Most patients respond to 10 to 15 mg daily. Safety of dosages greater than 20 mg daily hasn't been established.
➤ **Short-term treatment of acute manic episodes linked to bipolar I disorder**
Adults: Initially, 10 to 15 mg P.O. daily. Adjust dosage p.r.n. in 5-mg daily increments at intervals of 24 hours or more. Maximum, 20 mg P.O. daily. Duration of treatment is 3 to 4 weeks.
➤ **Short-term treatment, with lithium or valproate, of acute manic episodes linked to bipolar I disorder**
Adults: 10 mg P.O. once daily. Dosage range is 5 to 20 mg daily. Duration of treatment is 6 weeks.
➤ **Long-term treatment of bipolar I disorder**
Adults: 5 to 20 mg P.O. daily.
➤ **Adjunct to lithium or valproate to treat bipolar mania**
Adults: 10 mg P.O. daily. Usual range 5 to 20 mg daily.
Adjust-a-dose: In elderly or debilitated patients, those predisposed to hypotensive reactions, patients who may metabolize olanzapine more slowly than usual (nonsmoking women older than age 65) or may be more pharmacodynamically sensitive to olanzapine, initially, 5 mg P.O. Increase dose cautiously.
➤ **Agitation caused by schizophrenia and bipolar I mania**
Adults: 10 mg I.M. (range 2.5 to 10 mg). Subsequent doses of up to 10 mg may be given 2 hours after the first dose or 4 hours after the second dose, up to 30 mg I.M. daily. If maintenance therapy is required, convert patient to 5 to 20 mg P.O. daily.

Adjust-a-dose: In elderly patients, give 5 mg I.M. In debilitated patients, in those predisposed to hypotension, and in patients sensitive to effects of drug, give 2.5 mg I.M.

ACTION

May block dopamine and 5-HT_2 receptors.

Route	Onset	Peak	Duration
P.O.	Unknown	6 hr	Unknown
I.M.	Rapid	15–45 min	Unknown

Half-life: 21 to 54 hours.

ADVERSE REACTIONS

CNS: *somnolence, insomnia, parkinsonism, dizziness,* ***neuroleptic malignant syndrome, suicide attempt,*** abnormal gait, asthenia, personality disorder, akathisia, tremor, articulation impairment, tardive dyskinesia, fever, asthenia, somnolence, dizziness, tremor, parkinsonism, akathisia, extrapyramidal events (I.M.).
CV: orthostatic hypotension, tachycardia, chest pain, hypertension, ecchymosis, peripheral edema, hypotension (I.M.).
EENT: amblyopia, rhinitis, pharyngitis, conjunctivitis.
GI: *constipation, dry mouth, dyspepsia,* increased appetite, increased salivation, vomiting, thirst.
GU: hematuria, metrorrhagia, urinary incontinence, urinary tract infection, amenorrhea, vaginitis.
Hematologic: ***leukopenia.***
Metabolic: *hyperglycemia,* weight gain.
Musculoskeletal: joint pain, extremity pain, back pain, neck rigidity, twitching, hypertonia.
Respiratory: increased cough, dyspnea.
Skin: sweating, injection site pain (I.M.).
Other: flulike syndrome, injury.

INTERACTIONS

Drug-drug. *Antihypertensives:* May potentiate hypotensive effects. Monitor blood pressure closely.
Carbamazepine, omeprazole, rifampin: May increase clearance of olanzapine. Monitor patient.
Ciprofloxacin: May increase olanzapine level. Monitor patient for increased adverse effects.
Diazepam: May increase CNS effects. Monitor patient.
Dopamine agonists, levodopa: May cause antagonized activity of these drugs. Monitor patient.
Fluoxetine: May increase olanzapine level. Use together cautiously.
Fluvoxamine: May increase olanzapine level. May need to reduce olanzapine dose.
Drug-herb. *St. John's wort:* May decrease drug level. Discourage use together.
Drug-lifestyle. *Alcohol use:* May increase CNS effects. Discourage use together.
Smoking: May increase drug clearance. Urge patient to quit smoking.

EFFECTS ON LAB TEST RESULTS

- May increase AST, ALT, GGT, CK, triglyceride, and prolactin levels.
- May increase eosinophil count. May decrease WBC count.

CONTRAINDICATIONS & CAUTIONS

- Contraindicated in patients hypersensitive to drug.
- Use cautiously in patients with heart disease, cerebrovascular disease, conditions that predispose patient to hypotension, history of seizures or conditions that might lower the seizure threshold, and hepatic impairment.
- Use cautiously in elderly patients, those with a history of paralytic ileus, and those at risk for aspiration pneumonia, prostatic hyperplasia, or angle-closure glaucoma.

NURSING CONSIDERATIONS

- Inspect I.M. solution for particulate matter and discoloration before administration.
- To reconstitute I.M. injection, dissolve contents of one vial with 2.1 ml of sterile water for injection to yield a clear yellow 5 mg/ml solution. Store at room temperature and give within 1 hour of reconstitution. Discard any unused solution.
- Monitor patient for abnormal body temperature regulation, especially if he exercises, is exposed to extreme heat, takes anticholinergics, or is dehydrated.

- Obtain baseline and periodic liver function test results.
- Monitor patient for weight gain.
- ***Alert:*** Watch for evidence of neuroleptic malignant syndrome (hyperpyrexia, muscle rigidity, altered mental status, autonomic instability), which is rare but commonly fatal. Stop drug immediately; monitor and treat patient as needed.
- ***Alert:*** Drug may cause hyperglycemia. Monitor patients with diabetes regularly. In patients with risk factors for diabetes, obtain fasting blood glucose test results at baseline and periodically.
- ***Alert:*** Monitor patient for symptoms of metabolic syndrome (significant weight gain and increased BMI, hypertension, hyperglycemia, hypercholesterolemia, and hypertriglyceridemia).
- Monitor patient for tardive dyskinesia, which may occur after prolonged use. It may not appear until months or years later and may disappear spontaneously or persist for life, despite stopping drug.
- Periodically reevaluate the long-term usefulness of olanzapine.
- Drug may increase risk of stroke and death in elderly patients with dementia. Olanzapine isn't approved to treat patients with dementia-related psychosis.
- A patient who feels dizzy or drowsy after an I.M. injection should remain recumbent until he can be assessed for orthostatic hypotension and bradycardia. He should rest until the feeling passes.
- ***Look alike–sound alike:*** Don't confuse olanzapine with olsalazine or Zyprexa with Zyrtec.

PATIENT TEACHING

- Warn patient to avoid hazardous tasks until full effects of drug are known.
- Warn patient against exposure to extreme heat; drug may impair body's ability to reduce temperature.
- Inform patient that he may gain weight.
- Advise patient to avoid alcohol.
- Tell patient to rise slowly to avoid dizziness upon standing up quickly.
- Inform patient that orally disintegrating tablets contain phenylalanine.
- Drug may be taken without regard to food.
- Urge woman of childbearing age to notify prescriber if she becomes pregnant or plans or suspects pregnancy. Tell her not to breast-feed during therapy.

perphenazine

Apo-Perphenazine†, Trilafon

Pharmacologic class: phenothiazine
Pregnancy risk category C

AVAILABLE FORMS

Injection: 5 mg/ml
Oral concentrate: 16 mg/5 ml
Syrup: 2 mg/5 ml†
Tablets: 2 mg, 4 mg, 8 mg, 16 mg

INDICATIONS & DOSAGES

➤ **Psychosis in nonhospitalized patients**

Adults and children older than age 12: Initially, 4 to 8 mg P.O. t.i.d.; reduce as soon as possible to minimum effective dose.

➤ **Psychosis in hospitalized patients**

Adults and children older than age 12: Initially, 8 to 16 mg P.O. b.i.d., t.i.d., or q.i.d.; increase to 64 mg daily, p.r.n. Or, 5 to 10 mg I.M. q 6 hours, p.r.n. Maximum dose, 30 mg.

➤ **Severe nausea and vomiting**

Adults: 8 to 16 mg P.O. daily in divided doses to maximum of 24 mg. Or, 5 to 10 mg I.M., p.r.n. May be given I.V., diluted to 0.5 mg/ml with saline solution. Dose given I.V. shouldn't exceed 5 mg.

I.V. ADMINISTRATION

- I.V. use is intended for recumbent hospitalized patients only.
- For fractional injection, dilute to a concentration of 0.5 mg/ml with normal saline solution and give no more than 1 mg per injection at not less than 1- to 2-minute intervals.
- Drug may also be given by slow infusion.
- Monitor blood pressure and pulse continuously during infusion.

INCOMPATIBILITIES

Cefoperazone, midazolam hydrochloride, pentobarbital sodium.

ACTION

May exert antipsychotic effects by blocking postsynaptic dopamine receptors in the brain.

Route	Onset	Peak	Duration
P.O., I.V., I.M.	Unknown	Unknown	Unknown

Half-life: 9 to 12 hours.

ADVERSE REACTIONS

CNS: *extrapyramidal reactions, tardive dyskinesia,* ***seizures, neuroleptic malignant syndrome,*** sedation, pseudoparkinsonism, dizziness, drowsiness.
CV: *orthostatic hypotension,* tachycardia, ECG changes.
EENT: *blurred vision,* ocular changes, nasal congestion.
GI: *dry mouth, constipation,* nausea, vomiting, diarrhea.
GU: *urine retention,* dark urine, menstrual irregularities, inhibited ejaculation.
Hematologic: ***leukopenia, agranulocytosis, thrombocytopenia,*** eosinophilia, hemolytic anemia.
Hepatic: cholestatic jaundice.
Metabolic: weight gain.
Skin: *mild photosensitivity reactions,* allergic reactions, pain at I.M. injection site, sterile abscess.
Other: gynecomastia.

INTERACTIONS

Drug-drug. *Antacids:* May inhibit absorption of oral phenothiazines. Separate antacid and phenothiazine doses by at least 2 hours.
Barbiturates: May decrease phenothiazine effect. Monitor patient.
CNS depressants: May increase CNS depression. Use together cautiously.
Fluoxetine, paroxetine, sertraline, tricyclic antidepressants: May increase phenothiazine level. Monitor patient for increased adverse effects.
Lithium: May increase neurologic adverse effects. Monitor patient closely.
Drug-herb. *St. John's wort:* May cause photosensitivity reactions. Advise patient to avoid excessive sunlight exposure.
Drug-lifestyle. *Alcohol use:* May increase CNS depression, particularly psychomotor skills. Strongly discourage alcohol use.
Sun exposure: May increase risk of photosensitivity reactions. Advise patient to avoid excessive sunlight exposure.

EFFECTS ON LAB TEST RESULTS

- May decrease hemoglobin level and hematocrit.
- May increase liver function test values and eosinophil count. May decrease WBC, granulocyte, and platelet counts.
- May cause false-positive results for urinary porphyrin, urobilinogen, amylase, and 5-hydroxyindoleacetic acid tests and for urine pregnancy tests that use human chorionic gonadotropin.

CONTRAINDICATIONS & CAUTIONS

- Contraindicated in patients hypersensitive to drug and in those with CNS depression, blood dyscrasia, bone marrow depression, liver damage, or subcortical damage; also contraindicated in those experiencing coma or receiving large doses of CNS depressants.
- Use cautiously in elderly or debilitated patients and in those taking other CNS depressants or anticholinergics.
- Use cautiously in patients with alcohol withdrawal, psychotic depression, suicidal tendency, severe adverse reactions to other phenothiazines, renal impairment, CV disease, or respiratory disorders.

NURSING CONSIDERATIONS

- Obtain baseline blood pressure measurements before starting therapy and monitor pressure regularly. Watch for orthostatic hypotension, especially with parenteral administration. Keep patient supine for 1 hour after giving drug; tell him to change positions slowly.
- Protect drug from light. Slight yellowing of injection or concentrate is common and doesn't affect potency. Discard markedly discolored solutions.
- Wear gloves when preparing liquid forms to prevent contact dermatitis; keep drug away from skin and clothes.
- Dilute liquid concentrate with fruit juice, milk, carbonated beverage, or semisolid food just before giving. Don't use colas, black coffee, grape juice, apple juice, or tea because turbidity or precipitation may result.

• Give by deep I.M. injection only in upper outer quadrant of buttocks. Massage slowly afterward to prevent sterile abscess. Injection may sting.
• Monitor patient for tardive dyskinesia, which may occur after prolonged use. It may not appear until months or years later and may disappear spontaneously or persist for life, despite ending drug.
• **Alert:** Watch for evidence of neuroleptic malignant syndrome (extrapyramidal effects, hyperthermia, autonomic disturbance), which is rare but deadly.
• Monitor therapy with weekly bilirubin tests during first month, periodic blood tests (CBCs and liver function tests), and ophthalmic tests (long-term use).
• Withhold dose and notify prescriber if jaundice, symptoms of blood dyscrasia (fever, sore throat, infection, cellulitis, weakness), or persistent extrapyramidal reactions (longer than a few hours) develop.
• Don't withdraw drug abruptly unless severe adverse reactions occur.
• After abrupt withdrawal of long-term therapy, gastritis, nausea, vomiting, dizziness, tremor, feeling of warmth or cold, diaphoresis, tachycardia, headache, or insomnia may occur.

PATIENT TEACHING

• Tell patient which beverages he may use to dilute oral concentrate.
• Warn patient to avoid activities that require alertness or good coordination until effects of drug are known. Drowsiness and dizziness usually subside after a few weeks.
• Tell patient to avoid alcohol while taking drug.
• Advise patient to report signs of urine retention or constipation.
• Tell patient to use sunblock and wear protective clothing to avoid oversensitivity to the sun.
• Advise patient to relieve dry mouth with sugarless gum or hard candy.

quetiapine fumarate
Seroquel

Pharmacologic class: dibenzapine derivative
Pregnancy risk category C

AVAILABLE FORMS

Tablets: 25 mg, 100 mg, 200 mg, 300 mg

INDICATIONS & DOSAGES

✱ ***NEW INDICATION:*** **Depression associated with bipolar disorder**
Adults: Give drug P.O. once daily at bedtime to reach 300 mg/day by day 4. Day 1, give 50 mg; day 2, give 100 mg; day 3, give 200 mg; day 4, give 300 mg.

➤ **To manage signs and symptoms of psychotic disorders**
Adults: Initially, 25 mg P.O. b.i.d., with increases in increments of 25 to 50 mg b.i.d. or t.i.d. on days 2 and 3, as tolerated. Target range is 300 to 400 mg daily divided into two or three doses by day 4. Further dosage adjustments, if indicated, should occur at intervals of not less than 2 days. Dosage can be increased or decreased by 25 to 50 mg b.i.d. Antipsychotic effect generally occurs at 150 to 750 mg daily. Safety of dosages over 800 mg daily hasn't been evaluated.
Elderly patients: Give lower dosages, adjust more slowly, and monitor patient carefully in first dosing period.

➤ **Monotherapy and adjunct therapy with lithium or divalproex for the short-term treatment of acute manic episodes associated with bipolar I disorder**
Adults: Initially, 50 mg P.O. b.i.d. Increase dosage in increments of 100 mg daily in two divided doses up to 200 mg P.O. b.i.d. on day 4. May increase dosage in increments no greater than 200 mg daily up to 800 mg daily by day 6. Usual dose is 400 to 800 mg daily.
Elderly patients: Give lower dosages, adjust more slowly, and monitor patient carefully in first dosing period.
Adjust-a-dose: For debilitated patients and those with hypotension, consider lower dosages and slower adjustment. In patients with hepatic impairment, initial dose is 25 mg daily. Increase daily in

increments of 25 to 50 mg daily to an effective dose

ACTION

Unknown. A dibenzothiazepine derivative that may block dopamine receptors and serotonin 5-HT_2 receptors in the brain.

Route	Onset	Peak	Duration
P.O.	Unknown	1½ hr	Unknown

Half-life: 6 hours.

ADVERSE REACTIONS

CNS: *dizziness, headache, somnolence,* ***neuroleptic malignant syndrome, seizures,*** hypertonia, dysarthria, asthenia.
CV: orthostatic hypotension, tachycardia, palpitations, peripheral edema.
EENT: ear pain, pharyngitis, rhinitis.
GI: dry mouth, dyspepsia, abdominal pain, constipation, anorexia.
Hematologic: ***leukopenia.***
Metabolic: *weight gain,* hyperglycemia.
Musculoskeletal: back pain.
Respiratory: increased cough, dyspnea.
Skin: rash, diaphoresis.
Other: flulike syndrome.

INTERACTIONS

Drug-drug. *Antihypertensives:* May increase effects of antihypertensives. Monitor blood pressure.
Carbamazepine, glucocorticoids, phenobarbital, phenytoin, rifampin, thioridazine: May increase quetiapine clearance. May need to adjust quetiapine dosage.
CNS depressants: May increase CNS effects. Use together cautiously.
Dopamine agonists, levodopa: May antagonize the effects of these drugs. Monitor patient.
Erythromycin, fluconazole, itraconazole, ketoconazole: May decrease quetiapine clearance. Use together cautiously.
Lorazepam: May decrease lorazepam clearance. Monitor patient for increased CNS effects.
Drug-lifestyle. *Alcohol use:* May increase CNS effects. Discourage use together.

EFFECTS ON LAB TEST RESULTS

- May increase liver enzyme, cholesterol, triglyceride, and glucose levels. May decrease T_4 and thyroid-stimulating hormone levels.
- May decrease WBC count.

CONTRAINDICATIONS & CAUTIONS

- Contraindicated in patients hypersensitive to drug or its ingredients.
- Use cautiously in patients with CV disease, cerebrovascular disease, conditions that predispose to hypotension, a history of seizures or conditions that lower the seizure threshold, and conditions in which core body temperature may be elevated.
- Use cautiously in patients at risk for aspiration pneumonia.

NURSING CONSIDERATIONS

- Dispense lowest appropriate quantity of drug to reduce risk of overdose.
- ***Alert:*** Drug isn't indicated for use in elderly patients with dementia-related psychosis because of increased risk of death from CV disease or infection.
- ***Alert:*** Watch for evidence of neuroleptic malignant syndrome (extrapyramidal effects, hyperthermia, autonomic disturbance), which is rare but deadly.
- Monitor patient for tardive dyskinesia, which may occur after prolonged use. It may not appear until months or years later and may disappear spontaneously or persist for life, despite ending drug.
- Hyperglycemia may occur in patients taking drug. Monitor patients with diabetes regularly.
- Monitor patient for weight gain.
- ***Alert:*** Monitor patient for symptoms of metabolic syndrome (significant weight gain and increased BMI, hypertension, hyperglycemia, hypercholesterolemia, and hypertriglyceridemia).
- Drug use may cause cataract formation. Obtain baseline ophthalmologic examination and reassess every 6 months.

PATIENT TEACHING

- Advise patient about risk of dizziness upon standing up quickly. The risk is greatest during the 3- to 5-day period of first dosage adjustment, when resuming treatment, and when increasing dosages.
- Tell patient to avoid becoming overheated or dehydrated.
- Warn patient to avoid activities that require mental alertness until effects of drug

are known, especially during first dosage adjustment or dosage increases.
- Remind patient to have an eye examination at start of therapy and every 6 months during therapy to check for cataracts.
- Tell patient to notify prescriber about other prescription or over-the-counter drugs he's taking or plans to take.
- Tell woman of childbearing age to notify prescriber about planned, suspected, or known pregnancy.
- Advise her not to breast-feed during therapy.
- Advise patient to avoid alcohol while taking drug.
- Tell patient to take drug with or without food.

risperidone

Risperdal✐, Risperdal Consta, Risperdal M-Tab✐

Pharmacologic class: benzisoxazole derivative
Pregnancy risk category C

AVAILABLE FORMS

Injection: 25 mg, 37.5 mg, 50 mg
Solution: 1 mg/ml
Tablets: 0.25 mg, 0.5 mg, 1 mg, 2 mg, 3 mg, 4 mg
Tablets (orally disintegrating): 0.5 mg, 1 mg, 2 mg, 3 mg, 4 mg

INDICATIONS & DOSAGES

➤ Short-term (6 to 8 weeks) treatment of schizophrenia
Adults: Initially, 1 mg P.O. b.i.d. Increase by 1 mg b.i.d. on days 2 and 3 of treatment to a target dose of 3 mg b.i.d. Or, 1 mg P.O. on day 1, increase to 2 mg once daily on day 2, and 4 mg once daily on day 3. Wait at least 1 week before adjusting dosage further. Adjust doses by 1 to 2 mg. Maximum, 8 mg daily.

➤ To delay relapse in schizophrenia therapy lasting 1 to 2 years
Adults: Initially, 1 mg P.O. on day 1, increase to 2 mg once daily on day 2, and 4 mg once daily on day 3. Dosage range is 2 to 8 mg daily.

➤ Monotherapy or combination therapy with lithium or valproate for 3-week treatment of acute manic or mixed episodes from bipolar I disorder
Adults: 2 to 3 mg P.O. once daily. Adjust dose by 1 mg daily. Dosage range is 1 to 6 mg daily.
Adjust-a-dose: In elderly or debilitated patients, hypotensive patients, or those with severe renal or hepatic impairment, start with 0.5 mg P.O. b.i.d. Increase dosage by 0.5 mg b.i.d. Increase in dosages above 1.5 mg b.i.d. should occur at least 1 week apart. Subsequent switches to once-daily dosing may be made after patient is on a twice-daily regimen for 2 to 3 days at the target dose.

✷*NEW INDICATION:* Irritability, including aggression, self-injury, and temper tantrums, associated with an autistic disorder
Adolescents and children age 5 and older who weigh 20 kg (44 lb) or more: Initially, 0.5 mg P.O. once daily or divided b.i.d. After 4 days, increase dose to 1 mg. Increase dosage further in 0.5 mg increments at intervals of at least 2 weeks.
Children age 5 and older who weigh less than 20 kg: Initially, 0.25 mg P.O. once daily or divided b.i.d. After 4 days, increase dose to 0.5 mg. Increase dosage further in 0.25 mg increments at intervals of at least 2 weeks. Increase cautiously in children who weigh less than 15 kg (33 lb).

➤ 12-week therapy for schizophrenia
Adults: Establish tolerance to oral risperidone before giving I.M. Give 25 mg deep I.M. gluteal injection q 2 weeks; alternating injections between the two buttocks. Adjust dose no sooner than q 4 weeks. Maximum, 50 mg I.M. q 2 weeks. Continue oral antipsychotic for 3 weeks after first I.M. injection. Then stop oral therapy.

ACTION

Blocks dopamine and 5-HT_2 receptors in the brain.

Route	Onset	Peak	Duration
P.O.	Unknown	1 hr	Unknown
I.M.	3 wk	4–6 wk	7 wk

Half-life: 3 to 20 hours.

ADVERSE REACTIONS

CNS: *akathisia, somnolence, dystonia, headache, insomnia, agitation, anxiety, pain, parkinsonism,* ***neuroleptic malignant syndrome, suicide attempt,*** dizziness, fever, hallucination, mania, impaired concentration, abnormal thinking and dreaming, tremor, hypoesthesia, fatigue, depression, nervousness.
CV: tachycardia, chest pain, orthostatic hypotension, peripheral edema, syncope, hypertension.
EENT: *rhinitis,* sinusitis, pharyngitis, abnormal vision, ear disorder (I.M.).
GI: *constipation, nausea, vomiting, dyspepsia, abdominal pain,* anorexia, dry mouth, increased saliva, diarrhea.
GU: urinary incontinence, increased urination, abnormal orgasm, vaginal dryness.
Metabolic: *weight gain,* ***hyperglycemia,*** weight loss.
Musculoskeletal: arthralgia, back pain, leg pain, myalgia.
Respiratory: coughing, dyspnea, upper respiratory infection.
Skin: rash, dry skin, photosensitivity, acne, injection site pain (I.M.).
Other: tooth disorder, toothache, injury, decreased libido.

INTERACTIONS

Drug-drug. *Antihypertensives:* May enhance hypotensive effects. Monitor blood pressure.
Carbamazepine: May increase risperidone clearance and decrease effectiveness. Monitor patient closely.
Clozapine: May decrease risperidone clearance, increasing toxicity. Monitor patient closely.
CNS depressants: May cause additive CNS depression. Use together cautiously.
Dopamine agonists, levodopa: May antagonize effects of these drugs. Use together cautiously and monitor patient.
Fluoxetine, paroxetine: May increase the risk of risperidone's adverse effects, including serotonin syndrome. Monitor patient closely and adjust risperidone dose as needed.
Drug-lifestyle. *Alcohol use:* May cause additive CNS depression. Discourage use together.
Sun exposure: May increase risk of photosensitivity reactions. Advise patient to avoid excessive sunlight exposure.

EFFECTS ON LAB TEST RESULTS

- May increase prolactin level. May decrease hemoglobin level and hematocrit.

CONTRAINDICATIONS & CAUTIONS

- Contraindicated in patients hypersensitive to drug and in breast-feeding women.
- Use cautiously in patients with prolonged QT interval, CV disease, cerebrovascular disease, dehydration, hypovolemia, history of seizures, or conditions that could affect metabolism or hemodynamic responses.
- Use cautiously in patients exposed to extreme heat.
- Use caution in patients at risk for aspiration pneumonia.
- Use I.M. injection cautiously in those with hepatic or renal impairment.

NURSING CONSIDERATIONS

- ***Alert:*** Obtain baseline blood pressure measurements before starting therapy, and monitor pressure regularly. Watch for orthostatic hypotension, especially during first dosage adjustment.
- ***Alert:*** Fatal cerebrovascular adverse events (stroke, TIA) may occur in elderly patients with dementia. Drug isn't safe or effective in these patients.
- Monitor patient for tardive dyskinesia, which may occur after prolonged use. It may not appear until months or years later and may disappear spontaneously or persist for life, despite stopping drug.
- ***Alert:*** Watch for evidence of neuroleptic malignant syndrome (extrapyramidal effects, hyperthermia, autonomic disturbance), which is rare but can be fatal.
- Life-threatening hyperglycemia may occur in patients taking atypical antipsychotics. Monitor patients with diabetes regularly.
- ***Alert:*** Monitor patient for symptoms of metabolic syndrome (significant weight gain and increased BMI, hypertension, hyperglycemia, hypercholesterolemia, and hypertriglyceridemia).
- Periodically reevaluate drug's risks and benefits, especially during prolonged use.

• To reconstitute I.M. injection, inject premeasured diluent into vial and shake vigorously for at least 10 seconds. Suspension appears uniform, thick, and milky; particles are visible, but no dry particles remain. Drug should be used immediately, but may be refrigerated up to 6 hours of reconstitution. If more than 2 minutes pass before injection, shake vigorously again. See manufacturer's package insert for more detailed instructions.
• Refrigerate I.M. injection kit and protect it from light. Drug can be stored at temperature less than 77° F (25° C) for no more than 7 days before administration.
• Continue oral therapy for the first 3 weeks of I.M. injection therapy until injections take effect. Then stop oral therapy.
• Phenylalanine contents of orally disintegrating tablets are as follows: 0.5-mg tablet contains 0.14 mg phenylalanine; 1-mg tablet contains 0.28 mg phenylalanine; 2-mg tablet contains 0.56 mg phenylalanine; 3-mg tablet contains 0.63 mg phenylalanine; 4-mg tablet contains 0.84 mg phenylalanine.
• Monitor patient for weight gain.
• ***Look alike–sound alike:*** Don't confuse risperidone with reserpine.

PATIENT TEACHING
• Warn patient to avoid activities that require alertness until effects of drug are known.
• Warn patient to rise slowly, avoid hot showers, and use other precautions to avoid fainting when starting therapy.
• Advise patient to use caution in hot weather to prevent heatstroke.
• Tell patient to take drug with or without food.
• Instruct patient to keep the orally disintegrating tablet in the blister pack until just before taking it. After opening the pack, dissolve the tablet on tongue without cutting or chewing. Peel apart the foil to expose the tablet; don't attempt to push it through the foil.
• Tell patient to use sunblock and wear protective clothing outdoors.
• Advise women not to become pregnant or to breast-feed for 12 weeks after the last I.M. injection.
• Advise patient to avoid alcohol during therapy.

thioridazine hydrochloride

Pharmacologic class: phenothiazine
Pregnancy risk category C

AVAILABLE FORMS
Oral concentrate: 30 mg/ml, 100 mg/ml (3% to 4.2% alcohol)
Tablets: 10 mg, 15 mg, 25 mg, 50 mg, 100 mg, 150 mg, 200 mg

INDICATIONS & DOSAGES
➤ **Schizophrenia in patients who don't respond to treatment with at least two other antipsychotic drugs**
Adults: Initially, 50 to 100 mg P.O. t.i.d., increased gradually to 800 mg daily in divided doses, p.r.n.
Children age 2 to 12: Initially, 0.5 mg/kg daily in divided doses. Increase gradually to optimal therapeutic effect; maximum dose is 3 mg/kg daily.

ACTION
Unknown. A piperidine phenothiazine that probably blocks postsynaptic dopamine receptors in the brain.

Route	Onset	Peak	Duration
P.O.	Unknown	Unknown	Unknown

Half-life: 20 to 40 hours.

ADVERSE REACTIONS
CNS: *tardive dyskinesia, sedation,* ***neuroleptic malignant syndrome,*** EEG changes, dizziness.
CV: *orthostatic hypotension,* ***prolonged QTc interval, torsades de pointes,*** ECG changes, tachycardia.
EENT: *ocular changes, blurred vision,* retinitis pigmentosa.
GI: *dry mouth, constipation,* increased appetite.
GU: *urine retention,* dark urine, menstrual irregularities, inhibited ejaculation.
Hematologic: ***transient leukopenia, agranulocytosis,*** hyperprolactinemia.
Hepatic: cholestatic jaundice.
Metabolic: weight gain.

Skin: *mild photosensitivity reactions,* allergic reactions.
Other: gynecomastia, galactorrhea.

INTERACTIONS

Drug-drug. *Antacids:* May inhibit absorption of oral phenothiazines. Separate dosages by at least 2 hours.
antiarrhythmics (amiodarone, bretylium, disopyramide, dofetilide, procainamide, quinidine, sotalol), duloxetine, fluoxetine, fluvoxamine, paroxetine, pimozide, *pindolol, propranolol, other drugs that inhibit CYP2D6 enzyme,* ***quinolones:*** May inhibit metabolism of thioridazine; may cause arrhythmias resulting from QTc interval prolongation. Use together is contraindicated.
Barbiturates: May decrease phenothiazine effect. Monitor patient.
Centrally acting antihypertensives: May decrease antihypertensive effect. Monitor blood pressure.
Lithium: May decrease phenothiazine effect and increase neurologic adverse effects. Monitor patient closely.
Other CNS depressants: May increase CNS depression. Use together cautiously.
Drug-herb. *St. John's wort:* May cause photosensitivity reactions. Advise patient to avoid excessive sunlight exposure.
Drug-lifestyle. *Alcohol use:* May increase CNS depression, particularly psychomotor skills. Strongly discourage use together.
Sun exposure: May increase risk of photosensitivity reactions. Advise patient to avoid excessive sunlight exposure.

EFFECTS ON LAB TEST RESULTS

- May increase liver enzyme levels.
- May decrease granulocyte and WBC counts.
- May cause false-positive results for urinary porphyrin, urobilinogen, amylase, and 5-hydroxyindoleacetic acid tests and for urine pregnancy tests that use human chorionic gonadotropin.

CONTRAINDICATIONS & CAUTIONS

- Contraindicated in patients hypersensitive to drug and in those with CNS depression, coma, or severe hypertensive or hypotensive cardiac disease.
- Contraindicated in patients taking fluvoxamine, propranolol, pindolol, fluoxetine, drugs that inhibit the CYP2D6 enzyme, or drugs that prolong the QTc interval.
- Contraindicated in patients with reduced levels of CYP2D6 enzyme, those with congenital long QT interval syndrome, or those with history of cardiac arrhythmias.
- Use cautiously in elderly or debilitated patients and in patients with hepatic disease, CV disease, respiratory disorders, hypocalcemia, seizure disorders, or severe reactions to insulin or electroconvulsive therapy.
- Use cautiously in those exposed to extreme heat or cold (including antipyretic therapy) or organophosphate insecticides.

NURSING CONSIDERATIONS

- ***Alert:*** Before therapy, obtain baseline ECG and potassium level. Patients with a QTc interval greater than 450 msec shouldn't receive drug. Patients with a QTc interval greater than 500 msec should stop drug.
- ***Alert:*** Drug isn't used as first-line treatment of schizophrenia because of risk of life-threatening adverse reactions.
- ***Alert:*** Different liquid formulations have different concentrations. Check dosage carefully.
- Prevent contact dermatitis by keeping drug away from skin and clothes. Wear gloves when preparing liquid forms.
- Dilute liquid concentrate with water or fruit juice just before giving.
- Shake suspension well before using.
- Monitor patient for tardive dyskinesia, which may occur after prolonged use. It may not appear until months or years later and may disappear spontaneously or persist for life, despite ending drug.
- ***Alert:*** Watch for evidence of neuroleptic malignant syndrome (extrapyramidal effects, hyperthermia, autonomic disturbance), which is rare but commonly deadly.
- Monitor periodic blood tests (CBCs and liver function tests) and ophthalmic tests (long-term use).
- Withhold dose and notify prescriber if jaundice, blood dyscrasia (fever, sore

throat, infection, cellulitis, weakness), or persistent extrapyramidal reactions develop, especially in children or pregnant women.
- Don't stop drug abruptly unless required by severe adverse reactions.
- After abrupt withdrawal of long-term therapy, gastritis, nausea, vomiting, dizziness, tremor, feeling of warmth or cold, diaphoresis, tachycardia, headache, or insomnia may occur.
- ***Look alike–sound alike:*** Don't confuse thioridazine with Thorazine.

PATIENT TEACHING
- Tell patient to shake suspension before use.
- Warn patient to avoid activities that require alertness until effects of drug are known.
- Tell patient to watch for dizziness when standing quickly. Advise patient to change positions slowly.
- Instruct patient to report symptoms of dizziness, palpitations, or fainting to prescriber.
- Tell patient to avoid alcohol use.
- Have patient report signs of urine retention, constipation, or blurred vision.
- Tell patient that drug may discolor the urine.
- Advise patient to relieve dry mouth with sugarless gum or hard candy.
- Instruct patient to use sunblock and to wear protective clothing outdoors.

thiothixene
Navane

thiothixene hydrochloride
Navane*

Pharmacologic class: thioxanthene
Pregnancy risk category C

AVAILABLE FORMS
thiothixene
Capsules: 1 mg, 2 mg, 5 mg, 10 mg, 20 mg
thiothixene hydrochloride
Oral concentrate: 5 mg/ml*

INDICATIONS & DOSAGES
➤ Mild to moderate psychosis
Adults: Initially, 2 mg P.O. t.i.d. Increased gradually to 15 mg daily, p.r.n.
➤ Severe psychosis
Adults: Initially, 5 mg P.O. b.i.d. Increase gradually to 20 to 30 mg daily, p.r.n. Maximum dose is 60 mg daily.

ACTION
Unknown. A thioxanthene that probably blocks dopamine receptors in the brain.

Route	Onset	Peak	Duration
P.O.	Unknown	Unknown	Unknown

Half-life: 20 to 40 hours.

ADVERSE REACTIONS
CNS: *extrapyramidal reactions, drowsiness, tardive dyskinesia,* ***neuroleptic malignant syndrome,*** restlessness, agitation, insomnia, sedation, EEG changes, pseudoparkinsonism, dizziness.
CV: *hypotension,* tachycardia, ECG changes.
EENT: *blurred vision,* ocular changes, nasal congestion.
GI: *dry mouth, constipation.*
GU: *urine retention,* menstrual irregularities, inhibited ejaculation.
Hematologic: ***agranulocytosis, transient leukopenia,*** leukocytosis.
Hepatic: jaundice.
Metabolic: weight gain.
Skin: *mild photosensitivity reactions,* allergic reactions, exfoliative dermatitis.
Other: gynecomastia.

INTERACTIONS
Drug-drug. *CNS depressants:* May increase CNS depression. Use together cautiously.
Drug-lifestyle. *Alcohol use:* May increase CNS depression. Discourage use together.
Sun exposure: May increase risk of photosensitivity reactions. Advise patient to avoid excessive sunlight exposure.

EFFECTS ON LAB TEST RESULTS
- May increase liver enzyme levels.
- May increase or decrease WBC counts. May decrease granulocyte counts.
- May cause false-positive results for urinary porphyrin, urobilinogen, amylase,

and 5-hydroxyindoleacetic acid tests and for urine pregnancy tests that use human chorionic gonadotropin.

CONTRAINDICATIONS & CAUTIONS

- Contraindicated in patients hypersensitive to drug and in those with CNS depression, circulatory collapse, coma, or blood dyscrasia.
- Use with caution in patients with history of seizure disorder and in those undergoing alcohol withdrawal.
- Use cautiously in elderly or debilitated patients and in those with CV disease (may cause sudden drop in blood pressure), hepatic disease, heat exposure, glaucoma, or prostatic hyperplasia.

NURSING CONSIDERATIONS

- Prevent contact dermatitis by keeping drug off skin and clothes. Wear gloves when preparing liquid forms.
- Dilute liquid concentrate with fruit juice, milk, or semisolid food just before giving.
- Slight yellowing of injection or concentrate is common and doesn't affect potency. Discard markedly discolored solutions.
- Monitor patient for tardive dyskinesia, which may occur after prolonged use; it may not appear until months or years later, and may disappear spontaneously or persist for life, despite stopping drug.
- ***Alert:*** Watch for evidence of neuroleptic malignant syndrome (extrapyramidal effects, hyperthermia, autonomic disturbance), which is rare but deadly.
- Monitor periodic CBCs, liver function tests, and renal function tests; and ophthalmic tests for long-term use.
- Watch for orthostatic hypotension. Keep patient supine for 1 hour after drug administration, and tell him to change positions slowly.
- Withhold dose and notify prescriber if jaundice, blood dyscrasia (fever, sore throat, infection, cellulitis, weakness), or persistent extrapyramidal reactions develop, especially in pregnant women.
- Don't withdraw drug abruptly unless severe adverse reactions occur.
- After abrupt withdrawal of long-term therapy, gastritis, nausea, vomiting, dizziness, tremor, feeling of warmth or cold, diaphoresis, tachycardia, headache, or insomnia may occur.
- ***Look alike–sound alike:*** Don't confuse Navane with Nubain or Norvasc.

PATIENT TEACHING

- Warn patient to avoid activities that require alertness until effects of drug are known.
- Tell patient to watch for dizziness upon standing quickly. Advise him to change positions slowly.
- Instruct patient to dilute liquid appropriately.
- Tell patient to avoid alcohol use during therapy.
- Have patient report signs of urine retention, constipation, or blurred vision.
- Instruct patient to use sunblock and to wear protective clothing outdoors.

trifluoperazine hydrochloride

Apo-Trifluoperazine†, Novo-Trifluzine†, PMS Trifluoperazine†

Pharmacologic class: phenothiazine
Pregnancy risk category NR

AVAILABLE FORMS

Tablets (regular and film-coated): 1 mg, 2 mg, 5 mg, 10 mg

INDICATIONS & DOSAGES

➤ Anxiety states

Adults: 1 to 2 mg P.O. b.i.d. Maximum, 6 mg daily. Don't give drug for longer than 12 weeks for anxiety.

➤ Schizophrenia, other psychotic disorders

Adults: In outpatients, 1 to 2 mg P.O. b.i.d. In hospitalized patients, 2 to 5 mg P.O. b.i.d., gradually increased until therapeutic response occurs. Most patients respond to 15 to 20 mg P.O. daily, although some may need 40 mg daily or more.
Children ages 6 to 12: For hospitalized or closely supervised patients, 1 mg P.O. daily or b.i.d.; may increase gradually to 15 mg daily, if needed.

ACTION

Unknown. A piperazine phenothiazine that probably blocks dopamine receptors in the brain.

Route	Onset	Peak	Duration
P.O.	Unknown	Unknown	Unknown

Half-life: 20 to 40 hours.

ADVERSE REACTIONS

CNS: *extrapyramidal reactions, tardive dyskinesia,* ***neuroleptic malignant syndrome,*** pseudoparkinsonism, dizziness, drowsiness, insomnia, fatigue, headache.
CV: *orthostatic hypotension,* tachycardia, ECG changes.
EENT: *blurred vision,* ocular changes.
GI: *dry mouth, constipation,* nausea.
GU: *urine retention,* menstrual irregularities, inhibited ejaculation.
Hematologic: ***transient leukopenia, agranulocytosis.***
Hepatic: cholestatic jaundice.
Metabolic: weight gain.
Skin: *photosensitivity reactions,* allergic reactions, rash.
Other: gynecomastia.

INTERACTIONS

Drug-drug. *Antacids:* May inhibit absorption of oral phenothiazines. Separate antacid and phenothiazine doses by at least 2 hours.
Barbiturates, lithium: May decrease phenothiazine effect. Monitor patient.
Centrally acting antihypertensives: May decrease antihypertensive effect. Monitor blood pressure.
CNS depressants: May increase CNS depression. Use together cautiously.
Propranolol: May increase propranolol and trifluoperazine levels. Monitor patient.
Warfarin: May decrease effect of oral anticoagulants. Monitor PT and INR.
Drug-herb. *St. John's wort:* May cause photosensitivity reactions. Advise patient to avoid excessive sunlight exposure.
Drug-lifestyle. *Alcohol use:* May increase CNS depression, particularly psychomotor skills. Strongly discourage alcohol use.
Sun exposure: May increase risk of photosensitivity reactions. Advise patient to avoid excessive sunlight exposure.

EFFECTS ON LAB TEST RESULTS

- May increase liver enzyme levels.
- May decrease WBC and granulocyte counts.
- May cause false-positive results for urinary porphyrin, urobilinogen, amylase, and 5-hydroxyindoleacetic acid tests and for urine pregnancy tests that use human chorionic gonadotropin.

CONTRAINDICATIONS & CAUTIONS

- Contraindicated in patients hypersensitive to phenothiazines and in those with CNS depression, coma, bone marrow suppression, or liver damage.
- Use cautiously in elderly or debilitated patients and in patients with CV disease (may decrease blood pressure), seizure disorder, glaucoma, or prostatic hyperplasia; also, use cautiously in those exposed to extreme heat.
- Reserve use in children for those who are hospitalized or under close supervision.

NURSING CONSIDERATIONS

- Wear gloves when preparing liquid forms.
- Watch for orthostatic hypotension. Keep patient supine for 1 hour after giving drug, and tell him to change positions slowly.
- Monitor patient for tardive dyskinesia, which may occur after prolonged use. It may not appear until months or years later and may disappear spontaneously or persist for life, despite ending drug.
- ***Alert:*** Watch for evidence of neuroleptic malignant syndrome (extrapyramidal effects, hyperthermia, autonomic disturbance), which is rare but deadly
- Monitor periodic CBC and liver function tests, and ophthalmic tests (long-term use).
- Withhold dose and notify prescriber if jaundice, signs and symptoms of blood dyscrasia (fever, sore throat, infection, cellulitis, weakness), or persistent extrapyramidal reactions (longer than a few hours) develop, especially in children or pregnant women.
- Don't withdraw drug abruptly unless severe adverse reactions occur.
- After abrupt withdrawal of long-term therapy, gastritis, nausea, vomiting, dizziness, tremor, feeling of warmth or cold, diaphoresis, tachycardia, headache, in-

somnia, anorexia, muscle rigidity, altered mental status, or evidence of autonomic instability may occur.

• ***Look alike–sound alike:*** Don't confuse trifluoperazine with triflupromazine.

PATIENT TEACHING

• Warn patient to avoid activities that require alertness until effects of drug are known.
• Tell patient to avoid alcohol while taking drug.
• Instruct patient to properly dilute liquid.
• Tell patient to report signs of urine retention or constipation.
• Tell patient to use sunblock and to wear protective clothing outdoors.
• Advise patient to relieve dry mouth with sugarless gum or hard candy.

ziprasidone

Geodon

Pharmacologic class: benzisoxazole derivative
Pregnancy risk category C

AVAILABLE FORMS

Capsules: 20 mg, 40 mg, 60 mg, 80 mg
I.M. injection: 20 mg/ml single-dose vials (after reconstitution)

INDICATIONS & DOSAGES

➤ **Symptomatic treatment of schizophrenia**
Adults: Initially, 20 mg b.i.d. with food. Dosages are highly individualized. Adjust dosage, if necessary, no more frequently than q 2 days; to allow for lowest possible doses, the interval should be several weeks to assess symptom response. Effective dosage range is usually 20 to 80 mg b.i.d. Maximum dosage is 100 mg b.i.d.

➤ **Rapid control of acute agitation in schizophrenic patients**
Adults: 10 to 20 mg I.M. p.r.n., up to a maximum dose of 40 mg daily. Doses of 10 mg may be given q 2 hours; doses of 20 mg may be given q 4 hours.

➤ **Acute bipolar mania, including manic and mixed episodes, with or without psychotic features**
Adults: 40 mg P.O. b.i.d., with food, on day 1. Increase to 60 to 80 mg P.O. b.i.d., with food, on day 2; then adjust dosage based on patient response from 40 to 80 mg b.i.d., with food.

ACTION

May inhibit dopamine and serotonin-2 receptors, causing reduction in schizophrenia symptoms.

Route	Onset	Peak	Duration
P.O.	1–3 days	6–8 hr	12 hr
I.M.	Unknown	1 hr	Unknown

Half-life: 2¼ to 7 hours.

ADVERSE REACTIONS

CNS: *dizziness, headache, somnolence,* ***suicide attempt,*** akathisia, dizziness, extrapyramidal symptoms, hypertonia, asthenia, dystonia (P.O.), anxiety, insomnia, agitation, cogwheel rigidity, paresthesia, personality disorder, psychosis, speech disorder (I.M.).
CV: ***bradycardia, QT interval prolongation,*** orthostatic hypotension, tachycardia (P.O.), hypertension, vasodilation (I.M.).
EENT: rhinitis, abnormal vision (P.O.).
GI: *nausea,* constipation, dyspepsia, diarrhea, dry mouth, anorexia, abdominal pain, rectal hemorrhage, vomiting, dyspepsia, tooth disorder (I.M.).
GU: dysmenorrhea, priapism (I.M.).
Metabolic: hyperglycemia.
Musculoskeletal: myalgia (P.O.), back pain (I.M.).
Respiratory: cough (P.O.).
Skin: rash (P.O.), injection site pain, furunculosis, sweating (I.M.).
Other: flulike syndrome (I.M.).

INTERACTIONS

Drug-drug. ***Antiarrhythmics (amiodarone, bretylium, disopyramide, dofetilide, procainamide, quinidine, sotalol), arsenic trioxide, cisapride, dolasetron, droperidol, levomethadyl, mefloquine, pentamidine, phenothiazines, pimozide, quinolones, tacrolimus:*** May increase the risk of life-threatening arrhythmias. Use together is contraindicated.
Antihypertensives: May enhance hypotensive effects. Monitor blood pressure.
Carbamazepine: May decrease ziprasidone level. May need to increase ziprasidone dose to achieve desired effect.

Drugs that decrease potassium or magnesium such as diuretics: May increase risk of arrhythmias. Monitor potassium and magnesium levels if using these drugs together.
Itraconazole, ketoconazole: May increase ziprasidone level. May need to reduce ziprasidone dose to achieve desired effect.

EFFECTS ON LAB TEST RESULTS
None reported.

CONTRAINDICATIONS & CAUTIONS
- Contraindicated in patients hypersensitive to drug and in those with recent MI or uncompensated heart failure.
- Contraindicated in those with history of prolonged QT interval or congenital long QT interval syndrome and in those taking other drugs that prolong QT interval, such as dofetilide, sotalol, quinidine, other class IA and III antiarrhythmics, mesoridazine, thioridazine, chlorpromazine, droperidol, pimozide, sparfloxacin, gatifloxacin, moxifloxacin, halofantrine, mefloquine, pentamidine, arsenic trioxide, levomethadyl acetate, dolasetron mesylate, probucol, and tacrolimus.

P.O.
- Contraindicated in patients with a history of QT interval prolongation or congenital QT syndrome and in those taking other drugs that prolong QT interval.
- Use cautiously in patients with history of seizures, bradycardia, hypokalemia, or hypomagnesemia; in those with acute diarrhea; and in those with conditions that may lower the seizure threshold (such as Alzheimer dementia).
- Use cautiously in patients at risk for aspiration pneumonia.

I.M.
- Contraindicated in schizophrenic patients already taking P.O. ziprasidone.
- Use cautiously in elderly and renally or hepatically impaired patients.

NURSING CONSIDERATIONS
- ***Alert:*** In elderly patients with dementia-related psychosis, drug isn't indicated for use because of increased risk of death from CV events or infection.
- ***Alert:*** Hyperglycemia may occur. Monitor patients with diabetes regularly. Patients with risk factors for diabetes should undergo fasting blood glucose testing at baseline and periodically. Monitor all patients for symptoms of hyperglycemia, including excessive hunger or thirst, frequent urination, and weakness. Hyperglycemia may be reversible when drug is stopped.
- ***Alert:*** Monitor patient for symptoms of metabolic syndrome (significant weight gain and increased BMI, hypertension, hyperglycemia, hypercholesterolemia, and hypertriglyceridemia).

P.O.
- Stop drug in patients with a QTc interval more than 500 msec.
- Dizziness, palpitations, or syncope may be symptoms of a life-threatening arrhythmia such as torsades de pointes. Provide CV evaluation and monitoring in patients who experience these symptoms.
- Don't give to patients with electrolyte disturbances, such as hypokalemia or hypomagnesemia, because these increase the risk of arrhythmia.
- Patient taking an antipsychotic may develop life-threatening neuroleptic malignant syndrome (hyperpyrexia, muscle rigidity, altered mental status, and autonomic instability) or tardive dyskinesia. Assess abnormal involuntary movement before starting therapy, at dosage changes, and periodically thereafter, to monitor patient for tardive dyskinesia.
- Monitor patient for abnormal body temperature regulation, especially if he is exercising strenuously, is exposed to extreme heat, is also receiving anticholinergics, or is subject to dehydration.
- Symptoms may not improve for 4 to 6 weeks.
- Always give drug with food for optimal effect.
- Don't use drug in breast-feeding women.

I.M.
- To prepare I.M. ziprasidone, add 1.2 ml of sterile water for injection to the vial and shake vigorously until drug is completely dissolved.
- Don't mix injection with other medicinal products or solvents other than sterile water for injection.
- Inspect parenteral drug products for particulate matter and discoloration before administration, whenever possible.

• The effects of giving I.M. ziprasidone for more than 3 consecutive days are unknown. If long-term therapy of ziprasidone is necessary, switch to P.O. as soon as possible.
• Store injection at controlled room temperature, 59° to 86° F (15° to 30° C) in dry form, and protect from light. After reconstituting the drug, it may be stored away from light for up to 24 hours at 59° to 86° F (15° to 30° C) or up to 7 days refrigerated, 36° to 46° F (2° to 8° C).

PATIENT TEACHING

• Tell patient to take drug with food.
• Tell patient to immediately report to prescriber signs or symptoms of dizziness, fainting, irregular heartbeat, or relevant heart problems.
• Advise patient to report any recent episodes of diarrhea, abnormal movements, sudden fever, muscle rigidity, or change in mental status.
• Advise patient that symptoms may not improve for 4 to 6 weeks.

32

Central nervous system stimulants

dexmethylphenidate hydrochloride
dextroamphetamine sulfate
doxapram hydrochloride
methylphenidate hydrochloride
methylphenidate transdermal system
modafinil
phentermine hydrochloride

dexmethylphenidate hydrochloride
Focalin, Focalin XR

Pharmacologic class: methylphenidate derivative
Pregnancy risk category C
Controlled substance schedule II

AVAILABLE FORMS
Capsules (extended-release): 5 mg, 10 mg, 20 mg
Tablets: 2.5 mg, 5 mg, 10 mg

INDICATIONS & DOSAGES
➤Attention deficit hyperactivity disorder (ADHD)
immediate-release tablets
Adults and children age 6 and older: For patients who aren't now taking methylphenidate, initially, 2.5 mg P.O. b.i.d., given at least 4 hours apart. Increase weekly by 2.5 to 5 mg daily, up to a maximum of 20 mg daily in divided doses.

For patients who are now taking methylphenidate, initially give half the current methylphenidate dosage, up to a maximum of 20 mg P.O. daily in divided doses.
extended-release capsules
Adults: For patients who aren't now taking dexmethylphenidate or methylphenidate, or who are on stimulants other than methylphenidate, give 10 mg P.O. once daily in the morning. May adjust in weekly increments of 10 mg to a maximum dose of 20 mg daily.

For patients who are now taking methylphenidate, initially give half the total daily dose of methylphenidate. Patients who are now taking the immediate-release form of dexmethylphenidate may be switched to the same daily dose of extended-release form. Maximum daily dose is 20 mg.
Children ages 6 and older: For patients who aren't now taking dexmethylphenidate or methylphenidate, or who are on stimulants other than methylphenidate, give 5 mg P.O. once daily in the morning. May adjust in weekly increments of 5 mg to a maximum daily dose of 20 mg.

For patients who are now taking methylphenidate, initially give half the total daily dose of methylphenidate. Patients who are now taking the immediate-release form of dexmethylphenidate may be switched to the same daily dose of extended-release form. Maximum daily dose is 20 mg.

ACTION
Blocks presynaptic reuptake of norepinephrine and dopamine and increases their release, increasing concentration in the synapse.

Route	Onset	Peak	Duration
P.O. (immediate-release)	Unknown	1–1½ hr	Unknown
P.O. (extended-release)	Unknown	1–4 hr; 4½–7 hr	Unknown

ADVERSE REACTIONS
CNS: *headache, anxiety, feeling jittery,* nervousness, insomnia, fever, dizziness.
CV: tachycardia.
EENT: throat pain.
GI: *anorexia, abdominal pain,* nausea, dyspepsia, dry mouth.
Musculoskeletal: twitching (motor or vocal tics).
Other: hypersensitivity reactions.

INTERACTIONS
Drug-drug. *Antacids, acid suppressants:* May alter the release of extended-release form. Avoid using together.

Anticoagulants, phenobarbital, phenytoin, primidone, tricyclic antidepressants: May inhibit metabolism of these drugs. May need to decrease dosage of these drugs; monitor drug levels.
Antihypertensives: May decrease effectiveness of these drugs. Use together cautiously; monitor blood pressure.
Clonidine, other centrally acting alpha agonists: May cause serious adverse effects. Use together cautiously.
MAO inhibitors: May increase risk of hypertensive crisis. Using together within 14 days of MAO inhibitor therapy is contraindicated.

EFFECTS ON LAB TEST RESULTS
None reported.

CONTRAINDICATIONS & CAUTIONS
- Contraindicated in patients hypersensitive to methylphenidate or other components.
- Contraindicated in patients with severe anxiety, tension, or agitation; glaucoma; or motor tics or a family history or diagnosis of Tourette syndrome, or within 14 days of MAO inhibitor therapy.
- Use cautiously in patients with a psychiatric illness, bipolar disorder, depression, or family history of suicide; seizures, hypertension, hyperthyroidism, heart failure, recent MI, or a history of drug or alcohol abuse.
- Use in pregnant women only if the benefits outweigh the risks; drug may delay skeletal ossification, suppress weight gain, and impair organ development in the fetus.
- Use cautiously in breast-feeding women. It's unknown if drug appears in breast milk.
- Don't use in children or adolescents with structural cardiac abnormalities or other serious heart problems.

NURSING CONSIDERATIONS
- Diagnosis of ADHD must be based on complete history and evaluation of the patient by psychological and educational experts.
- Obtain a detailed patient history, including a family history for mental disorders, family suicide, ventricular arrhythmias, or sudden death.
- Refer patient for psychological, educational, and social support.
- Periodically reevaluate the long-term usefulness of the drug.
- Monitor CBC and differential and platelet counts during prolonged therapy.
- Don't use for severe depression or normal fatigue states.
- Stop treatment or reduce dosage if symptoms worsen or adverse reactions occur.
- Long-term stimulant use may temporarily suppress growth. Monitor children for growth and weight gain. If growth slows or weight gain is lower than expected, stop drug.
- Routinely monitor blood pressure and pulse.
- Monitor patient for signs of drug dependence or abuse.
- If seizures occur, stop drug.

PATIENT TEACHING
- Stress the importance of taking the correct dose of drug at the same time every day. Report accidental overdose immediately.
- ***Alert:*** Warn patient the misuse of amphetamines can have serious effects including sudden death.
- Advise patients unable to swallow capsules to empty the contents of the capsule onto a spoonful of applesauce and eat immediately.
- ***Alert:*** Tell patient not to cut, crush, or chew the contents of the extended-release beaded capsule.
- Advise parents to monitor child for medication abuse or sharing. Also inform parents to watch for increased aggression or hostility and to report worsening behavior.
- Advise parents to monitor child's height and weight and to tell the prescriber if they suspect growth is slowing.
- Caution patient to expect blurred vision or difficulty with accommodation and to exercise caution while performing activities that require a clear visual field. Advise patient to report blurred vision to the prescriber.

dextroamphetamine sulfate

Dexedrine*, Dexedrine Spansule, DextroStat

Pharmacologic class: amphetamine
Pregnancy risk category C
Controlled substance schedule II

AVAILABLE FORMS

Capsules (extended-release): 5 mg, 10 mg, 15 mg
Tablets: 5 mg, 10 mg

INDICATIONS & DOSAGES

➤Narcolepsy

Adults: 5 to 60 mg P.O. daily in divided doses.
Children ages 6 to 12: 5 mg P.O. daily. Increase by 5 mg at weekly intervals p.r.n.
Children age 12 and older: 10 mg P.O. daily. Increase by 10 mg at weekly intervals, p.r.n. Give first dose on awakening; additional doses (one or two) given at intervals of 4 to 6 hours.

➤Attention deficit hyperactivity disorder (ADHD)

Children age 6 and older: 5 mg P.O. once daily or b.i.d. Increase by 5 mg at weekly intervals, p.r.n. It's rarely necessary to exceed 40 mg/day.
Children ages 3 to 5: 2.5 mg P.O. daily. Increase by 2.5 mg at weekly intervals, p.r.n.

➤Short-term adjunct in exogenous obesity ♦

Adults and children age 12 and older: 5 to 30 mg P.O. daily 30 to 60 minutes before meals in divided doses of 5 to 10 mg. Or, 10- or 15-mg extended-release capsule daily in the morning.

ACTION

Unknown. Probably promotes nerve impulse transmission by releasing stored dopamine and norepinephrine from nerve terminals in the brain. Main sites of activity appear to be the cerebral cortex and the reticular activating system.

Route	Onset	Peak	Duration
P.O.	30–60 min	2 hr	4 hr
P.O. (extended)	60 min	2 hr	8 hr

Half-life: 10 to 12 hours.

ADVERSE REACTIONS

CNS: *insomnia, nervousness, restlessness,* tremor, dizziness, headache, chills, overstimulation, dysphoria, euphoria.
CV: *tachycardia, palpitations,* ***arrhythmias,*** hypertension.
GI: dry mouth, taste perversion, diarrhea, constipation, anorexia, other GI disturbances.
GU: impotence.
Metabolic: weight loss.
Skin: urticaria.
Other: increased libido.

INTERACTIONS

Drug-drug. *Acetazolamide, alkalizing drugs, antacids, sodium bicarbonate:* May increase renal reabsorption. Monitor patient for enhanced amphetamine effects.
Acidifying drugs, ammonium chloride, ascorbic acid: May decrease level and increase renal clearance of dextroamphetamine. Monitor patient for decreased amphetamine effects.
Adrenergic blockers: May inhibit adrenergic blocking effects. Avoid using together.
Chlorpromazine: May inhibit central stimulant effects of amphetamines. May use to treat amphetamine poisoning.
Insulin, oral antidiabetics: May decrease antidiabetic requirements. Monitor glucose level.
MAO inhibitors (MAOIs): May cause severe hypertension or hypertensive crisis. Avoid using within 14 days of MAOI therapy.
Meperidine: May potentiate analgesic effect. Use together cautiously.
Methenamine: May increase urinary excretion of amphetamines and reduce effectiveness. Monitor drug effects.
Norepinephrine: May enhance adrenergic effect of norepinephrine. Monitor patient.
Phenobarbital, phenytoin: May delay absorption of these drugs. Monitor patient closely.
Drug-food. *Caffeine:* May increase amphetamine and related amine effects. Urge caution.

EFFECTS ON LAB TEST RESULTS

- May increase corticosteroid level.

CONTRAINDICATIONS & CAUTIONS

- Contraindicated in patients hypersensitive to or with idiosyncratic reactions to sympathomimetic amines and in those with hyperthyroidism, moderate to severe hypertension, symptomatic CV disease, glaucoma, advanced arteriosclerosis, or history of drug abuse.
- Contraindicated as first-line treatment for obesity or within 14 days of MAOI therapy.
- Use cautiously in agitated patients and patients with motor tics, phonic tics, or Tourette syndrome. Also use cautiously in patients whose underlying condition may be worsened by an increase in blood pressure or heart rate (pre-existing hypertension, heart failure, recent MI); patients with a psychiatric illness, bipolar disorder, depression, or family history of suicide; those with a seizure disorder.
- Don't use in children or adolescents with structural cardiac abnormalities or other serious heart problems.

NURSING CONSIDERATIONS

- Obtain a detailed patient history, including a family history for mental disorders, family suicide, ventricular arrhythmias, or sudden death.
- Drug shouldn't be used to prevent fatigue.
- Obese patients should follow a weight-reduction program.
- Drug has a high abuse potential and may cause dependence.
- Certain formulations may contain tartrazine.
- ***Alert:*** Overdose may cause seizures.
- If tolerance to anorexigenic effect develops, stop drug and notify prescriber.
- ***Look alike–sound alike:*** Don't confuse Dexedrine with dextran or Excedrin.

PATIENT TEACHING

- ***Alert:*** Warn patient the misuse of amphetamines can cause serious cardiovascular adverse events including sudden death.
- Tell patient to take drug 30 to 60 minutes before meals if used for weight reduction and at least 6 hours before bedtime to avoid sleep interference.
- Warn patient to avoid activities that require alertness, a clear visual field, or good coordination until CNS effects of drug are known.
- Tell patient he may get tired as drug effects wear off.
- Ask patient to report signs and symptoms of excessive stimulation.
- Inform parents children may show increased aggression or hostility and to report and worsening of behavior.
- Advise patient to consume caffeine-containing products cautiously.
- Warn patient with a seizure disorder that drug may decrease seizure threshold. Instruct him to notify prescriber if seizures occur.

doxapram hydrochloride

Dopram

Pharmacologic class: analeptic
Pregnancy risk category B

AVAILABLE FORMS

Injection: 20 mg/ml (benzyl alcohol 0.9%)

INDICATIONS & DOSAGES

➤ **Postanesthesia respiratory stimulation**

Adults: 0.5 to 1 mg/kg as a single I.V. injection (not to exceed 1.5 mg/kg) or as multiple injections q 5 minutes, total not to exceed 2 mg/kg. Or, 250 mg in 250 ml of normal saline solution or D_5W infused at initial rate of 5 mg/minute I.V. until satisfactory response is achieved. Maintain at 1 to 3 mg/minute. Don't exceed total dose for infusion of 4 mg/kg.

➤ **Drug-induced CNS depression**

Adults: For injection, priming dose of 2 mg/kg I.V., repeated in 5 minutes and again q 1 to 2 hours until patient awakens (and if relapse occurs). Maximum daily dose is 3 g.

For infusion, priming dose of 2 mg/kg I.V., repeated in 5 minutes and again in 1 to 2 hours, if needed. If response occurs, give I.V. infusion (1 mg/ml) at 1 to 3 mg/minute until patient awakens. Don't infuse for longer than 2 hours or give more than 3 g/day. May resume I.V. infusion after rest period of 30 minutes to 2 hours, if needed.

➤ **Chronic pulmonary disease related to acute hypercapnia**
Adults: 1 to 2 mg/minute by I.V. infusion using 2 mg/ml solution. Maximum, 3 mg/minute for up to 2 hours.

I.V. ADMINISTRATION

- Drug is compatible with D_5W, dextrose 10% in water, and normal saline solution.
- Give slowly; rapid infusion may cause hemolysis.
- Watch for irritation and infiltration; it can cause tissue damage and necrosis.

INCOMPATIBILITIES

Aminophylline, ascorbic acid, cefoperazone, cefotaxime, cefuroxime sodium, dexamethasone sodium phosphate, diazepam, digoxin, dobutamine, folic acid, furosemide, hydrocortisone sodium phosphate, hydrocortisone sodium succinate, ketamine, methylprednisolone sodium succinate, minocycline, sodium bicarbonate, thiopental, ticarcillin disodium.

ACTION

Not clearly defined. Directly stimulates the central respiratory centers in the medulla and may indirectly act on carotid, aortic, or other peripheral chemoreceptors.

Route	Onset	Peak	Duration
I.V.	20–40 sec	1–2 min	5–12 min

Half-life: 2½ to 4 hours.

ADVERSE REACTIONS

CNS: *headache, dizziness,* ***seizures,*** apprehension, disorientation, hyperactivity, bilateral Babinski's signs, paresthesia.
CV: *chest pain and tightness, variations in heart rate, hypertension,* ***arrhythmias,*** T-wave depression on ECG, flushing.
EENT: ***laryngospasm,*** sneezing.
GI: nausea, vomiting, diarrhea.
GU: urine retention, bladder stimulation with incontinence, albuminuria.
Musculoskeletal: muscle spasms.
Respiratory: ***bronchospasm,*** cough, dyspnea, rebound hypoventilation, hiccups.
Skin: pruritus, diaphoresis.

INTERACTIONS

Drug-drug. *General anesthetics:* May cause self-limiting arrhythmias. Avoid using doxapram within 10 minutes of an anesthetic that sensitizes the myocardium to catecholamines.
MAO inhibitors, sympathomimetics: May increase adverse CV effects. Use together cautiously.

EFFECTS ON LAB TEST RESULTS

- May increase BUN level. May decrease hemoglobin level and hematocrit.
- May decrease erythrocyte, RBC, and WBC counts.

CONTRAINDICATIONS & CAUTIONS

- Contraindicated in patients with seizure disorders; head injury; CV disorders; frank, uncompensated heart failure; severe hypertension; stroke; respiratory failure or incompetence secondary to neuromuscular disorders, muscle paresis, flail chest, obstructed airway, pulmonary embolism, pneumothorax, restrictive respiratory disease, acute bronchial asthma, or extreme dyspnea; or hypoxia unrelated to hypercapnia.
- Use cautiously in patients with bronchial asthma, severe tachycardia or arrhythmias, cerebral edema, increased intracranial pressure, hyperthyroidism, pheochromocytoma, or metabolic disorders.

NURSING CONSIDERATIONS

- Drug is used only in surgical or emergency department situations.
- Separate end of anesthetic treatment and start of this drug by at least 10 minutes.
- ***Alert:*** Establish an adequate airway before giving drug. Prevent patient from aspirating vomitus by placing him on his side.
- Monitor blood pressure, heart rate, deep tendon reflexes, and arterial blood gases before giving drug and every 30 minutes afterward.
- Monitor patient for evidence of overdose, such as hypertension, tachycardia, arrhythmias, skeletal muscle hyperactivity, and dyspnea. Hold drug and notify prescriber if patient needs mechanical ventilation or shows signs of increased arterial carbon dioxide or oxygen tension.

• ***Look alike–sound alike:*** Don't confuse doxapram with doxorubicin, doxepin, or doxazosin.

PATIENT TEACHING
• Inform family and patient about need for drug.
• Answer patient's questions and address his concerns.

methylphenidate hydrochloride
Concerta✐, Metadate CD, Metadate ER, Methylin, Methylin ER, Ritalin✐, Ritalin LA, Ritalin-SR✐

methylphenidate transdermal system
Daytrana

Pharmacologic class: piperidine derivative
Pregnancy risk category NR; C (for Concerta, Daytrana, Metadate CD, Ritalin LA)
Controlled substance schedule II

AVAILABLE FORMS
Oral solution (Methylin): 5 mg/5 ml, 10 mg/5 ml
Tablets (chewable): 2.5 mg, 5 mg, 10 mg
Tablets (Ritalin, Methylin): 5 mg, 10 mg, 20 mg
Extended-release
Capsules (Metadate CD): 10 mg, 20 mg, 30 mg
Capsules (Ritalin LA): 20 mg, 30 mg, 40 mg
Tablets (Concerta): 18 mg, 27 mg, 36 mg, 54 mg
Tablets (Metadate ER, Methylin ER): 10 mg, 20 mg
Sustained-release
Tablets (Ritalin-SR): 20 mg
Transdermal system
Patch: 10 mg, 15 mg, 20 mg, 30 mg

INDICATIONS & DOSAGES
➤ **Attention deficit hyperactivity disorder (ADHD)**
Children age 6 and older: Initially, 5 mg P.O. b.i.d. immediate-release form before breakfast and lunch, increasing by 5 to 10 mg at weekly intervals, p.r.n., until an optimum daily dose of 2 mg/kg is reached, not to exceed 60 mg/day. To use Ritalin-SR, Metadate ER, and Methylin ER tablets in place of immediate-release methylphenidate tablets, calculate methylphenidate dosage in 8-hour intervals.
Concerta
Adolescents age 13 to 17 not currently taking methylphenidate, or for patients taking other stimulants: 18 mg P.O. extended-release Concerta once daily in the morning. Adjust dosage by 18 mg at weekly intervals to a maximum of 72 mg P.O. (not to exceed 2 mg/kg) once daily in the morning.
Children age 6 to 12 not currently taking methylphenidate or patients taking stimulants other than methylphenidate: 18 mg extended-release P.O. once daily q morning. Adjust dosage by 18 mg at weekly intervals to a maximum of 54 mg daily q morning.
Adolescents and children age 6 and older currently taking methylphenidate: If previous methylphenidate dosage was 5 mg b.i.d. or t.i.d. or 20 mg sustained-release, give 18 mg P.O. q morning. If previous dosage was 10 mg b.i.d. or t.i.d. or 40 mg sustained-release, give 36 mg P.O. q morning. If previous dosage was 15 mg b.i.d. or t.i.d. or 60 mg sustained-release, give 54 mg P.O. q morning. Maximum conversion daily dose is 54 mg. Once conversion complete, adjust adolescents age 13 to 17 to maximum dose of 72 mg once daily (not to exceed 2 mg/kg).
Metadate CD
Children age 6 and older: Initially, 20 mg P.O. daily before breakfast, increasing by 10 to 20 mg at weekly intervals to a maximum of 60 mg daily.
Ritalin LA
Children age 6 and older: 20 mg P.O. once daily. Increase by 10 mg at weekly intervals to a maximum of 60 mg daily. If previous methylphenidate dosage was 10 mg b.i.d. or 20 mg sustained-release, give 20 mg P.O. once daily. If previous methylphenidate dosage was 15 mg b.i.d., give 30 mg P.O. once daily. If previous methylphenidate dosage was 20 mg b.i.d. or 40 mg sustained-release, give 40 mg P.O. once daily. If previous methylphenidate

dosage was 30 mg b.i.d. or 60 mg sustained-release, give 60 mg P.O. once daily.

Daytrana

Children age 6 to 12: Initially, apply one 10-mg patch to clean, dry, nonirritated skin on the hip, alternating sites daily. Avoid the waistline or where tight clothing may rub it off. Apply 2 hours before desired effect and remove 9 hours later. Increase dose weekly as needed to a maximum of 30 mg daily. Base final dose and wear time on patient response.

➤ Narcolepsy

Adults: 10 mg P.O. b.i.d. or t.i.d. immediate-release, 30 to 45 minutes before meals. Dosage varies; average is 40 to 60 mg/day. To use Ritalin-SR, Metadate ER, or Methylin ER tablets in place of immediate-release methylphenidate tablets, calculate the dose of methylphenidate in 8-hour intervals.

ACTION

Releases nerve terminal stores of norepinephrine, promoting nerve impulse transmission. At high doses, effects are mediated by dopamine.

Route	Onset	Peak	Duration
P.O. (Methylin, Ritalin)	Unknown	2 hr	Unknown
P.O. (Methylin ER, Ritalin-SR)	Unknown	5 hr	8 hr
P.O. (Metadate CD)	Unknown	1½ hr; 4½ hr	Unknown
P.O. (Ritalin LA)	Unknown	1–3 hr; 4–7 hr	Unknown
P.O. (Concerta)	Unknown	6–8 hr	Unknown
Transdermal	2 hr	Variable	14 hr

Half-life: Conventional, 3 to 6 hours; extended-release (Metadate ER, Methylin ER, Ritalin SR), 3 to 8 hours, (Concerta, Metadate CD, Ritalin LA) 8 to 12 hours; transdermal, 3 to 4 hours.

ADVERSE REACTIONS

CNS: *nervousness, headache, insomnia,* ***seizures,*** tics, dizziness, akathisia, dyskinesia, drowsiness, mood swings.
CV: *palpitations, tachycardia,* ***arrhythmias,*** hypertension.
EENT: pharyngitis, sinusitis.
GI: *nausea, abdominal pain, anorexia, decreased appetite, vomiting.*
Hematologic: ***thrombocytopenia, thrombocytopenic purpura, leukopenia,*** anemia.
Metabolic: weight loss.
Respiratory: cough, upper respiratory tract infection.
Skin: *exfoliative dermatitis,* ***erythema multiforme,*** rash, urticaria, application site irritation (redness, swelling, papules).
Other: *viral infection.*

INTERACTIONS

Drug-drug. *Anticonvulsants (such as phenobarbital, phenytoin, primidone), SSRIs, tricyclic antidepressants (imipramine, clomipramine, desipramine), warfarin:* May increase levels of these drugs. Monitor patient for adverse reactions and decrease dose of these drugs as needed. Monitor drug levels (or coagulation times if patient is also taking warfarin).
Centrally acting $alpha_2$ agonists, clonidine: May cause serious adverse events. Avoid using together.
Centrally acting antihypertensives: May decrease antihypertensive effect. Monitor blood pressure.
MAO inhibitors: May cause severe hypertension or hypertensive crisis. Avoid using within 14 days of MAO inhibitor therapy.
Drug-food. *Caffeine:* May increase amphetamine and related amine effects. Discourage use together.

EFFECTS ON LAB TEST RESULTS

- May decrease hemoglobin level and hematocrit.
- May decrease platelet and WBC counts.

CONTRAINDICATIONS & CAUTIONS

- Contraindicated in patients hypersensitive to drug and in those with glaucoma, motor tics, family history or diagnosis of Tourette syndrome, or history of marked anxiety, tension, or agitation. Also contraindicated within 14 days of MAO inhibitor therapy. Avoid use in patients with structural cardiac abnormalities.
- Because it doesn't dissolve, Concerta isn't recommended in patients with a history of peritonitis or with severe GI narrowing (such as small bowel inflammatory

disease, short-gut syndrome caused by adhesions or decreased transit time, cystic fibrosis, chronic intestinal pseudoobstruction, or Meckel diverticulum).
- Use cautiously in patients with a history of seizures, EEG abnormalities, or hypertension, and in patients whose underlying medical conditions might be compromised by increases in blood pressure or heart rate, such as those with preexisting hypertension, heart failure, recent MI, or hyperthyroidism.
- Use cautiously in patients who are emotionally unstable or who have a history of drug dependence or alcoholism.

NURSING CONSIDERATIONS
- Don't use drug to prevent fatigue or treat severe depression.
- Drug may trigger Tourette syndrome in children. Monitor patient, especially at start of therapy.
- Observe patient for signs of excessive stimulation. Monitor blood pressure.
- Check CBC, differential, and platelet counts with long-term use, particularly if patient shows signs or symptoms of hematologic toxicity (fever, sore throat, easy bruising).
- Monitor height and weight in children on long-term therapy. Drug may delay growth spurt, but children will attain normal height when drug is stopped.
- Monitor patient for tolerance or psychological dependence.
- Chewable tablets contain phenylalanine.
- ***Look alike–sound alike:*** Don't confuse Ritalin with Rifadin.

PATIENT TEACHING
- Tell patient or caregiver to give last daily dose at least 6 hours before bedtime to prevent insomnia and after meals to reduce appetite-suppressant effects.
- Warn patient against chewing sustained-release tablets.
- Metadate CD or Ritalin LA may be swallowed whole, or the contents of the capsule may be sprinkled onto a small amount of cool applesauce and taken immediately.
- ***Alert:*** Warn patient to take chewable tablet with at least 8 ounces of water. Not using enough water to swallow tablet may cause the tablet to swell and block the throat, causing choking.
- Caution patient to avoid activities that require alertness or good psychomotor coordination until CNS effects of drug are known.
- Warn patient with seizure disorder that drug may decrease seizure threshold. Urge him to notify prescriber if seizure occurs.
- Advise patient to avoid beverages containing caffeine while taking drug.
- Tell parent to apply patch immediately after opening; don't use if pouch seal is broken. Press firmly in place for about 30 seconds using the palm of your hand, being sure there is good contact with the skin—especially around the edges. Once applied correctly, the child may shower, bathe, or swim as usual.
- Inform parent if patch comes off, a new one may be applied on a different site, but the total wear time for that day should be 9 hours. Upon removal, fold patch in half so the sticky sides adhere to itself, then flush down toilet or dispose of in a lidded container.
- Tell parent, if the applied patch is missing, to ask the child when or how the patch came off.
- Encourage parent to use the application chart provided with patch carton to keep track of application and removal.
- Tell parent to remove patch sooner than 9 hours if the child has decreased evening appetite or has difficulty sleeping.
- Tell parent the effects of the patch lasts for several hours after its removal.
- Warn parent and patient to avoid exposing patch to direct external heat sources, such as heating pads, electric blankets, and heated water beds.
- Tell parent to notify prescriber if the child develops bumps, swelling, or blistering at the application site or is experiencing blurred vision or other serious side effects.

modafinil
Provigil

Pharmacologic class: analeptic
Pregnancy risk category C
Controlled substance schedule IV

AVAILABLE FORMS
Tablets: 100 mg, 200 mg

INDICATIONS & DOSAGES
➤ **To improve wakefulness in patients with excessive daytime sleepiness caused by narcolepsy, obstructive sleep apnea-hypoapnea syndrome, and shift-work sleep disorder**
Adults: 200 mg P.O. daily, as single dose in the morning. Patients with shift-work sleep disorder should take dose about 1 hour before the start of their shift.
Adjust-a-dose: In patients with severe hepatic impairment, give 100 mg P.O. daily, as single dose in the morning.

ACTION
Unknown. Similar to action of sympathomimetics, including amphetamines, but drug is structurally distinct from amphetamines and doesn't alter release of dopamine or norepinephrine to produce CNS stimulation.

Route	Onset	Peak	Duration
P.O.	Unknown	2–4 hr	Unknown

Half-life: 15 hours.

ADVERSE REACTIONS
CNS: *headache, nervousness, dizziness, insomnia,* fever, depression, anxiety, cataplexy, paresthesia, dyskinesia, hypertonia, confusion, syncope, amnesia, emotional lability, ataxia, tremor.
CV: ***arrhythmias,*** hypotension, hypertension, vasodilation, chest pain.
EENT: *rhinitis,* pharyngitis, epistaxis, amblyopia, abnormal vision.
GI: *nausea,* diarrhea, dry mouth, anorexia, vomiting, mouth ulcer, gingivitis, thirst.
GU: abnormal urine, urine retention, abnormal ejaculation, albuminuria.
Hematologic: eosinophilia.
Metabolic: hyperglycemia.
Musculoskeletal: joint disorder, neck pain, neck rigidity.
Respiratory: asthma, dyspnea, lung disorder.
Skin: sweating.
Other: herpes simplex, chills.

INTERACTIONS
Drug-drug. *Carbamazepine, phenobarbital, rifampin, and other inducers of CYP3A4:* May alter modafinil level. Monitor patient closely.
Cyclosporine, theophylline: May reduce levels of these drugs. Use together cautiously.
Diazepam, phenytoin, propranolol, other drugs metabolized by CYP2C19: May inhibit CYP2C19 and lead to higher levels of drugs metabolized by this enzyme. Use together cautiously; adjust dosage as needed.
Hormonal contraceptives: May reduce contraceptive effectiveness. Advise patient to use alternative or additional method of contraception during modafinil therapy and for 1 month after drug is stopped.
Itraconazole, ketoconazole, other inhibitors of CYP3A4: May alter modafinil level. Monitor patient closely.
Methylphenidate: May cause 1-hour delay in modafinil absorption. Separate dosage times.
Phenytoin, warfarin: May inhibit CYP2C9 and increase phenytoin and warfarin levels. Monitor patient closely for toxicity.
Tricyclic antidepressants (such as clomipramine, desipramine): May increase tricyclic antidepressant level. Reduce dosage of these drugs.

EFFECTS ON LAB TEST RESULTS
- May increase glucose, GGT, and AST levels.
- May increase eosinophil count.

CONTRAINDICATIONS & CAUTIONS
- Contraindicated in patients hypersensitive to drug and in those with a history of left ventricular hypertrophy or ischemic ECG changes, chest pain, arrhythmias, or other evidence of mitral valve prolapse linked to CNS stimulant use.

- Use cautiously in patients with recent MI or unstable angina and in those with history of psychosis.
- Use cautiously and give reduced dosage to patients with severe hepatic impairment, with or without cirrhosis.
- Use cautiously in patients taking MAO inhibitors.
- Safety and efficacy in patients with severe renal impairment haven't been determined.

NURSING CONSIDERATIONS

- Monitor hypertensive patients closely.
- Although single daily 400-mg doses have been well tolerated, the larger dose is no more beneficial than the 200-mg dose.
- Food has no effect on overall bioavailability but may delay absorption of drug by 1 hour.

PATIENT TEACHING

- Advise woman to notify prescriber about planned, suspected, or known pregnancy, or if she's breast-feeding.
- Caution patient that use of hormonal contraceptives (including depot or implantable contraceptives) together with modafinil tablets may reduce contraceptive effectiveness. Recommend an alternative method of contraception during modafinil therapy and for 1 month after drug is stopped.
- Instruct patient to confer with prescriber before taking prescription or OTC drugs to avoid drug interactions.
- Tell patient to avoid alcohol while taking drug.
- Warn patient to avoid activities that require alertness or good coordination until CNS effects of drug are known.

phentermine hydrochloride

Adipex-P, Duromine‡, Ionamin

Pharmacologic class: sympathomimetic amine
Pregnancy risk category NR
Controlled substance schedule IV

AVAILABLE FORMS

Capsules: 18.75 mg, 30 mg, 37.5 mg
Capsules (resin complex, sustained-release): 15 mg, 30 mg
Tablets: 8 mg, 30 mg, 37.5 mg

INDICATIONS & DOSAGES

➤ Short-term adjunct in exogenous obesity

Adults: 8 mg P.O. t.i.d. 30 minutes before meals. Or, 15 to 37.5 mg or 15 to 30 mg (as resin complex) P.O. daily as a single dose in the morning. Give Pro-Fast HS and Pro-Fast SR 2 hours after breakfast. Give Adipex-P before breakfast or 1 to 2 hours after breakfast.

ACTION

Unknown. Probably promotes nerve impulse transmission by releasing stored norepinephrine from nerve terminals in the brain, especially in the cerebral cortex and reticular activating system.

Route	Onset	Peak	Duration
P.O.	Unknown	Unknown	12–14 hr

Half-life: 19 to 24 hours.

ADVERSE REACTIONS

CNS: *insomnia,* overstimulation, headache, euphoria, dysphoria, dizziness.
CV: *palpitations, tachycardia,* increased blood pressure.
GI: dry mouth, dysgeusia, constipation, diarrhea, unpleasant taste, other GI disturbances.
GU: impotence.
Skin: urticaria.
Other: altered libido.

INTERACTIONS

Drug-drug. *Acetazolamide, antacids, sodium bicarbonate:* May increase renal reabsorption. Monitor patient for enhanced effects.
Ammonium chloride, ascorbic acid: May decrease level and increase renal excretion of phentermine. Monitor patient for decreased phentermine effects.
Insulin, oral antidiabetics: May alter antidiabetic requirements. Monitor glucose level.
MAO inhibitors (MAOI): May cause severe hypertension or hypertensive crisis. Avoid using within 14 days of MAOI therapy.

Drug-food. *Caffeine:* May increase CNS stimulation. Discourage use together.

EFFECTS ON LAB TEST RESULTS
None reported.

CONTRAINDICATIONS & CAUTIONS
- Contraindicated in patients hypersensitive to sympathomimetic amines, in those with idiosyncratic reactions to them, in agitated patients, and in those with hyperthyroidism, moderate-to-severe hypertension, advanced arteriosclerosis, symptomatic CV disease, or glaucoma.
- Contraindicated within 14 days of MAOI therapy.
- Use cautiously in patients with mild hypertension.

NURSING CONSIDERATIONS
- Use drug with a weight-reduction program.
- Monitor patient for tolerance or dependence.
- ***Look alike–sound alike:*** Don't confuse phentermine with phentolamine.

PATIENT TEACHING
- Tell patient to take drug at least 10 hours before bedtime to avoid sleep interference.
- Advise patient to avoid products that contain caffeine. Tell him to report evidence of excessive stimulation.
- Warn patient that fatigue may result as drug effects wear off and that he'll need more rest.
- Warn patient that drug may lose its effectiveness over time.

33

Antiparkinsonians

amantadine hydrochloride
apomorphine hydrochloride
benztropine mesylate
bromocriptine mesylate
entacapone
levodopa
levodopa and carbidopa
levodopa, carbidopa, and entacapone
pramipexole dihydrochloride
rasagiline mesylate
ropinirole hydrochloride
selegiline
selegiline hydrochloride
tolcapone

amantadine hydrochloride

Symmetrel

Pharmacologic class: synthetic cyclic primary amine
Pregnancy risk category C

AVAILABLE FORMS

Syrup: 50 mg/5 ml
Tablets: 100 mg

INDICATIONS & DOSAGES

➤ Parkinson disease

Adults: Initially, if used as monotherapy, 100 mg P.O. b.i.d. In patients with serious illness or in those already receiving high doses of other antiparkinsonians, begin dose at 100 mg P.O. once daily. Increase to 100 mg b.i.d. if needed after at least 1 week. Some patients may benefit from 400 mg daily in divided doses.

➤ To prevent or treat symptoms of influenza type A virus and respiratory tract illnesses

Children age 13 or older and adults up to age 65: 200 mg P.O. daily in a single dose or 100 mg P.O. b.i.d.
Children ages 9 to 12: 100 mg P.O. b.i.d.
Children ages 1 to 8 or who weigh less than 45 kg (99 lb): 4.4 to 8.8 mg/kg P.O. as a total daily dose given once daily or divided equally b.i.d. Maximum daily dose is 150 mg.
Elderly patients: 100 mg P.O. once daily in patients older than age 65 with normal renal function.

Begin treatment within 24 to 48 hours after symptoms appear and continue for 24 to 48 hours after symptoms disappear (usually 2 to 7 days). Start prophylaxis as soon as possible after exposure and continue for at least 10 days after exposure. May continue prophylactic treatment up to 90 days for repeated or suspected exposures if influenza vaccine is unavailable. If used with influenza vaccine, continue dose for 2 to 3 weeks until antibody response to vaccine has developed.
Adjust-a-dose: For patients with creatinine clearance of 30 to 50 ml/minute, give 200 mg the first day and 100 mg thereafter; if clearance is 15 to 29 ml/minute, give 200 mg the first day and then 100 mg on alternate days; if clearance is less than 15 ml/minute or if patient is receiving hemodialysis, give 200 mg q 7 days.

ACTION

May exert its antiparkinsonian effect by causing the release of dopamine in the substantia nigra. As an antiviral, may prevent release of viral nucleic acid into the host cell, reducing duration of fever and other systemic symptoms.

Route	Onset	Peak	Duration
P.O.	Unknown	1–4 hr	Unknown

Half-life: About 24 hours; with renal dysfunction, as long as 10 days.

ADVERSE REACTIONS

CNS: *dizziness, insomnia, irritability, light-headedness,* depression, fatigue, confusion, hallucinations, anxiety, ataxia, headache.
CV: ***heart failure,*** peripheral edema, orthostatic hypotension.
EENT: blurred vision.
GI: *nausea,* anorexia, constipation, vomiting, dry mouth.
Skin: livedo reticularis.

INTERACTIONS

Drug-drug. *Anticholinergics:* May increase anticholinergic effects. Use together cautiously; reduce dosage of anticholinergic before starting amantadine.
CNS stimulants: May increase CNS stimulation. Use together cautiously.
Co-trimoxazole, quinidine, thiazide diuretics, triamterene: May increase amantadine level, increasing the risk of toxicity. Use cautiously.
Thioridazine: May worsen Parkinson disease tremor. Monitor patient closely.
Drug-herb. *Jimsonweed:* May adversely affect CV function. Discourage use together.
Drug-lifestyle. *Alcohol use:* May increase CNS effects, including dizziness, confusion, and orthostatic hypotension. Discourage use together.

EFFECTS ON LAB TEST RESULTS

- May increase CK, BUN, creatinine, alkaline phosphatase, LDH, bilirubin, GGT, AST, and ALT levels.

CONTRAINDICATIONS & CAUTIONS

- Contraindicated in patients hypersensitive to drug.
- Use cautiously in elderly patients and in patients with seizure disorders, heart failure, peripheral edema, hepatic disease, mental illness, eczematoid rash, renal impairment, orthostatic hypotension, and CV disease. Monitor renal and liver function tests.

NURSING CONSIDERATIONS

- Patients with Parkinson disease who don't respond to anticholinergics may respond to this drug.
- Begin treatment for influenza within 24 to 48 hours after symptoms appear and continue for 24 to 48 hours after symptoms disappear (usually 2 to 7 days of therapy).
- Start influenza prophylaxis as soon as possible after first exposure and continue for at least 10 days after exposure. For repeated or suspected exposures, if influenza vaccine is unavailable, may continue prophylaxis for up to 90 days. If used with influenza vaccine, continue dose for 2 to 3 weeks until antibody response to vaccine has developed.
- ***Alert:*** Elderly patients are more susceptible to adverse neurologic effects. Monitor patient for mental status changes.
- Suicidal ideation and attempts may occur in any patient, regardless of psychiatric history.
- Drug can worsen mental problems in patients with a history of psychiatric disorders or substance abuse.
- ***Look alike–sound alike:*** Don't confuse amantadine with rimantadine.

PATIENT TEACHING

- ***Alert:*** Tell patient to take drug exactly as prescribed because not doing so may result in serious adverse reactions or death.
- If insomnia occurs, tell patient to take drug several hours before bedtime.
- If patient gets dizzy when he stands up, instruct him not to stand or change positions too quickly.
- Instruct patient to notify prescriber of adverse reactions, especially dizziness, depression, anxiety, nausea, and urine retention.
- Caution patient to avoid activities that require mental alertness until effects of drug are known.
- Encourage patient with Parkinson disease to gradually increase his physical activity as his symptoms improve.
- Advise patient to avoid alcohol while taking drug.

apomorphine hydrochloride

Apokyn

Pharmacologic class: nonergot-derivative dopamine agonist
Pregnancy risk category C

AVAILABLE FORMS

Solution for injection: 10 mg/ml (contains benzyl alcohol)

INDICATIONS & DOSAGES

➤ **Intermittent hypomobility, "off" episodes caused by advanced Parkinson disease (given with an antiemetic)**
Adults: Initially, give a 0.2-ml subcutaneous test dose. Measure supine and standing blood pressure q 20 minutes for the first hour. If patient tolerates and responds

to drug, start with 0.2 ml subcutaneously p.r.n. as outpatient. Separate doses by at least 2 hours. Increase by 0.1 ml every few days, p.r.n.

If initial 0.2-ml dose is ineffective but tolerated, give 0.4 ml at next "off" period, measuring supine and standing blood pressure q 20 minutes for the first hour. If drug is tolerated, start with 0.3 ml subcutaneously as outpatient. If needed, increase by 0.1 ml every few days.

If patient doesn't tolerate 0.4-ml dose, give 0.3 ml as a test dose at the next "off" period, measuring supine and standing blood pressure q 20 minutes for the first hour. If drug is tolerated, give 0.2 ml as outpatient. Increase by 0.1 ml every few days, p.r.n.; doses higher than 0.4 ml usually aren't tolerated if 0.2 ml is the starting dose.

Maximum recommended dose is usually 0.6 ml p.r.n. Most patients use drug t.i.d. Experience is limited at more than five times daily or more than 2 ml daily.

Adjust-a-dose: In patients with mild to moderate renal impairment, give test and starting doses of 0.1 ml subcutaneously.

ACTION

Thought to improve motor function by stimulating dopamine D2 receptors in the brain.

Route	Onset	Peak	Duration
SubQ	20 min	10–60 min	2 hr

Half-life: About 30 to 60 minutes in patients with normal or impaired renal function.

ADVERSE REACTIONS

CNS: *confusion, dizziness, drowsiness, hallucinations, somnolence,* aggravated Parkinson disease, anxiety, depression, fatigue, headache, insomnia, syncope, weakness.
CV: *angina, chest pain, chest pressure, edema, hypotension, orthostatic hypotension,* ***cardiac arrest, heart failure, MI,*** flushing.
EENT: *rhinorrhea.*
GI: *nausea, vomiting,* constipation, diarrhea.
GU: UTI.
Respiratory: dyspnea, pneumonia.
Metabolic: dehydration.
Musculoskeletal: *dyskinesias,* arthralgia, back pain, limb pain.
Skin: bruising, injection site reaction, pallor, sweating.
Other: *falls, yawning.*

INTERACTIONS

Drug-drug. *Antihypertensives, vasodilators:* May increase risk of hypotension, MI, pneumonia, falls, and joint injury. Use together cautiously.
Dopamine antagonists, metoclopramide: May reduce apomorphine's effectiveness. Use together cautiously.
Drugs that prolong the QTc interval: May further prolong the QTc interval. Use together cautiously.
5-HT_3 antagonists (alosetron, dolasetron, granisetron, ondansetron, palonosetron): May cause serious hypotension and loss of consciousness. Don't use together.
Drug-lifestyle. *Alcohol use:* May increase risk of sedation and hypotension. Discourage use together.

EFFECTS ON LAB TEST RESULTS

None reported.

CONTRAINDICATIONS & CAUTIONS

- Contraindicated in patients allergic to apomorphine or its ingredients, including sulfites, and in patients who take 5-HT_3 antagonists.
- Use cautiously in patients at risk for prolonged QTc interval, such as those with hypokalemia, hypomagnesemia, bradycardia, or genetic predisposition.
- Use cautiously in patients with CV or cerebrovascular disease and in those with renal or hepatic impairment.

NURSING CONSIDERATIONS

- ***Alert:*** Drug is for subcutaneous injection only. Avoid I.V. use.
- Give with an antiemetic to avoid severe nausea and vomiting. Start with trimethobenzamide 300 mg P.O. t.i.d. 3 days before starting apomorphine, and continue antiemetic at least 2 months.
- ***Alert:*** The prescribed dose should always be specified in milliliters rather than milligrams to avoid confusion; the dosing pen is marked in milliliters.
- Give test dose in a medically supervised setting to determine tolerability and effect.

• Monitor supine and standing blood pressure every 20 minutes for the first hour after starting doses or dosage changes.
• When programming the dosing pen, it's possible to select the appropriate dose even though insufficient drug remains in the pen. To avoid insufficient dosing, track the amount of drug received at each dose and change the cartridge before drug runs out.
• ***Alert:*** Monitor patient for drowsiness or sleepiness, which may occur well after treatment starts. Stop drug if patient develops significant daytime sleepiness that interferes with activities of daily living.
• Watch for evidence of coronary or cerebral ischemia, and stop drug if it occurs.
• Adverse effects are more likely in elderly patients, particularly hallucinations, falls, CV events, respiratory problems, and GI effects.

PATIENT TEACHING
• Tell patient to avoid sudden position changes, especially rising too quickly from lying down. A sudden drop in blood pressure, dizziness, or fainting can occur.
• Urge patient to keep taking the prescribed antiemetic because nausea and vomiting are likely.
• Instruct patient or caregiver to document each dose to make sure enough drug remains in the cartridge to provide a full next dose.
• Tell patient or caregiver to wait at least 2 hours between doses.
• ***Alert:*** Show patient or caregiver how to read the dosing pen, and make sure he understands that it's marked in milliliters and not milligrams.
• Tell patient or caregiver to rotate injection sites and to wash hands before each injection. Applying ice to the site before and after the injection may reduce soreness, redness, pain, itching, swelling, or bruising at the site.
• Explain that hallucinations (either visual or auditory) may occur, and urge patient or caregiver to report them immediately.
• Explain that headaches may occur and tell patient to notify prescriber if they become severe or don't go away.
• Advise patient to avoid hazardous activities that require alertness until drug effects are known.
• Caution patient to avoid consuming alcohol.

benztropine mesylate
Apo-Benztropine†, Cogentin, PMS Benztropine†

Pharmacologic class: anticholinergic
Pregnancy risk category C

AVAILABLE FORMS
Injection: 1 mg/ml in 2-ml ampules
Tablets: 0.5 mg, 1 mg, 2 mg

INDICATIONS & DOSAGES
➤ **Drug-induced extrapyramidal disorders (except tardive dyskinesia)**
Adults: 1 to 4 mg P.O. or I.M. once or twice daily.
➤ **Acute dystonic reaction**
Adults: 1 to 2 mg I.V. or I.M.; then 1 to 2 mg P.O. b.i.d. to prevent recurrence.
➤ **Parkinsonism**
Adults: 0.5 to 6 mg P.O. or I.M. daily. First dosage is 0.5 mg to 1 mg, increased by 0.5 mg q 5 to 6 days. Adjust dosage to meet individual requirements. Maximum, 6 mg daily.

I.V. ADMINISTRATION
• Reserve I.V. delivery for emergencies, such as acute dystonic reactions.
• The I.V. form is seldom used because no significant difference exists between it and the I.M. form.

INCOMPATIBILITIES
Haloperidol lactate.

ACTION
Unknown. May block central cholinergic receptors, helping to balance cholinergic activity in the basal ganglia.

Route	Onset	Peak	Duration
P.O.	1–2 hr	Unknown	24 hr
I.V., I.M.	15 min	Unknown	24 hr

Half-life: Unknown.

ADVERSE REACTIONS
CNS: confusion, memory impairment, nervousness, depression, disorientation, hallucinations, toxic psychosis.
CV: tachycardia.
EENT: dilated pupils, blurred vision.
GI: *dry mouth, constipation,* nausea, vomiting, paralytic ileus.
GU: urine retention, dysuria.
Skin: decreased sweating.

INTERACTIONS
Drug-drug. *Amantadine, phenothiazines, tricyclic antidepressants:* May cause additive anticholinergic adverse reactions, such as confusion and hallucinations. Reduce dosage before giving.
Cholinergics (donepezil, galantamine, rivastigmine, tacrine): May antagonize the therapeutic effects of these drugs. If used together, monitor patient for therapeutic effect.

EFFECTS ON LAB TEST RESULTS
None reported.

CONTRAINDICATIONS & CAUTIONS
- Contraindicated in patients hypersensitive to drug or its components, in those with angle-closure glaucoma, and in children younger than age 3.
- Use cautiously in hot weather, in patients with mental disorders, in elderly patients, and in children age 3 and older.
- Use cautiously in patients with prostatic hyperplasia, arrhythmias, or seizure disorders.

NURSING CONSIDERATIONS
- Monitor vital signs carefully. Watch closely for adverse reactions, especially in elderly or debilitated patients. Call prescriber promptly if adverse reactions occur.
- At certain doses, drug produces atropine-like toxicity, which may aggravate tardive dyskinesia.
- Watch for intermittent constipation and abdominal distention and pain, which may indicate onset of paralytic ileus.
- Monitor elderly patients closely as they are more prone to severe adverse effects.
- ***Alert:*** Never stop drug abruptly. Reduce dosage gradually.
- ***Look alike–sound alike:*** Don't confuse benztropine with bromocriptine.

PATIENT TEACHING
- Warn patient to avoid activities that require alertness until CNS effects of drug are known.
- If patient takes a single daily dose, tell him to do so at bedtime.
- Advise patient to report signs and symptoms of urinary hesitancy or urine retention.
- Tell patient to relieve dry mouth with cool drinks, ice chips, sugarless gum, or hard candy.
- Advise patient to limit hot weather activities because drug-induced lack of sweating may cause overheating.

bromocriptine mesylate
Parlodel

Pharmacologic class: dopamine receptor agonist
Pregnancy risk category B

AVAILABLE FORMS
Capsules: 5 mg
Tablets: 2.5 mg

INDICATIONS & DOSAGES
➤ **Parkinson disease**
Adults: 1.25 mg P.O. b.i.d. with meals. Increase dosage by 2.5 mg/day q 14 to 28 days, up to 100 mg daily.
➤ **Amenorrhea and galactorrhea from hyperprolactinemia; hypogonadism, infertility**
Adults: 0.5 to 2.5 mg P.O. daily, increased by 2.5 mg daily at 3- to 7-day intervals until desired effect occurs. Therapeutic daily dose is 2.5 to 15 mg.
➤ **Acromegaly**
Adults: 1.25 to 2.5 mg P.O. with bedtime snack for 3 days. Another 1.25 to 2.5 mg may be added q 3 to 7 days until therapeutic benefit occurs. Maximum, 100 mg daily.
➤ **Neuroleptic malignant syndrome** ♦
Adults: 2.5 to 5 mg P.O. two to six times daily.

ACTION
Inhibits secretion of prolactin and acts as a dopamine-receptor agonist by activating postsynaptic dopamine receptors.

Route	Onset	Peak	Duration
P.O.	2 hr	8 hr	24 hr

Half-life: 15 hours.

ADVERSE REACTIONS
CNS: *dizziness, headache, fatigue,* ***seizures, stroke,*** mania, light-headedness, drowsiness, delusions, nervousness, insomnia, depression.
CV: *hypotension,* ***acute MI.***
EENT: nasal congestion, blurred vision.
GI: *nausea, abdominal cramps, constipation,* diarrhea, vomiting, anorexia.
GU: urine retention, urinary frequency.
Skin: coolness and pallor of fingers and toes.

INTERACTIONS
Drug-drug. *Amitriptyline, haloperidol, imipramine, loxapine, MAO inhibitors, methyldopa, metoclopramide, phenothiazines, reserpine:* May interfere with bromocriptine's effects. Bromocriptine dosage may need to be increased.
Antihypertensives: May increase hypotensive effects. Adjust dosage of antihypertensive.
Erythromycin: May increase bromocriptine level and risk of adverse reactions. Use together cautiously.
Estrogens, hormonal contraceptives, progestins: May interfere with effects of bromocriptine. Avoid using together.
Levodopa: May have additive effects. Adjust dosage of levodopa, if needed.
Drug-lifestyle. *Alcohol use:* May cause disulfiram-like reaction. Discourage use together.

EFFECTS ON LAB TEST RESULTS
- May increase alkaline phosphatase, ALT, AST, BUN, CK, and uric acid levels.

CONTRAINDICATIONS & CAUTIONS
- Contraindicated in patients hypersensitive to ergot derivatives and in those with uncontrolled hypertension, toxemia of pregnancy, severe ischemic heart disease, or peripheral vascular disease.
- Use cautiously in patients with impaired renal or hepatic function and in those with a history of MI with residual arrhythmias.

NURSING CONSIDERATIONS
- For Parkinson disease, bromocriptine usually is given with levodopa or levodopa and carbidopa. The levodopa and carbidopa may need to be reduced.
- Adverse reactions may be minimized if drug is given in the evening with food.
- ***Alert:*** Monitor patient for adverse reactions, which occur in 68% of patients, particularly at start of therapy. Most reactions are mild to moderate; nausea is most common. Minimize adverse reactions by gradually adjusting dosages to effective levels. Adverse reactions are more common when drug is used for Parkinson disease.
- Baseline and periodic evaluations of cardiac, hepatic, renal, and hematopoietic function are recommended during prolonged therapy.
- Drug may lead to early postpartum conception. After menses resumes, test for pregnancy every 4 weeks or as soon as a period is missed.
- ***Look alike–sound alike:*** Don't confuse bromocriptine with benztropine or brimonidine, or Parlodel with pindolol.

PATIENT TEACHING
- Instruct patient to take drug with meals.
- Advise patient to use contraceptive methods during treatment other than oral contraceptives or subdermal implants.
- Instruct patient to avoid dizziness and fainting by rising slowly to an upright position and avoiding sudden position changes.
- Inform patient that it may take 8 weeks or longer for menses to resume and excess production of milk to slow down.
- Advise patient to avoid alcohol while taking drug.

entacapone
Comtan

Pharmacologic class: catechol-O-methyltransferase (COMT) inhibitor
Pregnancy risk category C

AVAILABLE FORMS
Tablets: 200 mg

INDICATIONS & DOSAGES
➤ **Adjunct to levodopa and carbidopa for treatment of idiopathic Parkinson disease in patients with signs and symptoms of end-of-dose wearing off**
Adults: 200 mg P.O. with each dose of levodopa and carbidopa, up to eight times daily. Maximum, 1,600 mg daily. May need to reduce daily levodopa dose or extend the interval between doses to optimize patient's response.

ACTION
A reversible COMT inhibitor given with levodopa and carbidopa. The combination is thought to cause higher levels of levodopa and optimal control of parkinsonian symptoms.

Route	Onset	Peak	Duration
P.O.	1 hr	1 hr	6 hr

Half-life: About ½ to ¾ hour for first phase and about 2½ hours for second phase.

ADVERSE REACTIONS
CNS: *dyskinesia, hyperkinesia,* hypokinesia, dizziness, anxiety, somnolence, agitation, fatigue, asthenia, hallucinations.
GI: *nausea, diarrhea,* abdominal pain, constipation, vomiting, dry mouth, dyspepsia, flatulence, gastritis, taste perversion.
GU: *urine discoloration.*
Hematologic: purpura.
Musculoskeletal: back pain.
Respiratory: dyspnea.
Skin: sweating.
Other: bacterial infection.

INTERACTIONS
Drug-drug. *Ampicillin, chloramphenicol, cholestyramine, erythromycin, probenecid:* May block biliary excretion, resulting in higher levels of entacapone. Use together cautiously.
CNS depressants: May cause additive effect. Use together cautiously.
Drugs metabolized by COMT (dobutamine, dopamine, epinephrine, isoetharine, isoproterenol, norepinephrine): May cause higher levels of these drugs, resulting in increased heart rate, changes in blood pressure, or arrhythmias. Use together cautiously.
Nonselective MAO inhibitors (such as phenelzine, tranylcypromine): May inhibit normal catecholamine metabolism. Avoid using together.
Drug-lifestyle. *Alcohol use:* May cause additive CNS effects. Discourage use together.

EFFECTS ON LAB TEST RESULTS
None reported.

CONTRAINDICATIONS & CAUTIONS
- Contraindicated in patients hypersensitive to drug.
- Use cautiously in patients with hepatic impairment, biliary obstruction, or orthostatic hypotension.

NURSING CONSIDERATIONS
- Use drug only with levodopa and carbidopa; no antiparkinsonian effects occur when drug is given as monotherapy.
- Levodopa and carbidopa dosage requirements are usually lower when drug is given with entacapone; lower levodopa and carbidopa dose or increase dosing interval to avoid adverse effects.
- Drug may cause or worsen dyskinesia, even if levodopa dose is lowered.
- Hallucinations may occur or worsen during therapy with this drug.
- Monitor blood pressure closely, and watch for orthostatic hypotension.
- Diarrhea most often begins within 4 to 12 weeks of starting therapy but may begin as early as 1 week or as late as many months after starting treatment.
- Drug may discolor urine.
- Rarely, rhabdomyolysis has occurred with drug use.
- Rapid withdrawal or abrupt reduction in dose could lead to signs and symptoms of Parkinson disease; it may also lead to

hyperpyrexia and confusion, a group of symptoms resembling neuroleptic malignant syndrome. Stop drug gradually, and monitor patient closely. Adjust other dopaminergic treatments, as needed.
• Drug can be given with immediate or sustained-release levodopa and carbidopa and can be taken with or without food.

PATIENT TEACHING
• Instruct patient not to crush or break tablet and to take it at same time as levodopa and carbidopa.
• Warn patient to avoid hazardous activities until CNS effects of drug are known.
• Advise patient to avoid alcohol during treatment.
• Instruct patient to use caution when standing after a prolonged period of sitting or lying down because dizziness may occur. This effect is more common during initial therapy.
• Warn patient that hallucinations, increased difficulty with voluntary movements, nausea, and diarrhea could occur.
• Inform patient that drug may turn urine brownish orange.
• Advise patient to notify prescriber about planned, suspected, or known pregnancy, and to notify prescriber if she's breast-feeding.

levodopa
Larodopa

Pharmacologic class: dopamine precursor
Pregnancy risk category NR

AVAILABLE FORMS
Capsules: 100 mg, 250 mg, 500 mg
Tablets: 100 mg, 250 mg, 500 mg

INDICATIONS & DOSAGES
➤**Idiopathic parkinsonism, postencephalitic parkinsonism, and symptomatic parkinsonism after carbon monoxide or manganese intoxication or with cerebral arteriosclerosis**
Adults and children age 12 or older: Initially, 0.5 to 1 g P.O. daily, divided in two or more doses with food; increase by no more than 0.75 g daily q 3 to 7 days until maximal response is achieved. Don't exceed 8 g daily. Adjust dosage to patient requirements, tolerance, and response. Higher dosage needs close supervision.

ACTION
Unknown. May be decarboxylated to dopamine, countering the depletion of striatal dopamine in extrapyramidal centers; this depletion is thought to produce parkinsonism.

Route	Onset	Peak	Duration
P.O.	Unknown	1–3 hr	5 hr

Half-life: 1 to 3 hours.

ADVERSE REACTIONS
CNS: *aggressive behavior, involuntary grimacing, head movements, myoclonic body jerks, ataxia, tremor, muscle twitching, bradykinetic episodes, psychiatric disturbances, mood changes, nervousness, anxiety, disturbing dreams, euphoria, malaise, fatigue, severe depression, dementia, delirium, hallucinations, choreiform, dystonic, and dyskinetic movements,* ***suicidal tendencies, seizures.***
CV: *orthostatic hypotension,* phlebitis, cardiac irregularities.
EENT: blepharospasm, blurred vision, diplopia, mydriasis or miosis, activation of latent Horner syndrome, oculogyric crises.
GI: *anorexia, nausea, vomiting,* dry mouth, bitter taste, constipation, flatulence, diarrhea, abdominal pain, excessive salivation.
GU: urinary frequency, urine retention, incontinence, darkened urine, priapism.
Hematologic: ***leukopenia, agranulocytosis,*** hemolytic anemia.
Hepatic: ***hepatotoxicity.***
Metabolic: weight loss.
Respiratory: hiccups, hyperventilation.
Skin: dark perspiration.

INTERACTIONS
Drug-drug. *Antacids:* May increase absorption of levodopa. Give antacids 1 hour after levodopa.
Furazolidone, MAO inhibitors (phenelzine, tranylcypromine), procarbazine: May cause severe hypertension. Avoid using together.

Inhaled anesthetics, sympathomimetics: May increase risk of arrhythmias. Monitor patient closely.
Iron salts: May reduce bioavailability of levodopa. Separate dosage times.
Metoclopramide: May accelerate gastric emptying of levodopa. Give metoclopramide 1 hour after levodopa.
Phenothiazines, other antipsychotics, phenytoin, rauwolfia alkaloids: May decrease levodopa effect. Avoid using together.
Pyridoxine (vitamin B_6): May decrease the effectiveness of levodopa; has little to no effect on the combination drug levodopa and carbidopa. Avoid using pyridoxine with levodopa.
Drug-herb. *Kava:* May increase parkinsonism symptoms. Discourage kava use altogether.
Drug-food. *Foods high in protein:* May decrease levodopa absorption. Discourage use together.
Drug-lifestyle. *Cocaine use:* May increase risk of arrhythmias. Inform patient of this interaction.

EFFECTS ON LAB TEST RESULTS

- May increase BUN, ALT, AST, alkaline phosphatase, LDH, and bilirubin levels; may cause transient elevations in protein-bound iodine levels. May decrease hemoglobin level and hematocrit.
- May decrease WBC and granulocyte counts.
- May falsely elevate levels of colorimetric test for uric acid and urinary catecholamine, and may falsely decrease urinary vanillylmandelic acid levels. May cause false-positive Coombs test result during extended therapy. May cause false-positive results for urine glucose using copper-reduction method; and false-negative results using glucose oxidase method. May interfere with tests for urine ketones. May interfere with urine screening tests for phenylketonuria.

CONTRAINDICATIONS & CAUTIONS

- Contraindicated in patients hypersensitive to drug and in those with acute angle-closure glaucoma, melanoma, or undiagnosed skin lesions; also contraindicated within 14 days of MAO inhibitor therapy.
- Use cautiously in patients with severe CV, renal, hepatic, and pulmonary disorders; peptic ulcer; psychiatric illness; MI with residual arrhythmias; bronchial asthma; emphysema; and endocrine disease.

NURSING CONSIDERATIONS

- Capsules may contain tartrazine.
- Patients who need surgery should continue levodopa therapy as long as oral intake is permitted, usually until 6 to 24 hours before surgery. Resume therapy as soon as patient can take drug orally.
- ***Alert:*** Because of risk of triggering a symptom complex resembling neuroleptic malignant syndrome, observe patient closely if levodopa dosage is reduced abruptly or stopped.
- Giving levodopa and carbidopa together typically decreases amount of levodopa needed by 75%, reducing risk of adverse reactions.
- Monitor vital signs, especially while adjusting dosage. Report changes.
- ***Alert:*** Watch for muscle twitching and blepharospasm, which may be early signs of drug overdose; report immediately.
- ***Alert:*** Hallucinations may require reduction or withdrawal of drug.
- An accurate measure for urine glucose can be obtained if paper strip is partially immersed in the urine sample. Urine migrates up the strip, as with an ascending chromatographic system. Read only the top of the strip.
- Test patients receiving long-term therapy regularly for diabetes and acromegaly; also periodically monitor renal, hepatic, and hematopoietic function.

PATIENT TEACHING

- Tell patient to take drug with food to minimize GI upset, but tell him high-protein meals can impair absorption and reduce effectiveness.
- If patient has trouble swallowing pills, tell him or caregiver to crush tablets and mix with applesauce or pureed fruit.
- Warn patient or caregiver not to increase dosage unless ordered. Daily dose shouldn't exceed 8 g.
- Tell patient to protect drug from heat, light, and moisture. If preparation darkens, it has lost potency; tell him to discard it.

• Warn patient about possible dizziness upon standing quickly, especially at start of therapy. Tell him to change positions slowly and dangle legs before rising. Elastic stockings may control these adverse reactions.
• Advise patient and caregivers that multivitamin preparations, fortified cereals, and certain OTC drugs may contain pyridoxine (vitamin B_6), which can block the effects of levodopa by enhancing its peripheral metabolism.

levodopa and carbidopa
Parcopa, Sinemet✐, Sinemet CR✐

Pharmacologic class: decarboxylase inhibitor and dopamine precursor
Pregnancy risk category C

AVAILABLE FORMS
Tablets: 100 mg levodopa with 10 mg carbidopa (Sinemet 10-100), 100 mg levodopa with 25 mg carbidopa (Sinemet 25-100), 250 mg levodopa with 25 mg carbidopa (Sinemet 25-250)
Tablets (extended-release): 200 mg levodopa with 50 mg carbidopa (Sinemet CR), 100 mg levodopa with 25 mg carbidopa
Tablets (orally disintegrating): 100 mg levodopa with 10 mg carbidopa, 100 mg levodopa with 25 mg carbidopa, 250 mg levodopa with 25 mg carbidopa

INDICATIONS & DOSAGES
➤ **Idiopathic Parkinson disease, postencephalitic parkinsonism, and symptomatic parkinsonism resulting from carbon monoxide or manganese intoxication**
Adults: 1 tablet of 100 mg levodopa with 25 mg carbidopa P.O. t.i.d.; then increased by 1 tablet daily or every other day, p.r.n., to maximum daily dose of 8 tablets. May use 250 mg levodopa with 25 mg carbidopa or 100 mg levodopa with 10 mg carbidopa tablets, as directed, to obtain maximal response. Optimum daily dose must be determined by careful adjustment for each patient.

Patients given conventional tablets may receive extended-release tablets; dosage is calculated on current levodopa intake. Extended-release tablets should provide 10% more levodopa daily, increased p.r.n. and as tolerated to 30% more levodopa daily. Give in divided doses at intervals of 4 to 8 hours.

ACTION
Levodopa, a dopamine precursor, relieves parkinsonian symptoms by being converted to dopamine in the brain. Carbidopa inhibits the decarboxylation of peripheral levodopa, which allows more intact levodopa to travel to the brain.

Route	Onset	Peak	Duration
P.O.	Unknown	40–150 min	Unknown

Half-life: 1 to 2 hours.

ADVERSE REACTIONS
CNS: *choreiform, dystonic, dyskinetic movements, involuntary grimacing, head movements, myoclonic body jerks, ataxia,* ***suicidal tendencies,*** tremor, muscle twitching, bradykinetic episodes, psychiatric disturbances, anxiety, disturbing dreams, euphoria, malaise, fatigue, severe depression, dementia, delirium, hallucinations, confusion, insomnia, agitation.
CV: *orthostatic hypotension,* cardiac irregularities, phlebitis.
EENT: blepharospasm, blurred vision, diplopia, mydriasis or miosis, oculogyric crises, excessive salivation.
GI: *dry mouth, nausea, vomiting, anorexia,* bitter taste, constipation, flatulence, diarrhea, abdominal pain.
GU: urinary frequency, urine retention, urinary incontinence, darkened urine, priapism.
Hematologic: ***thrombocytopenia, leukopenia, agranulocytosis,*** hemolytic anemia.
Hepatic: ***hepatotoxicity.***
Metabolic: weight loss.
Respiratory: hiccups, hyperventilation.
Skin: dark perspiration.

INTERACTIONS
Drug-drug. *Antihypertensives:* May cause additive hypotensive effects. Use together cautiously.
Iron salts: May reduce bioavailability of levodopa and carbidopa. Give iron 1 hour before or 2 hours after Sinemet.

MAO inhibitors: May cause risk of severe hypertension. Avoid using together.
Papaverine, phenytoin: May antagonize antiparkinsonian actions. Avoid using together.
Phenothiazines, other antipsychotics: May antagonize antiparkinsonian actions. Use together cautiously.
Drug-herb. *Kava:* May decrease action of drug. Discourage kava use altogether.
Octacosanol: May worsen dyskinesias. Discourage use together.
Drug-food. *Foods high in protein:* May decrease levodopa absorption. Don't give levodopa with high-protein foods.

EFFECTS ON LAB TEST RESULTS

- May increase uric acid, ALT, AST, alkaline phosphatase, LDH, and bilirubin levels. May decrease hemoglobin level and hematocrit.
- May decrease WBC, granulocyte, and platelet counts.
- May falsely increase urinary catecholamine level and serum and urinary uric acid levels in colorimetric tests. May falsely decrease urinary vanillylmandelic acid level. May cause false-positive results in urine ketone tests using sodium nitroprusside reagent and in urinary glucose tests using cupric sulfate reagent. May cause false-negative results in tests using glucose oxidase. May alter results of urine screening tests for phenylketonuria.

CONTRAINDICATIONS & CAUTIONS

- Contraindicated in patients hypersensitive to drug and in those with angle-closure glaucoma, melanoma, or undiagnosed skin lesions.
- Contraindicated within 14 days of MAO inhibitor therapy.
- Use cautiously in patients with severe CV, renal, hepatic, endocrine, or pulmonary disorders; history of peptic ulcer; psychiatric illness; MI with residual arrhythmias; bronchial asthma; emphysema; or well-controlled, chronic open-angle glaucoma.

NURSING CONSIDERATIONS

- If patient takes levodopa, stop drug at least 8 hours before starting levodopa-carbidopa.
- Giving levodopa and carbidopa together typically decreases amount of levodopa needed by 75%, reducing risk of adverse reactions.
- Therapeutic and adverse reactions occur more rapidly with levodopa and carbidopa than with levodopa alone. Observe patient and monitor vital signs, especially while adjusting dosage. Report significant changes.
- ***Alert:*** Because of risk of precipitating a symptom complex resembling neuroleptic malignant syndrome, observe patient closely if levodopa dosage is reduced abruptly or stopped.
- Hallucinations may require reduction or withdrawal of drug.
- ***Alert:*** Muscle twitching and blepharospasm may be early signs of drug overdose; report immediately.
- Test patients receiving long-term therapy regularly for diabetes and acromegaly, and periodically for hepatic, renal, and hematopoietic function.

PATIENT TEACHING

- Tell patient to take drug with food to minimize GI upset; however, high-protein meals can impair absorption and reduce effectiveness.
- Tell patient not to chew or crush extended-release form.
- Warn patient and caregivers not to increase dosage without prescriber's orders.
- Caution patient about possible dizziness when standing up quickly, especially at start of therapy. Tell him to change positions slowly and dangle his legs before getting out of bed. Elastic stockings may control these adverse reactions in some patients.
- Instruct patient to report adverse reactions and therapeutic effects.
- Inform patient that pyridoxine (vitamin B_6) doesn't reverse beneficial effects of levodopa and carbidopa. Multivitamins can be taken without reversing levodopa's effects.

levodopa, carbidopa, and entacapone

Stalevo

Pharmacologic class: dopamine precursor, decarboxylase inhibitor, and catecholamine-*O*-methyltransferase (COMT) inhibitor
Pregnancy risk category C

AVAILABLE FORMS

Tablets (film-coated): 50 mg levodopa, 12.5 mg carbidopa, 200 mg entacapone; 100 mg levodopa, 25 mg carbidopa, 200 mg entacapone; 150 mg levodopa, 37.5 mg carbidopa, 200 mg entacapone

INDICATIONS & DOSAGES

➤ **Idiopathic Parkinson disease, to replace (with equivalent strengths) levodopa, carbidopa, and entacapone given individually or to replace immediate-release levodopa and carbidopa for a patient who has end-of-dose "wearing off," who's taking a total daily levodopa dose of 600 mg or less and who has no dyskinesia**

Adults: 1 tablet P.O.; determine dose and interval by therapeutic response. Maximum, 8 tablets daily.

ACTION

Levodopa, a dopamine precursor, relieves parkinsonian symptoms by converting to dopamine in the brain. Carbidopa inhibits the decarboxylation of peripheral levodopa, which allows more intact levodopa to travel to the brain. Entacapone is a reversible COMT inhibitor that increases levodopa level.

Route	Onset	Peak	Duration
P.O.	Unknown	1½ hr	Unknown

Half-life: 1½ to 2 hours carbidopa, 1 to 5 hours levodopa, and 1 to 4 hours entacapone.

ADVERSE REACTIONS

levodopa and carbidopa

CNS: ***neuroleptic malignant syndrome,*** agitation, asthenia, confusion, delusions, dementia, depression, dizziness, dyskinesia, hallucinations, headache, increased libido, insomnia, nightmares, paranoid ideation, paresthesias, psychosis, somnolence, syncope.
CV: cardiac irregularities, chest pain, hypertension, hypotension, orthostatic hypotension, palpitations, phlebitis.
GI: anorexia, constipation, dark saliva, diarrhea, dry mouth, duodenal ulcer, dyspepsia, GI bleeding, nausea, taste alterations, vomiting.
GU: dark urine, urinary frequency, UTI.
Hematologic: ***agranulocytosis, leukopenia, thrombocytopenia,*** anemia.
Musculoskeletal: back pain, muscle cramps, shoulder pain.
Respiratory: dyspnea, upper respiratory infection.
Skin: alopecia, bullous lesions, dark sweat, Henoch-Schönlein purpura, increased sweating, pruritus, rash, urticaria.
Other: ***angioedema.***

entacapone

CNS: *dyskinesia, hyperkinesia,* agitation, anxiety, asthenia, dizziness, fatigue, hypokinesia, somnolence.
GI: *diarrhea, nausea,* abdominal pain, constipation, dry mouth, dyspepsia, flatulence, gastritis, taste perversion, vomiting.
GU: *urine discoloration.*
Musculoskeletal: back pain.
Respiratory: dyspnea.
Skin: increased sweating, purpura.
Other: bacterial infection.

INTERACTIONS

Drug-drug. *Ampicillin, chloramphenicol, cholestyramine, erythromycin, probenecid, rifampicin:* May interfere with entacapone excretion. Use together cautiously.
Antihypertensives: May cause orthostatic hypotension. Adjust antihypertensive dosage as needed.
CNS depressants: Additive effects. Use together cautiously.
Dopamine (D2) receptor antagonists such as butyrophenones, iron salts, isoniazid, metoclopramide, phenothiazines, phenytoin, risperidone: May decrease levodopa, carbidopa, and entacapone effects. Monitor patient for effectiveness.
Drugs metabolized by COMT, such as alpha-methyldopa, apomorphine, dobutamine, dopamine, epinephrine, isoproterenol, isoetharine, norepinephrine: May increase heart rate, arrhythmias, and ex-

cessive blood pressure changes. Use together cautiously.
Metoclopramide: May increase availability of levodopa and carbidopa by increasing gastric emptying. Monitor patient for adverse effects.
Nonselective MAO inhibitor: May disrupt catecholamine metabolism. Avoid using together.
Selegiline: May cause severe hypotension. Use together cautiously, and monitor blood pressure.
Tricyclic antidepressants: May increase risk of hypertension and dyskinesia. Monitor patient closely.

EFFECTS ON LAB TEST RESULTS
- May increase alkaline phosphatase, AST, ALT, LDH, glucose, BUN, and bilirubin levels. May decrease hemoglobin level and hematocrit.
- May decrease platelet and WBC counts.
- May cause false-positive reaction for urinary ketone bodies on a test tape. May cause false-negative result for glucosuria with glucose oxidase testing methods.

CONTRAINDICATIONS & CAUTIONS
- Contraindicated in patients hypersensitive to drug or its ingredients.
- Contraindicated in patients with angle-closure glaucoma, suspicious undiagnosed skin lesions, or a history of melanoma.
- Contraindicated within 2 weeks of MAO inhibitor therapy.
- Use cautiously in patients with past or current psychosis and in patients with severe cardiovascular or pulmonary disease, bronchial asthma, biliary obstruction, or renal, hepatic, or endocrine disease.
- Use cautiously in patients with chronic open-angle glaucoma or a history of MI and residual atrial, nodal, or ventricular arrhythmias.

NURSING CONSIDERATIONS
- Certain CNS effects, such as dyskinesia, may occur at lower dosages and sooner with levodopa, carbidopa, and entacapone than with levodopa alone. Dyskinesia may require a reduced dosage.
- During the first adjustment period, monitor a patient with CV disease carefully and in a facility equipped to provide intensive cardiac care.
- Neuroleptic malignant syndrome may develop when levodopa and carbidopa are reduced or stopped, especially in patients taking antipsychotic drugs. Watch patient carefully for fever, hyperthermia, muscle rigidity, involuntary movements, altered consciousness, mental status changes, and autonomic dysfunction.
- During extended therapy, periodically monitor hepatic, hematopoietic, CV, and renal function.
- Diarrhea is common; it usually develops 4 to 12 weeks after treatment starts but may appear as early as the first week or as late as many months after treatment starts.
- Monitor patient for hallucinations, depression, and suicidal tendencies.

PATIENT TEACHING
- Advise patient to take drug exactly as prescribed.
- Tell patient to report a "wearing-off" effect, which may occur at the end of the dosing interval.
- Tell patient that urine, sweat, and saliva may turn dark (red, brown, or black) during treatment.
- Advise patient to notify the prescriber if problems making voluntary movements increase.
- Tell patient that diarrhea is common with this treatment.
- Inform patient that hallucinations may occur.
- Urge patient to immediately report depression or suicidal thoughts.
- Explain that he may become dizzy if he rises quickly. Urge patient to use caution when rising.
- Tell patient that a high-protein diet, excessive acidity, and iron salts may reduce the drug's effectiveness.
- Urge patient to avoid hazardous activities until the CNS effects of the drug are known.
- Advise patient to notify prescriber if she becomes pregnant.

pramipexole dihydrochloride
Mirapex

Pharmacologic class: nonergot dopamine agonist
Pregnancy risk category C

AVAILABLE FORMS
Tablets: 0.125 mg, 0.25 mg, 0.5 mg, 1 mg, 1.5 mg

INDICATIONS & DOSAGES
➤ **Signs and symptoms of idiopathic Parkinson disease**
Adults: Initially, 0.375 mg P.O. daily in three divided doses. Adjust doses slowly (not more often than q 5 to 7 days) over several weeks until desired therapeutic effect is achieved. Maintenance dosage is 1.5 to 4.5 mg daily in three divided doses.
Adjust-a-dose: For patients with creatinine clearance over 60 ml/minute, first dosage is 0.125 mg P.O. t.i.d., up to 1.5 mg t.i.d. For those with clearance of 35 to 59 ml/minute, first dosage is 0.125 mg P.O. b.i.d., up to 1.5 mg b.i.d. For those with clearance of 15 to 34 ml/minute, first dosage is 0.125 mg P.O. daily, up to 1.5 mg daily.

ACTION
Nonergot dopamine receptor agonist thought to stimulate dopamine receptors.

Route	Onset	Peak	Duration
P.O.	Rapid	2 hr	8–12 hr

Half-life: 8 to 12 hours.

ADVERSE REACTIONS
CNS: *asthenia, confusion, dizziness, dream abnormalities, dyskinesia, extrapyramidal syndrome, hallucinations, insomnia, somnolence,* amnesia, akathisia, drowsiness, delusions, dystonia, gait abnormalities, hypoesthesia, hypertonia, myoclonus, paranoid reaction, malaise, sleep disorders, thought abnormalities, fever.
CV: *orthostatic hypotension,* chest pain, peripheral edema.
EENT: accommodation abnormalities, diplopia, rhinitis, vision abnormalities.
GI: *constipation, nausea,* dry mouth, anorexia, dysphagia.
GU: impotence, urinary frequency, UTI, urinary incontinence.
Metabolic: weight loss.
Musculoskeletal: arthritis, bursitis, myasthenia, twitching.
Respiratory: dyspnea, pneumonia.
Skin: skin disorders.
Other: *accidental injury,* decreased libido, general edema.

INTERACTIONS
Drug-drug. *Cimetidine, diltiazem, quinidine, quinine, ranitidine, triamterene, verapamil:* May decrease pramipexole clearance. Adjust dosage as needed.
Dopamine antagonists: May reduce pramipexole effectiveness. Monitor patient closely.

EFFECTS ON LAB TEST RESULTS
None reported.

CONTRAINDICATIONS & CAUTIONS
- Contraindicated in patients hypersensitive to drug or its components.
- Use cautiously in renally impaired patients.
- Use cautiously in breast-feeding women. It's unknown if drug appears in breast milk.

NURSING CONSIDERATIONS
- If drug must be stopped, withdraw over 1 week.
- Drug may cause orthostatic hypotension, especially during dosage increases. Monitor patient carefully.
- Adjust dosage gradually to achieve maximal therapeutic effect, balanced against the main adverse effects of dyskinesia, hallucinations, somnolence, and dry mouth.

PATIENT TEACHING
- Instruct patient not to rise rapidly after sitting or lying down because of risk of dizziness.
- Caution patient to avoid hazardous activities until CNS response to drug is known.
- Tell patient to use caution before taking drug with other CNS depressants.
- Tell patient (especially elderly patient) that hallucinations may occur.
- Advise patient to take drug with food if nausea develops.
- Tell woman to notify prescriber if she is breast-feeding or intends to do so.

• Advise patient that it may take 4 weeks for effects of drug to be noticed because of slow adjustment schedule.

✱ NEW DRUG

rasagiline mesylate
Azilect

Pharmacologic class: irreversible, selective MAO inhibitor type B
Pregnancy risk category C

AVAILABLE FORMS
Tablets: 0.5 mg, 1 mg

INDICATIONS & DOSAGES
➤ **Idiopathic Parkinson disease, as monotherapy or with levodopa**
Adults: As monotherapy, 1 mg P.O. once daily. With levodopa, 0.5 mg P.O. once daily; increase to 1 mg once daily p.r.n. If patient taking both drugs has hallucinations or dyskinesia, reduce levodopa dosage.
Adjust-a-dose: If patient has mild hepatic impairment or takes a CYP1A2 inhibitor such as ciprofloxacin, give 0.5 mg once daily.

ACTION
May increase extracellular dopamine level in the CNS, improving neurotransmission and relieving signs and symptoms of Parkinson disease

Route	Onset	Peak	Duration
P.O.	Variable	1 hr	1 wk

Half-life: 3 hours.

ADVERSE REACTIONS
Monotherapy
CNS: *dizziness, falls, headache,* depression, fever, hallucinations, malaise, paresthesia, syncope, vertigo.
CV: *chest pain,* angina pectoris, postural hypotension.
EENT: gingivitis.
GI: anorexia, diarrhea, dyspepsia, gastroenteritis, vomiting.
GU: albuminuria, impotence.
Hematologic: ***leukopenia.***
Musculoskeletal: arthralgia, arthritis, neck pain.
Respiratory: asthma, flu syndrome, rhinitis.
Skin: alopecia, carcinoma, ecchymosis, vesiculobullous rash.
Other: allergic reaction, decreased libido.
Combined with levodopa
CNS: *confusion, falls, headache,* abnormal dreams, amnesia, ataxia, dyskinesia, dystonia, hallucinations, paresthesia, somnolence, sweating.
EENT: epistaxis, gingivitis.
GI: *nausea,* abdominal pain, anorexia, constipation, diarrhea, dry mouth, dyspepsia, dysphagia, vomiting, weight loss.
GU: albuminuria.
Hematologic: ***hemorrhage,*** anemia.
Musculoskeletal: arthralgia, arthritis, bursitis, hernia, leg cramps, myasthenia, neck pain, tenosynovitis.
Respiratory: dyspnea.
Skin: carcinoma, ecchymosis, pruritus, rash, ulcer.
Other: infection.

INTERACTIONS
Drug-drug. *Ciprofloxacin and other CYP1A2 inhibitors:* May double rasagiline level. Decrease rasagiline dosage to 0.5 mg daily.
Levodopa: : May increase rasagiline level. Watch for dyskinesia, dystonia, hallucinations, and hypotension, and reduce levodopa dosage if needed.
SSRIs, serotonin-norepinephrine reuptake inhibitors, tricyclic antidepressants: : May cause severe or fatal CNS toxicity. Stop rasagiline for at least 14 days before starting an antidepressant. Stop fluoxetine for 5 weeks before starting rasagiline.
Drug-herb. *St. John's wort: :* May cause severe reaction. Strongly discourage use together.
Drug-food. *Tyramine-rich foods and supplements:* May cause hypertensive crisis. Urge patient to avoid tyramine-rich foods, such as aged meat, salami, pickled herring, aged cheese, unpasteurized beer, red wine, fava beans, sauerkraut, soybean products, and concentrated yeast extract.

EFFECTS ON LAB TEST RESULTS
• May increase liver enzyme levels.
• May decrease WBC count.

CONTRAINDICATIONS & CAUTIONS

- Contraindicated in patients with pheochromocytoma, those with moderate to severe hepatic impairment, and those taking amphetamines, cold products, dextromethorphan, ephedrine, MAO inhibitors, meperidine, methadone, phenylephrine, propoxyphene, pseudoephedrine, sympathomimetic amines, or tramadol.
- Use cautiously in patients with mild hepatic impairment and in pregnant or breast-feeding women.

NURSING CONSIDERATIONS

- Postural hypotension may occur during first 2 months of therapy; assist patient when rising from a reclining position.
- Notify prescriber if patient is experiencing adverse effects; a reduced levodopa dose may be needed.
- Examine the patient's skin periodically for possible melanoma.
- Notify prescriber if patient is having elective surgery, drug should be stopped at least 2 weeks beforehand.

PATIENT TEACHING

- Explain the risk of hypertensive crisis if patient ingests tyramine while taking rasagiline. Give patient a list of foods and products containing tyramine
- Tell patient to contact prescriber if hallucinations occur.
- Urge patient to watch for skin changes that could suggest melanoma and to have periodic skin examinations by a health professional.
- Instruct patient to maintain his usual dosage schedule if he misses a dose and not to double the next dose to make up for a missed one.

ropinirole hydrochloride
Requip

Pharmacologic class: nonergot dopamine agonist
Pregnancy risk category C

AVAILABLE FORMS

Tablets: 0.25 mg, 0.5 mg, 1 mg, 2 mg, 3 mg, 4 mg, 5 mg.

INDICATIONS & DOSAGES

➤Idiopathic Parkinson disease
Adults: Initially, 0.25 mg P.O., t.i.d. Increase dose by 0.25 mg t.i.d. at weekly intervals for 4 weeks. After week 4, dosage may be increased by 1.5 mg daily divided t.i.d.; at weekly intervals, up to 9 mg daily divided t.i.d.; then dosage may be increased by up to 3 mg daily divided t.i.d.; at weekly intervals, up to 24 mg daily divided t.i.d.
Elderly patients: Adjust dosages individually, according to patient response; clearance is reduced in these patients.

➤Moderate to severe restless leg syndrome
Adults: Initially, 0.25 mg P.O. 1 to 3 hours before bedtime. May increase dose as needed and tolerated after 2 days to 0.5 mg, then to 1 mg by the end of the first week. May further increase dose as needed and tolerated as follows: week 2, give 1 mg once daily. Week 3, give 1.5 mg once daily. Week 4, give 2 mg once daily. Week 5, give 2.5 mg once daily. Week 6, give 3 mg once daily. And week 7, give 4 mg once daily. All doses should be taken 1 to 2 hours before bedtime.

ACTION

Nonergot-derivative dopamine agonist thought to stimulate dopamine (D2) receptors.

Route	Onset	Peak	Duration
P.O.	Unknown	1–2 hr	6 hr

Half-life: 6 hours.

ADVERSE REACTIONS

Early Parkinson disease (without levodopa)
CNS: *dizziness, fatigue, somnolence, syncope,* hallucinations, aggravated Parkinson disease, headache, confusion, hyperkinesia, hypoesthesia, vertigo, amnesia, impaired concentration, malaise, asthenia.
CV: orthostatic hypotension, orthostatic symptoms, hypertension, edema, chest pain, extrasystoles, atrial fibrillation, palpitations, tachycardia, flushing.
EENT: pharyngitis, abnormal vision, eye abnormality, xerophthalmia, rhinitis, sinusitis.

GI: *nausea, vomiting, dyspepsia,* dry mouth, flatulence, abdominal pain, anorexia, constipation.
GU: UTI, impotence.
Respiratory: bronchitis, dyspnea, yawning.
Other: *viral infection,* pain, increased sweating, peripheral ischemia.
Advanced Parkinson disease (with levodopa)
CNS: *dizziness, somnolence, headache, hallucinations,* aggravated parkinsonism, insomnia, abnormal dreaming, confusion, tremor, anxiety, nervousness, amnesia, paresis, paresthesia, syncope.
CV: hypotension.
EENT: diplopia.
GI: *nausea,* abdominal pain, dry mouth, vomiting, constipation, diarrhea, dysphagia, flatulence, increased saliva.
GU: UTI, pyuria, urinary incontinence.
Hematologic: anemia.
Metabolic: weight decrease, suppressed prolactin.
Musculoskeletal: *dyskinesia,* arthralgia, arthritis, hypokinesia.
Respiratory: upper respiratory tract infection, dyspnea.
Skin: increased sweating.
Other: *falls,* injury, viral infection, pain.
Restless leg syndrome
CNS: *fatigue, somnolence, dizziness,* vertigo, paresthesia.
CV: peripheral edema.
EENT: *nasopharyngitis,* nasal congestion.
GI: *nausea, vomiting,* diarrhea, dyspepsia, dry mouth.
Musculoskeletal: arthralgia, muscle cramps, extremity pain.
Respiratory: cough.
Skin: increased sweating.
Other: influenza.

INTERACTIONS

Drug-drug. *Cimetidine, ciprofloxacin, fluvoxamine, inhibitors or substrates of CYP1A2, ritonavir:* May alter ropinirole clearance. Adjust ropinirole dose if other drugs are started or stopped during treatment.
CNS depressants: May increase CNS effects. Use together cautiously.
Dopamine antagonists (neuroleptics), metoclopramide: May decrease ropinirole effects. Avoid using together.
Estrogens: May decrease ropinirole clearance. Adjust ropinirole dosage if estrogen therapy is started or stopped during treatment.
Drug-lifestyle. *Alcohol use:* May increase sedative effect. Advise patient to use cautiously.
Smoking: May increase drug clearance. Discourage use together.

EFFECTS ON LAB TEST RESULTS

- May increase BUN and alkaline phosphatase levels. May decrease hemoglobin level.

CONTRAINDICATIONS & CAUTIONS

- Contraindicated in patients hypersensitive to drug.
- Use cautiously in patients with severe hepatic or renal impairment.

NURSING CONSIDERATIONS

- ***Alert:*** Monitor patient carefully for orthostatic hypotension, especially during dosage increases.
- Drug may potentiate the adverse effects of levodopa and may cause or worsen dyskinesia. Dosage may be decreased.
- Although not reported with ropinirole, other adverse reactions reported with dopaminergic therapy include hyperpyrexia, fibrotic complications, and confusion, which may occur with rapid dosage reduction or withdrawal of drug.
- Patient may have syncope, with or without bradycardia. Monitor patient carefully, especially for 4 weeks after start of therapy and with dosage increases.
- When used for Parkinson disease, withdraw drug gradually over 7 days.
- When used for restless leg syndrome, stop drug without tapering.

PATIENT TEACHING

- Advise patient to take drug with food if nausea occurs.
- Inform patient (especially elderly patient) that hallucinations can occur.
- Instruct patient not to rise rapidly after sitting or lying down because of risk of dizziness, which may occur more fre-

quently early in therapy or when dosage increases.
- Sleepiness can occur early in therapy. Warn patient to minimize hazardous activities until CNS effects of drug are known.
- Advise patient to avoid alcohol.
- Tell woman to notify prescriber about planned, suspected, or known pregnancy; also tell her to inform prescriber if she's breast-feeding.

selegiline
Emsam

selegiline hydrochloride (L-deprenyl hydrochloride)
Eldepryl, Zelapar

Pharmacologic class: MAO inhibitor
Pregnancy risk category C

AVAILABLE FORMS
selegiline
Transdermal system: 6 mg/24 hours, 9 mg/24 hours, 12 mg/24 hours
selegiline hydrochloride
Capsules: 5 mg
Orally disintegrating tablets (ODTs): 1.25 mg
Tablets: 5 mg

INDICATIONS & DOSAGES
➤ **Adjunctive treatment with levodopa and carbidopa in managing signs and symptoms of Parkinson disease**
Adults: 10 mg P.O. daily divided as 5 mg at breakfast and 5 mg at lunch. After 2 or 3 days, gradual decrease of levodopa and carbidopa dosage may be needed. Or, if using ODTs, start with 1.25 mg P.O. once daily before breakfast and without liquid. Increase to 2.5 mg daily after at least 6 weeks, if needed.
➤ **Major depressive disorder**
Adults: Apply one patch daily to dry intact skin on the upper torso, upper thigh, or upper arm. Initially, use 6 mg/day. Increase, if needed, in increments of 3 mg/day at intervals of 2 or more weeks. Maximum daily dose, 12 mg.
Elderly patients: 6 mg daily.

ACTION
May inhibit MAO type B (mainly found in the brain) and dopamine metabolism. At higher-than-recommended doses, drug nonselectively inhibits MAO, including MAO type A (mainly found in the intestine). May also directly increase dopaminergic activity by decreasing the reuptake of dopamine into nerve cells.

Route	Onset	Peak	Duration
P.O.	Unknown	30–120 min	Unknown
Transdermal	Unknown	Unknown	24 hr

Half-life: selegiline, 2 to 10 hours; N-desmethyldeprenyl, 2 hours; L-amphetamine, 17¾ hours; L-methamphetamine, 20½ hours

ADVERSE REACTIONS
transdermal form
CNS: *headache, insomnia.*
CV: chest pain, low blood pressure, orthostatic blood pressure.
GI: diarrhea, dry mouth, dyspepsia.
Metabolic: weight gain, weight loss.
Respiratory: pharyngitis, sinusitis.
Skin: *application site reaction,* rash.
oral form
CNS: *dizziness,* agitation, delusions, loss of balance, depression, increased bradykinesia, involuntary movements, headache, confusion, hallucinations, vivid dreams, insomnia, syncope.
CV: ***arrhythmias,*** orthostatic hypotension, hypertension, new or increased angina.
GI: *nausea,* dry mouth, abdominal pain.

INTERACTIONS
Drug-drug. *Citalopram, duloxetine, fluoxetine, fluvoxamine, nefazodone, paroxetine, sertraline, venlafaxine:* May cause serotonin syndrome (CNS irritability, shivering, and altered consciousness). Separate use by at least 2 weeks (5 weeks if switching to or from fluoxetine).
Bupropion, cyclobenzaprine, dextromethorphan, meperidine, methadone, mirtazapine, MAO inhibitors, propoxyphene, sympathomimetic amines, including amphetamines, cold products and weight loss preparations containing vasoconstrictors, tramadol, tricyclic antidepressants: May cause hypertensive crisis. Separate use by at least 2 weeks.

carbamazepine, oxcarbazepine: May increase selegiline levels. Use together is contraindicated.
Drug-herb. *Ginseng:* May cause headache, tremors, or mania. Discourage use together.
St. John's wort: May cause increased serotonergic effects. Warn patient against use together.
Drug-food. *Foods high in tyramine:* May cause hypertensive crisis especially at increased doses. Provide patient with a list of foods to avoid.

EFFECTS ON LAB TEST RESULTS
- May cause positive result for amphetamine on urine drug screen.

CONTRAINDICATIONS & CAUTIONS
- Contraindicated in patients hypersensitive to drug, in patients with pheochromocytoma, and in those taking bupropion, carbamazepine, cyclobenzaprine, dextromethorphan, duloxetine, methadone, meperidine, mirtazapine, MAO inhibitors, oxcarbazepine, propoxyphene, SSRIs, sympathomimetics, tramadol, tricyclic antidepressants, venlafaxine. Don't use oral drug with the transdermal system.

NURSING CONSIDERATIONS
- ***Alert:*** Some patients experience increased levodopa adverse reactions when it's used with selegiline and need a 10% to 30% reduction of levodopa and carbidopa dosage.
- ***Look alike–sound alike:*** Don't confuse selegiline with Stelazine or Eldepryl with enalapril.
- ***Alert:*** Drug may increase the risk of suicidal thinking in children and adolescents. Drug isn't approved for use in children.
- Monitor patients with major depressive disorder for worsening of symptoms and of suicidal behavior, especially during the first few weeks of treatment and during dosage changes.

PATIENT TEACHING
- Warn patient to move cautiously or change positions slowly at start of therapy because he may become dizzy or light-headed.
- Caution patient to avoid driving and other hazardous activities that require mental alertness until the drug's effects are known.
- Advise patient not to take drug in the evening because doing so may cause insomnia.
- Advise patient not to overindulge in tyramine-rich foods or beverages. If using a 9 mg/day or higher transdermal system, avoid these products all together.
- Advise patient to avoid liquids for 5 minutes before and after taking ODTs.
- ***Alert:*** Warn patient about the many drugs, including OTC drugs, that may interact with this drug and about the need to consult a pharmacist or his prescriber before using them.
- Teach patient and family the signs and symptoms of hypertensive crisis including severe headache, sore or stiff neck, nausea, vomiting, sweating, rapid heartbeat, dilated pupils, and photophobia.
- ***Alert:*** Advise family members to watch patient for anxiety, agitation, insomnia, irritability, hostility, and aggressiveness and to report these immediately to prescriber.
- Tell patient to avoid exposing transdermal system to direct external heat sources, such as heating pads, electric blankets, hot tubs, heated water beds, and prolonged sunlight.
- Tell patient to stop using the transdermal system 10 days before having surgery requiring general anesthesia.
- Tell patient not to cut the transdermal system into smaller pieces.
- Advise woman planning pregnancy or breast-feeding to first contact her prescriber.

tolcapone
Tasmar

Pharmacologic class: catechol-O-methyltransferase (COMT) inhibitor
Pregnancy risk category C

AVAILABLE FORMS
Tablets: 100 mg, 200 mg

INDICATIONS & DOSAGES
➤ **Adjunct to levodopa and carbidopa for signs and symptoms of idi-**

opathic Parkinson disease in patients who have symptom fluctuation or haven't responded to other adjunctive treatment
Adults: Initially, 100 mg P.O. t.i.d. with levodopa and carbidopa. Recommended daily dosage is 100 mg P.O. t.i.d. Levodopa dosage may need to be reduced by 20% to 30% to minimize risk of dyskinesias. Maximum, 600 mg daily. Stop drug if patient shows no benefit within 3 weeks.

ACTION
May reversibly inhibit COMT when given with levodopa and carbidopa, increasing levodopa bioavailability. This causes a more constant dopaminergic stimulation in the brain.

Route	Onset	Peak	Duration
P.O.	Unknown	2 hr	Unknown

Half-life: 2 to 3 hours.

ADVERSE REACTIONS
CNS: *dyskinesia, sleep disorder, dystonia, excessive dreaming, somnolence, confusion, headache, hallucinations,* dizziness, fever, hyperkinesia, hypertonia, fatigue, falling, syncope, balance loss, depression, tremor, speech disorder, paresthesia, agitation, irritability, mental deficiency, hyperactivity, hypokinesia.
CV: *orthostatic complaints,* chest pain, chest discomfort, palpitations, hypotension.
EENT: pharyngitis, tinnitus, sinus congestion.
GI: *nausea, anorexia, diarrhea, vomiting,* flatulence, constipation, abdominal pain, dyspepsia, dry mouth.
GU: UTI, urine discoloration, hematuria, micturition disorder, urinary incontinence, impotence.
Hematologic: bleeding.
Hepatic: ***hepatotoxicity.***
Musculoskeletal: *muscle cramps,* stiffness, arthritis, neck pain.
Respiratory: bronchitis, dyspnea, upper respiratory tract infection.
Skin: increased sweating, rash.
Other: influenza.

INTERACTIONS
Drug-drug. *CNS depressants:* May cause additive effects. Monitor patient closely.
Desipramine, SSRIs, tricyclic antidepressants: May increase risk of adverse effects. Use together cautiously.
Nonselective MAO inhibitors (phenelzine, tranylcypromine): May cause hypertensive crisis. Avoid using together.
Warfarin: May cause increased warfarin level. Monitor INR and adjust warfarin dosage as needed.

EFFECTS ON LAB TEST RESULTS
- May increase liver function test values.

CONTRAINDICATIONS & CAUTIONS
- Contraindicated in patients hypersensitive to drug or its components and in those with hepatic disease, elevated ALT or AST levels, or history of drug-related confusion and nontraumatic rhabdomyolysis or hyperpyrexia.
- Contraindicated in those previously withdrawn from drug because of drug-induced hepatocellular injury.
- Use cautiously in patients with severe renal impairment and in breast-feeding women.

NURSING CONSIDERATIONS
- Because of risk of liver toxicity, stop treatment if patient shows no benefit within 3 weeks.
- Because of fatal hepatic failure risk, use drug only in patients taking levodopa and carbidopa who don't respond to or who aren't appropriate candidates for other adjunctive therapies.
- ***Alert:*** Make sure patient provides written informed consent before taking drug.
- Monitor liver function test results before starting drug, every 2 to 4 weeks for the first 6 months of therapy, then as indicated. If the dose is increased to 200 mg t.i.d., resume monitoring as described. Stop drug if AST or ALT exceeds two times the upper limit of normal or if patient shows signs or symptoms of hepatic dysfunction.
- Because drug is highly protein bound, it isn't significantly removed during dialysis.
- Monitor patient for orthostatic hypotension and syncope.

• Give first dose of the day with first daily dose of levodopa and carbidopa.

PATIENT TEACHING

• Advise patient to take drug exactly as prescribed.
• Teach patient to immediately report the signs and symptoms of liver injury (yellow eyes or skin, fatigue, loss of appetite, persistent nausea, itching, dark urine, or right upper abdominal tenderness).
• Warn patient about risk of dizziness upon standing up quickly; tell him to stand up cautiously.
• Advise patient to avoid hazardous activities until CNS effects of drug are known.
• Tell patient that nausea may occur early in therapy.
• Inform patient that diarrhea is common, sometimes occurring 2 to 12 weeks after therapy begins, and usually resolves when therapy stops.
• Advise patient about risk of increased problems making voluntary movements or impaired muscle tone.
• Inform patient that hallucinations may occur.
• Tell woman to notify prescriber about planned, suspected, or known pregnancy.
• Inform patient that drug may be taken without regard to meals.

34

Miscellaneous central nervous system drugs

almotriptan malate
atomoxetine hydrochloride
donepezil hydrochloride
droperidol
eletriptan hydrobromide
frovatriptan succinate
galantamine hydrobromide
lithium carbonate
lithium citrate
memantine hydrochloride
naratriptan hydrochloride
propofol
rivastigmine tartrate
rizatriptan benzoate
sibutramine hydrochloride monohydrate
sumatriptan succinate
zolmitriptan

almotriptan malate

Axert

Pharmacologic class: serotonin $5\text{-}HT_1$ receptor agonist
Pregnancy risk category C

AVAILABLE FORMS

Tablets: 6.25 mg, 12.5 mg

INDICATIONS & DOSAGES

➤ **Acute migraine with or without aura**

Adults: Give 6.25-mg or 12.5-mg tablet P.O., with one additional dose after 2 hours if headache is unresolved or recurs. Maximum, two doses within 24 hours.

Adjust-a-dose: For patients with hepatic or renal impairment, initially 6.25 mg, with maximum daily dose of 12.5 mg.

ACTION

Not fully understood. Believed to relieve migraine through selective vasoconstriction of certain cranial blood vessels, inhibition of neuropeptide release, and reduced pain transmission down trigeminal pathway.

Route	Onset	Peak	Duration
P.O.	1–3 hr	1–3 hr	3–4 hr

Half-life: 3 to 4 hours.

ADVERSE REACTIONS

CNS: paresthesia, headache, dizziness, somnolence.
CV: ***coronary artery vasospasm, transient myocardial ischemia, MI, ventricular tachycardia, ventricular fibrillation.***
GI: nausea, dry mouth.

INTERACTIONS

Drug-drug. *MAO inhibitors, verapamil:* May increase almotriptan level. No dose adjustment is necessary.
CYP3A4 inhibitors such as ketoconazole: May increase almotriptan level. Monitor patient for potential adverse reaction. May need to reduce dosage.
Ergot-containing drugs, serotonin $5\text{-}HT_{1B/1D}$ agonists: May cause additive effects. Avoid using within 24 hours of almotriptan.
SSRIs: May cause additive serotonin effects, resulting in weakness, hyperreflexia, or incoordination. Monitor patient closely if given together.

EFFECTS ON LAB TEST RESULTS

None reported.

CONTRAINDICATIONS & CAUTIONS

- Contraindicated in patients hypersensitive to drug.
- Contraindicated in those with angina pectoris, history of MI, silent ischemia, coronary artery vasospasm, Prinzmetal variant angina, or other CV disease; uncontrolled hypertension; and hemiplegic or basilar migraine.
- Don't give within 24 hours after treatment with other $5\text{-}HT_{1B/1D}$ agonists or ergot derivatives.
- Use cautiously in patients with renal or hepatic impairment and in those with cataracts because of the potential for corneal opacities.

• Use cautiously in patients with risk factors for coronary artery disease (CAD), such as obesity, diabetes, and family history of CAD.

NURSING CONSIDERATIONS

• Patients with poor renal or hepatic function should receive a reduced dosage.
• Repeat dose after 2 hours, if needed, and don't give more than two doses within 24 hours.
• ***Alert:*** Combining triptans with SSRIs or selective serotonin-norepinephrine reuptake inhibitors (SNRIs) may cause serotonin syndrome. Signs and symptoms include restlessness, hallucinations, loss of coordination, rapid heart beat, rapid changes in blood pressure, increased body temperature, overactive reflexes, nausea, vomiting, and diarrhea. Serotonin syndrome occurs more often when starting or increasing the dose of a triptan, SSRI, or SNRI.
• ***Look alike–sound alike:*** Don't confuse Axert with Antivert.

PATIENT TEACHING

• Tell patient that drug can be taken with or without food.
• Advise patient to take drug only when he's having a migraine; explain that drug isn't taken on a regular schedule.
• Advise patient to use only one repeat dose within 24 hours, no sooner than 2 hours after first dose.
• Advise patient that other commonly prescribed migraine drugs can interact with almotriptan.
• Advise patient to report chest or throat tightness, pain, or heaviness.
• Teach patient to avoid possible migraine triggers, such as cheese, chocolate, citrus fruits, caffeine, and alcohol.

atomoxetine hydrochloride

Strattera

Pharmacologic class: selective norepinephrine reuptake inhibitor
Pregnancy risk category C

AVAILABLE FORMS

Capsules: 10 mg, 18 mg, 25 mg, 40 mg, 60 mg, 80 mg, 100 mg

INDICATIONS & DOSAGES

➤ Attention-deficit hyperactivity disorder (ADHD)

Adults, children, and adolescents who weigh more than 70 kg (154 lb): Initially, 40 mg P.O. daily; increase after at least 3 days to a total of 80 mg/day P.O., as a single dose in the morning or two evenly divided doses in the morning and late afternoon or early evening. After 2 to 4 weeks, increase total dose to a maximum of 100 mg, if needed.
Children who weigh 70 kg or less: Initially, 0.5 mg/kg P.O. daily; increase after a minimum of 3 days to a target total daily dose of 1.2 mg/kg P.O. as a single dose in the morning or two evenly divided doses in the morning and late afternoon or early evening. Don't exceed 1.4 mg/kg or 100 mg daily, whichever is less.
Adjust-a-dose: In patients with moderate hepatic impairment, reduce to 50% of the normal dose; in those with severe hepatic impairment, reduce to 25% of the normal dose. Poor metabolizers of CYP2D6 may require a reduced dose. In children who weigh less than 70 kg, adjust dosage to 0.5 mg/kg daily and increase to 1.2 mg/kg daily if symptoms don't improve after 4 weeks and if first dose is tolerated. In children and adults who weigh more than 70 kg, start at 40 mg daily and increase to 80 mg daily if symptoms don't improve after 4 weeks and if first dose is tolerated.

ACTION

May be related to selective inhibition of the presynaptic norepinephrine transporter.

Route	Onset	Peak	Duration
P.O.	Rapid	1–2 hr	Unknown

Half-life: 21½ hours.

ADVERSE REACTIONS

CNS: *headache, insomnia,* dizziness, somnolence, crying, irritability, mood swings, pyrexia, fatigue, sedation, depression, tremor, early-morning awakening, paresthesia, abnormal dreams, sleep disorder.
CV: orthostatic hypotension, tachycardia, hypertension, palpitations, hot flashes.

EENT: ear infection, rhinorrhea, sore throat, nasal congestion, nasopharyngitis, sinus congestion, mydriasis, sinusitis.
GI: *abdominal pain, constipation,* dyspepsia, *nausea, vomiting, decreased appetite,* gastroenteritis, *dry mouth,* flatulence.
GU: urinary retention, urinary hesitation, ejaculatory problems, difficulty in micturition, dysmenorrhea, erectile disturbance, impotence, delayed menses, menstrual disorder, prostatitis.
Metabolic: weight loss.
Musculoskeletal: arthralgia, myalgia.
Respiratory: *cough,* upper respiratory tract infection.
Skin: *dermatitis, pruritus, increased sweating.*
Other: influenza, decreased libido, rigors.

INTERACTIONS

Drug-drug. *Albuterol:* May increase CV effects. Use together cautiously.
MAO inhibitors: May cause hyperthermia, rigidity, myoclonus, autonomic instability with possible rapid fluctuations of vital signs, and mental status changes. Avoid use within 2 weeks of MAO inhibitor.
Pressor agents: May increase blood pressure. Use together cautiously.
Strong CYP2D6 inhibitors (paroxetine, fluoxetine, quinidine): May increase atomoxetine level. Reduce first dose.

EFFECTS ON LAB TEST RESULTS

None reported.

CONTRAINDICATIONS & CAUTIONS

- Contraindicated in patients hypersensitive to atomoxetine or to components of drug, in those who have taken an MAO inhibitor within the past 2 weeks, and in those with angle-closure glaucoma.
- Use cautiously in patients with hypertension, tachycardia, or CV or cerebrovascular disease, and in pregnant or breast-feeding women.
- Safety and efficacy haven't been established in patients younger than age 6.

NURSING CONSIDERATIONS

- Use drug as part of a total treatment program for ADHD, including psychological, educational, and social intervention.
- ***Alert:*** Monitor children and adolescents closely for worsening of condition, agitation, irritability, suicidal thinking or behaviors, and unusual changes in behavior, especially the first few months of therapy or when the dosage is increased or decreased.
- Patients taking drug for extended periods must be reevaluated periodically to determine drug's usefulness.
- Monitor growth during treatment. If growth or weight gain is unsatisfactory, consider interrupting therapy.
- ***Alert:*** Severe liver injury may occur and progress to liver failure. Notify prescriber at any sign of liver injury: yellowing of the skin or the sclera of the eyes, pruritus, dark urine, upper right-sided tenderness or unexplained flulike syndrome.
- Monitor blood pressure and pulse at baseline, after each dose increase, and during treatment periodically.
- Monitor for urinary hesitancy or retention and sexual dysfunction.
- Patient can stop drug without tapering off.

PATIENT TEACHING

- ***Alert:*** Advise parents to call prescriber immediately about unusual behavior or suicidal thoughts.
- Tell pregnant women, women planning to become pregnant, and breast-feeding women to consult prescriber before taking atomoxetine.
- Tell patient to use caution when operating a vehicle or machinery until the effects of drug are known.

donepezil hydrochloride

Aricept, Aricept ODT

Pharmacologic class: cholinesterase inhibitor
Pregnancy risk category C

AVAILABLE FORMS

Orally disintegrating tablets (ODTs): 5 mg, 10 mg
Tablets: 5 mg, 10 mg

INDICATIONS & DOSAGES

➤ Mild to severe Alzheimer dementia

Adults: Initially, 5 mg P.O. daily at bedtime. After 4 to 6 weeks, increase to 10 mg daily, if needed.

ACTION

Thought to increase acetylcholine concentration by inhibiting the cholinesterase enzyme, which causes hydrolysis of acetylcholine. May improve cognitive function in patients with mild to moderate Alzheimer disease.

Route	Onset	Peak	Duration
P.O.	Unknown	3–4 hr	Unknown

Half-life: 70 hours.

ADVERSE REACTIONS

CNS: *headache, insomnia,* ***seizures,*** dizziness, fatigue, depression, abnormal dreams, somnolence, tremor, irritability, paresthesia, aggression, vertigo, ataxia, restlessness, abnormal crying, nervousness, aphasia, syncope, pain.
CV: chest pain, hypertension, vasodilation, atrial fibrillation, hot flashes, hypotension.
EENT: cataract, blurred vision, eye irritation, sore throat.
GI: *nausea, diarrhea,* vomiting, anorexia, fecal incontinence, GI bleeding, bloating, epigastric pain.
GU: urinary frequency.
Metabolic: weight loss, dehydration.
Musculoskeletal: muscle cramps, arthritis, bone fracture.
Respiratory: dyspnea, bronchitis.
Skin: pruritus, urticaria, diaphoresis, ecchymoses.
Other: toothache, influenza, increased libido.

INTERACTIONS

Drug-drug. *Anticholinergics:* May decrease donepezil effects. Avoid using together.
Anticholinesterases, cholinomimetics: May have synergistic effect. Monitor patient closely.
Bethanechol, succinylcholine: May have additive effects. Monitor patient closely.
Carbamazepine, dexamethasone, phenobarbital, phenytoin, rifampin: May increase rate of donepezil elimination. Monitor patient.

EFFECTS ON LAB TEST RESULTS

None reported.

CONTRAINDICATIONS & CAUTIONS

- Contraindicated in patients hypersensitive to drug or piperidine derivatives and in breast-feeding women.
- Use cautiously in pregnant women and in patients who take NSAIDs or have CV disease, asthma, obstructive pulmonary disease, urinary outflow impairment, or history of ulcer disease.

NURSING CONSIDERATIONS

- Monitor patient for evidence of active or occult GI bleeding.
- ***Look alike–sound alike:*** Don't confuse Aricept with Ascriptin.

PATIENT TEACHING

- Stress that drug doesn't alter underlying degenerative disease but can temporarily stabilize or relieve symptoms. Effectiveness depends on taking drug at regular intervals.
- Tell caregiver to give drug just before patient's bedtime.
- ODTs may be taken with or without food. Have patient allow tablet to dissolve on his tongue, then swallow with a sip of water.
- Advise patient and caregiver to report immediately significant adverse effects or changes in overall health status and to inform health care team that patient is taking drug before he receives anesthesia.
- Tell patient to avoid OTC cold or sleep remedies because of risk of increased anticholinergic effects.

droperidol

Inapsine

Pharmacologic class: butyrophenone derivative
Pregnancy risk category C

AVAILABLE FORMS

Injection: 2.5 mg/ml in 1-, 2-, and 5-ml ampules and 2-, 5-, and 10-ml vials

INDICATIONS & DOSAGES

➤ **To prevent nausea and vomiting from surgical or diagnostic procedures**

Adults and children older than age 12: Maximum first dose, 2.5 mg I.M. or slow

I.V. Give additional 1.25 mg cautiously, if needed. Give additional doses only if benefit outweighs risk.
Children ages 2 to 12: Maximum first dose, 0.1 mg/kg, considering patient's age and other factors. Give additional doses cautiously and only if benefit outweighs risk.
Adjust-a-dose: In elderly or debilitated patients and those who have received other CNS depressant drugs, give reduced dosage.

➤ **Breakthrough, chemotherapy-induced nausea and vomiting ♦**
Adults: 0.5 to 2 mg I.V. or I.M. every 3 or 4 hours, p.r.n. For acute treatment, give 0.5 to 2 mg I.V. or I.M. before chemotherapy.

I.V. ADMINISTRATION
- Give dose slowly.
- For high-risk patients, dilute calculated dose in D_5W or lactated Ringer injection, and give as a slow I.V. infusion.

INCOMPATIBILITIES
Allopurinol, barbiturates, cefepime, fluorouracil, foscarnet, furosemide, heparin, leucovorin, methotrexate sodium, nafcillin, piperacillin with tazobactam.

ACTION
Unknown. Tranquilizes, sedates, and provides antiemetic effects without affecting reflex alertness; also causes mild alpha blockade.

Route	Onset	Peak	Duration
I.V., I.M.	3–10 min	30 min	2–4 hr

Half-life: Unknown.

ADVERSE REACTIONS
CNS: *drowsiness,* ***neuroleptic malignant syndrome,*** restlessness, hyperactivity, anxiety, extrapyramidal symptoms, dizziness, hallucinations, dysphoria.
CV: hypotension, tachycardia.
Respiratory: ***laryngospasm, bronchospasm.***
Other: chills, shivering.

INTERACTIONS
Drug-drug. *CNS depressants:* May cause additive CNS effects. Adjust dosage, as needed.
Cyclobenzaprines: May have additive effects on prolonging QT interval. Monitor patient closely.
Fentanyl citrate: May cause hypertension and respiratory depression. Use together cautiously.

EFFECTS ON LAB TEST RESULTS
None reported.

CONTRAINDICATIONS & CAUTIONS
- Contraindicated in patients hypersensitive to drug.
- Contraindicated in patients with prolonged QT interval, including patients with congenital long QT-interval syndrome.
- Use cautiously in those at risk for prolonged QT-interval syndrome (those with heart failure, bradycardia, cardiac hypertrophy, hypokalemia, or hypomagnesemia and those taking drugs that prolong QT interval or worsen hypokalemia or hypomagnesemia).
- Use cautiously in patients with hepatic or renal dysfunction and in breast-feeding woman.
- Use with caution in patients with suspected or diagnosed pheochromocytoma because severe hypertension and tachycardia can occur.

NURSING CONSIDERATIONS
- When used for induction of general anesthesia, give drug with an analgesic.
- If used in procedures such as bronchoscopy, topical anesthesia is still needed.
- ***Alert:*** Keep fluids and other measures to manage hypotension readily available.
- Monitor patient for signs and symptoms of neuroleptic malignant syndrome (fever, altered consciousness, extrapyramidal symptoms, tachycardia).
- ***Look alike–sound alike:*** Don't confuse droperidol with dronabinol.

PATIENT TEACHING
- Warn patient to rise slowly to minimize dizziness.
- Advise patient to avoid alcohol for 24 hours after receiving drug.

eletriptan hydrobromide
Relpax

Pharmacologic class: serotonin 5-HT_1 receptor agonist
Pregnancy risk category C

AVAILABLE FORMS
Tablets: 20 mg, 40 mg

INDICATIONS & DOSAGES
➤ **Acute migraine with or without aura**
Adults: 20 to 40 mg P.O. at first migraine symptom. If headache recurs, dose may be repeated at least 2 hours later to a maximum of 80 mg daily.

ACTION
Binds to 5-HT_1 receptors and may constrict intracranial blood vessels and inhibit proinflammatory neuropeptide release.

Route	Onset	Peak	Duration
P.O.	½ hr	1½–2 hr	Unknown

Half-life: About 4 hours.

ADVERSE REACTIONS
CNS: *asthenia,* dizziness, headache, hypertonia, hypesthesia, pain, paresthesia, somnolence, vertigo.
CV: chest tightness, pain, and pressure, flushing, palpitations.
EENT: pharyngitis.
GI: abdominal pain, discomfort or cramps, dry mouth, dyspepsia, dysphagia, nausea.
Musculoskeletal: back pain.
Skin: increased sweating.
Other: chills.

INTERACTIONS
Drug-drug. *CYP3A4 inhibitors (such as clarithromycin, itraconazole, ketoconazole, nefazodone, nelfinavir, ritonavir, troleandomycin):* May decrease eletriptan metabolism. Avoid use within 72 hours of these drugs.
Ergotamine-containing or ergot-type drugs (such as dihydroergotamine or methysergide), other triptans: May prolong vasospastic reactions. Avoid use within 24 hours of these drugs.
SSRIs: May increase the risk of serotonin syndrome (weakness, hyperreflexia, and incoordination). If used together, observe patient closely.

EFFECTS ON LAB TEST RESULTS
None known.

CONTRAINDICATIONS & CAUTIONS
- Contraindicated in patients hypersensitive to drug or its components and in those with severe hepatic impairment; ischemic heart disease, such as angina pectoris, a history of MI, or silent ischemia; coronary artery vasospasm, including Prinzmetal variant angina; and other significant CV conditions.
- Contraindicated in patients with cerebrovascular syndromes, such as stroke or transient ischemic attack; peripheral vascular disease, including ischemic bowel disease; uncontrolled hypertension; or hemiplegic or basilar migraine.
- Contraindicated within 24 hours of another 5-HT_1 agonist, drugs containing ergotamine, or ergot-type drug.
- Contraindicated in patients with risk factors for coronary artery disease (CAD), such as hypertension, hypercholesterolemia, smoking, obesity, diabetes, strong family history of CAD, postmenopausal women, or men older than age 40, unless patient is free from cardiac disease. Monitor patient closely after first dose.

NURSING CONSIDERATIONS
- Drug isn't intended for migraine prevention.
- ***Alert:*** Combining triptans with SSRIs or selective serotonin-norepinephrine reuptake inhibitors (SNRIs) may cause serotonin syndrome. Signs and symptoms may include restlessness, hallucinations, loss of coordination, fast heart beat, rapid changes in blood pressure, increased body temperature, hyperreflexia, nausea, vomiting, and diarrhea. Serotonin syndrome may be more likely to occur when starting or increasing the dose of a triptan, SSRI, or SNRI.
- Safety of treating more than three migraine headaches in 30 days hasn't been established.
- Use drug only when patient has a clear diagnosis of migraine. If the first use pro-

duces no response, reconsider the migraine diagnosis.
• *Alert:* Serious cardiac events including acute MI, arrhythmias, and death occur rarely within a few hours after use of 5-HT_1 agonists.
• Ophthalmologic effects may occur with long-term use.
• Older patients may develop higher blood pressure than younger patients after taking drug.

PATIENT TEACHING
• Instruct patient to take dose at the first sign of a migraine headache. If the headache comes back after the first dose, he may take a second dose after 2 hours. Caution patient not to take more than 80 mg in 24 hours.
• Warn patient to avoid driving and operating machinery if he feels dizzy or fatigued after taking the drug.
• Tell patient to immediately report pain, tightness, heaviness, or pressure in the chest, throat, neck, or jaw.

frovatriptan succinate
Frova

Pharmacologic class: serotonin 5-HT_1 receptor agonist
Pregnancy risk category C

AVAILABLE FORMS
Tablets: 2.5 mg

INDICATIONS & DOSAGES
➤ **Acute treatment of migraine attacks with or without aura**
Adults: 2.5 mg P.O. taken at the first sign of migraine attack. If the headache recurs, a second tablet may be taken at least 2 hours after the first dose. The total daily dose shouldn't exceed 7.5 mg.

ACTION
May inhibit excessive dilation of extracerebral and intracranial arteries during migraine headaches.

Route	Onset	Peak	Duration
P.O.	Unknown	2–4 hr	Unknown

Half-life: 26 hours.

ADVERSE REACTIONS
CNS: dizziness, headache, fatigue, paresthesia, insomnia, anxiety, somnolence, dysesthesia, hypoesthesia, hot or cold sensation, pain.
CV: ***coronary artery vasospasm, transient myocardial ischemia, MI, ventricular tachycardia, ventricular fibrillation,*** chest pain, palpitations, flushing.
EENT: abnormal vision, tinnitus, sinusitis, rhinitis.
GI: dry mouth, dyspepsia, vomiting, abdominal pain, diarrhea, nausea.
Musculoskeletal: skeletal pain.
Skin: increased sweating.

INTERACTIONS
Drug-drug. *5-HT_1 agonists:* May cause additive effects. Separate doses by 24 hours.
Ergotamine-containing or ergot-type drugs (such as dihydroergotamine or methysergide): May cause prolonged vasospastic reactions. Separate doses by 24 hours.
SSRIs (such as citalopram, fluoxetine, fluvoxamine, paroxetine, sertraline): May cause weakness, hyperreflexia, and incoordination. Monitor patient closely.

EFFECTS ON LAB TEST RESULTS
None reported.

CONTRAINDICATIONS & CAUTIONS
• Contraindicated in patients hypersensitive to drug or any of its components.
• Contraindicated in patients with history or symptoms of ischemic heart disease or coronary artery vasospasm, including Prinzmetal variant angina; in those with cerebrovascular or peripheral vascular disease, including ischemic bowel disease; in those with uncontrolled hypertension; and in those with hemiplegic or basilar migraine.
• Contraindicated within 24 hours of another triptan, drug containing ergotamine, or ergot-type drug.
• Contraindicated in patients with risk factors for coronary artery disease (CAD), such as hypertension, hypercholesterolemia, smoking, obesity, diabetes, strong family history of CAD, postmenopausal women, or men older than age 40, unless patient is free from cardiac disease. If

drug is used in such a patient, monitor patient closely and consider obtaining an ECG after the first dose. Intermittent, long-term users of triptans or those with risk factors should undergo periodic cardiac evaluation while using drug.
- Use cautiously in breast-feeding women. It's unknown if drug appears in breast milk.

NURSING CONSIDERATIONS

- ***Alert:*** Serious cardiac events, including acute MI, life-threatening cardiac arrhythmias, and death may occur within a few hours of taking a triptan.
- Use drug only when patient has a clear diagnosis of migraine. If a patient has no response for the first migraine attack treated with frovatriptan, reconsider the diagnosis of migraine.
- The safety of treating an average of more than four migraine headaches in a 30-day period hasn't been established.
- ***Alert:*** Combining a triptan with SSRIs or selective serotonin-norepinephrine reuptake inhibitors (SNRIs) may cause serotonin syndrome. Symptoms may include restlessness, hallucinations, loss of coordination, fast heart beat, rapid changes in blood pressure, increased body temperature, hyperreflexia, nausea, vomiting, and diarrhea. Serotonin syndrome is more likely to occur when starting or increasing the dose of a triptan, SSRI, or SNRI.

PATIENT TEACHING

- Instruct patient to take dose at first sign of migraine headache. If headache comes back after first dose, he may take a second dose after 2 hours. Tell patient not to take more than 3 tablets in 24 hours.
- Caution patient to take extra care or avoid driving and operating machinery if dizziness or fatigue develops after taking drug.
- Stress importance of immediately reporting pain, tightness, heaviness, or pressure in chest, throat, neck, or jaw, or rash or itching after taking drug.
- Instruct the patient not to take drug within 24 hours of taking another serotonin-receptor agonist or ergot-type drug.

galantamine hydrobromide

Razadyne, Razadyne ER

Pharmacologic class: cholinesterase inhibitor
Pregnancy risk category B

AVAILABLE FORMS

Capsules (extended-release): 8 mg, 16 mg, 24 mg
Oral solution: 4 mg/ml
Tablets: 4 mg, 8 mg, 12 mg

INDICATIONS & DOSAGES

➤ **Mild to moderate Alzheimer dementia**

Adults: Initially, 4 mg b.i.d., preferably with morning and evening meals. If dose is well tolerated after minimum of 4 weeks of therapy, increase dosage to 8 mg b.i.d. A further increase to 12 mg b.i.d. may be attempted, but only after at least 4 weeks of therapy at the previous dosage. Dosage range is 16 to 24 mg daily in two divided doses.

Or, 8 mg extended-release capsule P.O. once daily in the morning with food. Increase to 16 mg P.O. once daily after a minimum of 4 weeks. May further increase to 24 mg once daily after a minimum of 4 weeks, based upon patient response and tolerability.

Adjust-a-dose: For patients with Child-Pugh score of 7 to 9, dosage usually shouldn't exceed 16 mg daily. Drug isn't recommended for patients with Child-Pugh score of 10 to 15. For patients with moderate renal impairment, dosage usually shouldn't exceed 16 mg daily. For patients with creatinine clearance less than 9 ml/minute, drug isn't recommended.

ACTION

A competitive and reversible inhibitor of acetylcholinesterase, which is believed to enhance cholinergic function by increasing the level of acetylcholine in the brain.

Route	Onset	Peak	Duration
P.O.	Unknown	1 hr	Unknown

Half-life: About 7 hours.

ADVERSE REACTIONS

CNS: depression, dizziness, headache, tremor, insomnia, somnolence, fatigue, syncope.
CV: ***bradycardia.***
EENT: rhinitis.
GI: *diarrhea, nausea, vomiting,* anorexia, abdominal pain, dyspepsia, anorexia.
GU: UTI, hematuria.
Hematologic: anemia.
Metabolic: weight loss.

INTERACTIONS

Drug-drug. *Amitriptyline, fluoxetine, fluvoxamine, quinidine:* May decrease galantamine clearance. Monitor patient closely.
Anticholinergics: May antagonize anticholinergic activity. Monitor patient.
Cholinergics (such as bethanechol, succinylcholine): May have synergistic effect. Monitor patient closely. May need to avoid use before procedures using general anesthesia with succinylcholine-type neuromuscular blockers.
Cimetidine, clarithromycin, erythromycin, ketoconazole, paroxetine: May increase galantamine bioavailability. Monitor patient closely.

EFFECTS ON LAB TEST RESULTS

None reported.

CONTRAINDICATIONS & CAUTIONS

- Contraindicated in patients hypersensitive to drug or its components.
- Use cautiously in patients with supraventricular cardiac conduction disorders and in those taking other drugs that significantly slow heart rate.
- Use cautiously during or before procedures involving anesthesia using succinylcholine-type or similar neuromuscular blockers.
- Use cautiously in patients with history of peptic ulcer disease and in those taking NSAIDs. Because of the potential for cholinomimetic effects, use cautiously in patients with bladder outflow obstruction, seizures, asthma, or COPD.

NURSING CONSIDERATIONS

- ***Alert:*** Razadyne tablets should be given twice daily; Razadyne ER capsules should be given once daily. To avoid possible dosing errors, verify any prescription that suggests a different dosing schedule.
- Drug may cause bradycardia and heart block. Consider all patients at risk for adverse effects on cardiac conduction.
- Give drug with food and antiemetics and ensure adequate fluid intake to decrease the risk of nausea and vomiting.
- ***Alert:*** The original trade name for galantamine, "Reminyl," was changed to "Razadyne" because of name confusion with the antidiabetic Amaryl.
- Use proper technique when dispensing the oral solution with the pipette. Dispense measured amount into a beverage and give right away.
- If drug is stopped for several days or longer, restart at the lowest dose and gradually increase, at 4-week or longer intervals, to the previous dosage level.
- Because of the risk of increased gastric acid secretion, monitor patients closely for symptoms of active or occult GI bleeding, especially those with an increased risk of developing ulcers.

PATIENT TEACHING

- Advise caregiver to give drug with morning and evening meals (for the conventional form), or only in the morning (for the extended-release form).
- Inform patient that nausea and vomiting are common adverse effects.
- Teach caregiver the proper technique when measuring the oral solution with the pipette. Tell her to place measured amount in a nonalcoholic beverage and have patient drink right away.
- Urge patient or caregiver to report slow heartbeat immediately.
- Advise patient and caregiver that although drug may improve cognitive function, it doesn't alter the underlying disease process.

lithium carbonate
Carbolith†, Duralith†, Eskalith, Eskalith CR, Lithane, Lithicarb‡, Lithizine†, Lithobid, Lithonate, Lithotabs, Quilonum SR‡

lithium citrate
Cibalith-S*

Pharmacologic class: alkali metal
Pregnancy risk category D

AVAILABLE FORMS
lithium carbonate
Capsules: 150 mg, 300 mg, 600 mg
Tablets: 250 mg‡, 300 mg (300 mg equals 8.12 mEq lithium)
Tablets (controlled-release): 300 mg, 450 mg
lithium citrate
Syrup (sugarless): 8 mEq lithium/5 ml. 5 ml lithium citrate liquid contains 8 mEq lithium, equal to 300 mg lithium carbonate

INDICATIONS & DOSAGES
➤ To prevent or control mania
Adults: 300 to 600 mg P.O. up to q.i.d. Or, 900-mg controlled-release tablets P.O. q 12 hours. Increase dosage based on blood levels to achieve optimal dosage. Recommended therapeutic lithium levels are 1 to 1.5 mEq/L for acute mania and 0.6 to 1.2 mEq/L for maintenance therapy.

ACTION
Probably alters chemical transmitters in the CNS, possibly by interfering with ionic pump mechanisms in brain cells, and may compete with or replace sodium ions.

Route	Onset	Peak	Duration
P.O.	Unknown	30 min–3 hr	Unknown

Half-life: 18 hours (adolescents) to 36 hours (elderly).

ADVERSE REACTIONS
CNS: *fatigue, lethargy,* ***coma, epileptiform seizures,*** tremors, drowsiness, headache, confusion, restlessness, dizziness, psychomotor retardation, blackouts, EEG changes, worsened organic mental syndrome, impaired speech, ataxia, incoordination.
CV: ***arrhythmias, bradycardia,*** reversible ECG changes, hypotension.
EENT: tinnitus, blurred vision.
GI: *vomiting, anorexia, diarrhea, thirst,* nausea, metallic taste, dry mouth, abdominal pain, flatulence, indigestion.
GU: *polyuria,* ***renal toxicity with long-term use,*** glycosuria, decreased creatinine clearance, albuminuria.
Hematologic: *leukocytosis with leukocyte count of 14,000 to 18,000/mm³.*
Metabolic: transient hyperglycemia, goiter, hypothyroidism, hyponatremia.
Musculoskeletal: *muscle weakness.*
Skin: pruritus, rash, diminished or absent sensation, drying and thinning of hair, psoriasis, acne, alopecia.
Other: ankle and wrist edema.

INTERACTIONS
Drug-drug. *ACE inhibitors:* May increase lithium level. Monitor lithium level; adjust lithium dosage, as needed.
Aminophylline, sodium bicarbonate, urine alkalinizers: May increase lithium excretion. Avoid excessive salt, and monitor lithium levels.
Calcium channel blockers (verapamil): May decrease lithium levels and may increase risk of neurotoxicity. Use together cautiously.
Carbamazepine, fluoxetine, methyldopa, NSAIDs, probenecid: May increase effect of lithium. Monitor patient for lithium toxicity.
Neuromuscular blockers: May cause prolonged paralysis or weakness. Monitor patient closely.
Thiazide diuretics: May increase reabsorption of lithium by kidneys, with possible toxic effect. Use with caution, and monitor lithium and electrolyte levels (especially sodium).
Drug-food. *Caffeine:* May decrease lithium level and drug effect. Advise patient who ingests large amounts of caffeine to tell prescriber before stopping caffeine. Adjust lithium dosage, as needed.

EFFECTS ON LAB TEST RESULTS
- May increase glucose and creatinine levels. May decrease sodium, T_3, T_4, and protein-bound iodine levels.

• May increase ^{131}I uptake and WBC and neutrophil counts.

CONTRAINDICATIONS & CAUTIONS
• Contraindicated if therapy can't be closely monitored.
• Avoid using in pregnant patient unless benefits outweigh risks.
• Use with caution in patients receiving neuromuscular blockers and diuretics; in elderly or debilitated patients; and in patients with thyroid disease, seizure disorder, infection, renal or CV disease, severe debilitation or dehydration, or sodium depletion.

NURSING CONSIDERATIONS
• Lithane may contain tartrazine.
• ***Alert:*** Drug has a narrow therapeutic margin of safety. Determining drug level is crucial to safe use of drug. Don't use drug in patients who can't have regular tests. Monitor level 8 to 12 hours after first dose, the morning before second dose is given, two or three times weekly for the first month, and then weekly to monthly during maintenance therapy.
• When drug level is less than 1.5 mEq/L, adverse reactions are usually mild.
• Monitor baseline ECG, thyroid studies, renal studies, and electrolyte levels.
• Check fluid intake and output, especially when surgery is scheduled.
• Weigh patient daily; check for edema or sudden weight gain.
• Adjust fluid and salt ingestion to compensate if excessive loss occurs from protracted diaphoresis or diarrhea. Under normal conditions, patient fluid intake should be 2½ to 3 L daily, and he should follow a balanced diet with adequate salt intake.
• Check urine specific gravity and report level below 1.005, which may indicate diabetes insipidus.
• Drug alters glucose tolerance in diabetics. Monitor glucose level closely.
• Perform outpatient follow-up of thyroid and renal functions every 6 to 12 months. Palpate thyroid to check for enlargement.
• ***Look alike–sound alike:*** Don't confuse Lithobid with Levbid, Lithonate with Lithostat, or Lithotabs with Lithobid or Lithostat.

PATIENT TEACHING
• Tell patient to take drug with plenty of water and after meals to minimize GI upset.
• Explain the importance of having regular blood tests to determine drug levels; even slightly high values can be dangerous.
• Warn patient and caregivers to expect transient nausea, large amounts of urine, thirst, and discomfort during first few days of therapy and to watch for evidence of toxicity (diarrhea, vomiting, tremor, drowsiness, muscle weakness, incoordination).
• Instruct patient to withhold one dose and call prescriber if signs and symptoms of toxicity appear, but not to stop drug abruptly.
• Warn patient to avoid hazardous activities that require alertness and good psychomotor coordination until CNS effects of drug are known.
• Tell patient not to switch brands or take other prescription or OTC drugs without prescriber's guidance.
• Tell patient to wear or carry medical identification at all times.

memantine hydrochloride
Namenda

Pharmacologic class: N-methyl-D-aspartate (NMDA) receptor antagonist
Pregnancy risk category B

AVAILABLE FORMS
Oral solution: 2 mg/ml
Tablets: 5 mg, 10 mg

INDICATIONS & DOSAGES
➤ **Moderate to severe Alzheimer dementia**
Adults: Initially, 5 mg P.O. once daily. Increase by 5 mg/day q week until target dose is reached. Maximum, 10 mg P.O. b.i.d. Doses greater than 5 mg should be divided b.i.d.
Adjust-a-dose: Reduce dosage in patients with moderate renal impairment.

ACTION

Antagonizes N-methyl-D-aspartate (NMDA) receptors, the persistent activation of which seems to increase Alzheimer symptoms.

Route	Onset	Peak	Duration
P.O.	Unknown	3–7 hr	Unknown

Half-life: 60 to 80 hours.

ADVERSE REACTIONS

CNS: ***stroke,*** aggressiveness, agitation, anxiety, ataxia, confusion, depression, dizziness, fatigue, hallucinations, headache, hypokinesia, insomnia, pain, somnolence, syncope, transient ischemic attack, vertigo.
CV: ***heart failure,*** edema, hypertension.
EENT: cataracts, conjunctivitis.
GI: anorexia, constipation, diarrhea, nausea, vomiting.
GU: incontinence, urinary frequency, UTI.
Hematologic: anemia.
Metabolic: weight loss.
Musculoskeletal: arthralgia, back pain.
Respiratory: bronchitis, coughing, dyspnea, flulike symptoms, pneumonia, upper respiratory tract infection.
Skin: rash.
Other: abnormal gait, falls, injury.

INTERACTIONS

Drug-drug. *Cimetidine, hydrochlorothiazide, quinidine, ranitidine, triamterene:* May alter levels of both drugs. Monitor patient.
NMDA antagonists (amantadine, dextromethorphan, ketamine): Combined use unknown. Use together cautiously.
Urine alkalinizers (carbonic anhydrase inhibitors, sodium bicarbonate): May decrease memantine clearance. Monitor patient for adverse effects.
Drug-herb. *Herbs that alkalinize urine:* May increase drug level and adverse effects. Use together cautiously.
Drug-food. *Foods that alkalinize urine:* May increase drug level and adverse effects. Use together cautiously.
Drug-lifestyle. *Alcohol use:* May alter drug adherence, decrease its effectiveness, or increase adverse effects. Discourage use together.
Nicotine: May alter levels of drug and nicotine. Discourage use together.

EFFECTS ON LAB TEST RESULTS

- May increase alkaline phosphatase level. May decrease hemoglobin level and hematocrit.

CONTRAINDICATIONS & CAUTIONS

- Contraindicated in patients allergic to drug or its components.
- Not recommended for patients with severe renal impairment.
- Use cautiously in patients with seizures, hepatic impairment, or moderate renal impairment.
- Use cautiously in patients who may have an increased urine pH (from drugs, diet, renal tubular acidosis, or severe UTI, for example).

NURSING CONSIDERATIONS

- Drug isn't indicated for mild Alzheimer disease or other types of dementia.
- In elderly patients, even those with a normal creatinine level, use of this drug may impair renal function. Estimate creatinine clearance; reduce dosage in patients with moderate renal impairment. Don't give drug to patients with severe renal impairment.

PATIENT TEACHING

- Explain that drug doesn't cure Alzheimer disease, but may improve the symptoms.
- Tell patient to report adverse effects.
- Urge patient to avoid alcohol during treatment.
- To avoid possible interactions, advise patient not to take herbal or OTC products without consulting prescriber.

naratriptan hydrochloride

Amerge, Naramig‡

Pharmacologic class: serotonin 5-HT_1 receptor agonist
Pregnancy risk category C

AVAILABLE FORMS

Tablets: 1 mg, 2.5 mg

INDICATIONS & DOSAGES

➤ Acute migraine attacks with or without aura

Adults: 1 or 2.5 mg P.O. as a single dose. If headache returns or responds only partially, dose may be repeated after 4 hours. Maximum, 5 mg in 24 hours.

Adjust-a-dose: For patients with mild to moderate renal or hepatic impairment, reduce dosage. Maximum, 2.5 mg in 24 hours.

ACTION

May selectively activate serotonin receptors in intracranial blood vessels, resulting in vasoconstriction and migraine headache relief. Or, may inhibit neuropeptide release, reducing pain transmission in the trigeminal pathways.

Route	Onset	Peak	Duration
P.O.	Unknown	2–3 hr	Unknown

Half-life: 6 hours.

ADVERSE REACTIONS

CNS: paresthesia, dizziness, drowsiness, malaise, fatigue, vertigo, syncope.
CV: ***tachyarrhythmias, abnormal ECG changes, coronary artery vasospasm, transient myocardial ischemia, MI, ventricular tachycardia, ventricular fibrillation,*** palpitations, increased blood pressure.
EENT: ear, nose, and throat infections, photophobia.
GI: nausea, hyposalivation, vomiting.
Other: sensations of warmth, cold, pressure, tightness, or heaviness.

INTERACTIONS

Drug-drug. *Ergot-containing or ergot-type drugs (dihydroergotamine, methysergide), other 5-HT_1 agonists:* May prolong vasospastic reactions. Avoid using within 24 hours of naratriptan.
Hormonal contraceptives: May slightly increase naratriptan level. Monitor patient.
SSRIs (fluoxetine, fluvoxamine, paroxetine, sertraline): May cause weakness, hyperreflexia, and incoordination. Monitor patient.
Drug-herb. *St. John's wort:* May increase serotonergic effect. Discourage use together.
Drug-lifestyle. *Smoking:* May increase naratriptan clearance. Discourage smoking.

EFFECTS ON LAB TEST RESULTS

None reported.

CONTRAINDICATIONS & CAUTIONS

- Contraindicated in patients hypersensitive to drug or its components, in those with prior or current cardiac ischemia, in those with cerebrovascular or peripheral vascular syndromes, and in those with uncontrolled hypertension.
- Contraindicated in elderly patients, patients with creatinine clearance below 15 ml/minute, patients with Child-Pugh grade C, and patients who have used ergot-containing, ergot-type, or other 5-HT_1 agonists within 24 hours.
- Use cautiously in patients with risk factors for coronary artery disease (CAD), such as hypertension, hypercholesterolemia, obesity, diabetes, smoking, strong family history of CAD, postmenopausal women, and men older than age 40, unless patient is free from cardiac disease. Monitor patient closely after first dose.
- Use cautiously in patients with renal or hepatic impairment.

NURSING CONSIDERATIONS

- Assess cardiac status in patients who develop risk factors for CAD.
- ***Alert:*** Drug can cause coronary artery vasospasm and increased risk of cerebrovascular events.
- Drug isn't intended to prevent migraines or manage hemiplegic or basilar migraine.
- Safety and effectiveness of treating cluster headaches or more than four headaches in a 30-day period haven't been established.
- Use drug only when patient has a clear diagnosis of migraine.
- ***Alert:*** Combining drug with an SSRI or a selective serotonin-norepinephrine reuptake inhibitor (SNRI) may cause serotonin syndrome. Symptoms include restlessness, hallucinations, loss of coordination, fast heart beat, rapid changes in blood pressure, increased body temperature, hyperreflexia, nausea, vomiting, and diarrhea. Serotonin syndrome is more

likely to occur when starting or increasing the dose of naratriptan, the SSRI, or the SNRI.

PATIENT TEACHING

- Instruct patient to take drug only as prescribed and to read the accompanying patient instruction leaflet before using drug.
- Tell patient that drug is intended to relieve, not prevent, migraines.
- Instruct patient to take dose soon after headache starts. If no response occurs with first tablet, tell him to seek medical approval before taking second tablet. Tell patient that if more relief is needed after first tablet (if a partial response occurs or headache returns), and prescriber has approved a second dose, he may take a second tablet (but not sooner than 4 hours after first tablet). Tell him not to exceed 2 tablets within 24 hours.
- Advise patient to increase fluid intake.
- Advise patient not to use drug if she suspects or knows that she's pregnant.
- Tell patient to alert prescriber about bothersome adverse effects.

SAFETY ALERT!

propofol
Diprivan

Pharmacologic class: phenol derivative
Pregnancy risk category B

AVAILABLE FORMS

Injection: 10 mg/ml in 20-ml ampules; 50-ml prefilled syringes; 50-ml and 100-ml infusion vials

INDICATIONS & DOSAGES

➤ To induce anesthesia

Adults younger than age 55 classified as American Society of Anesthesiologists (ASA) Physical Status (PS) category I or II: Give 2 to 2.5 mg/kg. Give in 40-mg boluses q 10 seconds until desired response is achieved.
Children ages 3 to 16 classified as ASA I or II: Give 2.5 to 3.5 mg/kg over 20 to 30 seconds.
Adjust-a-dose: In geriatric, debilitated, hypovolemic, or ASA PS III or IV patients, give half the usual induction dose, in 20-mg boluses, q 10 seconds. For cardiac anesthesia, give 20 mg (0.5 to 1.5 mg/kg) q 10 seconds until desired response is achieved. For neurosurgical patients, give 20 mg (1 to 2 mg/kg) q 10 seconds until desired response is achieved.

➤ To maintain anesthesia

Healthy adults younger than age 55: Give 0.1 to 0.2 mg/kg/minute (6 to 12 mg/kg/hour). Or, give in 20- to 50-mg intermittent boluses, p.r.n.
Healthy children ages 2 months to 16 years: Give 125 to 300 mcg/kg/minute (7.5 to 18 mg/kg/hour).
Adjust-a-dose: In geriatric, debilitated, hypovolemic, or ASA PS III or IV patients, give half the usual maintenance dose (0.05 to 0.1 mg/kg/minute or 3 to 6 mg/kg/hour). For cardiac anesthesia with secondary opioid, 100 to 150 mcg/kg/minute; low dose with primary opioid, 50 to 100 mcg/kg/minute. For neurosurgical patients, 100 to 200 mcg/kg/minute (6 to 12 mg/kg/hour).

➤ Monitored anesthesia care

Healthy adults younger than age 55: Initially, 100 to 150 mcg/kg/minute (6 to 9 mg/kg/hour) for 3 to 5 minutes or a slow injection of 0.5 mg/kg over 3 to 5 minutes. For maintenance dose, give infusion of 25 to 75 mcg/kg/minute (1.5 to 4.5 mg/kg/hour), or incremental 10- or 20-mg boluses.
Adjust-a-dose: In geriatric, debilitated, or ASA PS III or IV patients, give 80% of usual adult maintenance dose. Don't use rapid bolus.

➤ To sedate intubated intensive care unit (ICU) patients

Adults: Initially, 5 mcg/kg/minute (0.3 mg/kg/hour) for 5 minutes. Increments of 5 to 10 mcg/kg/minute (0.3 to 0.6 mg/kg/hour) over 5 to 10 minutes may be used until desired sedation is achieved. Maintenance rate, 5 to 50 mcg/kg/minute (0.3 to 3 mg/kg/hour).

I.V. ADMINISTRATION

- Maintain aseptic technique when handling the solution. Drug can support the growth of microorganisms; don't use if solution might be contaminated.
- Protect drug from light. Shake well.

- Dilute only with D_5W. Don't dilute to less than 2 mg/ml.
- Don't use if emulsion shows evidence of separation.
- Don't infuse through a filter with a pore size smaller than 5 microns. Give via larger veins in arms to decrease injection site pain.
- Titrate drug daily to maintain minimum effective level. Allow 3 to 5 minutes between dosage adjustments to assess effects.
- Discard tubing and unused portions of drug after 12 hours.

INCOMPATIBILITIES

Other I.V. drugs, blood, and plasma.

ACTION

Unknown. Rapid-acting I.V. sedative-hypnotic.

Route	Onset	Peak	Duration
I.V.	< 40 sec	Unknown	10–15 min

Half-life: Initial (distribution) phase, about 2 to 10 minutes; second (redistribution) phase, 21 to 70 minutes; terminal (elimination) phase is 1½ to 31 hours.

ADVERSE REACTIONS

CNS: dystonic or choreiform movement.
CV: ***bradycardia, hypotension,*** hypertension, decreased cardiac output.
Metabolic: hyperlipemia.
Respiratory: APNEA, respiratory acidosis.
Skin: rash.
Other: *burning or stinging at injection site.*

INTERACTIONS

Drug-drug. *Inhaled anesthetics (such as enflurane, halothane, isoflurane), opioids (alfentanil, fentanyl, meperidine, morphine), sedatives (such as barbiturates, benzodiazepines, chloral hydrate, droperidol):* May increase anesthetic and sedative effects and further decrease blood pressure and cardiac output. Monitor patient closely.
Drug-herb. *St. John's wort:* May prolong anesthetic effects. Advise patient to stop using herb 5 days before surgery.

EFFECTS ON LAB TEST RESULTS

- May increase lipid levels.

CONTRAINDICATIONS & CAUTIONS

- Contraindicated in patients hypersensitive to drug or its components (including egg lecithin, soybean oil, and glycerol), in pregnant women (because it may cause fetal depression), and in those unable to undergo general anesthesia or sedation.
- Use cautiously in patients who are hemodynamically unstable or who have seizures, disorders of lipid metabolism, or increased intracranial pressure.
- Because drug appears in breast milk, avoid using in breast-feeding women.

NURSING CONSIDERATIONS

- If drug is used for prolonged sedation in ICU, urine may turn green.
- For general anesthesia or monitored anesthesia care sedation, trained staff not involved in the surgical or diagnostic procedure should give drug. For ICU sedation, persons skilled in managing critically ill patients and trained in cardiopulmonary resuscitation and airway management should give drug.
- Continuously monitor vital signs.
- Monitor patient at risk for hyperlipidemia for elevated triglyceride levels.
- Drug contains 0.1 g of fat (1.1 kcal)/ml. Reduce other lipid products if given together.
- Drug contains ethylenediaminetetraacetic acid, a strong metal chelator. Consider supplemental zinc during prolonged therapy.
- When giving drug in the ICU, assess patient's CNS function daily to determine minimum dose needed.
- Stop drug gradually to prevent abrupt awakening and increased agitation.
- ***Look alike–sound alike:*** Don't confuse Diprivan with Ditropan or Dipivefrin.

PATIENT TEACHING

- Advise patient that performance of activities requiring mental alertness may be impaired for some time after drug use.

rivastigmine tartrate
Exelon
Pharmacologic class: cholinesterase inhibitor
Pregnancy risk category B

AVAILABLE FORMS
Capsules: 1.5 mg, 3 mg, 4.5 mg, 6 mg

INDICATIONS & DOSAGES
➤ **Mild to moderate Alzheimer dementia**
Adults: Initially, 1.5 mg P.O. b.i.d. with food. If tolerated, may increase to 3 mg b.i.d. after 2 weeks. After 2 weeks at this dose, may increase to 4.5 mg b.i.d. and 6 mg b.i.d., as tolerated. Effective dosage range is 6 to 12 mg daily; maximum, 12 mg daily.
✷ ***NEW INDICATION:*** **Mild to moderate dementia associated with Parkinson disease**
Adults: Initially, 1.5 mg P.O. b.i.d. May increase, as tolerated, to 3 mg b.i.d., then 4.5 mg b.i.d., and finally to 6 mg b.i.d. after a minimum of 4 weeks at each dose.

ACTION
Thought to increase acetylcholine level by inhibiting the cholinesterase enzyme, which causes acetylcholine hydrolysis, which may lead to some memory improvement.

Route	Onset	Peak	Duration
P.O.	Unknown	1 hr	12 hr

Half-life: About 1½ hours in patients with normal renal function.

ADVERSE REACTIONS
CNS: *headache, dizziness,* syncope, fatigue, asthenia, malaise, somnolence, tremor, insomnia, confusion, depression, anxiety, hallucinations, aggressive reaction, vertigo, agitation, nervousness, delusion, paranoid reaction.
CV: hypertension, chest pain, peripheral edema.
EENT: rhinitis, pharyngitis.
GI: *nausea, vomiting, diarrhea, anorexia, abdominal pain,* dyspepsia, constipation, flatulence, eructation.
GU: UTI, incontinence.
Metabolic: weight loss.
Musculoskeletal: back pain, arthralgia, bone fracture.
Respiratory: upper respiratory tract infection, cough, bronchitis.
Skin: increased sweating, rash.
Other: *accidental trauma,* flulike symptoms, pain.

INTERACTIONS
Drug-drug. *Bethanechol, succinylcholine, other neuromuscular-blocking drugs or cholinergic antagonists:* May have synergistic effect. Monitor patient closely.
Drug-lifestyle. *Smoking:* May increase drug clearance. Discourage smoking.

EFFECTS ON LAB TEST RESULTS
None reported.

CONTRAINDICATIONS & CAUTIONS
- Contraindicated in patients hypersensitive to drug, other carbamate derivatives, or other components of the drug.

NURSING CONSIDERATIONS
- Expect significant GI adverse effects (such as nausea, vomiting, anorexia, and weight loss). These effects are less common during maintenance doses.
- Monitor patient for evidence of active or occult GI bleeding.
- Dramatic memory improvement is unlikely. As disease progresses, the benefits of drug may decline.
- Monitor patient for severe nausea, vomiting, and diarrhea, which may lead to dehydration and weight loss.
- Carefully monitor patient with a history of GI bleeding, NSAID use, arrhythmias, seizures, or pulmonary conditions for adverse effects.

PATIENT TEACHING
- Tell caregiver to give rivastigmine with food in the morning and evening.
- Advise patient that memory improvement may be subtle and that drug more likely slows future memory loss.
- Tell patient to report nausea, vomiting, or diarrhea.
- Tell patient to consult prescriber before using OTC drugs.

rizatriptan benzoate
Maxalt, Maxalt-MLT

Pharmacologic class: serotonin 5-HT_1 receptor agonist
Pregnancy risk category C

AVAILABLE FORMS
Tablets: 5 mg, 10 mg
Tablets (orally disintegrating): 5 mg, 10 mg

INDICATIONS & DOSAGES
➤ **Acute migraine headaches with or without aura**
Adults: Initially, 5 or 10 mg P.O. If first dose is ineffective, may give another dose at least 2 hours after first dose; maximum, 30 mg in 24 hours. For patients receiving propranolol, 5 mg P.O.; maximum, 15 mg in 24 hours.

ACTION
May act as an agonist at serotonin receptors on extracerebral intracranial blood vessels, which constricts the affected vessels, inhibits neuropeptide release, and reduces pain transmission in the trigeminal pathways.

Route	Onset	Peak	Duration
P.O.	Unknown	60–90 min	Unknown

Half-life: 2 to 3 hours.

ADVERSE REACTIONS
CNS: dizziness, headache, somnolence, paresthesia, asthenia, fatigue, decreased mental acuity, euphoria, tremor, pain.
CV: ***coronary artery vasospasm; transient myocardial ischemia; MI; ventricular tachycardia; ventricular fibrillation;*** chest pain, pressure, or heaviness; palpitations; flushing.
EENT: neck, throat, and jaw pain.
GI: dry mouth, nausea, diarrhea, vomiting.
Respiratory: dyspnea.
Other: hot flashes, warm or cold feelings.

INTERACTIONS
Drug-drug. *Ergot-containing or ergot-type drugs (dihydroergotamine, methysergide), other 5-HT_1 agonists:* May prolong vasospastic reactions. Avoid using within 24 hours of rizatriptan.
MAO inhibitors: May increase rizatriptan level. Avoid using within 2 weeks of MAO inhibitor.
Propranolol: May increase rizatriptan level. Reduce rizatriptan dose to 5 mg.
SSRIs (fluoxetine, fluvoxamine, paroxetine, sertraline): May cause weakness, hyperreflexia, and incoordination. Monitor patient.

EFFECTS ON LAB TEST RESULTS
None reported.

CONTRAINDICATIONS & CAUTIONS
- Contraindicated in patients hypersensitive to drug or its components and in those with a history or symptoms of ischemic heart disease, coronary artery vasospasm (Prinzmetal variant angina), or other significant underlying CV disease.
- Contraindicated in patients with uncontrolled hypertension; within 24 hours of another 5-HT_1 agonist, drug containing ergotamine, or ergot-type drug, such as dihydroergotamine or methysergide; or within 2 weeks of MAO inhibitor.
- Contraindicated in patients with hemiplegic or basilar migraine.
- Use cautiously in patients with risk factors for coronary artery disease (CAD), such as hypertension, hypercholesterolemia, smoking, obesity, diabetes, strong family history of CAD, postmenopausal women, or men older than age 40, unless patient is free from cardiac disease. Monitor patient closely after first dose.
- Use cautiously in patients with hepatic or renal impairment.

NURSING CONSIDERATIONS
- Assess CV status in patients who develop risk factors for CAD during treatment.
- Use drug only when patient has a clear diagnosis of migraine.
- Safety of treating more than four headaches in a 30-day period hasn't been established.
- Don't use drug to prevent migraines or to treat hemiplegic or basilar migraine or cluster headaches.

• *Alert:* Combining drug with an SSRI or a selective serotonin-norepinephrine reuptake inhibitor (SNRI) may cause serotonin syndrome. Symptoms include restlessness, hallucinations, loss of coordination, fast heart beat, rapid changes in blood pressure, increased body temperature, hyperreflexia, nausea, vomiting, and diarrhea. Serotonin syndrome is more likely to occur when starting or increasing the dose of this drug, the SSRI, or the SNRI.
• The orally disintegrating tablets contain phenylalanine.
• Safety and effectiveness in children are unknown.

PATIENT TEACHING

• Inform patient that drug doesn't prevent migraine headache.
• For Maxalt-MLT, tell patient to remove blister pack from pouch and remove drug from blister pack immediately before use. Tablet shouldn't be popped out of blister pack; tell patient to carefully peel away package with dry hands, place tablet on tongue, and allow tablet to dissolve. Tablet is then swallowed with saliva. No water is needed or recommended. Tell patient that orally dissolving tablet doesn't relieve headache more quickly.
• Advise patient that, if headache returns after first dose, he may take a second dose at least 2 hours after the first dose. Warn against taking more than 30 mg in a 24-hour period.
• Inform patient that drug may cause sleepiness and dizziness, and warn him to avoid hazardous activities until effects are known.
• Tell patient that food may delay onset of drug action.
• Advise patient to notify prescriber about suspected or known pregnancy.
• Instruct patient not to breast-feed during therapy because effects on the infant are unknown.

sibutramine hydrochloride monohydrate

Meridia

Pharmacologic class: norepinephrine, serotonin, and dopamine reuptake inhibitor
Pregnancy risk category C
Controlled substance schedule IV

AVAILABLE FORMS

Capsules: 5 mg, 10 mg, 15 mg

INDICATIONS & DOSAGES

➤ To manage obesity
Adults: 10 mg P.O. given once daily with or without food. May increase to 15 mg P.O. daily after 4 weeks if weight loss is inadequate. Patients who don't tolerate 10 mg daily may receive 5 mg P.O. daily. Don't exceed 15 mg daily.

ACTION

Inhibits reuptake of norepinephrine and, to a lesser extent, serotonin and dopamine.

Route	Onset	Peak	Duration
P.O.	Unknown	3–4 hr	Unknown

Half-life: About 15 hours.

ADVERSE REACTIONS

CNS: *headache, insomnia,* dizziness, nervousness, anxiety, depression, paresthesia, somnolence, CNS stimulation, emotional lability, asthenia, migraine.
CV: tachycardia, vasodilation, hypertension, palpitations, chest pain.
EENT: *rhinitis, pharyngitis,* sinusitis, ear disorder, ear pain.
GI: *anorexia, constipation, dry mouth,* thirst, increased appetite, nausea, dyspepsia, gastritis, vomiting, taste perversion, abdominal pain, rectal disorder.
GU: dysmenorrhea, UTI, vaginal candidiasis, metrorrhagia.
Musculoskeletal: arthralgia, myalgia, tenosynovitis, joint disorder, neck or back pain.
Respiratory: increased cough, laryngitis.
Skin: rash, sweating, acne.
Other: herpes simplex, flulike syndrome, accidental injury, allergic reaction, generalized edema.

INTERACTIONS

Drug-drug. *CNS depressants:* May enhance CNS depression. Use together cautiously.
Dextromethorphan, dihydroergotamine, fentanyl, fluoxetine, fluvoxamine, lithium, MAO inhibitors, meperidine, paroxetine, pentazocine, sertraline, sumatriptan, tryptophan, venlafaxine: May cause hyperthermia, tachycardia, and loss of consciousness. Avoid using together.
Ephedrine, pseudoephedrine: May increase blood pressure or heart rate. Use together cautiously.
Drug-lifestyle. *Alcohol use:* May enhance CNS depression. Discourage use together.

EFFECTS ON LAB TEST RESULTS

- May increase ALT, AST, GGT, LDH, alkaline phosphatase, and bilirubin levels.

CONTRAINDICATIONS & CAUTIONS

- Contraindicated in patients hypersensitive to drug or its active ingredients, in those taking MAO inhibitors or other centrally acting appetite suppressants, and in those with anorexia nervosa.
- Contraindicated in patients with severe renal or hepatic dysfunction, history of hypertension, coronary artery disease, heart failure, arrhythmias, or stroke.
- Contraindicated in elderly patients.
- Use cautiously in patients with history of seizures or angle-closure glaucoma.

NURSING CONSIDERATIONS

- Measure blood pressure and pulse before starting therapy, with dosage changes, and at regular intervals during therapy.
- Use drug in obese patients with a body mass index of 30 or more (27 or more if patient has other risk factors, such as hypertension, diabetes, or dyslipidemia).
- Avoid using within 2 weeks of MAO inhibitor.
- ***Alert:*** Combining this drug with triptans, SSRIs or SNRIs may cause serotonin syndrome. Symptoms include restlessness, hallucinations, loss of coordination, fast heart beat, rapid changes in blood pressure, increased body temperature, hyperreflexia, nausea, vomiting, and diarrhea. The syndrome is more likely to occur when starting or increasing the dose of the triptan, SSRI, or SNRI.

PATIENT TEACHING

- Advise patient to report rash, hives, or other allergic reactions immediately.
- Instruct patient to notify prescriber before taking other prescription or OTC drugs.
- Advise patient to have blood pressure and pulse monitored at regular intervals. Stress importance of regular follow-up visits with prescriber.
- Advise patient to follow a reduced-calorie diet.
- Tell patient that weight loss can cause gallstones. Teach signs and symptoms, and tell patient to notify prescriber promptly if they occur.

sumatriptan succinate

Imitrex✐

Pharmacologic class: serotonin 5-HT_1 receptor agonist
Pregnancy risk category C

AVAILABLE FORMS

Injection: 6 mg/0.5 ml (12 mg/ml) in 0.5-ml prefilled syringes and vials
Nasal solution: 5 mg/0.1 ml, 20 mg/0.1 ml
Tablets: 25 mg, 50 mg, 100 mg (base)†

INDICATIONS & DOSAGES

➤ Acute migraine attacks (with or without aura)

Adults: For injection, 6 mg subcutaneously; maximum dose is two 6-mg injections in 24 hours, separated by at least 1 hour.

For tablets, 25 to 100 mg P.O., initially. If desired response isn't achieved in 2 hours, may give second dose of 25 to 100 mg. Additional doses may be used in at least 2-hour intervals. Maximum daily dose, 200 mg.

For nasal spray, give 5 mg, 10 mg, or 20 mg once in one nostril; may repeat once after 2 hours, for maximum daily dose of 40 mg. A 10-mg dose may be achieved by giving a 5-mg dose in each nostril.

➤ Cluster headache

Adults: 6 mg subcutaneously. Maximum recommended dose is two 6-mg injections in 24 hours, separated by at least 1 hour.

Adjust-a-dose: In patients with hepatic impairment, the maximum single oral dose shouldn't exceed 50 mg.

ACTION

May act as an agonist at serotonin receptors on extracerebral intracranial blood vessels, which constricts the affected vessels, inhibits neuropeptide release, and reduces pain transmission in the trigeminal pathways.

Route	Onset	Peak	Duration
P.O.	30 min	90 min	Unknown
SubQ	10 min	12 min	Unknown
Intranasal	Rapid	1–2 hr	Unknown

Half-life: About 2 hours.

ADVERSE REACTIONS

CNS: *dizziness, vertigo,* drowsiness, headache, anxiety, malaise, fatigue.
CV: ***atrial fibrillation, ventricular fibrillation, ventricular tachycardia, coronary artery vasospasm, transient myocardial ischemia, MI,*** pressure or tightness in chest.
EENT: discomfort of throat, nasal cavity or sinus, mouth, jaw, or tongue, altered vision.
GI: abdominal discomfort, dysphagia, diarrhea, nausea, vomiting, unusual or bad taste (nasal spray).
Musculoskeletal: myalgia, muscle cramps, neck pain.
Respiratory: upper respiratory inflammation and dyspnea (P.O.).
Skin: *injection site reaction, tingling,* diaphoresis, flushing.
Other: *warm or hot sensation, burning sensation,* heaviness, pressure or tightness, tight feeling in head, cold sensation, numbness.

INTERACTIONS

Drug-drug. *Ergot and ergot derivatives, other 5-HT_1 agonists:* May prolong vasospastic effects. Don't use within 24 hours of sumatriptan therapy.
MAO inhibitors: May reduce sumatriptan clearance. Avoid using within 2 weeks of MAO inhibitor. Use injection cautiously and decrease sumatriptan dose.
SSRIs: May cause weakness, hyperreflexia, and incoordination. Monitor patient closely if use together can't be avoided.
Drug-herb. *Horehound:* May enhance serotonergic effects. Discourage use together.

EFFECTS ON LAB TEST RESULTS

- May increase liver enzyme levels.

CONTRAINDICATIONS & CAUTIONS

- Contraindicated in patients with hypersensitivity to drug or its components; those with history, symptoms, or signs of ischemic cardiac, cerebrovascular (such as stroke or transient ischemic attack), or peripheral vascular syndromes (such as ischemic bowel disease); significant underlying CV diseases, including angina pectoris, MI, and silent myocardial ischemia; uncontrolled hypertension; or severe hepatic impairment.
- Contraindicated within 24 hours of another 5-HT_1 agonist or drug containing ergotamine and within 2 weeks of MAO inhibitor.

NURSING CONSIDERATIONS

- Use cautiously in woman who is or may become pregnant.
- Use cautiously in patient with risk factors for coronary artery disease (CAD), such as postmenopausal women, men older than age 40, or patients with hypertension, hypercholesterolemia, obesity, diabetes, smoking, or family history of CAD.
- ***Alert:*** When giving drug to patient at risk for CAD, give first dose in presence of other medical personnel. Rarely, serious adverse cardiac effects can follow administration.
- ***Alert:*** Combining drug with an SSRI or a selective serotonin-norepinephrine reuptake inhibitor (SNRI) may cause serotonin syndrome. Symptoms include restlessness, hallucinations, loss of coordination, fast heart beat, rapid changes in blood pressure, increased body temperature, hyperreflexia, nausea, vomiting, and diarrhea. Serotonin syndrome may occur when starting or increasing the dose of drug, SSRI, or SNRI.
- After subcutaneous injection, most patients experience relief in 1 to 2 hours.

- Redness or pain at injection site should subside within 1 hour after injection.
- ***Look alike–sound alike:*** Don't confuse sumatriptan with somatropin.

PATIENT TEACHING

- Inform patient that drug is intended only to treat migraine attacks, not to prevent them or reduce their occurrence.
- If patient is pregnant or may become pregnant, tell her not to use drug but to discuss with prescriber the risks and benefits of using drug during pregnancy.
- Tell patient that drug may be taken any time during a migraine attack, as soon as signs or symptoms appear.
- Review information about drug's injectable form, which is available in a spring-loaded injector system for easier patient use. Make sure patient understands how to load the injector, give the injection, and dispose of used syringes.
- ***Alert:*** Tell patient to tell prescriber immediately about persistent or severe chest pain. Warn him to stop using drug and to call prescriber if he develops pain or tightness in the throat, wheezing, heart throbbing, rash, lumps, hives, or swollen eyelids, face, or lips.

zolmitriptan
Zomig, Zomig ZMT

Pharmacologic class: serotonin 5-HT_1 receptor agonist
Pregnancy risk category C

AVAILABLE FORMS

Nasal spray: 5 mg
Tablets (immediate-release): 2.5 mg, 5 mg
Tablets (oral disintegrating): 2.5 mg, 5 mg

INDICATIONS & DOSAGES

➤ **Acute migraine headaches**

Adults: Initially, 2.5 mg or less P.O. Break a 2.5-mg immediate-release tablet in half if a lower dose is needed. Increase to 5 mg per dosage, p.r.n. If using orally disintegrating tablets, initially, 2.5 mg P.O. Don't break orally disintegrating tablets in half. Or, 1 spray (5 mg) into nostril. If headache returns after first dose, give a second dose at least 2 hours after the first dose. Maximum dosage is 10 mg in 24 hours.

Adjust-a-dose: In patients with hepatic disease, use doses less than 2.5 mg. Don't use orally disintegrating tablets because they shouldn't be broken in half, or nasal spray because 5 mg is the lowest deliverable dose.

ACTION

May act as an agonist at serotonin receptors on extracerebral intracranial blood vessels, which constricts the affected vessels, inhibits neuropeptide release, and reduces pain transmission in the trigeminal pathways.

Route	Onset	Peak	Duration
P.O.	Unknown	2 hr	3 hr
Nasal	5 min	3 hr	Unknown

Half-life: 3 hours.

ADVERSE REACTIONS

CNS: *dizziness,* somnolence, vertigo, hypesthesia, paresthesia, asthenia, pain.
CV: ***coronary artery vasospasm, transient myocardial ischemia, MI, ventricular tachycardia, ventricular fibrillation,*** palpitations, pain, tightness, pressure, or heaviness in chest.
EENT: *pain, tightness, or pressure in the neck, throat, or jaw.*
GI: dry mouth, dyspepsia, dysphagia, nausea.
Musculoskeletal: myalgia, myasthenia.
Skin: sweating.
Other: warm or cold sensations.

INTERACTIONS

Drug-drug. *Cimetidine:* May double half-life of zolmitriptan. Monitor patient closely.
Ergot-containing drugs, other triptans: May cause additive effects. Avoid using within 24 hours of almotriptan.
Hormonal contraceptives, propranolol: May increase zolmitriptan level. Monitor patient closely.
MAO inhibitors: May increase zolmitriptan level. Avoid using within 2 weeks of MAO inhibitor.
SSRIs: May cause additive serotonin effects, resulting in weakness, hyperreflexia, or incoordination. Monitor patient closely if given together.

EFFECTS ON LAB TEST RESULTS

- May increase glucose levels.

CONTRAINDICATIONS & CAUTIONS

- Contraindicated in patients hypersensitive to drug or its components, pregnant or breast-feeding patients, and those with uncontrolled hypertension, hemiplegic or basilar migraine, ischemic heart disease (angina pectoris, history of MI or documented silent ischemia), symptoms of ischemic heart disease (coronary artery vasospasm, including Prinzmetal variant angina), or other significant heart disease.
- Contraindicated within 24 hours of other triptans or drugs containing ergot or within 2 weeks of stopping MAO inhibitor.
- Use cautiously in patients with liver disease and in those who may be at risk for coronary artery disease (such as postmenopausal women or men older than age 40) or those with risk factors, such as hypertension, hypercholesterolemia, obesity, diabetes, smoking, or family history.

NURSING CONSIDERATIONS

- Drug isn't intended for preventing migraines or treating hemiplegic or basilar migraines.
- Safety of drug hasn't been established for cluster headaches.
- ***Alert:*** Combining drug with an SSRI or a selective serotonin-norepinephrine reuptake inhibitor (SNRI) may cause serotonin syndrome. Signs and symptoms may include restlessness, hallucinations, loss of coordination, fast heart beat, rapid changes in blood pressure, increased body temperature, overactive reflexes, nausea, vomiting, and diarrhea. Serotonin syndrome may be more likely to occur when starting or increasing the dose of drug, SSRI, or SNRI.

PATIENT TEACHING

- Tell patient that drug is intended to relieve, not prevent, signs and symptoms of migraine.
- Advise patient to take drug as prescribed and not to take a second dose unless instructed by prescriber. Tell patient if a second dose is indicated and permitted, he should take it 2 hours after first dose.
- Instruct patient to release the orally disintegrating tablets from the blister pack just before taking; tablet should dissolve on tongue.
- Advise patient not to break the orally disintegrating tablets in half.
- Advise patient to immediately report pain or tightness in the chest or throat, heart throbbing, rash, skin lumps, or swelling of the face, lips, or eyelids.
- Tell woman not to take drug if she is or may become pregnant.

35

Cholinergics (parasympathomimetics)

bethanechol chloride
cevimeline hydrochloride
neostigmine bromide
neostigmine methylsulfate
physostigmine salicylate
pilocarpine hydrochloride
pyridostigmine bromide

bethanechol chloride

Duvoid, Urabeth, Urocarb‡, Urecholine

Pharmacologic class: cholinergic agonist
Pregnancy risk category C

AVAILABLE FORMS
Injection: 5 mg/ml
Tablets: 5 mg, 10 mg, 25 mg, 50 mg

INDICATIONS & DOSAGES
➤ **Acute postoperative and postpartum nonobstructive (functional) urine retention, neurogenic atony of urinary bladder with urine retention**
Adults: 10 to 50 mg P.O. t.i.d. to q.i.d. Or, 2.5 to 5 mg subcutaneously. Never give I.V. or I.M.

Test dosage is 2.5 mg subcutaneously, repeated at 15- to 30-minute intervals to total of four doses to determine the minimum effective dose; then, minimum effective dose used q 6 to 8 hours. All doses must be adjusted individually.

ACTION
Directly stimulates muscarinic cholinergic receptors, mimicking acetylcholine action, increasing GI tract tone and peristalsis and contraction of the detrusor muscle of the urinary bladder.

Route	Onset	Peak	Duration
P.O.	30–90 min	1 hr	6 hr
SubQ	5–15 min	15–30 min	2 hr

Half-life: Unknown.

ADVERSE REACTIONS
CNS: headache, malaise.
CV: ***bradycardia,*** profound hypotension with reflexive tachycardia, flushing.
EENT: lacrimation, miosis.
GI: *abdominal cramps, diarrhea,* excessive salivation, nausea, belching, borborygmus.
GU: urinary urgency.
Respiratory: ***bronchoconstriction,*** increased bronchial secretions.
Skin: diaphoresis.

INTERACTIONS
Drug-drug. *Anticholinergics, atropine, belladonna alkaloids, procainamide, quinidine:* May reverse cholinergic effects. Observe patient for lack of drug effect.
Cholinesterase inhibitors (donepezil), cholinergic agonists: May cause additive effects or increase toxicity. Avoid using together.
Ganglionic blockers: May cause critical drop in blood pressure, usually preceded by severe abdominal pain. Avoid using together.

EFFECTS ON LAB TEST RESULTS
- May increase amylase, lipase, and liver enzyme levels.

CONTRAINDICATIONS & CAUTIONS
- Contraindicated in patients hypersensitive to drug or its components and in those with uncertain strength or integrity of bladder wall, mechanical obstruction of GI or urinary tract, hyperthyroidism, peptic ulceration, latent or active bronchial asthma, obstructive pulmonary disease, pronounced bradycardia or hypotension, vasomotor instability, cardiac or coronary artery disease, AV conduction defects, hypertension, seizure disorder, Parkinson disease, spastic GI disturbances, acute inflammatory lesions of the GI tract, peritonitis, or marked vagotonia.
- Contraindicated for I.V. or I.M. use and when increased muscular activity of the GI or urinary tract is harmful.

• Use cautiously in pregnant or breast-feeding women.

NURSING CONSIDERATIONS
• Give drug 1 hour before or 2 hours after meals because it may cause nausea and vomiting if taken soon after eating.
• Adverse effects are rare with P.O. use.
• ***Alert:*** Never give I.V. or I.M. because of possible circulatory collapse, hypotension, severe abdominal cramping, bloody diarrhea, shock, or cardiac arrest.
• Monitor vital signs frequently, especially respirations. Always have atropine injection available, and be prepared to give 0.6 mg subcutaneously or by slow I.V. push. Provide respiratory support, if needed.
• Monitor patient for orthostatic hypotension.
• Watch for toxicity, especially with subcutaneous use.
• Watch closely for adverse reactions that may indicate drug toxicity.
• Oral drug absorption is poor and variable, requiring larger oral doses. Oral and subcutaneous doses aren't interchangeable.

PATIENT TEACHING
• Tell patient to take oral form on an empty stomach and at regular intervals.
• Inform patient that drug is usually effective 30 to 90 minutes after oral use and 5 to 15 minutes after subcutaneous use.

cevimeline hydrochloride
Evoxac

Pharmacologic class: cholinergic agonist
Pregnancy risk category C

AVAILABLE FORMS
Capsules: 30 mg

INDICATIONS & DOSAGES
➤ **Dry mouth in patients with Sjögren syndrome**
Adults: 30 mg P.O. t.i.d.

ACTION
Stimulates the muscarinic receptors of the exocrine glands (salivary, sweat) and increases GI and urinary smooth muscle tone.

Route	Onset	Peak	Duration
P.O.	Unknown	1½–2 hr	Unknown

Half-life: 4 to 6 hours.

ADVERSE REACTIONS
CNS: *headache,* anxiety, depression, fever, dizziness, fatigue, hypoesthesia, insomnia, migraine, pain, tremor, vertigo.
CV: chest pain, palpitations, peripheral edema.
EENT: *rhinitis, sinusitis,* abnormal vision, conjunctivitis, earache, epistaxis, eye infection, eye pain, otitis media, pharyngitis, xerophthalmia, eye abnormality.
GI: *diarrhea, nausea,* abdominal pain, anorexia, constipation, dry mouth, eructation, excessive salivation, flatulence, gastroesophageal reflux, salivary gland enlargement and pain, salivary calculi, ulcerative stomatitis, vomiting, dyspepsia, increased amylase.
GU: cystitis, candidiasis, UTI, vaginitis.
Hematologic: anemia.
Musculoskeletal: arthralgia, back pain, hypertonia, hyporeflexia, leg cramps, myalgia, rigors, skeletal pain.
Respiratory: *upper respiratory tract infection,* bronchitis, pneumonia, coughing, hiccups.
Skin: *excessive sweating,* rash, pruritus, skin disorder, erythematous rash.
Other: fungal infections, flulike symptoms, injury, hot flushes, tooth disorder, toothache, postoperative pain, allergic reaction, infection, abscess.

INTERACTIONS
Drug-drug. *Antimuscarinics:* May cause antagonistic effects. Monitor patient for effectiveness.
Beta blockers: May cause conduction disturbances. Use together cautiously.
CYP inhibitors: May inhibit metabolism of cevimeline. Monitor patient closely.
Parasympathomimetics: May have additive effects. Use together cautiously.

EFFECTS ON LAB TEST RESULTS
• May increase amylase level. May decrease hemoglobin level.

CONTRAINDICATIONS & CAUTIONS

- Contraindicated in patients hypersensitive to drug and in those for whom miosis is undesirable (as in those who have acute iritis or angle-closure glaucoma).
- Contraindicated in patients with uncontrolled asthma.
- Use cautiously in patients with significant CV disease, controlled asthma, chronic bronchitis, or COPD and in those with a history of kidney stones or gallstones.

NURSING CONSIDERATIONS

- Monitor patients with a history of asthma, COPD, or chronic bronchitis for an increase in signs or symptoms, such as wheezing, increased sputum production, or cough.
- Monitor patients with a history of cardiac disease for changes in heart rate or increased frequency, severity, or duration of angina.
- Monitor elderly patients closely because they have an increased risk of impaired renal, hepatic, and cardiac function.

PATIENT TEACHING

- Advise patient not to interrupt or stop treatment without consulting prescriber.
- Tell patient that sweating is a common adverse effect. Urge adequate fluid intake to prevent dehydration.
- Inform patient that drug may cause visual disturbances that can impair driving ability, especially at night.

---

neostigmine bromide
Prostigmin

neostigmine methylsulfate
Prostigmin

Pharmacologic class: cholinesterase inhibitor
Pregnancy risk category C

AVAILABLE FORMS

neostigmine bromide
Tablets: 15 mg
neostigmine methylsulfate
Injection: 0.25 mg/ml, 0.5 mg/ml, 1 mg/ml

INDICATIONS & DOSAGES

➤ To control myasthenia gravis symptoms
Adults: Initially, 15 mg P.O. t.i.d.; increase gradually, p.r.n. Range is 15 to 375 mg/day. Average dosage is 150 mg/day with intervals individualized. Or, 0.5 mg I.M. or subcutaneously; base subsequent parenteral doses on patient's response.
Children: 2 mg/kg/day P.O. divided q 3 to 4 hours, or 0.01 to 0.04 mg/kg/dose I.M. or subcutaneously q 2 to 3 hours, p.r.n.
Neonates: 0.1 to 0.2 mg subcutaneously, or 0.03 mg/kg I.M. q 2 to 4 hours. Or, 1 to 4 mg P.O. q 2 to 3 hours. Gradually reduce dose until drug can be withdrawn.

➤ To prevent and treat postoperative distention and urine retention
Adults: For prevention, 0.25 mg I.M. or subcutaneously as soon as possible after surgery; then q 4 to 6 hours for 2 to 3 days. For treatment, 0.5 mg I.M. or subcutaneously. If urination hasn't occurred in 1 hour, catheterize. Continue 0.5-mg injections q 3 hours for at least 5 doses.

➤ Antidote for nondepolarizing neuromuscular blockers
Adults: 0.5 to 2 mg I.V. slowly. Repeat, p.r.n., to total of 5 mg. Before antidote dose, give 0.6 to 1.2 mg atropine sulfate I.V. if patient is bradycardic.

➤ Supraventricular tachycardia from tricyclic antidepressant overdose ♦
Children: 0.5 to 1 mg slow I.V. injection, followed by 0.25 to 0.5 mg q 1 to 3 hours, p.r.n.

I.V. ADMINISTRATION

- Give as a slow I.V. injection.
- If patient's muscle weakness is severe, prescriber will determine if it's from drug toxicity or worsening myasthenia gravis. Test dose of edrophonium I.V. will aggravate drug-induced weakness but will temporarily relieve disease-induced weakness.

INCOMPATIBILITIES

None reported.

ACTION

Inhibits acetylcholinesterase, blocking destruction of acetylcholine from the parasympathetic and somatic efferent nerves.

Acetylcholine accumulates, promoting increased stimulation of the receptors.

Route	Onset	Peak	Duration
P.O.	45–75 min	1–2 hr	2–4 hr
I.V.	4–8 min	1–2 hr	2–4 hr
I.M., SubQ	20–30 min	1–2 hr	2–4 hr

Half-life: About 53 minutes.

ADVERSE REACTIONS

CNS: ***seizures,*** dizziness, headache, muscle weakness, loss of consciousness, drowsiness, syncope.
CV: ***bradycardia, AV block, cardiac arrest,*** hypotension, tachycardia, flushing, thrombophlebitis (I.V.).
EENT: blurred vision, lacrimation, miosis.
GI: *nausea, vomiting, diarrhea, abdominal cramps,* excessive salivation, flatulence, increased peristalsis.
GU: urinary frequency, incontinence, urinary urgency.
Musculoskeletal: *muscle cramps,* muscle weakness, muscle fasciculations, arthralgia.
Respiratory: ***bronchospasm, respiratory depression, respiratory arrest, laryngospasm, paralysis of respiratory muscles, central respiratory paralysis,*** dyspnea, increased secretions.
Skin: rash, urticaria, diaphoresis.
Other: ***anaphylaxis,*** hypersensitivity reactions.

INTERACTIONS

Drug-drug. *Aminoglycosides, anticholinergics, atropine, local and general anesthetics, magnesium sulfate, procainamide, quinidine:* May reverse cholinergic effects; watch for lack of drug effect. Stop all other cholinergics before giving this drug.
Corticosteroids: May antagonize the effects of cholinesterase inhibitors in myasthenia gravis. Monitor patient for severe muscle deterioration.
Other cholinesterase inhibitors: May cause cholinergic crisis; myasthenic weakness may mimic symptoms of cholinesterase inhibitor overdose in myasthenia gravis patients. Monitor patient.
Succinylcholine: May worsen blockade produced by succinylcholine when used to reverse the effects of nondepolarizing neuromuscular blockers in surgical patients. Monitor patient.

EFFECTS ON LAB TEST RESULTS

None reported.

CONTRAINDICATIONS & CAUTIONS

- Contraindicated in patients hypersensitive to cholinergics or bromides and in those with peritonitis or mechanical obstruction of the intestinal or urinary tract.
- Don't give if patient has received high concentrations of halothane or cyclopropane.
- Use cautiously in patients with bronchial asthma, bradycardia, seizure disorders, recent coronary occlusion, vagotonia, hyperthyroidism, arrhythmias, and peptic ulcer.

NURSING CONSIDERATIONS

- Dosage for the treatment of myasthenia gravis must be highly individualized, depending on response and tolerance of adverse effects. Therapy may be needed day and night.
- For myasthenia gravis, schedule doses before periods of fatigue. For example, if patient has difficulty swallowing, schedule dose 30 minutes before each meal.
- ***Alert:*** Monitor vital signs frequently, especially respirations. Keep atropine injection available, and provide respiratory support, as needed.
- ***Look alike–sound alike:*** Don't confuse neostigmine vials with etomidate vials, which look similar.
- Monitor and document patient's response after each dose. Ideal dosage is difficult to judge. Watch closely for improvement in strength, vision, and ptosis 45 to 60 minutes after each dose.
- When drug is used to prevent abdominal distention and GI distress, inserting a rectal tube may help passage of gas.
- When drug is given for postoperative abdominal distention and bladder atony, rule out mechanical obstruction before dose is given. If no response within 1 hour after first dose, catheterize patient.
- Patient may develop resistance to drug.
- Many patients with long-standing disease insist on self-administration. Provide bedside supply of tablets.

PATIENT TEACHING

- Tell patient to take drug with food or milk to reduce adverse GI reactions.
- When giving drug for myasthenia gravis, explain that it will relieve ptosis, double vision, chewing and swallowing problems, and trunk and limb weakness. Stress the importance of taking drug exactly as prescribed, including nighttime doses. Explain that patient may need to take drug for life.
- Teach patient how to observe and record variations in muscle strength.
- Advise patient to wear or carry medical identification.

physostigmine salicylate (eserine salicylate)

Antilirium

Pharmacologic class: cholinesterase inhibitor
Pregnancy risk category C

AVAILABLE FORMS

Injection: 1 mg/ml

INDICATIONS & DOSAGES

➤ Reversal of drug-induced anticholinergic effects
Adults: 0.5 to 2 mg slow I.V. or I.M. not to exceed 1 mg/minute I.V. repeated q 20 minutes p.r.n. until patient responds or develops adverse cholinergic effects. Give additional 1 to 4 mg I.V. or I.M. q 30 to 60 minutes if life-threatening problems, such as coma, seizures, and arrhythmias recur.
Children: Only for life-threatening situations. Give 0.02 mg/kg I.M. or slow I.V. at 0.5 mg/minute or slower, and repeat q 5 to 10 minutes until patient responds, adverse anticholinergic reactions develop, or a total dose of 2 mg has been given. Or, give 0.03 mg/kg or 0.9 mg/m^2, as needed.

➤ Alzheimer dementia ♦
Adults: Initially, 0.5 mg P.O. q 2 hours six to seven times daily; may increase to 2 to 2.5 mg q 2 hours six or seven times daily. Maximum, 16 mg P.O. daily.

I.V. ADMINISTRATION

- Position patient to ease breathing. Keep atropine injection available, and give 0.5 mg by slow I.V. push or subcutaneously.
- Give drug at controlled rate; use direct injection at no more than 1 mg/minute in adults or 0.5 mg/minute in children.
- Monitor vital signs frequently, especially respirations. Provide respiratory support, as needed.

INCOMPATIBILITIES

None reported.

ACTION

Inhibits acetylcholinesterase, blocking destruction of acetylcholine from the parasympathetic and somatic efferent nerves. Acetylcholine accumulates, promoting increased stimulation of the receptors.

Route	Onset	Peak	Duration
I.V.	3–5 min	5 min	30 min–5 hr
I.M.	3–5 min	20–30 min	30 min–5 hr

Half-life: 1 to 2 hours.

ADVERSE REACTIONS

CNS: *restlessness, excitability,* ***seizures,*** muscle weakness.
CV: ***bradycardia,*** hypotension, palpitations, irregular pulse.
EENT: miosis, lacrimation.
GI: *diarrhea, excessive salivation,* nausea, vomiting, epigastric pain.
GU: urinary urgency.
Respiratory: ***bronchospasm, bronchial constriction, respiratory paralysis,*** dyspnea.
Skin: diaphoresis.

INTERACTIONS

Drug-drug. *Anticholinergics, atropine, local and general anesthetics, procainamide, quinidine:* May reverse cholinergic effects. Observe patient for lack of drug effect.
Ganglionic blockers: May decrease blood pressure. Avoid using together.
Neuromuscular blockers (succinylcholine): May increase neuromuscular blockade, respiratory depression. Use together cautiously.
Drug-herb. *Jaborandi tree, pill-bearing spurge:* May have additive effect. Ask patient about use of herbal remedies, and recommend caution.

EFFECTS ON LAB TEST RESULTS
None reported.

CONTRAINDICATIONS & CAUTIONS
- Contraindicated in patients with mechanical obstruction of the intestine or urogenital tract; in patients with asthma, gangrene, diabetes, CV disease, or vagotonia; and in patients receiving choline esters or depolarizing neuromuscular blockers.
- Use cautiously in pregnant patients and those with epilepsy, parkinsonism, or bradycardia.

NURSING CONSIDERATIONS
- Use only clear solution. Darkening may indicate loss of potency.
- ***Alert:*** Watch closely for adverse reactions, particularly CNS disturbances. Raise side rails of bed if patient becomes restless or hallucinates. Adverse reactions may indicate drug toxicity.
- Effectiveness is typically immediate and dramatic but may be short-lived. Patient may need repeated dosages.
- Drug contains benzyl alcohol and has been associated with fatal "gasping syndrome" in premature infants.
- Drug contains sulfites, which may cause an allergic reaction in susceptible people.

PATIENT TEACHING
- Inform patient of need for drug, explain its use and adverse reactions, and answer any questions or concerns.
- Tell patient to report adverse reactions promptly.
- Instruct patient to report discomfort at I.V. site.

pilocarpine hydrochloride
Salagen

Pharmacologic class: cholinergic agonist
Pregnancy risk category C

AVAILABLE FORMS
Tablets: 5 mg, 7.5 mg

INDICATIONS & DOSAGES
➤Xerostomia from salivary gland hypofunction caused by radiotherapy for cancer of head and neck
Adults: 5 mg P.O. t.i.d.; may increase to 10 mg P.O. t.i.d., p.r.n.
➤Dry mouth in patients with Sjögren syndrome
Adults: 5 mg P.O. q.i.d.
Adjust-a-dose: For patients with moderate hepatic impairment, initial dose is 5 mg P.O. b.i.d. Adjust dose based on tolerance.

ACTION
Cholinergic parasympathomimetic that increases secretion of salivary glands, eliminating dryness.

Route	Onset	Peak	Duration
P.O.	20 min	1 hr	3–5 hr

Half-life: 45 minutes to 1½ hours.

ADVERSE REACTIONS
CNS: *asthenia, dizziness, headache,* tremor.
CV: *flushing,* hypertension, tachycardia, edema.
EENT: *abnormal vision, rhinitis, sinusitis,* lacrimation, amblyopia, pharyngitis, voice alteration, conjunctivitis, epistaxis.
GI: *nausea,* dyspepsia, diarrhea, abdominal pain, vomiting, dysphagia, taste perversion.
GU: *urinary frequency.*
Musculoskeletal: myalgia.
Skin: *sweating,* rash, pruritus.
Other: *chills.*

INTERACTIONS
Drug-drug. *Beta blockers:* May increase risk of conduction disturbances. Use together cautiously.
Drugs with anticholinergic effects: May antagonize anticholinergic effects. Use together cautiously.
Drugs with parasympathomimetic effects: May result in additive pharmacologic effects. Monitor patient closely.
Drug-food. *High-fat meals:* May reduce drug absorption. Discourage patient from eating high-fat meals.

EFFECTS ON LAB TEST RESULTS
None reported.

CONTRAINDICATIONS & CAUTIONS
- Contraindicated in patients hypersensitive to pilocarpine, in breast-feeding women, in those with uncontrolled asthma, and in those for whom miosis is undesirable, as in acute iritis or angle-closure glaucoma.
- Use in severe hepatic insufficiency isn't recommended.
- Use cautiously in patients with CV disease, controlled asthma, chronic bronchitis, COPD, cholelithiasis, biliary tract disease, nephrolithiasis, cognitive or psychiatric disturbances, or in pregnant women.
- Safety and effectiveness of drug in children haven't been established.

NURSING CONSIDERATIONS
- Examine patient's fundus carefully before beginning therapy because retinal detachment may occur in patients with retinal disease.
- Monitor patient for signs and symptoms of toxicity: headache, visual disturbance, lacrimation, sweating, respiratory distress, GI spasm, nausea, vomiting, diarrhea, AV block, tachycardia, bradycardia, hypotension, hypertension, shock, mental confusion, arrhythmia, and tremors. Immediately notify prescriber of suspected toxicity.

PATIENT TEACHING
- Warn patient that driving ability may be impaired, especially at night, by drug-induced visual disturbances.
- Advise patient to drink plenty of fluids to prevent dehydration.
- Tell elderly patient with Sjögren syndrome that he may be especially prone to urinary frequency, diarrhea, and dizziness.
- Advise patient not to take drug with a high-fat meal.

pyridostigmine bromide
Mestinon*, Mestinon-SR†, Mestinon Timespans, Regonol

Pharmacologic class: cholinesterase inhibitor
Pregnancy risk category NR

AVAILABLE FORMS
Injection: 5 mg/ml in 2-ml ampules or 5-ml vials
Syrup: 60 mg/5 ml
Tablets: 30 mg (for military use only), 60 mg
Tablets (extended-release): 180 mg

INDICATIONS & DOSAGES
➤ Antidote for nondepolarizing neuromuscular blockers
Adults: 10 to 20 mg I.V., preceded by atropine sulfate 0.6 to 1.2 mg I.V.
➤ Myasthenia gravis
Adults: 60 to 120 mg P.O. q 3 or 4 hours. Average dosage is 600 mg daily, but dosages up to 1,500 mg daily may be needed. For I.M. or I.V. use, give 1/30 of oral dose. Dosage must be adjusted for each patient, based on response and tolerance. Or, 180 to 540 mg extended-release tablets P.O. b.i.d., with at least 6 hours between doses.
Children: 7 mg/kg or 200 mg/m^2 daily in five or six divided doses.
Neonates: 5 mg P.O. q 4 to 6 hours or 0.05 to 0.15 mg/kg I.M. q 4 to 6 hours.
➤ Preexposure prophylaxis against the deadly effects of nerve agent soman
Adults in military combat: 30 mg P.O. q 8 hours, starting at least several hours before soman exposure.
Adjust-a-dose: Smaller doses may be required in patients with renal disease. Adjust dosage to achieve desired effect.

I.V. ADMINISTRATION
- Position patient to ease breathing. Keep atropine injection available, and be prepared to give it immediately.
- Monitor vital signs frequently, especially respirations. Provide respiratory support as needed.

• Give injection no faster than 1 mg/minute. Rapid infusion may cause bradycardia and seizures.
• If patient's muscle weakness is severe, prescriber will determine if it results from drug toxicity or worsening myasthenia gravis. Test dose of edrophonium I.V. will aggravate drug-induced weakness but will temporarily relieve disease-induced weakness.

INCOMPATIBILITIES
Alkaline solutions.

ACTION
Inhibits acetylcholinesterase, blocking destruction of acetylcholine from the parasympathetic and somatic efferent nerves. Acetylcholine accumulates, promoting increased stimulation of the receptors.

Route	Onset	Peak	Duration
P.O.	20–30 min	2 hr	3–6 hr
P.O. (extended)	30–60 min	1–2 hr	6–12 hr
I.V.	2–5 min	Unknown	2–4 hr
I.M.	15 min	Unknown	2–4 hr

Half-life: 1 to 3 hours, depending on route.

ADVERSE REACTIONS
CNS: headache with high doses, weakness, syncope.
CV: ***bradycardia, cardiac arrest,*** hypotension, thrombophlebitis.
EENT: miosis, rhinorrhea.
GI: *nausea, vomiting,* abdominal cramps, diarrhea, excessive salivation, increased peristalsis.
GU: urinary frequency, urinary urgency.
Musculoskeletal: muscle cramps, muscle fasciculations, muscle weakness, tingling in extremities.
Respiratory: ***bronchospasm, bronchoconstriction,*** increased bronchial secretions.
Skin: rash, diaphoresis.

INTERACTIONS
Drug-drug. *Aminoglycosides:* May prolong or enhance muscle weakness. Use together cautiously.
Anticholinergics, atropine, corticosteroids, general or local anesthetics, magnesium, procainamide, quinidine: May antagonize cholinergic effects. Observe patient for lack of drug effect.
Ganglionic blockers: May increase risk of hypotension. Monitor patient closely.
Succinylcholine: May prolong the phase I block of the depolarizing muscle relaxant. Avoid use together.

EFFECTS ON LAB TEST RESULTS
None reported.

CONTRAINDICATIONS & CAUTIONS
• Contraindicated in patients hypersensitive to anticholinesterases or bromides and in those with mechanical obstruction of the intestinal or urinary tract.
• Use cautiously in patients with bronchial asthma, bradycardia, arrhythmias, epilepsy, recent coronary occlusion, vagotonia, renal impairment, hyperthyroidism, or peptic ulcer.
• Use cautiously in patients taking beta blockers for hypertension or glaucoma.
• Use cautiously in pregnant and breastfeeding women; drug appears in breast milk.

NURSING CONSIDERATIONS
• ***Alert:*** If taken immediately before or during soman exposure, drug may be ineffective and may worsen soman's effects. At the first sign of soman poisoning, stop drug and immediately start atropine and pralidoxime.
• Stop all other cholinergics before giving this drug.
• Don't crush extended-release tablets.
• If patient has trouble swallowing, give syrup form. If patient can't tolerate sweet flavor, give over ice chips.
• Monitor and document patient's response after each dose. Optimal dosage is difficult to judge.
• ***Alert:*** Regonol contains benzyl ethanol preservative, which may cause toxicity in neonates if given in high doses.
• Give hospitalized patient a bedside supply of tablets. Many patients with longstanding disease insist on self-administration.

PATIENT TEACHING
• When giving drug for myasthenia gravis, stress importance of taking exactly as prescribed, on time, in evenly spaced

doses. For extended-release tablets, tell patient to take at same time each day, at least 6 hours apart.

- Advise patient not to crush or chew extended-release tablets.
- Explain that patient may have to take drug for life.
- Advise patient to wear or carry medical identification that identifies his myasthenia gravis.
- Stress to military personnel importance of taking nerve agent antidotes, atropine and pralidoxime, rather than this drug at the first sign of nerve agent poisoning.

36

Anticholinergics

atropine sulfate
(See Chapter 19, ANTIARRHYTHMICS.)
dicyclomine hydrochloride
glycopyrrolate
hyoscyamine
L-hyoscyamine sulfate
scopolamine
scopolamine butylbromide
scopolamine hydrobromide

dicyclomine hydrochloride

Bentyl, Bentylol†, Formulex†, Spasmoban†

Pharmacologic class: anticholinergic, antimuscarinic
Pregnancy risk category NR

AVAILABLE FORMS

Capsules: 10 mg, 20 mg
Injection: 10 mg/ml
Syrup: 5 mg/5 ml‡, 10 mg/5 ml
Tablets: 10 mg‡, 20 mg

INDICATIONS & DOSAGES

➤ **Irritable bowel syndrome, other functional GI disorders**
Adults: Initially, 20 mg P.O. q.i.d., increased to 40 mg q.i.d. Or, 20 mg I.M. q.i.d.

ACTION

Inhibits action of acetylcholine on postganglionic, parasympathetic muscarinic receptors, decreasing GI motility. Also, possesses local anesthetic properties that may be partly responsible for spasmolysis.

Route	Onset	Peak	Duration
P.O., I.M.	Unknown	1–1½ hr	Unknown

Half-life: Initial, about 2 hours; secondary, 9 to 10 hours.

ADVERSE REACTIONS

CNS: *headache, dizziness,* fever, insomnia, light-headedness, drowsiness, nervousness, confusion, and excitement in elderly patients.
CV: *palpitations,* tachycardia.
EENT: blurred vision, increased intraocular pressure, mydriasis, photophobia.
GI: *constipation, dry mouth, thirst,* vomiting, nausea, abdominal distention, heartburn, paralytic ileus.
GU: *urinary hesitancy and retention,* impotence.
Skin: urticaria, decreased sweating or inability to sweat, local irritation.
Other: allergic reactions, heat prostration.

INTERACTIONS

Drug-drug. *Amantadine, antihistamines, antiparkinsonians, disopyramide, glutethimide, meperidine, phenothiazines, procainamide, quinidine, tricyclic antidepressants:* May have additive adverse effects. Avoid using together.
Antacids: May interfere with dicyclomine absorption. Give dicyclomine at least 1 hour before antacid.

EFFECTS ON LAB TEST RESULTS

None reported.

CONTRAINDICATIONS & CAUTIONS

- Contraindicated in patients hypersensitive to anticholinergics and in those with obstructive uropathy, obstructive disease of the GI tract, reflux esophagitis, severe ulcerative colitis, toxic megacolon, myasthenia gravis, unstable CV status in acute hemorrhage, tachycardia secondary to cardiac insufficiency or thyrotoxicosis, or glaucoma.
- Contraindicated in breast-feeding patients and in children younger than age 6 months.
- Use cautiously in patients with autonomic neuropathy, hyperthyroidism, coronary artery disease, arrhythmias, heart failure, hypertension, hiatal hernia, hepatic or renal disease, prostatic hyperplasia, known or suspected GI infection, and ulcerative colitis.

• Use cautiously in patients in hot or humid environments; drug can cause heatstroke.

NURSING CONSIDERATIONS

• Give drug 30 to 60 minutes before meals and at bedtime. Bedtime dose can be larger; give at least 2 hours after last meal of day.
• ***Alert:*** Don't give subcutaneously or I.V.
• Adjust dosage based on patient's needs and response. Dosages up to 40 mg P.O. q.i.d. have been used in adults, but safety and effectiveness for longer than 2 weeks haven't been established.
• Dicyclomine is a synthetic tertiary derivative that may have atropinelike adverse reactions.
• ***Alert:*** Overdose may cause curarelike effects such as respiratory paralysis. Keep emergency equipment available.
• Monitor patient's vital signs and urine output carefully.
• ***Alert:*** The dicyclomine labeling may be misleading. The ampule label reads 10 mg/ml but doesn't indicate that the ampule contains 2 ml of solution (20 mg of drug).
• ***Look alike–sound alike:*** Don't confuse dicyclomine with dyclonine or doxycycline; don't confuse Bentyl with Aventyl or Benadryl.

PATIENT TEACHING

• Tell patient when to take drug, and stress importance of doing so on time and at evenly spaced intervals.
• Advise patient to avoid driving and other hazardous activities if drowsiness, dizziness, or blurred vision occurs; to drink plenty of fluids to help prevent constipation; and to report rash or other skin eruption.

glycopyrrolate

Robinul, Robinul Forte

Pharmacologic class: anticholinergic, antimuscarinic
Pregnancy risk category B

AVAILABLE FORMS

Injection: 0.2 mg/ml in 1-, 2-, 5-, and 20-ml vials
Tablets: 1 mg, 2 mg

INDICATIONS & DOSAGES

➤ **To block adverse cholinergic effects caused by anticholinesterases used to reverse neuromuscular blockade**

Adults and children: 0.2 mg I.V. for each 1 mg of neostigmine or 5 mg of pyridostigmine. May be given I.V. without dilution or may be added to dextrose injection and given by infusion.

➤ **Preoperatively to diminish secretions and block cardiac vagal reflexes**

Adults and children age 2 and older: 0.004 mg/kg I.M. 30 to 60 minutes before anesthesia.
Children younger than age 2: 0.009 mg/kg I.M. 30 to 60 minutes before anesthesia.

➤ **Intraoperatively to diminish secretions and block cardiac vagal reflexes**

Adults: 0.1 mg I.V., may repeat q 2 to 3 minutes, p.r.n.
Children: 0.004 mg/kg (not to exceed 0.1 mg), may repeat q 2 to 3 minutes, p.r.n.

➤ **Adjunctive therapy in peptic ulcerations and other GI disorders**

Adults: 1 to 2 mg P.O. t.i.d. or 0.1 to 0.2 mg I.V. or I.M. q 4 hours, t.i.d., or q.i.d. daily. Individualize dosage. Maximum oral dose, 8 mg daily; maximum, four doses parenterally.

I.V. ADMINISTRATION

• Give by direct injection without dilution, or inject into tubing of a free-flowing I.V. solution.
• Concentration of 0.8 mg/L is stable at room temperature for 48 hours in D_5W, 5% dextrose and half-normal saline solution, normal saline solution, and lactated Ringer injection.

INCOMPATIBILITIES

Chloramphenicol sodium succinate, dexamethasone sodium phosphate, diazepam, dimenhydrinate, drugs with alkaline pH, methohexital, methylprednisolone sodium succinate, pentazocine lactate, pentobarbital sodium, secobarbital sodium, sodium bicarbonate, thiopental. Don't mix with solutions that contain sodium bicarbonate or alkaline solutions with a pH of 6 or higher.

ACTION

Inhibits cholinergic (muscarinic) actions of acetylcholine on autonomic effectors innervated by postganglionic cholinergic nerves. Diminishes the volume and free acidity of gastric secretion and controls excessive pharyngeal, tracheal, and bronchial secretions. Blocks cardiac vagal inhibitory reflexes.

Route	Onset	Peak	Duration
P.O.	Unknown	Unknown	8–12 hr
I.V.	1 min	Unknown	2–7 hr
I.M., SubQ	15–30 min	30–45 min	2–7 hr

Half-life: Unknown.

ADVERSE REACTIONS

CNS: fever, weakness, nervousness, insomnia, drowsiness, dizziness, headache, confusion, excitement.
CV: palpitations, tachycardia.
EENT: *dilated pupils, blurred vision,* photophobia, increased intraocular pressure.
GI: *constipation, dry mouth,* nausea, loss of taste, abdominal distention, vomiting, epigastric distress.
GU: urinary hesitancy and retention, impotence.
Skin: urticaria, decreased sweating or anhidrosis.
Other: ***anaphylaxis,*** allergic reactions, suppressed lactation.

INTERACTIONS

Drug-drug. *Amantadine, antihistamines, antiparkinsonians, disopyramide, glutethimide, meperidine, phenothiazines, procainamide, quinidine, tricyclic antidepressants:* May have additive adverse effects. Avoid using together.
Potassium chloride: May slow transit time and increase risk of potassium-induced GI lesions. Avoid wax-based potassium products.

EFFECTS ON LAB TEST RESULTS

None reported.

CONTRAINDICATIONS & CAUTIONS

- Contraindicated in patients hypersensitive to drug, in neonates, and in those with glaucoma, obstructive uropathy, obstructive disease of the GI tract, myasthenia gravis, paralytic ileus, intestinal atony, unstable CV status in acute hemorrhage, tachycardia secondary to cardiac insufficiency or thyrotoxicosis, severe ulcerative colitis, toxic megacolon, or known or suspected GI infection.
- Use cautiously in patients with autonomic neuropathy, hyperthyroidism, coronary artery disease, arrhythmias, heart failure, hypertension, hiatal hernia, hepatic or renal disease, ulcerative colitis, and known or suspected GI infection.
- Use cautiously in patients in hot or humid environments; drug can cause heatstroke.
- Not recommended for peptic ulcer in children younger than age 12.

NURSING CONSIDERATIONS

- Give oral form 30 to 60 minutes before meals.
- Injection contains benzyl alcohol; don't use in neonates younger than age 1 month.
- ***Alert:*** Check all dosages carefully; slight overdose can lead to toxicity.
- ***Alert:*** Overdose may cause curarelike effects, such as respiratory paralysis. Keep emergency equipment available.
- Monitor vital signs carefully. Watch closely for adverse reactions, especially in geriatric or debilitated patients. Call prescriber promptly if reactions occur.
- Elderly patients may be more susceptible to adverse effects and typically receive smaller doses.
- Monitor patient for diarrhea; it may be a sign of incomplete intestinal obstruction.

PATIENT TEACHING

- Tell patient to take oral drug 30 to 60 minutes before meals.
- Tell patient not to crush or chew extended-release products.
- Warn patient to avoid activities that require alertness until drug's CNS effects are known.
- Advise patient to report signs and symptoms of urinary hesitancy or retention.

hyoscyamine
Cystospaz, Hyospaz

L-hyoscyamine sulfate
Anaspaz, Cystospaz, Cystospaz-M, Gastrosed, Hyosol SL, IB-Stat, Levbid, Levsin*, Levsin Drops*, Levsin SL, Levsinex Timecaps, NuLev

Pharmacologic class: belladonna alkaloid, anticholinergic
Pregnancy risk category C

AVAILABLE FORMS
hyoscyamine
Tablets: 0.15 mg
L-hyoscyamine sulfate
Capsules (extended-release): 0.375 mg
Elixir: 0.125 mg/5 ml*
Injection: 0.5 mg/ml
Oral spray: 0.125 mg/ml*
Oral solution:* 0.125 mg/ml*
Tablets: 0.125 mg, 0.15 mg
Tablets (extended-release): 0.375 mg
Tablets (orally disintegrating): 0.125 mg
Tablets (S.L.): 0.125 mg

INDICATIONS & DOSAGES
➤ GI tract disorders caused by spasm; as adjunctive therapy for peptic ulcers, cystitis, renal colic; as drying agent to relieve symptoms of allergic rhinitis, parkinsonism
Adults and children age 12 and older: 0.125 to 0.25 mg P.O. or S.L. t.i.d. or q.i.d. before meals and at bedtime. Or, 0.375 to 0.75 mg extended-release form P.O. q 12 hours. Or, 0.25 to 0.5 mg I.V., I.M., or subcutaneously q 4 hours, b.i.d. to q.i.d. Substitute oral drug when symptoms are controlled. Maximum, 1.5 mg daily.
Children ages 2 to 12: Individualize dosage according to weight. Don't exceed 0.75 mg in 24 hours.
Children younger than age 2: Individualize dosage according to weight. Maximum dose is based on weight.
➤ To diminish secretions and block cardiac vagal reflexes preoperatively
Adults and children older than age 2: Give 0.005 mg/kg I.V., I.M., or subcutaneously 30 to 60 minutes before anesthesia. Intraoperatively, adults may receive 0.125 mg I.V. p.r.n. to reduce drug-induced bradycardia.
➤ Diagnostic procedures
Adults: 0.25 to 0.5 mg I.V., I.M., or subcutaneously 5 to 10 minutes before the procedure.
➤ To block adverse muscarinic effects of anticholinesterase agents
Adults: 0.3 to 0.6 mg I.V. for each 0.5 to 2 mg of neostigmine methylsulfate or physostigmine salicylate, or 10 to 20 mg of pyridostigmine bromide. Give hyoscyamine with or a few minutes before the anticholinesterase in a separate syringe.
➤ Organophosphate pesticide toxicity
Adults: Initially, 1 to 2 mg I.V. Additional 1 mg doses I.V. or I.M. q 3 to 10 minutes as needed; up to 25 mg may be needed in first 24 hours. Maintenance, 0.5 to 1 mg P.O. in intervals of several hours until symptoms are gone.

I.V. ADMINISTRATION
- Use when P.O. and S.L. routes aren't possible or when rapid effect is needed.

INCOMPATIBILITIES
None reported.

ACTION
Blocks acetylcholine action at muscarinic receptors, which decreases GI motility and inhibits gastric acid secretion.

Route	Onset	Peak	Duration
P.O.	20–30 min	½–1 hr	4–12 hr
P.O. (extended)	20–30 min	40–90 min	12 hr
I.V.	2–3 min	15–30 min	4 hr
I.M., SubQ	Unknown	15–30 min	4–12 hr
S.L.	5–20 min	½–1 hr	4 hr

Half-life: Conventional tablets, 2 to 3½ hours; extended-release capsules or tablets, 5 to 6 or 9 hours, respectively; I.M., 12½ hours or longer. Prolonged in patients with renal dysfunction.

ADVERSE REACTIONS
CNS: *confusion or excitement in elderly patients,* fever, headache, insomnia, drowsiness, dizziness, nervousness, weakness.
CV: *palpitations,* tachycardia.

EENT: *blurred vision,* mydriasis, increased intraocular pressure, cycloplegia, photophobia.
GI: *constipation, dry mouth, paralytic ileus,* dysphagia, heartburn, loss of taste, nausea, vomiting.
GU: *urinary hesitancy and retention,* impotence.
Skin: urticaria, decreased or lack of sweating.
Other: hypersensitivity reactions, fever (especially in children).

INTERACTIONS

Drug-drug. *Amantadine, antihistamines, antiparkinsonians, disopyramide, glutethimide, MAO inhibitors, meperidine, phenothiazines, procainamide, quinidine, tricyclic antidepressants:* May have additive adverse effects. Avoid using together.
Antacids: May decrease absorption of oral anticholinergics. Separate doses by 2 or 3 hours.
Ketoconazole: May interfere with ketoconazole absorption. Separate doses by 2 or 3 hours.

EFFECTS ON LAB TEST RESULTS

None reported.

CONTRAINDICATIONS & CAUTIONS

- Contraindicated in patients hypersensitive to anticholinergics and in those with glaucoma, obstructive uropathy, obstructive disease of the GI tract, severe ulcerative colitis, myasthenia gravis, paralytic ileus, intestinal atony, unstable CV status in acute hemorrhage, tachycardia secondary to cardiac insufficiency of thyrotoxicosis, or toxic megacolon.
- Use cautiously in patients with autonomic neuropathy, hyperthyroidism, coronary artery disease, arrhythmias, heart failure, hypertension, hiatal hernia with reflux esophagitis, hepatic or renal disease, known or suspected GI infection, and ulcerative colitis.
- Use cautiously in patients in hot or humid environments; drug can cause heatstroke.
- Use cautiously in children and the elderly because they may be more susceptible to adverse effects.

NURSING CONSIDERATIONS

- Give drug 30 minutes to 1 hour before meals and at bedtime. Bedtime dose can be larger; give at least 2 hours after last meal of day.
- ***Alert:*** Overdose may cause curarelike effects, such as respiratory paralysis. Keep emergency equipment available. Drug is dialyzable.
- Monitor patient's vital signs and urine output carefully.
- Injection contains sodium metabisulfite, which may cause allergic reaction in certain people.
- ***Look alike–sound alike:*** Don't confuse Anaspaz with Anaprox or Antispas.

PATIENT TEACHING

- Urge patient to take drug as prescribed.
- Caution patient not to crush or chew extended-release tablets.
- Advise patient to avoid driving and other hazardous activities if drowsiness, dizziness, or blurred vision occurs; to drink plenty of fluids to help prevent constipation; and to report rash or other skin eruption.
- Advise patient not to take any new drug or OTC preparation unless directed by prescriber.

scopolamine (hyoscine)

Transderm-Scop, Scopace

scopolamine butylbromide (hyoscine butylbromide)

Buscopan†

scopolamine hydrobromide (hyoscine hydrobromide)

Scopolamine Hydrobromide Injection

Pharmacologic class: belladonna alkaloid, antimuscarinic
Pregnancy risk category C

AVAILABLE FORMS

scopolamine
Tablets: 0.4 mg
Transdermal patch: 1.5 mg/2.5 cm^2 (1 mg/72 hours)

scopolamine butylbromide
Suppositories: 10 mg†
Tablets: 10 mg†
scopolamine hydrobromide
Injection: 0.4 mg, and 1 mg/ml

INDICATIONS & DOSAGES

➤Spastic states
Adults: 0.4 to 0.8 mg P.O.

➤Delirium, preanesthetic sedation, and obstetric amnesia with analgesics
Adults: 0.3 to 0.65 mg I.V., I.M., or subcutaneously. Dilute solution with sterile water for injection before giving I.V.
Children: 0.006 mg/kg I.V., I. M., or subcutaneously. Maximum dose, 0.3 mg. Dilute solution with sterile water for injection before giving I.V.

➤To prevent nausea and vomiting from motion sickness
Adults: One Transderm-Scop, formulated to deliver 1 mg scopolamine over 3 days, applied to the skin behind the ear at least 4 hours before antiemetic is needed. Or, 0.3 to 0.65 mg hydrobromide I.V., I.M. or subcutaneously. Or, 0.25 to 0.8 mg P.O. 1 hour before exposure to motion. Further doses of 0.25 to 0.8 mg may be given t.i.d., p.r.n.
Children: 6 mcg/kg or 200 mcg/m^2 hydrobromide I.V., I.M., or subcutaneously.

I.V. ADMINISTRATION

- For direct injection, dilute with sterile water and inject diluted drug at ordered rate through patent I.V. line. Intermittent and continuous infusions aren't recommended.
- Protect I.V. solutions from freezing and light, and store at room temperature.

INCOMPATIBILITIES

Alkalies, anticholinergics, methohexital.

ACTION

Inhibits muscarinic actions of acetylcholine on autonomic effectors innervated by postganglionic cholinergic neurons. May affect neural pathways originating in the inner ear to inhibit nausea and vomiting.

Route	Onset	Peak	Duration
P.O., I.M.	1 hr	1–2 hr	4–6 hr
I.V.	10 min	50–80 min	2 hr
Transdermal	4 hr	Unknown	72 hr
P.R., SubQ	Unknown	Unknown	Unknown

Half-life: 8 hours.

ADVERSE REACTIONS

CNS: disorientation, restlessness, irritability, dizziness, drowsiness, headache, confusion, hallucinations, delirium, impaired memory.
CV: ***paradoxical bradycardia,*** palpitations, tachycardia, flushing.
EENT: dilated pupils, blurred vision, photophobia, increased intraocular pressure, difficulty swallowing.
GI: *constipation, dry mouth, epigastric distress, nausea, vomiting.*
GU: urinary hesitancy, urine retention.
Respiratory: bronchial plugging, depressed respirations.
Skin: rash, dryness, contact dermatitis with transdermal patch.
Other: heat intolerance.

INTERACTIONS

Drug-drug. *Amantadine, antihistamines, antiparkinsonians, disopyramide, glutethimide, meperidine, phenothiazines, procainamide, quinidine, tricyclic antidepressants:* May increase risk of adverse CNS reactions. Avoid using together.
Antacids: May decrease oral absorption of anticholinergics. Separate doses by 2 or 3 hours.
Atenolol: May increase pharmacologic effects of atenolol. Monitor patient for adverse effects.
CNS depressants: May increase risk of CNS depression. Monitor patient closely.
Digoxin: May increase digoxin level. Monitor patient for digoxin toxicity.
Ketoconazole: May interfere with ketoconazole absorption. Separate doses by 2 or 3 hours.
Drug-herb. *Jaborandi tree:* May decrease drug effects. Discourage use together.
Pill-bearing spurge: May decrease drug effects. Inform patient of this interaction.

Squaw vine: May decrease metabolic breakdown. Discourage use together.
Drug-lifestyle. *Alcohol use:* May increase risk of CNS depression. Discourage use together.

EFFECTS ON LAB TEST RESULTS
None reported.

CONTRAINDICATIONS & CAUTIONS
- Contraindicated in patients with angle-closure glaucoma, obstructive uropathy, obstructive disease of the GI tract, asthma, chronic pulmonary disease, myasthenia gravis, paralytic ileus, intestinal atony, unstable CV status in acute hemorrhage, tachycardia from cardiac insufficiency, or toxic megacolon.
- Contraindicated in patients hypersensitive to belladonna or barbiturates.
- Use cautiously in patients with autonomic neuropathy, hyperthyroidism, coronary artery disease, arrhythmias, heart failure, hypertension, hiatal hernia with reflux esophagitis, hepatic or renal disease, known or suspected GI infection, or ulcerative colitis.
- Use cautiously in children.
- Use cautiously in patients in hot or humid environments; drug can cause heatstroke.

NURSING CONSIDERATIONS
- Raise side rails as a precaution because some patients become temporarily excited or disoriented and some develop amnesia or become drowsy. Reorient patient, as needed.
- Tolerance may develop when therapy is prolonged.
- Atropinelike toxicity may cause dose-related adverse reactions. Individual tolerance varies greatly.
- ***Alert:*** Overdose may cause curarelike effects such as respiratory paralysis. Keep emergency equipment available.

PATIENT TEACHING
- Advise patient to apply patch the night before a planned trip. Transdermal method releases a controlled therapeutic amount of drug. Transderm-Scop is effective if applied 2 or 3 hours before experiencing motion but is more effective if applied 12 hours before.
- Instruct patient to remove one patch before applying another.
- Instruct patient to wash and dry hands thoroughly before and after applying the transdermal patch (on dry skin behind the ear) and before touching the eye because pupil may dilate. Tell patient to discard patch after removing it and to wash application site thoroughly.
- Tell patient that if patch becomes displaced, he should remove it and apply another patch on a fresh skin site behind the ear.
- Alert patient to possible withdrawal signs or symptoms (nausea, vomiting, headache, dizziness) when transdermal system is used for longer than 72 hours.
- Advise patient that eyes may be more sensitive to light while wearing patch. Advise patient to wear sunglasses for comfort.
- Warn patient to avoid activities that require alertness until CNS effects of drug are known.
- Instruct patient to ask pharmacist for brochure that comes with the transdermal product.
- Urge patient to report urinary hesitancy or urine retention.

37

Adrenergics (sympathomimetics)

dobutamine hydrochloride
dopamine hydrochloride
norepinephrine bitartrate
phenylephrine hydrochloride

SAFETY ALERT!

dobutamine hydrochloride

Dobutrex

Pharmacologic class: adrenergic, $beta_1$ agonist
Pregnancy risk category B

AVAILABLE FORMS

Injection: 12.5 mg/ml in 20-ml vials (parenteral)
Dobutamine in 5% dextrose: 0.5 mg/ml (125 or 250 mg); 1 mg/ml (250 or 500 mg); 2 mg/ml (500 mg); 4 mg/ml (1,000 mg)

INDICATIONS & DOSAGES

➤ **Increased cardiac output in short-term treatment of cardiac decompensation caused by depressed contractility, such as during refractory heart failure; adjunctive therapy in cardiac surgery**
Adults: 0.5 to 1 mcg/kg/minute I.V. infusion, titrating to optimum dosage of 2 to 20 mcg/kg/minute. Usual effective range to increase cardiac output is 2.5 to 10 mcg/kg/minute. Rarely, rates up to 40 mcg/kg/minute may be needed.

I.V. ADMINISTRATION

- Dilute concentrate before injecting. Compatible solutions include D_5W, $D_{10}W$, half-normal or normal saline solution for injection, lactated Ringer injection, Isolyte-M with D_5W, Normosol-M in D_5W, and 20% Osmitrol.
- Diluting one vial (250 mg) with 1,000 ml of solution yields 250 mcg/ml. Diluting with 500 ml yields 500 mcg/ml. Diluting with 250 ml yields 1,000 mcg/ml.
- Oxidation may slightly discolor admixture. This doesn't indicate a significant loss of potency, provided drug is used within 24 hours of reconstitution.
- Give through a central venous catheter or large peripheral vein using an infusion pump.
- Titrate rate according to patient's condition. Don't exceed 5 mg/ml.
- Infusions lasting up to 72 hours produce no more adverse effects than shorter infusions.
- Watch for irritation and infiltration; extravasation can cause tissue damage and necrosis. Change I.V. sites regularly to avoid phlebitis.
- Solutions remain stable for 24 hours. Don't freeze.

INCOMPATIBILITIES

Acyclovir, alkaline solutions, alteplase, aminophylline, bretylium, bumetanide, calcium chloride, calcium gluconate, cefamandole, cefazolin, cefepime, diazepam, digoxin, ethacrynate, furosemide, heparin, hydrocortisone sodium succinate, indomethacin, insulin, magnesium sulfate, midazolam, penicillin, phenytoin, phytonadione, piperacillin with tazobactam, potassium chloride, sodium bicarbonate, thiopental, verapamil, warfarin. Don't give through same line with any other drugs.

ACTION

Stimulates heart's $beta_1$ receptors to increase myocardial contractility and stroke volume. At therapeutic dosages, drug increases cardiac output by decreasing peripheral vascular resistance, reducing ventricular filling pressure, and facilitating AV node conduction.

Route	Onset	Peak	Duration
I.V.	1–2 min	10 min	< 5 min after infusion

Half-life: 2 minutes.

ADVERSE REACTIONS

CNS: headache.
CV: *hypertension, increased heart rate,* angina, PVCs, phlebitis, nonspecific chest

pain, palpitations, ventricular ectopy, hypotension.
GI: nausea, vomiting.
Respiratory: ***asthma attack,*** shortness of breath.
Other: ***anaphylaxis,*** hypersensitivity reactions.

INTERACTIONS

Drug-drug. *Beta blockers:* May antagonize dobutamine effects. Avoid using together.
Bretylium: May increase risk of arrhythmias. Monitor ECG.
General anesthetics: May have greater risk of ventricular arrhythmias. Monitor ECG closely.
Guanethidine, oxytocic drugs: May increase pressor response, causing severe hypertension. Monitor blood pressure closely.
Tricyclic antidepressants: May potentiate pressor response and cause arrhythmias. Use together cautiously.
Drug-herb. *Rue:* May increase inotropic potential. Discourage use together.

EFFECTS ON LAB TEST RESULTS

- May decrease potassium level.

CONTRAINDICATIONS & CAUTIONS

- Contraindicated in patients hypersensitive to drug or its components and in those with idiopathic hypertrophic subaortic stenosis.
- Use cautiously in patients with history of hypertension because drug may increase pressor response.
- Use cautiously after acute MI.
- Use cautiously in patients with history of sulfite sensitivity.

NURSING CONSIDERATIONS

- Before starting therapy, give a plasma volume expander to correct hypovolemia and a cardiac glycoside.
- Because drug increases AV node conduction, patients with atrial fibrillation may develop a rapid ventricular rate.
- Continuously monitor ECG, blood pressure, pulmonary artery wedge pressure, cardiac output, and urine output.
- Monitor electrolyte levels. Drug may lower potassium level.
- ***Look alike–sound alike:*** Don't confuse dobutamine with dopamine.

PATIENT TEACHING

- Tell patient to report adverse reactions promptly, especially labored breathing and drug-induced headache.
- Instruct patient to report discomfort at I.V. insertion site.

SAFETY ALERT!

dopamine hydrochloride

Intropin

Pharmacologic class: adrenergic
Pregnancy risk category C

AVAILABLE FORMS

Injection: 40 mg/ml, 80 mg/ml, 160 mg/ml parenteral concentrate for injection for I.V. infusion; 0.8 mg/ml (200 or 400 mg) in D_5W; 1.6 mg/ml (400 or 800 mg) in D_5W; 3.2 mg/ml (800 mg) in D_5W parenteral injection for I.V. infusion

INDICATIONS & DOSAGES

➤ **To treat shock and correct hemodynamic imbalances; to improve perfusion to vital organs; to increase cardiac output; to correct hypotension**

Adults: Initially, 2 to 5 mcg/kg/minute by I.V. infusion. Titrate dosage to desired hemodynamic or renal response. Increase by 1 to 4 mcg/kg/minute at 10- to 30-minute intervals. In seriously ill patients, start with 5 mcg/kg/minute and increase gradually in increments of 5 to 10 mcg/kg/minute to a rate of 20 to 50 mcg/kg/minute, p.r.n.
Adjust-a-dose: In patients with occlusive vascular disease, initial dose is 1 mcg/kg/minute or less.

I.V. ADMINISTRATION

- Dilute with D_5W, normal saline solution, D_5W in normal saline or 0.45% saline, lactated Ringer, or D_5W in lactated Ringer. Mix just before use.
- Use a central line or large vein, as in the antecubital fossa, to minimize risk of extravasation.
- Use a continuous infusion pump to regulate flow rate.

• Watch infusion site carefully for extravasation; if it occurs, stop infusion immediately and call prescriber. You may need to infiltrate area with 5 to 10 mg phentolamine in 10 to 15 ml normal saline solution.
• Because solution will deteriorate rapidly, discard after 24 hours or earlier if it's discolored.

INCOMPATIBILITIES
Acyclovir sodium, additives with a dopamine and dextrose solution, alteplase, amphotericin B, cefepime, furosemide, gentamicin, indomethacin sodium trihydrate, iron salts, insulin, oxidizing agents, penicillin G potassium, sodium bicarbonate or other alkaline solutions, thiopental. Don't mix other drugs in I.V. container with dopamine.

ACTION
Stimulates dopaminergic and alpha and beta receptors of the sympathetic nervous system resulting in a positive inotropic effect and increased cardiac output. Action is dose-related; large doses cause mainly alpha stimulation.

Route	Onset	Peak	Duration
I.V.	5 min	Unknown	< 10 min after infusion

Half-life: 9 minutes.

ADVERSE REACTIONS
CNS: headache, anxiety.
CV: *hypotension,* ***ventricular arrhythmias (high doses),*** ectopic beats, tachycardia, angina, palpitations, vasoconstriction.
GI: nausea, vomiting.
Metabolic: azotemia, hyperglycemia.
Respiratory: ***asthmatic episodes,*** dyspnea.
Skin: necrosis and tissue sloughing with extravasation, piloerection.
Other: ***anaphylactic reactions.***

INTERACTIONS
Drug-drug. *Alpha and beta blockers:* May antagonize dopamine effects. Monitor patient closely.
Ergot alkaloids: May cause extremely high blood pressure. Avoid using together.
Inhaled anesthetics: May increase risk of arrhythmias or hypertension. Monitor patient closely.
MAO inhibitors (phenelzine, tranylcypromine): May cause fever, hypertensive crisis, and severe headache. Avoid using together; if patient received an MAO inhibitor in the past 2 to 3 weeks, initial dopamine dose is less than or equal to 10% of the usual dose.
Oxytocics: May cause severe, persistent hypertension. Use together cautiously.
Phenytoin: May cause severe hypotension, bradycardia, and cardiac arrest. Monitor patient carefully.
Tricyclic antidepressants: May decrease pressor response. Monitor patient closely.

EFFECTS ON LAB TEST RESULTS
• May increase catecholamine, glucose, and urine urea levels.

CONTRAINDICATIONS & CAUTIONS
• Contraindicated in patients with uncorrected tachyarrhythmias, pheochromocytoma, or ventricular fibrillation.
• Use cautiously in patients with occlusive vascular disease, cold injuries, diabetic endarteritis, and arterial embolism; in pregnant or breast-feeding women; in those with a history of sulfite sensitivity; and in those taking MAO inhibitors.

NURSING CONSIDERATIONS
• Most patients receive less than 20 mcg/kg/minute. Doses of 0.5 to 2 mcg/kg/minute mainly stimulate dopamine receptors and dilate the renal vasculature. Doses of 2 to 10 mcg/kg/minute stimulate beta receptors for a positive inotropic effect. Higher doses also stimulate alpha receptors, constricting blood vessels and increasing blood pressure.
• Drug isn't a substitute for blood or fluid volume deficit. If deficit exists, replace fluid before giving vasopressors.
• During infusion, frequently monitor ECG, blood pressure, cardiac output, central venous pressure, pulmonary artery wedge pressure, pulse rate, urine output, and color and temperature of limbs.
• If diastolic pressure rises disproportionately with a significant decrease in pulse pressure, decrease infusion rate, and watch carefully for further evidence of

predominant vasoconstrictor activity, unless such an effect is desired.
- Observe patient closely for adverse reactions; dosage may need to be adjusted or drug stopped.
- Check urine output often. If urine flow decreases without hypotension, notify prescriber because dosage may need to be reduced.
- ***Alert:*** After drug is stopped, watch closely for sudden drop in blood pressure. Taper dosage slowly to evaluate stability of blood pressure.
- Acidosis decreases effectiveness of drug.
- ***Look alike–sound alike:*** Don't confuse dopamine with dobutamine.

PATIENT TEACHING
- Tell patient to report adverse reactions promptly.
- Instruct patient to report discomfort at I.V. insertion site.

SAFETY ALERT!

norepinephrine bitartrate (levarterenol bitartrate, noradrenaline acid tartrate)
Levophed

Pharmacologic class: direct-acting adrenergic
Pregnancy risk category C

AVAILABLE FORMS
Injection: 1 mg/ml

INDICATIONS & DOSAGES
➤ To restore blood pressure in acute hypotension
Adults: Initially, 8 to 12 mcg/minute by I.V. infusion; then titrate to maintain systolic blood pressure at 80 to 100 mm Hg in previously normotensive patients and 30 to 40 mm Hg below preexisting systolic blood pressure in previously hypertensive patients. Average maintenance dose is 2 to 4 mcg/minute.
Children: 2 mcg/minute or 2 mcg/m^2/minute by I.V. infusion; adjust dosage based on patient response.

➤ Severe hypotension during cardiac arrest
Children: Initially, 0.1 mcg/kg/minute I.V. infusion. Titrate infusion rate based on patient response, up to 2 mcg/kg/minute.

I.V. ADMINISTRATION
- Use a central venous catheter or large vein, as in the antecubital fossa, to minimize risk of extravasation. Give in D_5W alone or D_5W in normal saline solution for injection. Use continuous infusion pump to regulate infusion flow rate and a piggyback setup so I.V. line stays open if norepinephrine is stopped.
- Never leave patient unattended during infusion. Check blood pressure every 2 minutes until stabilized; then check every 5 minutes.
- During infusion, frequently monitor ECG, cardiac output, central venous pressure, pulmonary artery wedge pressure, pulse rate, urine output, and color and temperature of limbs. Titrate infusion rate based on findings and prescriber guidelines.
- Check site frequently for extravasation. If they appear, stop infusion immediately and call prescriber. Infiltrate area with 5 to 10 mg phentolamine in 10 to 15 ml of normal saline solution to counteract effect of extravasation. Also, check for blanching along course of infused vein, which may progress to superficial sloughing.
- Protect drug from light. Discard discolored solution or solution that contains precipitate. Solution will deteriorate after 24 hours.
- If prolonged therapy is needed, change injection site frequently.

INCOMPATIBILITIES
Alkaline-buffered antibiotics, aminophylline, amobarbital, chlorothiazide, chlorpheniramine, insulin, lidocaine, pentobarbital sodium, phenobarbital sodium, phenytoin sodium, ranitidine hydrochloride, sodium bicarbonate, streptomycin, thiopental, whole blood. Avoid mixing with alkaline solutions, oxidizing drugs, or iron salts. The use of normal saline solution alone isn't recommended because of the lack of oxidation protection.

ACTION
Stimulates alpha and beta$_1$ receptors in the sympathetic nervous system, causing vasoconstriction and cardiac stimulation.

Route	Onset	Peak	Duration
I.V.	Immediate	Immediate	1–2 min after infusion

Half-life: About 1 minute.

ADVERSE REACTIONS
CNS: *headache,* anxiety, weakness, dizziness, tremor, restlessness, insomnia.
CV: ***bradycardia, severe hypertension, arrhythmias.***
Respiratory: ***asthma attacks,*** respiratory difficulties.
Skin: irritation with extravasation, necrosis and gangrene secondary to extravasation.
Other: ***anaphylaxis.***

INTERACTIONS
Drug-drug. *Alpha blockers:* May antagonize drug effects. Avoid using together.
Antihistamines, atropine, ergot alkaloids, guanethidine, MAO inhibitors, methyldopa, oxytocics: When given with sympathomimetics, may cause severe hypertension (hypertensive crisis). Avoid using together.
Inhaled anesthetics: May increase risk of arrhythmias. Monitor ECG.
Tricyclic antidepressants: May potentiate the pressor response and cause arrhythmias. Use together cautiously.

EFFECTS ON LAB TEST RESULTS
None reported.

CONTRAINDICATIONS & CAUTIONS
- Contraindicated in patients with mesenteric or peripheral vascular thrombosis, profound hypoxia, hypercarbia, or hypotension resulting from blood volume deficit.
- Contraindicated during cyclopropane and halothane anesthesia.
- Use cautiously in patients taking MAO inhibitors or tricyclic or imipramine-type antidepressants.
- Use cautiously in patients with sulfite sensitivity.

NURSING CONSIDERATIONS
- Drug isn't a substitute for blood or fluid replacement therapy. If patient has volume deficit, replace fluids before giving vasopressors.
- Keep emergency drugs on hand to reverse effects of drug: atropine for reflex bradycardia, phentolamine to decrease vasopressor effects, and propranolol for arrhythmias.
- Notify prescriber immediately of decreased urine output.
- When stopping drug, gradually slow infusion rate. Continue monitoring vital signs, watching for possible severe drop in blood pressure.
- ***Look alike–sound alike:*** Don't confuse norepinephrine with epinephrine.

PATIENT TEACHING
- Tell patient to report adverse reactions promptly.
- Advise patient to report discomfort at I.V. insertion site.

SAFETY ALERT!

phenylephrine hydrochloride
Neo-Synephrine

Pharmacologic class: adrenergic
Pregnancy risk category C

AVAILABLE FORMS
Injection: 10 mg/ml (1%)

INDICATIONS & DOSAGES
➤ Hypotensive emergencies during spinal anesthesia
Adults: Initially, 0.2 mg I.V.; don't let subsequent doses exceed the preceding dose by more than 0.2 mg. Maximum single dose is 0.5 mg.
➤ To maintain blood pressure during spinal or inhaled anesthesia
Adults: 2 to 3 mg I.M. or subcutaneously 3 to 4 minutes before anesthesia.
Children: 0.044 mg to 0.088 mg/kg I.M. or subcutaneously.
➤ To prolong spinal anesthesia
Adults: 2 to 5 mg added to anesthetic solution.

➤ **Prevention of hypotension during spinal anesthesia**
Adults: Give 2 to 3 mg I.M. or subcutaneously 3 to 4 minutes before injection of spinal anesthesia.
➤ **Hypotensive emergencies during spinal anesthesia**
Adults: 0.2 mg I.V.; subsequent doses should be no more than 0.1 to 0.2 mg over the previous dose; don't exceed 0.5 mg in a single dose.
Children: 0.044 to 0.088 mg/kg I.M. or subcutaneously.
➤ **Vasoconstrictor for regional anesthesia**
Adults: 1 mg phenylephrine added to each 20 ml local anesthetic.
➤ **Mild to moderate hypotension**
Adults: 2 to 5 mg I.M. (dose ranges from 1 to 10 mg) or subcutaneously; repeat in 1 or 2 hours as needed and tolerated. First dose shouldn't exceed 5 mg. Or, 0.1 to 0.5 mg slow I.V., not to be repeated more often than 10 to 15 minutes.
Children: 0.1 mg/kg or 3 mg/m^2 I.M. or subcutaneously; repeat in 1 or 2 hours as needed and tolerated.
➤ **Severe hypotension and shock (including drug-induced)**
Adults: 10 mg in 250 to 500 ml of D_5W or normal saline solution for injection. I.V. infusion started at 100 to 180 mcg/minute; then decrease to maintenance infusion of 40 to 60 mcg/minute when blood pressure stabilizes.
➤ **Paroxysmal supraventricular tachycardia**
Adults: Initially, 0.5 mg rapid I.V.; increase in increments of 0.1 to 0.2 mg. Use cautiously. Maximum single dose is 1 mg.

I.V. ADMINISTRATION

- For direct injection, dilute 10 mg (1 ml) with 9 ml sterile water for injection to provide 1 mg/ml. Infusions are usually prepared by adding 10 mg of drug to 500 ml of D_5W or normal saline solution for injection. The first I.V. infusion rate is usually 100 to 180 mcg/minute; maintenance rate is usually 40 to 60 mcg/minute.
- Use a central venous catheter or large vein, as in the antecubital fossa, to minimize risk of extravasation. Use a continuous infusion pump to regulate infusion flow rate.
- During infusion, frequently monitor ECG, blood pressure, cardiac output, central venous pressure, pulmonary artery wedge pressure, pulse rate, urine output, and color and temperature of limbs. Titrate infusion rate according to findings and prescriber guidelines. Maintain blood pressure slightly below patient's normal level. In previously normotensive patients, maintain systolic blood pressure at 80 to 100 mm Hg; in previously hypertensive patients, maintain systolic blood pressure at 30 to 40 mm Hg below usual level.
- Avoid abrupt withdrawal after prolonged I.V. infusions.
- To treat extravasation, infiltrate site promptly with 10 to 15 ml of normal saline solution for injection containing 5 to 10 mg phentolamine. Use a fine needle.

INCOMPATIBILITIES

Alkaline solutions, iron salts, other metals, phenytoin sodium, thiopental sodium.

ACTION

Stimulates alpha receptors in the sympathetic nervous system, causing vasoconstriction.

Route	Onset	Peak	Duration
I.V.	Immediate	Unknown	15–20 min
I.M.	10–15 min	Unknown	30–120 min
SubQ	10–15 min	Unknown	50–60 min

Half-life: Unknown.

ADVERSE REACTIONS

CNS: *headache,* excitability, restlessness, anxiety, nervousness, dizziness, weakness.
CV: ***bradycardia, arrhythmias,*** hypertension.
Respiratory: ***asthmatic episodes.***
Skin: tissue sloughing with extravasation.
Other: ***anaphylaxis,*** tachyphylaxis and decreased organ perfusion with continued use.

INTERACTIONS

Drug-drug. *Alpha blockers, phenothiazines:* May decrease pressor response. Monitor patient closely.
Atropine, guanethidine, oxytocics: May increase pressor response. Monitor patient.

Beta blockers: May block cardiostimulation. Monitor patient closely.
Halogenated hydrocarbon anesthetics, sympathomimetics: May cause serious arrhythmias. Use together with caution.
MAO inhibitors (phenelzine, tranylcypromine): May cause severe headache, hypertension, fever, and hypertensive crisis. Avoid using together.
Tricyclic antidepressants: May potentiate pressor response and cause arrhythmias. Use together cautiously.

EFFECTS ON LAB TEST RESULTS
None reported.

CONTRAINDICATIONS & CAUTIONS

- Contraindicated in patients hypersensitive to drug and in those with severe hypertension or ventricular tachycardia.
- Use with caution in elderly patients and in patients with heart disease, hyperthyroidism, severe atherosclerosis, bradycardia, partial heart block, myocardial disease, or sulfite sensitivity.

NURSING CONSIDERATIONS

- Drug causes little or no CNS stimulation.
- Drug may lower intraocular pressure in normal eyes or in open-angle glaucoma. It also may cause false-normal tonometry readings.
- Drug is used in eyedrops and OTC cold preparations for decongestant effects.

PATIENT TEACHING

- Tell patient to report adverse reactions promptly.
- Instruct patient to report discomfort at I.V. insertion site.

38
Skeletal muscle relaxants

baclofen
carisoprodol
cyclobenzaprine hydrochloride
dantrolene sodium
tizanidine hydrochloride

baclofen
Clofen‡, Kemstro, Lioresal, Lioresal Intrathecal

Pharmacologic class: chlorophenyl derivative
Pregnancy risk category C

AVAILABLE FORMS
Intrathecal injection: 50 mcg/ml, 500 mcg/ml, 2,000 mcg/ml
Tablets: 10 mg, 20 mg, 25 mg‡
Tablets (orally disintegrating): 10 mg, 20 mg

INDICATIONS & DOSAGES
➤ Spasticity in multiple sclerosis; spinal cord injury
Adults: Initially, 5 mg P.O. t.i.d. for 3 days; then 10 mg t.i.d. for 3 days, 15 mg t.i.d. for 3 days, 20 mg t.i.d. for 3 days. Increase daily dosage, based on response, to maximum of 80 mg.
Adjust-a-dose: For patients with psychiatric or brain disorders and for elderly patients, increase dose gradually.
➤ To manage severe spasticity in patients who don't respond to or can't tolerate oral baclofen therapy
Adults: For screening phase, after test dose to check responsiveness, give drug via implantable infusion pump. Give test dose of 1 ml of 50-mcg/ml dilution into intrathecal space by barbotage over 1 minute or longer. Significantly decreased severity or frequency of muscle spasm or reduced muscle tone should appear within 4 to 8 hours. If response is inadequate, give second test dose of 75 mcg/1.5 ml 24 hours after the first. If response is still inadequate, give final test dose of 100 mcg/2 ml after 24 hours. Patients unresponsive to the 100-mcg dose shouldn't be considered candidates for implantable pump.
Children: Initial test dose is the same as that of adults (50 mcg); very small children, initial dose is 25 mcg.
For maintenance therapy: Adjust first dose based on screening dose that elicited an adequate response. Double this effective dose and give over 24 hours. However, if screening dose effectiveness was maintained for 12 hours or longer, don't double the dose. After the first 24 hours, increase dose slowly as needed and tolerated by 10% to 30% increments at 24–hour intervals in spasticity of spinal cord origin. In children with spasticity of spinal cord origin and adults and children with spasticity of cerebral origin, increase by 5% to 15% increments at 24–hour intervals. During prolonged maintenance therapy, increase daily dose by 10% to 40% in spasticity of spinal cord origin, or increase daily dose by 5% to 15 % in spasticity of cerebral origin, if needed; if patient experiences adverse effects, decrease dose by 10% to 20%. Maintenance dosages range from 12 mcg to 2,000 mcg daily, but experience with dosages of more than 1,000 mcg daily is limited. Most patients need 300 to 800 mcg daily.
Adjust-a-dose: For patients with impaired renal function, decrease oral and intrathecal doses.

ACTION
Hyperpolarizes fibers to reduce impulse transmission. Appears to reduce transmission of impulses from the spinal cord to skeletal muscle, thus decreasing the frequency and amplitude of muscle spasms in patients with spinal cord lesions.

Route	Onset	Peak	Duration
P.O.	Unknown	2–3 hr	Unknown
P.O. (orally disintegrating)	Unknown	1½ hr	Unknown
Intrathecal	30 min–1 hr	4 hr	4–8 hr

Half-life: 2½ to 4 hours.

ADVERSE REACTIONS

CNS: *drowsiness,* ***high fever,*** *dizziness,* headache, *weakness, fatigue,* ***paresthesias,*** hypotonia, *confusion,* hallucinations, insomnia, dysarthria, ***seizures with intrathecal use.***
CV: hypotension, hypertension.
EENT: blurred vision, nasal congestion, slurred speech.
GI: *nausea,* constipation, *vomiting.*
GU: urinary frequency.
Metabolic: hyperglycemia, weight gain.
Musculoskeletal: muscle rigidity or spasticity, ***rhabdomyolysis,*** muscle weakness.
Respiratory: dyspnea.
Skin: rash, pruritus, excessive sweating.
Other: ***multiple organ-system failure.***

INTERACTIONS

Drug-drug. *CNS depressants:* May increase CNS depression. Avoid using together.
Drug-lifestyle. *Alcohol use:* May increase CNS depression. Discourage use together.

EFFECTS ON LAB TEST RESULTS

- May increase alkaline phosphatase, AST, CK, and glucose levels.

CONTRAINDICATIONS & CAUTIONS

- Contraindicated in patients hypersensitive to drug.
- Orally disintegrating tablets contraindicated in patients hypersensitive to aspartame or other components of the drug.
- Use cautiously in patients with impaired renal function or seizure disorder or when spasticity is used to maintain motor function.

NURSING CONSIDERATIONS

- Give oral form with meals or with milk to prevent GI distress.
- ***Alert:*** Don't use oral drug to treat muscle spasm caused by rheumatic disorders, cerebral palsy, Parkinson disease, or stroke because drug's effectiveness for these indications hasn't been established. Don't give intrathecal injection by I.V., I.M., subcutaneous, or epidural route.
- Watch for sensitivity reactions, such as fever, skin eruptions, and respiratory distress.
- Expect an increased risk of seizures in patients with seizure disorder.
- The amount of relief determines whether dosage (and drowsiness) can be reduced.
- Don't withdraw drug abruptly after long-term use unless severe adverse reactions demand it; doing so may precipitate seizures, hallucinations, or rebound spasticity.
- If patient suddenly requires a large intrathecal dose increase, check for a catheter complication, such as kinking or dislodgement.
- With long-term intrathecal use, about 5% of patients may develop tolerance to drug. In some cases, this may be treated by hospitalizing patient and slowly withdrawing drug over a 2-week period.
- ***Look alike–sound alike:*** Don't confuse baclofen with Bactroban.

PATIENT TEACHING

- Instruct patient to take oral form with meals or milk.
- Tell patients with phenylketonuria that orally disintegrating tablets contain phenylalanine (3.9 mg/10 mg tablet and 7.9 mg/20 mg tablet).
- Instruct patient to remove orally disintegrating tablet from blister pack and immediately place on the tongue to dissolve; then swallow with or without water.
- Tell patient to avoid activities that require alertness until CNS effects of drug are known. Drowsiness usually is transient.
- Tell patient to avoid alcohol and OTC antihistamines while taking drug.
- Advise patient to follow prescriber's orders regarding rest and physical therapy.

---

carisoprodol

Soma✐, Vanadom

Pharmacologic class: carbamate derivative
Pregnancy risk category NR

AVAILABLE FORMS

Tablets: 350 mg

INDICATIONS & DOSAGES

➤ **Adjunctive treatment for acute, painful musculoskeletal conditions**
Adults: 350 mg P.O. t.i.d. and at bedtime.

ACTION
May modify central perception of pain without modifying pain reflexes. Muscle relaxant effects may be related to sedative properties.

Route	Onset	Peak	Duration
P.O.	½ hr	4 hr	4–6 hr

Half-life: 8 hours.

ADVERSE REACTIONS
CNS: *drowsiness, dizziness,* vertigo, ataxia, tremor, agitation, irritability, headache, depressive reactions, fever, insomnia, syncope.
CV: *orthostatic hypotension,* tachycardia, facial flushing.
GI: nausea, vomiting, epigastric distress, hiccups.
Respiratory: ***asthmatic episodes,*** hiccups.
Skin: ***erythema multiforme,*** pruritus, rash.
Other: ***angioedema, anaphylaxis.***

INTERACTIONS
Drug-drug. *CNS depressants:* May increase CNS depression. Avoid using together.
Drug-lifestyle. *Alcohol use:* May increase CNS depression. Discourage use together.

EFFECTS ON LAB TEST RESULTS
- May increase eosinophil count.

CONTRAINDICATIONS & CAUTIONS
- Contraindicated in patients hypersensitive to related compounds (such as meprobamate or tybamate) and in those with intermittent porphyria.
- Use cautiously in patients with impaired hepatic or renal function.
- Safety and effectiveness in children younger than age 12 haven't been established.

NURSING CONSIDERATIONS
- ***Alert:*** Watch for idiosyncratic reactions after first to fourth doses (weakness, ataxia, visual and speech difficulties, fever, skin eruptions, and mental changes) and for severe reactions, including bronchospasm, hypotension, and anaphylactic shock. After unusual reactions, withhold dose and notify prescriber immediately.
- Record amount of relief to help prescriber determine whether dosage can be reduced.
- Don't stop drug abruptly, which may cause mild withdrawal effects, such as insomnia, headache, nausea, or abdominal cramps.
- Drug may be habit forming.

PATIENT TEACHING
- Warn patient to avoid activities that require alertness until CNS effects of drug are known. Drowsiness is transient.
- Advise patient to avoid combining drug with alcohol or other CNS depressants.
- Tell patient to ask prescriber before using OTC cold or hay fever remedies.
- Instruct patient to follow prescriber's orders regarding rest and physical therapy.
- Advise patient to avoid sudden changes in posture if dizziness occurs.
- Tell patient to take drug with food or milk if GI upset occurs.

cyclobenzaprine hydrochloride
Flexeril

Pharmacologic class: tricyclic-antidepressant derivative
Pregnancy risk category B

AVAILABLE FORMS
Tablets: 5 mg, 10 mg

INDICATIONS & DOSAGES
➤ **Adjunct to rest and physical therapy to relieve muscle spasm from acute, painful musculoskeletal conditions**
Adults: 5 mg P.O. t.i.d. Based on response, dose may be increased to 10 mg t.i.d. Don't exceed 60 mg/day. Use for longer than 2 or 3 weeks isn't recommended.
Adjust-a-dose: In elderly patients and in those with mild hepatic impairment, start with 5 mg and adjust slowly upward. Drug isn't recommended in patients with moderate to severe hepatic impairment.

ACTION
Unknown. Relieves skeletal muscle spasm of local origin without disrupting muscle function.

Route	Onset	Peak	Duration
P.O.	1 hr	4 hr	12–24 hr

Half-life: 1 to 3 days.

ADVERSE REACTIONS

CNS: *dizziness, drowsiness,* ***seizures,*** headache, insomnia, fatigue, asthenia, nervousness, confusion, paresthesia, depression, dysarthria, ataxia, syncope.
CV: ***arrhythmias,*** palpitations, hypotension, tachycardia, vasodilation.
EENT: visual disturbances, blurred vision.
GI: *dry mouth,* dyspepsia, abnormal taste, constipation, nausea.
GU: urine retention, urinary frequency.
Skin: rash, urticaria, pruritus, sweating.

INTERACTIONS

Drug-drug. *CNS depressants:* May increase CNS depression. Avoid using together.
Guanethidine: May block guanethidine's antihypertensive effect. Monitor patient's blood pressure.
MAO inhibitors: May cause hyperpyretic crisis, seizures, and death when MAO inhibitors are used with tricyclic antidepressants; may also occur with cyclobenzaprine. Avoid using within 2 weeks of MAO inhibitor therapy.
Naproxen: May increase drowsiness. Make patient aware of this interaction.
Tramadol: May increase risk for seizures. Use together cautiously.
Drug-lifestyle. *Alcohol use:* May increase CNS depression. Discourage use together.

EFFECTS ON LAB TEST RESULTS

None reported.

CONTRAINDICATIONS & CAUTIONS

- Contraindicated in patients hypersensitive to drug; in those with hyperthyroidism, heart block, arrhythmias, conduction disturbances, or heart failure; in those who have received MAO inhibitors within 14 days; and in those in the acute recovery phase of an MI.
- Use cautiously in elderly or debilitated patients and in those with a history of urine retention, acute angle-closure glaucoma, or increased intraocular pressure.
- Safety and effectiveness in children younger than age 15 haven't been established.

NURSING CONSIDERATIONS

- Cyclobenzaprine may cause toxic reactions similar to those of tricyclic antidepressants. Observe same precautions as when giving tricyclic antidepressants.
- Monitor patient for nausea, headache, and malaise, which may occur if drug is stopped abruptly after long-term use.
- ***Alert:*** Notify prescriber immediately of signs and symptoms of overdose, including cardiac toxicity.
- ***Look alike–sound alike:*** Don't confuse Flexeril with Floxin.

PATIENT TEACHING

- Advise patient to report urinary hesitancy or urine retention. If constipation is a problem, suggest that patient increase fluid intake and use a stool softener.
- Warn patient to avoid activities that require alertness until CNS effects of drug are known.
- Warn patient not to combine with alcohol or other CNS depressants, including OTC cold or allergy remedies.
- Instruct patient not to split the generic 10-mg tablets because of the high risk of inconsistent doses.

dantrolene sodium

Dantrium, Dantrium Intravenous

Pharmacologic class: hydantoin derivative
Pregnancy risk category C

AVAILABLE FORMS

Capsules: 25 mg, 50 mg, 100 mg
Injection: 20 mg/vial

INDICATIONS & DOSAGES

➤ **Spasticity and sequelae from severe chronic disorders, such as multiple sclerosis, cerebral palsy, spinal cord injury, stroke**
Adults: 25 mg P.O. daily. Increase by 25-mg increments, up to 100 mg t.i.d. to q.i.d. Maintain each dosage level for 7 days to determine response. Maximum, 400 mg daily.

Children: Initially, 0.5 mg/kg P.O. q.d. for 7 days; then 0.5 mg/kg t.i.d. for 7 days, 1 mg/kg t.i.d. for 7 days, and finally, 2 mg/kg, t.i.d. for 7 days. May increase up to 3 mg/kg b.i.d. to q.i.d. if necessary. Maximum, 100 mg q.i.d.

➤ **To manage malignant hyperthermic crisis**

Adults and children: Initially, 1 mg/kg I.V. push. Repeat, p.r.n., up to cumulative dose of 10 mg/kg.

➤ **To prevent or attenuate malignant hyperthermic crisis in susceptible patients who need surgery**

Adults and children: 4 to 8 mg/kg P.O. daily in three or four divided doses for 1 or 2 days before procedure. Give final dose 3 or 4 hours before procedure. Or, 2.5 mg/kg I.V. about 1 hour before anesthesia; infuse over 1 hour.

➤ **To prevent recurrence of malignant hyperthermic crisis**

Adults: 4 to 8 mg/kg P.O. daily in four divided doses for up to 3 days after hyperthermic crisis.

I.V. ADMINISTRATION

- Reconstitute drug by adding 60 ml of sterile water for injection and shaking vial until clear. Don't use a diluent that contains a bacteriostatic drug.
- Protect solution from light, and use within 6 hours.

INCOMPATIBILITIES

D_5W, normal saline solution, other I. V. drugs mixed in a syringe.

ACTION

Acts directly on skeletal muscle to decrease excitation and contraction coupling and reduce muscle strength by interfering with intracellular calcium movement.

Route	Onset	Peak	Duration
P.O.	Unknown	5 hr	Unknown
I.V.	Unknown	Unknown	3 hr after infusion

Half-life: P.O., 9 hours; I.V., 4 to 8 hours.

ADVERSE REACTIONS

CNS: *drowsiness, dizziness, malaise, fatigue,* ***seizures,*** headache, lightheadedness, confusion, nervousness, insomnia, fever, depression.
CV: tachycardia, blood pressure changes, phlebitis, thrombophlebitis, heart failure.
EENT: excessive lacrimation, speech disturbance, diplopia, visual disturbances.
GI: anorexia, constipation, cramping, dysphagia, metallic taste, severe diarrhea, GI bleeding, vomiting.
GU: urinary frequency, hematuria, incontinence, nocturia, dysuria, crystalluria, difficult erection, urine retention.
Hematologic: ***leukopenia, thrombocytopenia, lymphocytic lymphoma,*** anemia.
Hepatic: ***hepatitis.***
Musculoskeletal: *muscle weakness,* myalgia, back pain.
Respiratory: pleural effusion with pericarditis, pulmonary edema.
Skin: eczematous eruption, pruritus, urticaria, abnormal hair growth, diaphoresis, photosensitivity.
Other: chills.

INTERACTIONS

Drug-drug. *Clofibrate, warfarin:* May decrease protein binding of dantrolene. Use together cautiously.
CNS depressants: May increase CNS depression. Avoid using together.
Estrogens: May increase risk of hepatotoxicity. Use together cautiously.
I.V. verapamil and other calcium channel blockers: May cause hyperkalemia, ventricular fibrillation, and myocardial depression. Stop verapamil before giving I.V. dantrolene.
Vecuronium: May increase neuromuscular blockade effect. Use together cautiously.
Drug-lifestyle. *Alcohol use:* May increase CNS depression. Discourage use together.
Sun exposure: May cause photosensitivity reactions. Advise patient to avoid excessive sunlight exposure.

EFFECTS ON LAB TEST RESULTS

- May increase ALT, AST, alkaline phosphatase, LDH, bilirubin, and BUN levels.

CONTRAINDICATIONS & CAUTIONS

- Contraindicated for spasms in rheumatic disorders and when spasticity is used to maintain motor function.

• Contraindicated in breast-feeding patients and patients with upper motor neuron disorders or active hepatic disease.
• Use cautiously in women, patients older than age 35, and patients with hepatic disease (such as cirrhosis or hepatitis) or severely impaired cardiac or pulmonary function.

NURSING CONSIDERATIONS
• Start therapy as soon as malignant hyperthermia reaction is recognized.
• Liver damage may occur with long-term use. If benefits don't occur within 45 days, stop therapy.
• Obtain liver function test results at start of therapy.
• Prepare oral suspension for single dose by dissolving capsule contents in juice or other liquid. For multiple doses, use acid vehicle, and refrigerate. Use within several days.
• ***Alert:*** Watch for fever, jaundice, severe diarrhea, weakness, and sensitivity reactions, including skin eruptions. Withhold dose and notify prescriber.
• ***Look alike–sound alike:*** Don't confuse Dantrium with Daraprim.

PATIENT TEACHING
• Instruct patient to take drug with meals or milk in four divided doses.
• Tell patient to eat carefully to avoid choking. Some patients may have trouble swallowing during therapy.
• Warn patient to avoid driving and other hazardous activities until CNS effects of drug are known.
• Advise patient to avoid combining drug with alcohol or other CNS depressants.
• Advise patient to notify prescriber if skin or eyes turn yellow, skin itches, or fever develops.
• Tell patient to avoid photosensitivity reactions by using sunblock and wearing protective clothing, to report abdominal discomfort or GI problems immediately, and to follow prescriber's orders regarding rest and physical therapy.

tizanidine hydrochloride
Zanaflex

Pharmacologic class: imidazoline derivative, centrally acting alpha$_2$-adrenergic agonist
Pregnancy risk category C

AVAILABLE FORMS
Capsules: 2 mg, 4 mg, 6 mg
Tablets: 2 mg, 4 mg

INDICATIONS & DOSAGES
➤ **Acute and intermittent management of increased muscle tone with spasticity**
Adults: Initially, 4 mg P.O. q 6 to 8 hours, p.r.n., to maximum of three doses in 24 hours. Dosage can be increased gradually in 2- to 4-mg increments, reaching optimum dose over 2 to 4 weeks. Maximum, 36 mg daily.
Adjust-a-dose: For patients with renal insufficiency, reduce dosage. If higher dosages are needed, increase individual doses rather than frequency.

ACTION
Unknown. Acts as an alpha$_2$ agonist. May reduce spasticity by increasing presynaptic inhibition of motor neurons at the level of the spinal cord.

Route	Onset	Peak	Duration
P.O.	Unknown	1–2 hr	3–6 hr

Half-life: 2½ hours; metabolites, 20 to 40 hours.

ADVERSE REACTIONS
CNS: *somnolence, sedation, asthenia, dizziness,* speech disorder, dyskinesia, nervousness, hallucinations.
CV: *hypotension,* ***bradycardia.***
EENT: amblyopia, pharyngitis, rhinitis.
GI: *dry mouth,* constipation, vomiting.
GU: *UTI,* urinary frequency.
Hepatic: hepatic injury.
Other: infection, flulike syndrome.

INTERACTIONS
Drug-drug. *Acetaminophen:* May delay acetaminophen absorption time. Monitor patient for clinical effect.

Antihypertensives, other alpha agonists such as clonidine: May cause hypotension; monitor patient closely. Avoid using together.
Baclofen, benzodiazepines, other CNS depressants: May have additive CNS depressant effects. Avoid using together.
CYP1A2 inhibitors (amiodarone, acyclovir, cimetidine, ciprofloxacin, famotidine, fluoroquinolones, fluvoxamine, mexiletine, propafenone, ticlodipine, verapamil, zileuton): May cause significant increases in tizanidine levels. Use together should be avoided; use of ciprofloxacin or fluvoxamine with tizanidine is contraindicated.
Oral contraceptives: May decrease tizanidine clearance. Reduce tizanidine dosage.
Drug-lifestyle. *Alcohol use:* May increase CNS depression. Discourage use together.

EFFECTS ON LAB TEST RESULTS
- May increase AST and ALT levels.

CONTRAINDICATIONS & CAUTIONS
- Contraindicated in patients hypersensitive to drug.
- Use of potent CYP1A2 inhibitors ciprofloxacin and fluvoxamine with tizanidine is contraindicated.
- Use cautiously in patients who are taking antihypertensives, in those with renal and hepatic impairment, in pregnant or breast-feeding women, and in elderly patients.
- Safety and effectiveness in children haven't been established.

NURSING CONSIDERATIONS
- ***Look alike–sound alike:*** Don't confuse tizanidine with tiagabine; both have 4-mg starting doses.
- ***Alert:*** The capsules and tablets are bioequivalent only if taken on an empty stomach.
- Obtain liver function test results before treatment; during treatment at 1, 3, and 6 months; and then periodically thereafter.

PATIENT TEACHING
- Caution patient to avoid alcohol and activities that require alertness. Drug may cause drowsiness.
- Inform patient that dizziness upon standing quickly can be minimized by rising slowly and avoiding sudden position changes.

39

Neuromuscular blockers

atracurium besylate
cisatracurium besylate
pancuronium bromide
rocuronium bromide
succinylcholine chloride
vecuronium bromide

SAFETY ALERT!

atracurium besylate

Tracrium

Pharmacologic class: nondepolarizing neuromuscular blocker
Pregnancy risk category C

AVAILABLE FORMS

Injection: 10 mg/ml

INDICATIONS & DOSAGES

➤ **Adjunct to general anesthesia to facilitate endotracheal intubation and relax skeletal muscles during surgery or mechanical ventilation**

Adults and children age 2 or older: 0.4 to 0.5 mg/kg by I.V. bolus. Give maintenance dose of 0.08 to 0.1 mg/kg within 20 to 45 minutes during prolonged surgery. Give maintenance doses q 15 to 25 minutes in patients receiving balanced anesthesia. For prolonged procedures, use a constant infusion at an initial rate of 9 to 10 mcg/kg/minute, then reduce to 5 to 9 mcg/kg/minute.

Children ages 1 month to 2 years: First dose, 0.3 to 0.4 mg/kg I.V. for children under halothane anesthesia. Frequent maintenance doses may be needed.

Adjust-a-dose: In adults receiving enflurane or isoflurane at the same time, reduce initial atracurium dose by 33% (0.25 to 0.35 mg/kg). In adults receiving atracurium following succinylcholine, initial dose is 0.3 to 0.4 mg/kg.

I.V. ADMINISTRATION

- Use drug only under direct supervision by medical staff skilled in using neuromuscular blockers and maintaining patent airway. Keep available emergency respiratory support (endotracheal equipment, ventilator, oxygen, atropine, edrophonium, neostigmine, and epinephrine).
- Give sedatives or general anesthetics before neuromuscular blockers, which don't reduce consciousness or alter pain threshold.
- Drug usually is given by rapid I.V. bolus injection but may be given by intermittent infusion or continuous infusion.
- At concentrations of 0.2 mg/ml to 0.5 mg/ml, drug is compatible in D_5W, normal saline solution for injection, or dextrose 5% in normal saline solution for injection for 24 hours (at room temperature or refrigerated).
- Stable if undiluted for 6 weeks.
- Store in refrigerator. Don't freeze. Once removed, use within 14 days.

INCOMPATIBILITIES

Alkaline solutions (such as barbiturates), lactated Ringer solution.

ACTION

A nondepolarizing drug that keeps acetylcholine from binding to receptors on motor end plate, thus blocking neuromuscular transmission.

Route	Onset	Peak	Duration
I.V.	2 min	3–5 min	35–70 min

Half-life: 20 minutes.

ADVERSE REACTIONS

CV: ***bradycardia,*** hypotension, tachycardia.
Respiratory: ***prolonged, dose-related apnea, bronchospasm, laryngospasm,*** wheezing, increased bronchial secretions, dyspnea.
Skin: *skin flushing,* erythema, pruritus, urticaria, rash.
Other: ***anaphylaxis.***

INTERACTIONS

Drug-drug. *Amikacin, gentamicin, neomycin, streptomycin, tobramycin:* May increase the effects of nondepolarizing

muscle relaxant including prolonged respiratory depression. Use together cautiously. May reduce nondepolarizing muscle relaxant dose.
Carbamazepine, phenytoin, theophylline: May reverse, or cause resistance to, neuromuscular blockade. May need to increase atracurium dose.
Clindamycin, general anesthetics (enflurane, halothane, isoflurane), kanamycin, polymyxin antibiotics (colistin, polymyxin B sulfate), procainamide, quinidine, quinine, thiazide and loop diuretics, trimethaphan, verapamil: May enhance neuromuscular blockade, increasing skeletal muscle relaxation and prolonging effect of atracurium. Use together cautiously during and after surgery.
Corticosteroids: May cause prolonged weakness. Monitor patient closely.
Edrophonium, neostigmine, pyridostigmine: May inhibit drug and reverse neuromuscular block. Monitor patient closely.
Lithium, magnesium salts, opioid analgesics: May enhance neuromuscular blockade, increasing skeletal muscle relaxation and possibly causing respiratory paralysis. Reduce atracurium dosage.
Succinylcholine: May cause quicker onset of atracurium; may increase depth of neuromuscular blockade. Monitor patient.

EFFECTS ON LAB TEST RESULTS

None reported.

CONTRAINDICATIONS & CAUTIONS

- Contraindicated in patients hypersensitive to drug.
- Use cautiously in elderly or debilitated patients and in those with CV disease; severe electrolyte disorder; bronchogenic carcinoma; hepatic, renal, or pulmonary impairment; neuromuscular disease; or myasthenia gravis.

NURSING CONSIDERATIONS

- Dosage depends on anesthetic used, individual needs, and response. Recommended dosages must be individually adjusted.
- Resistance may develop in burn patients; increase dosage if needed.
- Give analgesics for pain. Patient may have pain but may be unable to express it.
- Don't give drug by I.M. injection.
- Once spontaneous recovery starts, reverse atracurium-induced neuromuscular blockade with an anticholinesterase (such as neostigmine or edrophonium), usually given with an anticholinergic such as atropine. Complete reversal of neuromuscular blockade is usually achieved within 8 to 10 minutes after using an anticholinesterase.
- Monitor respirations and vital signs closely until patient has fully recovered from neuromuscular blockade, as indicated by tests of muscle strength (hand grip, head lift, and ability to cough).
- A nerve stimulator and train-of-four monitoring are recommended to confirm antagonism of neuromuscular blockade and recovery of muscle strength. Make sure spontaneous recovery is evident before attempting reversal with neostigmine.
- Prior use of succinylcholine doesn't prolong duration of action, but quickens onset and may deepen neuromuscular blockade.
- ***Alert:*** Careful dosage calculation is essential. Always verify dosage with another health care professional.

PATIENT TEACHING

- Explain all events and procedures to patient because he can still hear.

SAFETY ALERT!

cisatracurium besylate

Nimbex

Pharmacologic class: nondepolarizing neuromuscular blocker
Pregnancy risk category B

AVAILABLE FORMS

Injection: 2 mg/ml, 10 mg/ml

INDICATIONS & DOSAGES

➤Adjunct to general anesthesia to facilitate endotracheal intubation and relax skeletal muscles during surgery
Adults: First dose of 0.15 mg/kg I.V.; then maintenance dosages of 0.03 mg/kg I.V. q 40 to 50 minutes, p.r.n. Or, first dose of 0.2 mg/kg I.V.; then maintenance dosages of 0.03 mg/kg I.V. q 50 to 60 min-

utes, p.r.n. Or, after first dose, give a maintenance infusion at 3 mcg/kg/minute and reduce to 1 to 2 mcg/kg/minute, p.r.n.
Children ages 2 to 12: 0.1 mg/kg I.V. over 5 to 10 seconds. After first dose, give a maintenance infusion of 3 mcg/kg/minute, then reduce to 1 to 2 mcg/kg/minute, p.r.n.
Adjust-a-dose: During coronary artery bypass surgery with induced hypothermia, reduce infusion rate by 50%.

➤ **To maintain neuromuscular blockade during mechanical ventilation in intensive care unit (ICU)**
Adults: Principles for infusion in operating room apply to use in ICU. After first dose, give 3 mcg/kg/minute by I.V. infusion. Range, 0.5 to 5 mcg/kg/minute.
Adjust-a-dose: In patients with neuromuscular disease, such as myasthenia gravis or Eaton-Lambert syndrome, don't exceed 0.02 mg/kg. Patients with burns may need increased amount.

I.V. ADMINISTRATION

- Drug is colorless to slightly yellow or green-yellow. Inspect vials for particulates and discoloration before use. Don't use unclear solutions or those with visible particulates.
- The 20-ml vial is intended for use only in the ICU.
- Use only under direct supervision of medical staff skilled in using neuromuscular blockers and maintaining airway patency. Don't give drug unless resources for intubation, mechanical ventilation, and oxygen therapy are within reach.
- Keep refrigerated; don't freeze. Use drug within 21 days after removing from refrigeration.
- Use drug within 24 hours when diluted to a concentration of 0.1 mg/ml in D_5W, normal saline solution (NSS), or 5% dextrose and NSS.

INCOMPATIBILITIES

Acyclovir, alkaline solutions with pH higher than 8.5, aminophylline, amphotericin B, amphotericin B cholesteryl sulfate complex, ampicillin, ampicillin sodium and sulbactam sodium, cefazolin, cefoperazone, cefotaxime, cefoxitin, ceftazidime, ceftizoxime, cefuroxime, diazepam, furosemide, ganciclovir, heparin sodium, ketorolac, lactated Ringer injection, methylprednisolone sodium succinate, piperacillin, piperacillin sodium and tazobactam sodium, propofol, sodium bicarbonate, sodium nitroprusside, thiopental sodium, ticarcillin disodium and clavulanate potassium, trimethoprim and sulfamethoxazole.

ACTION

Nondepolarizing drug that binds to cholinergic receptors on the motor end plate, antagonizing acetylcholine and blocking neuromuscular transmission.

Route	Onset	Peak	Duration
I.V.	1–2 min	2–5 min	25–44 min

Half-life: 22 to 29 minutes; about 3 hours for laudanosine.

ADVERSE REACTIONS

CV: ***bradycardia,*** hypotension, flushing.
Respiratory: ***bronchospasm, prolonged apnea.***
Skin: rash.

INTERACTIONS

Drug-drug. *Aminoglycosides, bacitracin, clindamycin, colistimethate sodium, colistin, lithium, local anesthetics, magnesium salts, polymyxins, procainamide, quinidine, quinine, tetracyclines:* May enhance neuromuscular blocking action of cisatracurium. Use together cautiously.
Carbamazepine, phenytoin: May decrease the effects of cisatracurium. May need to increase cisatracurium dose.
Enflurane or isoflurane given with nitrous oxide or oxygen: May prolong cisatracurium duration of action. Patient may need less frequent maintenance doses, lower maintenance doses, or reduced infusion rate of cisatracurium.
Succinylcholine: May shorten time to onset of maximal neuromuscular block. Monitor patient.

EFFECTS ON LAB TEST RESULTS

None reported.

CONTRAINDICATIONS & CAUTIONS

- Contraindicated in patients who are hypersensitive to drug, to other bis-

benzylisoquinolinium drugs, or to benzyl alcohol (found in 10-ml vial).
- Use cautiously in pregnant or breast-feeding women.

NURSING CONSIDERATIONS
- Drug isn't recommended for rapid-sequence endotracheal intubation because of its intermediate onset.
- Dosage requirements vary widely among patients.
- ***Alert:*** Drug has no known effect on consciousness, pain threshold, or cerebration. To avoid patient distress, don't induce neuromuscular block before unconsciousness.
- Monitor neuromuscular function with nerve stimulator during drug administration. If stimulation doesn't elicit a response, stop infusion until response returns.
- To avoid inaccurate dosing, perform neuromuscular monitoring on a nonparetic arm or leg in patients with hemiparesis or paraparesis.
- Monitor acid-base balance and electrolyte levels. Abnormalities may potentiate or antagonize the action of cisatracurium.
- Monitor patient for malignant hyperthermia.
- Give analgesics, if indicated. Patient can feel pain but can't indicate its presence.
- ***Alert:*** Careful dosage calculation is essential. Always verify dosage with another health care professional.

PATIENT TEACHING
- Explain purpose of drug.
- Assure patient that monitoring will be continuous.
- Explain all procedures and events because patient can still hear.

SAFETY ALERT!

pancuronium bromide

Pharmacologic class: nondepolarizing neuromuscular blocker
Pregnancy risk category C

AVAILABLE FORMS
Injection: 1 mg/ml, 2 mg/ml

INDICATIONS & DOSAGES
➤Adjunct to anesthesia to relax skeletal muscle, facilitate intubation, assist with mechanical ventilation
Adults and children age 1 month and older: Initially, 0.04 to 0.1 mg/kg I.V.; then 0.01 mg/kg q 30 to 60 minutes.
Neonates: Individualize dosage.

I.V. ADMINISTRATION
- Drug has no known effect on consciousness, pain threshold, or cerebration. To avoid patient distress, don't induce neuromuscular block before unconsciousness.
- Keep endotracheal equipment, ventilator, oxygen, atropine, edrophonium, epinephrine, and neostigmine immediately available.
- Store in refrigerator. Don't store in plastic containers or syringes, although plastic syringes may be used for administration.

INCOMPATIBILITIES
Alkaline solutions, barbiturates, diazepam, thiopental sodium.

ACTION
Nondepolarizing drug that prevents acetylcholine from binding to receptors on the motor end plate, blocking neuromuscular transmission.

Route	Onset	Peak	Duration
I.V.	30–45 sec	3–4½ min	35–65 min

Half-life: About 2 hours.

ADVERSE REACTIONS
CV: tachycardia, increased blood pressure.
EENT: excessive salivation.
Musculoskeletal: residual muscle weakness.
Respiratory: ***prolonged respiratory insufficiency or apnea.***
Skin: transient rashes.
Other: ***allergic or idiosyncratic hypersensitivity reactions.***

INTERACTIONS
Drug-drug. *Aminoglycosides (amikacin, gentamicin, neomycin, streptomycin, tobramycin):* May increase the effects of

nondepolarizing muscle relaxant, including prolonged respiratory depression. Use together only when necessary. Dose of nondepolarizing muscle relaxant may need to be reduced.
Azathioprine: May reverse neuromuscular blockade induced by pancuronium. Monitor patient.
Beta blockers, clindamycin, general anesthetics (such as enflurane, halothane, isoflurane), ketamine, lincomycin, magnesium sulfate, polymyxin antibiotics (colistin, polymyxin B sulfate), quinidine, quinine, verapamil: May enhance neuromuscular blockade, increasing skeletal muscle relaxation and prolonging effect of pancuronium. Use together cautiously during and after surgery.
Carbamazepine, phenytoin: May decrease effects of pancuronium. May need to increase pancuronium dose.
Diuretics: May cause electrolyte imbalance, or alter neuromuscular blockade. Monitor electrolytes before giving drug.
Lithium, opioid analgesics: May enhance neuromuscular blockade, increasing skeletal muscle relaxation and possibly causing respiratory paralysis. Use cautiously, and reduce dose of pancuronium.
Succinylcholine: May increase intensity and duration of neuromuscular blockade. Allow effects of succinylcholine to subside before giving pancuronium.
Theophylline: May produce a dose-dependent reversal of neuromuscular blocking effects. Monitor patient for clinical effect.
Tricyclic antidepressants (TCAs): May increase risk for ventricular arrhythmias in patients anesthetized with both halothane and pancuronium. Monitor ECG closely in patients taking TCAs before surgery.

EFFECTS ON LAB TEST RESULTS

None reported.

CONTRAINDICATIONS & CAUTIONS

- Contraindicated in patients hypersensitive to bromides, those with tachycardia, and those for whom even a minor increase in heart rate is undesirable.
- Use cautiously in elderly or debilitated patients; in patients with renal, hepatic, or pulmonary impairment; and in those with respiratory depression, myasthenia gravis, myasthenic syndrome related to lung cancer, dehydration, thyroid disorders, CV disease, collagen diseases, porphyria, electrolyte disturbances, hyperthermia, and toxemic states. Also, use large doses cautiously in patients undergoing cesarean section.

NURSING CONSIDERATIONS

- Dosage depends on anesthetic used, individual needs, and response. Dosages are representative and must be adjusted.
- Only staff skilled in airway management should use drug.
- Allow succinylcholine effects to subside before giving this drug.
- Monitor baseline electrolyte determinations (electrolyte imbalance can potentiate neuromuscular effects) and vital signs, especially respirations and heart rate.
- Measure fluid intake and output; renal dysfunction may prolong duration of action because 25% of drug is excreted unchanged in the urine.
- A nerve stimulator and train-of-four monitoring are recommended to confirm antagonism of neuromuscular blockade and recovery of muscle strength. Make sure there is some evidence of spontaneous recovery before attempting pharmacologic reversal with neostigmine.
- Monitor respirations closely until patient recovers fully from neuromuscular blockade, as indicated by tests of muscle strength (hand grip, head lift, and ability to cough).
- Once spontaneous recovery starts, neuromuscular blockade may be reversed with an anticholinesterase (such as neostigmine or edrophonium), which is usually given with an anticholinergic (such as atropine).
- Drug doesn't cause histamine release or hypotension, but it may raise heart rate and blood pressure.
- Give analgesics for pain.
- ***Alert:*** Careful dosage calculation is essential. Always verify dosage with another health care professional.

PATIENT TEACHING

- Explain all events and procedures to patient because he can still hear.

SAFETY ALERT!

rocuronium bromide
Zemuron

Pharmacologic class: nondepolarizing neuromuscular blocker
Pregnancy risk category C

AVAILABLE FORMS
Injection: 10 mg/ml

INDICATIONS & DOSAGES
➤**Adjunct to general anesthesia to facilitate endotracheal intubation and relax skeletal muscles during surgery or mechanical ventilation**
Adults: Initially, 0.6 mg/kg to 1.2 mg/kg I.V. bolus. In most patients, tracheal intubation may be performed within 2 minutes; muscle paralysis should last about 31 minutes. A maintenance dosage of 0.1 mg/kg should provide an additional 12 minutes (average) of muscle relaxation; 0.15 mg/kg will add 17 minutes (average); or 0.2 mg/kg will add 24 minutes (average) to the duration of effect. Or, maintenance doses may be maintained using a continuous infusion at a rate of 4 to 16 mcg/kg/minute.
Children ages 3 months to 12 years receiving halothane anesthesia: Initially, 0.6 mg/kg I.V. bolus. In most patients, tracheal intubation may be performed within 1 minute; muscle paralysis should last about 41 minutes in children ages 3 to 12 months and 27 minutes in children ages 13 months to 12 years. A maintenance dose of 0.075 to 0.125 mg/kg should provide an additional 7 to 10 minutes of muscle relaxation.

I.V. ADMINISTRATION
- Keep airway clear. Keep emergency respiratory support (endotracheal equipment, ventilator, oxygen, atropine, edrophonium, epinephrine, and neostigmine) readily available.
- Give by rapid I.V. injection or by continuous I.V. infusion. Infusion rates are highly individualized. Compatible solutions include D_5W, normal saline solution for injection, dextrose 5% in normal saline solution for injection, sterile water for injection, and lactated Ringer injection.
- Store vials at room temperature for up to 60 days. Use open vials within 30 days. Use diluted infusion solutions within 24 hours.

INCOMPATIBILITIES
Alkaline solutions such as barbiturates, other I.V. drugs.

ACTION
Nondepolarizing drug that prevents acetylcholine from binding to receptors on the motor end plate, thus blocking neuromuscular transmission.

Route	Onset	Peak	Duration
I.V.	1 min	2 min	20–60 min

Half-life: 14 to 18 minutes in adults; ¾ to 1¼ hours in children.

ADVERSE REACTIONS
CV: tachycardia, abnormal ECG, transient hypotension, hypertension, edema.
GI: nausea, vomiting.
Respiratory: ***apnea, respiratory insufficiency,*** asthma, hiccups.
Skin: rash, pruritus, injection site edema.

INTERACTIONS
Drug-drug. *Aminoglycosides (amikacin, gentamicin, neomycin, streptomycin, tobramycin):* May increase the effects of nondepolarizing muscle relaxant including prolonged respiratory depression. Use together only when necessary. May need to reduce nondepolarizing muscle relaxant dose.
Anticonvulsants, beta blockers, clindamycin, general anesthetics (enflurane, halothane, isoflurane), ketamine, magnesium salts, opiate analgesics, polymyxin antibiotics (colistin, polymyxin B sulfate), quinidine, quinine, succinylcholine, tetracyclines, verapamil: May enhance neuromuscular blockade, increasing skeletal muscle relaxation and potentiating effect. Reduce rocuronium if needed. Use together cautiously during and after surgery.
Azathioprine, carbamazepine, phenytoin, theophylline: May decrease effect of rocuronium. May need to increase rocuronium dose.

EFFECTS ON LAB TEST RESULTS
None reported.

CONTRAINDICATIONS & CAUTIONS
• Contraindicated in patients hypersensitive to drug or to bromides.
• Use cautiously in patients with hepatic disease, severe obesity, bronchogenic carcinoma, electrolyte disturbances, neuromuscular disease, and an altered circulation time caused by CV disease, old age, or edema.
• Drug isn't recommended for use during rapid sequence induction for cesarean section.

NURSING CONSIDERATIONS
• ***Alert:*** Drug has no known effect on consciousness, pain threshold, or cerebration. To avoid patient distress, don't induce neuromuscular block before unconsciousness.
• Dosage depends on anesthetic used, individual needs, and response. Recommended dosages must be individually adjusted.
• In obese patients, base the initial dose on the patient's actual body weight.
• Only staff skilled in airway management should use drug.
• Drug allows intubation within 3 minutes.
• A nerve stimulator and train-of-four monitoring are recommended to confirm antagonism of neuromuscular blockade and recovery of muscle strength. Make sure there is some evidence of spontaneous recovery before attempting pharmacologic reversal with neostigmine.
• Prior use of succinylcholine may enhance neuromuscular-blocking effect and duration of action.
• Monitor patients with liver disease because they may need higher doses to achieve adequate muscle relaxation. However, such patients have prolonged drug effects.
• Monitor respirations closely until patient recovers fully from neuromuscular blockade, as indicated by tests of muscle strength (hand grip, head lift, and ability to cough).
• In patients with renal failure, drug is well tolerated.
• Give analgesics for pain.
• ***Alert:*** Careful drug calculation is essential. Always verify dosage with another health care professional.

PATIENT TEACHING
• Explain all events and procedures to patient because he can still hear.

SAFETY ALERT!

succinylcholine chloride (suxamethonium chloride)
Anectine, Anectine Flo-Pack, Quelicin, Scoline‡

Pharmacologic class: depolarizing neuromuscular blocker
Pregnancy risk category C

AVAILABLE FORMS
Injection: 20 mg/ml, 50 mg/ml, 100 mg/ml
Powder for infusion: 500-mg vial, 1-g vial

INDICATIONS & DOSAGES
➤ **Adjunct to anesthesia to relax skeletal muscles for surgery and orthopedic manipulations; to facilitate intubation and assist with mechanical ventilation; to lessen muscle contractions in pharmacologically or electrically induced seizures**
Adults: 0.6 mg/kg I.V. given over 10 to 30 seconds. Dosage range is 0.3 to 1.1 mg/kg. For longer response, give continuous infusion at 0.5 to 10 mg/minute, or give 0.04 to 0.07 mg/kg intermittently, p.r.n., to maintain relaxation. Or, 2.5 to 4 mg/kg I.M. Maximum I.M. dose is 150 mg.
Children: 1 to 2 mg/kg I.V. or 3 to 4 mg/kg I.M. Maximum I.M. dose is 150 mg.

I.V. ADMINISTRATION
• Drug may contain benzyl alcohol. Avoid use in neonates.
• Drug has no known effect on consciousness, pain threshold, or cerebration. To avoid patient distress, don't induce neuromuscular block before unconsciousness.
• Give test dose of 5 to 10 mg after patient has been anesthetized. No respiratory depression or transient depression for up to 5 minutes indicates patient can metabolize drug, and it's OK to give. Don't give

if patient develops respiratory paralysis sufficient to permit endotracheal intubation. (Recovery should occur within 30 to 60 minutes.)
- Use within 24 hours after reconstitution.
- Store injectable form in refrigerator. Store powder form at room temperature in tightly closed container.

INCOMPATIBILITIES

Alkaline solutions, barbiturates, nafcillin, sodium bicarbonate, solutions with pH above 4.5, thiopental sodium.

ACTION

Binds with a high affinity to cholinergic receptors, prolonging depolarization of the motor end plate and ultimately producing muscle paralysis.

Route	Onset	Peak	Duration
I.V.	30–60 sec	1–2 min	4–10 min
I.M.	2–3 min	Unknown	10–30 min

Half-life: Unknown.

ADVERSE REACTIONS

CV: ***arrhythmias, bradycardia, cardiac arrest,*** tachycardia, hypertension, hypotension, flushing.
EENT: increased intraocular pressure.
GI: excessive salivation.
Metabolic: hyperkalemia.
Musculoskeletal: *postoperative muscle pain,* muscle fasciculation, jaw rigidity.
Respiratory: ***apnea, bronchoconstriction, prolonged respiratory depression.***
Skin: rash.
Other: ***allergic or idiosyncratic hypersensitivity reactions, anaphylaxis, malignant hyperthermia, rhabdomyolysis with acute renal failure.***

INTERACTIONS

Drug-drug. *Aminoglycosides, anticholinesterases (such as echothiophate, edrophonium, neostigmine, physostigmine, pyridostigmine), aprotinin, general anesthetics (such as enflurane, halothane, isoflurane), glucocorticoids, hormonal contraceptives, lidocaine, lithium, magnesium, oxytocin, polymyxin antibiotics, such as colistin, polymyxin B sulfate, procainamide, quinine:* May enhance neuromuscular blockade, increasing skeletal muscle relaxation and potentiating effect. Use together cautiously during and after surgery.
Cardiac glycosides: May cause arrhythmias. Use together cautiously.
Cyclophosphamide, lithium, MAO inhibitors: May enhance neuromuscular blockade and prolong apnea. Use together cautiously.
Opioid analgesics: May enhance neuromuscular blockade, increasing skeletal muscle relaxation and possibly causing respiratory paralysis. Use together cautiously.
Parenteral magnesium sulfate: May enhance neuromuscular blockade, may increase skeletal muscle relaxation, and may cause respiratory paralysis. Use together cautiously, preferably at reduced doses.
Drug-herb. *Melatonin:* May potentiate blocking properties of drug. Ask patient about herbal remedy use, and recommend caution.

EFFECTS ON LAB TEST RESULTS

- May increase myoglobin and potassium levels.

CONTRAINDICATIONS & CAUTIONS

- Contraindicated in patients hypersensitive to drug and in those with abnormally low plasma pseudocholinesterase levels, angle-closure glaucoma, personal or family history of malignant hyperthermia, myopathies with elevated CK levels, acute major burns, multiple trauma, skeletal muscle denervation, upper motor neuron injury, or penetrating eye injuries.
- Use cautiously in elderly or debilitated patients; in patients receiving quinidine or cardiac glycoside therapy; in patients with hepatic, renal, or pulmonary impairment; in those with respiratory depression, severe burns or trauma, electrolyte imbalances, hyperkalemia, paraplegia, spinal CNS injury, stroke, degenerative or dystrophic neuromuscular disease, myasthenia gravis, myasthenic syndrome related to lung cancer, dehydration, thyroid disorders, collagen diseases, porphyria, fractures, muscle spasms, eye surgery, and pheochromocytoma. Also, use large doses cautiously in patients undergoing cesarean section.

NURSING CONSIDERATIONS

- Dosage depends on anesthetic used, individual needs, and response. Recommended dosages must be individually adjusted.
- Children may be less sensitive to drug than adults.
- Succinylcholine is the drug of choice for procedures less than 3 minutes and for orthopedic manipulations; use cautiously with fractures or dislocations.
- Only staff skilled in airway management should use drug.
- If giving I.M., inject deeply and preferably high into deltoid muscle.
- Monitor baseline electrolyte determinations and vital signs. Check respirations every 5 to 10 minutes during infusion.
- Monitor respirations closely until tests of muscle strength (hand grip, head lift, and ability to cough) indicate full recovery from neuromuscular blockade.
- ***Alert:*** Don't use reversing drugs. Unlike nondepolarizing drugs, neostigmine or edrophonium may worsen neuromuscular blockade.
- Repeated or continuous infusions aren't advisable; they may cause reduced response or prolonged muscle relaxation and apnea.
- Give analgesics for pain.
- Keep airway clear. Have emergency respiratory support equipment (endotracheal equipment, ventilator, oxygen, atropine, and epinephrine) immediately available.
- ***Alert:*** Careful dosage calculation is essential. Always verify dosage with another health care professional.

PATIENT TEACHING

- Explain all events and procedures to patient because he can still hear.
- Reassure patient that postoperative stiffness is normal and will soon subside.

SAFETY ALERT!

vecuronium bromide

Pharmacologic class: nondepolarizing neuromuscular blocker
Pregnancy risk category C

AVAILABLE FORMS

Injection: 10-mg vial, 20-mg vial

INDICATIONS & DOSAGES

➤ Adjunct to general anesthesia to facilitate endotracheal intubation and relax skeletal muscles during surgery or mechanical ventilation

Adults and children age 10 or older: Initially, 0.08 to 0.1 mg/kg I.V. bolus. Give maintenance doses of 0.01 to 0.015 mg/kg within 25 to 40 minutes of first dose during prolonged surgical procedures. Maintenance doses may be given q 12 to 15 minutes in patients receiving balanced anesthesia. Or, continuous infusion at a rate of 1 mcg/kg/minute 20 to 40 minutes after bolus dose.

Children ages 1 to 9: May need a slightly higher first dose and slightly more frequent supplementation than adults. Or, may give continuous I.V. infusion of 1 mcg/kg/minute initially; then 0.8 to 1.2 mcg/kg/minute.

Children ages 7 weeks to 1 year: Doses comparable to those used in adults, possibly with less frequent use of maintenance doses.

Adjust-a-dose: In adults receiving enflurane, isoflurane, or halothane, reduce initial dose by 15% (0.06 to 0.085 mg/kg). In adults receiving succinylcholine, reduce initial dose to 0.05 to 0.06 mg/kg with balanced anesthesia, or 0.04 to 0.06 mg/kg with inhalation anesthesia.

I.V. ADMINISTRATION

- Keep airway clear. Keep emergency respiratory support (endotracheal equipment, ventilator, oxygen, atropine, edrophonium, epinephrine, and neostigmine) readily available.
- In neonates, don't use solutions reconstituted with bacteriostatic water for injection containing benzyl alcohol.
- Don't mix with barbiturates or other alkaline solutions because a precipitate will form. Use only fresh solutions, and discard if discolored.
- Give over 60 to 90 seconds.
- Solutions reconstituted with sterile water for injection to a concentration of 2 mg/ml are stable under refrigeration or at room temperature for 24 hours if stored in original container.
- Solutions reconstituted with normal saline solution, D_5W, 5% dextrose in normal saline solution, or lactated Ringer are

stable for 24 hours if refrigerated in the original container. Discard unused portion.
• Solutions reconstituted with bacteriostatic water for injection containing benzyl alcohol are stable for 5 days under refrigeration or at room temperature if stored in original container.

INCOMPATIBILITIES
Alkaline solutions, amphotericin B, diazepam, furosemide, thiopental.

ACTION
Nondepolarizing drug that prevents acetylcholine from binding to receptors on the motor end plate, thus blocking neuromuscular transmission.

Route	Onset	Peak	Duration
I.V.	1 min	3–5 min	15–25 min

Half-life: 20 minutes.

ADVERSE REACTIONS
Musculoskeletal: skeletal muscle weakness.
Respiratory: ***prolonged respiratory insufficiency or apnea.***

INTERACTIONS
Drug-drug. *Aminoglycosides (amikacin, gentamicin, neomycin, streptomycin, tobramycin):* May increase the effects of nondepolarizing muscle relaxant, including prolonged respiratory depression. Use together only when necessary. May need to reduce nondepolarizing muscle relaxant dose.
Bacitracin, beta blockers, clindamycin, general anesthetics (enflurane, halothane, isoflurane), magnesium salts, other skeletal muscle relaxants, polymyxin antibiotics (colistin, polymyxin B sulfate), quinidine, quinine, succinylcholine, tetracyclines: May enhance neuromuscular blockade, increasing skeletal muscle relaxation and potentiating effect. Use together cautiously during and after surgery.
Carbamazepine, phenytoin: May decrease effects of vecuronium. May need to increase vecuronium dose.

EFFECTS ON LAB TEST RESULTS
None reported.

CONTRAINDICATIONS & CAUTIONS
• Contraindicated in patients hypersensitive to drug or to bromides.
• Use cautiously in elderly patients; in patients with altered circulation caused by CV disease or edema; and in those with hepatic disease, severe obesity, bronchogenic carcinoma, electrolyte disturbances, and neuromuscular disease.
• Not recommended for use in infants younger than age 7 weeks.

NURSING CONSIDERATIONS
• ***Alert:*** Drug has no known effect on consciousness, pain threshold, or cerebration. To avoid patient distress, don't induce neuromuscular block before unconsciousness.
• Dosage depends on anesthetic used, individual needs, and response. Recommended dosages must be individually adjusted.
• Only staff skilled in airway management should use drug.
• A nerve stimulator and train-of-four monitoring are recommended to confirm antagonism of neuromuscular blockade and recovery of muscle strength. Make sure there is some evidence of spontaneous recovery before attempting reversal with neostigmine.
• Monitor respirations closely until patient recovers fully from neuromuscular blockade, as indicated by tests of muscle strength (hand grip, head lift, and ability to cough).
• Previous use of succinylcholine may enhance the neuromuscular-blocking effect and duration of action.
• Patients with renal failure tolerate drug well.
• Give analgesics for pain.
• ***Alert:*** Careful dosage calculation is essential. Always verify dosage with another health care professional.

PATIENT TEACHING
• Explain all events and procedures to patient because he can still hear.

40

Antihistamines

cetirizine hydrochloride
chlorpheniramine maleate
clemastine fumarate
desloratadine
diphenhydramine hydrochloride
fexofenadine hydrochloride
loratadine
promethazine hydrochloride

cetirizine hydrochloride

Zyrtec✐

Pharmacologic class: piperazine derivative
Pregnancy risk category B

AVAILABLE FORMS

Oral solution: 5 mg/5 ml
Tablets: 5 mg, 10 mg
Tablets (chewable): 5 mg, 10 mg

INDICATIONS & DOSAGES

➤ **Seasonal allergic rhinitis**

Adults and children age 6 and older: 5 to 10 mg P.O. once daily.
Children ages 2 to 5: 2.5 mg P.O. once daily. Maximum daily dose is 5 mg.

➤ **Perennial allergic rhinitis, chronic urticaria**

Adults and children age 6 and older: 5 to 10 mg P.O. once daily.
Children ages 6 months to 5 years: 2.5 mg P.O. once daily; in children ages 1 to 5, increase to maximum of 5 mg daily in two divided doses.

Adjust-a-dose: In adults and children age 6 and older receiving hemodialysis, those with hepatic impairment, and those with creatinine clearance less than 31 ml/minute, give 5 mg P.O. daily. Don't use in children younger than age 6 with renal or hepatic impairment.

ACTION

A long-acting, nonsedating antihistamine that selectively inhibits peripheral H_1 receptors.

Route	Onset	Peak	Duration
P.O.	20–60 min	30–90 min	24 hr

Half-life: About 8 hours.

ADVERSE REACTIONS

CNS: *somnolence,* fatigue, dizziness, headache.
EENT: pharyngitis.
GI: dry mouth, nausea, vomiting, abdominal distress.

INTERACTIONS

Drug-drug. *CNS depressants:* May cause additive effect. Avoid using together.
Theophylline: May decrease cetirizine clearance. Monitor patient closely.
Drug-lifestyle. *Alcohol use:* May cause additive effect. Discourage use together.

EFFECTS ON LAB TEST RESULTS

- May prevent, reduce, or mask positive result in diagnostic skin test.

CONTRAINDICATIONS & CAUTIONS

- Contraindicated in patients hypersensitive to drug or to hydroxyzine and in breast-feeding women.
- Use cautiously in patients with renal or hepatic impairment.

NURSING CONSIDERATIONS

- Stop drug 4 days before diagnostic skin testing because antihistamines can prevent, reduce, or mask positive skin test response.
- ***Look alike–sound alike:*** Don't confuse Zyrtec with Zyprexa or Zantac.

PATIENT TEACHING

- Warn patient not to perform hazardous activities until CNS effects of drug are known. Somnolence is a common adverse reaction.
- Advise patient not to use alcohol or other CNS depressants while taking drug.
- Tell patient that coffee or tea may reduce drowsiness.

• Inform patient that sugarless gum, hard candy, or ice chips may relieve dry mouth.

chlorpheniramine maleate

Aller-Chlor, Allergy, Chlo-Amine, Chlor-Trimeton Allergy 4 hour, Chlor-Trimeton Allergy 8 hour, Chlor-Trimeton Allergy 12 hour, Chlor-Tripolon†

Pharmacologic class: alkylamine
Pregnancy risk category C

AVAILABLE FORMS

Capsules (sustained-release) ◊ †: 8 mg, 12 mg
Syrup ◊ : 2 mg/5 ml*
Tablets ◊ : 4 mg
Tablets (chewable) ◊ : 2 mg
Tablets (extended-release) ◊ : 8 mg, 12 mg

INDICATIONS & DOSAGES

➤Rhinitis, allergy symptoms
Adults and children age 12 and older: 4 mg P.O. q 4 to 6 hours, not to exceed 24 mg daily. Or, 8 to 12 mg timed-release P.O. q 8 to 12 hours, not to exceed 24 mg daily.
Children ages 6 to 12: 2 mg P.O. q 4 to 6 hours, not to exceed 12 mg daily. Or, 8 mg timed-release P.O. at bedtime.
Children ages 2 to 5: 1 mg P.O. q 4 to 6 hours, not to exceed 4 mg daily.
Children younger than age 2: 0.35 mg/kg daily in divided doses q 4 to 6 hours.

ACTION

Competes with histamine for H_1-receptor sites on effector cells. Drug prevents, but doesn't reverse, histamine-mediated responses.

Route	Onset	Peak	Duration
P.O.	15–60 min	2–6 hr	24 hr

Half-life: Adults with normal renal and hepatic function, 12 to 43 hours; children with normal renal and hepatic function, 9½ to 13 hours; chronic renal failure on hemodialysis, 11½ to 13¾ days.

ADVERSE REACTIONS

CNS: *drowsiness, stimulation,* sedation, excitability in children.
CV: hypotension, palpitations, weak pulse.
GI: *dry mouth,* epigastric distress.
GU: urine retention.
Respiratory: thick bronchial secretions.
Skin: rash, urticaria, pallor.

INTERACTIONS

Drug-drug. *CNS depressants:* May increase sedation. Use together cautiously.
MAO inhibitors: May increase anticholinergic effects. Avoid using together.
Drug-lifestyle. *Alcohol use:* May increase CNS depression. Discourage use together.

EFFECTS ON LAB TEST RESULTS

• May prevent, reduce, or mask positive result in diagnostic skin test.

CONTRAINDICATIONS & CAUTIONS

• Contraindicated in patients having acute asthmatic attacks and in those with angle-closure glaucoma, symptomatic prostatic hyperplasia, pyloroduodenal obstruction, or bladder neck obstruction.
• Contraindicated in breast-feeding women and in patients taking MAO inhibitors.
• Use cautiously in elderly patients and in those with increased intraocular pressure, hyperthyroidism, CV or renal disease, hypertension, bronchial asthma, urine retention, prostatic hyperplasia, and stenosing peptic ulcerations.

NURSING CONSIDERATIONS

• Stop drug 4 days before diagnostic skin testing because antihistamines can prevent, reduce, or mask positive skin test response.

PATIENT TEACHING

• Warn patient to avoid alcohol and hazardous activities that require alertness until CNS effects of drug are known.
• Tell patient that coffee or tea may reduce drowsiness.
• Inform patient that sugarless gum, hard candy, or ice chips may relieve dry mouth.
• Instruct patient to notify prescriber if tolerance develops because a different antihistamine may need to be prescribed.
• Advise patient that extended-release tablets should be swallowed whole and not crushed, chewed, or divided.

clemastine fumarate

Dayhist-1 ◇, Tavist Allergy ◇

Pharmacologic class: ethanolamine-derivative
Pregnancy risk category B

AVAILABLE FORMS

Syrup: 0.67 mg (equivalent to 0.5 mg clemastine)/5 ml*
Tablets: 1.34 mg (equivalent to 1 mg clemastine) ◇, 2.68 mg (equivalent to 2 mg clemastine)

INDICATIONS & DOSAGES

➤ **Rhinitis, allergy symptoms**
Adults and children age 12 and older: 1.34 mg P.O. b.i.d.; not to exceed 8.04 mg/day for syrup and 2.68 mg/day for tablets.
Children ages 6 to 11: Give 0.67 mg syrup P.O. b.i.d.; not to exceed 4.02 mg/day.

➤ **Allergic skin manifestation of urticaria and angioedema**
Adults and children age 12 and older: 2.68 mg P.O. b.i.d.; not to exceed 8.04 mg daily.
Children ages 6 to 11: Give 1.34 mg syrup P.O. b.i.d.; not to exceed 4.02 mg/day.

ACTION

Competes with histamine for H_1-receptor sites effector cells. Drug prevents, but doesn't reverse, histamine-mediated responses.

Route	Onset	Peak	Duration
P.O.	15–60 min	5–7 hr	12 hr

Half-life: Unknown.

ADVERSE REACTIONS

CNS: *incoordination, dizziness, sleepiness, sedation, drowsiness,* ***seizures,*** nervousness, tremor, confusion, restlessness, vertigo, headache, fatigue.
CV: hypotension, palpitations, tachycardia.
GI: *dry mouth, epigastric distress,* anorexia, diarrhea, nausea, vomiting, constipation.
GU: urine retention, urinary frequency.
Hematologic: hemolytic anemia, ***thrombocytopenia, agranulocytosis.***
Respiratory: *thick bronchial secretions.*
Skin: rash, urticaria, photosensitivity, diaphoresis.
Other: ***anaphylactic shock.***

INTERACTIONS

Drug-drug. *CNS depressants:* May increase sedation. Use together cautiously.
MAO inhibitors: May increase anticholinergic effects. Avoid using together.
Drug-lifestyle. *Alcohol use:* May increase CNS depression. Discourage use together.
Sun exposure: May cause photosensitivity reactions. Advise patient to avoid extensive sunlight exposure.

EFFECTS ON LAB TEST RESULTS

- May decrease hemoglobin level and hematocrit.
- May decrease granulocyte and platelet counts.
- May prevent, reduce, or mask positive result in diagnostic skin test.

CONTRAINDICATIONS & CAUTIONS

- Contraindicated in patients hypersensitive to drug or other antihistamines of similar chemical structure, in those taking MAO inhibitors, and in those with acute asthma, angle-closure glaucoma, stenosing peptic ulcer, symptomatic prostatic hyperplasia, bladder neck obstruction, or pyloroduodenal obstruction.
- Contraindicated in neonates, premature infants, and breast-feeding women.
- Use cautiously in elderly patients and in those with increased intraocular pressure, hyperthyroidism, CV disease, hypertension, bronchial asthma, and prostatic hyperplasia.
- Use in children younger than age 12 only as directed by prescriber.

NURSING CONSIDERATIONS

- Stop drug 4 days before diagnostic skin testing because antihistamines can prevent, reduce, or mask positive skin test result.
- Monitor blood counts during long-term therapy; observe for signs of blood dyscrasias.

PATIENT TEACHING

- Warn patient to avoid alcohol and hazardous activities that require alertness until CNS effects of drug are known.

- Tell patient that coffee or tea may reduce drowsiness. Urge caution if palpitations develop.
- Inform patient that sugarless gum, hard candy, or ice chips may relieve dry mouth.
- Warn patient of possible photosensitivity reactions. Advise use of a sunblock.
- Tell patient to notify prescriber if tolerance develops because a different antihistamine may need to be prescribed.

desloratadine

Clarinex✐, Clarinex Reditabs

Pharmacologic class: piperidine
Pregnancy risk category C

AVAILABLE FORMS

Tablets: 5 mg
Tablets (orally disintegrating): 2.5 mg, 5 mg
Syrup: 2.5 mg/5 ml

INDICATIONS & DOSAGES

➤ **Seasonal allergic rhinitis (patients age 2 and older); perennial allergic rhinitis; chronic idiopathic urticaria**
Adults and children age 12 and older: 5 mg P.O. tablets or syrup once daily.
Children ages 6 to 11: Give 2.5 mg orally disintegrating tablet (ODT) or syrup P.O. once daily.
Children ages 12 months to 5 years: 1.25 mg (2.5 ml syrup) P.O. once daily.
Infants ages 6 to 11 months: 1 mg (2 ml syrup) P.O. once daily.
Adjust-a-dose: In patients with hepatic or renal impairment, start dosage at 5 mg P.O. every other day.

ACTION

Long-acting tricyclic antihistamine with selective H_1-receptor histamine antagonist activity. It inhibits histamine release from human mast cells in vitro. Drug doesn't cross the blood-brain barrier.

Route	Onset	Peak	Duration
P.O.	Unknown	3 hr	Unknown
P.O. (orally disintegrating)	Unknown	2½–4 hr	Unknown

Half-life: 27 hours.

ADVERSE REACTIONS

CNS: *headache,* somnolence, fatigue, dizziness.
EENT: pharyngitis, dry throat.
GI: nausea, dry mouth.
Musculoskeletal: myalgia.
Other: flulike symptoms.

INTERACTIONS

None reported.

EFFECTS ON LAB TEST RESULTS

- May increase bilirubin and liver enzyme levels.
- May prevent, reduce, or mask positive result in diagnostic skin test.

CONTRAINDICATIONS & CAUTIONS

- Contraindicated in breast-feeding women and in patients hypersensitive to drug, to any of its components, or to loratadine.
- Use cautiously in elderly patients because of the greater likelihood of decreased hepatic, renal, or cardiac function, and concomitant disease or other drug therapy.

NURSING CONSIDERATIONS

- Stop drug 4 days before diagnostic skin testing because antihistamines can prevent, reduce, or mask positive skin test response.
- Store tablets at 36° to 86° F (2° to 30° C); store ODTs at 59° to 86° F (15° to 30° C).

PATIENT TEACHING

- Advise patient not to exceed recommended dosage. Higher doses don't increase effectiveness and may cause somnolence.
- Tell patient that drug can be taken without regard to meals.
- Instruct patient to remove ODTs from blister pack and place on tongue immediately to dissolve.
- ODTs may be taken with or without water.
- Tell patient to report adverse effects.

diphenhydramine hydrochloride

Allerdryl † ◊, AllerMax Allergy and Cough Formula, AllerMax Caplets ◊, Aller-med ◊, Banophen ◊, Banophen Caplets ◊, Benadryl ◊, Benadryl Allergy, Benylin Cough ◊, Bydramine Cough ◊, Compoz ◊, Diphen Cough ◊, Diphenhist ◊, Diphenhist Captabs ◊, Dormarex 2 ◊, Genahist ◊, Hydramine ◊, Hydramine Cough ◊, Nervine Nighttime Sleep-Aid ◊, Nordryl Cough ◊, Sleep-Eze 3 ◊, Sominex ◊, Tusstat ◊, Twilite Caplets ◊, Uni-Bent Cough ◊

Pharmacologic class: ethanolamine-derivative
Pregnancy risk category B

AVAILABLE FORMS

Capsules: 25 mg ◊, 50 mg ◊
Elixir: 12.5 mg/5 ml* ◊
Injection: 10 mg/ml, 50 mg/ml
Syrup: 12.5 mg/5 ml* ◊
Tablets: 25 mg ◊, 50 mg ◊
Tablets (chewable): 12.5 mg ◊

INDICATIONS & DOSAGES

➤ **Rhinitis, allergy symptoms, motion sickness, Parkinson disease**
Adults and children age 12 and older: 25 to 50 mg P.O. t.i.d. or q.i.d. Maximum, 300 mg P.O. daily. Or, 10 to 50 mg I.V. or deep I.M. Maximum I.V. or I.M. dosage, 400 mg daily.
Children younger than age 12: 5 mg/kg/day P.O., I.V., or deep I.M. in divided doses q.i.d. Maximum, 300 mg daily.

➤ **Sedation**
Adults: 25 to 50 mg P.O. or deep I.M., p.r.n.

➤ **Nighttime sleep aid**
Adults: 25 to 50 mg P.O. at bedtime.

➤ **Nonproductive cough (syrup only)**
Adults and children age 12 and older: 25 mg P.O. q 4 to 6 hours. Don't exceed 150 mg daily.
Children ages 6 to 11: 12.5 mg P.O. q 4 to 6 hours. Don't exceed 75 mg daily.
Children ages 2 to 5: 6.25 mg P.O. q 4 to 6 hours. Don't exceed 25 mg daily.

I.V. ADMINISTRATION

- Make sure site is patent. Infiltration causes tissue irritation.
- Don't exceed 25 mg/minute.

INCOMPATIBILITIES

Allopurinol, amobarbital, amphotericin B, cefepime, dexamethasone, foscarnet, haloperidol lactate, pentobarbital, phenobarbital, phenytoin, thiopental.

ACTION

Competes with histamine for H_1-receptor sites. Prevents, but doesn't reverse, histamine-mediated responses, particularly those of the bronchial tubes, GI tract, uterus, and blood vessels. Structurally related to local anesthetics, drug provides local anesthesia and suppresses cough reflex.

Route	Onset	Peak	Duration
P.O.	15 min	1–4 hr	6–8 hr
I.V.	Immediate	1–4 hr	6–8 hr
I.M.	Unknown	1–4 hr	6–8 hr

Half-life: About 3½ hours.

ADVERSE REACTIONS

CNS: *drowsiness, sedation, sleepiness, dizziness, incoordination,* ***seizures,*** confusion, insomnia, headache, vertigo, fatigue, restlessness, tremor, nervousness.
CV: palpitations, hypotension, tachycardia.
EENT: diplopia, blurred vision, nasal congestion, tinnitus.
GI: *dry mouth, nausea, epigastric distress,* vomiting, diarrhea, constipation, anorexia.
GU: dysuria, urine retention, urinary frequency.
Hematologic: ***thrombocytopenia, agranulocytosis,*** hemolytic anemia.
Respiratory: *thickening of bronchial secretions.*
Skin: urticaria, photosensitivity, rash.
Other: ***anaphylactic shock.***

INTERACTIONS

Drug-drug. *CNS depressants:* May increase sedation. Use together cautiously.
MAO inhibitors: May increase anticholinergic effects. Avoid using together.
Other products that contain diphenhydramine (including topical therapy): May in-

crease risk of adverse reactions. Avoid using together.
Drug-lifestyle. *Alcohol use:* May increase CNS depression. Discourage use together.
Sun exposure: May cause photosensitivity reactions. Advise patient to avoid extensive sunlight exposure.

EFFECTS ON LAB TEST RESULTS
- May decrease hemoglobin level and hematocrit.
- May decrease granulocyte and platelet counts.
- May prevent, reduce, or mask positive result in diagnostic skin test.

CONTRAINDICATIONS & CAUTIONS
- Contraindicated in patients hypersensitive to drug; newborns; premature neonates; breast-feeding women; patients with angle-closure glaucoma, stenosing peptic ulcer, symptomatic prostatic hyperplasia, bladder neck obstruction, or pyloroduodenal obstruction; and those having an acute asthmatic attack.
- Avoid use in patients taking MAO inhibitors.
- Use with caution in patients with prostatic hyperplasia, asthma, COPD, increased intraocular pressure, hyperthyroidism, CV disease, and hypertension.
- Children younger than age 12 should use drug only as directed by prescriber.

NURSING CONSIDERATIONS
- Stop drug 4 days before diagnostic skin testing.
- Alternate injection sites to prevent irritation. Give I.M. injection deep into large muscle.
- Dizziness, excessive sedation, syncope, toxicity, paradoxical stimulation, and hypotension are more likely to occur in the elderly.
- ***Look alike–sound alike:*** Don't confuse diphenhydramine with dimenhydrinate; don't confuse Benadryl with Bentyl, or benazepril.

PATIENT TEACHING
- Warn patient not to take this drug with any other products that contain diphenhydramine (including topical therapy) because of increased adverse reactions.
- Instruct patient to take drug 30 minutes before travel to prevent motion sickness.
- Tell patient to take diphenhydramine with food or milk to reduce GI distress.
- Warn patient to avoid alcohol and hazardous activities that require alertness until CNS effects of drug are known.
- Tell patient that coffee or tea may reduce drowsiness. Urge caution if palpitations develop.
- Inform patient that sugarless gum, hard candy, or ice chips may relieve dry mouth.
- Tell patient to notify prescriber if tolerance develops because a different antihistamine may need to be prescribed.
- Drug is in many OTC sleep and cold products. Advise patient to consult prescriber before using these products.
- Warn patient of possible photosensitivity reactions. Advise use of a sunblock.

fexofenadine hydrochloride
Allegra✐, Telfast‡

Pharmacologic class: piperidine
Pregnancy risk category C

AVAILABLE FORMS
Capsules: 60 mg
Oral suspension: 30 mg/5 ml
Tablets: 30 mg, 60 mg, 120 mg‡, 180 mg

INDICATIONS & DOSAGES
➤ **Seasonal allergic rhinitis**
Adults and children age 12 and older: 60 mg P.O. b.i.d. or 180 mg P.O. once daily.
Children ages 2 to 11: Give 30 mg P.O. b.i.d. either as a tablet or 5-ml oral suspension.
➤ **Chronic idiopathic urticaria**
Adults and children age 12 and older: 60 mg P.O. b.i.d. or 180 mg P.O. once daily.
Children ages 2 to 11: Give 30 mg P.O. b.i.d. either as a tablet or 5-ml oral suspension.
Children ages 6 months to 2 years: 15 mg (2.5 ml) P.O. b.i.d.
Adjust-a-dose: For patients with impaired renal function or a need for dialysis, give adults 60 mg daily, children ages 2 to 11, 30 mg daily, and children ages 6 months to 2 years, 15 mg daily.

ACTION
A long-acting nonsedating antihistamine that selectively inhibits peripheral H_1 receptors.

Route	Onset	Peak	Duration
P.O.	Rapid	3 hr	14 hr

Half-life: 14½ hours.

ADVERSE REACTIONS
CNS: fatigue, drowsiness, headache.
GI: nausea, dyspepsia.
GU: dysmenorrhea.
Other: viral infection.

INTERACTIONS
Drug-drug. *Aluminum or magnesium antacids:* May decrease fexofenadine level. Separate dosage times.
Erythromycin, ketoconazole: May increase fexofenadine level. Monitor patient for side effects.
Drug-food. *Apple juice, grapefruit juice, orange juice:* May decrease drug effects. Patients should take drug with liquid other than these juices.
Drug-lifestyle. *Alcohol use:* May increase CNS depression. Discourage use together.

EFFECTS ON LAB TEST RESULTS
- May prevent, reduce, or mask positive result in diagnostic skin test.

CONTRAINDICATIONS & CAUTIONS
- Contraindicated in patients hypersensitive to drug or its components.
- Use cautiously in patients with impaired renal function.

NURSING CONSIDERATIONS
- Stop drug 4 days before patient undergoes diagnostic skin tests because drug can prevent, reduce, or mask positive skin test response.
- It's unknown if drug appears in breast milk; use caution when using drug in breast-feeding woman.

PATIENT TEACHING
- Instruct patient or parent not to exceed prescribed dosage and to use drug only when needed.
- Warn patient to avoid alcohol and hazardous activities that require alertness until CNS effects of drug are known. Explain that drug may cause drowsiness.
- Tell patient not to take antacids within 2 hours of this drug.
- Advise patient with dry mouth to try sugarless gum, hard candy, or ice chips.
- Tell parents to keep the oral solution in a cool, dry place, tightly closed, and to shake well before using.

loratadine
Alavert ◇, Claratyne‡, Clarinase‡, Claritin ◇, Claritin Reditabs ◇, Claritin Syrup ◇, Tavist ND Allergy ◇

Pharmacologic class: piperidine
Pregnancy risk category B

AVAILABLE FORMS
Syrup: 1 mg/ml ◇
Tablets: 10 mg ◇
Tablets (chewable): 5 mg
Tablets (rapidly disintegrating): 10 mg ◇

INDICATIONS & DOSAGES
➤Hay fever or other upper respiratory allergies; chronic idiopathic urticaria
Adults and children age 6 and older: 10 mg P.O. daily.
Children ages 2 to 5 years: 5 mg P.O. daily.
Adjust-a-dose: In adults and children age 6 and older with hepatic failure or creatinine clearance less than 30 ml/minute, give 10 mg every other day. In children ages 2 to 5 years with hepatic failure or renal insufficiency, give 5 mg every other day.

ACTION
Blocks effects of histamine at H_1-receptor sites. Drug is a nonsedating antihistamine; its chemical structure prevents entry into the CNS.

Route	Onset	Peak	Duration
P.O.	1–3 hr	8–10 hr	24 hr

Half-life: 8½ hours.

ADVERSE REACTIONS

CNS: *headache,* drowsiness, fatigue, insomnia, nervousness.
GI: dry mouth.

INTERACTIONS

Drug-drug. *Cimetidine, ketoconazole, macrolide antibiotics (clarithromycin, erythromycin, troleandomycin):* May increase loratadine level. Monitor patient closely.
Drug-lifestyle. *Alcohol use:* May increase CNS depression. Discourage use together.

EFFECTS ON LAB TEST RESULTS

- May prevent, reduce, or mask positive result in diagnostic skin test.

CONTRAINDICATIONS & CAUTIONS

- Contraindicated in patients hypersensitive to drug.
- Use cautiously in patients with hepatic or renal impairment and in breast-feeding women.

NURSING CONSIDERATIONS

- Stop drug 4 days before patient undergoes diagnostic skin tests because drug can prevent, reduce, or mask positive skin test response.

PATIENT TEACHING

- Make sure patient understands to take drug once daily. If symptoms persist or worsen, tell him to contact prescriber.
- Tell patient taking Claritin Reditabs to use tablet immediately after opening individual blister.
- Advise patient taking Claritin Reditabs to place tablet on the tongue, where it disintegrates within a few seconds. It can be swallowed with or without water.
- Warn patient to avoid alcohol and hazardous activities that require alertness until CNS effects of drug are known.
- Tell patient that dry mouth can be relieved with sugarless gum, hard candy, or ice chips.

promethazine hydrochloride

Phenadoz, Phenergan*

Pharmacologic class: phenothiazine derivative
Pregnancy risk category C

AVAILABLE FORMS

Injection: 25 mg/ml, 50 mg/ml
Suppositories: 12.5 mg, 25 mg, 50 mg
Syrup: 6.25 mg/5 ml*
Tablets: 12.5 mg, 25 mg, 50 mg

INDICATIONS & DOSAGES

➤ Motion sickness
Adults: 25 mg P.O. or P.R. taken 30 minutes to 1 hour before departure. May repeat dose 8 to 12 hours later, if needed.
Children older than age 2: 12.5 to 25 mg P.O. or P.R. 30 minutes to 1 hour before departure. May repeat dose 8 to 12 hours later, if needed.
➤ Nausea and vomiting
Adults: 12.5 to 25 mg P.O., I.M., or P.R. q 4 to 6 hours, p.r.n.
Children older than age 2: 12.5 to 25 mg P.O. or P.R. q 4 to 6 hours, p.r.n. Or, 6.25 to 12.5 mg I.M. q 4 to 6 hours, p.r.n.
➤ Rhinitis, allergy symptoms
Adults: 12.5 mg P.O. or P.R. q.i.d.; or 25 mg P.O. or P.R. at bedtime.
Children older than age 2: 6.25 to 12.5 mg P.O. or P.R. t.i.d., or 25 mg P.O. or P.R. at bedtime.
➤ Nighttime sedation
Adults: 25 to 50 mg P.O., I.V., I.M., or P.R. at bedtime.
Children older than age 2: 12.5 to 25 mg P.O., I.M., or P.R. at bedtime.
➤ Adjunct to analgesics for routine preoperative or postoperative sedation
Adults: 25 to 50 mg I.V. or I.M., or 25 to 50 mg P.O. or P.R.
Children older than age 2: 0.5 to 1.1 mg/kg P.O., I.M., or P.R.

I.V. ADMINISTRATION

- If solution is discolored or contains a precipitate, discard.
- Give injection through a free-flowing I.V. line.
- Don't give at a concentration above 25 mg/ml or a rate above 25 mg/minute.

INCOMPATIBILITIES

Aldesleukin, allopurinol, aminophylline, amphotericin B, cephalosporins, chloramphenicol sodium succinate, chloroquine phosphate, chlorothiazide, diatrizoate, dimenhydrinate, doxorubicin liposomal, foscarnet, furosemide, heparin sodium, hydrocortisone sodium succinate, iodipamide meglumine (52%), iothalamate, ketorolac, methohexital, morphine, nalbuphine, penicillin G potassium and sodium, pentobarbital sodium, phenobarbital sodium, phenytoin sodium, thiopental, vitamin B complex.

ACTION

Phenothiazine derivative that competes with histamine for H_1-receptor sites on effector cells. Prevents, but doesn't reverse, histamine-mediated responses. At high doses, drug also has local anesthetic effects.

Route	Onset	Peak	Duration
P.O.	15–60 min	Unknown	< 12 hr
I.V.	3–5 min	Unknown	< 12 hr
I.M., P.R.	20 min	Unknown	< 12 hr

Half-life: Unknown.

ADVERSE REACTIONS

CNS: *drowsiness, sedation,* confusion, sleepiness, dizziness, disorientation, extrapyramidal symptoms.
CV: hypotension, hypertension.
EENT: *dry mouth,* blurred vision.
GI: nausea, vomiting.
GU: urine retention.
Hematologic: ***leukopenia, agranulocytosis, thrombocytopenia.***
Metabolic: hyperglycemia.
Respiratory: ***respiratory depression, apnea.***
Skin: photosensitivity, rash.

INTERACTIONS

Drug-drug. *Anticholinergics, tricyclic antidepressants:* May increase anticholinergic effects. Avoid using together.
CNS depressants: May increase sedation. Use together cautiously.
Epinephrine: May block or reverse effects of epinephrine. Use other pressor drugs instead.
Levodopa: May decrease antiparkinsonian action of levodopa. Avoid using together.
Lithium: May reduce GI absorption or enhance renal elimination of lithium. Avoid using together.
MAO inhibitors: May increase extrapyramidal effects. Avoid using together.
Quinolones: May cause life-threatening arrhythmias. Avoid using together.
Drug-herb. *Yohimbe:* May increase risk of herb toxicity. Ask patient about use of herbal remedies, and recommend caution.
Drug-lifestyle. *Alcohol use:* May increase sedation. Discourage use together.
Sun exposure: May cause photosensitivity reactions. Advise patient to avoid extensive sunlight exposure and to use sunblock.

EFFECTS ON LAB TEST RESULTS

- May increase hemoglobin level and hematocrit.
- May decrease WBC, platelet, and granulocyte counts.
- May prevent, reduce, or mask positive result in diagnostic skin test. May cause false-positive or false-negative pregnancy test result. May interfere with blood grouping in the ABO system.

CONTRAINDICATIONS & CAUTIONS

- Contraindicated in patients hypersensitive to drug, those who have experienced adverse reactions to phenothiazines, breast-feeding women, children younger than age 2, and acutely ill or dehydrated children.
- Use cautiously in patients with asthma or pulmonary, hepatic, or CV disease and in those with intestinal obstruction, prostatic hyperplasia, bladder-neck obstruction, angle-closure glaucoma, seizure disorders, coma, CNS depression, and stenosing or peptic ulcerations.

NURSING CONSIDERATIONS

- Monitor patient for neuroleptic malignant syndrome: altered mental status, autonomic instability, muscle rigidity, and hyperpyrexia.
- Stop drug 4 days before diagnostic skin testing because antihistamines can prevent, reduce, or mask positive skin test response.

- Drug is used as an adjunct to analgesics, usually to increase sedation; it has no analgesic activity.
- Reduce GI distress by giving drug with food or milk.
- I.M. injection is the preferred parenteral route. Inject deep I.M. into large muscle mass. Rotate injection sites.
- ***Alert:*** Don't give subcutaneously.
- Drug may be mixed with meperidine in same syringe.
- In patients scheduled for a myelogram, stop drug 48 hours before procedure. Don't resume drug until 24 hours after procedure because of the risk of seizures.
- ***Look alike–sound alike:*** Don't confuse promethazine with promazine.

PATIENT TEACHING

- Tell patient to take oral form with food or milk.
- When treating motion sickness, tell patient to take first dose 30 to 60 minutes before travel; dose may be repeated in 8 to 12 hours if necessary. On succeeding days of travel, patient should take dose upon arising and with evening meal.
- Warn patient to avoid alcohol and hazardous activities that require alertness until CNS effects of drug are known.
- Inform patient that sugarless gum, hard candy, or ice chips may relieve dry mouth.
- Warn patient about possible photosensitivity reactions. Advise use of a sunblock.

41

Bronchodilators

albuterol sulfate
arformoterol tartrate
atropine sulfate
(See Chapter 19, ANTIARRHYTHMICS.)
ephedrine sulfate
epinephrine
epinephrine bitartrate
epinephrine hydrochloride
formoterol fumarate inhalation powder
ipratropium bromide
isoproterenol hydrochloride
levalbuterol hydrochloride
pirbuterol acetate
salmeterol xinafoate
terbutaline sulfate
theophylline
tiotropium bromide

albuterol sulfate

AccuNeb, Proventil, Proventil HFA, Ventolin, Ventolin HFA, VoSpire ER

Pharmacologic class: adrenergic
Pregnancy risk category C

AVAILABLE FORMS

Solution for inhalation: 0.083%, 0.5%, 0.63 mg/ml, 1.25 mg/3 ml
Syrup: 2 mg/5 ml
Tablets: 2 mg, 4 mg
Tablets (extended-release): 4 mg, 8 mg

INDICATIONS & DOSAGES

➤ To prevent or treat bronchospasm in patients with reversible obstructive airway disease

Tablets (extended-release)
Adults and children age 12 and older: 4 to 8 mg P.O. q 12 hours. Maximum, 16 mg b.i.d.
Children ages 6 to 12: 4 mg P.O. q 12 hours. Maximum, 12 mg b.i.d.

Tablets
Adults and children age 12 and older: 2 to 4 mg P.O. t.i.d. or q.i.d. Maximum, 8 mg q.i.d.
Children ages 6 to 12: 2 mg P.O. t.i.d. or q.i.d. Maximum, 6 mg q.i.d.

Solution for inhalation
Adults and children age 12 and older: 2.5 mg t.i.d. or q.i.d. by nebulizer, given over 5 to 15 minutes. To prepare solution, use 0.5 ml of 0.5% solution diluted with 2.5 ml of normal saline solution. Or, use 3 ml of 0.083% solution.
Children ages 2 to 12: Initially, 0.1 to 0.15 mg/kg by nebulizer given over 5 to 15 minutes, with subsequent doses adjusted to response. Don't exceed 2.5 mg t.i.d. or q.i.d. by nebulization.

Syrup
Adults and children older than age 12: 2 to 4 mg (1 to 2 tsp) P.O. t.i.d. or q.i.d. Maximum, 8 mg q.i.d.
Children ages 6 to 12: 2 mg (1 tsp) P.O. t.i.d. or q.i.d. Maximum, 24 mg daily in divided doses.
Children ages 2 to 6: Initially, 0.1 mg/kg P.O. t.i.d. Starting dose shouldn't exceed 2 mg (1 tsp) t.i.d. Maximum, 4 mg (2 tsp) t.i.d.

Adjust-a-dose: For elderly patients and those sensitive to sympathomimetic amines, 2 mg P.O. t.i.d. or q.i.d. as oral tablets or syrup. Maximum, 8 mg t.i.d. or q.i.d.

➤ To prevent exercise-induced bronchospasm

Adults and children age 4 and older: 2 inhalations using the metered-dose inhaler (MDI) 15 minutes before exercise; up to 12 inhalations may be taken in 24 hours.

ACTION

Relaxes bronchial, uterine, and vascular smooth muscle by stimulating $beta_2$ receptors.

Route	Onset	Peak	Duration
P.O.	15–30 min	2–3 hr	6–12 hr
P.O. (extended)	Unknown	Unknown	12 hr
Inhalation	5–15 min	30–120 min	2–6 hr

Half-life: About 4 hours.

ADVERSE REACTIONS

CNS: *tremor, nervousness, headache, hyperactivity,* insomnia, dizziness, weakness, CNS stimulation, malaise.
CV: *tachycardia, palpitations,* hypertension.
EENT: dry and irritated nose and throat with inhaled form, nasal congestion, epistaxis, hoarseness.
GI: *nausea, vomiting,* heartburn, anorexia, altered taste, increased appetite.
Metabolic: hypokalemia.
Musculoskeletal: muscle cramps.
Respiratory: ***bronchospasm,*** cough, wheezing, dyspnea, bronchitis, increased sputum.
Other: hypersensitivity reactions.

INTERACTIONS

Drug-drug. *CNS stimulants:* May increase CNS stimulation. Avoid using together.
Digoxin: May decrease digoxin level. Monitor digoxin level closely.
MAO inhibitors, tricyclic antidepressants: May increase adverse CV effects. Monitor patient closely.
Propranolol and other beta blockers: May cause mutual antagonism. Monitor patient carefully.

EFFECTS ON LAB TEST RESULTS

- May decrease potassium level.

CONTRAINDICATIONS & CAUTIONS

- Contraindicated in patients hypersensitive to drug or its ingredients.
- Use cautiously in patients with CV disorders (including coronary insufficiency and hypertension), hyperthyroidism, or diabetes mellitus and in those who are unusually responsive to adrenergics.
- Use extended-release tablets cautiously in patients with GI narrowing.

NURSING CONSIDERATIONS

- Drug may decrease sensitivity of spirometry used for diagnosis of asthma.
- When switching patient from regular to extended-release tablets, remember that a regular 2-mg tablet every 6 hours is equivalent to an extended-release 4-mg tablet every 12 hours.
- Syrup contains no alcohol or sugar and may be taken by children as young as age 2.
- In children, syrup may rarely cause erythema multiforme or Stevens-Johnson syndrome.
- The HFA form uses the propellant hydrofluroalkane (HFA) instead of chlorofluorocarbons.
- ***Alert:*** Patient may use tablets and aerosol together. Monitor these patients closely for signs and symptoms of toxicity.
- ***Look alike–sound alike:*** Don't confuse albuterol with atenolol or Albutein.

PATIENT TEACHING

- Warn patient about risk of paradoxical bronchospasm and to stop drug immediately if it occurs.
- Teach patient to perform oral inhalation correctly. Give the following instructions for using the MDI:
  - Shake the inhaler.
  - Clear nasal passages and throat.
  - Breathe out, expelling as much air from lungs as possible.
  - Place mouthpiece well into mouth, seal lips around mouthpiece, and inhale deeply as you release a dose from inhaler. Or, hold inhaler about 1 inch (two finger-widths) from open mouth; inhale while dose is released.
  - Hold breath for several seconds, remove mouthpiece, and exhale slowly.
- If prescriber orders more than 1 inhalation, tell patient to wait at least 2 minutes before repeating procedure.
- Tell patient that use of a spacer device may improve drug delivery to lungs.
- If patient is also using a corticosteroid inhaler, instruct him to use the bronchodilator first and then to wait about 5 minutes before using the corticosteroid. This lets the bronchodilator open the air passages for maximum effectiveness of the corticosteroid.
- Tell patient to remove canister and wash inhaler with warm, soapy water at least once a week.
- Advise patient not to chew or crush extended-release tablets or mix them with food.

✱ NEW DRUG

arformoterol tartrate
Brovana

Pharmacologic class: long-acting selective $beta_2$ agonist.
Pregnancy risk category C

AVAILABLE FORMS
Solution for inhalation: 15 mcg/2 ml vials

INDICATIONS & DOSAGES
➤ **Long-term maintenance treatment of bronchoconstriction in patients with COPD, including chronic bronchitis and emphysema**
Adults: 15 mcg, inhaled b.i.d. (morning and evening) via nebulizer.

ACTION
Relaxes bronchial and cardiac smooth muscle by acting on $beta_2$ adrenergic receptors; stimulates the enzyme adenyl cyclase which catalyzes the conversion from ATP to cAMP. This further relaxes bronchial smooth muscle and inhibits release of mediators (such as histamine and leukotrienes) from mast cells.

Route	Onset	Peak	Duration
Inhalation	Rapid	30 min	Unknown

Half-life: 26 hours.

ADVERSE REACTIONS
CV: *chest pain,* ***AV block, atrial flutter, heart failure, MI, prolonged QT interval, supraventricular tachycardia, inverted T-wave,*** peripheral edema.
EENT: sinusitis.
GI: diarrhea.
Metabolic: ***hypoglycemia, hypokalemia.***
Musculoskeletal: back pain, leg cramps.
Respiratory: dyspnea, pulmonary or congestion, ***bronchospasm.***
Skin: rash.
Other: ***hypersensitivity reaction,*** *pain,* flu syndrome.

INTERACTIONS
Drug-drug. *Aminophylline, corticosteroids (such as dexamethasone, prednisone), theophylline:* May increase the risk for hypokalemia. Monitor patient's potassium level.
Beta blockers (such as metoprolol, atenolol): May decrease effectiveness of arformoterol and increase risk of bronchospasm. Avoid use together, if possible; otherwise, use with extreme caution.
Non-potassium sparing diuretics (such as furosemide, hydrochlorothiazide): May increase the risk of hypokalemia and ECG changes. Use cautiously together and monitor patient's ECG and potassium level.
Other $beta_2$ adrenergics (such as albuterol, formoterol): May cause additive effects. Avoid use together.
QT interval–prolonging drugs (such as MAO inhibitors, tricyclic antidepressants): May increase risk of ventricular arrhythmias. Use cautiously together.

EFFECTS ON LAB TEST RESULTS
- May increase PSA levels. May decrease potassium levels. May increase or decrease glucose levels.

CONTRAINDICATIONS & CAUTIONS
- Contraindicated in patients hypersensitive to drug, formoterol, or any other components of this drug.
- Don't use in patients with acutely deteriorating COPD.
- Use cautiously in patients with seizure disorder, thyrotoxicosis, hepatic insufficiency, preexisting cardiovascular disease, including coronary insufficiency, arrhythmias and hypertension; or in those unresponsive to sympathomimetic amines.

NURSING CONSIDERATIONS
- Don't mix with other drugs in the nebulizer.
- Drug may increase the risk of asthma-related death.
- Drug is twice as potent as formoterol inhaler.
- ***Alert:*** Be sure patient has a rescue inhaler, such as albuterol, to treat an acute asthma attack or bronchospasm.
- ***Alert:*** Notify prescriber if patient experiences decreasing control of symptoms or begins using his short-acting $beta_2$ agonist more often.
- If paradoxical bronchospasm occurs, stop drug immediately.

• Monitor blood pressure, pulse and ECG, as indicated.

PATIENT TEACHING

• Tell patient to store vials in the foil pouches in the refrigerator and use immediately after opening.
• Tell patient to use only the recommended nebulizer and compressor for treatment and not to mix drug with other inhaled drugs or solutions.
• ***Alert:*** Warn patient that drug is for maintenance treatment only and shouldn't be used to stop an asthma attack or bronchospasm. For emergency treatment, use a short-acting rescue inhaler, such as albuterol.
• Educate patient using a short-acting bronchodilator on a scheduled basis to stop scheduled use and use only for rescue therapy.
• ***Alert:*** Warn patient that serious adverse effects, including death, can occur at higher than recommended doses and not to take more inhalations than prescribed.
• Tell patient to stop drug immediately and obtain medical help if life-threatening bronchospasm, severe rash, or swelling in throat occurs.
• Inform patient that he may experience palpitations, chest pain, rapid heart beat, tremors, or nervousness.
• Tell patient not to swallow the inhalation solution.
• Caution patient to notify prescriber if he notices a decrease in symptom control or more frequent use of his rescue inhaler.

SAFETY ALERT!

ephedrine sulfate

Pharmacologic class: adrenergic
Pregnancy risk category C

AVAILABLE FORMS

Capsules: 25 mg, 50 mg
Injection: 25 mg/ml, 50 mg/ml

INDICATIONS & DOSAGES

➤ **Bronchodilation**

Adults and children older than age 12: 12.5 to 25 mg P.O. q 4 hours, p.r.n., not to exceed 150 mg in 24 hours.
Children age 2 to 12: 2 to 3 mg/kg or 100 mg/m^2 P.O. daily in four to six divided doses. Or, for children ages 6 to 12, 6.25 to 12.5 mg P.O. q 4 hours, not to exceed 75 mg in 24 hours.

➤ **Hypotension**

Adults: 25 mg P.O. once daily to q.i.d. Or, 5 to 25 mg I.V., p.r.n., to maximum of 150 mg/24 hours. Or, 25 to 50 mg I.M. or subcutaneously.
Children: 3 mg/kg P.O. or 0.5 mg/kg or 16.7 mg/m^2 subcutaneously or I.M. q 4 to 6 hours.

I.V. ADMINISTRATION

• Drug is compatible with most common solutions.
• Give slowly by direct injection.
• If needed, repeat in 5 to 10 minutes.

INCOMPATIBILITIES

Fructose 10% in normal saline solution; hydrocortisone sodium succinate; Ionosol B, D-CM, and D solutions; pentobarbital sodium; phenobarbital sodium; thiopental.

ACTION

Relaxes bronchial smooth muscle by stimulating beta$_2$ receptors; also stimulates alpha and beta receptors and is a direct- and indirect-acting sympathomimetic.

Route	Onset	Peak	Duration
P.O.	15–60 min	Unknown	3–5 hr
I.V.	5 min	Unknown	60 min
I.M., SubQ	10–20 min	Unknown	30–60 min

Half-life: 3 to 6 hours.

ADVERSE REACTIONS

CNS: *insomnia, nervousness,* ***cerebral hemorrhage,*** dizziness, headache, muscle weakness, euphoria, confusion, delirium, tremor.
CV: *palpitations,* ***arrhythmias,*** tachycardia, hypertension, precordial pain.
EENT: dry nose and throat.
GI: nausea, vomiting, anorexia.
GU: urine retention, painful urination from visceral sphincter spasm.
Skin: diaphoresis.

INTERACTIONS

Drug-drug. *Acetazolamide:* May increase ephedrine level. Monitor patient for toxicity.
Alpha blockers: May reduce vasopressor response. Monitor patient closely.
Antihypertensives: May decrease effects. Monitor blood pressure.
Beta blockers: May block the effects of ephedrine. Monitor patient closely.
Cardiac glycosides, general anesthetics (halogenated hydrocarbons): May increase risk of ventricular arrhythmias. Monitor ECG closely.
Guanethidine: May decrease pressor effects of ephedrine. Monitor patient closely.
MAO inhibitors (phenelzine, tranylcypromine): May cause severe headache, hypertension, fever, and hypertensive crisis. Avoid using together.
Methyldopa, reserpine: May inhibit ephedrine effects. Use together cautiously.
Oxytocics: May cause severe hypertension. Avoid using together.
Tricyclic antidepressants: May decrease pressor response. Monitor patient closely.

EFFECTS ON LAB TEST RESULTS

None reported.

CONTRAINDICATIONS & CAUTIONS

- Contraindicated in patients hypersensitive to ephedrine and other sympathomimetics and in those with porphyria, severe coronary artery disease, arrhythmias, angle-closure glaucoma, psychoneurosis, angina pectoris, substantial organic heart disease, or CV disease.
- Contraindicated in those receiving MAO inhibitors or general anesthesia with cyclopropane or halothane.
- Use with caution in elderly patients and in those with hypertension, hyperthyroidism, nervous or excitable states, diabetes, or prostatic hyperplasia.

NURSING CONSIDERATIONS

- ***Alert:*** Hypoxia, hypercapnia, and acidosis must be identified and corrected before or during therapy because they may reduce effectiveness or increase adverse reactions.
- Drug isn't a substitute for blood or fluid volume replenishment. Volume deficit must be corrected before giving vasopressors.
- To prevent insomnia, avoid giving drug within 2 hours of bedtime.
- Effectiveness decreases after 2 to 3 weeks as tolerance develops. Prescriber may increase dosage. Drug isn't addictive.
- In children younger than age 12, use only under direction of prescriber.
- ***Look alike–sound alike:*** Don't confuse ephedrine with epinephrine.

PATIENT TEACHING

- Tell patient taking oral form of drug at home to take last dose of day at least 2 hours before bedtime.
- Warn patient not to take OTC drugs or herbs that contain ephedrine without consulting prescriber.

SAFETY ALERT!

epinephrine (adrenaline)

Bronkaid Mistometer†, Primatene Mist ◊

epinephrine bitartrate

AsthmaHaler Mist ◊, Primatene Mist*

epinephrine hydrochloride

Adrenalin Chloride, AsthmaNefrin ◊, EpiPen, EpiPen Jr, Nephron ◊, Vaponefrin

Pharmacologic class: adrenergic
Pregnancy risk category C

AVAILABLE FORMS

Aerosol inhaler: 160 mcg ◊, 200 mcg ◊, 220 mcg ◊
Injection: 0.01 mg/ml (1:100,000), 0.1 mg/ml (1:10,000), 0.5 mg/ml (1:2,000), 1 mg/ml (1:1,000) parenteral; 5 mg/ml (1:200) parenteral suspension
Nebulizer inhaler: 1% (1:100)† ◊, 1.25%† ◊, 2.25%† ◊

INDICATIONS & DOSAGES

➤ **Bronchospasm, hypersensitivity reactions, anaphylaxis**
Adults: 0.1 to 0.5 ml of 1:1,000 solution I.M. or subcutaneously. Repeat q 10 to 15 minutes, p.r.n. Or, 0.1 to 0.25 ml of 1:1,000 solution I.V. slowly over 5 to

10 minutes (1 to 2.5 ml of a commercially available 1:10,000 injection or of a 1:10,000 dilution prepared by diluting 1 ml of a commercially available 1:1,000 injection with 10 ml of water for injection or normal saline solution for injection). May repeat q 5 to 15 minutes, p.r.n., or follow with a continuous I.V. infusion, starting at 1 mcg/minute and increasing to 4 mcg/minute, p.r.n.
Children: 0.01 ml/kg (10 mcg) of 1:1,000 solution subcutaneously; repeat q 20 minutes to 4 hours, p.r.n. Maximum single dose shouldn't exceed 0.5 mg.

➤ **Hemostasis**
Adults: 1:50,000 to 1:1,000, sprayed or applied topically.

➤ **Acute asthma attacks**
Adults and children age 4 and older: One inhalation, repeated once if needed after at least 1 minute; don't give subsequent doses for at least 3 hours. Or, 1 to 3 deep inhalations using a hand-bulb nebulizer containing 1% (1:100) solution of epinephrine or 2.25% solution of racepinephrine, repeated q 3 hours, p.r.n.

➤ **To prolong local anesthetic effect**
Adults and children: With local anesthetics, may be used in concentrations of 1:500,000 to 1:50,000; most commonly, 1:200,000.

➤ **To restore cardiac rhythm in cardiac arrest**
Adults: 0.5 to 1 mg I.V., repeated q 3 to 5 minutes, if needed. A higher dose may be used if 1 mg fails: 3 to 5 mg (about 0.1 mg/kg); repeat q 3 to 5 minutes.
Children: 0.01 mg/kg (0.1 ml/kg of 1:10,000 injection) I.V. First endotracheal dose is 0.1 mg/kg (0.1 ml/kg of a 1:1,000 injection) diluted in 1 to 2 ml of half-normal or normal saline solution. Give subsequent I.V. or intratracheal doses from 0.1 to 0.2 mg/kg (0.1 to 0.2 ml/kg of a 1:1,000 injection), repeated q 3 to 5 minutes, if needed.

I.V. ADMINISTRATION

- Keep solution in light-resistant container, and don't remove before use.
- Just before use, mix with D_5W, normal saline solution for injection, lactated Ringer injection, or combinations of dextrose in saline solution.
- Monitor blood pressure, heart rate, and ECG when therapy starts and frequently thereafter.
- Discard solution if it's discolored or contains precipitate or after 24 hours.

INCOMPATIBILITIES

Aminophylline; ampicillin sodium; furosemide; hyaluronidase; Ionosol D-CM, PSL, and T solutions with D_5W; mephentermine; thiopental sodium. Compatible with most other I.V. solutions. Rapidly destroyed by alkalies or oxidizing drugs, including halogens, nitrates, nitrites, permanganates, sodium bicarbonate, and salts of easily reducible metals, such as iron, copper, and zinc. Don't mix with alkaline solutions.

ACTION

Relaxes bronchial smooth muscle by stimulating $beta_2$ receptors and alpha and beta receptors in the sympathetic nervous system.

Route	Onset	Peak	Duration
I.V.	Immediate	5 min	Short
I.M.	Variable	Unknown	1–4 hr
SubQ	5–15 min	30 min	1–4 hr
Inhalation	1–5 min	Unknown	1–3 hr

Half-life: Unknown.

ADVERSE REACTIONS

CNS: *drowsiness, headache, nervousness, tremor,* ***cerebral hemorrhage, stroke,*** vertigo, pain, disorientation, agitation, fear, dizziness, weakness.
CV: *palpitations,* ***ventricular fibrillation, shock,*** widened pulse pressure, hypertension, tachycardia, anginal pain, altered ECG (including a decreased T-wave amplitude).
GI: *nausea, vomiting.*
Respiratory: dyspnea.
Skin: urticaria, hemorrhage at injection site, pallor.
Other: tissue necrosis.

INTERACTIONS

Drug-drug. *Alpha blockers:* May cause hypotension from unopposed beta-adrenergic effects. Avoid using together.
Antihistamines, thyroid hormones: When given with sympathomimetics, may cause

severe adverse cardiac effects. Avoid using together.
Cardiac glycosides, general anesthetics (halogenated hydrocarbons): May increase risk of ventricular arrhythmias. Monitor ECG closely.
Carteolol, nadolol, penbutolol, pindolol, propranolol, timolol: May cause hypertension followed by bradycardia. Stop beta blocker 3 days before starting epinephrine.
Doxapram, methylphenidate: May enhance CNS stimulation or pressor effects. Monitor patient closely.
Ergot alkaloids: May decrease vasoconstrictor activity. Monitor patient closely.
Guanadrel, guanethidine: May enhance pressor effects of epinephrine. Monitor patient closely.
Levodopa: May enhance risk of arrhythmias. Monitor ECG closely.
MAO inhibitors: May increase risk of hypertensive crisis. Monitor blood pressure closely.
Tricyclic antidepressants: May potentiate the pressor response and cause arrhythmias. Use together cautiously.

EFFECTS ON LAB TEST RESULTS
- May increase BUN, glucose, and lactic acid levels.

CONTRAINDICATIONS & CAUTIONS
- Contraindicated in patients with angle-closure glaucoma, shock (other than anaphylactic shock), organic brain damage, cardiac dilation, arrhythmias, coronary insufficiency, or cerebral arteriosclerosis.
- Contraindicated in patients receiving general anesthesia with halogenated hydrocarbons or cyclopropane and in patients in labor (may delay second stage).
- Commercial products containing sulfites contraindicated in patients with sulfite allergies, except when epinephrine is being used to treat serious allergic reactions or other emergency situations.
- Contraindicated for use in fingers, toes, ears, nose, or genitalia when used with local anesthetic.
- Use cautiously in patients with long-standing bronchial asthma or emphysema who have developed degenerative heart disease.
- Use cautiously in elderly patients and in those with hyperthyroidism, CV disease, hypertension, psychoneurosis, and diabetes.

NURSING CONSIDERATIONS
- In patients with Parkinson disease, drug increases rigidity and tremor.
- Drug interferes with tests for urinary catecholamines.
- One mg equals 1 ml of 1:1,000 solution or 10 ml of 1:10,000 solution.
- Epinephrine is drug of choice in emergency treatment of acute anaphylactic reactions.
- ***Alert:*** Avoid I.M. use of parenteral suspension into buttocks. Gas gangrene may occur because drug reduces oxygen tension of the tissues, encouraging growth of contaminating organisms.
- Massage site after I.M. injection to counteract vasoconstriction. Repeated local injection can cause necrosis at injection site.
- Observe patient closely for adverse reactions. Notify prescriber if adverse reactions develop; adjusting dosage or stopping drug may be necessary.
- If blood pressure increases sharply, give rapid-acting vasodilators, such as nitrates and alpha blockers, to counteract the marked pressor effect of large doses.
- Drug is rapidly destroyed by oxidizing products, such as iodine, chromates, nitrites, oxygen, and salts of easily reducible metals (such as iron).
- ***Look alike–sound alike:*** Don't confuse epinephrine with ephedrine or norepinephrine.
- When treating patient with reactions caused by other drugs given I.M. or subcutaneously, inject this drug into the site where the other drug was given to minimize further absorption.

PATIENT TEACHING
- Teach patient to perform oral inhalation correctly. Give the following instructions for using a metered-dose inhaler:
  - Shake canister.
  - Clear nasal passages and throat.
  - Breathe out, expelling as much air from lungs as possible.
  - Place mouthpiece well into mouth, and inhale deeply as you release dose from inhaler. Or, hold inhaler about 1 inch (two

fingerwidths) from open mouth, and inhale while releasing dose.
– Hold breath for several seconds, remove mouthpiece, and exhale slowly.
- If more than one inhalation is prescribed, advise patient to wait at least 2 minutes before repeating procedure.
- Tell patient that use of a spacer device may improve drug delivery to lungs.
- If patient is also using a corticosteroid inhaler, instruct him to use the bronchodilator first and then to wait about 5 minutes before using the corticosteroid. This lets the bronchodilator open the air passages for maximal effectiveness.
- Instruct patient to remove canister and wash inhaler with warm, soapy water at least once weekly.
- If patient has acute hypersensitivity reactions (such as to bee stings), you may need to teach him to self-inject drug.

formoterol fumarate inhalation powder

Foradil Aerolizer

Pharmacologic class: selective $beta_2$-adrenergic agonist
Pregnancy risk category C

AVAILABLE FORMS

Capsules for inhalation: 12 mcg

INDICATIONS & DOSAGES

➤ **Maintenance treatment and prevention of bronchospasm in patients with reversible obstructive airway disease or nocturnal asthma, who usually require treatment with short-acting inhaled $beta_2$ agonists**
Adults and children age 5 and older: One 12-mcg capsule by inhalation via Aerolizer inhaler q 12 hours. Total daily dosage shouldn't exceed 1 capsule b.i.d. (24 mcg/day). If symptoms occur between doses, use a short-acting $beta_2$ agonist for immediate relief.

➤ **To prevent exercise-induced bronchospasm**
Adults and children age 5 and older: One 12-mcg capsule by inhalation via Aerolizer inhaler at least 15 minutes before exercise, p.r.n. Don't give additional doses within 12 hours of first dose.

ACTION

Long-acting selective $beta_2$ agonist that causes bronchodilation. It ultimately increases cAMP, leading to relaxation of bronchial smooth muscle and inhibition of mediator release from mast cells.

Route	Onset	Peak	Duration
Inhalation	15 min	1–3 hr	12 hr

Half-life: Unknown.

ADVERSE REACTIONS

CNS: tremor, dizziness, insomnia, nervousness, headache, fatigue, malaise.
CV: ***arrhythmias,*** chest pain, angina, hypertension, hypotension, tachycardia, palpitations.
EENT: dry mouth, tonsillitis, dysphonia.
GI: nausea.
Metabolic: ***metabolic acidosis,*** hypokalemia, hyperglycemia.
Musculoskeletal: muscle cramps.
Respiratory: bronchitis, chest infection, dyspnea.
Skin: rash.
Other: viral infection.

INTERACTIONS

Drug-drug. *Adrenergics:* May potentiate sympathetic effects of formoterol. Use together cautiously.
Beta blockers: May antagonize effects of beta agonists, causing bronchospasm in asthmatic patients. Avoid use except when benefit outweighs risks. Use cardioselective beta blockers with caution to minimize risk of bronchospasm.
Diuretics, steroids, xanthine derivatives: May increase hypokalemic effect of formoterol. Use together cautiously.
MAO inhibitors, tricyclic antidepressants, other drugs that prolong QT interval: May increase risk of ventricular arrhythmias. Use together cautiously.
Non–potassium-sparing diuretics, such as loop or thiazide diuretics: May worsen ECG changes or hypokalemia. Use together cautiously, and monitor patient for toxicity.

EFFECTS ON LAB TEST RESULTS

- May increase glucose level. May decrease potassium level.

CONTRAINDICATIONS & CAUTIONS

• Contraindicated in patients hypersensitive to drug or its components.
• Use cautiously in patients with CV disease, especially coronary insufficiency, cardiac arrhythmias, and hypertension, and in those who are unusually responsive to sympathomimetic amines.
• Use cautiously in patients with diabetes mellitus because hyperglycemia and ketoacidosis have occurred rarely with the use of beta agonists.
• Use cautiously in patients with seizure disorders or thyrotoxicosis and in breast-feeding women.

NURSING CONSIDERATIONS

• Drug isn't indicated for patients who can control asthma symptoms with just occasional use of inhaled, short-acting beta$_2$ agonists or for treatment of acute bronchospasm requiring immediate reversal with short-acting beta$_2$ agonists or in patients with rapidly deteriorating or significantly worsening asthma.
• Drug may be used along with short-acting beta agonists, inhaled corticosteroids, and theophylline therapy for asthma management.
• ***Alert:*** Drug isn't a substitute for short-acting beta$_2$ agonists for immediate relief of bronchospasm or as substitute for inhaled or oral corticosteroids.
• Patients using drug twice daily shouldn't take additional doses to prevent exercise-induced bronchospasm.
• For patients formerly using regularly scheduled short-acting beta$_2$ agonists, decrease use of the short-acting drug to an as-needed basis when starting long-acting formoterol.
• ***Alert:*** As with all beta$_2$ agonists, drug may produce life-threatening paradoxical bronchospasm. If bronchospasm occurs, notify prescriber immediately.
• ***Alert:*** If patient develops tachycardia, hypertension, or other CV adverse effects, drug may need to be stopped.
• Watch for immediate hypersensitivity reactions, such as anaphylaxis, urticaria, angioedema, rash, and bronchospasm.
• Give Foradil capsules only by oral inhalation and only with the Aerolizer inhaler. They aren't for oral ingestion. Patient shouldn't exhale into the device. Capsules should remain in the unopened blister until administration time and only be removed immediately before use.
• Pierce capsules only once. In rare instances, the gelatin capsule may break into small pieces and get delivered to the mouth or throat upon inhalation. The Aerolizer contains a screen that should catch any broken pieces before they leave the device. To minimize the possibility of shattering the capsule, strictly follow storage and use instructions.
• ***Look alike–sound alike:*** Don't confuse Foradil with Toradol.

PATIENT TEACHING

• Tell patient not to increase the dosage or frequency of use without medical advice.
• Warn patient not to stop or reduce other medication taken for asthma.
• Advise patient that drug isn't to be used for acute asthmatic episodes. Prescriber should give a short-acting beta$_2$ agonist for this use.
• Advise patient to report worsening symptoms, treatment that becomes less effective, or increased use of short-acting beta agonists.
• Tell patient to report nausea, vomiting, shakiness, headache, fast or irregular heartbeat, or sleeplessness.
• Tell patient using drug for exercise-induced bronchospasm to take it at least 15 minutes before exercise and to wait 12 hours before taking additional doses.
• Tell patient not to use the Foradil Aerolizer with a spacer device or to exhale or blow into the Aerolizer.
• Advise patient to avoid washing the Aerolizer and to always keep it dry. Each refill contains a new device to replace the old one.
• Tell patient to avoid exposing capsules to moisture and to handle them only with dry hands.
• Advise woman to notify prescriber if she becomes pregnant or is breast-feeding.

ipratropium bromide

Atrovent, Atrovent HFA

Pharmacologic class: anticholinergic
Pregnancy risk category B

AVAILABLE FORMS

Inhaler: 18 mcg/metered dose (Atrovent), 17 mcg/metered dose (Atrovent HFA)
Nasal spray: 0.03% (21 mcg/metered dose), 0.06% (42 mcg/metered dose)
Solution (for inhalation): 0.02% (500 mcg/vial)

INDICATIONS & DOSAGES

➤ **Bronchospasm in chronic bronchitis and emphysema**
Adults: Usually, 2 inhalations q.i.d.; patient may take additional inhalations p.r.n. but shouldn't exceed 12 inhalations in 24 hours. Or 250 to 500 mcg q 6 to 8 hours via oral nebulizer.

➤ **Rhinorrhea caused by allergic and nonallergic perennial rhinitis**
Adults and children age 6 and older: Two 0.03% nasal sprays (42 mcg) per nostril b.i.d. or t.i.d.

➤ **Rhinorrhea caused by the common cold**
Adults and children age 12 and older: Two 0.06% nasal sprays (84 mcg) per nostril t.i.d. or q.i.d.
Children ages 5 to 11: Two 0.06% nasal sprays (84 mcg) per nostril t.i.d.

➤ **Rhinorrhea caused by seasonal allergic rhinitis**
Adults and children age 5 and older: Two 0.06% nasal sprays (84 mcg) per nostril q.i.d.

ACTION

Inhibits vagally mediated reflexes by antagonizing acetylcholine at muscarinic receptors on bronchial smooth muscle.

Route	Onset	Peak	Duration
Inhalation	5–15 min	1–2 hr	3–6 hr

Half-life: About 2 hours.

ADVERSE REACTIONS

CNS: dizziness, pain, headache, nervousness.
CV: palpitations, hypertension, chest pain.
EENT: blurred vision, rhinitis, pharyngitis, sinusitis, epistaxis.
GI: nausea, GI distress, dry mouth.
Musculoskeletal: back pain.
Respiratory: *upper respiratory tract infection, bronchitis,* ***bronchospasm,*** cough, dyspnea, increased sputum.
Skin: rash.
Other: flulike symptoms, hypersensitivity reactions.

INTERACTIONS

Drug-drug. *Anticholinergics:* May increase anticholinergic effects. Avoid using together.
Drug-herb. *Jaborandi tree:* May decrease effect of drug. Advise patient to use cautiously.
Pill-bearing spurge: May decrease effect of drug. Advise patient to use cautiously.

EFFECTS ON LAB TEST RESULTS

None reported.

CONTRAINDICATIONS & CAUTIONS

- Contraindicated in patients hypersensitive to drug, atropine, or its derivatives and in those hypersensitive to soy lecithin or related food products, such as soybeans and peanuts.
- Use cautiously in patients with angle-closure glaucoma, prostatic hyperplasia, or bladder-neck obstruction.
- Safety and effectiveness of nebulization or inhaler in children younger than age 12 haven't been established.

NURSING CONSIDERATIONS

- If patient uses a face mask for a nebulizer, take care to prevent leakage around the mask because eye pain or temporary blurring of vision may occur.
- Safety and effectiveness of use beyond 4 days in patients with a common cold haven't been established.
- ***Alert:*** Patient with a severe peanut allergy could have an anaphylactic reaction after using Atrovent inhalation aerosol metered-dose inhaler (MDI). Get a thorough allergy history from patient before giving any drug.
- ***Look alike–sound alike:*** Don't confuse Atrovent with Alupent.

PATIENT TEACHING
- Warn patient that drug isn't effective for treating acute episodes of bronchospasm when rapid response is needed.
- Teach patient to perform oral inhalation correctly. Give the following instructions for using an MDI:
  - Shake canister. The HFA form doesn't need to be shaken.
  - Clear nasal passages and throat.
  - Breathe out, expelling as much air from lungs as possible.
  - Place mouthpiece well into mouth, and inhale deeply as you release dose from inhaler. (Patient should close his eyes.)
  - Hold breath for several seconds, remove mouthpiece, and exhale slowly.
- Inform patient that use of a spacer device with MDI may improve drug delivery to lungs.
- Warn patient to avoid accidentally spraying drug into eyes. Temporary blurring of vision may result.
- If more than 1 inhalation is prescribed, tell patient to wait at least 2 minutes before repeating procedure.
- Instruct patient to remove canister and wash inhaler in warm, soapy water at least once weekly.
- If patient is also using a corticosteroid inhaler, instruct him to use ipratropium first and then to wait about 5 minutes before using the corticosteroid. This lets the bronchodilator open air passages for maximal effectiveness of the corticosteroid.

isoproterenol hydrochloride
Isuprel

Pharmacologic class: nonselective beta-adrenergic agonist
Pregnancy risk category C

AVAILABLE FORMS
Injection: 20 mcg/ml in 10-ml prefilled syringes, 200 mcg/ml in 1- and 5-ml ampules and 5- and 10-ml vials

INDICATIONS & DOSAGES
➤ **Bronchospasm during anesthesia**
Adults: Dilute 1 ml of a 1:5,000 solution with 10 ml of normal saline or D_5W. Give 0.01 to 0.02 mg I.V. and repeat as necessary. Or, give 1:50,000 solution undiluted using same dose.
➤ **Heart block, ventricular arrhythmias**
Adults: Initially, 0.02 to 0.06 mg I.V.; then 0.01 to 0.2 mg I.V. or 5 mcg/minute I.V. Or, initially, 0.2 mg I.M.; then 0.02 to 1 mg I.M., p.r.n.
Children: Initial I.V. infusion of 0.1 mcg/kg/minute. Adjust dosage based on patient's response. Usual dosage range is 0.1 to 1 mcg/kg/minute.
➤ **Shock**
Adults and children: 0.5 to 5 mcg/minute isoproterenol hydrochloride by continuous I.V. infusion. Usual concentration is 1 mg or 5 ml in 500 ml D_5W. Titrate infusion rate according to heart rate, central venous pressure, blood pressure, and urine flow.
➤ **Postoperative cardiac patients with bradycardia ♦**
Children: I.V. infusion of 0.029 mcg/kg/minute.
➤ **As an aid in diagnosing the cause of mitral regurgitation ♦**
Adults: 4 mcg/minute I.V. infusion.
➤ **As an aid in diagnosing coronary artery disease or lesions ♦**
Adults: 1 to 3 mcg/minute I.V. infusion.

I.V. ADMINISTRATION
- For infusion, dilute with most common I.V. solutions, but don't use with sodium bicarbonate injection; drug decomposes rapidly in alkaline solutions.
- Give by direct injection or I.V. infusion.
- For shock, closely monitor blood pressure, central venous pressure, ECG, arterial blood gas measurements, and urine output. Carefully titrate infusion rate according to these measurements. Use a continuous infusion pump to regulate flow rate.
- Store at room temperature. Protect from light.

INCOMPATIBILITIES
Alkalies, aminophylline, furosemide, metals, sodium bicarbonate.

ACTION
Relaxes bronchial smooth muscle by stimulating $beta_2$ receptors. As a cardiac

stimulant, acts on $beta_1$ receptors in the heart.

Route	Onset	Peak	Duration
I.V.	Immediate	Unknown	< 60 min

Half-life: Unknown.

ADVERSE REACTIONS

CNS: headache, mild tremor, weakness, dizziness, nervousness, insomnia, anxiety.
CV: *palpitations, rapid rise and fall in blood pressure, tachycardia, angina,* ***arrhythmias, cardiac arrest.***
GI: nausea, vomiting.
Metabolic: hyperglycemia.
Skin: diaphoresis.
Other: swelling of parotid glands with prolonged use.

INTERACTIONS

Drug-drug. *Epinephrine, other sympathomimetics:* May increase risk of arrhythmias. Use together cautiously. If used together, give at least 4 hours apart.
Halogenated general anesthetics or cyclopropane: May increase risk of arrhythmias. Avoid using together.
Propranolol, other beta blockers: May block bronchodilating effect of isoproterenol. Monitor patient carefully.

EFFECTS ON LAB TEST RESULTS

- May increase glucose level.

CONTRAINDICATIONS & CAUTIONS

- Contraindicated in patients with tachycardia or AV block caused by digoxin intoxication, arrhythmias other than those that may respond to drug, angina pectoris, or angle-closure glaucoma.
- Contraindicated when used with general anesthetics with halogenated drugs or cyclopropane.
- Use cautiously in elderly patients and in those with renal or CV disease, coronary insufficiency, diabetes, hyperthyroidism, or history of sensitivity to sympathomimetic amines.

NURSING CONSIDERATIONS

- Correct volume deficit before giving vasopressors.
- Don't use solution if it's discolored or contains precipitate.
- ***Alert:*** If heart rate exceeds 110 beats/minute during I.V. infusion, notify prescriber. Doses that increase the heart rate to more than 130 beats/minute may induce ventricular arrhythmias.
- Drug may cause a slight increase in systolic blood pressure and a slight to marked decrease in diastolic blood pressure.
- Monitor patient for adverse reactions.
- ***Look alike–sound alike:*** Don't confuse Isuprel with Isordil.

PATIENT TEACHING

- Tell patient to report chest pain, fluttering in chest, or other adverse reactions.
- Remind patient to report pain at the I.V. injection site.

levalbuterol hydrochloride

Xopenex, Xopenex HFA

Pharmacologic class: $beta_2$ agonist
Pregnancy risk category C

AVAILABLE FORMS

Solution for inhalation: 0.31 mg, 0.63 mg, or 1.25 mg in 3-ml vials
Inhalation aerosol: 15 g containing 200 actuations

INDICATIONS & DOSAGES

➤ To prevent or treat bronchospasm in patients with reversible obstructive airway disease
Adults and adolescents age 12 and older: 0.63 mg given t.i.d. q 6 to 8 hours, by oral inhalation via a nebulizer. Patients with more severe asthma who don't respond adequately to 0.63 mg t.i.d. may benefit from 1.25 mg t.i.d.
Children ages 6 to 11: 0.31 mg inhaled t.i.d. by nebulizer. Routine dosage shouldn't exceed 0.63 mg t.i.d.
Adults and children age 4 and older: 2 inhalations Xopenex HFA (90 mcg) q 4 to 6 hours. In some patients, 1 inhalation q 4 hours is sufficient.

ACTION

Relaxes bronchial smooth muscle by stimulating $beta_2$ receptors; also, inhibits release of mediators from mast cells in the airway.

Route	Onset	Peak	Duration
Inhalation	10–17 min	1½ hr	5–8 hr

Half-life: 3¼ to 4 hours.

ADVERSE REACTIONS

CNS: dizziness, migraine, nervousness, pain, tremor, anxiety.
CV: tachycardia.
EENT: *rhinitis,* sinusitis, turbinate edema.
GI: dyspepsia.
Musculoskeletal: leg cramps.
Respiratory: increased cough.
Other: *viral infection,* flulike syndrome, accidental injury.

INTERACTIONS

Drug-drug. *Beta blockers:* May block pulmonary effect of the drug and cause severe bronchospasm. Avoid using together, if possible. If use together is unavoidable, consider a cardioselective beta blocker, but use cautiously.
Digoxin: May decrease digoxin level up to 22%. Monitor digoxin level.
Loop or thiazide diuretics: May cause ECG changes and hypokalemia. Use together cautiously.
MAO inhibitors, tricyclic antidepressants: May potentiate action of levalbuterol on the vascular system. Avoid using within 2 weeks of MAO inhibitor or tricyclic antidepressant therapy.
Other short-acting sympathomimetic aerosol bronchodilators, epinephrine: May increase adrenergic adverse effects. Use together cautiously.

EFFECTS ON LAB TEST RESULTS

None reported.

CONTRAINDICATIONS & CAUTIONS

- Contraindicated in patients hypersensitive to drug or to racemic albuterol.
- Use cautiously in patients with CV disorders (especially coronary insufficiency, hypertension, and arrhythmias), seizure disorders, hyperthyroidism, or diabetes mellitus, and in those who are unusually responsive to sympathomimetic amines.

NURSING CONSIDERATIONS

- ***Alert:*** As with other inhaled beta agonists, drug can produce paradoxical bronchospasm or life-threatening CV effects. If this occurs, stop drug immediately and notify prescriber.
- Drug may worsen diabetes mellitus and ketoacidosis.
- Drug may temporarily decrease potassium level, but potassium supplementation is usually unnecessary.
- The compatibility of levalbuterol mixed with other drugs in a nebulizer hasn't been established.

PATIENT TEACHING

- Warn patient that he may experience worsened breathing. Tell him to stop drug and contact prescriber immediately if this occurs.
- Tell patient not to increase dosage without consulting prescriber.
- Urge patient to seek medical attention immediately if levalbuterol becomes less effective, if signs and symptoms become worse, or if he's using drug more frequently than usual.
- Tell patient that the effects of levalbuterol may last up to 8 hours.
- Tell patient not to double the next dose if he misses a dose. Tell him to take doses at least 6 hours apart.
- Advise patient to use other inhalations and antiasthmatics only as directed while taking levalbuterol.
- Inform patient that common adverse reactions include palpitations, rapid heart rate, headache, dizziness, tremor, and nervousness.
- Encourage woman to contact prescriber if she becomes pregnant or is breastfeeding.
- Tell patient to keep unopened vials in foil pouch. Once the foil pouch is opened, vials must be used within 2 weeks. Inform patient that vials removed from the pouch, if not used immediately, should be protected from light and excessive heat and used within 1 week.
- Teach patient to use drug correctly when inhaling by nebulizer.
- Instruct patient to breathe as calmly, deeply, and evenly as possible until no more mist is formed in the nebulizer reservoir (5 to 15 minutes).
- Tell patient using the inhaler to release 4 test sprays into the air away from the

face before the first use or if it hasn't been used for more than 3 days.

pirbuterol acetate
Maxair Autohaler

Pharmacologic class: beta agonist
Pregnancy risk category C

AVAILABLE FORMS
Inhaler: 0.2 mg/metered dose

INDICATIONS & DOSAGES
➤To prevent and reverse bronchospasm; asthma
Adults and children age 12 and older: 1 or 2 inhalations (0.2 to 0.4 mg), repeated q 4 to 6 hours. Don't exceed 12 inhalations daily.

ACTION
Relaxes bronchial smooth muscle by stimulating $beta_2$ receptors.

Route	Onset	Peak	Duration
Inhalation	5 min	30–60 min	5 hr

Half-life: About 2 hours.

ADVERSE REACTIONS
CNS: tremor, nervousness, dizziness, insomnia, headache, vertigo.
CV: tachycardia, palpitations, chest tightness.
EENT: dry or irritated throat.
GI: nausea, vomiting, diarrhea, dry mouth.
Respiratory: cough.

INTERACTIONS
Drug-drug. *Beta blockers, propranolol:* May decrease bronchodilating effects. Avoid using together.
MAO inhibitors, tricyclic antidepressants: May potentiate action of beta agonist on vascular system. Use together cautiously.

EFFECTS ON LAB TEST RESULTS
None reported.

CONTRAINDICATIONS & CAUTIONS
- Contraindicated in patients hypersensitive to drug.
- Use cautiously in patients unusually responsive to sympathomimetic amines and patients with CV disorders, hyperthyroidism, diabetes, and seizure disorders.

NURSING CONSIDERATIONS
- Monitor patient for increased pulse or blood pressure during therapy.
- Stop drug immediately and notify prescriber if paradoxical bronchospasm occurs.
- The likelihood of paradoxical bronchospasm is increased with the first use of a new canister.
- Notify prescriber of decreasing effectiveness of the drug.

PATIENT TEACHING
- Give the following instructions for using Autohaler:
  - –Remove mouthpiece cover by pulling down lip on back cover. Inspect mouthpiece for foreign objects. Locate "Up" arrows and air vents.
  - –Hold Autohaler upright so that arrows point up; raise lever until it snaps into place.
  - –Hold Autohaler around the middle, and shake gently several times.
  - –Continue to hold upright, and be careful not to block air vents at bottom. Exhale normally before use.
  - –Seal lips around mouthpiece. Inhale deeply through mouthpiece with steady, moderate force to trigger release of the drug. You'll hear a click and feel a soft puff when drug is released. Continue to take a full, deep breath.
  - –Take Autohaler away from mouth when done inhaling. Hold breath for 10 seconds; then exhale slowly.
  - –Continue to hold Autohaler upright while lowering lever. Lower lever after each puff. If additional puffs are ordered, wait 1 minute before repeating process to obtain the next puff.
- Have patient clean inhaler per manufacturer's instructions.
- If patient also uses a corticosteroid inhaler, tell him to use the bronchodilator first, and then wait about 5 minutes before using the corticosteroid. This allows the bronchodilator to open air passages for maximal effectiveness of the corticosteroid.

• Instruct patient to call prescriber if bronchospasm increases after using drug.
• Advise patient to seek medical attention if a previously effective dosage doesn't control symptoms; this change may signal worsening of disease.

salmeterol xinafoate
Serevent Diskus

Pharmacologic class: selective $beta_2$ agonist
Pregnancy risk category C

AVAILABLE FORMS
Inhalation powder: 50 mcg/blister

INDICATIONS & DOSAGES
➤ **Long-term maintenance of asthma; to prevent bronchospasm in patients with nocturnal asthma or reversible obstructive airway disease who need regular treatment with short-acting beta agonists**
Adults and children age 4 and older: 1 inhalation (50 mcg) q 12 hours, morning and evening.
➤ **To prevent exercise-induced bronchospasm**
Adults and children age 4 and older: 1 inhalation (50 mcg) at least 30 minutes before exercise. Additional doses shouldn't be taken for at least 12 hours.
➤ **COPD or emphysema**
Adults: 1 inhalation (50 mcg) b.i.d. in the morning and evening, about 12 hours apart.

ACTION
Unclear. Selectively activates $beta_2$ receptors, which results in bronchodilation; also, blocks the release of allergic mediators from mast cells lining the respiratory tract.

Route	Onset	Peak	Duration
Inhalation	10–20 min	3 hr	12 hr

Half-life: 5½ hours; xinafoate salt, 11 days.

ADVERSE REACTIONS
CNS: headache, sinus headache, tremor, nervousness, giddiness, dizziness.
CV: ***ventricular arrhythmias,*** tachycardia, palpitations.
EENT: *nasopharyngitis,* pharyngitis, nasal cavity or sinus disorder.
GI: nausea, vomiting, diarrhea, heartburn.
Musculoskeletal: joint and back pain, myalgia.
Respiratory: *upper respiratory tract infection,* ***bronchospasm,*** cough, lower respiratory tract infection.
Other: hypersensitivity reactions.

INTERACTIONS
Drug-drug. *Beta agonists, other methylxanthines, theophylline:* May cause adverse cardiac effects with excessive use. Monitor patient.
MAO inhibitors: May cause risk of severe adverse CV effects. Avoid use within 14 days of MAO inhibitor therapy.
Tricyclic antidepressants: May cause risk of moderate to severe adverse CV effects. Use together with caution.

EFFECTS ON LAB TEST RESULTS
None reported.

CONTRAINDICATIONS & CAUTIONS
• Contraindicated in patients hypersensitive to drug or its ingredients.
• Use cautiously in patients unusually responsive to sympathomimetics and those with coronary insufficiency, arrhythmias, hypertension, other CV disorders, thyrotoxicosis, or seizure disorders.

NURSING CONSIDERATIONS
• Drug isn't indicated for acute bronchospasm.
• ***Alert:*** Monitor patient for rash and urticaria, which may signal a hypersensitivity reaction.
• ***Look alike–sound alike:*** Don't confuse Serevent with Serentil.

PATIENT TEACHING
• Remind patient to take drug at about 12-hour intervals for optimum effect and to take drug even when feeling better.
• If patient is taking drug to prevent exercise-induced bronchospasm, tell him to take it 30 to 60 minutes before exercise.
• ***Alert:*** Tell patient drug shouldn't be used to treat acute bronchospasm. He must use

a short-acting beta agonist, such as albuterol, to treat worsening symptoms.
- ***Alert:*** Rare serious asthma episodes or asthma-related deaths may occur in patients using salmeterol. Black patients may be at greater risk.
- Tell patient to contact prescriber if the short-acting agonist no longer provides sufficient relief or if he needs more than 4 inhalations daily. This may be a sign that the asthma symptoms are worsening. Tell him not to increase the dosage of salmeterol.
- If patient takes an inhaled corticosteroid, he should continue to use it regularly. Warn patient not to take other drugs without prescriber's consent.
- If patient takes the inhalation powder (in a multidose inhaler), instruct him not to exhale into the device. He should activate and use it only in a level, horizontal position.
- Tell patient not to use the dry-powder multidose inhaler with a spacer.
- Instruct patient never to wash the mouthpiece or any part of the dry-powder multidose inhaler; it must be kept dry.

terbutaline sulfate

Brethine

Pharmacologic class: beta$_2$ agonist
Pregnancy risk category B

AVAILABLE FORMS

Injection: 1 mg/ml
Tablets: 2.5 mg, 5 mg

INDICATIONS & DOSAGES

➤ Bronchospasm in patients with reversible obstructive airway disease

Adults and children age 12 and older: 0.25 mg subcutaneously. Repeat in 15 to 30 minutes, p.r.n. Maximum, 0.5 mg in 4 hours.

Adults and adolescents older than age 15: Give 2.5 to 5 mg P.O. t.i.d. q 6 hours while awake. Maximum, 15 mg daily.

Children ages 12 to 15: Give 2.5 mg P.O. t.i.d. q 6 hours while awake. Maximum, 7.5 mg daily.

ACTION

Relaxes bronchial smooth muscle by stimulating beta$_2$ receptors.

Route	Onset	Peak	Duration
P.O.	30 min	2–3 hr	4–8 hr
SubQ	15 min	30 min	1½–4 hr

Half-life: Unknown.

ADVERSE REACTIONS

CNS: *nervousness, tremor, drowsiness, dizziness, headache,* weakness.
CV: *palpitations,* ***arrhythmias,*** tachycardia, flushing.
GI: *vomiting, nausea,* heartburn.
Metabolic: hypokalemia.
Respiratory: ***paradoxical bronchospasm with prolonged use,*** dyspnea.
Skin: diaphoresis.

INTERACTIONS

Drug-drug. *Cardiac glycosides, cyclopropane, halogenated inhaled anesthetics, levodopa:* May increase risk of arrhythmias. Monitor patient closely, and avoid using together with levodopa.
CNS stimulants: May increase CNS stimulation. Avoid using together.
MAO inhibitors: When given with sympathomimetics, may cause severe hypertension (hypertensive crisis). Avoid using together.
Propranolol, other beta blockers: May block bronchodilating effects of terbutaline. Avoid using together.

EFFECTS ON LAB TEST RESULTS

- May decrease potassium level.

CONTRAINDICATIONS & CAUTIONS

- Contraindicated in patients hypersensitive to drug or sympathomimetic amines.
- Use cautiously in patient with CV disorders, hyperthyroidism, diabetes, or seizure disorders.

NURSING CONSIDERATIONS

- Give subcutaneous injections in the side of the deltoid.
- Protect drug from light. Don't use if discolored.
- Drug may reduce the sensitivity of spirometry for the diagnosis of bronchospasm.

• ***Look alike–sound alike:*** Don't confuse terbutaline with tolbutamide or terbinafine.

PATIENT TEACHING

• Make sure patient and caregivers understand why patient needs drug.
• Remind patient to separate oral doses by 6 hours.

theophylline

Immediate-release liquids
Accurbron*, Aerolate, Asmalix*, Bronkodyl*, Elixomin*, Elixophyllin*, Lanophyllin*, Theolair Liquid

Immediate-release tablets and capsules
Bronkodyl, Elixophyllin, Nuelin‡, Quibron T Dividose

Timed-release tablets
Quibron-T/SR, Theochron, Theolair-SR, T-Phyl, Uniphyl

Timed-release capsules
Aerolate, Elixophyllin, Nuelin-SR‡, Slo-bid Gyrocaps, Theobid Duracaps, Theochron, Theo-24

Pharmacologic class: xanthine derivative
Pregnancy risk category C

AVAILABLE FORMS

Capsules: 100 mg, 200 mg
Capsules (extended-release): 100 mg, 125 mg, 200 mg, 300 mg
D_5W injection: 200 mg in 50 ml or 100 ml; 400 mg in 100 ml, 250 ml, 500 ml, or 1,000 ml; 800 mg in 500 ml or 1,000 ml
Elixir: 27 mg/5 ml*
Syrup: 50 mg/5 ml
Tablets: 100 mg, 125 mg, 200 mg, 300 mg
Tablets (extended-release): 100 mg, 200 mg, 300 mg, 400 mg, 450 mg, 600 mg

INDICATIONS & DOSAGES

Extended-release preparations shouldn't be used to treat acute bronchospasm.

➤ **Oral theophylline for acute bronchospasm in patients not currently receiving theophylline**
Adult nonsmokers and children older than age 16: 5 mg/kg P.O., then 3 mg/kg q 6 hours for two doses. Maintenance dosage is 3 mg/kg q 8 hours.
Children ages 9 to 16: 5 mg/kg P.O.; then 3 mg/kg q 4 hours for three doses. Maintenance dosage is 3 mg/kg q 6 hours.
Children ages 6 months to 9 years: 5 mg/kg P.O.; then 4 mg/kg q 4 hours for three doses. Maintenance dosage is 4 mg/kg q 6 hours.
Adjust-a-dose: For otherwise healthy adult smokers, 5 mg/kg P.O.; then 3 mg/kg q 4 hours for three doses. Maintenance dosage is 3 mg/kg q 6 hours. For older adults and patients with cor pulmonale, 5 mg/kg P.O.; then 2 mg/kg q 6 hours for two doses. Maintenance dosage is 2 mg/kg q 8 hours. For adults with heart failure or liver disease, 5 mg/kg P.O.; then 2 mg/kg q 8 hours for two doses. Maintenance dosage is 1 to 2 mg/kg q 12 hours.

➤ **Parenteral theophylline for patients not currently receiving theophylline**
Loading dose: 4.7 mg/kg I.V. slowly; then maintenance infusion.
Adult nonsmokers and children older than age 16: 0.55 mg/kg/hour I.V. for 12 hours; then 0.39 mg/kg/hour.
Children ages 9 to 16: 0.79 mg/kg/hour I.V. for 12 hours; then 0.63 mg/kg/hour.
Children ages 6 months to 9 years: 0.95 mg/kg/hour I.V. for 12 hours; then 0.79 mg/kg/hour.
Adjust-a-dose: For otherwise healthy adult smokers, 0.79 mg/kg/hour I.V. for 12 hours; then 0.63 mg/kg/hour. For older adults and patients with cor pulmonale, 0.47 mg/kg/hour I.V. for 12 hours; then 0.24 mg/kg/hour. For adults with heart failure or liver disease, 0.39 mg/kg/hour I.V. for 12 hours; then 0.08 to 0.16 mg/kg/hour.

➤ **Oral and parenteral theophylline for acute bronchospasm in patients currently receiving theophylline**
Adults and children: Ideally, dose is based on current theophylline level. Each 0.5 mg/kg I.V. or P.O. loading dose will increase drug level by 1 mcg/ml. In emergencies, when theophylline level can't be

readily obtained, some prescribers recommend a 2.5-mg/kg P.O. dose of rapidly absorbed form if patient develops no obvious signs or symptoms of theophylline toxicity.

➤**Chronic bronchospasm**
Adults and children: Initially, 16 mg/kg or 400 mg P.O. daily, whichever is less, given in three or four divided doses at 6- to 8-hour intervals. Or, 12 mg/kg or 400 mg P.O. daily, whichever is less, in an extended-release preparation given in two or three divided doses at 8- or 12-hour intervals. Dosage may be increased, as tolerated, at 2- to 3-day intervals to the following maximums: adults and children older than age 16, 13 mg/kg or 900 mg P.O. daily, whichever is less; children ages 12 to 16, 18 mg/kg P.O. daily; children ages 9 to 12, 20 mg/kg P.O. daily; children younger than age 9, 24 mg/kg P.O. daily.

I.V. ADMINISTRATION
- Use commercially available infusion solution, or mix in D_5W solution.
- Use infusion pump for continuous infusion.

INCOMPATIBILITIES
Ascorbic acid, ceftriaxone, cimetidine, hetastarch, phenytoin.

ACTION
Inhibits phosphodiesterase, the enzyme that degrades cAMP, resulting in relaxation of smooth muscle of the bronchial airways and pulmonary blood vessels.

Route	Onset	Peak	Duration
P.O.	15–60 min	1–2 hr	Unknown
P.O. (extended)	15–60 min	4–7 hr	Unknown
I.V.	15 min	15–30 min	Unknown

Half-life: Adults, 7 to 9 hours; smokers, 4 to 5 hours; children, 3 to 5. hours; premature infants, 20 to 30 hours.

ADVERSE REACTIONS
CNS: *restlessness, dizziness, insomnia,* ***seizures,*** headache, irritability, muscle twitching.
CV: *palpitations, sinus tachycardia,* ***arrhythmias,*** extrasystoles, flushing, marked hypotension.
GI: *nausea, vomiting,* diarrhea, epigastric pain.
Metabolic: urinary catecholamines.
Respiratory: ***respiratory arrest,*** tachypnea.

INTERACTIONS
Drug-drug. *Adenosine:* May decrease antiarrhythmic effect. Higher doses of adenosine may be needed.
Allopurinol, calcium channel blockers, ***cimetidine,*** *disulfiram, influenza virus vaccine, interferon,* ***macrolides (such as erythromycin),*** *methotrexate,* ***mexiletine,*** *oral contraceptives,* ***quinolones (such as ciprofloxacin):*** May decrease hepatic clearance of theophylline; may increase theophylline level. Monitor levels closely and adjust theophylline dose.
Barbiturates, ketoconazole, nicotine, ***phenytoin, rifamycins:*** May enhance metabolism and decrease theophylline level; may increase phenytoin metabolism. Monitor patient for decreased therapeutic effect; monitor levels and adjust dosage.
Carbamazepine, isoniazid, loop diuretics: May increase or decrease theophylline level. Monitor theophylline level.
Carteolol, pindolol, propranolol, timolol: May act antagonistically, reducing the effects of one or both drugs; may reduce elimination of theophylline. Monitor theophylline level and patient closely.
Ephedrine, other sympathomimetics: May exhibit synergistic toxicity with these drugs, predisposing patient to arrhythmias. Monitor patient closely.
Lithium: May increase lithium excretion. Monitor patient closely.
Tetracyclines: May enhance the adverse effects of theophylline. Monitor patient closely.
Drug-herb. *Cacao tree:* May inhibit drug metabolism. Discourage use together.
Cayenne: May increase risk of drug toxicity. Advise patient to use together cautiously.
Ephedra: May increase risk of adverse reactions. Discourage use together.
Guarana: May cause additive CNS and CV effects. Discourage use together.
Ipriflavone: May increase risk of drug toxicity. Advise patient to use together cautiously.

St. John's wort: May decrease drug level. Discourage use together.
Drug-food. *Any food:* May cause accelerated drug release from extended-release products. Tell patient to take extended-release products on an empty stomach.
Caffeine: May decrease hepatic clearance of drug and increase drug level. Monitor patient for toxicity.
Drug-lifestyle. *Smoking:* May increase elimination of drug, increasing dosage requirements. Monitor drug response and level.

EFFECTS ON LAB TEST RESULTS

- May increase free fatty acid level and blood glucose.
- May falsely elevate theophylline level in the presence of acetaminophen, furosemide, phenylbutazone, probenecid, theobromine, caffeine, tea, chocolate, and cola, depending on assay used.

CONTRAINDICATIONS & CAUTIONS

- Contraindicated in patients hypersensitive to xanthine compounds (caffeine, theobromine) and in those with active peptic ulcer or poorly controlled seizure disorders.
- Use cautiously in young children, infants, neonates, elderly patients, and those with COPD, cardiac failure, cor pulmonale, renal or hepatic disease, peptic ulceration, hyperthyroidism, diabetes mellitus, glaucoma, severe hypoxemia, hypertension, compromised cardiac or circulatory function, angina, acute MI, or sulfite sensitivity.

NURSING CONSIDERATIONS

- Dosage may need to be increased in cigarette smokers and in habitual marijuana smokers because smoking causes drug to be metabolized faster.
- Give drug around the clock, using extended-release product at bedtime.
- Monitor vital signs; measure and record fluid intake and output. Expect improved quality of pulse and respirations.
- Patients metabolize xanthines at different rates; dosage is determined by monitoring response, tolerance, pulmonary function, and drug level. Drug levels range from 10 to 20 mcg/ml; toxicity may occur at levels above 20 mcg/ml.
- ***Alert:*** Evidence of toxicity includes tachycardia, anorexia, nausea, vomiting, diarrhea, restlessness, irritability, and headache. If these signs occur, check drug level and adjust dosage, as indicated.
- ***Look alike–sound alike:*** Don't confuse extended-release form with regular-release form.
- ***Look alike–sound alike:*** Don't confuse Theolair with Thyrolar.

PATIENT TEACHING

- Supply instructions for home care and dosage schedule.
- Warn patient not to dissolve, crush, or chew extended-release products. Small children unable to swallow these can ingest (without chewing) the contents of capsules sprinkled over soft food.
- Tell patient to relieve GI symptoms by taking oral drug with full glass of water after meals, although food in stomach delays absorption.
- Warn patient to take drug regularly, only as directed. Patients tend to want to take extra "breathing pills."
- Inform elderly patient that dizziness is common at start of therapy.
- Urge patient to tell prescriber about any other drugs taken. OTC drugs or herbal remedies may contain ephedrine or theophylline salts; excessive CNS stimulation may result.
- If a smoker quits, tell him to inform prescriber. Dosage reduction may be needed to prevent toxicity.

tiotropium bromide

Spiriva

Pharmacologic class: anticholinergic
Pregnancy risk category C

AVAILABLE FORMS

Capsules for inhalation: 18 mcg

INDICATIONS & DOSAGES

➤ **Maintenance treatment of bronchospasm in COPD, including chronic bronchitis and emphysema**
Adults: 1 capsule (18 mcg) inhaled orally once daily using the HandiHaler inhalation device.

ACTION

Competitive, reversible inhibition of muscarinic receptors leads to bronchodilation.

Route	Onset	Peak	Duration
Inhalation	30 min	3 hr	> 24 hr

Half-life: 5 to 6 days.

ADVERSE REACTIONS

CNS: depression, paresthesia.
CV: ***angina pectoris,*** chest pain, edema.
EENT: *sinusitis,* cataract, dysphonia, epistaxis, glaucoma, laryngitis, pharyngitis, rhinitis.
GI: *dry mouth,* abdominal pain, constipation, dyspepsia, gastroesophageal reflux, stomatitis, vomiting.
GU: UTI.
Metabolic: hypercholesterolemia, hyperglycemia.
Musculoskeletal: arthritis, leg pain, myalgia, skeletal pain.
Respiratory: *upper respiratory tract infection,* cough.
Skin: rash.
Other: *accidental injury,* allergic reaction, candidiasis, flulike syndrome, herpes zoster, infections.

INTERACTIONS

Drug-drug. *Anticholinergics:* May increase the risk of adverse reactions. Avoid using together.

EFFECTS ON LAB TEST RESULTS

- May increase cholesterol and glucose levels.

CONTRAINDICATIONS & CAUTIONS

- Contraindicated in patients hypersensitive to atropine, its derivatives, ipratropium, or any component of the product.
- Use cautiously in women who are pregnant or breast-feeding, patients with creatinine clearance of 50 ml/minute or less, or patients with angle-closure glaucoma, prostatic hyperplasia, or bladder neck obstruction.

NURSING CONSIDERATIONS

- ***Alert:*** Use drug for maintenance treatment of COPD, not for acute bronchospasm.
- Capsules aren't for oral ingestion. Give them only by oral inhalation with the HandiHaler device.
- Watch for evidence of hypersensitivity (especially angioedema) and paradoxical bronchospasm.

PATIENT TEACHING

- Inform patient that drug is for maintenance treatment of COPD and not for immediate relief of breathing problems.
- ***Alert:*** Explain that capsules are for inhalation and shouldn't be swallowed.
- Provide full instructions for the HandiHaler device.
- Tell patient not to get powder in his eyes.
- Review signs and symptoms of hypersensitivity (especially angioedema) and paradoxical bronchospasm. Tell patient to stop the drug and contact the prescriber if they occur.
- Advise patient to report eye pain, blurred vision, visual halos, colored images, or red eyes immediately.
- Tell patient to keep capsules in sealed blisters and to remove each capsule just before use. Caution against storing capsules in the HandiHaler device.
- Instruct patient to store capsules at 77° F (25° C) and not to expose them to extreme temperatures or moisture.

42

Expectorants and antitussives

benzonatate
codeine phosphate
(See Chapter 26, OPIOID ANALGESICS.)
codeine sulfate
(See Chapter 26, OPIOID ANALGESICS.)
dextromethorphan hydrobromide
diphenhydramine hydrochloride
(See Chapter 40, ANTIHISTAMINES.)
guaifenesin

benzonatate

Tessalon, Tessalon Perles

Pharmacologic class: local anesthetic
Pregnancy risk category C

AVAILABLE FORMS

Capsules: 100 mg, 200 mg

INDICATIONS & DOSAGES

➤ **Symptomatic relief of cough**
Adults and children older than age 10: 100 to 200 mg P.O. t.i.d.; up to 600 mg daily.

ACTION

Chemical relative of tetracaine that suppresses the cough reflex by direct action on the cough center in the medulla and through an anesthetic action on stretch receptors of vagal afferent fibers in the respiratory passages, lungs, and pleura.

Route	Onset	Peak	Duration
P.O.	15–20 min	Unknown	3–8 hr

Half-life: Unknown.

ADVERSE REACTIONS

CNS: dizziness, headache, sedation.
EENT: nasal congestion, burning sensation in eyes.
GI: nausea, constipation, GI upset.
Other: chills, hypersensitivity reactions.

INTERACTIONS

None significant.

EFFECTS ON LAB TEST RESULTS

None reported.

CONTRAINDICATIONS & CAUTIONS

- Contraindicated in patients hypersensitive to drug or related compounds.
- Use cautiously in patients hypersensitive to PABA anesthetics (procaine, tetracaine) because cross-sensitivity reactions may occur.

NURSING CONSIDERATIONS

- Don't use drug when cough is a valuable diagnostic sign or is beneficial (such as after thoracic surgery).
- Monitor cough type and frequency.
- Use with percussion and chest vibration.

PATIENT TEACHING

- Warn patient not to chew capsules or dissolve in mouth, which produces either local anesthesia that may result in aspiration, or CNS stimulation that may cause restlessness, tremor, and seizures.
- Instruct patient to report adverse reactions.
- Instruct patient to protect drug from light and moisture.
- Tell patient to contact his prescriber if cough lasts longer than 1 week, recurs frequently, or is accompanied by high fever, rash, or severe headache.

dextromethorphan hydrobromide

Balminil DM◇, Benylin DM◇, Buckley's DM, Children's Hold◇, Delsym, Hold◇, Pertussin CS◇, Pertussin ES◇, Robitussin Pediatric◇, St. Joseph Cough Suppressant for Children◇, Trocal◇, Vicks Formula 44e Pediatric◇

Commonly available in combination products, such as
Anti-Tuss DM Expectorant ◇, Benylin Expectorant ◇, Cheracol D Cough ◇, DexAlone ◇, Glycotuss-dM, Guiamid D.M. Liquid ◇, Guiatuss-DM ◇, Halotussin-DM ◇, Kolephrin GG/DM ◇, Mytussin DM ◇, Naldecon Senior DX ◇, Pertussin CS ◇, Rhinosyn-DMX Expectorant ◇, Robitussin-DM ◇, Scot-Tussin DM Cough Chasers ◇, Tolu-Sed DM ◇, Tuss-DM ◇, Unproco ◇

Pharmacologic class: levorphanol derivative
Pregnancy risk category C

AVAILABLE FORMS

Gelcaps: 30 mg ◇
Liquid (extended-release): 30 mg/5 ml ◇
Lozenges: 5 mg ◇, 7.5 mg ◇, 15 mg ◇
Solution: 3.5 mg/5 ml, 5 mg/5 ml* ◇, 7.5 mg/5 ml ◇, 10 mg/5 ml* ◇, 15 mg/5 ml* ◇, 15 mg/15 ml* ◇, 12.5 mg/5 ml

INDICATIONS & DOSAGES

➤Nonproductive cough
Adults and children age 12 and older: 10 to 20 mg P.O. q 4 hours, or 30 mg q 6 to 8 hours. Or, 60 mg extended-release liquid b.i.d. Maximum, 120 mg daily.
Children ages 6 to 11: Give 5 to 10 mg P.O. q 4 hours, or 15 mg q 6 to 8 hours. Or, 30 mg extended-release liquid b.i.d. Maximum, 60 mg daily.
Children ages 2 to 5: Give 2.5 to 5 mg P.O. q 4 hours, or 7.5 mg q 6 to 8 hours. Or, 15 mg extended-release liquid b.i.d. Maximum, 30 mg daily.
Children younger than age 2: Individualize dosages.

ACTION

Suppresses the cough reflex by direct action on the cough center in the medulla.

Route	Onset	Peak	Duration
P.O.	< 30 min	Unknown	3–6 hr

Half-life: About 11 hours.

ADVERSE REACTIONS

CNS: drowsiness, dizziness.
GI: nausea, vomiting, stomach pain.

INTERACTIONS

Drug-drug. *MAO inhibitors:* May cause risk of hypotension, coma, hyperpyrexia, and death. Avoid using together.
Quinidine: May increase the risk of dextromethorphan adverse effects. Consider decreasing dextromethorphan dose if needed.
Drug-herb. *Parsley:* May promote or produce serotonin syndrome. Discourage use together.

EFFECTS ON LAB TEST RESULTS

None reported.

CONTRAINDICATIONS & CAUTIONS

- Contraindicated in patients currently taking MAO inhibitors or within 2 weeks of stopping MAO inhibitors.
- Use cautiously in atopic children, sedated or debilitated patients, and patients confined to the supine position.
- Use cautiously in patients sensitive to aspirin or tartrazine dyes.

NURSING CONSIDERATIONS

- Don't use dextromethorphan when cough is a valuable diagnostic sign or is beneficial (such as after thoracic surgery).
- 15 to 30 mg is equivalent to 8 to 15 mg codeine as an antitussive.
- Drug produces no analgesia or addiction and little or no CNS depression.
- Use drug with chest percussion and vibration.
- Monitor cough type and frequency.

PATIENT TEACHING

- Instruct patient to take drug exactly as prescribed.
- Tell patient to report adverse reactions.
- Tell patient to contact his health care provider if cough lasts longer than 1 week, recurs frequently, or is accompanied by high fever, rash, or severe headache.

guaifenesin (glyceryl guaiacolate)

Allfen Jr, Anti-Tuss* ◇, Diabetic Tussin ◇, Ganidin NR, Guiatuss* ◇, Hytuss ◇, Hytuss 2X ◇, Mucinex ◇, Naldecon Senior EX ◇, Robitussin* ◇, Scot-Tussin Expectorant ◇

Pharmacologic class: propanediol derivative
Pregnancy risk category C

AVAILABLE FORMS

Capsules: 200 mg ◇
Liquid: 100 mg/5 ml* ◇, 200 mg/5 ml ◇
Syrup: 100 mg/5 ml ◇
Tablets: 100 mg ◇, 200 mg ◇, 400 mg
Tablets (extended-release): 600 mg ◇, 1,200 mg ◇

INDICATIONS & DOSAGES

➤ **Expectorant**
Adults and children age 12 and older: 200 to 400 mg P.O. q 4 hours, or 600 to 1,200 mg extended-release capsules or tablets q 12 hours. Maximum, 2,400 mg daily.
Children ages 6 to 11: 100 to 200 mg P.O. q 4 hours. Maximum, 1,200 mg daily.
Children ages 2 to 5: 50 to 100 mg P.O. q 4 hours. Maximum, 600 mg daily.

ACTION

Increases production of respiratory tract fluids to help liquefy and reduce the viscosity of tenacious secretions.

Route	Onset	Peak	Duration
P.O.	Unknown	Unknown	Unknown

Half-life: Unknown.

ADVERSE REACTIONS

CNS: dizziness, headache.
GI: vomiting, nausea.
Skin: rash.

INTERACTIONS

None significant.

EFFECTS ON LAB TEST RESULTS

- May interfere with uric acid level determination and with 5-hydroxyindoleacetic acid and vanillylmandelic tests.

CONTRAINDICATIONS & CAUTIONS

- Contraindicated in patients hypersensitive to drug.

NURSING CONSIDERATIONS

- Drug is used to liquefy thick, tenacious sputum. Evidence suggests that guaifenesin is effective as an expectorant, but no evidence exists to support its role as an antitussive.
- Monitor cough type and frequency.
- ***Look alike–sound alike:*** Don't confuse guaifenesin with guanfacine.

PATIENT TEACHING

- Tell patient to contact his health care provider if cough lasts longer than 1 week, recurs frequently, or is accompanied by high fever, rash, or severe headache.
- Inform patient that drug shouldn't be used for chronic or persistent cough, such as with smoking, asthma, chronic bronchitis, or emphysema.
- Advise patient to take each dose with one glass of water; increasing fluid intake may prove beneficial.
- Encourage deep-breathing exercises.

43

Miscellaneous respiratory tract drugs

acetylcysteine
beclomethasone dipropionate
beractant
budesonide
calfactant
dornase alfa
flunisolide
flunisolide hemihydrate
fluticasone propionate
fluticasone propionate and salmeterol inhalation powder
mometasone furoate
montelukast sodium
omalizumab
palivizumab
triamcinolone acetonide
zafirlukast

acetylcysteine

Acetadote, Mucomyst, Mucosil-10, Mucosil-20

Pharmacologic class: L-cysteine derivative
Pregnancy risk category B

AVAILABLE FORMS

Solution: 10%, 20%
I.V. injection: 200 mg/ml

INDICATIONS & DOSAGES

➤ **Adjunct therapy for abnormal viscid or thickened mucous secretions in patients with pneumonia, bronchitis, bronchiectasis, primary amyloidosis of the lung, tuberculosis, cystic fibrosis, emphysema, atelectasis, pulmonary complications of thoracic surgery, or CV surgery**

Adults and children: 1 to 2 ml 10% or 20% solution by direct instillation into trachea as often as q hour. Or, 1 to 10 ml of 20% solution or 2 to 20 ml of 10% solution by nebulization q 2 to 6 hours, p.r.n.

➤ **Acetaminophen toxicity**

Adults and children: Initially, 140 mg/kg P.O.; then 70 mg/kg P.O. q 4 hours for 17 doses (total). Or, a loading dose of 150 mg/kg I.V. over 60 minutes; then I.V. maintenance dose of 50 mg/kg infused over 4 hours, followed by 100 mg/kg infused over 16 hours.

I.V. ADMINISTRATION

- Drug may turn from a colorless liquid to a slight pink or purple color once the stopper is punctured. This color change doesn't affect the drug.
- Drug is hyperosmolar and is compatible with D_5W, half-normal saline, and sterile water for injection.
- Adjust total volume given for patients who weigh less than 40 kg or who are fluid restricted.
- For patients who weigh 40 kg (88 lb) or more, dilute loading dose in 200 ml of D_5W, the second dose in 500 ml, and the third dose in 1,000 ml.
- For patients who weigh 25 to 40 kg (55 to 88 lb), dilute loading dose in 100 ml, second dose in 250 ml, and third dose in 500 ml.
- For patients who weigh 20 kg (44 lb), dilute loading dose in 60 ml, second dose in 140 ml, and third dose in 280 ml.
- For patients who weigh 15 kg (33 lb), dilute loading dose in 45 ml, second dose in 105 ml, and third dose in 210 ml.
- For patients who weigh 10 kg (22 lb), dilute loading dose in 30 ml, second dose in 70 ml, and third dose in 140 ml.
- Reconstituted solution is stable for 24 hours at room temperature.
- Vials contain no preservatives; discard after opening.

INCOMPATIBILITIES

Incompatible with rubber and metals, especially iron, copper, and nickel.

ACTION

Mucolytic that reduces the viscosity of pulmonary secretions by splitting disulfide linkages between mucoprotein molecular complexes. Also, restores liver stores

- Tell patient it may take up to 4 weeks to feel the full benefit of the drug.
- Tell patient to keep inhaler clean by wiping it weekly with a dry tissue or cloth; don't get it wet.
- Advise patient to prevent oral fungal infections by gargling or rinsing his mouth with water after each use. Caution him not to swallow the water.
- Tell patient to report evidence of corticosteroid withdrawal, including fatigue, weakness, arthralgia, orthostatic hypotension, and dyspnea.
- Instruct patient to store drug at 77° F (25° C). Advise patient to ensure delivery of proper dose by gently warming canister to room temperature before using.

beractant (natural lung surfactant)

Survanta

Pharmacologic class: bovine lung extract
Pregnancy risk category NR

AVAILABLE FORMS

Suspension for intratracheal instillation: 25 mg/ml

INDICATIONS & DOSAGES

➤ **To prevent respiratory distress syndrome (RDS), also known as hyaline membrane disease, in premature neonates weighing 1,250 g (2 lb, 12 ounces) or less at birth, or having symptoms consistent with surfactant deficiency**

Neonates: 4 ml/kg intratracheally. Divide each dose into four quarter-doses and give each quarter-dose with infant in a different position to ensure even distribution of drug; between quarter-doses, use a handheld resuscitation bag at 60 breaths/minute and sufficient oxygen to prevent cyanosis. Give drug as soon as possible, preferably within 15 minutes of birth. Repeat in 6 hours if respiratory distress continues. Give no more than four doses in 48 hours.

➤ **Rescue treatment of RDS in premature infants**

Neonates: 4 ml/kg intratracheally; before giving, increase ventilator rate to 60 breaths/minute with an inspiratory time of 0.5 second and a fraction of inspired oxygen of 1. Divide each dose into four quarter-doses and give each quarter-dose with infant in a different position to ensure even distribution of drug; between quarter-doses, continue mechanical ventilation for at least 30 seconds or until stable. Give dose as soon as RDS is confirmed by X-ray, preferably within 8 hours of birth. Repeat in 6 hours if respiratory distress continues. Give no more than four doses in 48 hours.

ACTION

Lowers alveolar surface tension during respiration and stabilizes alveoli against collapse. Drug contains neutral lipids, fatty acids, surfactant-related proteins, and phospholipids that mimic naturally occurring surfactant.

Route	Onset	Peak	Duration
Intra-tracheal	30–120 min	Unknown	2–3 days

Half-life: Unknown.

ADVERSE REACTIONS

CV: TRANSIENT BRADYCARDIA, hypotension, vasoconstriction.
Hematologic: decreased oxygen saturation, hypercapnia, hypocapnia.
Respiratory: ***apnea, endotracheal tube reflux or blockage.***
Skin: pallor.

INTERACTIONS

None significant.

EFFECTS ON LAB TEST RESULTS

None reported.

CONTRAINDICATIONS & CAUTIONS

- In infants who weigh less than 600 g at birth or more than 1,750 g at birth, use hasn't been studied.

NURSING CONSIDERATIONS

- Only staff experienced in treating clinically unstable premature neonates, including neonatal intubation and airway management, should give drug.
- Accurate weight determination is essential for proper measurement of dosage.

• Continuously monitor neonate before, during, and after giving beractant. The endotracheal tube may be suctioned before giving drug; allow neonate to stabilize before proceeding with administration.
• Refrigerate at 36° to 46° F (2° to 8° C). Warm before use by allowing drug to stand at room temperature for at least 20 minutes or by holding in hand for at least 8 minutes. Don't use artificial warming methods. Unopened vials that have been warmed to room temperature may be returned to the refrigerator within 24 hours; however, warm and return drug to the refrigerator only once. Vials are for single use only; discard unused drug.
• Beractant doesn't need sonication or reconstitution before use. Inspect contents before giving; make sure color is off-white to light brown and that contents are uniform. If settling occurs, swirl vial gently; don't shake. Some foaming is normal.
• Use a 20G or larger needle to draw up drug; don't use a filter. Give drug using a #5 French end-hole catheter. Premeasure and shorten catheter before use. Fill catheter with beractant and discard excess drug so that only total dose to be given remains in the syringe. Insert catheter into neonate's endotracheal tube; make sure catheter tip protrudes just beyond end of tube above neonate's carina. Don't instill drug into a mainstream bronchus.
• Even distribution of drug is important. Give each dose in four quarter-doses, with each quarter-dose being given over 2 to 3 seconds and with the patient positioned differently after each use. Between giving quarter-doses, remove the catheter and ventilate the patient. Give the first quarter-dose with the patient's head and body inclined slightly downward, and the head turned to the right. Give the second quarter-dose with the head turned to the left. Then, incline the head and body slightly upward with the head turned to the right to give the third quarter-dose. Turn the head to the left for the fourth quarter-dose.
• Immediately after giving, moist breath sounds and crackles can occur. Don't suction the neonate for 1 hour unless he has other signs or symptoms of airway obstruction.
• Continuous monitoring of ECG and transcutaneous oxygen saturation are essential; frequent arterial blood pressure monitoring and frequent arterial blood gas sampling are highly desirable.
• Transient bradycardia and oxygen desaturation are common after dosing.
• ***Alert:*** Drug can rapidly affect oxygenation and lung compliance. Peak ventilator inspiratory pressures may need to be adjusted if chest expansion improves substantially after drug administration. Notify prescriber and adjust immediately as directed because failing to do so may cause lung overdistention and fatal pulmonary air leakage.
• Review manufacturer's audiovisual materials that describe dosage and usage procedures.
• ***Look alike–sound alike:*** Don't confuse Survanta with Sufenta.

PATIENT TEACHING

• Inform parents of neonate's need for drug, and explain drug action and use.
• Encourage parents to ask questions, and address their concerns.

budesonide

Pulmicort Respules, Pulmicort Turbuhaler

Pharmacologic class: corticosteroid
Pregnancy risk category B

AVAILABLE FORMS

Dry powder inhaler: 200 mcg/dose
Inhalation suspension: 0.25 mg, 0.5 mg

INDICATIONS & DOSAGES

➤ **As a preventative in maintenance of asthma**

All patients: Use lowest effective dose after stabilizing asthma.
Adults previously taking bronchodilator alone: Initially, inhaled dose of 200 to 400 mcg b.i.d. to maximum of 400 mcg b.i.d.
Adults previously taking inhaled corticosteroid: Initially, inhaled dose of 200 to 400 mcg b.i.d. to maximum of 800 mcg b.i.d.
Adults previously taking oral corticosteroid: Initially, inhaled dose of 400 to

800 mcg b.i.d. to maximum of 800 mcg b.i.d.
Children older than age 6 previously taking bronchodilator alone or inhaled corticosteroid: Initially, inhaled dose of 200 mcg b.i.d. to maximum of 400 mcg b.i.d.
Children older than age 6 previously taking oral corticosteroid: 400 mcg b.i.d., maximum.
Children ages 1 to 8: 0.25 mg Respules via jet nebulizer with compressor once daily. Increase to 0.5 mg daily or 0.25 mg b.i.d. in child not receiving systemic or inhaled corticosteroid or 1 mg daily or 0.5 mg b.i.d. in child receiving oral corticosteroid.

ACTION

Anti-inflammatory corticosteroid that exhibits potent glucocorticoid activity and weak mineralocorticoid activity. Drug inhibits mast cells, macrophages, and mediators (such as leukotrienes) involved in inflammation.

Route	Onset	Peak	Duration
Inhalation powder	24 hr	1–2 wk	Unknown
Respules	2–8 days	4–6 wk	Unknown

Half-life: About 2 hours.

ADVERSE REACTIONS

CNS: *headache,* asthenia, fever, hypertonia, insomnia, pain, syncope.
EENT: *sinusitis, pharyngitis,* rhinitis, voice alteration.
GI: abdominal pain, dry mouth, dyspepsia, gastroenteritis, nausea, oral candidiasis, taste perversion, vomiting.
Metabolic: weight gain.
Musculoskeletal: back pain, fractures, myalgia.
Respiratory: *respiratory tract infection,* ***bronchospasm,*** increased cough.
Skin: ecchymoses.
Other: flulike symptoms, hypersensitivity reactions.

INTERACTIONS

Drug-drug. *Ketoconazole:* May inhibit metabolism and increase level of budesonide. Monitor patient.

EFFECTS ON LAB TEST RESULTS

None reported.

CONTRAINDICATIONS & CAUTIONS

- Contraindicated in patients hypersensitive to drug and in those with status asthmaticus or other acute asthma episodes.
- Use cautiously, if at all, in patients with active or inactive tuberculosis, ocular herpes simplex, or untreated systemic fungal, bacterial, viral, or parasitic infections.

NURSING CONSIDERATIONS

- When transferring from systemic corticosteroid to this drug, use caution and gradually decrease corticosteroid dose to prevent adrenal insufficiency.
- Drug doesn't remove the need for systemic corticosteroid therapy in some situations.
- If bronchospasm occurs after use, stop therapy and treat with a bronchodilator.
- Lung function may improve within 24 hours of starting therapy, but maximum benefit may not be achieved for 1 to 2 weeks or longer.
- For Pulmicort Respules, lung function improves in 2 to 8 days, but maximum benefit may not be seen for 4 to 6 weeks.
- Watch for *Candida* infections of the mouth or pharynx.
- ***Alert:*** Corticosteroids may increase risk of developing serious or fatal infections in patients exposed to viral illnesses, such as chickenpox or measles.
- In rare cases, inhaled corticosteroids have been linked to increased intraocular pressure and cataract development. Stop drug if local irritation occurs.

PATIENT TEACHING

- Tell patient that budesonide inhaler isn't a bronchodilator and isn't intended to treat acute episodes of asthma.
- Instruct patient to use the inhaler at regular intervals because effectiveness depends on twice-daily use on a regular basis, by following these instructions:
  –Keep Pulmicort Turbuhaler upright (mouthpiece on top) during loading, to provide the correct dose.
  –Prime Turbuhaler when using it for the first time. To prime, hold unit upright and turn brown grip fully to the right, then

fully to the left until it clicks. Repeat priming.
–Load first dose by holding unit upright and turning brown grip to the right and then to the left until it clicks.
–Turn your head away from the inhaler and breathe out.
–During inhalation, Turbuhaler must be in the upright or horizontal position.
–Don't shake inhaler.
–Place mouthpiece between lips and to inhale forcefully and deeply.
–You may not taste the drug or sense it entering your lungs, but this doesn't mean it isn't effective.
–Don't exhale through the Turbuhaler. If more than one dose is required, repeat steps.
–Rinse your mouth with water and then spit out the water after each dose to decrease the risk of developing oral candidiasis.
–When 20 doses remain in the Turbuhaler, a red mark appears in the indicator window. When red mark reaches the bottom, the unit's empty.
–Don't use Turbuhaler with a spacer device and don't chew or bite the mouthpiece.
–Replace mouthpiece cover after use and always keep it clean and dry.

- Tell patient that improvement in asthma control may be seen within 24 hours, although the maximum benefit may not appear for 1 to 2 weeks. If signs or symptoms worsen during this time, instruct patient to contact prescriber.
- Advise patient to avoid exposure to chickenpox or measles and to contact prescriber if exposure occurs.
- Instruct patient to carry or wear medical identification indicating need for supplementary corticosteroids during periods of stress or an asthma attack.
- Advise patient that unused Respules are good for 2 weeks after the foil envelope has been opened; however, unused Respules should be returned to the envelope to protect them from light.
- Tell patient to read and follow the patient information leaflet contained in the package.

calfactant

Infasurf

Pharmacologic class: bovine lung extract
Pregnancy risk category NR

AVAILABLE FORMS

Intratracheal suspension: 35 mg phospholipids and 0.65 mg proteins/ml; 6-ml vial

INDICATIONS & DOSAGES

➤ To prevent respiratory distress syndrome (RDS) in premature infants under 29 weeks' gestational age at high risk for RDS; to treat infants younger than 72 hours of age, who develop RDS (confirmed by clinical and radiologic findings) and need an endotracheal tube (ETT)
Newborns: 3 ml/kg of body weight at birth intratracheally, given in two aliquots of 1.5 ml/kg each, q 12 hours for total of three doses.

ACTION

Nonpyrogenic lung surfactant that modifies alveolar surface tension, which stabilizes the alveoli.

Route	Onset	Peak	Duration
Intratracheal	Unknown	Unknown	Unknown

Half-life: Unknown.

ADVERSE REACTIONS

CV: BRADYCARDIA.
Respiratory: AIRWAY OBSTRUCTION, APNEA, *cyanosis, hypoventilation.*
Other: ***reflux of drug into endotracheal tube,*** dislodgment of endotracheal tube.

INTERACTIONS

None significant.

EFFECTS ON LAB TEST RESULTS

None reported.

CONTRAINDICATIONS & CAUTIONS

- None known..

NURSING CONSIDERATIONS

- Give drug under supervision of medical staff experienced in the acute care of newborn infants with respiratory failure who need intubation.

- Store drug at 36° to 46° F (2° to 8° C). It isn't necessary to warm drug before use.
- Unopened, unused vials that have warmed to room temperature can be re-refrigerated within 24 hours for future use. Avoid repeated warming to room temperature.
- Suspension settles during storage. Gentle swirling or agitation of the vial is commonly needed for redispersion. Don't shake vial. Visible flecks in the suspension and foaming at the surface are normal.
- ***Alert:*** Drug intended only for intratracheal use; to prevent RDS, give to infant as soon as possible after birth, preferably within 30 minutes.
- Withdraw dose into a syringe from single-use vial using a 20G or larger needle; avoid excessive foaming.
- Give through a side-port adapter into the ETT. Make sure two medical staff are present while giving dose. Give dose in two aliquots of 1.5 ml/kg each. Place infant on one side after first aliquot and other side after second aliquot. Give while ventilation is continued over 20 to 30 breaths for each aliquot, with small bursts timed only during the inspiratory cycles. Evaluate respiratory status and reposition infant between each aliquot.
- Monitor patient for reflux of drug into ETT, cyanosis, bradycardia, or airway obstruction during the procedure. If these occur, stop drug and take appropriate measures to stabilize infant. After infant is stable, resume drug with appropriate monitoring.
- After giving drug, carefully monitor infant so that oxygen therapy and ventilatory support can be modified in response to improvements in oxygenation and lung compliance.
- Enter each single-use vial only once; discard unused material.

PATIENT TEACHING

- Explain to parents the function of drug in preventing and treating RDS.
- Notify parents that, although infant may improve rapidly after treatment, he may continue to need intubation and mechanical ventilation.
- Notify parents of possible adverse effects of drug, including bradycardia, reflux into ETT, airway obstruction, cyanosis, dislodgment of ETT, and hypoventilation.
- Reassure parents that infant will be carefully monitored.

dornase alfa

Pulmozyme

Pharmacologic class: recombinant human deoxycarbonuclease 1
Pregnancy risk category B

AVAILABLE FORMS

Inhalation solution: 2.5-mg ampule (1 mg/ml)

INDICATIONS & DOSAGES

➤ **To improve pulmonary function and decrease the frequency of moderate to severe respiratory tract infections in patients with cystic fibrosis (CF)**

Adults and children age 5 and older: 1 ampule or 2.5 mg inhaled once daily. Treatment usually takes 10 to 15 minutes. Use drug only with an approved nebulizer.

ACTION

Hydrolyzes DNA in sputum of CF patients, causing decreased viscosity and elasticity of pulmonary secretions.

Route	Onset	Peak	Duration
Inhalation	Unknown	Unknown	Unknown

Half-life: Unknown.

ADVERSE REACTIONS

CV: *chest pain.*
EENT: *pharyngitis, voice alteration,* conjunctivitis, laryngitis.
Skin: *rash,* urticaria.

INTERACTIONS

None significant.

EFFECTS ON LAB TEST RESULTS

None reported.

CONTRAINDICATIONS & CAUTIONS

- Contraindicated in patients hypersensitive to drug or to products derived from Chinese hamster ovary cells.
- Safety and effectiveness haven't been established for use longer than 12 months, for children younger than age 5, and for children with forced vital capacity below 40% of normal value.

NURSING CONSIDERATIONS

- Drug is used with other standard therapies for CF.
- Patients older than age 21 and those with a forced vital capacity over 85% may benefit from twice-daily use.
- ***Alert:*** Give only with the Hudson T Updraft II disposable jet nebulizer, the Marquest Acorn II disposable jet nebulizer along with Pulmo-Aide compressor, or the LC Jet+ reusable nebulizer or the Pari Baby along with the Pari Proneb compressor, or the Durable sidestream with either the Mobilairé or Porta Neb compressors.
- Discard cloudy or discolored solution.
- Don't mix with other drugs in the nebulizer. Mixing could lead to a physical or chemical reaction that may inactivate dornase alfa.
- Refrigerate drug in its protective foil pouch to protect it from strong light.
- Once opened, the entire ampule must be used or discarded.

PATIENT TEACHING

- Teach patient how to use drug at home.
- Remind patient to breathe only through his mouth when using the nebulizer. If this is difficult, suggest that he use a nose clip.
- Tell patient that if he begins coughing during treatment, he should turn off nebulizer without spilling drug. To resume, he should turn on nebulizer and continue breathing through the mouthpiece until the nebulizer cup is empty or mist is no longer produced.

flunisolide

AeroBid, AeroBid-M, Bronalide†, Nasalide, Nasarel

flunisolide hemihydrate

AeroSpan HFA

Pharmacologic class: glucocorticoid
Pregnancy risk category C

AVAILABLE FORMS

flunisolide
Nasal solution: 25 mcg/metered spray
Oral inhalant: 250 mcg/metered spray (at least 100 metered inhalations/container)
flunisolide hemihydrate
Oral inhalant in a hydrofluoroalkane (HFA) inhaler: 80 mcg/metered dose

INDICATIONS & DOSAGES

➤ **Chronic asthma**

Adults and adolescents older than age 15: Give 2 inhalations (500 mcg) with chlorofluorocarbon (CFC) inhaler b.i.d. Maximum, 8 inhalations (2,000 mcg) daily.
Children ages 6 to 15: Give 2 inhalations (500 mcg) with CFC inhaler b.i.d. Maximum, 1,000 mcg daily.

➤ **Chronic asthma**

Adults and children age 12 and older: Give 2 inhalations (160 mcg) with HFA inhaler b.i.d. Don't exceed 320 mcg twice daily.
Children ages 6 to 11: Give 1 inhalation (80 mcg) with HFA inhaler b.i.d. Don't exceed 160 mcg twice daily.

➤ **Seasonal or perennial rhinitis**

Adults and adolescents older than age 14: Give 2 sprays (50 mcg) in each nostril b.i.d. May be increased to t.i.d., p.r.n. Maximum dose is 8 sprays in each nostril daily (400 mcg).
Children ages 6 to 14: Give 1 spray (25 mcg) in each nostril t.i.d. or 2 sprays (50 mcg) in each nostril b.i.d. Maximum dose is 4 sprays in each nostril daily (200 mcg).

ACTION

A corticosteroid that may decrease inflammation of asthma by inhibiting macrophages, T-cells, eosinophils, and mediators such as leukotrienes, while reducing the number of mast cells within the airway.

Route	Onset	Peak	Duration
Inhalation (nasal)	< 3 wk	Unknown	Unknown
Inhalation (oral)	1–4 wk	Unknown	Unknown

Half-life: Unknown.

ADVERSE REACTIONS

CNS: *headache,* dizziness, fever, irritability, nervousness.
CV: chest pain, edema, palpitations.
EENT: *nasal congestion, sore throat,* altered taste, hoarseness, nasal burning or stinging, nasal irritation, nasopharyngeal fungal infections, throat irritation.
GI: *diarrhea, nausea, unpleasant taste, upset stomach, vomiting,* abdominal pain, decreased appetite, dry mouth.
Respiratory: *cold symptoms, upper respiratory tract infection.*
Skin: pruritus, rash.
Other: *influenza.*

INTERACTIONS

None significant.

EFFECTS ON LAB TEST RESULTS

None reported.

CONTRAINDICATIONS & CAUTIONS

- Contraindicated in patients hypersensitive to drug and in those with status asthmaticus or respiratory tract infections.
- Drug isn't recommended in patients with nonasthmatic bronchial diseases or with asthma controlled by bronchodilator or other noncorticosteroid alone.

NURSING CONSIDERATIONS

- All patients with asthma should have routine tests of adrenal cortical function, including measurement of early morning resting cortisol levels to establish a baseline in the event of an emergency.
- ***Alert:*** Withdraw drug slowly in patients who have received long-term oral corticosteroid therapy.
- After withdrawing systemic corticosteroids, patient may need supplemental systemic corticosteroids if stress (trauma, surgery, or infection) causes adrenal insufficiency.
- Store drug at room temperature.
- ***Look alike–sound alike:*** Don't confuse flunisolide with fluocinonide.
- Stop nasal spray after 3 weeks if symptoms don't improve.

PATIENT TEACHING

Oral inhalant

- Warn patient that drug doesn't relieve acute asthma attacks.
- ***Alert:*** Instruct patient to immediately contact prescriber if asthma episodes unresponsive to bronchodilators occur during treatment.
- Advise patient to ensure delivery of proper dose by gently warming the canister to room temperature before using. Some patients carry the canister in a pocket to keep it warm.
- Tell patient who also is using a bronchodilator to use it several minutes before beginning flunisolide treatment.
- Instruct patient to begin inhaling immediately before activating the canister to get the full dose.
- Instruct patient to allow 1 minute to elapse before repeating inhalations and to hold his breath for a few seconds to enhance drug action.
- Teach patient to keep inhaler clean and unobstructed. If he's using a CFC inhaler, tell him to wash it with warm water and dry it thoroughly after use. The HFA inhaler doesn't need cleaning during normal use.
- Teach patient to check mucous membranes frequently for signs and symptoms of fungal infection.
- Advise patient to prevent oral fungal infections by gargling or rinsing mouth with water after each inhaler use. Caution him not to swallow the water.
- Warn patient to avoid exposure to chickenpox or measles. If exposed, contact prescriber immediately.
- Advise parents of a child receiving long-term therapy that the child should have periodic growth measurements and be checked for evidence of hypothalamic-pituitary-adrenal axis suppression.

Nasal spray

- Tell patient to prime the nasal inhaler (5 to 6 sprays) before first use and after long periods of no use.

- Advise patient to clear nasal passageways before use.
- Patient should follow manufacturer's instructions for use and cleaning. Tell him to discard open containers after 3 months.
- Advise patient that therapeutic results may take several weeks.

fluticasone propionate

Flonase, Flovent Diskus†, Flovent HFA

Pharmacologic class: corticosteroid
Pregnancy risk category C

AVAILABLE FORMS

Nasal spray: 50 mcg/metered spray
Oral inhalation aerosol: 44 mcg, 110 mcg, 220 mcg
Oral inhalation powder†: 50 mcg, 100 mcg, 250 mcg

INDICATIONS & DOSAGES

➤As preventative in maintenance of chronic asthma in patients requiring oral corticosteroid

Flovent Diskus†

Adults and children ages 12 and older: In patients previously taking bronchodilators alone, initially, inhaled dose of 100 mcg b.i.d. to maximum of 500 mcg b.i.d.

Adults and children age 12 and older previously taking inhaled corticosteroids: Initially, inhaled dose of 100 to 250 mcg b.i.d. to maximum of 500 mcg b.i.d.

Adults and children ages 12 and older previously taking oral corticosteroids: Inhaled dose of 500 to 1,000 mcg b.i.d. Maximum dose, 1,000 mcg b.i.d.

Children ages 4 to 11: For patients previously on bronchodilators alone or on inhaled corticosteroids, initially, inhaled dose of 50 mcg b.i.d. to maximum of 100 mcg b.i.d.

Flovent HFA

Adults and children age 12 and older: In those previously taking bronchodilators alone, initially, inhaled dose of 88 mcg b.i.d. to maximum of 440 mcg b.i.d.

Adults and children age 12 and older previously taking inhaled corticosteroids: Initially, inhaled dose of 88 to 220 mcg b.i.d. to maximum of 440 mcg b.i.d.

Adults and children age 12 and older previously taking oral corticosteroids: Initially, inhaled dose of 440 mcg b.i.d. to maximum of 880 mcg b.i.d.

Children ages 4 to 11: 88 mcg inhaled b.i.d. regardless of prior therapy.

➤Nasal symptoms of seasonal and perennial allergic and nonallergic rhinitis

Flonase

Adults: Initially, 2 sprays (100 mcg) in each nostril daily or 1 spray b.i.d. Once symptoms are controlled, decrease to 1 spray in each nostril daily. Or, for seasonal allergic rhinitis, 2 sprays in each nostril once daily, as needed, for symptom control.

Adolescents and children age 4 and older: Initially, 1 spray (50 mcg) in each nostril daily. If not responding, increase to 2 sprays in each nostril daily. Once symptoms are controlled, decrease to 1 spray in each nostril daily. Maximum dose is 2 sprays in each nostril daily.

ACTION

Anti-inflammatory and vasoconstrictor that may decrease inflammation by inhibiting mast cells, macrophages, and mediators such as leukotrienes.

Route	Onset	Peak	Duration
Inhalation (nasal)	12 hr	Several days	1–2 wk
Inhalation (oral)	24 hr	Several days	1–2 wk

Half-life: 3 hours.

ADVERSE REACTIONS

CNS: *headache,* dizziness, fever, migraine, nervousness.
EENT: *pharyngitis,* blood in nasal mucus, cataracts, conjunctivitis, dry eye, dysphonia, epistaxis, eye irritation, hoarseness, laryngitis, nasal burning or irritation, nasal discharge, rhinitis, sinusitis.
GI: *oral candidiasis,* abdominal discomfort, abdominal pain, diarrhea, mouth irritation, nausea, viral gastroenteritis, vomiting.
GU: UTI.
Metabolic: cushingoid features, growth retardation in children, hyperglycemia, weight gain.

Musculoskeletal: aches and pains, disorder or symptoms of neck sprain or strain, joint pain, muscular soreness, osteoporosis.
Respiratory: *upper respiratory tract infection,* ***bronchospasm,*** asthma symptoms, bronchitis, chest congestion, cough, dyspnea.
Skin: dermatitis, urticaria.
Other: ***angioedema, eosinophilia,*** influenza, viral infections.

INTERACTIONS

Drug-drug. *Ketoconazole and other cytochrome P-450 3A4 inhibitors:* May increase mean fluticasone level. Use together cautiously.
Ritonavir: May cause systemic corticosteroid effects, such as Cushing syndrome and adrenal suppression. Avoid using together.

EFFECTS ON LAB TEST RESULTS

- May cause an abnormal response to the 6-hour cosyntropin stimulation test in patients taking high doses of fluticasone.

CONTRAINDICATIONS & CAUTIONS

- Contraindicated in patients hypersensitive to ingredients in these preparations.
- Contraindicated as primary treatment of patients with status asthmaticus or other acute, intense episodes of asthma.
- Use cautiously in breast-feeding women.

NURSING CONSIDERATIONS

- Because of risk of systemic absorption of inhaled corticosteroids, observe patient carefully for evidence of systemic corticosteroid effects.
- Monitor patient, especially postoperatively or during periods of stress, for evidence of inadequate adrenal response.
- During withdrawal from oral corticosteroids, some patients may experience signs and symptoms of systemically active corticosteroid withdrawal, such as joint or muscle pain, lassitude, and depression, despite maintenance or even improvement of respiratory function.
- For patients starting therapy who are currently receiving oral corticosteroid therapy, reduce dose of prednisone to no more than 2.5 mg/day on a weekly basis, beginning after at least 1 week of therapy with fluticasone.
- ***Alert:*** As with other inhaled asthma drugs, bronchospasm may occur with an immediate increase in wheezing after a dose. If bronchospasm occurs after a dose of inhalation aerosol, treat immediately with a fast-acting inhaled bronchodilator.

PATIENT TEACHING

- Tell patient that drug isn't indicated for the relief of acute bronchospasm.
- For proper use of drug and to attain maximum improvement, tell patient to carefully follow the accompanying patient instructions.
- Advise patient to use drug at regular intervals, as directed.
- Instruct patient to contact prescriber if nasal spray doesn't improve condition after 4 days of treatment.
- Instruct patient to immediately contact prescriber if asthma episodes unresponsive to bronchodilators occur during treatment with fluticasone. During such episodes, patient may need therapy with oral corticosteroids.
- Warn patient to avoid exposure to chickenpox or measles and, if exposed, to consult prescriber immediately.
- Tell patient to carry or wear medical identification indicating that he may need supplementary corticosteroids during stress or a severe asthma attack.
- During periods of stress or a severe asthma attack, instruct patient who has been withdrawn from systemic corticosteroids to resume prescribed oral corticosteroids immediately and to contact prescriber for further instruction.
- Tell patient to prime inhaler with 4 test sprays (away from his face) before first use, shaking well before each spray. Also, prime with 1 spray if inhaler has been dropped or not used for 1 week or longer.
- Advise patient to avoid spraying inhalation aerosol into eyes.
- Instruct patient to shake canister well before using inhalation aerosol.
- Instruct patient to rinse his mouth and spit water out after inhalation.
- Advise patient to store fluticasone powder in a dry place.

Flonase nasal spray

- Tell patient to prime the nasal inhaler before first use or after 1 week or longer of nonuse.
- Have patient clear nasal passages before use.
- Advise patient to follow manufacturer's recommendations for use and cleaning.
- Advise patient to use at regular intervals for full benefit.
- Tell patient to contact provider if signs or symptoms don't improve within 4 days or if signs or symptoms worsen.
- Tell patient that the correct amount of spray can't be guaranteed after 120 sprays, even though the bottle may not be completely empty.

fluticasone propionate and salmeterol inhalation powder

Advair Diskus 100/50, Advair Diskus 250/50, Advair Diskus 500/50

Pharmacologic class: corticosteroid, long-acting beta$_2$ adrenergic agonist
Pregnancy risk category C

AVAILABLE FORMS

Inhalation powder: 100 mcg fluticasone and 50 mcg salmeterol, 250 mcg fluticasone and 50 mcg salmeterol, 500 mcg fluticasone and 50 mcg salmeterol

INDICATIONS & DOSAGES

➤Long-term maintenance of asthma

Adults and children age 12 and older: 1 inhalation b.i.d., at least 12 hours apart.
Adults and children age 12 and older not currently taking an inhaled corticosteroid: 1 inhalation of Advair Diskus 100/50 b.i.d.
Adults and children age 12 and older currently taking beclomethasone dipropionate: If beclomethasone dipropionate daily dose is 420 mcg or less, start with 1 inhalation of Advair Diskus 100/50 b.i.d. If beclomethasone dipropionate daily dose is 462 to 840 mcg, start with 1 inhalation of Advair Diskus 250/50 b.i.d.
Adults and children age 12 and older currently taking budesonide: If budesonide daily dose is 400 mcg or less, start with 1 inhalation of Advair Diskus 100/50 b.i.d. If budesonide daily dose is 800 to 1,200 mcg, start with 1 inhalation of Advair Diskus 250/50 b.i.d. If budesonide daily dose is 1,600 mcg, start with 1 inhalation of Advair Diskus 500/50 b.i.d.
Adults and children age 12 and older currently taking flunisolide: If flunisolide daily dose is 1,000 mcg or less, start with 1 inhalation of Advair Diskus 100/50 b.i.d. If flunisolide daily dose is 1,250 to 2,000 mcg, start with 1 inhalation of Advair Diskus 250/50 b.i.d.
Adults and children age 12 and older currently taking fluticasone propionate inhalation aerosol: If fluticasone propionate inhalation aerosol daily dose is 176 mcg or less, start with 1 inhalation of Advair Diskus 100/50 b.i.d. If fluticasone propionate inhalation aerosol daily dose is 440 mcg, start with 1 inhalation of Advair Diskus 250/50 b.i.d. If fluticasone propionate inhalation aerosol daily dose is 660 to 880 mcg, start with 1 inhalation of Advair Diskus 500/50 b.i.d.
Adults and children age 12 and older currently taking fluticasone propionate inhalation powder: If fluticasone propionate inhalation powder daily dose is 200 mcg or less, start with 1 inhalation of Advair Diskus 100/50 b.i.d. If fluticasone propionate inhalation powder daily dose is 500 mcg, start with 1 inhalation of Advair Diskus 250/50 b.i.d. If fluticasone propionate inhalation powder daily dose is 1,000 mcg, start with 1 inhalation of Advair Diskus 500/50 b.i.d.
Adults and children age 12 and older currently taking triamcinolone acetonide: If triamcinolone acetonide daily dose is 1,000 mcg or less, start with 1 inhalation of Advair Diskus 100/50 b.i.d. If triamcinolone acetonide daily dose is 1,100 to 1,600 mcg, start with 1 inhalation of Advair Diskus 250/50 b.i.d.
For patients already using an inhaled corticosteroid: Maximum inhalation of Advair Diskus is 500/50 b.i.d.

➤Asthma in children who remain symptomatic while taking an inhaled corticosteroid

Children ages 4 to 11: 1 inhalation (100 mg fluticasone and 50 mg salmeterol) b.i.d., morning and evening, about 12 hours apart.

➤ Maintenance therapy for airflow obstruction in patients with COPD from chronic bronchitis
Adults: 1 inhalation of Advair Diskus 250/50 only, b.i.d., about 12 hours apart.

ACTION

Fluticasone is a synthetic corticosteroid with potent anti-inflammatory activity.

Salmeterol xinafoate, a long-acting beta agonist, relaxes bronchial smooth muscle and inhibits release of mediators.

Route	Onset	Peak	Duration
Inhalation (fluticasone)	Unknown	1–2 hr	Unknown
Inhalation (salmeterol)	Unknown	5 min	Unknown

Half-life: Fluticasone: 8 hours; salmeterol: 5½ hours.

ADVERSE REACTIONS

CNS: *headache,* compressed nerve syndromes, hypnagogic effects, sleep disorders, tremors.
CV: pain, palpitations.
EENT: *pharyngitis,* blood in nasal mucosa, congestion, conjunctivitis, dental discomfort and pain, eye redness, hoarseness or dysphonia, keratitis, nasal irritation, oral candidiasis, rhinorrhea, rhinitis, sinusitis, sneezing, viral eye infections.
GI: abdominal pain and discomfort, appendicitis, constipation, diarrhea, gastroenteritis, nausea, oral discomfort and pain, oral erythema and rashes, oral ulcerations, unusual taste, vomiting.
Musculoskeletal: arthralgia, articular rheumatism, bone and cartilage disorders, muscle pain, muscle stiffness, rigidity, tightness.
Respiratory: *upper respiratory tract infection,* bronchitis, cough, lower respiratory tract infections, pneumonia.
Skin: disorders of sweat and sebum, infection, skin flakiness, sweating, urticaria.
Other: allergic reactions, chest symptoms, fluid retention, viral or bacterial infections.

INTERACTIONS

Drug-drug. *Beta blockers:* Blocked pulmonary effect of salmeterol may produce severe bronchospasm in patients with asthma. Avoid using together. If necessary, use a cardioselective beta blocker cautiously.
Ketoconazole, other inhibitors of cytochrome P-450: May increase fluticasone level and adverse effects. Use together cautiously.
Loop diuretics, thiazide diuretics: Potassium-wasting diuretics may cause or worsen ECG changes or hypokalemia. Use together cautiously.
MAO inhibitors, tricyclic antidepressants: May potentiate the action of salmeterol on the vascular system. Separate doses by 2 weeks.

EFFECTS ON LAB TEST RESULTS

- May increase liver enzyme levels.

CONTRAINDICATIONS & CAUTIONS

- Contraindicated in patients hypersensitive to drug or its components.
- Contraindicated as primary treatment of status asthmaticus or other acute asthmatic episodes.
- Use cautiously, if at all, in patients with active or quiescent respiratory tuberculosis infection; untreated systemic fungal, bacterial, viral, or parasitic infection; or ocular herpes simplex.
- Use cautiously in patients with CV disorders, seizure disorders or thyrotoxicosis; in patients unusually responsive to sympathomimetic amines; and in patients with hepatic impairment.

NURSING CONSIDERATIONS

- ***Alert:*** Patient shouldn't be switched from systemic corticosteroids to Advair Diskus because of hypothalamic-pituitary-adrenal axis suppression. Death from adrenal insufficiency can occur. Several months are required for recovery of hypothalamic-pituitary-adrenal function after withdrawal of systemic corticosteroids.
- Don't start therapy during rapidly deteriorating or potentially life-threatening episodes of asthma. Serious acute respiratory events, including fatality, can occur.
- The benefit of Advair 250/50 in treating patients with COPD for more than 6 months is unknown. If drug is used for longer than 6 months, periodically reevaluate patient to assess for benefits or risks of therapy.

- Monitor patient for urticaria, angioedema, rash, bronchospasm, or other signs of hypersensitivity.
- Don't use Advair Diskus to stop an asthma attack. Patients using Advair Diskus should carry an inhaled, short-acting $beta_2$ agonist (such as albuterol) for acute symptoms.
- If Advair Diskus causes paradoxical bronchospasm, treat immediately with a short-acting inhaled bronchodilator (such as albuterol), and notify prescriber.
- ***Alert:*** Rare, serious asthma episodes or asthma-related deaths have occurred in patients taking salmeterol; black patients may be at a greater risk.
- Monitor patient for increased use of inhaled short-acting $beta_2$-agonist. The dose of Advair Diskus may need to be increased.
- Closely monitor children for growth suppression.

PATIENT TEACHING

- Instruct patient on proper use of the dry-powder multidose inhaler to provide effective treatment.
- Tell patient to avoid exhaling into the dry-powder multidose inhaler, to activate and use the dry-powder multidose inhaler in a level, horizontal position and not to use Advair Diskus with a spacer device.
- Instruct patient to keep the dry-powder multidose inhaler in a dry place, away from direct heat or sunlight, to avoid washing the mouthpiece or other parts of the device. Patient should discard device 1 month after removal from the moisture-protective overwrap pouch or after every blister has been used, whichever comes first. He shouldn't attempt to take device apart.
- Instruct patient to rinse mouth after inhalation to prevent oral candidiasis.
- Inform patient that improvement may occur within 30 minutes after dose, but the full benefit may not occur for 1 week or more.
- Advise patient not to exceed recommended prescribing dose.
- Instruct patient not to relieve acute symptoms with Advair Diskus. Treat acute symptoms with an inhaled short-acting $beta_2$ agonist.
- Instruct patient to report decreasing effects or use of increasing doses of their short-acting inhaled $beta_2$ agonist.
- Tell patient to report palpitations, chest pain, rapid heart rate, tremor, or nervousness.
- Instruct patient to call immediately if exposed to chickenpox or measles.

mometasone furoate

Asmanex Twisthaler

Pharmacologic class: glucocorticoid
Pregnancy risk category C

AVAILABLE FORMS

Inhalation powder: 220 mcg/inhalation

INDICATIONS & DOSAGES

➤ Maintenance therapy for asthma; asthma in patients who take an oral corticosteroid

Adults and children age 12 and older who use a bronchodilator or inhale a corticosteroid: Initially, 220 mcg by oral inhalation q day in the evening. Maximum, 440 mcg/day.

Adults and children age 12 and older who take an oral corticosteroid: 440 mcg b.i.d. by oral inhalation. Maximum, 880 mcg/day. Reduce oral corticosteroid dosage by no more than 2.5 mg/day at weekly intervals, beginning at least 1 week after starting mometasone. After stopping oral corticosteroid, reduce mometasone dose to lowest effective amount.

ACTION

Unknown, although corticosteroids inhibit many cells and mediators involved in inflammation and the asthmatic response.

Route	Onset	Peak	Duration
P.O.	Unknown	Unknown	Unknown

Half-life: Unknown.

ADVERSE REACTIONS

CNS: *headache,* depression, fatigue, insomnia.
EENT: *allergic rhinitis, pharyngitis,* dry throat, dysphonia, earache, epistaxis, nasal irritation, sinus congestion, sinusitis.

GI: abdominal pain, anorexia, dyspepsia, flatulence, gastroenteritis, nausea, oral candidiasis, vomiting.
GU: dysmenorrhea, menstrual disorder, UTI.
Musculoskeletal: arthralgia, back pain, myalgia, pain.
Respiratory: *upper respiratory tract infection,* respiratory disorder.
Other: accidental injury, flulike symptoms, infection.

INTERACTIONS

Drug-drug. *Ketoconazole:* May increase mometasone level. Use together cautiously.

EFFECTS ON LAB TEST RESULTS

None reported.

CONTRAINDICATIONS & CAUTIONS

- Contraindicated in patients hypersensitive to drug or its ingredients and in those with status asthmaticus or other acute forms of asthma or bronchospasm (as primary treatment).
- Use cautiously in patients at high risk for decreased bone mineral content (those with a family history of osteoporosis, prolonged immobilization, long-term use of drugs that reduce bone mass), patients switching from a systemic to an inhaled corticosteroid, and patients with active or dormant tuberculosis, untreated systemic infections, ocular herpes simplex, or immunosuppression.
- Use cautiously in breast-feeding women.

NURSING CONSIDERATIONS

- ***Alert:*** Don't use for acute bronchospasm.
- Wean patient slowly from a systemic corticosteroid after he switches to mometasone. Monitor lung function tests, beta-agonist use, and asthma symptoms.
- ***Alert:*** If patient is switching from an oral corticosteroid to an inhaled form, watch closely for evidence of adrenal insufficiency, such as fatigue, lethargy, weakness, nausea, vomiting, and hypotension.
- After an oral corticosteroid is withdrawn, hypothalamic-pituitary-adrenal (HPA) function may not recover for months. If patient has trauma, stress, infection, or surgery during this HPA recovery period, he is particularly vulnerable to adrenal insufficiency or adrenal crisis.
- Because an inhaled corticosteroid can be systemically absorbed, watch for cushingoid effects.
- Assess patient for bone loss during long-term use.
- Watch for evidence of localized mouth infections, glaucoma, and immunosuppression.
- Use drug only if benefits to mother justify risks to fetus. If a woman takes a corticosteroid during pregnancy, monitor newborn for hypoadrenalism.
- Monitor elderly patients for increased sensitivity to drug effects.

PATIENT TEACHING

- Tell patient to use drug regularly and at the same time each day. If he uses it only once daily, tell him to do so in the evening.
- Caution patient not to use drug for immediate relief of an asthma attack or bronchospasm.
- Inform patient that maximum benefits might not occur for 1 to 2 weeks or longer after therapy starts; instruct him to notify his prescriber if his condition fails to improve or worsens.
- Tell patient that if he has bronchospasm after taking drug, he should immediately use a fast-acting bronchodilator. Urge him to contact prescriber immediately if bronchospasm doesn't respond to the fast-acting bronchodilator.
- ***Alert:*** If patient has been weaned from an oral corticosteroid, urge him to contact prescriber immediately if an asthma attack occurs or if he is experiencing a period of stress. The oral corticosteroid may need to be resumed.
- Warn patient to avoid exposure to chickenpox or measles and to notify prescriber if such contact occurs.
- Long-term use of an inhaled corticosteroid may increase the risk of cataracts or glaucoma; tell patient to report vision changes.
- Advise patient to write the date on a new inhaler on the day he opens it and to discard the inhaler after 45 days or when the dose counter reads "00."
- Instruct patient on proper use and routine care of the inhaler.

montelukast sodium

Singulair

Pharmacologic class: leukotriene receptor antagonist
Pregnancy risk category B

AVAILABLE FORMS

Oral granules: 4-mg packet
Tablets (chewable): 4 mg, 5 mg
Tablets (film-coated): 10 mg

INDICATIONS & DOSAGES

➤ **Asthma, seasonal allergic rhinitis, perennial allergic rhinitis**

Adults and children age 15 and older: Give 10 mg P.O. once daily in evening.
Children ages 6 to 14: Give 5 mg chewable tablet P.O. once daily in evening.
Children ages 2 to 5: Give 4 mg chewable tablet or 1 packet of 4-mg oral granules P.O. once daily in the evening.
Children ages 12 to 23 months (asthma only): Give 1 packet of 4-mg oral granules P.O. once daily in the evening.
Children ages 6 to 23 months (perennial allergic rhinitis only): Give 1 packet of 4-mg oral granules P.O. once daily in the evening.

ACTION

Selective, competitive leukotriene-receptor antagonist that reduces early and late-phase bronchoconstriction from antigen challenge.

Route	Onset	Peak	Duration
P.O. (chewable, granules)	Unknown	2–2½ hr	24 hr
P.O. (film-coated)	Unknown	3–4 hr	24 hr

Half-life: 2¾ to 5½ hours.

ADVERSE REACTIONS

CNS: *headache,* asthenia, dizziness, fatigue, fever.
EENT: dental pain, nasal congestion.
GI: abdominal pain, dyspepsia, infectious gastroenteritis.
GU: pyuria.
Respiratory: cough.
Skin: rash.
Other: *systemic eosinophilia,* influenza, trauma.

INTERACTIONS

Drug-drug. *Phenobarbital, rifampin:* May decrease bioavailability of montelukast because of hepatic metabolism induction. Monitor patient for effectiveness.

EFFECTS ON LAB TEST RESULTS

- May increase ALT and AST levels.

CONTRAINDICATIONS & CAUTIONS

- Contraindicated in patients hypersensitive to drug or its ingredients.
- Use cautiously and with appropriate monitoring in patients whose dosages of systemic corticosteroids are reduced.

NURSING CONSIDERATIONS

- Assess patient's underlying condition, and monitor patient for effectiveness.
- ***Alert:*** Don't abruptly substitute drug for inhaled or oral corticosteroids. Dose of inhaled corticosteroids may be reduced gradually.
- Drug isn't indicated for use in patients with acute asthmatic attacks, status asthmaticus, or as monotherapy for management of exercise-induced bronchospasm. Continue appropriate rescue drug for acute worsening.
- Don't dissolve oral granules in liquid; let the patient take a drink after receiving the granules.
- Oral granules may be given without regard to meals.

PATIENT TEACHING

- Inform caregiver that the oral granules may be given directly into the child's mouth, dissolved in 1 teaspoon of cold or room temperature baby formula or breast milk, or mixed in a spoonful of applesauce, carrots, rice, or ice cream.
- Tell caregiver not to open packet until ready to use and after opening, to give the full dose within 15 minutes. Tell her that if she's mixing the drug with food, not to store excess for future use and to discard the unused portion.
- Advise patient to take drug daily, even if asymptomatic, and to contact his prescriber if asthma isn't well controlled.

• Warn patient not to reduce or stop taking other prescribed antasthmatics without prescriber's approval.
• Advise patient to seek medical attention if short-acting inhaled bronchodilators are needed more often than usual during drug therapy.
• Warn patient that drug isn't beneficial in acute asthma attacks or in exercise-induced bronchospasm, and advise him to keep appropriate rescue drugs available.
• Advise patient with known aspirin sensitivity to continue to avoid using aspirin and NSAIDs during drug therapy.
• Advise patient with phenylketonuria that chewable tablet contains phenylalanine.

omalizumab
Xolair

Pharmacologic class: DNA-derived humanized immunoglobulin monoclonal antibody
Pregnancy risk category B

AVAILABLE FORMS
Powder for injection: 150 mg in 5-ml vial

INDICATIONS & DOSAGES
➤ **Moderate to severe persistent asthma in patients with positive skin test or in vitro reactivity to a perennial aeroallergen and whose symptoms aren't adequately controlled by inhaled corticosteroids**
Adults and adolescents age 12 and older: 150 to 375 mg subcutaneously q 2 or 4 weeks. Dose and frequency vary with pretreatment immunoglobulin E (IgE) level (international unit/ml) and patient. Divide doses larger than 150 mg among more than one injection site.

ACTION
Inhibits binding of IgE to the high-affinity receptor (FceRI) on the surface of mast cells and basophils, which limits release of allergic response mediators; also reduces number of FceRI receptors on basophils in atopic patients.

Route	Onset	Peak	Duration
SubQ	Unknown	7–8 days	Unknown

Half-life: About 26 days.

ADVERSE REACTIONS
CNS: *headache,* dizziness, fatigue, pain.
EENT: *pharyngitis, sinusitis,* earache.
Musculoskeletal: arm pain, arthralgia, fracture, leg pain.
Respiratory: *upper respiratory tract infection.*
Skin: *injection site reaction,* dermatitis, pruritus.
Other: *viral infections.*

INTERACTIONS
None reported.

EFFECTS ON LAB TEST RESULTS
• May increase IgE level.

CONTRAINDICATIONS & CAUTIONS
• Contraindicated in patients severely hypersensitive to drug.
• Safety and effectiveness haven't been established in children younger than age 12.

NURSING CONSIDERATIONS
• ***Alert:*** Don't use this drug to treat acute bronchospasm or status asthmaticus.
• Don't abruptly stop systemic or inhaled corticosteroid when omalizumab therapy starts; taper the dose gradually and under supervision.
• Because the solution is slightly viscous, it may take 5 to 10 seconds to give.
• Injection site reactions may occur, such as bruising, redness, warmth, burning, stinging, itching, hives, pain, induration, and inflammation. Most occur within 1 hour after the injection, last fewer than 8 days, and decrease in frequency with subsequent injections.
• ***Alert:*** Observe patient after the injection, and keep drugs available to respond to anaphylactic reactions. If the patient has a severe hypersensitivity reaction, stop treatment.
• Drug increases IgE level, so it can't be used to determine appropriate dosage during therapy or for 1 year after therapy ends.

PATIENT TEACHING

- Tell patients not to stop or reduce the dosage of any other asthma drugs unless directed by the prescriber.
- Explain that patient may not notice an immediate improvement in asthma after omalizumab therapy starts.

palivizumab

Synagis

Pharmacologic class: recombinant monoclonal antibody
Pregnancy risk category C

AVAILABLE FORMS

Injection: 50-mg vial, 100-mg vial

INDICATIONS & DOSAGES

➤ **To prevent serious lower respiratory tract disease caused by respiratory syncytial virus (RSV) in children at high risk**

Children: 15 mg/kg I.M. monthly throughout RSV season (November to April in the northern hemisphere). Give first dose before start of RSV season.

ACTION

Exhibits neutralizing and fusion-inhibitory activity against RSV, which inhibits RSV replication.

Route	Onset	Peak	Duration
I.M.	Unknown	Unknown	Unknown

Half-life: About 18 days.

ADVERSE REACTIONS

CNS: nervousness, pain.
EENT: *otitis media, rhinitis,* conjunctivitis, pharyngitis, sinusitis.
GI: diarrhea, gastroenteritis, oral candidiasis, vomiting.
Hematologic: anemia.
Respiratory: *upper respiratory tract infection,* ***apnea,*** asthma, bronchiolitis, bronchitis, cough, croup, dyspnea, pneumonia, wheeze.
Skin: *rash,* eczema, fungal dermatitis, seborrhea.
Other: ***failure to thrive,*** flu syndrome, hernia, injection site reaction, viral infection.

INTERACTIONS

None significant.

EFFECTS ON LAB TEST RESULTS

- May increase ALT and AST levels. May decrease hemoglobin level and hematocrit.

CONTRAINDICATIONS & CAUTIONS

- Contraindicated in children hypersensitive to drug or its components.
- Use cautiously in patients with thrombocytopenia or other coagulation disorders.

NURSING CONSIDERATIONS

- Patients should receive monthly doses throughout RSV season, even if RSV infection develops. In the northern hemisphere, RSV season typically lasts from November to April.
- To reconstitute, slowly add 1 ml of sterile water for injection into a 100-mg vial or 0.6 ml of sterile water for injection into a 50-mg vial. Gently swirl the vial for 30 seconds to avoid foaming. Don't shake vial. Let reconstituted solution stand at room temperature for 20 minutes until the solution clears. Give within 6 hours of reconstitution.
- Give drug into anterolateral aspect of thigh. Don't use gluteal muscle routinely as an injection site because of risk of damage to sciatic nerve. Give injection volumes over 1 ml as a divided dose.
- ***Alert:*** Rarely, patient may have an anaphylactoid reaction after using this drug. If anaphylaxis or severe allergic reaction occurs, give epinephrine (1:1,000), and provide supportive care as needed. If reaction is mild, use caution when giving again; if severe, stop therapy.

PATIENT TEACHING

- Explain to parent or caregiver that drug is used to prevent RSV and not to treat it.
- Advise parent that monthly injections are recommended throughout RSV season (November to April in the northern hemisphere).
- Tell parent to immediately report adverse reactions or any unusual bruising, bleeding, or weakness.

triamcinolone acetonide

Azmacort, Nasacort AQ, Nasacort HFA

Pharmacologic class: glucocorticoid
Pregnancy risk category C

AVAILABLE FORMS

Inhalation aerosol: 100 mcg/metered spray
Nasal spray: 55 mcg/metered spray, 50 mcg/metered spray

INDICATIONS & DOSAGES

➤ **Persistent asthma**

Adults and children older than age 12: Give 2 inhalations t.i.d. to q.i.d. Maximum, 16 inhalations daily. In some patients, maintenance can be achieved when total daily dose is given b.i.d.
Children ages 6 to 12: Give 1 to 2 inhalations t.i.d. to q.i.d. Maximum, 12 inhalations daily.

➤ **Nasal treatment of symptoms of seasonal and perennial allergic rhinitis**

Adults and children older than age 12: Give 2 sprays Nasacort AQ in each nostril daily; may decrease to 1 spray per nostril daily. Or, 2 sprays Nasacort HFA in each nostril once daily. May increase to 4 sprays into each nostril once daily. Adjust to minimum effective dosage.
Children ages 6 to 12: Initially, give 1 spray Nasacort AQ in each nostril daily. If no response occurs, increase to 2 sprays in each nostril daily. Or, 2 sprays Nasacort HFA into each nostril once daily. Adjust to minimum effective dosage.

ACTION

May decrease inflammation through inhibitory activities against cell types such as mast cells and macrophages and against mediators such as leukotrienes.

Route	Onset	Peak	Duration
Inhalation (nasal)	12–24 hr	Several days	1–2 wk
Inhalation (oral)	1–4 wk	Unknown	Unknown

Half-life: 18 to 36 hours; 5.4 hours (HFA).

ADVERSE REACTIONS

CNS: *headache.*
EENT: *pharyngitis, sneezing,* dry or irritated nose or throat, hoarseness, rhinitis.
GI: dry or irritated tongue or mouth, oral candidiasis.
Metabolic: adrenal insufficiency, hypothalamic-pituitary-adrenal function suppression.
Respiratory: cough, wheezing.
Other: facial edema.

INTERACTIONS

None significant.

EFFECTS ON LAB TEST RESULTS

None reported.

CONTRAINDICATIONS & CAUTIONS

- Contraindicated in patients hypersensitive to drug or its ingredients and in those with status asthmaticus.
- Use with extreme caution, if at all, in patients with tuberculosis of the respiratory tract, ocular herpes simplex, or untreated fungal, bacterial, or systemic viral infections.
- Because of risk of severe adverse effects, don't use in breast-feeding women. It's unknown if drug appears in breast milk.

NURSING CONSIDERATIONS

- Unlike other corticosteroids, drug has a spacer built into the drug-delivery device.
- Use cautiously in patients receiving systemic corticosteroids.
- Most adverse reactions to corticosteroids are dose- or duration-dependent.
- Patients who have recently been switched from systemic corticosteroids to oral inhaled corticosteroids may need to resume systemic corticosteroid therapy during periods of stress or severe asthma attacks.
- Taper oral therapy slowly.
- Store drug between 59° and 86° F (15° and 30° C).
- For nasal spray, if symptoms don't improve after 2 to 3 weeks, reevaluate the patient.
- ***Look alike–sound alike:*** Don't confuse triamcinolone with Triaminicin.

PATIENT TEACHING

Inhalation aerosol

- Inform patient that inhaled corticosteroids don't relieve emergency asthma attacks.
- Advise patient to warm canister to room temperature before using. Some patients carry canister in a pocket to keep it warm.
- If patient needs a bronchodilator, tell him to use it several minutes before triamcinolone. Tell patient to allow 1 minute to elapse before repeat inhalations and to hold his breath for a few seconds to enhance drug action.
- Teach patient to check mucous membranes frequently for evidence of fungal infection. Advise patient to avoid exposure to chickenpox or measles and to contact provider if exposure occurs.
- Tell patient to prevent oral fungal infections by gargling or rinsing mouth with water after each use of the inhaler. Remind him not to swallow the water.
- Tell patient to keep inhaler clean and unobstructed and to wash it with warm water and dry it thoroughly after use.
- Instruct patient to contact prescriber if response to therapy decreases; dosage may need adjustment. Tell him not to exceed recommended dosage on his own.
- Instruct patient to wear or carry medical identification indicating his need for supplemental systemic glucocorticoids during periods of stress.

Nasal spray

- Advise patient to use at regular intervals for full therapeutic effect.
- Advise patient to clear nasal passages before use.
- Have patient follow manufacturer's recommendations for use and cleaning.

zafirlukast

Accolate

Pharmacologic class: leukotriene receptor antagonist
Pregnancy risk category B

AVAILABLE FORMS

Tablets: 10 mg, 20 mg

INDICATIONS & DOSAGES

➤ Prevention and long-term treatment of asthma

Adults and children age 12 and older: Give 20 mg P.O. b.i.d. taken 1 hour before or 2 hours after meals.
Children ages 5 to 11: Give 10 mg P.O. b.i.d. taken 1 hour before or 2 hours after meals.

ACTION

Selectively competes for leukotriene receptor sites, blocking inflammatory action.

Route	Onset	Peak	Duration
P.O.	Rapid	3 hr	Unknown

Half-life: 10 hours.

ADVERSE REACTIONS

CNS: *headache,* asthenia, dizziness, pain.
GI: abdominal pain, diarrhea, dyspepsia, gastritis, nausea, vomiting.
Musculoskeletal: back pain, myalgia.
Other: accidental injury, fever, infection.

INTERACTIONS

Drug-drug. *Aspirin:* May increase zafirlukast level. Monitor patient for adverse effects.
Erythromycin, theophylline: May decrease zafirlukast level. Monitor patient for decreased effectiveness.
Warfarin: May increase PT. Monitor PT and INR, and adjust anticoagulant dosage.
Drug-food. *Food:* May reduce rate and extent of drug absorption. Give 1 hour before or 2 hours after a meal.

EFFECTS ON LAB TEST RESULTS

- May increase liver enzyme levels.

CONTRAINDICATIONS & CAUTIONS

- Contraindicated in patients hypersensitive to drug.
- Give cautiously to elderly patients and those with hepatic impairment.
- Give to pregnant women only if clearly needed. Don't use in breast-feeding women.

NURSING CONSIDERATIONS

- ***Alert:*** Reducing oral corticosteroid dose has been followed in rare cases by eosino-

philia, vasculitic rash, worsening pulmonary symptoms, cardiac complications, or neuropathy, sometimes as Churg-Strauss syndrome.
- Drug isn't indicated to reverse bronchospasm in acute asthma attacks.

PATIENT TEACHING
- Tell patient that drug is used for long-term treatment of asthma and to keep taking it even if symptoms resolve.
- Advise patient to continue taking other antiasthmatics, as prescribed.
- Instruct patient to take drug 1 hour before or 2 hours after meals.

44

Antacids, adsorbents, and antiflatulents

aluminum hydroxide
calcium carbonate
magnesium hydroxide
(See Chapter 47, LAXATIVES.)
magnesium oxide
simethicone
sodium bicarbonate
(See Chapter 62, ACIDIFIERS AND ALKALINIZERS.)

aluminum hydroxide

AlternaGEL ◊, Alu-Cap ◊, Aluminum Hydroxide Gel ◊, Aluminum Hydroxide Gel Concentrated ◊, Alu-Tab ◊, Amphojel ◊, Dialume ◊

Pharmacologic class: aluminum salt
Pregnancy risk category C

AVAILABLE FORMS

Capsules: 400 mg ◊, 500 mg ◊
Liquid: 600 mg/5 ml ◊
Oral suspension: 320 mg/5 ml ◊, 450 mg/5 ml ◊, 675 mg/5 ml ◊
Tablets: 500 mg ◊, 600 mg ◊

INDICATIONS & DOSAGES

➤ Acid indigestion

Adults: 500 to 1,500 mg P.O. 3 to 6 times daily between meals and at bedtime. Or, 5 to 10 ml of liquid formulation or 5 to 30 ml of oral suspension between meals and at bedtime or as directed by prescriber.

ACTION

Reduces total acid load in GI tract, elevates gastric pH to reduce pepsin activity, strengthens gastric mucosal barrier, and increases esophageal sphincter tone.

Route	Onset	Peak	Duration
P.O.	Variable	Unknown	20–180 min

Half-life: Unknown.

ADVERSE REACTIONS

CNS: ***encephalopathy.***
GI: *constipation,* ***intestinal obstruction.***
Metabolic: hypophosphatemia.
Musculoskeletal: osteomalacia.

INTERACTIONS

Drug-drug. *Allopurinol, antibiotics (tetracyclines), corticosteroids, diflunisal, digoxin, ethambutol, H_2-receptor antagonists, iron salts, isoniazid, penicillamine, phenothiazines, thyroid hormones, ticlopidine:* May decrease effect of these drugs by impairing absorption. Separate doses by 1 to 2 hours.
Ciprofloxacin, levofloxacin, lomefloxacin, moxifloxacin, norfloxacin, ofloxacin: May decrease quinolone effect. Give antacid at least 6 hours before or 2 hours after quinolone.
Enteric-coated drugs: May be released prematurely in stomach. Separate doses by at least 1 hour.

EFFECTS ON LAB TEST RESULTS

- May increase gastrin level. May decrease phosphate level.

CONTRAINDICATIONS & CAUTIONS

- No known contraindications.
- Use cautiously in patients with chronic renal disease.

NURSING CONSIDERATIONS

- When giving through nasogastric tube, make sure tube is placed correctly and is patent; after instilling drug, flush tube with water to ensure passage to stomach and to clear tube.
- ***Alert:*** Monitor long-term, high-dose use in patient on restricted sodium intake. Each tablet, capsule, or 5 ml of suspension may contain 2 or 3 mg of sodium. Refer to manufacturer's label for specific sodium content.
- Record amount and consistency of stools. Manage constipation with laxatives or stool softeners; alternate with magnesium-containing antacids (if patient doesn't have renal disease).

• Monitor phosphate level.
• Watch for evidence of hypophosphatemia (anorexia, malaise, and muscle weakness) with prolonged use; also can lead to resorption of calcium and bone demineralization.
• Aluminum hydroxide therapy may interfere with imaging techniques using sodium pertechnetate Tc-99m, and thus impair evaluation of Meckel's diverticulum. It also may interfere with reticuloendothelial imaging of liver, spleen, or bone marrow using technetium-99m sulfur colloid. It may antagonize effect of pentagastrin during gastric acid secretion tests.
• Because drug contains aluminum, it's used in patients with renal failure to help control hyperphosphatemia by binding with phosphate in the GI tract.

PATIENT TEACHING
• Instruct patient to shake suspension well and to follow with a small amount of milk or water to facilitate passage.
• Advise patient not to take aluminum hydroxide indiscriminately or to switch antacids without prescriber's advice.
• Urge patient to notify prescriber about signs and symptoms of GI bleeding, such as tarry stools or coffee-ground vomitus.
• Instruct pregnant patient to seek medical advice before taking drug.

calcium carbonate

Alka-Mints ◇, Amitone ◇, Calci-Chew, Cal-Supp‡, Caltrate, Chooz ◇, Dicarbosil ◇, Maalox Antacid Caplets ◇, Oscal, Rolaids Calcium Rich ◇, Tums ◇, Tums E-X ◇, Tums Ultra ◇, Viactiv ◇

Pharmacologic class: calcium salt
Pregnancy risk category C

AVAILABLE FORMS
Calcium carbonate contains 40% calcium; 20 mEq calcium per gram.
Chewing gum: 500 mg/piece
Lozenges: 600 mg ◇
Oral suspension: 1,250 mg/5 ml
Tablets: 500 mg ◇, 600 mg ◇, 650 mg ◇, 1,000 mg ◇, 1,250 mg ◇
Tablets (chewable): 350 mg ◇, 420 mg ◇, 500 mg ◇, 750 mg, 850 mg, 1,000 mg, 1,250 mg‡

INDICATIONS & DOSAGES
➤ Acid indigestion, calcium supplement
Adults: 350 mg to 1.5 g P.O. or two pieces of chewing gum 1 hour after meals and at bedtime, p.r.n.

ACTION
Reduces total acid load in GI tract, elevates gastric pH to reduce pepsin activity, strengthens gastric mucosal barrier, and increases esophageal sphincter tone.

Route	Onset	Peak	Duration
P.O.	20 min	Unknown	20–180 min

Half-life: Unknown.

ADVERSE REACTIONS
CNS: headache, irritability, weakness.
GI: *nausea,* constipation, flatulence, rebound hyperacidity.

INTERACTIONS
Drug-drug. *Antibiotics (tetracyclines), hydantoins, iron salts, isoniazid, salicylates:* May decrease effect of these drugs because may impair absorption. Separate doses by 2 hours.
Ciprofloxacin, levofloxacin, lomefloxacin, moxifloxacin, norfloxacin, ofloxacin: May decrease quinolone effects. Give antacid at least 6 hours before or 2 hours after quinolone.
Enteric-coated drugs: May be released prematurely in stomach. Separate doses by at least 1 hour.
Drug-food. *Milk, other foods high in vitamin D:* May cause milk-alkali syndrome (headache, confusion, distaste for food, nausea, vomiting, hypercalcemia, hypercalciuria). Discourage use together.

EFFECTS ON LAB TEST RESULTS
• May decrease phosphate level.

CONTRAINDICATIONS & CAUTIONS
• Contraindicated in patients with ventricular fibrillation or hypercalcemia.

- Use cautiously, if at all, if patient takes a cardiac glycoside or has sarcoidosis or renal or cardiac disease.

NURSING CONSIDERATIONS
- Record amount and consistency of stools. Manage constipation with laxatives or stool softeners.
- Monitor calcium level, especially in patients with mild renal impairment.
- Watch for evidence of hypercalcemia (nausea, vomiting, headache, confusion, and anorexia).

PATIENT TEACHING
- Advise patient not to take calcium carbonate indiscriminately or to switch antacids without prescriber's advice.
- Tell patient who takes chewable tablets to chew thoroughly before swallowing and to follow with a glass of water.
- Tell patient who uses suspension form to shake well and take with a small amount of water to facilitate passage.
- Urge patient to notify prescriber about signs and symptoms of GI bleeding, such as tarry stools, or coffee-ground vomitus.

magnesium oxide
Mag-Ox 400 ◇, Maox ◇, Uro-Mag ◇

Pharmacologic class: magnesium salt
Pregnancy risk category B

AVAILABLE FORMS
Capsules: 140 mg ◇
Tablets: 400 mg ◇, 420 mg ◇, 500 mg

INDICATIONS & DOSAGES
➤ **Acid indigestion**
Adults: 140 mg P.O. with water or milk after meals and at bedtime.
➤ **Oral replacement therapy in mild hypomagnesemia**
Adults: 400 to 840 mg P.O. daily. Monitor magnesium level.

ACTION
Reduces total acid load in GI tract, elevates gastric pH to reduce pepsin activity, strengthens gastric mucosal barrier, and increases esophageal sphincter tone.

Route	Onset	Peak	Duration
P.O.	20 min	Unknown	20–180 min

Half-life: Unknown.

ADVERSE REACTIONS
GI: *diarrhea,* abdominal pain, nausea.
Metabolic: hypermagnesemia.

INTERACTIONS
Drug-drug. *Allopurinol, antibiotics, digoxin, iron salts, penicillamine, phenothiazines:* May decrease effects of these drugs because may impair absorption. Separate doses by 1 to 2 hours.
Enteric-coated drugs: May be released prematurely in stomach. Separate doses by at least 1 hour.

EFFECTS ON LAB TEST RESULTS
- May increase magnesium level.

CONTRAINDICATIONS & CAUTIONS
- Contraindicated in patients with severe renal disease.
- Use cautiously in patients with mild renal impairment.

NURSING CONSIDERATIONS
- ***Alert:*** Monitor magnesium level. With prolonged use and renal impairment, watch for evidence of hypermagnesemia (hypotension, nausea, vomiting, depressed reflexes, respiratory depression, and coma).
- If diarrhea occurs, use a different drug.

PATIENT TEACHING
- Advise patient not to take drug indiscriminately or to switch antacids without prescriber's advice.
- Urge patient to report signs of GI bleeding, such as tarry stools, or coffee-ground vomitus.

simethicone

Flatulex ◊, Gas Relief ◊, Gas-X ◊, Gas-X Extra Strength ◊, Maalox Anti-Gas Extra Strength ◊, Maalox Anti-Gas Regular Strength ◊, Mylanta Gas ◊, Mylanta Anti-Gas Extra Strength ◊, Mylicon ◊, Ovol†, Ovol-40†, Ovol-80†, Phazyme ◊, Phazyme 95 ◊, Phazyme-125 ◊, Phazyme-166 Maximum Strength ◊

Pharmacologic class: polydimethylsiloxanes
Pregnancy risk category C

AVAILABLE FORMS
Capsules: 125 mg, 166 mg
Drops: 40 mg/0.6 ml ◊
Tablets: 40 mg ◊, 55 mg† ◊, 60 mg ◊, 80 mg ◊, 95 mg ◊, 125 mg ◊
Tablets (chewable): 80 mg ◊, 125 mg ◊, 150 mg ◊, 166 mg ◊

INDICATIONS & DOSAGES
➤ Flatulence, functional gastric bloating
Adults and children older than age 12: Give 40 to 125 mg P.O. after each meal and at bedtime, up to 500 mg daily. For drops, 40 to 80 mg P.O. after each meal and at bedtime, up to 500 mg daily.
Children ages 2 to 12: 40 mg after meals and at bedtime, up to 240 mg daily.
Children younger than age 2: Give 20 mg after meals and at bedtime, up to 240 mg daily.

ACTION
Disperses or prevents formation of mucus-surrounded gas pockets in the GI tract.

Route	Onset	Peak	Duration
P.O.	Immediate	Immediate	Unknown

Half-life: Unknown.

ADVERSE REACTIONS
GI: belching, flatus.

INTERACTIONS
None significant.

EFFECTS ON LAB TEST RESULTS
None reported.

CONTRAINDICATIONS & CAUTIONS
- Contraindicated in patients hypersensitive to drug.
- For infant colic, safety is unknown. .

NURSING CONSIDERATIONS
- Drug doesn't prevent gas formation.
- ***Look alike–sound alike:*** Don't confuse simethicone with cimetidine.

PATIENT TEACHING
- Tell patient to chew tablet before swallowing.
- Tell parent that drops may be mixed with 1 ounce of cool water, infant formula, or juice.
- Advise patient that changing positions often and walking will help pass flatus.

45

Digestive enzymes and gallstone solubilizers

pancreatin
pancrelipase
ursodiol

pancreatin

Donnazyme, Kutrase, Ku-Zyme, Pancreatin 4X ◊, Pancreatin 8X ◊

Pharmacologic class: pancreatic enzyme
Pregnancy risk category C

AVAILABLE FORMS

Donnazyme
Tablets: 1,000 units lipase, 12,500 units protease, 12,500 units amylase
Kutrase
Capsules: 2,400 units lipase, 30,000 units protease, 30,000 units amylase
Ku-Zyme
Capsules: 1,200 units lipase, 15,000 units protease, 15,000 units amylase
Pancreatin 4X ◊
Tablets : 12,000 units lipase, 60,000 units protease, and 60,000 units amylase ◊
Pancreatin 8X ◊
Tablets: 22,500 units lipase, 180,000 units protease, and 180,000 units amylase ◊

INDICATIONS & DOSAGES

➤ **Exocrine pancreatic secretion insufficiency; digestive aid in diseases related to deficiency of pancreatic enzymes, such as cystic fibrosis**
Adults and children: Dosage varies with condition treated. Usual first dose is 8,000 to 24,000 units of lipase activity P.O. before or with each meal or snack. Total daily dose also may be given in divided doses q 1 to 2 hours throughout.

ACTION

Replaces endogenous exocrine pancreatic enzymes and aids digestion of starches, fats, and proteins.

Route	Onset	Peak	Duration
P.O.	Unknown	Unknown	1–2 hr

Half-life: Unknown.

ADVERSE REACTIONS

GI: diarrhea with high doses, nausea.
Skin: perianal irritation.
Other: allergic reactions.

INTERACTIONS

Drug-drug. *Antacids:* May counteract pancreatin's beneficial effect. Avoid using together.
Oral iron supplement: May reduce oral iron supplement level. Separate doses.

EFFECTS ON LAB TEST RESULTS

- May increase uric acid level.

CONTRAINDICATIONS & CAUTIONS

- Contraindicated in patients hypersensitive to drug, pork protein, or pork enzymes and in those with acute pancreatitis or acute worsening of chronic pancreatitis.
- Use with caution in pregnant or breast-feeding women.

NURSING CONSIDERATIONS

- The different available products aren't interchangeable.
- To avoid indigestion, monitor patient's diet to ensure proper balance of fat, protein, and starch. Dosage varies according to degree of maldigestion and malabsorption, amount of fat in diet, and enzyme activity of individual preparations.
- Fewer bowel movements and improved stool consistency indicate effective therapy.
- Drug isn't effective in GI disorders unrelated to pancreatic enzyme deficiency.
- Enteric coating on some products may reduce available enzyme in upper portion of jejunum.

PATIENT TEACHING

- Instruct patient to take drug before or with meals and snacks.
- Tell patient not to crush or chew enteric-coated forms. Capsules containing enteric-coated microspheres may be opened and sprinkled on a small quantity of cool, soft food. Stress importance of swallowing immediately, without chewing, and following with a glass of water or juice.
- Warn patient not to inhale powder form or powder from capsules; it may irritate skin or mucous membranes.
- Tell patient to store drug in airtight container at room temperature.
- Instruct patient not to change brands without consulting prescriber.

pancrelipase

Creon 5, Creon 10, Creon 20, Ku-Zyme HP, Lipram 4500, Lipram-CR5, Lipram-CR10, Lipram-CR20, Lipram-PN10, Lipram-PN16, Lipram-PN20, Lipram-UL12, Lipram-UL18, Lipram-UL20, Pancrease, Pancrease MT4, Pancrease MT10, Pancrease MT 16, Pancrease MT 20, Pancrecarb MS4, Pancrecarb MS8, Panokase, Plaretase 8000, Ultrase MT12, Ultrase, Ultrase MT18, Ultrase MT20, Viokase, Viokase 8, Viokase 16, Viokase Powder, Viokase Tablets

Pharmacologic class: pancreatic enzyme
Pregnancy risk category C; B for Pancrease and Pancrease MT

AVAILABLE FORMS

Creon 5, Lipram-CR5
Capsules (enteric-coated microspheres): 5,000 units lipase, 18,750 units protease, and 16,600 units amylase
Creon 10, Lipram-CR10
Capsules (enteric-coated microspheres): 10,000 units lipase, 37,500 units protease, and 33,200 units amylase
Creon 20, Lipram-CR20
Capsules (enteric-coated microspheres): 20,000 units lipase, 75,000 units protease, and 66,400 units amylase
Ku-Zyme HP, PanoKase, Plaretase 8000, Viokase 8
Capsules or tablets: 8,000 units lipase, 30,000 units protease, and 30,000 units amylase
Lipram-PN10, Pancrease MT10
Capsules (enteric-coated contents): 10,000 units lipase, 30,000 units protease, and 30,000 units amylase
Lipram-PN16, Pancrease MT16
Capsules (enteric-coated contents): 16,000 units lipase, 48,000 units protease, and 48,000 units amylase
Lipram-PN20, Pancrease MT20
Capsules (enteric-coated contents): 20,000 units lipase, 44,000 units protease, and 56,000 units amylase
Lipram-UL12, Ultrase MT12
Capsules (enteric-coated contents): 12,000 units lipase, 39,000 units protease, and 39,000 units amylase
Lipram-UL18, Ultrase MT18
Capsules (enteric-coated contents): 18,000 units lipase, 58,500 units protease, and 58,500 units amylase
Lipram-UL20, Ultrase MT20
Capsules (enteric-coated contents): 20,000 units lipase, 65,000 units protease, and 65,000 units amylase
Pancrease, Lipram 4,500, Ultrase
Capsules (enteric-coated microspheres): 4,500 units lipase, 25,000 units protease, and 20,000 units amylase
Pancrease MT4
Capsules (enteric-coated microtablets): 4,000 units lipase, 12,000 units protease, and 12,000 units amylase
Pancrecarb MS4
Capsules (enteric-coated microspheres): 4,000 units lipase; 25,000 units protease; 25,000 units amylase
Pancrecarb MS8
Capsules (enteric-coated microspheres): 8,000 units lipase; 45,000 units protease; 40,000 units amylase
Viokase
Powder: 16,800 units lipase, 70,000 units protease, and 70,000 units amylase per 0.7 g powder
Viokase 16
Tablets: 16,000 units lipase, 60,000 units protease, and 60,000 units amylase

INDICATIONS & DOSAGES

➤ **Exocrine pancreatic secretion insufficiency; cystic fibrosis in adults and children; steatorrhea and other disorders of fat metabolism caused by insufficient pancreatic enzymes**
Adults and children older than age 12: Adjust dosage to patient's response. Usual first dosage 4,000 to 48,000 units of lipase with each meal.
Children ages 7 to 12: Give 4,000 to 12,000 units of lipase activity with each meal or snack. More can be taken, if needed.
Children ages 1 to 6: Give 4,000 to 8,000 units of lipase with each meal and 4,000 units of lipase with each snack.
Children ages 6 months to 11 months: Give 2,000 units of lipase with each meal.

ACTION

Replaces endogenous exocrine pancreatic enzymes and aids digestion of starches, fats, and proteins.

Route	Onset	Peak	Duration
P.O.	Variable	Variable	Variable

Half-life: Unknown.

ADVERSE REACTIONS

GI: *nausea,* cramping, diarrhea with high doses.

INTERACTIONS

Drug-drug. *Antacids:* May destroy enteric coating and enhance degradation of pancrelipase. Avoid using together.
Oral iron supplement: May decrease iron response. Monitor patient for decreased effectiveness.

EFFECTS ON LAB TEST RESULTS

- May increase uric acid level.

CONTRAINDICATIONS & CAUTIONS

- Contraindicated in patients with severe hypersensitivity to pork and in those with acute pancreatitis or acute worsening of chronic pancreatic diseases.

NURSING CONSIDERATIONS

- ***Alert:*** Use drug only for confirmed exocrine pancreatic insufficiency. It isn't effective in GI disorders unrelated to enzyme deficiency.
- Lipase activity is greater than with other pancreatic enzymes.
- For infants, mix powder with applesauce and give with meals. Avoid contact with or inhalation of powder because it may be highly irritating. Older children may take capsules with food.
- Monitor patient's stools. Adequate replacement decreases number of bowel movements and improves stool consistency.
- Individual products aren't bioequivalent and shouldn't be interchanged without prescriber supervision.
- Dosage varies with degree of maldigestion and malabsorption, amount of fat in diet, and enzyme activity of individual preparations.
- Enteric coating on some products may reduce available enzyme in upper portion of jejunum.

PATIENT TEACHING

- Instruct patient to take drug before or with meals and snacks.
- Advise patient not to crush or chew enteric-coated forms. Capsules containing enteric-coated microspheres may be opened and sprinkled on a small quantity of cool, soft food. Stress importance of swallowing immediately, without chewing, and following with glass of water or juice.
- Warn patient not to inhale powder form or powder from capsules; it may irritate skin or mucous membranes.
- Tell patient to store drug in airtight container at room temperature.
- Instruct patient not to change brands without consulting prescriber.

ursodiol

Actigall, Urso, Urso Forte

Pharmacologic class: ursodeoxycholic acid, bile acid
Pregnancy risk category B

AVAILABLE FORMS

Capsules: 300 mg
Tablets: 250 mg, 500 mg

INDICATIONS & DOSAGES

➤Dissolution of gallstones less than 20 mm in diameter when surgery is prohibited

Adults: 8 to 10 mg/kg P.O. daily in two or three divided doses.

➤To prevent gallstone formation in obese patients experiencing rapid weight loss

Adults: 300 mg P.O. b.i.d.

ACTION

Probably suppresses hepatic synthesis, cholesterol secretion, and intestinal cholesterol absorption. With long-term use, drug solubilizes cholesterol from gallstones.

Route	Onset	Peak	Duration
P.O.	Unknown	1–3 hr	Unknown

Half-life: Unknown.

ADVERSE REACTIONS

CNS: *dizziness, headache,* anxiety, depression, fatigue, sleep disorders.
EENT: rhinitis.
GI: *abdominal pain, constipation, diarrhea, dyspepsia, nausea, vomiting,* biliary pain, cholecystitis, flatulence, metallic taste, stomatitis.
GU: *UTI.*
Musculoskeletal: *back pain,* arthralgia, myalgia.
Respiratory: cough.
Skin: diaphoresis, dry skin, hair thinning, pruritus, rash, urticaria.

INTERACTIONS

Drug-drug. *Antacids containing aluminum, cholestyramine, colestipol:* May bind ursodiol, preventing its absorption. Avoid using together.
Clofibrate, estrogens, hormonal contraceptives: May increase hepatic cholesterol secretion; may counteract ursodiol effect. Avoid using together.

EFFECTS ON LAB TEST RESULTS

None reported.

CONTRAINDICATIONS & CAUTIONS

- Contraindicated in patients hypersensitive to drug or other bile acids and in those with chronic hepatic disease, unremitting acute cholecystitis, cholangitis, biliary obstruction, gallstone-induced pancreatitis, or biliary fistula. Capsules are contraindicated in patients with calcified cholesterol stones, radiopaque stones, or radiolucent bile pigment stones.

NURSING CONSIDERATIONS

- Drug won't dissolve calcified cholesterol stones, radiolucent bile pigment stones, or radiopaque stones.
- ***Alert:*** Monitor liver function test results, including AST and ALT levels, at the start of therapy and after 1 month, 3 months, and then every 6 months during therapy. Abnormal test results may indicate worsening of the disease. A hepatotoxic metabolite of drug may form in some patients.
- Therapy usually is long term, with an ultrasound done every 6 months. If stones don't partially dissolve in 12 months, success is unlikely. Safety of use for longer than 2 years hasn't been established.

PATIENT TEACHING

- Advise patient of other therapies, including watchful waiting with no intervention and cholecystectomy because the relapse rate of drug may be as high as 50% after 5 years.
- Tell patient to report adverse effects.
- Advise patient that dissolution of gallstones requires months of treatment.

46
Antidiarrheals

bismuth subsalicylate
calcium polycarbophil
(See Chapter 47, LAXATIVES.)
diphenoxylate hydrochloride and atropine sulfate
loperamide
octreotide acetate
rifaximin

bismuth subsalicylate

Bismatrol ◊, Bismatrol Extra Strength ◊, Children's Kaopectate ◊, Extra Strength Kaopectate ◊, Kaopectate ◊, Pepto-Bismol ◊, Pepto-Bismol Maximum Strength Liquid ◊, Pink Bismuth ◊

Pharmacologic class: adsorbent
Pregnancy risk category NR

AVAILABLE FORMS

Caplets: 262 mg
Oral suspension: 262 mg/15 ml ◊, 524 mg/15 ml ◊, 130 mg/15 ml
Tablets (chewable): 262 mg ◊
Liquid: 87 mg/5 ml ◊, 87.3 mg/5 ml ◊, 175 mg/5 ml ◊

INDICATIONS & DOSAGES

➤ **Mild, nonspecific diarrhea**
Adults and children age 12 and older : 30 ml or 2 tablets P.O. q 30 minutes to 1 hour, up to maximum of eight doses and for no longer than 2 days.
Children ages 9 to 12: 15 ml or 1 tablet P.O. q 30 minutes to 1 hour, up to maximum of eight doses and for no longer than 2 days.
Children ages 6 to 9: 10 ml or ⅔ tablet P.O. q 30 minutes to 1 hour, up to maximum of eight doses and for no longer than 2 days.
Children ages 3 to 6: 5 ml or ⅓ tablet P.O. q 30 minutes to 1 hour, up to maximum of eight doses and for no longer than 2 days.

➤ **Traveler's diarrhea**
Adults: 2 tablets P.O. q.i.d., before meals and h.s. for up to 3 weeks when traveling in high-risk areas during instances of high risk.

ACTION

May have antisecretory, antimicrobial, and anti-inflammatory effects against bacterial and viral enteropathogens.

Route	Onset	Peak	Duration
P.O.	1 hr	Unknown	Unknown

Half-life: Unknown.

ADVERSE REACTIONS

GI: temporary darkening of tongue and stools.
Other: salicylism with high doses.

INTERACTIONS

Drug-drug. *Aspirin, other salicylates:* May cause salicylate toxicity. Monitor patient.
Oral anticoagulants, oral antidiabetics: May increase effects of these drugs after high doses of bismuth subsalicylate. Monitor patient closely.
Tetracycline: May decrease tetracycline absorption. Separate doses by at least 2 hours.

EFFECTS ON LAB TEST RESULTS

None reported.

CONTRAINDICATIONS & CAUTIONS

- Contraindicated in patients hypersensitive to salicylates.
- Use cautiously in patients taking aspirin. Stop therapy if tinnitus occurs.
- Use cautiously in children and in patients with bleeding disorders or salicylate sensitivity.

NURSING CONSIDERATIONS

- Avoid use before GI radiologic procedures because drug is radiopaque and may interfere with X-rays.

PATIENT TEACHING

- Advise patient that drug contains salicylate. Each tablet has 102 mg salicylate. Regular-strength liquid has 130 mg/15 ml. Extra-strength liquid has 230 mg/15 ml.
- Instruct patient to shake liquid before measuring dose and to chew tablets well before swallowing.
- Tell patient to call prescriber if diarrhea lasts longer than 2 days or is accompanied by high fever.
- Advise patient to drink plenty of clear fluids to help prevent dehydration, which may accompany diarrhea.
- Tell patient that tongue and stools may temporarily turn gray-black.
- Urge patient to consult with prescriber before giving drug to children or teenagers during or after recovery from the flu or chickenpox.
- Inform patient that all forms of drug are effective against traveler's diarrhea. Tablets and caplets may be more convenient to carry.

diphenoxylate hydrochloride and atropine sulfate

Logen, Lomanate, Lomotil*, Lonox

Pharmacologic class: opioid
Pregnancy risk category C
Controlled substance schedule V

AVAILABLE FORMS

Liquid: 2.5 mg/5 ml (with atropine sulfate 0.025 mg/5 ml)*
Tablets: 2.5 mg (with atropine sulfate 0.025 mg)

INDICATIONS & DOSAGES

➤ **Acute, nonspecific diarrhea**

Adults and children older than age 12: Initially, give 5 mg P.O. q.i.d.; then adjusted, p.r.n. Maximum dosage 20 mg/day.
Children ages 2 to 12: Give 0.3 to 0.4 mg/kg liquid form P.O. daily in four divided doses. For maintenance, reduce first dose p.r.n., up to 75%. Maximum dosage 20 mg/day.

ACTION

Probably increases smooth muscle tone in GI tract, inhibits motility and propulsion, and diminishes secretions.

Route	Onset	Peak	Duration
P.O.	45–60 min	3 hr	3–4 hr

Half-life: Diphenoxylate, 2½ hours; its major metabolite, diphenoxylic acid, 4½ hours; atropine, 2½ hours.

ADVERSE REACTIONS

CNS: *dizziness, sedation,* confusion, depression, drowsiness, euphoria, headache, lethargy, malaise, numbness in limbs, restlessness.
CV: tachycardia.
EENT: blurred vision.
GI: *dry mouth,* ***pancreatitis, paralytic ileus,*** abdominal discomfort or distention, anorexia, fluid retention in bowel or megacolon, nausea, swollen gums, vomiting.
GU: urine retention.
Respiratory: ***respiratory depression.***
Skin: dry skin, pruritus, rash.
Other: ***anaphylaxis, angioedema,*** possible physical dependence with long-term use.

INTERACTIONS

Drug-drug. *Barbiturates, CNS depressants, opioids, tranquilizers:* May enhance CNS depression. Monitor patient closely.
MAO inhibitors: May cause hypertensive crisis. Avoid using together.
Drug-lifestyle. *Alcohol use:* May enhance CNS depression. Discourage use together.

EFFECTS ON LAB TEST RESULTS

None reported.

CONTRAINDICATIONS & CAUTIONS

- Contraindicated in children younger than age 2 and in patients hypersensitive to diphenoxylate or atropine, in those with obstructive jaundice, and with acute diarrhea resulting from poison, organisms that penetrate intestinal mucosa, or antibiotic-induced pseudomembranous enterocolitis.
- Use cautiously in children age 2 and older; in patients with hepatic disease, opioid dependence, or acute ulcerative colitis; and in pregnant women.

NURSING CONSIDERATIONS

- ***Alert:*** Monitor fluid and electrolyte balance. Correct fluid and electrolyte disturbances before starting drug. Dehydration, especially in young children, may in-

crease risk of delayed toxicity. Fluid retention in bowel or megacolon may occur with drug use and may mask depletion of extracellular fluid and electrolytes, especially in young children treated for acute gastroenteritis.
- Stop therapy immediately and notify prescriber if abdominal distention or other signs or symptoms of toxic megacolon develop.
- Don't use for antibiotic-induced diarrhea.
- Drug is unlikely to be effective if no response occurs within 48 hours.
- Risk of physical dependence increases with high dosage and long-term use. Atropine sulfate helps discourage abuse.
- Monitor for signs of overdose, which may include restlessness, flushing, hyperthermia, and tachycardia, initially, followed by lethargy, coma, pinpoint pupils, hypotonicity, and respiratory depression.
- ***Look alike–sound alike:*** Don't confuse Lomotil with Lamictal.

PATIENT TEACHING
- Tell patient not to exceed recommended dosage.
- Warn patient not to use drug to treat acute diarrhea for longer than 2 days and to seek medical attention if diarrhea continues.
- Advise patient to avoid hazardous activities, such as driving, until CNS effects of drug are known.

loperamide
Imodium, Imodium A-D ◊, Kaopectate II Caplets ◊, Maalox Anti-Diarrheal Caplets ◊, Pepto Diarrhea Control ◊

Pharmacologic class: piperidine derivative
Pregnancy risk category B

AVAILABLE FORMS
Tablets: 2 mg ◊
Capsules: 2 mg
Oral liquid: 1 mg/5 ml ◊

INDICATIONS & DOSAGES
➤ Acute, nonspecific diarrhea
Adults and children older than age 12: Initially, give 4 mg P.O.; then 2 mg after each unformed stool. Maximum, 8 mg daily, unless otherwise directed.
Children ages 8 to 12: Give 2 mg P.O. t.i.d. on first day. Subsequent dosages of 5 ml or 0.1 mg/kg of body weight may be given after each unformed stool. Maximum, 6 mg daily.
Children ages 6 to 8: Give 2 mg P.O. b.i.d. on first day. If diarrhea persists, contact prescriber. Maximum, 4 mg daily.
Children ages 2 to 5: Give 1 mg P.O. t.i.d. on first day. If diarrhea persists, contact prescriber.
➤ Chronic diarrhea
Adults: Initially, give 4 mg P.O.; then 2 mg after each unformed stool until diarrhea subsides. Adjust dosage to individual response.

ACTION
Inhibits peristalsis.

Route	Onset	Peak	Duration
P.O.	Unknown	2½–5 hr	24 hr

Half-life: 9 to 14½ hours.

ADVERSE REACTIONS
CNS: dizziness, drowsiness, fatigue.
GI: *constipation,* abdominal pain, distention or discomfort, dry mouth, nausea, vomiting.
Skin: hypersensitivity reactions, rash.

INTERACTIONS
Drug-drug. *Saquinavir:* May increase loperamide levels and decrease saquinavir levels. Avoid using together.

EFFECTS ON LAB TEST RESULTS
None reported.

CONTRAINDICATIONS & CAUTIONS
- Contraindicated in patients hypersensitive to drug and in those who must avoid constipation.
- Contraindicated in patients with bloody diarrhea or diarrhea with fever greater than 101° F (38° C), in breast-feeding women, and in children younger than age 2.

- Use cautiously in patients with hepatic disease.

NURSING CONSIDERATIONS

- If symptoms don't improve within 48 hours, stop therapy and consider another drug.
- Drug produces antidiarrheal action similar to that of diphenoxylate but without as many adverse CNS effects.
- ***Alert:*** Monitor children closely for CNS effects; children may be more sensitive to these effects than adults.
- ***Look alike–sound alike:*** Don't confuse Imodium with Ionamin.

PATIENT TEACHING

- Advise patient not to exceed recommended dosage.
- Tell patient with acute diarrhea to stop drug and seek medical attention if no improvement occurs within 48 hours. In chronic diarrhea, tell patient to notify prescriber and to stop drug if no improvement occurs after taking 16 mg daily for at least 10 days.
- Advise patient with acute colitis to stop drug immediately and notify prescriber about abdominal distention.
- Warn patient to avoid activities that require mental alertness until CNS effects of drug are known.
- Tell patient to report nausea, abdominal pain, or abdominal discomfort.
- Advise patient to relieve dry mouth with ice chips or sugarless gum.
- Advise breast-feeding women to avoid use.

octreotide acetate

Sandostatin, Sandostatin LAR

Pharmacologic class: synthetic octapeptide
Pregnancy risk category B

AVAILABLE FORMS

Injection ampules: 0.05 mg/ml, 0.1 mg/ml, 0.2 mg/ml, 0.5 mg/ml, 1.0 mg/ml
Injection (long-acting): 10 mg, 20 mg, 30 mg
Injection (multidose vials): 0.2 mg/ml, 1 mg/ml

INDICATIONS & DOSAGES

➤ **Flushing and diarrhea from carcinoid tumors**
Adults: 0.1 to 0.6 mg daily subcutaneously in two to four divided doses for first 2 weeks of therapy. Usual daily dosage is 0.3 mg. Base subsequent dosage on individual response.

➤ **Watery diarrhea from vasoactive intestinal polypeptide-secreting tumors (VIPomas)**
Adults: 0.2 to 0.3 mg daily subcutaneously in two to four divided doses for first 2 weeks of therapy. Base subsequent dosage on individual response but usually shouldn't exceed 0.45 mg daily.

➤ **Acromegaly**
Adults: Initially, 50 mcg subcutaneously t.i.d.; then adjust based on somatomedin C levels q 2 weeks. If Sandostatin LAR is used, give 20 mg I.M. (intragluteally) at 4-week intervals.

➤ **Carcinoid crisis including hypotension ♦**
Adults: 50 to 500 mcg by rapid I.V. injection. Repeat dose as needed. Or, 50 mcg/hour I.V. infusion for 8 to 24 hours.

➤ **GI fistula ♦**
Adults: 50 to 200 mcg subcutaneously q 8 hours.

➤ **Variceal bleeding ♦**
Adults: 25 to 50 mcg/hour via continuous I.V. infusion, over 18 hours to 5 days.

➤ **AIDS-related diarrhea ♦**
Adults: 100 to 500 mcg subcutaneously t.i.d.

➤ **Short-bowel syndrome ♦**
Adults: I.V. infusion of 25 mcg/hour or 50 mcg subcutaneously b.i.d.

➤ **Diarrhea caused by chemotherapy or radiation therapy ♦**
Adults: 50 to 100 mcg subcutaneously t.i.d. for 1 to 3 days.

➤ **Pancreatic fistula ♦**
Adults: 50 to 200 mcg q 8 hours.

➤ **Irritable bowel syndrome ♦**
Adults: Initially, 100 mcg subcutaneously as single dose; maximum, 125 mcg subcutaneously b.i.d.

I.V. ADMINISTRATION

- For emergency management of carcinoid crisis, give undiluted by rapid I.V. push.

• For other uses, dilute in 50 to 200 ml D_5W or normal saline solution and infuse over 15 to 30 minutes.
• Solution stable for 24 hours.

INCOMPATIBILITIES
Total parenteral nutrition.

ACTION
Mimics action of naturally occurring somatostatin.

Route	Onset	Peak	Duration
SubQ	30 min	30 min	< 12 hr
I.V.	Rapid	30 min	< 12 hr

Half-life: About 1½ hours.

ADVERSE REACTIONS
CNS: dizziness, fatigue, headache, lightheadedness.
CV: ***arrhythmias, bradycardia,*** conduction abnormalities, edema.
EENT: blurred vision.
GI: *abdominal pain or discomfort, diarrhea, gallbladder abnormalities, loose stools, nausea,* **pancreatitis,** constipation, fat malabsorption, flatulence, vomiting.
GU: pollakiuria, UTI.
Metabolic: ***hypoglycemia,*** hyperglycemia, hypothyroidism, suppressed secretion of growth hormone and gastroenterohepatic peptides (gastrin, vasoactive intestinal polypeptide, insulin, glucagon, secretin, motilin, and pancreatic polypeptide).
Musculoskeletal: backache, joint pain.
Skin: alopecia, erythema or pain at injection site, flushing, wheal.
Other: cold symptoms, flulike symptoms, pain or burning at subcutaneous injection site.

INTERACTIONS
Drug-drug. *Cyclosporine:* May decrease cyclosporine level. Monitor patient closely.

EFFECTS ON LAB TEST RESULTS
• May decrease vitamin B_{12} level. May increase or decrease glucose level.
• May alter liver function test values.

CONTRAINDICATIONS & CAUTIONS
• Contraindicated in patients hypersensitive to drug or its components.

NURSING CONSIDERATIONS
• ***Look alike–sound alike:*** To avoid giving drug by the wrong route, don't confuse octreotide acetate injection with injectable depot suspension product.
• Monitor baseline thyroid function tests.
• Monitor IGF-I (somatomedin C) levels every 2 weeks. Dosage adjustments are based on this level.
• Periodically monitor laboratory tests, such as thyroid function, glucose, urine 5-hydroxyindoleacetic acid, plasma serotonin, and plasma substance P (for carcinoid tumors).
• Monitor patient regularly for gallbladder disease. Therapy may be related to the development of cholelithiasis because of its effect on gallbladder motility or fat absorption.
• Monitor patient closely for signs and symptoms of glucose imbalance. Patients with type 1 diabetes mellitus and those receiving oral antidiabetics or oral diazoxide may need dosage adjustments during therapy. Monitor glucose level.
• Drug may alter fluid and electrolyte balance; other therapies may need adjusting.
• Half-life may be altered in patients with end-stage renal failure who are receiving dialysis.
• ***Look alike–sound alike:*** Don't confuse Sandostatin with Sandimmune or Sandoglobulin.

PATIENT TEACHING
• Urge patient to report signs and symptoms of abdominal discomfort immediately.
• Stress importance of the need for periodic laboratory testing during octreotide therapy.

rifaximin
Xifaxan

Pharmacologic class: rifamycin antibacterial
Pregnancy risk category C

AVAILABLE FORMS
Tablets: 200 mg

INDICATIONS & DOSAGES
➤ **Traveler's diarrhea from noninvasive strains of *Escherichia coli***
Adults and children age 12 and older: 200 mg P.O. t.i.d. for 3 days.

ACTION
Drug binds to the beta-subunit of bacterial DNA-dependent RNA polymerase, which inhibits bacterial RNA synthesis and kills *E. coli*.

Route	Onset	Peak	Duration
P.O.	Unknown	Unknown	Unknown

Half-life: Unknown.

ADVERSE REACTIONS
CNS: fever, headache.
GI: abdominal pain, constipation, defecation urgency, flatulence, nausea, rectal tenesmus, vomiting.

INTERACTIONS
None significant.

EFFECTS ON LAB TEST RESULTS
None reported.

CONTRAINDICATIONS & CAUTIONS
- Contraindicated in patients hypersensitive to rifaximin or any rifamycin antibacterial.

NURSING CONSIDERATIONS
- Don't use drug in patients whose illness may be caused by *Campylobacter jejuni, Shigella,* or *Salmonella.*
- ***Alert:*** Don't use drug in patients with blood in the stool, diarrhea with fever, or diarrhea from pathogens other than *E. coli.*
- Stop drug if diarrhea worsens or lasts longer than 24 to 48 hours. The patient may need a different antibiotic.
- Patients who have diarrhea after antibiotic therapy may have pseudomembranous colitis, which may range from mild to life-threatening.
- Monitor patient for overgrowth of nonsusceptible organisms.

PATIENT TEACHING
- Explain that drug may be taken with or without food.
- Tell patient to take all the prescribed drug, even if he feels better before the drug is finished.
- Advise patient to notify his prescriber if diarrhea worsens or lasts longer than 1 or 2 days after starting treatment. A different treatment may be needed.
- Tell patient to call the prescriber if he develops a fever or has blood in his stool.
- Explain that this drug is only for treating diarrhea caused by contaminated foods or beverages while traveling and not for any other type of infection.
- Caution patient not to share this drug with others.

47 Laxatives

bisacodyl
calcium polycarbophil
docusate calcium
docusate sodium
glycerin
lactulose
magnesium citrate
magnesium hydroxide
magnesium sulfate
polyethylene glycol
polyethylene glycol and electrolyte solution
sodium phosphates
sodium phosphate monohydrate and sodium phosphate dibasic anhydrous

bisacodyl

Bisacolax‡ ◊, Bisalax‡, Bisco-Lax ◊, Correctol, Dulcolax ◊, Durolax‡, Feen-a-Mint, Fleet Bisacodyl ◊, Fleet Bisacodyl Enema ◊, Fleet Laxatives ◊, Laxit† ◊

Pharmacologic class: diphenylmethane derivative
Pregnancy risk category B

AVAILABLE FORMS

Enema: 0.33 mg/ml ◊, 10 mg/5 ml (microenema)‡
Powder for rectal solution (bisacodyl tannex): 1.5 mg bisacodyl and 2.5 g tannic acid
Suppositories: 5 mg ◊, 10 mg ◊
Tablets (enteric-coated): 5 mg ◊

INDICATIONS & DOSAGES

➤ **Chronic constipation; preparation for childbirth, surgery, or rectal or bowel examination**

Adults and children age 12 and older: Give 10 to 15 mg P.O. in evening or before breakfast. Up to 30 mg P.O., p.r.n. Or, 10 mg P.R. for evacuation before examination or surgery.

Children ages 6 to 11: Give 5 mg P.O. or P.R. at bedtime or before breakfast. Oral dose isn't recommended if child can't swallow tablet whole.

ACTION

Unknown. Stimulant laxative that increases peristalsis, probably by direct effect on smooth muscle of the intestine, by irritating the muscle or stimulating the colonic intramural plexus. Drug also promotes fluid accumulation in colon and small intestine.

Route	Onset	Peak	Duration
P.O.	6–12 hr	Variable	Variable
P.R.	15–60 min	Variable	Variable

Half-life: Unknown.

ADVERSE REACTIONS

CNS: dizziness, faintness, muscle weakness with excessive use.
GI: *abdominal cramps, burning sensation in rectum with suppositories, nausea, vomiting,* diarrhea with high doses, laxative dependence with long-term or excessive use, protein-losing enteropathy with excessive use.
Metabolic: alkalosis, fluid and electrolyte imbalance, hypokalemia.
Musculoskeletal: tetany.

INTERACTIONS

Drug-drug. *Antacids:* May cause gastric irritation or dyspepsia from premature dissolution of enteric coating. Separate doses by at least 1 or 2 hours.
Drug-food. *Milk:* May cause gastric irritation or dyspepsia from premature dissolution of enteric coating. Don't use within 1 or 2 hours of drinking milk.

EFFECTS ON LAB TEST RESULTS

• May increase phosphate and sodium levels. May decrease calcium, magnesium, and potassium levels.

CONTRAINDICATIONS & CAUTIONS

• Contraindicated in patients hypersensitive to drug or its components and in those with rectal bleeding, gastroenteritis, intes-

Nursing2008 Drug Handbook Photoguide to tablets and capsules

This photoguide presents nearly 400 tablets and capsules, representing the most commonly prescribed generic and trade name drugs. These drugs, organized alphabetically by generic name, are shown in actual size and color with cross-references to drug information. Each product is labeled with its trade name and its strength.

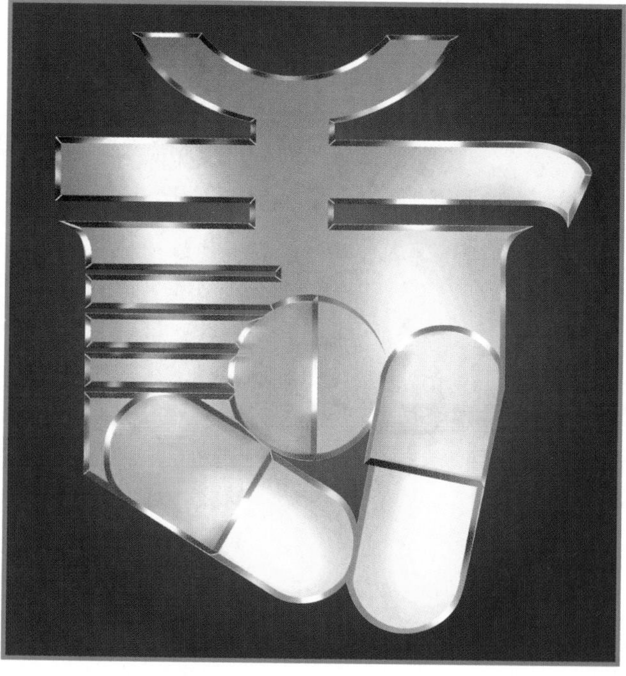

Adapted from Facts & Comparisons, St. Louis, Missouri.

For the list of companies permitting use of these photographs, see pages 1375–1376.

ACAMPROSATE CALCIUM

Campral
(page 1249)

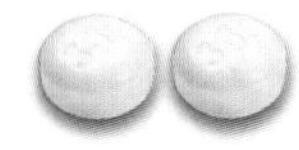

333 mg

ACETAMINOPHEN WITH CODEINE

Tylenol with Codeine No. 3
(page 1331)

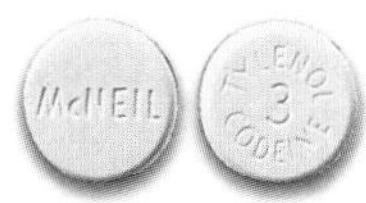

300 mg/30 mg

ACYCLOVIR

Zovirax
(page 152)

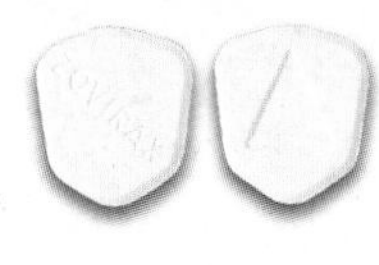

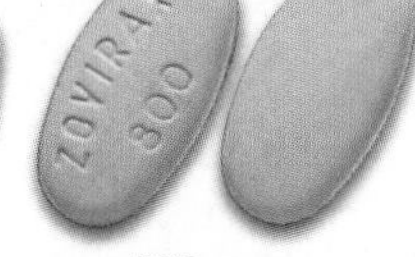

400 mg | 800 mg

ALENDRONATE SODIUM

Fosamax
(page 849)

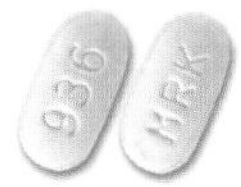

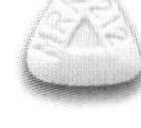

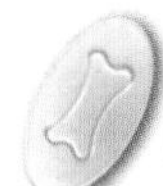

10 mg | 40 mg | 70 mg

ALFUZOSIN HYDROCHLORIDE

Uroxatral
(page 1271)

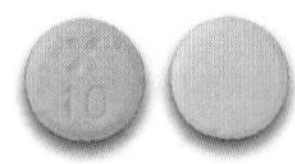

10 mg

ALOSETRON HYDROCHLORIDE

Lotronex
(page 733)

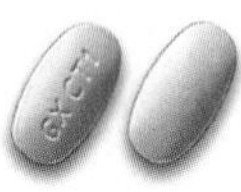

1 mg

ALPRAZOLAM

Xanax
(page 489)

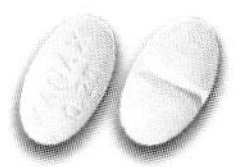
0.25 mg

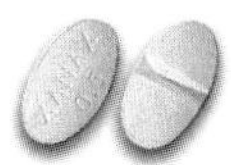
0.5 mg

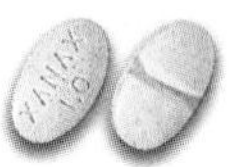
1 mg

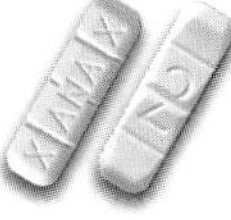
2 mg

AMLODIPINE BESYLATE

Norvasc
(page 265)

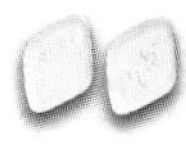
2.5 mg

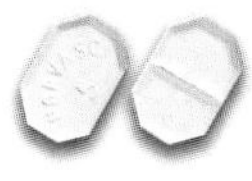
5 mg

ANASTROZOLE

Arimidex
(page 988)

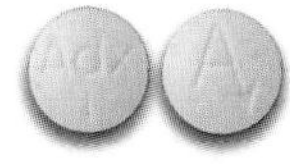
1 mg

ARIPIPRAZOLE

Abilify
(page 501)

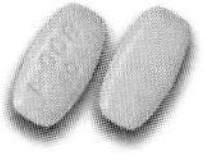

10 mg

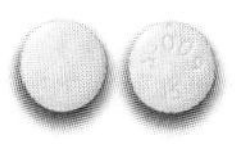
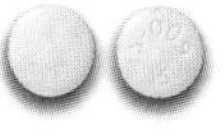
15 mg

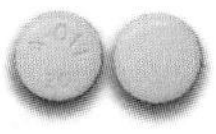
30 mg

ATAZANAVIR SULFATE

Reyataz
(page 157)

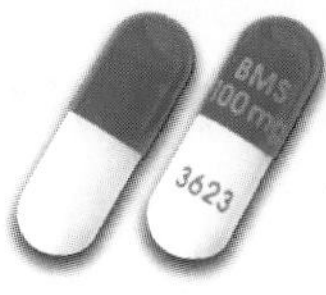

100 mg

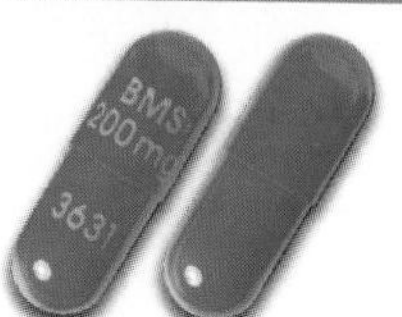

200 mg

ATENOLOL

Tenormin
(page 282)

25 mg

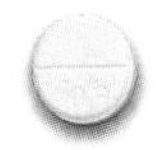
50 mg

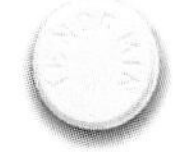
100 mg

ATOMOXETINE HYDROCHLORIDE

Strattera
(page 562)

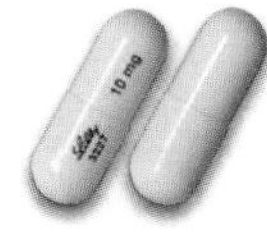
10 mg

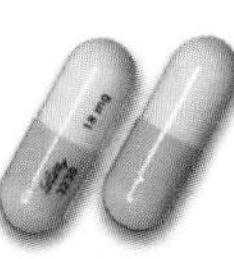
18 mg

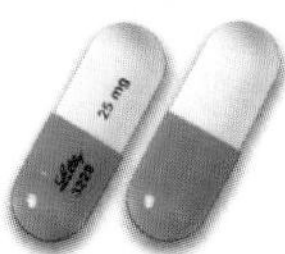
25 mg

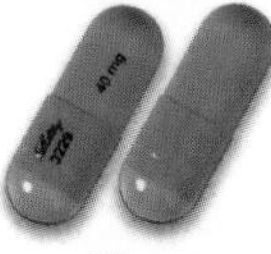
40 mg

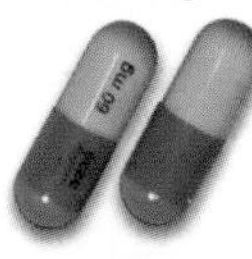
60 mg

ATORVASTATIN CALCIUM

Lipitor
(page 330)

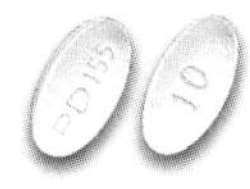

10 mg

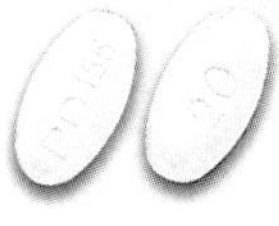

20 mg

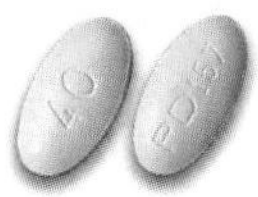

40 mg

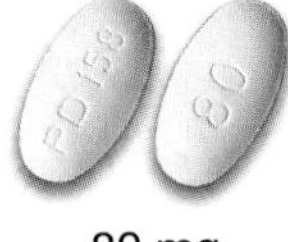

80 mg

AZITHROMYCIN

Zithromax
(page 205)

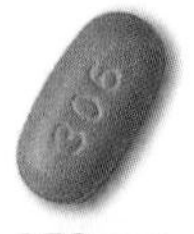

250 mg

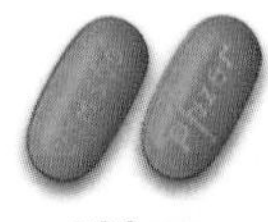

500 mg

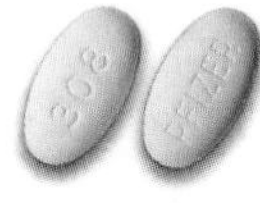

600 mg

BENAZEPRIL HYDROCHLORIDE

Lotensin
(page 284)

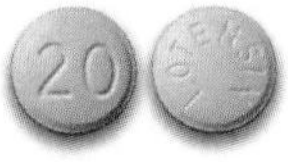

20 mg

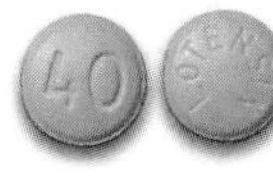

40 mg

BUMETANIDE

Bumex
(page 864)

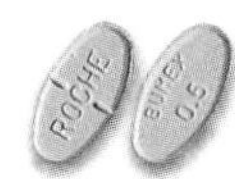

0.5 mg

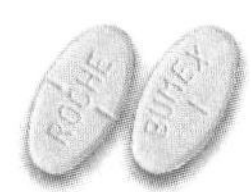

1 mg

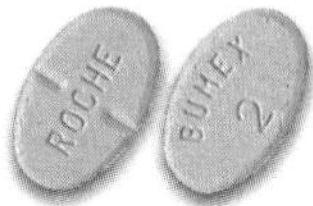

2 mg

BUPROPION HYDROCHLORIDE

Wellbutrin
(page 461)

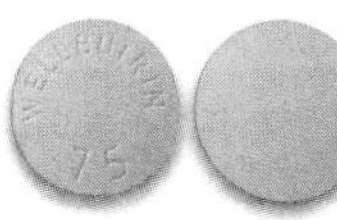

75 mg

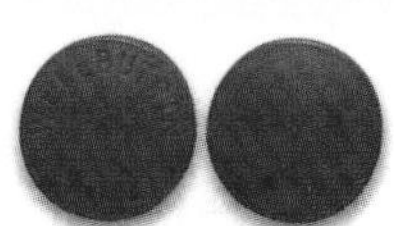
100 mg

Wellbutrin SR
(page 461)

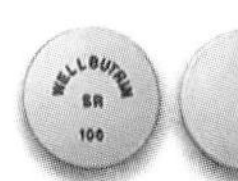

100 mg

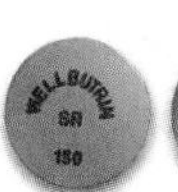

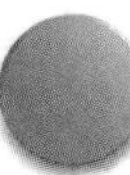
150 mg

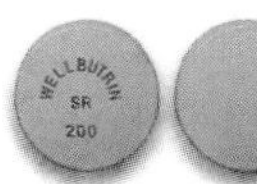

200 mg

Zyban
(page 461)

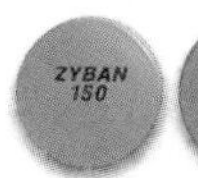

150 mg

BUSPIRONE HYDROCHLORIDE

BuSpar
(page 490)

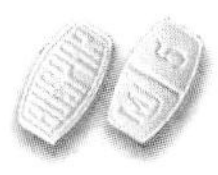

5 mg

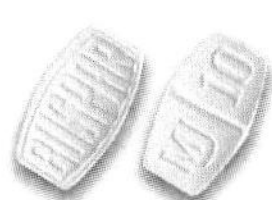

10 mg

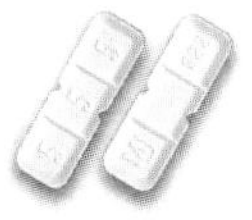
15 mg

CAPTOPRIL

Capoten
(page 286)

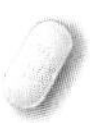
12.5 mg

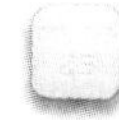
25 mg

CARISOPRODOL

Soma
(page 607)

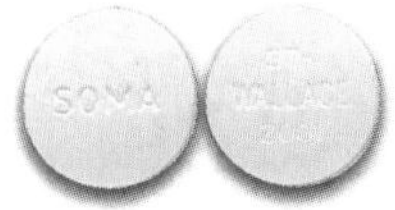

350 mg

CEFADROXIL

Duricef
(page 99)

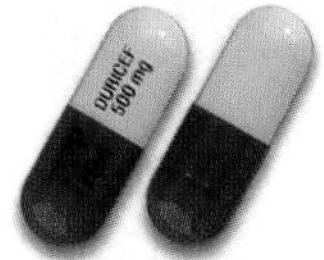

500 mg

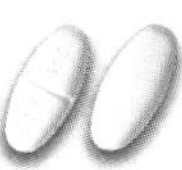

1,000 mg

CEFPROZIL

Cefzil
(page 113)

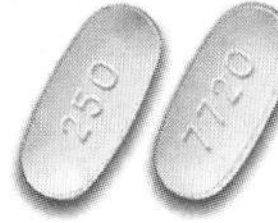

250 mg

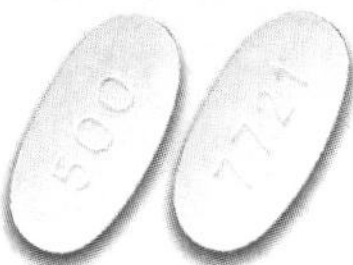

500 mg

CELECOXIB

Celebrex
(page 373)

100 mg

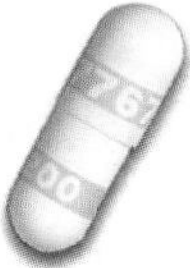

200 mg

CETIRIZINE HYDROCHLORIDE

Zyrtec
(page 623)

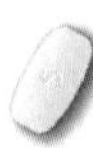

5 mg

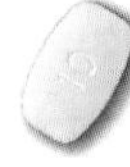

10 mg

CIPROFLOXACIN

Cipro
(page 138)

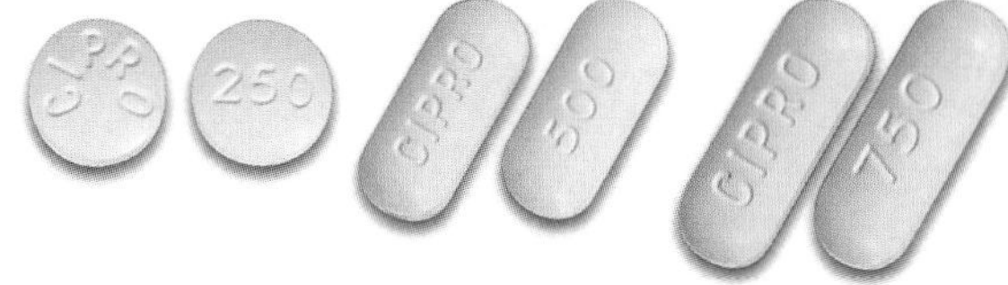

250 mg | 500 mg | 750 mg

CITALOPRAM HYDROBROMIDE

Celexa
(page 463)

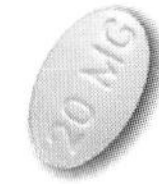

20 mg | 40 mg

CLARITHROMYCIN

Biaxin
(page 207)

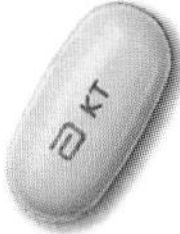

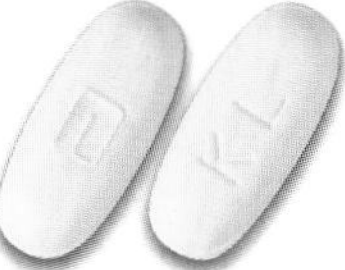

250 mg | 500 mg

Biaxin XL
(page 207)

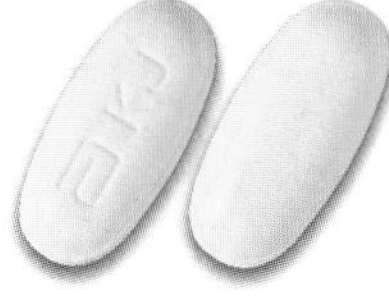

500 mg

CLONAZEPAM

Klonopin
(page 433)

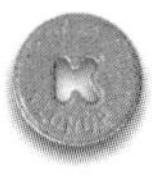

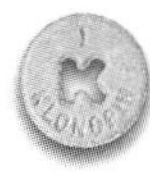

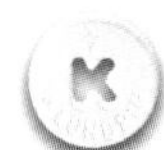

0.5 mg | 1 mg | 2 mg

CO-TRIMOXAZOLE

Bactrim DS
(page 132)

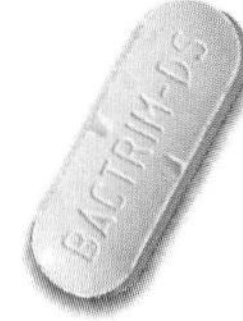

160 mg/800 mg

DARIFENACIN HYDROBROMIDE

Enablex
(page 1238)

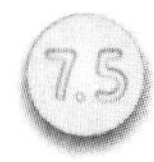

7.5 mg

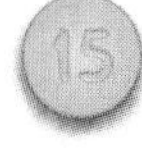

15 mg

DESLORATADINE

Clarinex
(page 626)

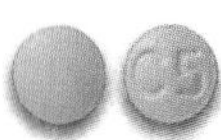

5 mg

DIAZEPAM

Valium
(page 493)

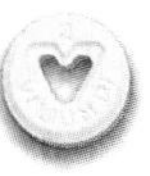

2 mg

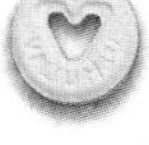

5 mg

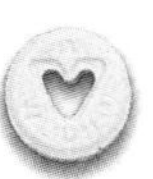

10 mg

DIGOXIN

Lanoxin
(page 232)

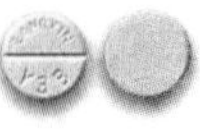

0.125 mg

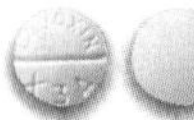

0.25 mg

DILTIAZEM HYDROCHLORIDE

Cardizem
(page 266)

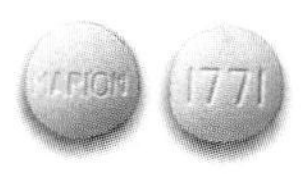

30 mg

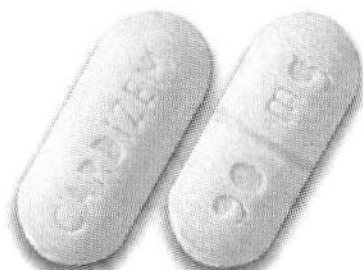
90 mg

Cardizem CD
(page 266)

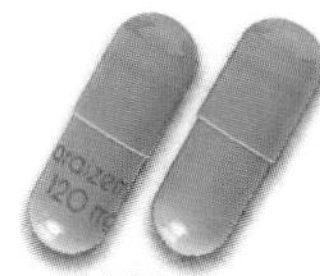
120 mg

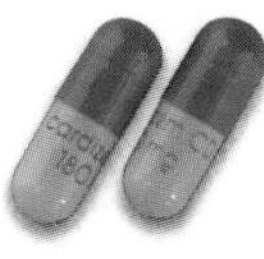
180 mg

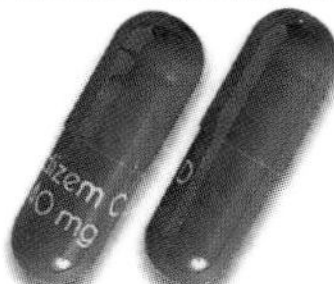
240 mg

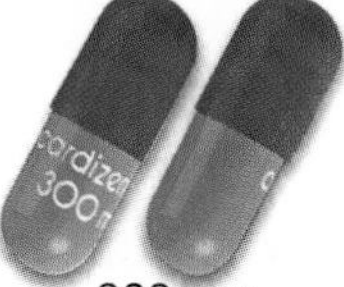
300 mg

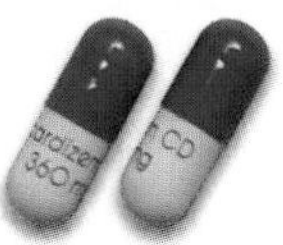
360 mg

Cardizem LA
(page 266)

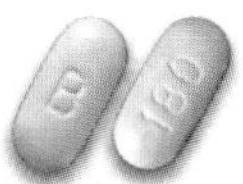
180 mg

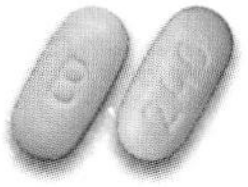
240 mg

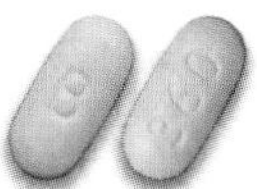
360 mg

DIVALPROEX SODIUM

Depakote
(page 455)

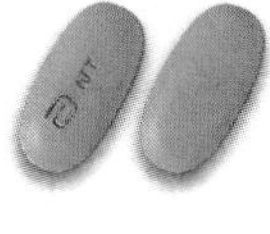
125 mg

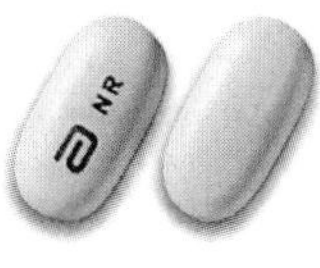

250 mg

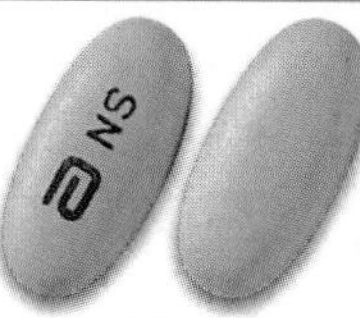

500 mg

Depakote Sprinkle
(page 455)

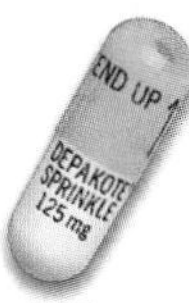

125 mg

DOXAZOSIN MESYLATE

Cardura
(page 292)

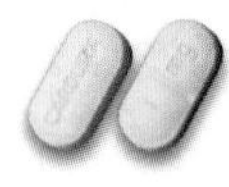

1 mg

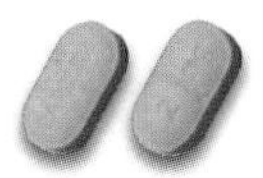

2 mg

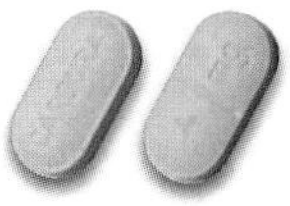

4 mg

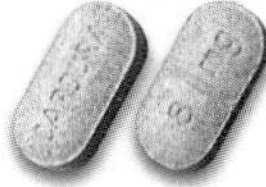

8 mg

DULOXETINE HYDROCHLORIDE

Cymbalta
(page 469)

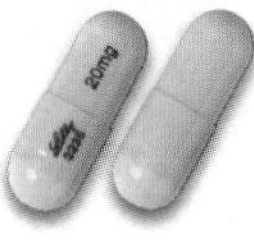

20 mg

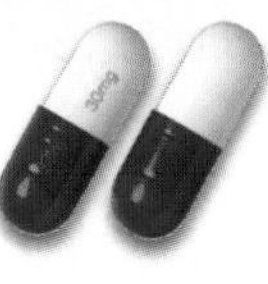

30 mg

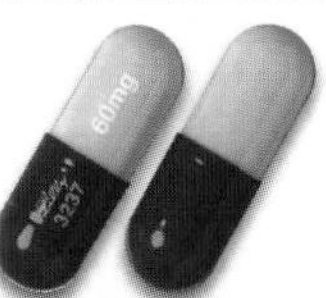

60 mg

ELETRIPTAN HYDROBROMIDE

Relpax
(page 566)

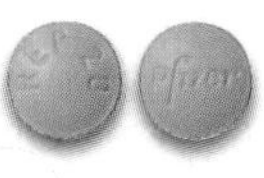

20 mg

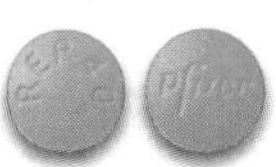

40 mg

ENALAPRIL MALEATE

Vasotec
(page 293)

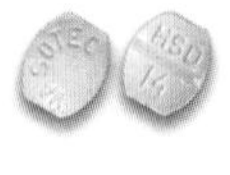

2.5 mg

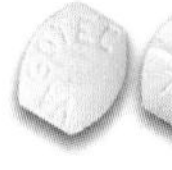

5 mg

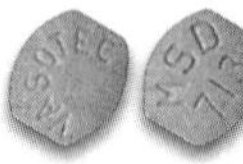

10 mg

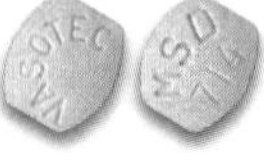

20 mg

ERYTHROMYCIN BASE

E-Mycin
(page 209)

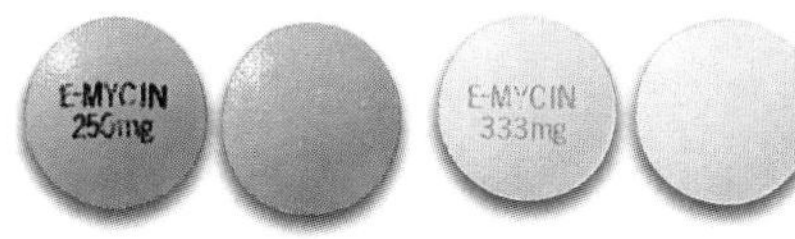

250 mg 333 mg

Eryc
(page 209)

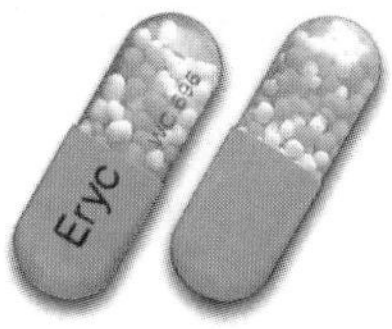

250 mg

Ery-Tab
(page 209)

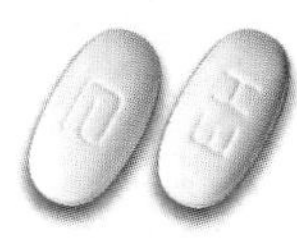

333 mg

ESCITALOPRAM OXALATE

Lexapro
(page 470)

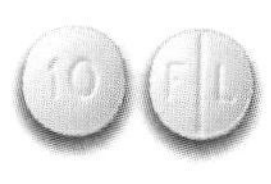

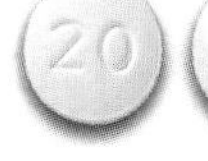

10 mg 20 mg

ESTRADIOL

Estrace
(page 769)

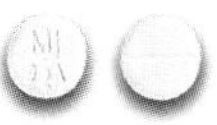

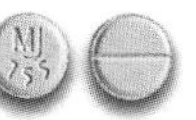

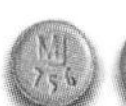

0.5 mg 1 mg 2 mg

ESZOPICLONE

Lunesta
(page 421)

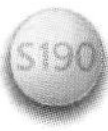

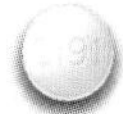

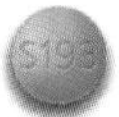

1 mg 2 mg 3 mg

ETHINYL ESTRADIOL AND ETHYNODIOL DIACETATE

Demulen
(page 780)

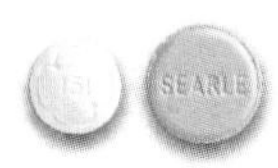

1 mg/35 mcg

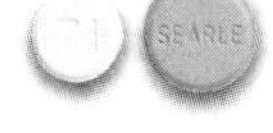

1 mg/50 mcg

EZETIMIBE

Zetia
(page 334)

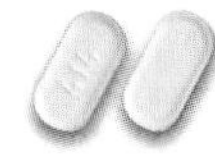

10 mg

FAMOTIDINE

Pepcid
(page 721)

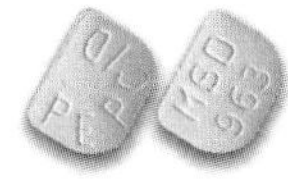

20 mg

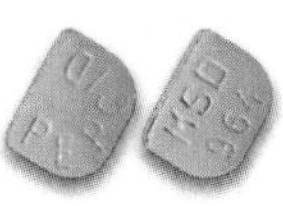

40 mg

FEXOFENADINE HYDROCHLORIDE

Allegra
(page 628)

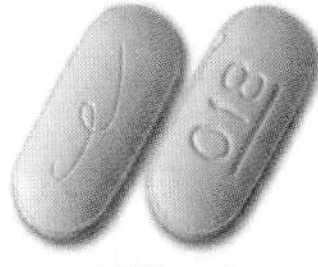

180 mg

FLUCONAZOLE

Diflucan
(page 39)

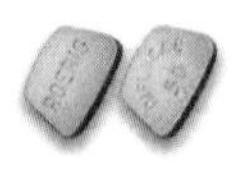

50 mg

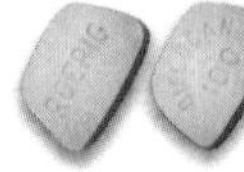

100 mg

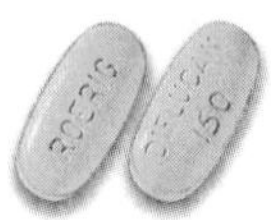

150 mg

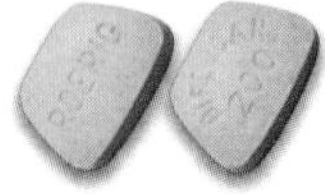

200 mg

FLUOXETINE HYDROCHLORIDE

Prozac
(page 472)

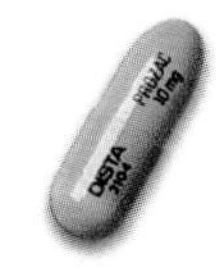

10 mg

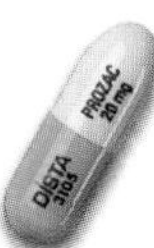

20 mg

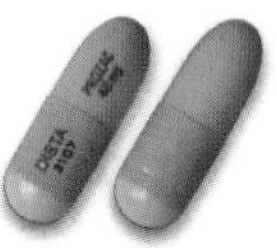
40 mg

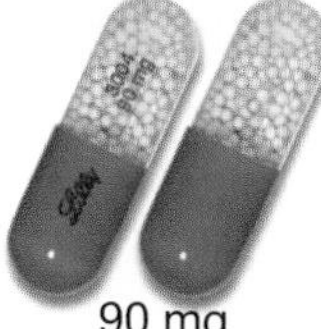
90 mg

Sarafem
(page 472)

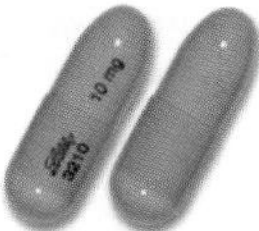

10 mg

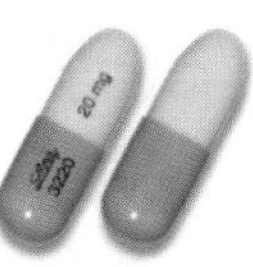

20 mg

FLUVASTATIN SODIUM

Lescol
(page 336)

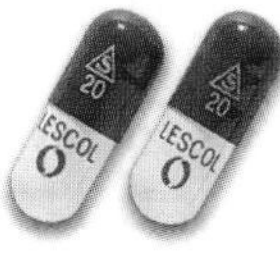

20 mg

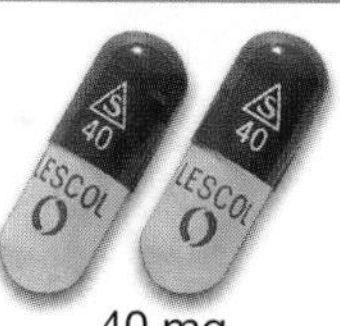

40 mg

FOSINOPRIL SODIUM

Monopril
(page 299)

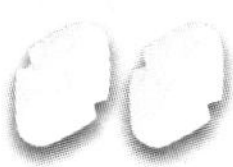
10 mg

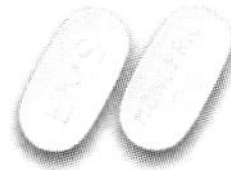
20 mg

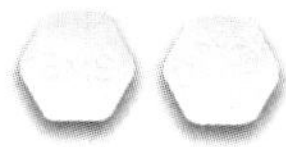
40 mg

FROVATRIPTAN SUCCINATE

Frova
(page 567)

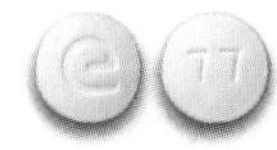

2.5 mg

FUROSEMIDE

Lasix
(page 866)

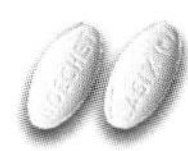

20 mg

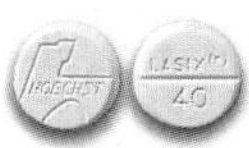

40 mg

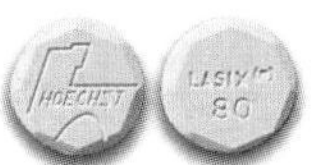

80 mg

GABAPENTIN

Neurontin
(page 437)

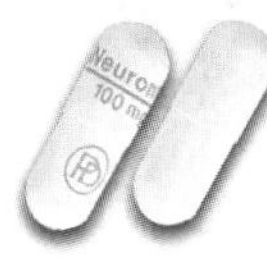

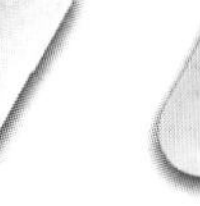

100 mg

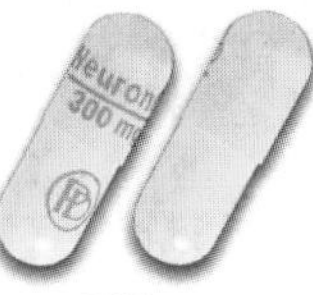

300 mg

400 mg

GEMFIBROZIL

Lopid
(page 338)

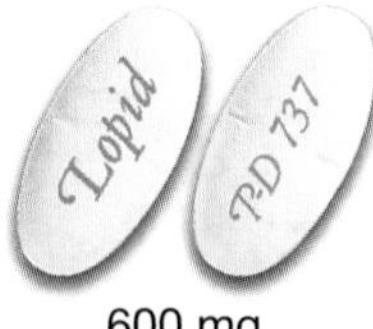

600 mg

GLIPIZIDE

Glucotrol

(page 801)

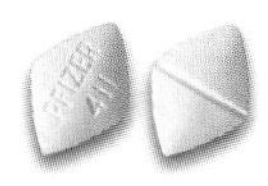

5 mg

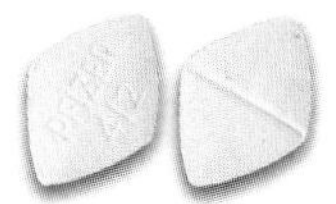

10 mg

Glucotrol XL

(page 801)

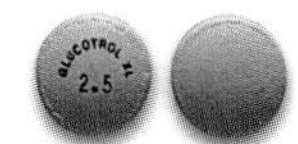

2.5 mg

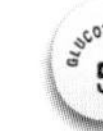

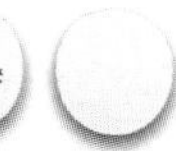

5 mg

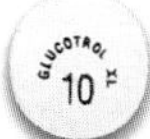

10 mg

GLYBURIDE

DiaBeta

(page 803)

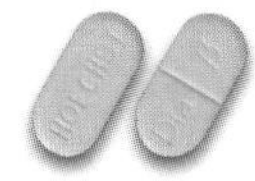

1.25 mg

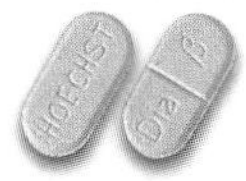

2.5 mg

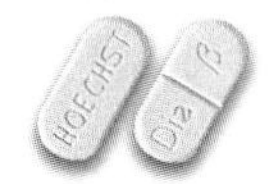

5 mg

Micronase

(page 803)

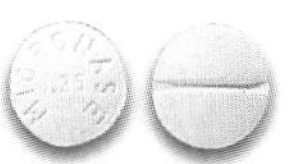

1.25 mg

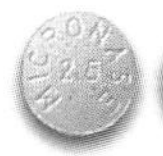

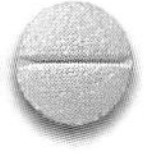

2.5 mg

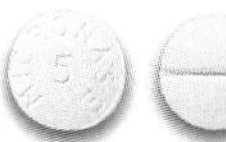

5 mg

HYDROCHLOROTHIAZIDE

HydroDIURIL

(page 868)

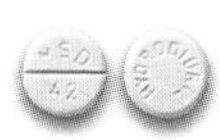

25 mg

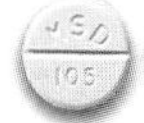

50 mg

HYDROCODONE BITARTRATE AND ACETAMINOPHEN

Lortab

(page 1329)

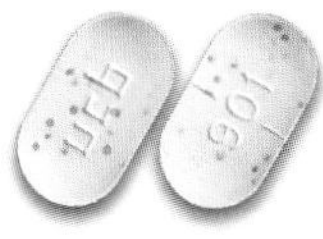

2.5 mg/500 mg

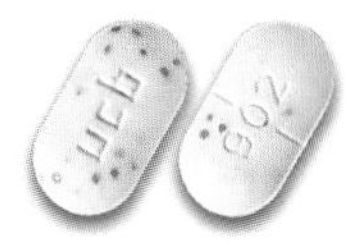

5 mg/500 mg

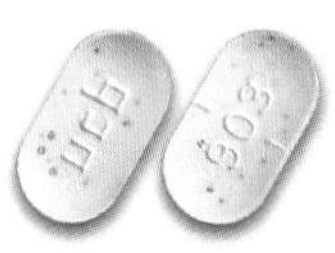

7.5 mg/500 mg

HYDROCODONE BITARTRATE AND ACETAMINOPHEN *(continued)*

Vicodin
(page 1327)

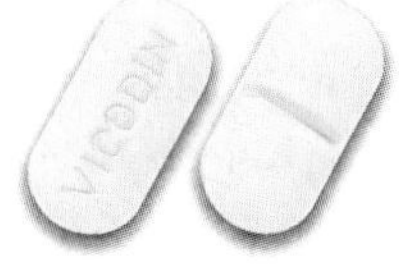

5 mg/500 mg

Vicodin ES
(page 1331)

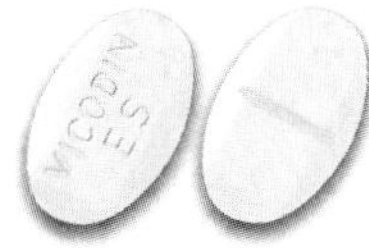

7.5 mg/750 mg

IBUPROFEN

Motrin
(page 378)

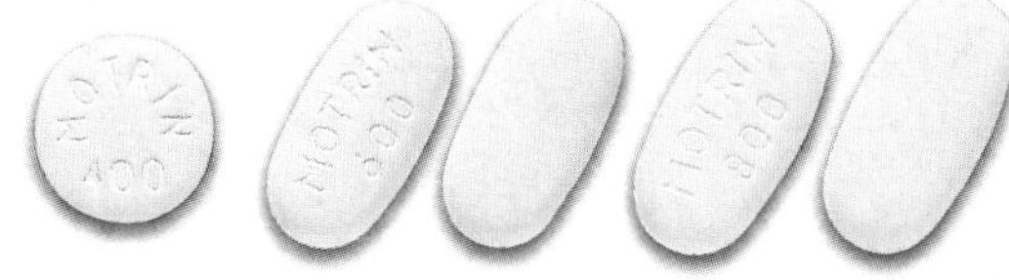

400 mg 600 mg 800 mg

INDINAVIR SULFATE

Crixivan
(page 178)

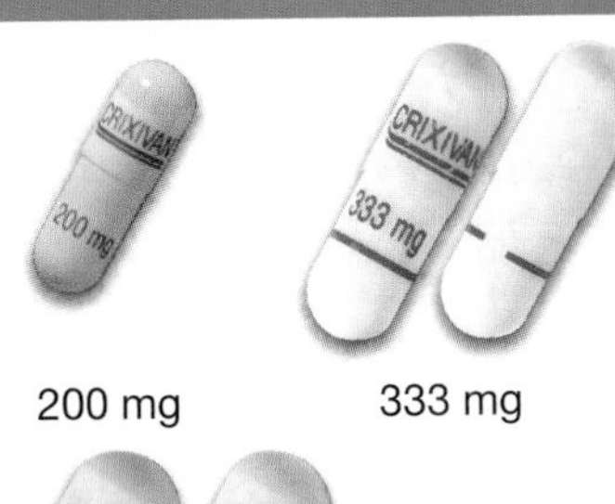

200 mg 333 mg

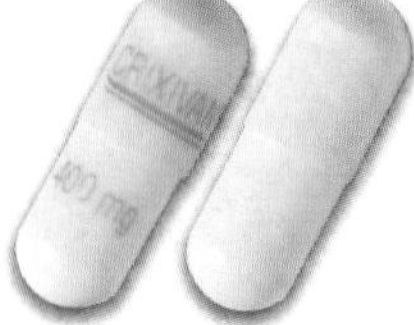

400 mg

LAMIVUDINE AND ZIDOVUDINE

Combivir
(page 1332)

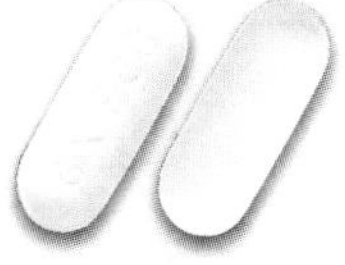

150 mg/300 mg

LANSOPRAZOLE

Prevacid
(page 722)

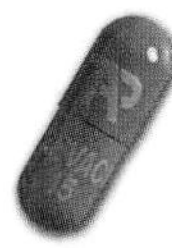

15 mg

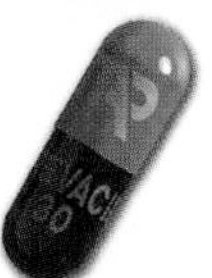

30 mg

LEVODOPA AND CARBIDOPA

Sinemet
(page 549)

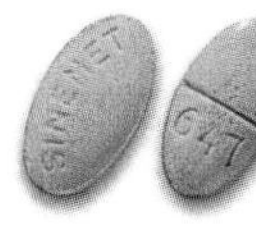

10 mg/100 mg

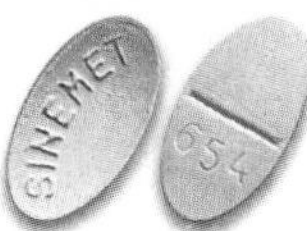

25 mg/250 mg

Sinemet CR
(page 549)

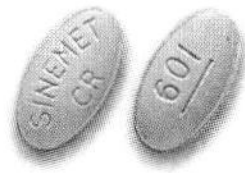

25 mg/100 mg

LEVODOPA, CARBIDOPA, AND ENTACAPONE

Stalevo
(page 551)

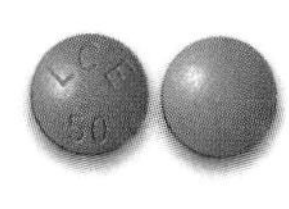

50 mg

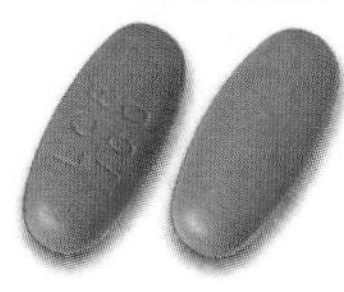

100 mg

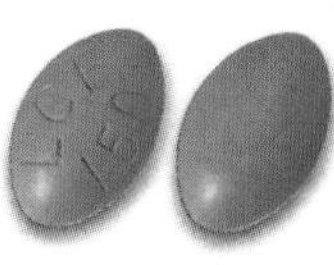

150 mg

LEVOFLOXACIN

Levaquin
(page 142)

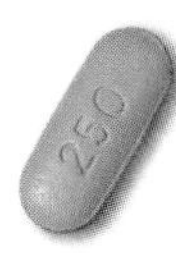

250 mg

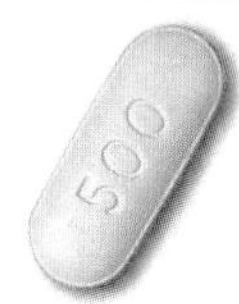

500 mg

LEVOTHYROXINE SODIUM

Levoxyl

(page 829)

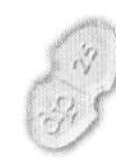
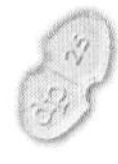

25 mcg 50 mcg 75 mcg

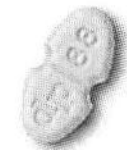
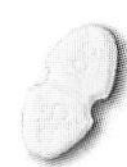

88 mcg 100 mcg 112 mcg

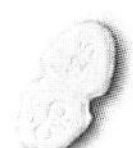
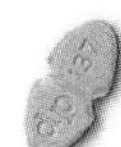

125 mcg 137 mcg 150 mcg

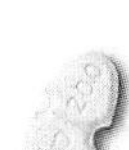
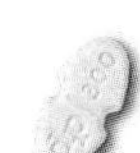

175 mcg 200 mcg 300 mcg

Synthroid

(page 829)

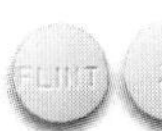
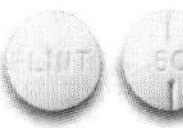

25 mcg 50 mcg 75 mcg

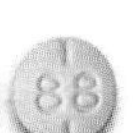
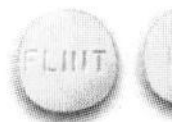

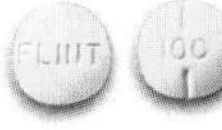
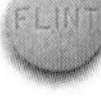

88 mcg 100 mcg 112 mcg

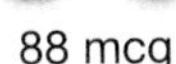
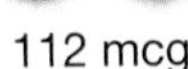

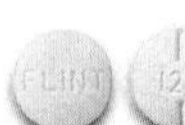
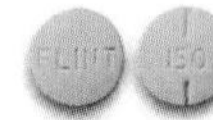
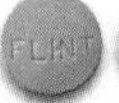
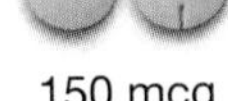

125 mcg 150 mcg 175 mcg

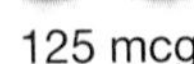

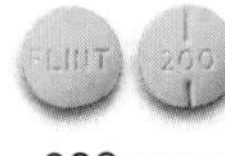
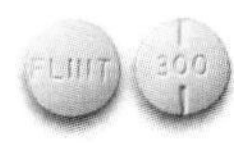

200 mcg 300 mcg

LISINOPRIL

Prinivil
(page 305)

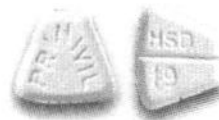
5 mg

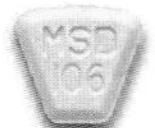

10 mg

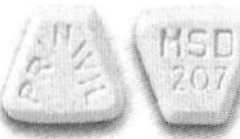

20 mg

Zestril
(page 305)

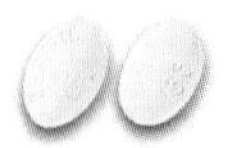
2.5 mg

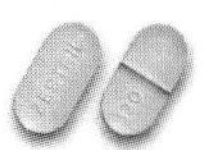
5 mg

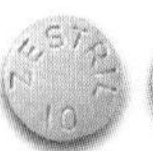

10 mg

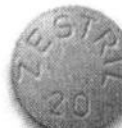

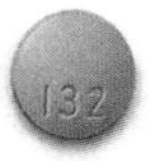

20 mg

40 mg

LOPINAVIR AND RITONAVIR

Kaletra
(page 182)

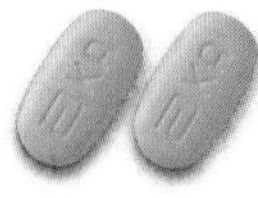
200 mg/50 mg

LOSARTAN POTASSIUM

Cozaar
(page 307)

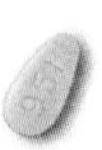

25 mg

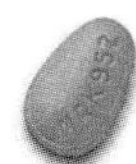

50 mg

LOVASTATIN

Mevacor
(page 339)

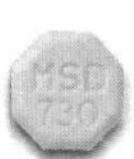

10 mg

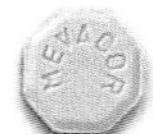

20 mg

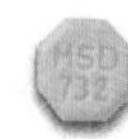

40 mg

LUBIPROSTONE

Amitiza
(page 735)

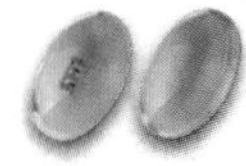

24 mcg

MEDROXYPROGESTERONE ACETATE

Provera
(page 787)

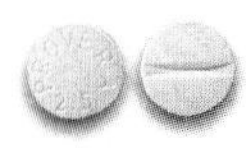

2.5 mg

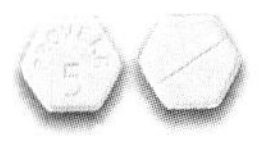

5 mg

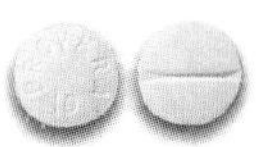

10 mg

MEPERIDINE HYDROCHLORIDE

Demerol
(page 403)

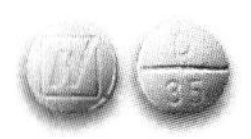

50 mg

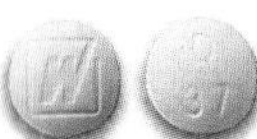

100 mg

METFORMIN HYDROCHLORIDE

Glucophage
(page 817)

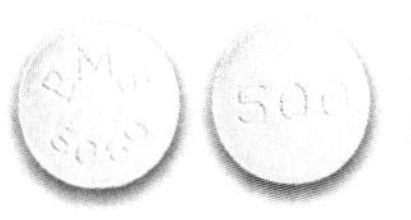

500 mg

850 mg

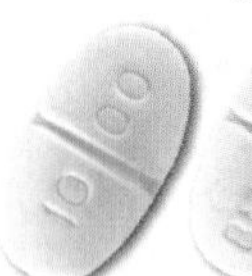

1,000 mg

Glucophage XR
(page 817)

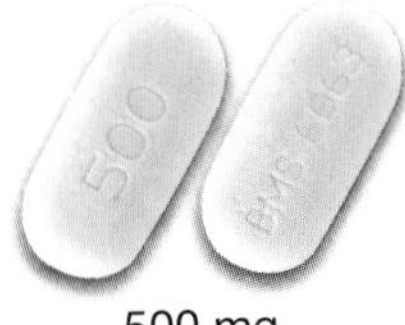

500 mg

METHYLPHENIDATE HYDROCHLORIDE

Concerta
(page 534)

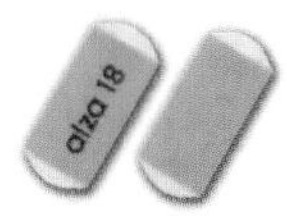

18 mg

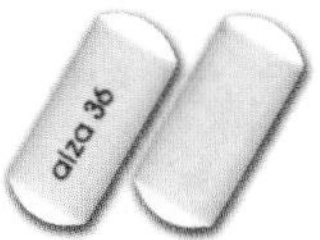

36 mg

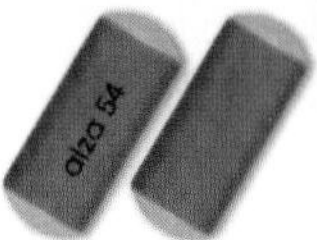

54 mg

Ritalin
(page 534)

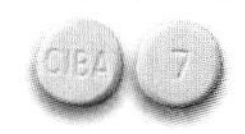

5 mg

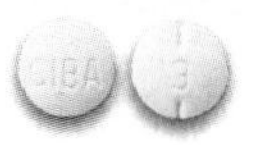

10 mg

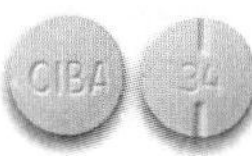

20 mg

Ritalin-SR
(page 534)

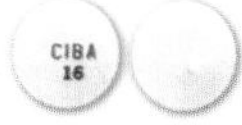

20 mg

METHYLPREDNISOLONE

Medrol
(page 748)

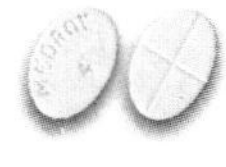
4 mg

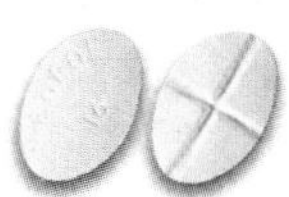
16 mg

METOPROLOL SUCCINATE

Toprol-XL
(page 310)

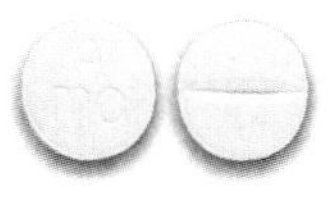
50 mg

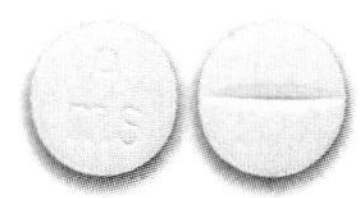
100 mg

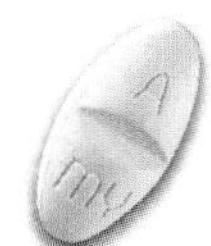
200 mg

MONTELUKAST SODIUM

Singulair
(page 672)

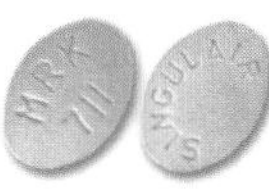

4 mg

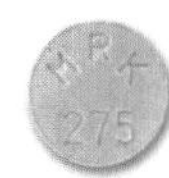

5 mg

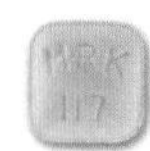
10 mg

NAPROXEN

Naprosyn
(page 389)

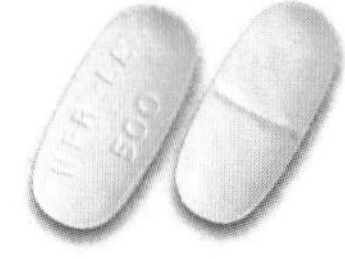

500 mg

NIFEDIPINE

Procardia XL
(page 272)

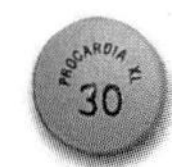

30 mg

60 mg

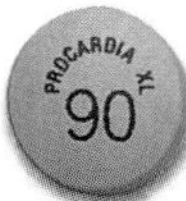

90 mg

NITROFURANTOIN MACROCRYSTALS

Macrobid
(page 225)

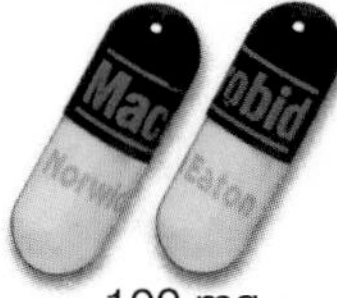

100 mg

NITROGLYCERIN

Nitrostat
(page 273)

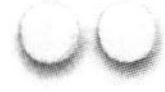

0.4 mg

NORTRIPTYLINE HYDROCHLORIDE

Pamelor
(page 480)

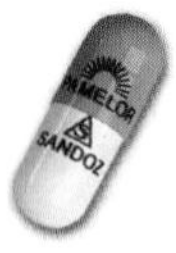

10 mg

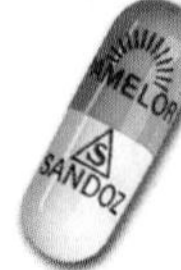

25 mg

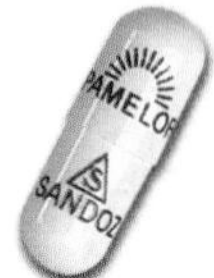

50 mg

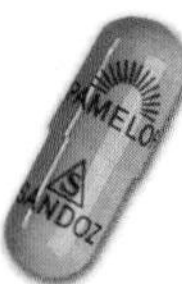

75 mg

OFLOXACIN

Floxin
(page 148)

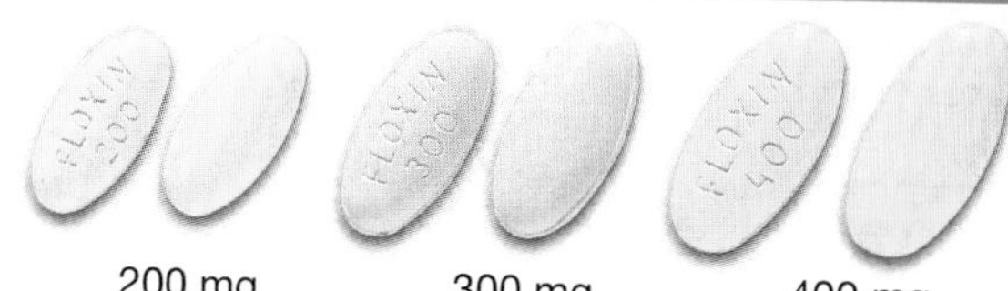

200 mg 300 mg 400 mg

OLMESARTAN MEDOXOMIL

Benicar
(page 316)

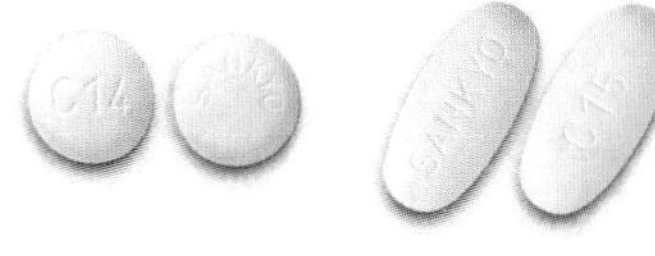

20 mg 40 mg

OMEPRAZOLE

Prilosec
(page 725)

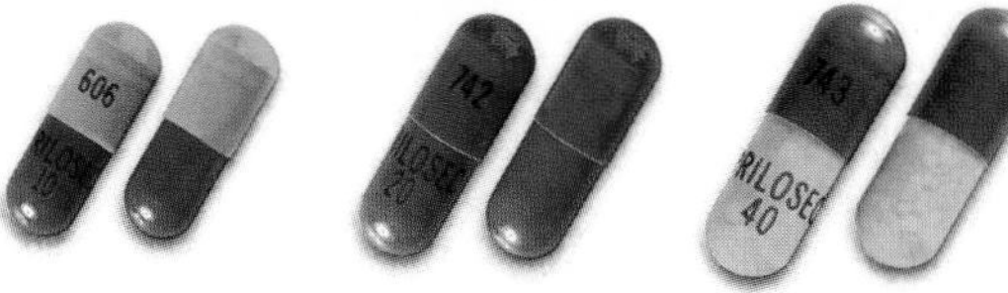

10 mg 20 mg 40 mg

OXYCODONE HYDROCHLORIDE

OxyContin
(page 411)

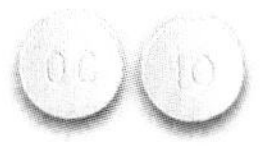

10 mg

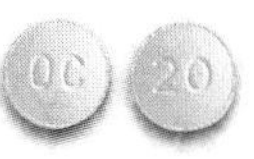

20 mg

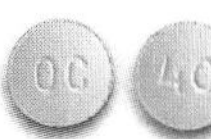

40 mg

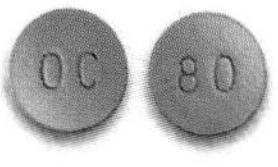

80 mg

PENTOXIFYLLINE

Trental
(page 359)

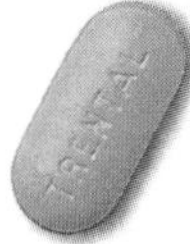

400 mg

PHENYTOIN SODIUM

Dilantin Kapseals
(page 448)

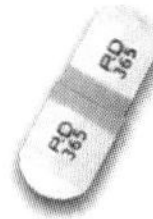

30 mg

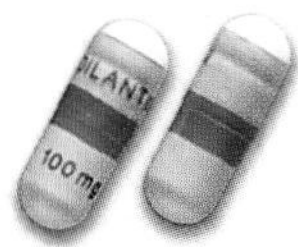

100 mg

POTASSIUM CHLORIDE

K-Dur 20
(page 885)

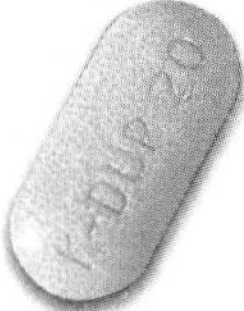

20 mEq

PRAVASTATIN SODIUM

Pravachol
(page 341)

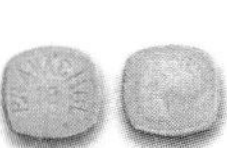
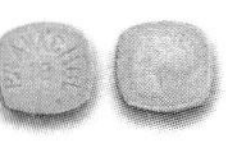

10 mg

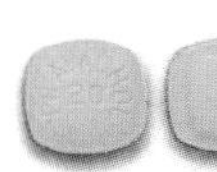
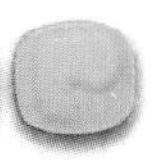

20 mg

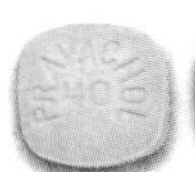

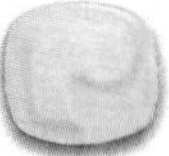

40 mg

PROPRANOLOL HYDROCHLORIDE

Inderal
(page 276)

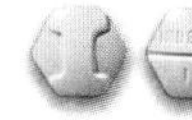
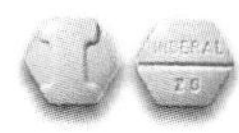
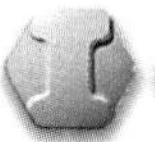
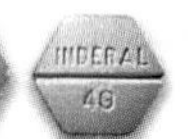

10 mg 20 mg 40 mg

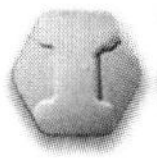
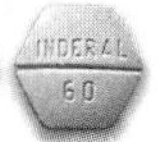
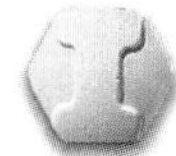
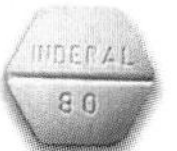

60 mg 80 mg

Inderal LA
(page 276)

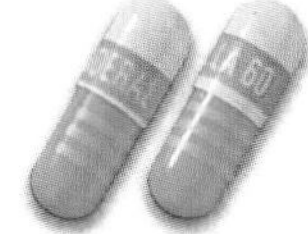
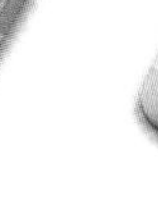
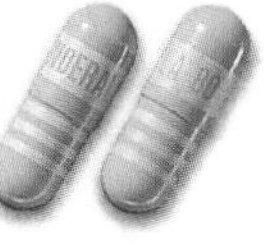
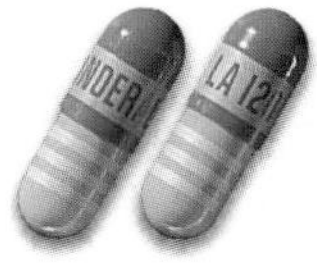

60 mg 80 mg 120 mg

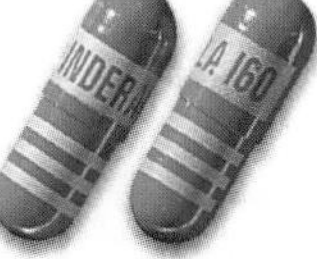

160 mg

QUINAPRIL HYDROCHLORIDE

Accupril
(page 321)

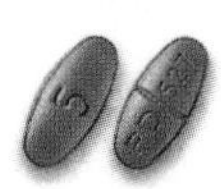
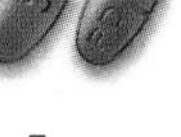
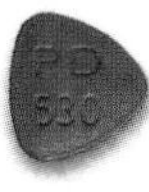
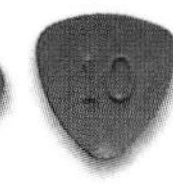
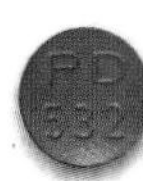
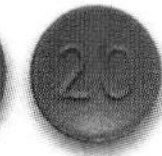

5 mg 10 mg 20 mg

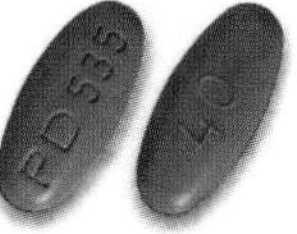

40 mg

RALOXIFENE HYDROCHLORIDE

Evista
(page 1293)

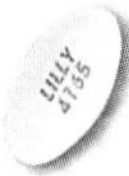

60 mg

RANITIDINE HYDROCHLORIDE

Zantac
(page 729)

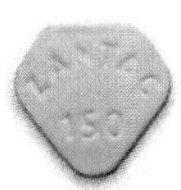
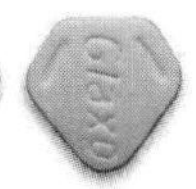

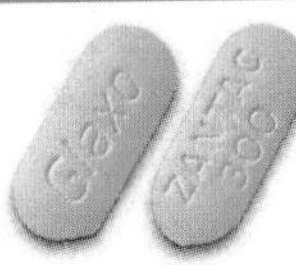

150 mg 300 mg

RANOLAZINE

Ranexa
(page 278)

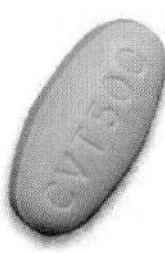

500 mg

RASAGILINE

Azilect
(page 554)

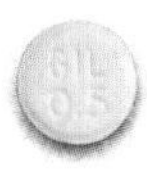
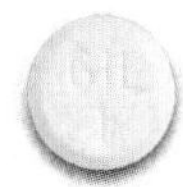

0.5 mg 1 mg

RISEDRONATE SODIUM

Actonel
(page 857)

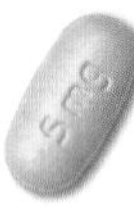

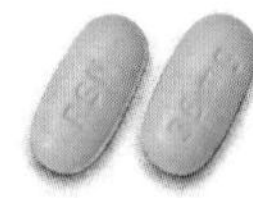

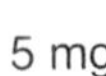

5 mg 35 mg

RISPERIDONE

Risperdal
(page 519)

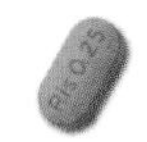

0.25 mg

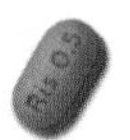

0.5 mg

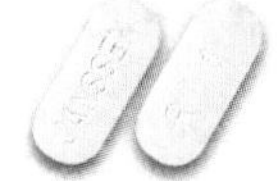

1 mg

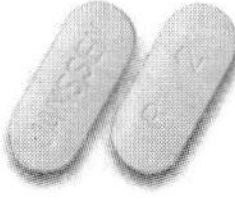

2 mg

3 mg

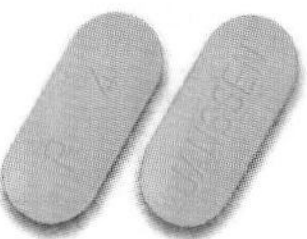

4 mg

Risperdal M-Tab
(page 519)

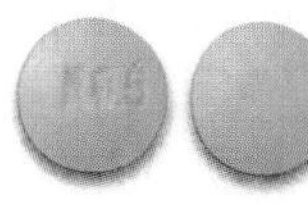

0.5 mg

ROSIGLITAZONE MALEATE

Avandia
(page 826)

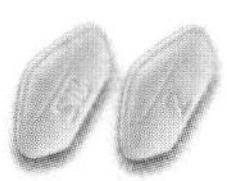

2 mg

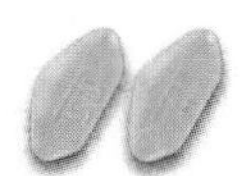

4 mg

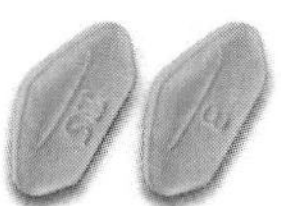

8 mg

ROSUVASTATIN CALCIUM

Crestor
(page 343)

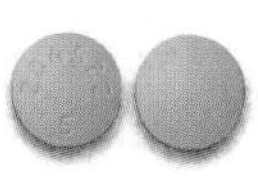

5 mg

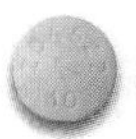

10 mg

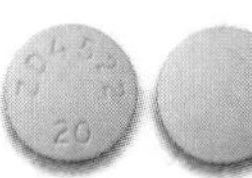

20 mg

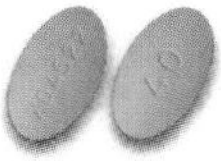

40 mg

SERTRALINE HYDROCHLORIDE

Zoloft
(page 484)

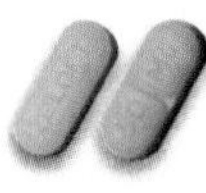

50 mg

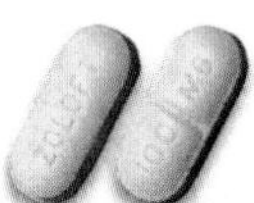

100 mg

SILDENAFIL CITRATE

Viagra
(page 1296)

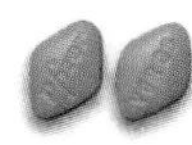

25 mg

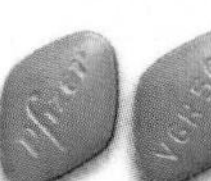

50 mg

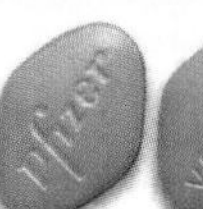

100 mg

SIMVASTATIN

Zocor
(page 344)

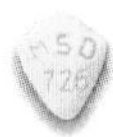

5 mg

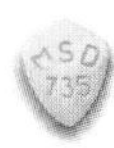

10 mg

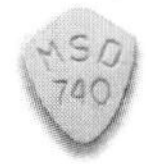

20 mg

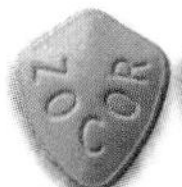

40 mg

SITAGLIPTIN PHOSPHATE

Januvia
(page 828)

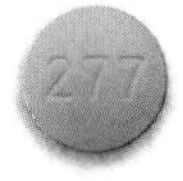

100 mg

SORAFENIB

Nexavar
(page 1036)

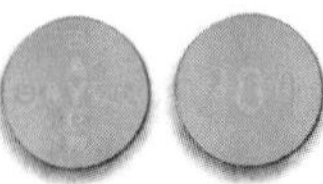

200 mg

SUCRALFATE

Carafate
(page 731)

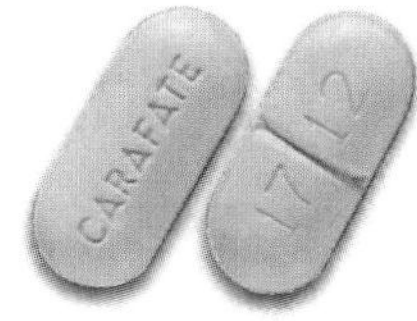

1 g

SUMATRIPTAN SUCCINATE

Imitrex
(page 579)

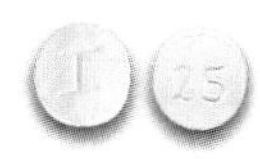

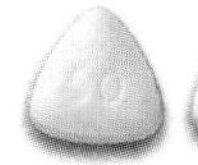

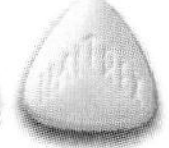

25 mg

50 mg

SUNITINIB

Sutent
(page 1038)

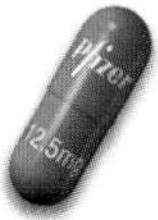

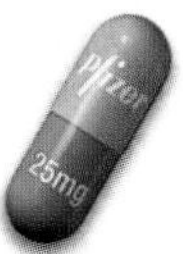

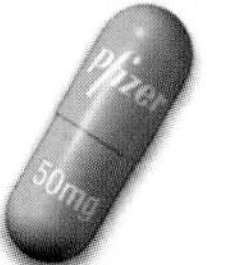

12.5 mg

25 mg

50 mg

TEMAZEPAM

Restoril
(page 426)

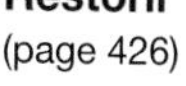

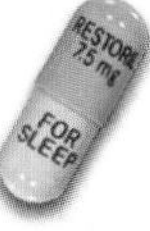

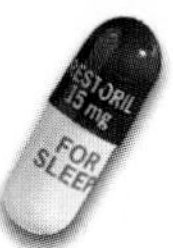

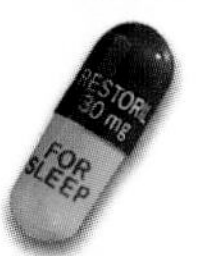

7.5 mg

15 mg

30 mg

TENOFOVIR DISOPROXIL FUMARATE

Viread
(page 195)

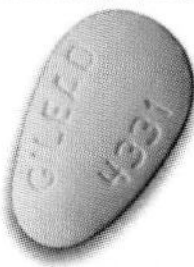

300 mg

TERAZOSIN HYDROCHLORIDE

Hytrin
(page 325)

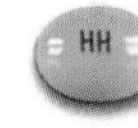
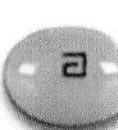

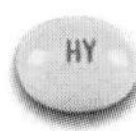
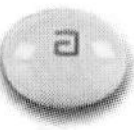

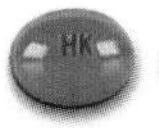
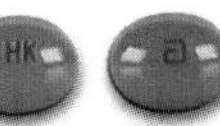

1 mg 2 mg 5 mg

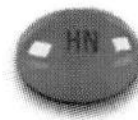
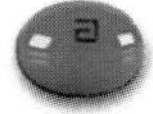

10 mg

TICLOPIDINE HYDROCHLORIDE

Ticlid
(page 361)

250 mg

TOLTERODINE TARTRATE

Detrol
(page 1243)

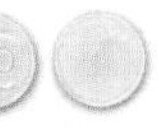
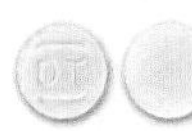

1 mg 2 mg

TRAMADOL HYDROCHLORIDE AND ACETAMINOPHEN

Ultracet
(page 1331)

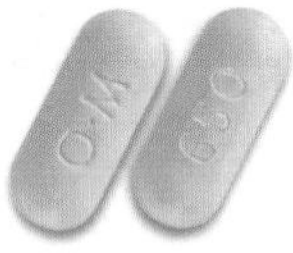

37.5 mg/325 mg

VARDENAFIL HYDROCHLORIDE

Levitra
(page 1302)

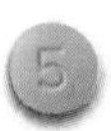

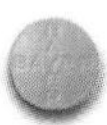
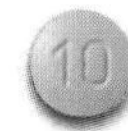

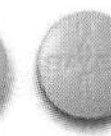
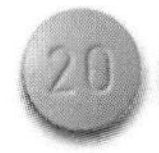

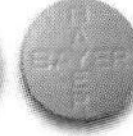

5 mg 10 mg 20 mg

VARENICLINE

Chantix
(page 1303)

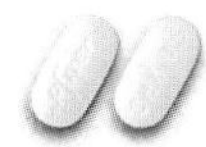
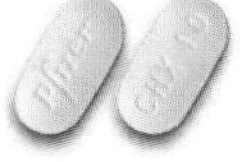

0.5 mg 1 mg

VENLAFAXINE HYDROCHLORIDE

Effexor
(page 487)

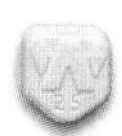
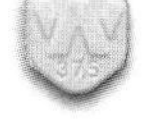
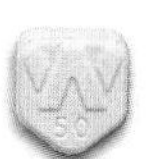

25 mg 37.5 mg 50 mg

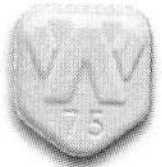
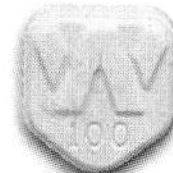

75 mg 100 mg

Effexor XR
(page 487)

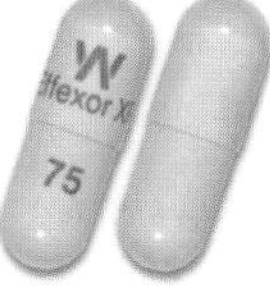

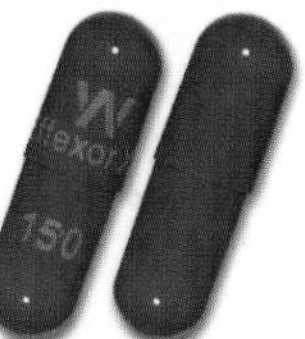

75 mg 150 mg

VERAPAMIL HYDROCHLORIDE

Calan
(page 279)

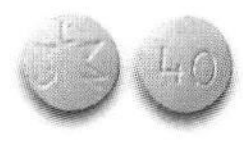

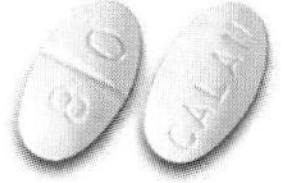

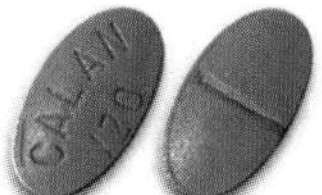

40 mg 80 mg 120 mg

Isoptin SR
(page 279)

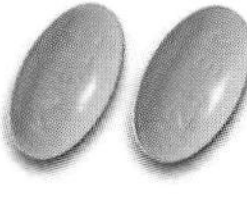
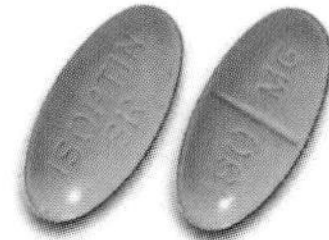
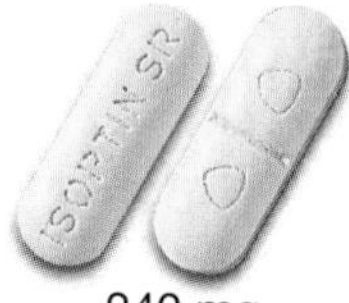

120 mg 180 mg 240 mg

VERAPAMIL HYDROCHLORIDE *(continued)*

Verelan
(page 279)

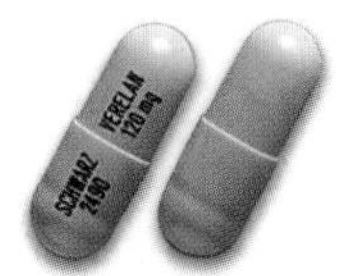

120 mg

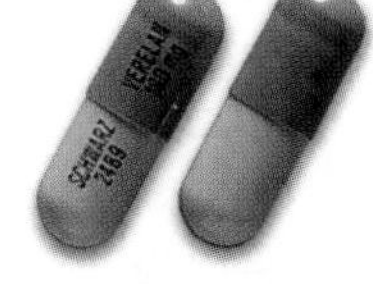
180 mg

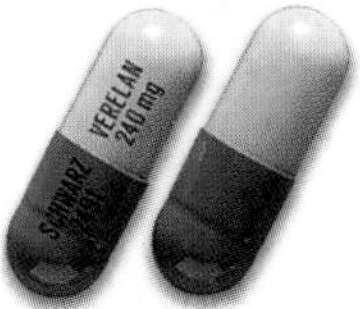

240 mg

WARFARIN SODIUM

Coumadin
(page 915)

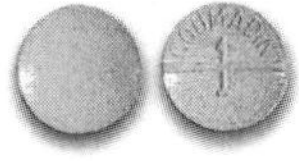
1 mg

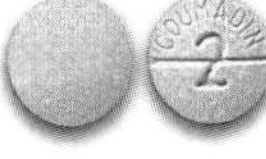
2 mg

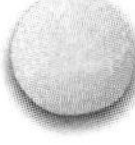
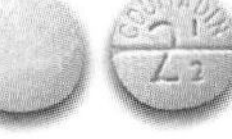
2.5 mg

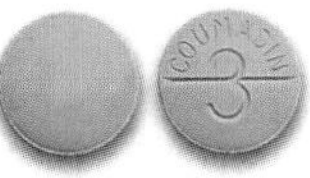
3 mg

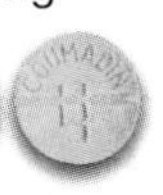
4 mg

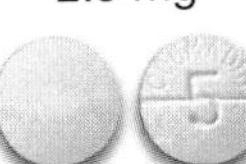
5 mg

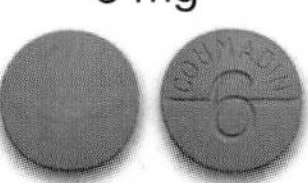
6 mg

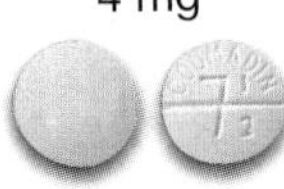
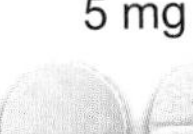
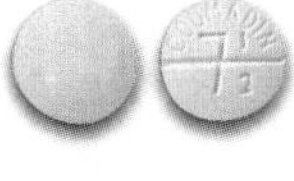
7.5 mg

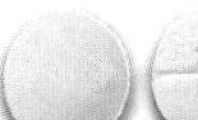
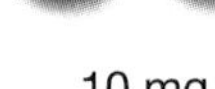
10 mg

ZIDOVUDINE

Retrovir
(page 202)

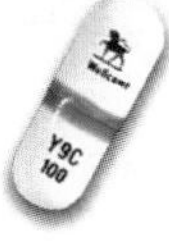

100 mg

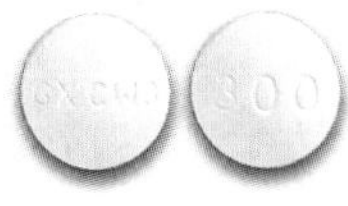
300 mg

ZOLPIDEM TARTRATE

Ambien
(page 430)

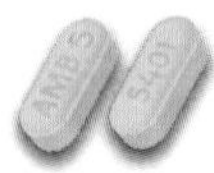
5 mg

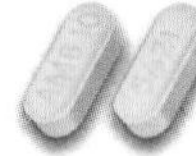
10 mg

tinal obstruction, abdominal pain, nausea, vomiting, or other symptoms of appendicitis or acute surgical abdomen.

NURSING CONSIDERATIONS

- Give drug at times that don't interfere with scheduled activities or sleep. Soft, formed stools are usually produced 15 to 60 minutes after rectal use.
- Before giving for constipation, determine whether patient has adequate fluid intake, exercise, and diet.
- Tablets and suppositories are used together to clean the colon before and after surgery and before barium enema.
- Insert suppository as high as possible into the rectum, and try to position suppository against the rectal wall. Avoid embedding within fecal material because doing so may delay onset of action.
- Bisco-Lax may contain tartrazine.

PATIENT TEACHING

- Advise patient to swallow enteric-coated tablet whole to avoid GI irritation. Instruct him not to take within 1 hour of milk or antacid.
- Tell patient that drug is for 1-week treatment only. (Stimulant laxatives are often abused.) Discourage excessive use.
- Advise patient to report adverse effects to prescriber.
- Teach patient about dietary sources of bulk, including bran and other cereals, fresh fruit, and vegetables.
- Tell patient to take drug with a full glass of water or juice.

calcium polycarbophil

Equalactin ◇, Fiberall ◇, FiberCon ◇, Fiber-Lax ◇, Konsyl Fiber ◇, Phillips' Fibercaps

Pharmacologic class: hydrophilic drug
Pregnancy risk category A

AVAILABLE FORMS

Tablets: 500 mg ◇, 625 mg ◇
Tablets (chewable): 500 mg ◇

INDICATIONS & DOSAGES

➤ **Constipation**

Adults and children older than age 12: 1 g P.O. once daily to q.i.d., p.r.n. Maximum, 4 g in 24 hours.
Children ages 7 to 12: 500 mg P.O. once daily to t.i.d., p.r.n. Maximum, 2 g in 24 hours.

➤ **Diarrhea from irritable bowel syndrome; acute, nonspecific diarrhea**

Adults and children older than age 12: 1 g P.O. once daily to q.i.d., p.r.n. Maximum, 4 g in 24 hours.
Children ages 7 to 12: 500 mg P.O. once daily to t.i.d., p.r.n. Maximum, 2 g in 24 hours.

ACTION

Bulk-forming laxative that absorbs water and expands to increase bulk and moisture content of stools. The increased bulk encourages peristalsis and bowel movement. As an antidiarrheal, drug absorbs free fecal water, thereby producing formed stools.

Route	Onset	Peak	Duration
P.O.	12–24 hr	3 days	Variable

Half-life: Unknown.

ADVERSE REACTIONS

GI: ***intestinal obstruction,*** abdominal fullness and increased flatus.
Other: laxative dependence with long-term or excessive use.

INTERACTIONS

Drug-drug. *Tetracyclines:* May impair tetracycline absorption. Avoid using together.

EFFECTS ON LAB TEST RESULTS

None reported.

CONTRAINDICATIONS & CAUTIONS

- Contraindicated in patients with signs or symptoms of GI obstruction or those with swallowing difficulty.

NURSING CONSIDERATIONS

- Before giving drug for constipation, determine whether patient has adequate fluid intake, exercise, and diet.

• In children younger than age 6, use must be directed by prescriber.
• ***Alert:*** Rectal bleeding or failure to respond to therapy may indicate need for surgery.

PATIENT TEACHING

• Full benefit of drug may take 1 to 3 days.
• Advise patient to chew Equalactin tablets thoroughly before swallowing and to drink an 8-ounce glass of water with each dose. When drug is used as an antidiarrheal, tell patient not to drink the glass of water.
• Advise patient to seek medical attention if he experiences vomiting, chest pain, or difficulty breathing or swallowing after taking medication.
• Teach patient about dietary sources of fiber, including bran and other cereals, fresh fruit, and vegetables.
• For severe diarrhea, advise patient to repeat dose every 30 minutes, but not to exceed maximum daily dose. Tell patient not to use for longer than 2 days, unless directed by a prescriber.

docusate calcium (dioctyl calcium sulfosuccinate)

DC Softgels◊, Surfak◊

docusate sodium (dioctyl sodium sulfosuccinate)

Colace◊, Coloxyl‡, Coloxyl Enema Concentrate‡, Diocto◊, Dioeze◊, D.O.S◊, D-S-S◊, Dulcolax Stool Softener◊, Duosol◊, Ex-Lax Stool Softener Caplets, Modane Soft◊, Phillips' Liqui-Gels, Regulax SS◊, Regulex†◊

Pharmacologic class: surfactant
Pregnancy risk category C

AVAILABLE FORMS

docusate calcium
Capsules: 240 mg◊
docusate sodium
Capsules: 50 mg◊, 100 mg◊, 240 mg◊, 250 mg◊
Enema concentrate: 18 g/100 ml (must be diluted)‡
Oral liquid: 150 mg/15 ml◊
Oral solution: 10 mg/ml◊, 50 mg/ml◊
Syrup: 20 mg/5 ml, 50 mg/15 ml◊, 60 mg/15 ml◊
Tablets: 50 mg◊, 100 mg◊

INDICATIONS & DOSAGES

➤ Stool softener
Adults and children older than age 12: 50 to 500 mg docusate calcium or sodium P.O. daily until bowel movements are normal. Or, give enema. Dilute 1:24 with sterile water before use, and give 100 to 150 ml retention enema, 300 to 500 ml evacuation enema, or 0.5 to 1.5 L flushing enema P.R.
Children ages 7 to 12: 40 to 120 mg docusate sodium P.O. daily.
Children ages 3 to 6: 20 to 60 mg docusate sodium P.O. daily.
Children younger than age 3: 10 to 40 mg docusate sodium P.O. daily.

Higher dosage is used for initial therapy. Adjust dosage to individual response.

ACTION

Stool softener that reduces surface tension of interfacing liquid contents of the bowel. This detergent activity promotes incorporation of additional liquid into stools, thus forming a softer mass.

Route	Onset	Peak	Duration
P.O.	1–3 days	Unknown	Unknown
P.R.	Unknown	Unknown	Unknown

Half-life: Unknown.

ADVERSE REACTIONS

GI: bitter taste, mild abdominal cramping, diarrhea.
Other: laxative dependence with long-term or excessive use.

INTERACTIONS

Drug-drug. *Mineral oil:* May increase mineral oil absorption and cause toxicity and lipid pneumonia. Separate doses.

EFFECTS ON LAB TEST RESULTS

None reported.

CONTRAINDICATIONS & CAUTIONS

• Contraindicated in patients hypersensitive to drug and in those with intestinal obstruction or signs and symptoms of appendicitis, fecal impaction, or acute surgical abdomen, such as undiagnosed abdominal pain or vomiting.

NURSING CONSIDERATIONS
- Drug isn't used to treat existing constipation but prevents constipation from developing.
- Before giving drug, determine whether patient has adequate fluid intake, exercise, and diet.
- Give liquid (not syrups) in milk, fruit juice, or infant formula to mask bitter taste.
- Drug is laxative of choice for patients who shouldn't strain during defecation, including patients recovering from MI or rectal surgery, those with rectal or anal disease that makes passage of firm stools difficult, and those with postpartum constipation.
- Store drug at 59° to 86° F (15° to 30° C), and protect liquid from light.

PATIENT TEACHING
- Teach patient about dietary sources of fiber, including bran and other cereals, fresh fruit, and vegetables.
- Instruct patient to use drug only occasionally and not for longer than 1 week without prescriber's knowledge.
- Tell patient to stop drug and notify prescriber if severe cramping occurs.
- Notify patient that it may take from 1 to 3 days to soften stools.

glycerin
Fleet Babylax ◊, Sani-Supp ◊

Pharmacologic class: trihydric alcohol
Pregnancy risk category NR

AVAILABLE FORMS
Enema (pediatric): 4 ml/applicator ◊
Suppositories: Adult, children, and infant sizes ◊

INDICATIONS & DOSAGES
➤ **Constipation**
Adults and children age 6 and older: Give 2 to 3 g as rectal suppository; or 5 to 15 ml as enema.
Children ages 2 to 6: Give 1 to 1.7 g as rectal suppository; or 2 to 5 ml as enema.

ACTION
Hyperosmolar laxative that draws water from the tissues into the feces, thus stimulating evacuation.

Route	Onset	Peak	Duration
P.R.	15–30 min	Unknown	Unknown

Half-life: Unknown.

ADVERSE REACTIONS
GI: *cramping pain,* hyperemia of rectal mucosa, rectal discomfort.

INTERACTIONS
None significant.

EFFECTS ON LAB TEST RESULTS
None reported.

CONTRAINDICATIONS & CAUTIONS
- Contraindicated in patients hypersensitive to drug and in those with intestinal obstruction or signs and symptoms of appendicitis, fecal impaction, or acute surgical abdomen, such as undiagnosed abdominal pain or vomiting.

NURSING CONSIDERATIONS
- Drug is used mainly to reestablish proper toilet habits in laxative-dependent patients.

PATIENT TEACHING
- Tell patient that drug must be retained for at least 15 minutes and that it usually acts within 1 hour. Entire suppository need not melt to be effective.
- Warn patient about adverse GI reactions.

lactulose
Cephulac, Cholac, Chronulac, Constilac, Constulose, Duphalac, Enulose, Kristalose, Lactulax†

Pharmacologic class: disaccharide
Pregnancy risk category B

AVAILABLE FORMS
Packets: 10 g, 20 g
Syrup: 10 g/15 ml

INDICATIONS & DOSAGES

➤ **Constipation**

Adults: 10 to 20 g or 15 to 30 ml P.O. daily, increased to 60 ml/day, if needed.

➤ **To prevent and treat hepatic encephalopathy, including hepatic precoma and coma in patients with severe hepatic disease**

Adults: Initially, 20 to 30 g or 30 to 45 ml P.O. t.i.d. or q.i.d., until two or three soft stools are produced daily. Usual dose is 60 to 100 g daily in divided doses. Or, 200 g or 300 ml diluted with 700 ml of water or normal saline solution and given as retention enema P.R. q 4 to 6 hours, p.r.n.

ACTION

Produces an osmotic effect in colon; resulting distention promotes peristalsis. Also decreases ammonia, probably as a result of bacterial degradation, which lowers the pH of colon contents.

Route	Onset	Peak	Duration
P.O.	24–48 hr	Variable	Variable
P.R.	Unknown	Unknown	Unknown

Half-life: Unknown.

ADVERSE REACTIONS

GI: *abdominal cramps, belching, diarrhea, flatulence, gaseous distention,* nausea, vomiting.

INTERACTIONS

Drug-drug. *Antacids, antibiotics, oral neomycin:* May decrease lactulose effectiveness. Avoid using together.

EFFECTS ON LAB TEST RESULTS

None reported.

CONTRAINDICATIONS & CAUTIONS

- Contraindicated in patients on a low-galactose diet.
- Use cautiously in patients with diabetes mellitus.

NURSING CONSIDERATIONS

- To minimize sweet taste, dilute with water or fruit juice or give with food.
- Prepare enema (not commercially available) by adding 200 g (300 ml) to 700 ml of water or normal saline solution. The diluted solution is given as retention enema for 30 to 60 minutes. Use a rectal balloon.
- If enema isn't retained for at least 30 minutes, repeat dose.
- Monitor sodium level for hypernatremia, especially when giving in higher doses to treat hepatic encephalopathy.
- Monitor mental status and potassium levels when giving to patients with hepatic encephalopathy.
- Replace fluid loss.
- ***Look alike–sound alike:*** Don't confuse lactulose with lactose.

PATIENT TEACHING

- Show home care patient how to mix and use drug.
- Inform patient about adverse reactions and tell him to notify prescriber if reactions become bothersome or if diarrhea occurs.
- Instruct patient not to take other laxatives during lactulose therapy.

magnesium citrate (citrate of magnesia)

Citroma ◊, Citro-Mag†

magnesium hydroxide (milk of magnesia)

Milk of Magnesia ◊, Milk of Magnesia-Concentrated ◊, Phillips' Milk of Magnesia ◊

magnesium sulfate ◊ (Epsom salts) ◊)

Pharmacologic class: magnesium salt
Pregnancy risk category B

AVAILABLE FORMS

magnesium citrate
Oral solution: About 168 mEq magnesium/240 ml ◊

magnesium hydroxide
Chewable tablets: 300 mg, 600 mg
Oral suspension: 400 mg/5 ml, 800 mg/5 ml

magnesium sulfate
Granules: About 40 mEq magnesium/5 g ◊

INDICATIONS & DOSAGES

➤Constipation, to evacuate bowel before surgery

Adults and children age 12 and older: 11 to 25 g magnesium citrate P.O. daily as a single or divided dose. Or, 2.4 to 4.8 g or 30 to 60 ml magnesium hydroxide P.O. (2 to 4 tablespoons at bedtime or upon arising, followed by 8 ounces of liquid) daily as a single dose or divided. Or, 10 to 30 g magnesium sulfate P.O. daily as a single or divided dose.

Children ages 6 to 11: 5.5 to 12.5 g magnesium citrate P.O. daily as a single or divided dose. Or, 1.2 to 2.4 g or 15 to 30 ml magnesium hydroxide P.O. (1 to 2 tablespoons, followed by 8 ounces of liquid) daily as a single or divided dose. Or, 5 to 10 g magnesium sulfate P.O. daily as a single or divided dose. Don't use dosage cup.

Children ages 2 to 5: 2.7 to 6.25 g magnesium citrate P.O. daily as a single or divided dose. Or, 0.4 to 1.2 g or 5 to 15 ml magnesium hydroxide P.O. (1 to 3 tsp, followed by 8 ounces of liquid) daily as a single or divided dose. Or, 2.5 to 5 g magnesium sulfate P.O. daily as a single or divided dose. Don't use dosage cup.

➤Acid indigestion

Adults and children age 12 and older: 1 to 3 tsp with a little water, up to four times a day, or as directed. Don't use dosage cup.

ACTION

Saline laxative that produces an osmotic effect in the small intestine by drawing water into the intestinal lumen.

Route	Onset	Peak	Duration
P.O.	30 min–3 hr	Variable	Variable

Half-life: Unknown.

ADVERSE REACTIONS

GI: *abdominal cramping, diarrhea, nausea.*

Metabolic: fluid and electrolyte disturbances with daily use.

Other: laxative dependence with long-term or excessive use.

INTERACTIONS

Drug-drug. *Oral drugs:* May impair absorption. Separate doses.

EFFECTS ON LAB TEST RESULTS

- May alter fluid and electrolyte levels with prolonged use.

CONTRAINDICATIONS & CAUTIONS

- Contraindicated in pregnant patients about to deliver and in patients with myocardial damage, heart block, fecal impaction, rectal fissures, intestinal obstruction or perforation, renal disease, or signs and symptoms of appendicitis or acute surgical abdomen, such as abdominal pain, nausea, or vomiting.
- Use cautiously in patients with rectal bleeding.

NURSING CONSIDERATIONS

- Give drug at times that don't interfere with scheduled activities or sleep. Drug produces watery stools in 3 to 6 hours.
- Before giving drug for constipation, determine whether patient has adequate fluid intake, exercise, and diet.
- Chill magnesium citrate before use to improve its palatability.
- Shake suspension well; give with a large amount of water when used as laxative. When giving by nasogastric tube, make sure tube is placed properly and is patent. After instilling drug, flush tube with water to ensure passage to stomach and maintain tube patency.
- ***Alert:*** Monitor electrolyte levels during prolonged use. Magnesium may accumulate if patient has renal insufficiency.
- Drug is recommended for short-term use only.
- Magnesium sulfate is more potent than other saline laxatives.

PATIENT TEACHING

- Teach patient how to use drug.
- Teach patient about dietary sources of fiber, including bran and other cereals, fresh fruit, and vegetables.
- Warn patient that frequent or prolonged use as a laxative may cause dependence.

polyethylene glycol

GlycoLax, MiraLax

Pharmacologic class: osmotic drug
Pregnancy risk category C

AVAILABLE FORMS

Powder: single-dose 17-g packets; 16-ounce (255-g), 24-ounce (527-g) containers

INDICATIONS & DOSAGES

➤ Short-term treatment of occasional constipation
Adults: 17 g (about 1 heaping tablespoon) powder P.O. daily, dissolved in 8 ounces (240 ml) of water, juice, soda, coffee, or tea.

ACTION

Causes water to be retained in stool.

Route	Onset	Peak	Duration
P.O.	48–96 hr	Unknown	Unknown

Half-life: Unknown.

ADVERSE REACTIONS

GI: abdominal bloating, cramping, diarrhea, excess stool frequency, flatulence, nausea.

INTERACTIONS

Drug-drug. *Drugs containing polyethylene glycol:* May cause urticaria. Monitor patient.

EFFECTS ON LAB TEST RESULTS

None reported.

CONTRAINDICATIONS & CAUTIONS

- Contraindicated in patients allergic to drug and those with known or suspected bowel obstruction.

NURSING CONSIDERATIONS

- Before giving, rule out bowel obstruction in patients who have nausea, vomiting, abdominal pain, or distension.
- It may take 2 to 4 days before a bowel movement occurs.
- Drug should be taken for 2 weeks or less to avoid the risk of laxative dependence.
- Occasional use as directed doesn't affect absorption or secretion of glucose or electrolytes.
- Prolonged, frequent, or excessive use may cause electrolyte imbalance and laxative dependence.
- Drug may be more likely to cause diarrhea in older patients.

PATIENT TEACHING

- Explain that proper eating habits and lifestyle changes may produce more regular bowel movements. Tell patient to eat adequate amounts of dietary fiber, drink ample fluids, and get appropriate exercise.
- If patient uses bottled form of drug, urge him to measure each 17-g dose using the measuring cup provided in the package. If patient uses drug packets, each one contains 17 g.
- Instruct patient to dissolve dose in 8 ounces of water, juice, soda, coffee, or tea.
- Inform patient that it may take 2 to 4 days to produce a bowel movement.
- Warn patient that taking more than the recommended dose can cause dehydration and severe diarrhea.
- Tell patient that drug should be used for 2 weeks or less to avoid the risk of laxative dependence.
- Urge patient to report unusual cramping, bloating, or diarrhea.

polyethylene glycol and electrolyte solution

Colyte, Glycoprep‡, Go-Evac, GoLYTELY, NuLYTELY, OCL

Pharmacologic class: polyethylene glycol nonabsorbable solution
Pregnancy risk category C

AVAILABLE FORMS

Powder for oral solution: PEG 3350 (227.1 g), sodium sulfate (21.5 g), sodium chloride (5.53 g), potassium chloride (2.82 g), sodium bicarbonate (6.36 g) per 4 L (Colyte); PEG 3350 (60 g), sodium chloride (1.46 g), potassium chloride (0.745 g), sodium bicarbonate

(1.68 g), sodium sulfate (5.68 g)/L (Co-Lav), PEG 3350 (60 g), sodium chloride (1.46 g), potassium chloride (745 mg), sodium bicarbonate (1.68 g), sodium sulfate (5.68 g)/L (Glycoprep)‡, PEG 3350 (420 g), sodium bicarbonate (5.72 g), sodium chloride (11.2 g), potassium chloride (1.48 g) per 4 L (NuLYTELY, TriLyte); PEG 3350 (6 g), sodium sulfate decahydrate (1.29 g), sodium chloride (146 mg), potassium chloride (75 mg), sodium bicarbonate (168 mg), polysorbate-80 (30 mg) per 100 ml (OCL)

INDICATIONS & DOSAGES

➤**Bowel preparation before GI examination**

Adults: 240 ml P.O. q 10 minutes until 4 L are consumed or until watery stool is clear. Typically, give 4 hours before examination, allowing 3 hours for drinking and 1 hour for bowel evacuation.

ACTION

PEG 3350, a nonabsorbable solution, acts as an osmotic product. Sodium sulfate greatly reduces sodium absorption. The electrolyte level causes virtually no net absorption or secretion of ions.

Route	Onset	Peak	Duration
P.O.	1 hr	Variable	Variable

Half-life: None.

ADVERSE REACTIONS

EENT: rhinorrhea.
GI: *abdominal fullness, bloating, cramps, nausea, vomiting.*
Skin: allergic reaction, anal irritation, dermatitis, urticaria.

INTERACTIONS

Drug-drug. *Oral drugs:* May decrease absorption if given within 1 hour of starting therapy. Give at least 2 to 3 hours before starting therapy.

EFFECTS ON LAB TEST RESULTS

None reported.

CONTRAINDICATIONS & CAUTIONS

- Contraindicated in patients with GI obstruction or perforation, gastric retention, toxic colitis, or megacolon.

NURSING CONSIDERATIONS

- Use tap water to reconstitute powder. Shake vigorously to dissolve all powder. Refrigerate reconstituted solution, but use within 48 hours.
- ***Alert:*** Don't add flavoring or additional ingredients to the solution or give chilled solution. Hypothermia has been reported after ingesting large amounts of chilled solution.
- Give solution early in the morning if patient is scheduled for a mid-morning examination. Oral solution induces diarrhea (onset 30 to 60 minutes) that rapidly cleans the bowel, usually within 4 hours.
- When using to prepare for barium enema, give solution the evening before the examination to avoid interfering with barium coating of the colonic mucosa.
- If given to semiconscious patient or to patient with impaired gag reflex, take care to prevent aspiration.
- No major shifts in fluid or electrolyte balance have been reported.
- Patient preparation for barium enema may be less satisfactory with this solution because it may interfere with the barium coating of the colonic mucosa using the double-contrast technique.

PATIENT TEACHING

- Tell patient to fast for 3 to 4 hours before taking the solution, and thereafter to drink only clear fluids until examination is complete.
- Warn patient about adverse reactions.

sodium phosphates

Fleet Enema ◇, Fleet Phospho-soda ◇

Pharmacologic class: acid salt
Pregnancy risk category NR

AVAILABLE FORMS

Enema: 160 mg/ml sodium phosphate and 60 mg/ml sodium biphosphate ◇
Liquid: 2.4 g/5 ml sodium phosphate and 900 mg sodium biphosphate/5 ml ◇

INDICATIONS & DOSAGES

➤**Constipation**

Adults and children age 12 and older: 20 to 45 ml solution mixed with 120 ml

cold water P.O. Or, 60 to 150 ml as an enema.
Children ages 10 to 11: 10 to 20 ml solution mixed with 120 ml cold water P.O.
Children ages 5 to 9: 5 to 10 ml solution mixed with 120 ml cold water P.O. Or, 30 to 60 ml as an enema.
Children ages 2 to 5: 60 ml P.R. as an enema.

ACTION

Saline laxative that produces an osmotic effect in the small intestine by drawing water into the intestinal lumen.

Route	Onset	Peak	Duration
P.O.	30–180 min	Variable	Variable
P.R.	5–10 min	With effect	With effect

Half-life: Unknown.

ADVERSE REACTIONS

GI: *abdominal cramping.*
Metabolic: fluid and electrolyte disturbances, such as hypernatremia and hyperphosphatemia, with daily use.
Other: laxative dependence with long-term or excessive use.

INTERACTIONS

None significant.

EFFECTS ON LAB TEST RESULTS

- May increase sodium and phosphate levels. May decrease electrolyte level with prolonged use.

CONTRAINDICATIONS & CAUTIONS

- Contraindicated in patients on sodium-restricted diets and in patients with intestinal obstruction, intestinal perforation, edema, heart failure, megacolon, impaired renal function, or signs and symptoms of appendicitis or acute surgical abdomen, such as abdominal pain, nausea, or vomiting.
- Use cautiously in patients with large hemorrhoids or anal abrasions.

NURSING CONSIDERATIONS

- Before giving drug for constipation, determine whether patient has adequate fluid intake, exercise, and diet.
- ***Alert:*** Up to 10% of sodium content of drug may be absorbed.
- ***Alert:*** Severe electrolyte imbalances may occur if recommended dosage is exceeded.

PATIENT TEACHING

- Teach patient about dietary sources of fiber, including bran and other cereals, fresh fruit, and vegetables.
- Warn patient about adverse reactions, and stress importance of using drug only for short-term therapy.

sodium phosphate monohydrate and sodium phosphate dibasic anhydrous

Visicol

Pharmacologic class: osmotic laxative
Pregnancy risk category C

AVAILABLE FORMS

Tablets: 1.5 g sodium phosphate (1.102 g sodium phosphate monohydrate and 0.398 g sodium phosphate dibasic anhydrous)

INDICATIONS & DOSAGES

➤ To cleanse the bowel before colonoscopy
Adults: 40 tablets taken in the following manner: The evening before the procedure, 3 tablets P.O. with at least 8 ounces of clear liquid q 15 minutes, for a total of 20 tablets. The last dose will be only 2 tablets. The day of the procedure, 3 tablets P.O. with at least 8 ounces of clear liquid q 15 minutes, for a total of 20 tablets, starting 3 to 5 hours before the procedure. The last dose will be only 2 tablets.

ACTION

Induces diarrhea by causing large amounts of water to be drawn into the colon, promoting rapid and effective evacuation.

Route	Onset	Peak	Duration
P.O.	Rapid	Varies	1–3 hr

Half-life: Unknown.

ADVERSE REACTIONS

CNS: dizziness, headache.

GI: abdominal bloating, abdominal pain, nausea, vomiting.

INTERACTIONS

Drug-drug. *Any drugs:* Reduces absorption of these drugs. Separate doses.

EFFECTS ON LAB TEST RESULTS

- May increase phosphorus level (typically normalizes 48 to 72 hours after giving drug). May decrease potassium and calcium levels.

CONTRAINDICATIONS & CAUTIONS

- Contraindicated in patients hypersensitive to sodium phosphate or any of its ingredients. Avoid giving drug to patients with heart failure, ascites, unstable angina, gastric retention, ileus, acute intestinal obstruction, pseudo-obstruction, severe chronic constipation, bowel perforation, acute colitis, toxic megacolon, or hypomotility syndrome (hypothyroidism, scleroderma).
- Use cautiously in patients with a history of electrolyte abnormalities, current electrolyte abnormalities, or impaired renal function. Also use cautiously in patients who take drugs that can induce electrolyte abnormalities or prolong the QT interval.
- Use cautiously in elderly patients because they may be more sensitive to drug effects.

NURSING CONSIDERATIONS

- Correct electrolyte imbalances before giving drug.
- As with other sodium phosphate cathartic preparations, this drug may induce colonic mucosal ulceration.
- Monitor patient for signs of dehydration.
- Don't repeat administration within 7 days.
- No enema or laxative is needed in addition to drug. Patients shouldn't take any additional purgatives, particularly those that contain sodium phosphate.
- ***Alert:*** Administration of other sodium phosphate products has caused death from significant fluid shifts, electrolyte abnormalities, and cardiac arrhythmias. Patients with electrolyte disturbances have an increased risk of prolonged QT interval. Use drug cautiously in patients who are taking other drugs known to prolong the QT interval.

PATIENT TEACHING

- Urge patient to drink at least 8 ounces of clear liquid with each dose. Inadequate fluid intake may lead to excessive fluid loss and hypovolemia.
- Tell patient to drink only clear liquids for at least 12 hours before starting the purgative regimen.
- Caution patient against taking an additional enema or laxative, particularly one that contains sodium phosphate.
- Tell patient that undigested or partially digested Visicol tablets and other drugs may appear in the stool.

48

Antiemetics

aprepitant
chlorpromazine hydrochloride
(See Chapter 31, ANTIPSYCHOTICS.)
dimenhydrinate
dolasetron mesylate
dronabinol
granisetron hydrochloride
meclizine hydrochloride
metoclopramide hydrochloride
nabilone
ondansetron hydrochloride
palonosetron hydrochloride
perphenazine
(See Chapter 31, ANTIPSYCHOTICS.)
prochlorperazine
prochlorperazine edisylate
prochlorperazine maleate
promethazine hydrochloride
(See Chapter 40, ANTIHISTAMINES.)
scopolamine
(See Chapter 36, ANTICHOLINERGICS.)
trimethobenzamide hydrochloride

aprepitant

Emend

Pharmacologic class: substance P and neurokinin-1 receptor antagonist
Pregnancy risk category B

AVAILABLE FORMS

Capsules: 40 mg, 80 mg, 125 mg

INDICATIONS & DOSAGES

➤To prevent nausea and vomiting after highly emetogenic chemotherapy (including cisplatin) and moderately emetogenic chemotherapy, with a 5-HT_3 antagonist and a corticosteroid

Adults: On day 1 of chemotherapy, 125 mg P.O. 1 hour before treatment. On days 2 and 3, 80 mg P.O. q morning.

***NEW INDICATION:* To prevent postoperative nausea and vomiting**

Adults: 40 mg P.O. within 3 hours before starting anesthesia.

ACTION

Selectively antagonizes substance P and neurokinin-1 receptors in the brain; appears to be synergistic with 5-HT_3 antagonists and corticosteroids.

Route	Onset	Peak	Duration
P.O.	Unknown	4 hr	Unknown

Half-life: 9 to 13 hours.

ADVERSE REACTIONS

CNS: *asthenia, fatigue,* dizziness, fever, headache, insomnia.
CV: ***bradycardia,*** hypertension, hypotension.
EENT: mucous membrane disorder, tinnitus.
GI: *anorexia, constipation, diarrhea, nausea,* abdominal pain, epigastric pain, flatulence, gastritis, heartburn, vomiting.
GU: UTI.
Hematologic: ***neutropenia,*** anemia.
Respiratory: *hiccups.*
Skin: pruritus.
Other: dehydration.

INTERACTIONS

Drug-drug. *Alprazolam, midazolam, triazolam:* May increase levels of these drugs. Watch for CNS effects, such as increased sedation. Decrease benzodiazepine dose by 50%.
Carbamazepine, phenytoin, rifampin, other CYP3A4 inducers: May decrease aprepitant level. Watch for decreased antiemetic effect.
Clarithromycin, diltiazem, erythromycin, itraconazole, ketoconazole, nefazodone, nelfinavir, ritonavir, troleandomycin, other CYP3A4 inhibitors: May increase aprepitant level and risk of toxicity. Use together cautiously.
Dexamethasone, methylprednisolone: May increase levels of these drugs and risk of toxicity. Decrease P.O. corticosteroid dose by 50%; decrease I.V. methylprednisolone dose by 25%.

Diltiazem: May increase diltiazem level. Monitor heart rate and blood pressure. Avoid using together.
Docetaxel, etoposide, ifosfamide, imatinib, irinotecan, paclitaxel, vinorelbine, vinblastine, vincristine: May increase levels and risk of toxicity of these drugs. Use together cautiously.
Hormonal contraceptives: May decrease contraceptive effectiveness. Tell women to use additional birth control method during therapy.
Paroxetine: May decrease paroxetine and aprepitant effects. Monitor patient for effectiveness.
Phenytoin: May decrease phenytoin level. Monitor level carefully. Avoid using together. Increase phenytoin dose as needed during therapy.
Pimozide: May increase pimozide level. Avoid using together.
Tolbutamide: May decrease tolbutamide effects. Monitor glucose level.
Warfarin: May decrease warfarin effectiveness. Monitor INR carefully for 2 weeks after each aprepitant treatment.
Drug-herb. *St. John's wort:* May decrease antiemetic effects by inducing CYP3A4. Discourage use together.
Drug-food. *Grapefruit juice:* May increase drug level and risk of toxicity. Discourage use together.

EFFECTS ON LAB TEST RESULTS

- May increase alkaline phosphatase, AST, ALT, BUN, creatinine, glucose, and urine protein levels. May decrease sodium level.
- May increase RBC and WBC counts. May decrease neutrophil count.

CONTRAINDICATIONS & CAUTIONS

- Contraindicated in patients hypersensitive to aprepitant or its components.
- Use cautiously in patients receiving chemotherapy drugs metabolized mainly via CYP3A4 and in those with severe hepatic disease.
- Use in pregnant women only when drug's benefit clearly outweighs its risk.
- Don't use in breast-feeding women; it's unknown if drug appears in breast milk.
- Safety and effectiveness haven't been established in children.

NURSING CONSIDERATIONS

- Avoid giving drug for more than 3 days per chemotherapy cycle.
- ***Alert:*** Before giving drug, screen patient carefully for possible drug and herb interactions.
- Don't give drug for existing nausea or vomiting.
- Expect to give drug with other antiemetics to treat breakthrough emesis.
- Monitor CBC, liver function test results, and creatinine level periodically during therapy.

PATIENT TEACHING

- Tell patient that drug is to be taken with other antiemetics and shouldn't be taken alone.
- If nausea or vomiting occurs, instruct patient to take breakthrough antiemetics rather than more aprepitant.
- Urge patient to report use of any other drugs or herbs.
- Caution patient against taking drug with grapefruit juice.
- Advise woman who takes a hormonal contraceptive to use an additional form of birth control.
- Tell patient who takes warfarin that PT and INR will be monitored closely for 2 weeks after therapy starts.

dimenhydrinate

Apo-Dimenhydrinate†, Calm-X ◊, Children's Dramamine* ◊, Dramamine* ◊, Dramamine Liquid* ◊, Dramanate, Dymenate, Gravol†, Gravol L/A†, Hydrate, PMS-Dimenhydrinate†, Traveltabs†, TripTone Caplets ◊

Pharmacologic class: anticholinergic
Pregnancy risk category B

AVAILABLE FORMS

Elixir: 15 mg/5 ml†
Injection: 50 mg/ml
Syrup: 12.5 mg/4 ml* ◊, 15.62 mg/5 ml
Tablets: 50 mg ◊
Tablets (chewable): 50 mg ◊

INDICATIONS & DOSAGES

➤ To prevent and treat motion sickness

Adults and children age 12 and older: Give 50 to 100 mg P.O. q 4 to 6 hours; 50 mg I.M., p.r.n.; or 50 mg I.V. diluted in 10 ml normal saline solution for injection, injected over 2 minutes. Maximum, 400 mg daily. For prevention, use drug 30 minutes before motion exposure.

Children ages 6 to 11: Give 25 to 50 mg P.O. q 6 to 8 hours, not to exceed 150 mg in 24 hours. Or, 1.25 mg/kg or 37.5 mg/m^2 I.M. or P.O. q.i.d. Maximum, 300 mg daily.

Children ages 2 to 5: Give 12.5 to 25 mg P.O. q 6 to 8 hours, not to exceed 75 mg in 24 hours. Or, 1.25 mg/kg or 37.5 mg/m^2 I.M. or P.O. q.i.d. Maximum, 300 mg daily.

I.V. ADMINISTRATION

- Dilute each milliliter (50 mg) of drug with 10 ml sterile water for injection, D_5W, or normal saline solution for injection.
- Give by direct injection over at least 2 minutes.

INCOMPATIBILITIES

Aminophylline, ammonium chloride, amobarbital, butorphanol, chlorpromazine, glycopyrrolate, heparin, hydrocortisone sodium succinate, hydroxyzine hydrochloride, midazolam, pentobarbital sodium, phenobarbital sodium, phenytoin, prochlorperazine edisylate, promazine, promethazine hydrochloride, and thiopental.

ACTION

May affect neural pathways originating in the labyrinth to inhibit nausea and vomiting.

Route	Onset	Peak	Duration
P.O.	15–30 min	Unknown	3–6 hr
I.V.	Immediate	Unknown	3–6 hr
I.M.	20–30 min	Unknown	3–6 hr

Half-life: Unknown.

ADVERSE REACTIONS

CNS: *drowsiness,* confusion, dizziness, excitation, headache, insomnia, lassitude, nervousness, tingling and weakness of hands, vertigo.

CV: hypotension, palpitations, tachycardia.

EENT: blurred vision, diplopia, dry respiratory passages, nasal congestion.

GI: anorexia, constipation, diarrhea, dry mouth, epigastric distress, nausea, vomiting.

GU: urine retention.

Respiratory: thickened bronchial secretions, wheezing.

Skin: photosensitivity, rash, urticaria.

Other: ***anaphylaxis,*** tightness of chest.

INTERACTIONS

Drug-drug. *CNS depressants:* May cause additive CNS depression. Avoid using together.

Ototoxic drugs: Dimenhydrinate may mask symptoms of ototoxicity. Use together cautiously.

Tricyclic antidepressants, other anticholinergics: May increase anticholinergic activity. Monitor patient.

Drug-lifestyle. *Alcohol use:* May cause additive CNS depression. Discourage use together.

EFFECTS ON LAB TEST RESULTS

- May prevent, reduce, or mask diagnostic skin test response. May alter xanthine (caffeine, aminophylline) test results.

CONTRAINDICATIONS & CAUTIONS

- Contraindicated in patients hypersensitive to drug or its components.
- Use cautiously in elderly patients, patients receiving ototoxic drugs, and patients with seizures, acute angle-closure glaucoma, or enlarged prostate gland.

NURSING CONSIDERATIONS

- Elderly patients may be more susceptible to adverse CNS effects.
- Undiluted solution irritates veins and may cause sclerosis.
- Stop drug 4 days before diagnostic skin tests to prevent falsifying test response.
- Dramamine may contain tartrazine.
- ***Alert:*** Drug may mask symptoms of ototoxicity, brain tumor, or intestinal obstruction.
- ***Look alike–sound alike:*** Don't confuse dimenhydrinate with diphenhydramine.

PATIENT TEACHING
- Advise patient to avoid activities that require alertness until CNS effects of drug are known.
- Instruct patient to report adverse reactions promptly.

dolasetron mesylate
Anzemet

Pharmacologic class: selective serotonin (5-HT_3) receptor antagonist
Pregnancy risk category B

AVAILABLE FORMS
Injection: 20 mg/ml as 12.5-mg/0.625-ml ampule or 100-mg/5-ml vial
Tablets: 50 mg, 100 mg

INDICATIONS & DOSAGES
➤**To prevent nausea and vomiting from cancer chemotherapy**
Adults: 100 mg P.O. given as a single dose 1 hour before chemotherapy. Or, 1.8 mg/kg or a fixed dose of 100 mg as a single I.V. dose given 30 minutes before chemotherapy.
Children ages 2 to 16: 1.8 mg/kg P.O. given 1 hour before chemotherapy. Or, 1.8 mg/kg as a single I.V. dose given 30 minutes before chemotherapy. Injectable formulation can be mixed with apple juice and given P.O. Maximum dose is 100 mg.
➤**To prevent postoperative nausea and vomiting**
Adults: 100 mg P.O. within 2 hours before surgery. Or, 12.5 mg as a single I.V. dose about 15 minutes before cessation of anesthesia or as soon as nausea or vomiting presents.
Children ages 2 to 16: 1.2 mg/kg P.O. given within 2 hours before surgery, to maximum of 100 mg. Or, 0.35 mg/kg, up to 12.5 mg given as a single I.V. dose about 15 minutes before stopping anesthesia or as soon as nausea or vomiting starts. I.V. form can be mixed with apple juice and given P.O.
➤**Postoperative nausea and vomiting**
Adults: 12.5 mg as a single I.V. dose as soon as nausea or vomiting occurs.
Children ages 2 to 16: 0.35 mg/kg, to maximum dosage of 12.5 mg, given as a single I.V. dose as soon as nausea or vomiting occurs.

I.V. ADMINISTRATION
- Drug can be injected as rapidly as 100 mg over 30 seconds or diluted in 50 ml of compatible solution and infused over 15 minutes.

INCOMPATIBILITIES
Other I.V. drugs.

ACTION
Blocks the action of serotonin and prevents serotonin from stimulating the vomiting reflex.

Route	Onset	Peak	Duration
P.O.	Rapid	1 hr	8 hr
I.V.	Rapid	36 min	7 hr

Half-life: 8 hours.

ADVERSE REACTIONS
CNS: *headache,* dizziness, drowsiness, fatigue, fever.
CV: ***arrhythmias,*** ECG changes, edema, hypertension, hypotension, tachycardia.
GI: *diarrhea,* abdominal pain, anorexia, constipation, dyspepsia.
GU: hematuria, polyuria, urine retention.
Skin: pruritus, rash.
Other: chills, pain at injection site.

INTERACTIONS
Drug-drug. *Drugs that prolong ECG intervals such as antiarrhythmics:* May increase risk of arrhythmia. Monitor patient closely.
Drugs that inhibit CYP enzymes such as cimetidine: May increase level of hydrodolasetron, an active metabolite of dolasetron. Monitor patient for adverse effects.
Drugs that induce CYP enzymes such as rifampin: May decrease level of hydrodolasetron, an active metabolite of dolasetron. Monitor patient for decreased effectiveness of antiemetic.

EFFECTS ON LAB TEST RESULTS
- May increase ALT and AST levels.
- May increase PTT.

CONTRAINDICATIONS & CAUTIONS

- Contraindicated in patients hypersensitive to drug.
- ***Alert:*** Give with caution in patients who have or may develop prolonged cardiac conduction intervals, such as those with electrolyte abnormalities, history of arrhythmia, and cumulative high-dose anthracycline therapy.
- Drug isn't recommended for use in children younger than age 2. Use cautiously in breast-feeding women.

NURSING CONSIDERATIONS

- Injection for oral use is stable in apple or apple-grape juice for 2 hours at room temperature.
- ***Look alike–sound alike:*** Don't confuse Anzemet with Aldomet or Avandamet.

PATIENT TEACHING

- Tell patient about possible adverse effects.
- Instruct patient to mix injection in juice for oral use immediately before giving.
- Tell patient to report nausea or vomiting.

dronabinol (delta-9-tetrahydrocannabinol)

Marinol

Pharmacologic class: cannabinoid
Pregnancy risk category C
Controlled substance schedule III

AVAILABLE FORMS

Capsules: 2.5 mg, 5 mg, 10 mg

INDICATIONS & DOSAGES

➤ Nausea and vomiting from cancer chemotherapy

Adults: 5 mg/m^2 P.O. 1 to 3 hours before chemotherapy session. Then, same dose q 2 to 4 hours after chemotherapy, for total of four to six doses daily. If needed, increase dosage in 2.5-mg/m^2 increments to maximum of 15 mg/m^2 per dose.

➤ Anorexia and weight loss in patients with AIDS

Adults: 2.5 mg P.O. b.i.d. before lunch and dinner. If patient can't tolerate it, decrease to 2.5 mg P.O. given as a single dose daily in evening or at bedtime. May gradually increase to maximum of 20 mg daily given in divided doses.

ACTION

Unknown. A derivative of marijuana.

Route	Onset	Peak	Duration
P.O.	30–60 min	2–4 hr	4–6 hr

Half-life: 1 to 1½ days.

ADVERSE REACTIONS

CNS: *ataxia, dizziness, drowsiness, euphoria, paranoia,* amnesia, asthenia, confusion, depersonalization, hallucinations, headache, muddled thinking, somnolence.
CV: orthostatic hypotension, palpitations, tachycardia, vasodilation.
EENT: visual disturbances.
GI: *abdominal pain, dry mouth, nausea, vomiting,* diarrhea.

INTERACTIONS

Drug-drug. *CNS depressants, psychomimetic substances, sedatives:* May cause additive CNS depression. Avoid using together.
Drug-lifestyle. *Alcohol use:* May cause additive CNS depression. Discourage use together.

EFFECTS ON LAB TEST RESULTS

None reported.

CONTRAINDICATIONS & CAUTIONS

- Contraindicated in patients hypersensitive to sesame oil or cannabinoids.
- Use cautiously in the elderly, in pregnant or breast-feeding women, and in those with heart disease, psychiatric illness, or history of drug abuse.

NURSING CONSIDERATIONS

- Expect drug to be prescribed only for patients who haven't responded satisfactorily to other antiemetics.
- ***Alert:*** Drug is the principal active substance in *Cannabis sativa* (marijuana), which can produce both physiological and psychological dependence and has a high risk of abuse.
- CNS effects are intensified at higher dosages.
- Drug effects may persist for days after treatment ends.

• ***Look alike–sound alike:*** Don't confuse dronabinol with droperidol.

PATIENT TEACHING

• Tell patient that drug may induce unusual changes in mood or other adverse behavioral effects.
• Advise patient against performing activities that require alertness until CNS effects of drug are known.
• Warn caregivers to supervise patient during and immediately after treatment.
• Advise patient to take drug 1 to 3 hours before chemotherapy use.

granisetron hydrochloride
Kytril

Pharmacologic class: selective serotonin (5-HT_3) receptor antagonist
Pregnancy risk category B

AVAILABLE FORMS

Injection: 1 mg/ml in 1-ml, single-dose, preservative-free vials and 4-ml multidose vials containing benzyl alcohol
Oral solution: 1 mg/5 ml
Tablets: 1 mg

INDICATIONS & DOSAGES

➤ **To prevent nausea and vomiting from emetogenic cancer chemotherapy**
Adults and children age 2 and older: 10 mcg/kg I.V. undiluted and given by direct injection over 30 seconds, or diluted and infused over 5 minutes. Start giving at least 30 minutes before chemotherapy.
Or, for adults, 1 mg P.O. up to 1 hour before chemotherapy and repeated 12 hours later. Or, for adults, 2 mg P.O. daily given up to 1 hour before chemotherapy.

➤ **To prevent nausea and vomiting from radiation, including total body irradiation and fractionated abdominal radiation**
Adults: 2 mg P.O. once daily within 1 hour of radiation.

➤ **Postoperative nausea and vomiting**
Adults: 1 mg I.V. undiluted and given over 30 seconds. For prevention, give before anesthesia induction or immediately before reversal.

I.V. ADMINISTRATION

• For direct injection, give drug undiluted over 30 seconds.
• For intermittent infusion, dilute with normal saline solution for injection or D_5W to a volume of 20 to 50 ml.
• Infuse over 5 minutes, starting within 30 minutes before chemotherapy and only on days chemotherapy is given.
• Diluted solutions are stable 24 hours at room temperature.
• Don't freeze vials.
• Once the multiuse vial is penetrated, use contents within 30 days.

INCOMPATIBILITIES

Other I.V. drugs.

ACTION

Selective antagonist of a specific type of serotonin receptor (5-HT_3) located in the CNS in the chemoreceptor trigger zone and in the peripheral nervous system on nerve terminals of the vagus nerve. Drug's blocking action may occur at both sites.

Route	Onset	Peak	Duration
P.O., I.V.	Unknown	Unknown	Unknown

Half-life: 5 to 9 hours.

ADVERSE REACTIONS

CNS: *asthenia, headache, fever,* agitation, anxiety, CNS stimulation, dizziness, insomnia, somnolence.
CV: ***bradycardia,*** hypertension, hypotension.
GI: *constipation, nausea, vomiting,* abdominal pain, decreased appetite, diarrhea, dyspepsia, flatulence, taste disorder.
GU: oliguria, UTI.
Hematologic: *anemia,* ***leukocytosis, leukopenia, thrombocytopenia.***
Respiratory: cough, increased sputum.
Skin: alopecia, rash, dermatitis.
Other: *pain,* ***hypersensitivity reactions (anaphylaxis, urticaria, dyspnea, hypotension),*** infection.

INTERACTIONS

None known.

EFFECTS ON LAB TEST RESULTS

• May increase ALT and AST levels. May decrease hemoglobin level and hemato-

crit. May alter fluid and electrolyte levels with prolonged use.
- May decrease platelet and WBC counts.

CONTRAINDICATIONS & CAUTIONS
- Contraindicated in patients hypersensitive to drug.

NURSING CONSIDERATIONS
- Drug regimen is given only on days when chemotherapy is given. Treatment at other times isn't useful.

PATIENT TEACHING
- Stress importance of taking second dose of oral drug 12 hours after the first for maximum effectiveness.
- Tell patient to report adverse reactions immediately.

meclizine hydrochloride (meclozine hydrochloride)

Antivert, Antivert/25 ◇, Antivert/50, Bonamine†, Bonine ◇, Dramamine Less Drowsy Formula

Pharmacologic class: anticholinergic
Pregnancy risk category B

AVAILABLE FORMS
Capsules: 25 mg, 30 mg ◇
Tablets: 12.5 mg, 25 mg ◇, 50 mg
Tablets (chewable): 25 mg ◇

INDICATIONS & DOSAGES
➤ **Vertigo**
Adults: 25 to 100 mg P.O. daily in divided doses. Dosage varies with response.
➤ **Motion sickness**
Adults and children age 12 and older: 25 to 50 mg P.O. 1 hour before travel; then daily for duration of trip.

ACTION
Unknown. May affect neural pathways originating in the labyrinth to inhibit nausea and vomiting.

Route	Onset	Peak	Duration
P.O.	1 hr	Unknown	8–24 hr

Half-life: About 6 hours.

ADVERSE REACTIONS
CNS: *drowsiness,* auditory and visual hallucinations, excitation, nervousness, restlessness.
CV: hypotension, palpitations, tachycardia.
EENT: blurred vision, diplopia, dry nose and throat, tinnitus.
GI: anorexia, constipation, diarrhea, dry mouth, nausea, vomiting.
GU: urinary frequency, urine retention.
Skin: rash, urticaria.

INTERACTIONS
Drug-drug. *CNS depressants:* May increase drowsiness. Use together cautiously.

EFFECTS ON LAB TEST RESULTS
- May prevent, reduce, or mask diagnostic skin test response.

CONTRAINDICATIONS & CAUTIONS
- Contraindicated in patients hypersensitive to drug.
- Use cautiously in patients with asthma, glaucoma, or prostatic hyperplasia.

NURSING CONSIDERATIONS
- Stop drug 4 days before diagnostic skin tests to avoid interference with test response.
- Drug may mask signs and symptoms of ototoxicity, brain tumor, or intestinal obstruction.
- ***Look alike–sound alike:*** Don't confuse Antivert with Axert.

PATIENT TEACHING
- Advise patient to avoid hazardous activities that require alertness until CNS effects of drug are known.
- Urge patient to report persistent or serious adverse reactions promptly.

metoclopramide hydrochloride

Apo-Metoclop†, Clopra, Maxeran†, Maxolon‡, Octamide PFS, Pramin‡, Reglan

Pharmacologic class: dopamine antagonist
Pregnancy risk category B

AVAILABLE FORMS
Injection: 5 mg/ml

Syrup: 5 mg/5 ml
Tablets: 5 mg, 10 mg

INDICATIONS & DOSAGES

➤ **To prevent or reduce nausea and vomiting from emetogenic cancer chemotherapy**
Adults: 1 to 2 mg/kg I.V. 30 minutes before chemotherapy; repeat q 2 hours for two doses, then q 3 hours for three doses.
➤ **To prevent or reduce postoperative nausea and vomiting**
Adults: 10 to 20 mg I.M. near end of surgical procedure; repeat q 4 to 6 hours, p.r.n.
➤ **To facilitate small-bowel intubation, to aid in radiologic examinations**
Adults and children older than age 14: 10 mg or 2 ml I.V. as a single dose over 1 to 2 minutes.
Children ages 6 to 14: 2.5 to 5 mg or 0.5 to 1 ml I.V.
Children younger than age 6: 0.1 mg/kg I.V.
➤ **Delayed gastric emptying secondary to diabetic gastroparesis**
Adults: 10 mg P.O. 30 minutes before each meal and at bedtime for mild symptoms. Give by slow I.V. infusion over 1 to 2 minutes 30 minutes before each meal and at bedtime for up to 10 days for severe symptoms; then P.O. dose may be started and continued for 2 to 8 weeks.
➤ **Gastroesophageal reflux disease**
Adults: 10 to 15 mg P.O. q.i.d., p.r.n., 30 minutes before meals and at bedtime.
Adjust-a-dose: For patients with creatinine clearance below 40 ml/minute, decrease dosage by half.
➤ **Emesis during pregnancy ♦**
Adults: 5 to 10 mg P.O. or 5 to 20 mg I.V. or I.M. t.i.d.

I.V. ADMINISTRATION

- Drug is compatible with D_5W, normal saline solution for injection, dextrose 5% in half-normal saline solution, Ringer injection, and lactated Ringer injection. Normal saline solution is the preferred diluent because drug is most stable in this solution.
- Give doses of 10 mg or less by direct injection over 1 to 2 minutes. Dilute doses larger than 10 mg in 50 ml of compatible diluent, and infuse over at least 15 minutes. Closely monitor blood pressure.
- No need to protect drug from light if infusion mixture is given within 24 hours. If protected from light and refrigerated, it's stable for 48 hours.

INCOMPATIBILITIES

Allopurinol, ampicillin, amphotericin B, calcium gluconate, cefepime, chloramphenicol sodium succinate, cisplatin, doxorubicin liposomal, erythromycin lactobionate, fluorouracil, furosemide, methotrexate sodium, penicillin G potassium, propofol, sodium bicarbonate.

ACTION

Stimulates motility of upper GI tract, increases lower esophageal sphincter tone, and blocks dopamine receptors at the chemoreceptor trigger zone.

Route	Onset	Peak	Duration
P.O.	30–60 min	1–2 hr	1–2 hr
I.V.	1–3 min	Unknown	1–2 hr
I.M.	10–15 min	Unknown	1–2 hr

Half-life: 4 to 6 hours.

ADVERSE REACTIONS

CNS: *anxiety, drowsiness, dystonic reactions, fatigue, lassitude, restlessness,* ***neuroleptic malignant syndrome, seizures, suicide ideation,*** akathisia, confusion, depression, dizziness, extrapyramidal symptoms, fever, hallucinations, headache, insomnia, tardive dyskinesia.
CV: ***bradycardia, supraventricular tachycardia,*** hypotension, transient hypertension.
GI: bowel disorders, diarrhea, nausea.
GU: incontinence, urinary frequency.
Hematologic: ***agranulocytosis, neutropenia.***
Skin: rash, urticaria.
Other: loss of libido, prolactin secretion.

INTERACTIONS

Drug-drug. *Anticholinergics, opioid analgesics:* May antagonize GI motility effects of metoclopramide. Use together cautiously.
CNS depressants: May cause additive CNS effects. Avoid using together.

Levodopa: Levodopa and metoclopramide have opposite effects on dopamine receptors. Avoid using together.
MAO inhibitors: May increase release of catecholamines in patients with hypertension. Use together cautiously.
Phenothiazines: May increase risk of extrapyramidal effects. Monitor patient closely.
Drug-lifestyle. *Alcohol use:* May cause additive CNS effects. Discourage use together.

EFFECTS ON LAB TEST RESULTS

- May increase liver function tests, aldosterone and prolactin levels.
- May decrease neutrophil and granulocyte counts.

CONTRAINDICATIONS & CAUTIONS

- Contraindicated in patients hypersensitive to drug and in those with pheochromocytoma or seizure disorders.
- Contraindicated in patients for whom stimulation of GI motility might be dangerous (those with hemorrhage, obstruction, or perforation).
- Use cautiously in patients with history of depression, Parkinson disease, or hypertension.

NURSING CONSIDERATIONS

- Monitor bowel sounds.
- Safety and effectiveness of drug haven't been established for therapy lasting longer than 12 weeks.
- ***Alert:*** Use 25 mg diphenhydramine I.V. to counteract extrapyramidal adverse effects from high doses.

PATIENT TEACHING

- Tell patient to avoid activities that require alertness for 2 hours after doses.
- Urge patient to report persistent or serious adverse reactions promptly.
- Advise patient not to drink alcohol during therapy.

NEW DRUG

nabilone

Cesamet

Pharmacologic class: cannabinoid
Pregnancy risk category C
Controlled substance schedule II

AVAILABLE FORMS

Capsules: 1 mg

INDICATIONS & DOSAGES

➤Chemotherapy-induced nausea and vomiting unresponsive to conventional antiemetics
Adults: Usual dose, 1 or 2 mg P.O. b.i.d. Give first dose 1 to 3 hours before chemotherapy starts and then two to three times daily throughout the cycle. If needed, start with 1 or 2 mg the night before chemotherapy starts and continue 48 hours after the cycle ends. Maximum daily dose is 6 mg, divided t.i.d.

ACTION

A synthetic cannabinoid, drug may exert effects by interacting with cannabinoid receptors in the CNS.

Route	Onset	Peak	Duration
P.O.	Rapid	2 hr	Unknown

Half-life: 2 hours for drug; 35 hours for metabolites.

ADVERSE REACTIONS

CNS: *ataxia, depression, difficulty concentrating, drowsiness, euphoria, sleep disturbance, vertigo,* anorexia, asthenia, headache, depersonalization, disorientation, dysphoria.
CV: hypotension, orthostatic hypotension, tachycardia.
EENT: *visual disturbance.*
GI: *dry mouth,* nausea, thirst.
Metabolic: increased appetite.

INTERACTIONS

Drug-drug. *Anticholinergics, sympathomimetics, tricyclic antidepressants:* May increase hypertension, tachycardia or drowsiness. Avoid using together if possible.

CNS depressants: May increase CNS depression. Use with extreme caution and monitor patient carefully.
Highly protein-bound drugs: May be displaced by nabilone. Monitor patient and drug levels, as needed. Dosages may need adjustment.
Drug-lifestyle. *Alcohol use:* May increase CNS depression. Caution patient to avoid alcohol.
Marijuana: May cause additive effects. Discourage use.

EFFECTS ON LAB TEST RESULTS
None reported.

CONTRAINDICATIONS & CAUTIONS
- Contraindicated in patients hypersensitive to cannabinoids.
- Use cautiously in elderly patients; those taking highly protein-bound drugs, sedatives, hypnotics, or other psychoactive drugs; and those with high blood pressure, heart disease, hepatic or renal impairment, or current or previous mental illness or substance abuse.

NURSING CONSIDERATIONS
- Because it may cause psychotic reactions, drug isn't a first-line treatment option.
- Obtain a detailed health history before therapy to rule out mental illness or substance abuse.
- ***Alert:*** Due to high abuse potential, prescription amount should be limited to the amount necessary for a single chemotherapy cycle.
- Monitor patient closely, especially when treatment starts or dosage changes.
- Check supine and standing pulse and blood pressure before and periodically during treatment.
- Be sure patient will remain under the supervision of a responsible adult during treatment.
- Watch for evidence of excessive use, abuse, or misuse.
- When stopping drug, monitor patient for evidence of withdrawal, including mental distress, insomnia, and autonomic hyperactivity (sweating, rhinorrhea, loose stools, hiccups). Psychiatric reactions can persist for up to 72 hours after treatment stops.
- Safety and effectiveness in children isn't known; use cautiously because of psychoactive effects.

PATIENT TEACHING
- Tell patient that drug commonly causes dizziness, euphoria, disorientation, and drowsiness. Explain that depression, hallucinations, and psychosis may occur.
- Stress that patient should remain under the supervision of a responsible adult, especially when treatment starts or dosage changes because of drug's psychoactive effects.
- Advise patient to rise slowly from a reclining position and to sit with his feet on the floor before standing until drug's effects are known.
- Urge patient to avoid alcohol, sedatives, and hypnotics because of the increased risk of adverse effects.
- Caution patient to avoid driving and other hazardous activities during treatment.
- Explain that drug has a high abuse potential and should be used only as prescribed.

ondansetron hydrochloride
Zofran, Zofran ODT

Pharmacologic class: selective serotonin (5-HT_3) receptor antagonist
Pregnancy risk category B

AVAILABLE FORMS
Injection: 2 mg/ml
Oral solution: 4 mg/5 ml
Orally disintegrating tablets (ODTs): 4 mg, 8 mg
Premixed injection: 32 mg/50 ml
Tablets: 4 mg, 8 mg, 24 mg

INDICATIONS & DOSAGES
➤ **To prevent nausea and vomiting from emetogenic chemotherapy**
Adults and children age 12 and older: 8 mg P.O. 30 minutes before chemotherapy. Then, 8 mg P.O. 8 hours after first dose. Then, 8 mg q 12 hours for 1 to 2 days. Or, a single dose of 32 mg by I.V. infusion over 15 minutes beginning 30 minutes before chemotherapy. Or, three doses of 0.15 mg/kg I.V. Give first dose

30 minutes before chemotherapy and subsequent doses 4 and 8 hours after first dose. Infuse drug over 15 minutes.
Children ages 4 to 12: 4 mg P.O. 30 minutes before chemotherapy. Then, 4 mg P.O. 4 and 8 hours after first dose. Then, 4 mg q 8 hours for 1 to 2 days.
Infants and children ages 6 months to 12 years: Three doses of 0.15 mg/kg I.V. Give first dose 30 minutes before chemotherapy; give subsequent doses 4 and 8 hours after first dose. Infuse drug over 15 minutes.

➤To prevent postoperative nausea and vomiting
Adults: 4 mg I.V. undiluted over 2 to 5 minutes. Or, 16 mg P.O. 1 hour before induction of anesthesia.
Children ages 1 month to 12 years who weigh more than 40 kg (88 lb): 4 mg I.V. as a single dose.
Children ages 1 month to 12 years who weigh 40 kg or less: 0.1 mg/kg I.V. as a single dose.

➤To prevent nausea and vomiting from radiation therapy in patients receiving total body irradiation, single high-dose fraction to abdomen, or daily fractions to abdomen
Adults: 8 mg P.O. t.i.d. For patients receiving total body irradiation, give 8 mg P.O. 1 to 2 hours before each fraction of radiation therapy each day. For patients receiving single high-dose fraction radiation therapy to the abdomen, give 8 mg P.O. 1 to 2 hours before therapy, then every 8 hours for 1 to 2 days after completion of therapy. For patients receiving daily fractionated radiation therapy, give 8 mg P.O. 1 to 2 hours before therapy, then every 8 hours for each day therapy is given.
Adjust-a-dose: For patients with severe hepatic impairment, total daily dose shouldn't exceed 8 mg.

I.V. ADMINISTRATION
- Dilute drug in 50 ml of D_5W injection or normal saline solution for injection.
- Drug is stable for up to 48 hours after dilution in D_5W, 5% dextrose in half-normal saline solution for injection, 5% dextrose in normal saline solution, and 3% sodium chloride solution for injection.
- Infuse over 15 minutes.

INCOMPATIBILITIES
Acyclovir sodium, allopurinol, aminophylline, amphotericin B, ampicillin sodium, ampicillin sodium and sulbactam sodium, cefepime, cefoperazone, dacarbazine with doxorubicin, dexamethasone sodium phosphate, droperidol, fluorouracil, furosemide, ganciclovir, lorazepam, meropenem, methylprednisolone sodium succinate, piperacillin sodium, sargramostim, sodium bicarbonate.

ACTION
Selective antagonist of 5-HT_3 located in the CNS at the chemoreceptor trigger zone and in the peripheral nervous system on nerve terminals of the vagus nerve. Drug's blocking action may occur at both sites.

Route	Onset	Peak	Duration
P.O., I.V.	Unknown	Unknown	Unknown

Half-life: 4 hours.

ADVERSE REACTIONS
CNS: *dizziness, fatigue, headache, malaise, sedation,* extrapyramidal syndrome, fever.
CV: ***arrhythmias,*** chest pain.
GI: *constipation, diarrhea,* abdominal pain, decreased appetite, xerostomia.
GU: gynecologic disorders, urine retention.
Musculoskeletal: *pain.*
Respiratory: hypoxia.
Skin: pruritus, rash.
Other: chills, injection site reaction.

INTERACTIONS
Drug-drug. *Drugs such as cimetidine that alter hepatic drug-metabolizing enzymes, phenobarbital, rifampin:* May change pharmacokinetics of ondansetron. No need to adjust dosage.
Drug-herb. *Horehound:* May enhance serotoninergic effects. Discourage use together.

EFFECTS ON LAB TEST RESULTS
- May increase ALT and AST levels.

CONTRAINDICATIONS & CAUTIONS
- Contraindicated in patients hypersensitive to drug.

• Use cautiously in patients with hepatic impairment.

NURSING CONSIDERATIONS
• ***Look alike–sound alike:*** Don't confuse Zofran with Zosyn, Zantac, or Zoloft.
• Monitor liver function test results. Don't exceed 8 mg in patients with hepatic impairment.

PATIENT TEACHING
• Instruct patient to immediately report difficulty breathing after drug administration.
• Tell patient receiving drug I.V. to report discomfort at insertion site.
• For patient taking ODTs, tell him to open blister just before use by peeling backing off and not by pushing through foil blister, and tell him that taking it with liquid isn't required.

palonosetron hydrochloride
Aloxi

Pharmacologic class: selective serotonin (5-HT_3) receptor antagonist
Pregnancy risk category B

AVAILABLE FORMS
Injection: 0.25 mg in 5-ml, single-use vial

INDICATIONS & DOSAGES
➤ **To prevent acute nausea and vomiting from moderately or highly emetogenic chemotherapy or delayed nausea and vomiting from moderately emetogenic chemotherapy**
Adults: 0.25 mg given I.V. over 30 seconds, 30 minutes before chemotherapy starts. Drug is given on the first day of each cycle, no more than q 7 days.

I.V. ADMINISTRATION
• Flush with normal saline solution before and after injection.
• Give by rapid I.V. injection over 30 seconds. Drug may be given through a peripheral or central I.V. line.

INCOMPATIBILITIES
Other I.V. drugs.

ACTION
Antagonizes 5-HT_3 receptors in the GI tract and brain, which inhibits emesis caused by chemotherapy.

Route	Onset	Peak	Duration
I.V.	30 min	Unknown	5 days

Half-life: 40 hours.

ADVERSE REACTIONS
CNS: anxiety, dizziness, headache, weakness.
CV: ***bradycardia, nonsustained ventricular tachycardia,*** hypotension.
GI: constipation, diarrhea.
Metabolic: ***hyperkalemia.***

INTERACTIONS
Drug-drug. *Antiarrhythmics or other drugs that prolong the QTc interval, diuretics that induce electrolyte abnormalities, high-dose anthracycline:* May increase risk of prolonged QTc interval. Use together cautiously.

EFFECTS ON LAB TEST RESULTS
• May increase potassium level.

CONTRAINDICATIONS & CAUTIONS
• Contraindicated in patents hypersensitive to palonosetron or its ingredients.
• Use cautiously in patients hypersensitive to other 5-HT_3 antagonists, in those taking drugs that affect cardiac conduction, and in those with cardiac conduction abnormalities, hypokalemia, or hypomagnesemia.
• Safety and efficacy in children haven't been established.

NURSING CONSIDERATIONS
• Before giving this drug, check patient's potassium level.
• Consider adding corticosteroids to the antiemetic regimen, particularly for patients receiving highly emetogenic chemotherapy.
• Make sure patient has additional antiemetics to take for breakthrough nausea or vomiting.
• If patient has cardiac conduction abnormalities, check the ECG before giving drug.

PATIENT TEACHING

- Advise patient to take a different antiemetic for breakthrough nausea or vomiting, at the first sign of nausea rather than waiting until symptoms are severe.
- Urge patient with a history of cardiac conduction abnormalities to report any changes in drug regimen such as adding or stopping an antiarrhythmic.

prochlorperazine

Compazine, Compro, PMS Prochlorperazine†, Stemetil†

prochlorperazine edisylate

Compazine, Compazine Syrup

prochlorperazine maleate

Compazine, Compazine Spansule, PMS Prochlorperazine†, Stemetil†

Pharmacologic class: dopamine antagonist
Pregnancy risk category C

AVAILABLE FORMS

prochlorperazine
Injection: 5 mg/ml
Suppositories: 2.5 mg, 5 mg, 25 mg
Tablets: 5 mg, 10 mg
prochlorperazine edisylate
Injection: 5 mg/ml
Syrup: 5 mg/5 ml
prochlorperazine maleate
Capsules (extended-release): 10 mg, 15 mg, 30 mg
Tablets: 5 mg, 10 mg, 25 mg

INDICATIONS & DOSAGES

➤ To control preoperative nausea
Adults: 5 to 10 mg I.M. 1 to 2 hours before induction of anesthesia; repeat once in 30 minutes, if needed. Or, 5 to 10 mg I.V. 15 to 30 minutes before induction of anesthesia; repeat once, if needed.

➤ Severe nausea and vomiting
Adults: 5 to 10 mg P.O., t.i.d. or q.i.d.; 15 mg sustained-release form P.O. on rising; 10 mg sustained-release form P.O. q 12 hours; 25 mg P.R., b.i.d.; or 5 to 10 mg I.M., repeated q 3 to 4 hours, p.r.n. Maximum I.M. dose is 40 mg daily. Or, 2.5 to 10 mg I.V. at no more than 5 mg/minute.
Children who weigh 18 to 39 kg (39 to 86 lb): 2.5 mg P.O. or P.R., t.i.d.; or 5 mg P.O. or P.R., b.i.d. Maximum, 15 mg daily. Or, 0.132 mg/kg by deep I.M. injection. Control is usually achieved with one dose.
Children who weigh 14 to 17 kg (30 to 38 lb): 2.5 mg P.O. or P.R., b.i.d. or t.i.d. Maximum, 10 mg daily. Or, 0.132 mg/kg by deep I.M. injection. Control is usually achieved with one dose.
Children who weigh 9 to 13 kg (20 to 29 lb): 2.5 mg P.O. or P.R. once daily or b.i.d. Maximum, 7.5 mg daily. Or, 0.132 mg/kg by deep I.M. injection. Control is usually achieved with one dose.

➤ To manage symptoms of psychotic disorders
Adults and children age 12 and older: Give 5 to 10 mg P.O., t.i.d. or q.i.d.
Children ages 2 to 12: Give 2.5 mg P.O. or P.R., b.i.d. or t.i.d. Don't exceed 10 mg on day 1. Increase dosage gradually to maximum, if needed. In children ages 2 to 5, maximum is 20 mg daily. In children ages 6 to 12, maximum is 25 mg daily.

➤ To manage symptoms of severe psychosis
Adults and children age 12 and older: 10 to 20 mg I.M., repeated in 1 to 4 hours, if needed. Rarely, patients may receive 10 to 20 mg q 4 to 6 hours. Start oral therapy after symptoms are controlled.
Children ages 2 to 12: 0.13 mg/kg I.M.

➤ Nonpsychotic anxiety
Adults: 5 to 10 mg P.O., t.i.d. or q.i.d. Or, 15 mg extended-release capsule once daily. Or, 10 mg extended-release capsule q 12 hours. Don't exceed 20 mg daily, and don't give for longer than 12 weeks.

I.V. ADMINISTRATION

- Add 20 mg of drug per liter of D_5W and normal saline solution, 15 to 30 minutes before induction of anesthesia.
- Infuse slowly; rate shouldn't exceed 5 mg/minute. Maximum parenteral dose is 40 mg daily.

INCOMPATIBILITIES

Aldesleukin, allopurinol, amifostine, aminophylline, amphotericin B, ampicillin sodium, aztreonam, calcium gluconate, chloramphenicol sodium succinate, chlorothiazide, dexamethasone sodium phosphate, dimenhydrinate, etoposide, filgrastim, fludarabine, foscarnet, furosemide, gemcitabine, heparin sodium, hydrocortisone sodium succinate, hydromorphone, ketorolac, solutions containing methylparabens, midazolam hydrochloride, morphine, penicillin G potassium, penicillin G sodium, pentobarbital, phenobarbital sodium, phenytoin sodium, piperacillin sodium and tazobactam sodium, solutions containing propylparabens, thiopental, vitamin B complex with C.

ACTION

Acts on the chemoreceptor trigger zone to inhibit nausea and vomiting; in larger doses, it partially depresses vomiting center.

Route	Onset	Peak	Duration
P.O.	30–40 min	Unknown	3–12 hr
P.O. (extended-release)	30–40 min	Unknown	10–12 hr
I.V.	Unknown	Unknown	Unknown
I.M.	10–20 min	Unknown	3–4 hr
P.R.	1 hr	Unknown	3–4 hr

Half-life: Unknown.

ADVERSE REACTIONS

CNS: *extrapyramidal reactions,* dizziness, EEG changes, pseudoparkinsonism, sedation.
CV: *orthostatic hypotension,* ECG changes, tachycardia.
EENT: *blurred vision, ocular changes.*
GI: *constipation, dry mouth,* increased appetite.
GU: *urine retention,* dark urine, inhibited ejaculation, menstrual irregularities.
Hematologic: ***agranulocytosis, transient leukopenia.***
Hepatic: cholestatic jaundice.
Metabolic: weight gain.
Skin: *mild photosensitivity,* allergic reactions, exfoliative dermatitis.
Other: gynecomastia, hyperprolactinemia.

INTERACTIONS

Drug-drug. *Antacids:* May inhibit absorption of oral phenothiazines. Separate antacid and phenothiazine doses by at least 2 hours.
Anticholinergics, including antidepressants and antiparkinsonians: May increase anticholinergic activity and may aggravate parkinsonian symptoms. Use together cautiously.
Barbiturates: May decrease phenothiazine effect. Monitor patient for decreased antiemetic effect.
Drug-herb. *Dong quai, St. John's wort:* May increase risk of photosensitivity. Advise patient to avoid excessive sun exposure.
Kava: May increase risk of dystonic reactions. Discourage use together.
Drug-lifestyle. *Alcohol use:* May increase CNS depression, particularly psychomotor skills. Strongly discourage use together.

EFFECTS ON LAB TEST RESULTS

- May decrease WBC and granulocyte counts.
- May cause false-positive results for urinary porphyrins, urobilinogen, amylase, and 5-hydroxyindoleacetic acid, and false-positive results in urine pregnancy tests using human chorionic gonadotropin. May cause abnormal liver function test results.

CONTRAINDICATIONS & CAUTIONS

- Contraindicated in patients hypersensitive to phenothiazines and in patients with CNS depression, including those in a coma.
- Contraindicated during pediatric surgery, when using spinal or epidural anesthetic or adrenergic blockers, and in children younger than age 2.
- Use cautiously in patients with impaired CV function, glaucoma, seizure disorders, and Parkinson disease; in those who have been exposed to extreme heat; and in children with acute illness.

NURSING CONSIDERATIONS

- Dilute oral solution with tomato juice, fruit juice, milk, coffee, carbonated beverage, tea, water, or soup. Or, mix with pudding.
- Watch for orthostatic hypotension, especially when giving drug I.V.
- For I.M. use, inject deeply into upper outer quadrant of gluteal region.
- Don't give by subcutaneous route or mix in syringe with another drug.
- To prevent contact dermatitis, avoid getting concentrate or injection solution on hands or clothing.

- Monitor CBC and liver function studies during long-term therapy.
- ***Alert:*** Use drug only when vomiting can't be controlled by other measures or when only a few doses are needed. If more than four doses are needed in 24 hours, notify prescriber.
- Store in light-resistant container. Slight yellowing doesn't affect potency; discard extremely discolored solutions.

PATIENT TEACHING
- Teach patient what to use to dilute oral solution.
- Advise patient to wear protective clothing when exposed to sunlight.
- Tell patient to call prescriber if more than four doses are needed within 24 hours.

trimethobenzamide hydrochloride

Tebamide, T-Gen, Ticon, Tigan, Triban, Trimazide

Pharmacologic class: anticholinergic
Pregnancy risk category C

AVAILABLE FORMS
Capsules: 250 mg, 300 mg
Injection: 100 mg/ml
Suppositories: 100 mg, 200 mg

INDICATIONS & DOSAGES
➤ **Nausea and vomiting**
Adults: 250 to 300 mg P.O. t.i.d. or q.i.d.; or 200 mg I.M. or P.R., t.i.d. or q.i.d.
Children who weigh 13 to 40 kg (29 to 88 lb): 100 to 200 mg P.O. or P.R., t.i.d. or q.i.d.
Children who weigh less than 13 kg: 100 mg P.R., t.i.d. or q.i.d.

ACTION
Probably acts on the chemoreceptor trigger zone to inhibit nausea and vomiting.

Route	Onset	Peak	Duration
P.O.	10–20 min	Unknown	3–4 hr
I.M.	15–35 min	Unknown	2–3 hr
P.R.	Unknown	Unknown	Unknown

Half-life: 7 to 9 hours.

ADVERSE REACTIONS
CNS: *drowsiness,* ***coma, seizures,*** depression, disorientation, dizziness with large doses, headache, parkinsonian-like symptoms.
CV: hypotension.
EENT: blurred vision.
GI: diarrhea.
Hepatic: jaundice.
Musculoskeletal: muscle cramps.
Other: hypersensitivity reactions.

INTERACTIONS
Drug-drug. *CNS depressants:* May cause additive CNS depression. Avoid using together.
Drug-lifestyle. *Alcohol use:* May cause additive CNS depression. Discourage use together.

EFFECTS ON LAB TEST RESULTS
None reported.

CONTRAINDICATIONS & CAUTIONS
- Contraindicated in patients hypersensitive to drug. Suppositories contraindicated in patients hypersensitive to benzocaine hydrochloride or similar local anesthetic.
- Use cautiously in children because drug may be linked to Reye syndrome.

NURSING CONSIDERATIONS
- For I.M. use, inject deep into upper outer quadrant of gluteal region to reduce pain and local irritation.
- Drug may mask signs and symptoms of toxic drug overdose, intestinal obstruction, brain tumor, or other conditions.
- Drug may cause pain, stinging, burning, redness, or swelling at I.M. injection site. Withhold drug if skin hypersensitivity reaction occurs.
- ***Look alike–sound alike:*** Don't confuse Tigan with Ticar.

PATIENT TEACHING
- Tell patient to refrigerate suppositories.
- Advise patient of possible drowsiness and dizziness; caution against performing hazardous activities requiring alertness until CNS effects of drug are known.

49
Antiulcer drugs

cimetidine
cimetidine hydrochloride
esomeprazole magnesium
esomeprazole sodium
famotidine
lansoprazole
misoprostol
omeprazole
omeprazole magnesium
pantoprazole sodium
rabeprazole sodium
ranitidine hydrochloride
sucralfate

cimetidine
Tagamet✐, Tagamet HB ◊

cimetidine hydrochloride
Tagamet

Pharmacologic class: H_2 receptor antagonist
Pregnancy risk category B

AVAILABLE FORMS
Injection: 300 mg/2 ml, 300 mg in 50 ml normal saline solution, 300 mg/2 ml ADD-Vantage vial
Oral liquid: 300 mg/5 ml*
Tablets: 200 mg ◊, 300 mg, 400 mg, 800 mg

INDICATIONS & DOSAGES
➤ **To prevent upper GI bleeding in critically ill patients**
Adults: 50 mg/hour by continuous I.V. infusion for up to 7 days; 25 mg/hour to patients with creatinine clearance below 30 ml/minute.
➤ **Short-term treatment of duodenal ulcer; maintenance therapy**
Adults and children age 16 and older: 800 mg P.O.at bedtime. Or, 400 mg P.O. b.i.d. or 300 mg q.i.d. (with meals and at bedtime). Or, 200 mg t.i.d. with a 400-mg bedtime dose. Treatment lasts 4 to 6 weeks unless endoscopy shows healing. For maintenance therapy, 400 mg at bedtime. For parenteral therapy, 300 mg diluted to 20 ml total volume with normal saline solution or other compatible I.V. solution by I.V. push over at least 5 minutes q 6 to 8 hours; or 300 mg diluted in 50 ml D_5W or other compatible I.V. solution by I.V. infusion over 15 to 20 minutes q 6 to 8 hours; or 300 mg I.M. q 6 to 8 hours (no dilution needed). To increase dosage, give 300-mg doses more frequently to maximum of 2,400 mg daily, p.r.n. Or, 900 mg/day (37.5 mg/hour) I.V. diluted in 100 to 1,000 ml of compatible solution by continuous I.V. infusion.
➤ **Active benign gastric ulceration**
Adults: 800 mg P.O. at bedtime or 300 mg P.O. q.i.d. (with meals and at bedtime) for up to 8 weeks.
➤ **Pathologic hypersecretory conditions, such as Zollinger-Ellison syndrome, systemic mastocytosis, and multiple endocrine adenomas**
Adults and children age 16 and older: 300 mg P.O. q.i.d. with meals and at bedtime; adjusted to patient needs. Maximum oral amount, 2,400 mg daily.

For parenteral therapy, 300 mg diluted to 20 ml with normal saline solution or other compatible I.V. solution by I.V. push over at least 5 minutes q 6 to 8 hours; or 300 mg diluted in 50 ml D_5W or other compatible I.V. solution by I.V. infusion over 15 to 20 minutes q 6 to 8 hours. Increase parenteral dosage by giving 300-mg doses more frequently to maximum of 2,400 mg daily, p.r.n.
➤ **Gastroesophageal reflux disease**
Adults: 800 mg P.O. b.i.d. or 400 mg q.i.d. before meals and at bedtime for up to 12 weeks.
Adjust-a-dose: In patients with renal impairment, decrease dosage to 300 mg P.O. or I.V. q 12 hours, increasing frequency to q 8 hours with caution. A renally impaired patient who also has liver dysfunction may require even further dose reduction.
➤ **Heartburn**
Adults: 200 mg Tagamet HB P.O. with water as symptoms occur, or as directed, up to b.i.d. For prevention, 200 mg right be-

fore or up to 30 minutes before eating food or drinking beverages that cause heartburn. Maximum, 400 mg daily. Drug shouldn't be taken daily for longer than 2 weeks.

I.V. ADMINISTRATION

- Drug is commonly added to total parenteral nutrition solutions, with or without fat emulsions.
- Dilute I.V. solutions with normal saline solution, D_5W, dextrose 10% in water (and combinations of these), lactated Ringer solution, or 5% sodium bicarbonate injection.
- For direct injection, give over 5 minutes. Rapid I.V. injection may result in arrhythmias and hypotension.
- For intermittent infusion, give drug over at least 30 minutes to minimize risk of adverse cardiac effects.
- For continuous infusion, if giving a total volume of 250 ml over 24 hours or less, use an infusion pump.

INCOMPATIBILITIES

Allopurinol, amphotericin B, barbiturates, cefazolin, cefepime, chlorpromazine, combination atropine sulfate and pentobarbital sodium, indomethacin sodium trihydrate, pentobarbital sodium, secobarbital, warfarin. Don't dilute with sterile water for injection.

ACTION

Competitively inhibits action of histamine on the H_2 receptor sites of parietal cells, decreasing gastric acid secretion.

Route	Onset	Peak	Duration
P.O.	Unknown	45–90 min	4–5 hr
I.V.	Unknown	Immediate	Unknown
I.M.	Unknown	Unknown	Unknown

Half-life: 2 hours.

ADVERSE REACTIONS

CNS: confusion, dizziness, hallucinations, headache, peripheral neuropathy, somnolence.
GI: mild and transient diarrhea.
GU: impotence.
Musculoskeletal: arthralgia, muscle pain.
Other: mild gynecomastia if used longer than 1 month, hypersensitivity reactions.

INTERACTIONS

Drug-drug. *Antacids:* May interfere with cimetidine absorption. Separate doses by at least 1 hour, if possible.
Carmustine: May enhance the bone marrow suppression effects of carmustine. Avoid using together.
Digoxin, fluconazole, indomethacin, iron salts, ketoconazole, tetracycline: May decrease drug absorption. Separate doses by at least 2 hours.
Fosphenytoin, phenytoin, some benzodiazepines, theophylline, warfarin: May inhibit hepatic microsomal enzyme metabolism of these drugs. Monitor drug level.
I.V. lidocaine: May decrease clearance of lidocaine, increasing the risk of toxicity. Consider using a different H_2 antagonist, if possible. Monitor lidocaine level closely.
Metoprolol, propranolol, timolol: May increase the effects of beta-blocker. Consider another H_2 agonist or decrease the dose of beta-blocker.
Procainamide: May increase procainamide level. Avoid this combination, if possible. Monitor procainamide level closely and adjust the dose as necessary.
Drug-herb. *Guarana:* May increase caffeine level or prolong caffeine half-life. Monitor patient.
Pennyroyal: May change rate at which herb's toxic metabolites form. Monitor patient.
Yerba maté: May decrease clearance of herb's methylxanthines and cause toxicity. Discourage use together.
Drug-lifestyle. *Alcohol use:* May increase blood alcohol level. Discourage use together.
Smoking: May decrease drug's ability to inhibit nocturnal gastric secretion. Urge patient to quit smoking.

EFFECTS ON LAB TEST RESULTS

- May increase ALT, AST, and creatinine levels.
- May antagonize pentagastrin's effect during gastric acid secretion tests. May cause false-negative results in skin tests using allergen extracts. May impair interpretation of Hemoccult and Gastroccult test results on gastric content aspirate because of FD&C blue dye number 2 used in tablets.

CONTRAINDICATIONS & CAUTIONS

- Contraindicated in patients hypersensitive to drug.
- Use cautiously in elderly or debilitated patients because they may be more susceptible to drug-induced confusion.

NURSING CONSIDERATIONS

- Assess patient for abdominal pain. Note blood in emesis, stool, or gastric aspirate.
- Identify tablet strength when obtaining a drug history.
- Schedule dose at end of hemodialysis treatment because hemodialysis reduces drug levels. Adjust dosage for patients with renal impairment.
- Wait at least 15 minutes after giving tablet before drawing sample for Hemoccult or Gastroccult test, and follow test manufacturer's instructions closely.
- I.M. injection may be given undiluted.
- Treatment of gastric ulcer isn't as effective as treatment of duodenal ulcer.
- ***Look alike–sound alike:*** Don't confuse cimetidine with simethicone.

PATIENT TEACHING

- Remind patient taking drug once daily to take it at bedtime and to take multiple daily doses with meals.
- Instruct patient taking Tagamet HB not to exceed recommended dosage and not to take daily for longer than 14 days.
- Warn patient receiving drug I.M. that injection may be painful.
- Urge patient to avoid cigarette smoking because it may increase gastric acid secretion and worsen disease.
- Advise patient to report abdominal pain and blood in stools or emesis.

esomeprazole magnesium

Nexium

esomeprazole sodium

Nexium I.V.

Pharmacologic class: proton pump inhibitor
Pregnancy risk category B

AVAILABLE FORMS

esomeprazole magnesium
Capsules (delayed-release): 20 mg, 40 mg

esomeprazole sodium
Powder for injection: 20 mg, 40 mg single-use vials

INDICATIONS & DOSAGES

➤ **Gastroesophageal reflux disease (GERD); to heal erosive esophagitis**
Adults: 20 or 40 mg P.O. daily for 4 to 8 weeks. Maintenance dose for healing erosive esophagitis is 20 mg P.O. for up to 6 months.
Children and adolescents age 12 to 17: For GERD only, 20 or 40 mg P.O. once daily for up to 8 weeks.

➤ **Symptomatic GERD**
Adults: 20 mg P.O. daily for 4 weeks. If symptoms are unresolved, may continue treatment for 4 more weeks.

➤ **Short-term therapy (up to 10 days) of GERD in patients with a history of erosive esophagitis who are unable to take drug orally.**
Adult: Reconstitute 20 or 40 mg with 5 ml of D_5W, normal saline solution, or lactated Ringer injection and give by I.V. bolus over 3 minutes. Or, further dilute to a total volume of 50 ml and give I.V. over 10 to 30 minutes. Switch patient to oral therapy as soon as he can tolerate it.

➤ **To reduce the risk of gastric ulcers in patients receiving continuous NSAID therapy**
Adults: 20 or 40 mg P.O. once daily for up to 6 months.

✱ ***NEW INDICATION:*** **Long-term treatment of pathological hypersecretory conditions, including Zollinger-Ellison syndrome**
Adults: 40 mg P.O. b.i.d. Adjust dosage based on patient response.

➤ **To eliminate *Helicobacter pylori***
Adults: 40 mg esomeprazole magnesium P.O. daily, 1,000 mg amoxicillin P.O. b.i.d., and 500 mg clarithromycin P.O. b.i.d., given together for 10 days to reduce duodenal ulcer recurrence.
Adjust-a-dose: For patient with severe hepatic failure, maximum daily dose is 20 mg.

I.V. ADMINISTRATION

- Flush I.V. line with D_5W, normal saline solution, or lactated Ringer injection before and after administration.

- Use reconstituted solution within 12 hours.
- Use admixture diluted with D_5W within 6 hours.
- If diluted with normal saline solution or lactated Ringer injection, use within 12 hours
- Store reconstituted solution and admixture at room temperature.

INCOMPATIBILITIES
Other I.V. drugs.

ACTION
Reduces gastric acid secretion and decreases gastric acidity.

Route	Onset	Peak	Duration
P.O.	Unknown	1½ hr	13–17 hr

Half-life: 1 to 1½ hours.

ADVERSE REACTIONS
CNS: headache.
GI: abdominal pain, constipation, diarrhea, dry mouth, flatulence, nausea, vomiting.

INTERACTIONS
Drug-drug. *Amoxicillin, clarithromycin:* May increase levels of esomeprazole. Monitor patient for toxicity.
Diazepam: May decrease clearance of diazepam. Monitor patient for diazepam toxicity.
Drugs metabolized by CYP2C19: May alter clearance of esomeprazole, especially in elderly patients or patients with hepatic insufficiency. Monitor patient for toxicity.
Warfarin: May prolong PT and INR, causing abnormal bleeding. Monitor the patient and his PT and INR.
Drug-food. *Any food:* May reduce drug level. Advise patient to take drug 1 hour before food.

EFFECTS ON LAB TEST RESULTS
None reported.

CONTRAINDICATIONS & CAUTIONS
- Contraindicated in patients hypersensitive to drug or components of esomeprazole or omeprazole (a drug similar to this one).
- Use cautiously in patients with hepatic insufficiency and in pregnant or breastfeeding women. It's unknown if this drug appears in breast milk, but omeprazole does.
- Patients receiving continuous NSAID therapy who are at increased risk for gastric ulcers include those age 60 and older or those with a history of gastric ulcers.

NURSING CONSIDERATIONS
- Give drug at least 1 hour before meals. If patient has difficulty swallowing the capsule, contents of the capsule can be emptied and mixed with 1 tablespoon of applesauce and swallowed (without chewing the enteric-coated pellets).
- If giving via nasogastric (NG) tube, open capsule and empty the granules into a 60-ml syringe. Mix with 50 ml of water. Replace the plunger and shake vigorously for 15 seconds. Flush NG tube with additional water after use. Don't give if pellets have dissolved or disintegrated.
- Antacids can be used while taking drug, unless otherwise directed by prescriber.
- Monitor patient for rash or signs and symptoms of hypersensitivity. Monitor GI symptoms for improvement or worsening. Monitor liver function tests, especially in patients with preexisting hepatic disease.
- Long-term therapy may cause atrophic gastritis.

PATIENT TEACHING
- Instruct patient to take drug exactly as prescribed.
- Tell patient to take drug at least 1 hour before a meal.
- Advise patient that antacids can be used while taking drug unless otherwise directed by prescriber.
- Warn patient not to chew or crush drug pellets because this inactivates the drug.
- If patient has difficulty swallowing capsule, tell him to mix contents of capsule with 1 tablespoon of soft applesauce and swallow immediately.
- Advise patient to store capsules at room temperature in a tight container.
- Tell patient to inform prescriber of worsening signs and symptoms or pain.

• Instruct patient to alert prescriber if rash or other signs and symptoms of allergy occur.

famotidine

Pepcid🖉, Pepcid AC◇, Pepcidine‡

Pharmacologic class: H_2 receptor antagonist
Pregnancy risk category B

AVAILABLE FORMS

Gelcaps: 10 mg◇
Injection: 10 mg/ml
Powder for oral suspension: 40 mg/5 ml after reconstitution
Premixed injection: 20 mg/50 ml in normal saline solution
Tablets: 10 mg◇, 20 mg◇, 40 mg
Tablets (chewable): 10 mg◇

INDICATIONS & DOSAGES

➤ **Short-term treatment for duodenal ulcer**
Adults: For acute therapy, 40 mg P.O. once daily at bedtime or 20 mg P.O. b.i.d. Healing usually occurs within 4 weeks. For maintenance therapy, 20 mg P.O. once daily at bedtime.

➤ **Short-term treatment for benign gastric ulcer**
Adults: 40 mg P.O. daily at bedtime for 8 weeks.
Children ages 1 to 16: 0.5 mg/kg/day P.O. at at bedtime or divided b.i.d., up to 40 mg daily.

➤ **Pathologic hypersecretory conditions (such as Zollinger-Ellison syndrome)**
Adults: 20 mg P.O. q 6 hours, up to 160 mg q 6 hours.

➤ **Hospitalized patients who can't take oral drug or who have intractable ulcers or hypersecretory conditions**
Adults: 20 mg I.V. q 12 hours.

➤ **Gastroesophageal reflux disease (GERD)**
Adults: 20 mg P.O. b.i.d. for up to 6 weeks. For esophagitis caused by GERD, 20 to 40 mg b.i.d. for up to 12 weeks.
Children ages 1 to 16: 1 mg/kg/day P.O. divided twice daily up to 40 mg b.i.d.

➤ **To prevent or treat heartburn**
Adults: 10 mg Pepcid AC P.O. 1 hour before meals to prevent symptoms, or 10 mg Pepcid AC P.O. with water when symptoms occur. Maximum daily dose is 20 mg. Drug shouldn't be taken daily for longer than 2 weeks.

Adjust-a-dose: For patients with creatinine clearance below 50 ml/minute, give half the dose, or increase dosing interval to q 36 to 48 hours.

I.V. ADMINISTRATION

• Compatible solutions include sterile water for injection, normal saline solution for injection, D_5W or dextrose 10% in water for injection, 5% sodium bicarbonate injection, and lactated Ringer injection. Drug also can be added to total parenteral nutrition solutions.
• For direct injection, dilute 2 ml (20 mg) with compatible solution to a total volume of either 5 or 10 ml.
• Inject over at least 2 minutes.
• For intermittent infusion, dilute 20 mg (2 ml) in 100-ml compatible solution. The premixed 50-ml solution doesn't need further dilution.
• Infuse over 15 to 30 minutes.
• After dilution, solution is stable 48 hours at 36° to 46° F (2° to 8° C).

INCOMPATIBILITIES

Amphotericin B cholesterol complex, azithromycin, cefepime, piperacillin with tazobactam.

ACTION

Competitively inhibits action of histamine on the H_2 at receptor sites of parietal cells, decreasing gastric acid secretion.

Route	Onset	Peak	Duration
P.O.	1 hr	1–3 hr	12 hr
I.V.	1 hr	1–4 hr	12 hr

Half-life: 2½ to 3½ hours.

ADVERSE REACTIONS

CNS: *headache,* dizziness, fever, malaise, paresthesia, vertigo.
CV: flushing, palpitations.
EENT: orbital edema, tinnitus.

GI: anorexia, constipation, diarrhea, dry mouth, taste perversion.
Musculoskeletal: bone and muscle pain.
Skin: acne, dry skin.
Other: transient irritation at I.V. site.

INTERACTIONS

None significant.

EFFECTS ON LAB TEST RESULTS

- May increase BUN, creatinine, and liver enzyme levels.
- May cause false-negative results in skin tests using allergen extracts. May antagonize pentagastrin in gastric acid secretion tests.

CONTRAINDICATIONS & CAUTIONS

- Contraindicated in patients hypersensitive to drug.

NURSING CONSIDERATIONS

- Assess patient for abdominal pain. Look for blood in emesis, stool, or gastric aspirate.
- Oral suspension must be reconstituted and shaken before use.
- Store reconstituted oral suspension below 86° F (30° C). Discard after 30 days.

PATIENT TEACHING

- Instruct patient in proper use of OTC product, if appropriate.
- Warn patient with phenylketonuria that Pepcid AC chewable tablets contain phenylalanine.
- Tell patient to take prescription drug with a snack, if desired.
- Remind patient that prescription drug is most effective if taken at bedtime. Tell patient taking 20 mg twice daily to take one dose at bedtime.
- Advise patient to limit use of prescription drug to no longer than 8 weeks, unless ordered by prescriber, and OTC drug to no longer than 2 weeks.
- With prescriber's knowledge, let patient take antacids together, especially at beginning of therapy when pain is severe.
- Urge patient to avoid cigarette smoking because it may increase gastric acid secretion and worsen disease.
- Advise patient to report abdominal pain or blood in stools or vomit.

lansoprazole

Prevacid, Prevacid I.V., Prevacid SoluTab

Pharmacologic class: proton pump inhibitor
Pregnancy risk category B

AVAILABLE FORMS

Capsules (delayed-release): 15 mg, 30 mg
Oral suspension (delayed-release): 15 mg/packet, 30 mg/packet
Orally disintegrating tablet (ODT)(delayed-release): 15 mg, 30 mg
Powder for injection: 30-mg single-use vial

INDICATIONS & DOSAGES

➤ **Short-term treatment of active duodenal ulcer**
Adults: 15 mg P.O. daily before eating for 4 weeks.

➤ **Maintenance of healed duodenal ulcers**
Adults: 15 mg P.O. daily.

➤ **Short-term treatment of active benign gastric ulcer**
Adults: 30 mg P.O. once daily for up to 8 weeks.

➤ **Short-term I.V. therapy for erosive esophagitis when patient can't take P.O. drug**
Adults: 30 mg I.V. daily over 30 minutes for up to 7 days. As soon as patient can take drug orally, switch to P.O. form and continue for 6 to 8 weeks.

➤ **Short-term treatment of erosive esophagitis**
Adults: 30 mg P.O. daily before eating for up to 8 weeks. If healing doesn't occur, 8 more weeks of therapy may be given. Maintenance dosage for healing is 15 mg P.O. daily.
Children ages 12 to 17: 30 mg P.O. once daily for up to 8 weeks.
Children ages 1 to 11 who weigh more than 30 kg (66 lb): 30 mg P.O. once daily for up to 12 weeks. Increase dosage up to 30 mg b.i.d. in patients who remain symptomatic after 2 weeks.
Children ages 1 to 1, who weigh 30 kg or less: 15 mg P.O. once daily for up to 12 weeks. Increase dosage up to 30 mg

b.i.d. in patients who remain symptomatic after 2 weeks.

➤ **Long-term treatment of pathologic hypersecretory conditions, including Zollinger-Ellison syndrome**

Adults: Initially, 60 mg P.O. once daily. Increase dosage, p.r.n. Give daily amounts above 120 mg in evenly divided doses.

➤ ***Helicobacter pylori* eradication to reduce risk of duodenal ulcer recurrence**

Adults: For patients receiving dual therapy, 30 mg P.O. lansoprazole with 1 g P.O. amoxicillin, each given t.i.d. for 14 days. For patients receiving triple therapy, 30 mg P.O. lansoprazole with 1 g P.O. amoxicillin and 500 mg P.O. clarithromycin, all given b.i.d. for 10 to 14 days.

➤ **Short-term treatment of symptomatic gastroesophageal reflux disease (GERD)**

Adults: 15 mg P.O. once daily for up to 8 weeks.

Children ages 12 to 17: 15 mg P.O. once daily for up to 8 weeks.

Children ages 1 to 11 who weigh more than 30 kg (66 lb): 30 mg P.O. once daily for up to 12 weeks. Dosage can be increased up to 30 mg b.i.d. in patients who remain symptomatic after 2 weeks.

Children ages 1 to 11, who weigh 30 kg or less: 15 mg P.O. once daily for up to 12 weeks. Dosage can be increased up to 30 mg b.i.d in patients who remain symptomatic after 2 weeks.

➤ **NSAID-related ulcer in patients who take NSAIDs**

Adults: 30 mg P.O. daily for 8 weeks.

➤ **To reduce risk of NSAID-related ulcer in patients with history of gastric ulcer who need NSAIDs**

Adults: 15 mg P.O. daily for up to 12 weeks.

I.V. ADMINISTRATION

- Reconstitute with 5 ml sterile water for injection only.
- Mix gently until powder is dissolved.
- Further dilute with 50 ml normal saline solution, lactated Ringer injection or D_5W
- Flush the I.V. line with normal saline solution, lactated Ringer injection, or D_5W before giving infusion.
- Infuse over 30 minutes using the 1.2 micron inline filter provided with drug.
- The inline filter will remove any precipitate that forms when reconstituted solution comes in contact with I.V. solutions.
- Solutions mixed with normal saline or lactated Ringer are stable at room temperature for 24 hours. Solutions mixed with D_5W are stable for 12 hours.
- Protect from light.

INCOMPATIBILITIES

Other I.V. drugs.

ACTION

Inhibits activity of proton pump and binds to hydrogen-potassium adenosine triphosphatase, located at secretory surface of gastric parietal cells, to block secretion of gastric acid.

Route	Onset	Peak	Duration
P.O.	1–3 hr	Unknown	24 hr
I.V.	Unknown	Unknown	24 hr

Half-life: Less than 2 hours.

ADVERSE REACTIONS

GI: abdominal pain, diarrhea, nausea.

INTERACTIONS

Drug-drug. *Ampicillin esters, digoxin, iron salts, ketoconazole:* May inhibit absorption of these drugs. Monitor patient closely.

Atazanavir: May reduce GI absorption of atazanavir, reducing antiviral activity. Don't use together.

Clarithromycin: May increase lansoprazole levels and adverse effects. Monitor patient.

Sucralfate: May cause delayed lansoprazole absorption. Give lansoprazole at least 30 minutes before sucralfate.

Theophylline: May mildly increase theophylline clearance. Adjust theophylline dosage when lansoprazole is started or stopped. Use together cautiously.

Drug-herb. *Male fern:* May inactivate herb. Discourage use together.

St. John's wort: May increase risk of sun sensitivity. Advise patient to avoid excessive sunlight exposure.

Drug-food. *Food:* May decrease rate and extent of GI absorption. Advise patient to take before meals.

EFFECTS ON LAB TEST RESULTS

None reported.

CONTRAINDICATIONS & CAUTIONS

- Contraindicated in patients hypersensitive to drug.

NURSING CONSIDERATIONS

- Patients with severe liver disease may need dosage adjustment, but don't adjust dosage for elderly patients or those with renal insufficiency.
- The contents of capsule can be mixed with 40 ml of apple juice in a syringe and given within 3 to 5 minutes via a nasogastric (NG) tube. Flush with additional apple juice to give entire dose and maintain patency of the tube.
- To give orally disintegrating tablets using an oral syringe, dissolve a 15-mg tablet in 4 ml water or a 30-mg tablet in 10 ml water and give within 15 minutes. Refill the syringe with about 2 ml (15-mg tablet) or 5 ml (30-mg tablet) of water, shake gently, and give any remaining contents.
- To give ODTs through an NG tube 8 French or larger, dissolve a 15-mg tablet in 4 ml water or a 30-mg tablet in 10 ml water and give within 15 minutes. Refill the syringe with about 5 ml of water, shake gently, and flush the NG tube.
- Orally disintegrating tablets contain 2.5 mg phenylalanine/15-mg tablet and 5.1 mg phenylalanine/30-mg tablet.
- Just because symptoms respond to therapy doesn't rule out gastric malignancy.
- It's unknown if drug appears in breast milk. Breast-feeding women should either stop breast-feeding or stop drug.
- ***Look alike–sound alike:*** Don't confuse Prevacid with Pepcid, Prilosec, or Prevpac.

PATIENT TEACHING

- For best effect, instruct patient to take drug no more than 30 minutes before eating.
- Tell patient he may mix the capsule's contents with a small amount (about 2 ounces) of apple, cranberry, grape, orange, pineapple, prune, tomato, or vegetable juice. The patient must drink the mixture within 30 minutes. To ensure complete delivery of the dose, the patient should fill the glass two or more times with juice and swallow the contents immediately.
- Contents of capsule can be mixed with 1 tablespoon of applesauce, Ensure, pudding, cottage cheese, yogurt, or strained pears and swallowed immediately. The granules shouldn't be chewed or crushed.
- For the oral suspension, instruct patient to empty packet contents into 30 ml of water, stir well, and drink immediately. Tell him not to crush or chew the granules and not to take with other liquids or food. If any material remains after drinking, tell him to add more water, stir, and drink immediately.
- Tell patient taking ODTs to allow tablet to dissolve on tongue until all particles can be swallowed.

misoprostol

Cytotec

Pharmacologic class: prostaglandin E_1 analogue
Pregnancy risk category X

AVAILABLE FORMS

Tablets: 100 mcg, 200 mcg

INDICATIONS & DOSAGES

➤ **To prevent NSAID-induced gastric ulcer in elderly or debilitated patients at high risk for complications from gastric ulcer and in patients with history of NSAID-induced ulcer**

Adults: 200 mcg P.O. q.i.d. with food; if not tolerated, decrease to 100 mcg P.O. q.i.d. Give dosage for duration of NSAID therapy. Give last dose at bedtime.

ACTION

A synthetic prostaglandin E_1 analogue that replaces gastric prostaglandins depleted by NSAID therapy, decreases basal and stimulated gastric acid secretion, and increases gastric mucus and bicarbonate production.

Route	Onset	Peak	Duration
P.O.	30 min	60–90 min	3 hr

Half-life: 20 to 40 minutes.

ADVERSE REACTIONS
CNS: headache.
GI: *abdominal pain, diarrhea,* constipation, dyspepsia, flatulence, nausea, vomiting.
GU: cramps, dysmenorrhea, hypermenorrhea, menstrual disorders, postmenopausal vaginal bleeding, spotting.

INTERACTIONS
Drug-food. *Any food:* May decrease absorption rate of drug. However, manufacturer recommends that patient take drug with food.

EFFECTS ON LAB TEST RESULTS
None reported.

CONTRAINDICATIONS & CAUTIONS
- Contraindicated in those allergic to prostaglandins. Drug shouldn't be taken by pregnant women to reduce the risk of NSAID-induced ulcers.
- Use with caution in patients with inflammatory bowel disease.

NURSING CONSIDERATIONS
- ***Alert:*** Take special precautions to prevent use of drug during pregnancy. Uterine rupture is linked to certain risk factors, including later trimester pregnancies, higher doses of the drug, prior cesarean delivery or uterine surgery, or five or more previous pregnancies. Make sure woman understands dangers of drug to herself and her fetus and that she receives both oral and written warnings about these dangers. Also, make sure she can comply with effective contraception and that the result of a pregnancy test performed within 2 weeks of starting therapy is negative. Don't resume therapy until woman is no longer breast-feeding.
- Drug causes modest decrease in basal pepsin secretion.
- ***Look alike–sound alike:*** Don't confuse misoprostol with mifepristone.

PATIENT TEACHING
- Instruct patient not to share drug.
- Remind pregnant woman that drug may cause miscarriage, often with potentially life-threatening bleeding.
- Advise woman not to begin therapy until second or third day of next normal menstrual period.
- Advise patient to take drug as prescribed for duration of NSAID therapy.
- Tell patient that diarrhea usually occurs early in the course of therapy and is usually self-limiting. Taking drug with food helps minimize the diarrhea.

---

omeprazole
Losec†‡, Prilosec🖉, Zegerid

omeprazole magnesium
Prilosec OTC ◊

Pharmacologic class: proton pump inhibitor
Pregnancy risk category C

AVAILABLE FORMS
Capsules (delayed-release): 10 mg, 20 mg, 40 mg
Powder for oral suspension: 20 mg/packet, 40 mg/packet
Tablets (delayed-release): 20 mg ◊

INDICATIONS & DOSAGES
➤ **Symptomatic gastroesophageal reflux disease (GERD) without esophageal lesions**
Adults: 20 mg P.O., as delayed-release or oral suspension, daily for 4 weeks for patients who respond poorly to customary medical treatment, usually including an adequate course of H_2-receptor antagonists.
➤ **Erosive esophagitis and accompanying symptoms caused by GERD**
Adults: 20 mg P.O. daily for 4 to 8 weeks.
➤ **Maintenance of healing erosive esophagitis**
Adults: 20 mg P.O., as delayed-release or oral suspension, daily.
➤ **Pathologic hypersecretory conditions (such as Zollinger-Ellison syndrome)**
Adults: Initially, 60 mg P.O. daily; adjust dosage based on patient response. If daily dose exceeds 80 mg, give in divided doses. Doses up to 120 mg t.i.d. have been given. Continue therapy as long as clinically indicated.

➤ **Duodenal ulcer (short-term treatment)**
Adults: 20 mg P.O., as delayed-release or oral suspension, daily for 4 to 8 weeks.
➤ ***Helicobacter pylori* infection and duodenal ulcer disease, to eradicate *H. pylori* with clarithromycin (dual therapy)**
Adults: 40 mg P.O. q morning with clarithromycin 500 mg P.O. t.i.d. for 14 days. For patients with an ulcer at start of therapy, give another 14 days of omeprazole 20 mg P.O. once daily.
➤ ***H. pylori* infection and duodenal ulcer disease, to eradicate *H. pylori* with clarithromycin and amoxicillin (triple therapy)**
Adults: 20 mg P.O. with clarithromycin 500 mg P.O. and amoxicillin 1,000 mg P.O., each given b.i.d. for 10 days. For patients with an ulcer at start of therapy, give another 18 days of omeprazole 20 mg P.O. once daily.
➤ **Short-term treatment of active benign gastric ulcer**
Adults: 40 mg P.O. once daily for 4 to 8 weeks.
➤ **Frequent heartburn (2 or more days a week)**
Adults: 20 mg P.O. Prilosec OTC once daily before breakfast for 14 days. May repeat the 14-day course q 4 months.

ACTION

Inhibits activity of acid (proton) pump and binds to hydrogen-potassium adenosine triphosphatase at secretory surface of gastric parietal cells to block formation of gastric acid.

Route	Onset	Peak	Duration
P.O.	1 hr	30 min–2 hr	< 3 days

Half-life: 30 to 60 minutes.

ADVERSE REACTIONS

CNS: asthenia, dizziness, headache.
GI: abdominal pain, constipation, diarrhea, flatulence, nausea, vomiting.
Musculoskeletal: back pain.
Respiratory: cough, upper respiratory tract infection.
Skin: rash.

INTERACTIONS

Drug-drug. *Ampicillin esters, iron derivatives, ketoconazole:* May cause poor bioavailability of these drugs because they need a low gastric pH for optimal absorption. Avoid using together.
Diazepam, fosphenytoin, phenytoin, warfarin: May decrease hepatic clearance, possibly leading to increased levels of these drugs. Monitor drug levels.
Drug-herb. *Ginkgo biloba:* May decrease therapeutic effects of drug. Discourage use together.
Male fern: May inactivate herb. Discourage use together.
Pennyroyal: May change rate at which herb's toxic metabolites form. Ask patient about the use of herb, and discourage use together.
St. John's wort: May increase risk of sun sensitivity. Advise patient to avoid excessive sunlight exposure.

EFFECTS ON LAB TEST RESULTS

None reported.

CONTRAINDICATIONS & CAUTIONS

- Contraindicated in patients hypersensitive to drug or its components.
- Zegerid is contraindicated in patients with metabolic alkalosis and hypocalcemia.
- Use cautiously in patients with Bartter syndrome, hypokalemia, and respiratory alkalosis.
- Long-term administration of bicarbonate with calcium or milk can cause milk-alkali syndrome.

NURSING CONSIDERATIONS

- Dosage adjustments may be necessary in Asians and patients with hepatic impairment.
- Drug increases its own bioavailability with repeated doses. Drug is unstable in gastric acid; less drug is lost to hydrolysis because drug increases gastric pH.
- Zegerid contains 460 mg sodium per dose in the form of sodium bicarbonate.
- ***Look alike–sound alike:*** Don't confuse Prilosec with Prozac, Prilocaine, or Prinivil.
- Gastrin level rises in most patients during the first 2 weeks of therapy.

PATIENT TEACHING

- Tell patient to swallow tablets or capsules whole and not to open, crush, or chew them.
- Warn patients that Zegerid contains 460 mg sodium bicarbonate per dose. Those following a sodium-restricted diet should be cautious.
- Tell patient to empty contents of Zegerid packet into a small cup containing 2 tablespoons of water. Instruct him not to use other liquids or foods. Stir contents and drink immediately. Refill cup with water and drink.
- Instruct patient to take drug 30 minutes before meals. Zegerid powder for oral suspension should be taken on an empty stomach at least 1 hour before a meal.
- Caution patient to avoid hazardous activities if he gets dizzy.
- Advise patient that Prilosec OTC isn't intended to treat infrequent heartburn (one episode of heartburn a week or less), or for those who want immediate relief of heartburn.
- Inform patient that Prilosec OTC may take 1 to 4 days for full effect, although some patients may get complete relief of symptoms within 24 hours.

pantoprazole sodium

Protonix, Protonix I.V.

Pharmacologic class: proton pump inhibitor
Pregnancy risk category B

AVAILABLE FORMS

Injection: 40 mg per vial
Tablet (delayed-release): 20 mg, 40 mg

INDICATIONS & DOSAGES

➤ **Erosive esophagitis with gastroesophageal reflux disease (GERD)**
Adults: 40 mg P.O. once daily for up to 8 weeks. For patients who haven't healed after 8 weeks of treatment, another 8-week course may be considered.

➤ **Short-term treatment of GERD in patients who can't take delayed-release tablets orally**
Adults: 40 mg I.V. daily for 7 to 10 days.

➤ **Short-term treatment of GERD linked to history of erosive esophagitis**
Adults: 40 mg I.V. once daily for 7 to 10 days. Switch to P.O. form as soon as patient is able to take orally.

➤ **Long-term maintenance of healing erosive esophagitis and reduction in relapse rates of daytime and nighttime heartburn symptoms in patients with GERD**
Adults: 40 mg P.O. once daily.

➤ **Short-term treatment of pathologic hypersecretion caused by Zollinger-Ellison syndrome or other neoplastic conditions**
Adults: Individualize dosage. Usual dose is 80 mg I.V. q 12 hours for no more than 6 days. For those needing a higher dose, 80 mg q 8 hours is expected to maintain acid output below 10 mEq/hour. Maximum daily dose is 240 mg/day.

➤ **Long-term treatment of pathologic hypersecretory conditions, including Zollinger-Ellison syndrome**
Adults: Individualize dosage. Usual starting dose is 40 mg P.O. b.i.d. Adjust dose to a maximum of 240 mg/day. Stop I.V. drug when P.O. drug is warranted.

I.V. ADMINISTRATION

- Safety and effectiveness of the I.V. form to start therapy for GERD are unknown.
- Reconstitute each vial with 10 ml of normal saline solution.
- Compatible diluents for infusion include normal saline solution, D_5W, or lactated Ringer solution for injection.
- For patients with GERD, further dilute with 100 ml of diluent to yield 0.4 mg/ml.
- For patients with hypersecretion, combine 2 reconstituted vials and further dilute with 80 ml of diluent to a total volume of 100 ml, to yield 0.8 mg/ml.
- Infuse diluted solutions over 15 minutes at a rate of about 7 ml/minute.
- For a 2-minute infusion, give the reconstituted vials (final yield of about 4 mg/ml) over at least 2 minutes.
- The reconstituted solution may be stored for up to 2 hours and the diluted solutions for up to 22 hours at room temperature.

INCOMPATIBILITIES
Midazolam, zinc-containing products or solutions. Don't give another infusion simultaneously through the same line.

ACTION
Inhibits proton pump activity by binding to hydrogen-potassium adenosine triphosphatase, located at secretory surface of gastric parietal cells, to suppress gastric acid secretion.

Route	Onset	Peak	Duration
P.O.	Unknown	2½ hr	> 24 hr
I.V.	15–30 min	Unknown	24 hr

Half-life: 1 hour.

ADVERSE REACTIONS
CNS: anxiety, asthenia, dizziness, headache, insomnia, migraine.
CV: chest pain.
EENT: pharyngitis, rhinitis, sinusitis.
GI: abdominal pain, constipation, diarrhea, dyspepsia, eructation, flatulence, gastroenteritis, GI disorder, nausea, rectal disorder, vomiting.
GU: urinary frequency, UTI.
Metabolic: hyperglycemia, hyperlipemia.
Musculoskeletal: arthralgia, back pain, hypertonia, neck pain.
Respiratory: bronchitis, dyspnea, increased cough, upper respiratory tract infection.
Skin: rash.
Other: flulike syndrome, infection, pain.

INTERACTIONS
Drug-drug. *Ampicillin esters, iron salts, ketoconazole:* May decrease absorption of these drugs. Monitor patient closely and separate doses.
Drug-herb. *St. John's wort:* May increase risk of sunburn. Advise patient to avoid excessive sunlight exposure.
Drug-lifestyle. *Sunlight:* May increase risk of sunburn. Advise patient to avoid excessive sunlight exposure.

EFFECTS ON LAB TEST RESULTS
- May increase glucose and lipid levels.
- May increase liver function test result values.

CONTRAINDICATIONS & CAUTIONS
- Contraindicated in patients hypersensitive to any component of the formulation.

NURSING CONSIDERATIONS
- ***Look alike–sound alike:*** Don't confuse Protonix with Prilosec, Prozac, or Prevacid.
- Drug can be given without regard to meals.
- Symptomatic response to therapy doesn't preclude the presence of gastric malignancy.

PATIENT TEACHING
- Instruct patient to take exactly as prescribed and at about the same time every day.
- Advise patient that drug can be taken without regard to meals.
- Tell patient to swallow tablet whole and not to crush, split, or chew it.
- Tell patient that antacids don't affect drug absorption.

rabeprazole sodium
Aciphex

Pharmacologic class: proton pump inhibitor
Pregnancy risk category B

AVAILABLE FORMS
Tablets (delayed-release): 20 mg

INDICATIONS & DOSAGES
➤ **Healing of erosive or ulcerative gastroesophageal reflux disease (GERD)**
Adults: 20 mg P.O. daily for 4 to 8 weeks. Additional 8-week course may be considered, if needed.
➤ **Maintenance of healing of erosive or ulcerative GERD**
Adults: 20 mg P.O. daily.
➤ **Healing of duodenal ulcers**
Adults: 20 mg P.O. daily after morning meal for up to 4 weeks.
➤ **Pathologic hypersecretory conditions, including Zollinger-Ellison syndrome**
Adults: 60 mg P.O. daily; may be increased, p.r.n., to 100 mg P.O. daily or 60 mg P.O. b.i.d.

➤ **Symptomatic GERD, including daytime and nighttime heartburn**
Adults: 20 mg P.O. daily for 4 weeks. Additional 4-week course may be considered, if needed.
➤ ***Helicobacter pylori* eradication, to reduce the risk of duodenal ulcer recurrence**
Adults: 20 mg P.O. b.i.d., combined with amoxicillin 1,000 mg P.O. b.i.d. and clarithromycin 500 mg P.O. b.i.d., for 7 days.

ACTION

Blocks proton pump activity and gastric acid secretion by inhibiting gastric hydrogen-potassium adenosine triphosphatase at secretory surface of gastric parietal cells.

Route	Onset	Peak	Duration
P.O.	< 1 hr	2–5 hr	> 24 hr

Half-life: 1 to 2 hours.

ADVERSE REACTIONS

CNS: headache.

INTERACTIONS

Drug-drug. *Clarithromycin:* May increase rabeprazole level. Monitor patient closely.
Cyclosporine: May inhibit cyclosporine metabolism. Use together cautiously.
Digoxin, ketoconazole, other gastric pH-dependent drugs: May decrease or increase drug absorption at increased pH values. Monitor patient closely.
Warfarin: May inhibit warfarin metabolism. Monitor PT and INR.

EFFECTS ON LAB TEST RESULTS

None reported.

CONTRAINDICATIONS & CAUTIONS

- Contraindicated in patients hypersensitive to drug, other benzimidazoles (lansoprazole, omeprazole), or components of these formulations.
- In *H. pylori* eradication, clarithromycin is contraindicated in pregnant women, patients hypersensitive to macrolides, and those taking pimozide; amoxicillin is contraindicated in patients hypersensitive to penicillin.
- Use cautiously in patients with severe hepatic impairment.

NURSING CONSIDERATIONS

- Consider additional courses of therapy if duodenal ulcer or GERD isn't healed after first course of therapy.
- If *H. pylori* eradication is unsuccessful, do susceptibility testing. If patient is resistant to clarithromycin or susceptibility testing isn't possible, expect to start therapy using a different antimicrobial.
- ***Alert:*** Amoxicillin may trigger anaphylaxis in patients with a history of penicillin hypersensitivity.
- Symptomatic response to therapy doesn't preclude presence of gastric malignancy.
- ***Alert:*** Patients treated for *H. pylori* eradication have developed pseudomembranous colitis with nearly all antibiotics, including clarithromycin and amoxicillin. Monitor patient closely.

PATIENT TEACHING

- Explain importance of taking drug exactly as prescribed.
- Advise patient to swallow delayed-release tablets whole and not to crush, chew, or split it.
- Inform patient that drug may be taken without regard to meals.

ranitidine hydrochloride

Apo-Ranitidine†, Zantac*, Zantac-C†, Zantac 75◇, Zantac 150◇, Zantac EFFERdose Tablets, Zantac 150 GELdose, Zantac 300✐, Zantac 300 GELdose

Pharmacologic class: H_2 receptor antagonist
Pregnancy risk category B

AVAILABLE FORMS

Granules (effervescent): 150 mg
Infusion: 1 mg/ml in 50-ml containers
Injection: 25 mg/ml
Syrup: 15 mg/ml*
Tablets: 75 mg◇, 150 mg◇, 300 mg
Tablets (dispersible): 150 mg‡
Tablets (effervescent): 25 mg, 150 mg

INDICATIONS & DOSAGES

➤ Active duodenal and gastric ulcer

Adults: 150 mg P.O. b.i.d. or 300 mg daily at bedtime. Or, 50 mg I.V. or I.M. q 6 to 8 hours. Maximum daily I.V. dose, 400 mg. Or, 150 mg by continuous infusion at 6.25 mg/hour over 24 hours.

Children ages 1 month to 16 years: For duodenal and gastric ulcers only, 2 to 4 mg/kg P.O. b.i.d., up to 300 mg/day.

➤ Maintenance therapy for duodenal or gastric ulcer

Adults: 150 mg P.O. at bedtime.

Children ages 1 month to 16 years: 2 to 4 mg/kg P.O. daily, up to 150 mg daily.

➤ Pathologic hypersecretory conditions, such as Zollinger-Ellison syndrome (ZES)

Adults: 150 mg P.O. b.i.d.; doses up to 6 g or more frequent intervals may be needed in patients with severe disease. Or, infuse continuously at 1 mg/kg/hour. After 4 hours, if patient remains symptomatic or gastric acid output is greater than 10 mEq/hour, increase dose in increments of 0.5 mg/kg/hour and recheck gastric acid output. Doses up to 2.5 mg/kg/hour and infusion rates up to 220 mg/hour have been used.

➤ Gastroesophageal reflux disease

Adults: 150 mg P.O. b.i.d.

Children ages 1 month to 16 years: 5 to 10 mg/kg P.O. daily given as two divided doses.

➤ Erosive esophagitis

Adults: 150 mg P.O. q.i.d. Maintenance dosage is 150 mg P.O. b.i.d.

Children ages 1 month to 16 years: 5 to 10 mg/kg P.O. daily given as two divided doses.

➤ Heartburn

Adults and children age 12 and older: 75 mg of Zantac 75 P.O. as symptoms occur, up to 150 mg daily, not to exceed 2 weeks of continuous treatment.

Adjust-a-dose: For patients with creatinine clearance below 50 ml/minute, 150 mg P.O. q 24 hours or 50 mg I.V. q 18 to 24 hours.

I.V. ADMINISTRATION

- To prepare I.V. injection, dilute 2 ml (50 mg) ranitidine with compatible I.V. solution to a total volume of 20 ml, and inject over at least 5 minutes. Compatible solutions include sterile water for injection, normal saline solution for injection, D_5W or lactated Ringer injection.
- To give drug by intermittent I.V. infusion, dilute 50 mg (2 ml) in 100 ml compatible solution and infuse at a rate of 5 to 7 ml/minute. The premixed solution is 50 ml and doesn't need further dilution. Infuse over 15 to 20 minutes.
- For continuous infusion to treat active duodenal or gastric ulcer, dilute 150 mg in 250 ml of D_5W. For hypersecretory conditions such as ZES, dilute with D_5W or other compatible solution to no more than 2.5 mg/ml
- After dilution, solution is stable for 48 hours at room temperature.
- Store I.V. injection at 39° to 86° F (4° to 30° C). Store premixed containers at 36° to 77° F (2° to 25° C).

INCOMPATIBILITIES

Amphotericin B, atracurium, cefazolin, cefoxitin, ceftazidime, cefuroxime, chlorpromazine, clindamycin phosphate, diazepam, ethacrynate sodium, hetastarch, hydroxyzine, insulin, methotrimeprazine, midazolam, norepinephrine, pentobarbital sodium, phenobarbital, phytonadione.

ACTION

Competitively inhibits action of histamine on the H_2 at receptor sites of parietal cells, decreasing gastric acid secretion.

Route	Onset	Peak	Duration
P.O.	1 hr	1–3 hr	13 hr
I.V.	Unknown	Unknown	Unknown

Half-life: 2 to 3 hours.

ADVERSE REACTIONS

CNS: headache, malaise, vertigo.
EENT: blurred vision.
Hepatic: jaundice.
Other: ***anaphylaxis, angioedema,*** burning and itching at injection site.

INTERACTIONS

Drug-drug. *Antacids:* May interfere with ranitidine absorption. Stagger doses, if possible.

Diazepam: May decrease absorption of diazepam. Monitor patient closely.

Glipizide: May increase hypoglycemic effect. Adjust glipizide dosage, as directed.
Procainamide: May decrease renal clearance of procainamide. Monitor patient closely for toxicity.
Warfarin: May interfere with warfarin clearance. Monitor patient closely.

EFFECTS ON LAB TEST RESULTS
- May increase creatinine and ALT levels.
- May cause false-positive results in urine protein tests using Multistix.

CONTRAINDICATIONS & CAUTIONS
- Contraindicated in patients hypersensitive to drug and those with acute porphyria.
- Use cautiously in patients with hepatic dysfunction. Adjust dosage in patients with impaired renal function.

NURSING CONSIDERATIONS
- Assess patient for abdominal pain. Note presence of blood in emesis, stool, or gastric aspirate.
- Drug may be added to total parenteral nutrition solutions.
- ***Look alike–sound alike:*** Don't confuse ranitidine with rimantadine; don't confuse Zantac with Xanax or Zyrtec.

PATIENT TEACHING
- Instruct patient on proper use of OTC preparation, as indicated.
- Remind patient to take once-daily prescription drug at bedtime for best results.
- Instruct patient to take without regard to meals because absorption isn't affected by food.
- Tell patient taking 150 mg EFFERdose to dissolve drug in 6 to 8 ounces of water before taking.
- Tell parent to dissolve 25 mg EFFERdose tablet in at least 5 ml of water and give with a dosing cup, medicine dropper, or oral syringe.
- Urge patient to avoid cigarette smoking because this may increase gastric acid secretion and worsen disease.
- Advise patient to report abdominal pain and blood in stool or emesis.
- Warn patients with phenylketonuria that EFFERdose granules and tablets contain aspartame.

sucralfate
Carafate✐

Pharmacologic class: pepsin inhibitor
Pregnancy risk category B

AVAILABLE FORMS
Suspension: 1 g/10 ml
Tablets: 1 g

INDICATIONS & DOSAGES
➤ **Short-term (up to 8 weeks) treatment of duodenal ulcer**
Adults: 1 g P.O. q.i.d. 1 hour before meals and at bedtime.
➤ **Maintenance therapy for duodenal ulcer**
Adults: 1 g P.O. b.i.d.

ACTION
Probably adheres to and protects surface of ulcer by forming a barrier.

Route	Onset	Peak	Duration
P.O.	Unknown	Unknown	6 hr

Half-life: 6 to 20 hours.

ADVERSE REACTIONS
CNS: dizziness, headache, sleepiness, vertigo.
GI: *constipation,* bezoar formation, diarrhea, dry mouth, flatulence, gastric discomfort, indigestion, nausea, vomiting.
Musculoskeletal: back pain.
Skin: pruritus, rash.

INTERACTIONS
Drug-drug. *Antacids:* May decrease binding of drug to gastroduodenal mucosa, impairing effectiveness. Separate doses by 30 minutes.
Cimetidine, digoxin, fosphenytoin, ketoconazole, phenytoin, quinidine, ranitidine, tetracycline, theophylline: May decrease absorption. Separate doses by at least 2 hours.
Ciprofloxacin, lomefloxacin, moxifloxacin, norfloxacin, ofloxacin: May decrease absorption of these drugs, reducing anti-infective response. If use together can't be avoided, give at least 6 hours apart.

EFFECTS ON LAB TEST RESULTS

None reported.

CONTRAINDICATIONS & CAUTIONS

- Use cautiously in patients with chronic renal failure.

NURSING CONSIDERATIONS

- Reconstitute drug before instillation through a nasogastric tube. Flush tube with water to ensure passage into stomach.
- Drug is minimally absorbed and causes few adverse reactions.
- Monitor patient for severe, persistent constipation.
- Drug is as effective as cimetidine in healing duodenal ulcer.
- Drug contains aluminum but isn't classified as an antacid. Monitor patient with renal insufficiency for aluminum toxicity.

PATIENT TEACHING

- Tell patient to take sucralfate on an empty stomach, 1 hour before each meal and at bedtime.
- Instruct patient to continue prescribed regimen to ensure complete healing. Pain and other ulcer signs and symptoms may subside within first few weeks of therapy.
- Urge patient to avoid cigarette smoking, which may increase gastric acid secretion and worsen disease.
- Antacids may be used while taking drug, but separate doses by 30 minutes.

50

Miscellaneous gastrointestinal tract drugs

alosetron hydrochloride
budesonide
lubiprostone
mesalamine
olsalazine sodium
sulfasalazine
tegaserod maleate

alosetron hydrochloride

Lotronex✐

Pharmacologic class: selective $5\text{-}HT_3$ receptor antagonist
Pregnancy risk category B

AVAILABLE FORMS

Tablets: 0.5 mg, 1 mg

INDICATIONS & DOSAGES

➤ **Severe diarrhea-predominant irritable bowel syndrome (IBS)**

Women: Give 0.5 mg P.O. b.i.d. with or without food. If, after 4 weeks, drug is well tolerated but doesn't adequately control IBS symptoms, increase to 1 mg b.i.d. After 4 weeks at this dosage, if symptoms aren't controlled, stop drug.

ACTION

Selectively inhibits $5\text{-}HT_3$ receptors in the GI tract, which blocks neuronal depolarization, resulting in less visceral pain, colonic transit, and GI secretions.

Route	Onset	Peak	Duration
P.O.	Unknown	1 hr	Variable

Half-life: 1½ hours.

ADVERSE REACTIONS

CNS: headache.
GI: CONSTIPATION, nausea, GI discomfort and pain, abdominal discomfort and pain, abdominal distention, hemorrhoids, regurgitation, reflux, ***ileus perforation, ischemic colitis, small bowel mesenteric ischemia, impaction, obstruction.***
Skin: rash.

INTERACTIONS

Drug-drug. *Hydralazine, isoniazid, and procainamide:* May cause slower metabolism of these drugs because of *N*-acetyltransferase inhibition. Monitor patient for toxicity.

EFFECTS ON LAB TEST RESULTS

- May increase ALT level.

CONTRAINDICATIONS & CAUTIONS

- Contraindicated in patients hypersensitive to drug or any of its components, and in those with a history of or current chronic or severe constipation, sequelae from constipation, intestinal obstruction, stricture, toxic megacolon, GI perforation, GI adhesions, ischemic colitis, impaired intestinal circulation, thrombophlebitis, or hypercoagulable state.
- Contraindicated in patients with a history of or current Crohn disease, ulcerative colitis, or diverticulitis and in those who are unable to understand or comply with the Patient-Physician Agreement.
- Don't use drug if predominant symptom is constipation.
- Use cautiously in patients with mild to moderate liver impairment; contraindicated in patients with severe liver impairment.
- Use cautiously in women who are pregnant, breast-feeding, or planning to become pregnant.
- Use in children younger than age 18 hasn't been studied.

NURSING CONSIDERATIONS

- Drug is only appropriate for women who experience symptoms for at least 6 months, have no anatomic or biochemical GI tract abnormalities, and haven't responded to other therapies.
- Diarrhea-predominant IBS is considered severe if one or more of the following accompanies the diarrhea:
  – frequent and severe abdominal pain or discomfort
  – frequent bowel urgency or fecal incontinence

–disability or restriction of daily activities
- ***Alert:*** Patients taking drug have developed ischemic colitis and serious complications of constipation, resulting in death. If patient develops ischemic colitis (acute colitis, rectal bleeding, or sudden worsening of abdominal pain) while taking drug, stop therapy.
- If patient taking drug develops constipation, stop drug until symptoms subside.
- Drug is approved for use only in women with IBS. This drug isn't indicated for use in men.
- Elderly people may be at greater risk for complications of constipation.

PATIENT TEACHING
- Have patient sign a Patient-Physician Agreement before starting therapy.
- Urge patient to read the Medication Guide before starting drug and each time she refills the prescription.
- Tell patient that this drug won't cure but may alleviate some IBS symptoms.
- Inform patient that most women notice their symptoms improving after about 1 week of therapy, but some may take up to 4 weeks to get relief from abdominal pain, discomfort, and diarrhea. Let patient know that symptoms usually return within 1 week after stopping the drug.
- Advise patient that drug may be taken with or without food.
- If constipation or signs of ischemic colitis occur (rectal bleeding, bloody diarrhea, or worsened abdominal pain or cramping), tell patient to stop the drug and consult prescriber immediately. Therapy can be resumed after the situation is discussed with prescriber and constipation resolves.
- Inform patient not to share drug with other people having similar symptoms. This drug hasn't been shown to be safe or effective for men.
- Tell woman to notify the prescriber immediately if she becomes pregnant.

budesonide

Entocort EC

Pharmacologic class: glucocorticoids
Pregnancy risk category B

AVAILABLE FORMS
Capsules: 3 mg

INDICATIONS & DOSAGES
➤ **Mild to moderate active Crohn disease involving the ileum, ascending colon, or both**
Adults: 9 mg P.O. once daily in morning for up to 8 weeks. For recurrent episodes of active Crohn disease, a repeat 8-week course may be given. Taper to 6 mg P.O. daily for 2 weeks before completely stopping.
➤ **To maintain remission in mild to moderate Crohn disease that involves the ileum or ascending colon**
Adults: 6 mg P.O. daily for up to 3 months. If symptom control is maintained at 3 months, taper dose to stop therapy. Therapy for longer than 3 months doesn't have added benefit.
Adjust-a-dose: In patients with moderate to severe liver disease who have increased signs or symptoms of hypercorticism, reduce dose.

ACTION
Significant glucocorticoid effects caused by drug's high affinity for glucocorticoid receptors.

Route	Onset	Peak	Duration
P.O.	Unknown	½–10 hr	Unknown

Half-life: About 2 hours.

ADVERSE REACTIONS
CNS: *headache,* dizziness, asthenia, hyperkinesia, paresthesia, tremor, vertigo, fatigue, malaise, agitation, confusion, insomnia, nervousness, somnolence.
CV: chest pain, hypertension, palpitations, tachycardia, flushing.
EENT: facial edema, ear infection, eye abnormality, abnormal vision, sinusitis.
GI: *nausea, diarrhea,* dyspepsia, abdominal pain, flatulence, vomiting, anal disorder, aggravated Crohn disease, enteritis,

epigastric pain, fistula, glossitis, hemorrhoids, intestinal obstruction, tongue edema, tooth disorder, increased appetite.
GU: dysuria, micturition frequency, nocturia, intermenstrual bleeding, menstrual disorder, hematuria, pyuria.
Hematologic: leukocytosis, anemia.
Metabolic: *hypercorticism,* dependent edema, hypokalemia, increased weight.
Musculoskeletal: back pain, aggravated arthritis, cramps, arthralgia, myalgia.
Respiratory: *respiratory tract infection,* bronchitis, dyspnea.
Skin: *acne,* alopecia, dermatitis, eczema, skin disorder, increased sweating.
Other: flulike disorder, sleep disorder, candidiasis, viral infection, pain.

INTERACTIONS

Drug-drug. *CYP inhibitors (erythromycin, indinavir, itraconazole, ketoconazole, ritonavir, saquinavir):* May increase effects of budesonide. If use together is unavoidable, reduce budesonide dosage.
Drug-food. *Grapefruit juice:* May increase drug effects. Discourage use together.

EFFECTS ON LAB TEST RESULTS

- May increase alkaline phosphatase and C-reactive protein levels. May decrease potassium and hemoglobin levels.
- May increase erythrocyte sedimentation rate and WBC count.

CONTRAINDICATIONS & CAUTIONS

- Contraindicated in patients hypersensitive to drug.
- Use cautiously in patients with tuberculosis, hypertension, diabetes mellitus, osteoporosis, peptic ulcer disease, glaucoma, or cataracts; those with a family history of diabetes or glaucoma; and those with any other condition in which glucocorticosteroids may have unwanted effects.
- Glucocorticoids appear in breast milk, and infants may have adverse reactions. Use cautiously in breast-feeding women only if benefits outweigh risks.

NURSING CONSIDERATIONS

- Reduced liver function affects elimination of this drug; systemic availability of drug may increase in patients with liver cirrhosis.
- Patients undergoing surgery or other stressful situations may need systemic glucocorticoid supplementation in addition to budesonide therapy.
- Carefully monitor patients transferred from systemic glucocorticoid therapy to budesonide for signs and symptoms of corticosteroid withdrawal. Watch for immunosuppression, especially in patients who haven't had diseases, such as chickenpox or measles; these can be fatal in patients who are immunosuppressed or receiving glucocorticoids.
- Replacement of systemic glucocorticoids with this drug may unmask allergies, such as eczema and rhinitis, which were previously controlled by systemic drug.
- Long-term use of drug may cause hypercorticism and adrenal suppression.

PATIENT TEACHING

- Tell patient to swallow capsules whole and not to chew or break them.
- Advise patient to avoid grapefruit juice while taking drug.
- Tell patient to notify prescriber immediately if he is exposed to or develops chickenpox or measles.

✱ *NEW DRUG*

lubiprostone

Amitiza

Pharmacologic class: chloride channel activator
Pregnancy risk category C

AVAILABLE FORMS

Capsules: 24 mcg

INDICATIONS & DOSAGES

➤ **Chronic idiopathic constipation**
Adults: 24 mcg P.O. b.i.d. with food.

ACTION

Increases intestinal fluid secretion by activating chloride channels, and increases intestinal motility.

Route	Onset	Peak	Duration
P.O.	Unknown	1 hr	Unknown

Half-life: Unknown; about 1 to 1½ hours for metabolite.

ADVERSE REACTIONS

CNS: *headache,* anxiety, depression, dizziness, fatigue, insomnia, pyrexia.
CV: chest pain, peripheral edema.
EENT: nasopharyngitis, pharyngolaryngeal pain, sinusitis.
GI: *diarrhea, nausea,* abdominal distension, abdominal pain or discomfort, constipation, dry mouth, dyspepsia, flatulence, gastroesophageal reflux disease, loose stools, stomach discomfort, viral gastroenteritis, vomiting.
GU: UTI.
Metabolic: weight gain.
Musculoskeletal: arthralgia, back pain, limb pain, muscle cramps.
Respiratory: bronchitis, cough, dyspnea, upper respiratory tract infection.
Other: influenza.

INTERACTIONS

None reported.

EFFECTS ON LAB TEST RESULTS

None reported.

CONTRAINDICATIONS & CAUTIONS

- Contraindicated in patients hypersensitive to drug or its components and in those with a history of mechanical GI obstruction.
- Use cautiously in women who are or may become pregnant.

NURSING CONSIDERATIONS

- Periodically assess patient's need for continued therapy.
- Monitor patient for diarrhea.
- Don't give drug to a patient with severe diarrhea.
- Safety and effectiveness in children haven't been established.

PATIENT TEACHING

- Tell patient to take drug with food.
- Explain to patient he may experience diarrhea; advise him not to take drug if he develops severe diarrhea.
- Advise patient about a proper diet and the need to drink plenty of fluids.

mesalamine

Asacol, Canasa, Mesasal, Pentasa, Rowasa, Salofalk

Pharmacologic class: salicylate
Pregnancy risk category B

AVAILABLE FORMS

Capsules (controlled-release): 250 mg
Rectal suspension: 4 g/60 ml
Suppositories: 1,000 mg
Tablets (delayed-release): 400 mg

INDICATIONS & DOSAGES

➤ **Active mild to moderate distal ulcerative colitis, proctitis, or proctosigmoiditis**
Adults: 800 mg P.O. (tablets) t.i.d. for total dose of 2.4 g/day for 6 weeks; or 1 g P.O. (capsules) q.i.d. for total dose of 4 g up to 8 weeks; or 1,000 mg suppository P.R., retained in the rectum for 1 to 3 hours or longer, once daily at bedtime; or 4 g retention enema once daily (preferably at bedtime). Patient should retain rectal dosage form overnight (for about 8 hours). Usual course of therapy for rectal form is 3 to 6 weeks.

ACTION

An active metabolite of sulfasalazine, drug probably acts topically by inhibiting prostaglandin production in the colon.

Route	Onset	Peak	Duration
P.O., P.R.	Unknown	3–12 hr	Unknown

Half-life: About 5 to 10 hours.

ADVERSE REACTIONS

CNS: *headache,* dizziness, fever, fatigue, malaise, asthenia.
CV: chest pain.
EENT: *pharyngitis.*
GI: abdominal pain, cramps, discomfort, flatulence, diarrhea, rectal pain, bloating, nausea, *pancolitis,* vomiting, constipation, eructation.
GU: interstitial nephritis, nephropathy, ***nephrotoxicity.***
Musculoskeletal: arthralgia, myalgia, back pain, hypertonia.
Respiratory: wheezing.

Skin: itching, rash, urticaria, hair loss.
Other: chills, acne.

INTERACTIONS
Drug-drug. *Lactulose:* May impair release of delayed or extended-release products. Monitor patient closely.
Omeprazole: May increase absorption of mesalamine. Monitor patient closely.

EFFECTS ON LAB TEST RESULTS
- May increase BUN, creatinine, AST, ALT, alkaline phosphatase, LDH, amylase, and lipase levels.

CONTRAINDICATIONS & CAUTIONS
- Contraindicated in children and in patients allergic to mesalamine, sulfites (including sulfasalazine), any salicylates, or any component of the preparation.
- Use cautiously in renally impaired, elderly, pregnant, and breast-feeding patients.

NURSING CONSIDERATIONS
- Shake suspension well before each use and remove sheath before inserting into rectum.
- Intact or partially intact tablets may be seen in stool. Notify prescriber if this occurs repeatedly.
- Monitor periodic renal function studies in patients on long-term therapy.
- Because the mesalamine rectal suspension contains potassium metabisulfite, it may cause hypersensitivity reactions in patients sensitive to sulfites.
- Absorption of drug may be nephrotoxic.
- ***Look alike–sound alike:*** Don't confuse Asacol with Os-Cal.

PATIENT TEACHING
- Instruct patient to carefully follow instructions supplied with drug and to swallow tablets whole without crushing or chewing.
- Advise patient to stop drug if fever or rash occurs. Patient intolerant of sulfasalazine may also be hypersensitive to mesalamine.
- Tell patient to remove foil wrapper from suppositories before inserting into rectum.
- Teach patient about proper use of retention enema.
- Tell patient that enema solution may stain bedsheets and clothing. Patient should use protective underpads and linens.

olsalazine sodium
Dipentum

Pharmacologic class: salicylate
Pregnancy risk category C

AVAILABLE FORMS
Capsules: 250 mg

INDICATIONS & DOSAGES
➤ **Maintenance of remission of ulcerative colitis in patients intolerant of sulfasalazine**
Adults: 500 mg P.O. b.i.d. with meals.

ACTION
Unknown. After oral use, converts to 5-aminosalicylic acid (5-ASA or mesalamine) in the colon, where it has local anti-inflammatory effect.

Route	Onset	Peak	Duration
P.O.	Unknown	1 hr	Unknown

Half-life: About 1 hour.

ADVERSE REACTIONS
CNS: headache, depression, vertigo, dizziness, fatigue.
GI: *diarrhea,* nausea, *abdominal pain,* dyspepsia, bloating, anorexia.
Musculoskeletal: arthralgia.
Skin: rash, itching.

INTERACTIONS
Drug-drug. *Anticoagulants:* May prolong PT or INR. Monitor bleeding study results.
Drug-food. *Any food:* May decrease GI irritation. Advise patient to take drug with food.

EFFECTS ON LAB TEST RESULTS
- May increase ALT and AST levels.

CONTRAINDICATIONS & CAUTIONS
- Contraindicated in patients hypersensitive to salicylates.

- Use cautiously in patients with renal disease.

NURSING CONSIDERATIONS
- Regularly monitor BUN and creatinine levels and urinalysis in patients with renal disease.
- Absorption of drug or its metabolites may cause renal tubular damage.
- Diarrhea sometimes occurs during therapy. Although diarrhea appears to be dose-related, it's difficult to distinguish from worsening of disease symptoms.
- Similar drugs have caused worsening of disease.
- ***Look alike–sound alike:*** Don't confuse olsalazine with olanzapine.

PATIENT TEACHING
- Teach patient to take drug in evenly divided doses and with food to minimize adverse GI reactions.
- Instruct patient to report persistent or severe adverse reactions promptly.

sulfasalazine (salazosulfapyridine, sulphasalazine)

Azulfidine, Azulfidine EN-tabs, PMS-Sulfasalazine E.C†, Salazopyrin†‡, Salazopyrin EN-Tabs†‡

Pharmacologic class: sulfonamide, salicylate
Pregnancy risk category B

AVAILABLE FORMS
Enteric-coated tablets: 500 mg
Tablets: 500 mg

INDICATIONS & DOSAGES
➤ **Mild to moderate ulcerative colitis, adjunctive therapy in severe ulcerative colitis, Crohn disease**
Adults: Initially, 3 to 4 g P.O. daily in evenly divided doses; usual maintenance dose is 2 g P.O. daily in divided doses q 6 hours. Dosage may be started with 1 to 2 g, with gradual increase to minimize adverse effects.
Children older than age 2: Initially, 40 to 60 mg/kg P.O. daily, divided into three to six doses; then 30 mg/kg daily in four doses. Dosage may be started at lower dose if GI intolerance occurs.
➤ **Rheumatoid arthritis in patients who have responded inadequately to salicylates or NSAIDs**
Adults: 2 g P.O. daily in evenly divided doses. To reduce possible GI intolerance, start at 0.5 to 1 g daily.
➤ **Polyarticular-course juvenile rheumatoid arthritis in patients who have responded inadequately to salicylates or other NSAIDs**
Children age 6 and older: 30 to 50 mg/kg P.O. daily in two divided doses. Maximum dose is 2 g daily. To reduce possible GI intolerance, start with one-quarter to one-third of planned maintenance dose and increase weekly until reaching maintenance dose at 1 month.

ACTION
Unknown.

Route	Onset	Peak	Duration
P.O.	Unknown	3–12 hr	Unknown

Half-life: 6 to 8 hours.

ADVERSE REACTIONS
CNS: *seizures,* headache, depression, hallucinations.
GI: *nausea, vomiting, diarrhea,* abdominal pain, anorexia, stomatitis.
GU: ***toxic nephrosis with oliguria and anuria,*** crystalluria, hematuria, oligospermia, infertility.
Hematologic: ***agranulocytosis, leukopenia, thrombocytopenia,*** aplastic anemia, megaloblastic anemia, hemolytic anemia.
Hepatic: ***hepatotoxicity,*** jaundice.
Skin: *generalized skin eruption,* ***erythema multiforme, Stevens-Johnson syndrome,*** epidermal necrolysis, exfoliative dermatitis, photosensitivity reaction, urticaria, pruritus.
Other: *serum sickness, drug fever,* ***anaphylaxis,*** hypersensitivity reactions.

INTERACTIONS
Drug-drug. *Antibiotics:* May alter action of sulfasalazine by changing intestinal flora. Monitor patient closely.
Digoxin: May reduce absorption of digoxin. Monitor patient closely.

Folic acid: May decrease absorption. Monitor patient.
Iron: May decrease levels of sulfasalazine caused by iron chelation. Monitor patient closely.
Methotrexate: May displace methotrexate from protein-binding sites and decrease renal clearance. Monitor patient for hematologic toxicity and adverse GI events, especially nausea.
Oral anticoagulants: May increase anticoagulant effect. Watch for bleeding.
Oral antidiabetics: May increase hypoglycemic effect. Monitor glucose levels.

EFFECTS ON LAB TEST RESULTS
- May increase ALT and AST levels. May decrease hemoglobin level.
- May decrease granulocyte, platelet, and WBC counts.

CONTRAINDICATIONS & CAUTIONS
- Contraindicated in patients hypersensitive to drug or its metabolites, in those with porphyria or intestinal and urinary obstruction, and in children younger than age 2.
- Use cautiously and in reduced doses in patients with impaired hepatic or renal function, severe allergy, bronchial asthma, or G6PD deficiency.

NURSING CONSIDERATIONS
- Therapeutic response in patients with rheumatoid arthritis may occur as soon as 4 weeks after starting therapy, but it may take up to 12 weeks in others.
- May cause urine discoloration.
- Give drug with food to decrease GI irritation.
- ***Alert:*** Stop drug immediately and notify prescriber if patient shows signs and symptoms of hypersensitivity.
- ***Look alike–sound alike:*** Don't confuse sulfasalazine with sulfisoxazole, salsalate, or sulfadiazine.

PATIENT TEACHING
- Instruct patient to take drug after eating and to space doses evenly.
- Warn patient to avoid ultraviolet light.
- Advise patient that drug may produce an orange-yellow discoloration of skin and urine and may cause contact lenses to turn yellow.
- Instruct patient that if his skin or urine is discolored, to notify prescriber immediately.
- Tell patient to drink plenty of water and to swallow tablets whole without crushing or chewing.

tegaserod maleate
Zelnorm

Pharmacologic class: 5-HT_4 receptor partial agonist
Pregnancy risk category B

AVAILABLE FORMS
Tablets: 2 mg, 6 mg

INDICATIONS & DOSAGES
➤ **Short-term treatment of women with irritable bowel syndrome, when the primary bowel symptom is constipation**
Women: 6 mg P.O. b.i.d. before meals for 4 to 6 weeks. May add another 4- to 6-week course for patients who respond to therapy at 4 to 6 weeks.
➤ **Chronic idiopathic constipation**
Men and women younger than age 65: 6 mg P.O. b.i.d. before meals.

ACTION
Binds with high affinity to 5-HT_4 receptors and acts as an agonist; stimulates the peristaltic reflex and intestinal secretion and inhibits visceral sensitivity.

Route	Onset	Peak	Duration
P.O.	Unknown	1 hr	Unknown

Half-life: Unknown.

ADVERSE REACTIONS
CNS: *headache,* dizziness, migraine.
GI: *abdominal pain,* diarrhea, nausea, flatulence.
Musculoskeletal: back pain, leg pain, arthropathy.
Other: accidental injury.

INTERACTIONS
Drug-drug. *Digoxin:* May reduce peak level and exposure of digoxin by 15%. No need to adjust digoxin dose.

Drug-food. *Food:* May reduce bioavailability of drug. Advise patient to take drug on an empty stomach.

EFFECTS ON LAB TEST RESULTS

None reported.

CONTRAINDICATIONS & CAUTIONS

- Contraindicated in patients hypersensitive to drug or its components and in those with severe renal impairment, moderate or severe hepatic impairment, a history of bowel obstruction, symptomatic gallbladder disease, suspected sphincter of Oddi dysfunction or abdominal adhesions, or frequently or currently occurring diarrhea.
- Use cautiously in patient who now has or often has diarrhea.

NURSING CONSIDERATIONS

- Stop drug if patient has new or sudden worsening of abdominal pain.
- Diarrhea sometimes develops during therapy, usually in the first week of treatment, and resolves as therapy continues.
- If serious diarrhea with hypovolemia, hypotension, and syncope occurs, stop drug. Don't start in patients with frequent diarrhea.
- Stop drug in patients who develop ischemic colitis or other forms of intestinal ischemia characterized by rectal bleeding, bloody diarrhea, or abdominal pain. Don't restart treatment with tegaserod if ischemic colitis has occurred.

PATIENT TEACHING

- Tell patient to take drug on an empty stomach, before a meal.
- Inform patient that diarrhea might develop during therapy.
- Tell patient to stop drug and consult prescriber if experiencing severe diarrhea, bloody diarrhea, or diarrhea with severe cramping, abdominal pain, or dizziness.
- Advise patient not to start therapy if he now has or often has diarrhea.
- Warn woman not to use during pregnancy or breast-feeding.

51 Corticosteroids

dexamethasone
dexamethasone acetate
dexamethasone sodium phosphate
fludrocortisone acetate
hydrocortisone
hydrocortisone acetate
hydrocortisone cypionate
hydrocortisone sodium phosphate
hydrocortisone sodium succinate
methylprednisolone
methylprednisolone acetate
methylprednisolone sodium succinate
prednisolone
prednisolone acetate
prednisolone sodium phosphate
prednisone
triamcinolone
triamcinolone acetonide
triamcinolone hexacetonide

dexamethasone
Decadron*, Dexameth*, Dexamethasone Elixir, Dexamethasone Intensol*, Dexamethasone Oral Solution, Dexone, Dexpak Taperpak, Hexadrol

dexamethasone acetate
Cortastat LA, Dalalone D.P., Decaject LA, Dexasone LA, Dexone LA, Solurex LA

dexamethasone sodium phosphate
Cortastat, Dalalone, Decadron Phosphate, Decaject, Dexasone, Hexadrol Phosphate, Solurex

Pharmacologic class: glucocorticoid
Pregnancy risk category C

AVAILABLE FORMS
dexamethasone
Elixir: 0.5 mg/5 ml*
Oral solution: 0.5 mg/5 ml, 0.5 mg/0.5 ml*
Tablets: 0.25 mg, 0.5 mg, 0.75 mg, 1 mg, 1.5 mg, 2 mg, 4 mg, 6 mg
dexamethasone acetate
Injection: 8 mg/ml, 16 mg/ml
dexamethasone sodium phosphate
Injection: 4 mg/ml, 10 mg/ml, 20 mg/ml, 24 mg/ml

INDICATIONS & DOSAGES

➤ **Cerebral edema**
Adults: Initially, 10 mg phosphate I.V.; then 4 mg I.M. q 6 hours until symptoms subside (usually 2 to 4 days); then taper over 5 to 7 days. Oral therapy (1 to 3 mg t.i.d.) should replace I.M. dosing as soon as possible.

➤ **Inflammatory conditions, allergic reactions, neoplasias**
Adults: 0.75 to 9 mg/day P.O. or 0.5 to 9 mg/day phosphate I.M., depending on size and location of affected area. Or, 8 to 16 mg acetate I.M. into joint or soft tissue q 1 to 3 weeks. Or, 0.8 to 1.6 mg acetate into lesions q 1 to 3 weeks.

➤ **Shock**
Adults: 20 mg phosphate as single first dose; then 3 mg/kg/24 hours via continuous I.V. infusion. Or, 1 to 6 mg/kg phosphate I.V. as single dose. Or, 40 mg phosphate I.V. q 2 to 6 hours, p.r.n., continued only until patient is stabilized (usually not longer than 48 to 72 hours).

➤ **Dexamethasone suppression test for Cushing syndrome**
Adults: Determine baseline 24-hour urine levels of 17-hydroxycorticosteroids; then, give 0.5 mg P.O. q 6 hours for 48 hours. Repeat 24-hour urine collection to determine 17-hydroxycorticosteroid excretion during second 24 hours of dexamethasone administration. Or, 1 mg P.O. as single dose at 11:00 p.m. with determination of plasma cortisol at 8 a.m. the next morning.

➤ **Adrenocortical insufficiency**
Children: 0.024 to 0.34 mg/kg or 0.66 to 10 mg/m² P.O. daily, in four divided doses.

➤ **Tuberculosis meningitis**
Adults: 8 to 12 mg phosphate I.M. daily, taper over 6 to 8 weeks.

➤Adjunctive treatment in bacterial meningitis ♦
Adults, children, infants: 0.15 mg/kg phosphate I.V. q.i.d. for the first 2 to 4 days of anti-infective therapy.

I.V. ADMINISTRATION

- For direct injection, inject undiluted over at least 1 minute.
- For intermittent or continuous infusion, dilute solution according to manufacturer's instructions, and give over prescribed duration.
- During continuous infusion, change solution every 24 hours.

INCOMPATIBILITIES

Ciprofloxacin, daunorubicin, diphenhydramine, doxapram, doxorubicin, glycopyrrolate, idarubicin, midazolam, vancomycin.

ACTION

Not clearly defined. Decreases inflammation, mainly by stabilizing leukocyte lysosomal membranes; suppresses immune response; stimulates bone marrow; and influences protein, fat, and carbohydrate metabolism.

Route	Onset	Peak	Duration
P.O.	1–2 hr	1–2 hr	2½ days
I.V.	1 hr	1 hr	Variable
I.M.	1 hr	1 hr	6 days
I.M. (acetate)	1 hr	8 hr	Unknown

Half-life: About 1 to 2 days.

ADVERSE REACTIONS

CNS: *euphoria, insomnia,* psychotic behavior, ***pseudotumor cerebri,*** vertigo, headache, paresthesia, ***seizures,*** depression.
CV: ***heart failure,*** hypertension, edema, ***arrhythmias,*** thrombophlebitis, ***thromboembolism.***
EENT: cataracts, glaucoma.
GI: *peptic ulceration,* GI irritation, increased appetite, ***pancreatitis,*** nausea, vomiting.
GU: menstrual irregularities, increased urine glucose and calcium levels.
Metabolic: hypokalemia, hyperglycemia, carbohydrate intolerance, hypercholesterolemia, hypocalcemia.
Musculoskeletal: growth suppression in children, muscle weakness, osteoporosis.
Skin: hirsutism, delayed wound healing, acne, various skin eruptions, atrophy at I.M. injection site.
Other: cushingoid state, susceptibility to infections, acute adrenal insufficiency after increased stress or abrupt withdrawal after long-term therapy.
After abrupt withdrawal: rebound inflammation, fatigue, weakness, arthralgia, fever, dizziness, lethargy, fainting, orthostatic hypotension, dyspnea, anorexia, ***hypoglycemia. After prolonged use, sudden withdrawal may be fatal.***

INTERACTIONS

Drug-drug. *Aminoglutethimide:* May cause loss of dexamethasone-induced adrenal suppression. Use together cautiously.
Antidiabetics, including insulin: May decrease response. May need dosage adjustment.
Aspirin, indomethacin, other NSAIDs: May increase risk of GI distress and bleeding. Use together cautiously.
Barbiturates, carbamazepine, phenytoin, rifampin: May decrease corticosteroid effect. Increase corticosteroid dosage.
Cardiac glycosides: May increase risk of arrhythmia resulting from hypokalemia. May need dosage adjustment.
Cyclosporine: May increase toxicity. Monitor patient closely.
Ephedrine: May cause decreased half-life and increased clearance of dexamethasone. Monitor patient.
Oral anticoagulants: May alter dosage requirements. Monitor PT and INR closely.
Potassium-depleting drugs such as thiazide diuretics: May enhance potassium-wasting effects of dexamethasone. Monitor potassium level.
Salicylates: May decrease salicylate level. Monitor patient for lack of salicylate effectiveness.
Skin-test antigens: May decrease response. Postpone skin testing until therapy is completed.
Toxoids, vaccines: May decrease antibody response and may increase risk of

neurologic complications. Avoid using together.
Drug-lifestyle. *Alcohol use:* May increase risk of gastric irritation and GI ulceration. Discourage use together.

EFFECTS ON LAB TEST RESULTS

- May increase cholesterol and glucose levels. May decrease calcium, potassium, T_3, and T_4 levels.
- May decrease ^{131}I uptake and protein-bound iodine levels in thyroid function tests. May cause false-negative results in nitroblue tetrazolium test for systemic bacterial infections. May alter reactions to skin tests.

CONTRAINDICATIONS & CAUTIONS

- Contraindicated in patients hypersensitive to drug or its ingredients, in those with systemic fungal infections, and in those receiving immunosuppressive doses together with live virus vaccines.
- Use with caution in patient with recent MI.
- Use cautiously in patients with GI ulcer, renal disease, hypertension, osteoporosis, diabetes mellitus, hypothyroidism, cirrhosis, diverticulitis, nonspecific ulcerative colitis, recent intestinal anastomoses, thromboembolic disorders, seizures, myasthenia gravis, heart failure, tuberculosis, active hepatitis, ocular herpes simplex, emotional instability, or psychotic tendencies and in women who are breast-feeding.
- Because some forms contain sulfite preservatives, also use cautiously in patients sensitive to sulfites.

NURSING CONSIDERATIONS

- Determine whether patient is sensitive to other corticosteroids.
- Most adverse reactions to corticosteroids are dose- or duration-dependent.
- For better results and less toxicity, give once-daily dose in morning.
- Give oral dose with food when possible. Patient may need drugs to prevent GI irritation.
- Give I.M. injection deeply into gluteal muscle. Rotate injection sites to prevent muscle atrophy. Avoid subcutaneous injection because atrophy and sterile abscesses may occur.
- Always adjust to lowest effective dose.
- Monitor patient's weight, blood pressure, and electrolyte levels.
- Monitor patient for cushingoid effects, including moon face, buffalo hump, central obesity, thinning hair, hypertension, and increased susceptibility to infection.
- Watch for depression or psychotic episodes, especially in high-dose therapy.
- Diabetic patient may need increased insulin; monitor glucose levels.
- Drug may mask or worsen infections, including latent amebiasis.
- Elderly patients may be more susceptible to osteoporosis with long-term use.
- Inspect patient's skin for petechiae.
- Gradually reduce dosage after long-term therapy.
- ***Look alike–sound alike:*** Don't confuse dexamethasone with desoximetasone.

PATIENT TEACHING

- Tell patient not to stop drug abruptly or without prescriber's consent.
- Instruct patient to take drug with food or milk.
- Teach patient signs and symptoms of early adrenal insufficiency: fatigue, muscle weakness, joint pain, fever, anorexia, nausea, shortness of breath, dizziness, and fainting.
- Instruct patient to carry medical identification indicating his need for supplemental systemic glucocorticoids during stress, especially when dosage is decreased. This card should contain prescriber's name and name and dosage of drug.
- Warn patient on long-term therapy about cushingoid effects (moon face, buffalo hump) and the need to notify prescriber about sudden weight gain or swelling.
- Warn patient about easy bruising.
- Advise patient receiving long-term therapy to consider exercise or physical therapy. Tell him to ask prescriber about vitamin D or calcium supplement.
- Instruct patient receiving long-term therapy to have periodic eye examinations.
- Advise patient to avoid exposure to infections (such as measles and chickenpox) and to notify prescriber if such exposure occurs.

fludrocortisone acetate

Florinef Acetate

Pharmacologic class: mineralocorticoid
Pregnancy risk category C

AVAILABLE FORMS

Tablets: 0.1 mg

INDICATIONS & DOSAGES

➤ **Salt-losing adrenogenital syndrome**
Adults: 0.1 to 0.2 mg P.O. daily.

➤ **Addison disease (adrenocortical insufficiency)**
Adults: 0.1 mg P.O. daily. Usual dosage range is 0.1 mg three times weekly to 0.2 mg daily. Decrease dosage to 0.05 mg daily if transient hypertension develops as a result of drug therapy.

➤ **Postural hypotension** ♦
Adults: 0.1 to 0.4 mg P.O. daily in patients with diabetes; 0.05 to 0.2 mg daily in patients with postural hypotension as a result of levodopa therapy.

ACTION

Increases sodium reabsorption and potassium and hydrogen secretion at the distal convoluted tubules of nephrons.

Route	Onset	Peak	Duration
P.O.	Variable	2 hr	1–2 days

Half-life: 18 to 36 hours.

ADVERSE REACTIONS

CV: ***heart failure,*** hypertension, cardiac hypertrophy, edema.
Hematologic: bruising.
Metabolic: *sodium and water retention,* hypokalemia.
Skin: diaphoresis, urticaria, allergic rash.

INTERACTIONS

Drug-drug. *Anabolic steroids, estrogen:* May increase fludrocortisone levels. Monitor patient for adverse effects.
Barbiturates, carbamazepine, fosphenytoin, phenytoin, rifampin: May increase clearance of fludrocortisone acetate. Monitor patient for possible diminished effect of corticosteroid. Corticosteroid dosage may need to be increased.
Digoxin: May increase the risk of digoxin toxicity associated with hypokalemia. Monitor potassium and digoxin levels.
Potassium-depleting drugs, such as amphotericin B, thiazide diuretics: May enhance potassium-wasting effects of fludrocortisone. Monitor potassium level.
Salicylates: May decrease salicylate effectiveness. Monitor patient for decreased effect.
Drug-food. *Sodium-containing drugs or foods:* May increase blood pressure. Sodium intake may need adjustment.

EFFECTS ON LAB TEST RESULTS

- May decrease potassium level.

CONTRAINDICATIONS & CAUTIONS

- Contraindicated in patients hypersensitive to drug and in those with systemic fungal infections.
- Use cautiously in patients with hypothyroidism, recent MI, cirrhosis, ocular herpes simplex, emotional instability, psychotic tendencies, diverticulitis, fresh intestinal anastomoses, active or latent peptic ulcer, renal insufficiency, hypertension, osteoporosis, myasthenia gravis, active hepatitis, active tuberculosis, or nonspecific ulcerative colitis. Also use cautiously in breast-feeding women.
- Patients shouldn't be vaccinated against smallpox while taking drug.

NURSING CONSIDERATIONS

- Drug is used with cortisone or hydrocortisone in adrenal insufficiency.
- Perform glucose tolerance tests only if needed because addisonian patients tend to develop severe hypoglycemia within 3 hours of the test.
- ***Alert:*** Monitor patient's blood pressure and electrolyte levels. If hypertension occurs, notify prescriber and expect dosage to be decreased by 50%.
- Weigh patient daily; notify prescriber about sudden weight gain.
- Unless contraindicated, give low-sodium diet that is high in potassium and protein. Potassium supplements may be needed.
- Drug may cause adverse effects similar to those of glucocorticoids.

PATIENT TEACHING

- Tell patient to notify prescriber if low blood pressure, weakness, cramping, or palpitations worsen, or if changes in mental status occur.
- Warn patient that mild swelling is common.
- Caution patient to avoid exposure to infections (such as chickenpox or measles) and to notify prescriber if such exposure occurs.

hydrocortisone
Aquacort†, Cortef, Cortenema, Hydrocortone

hydrocortisone acetate
Anucort-HC, Anusol-HC, Cortifoam, Proctocort, Hydrocortone Acetate

hydrocortisone cypionate
Cortef

hydrocortisone sodium phosphate
Hydrocortone Phosphate

hydrocortisone sodium succinate
A-Hydrocort, Solu-Cortef

Pharmacologic class: glucocorticoid
Pregnancy risk category C

AVAILABLE FORMS

hydrocortisone
Enema: 100 mg/60 ml
Tablets: 5 mg, 10 mg, 20 mg
hydrocortisone acetate
Injection: 25 mg/ml, 50 mg/ml suspension
Rectal aerosol foam: 10% aerosol foam (provides 90 mg/application)
Rectal suppository: 25 mg, 30 mg
hydrocortisone cypionate
Oral suspension: 2 mg/ml
hydrocortisone sodium phosphate
Injection: 50 mg/ml solution
hydrocortisone sodium succinate
Injection: 100-mg vial, 250-mg vial, 500-mg vial, 1,000-mg vial

INDICATIONS & DOSAGES

➤ **Severe inflammation, adrenal insufficiency**
Adults: 10 to 320 mg P.O. daily in three or four divided doses. Or, initially, 100 to 500 mg succinate I.M. or I.V.; repeat q 2 to 10 hours, as needed. Or, 15 to 240 mg phosphate I.M., subcutaneously, or I.V. daily in divided doses q 12 hours. Or, 5 to 75 mg acetate into joints or soft tissue repeated at 3 to 5 days for bursae and 1 to 4 weeks for joints. Dosage varies with size of joint. Local anesthetics commonly are injected with dose.

➤ **Shock**
Adults: Initially, 50 mg/kg succinate I.V., repeated in 4 hours. Repeat dosage q 24 hours, p.r.n. Or, 0.5 to 2 g q 2 to 6 hours, continued until patient is stabilized (usually not longer than 48 to 72 hours).
Children: Phosphate (I.M.) or succinate (I.M. or I.V.) 0.16 to 1 mg/kg or 6 to 30 mg/m^2 given once or twice daily.

➤ **Adjunct treatment for ulcerative colitis and proctitis**
Adults: 1 enema (100 mg) P.R. nightly for 21 days. Or, 1 applicatorful (90-mg foam) P.R. daily or b.i.d. for 14 to 21 days. Or, 25 mg rectal suppository b.i.d. for 2 weeks. For severe proctitis, 25 mg P.R. t.i.d. or 50 mg b.i.d.

I.V. ADMINISTRATION

- Don't use acetate or suspension form for I.V. route.
- Hydrocortisone sodium phosphate may be added directly to D_5W or normal saline solution for I.V. use.
- Reconstitute hydrocortisone sodium succinate with bacteriostatic water or bacteriostatic saline solution before adding to I.V. solutions. For direct injection, inject over 30 seconds to 10 minutes. For infusion, dilute with D_5W, normal saline solution, or dextrose 5% in normal saline solution to 1 mg/ml or less.

INCOMPATIBILITIES

Hydrocortisone sodium phosphate: doxapram, mitoxantrone, sargramostim. Hydrocortisone sodium succinate: amobarbital, ampicillin sodium, bleomycin, ciprofloxacin, colistimethate, cytarabine, dacarbazine, diazepam, dimenhydrinate, ephedrine, ergotamine, furosemide, heparin sodium, hydralazine, idarubicin, Ionosol B with invert sugar 10%, kanamycin, methylprednisolone sodium succinate, midazolam, nafcillin, pentobarbital sodium, phenobarbital sodium, phenytoin, prochlorperazine edisylate, promethazine hydrochloride, sargramostim, vancomycin, vitamin B complex with C.

ACTION

Not clearly defined. Decreases inflammation, mainly by stabilizing leukocyte lysosomal membranes; suppresses immune response; stimulates bone marrow; and influences protein, fat, and carbohydrate metabolism.

Route	Onset	Peak	Duration
P.O., I.V., I.M., P.R.	Variable	Variable	Variable

Half-life: 8 to 12 hours.

ADVERSE REACTIONS

CNS: *euphoria, insomnia,* psychotic behavior, ***pseudotumor cerebri,*** vertigo, headache, paresthesia, ***seizures.***
CV: ***heart failure,*** hypertension, edema, ***arrhythmias,*** thrombophlebitis, ***thromboembolism.***
EENT: cataracts, glaucoma.
GI: *peptic ulceration,* GI irritation, increased appetite, ***pancreatitis,*** nausea, vomiting.
GU: menstrual irregularities, increased urine calcium levels.
Hematologic: easy bruising.
Metabolic: hypokalemia, hyperglycemia, carbohydrate intolerance, hypercholesterolemia, hypocalcemia.
Musculoskeletal: growth suppression in children, muscle weakness, osteoporosis.
Skin: hirsutism, delayed wound healing, acne, skin eruptions.
Other: cushingoid state, susceptibility to infections, ***acute adrenal insufficiency after increased stress or abrupt withdrawal after long-term therapy.***
After abrupt withdrawal: rebound inflammation, fatigue, weakness, arthralgia, fever, dizziness, lethargy, depression, fainting, orthostatic hypotension, dyspnea, anorexia, ***hypoglycemia. After prolonged use, sudden withdrawal may be fatal.***

INTERACTIONS

Drug-drug. *Aspirin, indomethacin, other NSAIDs:* May increase risk of GI distress and bleeding. Use together cautiously.
Barbiturates, carbamazepine, fosphenytoin, phenytoin, rifampin: May decrease corticosteroid effect. Increase corticosteroid dosage.
Cyclosporine: May increase toxicity. Monitor patient closely.
Drugs that deplete potassium such as thiazide diuretics: May enhance potassium-wasting effects of hydrocortisone. Monitor potassium level.
Live attenuated virus vaccines, other toxoids and vaccines: May decrease antibody response and increase risk of neurologic complications. Avoid using together.
Oral anticoagulants: May alter dosage requirements. Monitor PT and INR closely.
Skin-test antigens: May decrease response. Postpone skin testing until after therapy.
Drug-herb. *Echinacea:* May increase immune-stimulating effects. Discourage use together.
Ginseng: May increase immune-modulating response. Discourage use together.

EFFECTS ON LAB TEST RESULTS

- May increase glucose and cholesterol levels. May decrease T_3, T_4, potassium, and calcium levels.
- May cause decreased ^{131}I uptake and protein-bound iodine levels in thyroid function tests. May cause false-negative results in nitroblue tetrazolium test for systemic bacterial infections. May alter reactions to skin tests.

CONTRAINDICATIONS & CAUTIONS

- Contraindicated in patients hypersensitive to drug or its ingredients, in those with systemic fungal infections, in those receiving immunosuppressive doses together with live virus vaccines, and in premature infants (succinate).
- Use with caution in patient with recent MI.
- Use cautiously in patients with GI ulcer, renal disease, hypertension, osteopo-

rosis, diabetes mellitus, hypothyroidism, cirrhosis, diverticulitis, nonspecific ulcerative colitis, active hepatitis, recent intestinal anastomoses, thromboembolic disorders, seizures, myasthenia gravis, heart failure, tuberculosis, ocular herpes simplex, emotional instability, and psychotic tendencies or in women who are breast-feeding.

NURSING CONSIDERATIONS

- Determine whether patient is sensitive to other corticosteroids.
- Most adverse reactions to corticosteroids are dose- or duration-dependent.
- For better results and less toxicity, give a once-daily dose in morning.
- Give oral dose with food when possible. Patient may need another drug to prevent GI irritation.
- ***Alert:*** Salts aren't interchangeable.
- Inject I.M. deeply into gluteal muscle. Rotate injection sites to prevent muscle atrophy. Avoid subcutaneous injection because atrophy and sterile abscesses may occur.
- Injectable forms aren't used for alternate-day therapy.
- ***Alert:*** Only hydrocortisone sodium phosphate and sodium succinate can be given I.V.
- Enema may produce same systemic effects as other forms of hydrocortisone. If enema therapy must exceed 21 days, taper off by giving every other night for 2 to 3 weeks.
- High-dose therapy usually isn't continued beyond 48 hours.
- Always adjust to lowest effective dose.
- Monitor patient's weight, blood pressure, and electrolyte level.
- Monitor patient for cushingoid effects, including moon face, buffalo hump, central obesity, thinning hair, hypertension, and increased susceptibility to infection.
- Unless contraindicated, give a low-sodium diet that is high in potassium and protein. Give potassium supplements.
- Drug may mask or worsen infections, including latent amebiasis.
- Stress (fever, trauma, surgery, and emotional problems) may increase adrenal insufficiency. Increase dosage.
- Watch for depression or psychotic episodes, especially during high-dose therapy.
- Inspect patient's skin for petechiae.
- Diabetic patient may need increased insulin; monitor glucose level.
- Periodic measurement of growth and development may be needed during high-dose or prolonged therapy in children.
- Elderly patients may be more susceptible to osteoporosis with prolonged use.
- Gradually reduce dosage after long-term therapy.
- ***Look alike–sound alike:*** Don't confuse Solu-Cortef with Solu-Medrol (methylprednisolone sodium succinate), or hydrocortisone with hydroxychloroquine.

PATIENT TEACHING

- Tell patient not to stop drug abruptly or without prescriber's consent.
- Instruct patient to take oral form of drug with milk or food.
- Warn patient on long-term therapy about cushingoid effects (moon face, buffalo hump) and the need to notify prescriber about sudden weight gain or swelling.
- Teach patient signs and symptoms of early adrenal insufficiency: fatigue, muscle weakness, joint pain, fever, anorexia, nausea, shortness of breath, dizziness, and fainting.
- Instruct patient to carry a card with his prescriber's name and name and dosage of drug, indicating his need for supplemental systemic glucocorticoids during stress.
- Warn patient about easy bruising.
- Urge patient receiving long-term therapy to consider exercise or physical therapy. Also, tell him to ask prescriber about vitamin D or calcium supplement.
- Advise patient receiving long-term therapy to have periodic eye examinations.
- Caution patient to avoid exposure to infections (such as chickenpox or measles) and to notify prescriber if such exposure occurs.

methylprednisolone
Medrol, Medrol Dosepak, Meprolone Unipak

methylprednisolone acetate
depMedalone 40, depMedalone 80, Depo-Medrol, Depopred-40, Depopred-80

methylprednisolone sodium succinate
A-Methapred, Solu-Medrol

Pharmacologic class: glucocorticoid
Pregnancy risk category C

AVAILABLE FORMS
methylprednisolone
Tablets: 2 mg, 4 mg, 8 mg, 16 mg, 24 mg, 32 mg
methylprednisolone acetate
Injection (suspension): 20 mg/ml, 40 mg/ml, 80 mg/ml
methylprednisolone sodium succinate
Injection: 40-mg vial, 125-mg vial, 500-mg vial, 1,000-mg vial, 2,000-mg vial

INDICATIONS & DOSAGES
➤Severe inflammation or immunosuppression
Adults: Give 2 to 60 mg base P.O. usually in four divided doses. Or, initially, 24 mg (six 4-mg tablets) on the first day; taper by 4 mg per day until 21 tablets have been given. Or, 10 to 80 mg acetate I.M. daily, or 10 to 250 mg succinate I.M. or I.V. up to six times daily. Or, 4 to 40 mg acetate into smaller joints or 20 to 80 mg acetate into larger joints. Intralesional use is usually 20 to 60 mg acetate. Repeat intralesional and intra-articular injections q 1 to 5 weeks.
Children: Give 0.117 to 1.66 mg/kg or 3.3 to 50 mg/m² P.O daily in three or four divided doses. Or, 0.03 to 0.2 mg/kg or 1 to 6.25 mg/m² succinate I.M. once daily or b.i.d.
➤Congenital adrenogenital syndrome
Children: 40 mg acetate I.M. q 2 weeks.
➤Shock
Adults: Give 100 to 250 mg succinate I.V. q 2 to 6 hours. Or, 30 mg/kg I.V. initially; repeat q 4 to 6 hours, as needed. Give over 3 to 15 minutes. Continue therapy for 2 to 3 days or until patient is stable.

I.V. ADMINISTRATION
- Use only methylprednisolone sodium succinate, never the acetate form.
- Reconstitute according to manufacturer's directions using supplied diluent, or use bacteriostatic water for injection with benzyl alcohol.
- Compatible solutions include D_5W, normal saline solution, and dextrose 5% in normal saline solution.
- For direct injection, inject diluted drug into vein or free-flowing compatible I.V. solution over at least 1 minute.
- For intermittent or continuous infusion, dilute solution according to manufacturer's instructions, and give over prescribed duration. If used for continuous infusion, change solution every 24 hours.
- For shock, give massive doses over at least 10 minutes to prevent arrhythmias and circulatory collapse.
- Discard reconstituted solution after 48 hours.

INCOMPATIBILITIES
Allopurinol, aminophylline, calcium gluconate, ciprofloxacin, cytarabine, diltiazem, docetaxel, doxapram, etoposide, filgrastim, gemcitabine, glycopyrrolate, nafcillin, ondansetron, paclitaxel, penicillin G sodium, potassium chloride, propofol, sargramostim, vinorelbine, vitamin B complex with C.

ACTION
Not clearly defined. Decreases inflammation, mainly by stabilizing leukocyte lysosomal membranes; suppresses immune response; stimulates bone marrow; and influences protein, fat, and carbohydrate metabolism.

Route	Onset	Peak	Duration
P.O.	Rapid	2–3 hr	30–36 hr
I.V.	Rapid	Immediate	1 wk
I.M.	6–48 hr	4–8 days	4–8 days
Intra-articular	Rapid	7 days	1–5 wk

Half-life: 18 to 36 hours.

ADVERSE REACTIONS

CNS: *euphoria, insomnia,* psychotic behavior, ***pseudotumor cerebri,*** vertigo, headache, paresthesia, ***seizures.***
CV: ***arrhythmias, heart failure,*** hypertension, edema, thrombophlebitis, ***thromboembolism, cardiac arrest, circulatory collapse after rapid use of large I.V. dose.***
EENT: cataracts, glaucoma.
GI: *peptic ulceration,* GI irritation, increased appetite, ***pancreatitis,*** nausea, vomiting.
GU: menstrual irregularities.
Metabolic: hypokalemia, hyperglycemia, carbohydrate intolerance, hypercholesterolemia, hypocalcemia.
Musculoskeletal: growth suppression in children, muscle weakness, osteoporosis.
Skin: hirsutism, delayed wound healing, acne, various skin eruptions.
Other: cushingoid state, susceptibility to infections, ***acute adrenal insufficiency after increased stress or abrupt withdrawal after long-term therapy.***
After abrupt withdrawal (may be fatal after prolonged use): rebound inflammation, fatigue, weakness, arthralgia, fever, dizziness, lethargy, depression, fainting, orthostatic hypotension, dyspnea, anorexia, hypoglycemia.

INTERACTIONS

Drug-drug. *Aspirin, indomethacin, other NSAIDs:* May increase risk of GI distress and bleeding. Use together cautiously.
Barbiturates, carbamazepine, phenytoin, rifampin: May decrease corticosteroid effect. Increase corticosteroid dosage.
Cyclosporine: May increase toxicity. Monitor patient closely.
Ketoconazole and macrolide antibiotics: May decrease methylprednisolone clearance. Decreased dose may be required.
Oral anticoagulants: May alter dosage requirements. Monitor PT and INR closely.
Potassium-depleting drugs such as thiazide diuretics: May enhance potassium-wasting effects of methylprednisolone. Monitor potassium level.
Salicylates: May decrease salicylate levels. Monitor patient for lack of salicylate effectiveness.
Skin-test antigens: May decrease response. Postpone skin testing until after therapy.
Toxoids, vaccines: May decrease antibody response and may increase risk of neurologic complications. Avoid using together.
Drug-herb. *Echinacea:* May increase immune-stimulating effects. Discourage use together.
Ginseng: May increase immune-regulating response. Discourage use together.

EFFECTS ON LAB TEST RESULTS

- May increase glucose and cholesterol levels and urine calcium levels. May decrease T_3, T_4, potassium, and calcium levels.
- May cause decreased ^{131}I uptake and protein-bound iodine levels in thyroid function tests. May cause false-negative results in nitroblue tetrazolium test for systemic bacterial infections. May alter reactions to skin tests.

CONTRAINDICATIONS & CAUTIONS

- Contraindicated in patients hypersensitive to drug or its ingredients, in those with systemic fungal infections, in premature infants (acetate and succinate), and in patients receiving immunosuppressive doses together with live virus vaccines.
- Use cautiously in patients with GI ulceration or renal disease, hypertension, osteoporosis, diabetes mellitus, hypothyroidism, cirrhosis, diverticulitis, nonspecific ulcerative colitis, recent intestinal anastomoses, thromboembolic disorders, seizures, active hepatitis, myasthenia gravis, heart failure, tuberculosis, ocular herpes simplex, emotional instability, and psychotic tendencies or in breast-feeding women.

NURSING CONSIDERATIONS

- Medrol may contain tartrazine. Watch for allergic reaction to tartrazine in patients with sensitivity to aspirin.
- Drug may be used for alternate-day therapy.
- Determine whether patient is sensitive to other corticosteroids. Most adverse reactions to corticosteroids are dose- or duration-dependent. For better results and less toxicity, give a once-daily dose in the morning.

- Give oral dose with food when possible. Critically ill patients may need to take drug with an antacid or H_2-receptor antagonist.
- ***Look alike–sound alike:*** Different salts aren't interchangeable.
- ***Alert:*** Don't give Solu-Medrol intrathecally because severe adverse reactions may occur.
- Give I.M. injection deeply into gluteal muscle. Avoid subcutaneous injection because atrophy and sterile abscesses may occur.
- Dermal atrophy may occur with large doses of acetate form. Use several small injections rather than a single large dose, and rotate injection sites.
- If immediate onset of action is needed, don't use acetate form.
- Always adjust to lowest effective dose.
- Monitor patient's weight, blood pressure, electrolyte level, and sleep patterns. Euphoria may initially interfere with sleep, but patients typically adjust to therapy in 1 to 3 weeks.
- Monitor patient for cushingoid effects, including moon face, buffalo hump, central obesity, thinning hair, hypertension, and increased susceptibility to infection.
- Measure growth and development periodically in children during high-dose or prolonged treatment.
- Drug may mask or worsen infections, including latent amebiasis.
- Watch for depression or psychotic episodes, especially in high-dose therapy.
- Diabetic patient may need increased insulin; monitor glucose level.
- Watch for an enhanced response to drug in patients with hypothyroidism or cirrhosis.
- Unless contraindicated, give low-sodium diet that's high in potassium and protein. Give potassium supplements, as needed.
- Elderly patients may be more susceptible to osteoporosis with prolonged use.
- Taper off dosage after long-term therapy.
- ***Look alike–sound alike:*** Don't confuse Solu-Medrol with Solu-Cortef or methylprednisolone with medroxyprogesterone.

PATIENT TEACHING

- Tell patient not to stop drug abruptly or without prescriber's consent.
- Instruct patient to take oral form of drug with milk or food.
- Teach patient signs and symptoms of early adrenal insufficiency: fatigue, muscle weakness, joint pain, fever, anorexia, nausea, shortness of breath, dizziness, and fainting.
- Instruct patient to carry or wear medical identification indicating his need for supplemental systemic glucocorticoids during stress. This card should contain prescriber's name, name of drug, and dosage taken.
- Warn patient on long-term therapy about cushingoid effects (moon face, buffalo hump) and the need to notify prescriber about sudden weight gain or swelling.
- Advise patient receiving long-term therapy to consider exercise or physical therapy. Also, tell patient to ask prescriber about vitamin D or calcium supplement.
- Instruct patient to avoid exposure to infections (such as chickenpox or measles) and to contact prescriber if such exposure occurs.

prednisolone

Delta-Cortef, Panafcortelone‡, Prelone

prednisolone acetate

Key-Pred 25, Key-Pred 50, Predalone 50, Predcor-50

prednisolone sodium phosphate

Hydeltrasol, Key-Pred-SP, Orapred, Orapred ODT, Pediapred, Predsol Retention Enema‡, Predsol Suppositories‡, Prelone

Pharmacologic class: glucocorticoid, mineralocorticoid
Pregnancy risk category C

AVAILABLE FORMS

prednisolone
Syrup: 5 mg/5 ml, 15 mg/5 ml*
Tablets: 1 mg‡, 5 mg, 25 mg‡
prednisolone acetate
Injection (suspension): 25 mg/ml, 50 mg/ml

prednisolone sodium phosphate
Injection: 20 mg/ml
Oral solution: 5 mg/5 ml, 20 mg/5 ml
Orally disintegrating tablets (ODTs): 10 mg, 15 mg, 30 mg
Retention enema: 20 mg/100 ml‡
Suppositories: 5 mg‡

INDICATIONS & DOSAGES

➤ **Severe inflammation, immunosuppression**
prednisolone
Adults: 2.5 to 15 mg P.O. b.i.d., t.i.d., or q.i.d.
Children: Initially, 0.14 to 2 mg/kg/day P.O. or 4 to 60 mg/m²/day, divided q.i.d.
prednisolone acetate
Adults: 2 to 30 mg I.M. q 12 hours. Intralesional, intra-articular, or soft-tissue injection, 4 to 100 mg.
Children: 0.04 to 0.25 mg/kg or 1.5 to 7.5 mg/m² I.M. once daily or b.i.d.
prednisolone sodium phosphate
Adults: 4 to 60 mg I.M., I.V., or P.O. daily.
Children: Initially, 0.14 to 2 mg/kg daily, or 4 to 60 mg/m² I.M., I.V., or P.O. daily, divided t.i.d. or q.i.d.

➤ **Uncontrolled asthma in those taking inhaled corticosteroids and long-acting bronchodilators**
Children: 1 to 2 mg/kg/day prednisolone sodium phosphate P.O. in single or divided doses. Continue short course (or "burst" therapy) until child achieves a peak expiratory flow rate of 80% of his personal best, or until symptoms resolve. This usually requires 3 to 10 days of treatment but can take longer. Tapering the dose after improvement doesn't necessarily prevent relapse.

➤ **Acute exacerbations of multiple sclerosis**
Adults and children: 200 mg/day prednisolone sodium phosphate P.O. as single or divided dose for 7 days; then 80 mg every other day for 1 month.

➤ **Nephrotic syndrome**
Children: 60 mg/m² daily prednisolone sodium phosphate P.O., divided t.i.d. for 4 weeks, followed by 4 weeks of single-dose alternate-day therapy at 40 mg/m²/day.

I.V. ADMINISTRATION

- Prednisolone sodium phosphate is the only I.V. form.
- For direct injection, inject undiluted over at least 1 minute.
- For intermittent or continuous infusion, dilute solution according to manufacturer's instructions, and give over prescribed duration.
- Use D_5W or normal saline solution as diluent for infusion.

INCOMPATIBILITIES

Calcium gluconate, dimenhydrinate, methotrexate sodium, polymyxin B, prochlorperazine edisylate, promazine, promethazine hydrochloride.

ACTION

Not clearly defined. Decreases inflammation, mainly by stabilizing leukocyte lysosomal membranes; suppresses immune response; stimulates bone marrow; and influences protein, fat, and carbohydrate metabolism.

Route	Onset	Peak	Duration
P.O.	Rapid	1–2 hr	3–36 hr
I.V.	Rapid	1 hr	Unknown
I.M.	Rapid	1 hr	4 wk
P.R.	Unknown	Unknown	Unknown
Intra-articular	1–2 days	Unknown	< 4 wk

Half-life: 18 to 36 hours.

ADVERSE REACTIONS

CNS: *euphoria, insomnia,* ***pseudotumor cerebri, seizures,*** psychotic behavior, vertigo, headache, paresthesia.
CV: ***arrhythmias, heart failure, thromboembolism,*** hypertension, edema, thrombophlebitis.
EENT: cataracts, glaucoma.
GI: *peptic ulceration,* ***pancreatitis,*** GI irritation, increased appetite, nausea, vomiting.
GU: menstrual irregularities, increased urine calcium levels.
Metabolic: hypokalemia, hyperglycemia, carbohydrate intolerance, hypercholesterolemia, hypocalcemia.
Musculoskeletal: growth suppression in children, muscle weakness, osteoporosis.

Skin: hirsutism, delayed wound healing, acne, various skin eruptions.
Other: ***acute adrenal insufficiency,*** susceptibility to infections, cushingoid state, after increased stress or abrupt withdrawal after long-term therapy.
After abrupt withdrawal: rebound inflammation, fatigue, weakness, arthralgia, fever, dizziness, lethargy, depression, fainting, orthostatic hypotension, dyspnea, anorexia, hypoglycemia., After prolonged use, sudden withdrawal may be fatal.

INTERACTIONS

Drug-drug. *Aspirin, indomethacin, other NSAIDs:* May increase risk of GI distress and bleeding. Use together cautiously.
Barbiturates, carbamazepine, fosphenytoin, phenytoin, rifampin: May decrease corticosteroid effect. Increase corticosteroid dosage.
Cyclosporine: May increase toxicity and risk of seizures. Monitor patient closely.
Drugs that deplete potassium, such as thiazide diuretics and amphotericin B: May enhance potassium-wasting effects of prednisolone. Monitor potassium level.
Oral anticoagulants: May alter dosage requirements. Monitor PT and INR closely.
Salicylates: May decrease salicylate level. Monitor patient for lack of salicylate effectiveness.
Skin-test antigens: May decrease response. Postpone skin testing until therapy is completed.
Toxoids, vaccines: May decrease antibody response and may increase risk of neurologic complications. Avoid using together.

EFFECTS ON LAB TEST RESULTS

- May increase glucose and cholesterol levels. May decrease T_3, T_4, potassium, and calcium levels.
- May decrease ^{131}I uptake and protein-bound iodine levels in thyroid function tests. May alter skin-test results.
- May cause false-negative results in nitroblue tetrazolium test for systemic bacterial infections.

CONTRAINDICATIONS & CAUTIONS

- Contraindicated in patients hypersensitive to drug or its ingredients, in those with systemic fungal infections, and in those receiving immunosuppressive doses together with live-virus vaccines.
- Use with caution in patients with recent MI.
- Use cautiously in patients with GI ulcer, renal disease, hypertension, osteoporosis, diabetes mellitus, hypothyroidism, cirrhosis, active hepatitis, diverticulitis, nonspecific ulcerative colitis, recent intestinal anastomoses, thromboembolic disorders, seizures, myasthenia gravis, heart failure, tuberculosis, ocular herpes simplex, emotional instability, and psychotic tendencies or in breast-feeding women.

NURSING CONSIDERATIONS

- Determine whether patient is sensitive to other corticosteroids.
- Always adjust to lowest effective dose.
- Drug may be used for alternate-day therapy.
- Most adverse reactions to corticosteroids are dose- or duration-dependent.
- Give oral dose with food, when possible, to reduce GI irritation. Patient may need a drug to prevent GI irritation.
- Give I.M. injection deeply into gluteal muscle. Rotate injection sites to prevent muscle atrophy. Avoid subcutaneous injection because atrophy and sterile abscesses may occur.
- ***Alert:*** Prednisolone acetate isn't for I.V. use.
- Monitor patient's weight, blood pressure, and electrolyte level.
- Monitor patient for cushingoid effects, including moon face, buffalo hump, central obesity, thinning hair, hypertension, and increased susceptibility to infection.
- Watch for depression or psychotic episodes, especially during high-dose therapy.
- Diabetic patient may need increased insulin; monitor glucose level.
- Give patient low-sodium diet that's high in potassium and protein. Give potassium supplements as needed.
- Drug may mask or worsen infections, including latent amebiasis.
- Elderly patients may be more susceptible to osteoporosis with long-term use.
- Gradually reduce dosage after long-term therapy.
- ***Look alike–sound alike:*** Don't confuse prednisolone with prednisone.

PATIENT TEACHING

- Tell patient not to stop drug abruptly or without prescriber's consent.
- Instruct patient to take oral form of drug with food or milk.
- Teach patient signs and symptoms of early adrenal insufficiency: fatigue, muscle weakness, joint pain, fever, anorexia, nausea, shortness of breath, dizziness, and fainting.
- Instruct patient to carry medical identification that includes prescriber's name and name and dosage of drug and indicates his need for supplemental systemic glucocorticoids during stress.
- Warn patient on long-term therapy about cushingoid effects and the need to notify prescriber about sudden weight gain or swelling.
- Tell patient to report slow healing.
- Advise patient receiving long-term therapy to consider exercise or physical therapy. Also, tell him to ask prescriber about vitamin D or calcium supplement.
- Instruct patient to avoid exposure to infections and to notify prescriber if exposure occurs.
- Tell patient to avoid immunizations while taking drug.
- ***Alert:*** Tell patient not to cut, crush, or chew ODTs.
- Instruct patient not to remove the ODT from the blister pack until he's ready to take it. The tablet can be swallowed whole or allowed to dissolve on the tongue with or without water.
- Tell patient to store Orapred in the refrigerator at 36° to 46° F.

---

prednisone

Apo-Prednisone†, Liquid Pred*, Meticorten, Orasone, Panafcort‡, Panasol-S, Prednicen-M, Prednisone Intensol*, Sterapred Unipak, Winpred†

Pharmacologic class: adrenocorticoid
Pregnancy risk category C

AVAILABLE FORMS

Oral solution: 5 mg/5 ml*, 5 mg/ml (concentrate)*
Syrup: 5 mg/5 ml*
Tablet: 1 mg, 2.5 mg, 5 mg, 10 mg, 20 mg, 50 mg
Tablet (film-coated): 5 mg

INDICATIONS & DOSAGES

➤ Severe inflammation, immunosuppression
Adults: 5 to 60 mg P.O. daily in single dose or as two to four divided doses. Maintenance dose given once daily or every other day. Dosage must be individualized.
Children: 0.14 to 2 mg/kg or 4 to 60 mg/m^2 daily P.O. in four divided doses.

➤ Contact dermatitis; poison ivy
Adults: Initially, 30 mg (six 5-mg tablets); taper by 5 mg daily until 21 tablets have been given.

➤ Acute exacerbations of multiple sclerosis
Adults: 200 mg P.O. daily for 7 days; then 80 mg P.O. every other day for 1 month.

➤ Advanced pulmonary tuberculosis
Adults: 40 to 60 mg P.O. daily; taper over 4 to 8 weeks.

➤ Tuberculosis meningitis
Adults: 1 mg/kg P.O. daily for 30 days; taper over several weeks.

➤ Adjunctive treatment in *Pneumocystis jiroveci (carinii)* pneumonia in patients with AIDS ♦
Adults and children age 13 and older: 40 mg P.O. b.i.d. for 5 days; then 40 mg P.O. daily for 5 days; then 20 mg P.O. daily for 11 days or until completion of anti-infective therapy.

ACTION

Not clearly defined. Decreases inflammation, mainly by stabilizing leukocyte lysosomal membranes; suppresses immune response; stimulates bone marrow; and influences protein, fat, and carbohydrate metabolism.

Route	Onset	Peak	Duration
P.O.	Variable	Variable	Variable

Half-life: 18 to 36 hours.

ADVERSE REACTIONS

CNS: *euphoria, insomnia,* psychotic behavior, ***pseudotumor cerebri,*** vertigo, headache, paresthesia, ***seizures.***

CV: ***heart failure,*** hypertension, edema, ***arrhythmias,*** thrombophlebitis, ***thromboembolism.***
EENT: cataracts, glaucoma.
GI: *peptic ulceration,* ***pancreatitis,*** GI irritation, increased appetite, nausea, vomiting.
GU: menstrual irregularities, increased urine calcium level.
Metabolic: hypokalemia, hyperglycemia, carbohydrate intolerance, hypercholesterolemia, hypocalcemia.
Musculoskeletal: growth suppression in children, muscle weakness, osteoporosis.
Skin: hirsutism, delayed wound healing, acne, various skin eruptions.
Other: cushingoid state, susceptibility to infections, ***acute adrenal insufficiency,*** after increased stress or abrupt withdrawal after long-term therapy.
After abrupt withdrawal: rebound inflammation, fatigue, weakness, arthralgia, fever, dizziness, lethargy, depression, fainting, orthostatic hypotension, dyspnea, anorexia, hypoglycemia. After prolonged use, sudden withdrawal may be fatal.

INTERACTIONS

Drug-drug. *Aspirin, indomethacin, other NSAIDs:* May increase risk of GI distress and bleeding. Use together cautiously.
Barbiturates, carbamazepine, fosphenytoin, phenytoin, rifampin: May decrease corticosteroid effect. Increase corticosteroid dosage.
Cyclosporine: May increase toxicity and cause seizures. Monitor patient closely.
Oral anticoagulants: May alter dosage requirements. Monitor PT and INR closely.
Potassium-depleting drugs, such as thiazide diuretics and amphotericin B: May enhance potassium-wasting effects of prednisone. Monitor potassium level.
Salicylates: May decrease salicylate level. Monitor patient for lack of salicylate effectiveness.
Skin-test antigens: May decrease response. Postpone skin testing until therapy is completed.
Toxoids, vaccines: May decrease antibody response and may increase risk of neurologic complications. Avoid using together.

EFFECTS ON LAB TEST RESULTS

- May increase glucose and cholesterol levels. May decrease T_3, T_4, potassium, and calcium levels.
- May decrease ^{131}I uptake and protein-bound iodine values in thyroid function tests. May cause false-negative results in nitroblue tetrazolium test for systemic bacterial infections. May alter reactions to skin tests.

CONTRAINDICATIONS & CAUTIONS

- Contraindicated in patients hypersensitive to drug or its ingredients, in those with systemic fungal infections, and in those receiving immunosuppressive doses together with live-virus vaccines.
- Use cautiously in patients with recent MI, GI ulcer, renal disease, hypertension, osteoporosis, diabetes mellitus, hypothyroidism, cirrhosis, active hepatitis, diverticulitis, nonspecific ulcerative colitis, recent intestinal anastomoses, thromboembolic disorders, seizures, myasthenia gravis, heart failure, tuberculosis, ocular herpes simplex, emotional instability, and psychotic tendencies or in breast-feeding women.

NURSING CONSIDERATIONS

- Determine whether patient is sensitive to other corticosteroids.
- Drug may be used for alternate-day therapy.
- Always adjust to lowest effective dose.
- Most adverse reactions to corticosteroids are dose- or duration-dependent.
- For better results and less toxicity, give a once-daily dose in the morning.
- Unless contraindicated, give oral dose with food when possible to reduce GI irritation. Patient may need medication to prevent GI irritation.
- The oral solution may be diluted in juice or other flavored diluent or semi-solid food such as applesauce before using.
- Monitor patient's blood pressure, sleep patterns, and potassium level.
- Weigh patient daily; report sudden weight gain to prescriber.
- Monitor patient for cushingoid effects, including moon face, buffalo hump, central obesity, thinning hair, hypertension, and increased susceptibility to infection.

• Watch for depression or psychotic episodes, especially during high-dose therapy.
• Diabetic patient may need increased insulin; monitor glucose level.
• Elderly patients may be more susceptible to osteoporosis with long-term use.
• Drug may mask or worsen infections, including latent amebiasis.
• Unless contraindicated, give low-sodium diet that's high in potassium and protein. Give potassium supplements, as needed.
• Gradually reduce dosage after long-term therapy.
• ***Look alike–sound alike:*** Don't confuse prednisone with prednisolone or primidone.

PATIENT TEACHING

• Tell patient not to stop drug abruptly or without prescriber's consent.
• Instruct patient to take drug with food or milk.
• Teach patient signs and symptoms of early adrenal insufficiency: fatigue, muscle weakness, joint pain, fever, anorexia, nausea, shortness of breath, dizziness, and fainting.
• Instruct patient to carry or wear medical identification indicating his need for supplemental systemic glucocorticoids during stress. It should include prescriber's name and name and dosage of drug.
• Warn patient on long-term therapy about cushingoid effects (moon face, buffalo hump) and the need to notify prescriber about sudden weight gain or swelling.
• Advise patient receiving long-term therapy to consider exercise or physical therapy. Also, tell patient to ask prescriber about vitamin D or calcium supplement.
• Tell patient to report slow healing.
• Advise patient receiving long-term therapy to have periodic eye examinations.
• Instruct patient to avoid exposure to infections and to contact prescriber if exposure occurs.

triamcinolone
Aristocort, Atolone, Kenacort

triamcinolone acetonide
Azmacort Oral Inhaler, Kenaject-40, Kenalog-10, Kenalog-40, Tac-3, Tac-40, Triam-A, Triamonide 40, Tri-Kort, Trilog

triamcinolone hexacetonide
Aristospan Intra-Articular, Aristospan Intralesional

Pharmacologic class: glucocorticoid
Pregnancy risk category C

AVAILABLE FORMS

triamcinolone
Tablets: 4 mg, 8 mg
triamcinolone acetonide
Injection (suspension): 3 mg/ml, 10 mg/ml, 40 mg/ml
Metered spray: 100 mcg/spray
triamcinolone hexacetonide
Injection (suspension): 5 mg/ml (intralesional); 20 mg/ml (intra-articular)

INDICATIONS & DOSAGES

➤ **Severe inflammation, immunosuppression**
Adults: 4 to 48 mg P.O. daily in single dose or divided doses. Or, 60 mg acetonide I.M., then 20 to 100 mg I.M. acetonide as needed q 6 weeks, if possible. Or, 1 mg acetonide into lesions. Or, initially, 2.5 to 15 mg acetonide into joints (depending on joint size) or soft tissue; then, may increase to 40 mg for larger areas. A local anesthetic is commonly injected with triamcinolone into the joint. For hexacetonide, up to 0.5 mg (of 5 mg/ml suspension) intralesional or sublesional injection per square inch of affected skin. Additional injections based on patient's response. Or, 2 to 20 mg (using the 20 mg/ml suspension) via intra-articular injection. Repeat q 3 to 4 weeks.
Children older than age 12: Initially, 60 mg acetonide I.M.; repeat with additional I.M. doses of 20 to 100 mg, as needed, at 6 week intervals, if possible.

Children ages 6 to 12: Give 0.03 to 0.2 mg/kg acetonide, or 1 to 6.25 mg/m^2 I.M. 1- to 7-day intervals.

➤**Asthma**

Adults and children age 12 and older: 2 inhalations t.i.d. or q.i.d. Maximum, 16 inhalations daily.

Children ages 6 to 12: Give 1 or 2 inhalations t.i.d. or q.i.d. Maximum, 12 inhalations daily.

ACTION

Not clearly defined. Decreases inflammation, mainly by stabilizing leukocyte lysosomal membranes; suppresses immune response; stimulates bone marrow; and influences protein, fat, and carbohydrate metabolism.

Route	Onset	Peak	Duration
P.O., I.M., I.D., inhalation, intra-articular, intralesional	Variable	Variable	Variable

Half-life: 18 to 36 hours; 5.4 hours (HFA).

ADVERSE REACTIONS

CNS: *euphoria, insomnia,* ***pseudotumor cerebri, seizures,*** headache, paresthesia, psychotic behavior, vertigo.
CV: ***arrhythmias, heart failure, thromboembolism,*** hypertension, edema, thrombophlebitis.
EENT: cataracts, glaucoma.
GI: ***pancreatitis,*** *peptic ulceration,* GI irritation, increased appetite, nausea, vomiting.
GU: menstrual irregularities, increased urine calcium level.
Metabolic: hypokalemia, hyperglycemia, and carbohydrate intolerance, hypercholesterolemia, hypokalemia, hypocalcemia.
Musculoskeletal: growth suppression in children, muscle weakness, osteoporosis.
Skin: hirsutism, delayed wound healing, acne, various skin eruptions.
Other: ***acute adrenal insufficiency,*** cushingoid state, susceptibility to infections, after increased stress or abrupt withdrawal after long-term therapy.
After abrupt withdrawal: After prolonged use, sudden withdrawal may be fatal, rebound inflammation, fatigue, weakness, arthralgia, fever, dizziness, lethargy, depression, fainting, orthostatic hypotension, dyspnea, anorexia, hypoglycemia.

INTERACTIONS

Drug-drug. *Aspirin, indomethacin, other NSAIDs:* May increase risk of GI distress and bleeding. Use together cautiously.
Barbiturates, carbamazepine, fosphenytoin, phenytoin, rifampin: May decrease corticosteroid effect. Increase corticosteroid dosage.
Cyclosporine: May increase toxicity and seizures. Monitor patient closely.
Oral anticoagulants: May alter dosage requirements. Monitor PT and INR closely.
Potassium-depleting drugs, such as thiazide diuretics, amphotericin B: May enhance potassium-wasting effects of triamcinolone. Monitor potassium level.
Salicylates: May decrease salicylate level. Monitor patient for lack of salicylate effectiveness.
Skin-test antigens: May decrease response. Postpone skin testing until after therapy.
Toxoids, vaccines: May decrease antibody response and increase risk of neurologic complications. Avoid using together.

EFFECTS ON LAB TEST RESULTS

- May increase glucose and cholesterol levels. May decrease potassium and calcium levels.
- May decrease ^{131}I uptake and protein-bound iodine values in thyroid function tests. May alter reactions to skin tests.
- May cause false-negative results in nitroblue tetrazolium test for systemic bacterial infections.

CONTRAINDICATIONS & CAUTIONS

- Contraindicated in patients hypersensitive to drug or its ingredients, in those with systemic fungal infections, and in those receiving immunosuppressive doses together with live-virus vaccines.
- Use cautiously in patients with recent MI, GI ulcer, renal disease, hypertension, osteoporosis, diabetes mellitus, hypothyroidism, cirrhosis, diverticulitis, nonspecific ulcerative colitis, recent intestinal anastomoses, thromboembolic disorders, seizures, myasthenia gravis, active hepatitis, lactation, heart failure, tuberculosis,

ocular herpes simplex, emotional instability, or psychotic tendencies.

NURSING CONSIDERATIONS

- Determine whether patient is sensitive to other corticosteroids.
- Kenacort may contain tartrazine.
- Drug isn't used for alternate-day therapy.
- Always adjust to lowest effective dose.
- Most adverse reactions to corticosteroids are dose- or duration-dependent.
- For better results and less toxicity, give a once-daily oral dose in the morning with food.
- ***Alert:*** Parenteral form isn't for I.V. use.
- ***Alert:*** Salts aren't interchangeable.
- Don't use 40 mg/ml strength for I.D. or intralesional use.
- Don't use 10 mg/ml strength for I.M. use.
- Don't use diluents that contain preservatives; flocculation may occur.
- Give I.M. deeply into gluteal muscle. Rotate injection sites to prevent muscle atrophy.
- Monitor patient's weight, blood pressure, and electrolyte level.
- Monitor patient for cushingoid effects, such as moon face, buffalo hump, central obesity, thinning hair, hypertension, and increased susceptibility to infection.
- Watch for allergic reaction to tartrazine in patients sensitive to aspirin.
- Watch for depression or psychotic episodes, especially during high-dose therapy.
- Diabetic patient may need increased insulin dosage; monitor glucose level.
- Drug may mask or worsen infections, including latent amebiasis.
- Elderly patients may be more susceptible to osteoporosis with long-term use.
- Unless contraindicated, give low-sodium diet that's high in potassium and protein. Give potassium supplements, as needed.
- Gradually reduce dosage after long-term therapy. Drug may affect patient's sleep.
- ***Look alike–sound alike:*** Don't confuse triamcinolone with Triaminicin or Triaminicol.

PATIENT TEACHING

- Tell patient not to stop drug abruptly or without prescriber's consent.
- Instruct patient to take drug with food or milk.
- Instruct patient on proper use of Azmacort inhaler.
- Teach patient signs and symptoms of early adrenal insufficiency: fatigue, muscle weakness, joint pain, fever, anorexia, nausea, shortness of breath, dizziness, and fainting.
- Instruct patient to carry medical identification that includes prescriber's name and drug's name and dosage and indicates his need for supplemental systemic glucocorticoids during stress.
- Warn patient on long-term therapy about cushingoid effects (moon face, buffalo hump) and the need to notify prescriber about sudden weight gain and swelling.
- Tell patient to report slow healing.
- Advise patient receiving long-term therapy to consider exercise or physical therapy. Also, tell patient to ask prescriber about vitamin D or calcium supplement.
- Instruct patient to avoid exposure to infections and to notify prescriber if exposure occurs.

52

Androgens and anabolic steroids

fluoxymesterone
methyltestosterone
testosterone
testosterone cypionate
testosterone enanthate
testosterone propionate
testosterone transdermal system

fluoxymesterone

Halotestin

Pharmacologic class: androgen
Pregnancy risk category X
Controlled substance schedule III

AVAILABLE FORMS

Tablets: 2 mg, 5 mg, 10 mg

INDICATIONS & DOSAGES

➤ Hypogonadism from testicular deficiency
Adults: 5 to 20 mg P.O. daily.

➤ Delayed puberty in boys
Adolescents: Highly individualized; usually 2.5 to 10 mg daily for 4 to 6 months.

➤ Palliation of breast cancer
Women: 10 to 40 mg P.O. daily in divided doses. Individualize and use lowest effective dose.

➤ Vasomotor symptoms associated with menopause in combination with estrogen therapy ♦
Women: 1 to 2 mg P.O. with 0.02 or 0.04 mg of ethinyl estradiol b.i.d. for 21 days, followed by 7 days without drugs. Repeat cycle as necessary.

ACTION

Stimulates target tissues to develop normally in androgen-deficient men. May have some antiestrogen properties, making it useful in treating certain estrogen-dependent breast cancers.

Route	Onset	Peak	Duration
P.O.	Unknown	Unknown	9 hr

Half-life: 9¼ hours.

ADVERSE REACTIONS

CNS: headache, anxiety, depression, paresthesia, sleep apnea.
CV: edema.
GI: nausea.
GU: decreased ejaculatory volume, oligospermia, priapism.
Hematologic: polycythemia, ***suppression of clotting factors.***
Hepatic: reversible jaundice.
Metabolic: hypercalcemia, hypernatremia, hyperkalemia, hyperphosphatemia.
Skin: hypersensitivity reactions.
Other: *hypoestrogenic effects in women,* excessive hormonal effects in men, androgenic effects in women, altered libido, male pattern baldness.

INTERACTIONS

Drug-drug. *Hepatotoxic drugs:* May increase risk of hepatotoxicity. Monitor liver function closely.
Insulin, oral antidiabetics: May alter dosage requirements. Monitor glucose levels in diabetic patients.
Oral anticoagulants: May increase sensitivity to oral anticoagulants; may alter dosage requirements. Monitor INR.

EFFECTS ON LAB TEST RESULTS

- May increase calcium, lipid, liver enzyme, phosphate, potassium, and sodium levels. May decrease thyroxine-binding globulin and total T_4 levels.
- May increase RBC count and resin uptake of T_3 and T_4.
- May cause abnormal glucose tolerance test results.

CONTRAINDICATIONS & CAUTIONS

- Contraindicated in patients hypersensitive to drug; in men with breast cancer or known or suspected prostate cancer; in patients with cardiac, hepatic, or renal decompensation; and in pregnant or breast-feeding women.
- Use cautiously in prepubertal boys or patients with benign prostatic hyperplasia or aspirin sensitivity.

NURSING CONSIDERATIONS

- ***Alert:*** Don't use in women of childbearing age until pregnancy is ruled out.
- Monitor INR in patients taking oral anticoagulants because dosage may need adjustment.
- Unless contraindicated, use with high-calorie, high-protein diet. Give small, frequent meals.
- Watch for evidence of jaundice, and periodically evaluate hepatic function. If liver function test results are abnormal, notify prescriber because therapy should be stopped.
- Edema can be controlled with sodium restriction or diuretics. Monitor weight routinely.
- Monitor boys and men for evidence of excessive hormonal effects. In prepubertal boys, watch for premature epiphyseal closure, acne, priapism, growth of body and facial hair, and phallic enlargement. If postpubertal men, watch for testicular atrophy, oligospermia, decreased ejaculatory volume, impotence, gynecomastia, and epididymitis.
- Evaluate semen routinely every 3 to 4 months, especially in adolescent boys.
- ***Alert:*** Hypercalcemia symptoms may be difficult to distinguish from those caused by the condition being treated, unless anticipated and thought of as a symptom cluster. Hypercalcemia is particularly likely to occur in immobilized patients and in women with metastatic breast cancer, and may indicate bone metastases.
- ***Alert:*** Don't give drug to enhance patient's athletic performance or physique.
- Watch for signs and symptoms of hypoglycemia in diabetic patients. Check glucose levels. Dosage of antidiabetic may need adjustment.
- When given for breast cancer, subjective effects may not occur for about 1 month; objective effects on clinical symptoms may take 3 months.
- Hypoestrogenic effects in women include flushing, diaphoresis, vaginal bleeding, nervousness, emotional lability, menstrual irregularities, and vaginitis, including itching, dryness, and burning.
- Halotestin may contain tartrazine.

PATIENT TEACHING

- If GI upset occurs, tell patient to take drug with food or meals.
- Make sure patient understands importance of using an effective nonhormonal contraceptive during therapy.
- Advise woman to wear cotton underwear and to wash after intercourse to decrease risk of vaginitis.
- Tell woman of childbearing age to report menstrual irregularities and to stop drug until she can be examined.
- Instruct woman to stop drug immediately and notify prescriber if pregnancy is suspected.
- Explain to woman taking drug for palliation of breast cancer that virilization usually occurs. Give emotional support. Tell her to immediately report androgenic effects (acne, swelling, weight gain, increased hair growth, hoarseness, clitoral enlargement, deepening voice, decreased breast size, changes in libido, male pattern baldness, and oily skin or hair).
- Tell patient that stopping drug prevents further androgenic changes but probably won't reverse existing effects.
- Warn patient with diabetes to be alert for signs and symptoms of hypoglycemia and to notify prescriber if these occur.
- Tell patient to report sudden weight gain.

methyltestosterone

Android, Metandren†, Testred, Virilon

Pharmacologic class: androgenic anabolic steroid hormone
Pregnancy risk category X
Controlled substance schedule III

AVAILABLE FORMS

Capsules: 10 mg
Tablets: 10 mg, 25 mg
Tablets (buccal): 10 mg

INDICATIONS & DOSAGES

➤ **Breast cancer**

Women 1 to 5 years after menopause: 50 to 200 mg P.O. daily or 25 to 100 mg buccally daily.

➤ **Hypogonadism**

Men: 10 to 50 mg P.O. daily or 5 to 25 mg buccally daily.

➤ Postpubertal cryptorchidism
Men: 30 mg P.O. daily or 15 mg buccally daily.

ACTION

Stimulates target tissues to develop normally in androgen-deficient men. May have some antiestrogen properties, making it useful in treating certain estrogen-dependent breast cancers. Action in postpartum breast engorgement isn't known because testosterone doesn't suppress lactation.

Route	Onset	Peak	Duration
P.O.	Unknown	2 hr	Unknown
Buccal	Unknown	1 hr	Unknown

Half-life: Unknown.

ADVERSE REACTIONS

CNS: headache, anxiety, depression, paresthesia.
CV: edema.
GI: irritation of oral mucosa with buccal administration, nausea.
GU: oligospermia, decreased ejaculatory volume, priapism.
Hematologic: ***suppression of clotting factors,*** polycythemia.
Hepatic: reversible jaundice, ***cholestatic hepatitis.***
Metabolic: hypernatremia, hyperkalemia, hyperphosphatemia, hypercholesterolemia, hypercalcemia.
Musculoskeletal: muscle cramps or spasms.
Skin: hypersensitivity reactions.
Other: androgenic effects in women, altered libido, *hypoestrogenic effects in women,* excessive hormonal effects in men, male pattern baldness.

INTERACTIONS

Drug-drug. *Hepatotoxic drugs:* May increase risk of hepatotoxicity. Monitor liver function closely.
Imipramine: May cause dramatic paranoid response. Monitor patient closely.
Insulin, oral antidiabetics: May decrease glucose level; may alter dosage requirements. Monitor glucose level in diabetic patients.
Oral anticoagulants: May increase sensitivity to oral anticoagulants; may alter dosage requirements. Monitor PT and INR.

EFFECTS ON LAB TEST RESULTS

- May increase sodium, potassium, phosphate, liver enzyme, lipid, and calcium levels. May decrease thyroxine-binding globulin and total T_4 levels.
- May increase RBC count and resin uptake of T_3 and T_4.

CONTRAINDICATIONS & CAUTIONS

- Contraindicated in pregnant or breast-feeding women and in men with breast or prostate cancer.
- Contraindicated in patients with cardiac, hepatic, or renal disease.
- Use cautiously in elderly patients; patients with cardiac, renal, or hepatic disease; and healthy males with delayed puberty.

NURSING CONSIDERATIONS

- Don't give to woman of childbearing age until pregnancy is ruled out.
- In children, obtain X-rays of wrist bones before therapy begins to establish bone maturation level. During treatment, bones may mature more rapidly than they grow in length. Periodically review X-rays to monitor bone maturation.
- Buccal tablets are twice as potent as oral tablets.
- Drug is typically used only for intermittent therapy. Because of potential hepatotoxicity, watch closely for jaundice.
- Promptly report evidence of virilization in women, such as deepening of the voice, increased hair growth, acne, or baldness.
- Watch for hypoestrogenic effects in women (flushing, diaphoresis, vaginal bleeding, nervousness, emotional lability, menstrual irregularities, and vaginitis, including itching, dryness, and burning).
- Watch for excessive hormonal effects in men. If patient is prepubertal, watch for premature epiphyseal closure, acne, priapism, growth of body and facial hair, and phallic enlargement. If he's postpubertal, watch for testicular atrophy, oligospermia, decreased ejaculatory volume, impotence, gynecomastia, and epididymitis.
- Unless contraindicated, use with high-calorie, high-protein diet. Give small, frequent meals.

• Periodically check cholesterol, calcium, and hemoglobin levels, hematocrit, and cardiac and liver function test results.
• Check weight regularly. Control edema with sodium restriction or diuretics.
• ***Alert:*** In breast cancer, therapeutic response usually occurs within 3 months. If disease appears to progress, stop drug.
• Report signs of hypercalcemia. In metastatic breast cancer, hypercalcemia may indicate progression of bone metastases.
• Evaluate semen every 3 to 4 months, especially in adolescent boys.
• ***Alert:*** Don't use to enhance athletic performance or physique.
• ***Look alike–sound alike:*** Testosterone and methyltestosterone aren't interchangeable. Don't confuse methyltestosterone with medroxyprogesterone.

PATIENT TEACHING
• Make sure patient understands importance of using effective contraception during therapy.
• Tell woman of childbearing age to report menstrual irregularities and to stop drug while awaiting examination.
• Instruct patient to stop drug immediately and notify prescriber if pregnancy is suspected.
• Tell patient to place buccal tablet in upper or lower buccal pouch between cheek and gum; tablet needs 30 to 60 minutes to dissolve. Tell patient not to eat, drink, chew, or smoke while buccal tablet is in place and not to swallow tablet.
• Instruct patient to change buccal tablet absorption site with each dose to minimize risk of irritation. Advise patient to rinse mouth after using buccal tablet.
• Tell woman to immediately report evidence of virilization, such as acne, swelling, weight gain, increased hair growth, hoarseness, clitoral enlargement, decreased breast size, deepening of voice, changes in libido, male pattern baldness, and oily skin or hair.
• Teach patient signs and symptoms of low glucose level (hypoglycemia) and method for checking glucose level; drug enhances hypoglycemia. Instruct patient to report signs or symptoms of hypoglycemia immediately.
• Advise woman to wear cotton underwear and to wash after intercourse to decrease risk of vaginitis.

testosterone
Striant, Testopel Pellets

testosterone cypionate
Depo-Testosterone

testosterone enanthate
Delatestryl

testosterone propionate
Malogen†

Pharmacologic class: androgen
Pregnancy risk category X
Controlled substance schedule III

AVAILABLE FORMS
testosterone
Blister packs (buccal; extended-release): 30 mg
Pellets (subcutaneous implant): 75 mg
testosterone cypionate
Injection (in oil): 100 mg/ml, 200 mg/ml
testosterone enanthate
Injection (in oil): 200 mg/ml
testosterone propionate
Injection (in oil): 100 mg/ml

INDICATIONS & DOSAGES
➤ Hypogonadism
Men: 10 to 25 mg propionate I.M. two to three times weekly; or 50 to 400 mg cypionate or enanthate I.M. q 2 to 4 weeks. Or, 75 to 150 mg enanthate I.M. q 7 to 10 days. Or, 150 to 450 mg (2 to 6 pellets) implanted subcutaneously q 3 to 6 months. Or, apply 1 buccal system (30 mg) to the gum region just above the incisor tooth on either side of the mouth, b.i.d., morning and evening about 12 hours apart. Alternate sides of the mouth with each application.
➤ Delayed puberty
Men and boys: 50 to 200 mg enanthate I.M. q 2 to 4 weeks for 4 to 6 months.
➤ Metastatic breast cancer
Women 1 to 5 years after menopause: 50 to 100 mg propionate I.M. three times weekly; or 200 to 400 mg cypionate or enanthate I.M. q 2 to 4 weeks.

ACTION

Stimulates target tissues to develop normally in androgen-deficient men. Because testosterone may have antiestrogen effects, it's used to treat estrogen-dependent breast cancer.

Route	Onset	Peak	Duration
I.M.	Unknown	10–100 min	Unknown
SubQ	Unknown	Unknown	3–6 mo
Buccal	Unknown	10–12 hr	2–4 hr

Half-life: 10 to 100 minutes.

ADVERSE REACTIONS

CNS: headache, anxiety, depression, paresthesia, sleep apnea.
CV: edema.
GI: nausea, gum or mouth irritation, bitter taste, gum pain, tenderness, or edema, taste perversion (with buccal application).
GU: amenorrhea, oligospermia, decreased ejaculatory volume, priapism.
Hematologic: polycythemia, ***suppression of clotting factors.***
Hepatic: reversible jaundice, ***cholestatic hepatitis.***
Metabolic: hypernatremia, hyperkalemia, hypercalcemia, hyperphosphatemia, hypercholesterolemia.
Skin: pain, induration at injection site, local edema, acne.
Other: androgenic effects in women, gynecomastia, hypersensitivity reactions, hypoestrogenic effects in women, excessive hormonal effects in men, male pattern baldness.

INTERACTIONS

Drug-drug. *Corticosteroids:* May increase risk of edema. Use together cautiously, especially in patients with cardiac or hepatic disease.
Hepatotoxic drugs: May increase risk of hepatotoxicity. Monitor liver function closely.
Insulin, oral antidiabetics: May decrease glucose level; may alter dosage requirements. Monitor glucose level in diabetic patients.
Oral anticoagulants: May increase sensitivity; may alter dosage requirements. Monitor PT and INR; decrease anticoagulant dose if necessary.
Oxyphenbutazone: May increase oxyphenbutazone level. Monitor patient.

EFFECTS ON LAB TEST RESULTS

- May increase sodium, potassium, phosphate, cholesterol, liver enzyme, calcium, and creatinine levels. May decrease thyroxine-binding globulin, total T_4 levels, serum creatinine, and 17-ketosteroid levels.
- May increase RBC count and resin uptake of T_3 and T_4.

CONTRAINDICATIONS & CAUTIONS

- Contraindicated in patients hypersensitive to drug and in those with hypercalcemia or cardiac, hepatic, or renal decompensation.
- Contraindicated in men with breast or prostate cancer and in pregnant or breast-feeding women.
- Use cautiously in elderly patients.

NURSING CONSIDERATIONS

- Don't give to woman of childbearing age until pregnancy is ruled out.
- Store I.M. preparations at room temperature. If crystals appear, warm and shake bottle to disperse them.
- Cypionate and enanthate are long-acting solutions.
- Inject deep into upper outer quadrant of gluteal muscle. Rotate injection sites; report soreness at site.
- Unless contraindicated, use with high-calorie, high-protein diet. Give small, frequent meals to help avoid nausea.
- Monitor patient's liver function test results.
- Testosterone may cause abnormal glucose tolerance test results.
- In patients with metastatic breast cancer, hypercalcemia usually indicates progression of bone metastases. Report signs and symptoms of hypercalcemia.
- Report evidence of virilization in women. Androgenic effects include acne, edema, weight gain, increased hair growth, hoarseness, clitoral enlargement, decreased breast size, changes in libido, male pattern baldness, and oily skin or hair.
- Watch for hypoestrogenic effects in women (flushing; diaphoresis; vaginitis,

including itching, drying, and burning; vaginal bleeding; menstrual irregularities).
- Watch for excessive hormonal effects in men and boys. In prepubertal boy, watch for premature epiphyseal closure, acne, priapism, growth of body and facial hair, and phallic enlargement. In postpubertal men, watch for testicular atrophy, oligospermia, decreased ejaculatory volume, impotence, gynecomastia, and epididymitis.
- Monitor patient's weight and blood pressure routinely.
- Monitor prepubertal boys by X-ray for rate of bone maturation.
- ***Alert:*** Therapeutic response in breast cancer is usually apparent within 3 months. If disease progresses, stop drug.
- Androgens may alter results of laboratory studies during therapy and for 2 to 3 weeks after therapy ends.
- ***Look alike–sound alike:*** Don't confuse testosterone with testolactone.
- ***Alert:*** Testosterone salts aren't interchangeable.

PATIENT TEACHING
- Make sure patient understands importance of using an effective nonhormonal contraceptive during therapy.
- Instruct patient to stop drug immediately and notify prescriber if pregnancy is suspected.
- Review signs and symptoms of virilization with woman, and instruct her to notify prescriber if they occur.
- Advise woman to wear cotton underwear and to wash after intercourse to decrease risk of vaginitis.
- Instruct man to notify prescriber about priapism, reduced ejaculatory volume, or gynecomastia.
- Warn diabetic patient to be alert for hypoglycemia and to notify prescriber if it occurs.
- Instruct boys using testosterone for delayed puberty to have X-rays of hand and wrist obtained every 6 months during treatment.
- Tell patient to report sudden weight gain.
- Warn patient that drug shouldn't be used to enhance athletic performance.
- Instruct patient how to use the buccal system.
- Advise patient to avoid dislodging buccal system and ensure that the system is in place after toothbrushing, use of mouthwash, and eating or drinking.
- Tell men not to chew or swallow buccal system.

testosterone transdermal system

Androderm, AndroGel, Testim

Pharmacologic class: androgen
Pregnancy risk category X
Controlled substance schedule III

AVAILABLE FORMS

1% gel: 25 mg, 50 mg per unit dose; 1.25 g per nonaerosol metered pump
Transdermal system: 2.5 mg/day, 5 mg/day

INDICATIONS & DOSAGES

➤ **Primary or hypogonadotropic hypogonadism**

Men: One or two Androderm patches applied to back, abdomen, arm, or thigh nightly for total dosage of 5 mg daily. Dose may be increased to 7.5 mg once daily or decreased to 2.5 mg once daily, depending upon a.m. serum testosterone levels. Or, initially, 50 mg applied q morning to shoulders, upper arms, or abdomen. Don't apply Testim to abdomen. Check testosterone level after about 2 weeks. If response is inadequate, may increase AndroGel to 75 mg daily. Then, adjust to 100 mg, (either gel) if needed. Or, for AndroGel pump, 5 g (4 pumps) applied q morning to shoulders, upper arms, or abdomen. Check testosterone level after about 2 weeks. If response is inadequate, may increase to 7.5 g (6 pumps) daily or from 7.5 g to 10 g (8 pumps) daily.

ACTION

Releases testosterone, which stimulates target tissues to develop normally in androgen-deficient men.

Route	Onset	Peak	Duration
Transdermal	Unknown	2–4 hr	2 hr after removal

Half-life: 10 to 100 minutes.

ADVERSE REACTIONS

CNS: ***stroke,*** asthenia, depression, headache.
GI: GI bleeding.
GU: prostatitis, prostate abnormalities, UTI.
Hepatic: ***cholestatic hepatitis,*** reversible jaundice.
Metabolic: hypernatremia, hyperkalemia, hypercalcemia, hyperphosphatemia, hypercholesterolemia.
Skin: *pruritus, blister under patch,* acne irritation, allergic contact dermatitis, burning.
Other: gynecomastia, breast tenderness, flulike syndrome.

INTERACTIONS

Drug-drug. *Insulin:* May alter insulin dosage requirements. Monitor glucose level.
Oral anticoagulants: May alter anticoagulant dosage requirements. Monitor PT and INR.

EFFECTS ON LAB TEST RESULTS

- May increase sodium, potassium, phosphate, cholesterol, liver enzyme, calcium, and creatinine levels.
- May increase RBC count.

CONTRAINDICATIONS & CAUTIONS

- Contraindicated in patients hypersensitive to drug, in women, in men with known or suspected breast or prostate cancer, and in patients with CV, renal, or hepatic disease.
- Use cautiously in elderly men.

NURSING CONSIDERATIONS

- Wear gloves when handling patches. Fold used patches with adhesive sides together to discard.
- Periodically assess liver function test results, lipid profiles, hemoglobin level, hematocrit (with long-term use), and levels of prostatic acid phosphatase and prostate-specific antigen.
- Watch for excessive hormonal effects.

PATIENT TEACHING

- Tell patient to fully prime the AndroGel pump by pumping three times before first use and discarding that gel.
- Tell patient to apply gel or patch to clean, dry, intact skin of the shoulders, upper arms, or abdomen only and not to scrotum or bony prominences. Testim shouldn't be applied to the abdomen. Tell him that he can first pump gel into his hand.
- Tell patient to wash his hands thoroughly with soap and water after applying.
- Instruct patient that patch must be changed every 24 hours.
- For best results, advise patient not to swim or shower for at least 5 hours after applying gel. Showering or swimming at least 1 hour after applying, if done infrequently, should have minimal effects on drug absorption.
- Tell patient that if the patch falls off, it may be reapplied. If patch falls off and can't be reapplied, and it has been worn at least 12 hours, a new patch may be applied at the next application time.
- Warn diabetic patient that drug may decrease glucose level and to be alert for hypoglycemia.
- Advise patient to report persistent erections, nausea, vomiting, changes in skin color, ankle swelling, or sudden weight gain to prescriber.
- Tell patient that drug may cause virilization in his female sexual partner, who should report acne or changes in body hair distribution.
- Tell patient that Androderm doesn't have to be removed during sexual intercourse or while showering.

53

Estrogens and progestins

drospirenone and ethinyl estradiol
esterified estrogens
estradiol
estradiol cypionate
estradiol gel
estradiol hemihydrate
estradiol valerate
estradiol and norethindrone acetate transdermal system
estrogens, conjugated
estropipate
ethinyl estradiol and desogestrel
ethinyl estradiol and ethynodiol diacetate
ethinyl estradiol and levonorgestrel
ethinyl estradiol and norethindrone
ethinyl estradiol and norethindrone acetate
ethinyl estradiol and norgestimate
ethinyl estradiol and norgestrel
ethinyl estradiol, norethindrone acetate, and ferrous fumarate
etonogestrel and ethinyl estradiol vaginal ring
medroxyprogesterone acetate
mestranol and norethindrone
norelgestromin and ethinyl estradiol transdermal system
norethindrone
norethindrone acetate

drospirenone and ethinyl estradiol

Yasmin, YAZ

Pharmacologic class: estrogenic and progestinic steroids
Pregnancy risk category X

AVAILABLE FORMS

Tablets: 3 mg drospirenone and 0.03 mg ethinyl estradiol as 21 yellow tablets and 7 white (inert) tablets (Yasmin); 3 mg drospirenone and 0.02 mg ethinyl estradiol as 24 light pink active tablets and four white (inert) tablets (YAZ)

INDICATIONS & DOSAGES

➤ Contraception

Women: 1 yellow Yasmin tablet P.O. daily for 21 days beginning on day 1 of menstrual cycle or the first Sunday after the onset of menstruation. Then 1 white inert tablet P.O. daily on days 22 through 28. Or 1 light pink YAZ tablet P.O. daily for 24 days beginning on day 1 of menstrual cycle or the first Sunday after the onset of menstruation. Then 1 white inert tablet P.O. daily on days 25 through 28. Begin the next and all subsequent 28-day regimens on the same day of the week that the first regimen began, following the same schedule. Restart yellow or light-pink tablets on the next day after the last white tablet.

ACTION

Reduces the chance for conception by inhibiting ovulation, inhibiting progression of sperm, and reducing chance of implantation.

Route	Onset	Peak	Duration
P.O.	Unknown	1–3 hr	Unknown

Half-life: drospirenone, 30 hours; ethinyl estradiol, 24 hours.

ADVERSE REACTIONS

CNS: ***cerebral hemorrhage, cerebral thrombosis,*** asthenia, depression, dizziness, emotional lability, headache, migraine, nervousness.
CV: ***arterial thromboembolism, mesenteric thrombosis, MI,*** hypertension, thrombophlebitis, fluid retention, edema.
EENT: cataracts, steepening of corneal curvature, intolerance to contact lenses, pharyngitis, retinal thrombosis, sinusitis.
GI: abdominal pain, abdominal cramping, bloating, changes in appetite, colitis, diarrhea, gastroenteritis, nausea, vomiting, gallbladder disease.
GU: amenorrhea, breakthrough bleeding, change in cervical erosion and secretion, change in menstrual flow, cystitis, cystitis-like syndrome, dysmenorrhea, ***hemolytic-***

uremic syndrome, impaired renal function, leukorrhea, menstrual disorder, premenstrual syndrome, spotting, temporary infertility after discontinuing treatment, UTI, vaginal candidiasis, vaginitis.
Hepatic: ***Budd-Chiari syndrome, hepatic adenomas,*** cholestatic jaundice, benign liver tumors.
Metabolic: reduced glucose tolerance, porphyria, weight change.
Musculoskeletal: back pain.
Respiratory: ***pulmonary embolism,*** bronchitis, upper respiratory tract infection.
Skin: ***erythema multiforme,*** acne, erythema nodosum, hemorrhagic eruption, hirsutism, loss of scalp hair, melasma, pruritus, rash.
Other: changes in libido.

INTERACTIONS

Drug-drug. *ACE inhibitors, aldosterone antagonists, angiotensin II receptor antagonists, NSAIDs, potassium-sparing diuretics:* May increase risk of hyperkalemia. Monitor potassium level.
Acetaminophen: May increase level of contraceptive and decrease effectiveness of acetaminophen. Monitor patient for adverse effects. Adjust acetaminophen dose as needed.
Ampicillin, griseofulvin, tetracycline: May decrease contraceptive effect. Advise patient to use additional method of birth control while taking the antibiotic.
Ascorbic acid, atorvastatin: May increase level of contraceptive. Monitor patient for adverse effects.
Carbamazepine, phenobarbital, phenytoin: May increase metabolism of ethinyl estradiol and decrease contraceptive effectiveness. Advise patient to use another method of birth control.
Clofibrate, morphine, salicylic acid, temazepam: May decrease levels and increase clearance of these drugs. Monitor patient for effectiveness.
Cyclosporine, prednisolone, theophylline: May increase levels of these drugs. Monitor patient for adverse effects and toxicity.
Phenylbutazone, rifampin: May decrease contraceptive effectiveness and increase menstrual irregularities. Advise patient to use another method of birth control.
Drug-herb. *St. John's wort:* May decrease contraceptive effectiveness and increase breakthrough bleeding. Discourage use together, or advise use of additional method of birth control.
Drug-lifestyle. *Smoking:* May increase risk of CV adverse effects. Advise patient to avoid smoking.

EFFECTS ON LAB TEST RESULTS

- May increase corticoid; factor VII, VIII, IX, and X; folate; prothrombin; thyroid-binding globulin; total circulating sex steroid; total thyroid hormone; and triglyceride levels. May decrease antithrombin III level.
- May increase norepinephrine-induced platelet aggregation. May decrease glucose tolerance and free T_3 resin uptake.

CONTRAINDICATIONS & CAUTIONS

- Contraindicated in women with hepatic dysfunction, tumor, or disease; renal or adrenal insufficiency; thrombophlebitis, thromboembolic disorders, or history of deep vein thrombosis or thromboembolic disorders; cerebrovascular or coronary artery disease; known or suspected breast cancer, endometrial cancer, or other estrogen-dependent neoplasia; abnormal genital bleeding; or cholestatic jaundice of pregnancy or jaundice with other contraceptive pill use.
- Contraindicated in women who are or may be pregnant and in women older than age 35 who smoke 15 or more cigarettes daily. Don't use in women age 65 or older.
- Use cautiously in patients with risk factors for CV disease, such as hypertension, hyperlipidemias, obesity, and diabetes.
- Use cautiously in patients with conditions aggravated by fluid retention.

NURSING CONSIDERATIONS

- The use of contraceptives causes increased risk of MI, thromboembolism, stroke, hepatic neoplasia, gallbladder disease, and hypertension. Risk increases in patients with hypertension, diabetes, hyperlipidemia, and obesity.
- Smoking increases the risk of serious CV adverse effects. The risk increases with age (especially age older than 35 years) and in patients who smoke 15 or more cigarettes daily.

• The relationship between the use of hormonal contraceptives and breast and cervical cancers is unclear. Encourage women to schedule a complete gynecologic examination at least yearly and to perform breast self-examinations monthly.
• In patients scheduled to have elective surgery that may increase the risk of thromboembolism, stop contraceptive use from at least 4 weeks before until 2 weeks after surgery. Also stop use during and after prolonged immobilization.
• Because of increased risk of thromboembolism in the postpartum period, don't start contraceptive earlier than 4 to 6 weeks after delivery.
• Stop use and evaluate patient if loss of vision, proptosis, diplopia, papilledema, or retinal vascular lesions occur. Recommend that contact lens wearers be evaluated by an ophthalmologist if visual changes or lens intolerance occurs.
• If patient misses two consecutive periods, she should obtain a negative pregnancy test result before continuing use of contraceptive.
• Immediately stop use if pregnancy is confirmed.
• Closely monitor patient with diabetes. Glucose intolerance may occur.
• Closely monitor patient with hypertension or a history of depression. Stop drug if these events occur.
• In patient taking medications that may increase potassium, check potassium level during the first treatment cycle.
• Stop drug and evaluate patient if persistent, severe headaches occur or if migraines occur or are worsened.
• Evaluate patient for malignancy or pregnancy if she experiences breakthrough bleeding or spotting.
• Closely monitor patient with hyperlipidemias.
• Stop use if jaundice occurs.

PATIENT TEACHING

• Advise patient to use additional method of birth control during the first 7 days of the first cycle of hormonal contraceptive.
• Inform patient that pills don't protect against sexually transmitted diseases, such as HIV.
• Advise patient of the dangers of smoking while taking hormonal contraceptives. Suggest smokers choose a different form of birth control.
• Tell patient to schedule gynecologic examinations yearly and perform breast self-examination monthly.
• Inform patient that spotting, light bleeding, or stomach upset may occur during the first 1 to 3 packs of pills. Tell her to continue taking the pills and to notify her health care provider if these symptoms persist.
• Tell patient to take the pill at the same time each day.
• Tell patient to immediately report sharp chest pain; coughing of blood or sudden shortness of breath; calf pain; crushing chest pain or chest heaviness; sudden severe headache or vomiting, dizziness or fainting, visual or speech disturbances, weakness or numbness in an arm or leg; vision loss; breast lumps; severe stomach pain or tenderness; difficulty sleeping, lack of energy, fatigue, or change in mood; jaundice with fever, fatigue, loss of appetite, dark urine, or light-colored bowel movements.
• Tell patient to notify health care provider if she wears contact lenses and notices a change in vision or has trouble wearing the lenses.
• Tell patient that the risk of pregnancy increases with each active yellow or light-pink tablet she forgets to take. Inform patient what to do if she misses pills.
• Tell patient to use an additional method of birth control and to notify health care provider if she isn't sure what to do about missed pills.
• Small amounts of hormonal contraceptives appear in breast milk. Yellow skin and eyes (jaundice) and breast enlargement may occur in breast-fed infants.

esterified estrogens
Estratab, Menest, Neo-Estrone†

Pharmacologic class: estrogen
Pregnancy risk category X

AVAILABLE FORMS

Tablets: 0.3 mg, 0.625 mg, 1.25 mg, 2.5 mg
Tablets (film-coated): 0.3 mg, 0.625 mg, 1.25 mg, 2.5 mg

INDICATIONS & DOSAGES

➤ **Inoperable prostate cancer**
Men: 1.25 to 2.5 mg P.O. t.i.d.

➤ **Palliative treatment for metastatic breast cancer**
Men and postmenopausal women: 10 mg P.O. t.i.d. for 3 or more months.

➤ **Hypogonadism**
Women: 2.5 to 7.5 mg daily in divided doses in cycles of 20 days on, 10 days off.

➤ **Castration, primary ovarian failure**
Women: 1.25 mg daily in cycles of 3 weeks on, 1 week off. Adjust for symptoms. Can be given continuously.

➤ **Vasomotor menopausal symptoms**
Women: 1.25 mg P.O. daily in cycles of 3 weeks on, 1 week off. Dosage may be increased to 2.5 to 3.75 mg P.O. daily if needed.

➤ **Atrophic vaginitis, atrophic urethritis**
Women: 0.3 to 1.25 mg or more P.O. daily in cycles of 3 weeks on, 1 week off.

ACTION

Increases synthesis of DNA, RNA, and protein in responsive tissues; reduces release of follicle-stimulating and luteinizing hormones from the pituitary gland.

Route	Onset	Peak	Duration
P.O.	Unknown	Unknown	Unknown

Half-life: Unknown.

ADVERSE REACTIONS

CNS: headache, dizziness, chorea, depression, ***stroke, seizures.***
CV: thrombophlebitis, ***thromboembolism,*** hypertension, *edema,* ***pulmonary embolism, MI.***
EENT: worsening myopia or astigmatism, intolerance of contact lenses.
GI: *nausea,* vomiting, abdominal cramps, bloating, anorexia, increased appetite, ***pancreatitis,*** increased risk of gallbladder disease.
GU: breakthrough bleeding, altered menstrual flow, dysmenorrhea, amenorrhea, ***increased risk of endometrial cancer,*** cervical erosion, altered cervical secretions, enlargement of uterine fibromas, vaginal candidiasis, testicular atrophy, impotence.
Hepatic: cholestatic jaundice, ***hepatic adenoma.***
Metabolic: hypercalcemia, weight changes.
Skin: melasma, rash, hirsutism or hair loss, erythema nodosum, dermatitis.
Other: *breast tenderness, enlargement, or secretion, gynecomastia,* ***increased risk of breast cancer.***

INTERACTIONS

Drug-drug. *Carbamazepine, fosphenytoin, phenobarbital, phenytoin, rifampin:* May decrease effectiveness of estrogen therapy. Monitor patient closely.
Corticosteroids: May enhance effects. Monitor patient closely.
Cyclosporine: May increase risk of toxicity. Use together with caution, and monitor cyclosporine level frequently.
Dantrolene, hepatotoxic drugs: May increase risk of hepatotoxicity. Monitor liver function closely.
Oral anticoagulants: May decrease anticoagulant effects. Adjust dosage if needed. Monitor PT and INR.
Tamoxifen: May interfere with tamoxifen effectiveness. Avoid using together.
Drug-herb. *St. John's wort:* May decrease effects of drug. Discourage use together.
Drug-food. *Caffeine:* May increase caffeine level. Urge caution.
Drug-lifestyle. *Smoking:* May increase risk of CV effects. If smoking continues, may need another form of therapy.

EFFECTS ON LAB TEST RESULTS

- May increase calcium and clotting factor VII, VIII, IX, and X levels.
- May increase norepinephrine-induced platelet aggregation and PT.
- May reduce metyrapone test results.

CONTRAINDICATIONS & CAUTIONS

- Contraindicated in pregnant women, in patients hypersensitive to drug, and in patients with breast cancer (except metastatic disease), estrogen-dependent neoplasia, active thrombophlebitis, thromboembolic disorders, undiagnosed abnormal genital bleeding, or history of thromboembolic disease.

- Use cautiously in patients with history of hypertension, mental depression, cardiac or renal dysfunction, liver impairment, bone disease, migraine, seizures, or diabetes.

NURSING CONSIDERATIONS
- When used for vasomotor symptoms in menstruating women, cyclic administration is started on day 5 of bleeding.
- Make sure patient has thorough physical examination before starting estrogen therapy. Patients receiving long-term therapy should have annual examinations. Periodically monitor body weight, blood pressure, lipid levels, and hepatic function.
- Notify pathologist about patient's estrogen therapy when sending specimens to laboratory for evaluation.
- Because of risk of thromboembolism, stop therapy at least 1 month before procedures that cause prolonged immobilization or increased risk of thromboembolism, such as knee or hip surgery.
- Glucose tolerance may be impaired. Monitor glucose level closely in patients with diabetes.
- ***Look alike–sound alike:*** Don't confuse Estratab with Estratest.

PATIENT TEACHING
- Tell patient to read package insert describing estrogen's adverse effects; also, give patient verbal explanation.
- Emphasize importance of regular physical examinations. Postmenopausal women who use estrogen replacement for longer than 5 years to treat menopausal symptoms may be at increased risk for endometrial cancer. This risk is reduced by using cyclic rather than continuous therapy and the lowest possible estrogen dosage. Adding progestins to the regimen decreases risk of endometrial hyperplasia; but it's unknown whether progestins affect risk of endometrial cancer.
- ***Alert:*** Warn patient to immediately report abdominal pain; pain, numbness, or stiffness in legs or buttocks; pressure or pain in chest or shortness of breath; severe headaches; visual disturbances, such as blind spots, flashing lights, or blurriness; vaginal bleeding or discharge; breast lumps; swelling of hands or feet; yellow skin or sclera; dark urine; or light-colored stools.
- Tell diabetic patient to report elevated glucose level so that antidiabetic dosage can be adjusted.
- Explain to woman receiving cyclic therapy for postmenopausal symptoms that she may experience withdrawal bleeding during week off drug. Tell her to report unusual vaginal bleeding.
- Teach woman to perform routine breast self-examination.
- Advise woman of childbearing age to consult prescriber before taking drug and to advise prescriber immediately if she becomes pregnant.
- Teach patient methods to decrease risk of blood clots.
- Encourage patient to stop smoking or reduce number of cigarettes smoked because of the risk of CV complications.

estradiol (oestradiol)
Alora, Climara, Esclim, Estrace🖉, Estrace Vaginal Cream, Estraderm, Estring Vaginal Ring, FemPatch, Femring, Gynodiol, Menostar, Vivelle, Vivelle-Dot

estradiol cypionate
depGynogen, Depo-Estradiol Cypionate, Depogen

estradiol gel
EstroGel

estradiol hemihydrate
Estrasorb, Vagifem

estradiol valerate (oestradiol valerate)
Delestrogen, Estra-L 40, Gynogen L.A, Primogyn Depot‡, Valergen

Pharmacologic class: estrogen
Pregnancy risk category X

AVAILABLE FORMS
estradiol
Tablets (micronized): 0.5 mg, 1 mg, 1.5 mg, 2 mg
Transdermal: 0.014 mg/24 hours, 0.025 mg/24 hours, 0.0375 mg/24 hours,

0.05 mg/24 hours, 0.06 mg/24 hours, 0.075 mg/24 hours, 0.1 mg/24 hours
Vaginal cream (in nonliquefying base): 0.1 mg/g
Vaginal ring: 0.0075 mg/24 hours; 0.05 mg/24 hours; 0.1 mg/24 hours
estradiol cypionate
Injection (in oil): 5 mg/ml
estradiol gel
Transdermal gel: 0.06% (1.25 g/metered dose)
estradiol hemihydrate
Topical emulsion: 0.25%
Vaginal tablets: 25 mcg
estradiol valerate
Injection (in oil): 10 mg/ml, 20 mg/ml, 40 mg/ml

INDICATIONS & DOSAGES

➤ Vasomotor menopausal symptoms, female hypogonadism, female castration, primary ovarian failure
Women: 0.5 to 2 mg P.O. estradiol daily in cycles of 21 days on and 7 days off or cycles of 5 days on and 2 days off. Or, for vasomotor symptoms, 1 to 5 mg cypionate I.M. once q 3 to 4 weeks; for female hypogonadism, 1.5 to 2 mg cypionate I.M. once q month.
Transdermal patch
Women: 0.025 mg/24 hours Esclim, 0.05 mg/24 hours Estraderm, 0.0375 mg/24 hours or 0.05 mg/24 hours twice weekly Vivelle, 0.05 mg/24 hours Climara, or 0.025 mg/24 hours FemPatch once weekly. Apply to clean, dry area of the trunk. Adjust dose if necessary after the first 2 or 3 weeks of therapy; then q 3 to 6 months, p.r.n. Rotate application sites weekly with an interval of at least 1 week between particular sites used. Adjust dosage, p.r.n.

➤ Postmenopausal urogenital symptoms
Women: One ring inserted into the upper third of the vagina. Ring is kept in place for 3 months.

➤ Atrophic vaginitis, kraurosis vulvae
Women: 0.05 mg/24 hours Estraderm applied twice weekly in a cyclic regimen. Or, 0.05 mg/24 hours Climara applied weekly in a cyclic regimen. Or, 2 to 4 g intravaginal applications of cream daily for 1 to 2 weeks. When vaginal mucosa is restored, maintenance dose is 1 g one to three times weekly in a cyclic regimen. If using Vagifem for atrophic vaginitis, give 1 tablet vaginally once daily for 2 weeks. Maintenance dose is 1 tablet inserted vaginally twice weekly. Or, 10 to 20 mg valerate I.M. q 4 weeks, p.r.n. Or, 1 to 5 mg estradiol cypionate I.M. once q 3 to 4 weeks.

➤ Moderate to severe vasomotor symptoms, as well as vulval and vaginal atrophy associated with menopause
Women: 1.25 g EstroGel applied once daily to skin in a thin layer from wrist to shoulder of one upper extremity.

➤ Palliative treatment of advanced, inoperable breast cancer
Men and postmenopausal women: 10 mg P.O. estradiol t.i.d. for 3 months.

➤ Palliative treatment of advanced, inoperable prostate cancer
Men: 30 mg valerate I.M. q 1 to 2 weeks, or 1 to 2 mg P.O. estradiol t.i.d.

➤ To prevent postmenopausal osteoporosis
Women: Place a 6.5-cm^2 (0.025 mg/24 hours) Climara patch once weekly on clean, dry skin of lower abdomen or upper quadrant of buttock. Or, place a 3.25-cm^2 (0.014 mg/24 hours) Menostar patch once weekly to clean, dry area of the lower abdomen. For each system, press firmly in place for about 10 seconds; ensure complete contact, especially around edges. Or, 0.025-mg/24 hours Vivelle, Vivelle-Dot, or Alora system applied to a clean, dry area of the trunk twice weekly. Or, 0.5 mg P.O. daily for 21 days, followed by 7 days without drug.

➤ Moderate to severe vasomotor symptoms from menopause
Women: Apply contents of two 1.74-g foil pouches (total 3.48 g) of Estrasorb daily. Open each pouch individually and use contents of one pouch for each leg. Rub emulsion into thigh and calf for 3 minutes until thoroughly absorbed; rub excess emulsion remaining on hands onto the buttocks. Allow areas to dry before covering with clothing. Wash hands with soap and water to remove excess drug.

ACTION

Increases synthesis of DNA, RNA, and protein in responsive tissues; reduces release of follicle-stimulating and luteinizing hormones from the pituitary gland.

Route	Onset	Peak	Duration
P.O., I.M., intravaginal	Unknown	Unknown	Unknown
Transdermal (Esclim)	Unknown	27–30 hr	Unknown
Transdermal (Estrasorb)	Immediate	Unknown	Unknown
Transdermal gel (EstroGel)	Immediate	1 hr	24–36 hr

Half-life: Unknown.

ADVERSE REACTIONS

CNS: ***stroke,*** *headache,* dizziness, chorea, depression, ***seizures,*** insomnia (Vagifem).
CV: thrombophlebitis, ***thromboembolism,*** hypertension, *edema,* ***pulmonary embolism (PE), MI.***
EENT: worsening myopia or astigmatism, intolerance of contact lenses, sinusitis (Vagifem).
GI: *nausea,* vomiting, abdominal cramps, bloating, increased appetite, ***pancreatitis,*** anorexia, gallbladder disease, dyspepsia (Vagifem).
GU: breakthrough bleeding, altered menstrual flow, dysmenorrhea, amenorrhea, ***increased risk of endometrial cancer,*** cervical erosion, abnormal Pap smear, altered cervical secretions, enlargement of uterine fibromas, vaginal candidiasis in women, testicular atrophy, impotence in men, genital pruritus, hematuria, vaginal discomfort, vaginitis (Vagifem).
Hepatic: cholestatic jaundice, ***hepatic adenoma.***
Metabolic: weight changes, hypothyroidism.
Respiratory: *upper respiratory tract infection,* allergy, bronchitis (Vagifem).
Skin: melasma, urticaria, erythema nodosum, dermatitis, hair loss, pruritus.
Other: *gynecomastia,* ***increased risk of breast cancer,*** hot flashes, pain (Vagifem), *breast tenderness, enlargement, or secretion,* flulike syndrome.

INTERACTIONS

Drug-drug. *Carbamazepine, fosphenytoin, phenobarbital, phenytoin, rifampin:* May decrease effectiveness of estrogen therapy. Monitor patient closely.
Corticosteroids: May enhance effects of corticosteroids. Monitor patient closely.
Cyclosporine: May increase risk of toxicity. Use together with caution and monitor cyclosporine level frequently.
Dantrolene, other hepatotoxic drugs: May increase risk of hepatotoxicity. Monitor liver function closely.
Oral anticoagulants: May decrease anticoagulant effect. Dosage adjustments may be needed. Monitor PT and INR.
Tamoxifen: May interfere with tamoxifen effectiveness. Avoid using together.
Drug-herb. *Black cohosh:* May increase drug's adverse effects. Discourage use together.
Saw palmetto: May negate drug's effects. Discourage use together.
St. John's wort: May decrease effects of drug. Discourage use together.
Drug-food. *Caffeine:* May increase caffeine level. Advise patient to avoid or minimize use of caffeine.
Grapefruit juice: May elevate drug level. Tell patient to take drug with liquid other than grapefruit juice.
Drug-lifestyle. *Smoking:* May increase risk of adverse CV effects. If smoking continues, may need another therapy.
Sunscreen use: May increase absorption of Estrasorb. Separate application times.

EFFECTS ON LAB TEST RESULTS

- May increase clotting factor VII, VIII, IX, and X; total T_4; thyroid-binding globulin; and triglyceride levels.
- May increase norepinephrine-induced platelet aggregation and PT.
- May decrease metyrapone test results.

CONTRAINDICATIONS & CAUTIONS

- Contraindicated in pregnant women and patients with thrombophlebitis or thromboembolic disorders, estrogen-dependent neoplasia, breast or reproductive organ cancer (except for palliative treatment), undiagnosed abnormal genital bleeding, or history of thrombophlebitis or thromboembolic disorders linked to previous estrogen use (except for palliative treatment of breast and prostate cancer).

• Contraindicated in patients with liver dysfunction or disease.
• Use cautiously in patients with cerebrovascular or coronary artery disease, asthma, bone disease, migraine, seizures, or cardiac or renal dysfunction.
• Use cautiously in women who have a strong family history (grandmother, mother, sister) of breast cancer, breast nodules, fibrocystic breasts, or abnormal mammogram findings.
• ***Alert:*** Postmenopausal women age 50 to 79 years old who are taking estrogen and progestin have an increased risk of MI, stroke, invasive breast cancer, pulmonary embolism, and thrombosis. Postmenopausal women age 65 or older also have an increased risk of dementia.

NURSING CONSIDERATIONS

• Ensure that patient has physical examination before starting therapy. Patients receiving long-term therapy should have yearly examinations. Monitor lipid levels, blood pressure, body weight, and hepatic function.
• Ask patient about allergies, especially to foods and plants. Estradiol is available as an aqueous solution or as a solution in peanut oil; estradiol cypionate, as a solution in cottonseed oil; estradiol valerate, as a solution in castor oil or sesame oil.
• To give I.M. injection, make sure drug is well dispersed by rolling vial between palms. Inject deep into large muscle. Rotate injection sites to prevent muscle atrophy. Never give drug I.V.
• Apply transdermal patch to clean, dry, hairless, intact skin on abdomen or buttock. Don't apply it to breasts, waistline, or other areas where clothing can loosen patch. When applying, ensure thorough contact between patch and skin, especially around edges, and hold in place for about 10 seconds. Apply patch immediately after opening and removing protective cover. Rotate application sites.
• ***Alert:*** EstroGel contains alcohol. Avoid fire, flame, or smoking until area dries in 2 to 5 minutes.
• In women also taking oral estrogen, treatment with the Estraderm transdermal patch can begin 1 week after withdrawal of oral therapy, or sooner if menopausal symptoms appear before the end of the week.
• Transdermal systems may be used continually rather than cyclically. Other alternative regimens are 1 to 5 mg cypionate I.M. q 3 to 4 weeks and 10 to 20 mg (valerate) I.M. q 4 weeks, p.r.n.
• Instruct patients using Vagifem who have severely atrophic vaginal mucosa to be careful when inserting the applicator. After gynecologic surgery, tell patient to use any vaginal applicator cautiously and only if clearly indicated.
• The prescriber should assess the patient's need to continue Vagifem therapy. Make attempts to stop or taper at 3- to 6-month intervals.
• Because of risk of thromboembolism, stop therapy at least 1 month before high-risk procedures or those that cause prolonged immobilization, such as knee or hip surgery.
• Glucose tolerance may be impaired. Monitor glucose level closely in patients with diabetes.
• Notify pathologist about estrogen therapy when sending specimens to laboratory for evaluation.
• Estrace may contain tartrazine.

PATIENT TEACHING

• Tell patient to read package insert describing estrogen's adverse effects and give verbal explanation.
• Emphasize importance of regular physical examinations. Postmenopausal women who use estrogen replacement for longer than 5 years may be at increased risk for endometrial cancer. Risk is reduced by using cyclic rather than continuous therapy and the lowest possible dosages of estrogen. Adding progestins to the regimen decreases risk of endometrial hyperplasia; however, it isn't known whether progestins affect risk of endometrial cancer. No increased risk of breast cancer has been reported.
• Teach woman how to use cream. She should wash vaginal area with soap and water before applying and insert cream high into the vagina (about two-thirds the length of the applicator). She should take drug at bedtime, or lie flat for 30 minutes after instillation to minimize drug loss.
• Tell patient using Estrasorb emulsion not to apply it with sunscreen.

• Tell patient to use transdermal system correctly, to rotate sites, to avoid breasts and waistline, and to reapply patch if it falls off.
• Teach patient using transdermal gel (EstroGel) to apply in a thin layer on one arm and allow to dry before smoking, nearing flames, dressing, or touching the arm. Recommend bathing prior to application to maintain full dosage.
• Tell patient to insert Vagifem by the applicator as far into vagina as it can comfortably go, without using force.
• ***Alert:*** Warn patient to immediately report abdominal pain, pressure or pain in chest, shortness of breath, severe headaches, visual disturbances, vaginal bleeding or discharge, breast lumps, swelling of hands or feet, yellow skin or sclera, dark urine, light-colored stools, and pain, numbness, or stiffness in legs or buttocks.
• Explain to patient receiving cyclic therapy for postmenopausal symptoms that withdrawal bleeding may occur during week off drug. Tell her to report unusual vaginal bleeding.
• Tell diabetic patient to report elevated glucose level so that antidiabetic dosage can be adjusted.
• Teach woman how to perform routine breast self-examination.
• Teach patient methods to decrease risk of blood clots.
• Advise woman not to become pregnant during estrogen therapy.
• Advise woman of childbearing age to consult prescriber before taking drug and to advise prescriber immediately if she becomes pregnant.
• Encourage patient to stop or reduce smoking because of the risk of CV complications.

estradiol and norethindrone acetate transdermal system
CombiPatch

Pharmacologic class: estrogen and progestin
Pregnancy risk category X

AVAILABLE FORMS
Transdermal: 9-cm² system releasing 0.05 mg estradiol and 0.14 mg norethindrone acetate daily; 16-cm² system releasing 0.05 mg estradiol and 0.25 mg norethindrone acetate daily

INDICATIONS & DOSAGES
➤ Moderate to severe vasomotor symptoms from menopause; vulval and vaginal atrophy; hypoestrogenemia from hypogonadism, castration, or primary ovarian failure in women with intact uterus
Continuous combined regimen
Women: Wear 9-cm² patch continuously on lower abdomen. Replace system twice weekly during 28-day cycle. May increase to 16-cm² patch.
Continuous sequential regimen
Women: For use in sequential regimen with an estradiol transdermal system (such as Alora, Esclim, Estraderm, Vivelle), wear 0.05-mg estradiol transdermal patch for first 14 days of 28-day cycle; replace system twice weekly. Wear 9-cm² patch system on lower abdomen for rest of 28-day cycle; replace system twice weekly. May increase to 16-cm² patch, p.r.n.

ACTION
A matrix transdermal system in which estradiol and norethindrone are released continuously. Estrogen replacement therapy can reduce menopausal symptoms and release of follicle-stimulating and luteinizing hormones in postmenopausal women.

Route	Onset	Peak	Duration
Transdermal	12–24 hr	Unknown	3–4 days

Half-life: 6 to 20 hours (estradiol); 5 to 14 hours (norethindrone).

ADVERSE REACTIONS
CNS: *asthenia,* ***stroke,*** depression, insomnia, nervousness, dizziness, *headache.*
CV: ***thromboembolism,*** thrombophlebitis, hypertension, *edema,* ***pulmonary embolism, MI.***
EENT: pharyngitis, *rhinitis, sinusitis.*
GI: *abdominal pain, diarrhea,* dyspepsia, changes in appetite, flatulence, *nausea,* constipation.
GU: *dysmenorrhea, leukorrhea, menstrual disorder,* suspicious Papanicolaou

smears, *vaginitis,* menorrhagia, vaginal hemorrhage.
Metabolic: weight changes.
Musculoskeletal: arthralgia, *back pain.*
Respiratory: *respiratory disorder,* bronchitis.
Skin: application site reactions, acne, melasma, chloasma.
Other: *accidental injury, flulike syndrome, pain, breast pain,* tooth disorder, peripheral edema, breast enlargement, infection.

INTERACTIONS

Drug-drug. *Carbamazepine, fosphenytoin, phenobarbital, phenytoin, rifampin:* May decrease estrogen therapy effectiveness. Monitor patient closely.
Corticosteroids: May enhance effects of corticosteroids. Monitor patient closely.
Cyclosporine: May increase risk of toxicity. Use together with caution; monitor cyclosporine level frequently.
Dantrolene, hepatotoxic drugs: May increase risk of hepatotoxicity. Monitor liver function closely.
Oral anticoagulants: May decrease effect of anticoagulant. May need to adjust dose. Monitor PT and INR.
Tamoxifen: May interfere with tamoxifen effectiveness. Avoid using together.
Drug-herb. *Black cohosh:* May increase adverse effects of drug. Discourage use together.
Saw palmetto: May cause antiestrogenic effects. Discourage use together.
St. John's wort: May decrease effects of drug. Discourage use together.
Drug-food. *Caffeine:* May increase caffeine level. Advise patient to avoid caffeine.
Grapefruit juice: May elevate estrogen level. Advise patient to take with liquid other than grapefruit juice.
Drug-lifestyle. *Smoking:* May increase risk of adverse CV effects. If smoking continues, may need alternative therapy.

EFFECTS ON LAB TEST RESULTS

- May increase T_3 and T_4 levels. May decrease HDL, LDL, total cholesterol, and triglyceride levels.
- May increase fibrinogen activity and platelet count. May decrease T_3 resin uptake. May alter activated PTT, INR, and platelet aggregation times.
- May reduce metyrapone test values. May alter glucose tolerance test results.

CONTRAINDICATIONS & CAUTIONS

- Contraindicated in women hypersensitive to estrogen, progestin, or any component of the patch; in pregnant women; and in patients with known or suspected breast cancer, known or suspected estrogen-dependent neoplasia, undiagnosed abnormal genital bleeding, active thrombophlebitis, thromboembolic disorders, or stroke.
- Use cautiously in breast-feeding women and in patients with impaired liver function, asthma, epilepsy, migraine, or cardiac or renal dysfunction.

NURSING CONSIDERATIONS

- Women not receiving continuous estrogen or combined estrogen and progestin therapy may start therapy at any time.
- Women receiving continuous hormone replacement therapy should complete the current cycle before starting therapy. Women commonly have withdrawal bleeding at completion of cycle; first day of withdrawal bleeding is appropriate time to start therapy.
- Store norethindrone patches in refrigerator before dispensing. Patient may then store patches at room temperature for up to 3 months.
- Reevaluate therapy at 3- to 6-month intervals.
- A combined estrogen and progestin regimen is indicated for a woman with an intact uterus. Progestins taken with estrogen significantly reduce, but don't eliminate, risk of endometrial cancer linked to use of estrogen alone.
- Blood pressure increases have been linked to estrogen use. Monitor patient's blood pressure regularly.
- Treatment of postmenopausal symptoms usually starts during menopausal stage when vasomotor symptoms occur.
- Apply patch system to a smooth (fold-free), clean, dry, nonirritated area of skin on lower abdomen, avoiding the waistline. Rotate application sites, with an interval of at least 1 week between applications to same site.

- Don't apply patch on or near breasts.
- Avoid applying to areas that may get prolonged sun exposure.
- Reapply patch, if needed, to another area of lower abdomen. If patch fails to adhere, replace with a new one.
- Monitor glucose level closely in patients with diabetes.
- ***Alert:*** Don't interchange CombiPatch with other estrogen patches. Verify therapy before application.

PATIENT TEACHING

- Teach woman how to apply patch properly. She should wear only one patch at any time during therapy. Tell her to apply patch immediately after opening protective cover.
- Tell patient an oil-based cream or lotion may help remove adhesive from the skin once patch has been removed and the area allowed to dry for 15 minutes.
- Advise woman not to use patch if she's pregnant or plans to become pregnant.
- Urge woman of childbearing age to consult prescriber before applying patch and to advise prescriber immediately if she becomes pregnant.
- Instruct patient that the continuous combined regimen may lead to irregular bleeding, particularly in the first 6 months, but that it usually decreases with time, and often stops completely.
- Tell patient that, for the continuous sequential regimen, monthly withdrawal bleeding is common.
- Advise patient to alert prescriber and remove patch at first sign of clotting disorders (thrombophlebitis, cerebrovascular disorders, and pulmonary embolism).
- Instruct patient to stop using patch and call prescriber about any loss of vision, sudden onset of protrusion of the eyeball (proptosis), double vision, or migraine.
- Encourage patient to stop or reduce smoking because of the risk of CV complications.
- Advise patient not to store patches where extreme temperatures can occur.

estrogens, conjugated (estrogenic substances, conjugated; oestrogens, conjugated)

C.E.S†, Cenestin, Premarin, Premarin Intravenous

Pharmacologic class: estrogen
Pregnancy risk category X

AVAILABLE FORMS

Injection: 25 mg/5 ml
Tablets: 0.3 mg, 0.45 mg, 0.625 mg, 0.9 mg, 1.25 mg
Vaginal cream: 0.625 mg/g

INDICATIONS & DOSAGES

➤ **Abnormal uterine bleeding (hormonal imbalance)**
Adults: 25 mg I.V. or I.M. Repeat dose in 6 to 12 hours, if necessary.

➤ **Vulvar or vaginal atrophy**
Adults: 0.5 to 2 g cream intravaginally once daily in cycles of 3 weeks on, 1 week off.

➤ **Castration and primary ovarian failure**
Adults: Initially, 1.25 mg Premarin P.O. daily in cycles of 3 weeks on, 1 week off. Adjust dose p.r.n.

➤ **Female hypogonadism**
Adults: 0.3 to 0.625 mg Premarin P.O. daily, given cyclically 3 weeks on, 1 week off.

➤ **Moderate to severe vasomotor symptoms with or without moderate to severe symptoms of vulvar and vaginal atrophy associated with menopause**
Adults: Initially, 0.3 mg Premarin P.O. daily, or cyclically 25 days on, 5 days off. Adjust dosage based on patient response.

➤ **Moderate to severe vasomotor symptoms from menopause**
Adults: 0.45 mg Cenestin P.O. daily. Adjust dose based on patient response.

➤ **Moderate to severe symptoms of vulvar and vaginal atrophy from menopause**
Adults: 0.3 mg Cenestin P.O. daily.

➤ **To prevent osteoporosis**
Adults: 0.3 mg Premarin P.O. daily, or cyclically, 25 days on, 5 days off. Adjust

dose based on response of bone mineral density testing.

➤ **Palliative treatment of inoperable prostatic cancer**

Adults: 1.25 to 2.5 mg Premarin P.O. t.i.d.

➤ **Palliative treatment of breast cancer**

Adults: 10 mg Premarin P.O. t.i.d. for at least 3 months.

I.V. ADMINISTRATION

- Reconstitute only with diluent provided. Agitate gently after adding diluent.
- Drug is compatible with normal saline, dextrose, or invert sugar solutions.
- Use reconstituted solution within a few hours. Don't use if solution darkens or precipitates.
- Give direct injection slowly to avoid flushing reaction.
- Refrigerate before reconstituting.

INCOMPATIBILITIES

Acidic solutions, ascorbic acid.

ACTION

Increases synthesis of DNA, RNA, and protein in responsive tissues. Also reduces release of follicle-stimulating and luteinizing hormones from the pituitary gland.

Route	Onset	Peak	Duration
P.O., I.V., I.M., intravaginal	Unknown	Unknown	Unknown

Half-life: Unknown.

ADVERSE REACTIONS

CNS: headache, dizziness, chorea, depression, ***stroke, seizures.***

CV: flushing with rapid I.V. administration, thrombophlebitis, ***thromboembolism,*** hypertension, *edema,* ***pulmonary embolism, MI.***

EENT: worsening myopia or astigmatism, intolerance of contact lenses.

GI: *nausea,* vomiting, abdominal cramps, bloating, anorexia, increased appetite, ***pancreatitis,*** gallbladder disease.

GU: breakthrough bleeding, altered menstrual flow, dysmenorrhea, amenorrhea, ***increased risk of endometrial cancer,*** cervical erosion, altered cervical secretions, enlargement of uterine fibromas, vaginal candidiasis, testicular atrophy, impotence.

Hepatic: cholestatic jaundice, ***hepatic adenoma.***

Metabolic: weight changes.

Skin: melasma, chloasma, urticaria, hirsutism or hair loss, erythema nodosum, dermatitis.

Other: *breast tenderness, enlargement, or secretion, gynecomastia,* ***increased risk of breast cancer.***

INTERACTIONS

Drug-drug. *Carbamazepine, fosphenytoin, phenobarbital, phenytoin, rifampin:* May decrease effectiveness of estrogen therapy. Monitor patient closely.

Corticosteroids: May enhance corticosteroid effects. Monitor patient closely.

Cyclosporine: May increase risk of toxicity. Use together with caution, and monitor cyclosporine level frequently.

Dantrolene, other hepatotoxic drugs: May increase risk of hepatotoxicity. Monitor liver function closely.

Oral anticoagulants: May decrease anticoagulant effects. May need to adjust dosage. Monitor PT and INR.

Tamoxifen: May interfere with tamoxifen effectiveness. Avoid using together.

Drug-herb. *Black cohosh:* May increase adverse effects of drug. Discourage use together.

Red clover: May interfere with hormonal therapies. Discourage use together.

Saw palmetto: May have antiestrogenic effects. Discourage use together.

St. John's wort: May decrease effects of drug. Discourage use together.

Drug-food. *Caffeine:* May increase caffeine level. Advise caution.

Drug-lifestyle. *Smoking:* May increase risk of adverse CV effects. If smoking continues, recommend nonhormonal contraception.

EFFECTS ON LAB TEST RESULTS

- May increase clotting factor VII, VIII, IX, and X; total T_4; phospholipid; thyroid-binding globulin; and triglyceride levels.
- May increase norepinephrine-induced platelet aggregation and PT.
- May cause a false-positive metyrapone test result.

CONTRAINDICATIONS & CAUTIONS

- Contraindicated in pregnant patients and in patients with thrombophlebitis, thromboembolic disorders, estrogen-dependent neoplasia, breast or reproductive cancer (except for palliative treatment), or undiagnosed abnormal genital bleeding.
- Use cautiously in patients with cerebrovascular or coronary artery disease, asthma, bone disease, migraine, seizures, or cardiac, hepatic, or renal dysfunction.
- Use cautiously in women who have a strong family history (mother, grandmother, sister) of breast or genital tract cancer, breast nodules, fibrocystic breasts, or abnormal mammogram findings.

NURSING CONSIDERATIONS

- Make sure patient has thorough physical exam before starting therapy, and patients receiving long-term therapy should have yearly exams. Periodically monitor lipid levels, blood pressure, body weight, and hepatic function.
- Rapid treatment of dysfunctional uterine bleeding or reduction of surgical bleeding usually requires delivery by I.V. or I.M. route.
- ***Alert:*** Don't use to prevent CV disease. In postmenopausal women receiving therapy for more than 5 years, drugs may increase risks of MI, stroke, invasive breast cancer, pulmonary emboli, and deep vein thrombosis. Use the lowest effective doses for the shortest time, considering the benefits and risks.
- ***Alert:*** In postmenopausal women receiving therapy for more than 5 years, drug may increase risk of endometrial cancer. Cyclic therapy and the lowest possible dose reduces risk. Adding progestins decreases risk of endometrial hyperplasia; but it's unknown whether they affect risk of endometrial cancer.
- When giving by I.M. injection, inject deep into large muscle. Rotate injection sites to prevent muscle atrophy.
- When used solely for the treatment of vulval and vaginal atrophy, topical products should be considered.
- Notify pathologist about estrogen therapy when sending specimens to laboratory for evaluation.
- Because of thromboembolism risk, stop therapy at least 1 month before procedures that prolong immobilization or raise the risk of thromboembolism, such as knee or hip surgery.
- Glucose tolerance may be impaired. Monitor glucose level closely in patients with diabetes.
- ***Look alike–sound alike:*** Don't confuse Premarin with Primaxin.

PATIENT TEACHING

- Tell patient to read package insert describing estrogen's adverse effects and to explain them back to you.
- Emphasize importance of regular physical exams.
- Teach woman how to use vaginal cream. Patient should wash the vaginal area with soap and water, insert about two-thirds the length of the applicator into the vagina, and release drug. Tell her to use drug at bedtime or to lie flat for 30 minutes after use to minimize drug loss.
- Explain to patient that cyclic therapy for postmenopausal symptoms may cause withdrawal bleeding during week off drug. Tell her to report unusual vaginal bleeding.
- ***Alert:*** Warn patient to immediately report abdominal pain; pain, numbness, or stiffness in legs or buttocks; pressure or pain in chest; shortness of breath; severe headaches; visual disturbances, such as blind spots, flashing lights, or blurriness; vaginal bleeding or discharge; breast lumps; swelling of hands or feet; yellow skin or sclera; dark urine; and light-colored stools.
- Tell diabetic patient to report elevated glucose level so that antidiabetic dosage can be adjusted.
- Teach woman how to perform routine breast self-examination.
- Advise woman not to become pregnant during estrogen therapy.
- Advise woman of childbearing age to consult prescriber before taking drug and to advise prescriber immediately if she becomes pregnant.
- Encourage patient to stop smoking or reduce number of cigarettes smoked because of the risk of CV complications.

estropipate (piperazine estrone sulfate)
Ogen, Ortho-Est

Pharmacologic class: estrogen
Pregnancy risk category X

AVAILABLE FORMS
Tablets: 0.75 mg, 1.5 mg, 3 mg, 6 mg
Vaginal cream: 1.5 mg/g

INDICATIONS & DOSAGES
➤ **Vulval and vaginal atrophy**
Women: 0.75 to 6 mg P.O. daily, 3 weeks on and 1 week off; or 2 to 4 g vaginal cream daily. Drug usually given on a cyclic, short-term basis but can be given continuously.
➤ **Primary ovarian failure, female castration, female hypogonadism**
Women: 1.5 to 9 mg P.O. daily for first 3 weeks; then a rest period of 8 to 10 days. If bleeding doesn't occur by end of rest period, cycle is repeated. Can be given continuously.
➤ **Vasomotor menopausal symptoms**
Women: 0.75 to 6 mg P.O. daily in cyclic method, 3 weeks on and 1 week off. Can be given continuously.
➤ **To prevent osteoporosis**
Women: 0.75 mg P.O. daily for 25 consecutive days of a 31-day cycle, followed by 6 days without drug. Repeat regimen, as indicated.

ACTION
Increases synthesis of DNA, RNA, and proteins in responsive tissues; reduces follicle-stimulating and luteinizing hormones.

Route	Onset	Peak	Duration
P.O., intravaginal	Unknown	Unknown	Unknown

Half-life: Unknown.

ADVERSE REACTIONS
CNS: depression, headache, dizziness, migraine, ***seizures, stroke.***
CV: *edema,* thrombophlebitis, ***pulmonary embolism (PE), MI, thromboembolism.***
GI: nausea, vomiting, gallbladder disease, abdominal cramps, bloating.
GU: increased size of uterine fibromas, ***endometrial cancer,*** vaginal candidiasis, cystitis-like syndrome, dysmenorrhea, amenorrhea, breakthrough bleeding, condition resembling premenstrual syndrome.
Hepatic: cholestatic jaundice, ***hepatic adenoma.***
Metabolic: weight changes.
Skin: hemorrhagic eruption, erythema nodosum, ***erythema multiforme,*** hirsutism or hair loss, melasma.
Other: breast engorgement or enlargement, ***breast cancer.***

INTERACTIONS
Drug-drug. *Carbamazepine, fosphenytoin, phenobarbital, phenytoin, rifampin:* May decrease estrogen effect. Monitor patient closely.
Corticosteroids: May enhance corticosteroid effect. Monitor patient closely.
Cyclosporine: May increase risk of toxicity. Use together with caution; frequently monitor cyclosporine level.
Dantrolene, other hepatotoxic drugs: May increase risk of hepatotoxicity. Monitor liver function closely.
Oral anticoagulants: May decrease anticoagulant effect. Dosage adjustments may be needed. Monitor PT and INR.
Tamoxifen: May interfere with tamoxifen effect. Avoid using together.
Drug-herb. *Black cohosh:* May increase adverse effects of estrogen. Discourage use together.
Red clover: May interfere with hormonal therapies. Discourage use together.
Saw palmetto: May have antiestrogenic effect. Discourage use together.
St. John's wort: May decrease estrogen effect. Discourage use together.
Drug-food. *Caffeine:* May increase caffeine level. Advise caution.
Drug-lifestyle. *Smoking:* May increase risk of adverse CV effects. If smoking continues, may need alternative therapy.

EFFECTS ON LAB TEST RESULTS
- May increase clotting factor VII, VIII, IX, and X; total T_4; phospholipid; thyroid-binding globulin; and triglyceride levels.

- May increase norepinephrine-induced platelet aggregation and PT.
- May reduce metyrapone test results.

CONTRAINDICATIONS & CAUTIONS

- Contraindicated in pregnant women and those with active thrombophlebitis, thromboembolic disorders, estrogen-dependent neoplasia, undiagnosed genital bleeding, and breast, reproductive organ, or genital cancer.
- Use cautiously in patients with cerebrovascular or coronary artery disease, asthma, mental depression, bone disease, migraine, seizures, or cardiac, hepatic, or renal dysfunction.
- Use cautiously in women who have a family history (mother, grandmother, sister) of breast or genital tract cancer, breast nodules, fibrocystic breasts, or abnormal mammogram findings.

NURSING CONSIDERATIONS

- Make sure patient has thorough physical examination before starting estrogen therapy. Patients receiving long-term therapy should have examinations yearly. Periodically monitor lipid levels, blood pressure, body weight, and hepatic function.
- ***Alert:*** Estrogens and progestins shouldn't be used to prevent CV disease. The Women's Health Initiative study reported increased risks of MI, stroke, invasive breast cancer, PE, and deep vein thrombosis in postmenopausal women during 5 years of combination therapy. Because of these risks, estrogens and progestins should be prescribed at the lowest effective doses and for the shortest duration consistent with treatment goals and risks for the individual woman.
- When used to treat hypogonadism, duration of therapy needed to produce withdrawal bleeding depends on patient's endometrial response to drug. If satisfactory withdrawal bleeding doesn't occur, an oral progestin is added to the regimen. Explain to patient that, despite return of withdrawal bleeding, pregnancy can't occur because she doesn't ovulate.
- Estropipate–estrone equivalents are:

0.75 mg estropipate = 0.625 mg estrone

1.5 mg estropipate = 1.25 mg estrone

3 mg estropipate = 2.5 mg estrone

6 mg estropipate = 5 mg estrone

- May give with meals to minimize GI upset.
- Because of risk of thromboembolism, stop therapy at least 1 month before procedures that prolong immobilization or raise the risk of thromboembolism, such as knee or hip surgery.
- Glucose tolerance may be impaired. Monitor glucose level closely in patients with diabetes.

PATIENT TEACHING

- Tell patient to read package insert describing estrogen's adverse effects; also explain effects verbally.
- Teach woman how to use vaginal cream. Patient should wash the vaginal area with soap and water and then insert vaginal cream high into the vagina (about two-thirds the length of the applicator). Tell her to use drug at bedtime or to lie flat for 30 minutes after application to minimize drug loss.
- Tell diabetic patient to report elevated glucose level to prescriber.
- Stress importance of regular physical examinations. Postmenopausal women who use estrogen replacement for longer than 5 years may have increased risk of endometrial cancer. Using cyclic therapy and lowest possible estrogen dosage reduces risk. Adding progestins to regimen decreases risk of endometrial hyperplasia; however, it isn't known whether progestins affect risk of endometrial cancer.
- ***Alert:*** Warn patient to immediately report abdominal pain; pain, stiffness, or numbness in legs or buttocks; pressure or pain in chest; shortness of breath; severe headaches; visual disturbances, such as blind spots or flashing lights; vaginal bleeding or discharge; breast lumps; swelling of hands or feet; yellow skin or sclera; dark urine; and light-colored stools.
- Teach woman how to perform routine breast self-examination.

- Advise woman not to become pregnant while on estrogen therapy.
- Encourage patient to stop or reduce smoking because of the risk of CV complications.
- Advise woman of childbearing age to consult prescriber before taking drug and to tell prescriber immediately if she becomes pregnant.

ethinyl estradiol and desogestrel

monophasic
Apri, Desogen, Ortho-Cept

biphasic
Kariva, Mircette

triphasic
Cyclessa, Velivet

ethinyl estradiol and ethynodiol diacetate

monophasic
Demulen 1/35✐, Demulen 1/50✐, Zovia 1/35E, Zovia 1/50E

ethinyl estradiol and levonorgestrel

monophasic
Alesse-21, Alesse-28, Aviane, Lessina, Levlen, Levlite, Levora-21, Levora-28, Nordette-21, Nordette-28, Portia-21, Portia-28, Seasonale

biphasic
Preven Emergency Contraceptive Kit, Seasonique

triphasic
Enpresse, Tri-Levlen, Triphasil, Trivora-28

ethinyl estradiol and norethindrone

monophasic
Brevicon, Genora 0.5/35, Genora 1/35, Junel 21-1/20, Junel 21-1.5/30, ModiCon, N.E.E. 1/35, Necon 1/35-21, Necon 1/35-28, Necon 0.5/35-21, Necon 0.5/35-28, Nelova 0.5/35E, Nelova 1/35E, Norethin 1/35E, Norinyl 1 + 35, Nortrel 0.5/35, Nortrel 1/35, Ortho-Novum 1/35, Ovcon-35, Ovcon-50

biphasic
Necon 10/11-21, Necon 10/11-28, Ortho-Novum 10/11

triphasic
Necon 7/7/7, Nortel 7/7/7, Ortho-Novum 7/7/7, Tri-Norinyl

ethinyl estradiol and norethindrone acetate

monophasic
Loestrin 1/20, Loestrin 1.5/30

triphasic
Estrostep

ethinyl estradiol and norgestimate

monophasic
MonoNessa, Ortho-Cyclen, Sprintec

triphasic
Ortho Tri-Cyclen, Ortho Tri-Cyclen Lo, Tri-Sprintec

ethinyl estradiol and norgestrel

monophasic
Cryselle, Lo/Ovral, Lo-Ogestrel, Ogestrel, Ovral

ethinyl estradiol, norethindrone acetate, and ferrous fumarate

monophasic
Loestrin Fe 1/20, Loestrin Fe 1.5/30, Microgesin Fe 1/20, Microgesin Fe 1.5/30

triphasic
Estrostep Fe

mestranol and norethindrone

monophasic
Genora 1/50, Necon 1/50-21, Necon 1/50-28, Nelova 1/50M, Norethin 1/50M, Norinyl 1+50, Ortho-Novum 1/50

Pharmacologic class: estrogenic and progestinic steroids
Pregnancy risk category X

AVAILABLE FORMS
monophasic hormonal contraceptives
ethinyl estradiol and desogestrel
Tablets: ethinyl estradiol 30 mcg and desogestrel 0.15 mg (Apri, Desogen, Ortho-Cept)
ethinyl estradiol and ethynodiol diacetate
Tablets: ethinyl estradiol 35 mcg and ethynodiol diacetate 1 mg (Demulen 1/35, Zovia 1/35E); ethinyl estradiol 50 mcg and ethynodiol diacetate 1 mg (Demulen 1/50, Zovia 1/50E)
ethinyl estradiol and levonorgestrel
Tablets: ethinyl estradiol 20 mcg and levonorgestrel 0.1 mg (Alesse-21, Alesse-28, Aviane, Lessina); ethinyl estradiol 30 mcg and levonorgestrel 0.15 mg (Levlen, Levlite, Levora, Nordette-21, Nordette-28, Portia, Seasonale); ethinyl estradiol 30 mcg and 0.15 mg levonorgestrel (84 tablets), and 10 mcg ethinyl estradiol (7 tablets) (Seasonique)
ethinyl estradiol and norethindrone
Tablets: ethinyl estradiol 35 mcg and norethindrone 0.4 mg (Ovcon-35); ethinyl estradiol 35 mcg and norethindrone 0.5 mg (Brevicon, Genora 0.5/35, Modi-Con, Necon 0.5/35-21, Necon 0.5/35-28, Nelova 0.5/35E, Nortel 0.5/35-28); ethinyl estradiol 35 mcg and norethindrone 1 mg (Genora 1/35, N.E.E. 1/35, Necon 1/35-21, Necon 1/35-28, Nelova 1/35E, Norethin 1/35E, Norinyl 1+35, Nortel 1/35-21, Ortho-Novum 1/35); ethinyl estradiol 50 mcg and norethindrone 1 mg (Ovcon-50)
ethinyl estradiol and norethindrone acetate
Tablets: ethinyl estradiol 20 mcg and norethindrone acetate 1 mg (Loestrin 1/20); ethinyl estradiol 30 mcg and norethindrone acetate 1.5 mg (Loestrin 1.5/30)
ethinyl estradiol and norgestimate
Tablets: ethinyl estradiol 35 mcg and norgestimate 0.25 mg (MonoNessa, Ortho-Cyclen, Sprintec)
ethinyl estradiol and norgestrel
Tablets: ethinyl estradiol 30 mcg and norgestrel 0.3 mg (Cryselle, Lo/Ovral, Lo-Ogestrel); ethinyl estradiol 50 mcg and norgestrel 0.5 mg (Ogestrel, Ovral)
ethinyl estradiol, norethindrone acetate, and ferrous fumarate
Tablets: ethinyl estradiol 20 mcg, norethindrone acetate 1 mg, and ferrous fumarate 75 mg (Loestrin Fe 1/20, Loestrin 24 Fe, Microgesin Fe 1/20); ethinyl estradiol 30 mcg, norethindrone acetate 1.5 mg, and ferrous fumarate 75 mg (Loestrin Fe 1.5/30, Microgesin Fe 1.5/30)
mestranol and norethindrone
Tablets: mestranol 50 mcg and norethindrone 1 mg (Genora 1/50, Nelova 1/50M, Norethin 1/50M, Norinyl 1/50, Ortho-Novum 1/50)
biphasic hormonal contraceptives
ethinyl estradiol and desogestrel
Tablets: ethinyl estradiol 20 mcg and desogestrel 0.15 mg (21 days), then inert tablets (2 days), then ethinyl estradiol 10 mcg (5 days) (Kariva, Mircette)
ethinyl estradiol and levonorgestrel
Tablets: ethinyl estradiol 50 mcg and levonorgestrel 0.25 mg (Preven Emergency Contraceptive Kit)
ethinyl estradiol and norethindrone
Tablets: ethinyl estradiol 35 mcg and norethindrone 0.5 mg (10 days); ethinyl estradiol 35 mcg and norethindrone 1 mg (11 days) (Necon 10/11-21, Necon 10/11-28, Ortho-Novum 10/11)
triphasic hormonal contraceptives
ethinyl estradiol and desogestrel
Tablets: 0.1 mg desogestrel with 25 mcg ethinyl estradiol (7 tablets); 0.125 mg desogestrel with 25 mcg ethinyl estradiol (7 tablets); 0.15 mg desogestrel with 25 mcg ethinyl estradiol (7 tablets) (Cyclessa, Velivet)
ethinyl estradiol and levonorgestrel
Tablets: ethinyl estradiol 30 mcg and levonorgestrel 0.05 mg (6 days); ethinyl estradiol 40 mcg and levonorgestrel 0.075 mg (5 days); ethinyl estradiol 30 mcg and levonorgestrel 0.125 mg

(10 days) (Enpresse, Tri-Levlen, Triphasil, Trivora-28)
ethinyl estradiol and norethindrone
Tablets: ethinyl estradiol 35 mcg and norethindrone 0.5 mg (7 days); ethinyl estradiol 35 mcg and norethindrone 1 mg (9 days); ethinyl estradiol 35 mcg and norethindrone 0.5 mg (5 days) (TriNorinyl); ethinyl estradiol 35 mcg and norethindrone 0.5 mg (7 days); ethinyl estradiol 35 mcg and norethindrone 0.75 mg (7 days); ethinyl estradiol 35 mcg and norethindrone 1 mg (7 days) (Necon 7/7/7, Nortel 7/7/7, Ortho-Novum 7/7/7)
ethinyl estradiol, norethindrone acetate, and ferrous fumarate
Tablets: ethinyl estradiol 20 mcg and norethindrone acetate 1 mg (5 days); ethinyl estradiol 30 mcg and norethindrone acetate 1 mg (7 days); ethinyl estradiol 35 mcg and norethindrone acetate 1 mg (9 days); and 75-mg ferrous fumarate tablets (7 days) (Estrostep Fe)
ethinyl estradiol and norgestimate
Tablets: ethinyl estradiol 25 mcg and norgestimate 0.18 mg (7 days); ethinyl estradiol 25 mcg and norgestimate 0.215 mg (7 days); ethinyl estradiol 25 mcg and norgestimate 0.25 mg (7 days) (Ortho Tri-Cyclen Lo); ethinyl estradiol 35 mcg and norgestimate 0.18 mg (7 days); ethinyl estradiol 35 mcg and norgestimate 0.215 mg (7 days); ethinyl estradiol 35 mcg and norgestimate 0.25 mg (7 days) (Ortho Tri-Cyclen, TriSprintec)

INDICATIONS & DOSAGES

➤ Contraception
Monophasic
Women: 1 tablet P.O. daily beginning on the first day of menstrual cycle or the first Sunday after menstrual cycle begins. With 20- and 21-tablet package, new cycle begins 7 days after last tablet taken. With 28-tablet package, dosage is 1 tablet daily without interruption; extra tablets taken on days 22 to 28 are placebos or contain iron. Or, for Seasonale, 1 pink tablet P.O. daily beginning on the first Sunday after menstrual cycle begins, for 84 consecutive days, followed by 7 days of white (inert) tablets.
Biphasic
Women: 1 color tablet P.O. daily for 10 days; then next color tablet for 11 days. With 21-tablet packages, new cycle begins 7 days after last tablet taken. With 28-tablet packages, dosage is 1 tablet daily without interruption. Or, for Seasonique, 1 light blue-green tablet P.O. once daily for 84 consecutive days followed by 1 yellow tablet for 7 consecutive days; then repeat cycle.
Triphasic
Women: 1 tablet P.O. daily in the sequence specified by the brand. With 21-tablet packages, new dosing cycle begins 7 days after last tablet taken. With 28-tablet packages, dosage is 1 tablet daily without interruption.

➤ To prevent pregnancy after unprotected intercourse
Women: For Preven Emergency Contraceptive Kit, 2 tablets P.O. within 72 hours of unprotected intercourse; take second dose 12 hours after the first dose.

➤ Moderate acne vulgaris in women age 15 and older who have no known contraindications to hormonal contraceptive therapy, who want oral contraception for at least 6 months, who have reached menarche, and who are unresponsive to topical antiacne drugs
Women age 15 and older: 1 tablet Ortho Tri-Cyclen P.O. daily (21 tablets contain active ingredients and 7 are inert).

ACTION

Hormonal contraceptives inhibit ovulation and also may prevent transport of the ovum (if ovulation should occur) through the fallopian tubes.

Estrogen suppresses follicle-stimulating hormone, blocking follicular development and ovulation.

Progestin suppresses luteinizing hormone so that ovulation can't occur even if the follicle develops; it also thickens cervical mucus, interfering with sperm migration, and prevents implantation of the fertilized ovum.

Route	Onset	Peak	Duration
P.O.	Unknown	½ hr–4 hr	Unknown

Half-life: 6 to 20 hours.

ADVERSE REACTIONS

CNS: *headache, dizziness,* depression, lethargy, migraine, ***stroke.***
CV: ***thromboembolism,*** hypertension, edema, ***pulmonary embolism.***
EENT: worsening myopia or astigmatism, intolerance of contact lenses, exophthalmos, diplopia.
GI: *nausea,* vomiting, abdominal cramps, bloating, anorexia, changes in appetite, gallbladder disease, ***pancreatitis.***
GU: *breakthrough bleeding, spotting,* granulomatous colitis, dysmenorrhea, amenorrhea, cervical erosion or abnormal secretions, enlargement of uterine fibromas, vaginal candidiasis.
Hepatic: cholestatic jaundice, ***liver tumors.***
Metabolic: weight gain.
Skin: rash, acne, ***erythema multiforme.***
Other: breast tenderness, enlargement, or secretion.

INTERACTIONS

Drug-drug. *Anti-infectives (chloramphenicol, griseofulvin, neomycin, nitrofurantoin, penicillins, sulfonamides, tetracyclines):* May decrease contraceptive effect. Advise patient to use another method of contraception.
Benzodiazepines: May decrease or increase benzodiazepine levels. Adjust dosage adjustment if necessary.
Beta blockers: May increase beta blocker level. Dosage adjustment may be necessary.
Carbamazepine, fosphenytoin, phenobarbital, phenytoin, rifampin: May decrease estrogen effect. Use together cautiously.
Corticosteroids: May enhance corticosteroid effect. Monitor patient closely.
Insulin, sulfonylureas: Glucose intolerance may decrease antidiabetic effects. Monitor these effects.
Nonnucleoside reverse transcriptase inhibitors, protease inhibitors: May decrease hormonal contraceptive effect. Avoid using together, if possible.
Oral anticoagulants: May decrease anticoagulant effect. Dosage adjustments may be needed. Monitor PT and INR.
Tamoxifen: May inhibit tamoxifen effect. Avoid using together.
Drug-herb. *Black cohosh:* May increase adverse effects of estrogen. Discourage use together.
Red clover: May interfere with drug. Discourage use together.
Saw palmetto: May have antiestrogenic effect. Discourage use together.
St. John's wort: May decrease drug effect because of increased hepatic metabolism. Discourage use together, or advise patient to use an additional method of contraception.
Drug-food. *Caffeine:* May increase caffeine level. Urge caution.
Grapefruit juice: May increase estrogen level. Advise patient to take with liquid other than grapefruit juice.
Drug-lifestyle. *Smoking:* May increase risk of adverse CV effects. If smoking continues, may need alternative therapy.

EFFECTS ON LAB TEST RESULTS

- May increase clotting factor II, VII, VIII, IX, X, and XII; fibrinogen; phospholipid; plasminogen; thyroid-binding globulin; total T_4; and triglyceride levels.
- May increase norepinephrine-induced platelet aggregation and PT.
- May reduce metyrapone test results. May cause false-positive result in nitroblue tetrazolium test.

CONTRAINDICATIONS & CAUTIONS

- Contraindicated in patients with thromboembolic disorders, cerebrovascular or coronary artery disease, diplopia or ocular lesions arising from ophthalmic vascular disease, classic migraine, MI, known or suspected breast cancer, known or suspected estrogen-dependent neoplasia, benign or malignant liver tumors, active liver disease or history of cholestatic jaundice with pregnancy or previous use of hormonal contraceptives, and undiagnosed abnormal vaginal bleeding.
- Contraindicated in women who are or may be pregnant or breast-feeding.
- Use cautiously in patients with hyperlipidemia, hypertension, migraines, seizure disorders, asthma, or cardiac, renal, or hepatic insufficiency.

NURSING CONSIDERATIONS

- Use estrogen-containing hormonal contraceptives cautiously in smokers.

• Triphasic hormonal contraceptives may cause fewer adverse reactions, such as breakthrough bleeding and spotting.
• The Centers for Disease Control and Prevention reports that use of hormonal contraceptives may decrease risk of ovarian and endometrial cancers and doesn't seem to increase risk of breast cancer. However, the FDA reports that hormonal contraceptives may be linked to an increase in cervical cancer.
• Monitor lipid levels, blood pressure, body weight, and hepatic function.
• ***Look alike–sound alike:*** Many hormonal contraceptives share similar names. Make sure to check the hormone strength for verification.
• Estrogens and progestins may alter glucose tolerance, thus changing dosage requirements for antidiabetics. Monitor glucose level.
• Stop hormonal contraceptives for a few weeks before adrenal function tests.
• Stop hormonal contraceptive and notify prescriber if patient develops granulomatous colitis.
• Stop drug at least 1 week before surgery to decrease risk of thromboembolism. Tell patient to use an alternative method of birth control.

PATIENT TEACHING

• Tell patient to take tablets at same time each day; nighttime doses may reduce nausea and headaches.
• Advise patient to use an additional method of birth control, such as condoms or a diaphragm with spermicide, for the first week of the first cycle.
• Tell patient that missing doses in midcycle greatly increases likelihood of pregnancy.
• Tell patient that missing a dose may cause spotting or light bleeding.
• Tell patient that hormonal contraceptives don't protect against HIV or other sexually transmitted diseases.
• Tell patient using Seasonale that there will be four planned menses per year, but spotting or bleeding between menses may occur.
• If 1 pill is missed, tell patient to take it as soon as possible (2 pills if remembered on the next day), and then to continue regular schedule. Advise an additional method of contraception for remainder of cycle. If 2 consecutive pills are missed, tell patient to take 2 pills a day for next 2 days and then resume regular schedule. Advise an additional method of contraception for the next 7 days or preferably for the remainder of cycle. If 2 consecutive pills are missed in the 3rd week or if patient misses 3 consecutive pills, tell patient to contact prescriber for instructions.
• Warn patient of common adverse effects, such as headache, nausea, dizziness, breast tenderness, spotting, and breakthrough bleeding, which usually diminish after 3 to 6 months.
• Instruct patient to weigh herself at least twice a week and to report any sudden weight gain or swelling to prescriber.
• Warn patient to avoid exposure to ultraviolet light or prolonged exposure to sunlight.
• ***Alert:*** Warn patient to immediately report abdominal pain; numbness, stiffness, or pain in legs or buttocks; pressure or pain in chest; shortness of breath; severe headache; visual disturbances such as blind spots, blurriness, or flashing lights; undiagnosed vaginal bleeding or discharge; two consecutive missed menstrual periods; lumps in the breast; swelling of hands or feet; or severe pain in the abdomen (tumor rupture in liver).
• Advise patient of increased risks created by simultaneous use of cigarettes and hormonal contraceptives.
• If one menstrual period is missed and tablets have been taken on schedule, tell patient to continue taking them. If two consecutive menstrual periods are missed, tell patient to stop drug and have pregnancy test. Progestins may cause birth defects if taken early in pregnancy.
• Advise patient not to take same drug for longer than 12 months without consulting prescriber. Stress importance of Pap tests and annual gynecologic examinations.
• Advise patient to check with prescriber about how soon pregnancy may be attempted after hormonal therapy is stopped. Many prescribers recommend that women not become pregnant within 2 months after stopping drug.
• Warn patient of possible delay in achieving pregnancy when drug is stopped.

• Teach woman how to perform routine breast self-examination.
• Teach patient methods to decrease risk of thromboembolism.
• Advise patient taking hormonal contraceptives to use additional form of birth control during concurrent treatment with certain antibiotics.
• Advise patient that hormonal contraceptives may change the fit of contact lenses.

etonogestrel and ethinyl estradiol vaginal ring
NuvaRing

Pharmacologic class: estrogenic and progestinic steroids
Pregnancy risk category X

AVAILABLE FORMS
Vaginal ring: Delivers 0.12 mg etonogestrel and 0.015 mg ethinyl estradiol daily

INDICATIONS & DOSAGES
➤ Contraception
Women: Insert one ring into the vagina and leave in place for 3 weeks. Insert new ring 1 week after the previous ring is removed.

ACTION
Suppresses gonadotropins, which inhibits ovulation, increases the viscosity of cervical mucus (decreasing the ability of sperm to enter the uterus), and alters the endometrial lining (reducing potential for implantation).

Route	Onset	Peak	Duration
Vaginal	Immediate	Unknown	Unknown

Half-life: ethinyl estradiol, 45 hours; etonogestrel, 29 hours.

ADVERSE REACTIONS
CNS: *headache,* emotional lability, ***cerebral thrombosis.***
CV: hypertension, ***thromboembolic events,*** coagulation abnormalities.
EENT: *sinusitis.*
GI: *nausea.*
GU: *vaginitis, leukorrhea,* device-related events (for example, foreign body sensation, coital difficulties, device expulsion), vaginal discomfort.
Hepatic: ***hepatic adenomas,*** benign liver tumors.
Metabolic: weight gain.
Respiratory: *upper respiratory tract infection.*

INTERACTIONS
Drug-drug. *Acetaminophen:* May decrease acetaminophen level and increase ethinyl estradiol level. Monitor patient for effects.
Ampicillin, barbiturates, carbamazepine, felbamate, griseofulvin, oxcarbazepine, phenylbutazone, phenytoin, rifampin, tetracyclines, topiramate: May decrease contraceptive effect and increase risk of pregnancy, breakthrough bleeding, or both. Tell patient to use an additional form of contraception while taking these drugs.
Ascorbic acid, atorvastatin, itraconazole: May increase ethinyl estradiol level. Monitor patient for adverse effects.
Clofibric acid, morphine, salicylic acid, temazepam: May increase clearance of these drugs. Monitor patient for effectiveness.
Cyclosporine, prednisolone, theophylline: May increase levels of these drugs. Monitor levels if appropriate and adjust dosage.
HIV protease inhibitors: May affect contraceptive effect. Refer to the specific protease inhibitor drug literature. May need to use a backup method of contraception.
Drug-herb. *St. John's wort:* May reduce drug effectiveness and increase the risk of breakthrough bleeding and pregnancy. Discourage use together.
Drug-lifestyle. *Smoking:* May increase risk of serious CV adverse effects, especially in those older than age 35 who smoke 15 or more cigarettes daily. Urge patient to avoid smoking.

EFFECTS ON LAB TEST RESULTS
• May increase clotting factor VII, VIII, IX, and X; prothrombin; thyroid-binding globulin (leading to increased circulating total thyroid hormone levels); sex hormone-binding globulin (and other binding proteins); and triglyceride levels. May decrease antithrombin III and folate levels.

• May increase norepinephrine-induced platelet aggregation. May decrease T_3 resin uptake.

CONTRAINDICATIONS & CAUTIONS

• Contraindicated in patients hypersensitive to any component of drug, patients who are or may be pregnant, patients older than age 35 who smoke 15 or more cigarettes daily, and patients with thrombophlebitis, thromboembolic disorder, history of deep vein thrombophlebitis, cerebral vascular or coronary artery disease (current or previous), valvular heart disease with complications, severe hypertension, diabetes with vascular complications, headache with focal neurologic symptoms, major surgery with prolonged immobilization, known or suspected cancer of the endometrium or breast, estrogen-dependent neoplasia, abnormal undiagnosed genital bleeding, jaundice related to pregnancy or previous use of hormonal contraceptive, active liver disease, or benign or malignant hepatic tumors.
• Use cautiously in patients with hypertension, hyperlipidemias, obesity, or diabetes.
• Use cautiously in patients with conditions that could be aggravated by fluid retention, and in patients with a history of depression.

NURSING CONSIDERATIONS

• ***Alert:*** Drug may increase the risk of MI, thromboembolism, stroke, hepatic neoplasia, and gallbladder disease.
• ***Alert:*** Cigarette smoking increases the risk of serious adverse cardiac effects. The risk increases with age and in patients who smoke 15 or more cigarettes daily.
• Stop drug at least 4 weeks before and for 2 weeks after procedures that may increase the risk of thromboembolism, and during and after prolonged immobilization.
• Stop drug and notify prescriber if patient develops unexplained partial or complete loss of vision, proptosis, diplopia, papilledema, retinal vascular lesions, migraines, depression, or jaundice.
• Monitor blood pressure closely if patient has hypertension or renal disease.
• Ring should remain in place continuously for a full 3 weeks to maintain effect. It's then removed for 1 week. During this time, withdrawal bleeding occurs (usually starting 2 or 3 days after removal). A new ring should be inserted 1 week after removal of the previous one, regardless of whether the patient is still menstruating.
• Rule out pregnancy if woman hasn't adhered to the prescribed regimen and a period is missed, if prescribed regimen has been adhered to and two periods are missed, or if the patient has retained the ring for longer than 4 weeks.

PATIENT TEACHING

• Stress importance of having regular annual physical examinations to check for adverse effects or developing contraindications.
• Tell patient that drug doesn't protect against HIV and other sexually transmitted diseases.
• Advise patient not to smoke while using contraceptive.
• Advise patient to use a backup method until ring has been used continuously for 7 days. Tell patient not to use a diaphragm if a backup method of birth control is needed.
• Tell patient who wears contact lenses to contact an ophthalmologist if vision or lens tolerance changes.
• Advise patient to follow the manufacturer's instructions for use if switching from a different form of hormonal contraceptive.
• Tell patient to insert ring into the vagina (using fingers) and keep it in place continuously for 3 weeks to maintain effect, saving the foil package for later disposal. Explain that it is then removed for 1 full week and that, during this time, withdrawal bleeding occurs (usually starting 2 or 3 days after removal). Tell patient to insert a new ring 1 week after removing the previous one, regardless of menstrual bleeding. Tell patient to reseal the ring in the package after removing it from the vagina.
• Advise patient that, if the ring is removed or expelled (such as while removing a tampon, straining, or moving bowels), it should be washed with cool to lukewarm (not hot) water and reinserted immediately. Stress that contraceptive ef-

fect may be compromised if the ring stays out for longer than 3 hours and that she should use a backup method of contraception until the newly reinserted ring is used continuously for 7 days.

medroxyprogesterone acetate

Amen, Cycrin, Depo-Provera†, Depo-subQ Provera 104, Provera

Pharmacologic class: progestin
Pregnancy risk category X

AVAILABLE FORMS

Tablets: 2.5 mg, 5 mg, 10 mg
Injection (suspension): 104 mg/0.65 ml, 150 mg/ml, 400 mg/ml

INDICATIONS & DOSAGES

➤ Abnormal uterine bleeding caused by hormonal imbalance
Women: 5 to 10 mg P.O. daily for 5 to 10 days beginning on day 16 of menstrual cycle. If patient also has received estrogen, give 10 mg P.O. daily for 10 days beginning on day 16 or 21 of cycle.
➤ Secondary amenorrhea
Women: 5 to 10 mg P.O. daily for 5 to 10 days. Start at any time during menstrual cycle (usually during latter half of cycle).
➤ Endometrial or renal cancer
Adults: 400 to 1,000 mg I.M. weekly. Dosage may be decreased to 400 mg/month when disease has stabilized.
➤ Contraception
Women: 150 mg (Depo-Provera) I.M. once q 3 months. Or, 104 mg Depo-subQ Provera subcutaneously once q. 3 months.
➤ Endometriosis
Adults: 104 mg Depo-subQ Provera subcutaneously once q 3 months. Therapy for longer than 2 years isn't recommended.

ACTION

Suppresses ovulation, possibly by inhibiting pituitary gonadotropin secretion, thus preventing follicular maturation and causing endometrial thinning.

Route	Onset	Peak	Duration
P.O.	Rapid	1 to 2 hr	3 to 5 days
I.M.	Rapid	24 hr	3 to 4 mo
SubQ	Unknown	Unknown	Unknown

Half-life: 2¼ to 9 hours P.O., 10 weeks I.M.

ADVERSE REACTIONS

CNS: depression, ***stroke,*** pain.
CV: thrombophlebitis, ***pulmonary embolism,*** edema, ***thromboembolism.***
EENT: exophthalmos, diplopia.
GI: *bloating, abdominal pain.*
GU: *breakthrough bleeding,* dysmenorrhea, *amenorrhea,* cervical erosion, abnormal secretions.
Hepatic: cholestatic jaundice.
Metabolic: weight changes.
Skin: rash, induration, sterile abscesses, acne, pruritus, melasma, alopecia, hirsutism.
Other: breast tenderness, enlargement, or secretion.

INTERACTIONS

Drug-drug. *Aminoglutethimide, carbamazepine, fosphenytoin, phenobarbital, phenytoin, rifampin:* May decrease progestin effects. Monitor patient for diminished therapeutic response. Tell patient to use a nonhormonal contraceptive during therapy with these drugs.
Drug-food. *Caffeine:* May increase caffeine level. Advise caution.
Drug-lifestyle. *Smoking:* May increase risk of adverse CV effects. If smoking continues, may need alternative therapy.

EFFECTS ON LAB TEST RESULTS

- May increase liver function test values.
- May reduce metyrapone test results. May cause abnormal thyroid function test results.

CONTRAINDICATIONS & CAUTIONS

- Contraindicated in patients hypersensitive to drug and in those with active thromboembolic disorders or history of thromboembolic disorders, cerebrovascular disease, apoplexy, breast cancer, undiagnosed abnormal vaginal bleeding, missed abortion, or hepatic dysfunction; also contraindicated during pregnancy. Tablets are contraindicated in patients with liver dysfunction or known or suspected malignant disease of genital organs.

- Use cautiously in patients with diabetes, seizures, migraine, cardiac or renal disease, asthma, or depression.

NURSING CONSIDERATIONS

- Drug shouldn't be used as test for pregnancy; it may cause birth defects and masculinization of female fetus.
- Depo-Provera and Depo-sub-Q Provera may cause a significant loss of bone mineral density.
- I.M. injection may be painful. Monitor sites for evidence of sterile abscess. Rotate injection sites to prevent muscle atrophy.
- Monitor patient for pain, swelling, warmth, or redness in calves; sudden, severe headaches; visual disturbances; numbness in extremities; signs of depression; signs of liver dysfunction (abdominal pain, dark urine, jaundice).

PATIENT TEACHING

- According to FDA regulations, patient must read package insert explaining possible adverse effects of progestins before receiving first dose. Also, give patient verbal explanation.
- Advise patient to take medication with food if GI upset occurs.
- ***Alert:*** Tell patient to report unusual symptoms immediately and to stop drug and notify prescriber about visual disturbances or migraine.
- Teach woman how to perform routine breast self-examination.
- Advise patient to immediately report to prescriber any breast abnormalities, vaginal bleeding, swelling, yellowed skin or eyes, dark urine, clay-colored stools, shortness of breath, chest pain, or pregnancy.
- Advise patient that injection must be given every 3 months to maintain adequate contraceptive effects.
- Tell woman to immediately report to prescriber a suspected pregnancy.

norelgestromin and ethinyl estradiol transdermal system

Ortho Evra

Pharmacologic class: estrogenic and progestogenic steroids
Pregnancy risk category X

AVAILABLE FORMS

Transdermal patch: norelgestromin 6 mg and ethinyl estradiol 0.75 mg per patch, delivering 150 mcg norelgestromin and 20 mcg ethinyl estradiol daily

INDICATIONS & DOSAGES

➤ Contraception

Women: Apply 1 patch weekly for 3 weeks. Apply each new patch on the same day of the week. Week 4 is patch free. On the day after week 4 ends, apply a new patch to start a new 4-week cycle. The patch-free interval between cycles should never be longer than 7 days.

ACTION

Combination hormonal contraceptives act by suppressing gonadotropins. The primary mechanism of this action is ovulation inhibition. However, changes in cervical mucus increase the difficulty of sperm entry into the uterus, and changes in the endometrium decrease the likelihood of implantation.

Route	Onset	Peak	Duration
Transdermal	Rapid	2 days	Unknown

Half-life: ethinyl estradiol, 6 to 45 hours; norelgestromin, 28 hours.

ADVERSE REACTIONS

CNS: *headache,* emotional lability.
CV: ***thromboembolic events, MI,*** hypertension, edema, ***cerebral hemorrhage.***
EENT: contact lens intolerance.
GI: *nausea, abdominal pain,* vomiting, gallbladder disease.
GU: *menstrual cramps,* changes in menstrual flow, vaginal candidiasis.
Hepatic: ***hepatic adenomas,*** benign liver tumors.
Metabolic: weight changes.
Respiratory: *upper respiratory tract infection.*

Skin: *application site reaction.*
Other: *breast tenderness, enlargement, or secretion.*

INTERACTIONS

Drug-drug. *Acetaminophen, clofibric acid, morphine, salicylic acid, temazepam:* May decrease levels or increase clearance of these drugs. Monitor patient for lack of effect.
Ampicillin, barbiturates, carbamazepine, felbamate, griseofulvin, oxcarbazepine, phenylbutazone, phenytoin, rifampin, tetracyclines, topiramate: May reduce contraceptive effectiveness, resulting in unintended pregnancy or breakthrough bleeding. Encourage backup method of contraception if used together.
Ascorbic acid, atorvastatin, itraconazole, ketoconazole: May increase hormone levels. Use together cautiously.
Cyclosporine, prednisolone, theophylline: May increase levels of these drugs. Monitor patient for adverse reactions.
HIV protease inhibitors: May affect contraceptive effectiveness and safety. Use together cautiously.
Drug-herb. *St. John's wort:* May reduce effectiveness of drug and cause breakthrough bleeding. Discourage use together.
Drug-lifestyle. *Smoking:* May increase risk of CV adverse effects, related to age and smoking 15 or more cigarettes daily. Urge patient not to smoke.

EFFECTS ON LAB TEST RESULTS

- May increase circulating total thyroid hormone, triglyceride, other binding protein, sex hormone-binding globulin, total circulating endogenous sex steroid, corticoid, and factor VII, VIII, IX, and X levels. May decrease antithrombin III and folate levels.
- May decrease free T_3 resin uptake and glucose tolerance.

CONTRAINDICATIONS & CAUTIONS

- Contraindicated in patients hypersensitive to any component of this drug and in those with past history of deep vein thrombosis or related disorder; current or past history of cerebrovascular or coronary artery disease; past or current known or suspected breast cancer, endometrial cancer or other known or suspected estrogen-dependent neoplasia; or hepatic adenoma or cancer; and in those who are or may be pregnant.
- Contraindicated in patients with thrombophlebitis, thromboembolic disorders, valvular heart disease with complications, severe hypertension, diabetes with vascular involvement, headaches with focal neurologic symptoms, major surgery with prolonged immobilization, undiagnosed abnormal genital bleeding, cholestatic jaundice of pregnancy or jaundice with previous hormonal contraceptive use, or acute or chronic hepatocellular disease with abnormal liver function.
- Use cautiously in patients with CV disease risk factors, with conditions that might be aggravated by fluid retention, or with a history of depression.

NURSING CONSIDERATIONS

- ***Alert:*** Patients taking combination hormonal contraceptives may be at increased risk for thrombophlebitis, venous thrombosis with or without embolism, pulmonary embolism, MI, cerebral hemorrhage, cerebral thrombosis, hypertension, gallbladder disease, hepatic adenomas, benign liver tumors, mesenteric thrombosis, and retinal thrombosis.
- Increased risk of MI occurs primarily in smokers and women with hypertension, hypercholesterolemia, morbid obesity, and diabetes.
- Encourage women with a history of hypertension or renal disease to use a different contraceptive. If this drug is used, monitor blood pressure closely and stop use if hypertension occurs.
- Drug may be less effective in women who weigh 90 kg (198 lb) or more.
- Cigarette smoking increases the risk of serious adverse cardiac effects. The risk increases with age and in those who smoke 15 or more cigarettes daily.
- The risk of thromboembolic disease increases if therapy is used postpartum or postabortion.
- Rule out pregnancy if withdrawal bleeding fails to occur for two consecutive cycles.
- If skin becomes irritated, the patch may be removed and a new patch applied at a different site.

• Stop drug and notify prescriber at least 4 weeks before and for 2 weeks after an elective surgery that increases the risk of thromboembolism, and during and after prolonged immobilization.
• Stop drug and notify prescriber if patient has headaches, vision loss, proptosis, diplopia, papilledema, retinal vascular lesions, jaundice, or depression.

PATIENT TEACHING
• Emphasize the importance of having regular annual physical examinations to check for adverse effects or developing contraindications.
• Tell patient that drug doesn't protect against HIV and other sexually transmitted diseases.
• Advise woman to apply patch on the first day of menstrual cycle or the first Sunday of menstrual cycle.
• Advise patient to use a backup method of contraception for the first 7 days.
• Tell patient switching from estrogen-progestin oral contraceptives to apply first patch on the first day of withdrawal bleeding. If no bleeding within 5 days of last hormonally active pill, advise patient to obtain a pregnancy test.
• Advise patient to immediately apply a new patch once the used patch is removed, on the same day of the week every 7 days for 3 weeks. Week 4 is patch free. Bleeding is expected to occur during this time.
• Tell patient to apply each patch to a clean, dry area of the skin on the buttocks, abdomen, upper outer arm, or upper torso. Tell patient not to apply to the breasts or to skin that is red, irritated, or cut.
• Tell patient to carefully fold the used patch in half so that it sticks to itself, before discarding.
• Tell woman to immediately stop use if pregnancy is confirmed.
• Tell patient who wears contact lenses to report visual changes or changes in lens tolerance.
• Advise patient not to smoke while using the patch.
• Stress that if woman isn't sure what to do about mistakes with patch use, she should use a backup method of birth control and contact her health care provider.

norethindrone
Camila, Errin, Jolivette, Micronor, Nora-BE, Nor-QD

norethindrone acetate
Aygestin

Pharmacologic class: progestin
Pregnancy risk category X

AVAILABLE FORMS
norethindrone
Tablets: 0.35 mg
norethindrone acetate
Tablets: 5 mg

INDICATIONS & DOSAGES
➤ **Amenorrhea, abnormal uterine bleeding**
Women: 2.5 to 10 mg norethindrone acetate P.O. daily for 5 to 10 days, beginning in the assumed latter half of the menstrual cycle.
➤ **Endometriosis**
Women: 5 mg norethindrone acetate P.O. daily for 14 days; then increased by 2.5 mg daily q 2 weeks, up to 15 mg daily.
➤ **Contraception**
Women: Initially, 0.35 mg norethindrone P.O. on first day of menstruation; then 0.35 mg daily.

ACTION
Suppresses ovulation, possibly by inhibiting pituitary gonadotropin secretion, and forms thick cervical mucus.

Route	Onset	Peak	Duration
P.O.	Unknown	Unknown	Unknown

Half-life: 5 to 14 hours.

ADVERSE REACTIONS
CNS: depression, ***stroke.***
CV: thrombophlebitis, ***pulmonary embolism,*** edema, ***thromboembolism.***
EENT: exophthalmos, diplopia.
GI: *bloating, abdominal pain or cramping.*
GU: *breakthrough bleeding,* dysmenorrhea, *amenorrhea,* cervical erosion, abnormal secretions.
Hepatic: cholestatic jaundice.
Metabolic: weight changes.

Skin: melasma, rash, acne, pruritus, alopecia, hirsutism, hemorrhagic skin eruptions.
Other: breast tenderness, enlargement, or secretion, premenstrual-like syndrome.

INTERACTIONS

Drug-drug. *Barbiturates, carbamazepine, fosphenytoin, phenytoin, rifampin:* May decrease progestin effects. Monitor patient for diminished therapeutic response.
Drug-food. *Caffeine:* May increase caffeine level. Urge caution.
Drug-lifestyle. *Smoking:* May increase risk of adverse CV effects. If smoking continues, may need alternative therapy.

EFFECTS ON LAB TEST RESULTS

- May increase liver function test values.
- May decrease metyrapone test results.

CONTRAINDICATIONS & CAUTIONS

- Contraindicated in pregnant women, patients hypersensitive to drug, and patients with breast cancer, undiagnosed abnormal vaginal bleeding, severe hepatic disease, missed abortion, or current or previous thromboembolic disorders.
- Use cautiously in patients with diabetes, seizures, migraines, cardiac or renal disease, asthma, and depression.

NURSING CONSIDERATIONS

- If switching from combined oral contraceptives to progestin-only pills (POPs), take the first POP the day after the last active combined pill.
- If switching from POPs to combined pills, take the first active combined pill on the first day of menstruation, even if the POP pack isn't finished.
- Norethindrone acetate is twice as potent as norethindrone. Norethindrone acetate shouldn't be used for contraception.
- Patients with menstrual disorders usually need preliminary estrogen treatment.
- Watch patient closely for signs of edema.
- Monitor blood pressure.
- ***Look alike–sound alike:*** Don't confuse Micronor with Micro K or Micronase.

PATIENT TEACHING

- According to FDA regulations, patient must read package insert explaining possible adverse effects before receiving first dose. Also, give patient verbal explanation.
- Tell patient to take drug at the same time every day when used as a contraceptive. If she is more than 3 hours late taking the pill or if she has missed a pill, she should take the pill as soon as she remembers, and then continue the normal schedule. Also tell her to use a backup method of contraception for the next 48 hours.
- ***Alert:*** Tell patient to report unusual symptoms immediately and to stop drug and notify prescriber about visual disturbances or migraine.
- Teach woman how to perform routine breast self-examination.
- Tell woman to report suspected pregnancy to prescriber.
- Encourage patient to stop or reduce smoking because of the risk of CV complications.

54

Gonadotropins

cetrorelix acetate
menotropins

cetrorelix acetate

Cetrotide

Pharmacologic class: gonadotropin-releasing hormone (GnRH) antagonist
Pregnancy risk category X

AVAILABLE FORMS

Powder for injection: 0.25 mg, 3 mg

INDICATIONS & DOSAGES

➤ To inhibit premature luteinizing hormone (LH) surges in women undergoing controlled ovarian stimulation

Women: 3 mg subcutaneously once during early to middle follicular phase, given when estradiol level indicates an appropriate stimulation response, usually on stimulation day 7 (range, days 5 to 9). If human chorionic gonadotropin (hCG) hasn't been given within 4 days after injection, give drug 0.25 mg subcutaneously once daily until the day of hCG administration. Or, give 0.25-mg multiple-dose regimen subcutaneously on stimulation day 5 (morning or evening) or day 6 (morning), and continue once daily until the day of hCG administration.

ACTION

Competes with natural GnRH for binding to membrane receptors on pituitary cells, which controls the release of LH and follicle-stimulating hormone (FSH).

Route	Onset	Peak	Duration
SubQ	1–2 hr	1–2 hr	> 4 days

Half-life: 62.8 hours (single 3-mg dose); 5 hours (single 0.25-mg dose); 20.6 hours (multiple 0.25-mg doses).

ADVERSE REACTIONS

CNS: headache.
GI: nausea.
GU: ovarian hyperstimulation syndrome.

INTERACTIONS

None reported.

EFFECTS ON LAB TEST RESULTS

- May increase alkaline phosphatase, ALT, AST, and GGT levels.

CONTRAINDICATIONS & CAUTIONS

- Contraindicated in patients hypersensitive to drug, extrinsic peptide hormones, mannitol, GnRH, or GnRH analogues.
- Contraindicated in patients with severe renal impairment.
- Contraindicated in pregnant and breast-feeding women, and in patients age 65 or older.

NURSING CONSIDERATIONS

- Rule out pregnancy before starting treatment.
- Prescriber should be experienced in fertility treatment.
- Adjust dose according to patient response.
- When ultrasound shows enough follicles of adequate size, give hCG to induce ovulation and maturation of oocytes.
- To reduce the risk of ovarian hyperstimulation syndrome, don't give hCG if ovaries show an excessive response to treatment.

PATIENT TEACHING

- Instruct patient to store 3-mg form at room temperature (77° F [25° C]) and 0.25-mg form in refrigerator (36° to 46° F [2° to 8° C]). Tell patient to keep this product away from children.
- Tell patient to report any adverse effects that become bothersome.
- Teach patient the importance of following the regimen exactly as prescribed to achieve optimal results.
- Instruct patient on proper administration technique, as follows: Wash hands thoroughly with soap and water. Flip off plastic cover of vial and wipe top with an alcohol swab. Attach needle with yellow

mark to prefilled syringe. Push needle through rubber stopper of vial and slowly inject liquid into vial. Leave syringe in place and gently swirl (don't shake) vial until solution is clear and without residue. Draw liquid from vial into syringe. If necessary, invert vial and pull needle back as far as needed to withdraw entire contents of vial. Detach needle with yellow mark from syringe and replace it with needle with gray mark. Invert syringe and push plunger until all air bubbles are gone.

- Tell patient to choose an injection site on lower abdomen, around the navel. If she receives a multiple-dose (0.25-mg) regimen, tell her to choose a different site each day to minimize local irritation. Instruct her to clean site with an alcohol swab and gently pinch a skinfold surrounding injection site. Instruct her to insert needle completely into skin at about a 45-degree angle and, once needle has been inserted completely, to release her grasp of skin. Tell her to gently pull back plunger of syringe to check for correct positioning of needle. If no blood appears, tell her to inject entire solution by slowly pushing plunger. She should then withdraw the needle and gently press an alcohol swab onto the injection site.
- If blood appears when patient pulls back on plunger, tell her to withdraw needle and gently press an alcohol swab onto injection site. Explain that she'll need to discard syringe and drug vial and repeat procedure using a new pack.
- Urge patient to use a syringe and needle only once and then to dispose of them properly, in a medical waste container, if available.

menotropins
Menopur, Repronex

Pharmacologic class: gonadotropin
Pregnancy risk category X

AVAILABLE FORMS
Injection: 75 international units of luteinizing hormone (LH) and 75 international units of follicle-stimulating hormone (FSH) activity per ampule; 150 international units of LH and 150 international units of FSH activity per ampule

INDICATIONS & DOSAGES
➤ Assisted reproductive technologies
Adults: Initially, 225 units subcutaneously (Menopur, Repronex) or I.M. (Repronex only) for patients who have received gonadotropin-releasing hormone (GnRH) agonist or antagonist pituitary suppression. Adjust dose based on ultrasound and estradiol levels not more frequently than q 2 days and not to exceed 75 to 150 units Repronex or 150 units Menopur per adjustment. Maximum daily dose is 450 units. Use for maximum of 12 days (Repronex) or 20 days (Menopur). Then, 5,000 to 10,000 units of human chorionic gonadotropin (hCG) after adequate follicular development.
➤ Infertility with oligoanovulation (Repronex)
Adults: Initially, 150 units subcutaneously or I.M. daily for 5 days in patients who have received GnRH agonist or antagonist pituitary suppression. Adjust based on response; 75 to 150 units per adjustment and not more frequently than q 2 days. Maximum daily dose is 450 units; don't use for more than 12 days. If patient response is adequate, 5,000 to 10,000 units of hCG, 1 day after the last dose. Hold hCG if estradiol level is greater than 2,000 picograms/ml.

ACTION
In women who haven't had primary ovarian failure, drug mimics FSH in inducing follicular growth and LH in aiding follicular maturation.

Route	Onset	Peak	Duration
I.M.; SubQ	9–12 days	12–18 hr	Unknown

Half-life: Menopur, 11 to 13 hours; Repronex, 54 to 60 hours.

ADVERSE REACTIONS
CNS: ***stroke,*** headache, migraine, malaise, fever, dizziness.
CV: tachycardia, venous thrombophlebitis, ***arterial occlusion, pulmonary embolism.***
GI: nausea, vomiting, diarrhea, abdominal cramps, bloating.
GU: *ovarian enlargement with pain and abdominal distention,* multiple births,

ovarian hyperstimulation syndrome, ovarian cysts, ectopic pregnancy, menstrual disorder.
Musculoskeletal: aches, back pain, joint pains.
Respiratory: ***acute respiratory distress syndrome, pulmonary infarction,*** atelectasis, dyspnea, tachypnea.
Skin: rash.
Other: *gynecomastia,* ***anaphylaxis,*** hypersensitivity reactions, injection site reaction, chills.

INTERACTIONS
None significant.

EFFECTS ON LAB TEST RESULTS
None reported.

CONTRAINDICATIONS & CAUTIONS
- Contraindicated in patients hypersensitive to drug and in those with primary ovarian failure, uncontrolled thyroid or adrenal dysfunction, pituitary tumor, abnormal uterine bleeding, uterine fibromas, ovarian cysts or enlargement not due to polycystic ovarian syndrome, sex hormone-dependent tumor of the reproductive tract (Menopur only), or any cause of infertility other than anovulation (Repronex only).
- Contraindicated in pregnant women.

NURSING CONSIDERATIONS
- Prescriber should be experienced in fertility treatment.
- Monitor woman closely to ensure adequate ovarian stimulation without hyperstimulation.
- ***Alert:*** Watch for ovarian hyperstimulation syndrome, which may rapidly progress to a life-threatening condition, characterized by dramatic increase in vascular permeability, which causes rapid accumulation of fluid in the peritoneal cavity, thorax, and pericardium. Signs and symptoms are hypovolemia, hemoconcentration, electrolyte imbalance, ascites, hemoperitoneum, pleural effusion, hydrothorax, and thromboembolism. Condition is common and severe if woman becomes pregnant.
- Refrigerate powder or store at room temperature.
- Reconstitute with 1 to 2 ml of sterile normal saline solution for injection. Use immediately.
- Rotate injection sites.

PATIENT TEACHING
- Tell woman about possibility of multiple births. (It occurs about 20% of the time.)
- In women being treated for infertility, encourage daily intercourse from day before hCG is given until ovulation occurs.
- Instruct patient to immediately report severe abdominal pain, bloating, swelling of hands or feet, nausea, vomiting, diarrhea, substantial weight gain, or shortness of breath.

55

Antidiabetics and glucagon

acarbose
chlorpropamide
exenatide
glimepiride
glipizide
glucagon
glyburide
insulin
insulin aspart injection
insulin aspart protamine suspension and insulin aspart
insulin detemir injection
insulin glargine injection
insulin glulisine injection
insulin inhalation powder
insulin lispro protamine and insulin lispro
isophane insulin suspension
isophane insulin suspension and insulin injection combinations
metformin hydrochloride
miglitol
nateglinide
pioglitazone hydrochloride
pramlintide acetate
repaglinide
rosiglitazone maleate
sitagliptin phosphate

SAFETY ALERT!

acarbose

Prandase†, Precose

Pharmacologic class: alpha-glucosidase inhibitor
Pregnancy risk category B

AVAILABLE FORMS

Tablets: 25 mg, 50 mg, 100 mg

INDICATIONS & DOSAGES

➤ **Adjunct to diet and exercise or with a sulfonylurea, metformin or insulin, to lower glucose level in patients with type 2 diabetes**

Adults: Individualized. Initially, 25 mg P.O. t.i.d. with first bite of each main meal. Adjust dosage q 4 to 8 weeks, based on 1-hour postprandial glucose level and tolerance. Maintenance dosage is 50 to 100 mg P.O. t.i.d.

Adjust-a-dose: For patients who weigh less than 60 kg (132 lb), don't exceed 50 mg P.O. t.i.d. For patients who weigh more than 60 kg, don't exceed 100 mg P.O. t.i.d.

ACTION

Delays digestion of carbohydrates, resulting in a smaller increase in glucose level after meals.

Route	Onset	Peak	Duration
P.O.	Unknown	1 hr	2–4 hr

Half-life: 2 hours.

ADVERSE REACTIONS

GI: *abdominal pain, diarrhea, flatulence.*
Metabolic: hypocalcemia.

INTERACTIONS

Drug-drug. *Calcium channel blockers, corticosteroids, estrogens, fosphenytoin, hormonal contraceptives, isoniazid, nicotinic acid, phenothiazine, phenytoin, sympathomimetics, thiazides and other diuretics, thyroid products:* May cause hyperglycemia when used together or hypoglycemia when withdrawn. Monitor glucose level.

Digestive enzyme preparations containing carbohydrate-splitting enzymes (such as amylase, pancreatin), intestinal adsorbents (such as activated charcoal): May reduce effect of acarbose. Avoid using together.

Digoxin: May reduce digoxin level. Monitor digoxin level.

EFFECTS ON LAB TEST RESULTS

• May increase ALT and AST levels. May decrease calcium, vitamin B_6, and hemoglobin levels and hematocrit.

CONTRAINDICATIONS & CAUTIONS

- Contraindicated in patients hypersensitive to drug and in those with diabetic ketoacidosis, cirrhosis, inflammatory bowel disease, colonic ulceration, renal impairment, partial intestinal obstruction, predisposition to intestinal obstruction, chronic intestinal disease with marked disorder of digestion or absorption, or conditions that may deteriorate because of increased intestinal gas formation.
- Contraindicated in pregnant or breast-feeding women and those with creatinine level greater than 2 mg/dl.
- Use cautiously in patients receiving a sulfonylurea or insulin.
- Safety and effectiveness of drug haven't been established in children.

NURSING CONSIDERATIONS

- Closely monitor patients receiving a sulfonylurea or insulin; drug may increase risk of hypoglycemia. If hypoglycemia occurs, give oral glucose (dextrose). Severe hypoglycemia may require I.V. glucose infusion or glucagon administration. Because dosage adjustments may be needed to prevent further hypoglycemia, report hypoglycemia and treatment required to prescriber.
- Insulin therapy may be needed during increased stress (infection, fever, surgery, or trauma). Monitor patient closely for hyperglycemia.
- Monitor patient's 1-hour postprandial glucose level to determine therapeutic effectiveness of drug and to identify appropriate dose. Report hyperglycemia to prescriber. Thereafter, measure glycosylated hemoglobin level every 3 months.
- Monitor transaminase level every 3 months in first year of therapy and periodically thereafter in patients receiving more than 50 mg three times a day. Report abnormalities; dosage adjustment or drug withdrawal may be needed.

PATIENT TEACHING

- Tell patient to take drug daily with first bite of each of three main meals.
- Explain that therapy relieves symptoms but doesn't cure disease.
- Stress importance of adhering to therapeutic regimen, specific diet, weight reduction, exercise, and hygiene programs. Show patient how to monitor glucose level and to recognize and treat hyperglycemia.
- Teach patient taking a sulfonylurea how to recognize hypoglycemia. Advise treating symptoms with a form of dextrose rather than with a product containing table sugar.
- Urge patient to wear or carry medical identification at all times.
- Advise patient that adverse reactions usually occur in the first few weeks of therapy and diminish over time.

SAFETY ALERT!

chlorpropamide
Apo-Chlorpropamide†, Diabinese

Pharmacologic class: sulfonylurea
Pregnancy risk category C

AVAILABLE FORMS

Tablets: 100 mg, 250 mg

INDICATIONS & DOSAGES

➤ **Adjunct to diet to lower glucose level in patients with type 2 diabetes**

Adults: Initially, 250 mg P.O. daily with breakfast. Increase first dose after 5 to 7 days because of extended duration of action; then increase q 3 to 5 days by 50 to 125 mg, if needed, to maximum of 750 mg daily. Some patients with mild diabetes respond well to 100 mg daily or less.
Patients older than age 65: Initially, 100 to 125 mg P.O. daily; then increase as with adult dose.
Adjust-a-dose: In patients with renal or hepatic impairment, use lower first doses, and increase dosage as tolerated.

➤ **To change from insulin to oral antidiabetic**

Adults: If insulin dosage is 40 units or less daily, stop insulin and start oral drug as above. If insulin dosage is more than 40 units daily, start oral drug as above with insulin reduced by 50%. Further reduce insulin dosage, according to response.

ACTION

Probably stimulates insulin release from pancreatic beta cells, reduces glucose output by the liver, increases peripheral sensitivity to insulin, and has an antidiuretic effect in patients with diabetes insipidus.

Route	Onset	Peak	Duration
P.O.	1 hr	2–4 hr	24–60 hr

Half-life: 36 hours.

ADVERSE REACTIONS

CNS: paresthesia, fatigue, dizziness, vertigo, malaise, headache.
CV: ***increased risk of CV death.***
EENT: tinnitus.
GI: nausea, heartburn, epigastric distress.
GU: tea-colored urine.
Hematologic: ***leukopenia, thrombocytopenia, aplastic anemia, agranulocytosis, pancytopenia,*** hemolytic anemia.
Hepatic: cholestatic jaundice.
Metabolic: ***prolonged hypoglycemia,*** dilutional hyponatremia.
Skin: rash, pruritus, erythema, urticaria, photosensitivity.
Other: *disulfiram-like reactions,* hypersensitivity reactions.

INTERACTIONS

Drug-drug. *Anabolic steroids, chloramphenicol, clofibrate, fluconazole, guanethidine, MAO inhibitors, miconazole, NSAIDs, probenecid,* **salicylates,** *sulfonamides:* May increase hypoglycemic activity. Monitor glucose level.
Beta blockers: May prolong hypoglycemic effect and mask symptoms of hypoglycemia. Use together cautiously.
Calcium channel blockers, Corticosteroids, glucagon, estrogen, phenothiazines, phenytoin, rifampin, sympathomimetics, thiazide diuretics: May decrease hypoglycemic response. Monitor glucose level.
Oral anticoagulants: May increase hypoglycemic activity or enhance anticoagulant effect. Monitor glucose level, PT, and INR.
Drug-herb. *Bitter melon (karela), burdock, dandelion, eucalyptus, ginkgo biloba, marshmallow:* May increase drug effects. Discourage use together.
Drug-lifestyle. *Alcohol use:* May alter glycemic control, most commonly causing hypoglycemia. May also cause a disulfiram-like reaction. Discourage use together.

EFFECTS ON LAB TEST RESULTS

- May increase alkaline phosphatase, AST, bilirubin, BUN, cholesterol, creatinine, and LDH levels. May decrease glucose, hemoglobin, and sodium levels.
- May decrease granulocyte, platelet, and WBC counts.

CONTRAINDICATIONS & CAUTIONS

- Contraindicated in pregnant or breastfeeding women, patients hypersensitive to drug, and those with type 2 diabetes complicated by ketosis, acidosis, diabetic coma, major surgery, severe infections, or severe trauma.
- Contraindicated for treating type 1 diabetes or diabetes that can be adequately controlled by diet.
- Use cautiously in patients with porphyria or impaired hepatic or renal function, or in debilitated, malnourished, or elderly patients.
- Use cautiously in patients allergic to sulfonamides.

NURSING CONSIDERATIONS

- Elderly patients may be more sensitive to therapeutic and adverse effects.
- Drug may accumulate in patients with renal insufficiency. Watch for and report signs of impending renal insufficiency, such as dysuria, anuria, and hematuria.
- ***Alert:*** Adverse effects of drug, especially hypoglycemia, may be more frequent, prolonged, or severe than with some other sulfonylureas because of drug's long duration of action. If hypoglycemia occurs, monitor patient closely for minimum of 3 to 5 days.
- Patients switching from another oral antidiabetic don't usually need a transition period.
- Patients may need hospitalization during transition from insulin to an oral antidiabetic. Monitor patient's glucose level at least three times daily before meals.

• ***Look alike–sound alike:*** Don't confuse chlorpropamide with chlorpromazine.

PATIENT TEACHING

• Teach patient about diabetes and importance of following therapeutic regimen, adhering to specific diet, losing weight, getting exercise, following personal hygiene programs, and avoiding infection. Explain how and when to monitor glucose level, and teach recognition of and intervention for both low and high glucose levels.
• Make sure patient understands that therapy relieves symptoms but doesn't cure the disease. He should also understand potential risks and advantages of taking drug and of other treatment methods.
• Advise woman planning pregnancy to consult prescriber before becoming pregnant. Insulin may be needed during pregnancy and breast-feeding.
• Tell patient not to change drug dosage without prescriber's consent and to report abnormal blood or urine glucose test results.
• Teach patient to carry candy or other simple sugars to treat mild low-glucose episodes. Patient experiencing severe episode may need hospital treatment.
• Advise patient not to take other drugs, including OTC drugs, without first checking with prescriber.
• ***Alert:*** Advise patient to avoid alcohol consumption. Signs and symptoms of chlorpropamide-alcohol flush are facial flushing, light-headedness, headache, and occasional breathlessness. Even very small amounts of alcohol can produce this reaction.
• Advise patient to carry medical identification at all times.
• ***Alert:*** Tell patient to report rash, skin eruptions, and other signs and symptoms of hypersensitivity to prescriber immediately.

SAFETY ALERT!

exenatide

Byetta

Pharmacologic class: incretin mimetic
Pregnancy risk category C

AVAILABLE FORMS

Injection: 5 mcg/dose in 1.2-ml prefilled pen (60 doses); 10 mcg/dose in 2.4-ml prefilled pen (60 doses)

INDICATIONS & DOSAGES

➤ **Adjunctive therapy to improve glycemic control in patients with type 2 diabetes who take metformin, a sulfonylurea, or both**
Adults: 5 mcg subcutaneously b.i.d. within 60 minutes before morning and evening meals. If needed, increase to 10 mcg b.i.d. after 1 month.

ACTION

Reduces fasting and postprandial glucose levels in type 2 diabetes by stimulating insulin production in response to elevated glucose levels, inhibiting glucagon release after meals, and slowing gastric emptying.

Route	Onset	Peak	Duration
SubQ	Unknown	2 hr	Unknown

Half-life: 2½ hours.

ADVERSE REACTIONS

CNS: dizziness, headache, jittery feeling.
GI: *diarrhea,* dyspepsia, *nausea, vomiting.*
Metabolic: ***hypoglycemia,*** immunogenicity.
Skin: excessive sweating.
Other: injection site reaction.

INTERACTIONS

Drug-drug. *Drugs that are rapidly absorbed:* May slow gastric emptying and reduce absorption of some oral drugs. Separate administration by 1 hour.
Oral drugs that need to maintain a threshold concentration to maintain effectiveness (antibiotics, hormonal contraceptives): May reduce rate and extent of

absorption of these drugs. Give these drugs at least 1 hour before giving exenatide.
Sulfonylureas: May increase the risk of hypoglycemia. Reduce sulfonylurea dose as needed, and monitor patient closely.

EFFECTS ON LAB TEST RESULTS
None reported.

CONTRAINDICATIONS & CAUTIONS
- Contraindicated in patients hypersensitive to drug or its components. Don't give to patients with type 1 diabetes or diabetic ketoacidosis. Avoid in patients with end-stage renal disease, creatinine clearance less than 30 ml/minute, or severe GI disease.
- Use cautiously in pregnant or breast-feeding women.

NURSING CONSIDERATIONS
- Assess GI function before and during treatment.
- Drug comes in two strengths; check cartridge carefully before use.
- Monitor glucose level regularly and glycosylated hemoglobin level periodically.
- ***Look alike–sound alike:*** Don't confuse exenatide with ezetimibe.
- Drug should be stored in refrigerator at 36° to 46° F (2° to 8° C).

PATIENT TEACHING
- Explain the risks of drug.
- Review proper use and storage of dosage pen, particularly the one-time setup for each new pen.
- Inform patient that prefilled pen doesn't include a needle; explain which needle length and gauge is appropriate.
- Instruct patient to inject drug in the thigh, abdomen, or upper arm within 60 minutes before morning and evening meals. Caution against injecting drug after a meal.
- Advise patient that drug may decrease appetite, food intake, and body weight and that these changes don't warrant a change in dosage.
- Review steps for managing hypoglycemia, especially if patient takes a sulfonylurea.
- Stress importance of proper storage (refrigerated), infection prevention, and timing of exenatide dose in relation to other oral drugs.

SAFETY ALERT!

glimepiride
Amaryl

Pharmacologic class: sulfonylurea
Pregnancy risk category C

AVAILABLE FORMS
Tablets: 1 mg, 2 mg, 4 mg

INDICATIONS & DOSAGES
➤ **Adjunct to diet and exercise to lower glucose level in patients with type 2 diabetes whose hyperglycemia can't be managed by diet and exercise alone**
Adults: Initially, 1 or 2 mg P.O. once daily with first main meal of day; usual maintenance dose is 1 to 4 mg P.O. once daily. After reaching 2 mg, dosage is increased in increments not exceeding 2 mg q 1 to 2 weeks, based on patient's glucose level response. Maximum dose is 8 mg daily.
➤ **Adjunct to diet and exercise in conjunction with insulin or metformin therapy in patients with type 2 diabetes whose hyperglycemia can't be managed with the maximum dosage of glimepiride alone**
Adults: 8 mg P.O. once daily with first main meal of day; used with low-dose insulin or metformin. Increase insulin or metformin dosage weekly, if needed, based on patient's glucose level response.
Adjust-a-dose: For patients with renal or hepatic impairment, initially, 1 mg P.O. once daily with first main meal of day; then adjust to appropriate dosage, if needed.

ACTION
Lowers glucose level, possibly by stimulating release of insulin from functioning pancreatic beta cells, and may lead to increased sensitivity of peripheral tissues to insulin.

Route	Onset	Peak	Duration
P.O.	1 hr	2–3 hr	> 24 hr

Half-life: 9 hours.

ADVERSE REACTIONS

CNS: dizziness, asthenia, headache.
EENT: changes in accommodation.
GI: nausea.
Hematologic: ***leukopenia,*** hemolytic anemia, ***agranulocytosis, thrombocytopenia, aplastic anemia, pancytopenia.***
Hepatic: cholestatic jaundice.
Metabolic: ***hypoglycemia,*** dilutional hyponatremia.
Skin: pruritus, erythema, urticaria, morbilliform or maculopapular eruptions, photosensitivity reactions.

INTERACTIONS

Drug-drug. *Beta blockers:* May mask symptoms of hypoglycemia. Monitor glucose level.
Drugs that tend to produce hyperglycemia (such as corticosteroids, estrogens, fosphenytoin, hormonal contraceptives, isoniazid, nicotinic acid, other diuretics, phenothiazines, phenytoin, thyroid products): May lead to loss of glucose control. Adjust dosage.
Insulin: May increase risk of hypoglycemia. Avoid using together.
NSAIDs, other drugs that are highly protein-bound (such as beta blockers, chloramphenicol, coumarin, MAO inhibitors, probenecid, sulfonamides): May increase hypoglycemic action of sulfonylureas such as glimepiride. Monitor glucose level carefully.
Rifamycins, thiazide diuretics: May increase risk of hyperglycemia. Monitor glucose level.
Salicylates: May increase hypoglycemic effects of sulfonylurea. Monitor glucose level.
Drug-herb. *Burdock, dandelion, eucalyptus, marshmallow:* May increase drug effects. Discourage use together.
Drug-lifestyle. *Alcohol use:* May alter glycemic control, most commonly causing hypoglycemia. May also cause disulfiram-like reaction. Discourage use together.

EFFECTS ON LAB TEST RESULTS

- May increase alkaline phosphatase, AST, BUN, and creatinine levels. May decrease glucose, hemoglobin, and sodium levels.
- May decrease granulocyte, platelet, RBC, and WBC counts.

CONTRAINDICATIONS & CAUTIONS

- Contraindicated in patients hypersensitive to drug and in those with diabetic ketoacidosis, which should be treated with insulin.
- Contraindicated in pregnant women or elderly patients and as sole therapy for type 1 diabetes.
- Contraindicated in breast-feeding women because it may cause hypoglycemia in breast-fed infants.
- Use cautiously in debilitated or malnourished patients and in those with adrenal, pituitary, hepatic, or renal insufficiency; these patients are more susceptible to the hypoglycemic action of glucose-lowering drugs.
- Use cautiously in patients allergic to sulfonamides.
- In children, safety and effectiveness haven't been established.

NURSING CONSIDERATIONS

- Glimepiride and insulin may be used together in patients who lose glucose control after first responding to therapy.
- Monitor fasting glucose level periodically to determine therapeutic response. Also monitor glycosylated hemoglobin level, usually every 3 to 6 months, to precisely assess long-term glycemic control.
- Use of oral hypoglycemics may carry higher risk of CV mortality than use of diet alone or of diet and insulin therapy.
- When changing patient from other sulfonylureas to glimepiride, a transition period isn't needed.
- ***Look alike–sound alike:*** Don't confuse glimepiride with glyburide or glipizide.

PATIENT TEACHING

- Tell patient to take drug with first meal of the day.
- Make sure patient understands that therapy relieves symptoms but doesn't cure the disease. He should also understand potential risks and advantages of taking drug and of other treatment methods.
- Stress importance of adhering to diet, weight reduction, exercise, and personal hygiene programs. Explain to patient and family how and when to monitor glucose level, and teach recognition of and intervention for signs and symptoms of high and low glucose levels.

- Advise patient to wear or carry medical identification at all times.
- Advise woman to consult prescriber before planning pregnancy. Insulin may be needed during pregnancy and breast-feeding.
- Advise patient to consult prescriber before taking any OTC products.
- Teach patient to carry candy or other simple sugars to treat mild episodes of low glucose level. Patient experiencing severe episode may need hospital treatment.
- Advise patient to avoid alcohol, which lowers glucose level.

SAFETY ALERT!

glipizide

Glucotrol, Glucotrol XL, Minidiab‡

Pharmacologic class: sulfonylurea
Pregnancy risk category C

AVAILABLE FORMS

Tablets (extended-release): 2.5 mg, 5 mg, 10 mg
Tablets (immediate-release): 5 mg, 10 mg

INDICATIONS & DOSAGES

➤ Adjunct to diet to lower glucose level in patients with type 2 (non–insulin-dependent) diabetes

Immediate-release tablets

Patients older than age 65: First dose is 2.5 mg P.O. daily.
Adults: Initially, 5 mg P.O. daily 30 minutes before breakfast. Maximum once-daily dose is 15 mg. Divide doses of more than 15 mg. Maximum daily dose is 40 mg.

Extended-release tablets

Adults: Initially, 5 mg P.O. with breakfast daily. Increase by 5 mg q 3 months, depending on level of glycemic control. Maximum daily dose is 20 mg.
Adjust-a-dose: For patients with liver disease, first dose is 2.5 mg P.O. daily.

➤ To replace insulin therapy

Adults: If insulin dosage is more than 20 units daily, start patient at usual dosage in addition to 50% of insulin. If insulin dosage is less than or equal to 20 units daily, insulin may be stopped when glipizide starts.

ACTION

Unknown. A sulfonylurea that probably stimulates insulin release from pancreatic beta cells, reduces glucose output by the liver, and increases peripheral sensitivity to insulin.

Route	Onset	Peak	Duration
P.O. (immediate-release)	15–30 min	1–3 hr	24 hr
P.O. (extended-release)	2–3 hr	6–12 hr	24 hr

Half-life: 2 to 4 hours.

ADVERSE REACTIONS

CNS: dizziness, drowsiness, headache, syncope.
GI: nausea, dyspepsia, flatulence, constipation, diarrhea.
GU: polyuria.
Hematologic: ***leukopenia,*** hemolytic anemia, ***agranulocytosis, thrombocytopenia, aplastic anemia.***
Hepatic: cholestatic jaundice.
Metabolic: ***hypoglycemia.***
Musculoskeletal: arthralgia, leg cramps.
Respiratory: rhinitis.
Skin: rash, pruritus, photosensitivity.

INTERACTIONS

Drug-drug. *Amantadine, anabolic steroids, antifungals, chloramphenicol, clofibrate, guanethidine, MAO inhibitors, probenecid,* ***salicylates,*** *sulfonamides:* May increase hypoglycemic activity. Monitor glucose level.
Beta blockers: May prolong hypoglycemic effect and mask symptoms of hypoglycemia. Use together cautiously.
Corticosteroids, glucagon, phenytoin, ***rifamycins, thiazide diuretics:*** May decrease hypoglycemic response. Monitor glucose level.
Oral anticoagulants: May increase hypoglycemic activity or enhance anticoagulant effect. Monitor glucose level, PT, and INR.
Drug-herb. *Burdock, dandelion, eucalyptus, marshmallow:* May increase drug effects. Discourage use together.
Drug-lifestyle. *Alcohol use:* May alter glycemic control, most commonly caus-

ing hypoglycemia. May cause disulfiram-like reaction. Discourage use together.

EFFECTS ON LAB TEST RESULTS
- May increase alkaline phosphatase, AST, LDH, BUN, cholesterol, and creatinine levels. May decrease glucose and hemoglobin levels.
- May decrease granulocyte, platelet, and WBC counts.

CONTRAINDICATIONS & CAUTIONS
- Contraindicated in patients hypersensitive to drug and in those with diabetic ketoacidosis with or without coma.
- Contraindicated in pregnant or breast-feeding women and as sole therapy in type 1 diabetes.
- Use cautiously in patients with renal or hepatic disease, in those allergic to sulfonamides, and in debilitated, malnourished, or elderly patients.

NURSING CONSIDERATIONS
- Give immediate-release tablet about 30 minutes before meals.
- Some patients may attain effective control on a once-daily regimen, whereas others respond better with divided dosing.
- Patient may switch from immediate-release dose to extended-release tablets at the nearest equivalent total daily dose.
- Glipizide is a second-generation sulfonylurea. The frequency of adverse reactions appears to be lower than with first-generation drugs such as chlorpropamide.
- During periods of increased stress, patient may need insulin therapy. Monitor patient closely for hyperglycemia in these situations.
- Patient switching from insulin therapy to an oral antidiabetic should check glucose level at least three times a day before meals. Patient may need hospitalization during transition.
- ***Look alike–sound alike:*** Don't confuse glipizide with glyburide or glimepiride.

PATIENT TEACHING
- Instruct patient about disease and importance of following therapeutic regimen, adhering to diet, losing weight, getting exercise, following personal hygiene programs, and avoiding infection. Explain how and when to monitor glucose level, and teach recognition of episodes of low and high glucose levels.
- Tell patient to carry candy or other simple sugars to treat mild low-glucose episodes. Patient experiencing severe episode may need hospital treatment.
- Instruct patient not to change drug dosage without prescriber's consent and to report abnormal blood or urine glucose test results.
- Tell patient not to take other drugs, including OTC drugs, without first checking with prescriber.
- Advise patient to wear or carry medical identification at all times.
- Advise woman planning pregnancy to first consult prescriber. Insulin may be needed during pregnancy and breast-feeding.
- Advise patient to avoid alcohol, which lowers glucose level.

glucagon
GlucaGen Diagnostic Kit, Glucagon Diagnostic Kit, Glucagon Emergency Kit

Pharmacologic class: antihypoglycemic
Pregnancy risk category B

AVAILABLE FORMS
Powder for injection: 1-mg (1-unit) vial

INDICATIONS & DOSAGES
➤ Hypoglycemia
Adults and children who weigh more than 20 kg (44 lb): 1 mg (1 unit) I.V., I.M., or subcutaneously.
Children who weigh 20 kg or less: 0.5 mg (0.5 units) or 20 to 30 mcg/kg I.V., I.M., or subcutaneously; maximum dose 1 mg. May repeat in 15 minutes, if needed. I.V. glucose must be given if patient fails to respond.
➤ Diagnostic aid for radiologic examination
Adults: 0.25 to 2 mg I.V. or 1 to 2 mg I.M. before radiologic examination.

I.V. ADMINISTRATION
- Reconstitute drug in 1-unit vial with 1 ml of diluent.

• Use only diluent supplied by manufacturer when preparing doses of 2 mg or less. For larger doses, dilute with sterile water for injection.
• Unstable hypoglycemic diabetic patients may not respond to glucagon; give dextrose I.V. instead.
• Store at room temperature before reconstituting. After reconstitution, use immediately.

INCOMPATIBILITIES
Sodium chloride solution, solutions with pH 3 to 9.5.

ACTION
Raises glucose level by promoting catalytic depolymerization of hepatic glycogen to glucose. Relaxes the smooth muscle of the stomach, duodenum, small bowel, and colon.

Route	Onset	Peak	Duration
I.V. (hyperglycemia)	Immediate	30 min	60–90 min
I.V. (gastric relaxation)	1 min	30 min	9–25 min
I.M.	4–10 min	13 min	12–32 min
SubQ	4–10 min	20 min	12–32 min

Half-life: 8 to 18 minutes.

ADVERSE REACTIONS
GI: nausea, vomiting.
Respiratory: ***bronchospasm, respiratory distress.***
Other: hypersensitivity reactions.

INTERACTIONS
Drug-drug. *Anticoagulants:* May enhance anticoagulant effect. Monitor prothrombin activity, and watch for signs of bleeding.

EFFECTS ON LAB TEST RESULTS
• May decrease potassium level.

CONTRAINDICATIONS & CAUTIONS
• Contraindicated in patients hypersensitive to drug and in those with pheochromocytoma.
• Use cautiously in patients with history of insulinoma or pheochromocytoma.

NURSING CONSIDERATIONS
• Use drug only in emergency situations.
• Monitor glucose level before, during, and after administration.
• ***Alert:*** Arouse patient from coma as quickly as possible, and give additional carbohydrates orally to prevent secondary hypoglycemic reactions.

PATIENT TEACHING
• Instruct patient and caregivers how to give glucagon and recognize a low glucose episode.
• Explain importance of calling prescriber at once in emergencies.
• Teach patient and caregivers how to prevent hypoglycemia.

SAFETY ALERT!

glyburide (glibenclamide)
DiaBeta✐, Euglucon†, Glynase PresTab, Micronase✐

Pharmacologic class: sulfonylurea
Pregnancy risk category B (Glynase, Micronase); C (Diabeta)

AVAILABLE FORMS
Tablets: 1.25 mg, 2.5 mg, 5 mg
Tablets (micronized): 1.5 mg, 3 mg, 4.5 mg, 6 mg

INDICATIONS & DOSAGES
➤ **Adjunct to diet to lower glucose level in patients with type 2 (non–insulin-dependent) diabetes**
Nonmicronized form
Adults: Initially, 2.5 to 5 mg P.O. once daily with breakfast or first main meal. Adjust to maintenance dose at no more than 2.5-mg increments at weekly intervals. Usual daily maintenance dose is 1.25 to 20 mg, in single dose or divided doses. Maximum daily dose is 20 mg P.O.
Micronized form
Adults: Initially, 1.5 to 3 mg daily with breakfast or first main meal. Adjust to maintenance dose at no more than 1.5-mg increments at weekly intervals. Usual daily maintenance dose is 0.75 to 12 mg. Dosages exceeding 6 mg daily may have better response with b.i.d. dosing. Maximum dose is 12 mg P.O. daily.

Adjust-a-dose: For patients who are more sensitive to antidiabetics and for those with adrenal or pituitary insufficiency, start with 1.25 mg daily. When using micronized tablets, patients who are more sensitive to antidiabetics should start with 0.75 mg daily.

➤**To replace insulin therapy**
Adults: If insulin dosage is less than 40 units/day, patient may be switched directly to glyburide when insulin is stopped. If insulin dose is less than 20 units/day, initial dose is 2.5 to 5 mg (1.5 to 3 mg micronized) P.O. daily. If insulin dose is 20 to 40 units/day, initial dose is 5 mg (3 mg micronized) P.O. daily. If insulin dosage is 40 or more units/day, initially, 5-mg (3-mg micronized) P.O. once daily in addition to 50% of insulin dose.

ACTION

Unknown. A sulfonylurea that probably stimulates insulin release from pancreatic beta cells, reduces glucose output by the liver, and increases peripheral sensitivity to insulin.

Route	Onset	Peak	Duration
P.O. (micronized)	1 hr	1 hr	12–24 hr
P.O. (nonmicronized)	2–4 hr	2–4 hr	16–24 hr

Half-life: 10 hours.

ADVERSE REACTIONS

EENT: changes in accommodation or blurred vision.
GI: nausea, epigastric fullness, heartburn.
Hematologic: ***leukopenia,*** hemolytic anemia, ***agranulocytosis, thrombocytopenia, aplastic anemia.***
Hepatic: cholestatic jaundice, ***hepatitis.***
Metabolic: ***hypoglycemia,*** hyponatremia.
Musculoskeletal: arthralgia, myalgia.
Skin: rash, pruritus, other allergic reactions.
Other: ***angioedema.***

INTERACTIONS

Drug-drug. *Anabolic steroids, chloramphenicol, clofibrate, fluoroquinolones, guanethidine, MAO inhibitors, probenecid, phenylbutazone,* **salicylates,** *sulfonamides:* May increase hypoglycemic activity. Monitor glucose level.
Beta blockers: May prolong hypoglycemic effect and mask symptoms of hypoglycemia. Use together cautiously.
Carbamazepine, corticosteroids, glucagon, ***rifamycins, thiazide diuretics:*** May decrease hypoglycemic response. Monitor glucose level.
Oral anticoagulants: May increase hypoglycemic activity or enhance anticoagulant effect. Monitor glucose level, PT, and INR.
Drug-herb. *Burdock, dandelion, eucalyptus, marshmallow:* May increase hypoglycemic effect. Discourage use together.
Drug-lifestyle. *Alcohol use:* May alter glycemic control, most commonly causing hypoglycemia. May cause disulfiram-like reaction. Discourage use together.

EFFECTS ON LAB TEST RESULTS

- May increase alkaline phosphatase, AST, ALT, bilirubin, BUN, and cholesterol levels. May decrease glucose, sodium, and hemoglobin levels.
- May decrease granulocyte, platelet, and WBC counts.

CONTRAINDICATIONS & CAUTIONS

- Contraindicated in patients hypersensitive to drug and in those with diabetic ketoacidosis with or without coma.
- Contraindicated as sole therapy for type 1 diabetes and in pregnant or breast-feeding women.
- Use cautiously in patients with hepatic or renal impairment; in debilitated, malnourished, or elderly patients; and in patients allergic to sulfonamides.

NURSING CONSIDERATIONS

- ***Alert:*** Micronized glyburide (Glynase PresTab) contains drug in a smaller particle size and isn't bioequivalent to regular glyburide tablets. In patients who have been taking Micronase or DiaBeta, adjust dosage.
- Although most patients may take drug once daily, those taking more than 10 mg daily may achieve better results with twice-daily dosage.
- Drug is a second-generation sulfonylurea. Adverse effects are less common with second-generation drugs than with

first-generation drugs such as chlorpropamide.
- During periods of increased stress, such as infection, fever, surgery, or trauma, patient may need insulin therapy. Monitor patient closely for hyperglycemia in these situations.
- Patient switching from insulin therapy to an oral antidiabetic should check glucose level at least three times a day before meals. Patient may need hospitalization during transition.
- ***Look alike–sound alike:*** Don't confuse glyburide with glimepiride or glipizide.
- DiaBeta may contain tartrazine.

PATIENT TEACHING
- Teach patient about diabetes and the importance of following therapeutic regimen, adhering to specific diet, losing weight, getting exercise, following personal hygiene programs, and avoiding infection. Explain how and when to monitor glucose level, and teach recognition of and intervention for low and high glucose levels.
- Tell patient not to change drug dosage without prescriber's consent and to report abnormal blood or urine glucose test results.
- Teach patient to carry candy or other simple sugars for mild low-glucose level. Patient experiencing severe episode may need hospital treatment.
- Advise patient not to take other drugs, including OTC drugs, without first checking with prescriber.
- Advise patient to wear or carry medical identification at all times.
- ***Alert:*** Instruct patient to report episodes of low glucose to prescriber immediately; a severely low glucose level is sometimes fatal in patients receiving as little as 2.5 to 5 mg daily.
- Advise patient to avoid alcohol, which may lower glucose level.

SAFETY ALERT!

insulin (regular)
Humulin R ◇, Humulin R Regular U-500 (concentrated), Novolin R ◇, Novolin R PenFill ◇, Novolin R Prefilled ◇

insulin (rDNA) inhalation powder
Exubera

insulin (lispro)
Humalog

insulin lispro protamine and insulin lispro
Humalog Mix 75/25

isophane insulin suspension (NPH)
Humulin N ◇, Novolin N ◇, Novolin N PenFill ◇, Novolin N Prefilled ◇

isophane insulin suspension and insulin injection combinations
Humulin 50/50 ◇, Humulin 70/30 ◇, Novolin 70/30 ◇, Novolin 70/30 PenFill ◇, Novolin 70/30 Prefilled ◇

Pharmacologic class: pancreatic hormone
Pregnancy risk category B; C (oral inhalation)

AVAILABLE FORMS
Available without a prescription
insulin (regular)
Injection (human): 100 units/ml (Humulin R, Novolin R, Novolin R PenFill, Novolin R Prefilled)
isophane insulin suspension (NPH)
Injection (human): 100 units/ml (Humulin N, Novolin N, Novolin N PenFill, Novolin N Prefilled)
isophane insulin suspension and insulin injection combinations
Injection (human): 100 units/ml (Humulin 50/50, Humulin 70/30, Novolin 70/30, Novolin 70/30 PenFill, Novolin 70/30 Prefilled)

Available by prescription only
insulin (regular)
Injection (human): 500 units/ml (Humulin R Regular U-500 [concentrated])
insulin (rDNA) inhalation powder
Dose blisters: 1 mg, 3 mg
insulin (lispro)
Injection (human): 100 units/ml (Humalog)
insulin lispro protamine and insulin lispro
Injection (human): 100 units/ml (Humalog Mix 75/25)

INDICATIONS & DOSAGES

➤ Moderate to severe diabetic ketoacidosis or hyperosmolar hyperglycemia
regular insulin
Adults older than age 20: Give loading dose of 0.15 units/kg I.V. by direct injection, followed by 0.1 unit/kg/hour as a continuous infusion. If glucose level doesn't fall by 50 mg/dl in the first hour, double the insulin infusion rate q hour until glucose level decreases steadily by 50 to 75 mg/dl. Decrease rate of insulin infusion to 0.05 to 0.1 unit/kg/hour when glucose level reaches 250 to 300 mg/dl. Start infusion of D_5W in half-normal saline solution separately from the insulin infusion when glucose level is 150 to 200 mg/dl in patients with diabetic ketoacidosis or 250 to 300 mg/dl in those with hyperosmolar hyperglycemia. Give dose of insulin subcutaneously 1 to 2 hours before stopping insulin infusion (intermediate-acting insulin is recommended).
Adults and children age 20 and younger: Loading dose isn't recommended. Begin therapy at 0.1 unit/kg/hour I.V. infusion. Once condition improves, decrease rate of insulin infusion to 0.05 unit/kg/hour. Start infusion of D_5W in half-normal saline solution separately from the insulin infusion when glucose level is 250 mg/dl.

➤ Mild diabetic ketoacidosis
regular insulin
Adults older than age 20: Give loading dose of 0.4 to 0.6 unit/kg divided in two equal parts, with half the dose given by direct I.V. injection and half given I.M. or subcutaneously. Subsequent doses can be based on 0.1 unit/kg/hour I.M. or subcutaneously.

➤ Newly diagnosed diabetes
regular insulin
Adults older than age 20: Individualize therapy. Initially, 0.5 to 1 unit/kg/day subcutaneously as part of a regimen with short-acting and long-acting insulin therapy.
Adults and children age 20 and younger: Individualize therapy. Initially, 0.1 to 0.25 unit/kg subcutaneously q 6 to 8 hours for 24 hours then adjust accordingly.

➤ Control of hyperglycemia with Humalog and longer-acting insulin in patients with type 1 diabetes
Adults: Dosage varies among patients and must be determined by prescriber familiar with patient's metabolic needs, eating habits, and other lifestyle variables. Inject subcutaneously within 15 minutes before or after a meal.

➤ Control of hyperglycemia with Humalog and sulfonylureas in patients with type 2 diabetes
Adults and children older than age 3: Dosage varies among patients and must be determined by prescriber familiar with patient's metabolic needs, eating habits, and other lifestyle variables. Inject subcutaneously within 15 minutes before or after a meal.

➤ For patients with type 1 or type 2 diabetes to control hyperglycemia with inhalation powder (Exubera)
Adults: Initially, 0.05 mg/kg Exubera oral inhalation per meal, rounded down to the nearest whole milligram. Give within 10 minutes of a meal. Adjust dosage based on patient's need and glucose response.

➤ Hyperkalemia ♦
Adults: 50 ml of dextrose 50% given over 5 minutes, followed by 5 to 10 units of regular insulin by I.V. push.

I.V. ADMINISTRATION

- Give only regular insulin I.V.
- Inject directly into vein or into a port close to I.V. access site. Intermittent infusion isn't recommended.
- For continuous infusion, dilute drug in normal saline solution and give at prescribed rate.

INCOMPATIBILITIES

Aminophylline, amobarbital, chlorothiazide, cytarabine, digoxin, diltiazem, dobutamine, dopamine, levofloxacin, methylprednisolone sodium succinate, nafcillin, norepinephrine, pentobarbital sodium, phenobarbital sodium, phenytoin sodium, ranitidine, sodium bicarbonate, thiopental.

ACTION

Increases glucose transport across muscle and fat cell membranes to reduce glucose level. Helps convert glucose to glycogen; triggers amino acid uptake and conversion to protein in muscle cells; stimulates triglyceride formation and inhibits release of free fatty acids from adipose tissue; and stimulates lipoprotein lipase activity, which converts circulating lipoproteins to fatty acids.

Route	Onset	Peak	Duration
I.V. (regular)	Immediate	Unknown	Unknown
SubQ (rapid)	½–1½ hr	2–3 hr	5–7 hr
SubQ (intermediate)	1–2½ hr	4–15 hr	24 hr
SubQ (long-acting)	4–8 hr	10–30 hr	36 hr
Oral inhalation	10–20 min	2 hr	6 hr

Half-life: About 9 minutes after I.V. use.

ADVERSE REACTIONS

EENT: blurred vision.
GI: *dry mouth.*
Metabolic: ***hypoglycemia,*** hyperglycemia, hypomagnesemia, hypokalemia.
Skin: rash, urticaria, pruritus, swelling, redness, stinging, warmth at injection site.
Respiratory: *increased cough, respiratory tract infection,* dyspnea, reduced pulmonary function.
Other: *lipoatrophy, lipohypertrophy,* ***anaphylaxis,*** hypersensitivity reactions.

INTERACTIONS

Drug-drug. *ACE inhibitors, anabolic steroids, antidiabetics, calcium, chloroquine, clofibrate, clonidine, disopyramide, fluoxetine, guanethidine, lithium,* ***MAO inhibitors,*** *mebendazole, octreotide, pentamidine, propoxyphene, pyridoxine, salicylates, sulfinpyrazone, sulfonamides, tetracyclines:* May enhance hypoglycemic effects of insulin. Monitor glucose level.
Acetazolamide, adrenocorticosteroids, albuterol, antiretrovirals, asparaginase, calcitonin, cyclophosphamide, danazol, diazoxide, diltiazem, diuretics, dobutamine, epinephrine, estrogens, ethacrynic acid, hormonal contraceptives containing estrogen, isoniazid, lithium, morphine, niacin, nicotine, phenothiazines, phenytoin, somatropin, terbutaline, thyroid hormones: May diminish insulin response. Monitor glucose level.
Bronchodilators and other inhaled drugs: May alter the absorption of inhaled insulin. Consistently time doses of other inhaled drugs with inhaled insulin, and monitor glucose level closely.
Carteolol, nadolol, pindolol, propranolol, timolol: May mask symptoms of hypoglycemia as a result of beta blockade (such as tachycardia). Use together cautiously in patients with diabetes.
Rosiglitazone: May cause fluid retention that may lead to or worsen heart failure. Monitor patient closely.
Drug-herb. *Basil, bay, bee pollen, burdock, ginseng, glucomannan, horehound, marshmallow, myrrh, sage:* May affect glycemic control. Discourage use together, and monitor glucose level carefully.
Drug-food. *Unregulated diet:* May cause hyperglycemia or hypoglycemia. Urge caution and monitor patient's diet.
Drug-lifestyle. *Alcohol use:* May cause hypoglycemic effect. Discourage use together.
Marijuana use: May increase glucose level. Inform patient of this interaction.
Smoking: May increase glucose level and decrease response to drug. Monitor glucose level.

EFFECTS ON LAB TEST RESULTS

- May decrease glucose, magnesium, and potassium levels.

CONTRAINDICATIONS & CAUTIONS

- Contraindicated in patients with history of systemic allergic reaction to pork when porcine-derived products are used or hypersensitivity to any component of preparation.
- Contraindicated during episodes of hypoglycemia.

• Inhaled form is contraindicated in patients who smoke, quit smoking within the past 6 months, have poorly controlled lung disease, or are allergic to any of its ingredients.

NURSING CONSIDERATIONS

• ***Alert:*** Regular insulin is for patients with circulatory collapse, diabetic ketoacidosis, or hyperkalemia. Don't use Humulin R (concentrated) U-500 I.V. Don't use intermediate or long-acting insulins for coma or other emergencies requiring rapid drug action. Also, ketosis-prone type 1, severely ill, and newly diagnosed diabetic patients with very high glucose levels may need hospitalization and I.V. treatment with regular fast-acting insulin.
• Injection dosage is expressed in USP units. Use only the syringes calibrated for that concentration of insulin.
• ***Alert:*** Some patients may develop insulin resistance and need large insulin doses to control symptoms of diabetes. U-500 insulin is available as Humulin R (concentrated) U-500 for such patients. Give pharmacy sufficient notice when requesting refill prescription. Never store U-500 insulin in same area with other insulin preparations because of the risk of severe overdose if accidentally given to the wrong patient.
• To mix insulin suspension, swirl vial gently or rotate between palms or between palm and thigh. Don't shake vigorously to avoid bubbling and air in syringe.
• Regular insulin may be mixed with NPH insulin in any proportion. When mixing regular insulin with NPH, always draw up regular insulin into syringe first.
• Switching from separate injections to a prepared mixture may alter patient response. When NPH is mixed with regular insulin in the same syringe, give immediately to avoid loss of potency.
• Lispro insulin may be mixed with Humulin N; give within 15 minutes before a meal to prevent a hypoglycemic reaction.
• Don't use insulin that changes color or becomes clumped or granular in appearance.
• Check expiration date on vial before using contents.
• Drug is usually given subcutaneously. To give, pinch a fold of skin with fingers at least 3 inches (7.6 cm) apart, and insert needle at a 45- to 90-degree angle.
• Press but don't rub site after injection. Rotate injection sites to avoid overuse of one area. Diabetic patients may achieve better control if injection site is rotated within same anatomic region.
• For a patient using inhaled insulin, obtain baseline and periodic pulmonary function tests. Carefully monitor glucose levels when switching from subcutaneous to inhaled insulin.
• Patients with type 1 diabetes should use inhaled form with a longer-acting insulin. Patients with type 2 diabetes may use inhaled form as monotherapy or with oral antidiabetics or longer-acting insulins.
• Monitor patient for hyperglycemia (rebound, or Somogyi effect).
• Store injectable insulin in cool area. Refrigeration is desirable but not essential, except with Humulin R (concentrated) U-500.

PATIENT TEACHING

• Make sure patient knows that drug relieves symptoms but doesn't cure disease.
• Instruct patient about the disease and importance of following therapeutic regimen, adhering to specific diet, losing weight, getting exercise, following personal hygiene program, and avoiding infection. Emphasize importance of timing injections with eating and of not skipping meals.
• Stress that accuracy of measurement is important, especially with concentrated regular insulin. A magnifying sleeve or dose magnifier may improve accuracy. Show patient and caregivers how to measure and give insulin.
• Advise patient not to change order in which insulins are mixed or model or brand of insulin, syringe, or needle. Be sure patient knows when mixing two insulins, always draw the regular into the syringe first.
• Teach patient that glucose level and urine ketone tests provide essential guides to dosage and success of therapy. It's important for patient to recognize symptoms of high and low glucose levels. Insulin-induced low glucose level is hazardous and may cause brain damage if prolonged; most adverse effects are temporary. Instruct patient on insulin peak times and their importance.

- Instruct patient on proper use of equipment for monitoring glucose level.
- Advise patient not to smoke within 30 minutes after insulin injection because smoking decreases amount of insulin absorbed subcutaneously.
- Advise patient to avoid vigorous exercise immediately after insulin injection, especially of the area where injection was given, because it increases absorption and risk of high glucose episodes.
- Teach patient to avoid alcohol because it lowers glucose level.
- Advise patient to wear or carry medical identification at all times, to carry ample insulin and syringes on trips, to keep carbohydrates (lump of sugar or candy) on hand for emergencies, and to note time zone changes for dosage schedule when traveling.
- Advise woman planning pregnancy to first consult prescriber.
- For patient using the inhaled form, make sure that he has a copy of the medication guide, detailing use, monitoring, care of the inhaler, and storage and that he understands the information.
- Advise patient to store injectable insulin at 36° to 46° F (2° to 8° C). Tell him not to freeze or expose vials to excessive heat or sunlight.

SAFETY ALERT!

insulin aspart (rDNA origin) injection
NovoLog

insulin aspart (rDNA origin) protamine suspension and insulin aspart (rDNA origin) injection
NovoLog 70/30

Pharmacologic class: human insulin analog
Pregnancy risk category C

AVAILABLE FORMS
PenFill cartridges: 3 ml
Prefilled syringes: 3 ml
Vial: 10 ml, containing 100 units of insulin aspart per ml (U-100)

INDICATIONS & DOSAGES
➤Control of hyperglycemia in patients with diabetes
NovoLog
Adults and children age 6 and older: Dosage is highly individualized. Typical daily insulin requirement is 0.5 to 1 unit/kg/day, divided in a meal-related treatment regimen. About 50% to 70% of dose is provided with NovoLog and the remainder by an intermediate- or long-acting insulin. Give 5 to 10 minutes before start of meal by subcutaneous injection in the abdominal wall, thigh, or upper arm. *External insulin infusion pumps:* initially, based on the total daily insulin dose of the previous regimen. Usually 50% of the total dose is given as meal-related boluses, and the remainder as basal infusion. Adjust dose if needed.

NovoLog may also be given as an I.V. infusion with close medical monitoring of glucose and potassium levels. Using a polypropylene bag, dilute insulin aspart to a concentration of 0.05 to 1 unit/ml in normal saline solution, D_5W, or 10% dextrose injection with 40 mEq/L of potassium chloride.
NovoLog 70/30
Adults: Dosage is individualized based on the needs of the patient. Doses are usually given twice daily within 15 minutes of meals.
➤Monotherapy in patients with type 1 or type 2 diabetes mellitus
Adults: 0.4 to 0.6 units/kg NovoLog 70/30 daily in two divided doses before the morning and evening meals. Adjust in increments of 2 to 4 units q 3 to 4 days, as needed. When used in combination with oral antidiabetics, initial dose is 0.2 to 0.3 units/kg daily.

ACTION
Regulates glucose metabolism. It has the same glucose-lowering effect as regular human insulin, but its effect is more rapid and of shorter duration.

Route	Onset	Peak	Duration
SubQ	15 min	1–3 hr	3–5 hr
SubQ (70/30)	Rapid	1–4 hr	≤ 24 hr

Half-life: 81 minutes.

ADVERSE REACTIONS

Metabolic: ***hypoglycemia,*** hypokalemia.
Skin: injection site reactions, lipodystrophy, pruritus, rash.
Other: ***allergic reactions.***

INTERACTIONS

Drug-drug. *ACE inhibitors, disopyramide, fibrates, fluoxetine, oral antidiabetics, propoxyphene, salicylates, somatostatin analogue (octreotide), sulfonamide antibiotics:* May enhance the glucose-lowering effect of insulin and potentiate hypoglycemia. Monitor glucose level, and watch for signs and symptoms of hypoglycemia. May need insulin dose adjustment.
Beta blockers, clonidine: May increase or decrease the glucose-lowering effect of insulin and cause hypoglycemia or hyperglycemia. May reduce or mask symptoms of hypoglycemia. Monitor glucose level.
Corticosteroids, danazol, diuretics, estrogens, isoniazid, niacin, phenothiazine derivatives, progestins (as in hormonal contraceptives), somatropin, sympathomimetics (epinephrine, salbutamol, terbutaline), thyroid hormones: May decrease the glucose-lowering effect of insulin and cause hyperglycemia. Monitor glucose level. May require insulin dose adjustment.
Crystalline zinc preparations: May be incompatible with NovoLog. Don't mix together.
Guanethidine, reserpine: May reduce or mask symptoms of hypoglycemia. Monitor glucose level.
Lithium salts, pentamidine: May increase or decrease glucose-lowering effect of insulin and may cause hypoglycemia or hyperglycemia. Pentamidine may cause hypoglycemia, sometimes followed by hyperglycemia. Monitor glucose level.
MAO inhibitors: May increase insulin's effects. Monitor patient and glucose level closely.
Drug-herb. *Burdock, dandelion, eucalyptus, marshmallow:* May increase drug's effects. Discourage use together.
Drug-lifestyle. *Alcohol use:* May increase or decrease drug effect, causing hypoglycemia or hyperglycemia. Advise patient to monitor glucose level.
Exercise: May alter the need for drug, requiring dose adjustment. Advise patient to report changes in physical activity.
Marijuana use: May increase glucose level. Inform patient of this interaction.
Smoking: May increase glucose level and decrease response to insulin. Monitor glucose level.

EFFECTS ON LAB TEST RESULTS

- May decrease glucose and potassium levels.

CONTRAINDICATIONS & CAUTIONS

- Contraindicated during episodes of hypoglycemia and in patients hypersensitive to NovoLog or one of its components.
- Use cautiously in patients susceptible to hypoglycemia and hypokalemia, such as those who have autonomic neuropathy or are fasting, taking potassium-lowering drugs, or taking drugs sensitive to potassium level.

NURSING CONSIDERATIONS

- Give NovoLog 5 to 10 minutes before the start of a meal. Give NovoLog 70/30 up to 15 minutes before the start of a meal. Because of its rapid onset of action and short duration of action, patients also may need longer-acting insulins to prevent hyperglycemia.
- Let insulin warm to room temperature before giving to minimize discomfort. Then give by subcutaneous injection into the abdominal wall, thigh, or upper arm. Rotate sites to minimize lipodystrophies.
- The time course of NovoLog action may vary among people or at different times in the same person and depends on the site of injection, blood supply, temperature, and physical activity.
- Adjustments in the dose of NovoLog or of any insulin may be needed with changes in physical activity or meal routine. Insulin requirements also may be altered during emotional disturbances, illness, or other stresses.
- When giving and mixing NovoLog with NPH human insulin, draw up NovoLog into syringe first and give immediately after dose is drawn up.
- Adjust dose regularly, according to patient's glucose measurements. Monitor glucose level regularly.

• Store drug between 36° and 46° F (2° and 8° C). Don't freeze. Don't expose vials to excessive heat or sunlight. Opened vials of NovoLog 70/30 and opened vials and cartridges of NovoLog are stable at room temperature for 28 days. Punctured cartridges of NovoLog 70/30 may be stored at room temperature up to 14 days; don't refrigerate punctured NovoLog 70/30 cartridges.
• ***Look alike–sound alike:*** Don't confuse NovoLog 70/30 with Novolin 70/30.
• Periodically monitor glycosylated hemoglobin level.
• Assess patient for rash (including pruritus) over whole body, shortness of breath, wheezing, hypotension, rapid pulse, or sweating, which may signify a generalized allergy to insulin. Severe cases, including anaphylactic reactions, may be life-threatening.
• Patients with renal dysfunction and hepatic impairment may need close glucose monitoring and dose adjustments of NovoLog.
• Observe injection sites for reactions, such as redness, swelling, itching, or burning. These reactions should resolve within a few days to a few weeks.
• ***Alert:*** Don't give 70/30 form I.V.
• Assess patient and notify prescriber for signs and symptoms of hypoglycemia (sweating, shaking, trembling, confusion, headache, irritability, hunger, rapid pulse, nausea) and hyperglycemia (drowsiness, fruity breath odor, frequent urination, thirst).
• Symptoms of hypoglycemia may occur in patients with diabetes, regardless of glucose value.
• Patients with long duration of diabetes, diabetic nerve disease, or intensified diabetes control may have different or less-pronounced early warning symptoms of hypoglycemia; severe hypoglycemia may occur in such patients with virtually no warning.
• Inspect insulin vials before use. NovoLog is a clear, colorless solution. It should never contain particulate matter or appear cloudy, viscous, or discolored. NovoLog 70/30 should appear uniformly white and cloudy and should never contain particulate matter or be discolored.

For external pump use with NovoLog
• Monitor patient with an external insulin pump for erythematous, pruritic, or thickened skin at injection site.
• ***Alert:*** Pump or infusion set malfunctions or insulin degradation can lead to hyperglycemia and ketosis in a short time because there is a subcutaneous depot of fast-acting insulin.
• Don't dilute or mix insulin aspart with any other insulin when using an external insulin pump.
• Teach patient how to properly use the external insulin pump.
• Insulin aspart is recommended for use with Disetronic H-TRON plus V100 with Disetronic 3.15 plastic cartridges and Classic or Tender infusion sets, Polyfin or Sof-set infusion sets, and MiniMed Models 505, 506, and 507 with MiniMed 3-ml syringes.
• Replace infusion sets, insulin aspart in the reservoir, and choose a new infusion site every 48 hours or less to avoid insulin degradation and infusion set malfunction.
• Discard insulin exposed to temperatures higher than 98.6° F (37° C). The temperature of the insulin may exceed ambient temperature when the pump housing, cover, tubing, or sport case is exposed to sunlight or radiant heat.

PATIENT TEACHING

• Tell patient not to stop insulin therapy without medical approval.
• Advise patient of the warning signs of low glucose level (shaking, sweating, moodiness, irritability, confusion, or agitation). Tell patient to carry sugar (candy, sugar packets) to counteract low glucose level.
• Instruct patient, to roll the cartridge or pen between his palms 10 times before inserting the Novolog Penfill cartridge into a compatible delivery device or using the Novolog FlexPen. Then, to turn the device upside down so the glass ball inside the cartridge or pen travels the length of the cartridge and to repeat this rolling and turning technique at least 10 times until the suspension is uniformly white and cloudy.
• Teach patient proper insulin injection technique and importance of timing dose to meals and adhering to meal plans.

- Tell patient to report swelling, redness, and itching at injection site, and instruct patient on the importance of rotating injection sites to avoid lipodystrophies.
- Instruct patient to use the same brand of insulin, especially if mixing insulin. Changing brands of insulin may necessitate dosage changes.
- Tell patient not to dilute or mix insulin aspart with any other insulin when using an external insulin pump.
- Instruct patient to monitor glucose level regularly.
- Advise patient to avoid vigorous exercise immediately after insulin injection, especially of the area where injection was given; it causes increased absorption and increased risk of high glucose level.
- Advise patient to store insulin at 36° to 46° F (2° to 8° C), and avoid freezing or excessive heat or sunlight.
- Advise woman to notify prescriber about planned, suspected, or known pregnancy.
- Urge patient to carry medical identification at all times.
- Instruct patient about the importance of diet and exercise. Explain long-term complications of diabetes and the importance of yearly eye and foot examinations.

SAFETY ALERT!

insulin detemir (rDNA origin) injection
Levemir

Pharmacologic class: insulin analog
Pregnancy risk category C

AVAILABLE FORMS
Injection: 100 units/ml in 10-ml vials, 3-ml cartridges (PenFill), 3-ml prefilled syringes (InnoLet, FlexPen)

INDICATIONS & DOSAGES
➤ **Hyperglycemia in patients with diabetes mellitus who need basal (long-acting) insulin**

Adults and children age 6 and older: Base dosage on patient response and glucose level. In insulin-naive patients with type 2 diabetes, start with 0.1 to 0.2 units/kg subcutaneously once daily in the evening or 10 units once or twice daily based on glucose level. Patients with type 1 or 2 diabetes already receiving basal-bolus treatment or basal insulin may switch to this drug on a unit-for-unit basis, adjusted to glycemic target.

ACTION
Regulates glucose metabolism by binding to insulin receptors, facilitating cellular uptake of glucose into muscle and fat, and inhibiting release of glucose from liver.

Route	Onset	Peak	Duration
SubQ	Unknown	6–8 hr	6–23 hr

Half-life: 5 to 7 hours.

ADVERSE REACTIONS
CV: edema.
Metabolic: HYPOGLYCEMIA, sodium retention, *weight gain.*
Skin: injection site reactions, lipodystrophy, pruritus, rash.
Other: ***allergic reactions.***

INTERACTIONS
Drug-drug. *ACE inhibitors, antidiabetic drugs, disopyramide, fibrates, fluoxetine,* ***MAO inhibitors,*** *octreotide, propoxyphene, salicylates, sulfonamides:* May increase the glucose-lowering effect of insulin and risk of hypoglycemia. Monitor glucose level carefully.
Beta blockers, clonidine, guanethidine, reserpine: May decrease or conceal signs of hypoglycemia. Avoid using together, if possible.
Clonidine, lithium salts: May increase or decrease glucose-lowering effect of insulin. Monitor glucose level carefully.
Corticosteroids, danazol, diuretics, estrogens, isoniazid, phenothiazines, progestogens, somatropin, sympathomimetics, thyroid hormones: May decrease glucose-lowering effect of insulin. Monitor glucose level carefully.
Other insulins: May alter the action of one or both insulins if mixed together. Don't mix or dilute insulin detemir with other insulins.
Pentamidine: May cause initial hypoglycemia followed by hyperglycemia. Use together cautiously.

Drug-lifestyle. *Alcohol use:* May increase or decrease effect of drug. Discourage use together.

EFFECTS ON LAB TEST RESULTS
- May decrease glucose level.

CONTRAINDICATIONS & CAUTIONS
- Contraindicated in patients hypersensitive to drug or its components. Don't give drug with an insulin infusion pump.
- Use cautiously in patients with hepatic or renal impairment; they may need dosage adjustment.

NURSING CONSIDERATIONS
- ***Alert:*** Don't give I.V. or I.M.
- ***Alert:*** Don't mix or dilute with other insulins.
- Monitor glucose level routinely in all patients receiving insulin.
- Measure patient's glycosylated hemoglobin level periodically.
- Watch for hyperglycemia, especially if patient's diet or exercise pattern changes.
- Assess patient for signs and symptoms of hypoglycemia. Insulin doses may need adjustment.
- Early warning symptoms of hypoglycemia may be less pronounced in patients who take beta blockers and those with longstanding diabetes, diabetic nerve disease, or intensified diabetes control. Monitor glucose level closely in these patients because severe hypoglycemia could develop before symptoms do.
- Insulin requirements may be altered during illness, emotional disturbance, or stress, or if patient changes his usual meal plan or exercise level.
- Starting dosage, increments of change, and maintenance dosage should be conservative in elderly patients as hypoglycemia may be harder to recognize.

PATIENT TEACHING
- Teach diabetes management, including glucose monitoring, injection techniques, and continuous rotation of injection sites.
- ***Alert:*** Urge patient not to mix with any other insulin or solution.
- Instruct patient to use only solution that's clear and colorless, with no visible particles.
- Tell patient to recognize and report signs and symptoms of hyperglycemia, such as nausea, vomiting, drowsiness, flushed dry skin, dry mouth, increased urination, thirst, and loss of appetite.
- Urge patient to check glucose level often to achieve control and avoid hyperglycemia and hypoglycemia.
- Teach patient to recognize and report signs and symptoms of hypoglycemia, such as sweating, dizziness, lightheadedness, headache, drowsiness, and irritability.
- Advise patient to carry a quick source of simple sugar, such as hard candy or glucose tablets, in case of hypoglycemia.
- Caution patient not to stop insulin abruptly or change the amount or type of insulin used without consulting prescriber.
- Advise patient to avoid alcohol because it lowers the glucose level.
- Caution woman to consult prescriber before trying to become pregnant.
- Tell patient to store unused vials, cartridges, and prefilled syringes in the refrigerator at 36° to 46° F (2° to 8° C).
- After initial use, vials may be refrigerated or stored at room temperature, below 86° F (30° C), away from direct heat and light, for up to 42 days. Cartridges or prefilled syringes may be stored at room temperature, below 86° F (30° C). Tell patient not to store or refrigerate insulin with a needle in place.
- Caution against freezing drug and against using drug that has been frozen.

SAFETY ALERT!

insulin glargine (rDNA origin) injection
Lantus

Pharmacologic class: pancreatic hormone
Pregnancy risk category C

AVAILABLE FORMS
Vial: 10 ml, containing 100 units of insulin glargine per ml (U-100)
Cartridge: 3 ml-cartridge for use in OptiClik device

INDICATIONS & DOSAGES

➤ To manage type 1 (insulin-dependent) diabetes in patients who need basal (long-acting) insulin to control hyperglycemia

Adults and children age 6 and older: Individualize dosage, and give subcutaneously once daily at the same time each day.

➤ To manage type 2 (non–insulin-dependent) diabetes in patients who need basal (long-acting) insulin to control hyperglycemia

Adults: Individualize dosage, and give subcutaneously once daily at the same time each day.

ACTION

Insulin glargine lowers glucose level by stimulating peripheral glucose uptake, especially by skeletal muscle and fat, and by inhibiting hepatic glucose production.

Route	Onset	Peak	Duration
SubQ	1 hr	None	24 hr

Half-life: Unknown.

ADVERSE REACTIONS

Metabolic: ***hypoglycemia.***
Skin: lipodystrophy, pruritus, rash.
Other: allergic reactions, pain at injection site.

INTERACTIONS

Drug-drug. *ACE inhibitors, disopyramide, fibrates, fluoxetine,* **MAO inhibitors,** *octreotide, oral antidiabetics, propoxyphene, salicylates, sulfonamide antibiotics:* May cause hypoglycemia and increase insulin effect. Monitor glucose level. May need to adjust dosage of insulin glargine.
Beta blockers, clonidine: May mask signs of hypoglycemia and may either increase or reduce insulin's glucose-lowering effect. Avoid using together, if possible. If used together, monitor glucose level carefully.
Corticosteroids, danazol, diuretics, estrogens, isoniazid, phenothiazines (such as prochlorperazine, promethazine hydrochloride), progestins (such as hormonal contraceptives), somatropin, sympathomimetics (such as albuterol, epinephrine, terbutaline), thyroid hormones: May reduce the glucose-lowering effect of insulin. Monitor glucose level. May need to adjust dosage of insulin glargine.
Guanethidine, reserpine: May mask the signs of hypoglycemia. Avoid using together, if possible. Monitor glucose level carefully.
Lithium: May either increase or decrease the glucose-lowering effect of insulin. Monitor glucose level. May require dosage adjustments of insulin glargine.
Pentamidine: May cause hypoglycemia, which may be followed by hyperglycemia. Avoid using together, if possible.
Drug-herb. *Burdock, dandelion, eucalyptus, marshmallow:* May increase hypoglycemic effects. Discourage use together.
Licorice root: May increase dosage requirements of insulin. Discourage use together.
Drug-lifestyle. *Alcohol use, emotional stress:* May increase or decrease the glucose-lowering effect of insulin. Advise patient to self-monitor glucose level.

EFFECTS ON LAB TEST RESULTS

- May decrease glucose level.

CONTRAINDICATIONS & CAUTIONS

- Contraindicated during hypoglycemic episodes and in patients hypersensitive to drug or its components.
- Use cautiously in patients with renal or hepatic impairment.

NURSING CONSIDERATIONS

- ***Alert:*** Don't give I.V.
- Because of prolonged duration, this isn't the insulin of choice for diabetic ketoacidosis.
- The rate of absorption, onset, and duration of action may be affected by exercise and other variables, such as illness and emotional stress.
- ***Alert:*** Insulin glargine must not be diluted or mixed with any other insulin or solution.
- As with any insulin therapy, lipodystrophy may occur at the injection site and delay insulin absorption. Reduce this risk by rotating the injection site with each injection.
- Hypoglycemia is the most common adverse effect of insulin. Early symptoms may be different or less pronounced in pa-

tients with long duration of diabetes, diabetic nerve disease, or intensified diabetes control. Monitor glucose level closely in these patients because severe hypoglycemia may result before the patient develops symptoms.
- ***Look alike–sound alike:*** Don't confuse Lente with Lantus.

PATIENT TEACHING
- Teach proper glucose monitoring, injection techniques, and diabetes management.
- Tell patient to take dose once daily at the same time each day.
- ***Alert:*** Educate diabetic patients about signs and symptoms of low glucose level, such as fatigue, weakness, confusion, headache, pallor, and profuse sweating.
- Urge patient to wear or carry medical identification at all times.
- Advise patient to treat mild hypoglycemia with oral glucose tablets. Encourage patient to always carry glucose tablets in case of a low-glucose episode.
- Educate patients on the importance of maintaining prescribed diet, and explain that adjustments in drug dosage, meal patterns, and exercise may be needed to regulate glucose.
- ***Alert:*** Advise patient not to dilute or mix any other insulin or solution with insulin glargine. If the solution is cloudy, urge patient to discard the vial. Use solution only if it is clear and colorless.
- ***Alert:*** Make any change of insulin cautiously and only under medical supervision. Changes in insulin type, strength, manufacturer, type (such as regular, NPH, or insulin analogues), species (animal, human), or method of manufacturer (rDNA versus animal source insulin) may require a change in dosage. Oral antidiabetic treatment taken at the same time may need to be adjusted.
- Tell patient to consult prescriber before using OTC medications.
- Inform patient to avoid alcohol, which lowers glucose level.
- Advise patient to avoid vigorous exercise immediately after insulin injection, especially of the area where injection was given; it causes increased absorption and increased risk of high glucose.
- Advise woman planning pregnancy to first consult prescriber.
- Advise patient that if OptiClik device malfunctions, drug may be drawn from the cartridge system into a U-100 syringe and injected.
- Advise patient on proper drug storage: store unopened insulin vials and 3-ml cartridge system in the refrigerator, opened vials may be stored at 86° F (30° C) or less and away from direct heat, discard opened vials or cartridge system after 28 days whether refrigerated or not, and don't freeze or refrigerate the open, in-use cartridge system if inserted in OptiClik.

SAFETY ALERT!

insulin glulisine (rDNA origin) injection
Apidra

Pharmacologic class: human insulin analog
Pregnancy risk category C

AVAILABLE FORMS
10-ml vial for injection: 100 units/ml

INDICATIONS & DOSAGES
➤ Diabetes mellitus
Adults: Individualize dosage. Give by subcutaneous injection within 15 minutes before a meal. If regimen also includes a longer-acting insulin or basal insulin analogue, give within 20 minutes after meal starts. Or, give drug as continuous subcutaneous infusion using an external infusion pump.

ACTION
Lowers glucose level by increasing peripheral glucose uptake and decreasing hepatic glucose production. When drug is given by subcutaneous injection, onset of action is more rapid and duration of action shorter than those of regular human insulin.

Route	Onset	Peak	Duration
SubQ	15 min	55 min	Unknown

Half-life: 42 minutes.

ADVERSE REACTIONS

Metabolic: ***hypoglycemia.***
Skin: *injection-site reactions,* lipodystrophy, pruritus, rash.
Other: allergic reactions, ***anaphylaxis,*** insulin antibody production.

INTERACTIONS

Drug-drug. *ACE inhibitors, disopyramide, fibrates, fluoxetine,* ***MAO inhibitors,*** *oral antidiabetics, pentoxifylline, propoxyphene, salicylates, sulfonamide antibiotics:* May increase glucose-lowering effects. Monitor glucose level, and watch for evidence of hypoglycemia.
Beta blockers, clonidine, lithium, pentamidine: May cause unpredictable response to insulin. Use together cautiously; monitor patient closely.
Clozapine, corticosteroids, danazol, diazoxide, diuretics, estrogens, glucagons, isoniazid, olanzapine, phenothiazines, progestogens, protease inhibitors, somatropin, sympathomimetics (such as epinephrine, albuterol, and terbutaline), thyroid hormone: May decrease glucose-lowering effects. Monitor glucose level carefully.
Drug-lifestyle. *Alcohol:* May potentiate or reduce insulin effects, resulting in either hypoglycemia or hyperglycemia. Discourage alcohol use.

EFFECTS ON LAB TEST RESULTS

- May decrease glucose level.

CONTRAINDICATIONS & CAUTIONS

- Contraindicated during periods of hypoglycemia and in patients hypersensitive to insulin glulisine or one of its ingredients.
- Use cautiously in patients with impaired renal or hepatic function and in pregnant or breast-feeding women.

NURSING CONSIDERATIONS

- Use with a longer-acting or basal insulin analogue.
- ***Alert:*** Drug has a more rapid onset and shorter duration of action than regular human insulin. Give within 15 minutes before or immediately after a meal.
- Don't mix drug in a syringe with any other insulin except NPH.
- When used in an external subcutaneous infusion pump, don't mix drug with any other insulin or diluent.
- Changes in insulin strength, manufacturer, type, or species may cause a need for dosage adjustment.
- Changes in physical activity or usual meal plan may cause a need for dosage adjustment.
- Insulin requirements may be altered during illness, emotional disturbances, or stress.
- Early warning signs of hypoglycemia may be different or less pronounced in patients who take beta blockers, who have had an oral antidiabetic added to the regimen, or who have long-term diabetes or diabetic nerve disease.
- Monitor patient for lipodystrophy at injection site; it may delay insulin absorption.
- Redness, swelling, or itching may occur at injection site.

PATIENT TEACHING

- Tell patient to take drug within 15 minutes before starting a meal to 20 minutes after starting a meal, depending on regimen.
- Teach patient how to give subcutaneous insulin injections.
- Tell patient not to mix insulin glulisine in a syringe with any insulin other than NPH.
- If patient is mixing insulin glulisine with NPH, tell patient to use U-100 syringes, to draw insulin glulisine into the syringe first, followed by NPH insulin, and to inject the mixture immediately.
- Instruct patient to rotate injection sites to avoid injection-site reactions.
- If patient is using an external infusion pump, teach proper use of the device. Tell patient not to mix insulin glulisine with any other insulin or diluents. Instruct patient to change the infusion set, reservoir with insulin, and infusion site at least every 48 hours.
- Teach patient the signs and symptoms of hypoglycemia (sweating, rapid pulse, trembling, confusion, headache, irritability, and nausea). Advise the patient to treat these symptoms by eating or drinking something containing sugar.

• Instruct the patient to contact a health care provider for possible dosage adjustments if hypoglycemia occurs frequently.
• Show patient how to monitor and log glucose levels to evaluate diabetes control.
• Explain the possible long-term complications of diabetes and the importance of regular preventive therapy. Urge patient to follow prescribed diet and exercise regimen. To further reduce the risk of heart disease, encourage patient to stop smoking and lose weight.
• Instruct patient to carry medical identification showing that he has diabetes.
• Tell patient to store unopened vials in the refrigerator and opened vials in the refrigerator or below 77° F (25° C). Opened vials should be used within 28 days. Protect from direct heat and light.

SAFETY ALERT!

metformin hydrochloride

Fortamet, Glucophage✐, Glucophage XR✐, Glumetza, Riomet

Pharmacologic class: biguanide
Pregnancy risk category B

AVAILABLE FORMS

Oral solution: 500 mg/5 ml
Tablets: 500 mg, 850 mg, 1,000 mg
Tablets (extended-release): 500 mg, 750 mg, 1,000 mg

INDICATIONS & DOSAGES

➤ Adjunct to diet to lower glucose level in patients with type 2 (non–insulin-dependent) diabetes

Adults: If using regular-release tablets or oral solution, initially 500 mg P.O. b.i.d. given with morning and evening meals, or 850 mg P.O. once daily given with morning meal. When 500-mg dose of regular-release form is used, may increase dosage by 500 mg weekly to maximum dose of 2,500 mg P.O. daily in divided doses. When 850-mg dose of regular-release form is used, may increase dosage by 850 mg every other week to maximum dose of 2,550 mg P.O. daily in divided doses. If using extended-release formulation, start therapy at 500 mg P.O. once daily with the evening meal. May increase dose weekly in increments of 500 mg daily, up to a maximum dose of 2,000 mg once daily. If higher doses are required, consider using the regular-release formulation up to its maximum dose.
Children ages 10 to 16: Give 500 mg P.O. b.i.d. using the regular-release formulation only. Increase dosage in increments of 500 mg weekly up to a maximum of 2,000 mg daily in divided doses.
Elderly patients: Dosage should be conservative because of potential decrease in renal function.
Adjust-a-dose: For debilitated patients, dosage should be conservative because of potential decrease in renal function.

➤ Adjunct to diet and exercise in type 2 diabetes as monotherapy or with a sulfonylurea or insulin (Fortamet)

Adults age 17 and older: Initially, 500 to 1,000 mg P.O. with evening meal. Increase dosage based on glucose level in increments of 500 mg weekly to a maximum of 2,500 mg daily. When used with a sulfonylurea or insulin, base dosage on glucose level and adjust slowly until desired therapeutic effect occurs. Decrease insulin dose by 10% to 25% when fasting blood glucose level is less than 120 mg/dl.
Elderly patients: Use conservative initial and maintenance dosage because of potential decrease in renal function. Adjust dosage carefully. Don't adjust to maximum dosage.

➤ Adjunct to diet and exercise in type 2 diabetes as monotherapy or with a sulfonylurea or insulin (Glumetza)

Adults: Initially, 1,000 mg P.O. once daily in the evening with food. Increase as needed in weekly increments of 500 mg, to a maximum of 2,000 mg daily. If glycemic control not attained at this dose, give 1,000 mg b.i.d.

When used with insulin or a sulfonylurea, base dosage on glucose level and adjust slowly until desired therapeutic effect occurs. For patients taking insulin, initial dose of Glumetza is 500 mg daily, increased in weekly increments of 500 mg, to a maximum of 2,000 mg daily. Decrease

insulin dose by 10% to 25%when fasting glucose level is less than 120 mg/dl.
Adjust-a-dose: For malnourished or debilitated patients, don't adjust to maximum dosage.

ACTION

Decreases hepatic glucose production and intestinal absorption of glucose and improves insulin sensitivity (increases peripheral glucose uptake and use).

Route	Onset	Peak	Duration
P.O. (conventional)	Unknown	2–4 hr	Unknown
P.O. (extended-release)	Unknown	4–8 hr	Unknown
P.O. (solution)	Unknown	2½ hr	Unknown

Half-life: About 6 hours.

ADVERSE REACTIONS

GI: *diarrhea, nausea, vomiting,* abdominal bloating, flatulence, anorexia, taste perversion.
Hematologic: megaloblastic anemia.
Metabolic: ***lactic acidosis,*** **HYPOGLYCEMIA.**

INTERACTIONS

Drug-drug. *Calcium channel blockers, corticosteroids, estrogens, fosphenytoin, hormonal contraceptives, isoniazid, nicotinic acid, phenothiazines, phenytoin, sympathomimetics, thiazide and other diuretics, thyroid drugs:* May produce hyperglycemia. Monitor patient's glycemic control. Metformin dosage may need to be increased.
Cationic drugs (such as amiloride, cimetidine, digoxin, morphine, procainamide, quinidine, quinine, ranitidine, triamterene, trimethoprim, vancomycin): May compete for common renal tubular transport systems, which may increase metformin level. Monitor glucose level.
Nifedipine: May increase metformin level. Monitor patient closely. Metformin dosage may need to be decreased.
Radiologic contrast dye: May cause acute renal failure. Withhold metformin for 24 hours before procedure.
Drug-herb. *Guar gum:* May decrease hypoglycemic effect. Discourage use together.
Drug-lifestyle. *Alcohol use:* May increase drug effects. Discourage use together.

EFFECTS ON LAB TEST RESULTS

- May decrease vitamin B_{12} and hemoglobin levels.

CONTRAINDICATIONS & CAUTIONS

- Contraindicated in patients hypersensitive to drug and in those with hepatic disease or metabolic acidosis.
- Contraindicated in patients with renal disease and in those with a creatinine clearance greater than or equal to 1.5 mg/dl (males) or greater than or equal to 1.4 mg/dl (females).
- Contraindicated in patients with heart failure requiring pharmacologic intervention and patients with conditions predisposing to renal dysfunction, CV collapse, MI, hypoxia, and septicemia. Temporarily withhold from patients having radiologic studies involving use of contrast media containing iodine.
- Contraindicated in patients older than age 80, unless creatinine clearance indicates normal renal function.
- Use caution when giving drug to elderly, debilitated, or malnourished patients and to those with adrenal or pituitary insufficiency because of increased risk of hypoglycemia.

NURSING CONSIDERATIONS

- Before therapy begins and at least annually thereafter, assess patient's renal function. If renal impairment is detected, a different antidiabetic may be indicated.
- Give with meals. Maximum doses may be better tolerated if total dose is divided into t.i.d. dosing and given with meals.
- When switching patients from chlorpropamide to metformin, take care during the first 2 weeks of metformin therapy because the prolonged retention of chlorpropamide increases the risk of hypoglycemia during this time.
- Monitor patient's glucose level regularly to evaluate effectiveness of therapy. Notify prescriber if glucose level increases despite therapy.

• If patient hasn't responded to 4 weeks of therapy with maximum dosage, an oral sulfonylurea can be added while keeping metformin at maximum dosage. If patient still doesn't respond after several months of therapy with both drugs at maximum dosage, prescriber may stop both and start insulin therapy.
• Monitor patient closely during times of increased stress, such as infection, fever, surgery, or trauma. Insulin therapy may be needed in these situations.
• Risk of drug-induced lactic acidosis is very low. Reported cases have occurred primarily in diabetic patients with significant renal insufficiency; in those with other medical or surgical problems; and in those with other drug regimens. Risk increases with degree of renal impairment and patient age.
• ***Alert:*** Stop drug immediately and notify prescriber if patient develops a condition related to hypoxemia or dehydration because of risk of lactic acidosis.
• Stop drug temporarily for surgical procedures (except minor procedures that don't restrict intake of food and fluids) and for patients undergoing radiologic studies involving use of contrast media containing iodine. Don't restart drug until patient's oral intake has resumed and renal function has been deemed normal by prescriber.
• Monitor patient's hematologic status for evidence of megaloblastic anemia. Patients with inadequate vitamin B_{12} or calcium intake or absorption appear to be predisposed to developing subnormal vitamin B_{12} level. These patients should have routine vitamin B_{12} level determinations every 2 to 3 years.
• ***Look alike–sound alike:*** Don't confuse Glucophage with Glucovance.

PATIENT TEACHING

• Instruct patient about nature of diabetes and importance of following therapeutic regimen, adhering to specific diet, losing weight, getting exercise, following personal hygiene programs, and avoiding infection. Explain how and when to monitor glucose level. Teach evidence of low and high glucose levels. Explain emergency measures.
• ***Alert:*** Instruct patient to stop drug and immediately notify prescriber about unexplained hyperventilation, muscle pain, malaise, dizziness, light-headedness, unusual sleepiness, unexplained stomach pain, feeling of coldness, slow or irregular heart rate, or other nonspecific symptoms of early lactic acidosis.
• Warn patient not to consume excessive alcohol while taking drug.
• Tell patient not to change drug dosage without prescriber's consent. Encourage patient to report abnormal glucose level test results.
• ***Alert:*** Advise patient not to cut, crush, or chew extended-release tablets; instead, he should swallow them whole.
• Advise patient not to take other drugs, including OTC drugs, without first checking with prescriber.
• Instruct patient to carry medical identification at all times.

SAFETY ALERT!

miglitol

Glyset

Pharmacologic class: alpha-glucosidase inhibitor
Pregnancy risk category B

AVAILABLE FORMS

Tablets: 25 mg, 50 mg, 100 mg

INDICATIONS & DOSAGES

➤ Adjunct to diet in patients with type 2 diabetes, alone or with a sulfonylurea

Adults: 25 mg P.O. t.i.d. with first bite of each main meal. May start with 25 mg P.O. daily and increase gradually to t.i.d. to minimize GI upset; dosage may be increased after 4 to 8 weeks to 50 mg P.O. t.i.d. Dosage may then be further increased after 3 months, based on glycosylated hemoglobin level, to maximum of 100 mg P.O. t.i.d.

ACTION

Lowers glucose level by inhibiting the alpha-glucosidases in the small intestine, which convert carbohydrates to glucose. Inhibiting these enzymes delays the digestion of carbohydrates after a meal, resulting in a smaller increase in postprandial glucose level.

Route	Onset	Peak	Duration
P.O.	Unknown	2–3 hr	Unknown

Half-life: About 2 hours.

ADVERSE REACTIONS

GI: *abdominal pain, diarrhea, flatulence.*
Skin: rash.

INTERACTIONS

Drug-drug. *Digoxin, propranolol, ranitidine:* May decrease bioavailability of these drugs. Watch for loss of effect of these drugs and adjust dosage.
Intestinal absorbents (such as charcoal), digestive enzyme preparations (such as amylase, pancreatin): May reduce effect of miglitol. Discourage use together.

EFFECTS ON LAB TEST RESULTS

- May decrease iron level.

CONTRAINDICATIONS & CAUTIONS

- Contraindicated in patients hypersensitive to drug or its components and in those with diabetic ketoacidosis, inflammatory bowel disease, colonic ulceration, partial intestinal obstruction, chronic intestinal diseases with marked disorders of digestion or absorption, or conditions that may deteriorate because of increased gas formation in the intestine.
- Contraindicated in those predisposed to intestinal obstruction and in those with creatinine level greater than 2 mg/dl.
- Use cautiously in patients also receiving insulin or a sulfonylurea because drug may increase hypoglycemic potential of these drugs.

NURSING CONSIDERATIONS

- In patients also taking insulin or a sulfonylurea, dosage adjustment of these drugs may be needed. Monitor patient for hypoglycemia.
- Diabetes management should include diet control, an exercise program, and regular testing of urine and glucose level.
- Monitor glucose level regularly, especially during situations of increased stress, such as infection, fever, surgery, or trauma.
- Monitor glycosylated hemoglobin level every 3 months to evaluate long-term glycemic control.
- Treat mild to moderate hypoglycemia with a ready form of sugar, such as glucose tablets or gel. Severe hypoglycemia may necessitate I.V. glucose or glucagon.
- Monitor patient for adverse GI effects.

PATIENT TEACHING

- Stress importance of adhering to diet, weight reduction, and exercise instructions. Urge patient to have glucose and glycosylated hemoglobin levels tested regularly.
- Inform patient that drug treatment relieves symptoms but doesn't cure diabetes.
- Teach patient how to recognize high and low glucose levels.
- Instruct patient to have a source of glucose readily available to treat hypoglycemia.
- Advise patient to seek medical advice promptly during periods of stress, such as fever, trauma, infection, or surgery, because dosage may have to be adjusted.
- Instruct patient to take drug three times daily with first bite of each main meal.
- Show patient how and when to monitor glucose level.
- Advise patient that sucrose (table sugar, cane sugar) or fruit juices shouldn't be used to treat low-glucose reactions with this drug. Oral glucose (dextrose) or glucagon is necessary to increase glucose.
- Advise patient that adverse GI effects are most common during first few weeks of therapy and should improve over time.
- Urge patient to carry medical identification at all times.

nateglinide
Starlix

Pharmacologic class: meglitinide derivative
Pregnancy risk category C

AVAILABLE FORMS

Tablets: 60 mg, 120 mg

INDICATIONS & DOSAGES

➤ Type 2 diabetes, as monotherapy, or with metformin or a thiazolidinedione

Adults: 120 mg P.O. t.i.d. taken 1 to 30 minutes before meals. Patients near goal HbA_{1c} when treatment is started may receive 60 mg P.O. t.i.d.

ACTION

Lowers glucose level by stimulating insulin secretion from pancreatic beta cells.

Route	Onset	Peak	Duration
P.O.	20 min	1 hr	4 hr

Half-life: About 1½ hours.

ADVERSE REACTIONS

CNS: dizziness.
GI: diarrhea.
Metabolic: ***hypoglycemia.***
Musculoskeletal: back pain, arthropathy.
Respiratory: *upper respiratory tract infection,* bronchitis, coughing.
Other: flulike symptoms, accidental trauma.

INTERACTIONS

Drug-drug. *Corticosteroids, rifamycins, sympathomimetics, thiazides, thyroid products:* May reduce hypoglycemic action of nateglinide. Monitor glucose level closely.
MAO inhibitors, nonselective beta blockers, NSAIDs, salicylates: May increase hypoglycemic action of nateglinide. Monitor glucose level closely.

EFFECTS ON LAB TEST RESULTS

- May decrease glucose level.

CONTRAINDICATIONS & CAUTIONS

- Contraindicated in patients hypersensitive to drug, in those with type 1 diabetes or diabetic ketoacidosis, and in breast-feeding patients.
- Use cautiously in patients with moderate to severe liver dysfunction or adrenal or pituitary insufficiency, and in elderly and malnourished patients.

NURSING CONSIDERATIONS

- Don't use with or as a substitute for glyburide or other oral antidiabetics; may use with metformin or a thiazolidinedione.
- Monitor glucose level regularly to evaluate drug's effectiveness.
- Observe patient for signs and symptoms of hypoglycemia. To minimize risk of hypoglycemia, make sure that patient has a meal immediately after dose. If hypoglycemia occurs and patient remains conscious, give him an oral form of glucose. If he's unconscious, treat with I.V. glucose.
- Risk of hypoglycemia increases with strenuous exercise, alcohol ingestion, or insufficient caloric intake.
- Symptoms of hypoglycemia may be masked in patients with autonomic neuropathy and in those who use beta blockers.
- Insulin therapy may be needed for glycemic control in patients with fever, infection, or trauma and in those undergoing surgery.
- Monitor glucose level closely when other drugs are started or stopped, to detect possible drug interactions.
- Periodically monitor HbA_{1c} level.
- Drug's effectiveness may decrease over time.
- No special dosage adjustments are usually necessary in elderly patients, but some elderly patients may have greater sensitivity to glucose-lowering effect.

PATIENT TEACHING

- Tell patient to take drug 1 to 30 minutes before a meal.
- Advise patient to skip the scheduled dose if he skips a meal to reduce risk of hypoglycemia.
- Instruct patient on risk of hypoglycemia, its signs and symptoms (sweating, rapid pulse, trembling, confusion, headache, irritability, and nausea), and ways to treat these symptoms by eating or drinking something containing sugar.
- Teach patient how to monitor and log glucose levels to evaluate diabetes control.
- Advise patient to notify prescriber for persistent low or high glucose level.
- Instruct patient to adhere to prescribed diet and exercise regimen.

• Explain possible long-term complications of diabetes and importance of regular preventive therapy.
• Encourage patient to wear a medical identification bracelet.

SAFETY ALERT!

pioglitazone hydrochloride
Actos

Pharmacologic class: thiazolidinedione
Pregnancy risk category C

AVAILABLE FORMS
Tablets: 15 mg, 30 mg, 45 mg

INDICATIONS & DOSAGES
➤ **Type 2 diabetes, alone or with a sulfonylurea, metformin, or insulin**
Adults: Initially, 15 or 30 mg P.O. once daily. Maximum daily dose, if used alone or in combination therapy, is 45 mg.
Adjust-a-dose: For patients taking pioglitazone with insulin, reduce insulin by 10% to 25% if patient reports hypoglycemia or if glucose level is less than 100 mg/dl.

ACTION
Lowers glucose level by decreasing insulin resistance and hepatic glucose production. Improves sensitivity of insulin in muscle and adipose tissue.

Route	Onset	Peak	Duration
P.O.	Unknown	≤ 2 hr	Unknown

Half-life: 3 to 7 hours.

ADVERSE REACTIONS
CNS: headache.
CV: *edema, **heart failure.***
EENT: sinusitis, pharyngitis.
Hematologic: anemia.
Metabolic: ***hypoglycemia with combination therapy,*** aggravated diabetes, weight gain.
Musculoskeletal: myalgia.
Respiratory: upper respiratory tract infection.
Other: tooth disorder.

INTERACTIONS
Drug-drug. *Ketoconazole:* May inhibit pioglitazone metabolism. Monitor glucose level more frequently.
Hormonal contraceptives: May decrease level of hormonal contraceptives, reducing contraceptive effectiveness. Advise patient taking drug and hormonal contraceptives to consider additional birth control measures.
Drug-herb. *Burdock, dandelion, eucalyptus, marshmallow:* May increase hypoglycemic effects. Discourage use together.
Drug-lifestyle. *Alcohol use:* May alter glycemic control and increase risk of hypoglycemia. Discourage use together.

EFFECTS ON LAB TEST RESULTS
• May increase ALT, HDL, LDL, and total cholesterol levels. May decrease glucose, triglyceride, and hemoglobin levels.

CONTRAINDICATIONS & CAUTIONS
• Contraindicated in patients hypersensitive to drug or its components and in those with type 1 diabetes, diabetic ketoacidosis, active liver disease, ALT level greater than two and a half times the upper limit of normal, New York Heart Association (NYHA) Class III or IV heart failure, and in those who experienced jaundice while taking troglitazone.
• Use cautiously in patients with edema or heart failure.

NURSING CONSIDERATIONS
• ***Alert:*** Measure liver enzyme levels at start of therapy, every 2 months for first year of therapy, and periodically thereafter. Obtain liver function test results in patients who develop signs and symptoms of liver dysfunction, such as nausea, vomiting, abdominal pain, fatigue, anorexia, or dark urine. Stop drug if patient develops jaundice or if liver function test results show ALT level greater than three times the upper limit of normal.
• Pioglitazone can cause fluid retention leading to or worsening heart failure. Monitor patients for signs or symptoms of heart failure and notify prescriber if cardiac status deteriorates.
• Hemoglobin level and hematocrit may drop, usually during first 4 to 12 weeks of therapy.

- Management of type 2 diabetes should include diet control. Because caloric restrictions, weight loss, and exercise help improve insulin sensitivity and help make drug therapy effective, these measures are essential for proper diabetes management.
- Watch for hypoglycemia, especially in patients receiving combination therapy. Dosage adjustments of these drugs may be needed.
- Monitor glucose level regularly, especially during situations of increased stress, such as infection, fever, surgery, and trauma.
- Safety and efficacy of drug in children haven't been evaluated.
- Use during pregnancy only if the benefit justifies risk to fetus; insulin is the preferred antidiabetic during pregnancy.
- ***Look alike–sound alike:*** Don't confuse pioglitazone with rosiglitazone.

PATIENT TEACHING

- Instruct patient to adhere to dietary instructions and to have glucose and glycosylated hemoglobin levels tested regularly.
- Teach patient taking pioglitazone with insulin or oral antidiabetics the signs and symptoms of hypoglycemia.
- Advise patient to notify prescriber during periods of stress, such as fever, trauma, infection, or surgery, because dosage may need adjustment.
- Instruct patient how and when to monitor glucose level.
- Notify patient that blood tests of liver function will be performed before therapy starts, every 2 months for the first year, and periodically thereafter.
- Tell patient to report unexplained nausea, vomiting, abdominal pain, fatigue, anorexia, and dark urine immediately because these symptoms may indicate liver problems.
- Warn patient to contact his health care provider if he has signs or symptoms of heart failure (unusually rapid increase in weight or swelling, shortness of breath).
- Advise anovulatory, premenopausal women with insulin resistance that therapy may cause resumption of ovulation; recommend using contraception.

SAFETY ALERT!

pramlintide acetate
Symlin

Pharmacologic class: human amylin analogue
Pregnancy risk category C

AVAILABLE FORMS

Injection: 0.6 mg/ml in 5-ml vials

INDICATIONS & DOSAGES

➤Adjunct to insulin in patients with type 1 diabetes

Adults: Initially, 15 mcg subcutaneously before meals of more than 250 calories or 30 g of carbohydrates. Reduce preprandial rapid-acting or short-acting insulin dose, including fixed-mix insulin such as 70/30, by 50%. Increase pramlintide dose by 15-mcg increments q 3 days if no nausea occurs to a maintenance dose of 30 to 60 mcg. Adjust insulin dose as needed.
Adjust-a-dose: If significant nausea at 45 or 60 mcg persists, decrease to 30 mcg. If nausea persists at 30 mcg, consider stopping.

➤Adjunct to insulin in patients with type 2 diabetes, with or without a sulfonylurea or metformin

Adults: Initially, 60 mcg subcutaneously immediately before major meals. Reduce preprandial rapid-acting or short-acting insulin dose, including fixed-mix insulin, by 50%. Increase pramlintide dose to 120 mcg if no significant nausea occurs for 3 to 7 days. Adjust insulin dose as needed.
Adjust-a-dose: If significant nausea persists at 120 mcg, decrease to 60 mcg.

ACTION

Slows rate at which food leaves the stomach, reducing the initial postprandial increase in glucose level. Decreases hyperglycemia by reducing postprandial glucagon level and reduces total caloric intake by reducing appetite.

Route	Onset	Peak	Duration
SubQ	Unknown	19–21 min	Unknown

Half-life: About 48 minutes each (parent drug and active metabolite).

ADVERSE REACTIONS

CNS: dizziness, fatigue, *headache.*
EENT: pharyngitis.
GI: abdominal pain, *anorexia, nausea, vomiting.*
Metabolic: ***hypoglycemia.***
Musculoskeletal: arthralgia.
Respiratory: cough.
Skin: injection site reaction.
Other: allergic reaction, *accidental injury.*

INTERACTIONS

Drug-drug. *ACE inhibitors, disopyramide, fibrates, fluoxetine, MAO inhibitors, oral antidiabetics, pentoxifylline, propoxyphene, salicylates, sulfonamide antibiotics:* May increase risk of hypoglycemia. Monitor glucose level closely.
Alpha glucosidase inhibitors (such as acarbose), anticholinergics (such as atropine, tricyclic antidepressants, benztropine): May alter GI motility. Avoid using together.
Beta blockers, clonidine, guanethidine, reserpine: May mask signs of hypoglycemia. Monitor glucose level closely.
Oral drugs dependent on rapid onset of action (such as analgesics): May delay absorption because of slowed gastric emptying. If rapid effect is needed, give oral drug 1 hour before or 2 hours after pramlintide.

EFFECTS ON LAB TEST RESULTS

None reported.

CONTRAINDICATIONS & CAUTIONS

- Contraindicated in patients hypersensitive to drug or its components, including metacresol, and in patients with gastroparesis or hypoglycemia unawareness.
- Don't use in patients noncompliant with current insulin and glucose monitoring regimen, patients with a glycosylated hemoglobin (HbA_{1c}) level greater than 9%, patients with severe hypoglycemia during the previous 6 months, and patients who take drugs that stimulate GI motility.
- Use cautiously in pregnant or breast-feeding women and in elderly patients.

NURSING CONSIDERATIONS

- Before starting drug, review patient's HbA_{1c} level, recent blood glucose monitoring data, hypoglycemic episodes, current insulin regimen, and body weight.
- To give drug, use a U-100 insulin syringe, preferably a 0.3-ml size.
- Give each dose subcutaneously into abdomen or thigh. Rotate injection sites, and use site separate from insulin site used at same time.
- ***Alert:*** Drug may increase the risk of insulin-induced severe hypoglycemia, particularly in patients with type 1 diabetes.
- The risk of severe hypoglycemia is highest within the first 3 hours after an injection.
- Symptoms of hypoglycemia may be masked in patients with a long history of diabetes, diabetic nerve disease, or intensified diabetes control.
- Notify prescriber of severe nausea and vomiting. A reduced dose may be needed.
- Don't mix drug with any type of insulin; give drug as separate injection.
- If patient has persistent nausea or recurrent, unexplained hypoglycemia that requires medical assistance, stop drug.
- If patient doesn't comply with glucose monitoring or drug dosage adjustments, stop drug.

PATIENT TEACHING

- Teach patient how to take drug exactly as prescribed, at mealtimes. Explain that it doesn't replace daily insulin but may lower the amount of insulin needed.
- Explain that a meal is considered more than 250 calories or 30 g of carbohydrates.
- Caution patient not to mix drug with insulin; instruct him to give the injections at separate sites.
- Instruct patient not to change doses of pramlintide or insulin without consulting prescriber.
- Tell patient to refrain from driving, operating heavy machinery, or performing other risky activities where he could hurt himself or others, until it's known how drug affects his glucose level.
- Caution patient about possibility of severe hypoglycemia, particularly within 3 hours after injection.
- Teach patient and family members the signs and symptoms of hypoglycemia, including hunger, headache, sweating, tremor, irritability, and difficulty concentrating.

- Instruct patient and family members what to do if patient develops hypoglycemia.
- Tell patient to report to prescriber severe nausea and vomiting.
- Advise women of childbearing age to tell the prescriber if they are, could be, or are planning to become pregnant.
- Teach patient how to handle unplanned situations, such as illness or stress, low or forgotten insulin dose, accidental use of too much insulin or drug, not enough food, or missed meals.
- Tell patient to refrigerate unopened and opened vials. Contents of opened vials should be used within 28 days and unopened vials before expiration date.

SAFETY ALERT!

repaglinide
Prandin

Pharmacologic class: meglitinide
Pregnancy risk category C

AVAILABLE FORMS
Tablets: 0.5 mg, 1 mg, 2 mg

INDICATIONS & DOSAGES
➤Type 2 diabetes alone or with metformin or a thiazolidinedione
Adults: For patients not previously treated or whose HbA_{1c} is below 8%, starting dose is 0.5 mg P.O. taken about 15 minutes before each meal. For patients previously treated with glucose-lowering drugs and whose HbA_{1c} is 8% or more, first dose is 1 to 2 mg P.O. with each meal. Recommended dosage range is 0.5 to 4 mg with meals b.i.d., t.i.d., or q.i.d. Maximum daily dose is 16 mg.

Determine dosage by glucose response. May double dosage up to 4 mg with each meal until satisfactory glucose response is achieved. At least 1 week should elapse between dosage adjustments to assess response to each dose.

Metformin may be added if repaglinide monotherapy is inadequate; no repaglinide dosage adjustment is necessary.
Adjust-a-dose: In patients with severe renal impairment, starting dose is 0.5 mg P.O. with meals.

ACTION
Stimulates insulin release from beta cells in the pancreas by closing ATP-dependent potassium channels in beta cell membranes, which causes calcium channels to open. Increased calcium influx induces insulin secretion; the overall effect is to lower glucose level.

Route	Onset	Peak	Duration
P.O.	30 min	1 hr	Unknown

Half-life: 1 hour.

ADVERSE REACTIONS
CNS: *headache,* paresthesia.
CV: angina.
EENT: rhinitis, sinusitis.
GI: constipation, diarrhea, dyspepsia, nausea, vomiting.
GU: UTI.
Metabolic: **HYPOGLYCEMIA,** hyperglycemia.
Musculoskeletal: arthralgia, back pain.
Respiratory: bronchitis, *upper respiratory tract infection.*
Other: tooth disorder.

INTERACTIONS
Drug-drug. *Barbiturates, carbamazepine, rifampin:* May increase repaglinide metabolism. Monitor glucose level.
Beta blockers, chloramphenicol, coumarin derivatives, MAO inhibitors, NSAIDs, other drugs that are highly protein-bound, probenecid, salicylates, sulfonamides: May increase hypoglycemic action of repaglinide. Monitor glucose level.
Calcium channel blockers, corticosteroids, estrogens, fosphenytoin, hormonal contraceptives, isoniazid, nicotinic acid, phenothiazines, phenytoin, sympathomimetics, thiazides and other diuretics, thyroid products: May produce hyperglycemia, resulting in a loss of glycemic control. Monitor glucose level.
Clarithromycin: May increase repaglinide levels. Adjust repaglinide dosage.
Erythromycin, itraconazole, ketoconazole, miconazole, similar inhibitors of CYP3A4: May inhibit repaglinide metabolism. Monitor glucose level.
Gemfibrozil: May increase repaglinide levels. Avoid using together, if possible.

Monitor glucose level and adjust repaglinide dosage, if indicated.
Drug-herb. *Burdock, dandelion, eucalyptus, marshmallow:* May increase hypoglycemic effects. Discourage use together.
Drug-food. *Grapefruit juice:* May inhibit metabolism of drug. Discourage use together.
Drug-lifestyle. *Alcohol use:* May alter glycemic control, most commonly causing hypoglycemia. Discourage use together.

EFFECTS ON LAB TEST RESULTS

- May increase or decrease glucose level.

CONTRAINDICATIONS & CAUTIONS

- Contraindicated in patients hypersensitive to drug or its inactive ingredients and in those with type 1 diabetes or diabetic ketoacidosis.
- Use cautiously in elderly, debilitated, or malnourished patients and in those with hepatic, adrenal, or pituitary insufficiency.

NURSING CONSIDERATIONS

- Increase dosage carefully in patients with impaired renal function or renal failure requiring dialysis.
- Metformin may be added if repaglinide alone is inadequate.
- Drug may increase CV mortality compared with diet alone or diet plus insulin.
- Monitor patient for loss of glycemic control, especially during stress, such as fever, trauma, infection, or surgery.
- Hypoglycemia may be difficult to recognize in elderly patients and in patients taking beta blockers.
- When switching to a different oral hypoglycemic, begin new drug on day after last dose of repaglinide.

PATIENT TEACHING

- Stress importance of diet and exercise with drug therapy.
- Discuss symptoms of hypoglycemia with patient and family.
- Encourage patient to keep regular appointments and have his HbA_{1c} level checked every 3 months to determine long-term glucose control.
- Tell patient to take drug before meals, usually 15 minutes before start of meal; however, time can vary from immediately preceding meal to up to 30 minutes before meal.
- Tell patient that, if a meal is skipped or added, he should skip dose or add an extra dose of drug for that meal, respectively.
- Instruct patient to monitor glucose level carefully and tell him what to do when he's ill, undergoing surgery, or under added stress.
- Advise woman planning pregnancy to first consult prescriber. Insulin may be needed during pregnancy and breastfeeding.
- Teach patient to carry candy or other simple sugars to treat mild hypoglycemia episodes. Patient experiencing severe episode may need emergency treatment.
- Advise patient to avoid alcohol, which lowers glucose level.

SAFETY ALERT!

rosiglitazone maleate

Avandia

Pharmacologic class: thiazolidinedione
Pregnancy risk category C

AVAILABLE FORMS

Tablets: 2 mg, 4 mg, 8 mg

INDICATIONS & DOSAGES

➤ Type 2 diabetes, alone or with a sulfonylurea, metformin, or insulin
Adults: Initially, 4 mg P.O. daily in the morning or in divided doses b.i.d. (morning and evening). Increase to 8 mg P.O. daily or in divided doses b.i.d. if fasting glucose level doesn't improve after 12 weeks of treatment.
Adjust-a-dose: For patients stabilized on insulin, continue the insulin dose when rosiglitazone therapy starts. Don't use rosiglitazone doses greater than 4 mg daily with insulin. Decrease insulin dose by 10% to 25% if patient reports hypoglycemia or if fasting glucose level falls to below 100 mg/dl. Adjust based on glucose-lowering response.

ACTION

Lowers glucose level by improving insulin sensitivity.

Route	Onset	Peak	Duration
P.O.	Unknown	1 hr	Unknown

Half-life: 3 to 4 hours.

ADVERSE REACTIONS
CNS: headache, fatigue.
CV: edema.
EENT: sinusitis.
GI: diarrhea.
Hematologic: anemia.
Metabolic: hyperglycemia.
Musculoskeletal: back pain.
Respiratory: upper respiratory tract infection.
Other: accidental injury.

INTERACTIONS
Drug-drug. *Gemfibrozil, ketoconazole:* May increase rosiglitazone levels. Monitor glucose; dosage adjustment may be necessary.
Rifampin: May decrease rosiglitazone levels. Monitor glucose; dosage adjustment may be necessary.

EFFECTS ON LAB TEST RESULTS
- May increase glucose, HDL, LDL, total cholesterol, and ALT levels. May decrease hemoglobin level and hematocrit.

CONTRAINDICATIONS & CAUTIONS
- Contraindicated in patients hypersensitive to drug or its components and in those with New York Heart Association Class III or IV cardiac status unless expected benefits outweigh risks.
- Contraindicated in patients with active liver disease, increased baseline liver enzyme levels (ALT level greater than two and a half times upper limit of normal), type 1 diabetes, or diabetic ketoacidosis and in those who experienced jaundice while taking troglitazone.
- Use cautiously in patients with edema or heart failure.

NURSING CONSIDERATIONS
- ***Alert:*** Check liver enzyme levels before therapy starts. Don't use drug in patients with increased baseline liver enzyme levels. Monitor these levels every 2 months for first 12 months and periodically thereafter. If ALT level becomes elevated, recheck as soon as possible. Stop drug if levels remain elevated.
- Drug can cause fluid retention leading to or worsening heart failure. Monitor patients for signs or symptoms of heart failure. Notify prescriber if any deterioration in cardiac status occurs.
- Management of type 2 diabetes should include diet control. Because caloric restriction, weight loss, and exercise help improve insulin sensitivity and improve effectiveness of drug therapy, these measures are essential to proper diabetes treatment.
- Check glucose and glycosylated hemoglobin levels periodically to monitor therapeutic response to drug.
- Hemoglobin level and hematocrit may drop during therapy, usually during first 4 to 8 weeks. Increases in total cholesterol, low-density lipoprotein, and high-density lipoprotein levels and decreases in free fatty acid level also may occur.
- For patients inadequately controlled with a maximum dose of a sulfonylurea or metformin, add rosiglitazone to, rather than substitute it for, a sulfonylurea or metformin.
- ***Look alike–sound alike:*** Don't confuse rosiglitazone with pioglitazone.

PATIENT TEACHING
- Advise patient that drug can be taken with or without food.
- Notify patient that blood will be tested to check liver function before therapy starts, every 2 months for first 12 months, and then periodically thereafter.
- Tell patient to immediately notify prescriber about unexplained signs and symptoms, such as nausea, vomiting, abdominal pain, fatigue, anorexia, or dark urine; these may indicate liver problems.
- Warn patient to contact his health care provider about signs or symptoms of heart failure (unusually rapid increase in weight or swelling, shortness of breath).
- Recommend use of contraceptives to premenopausal, anovulatory women with insulin resistance because ovulation may resume with therapy.
- Advise patient that management of diabetes includes diet control, calorie restriction, weight loss, and exercise, and that

these measures improve effectiveness of drug therapy.

- Instruct patient to monitor glucose level carefully and tell him what to do when he's ill, undergoing surgery, or under added stress.

✷ NEW DRUG

sitagliptin phosphate
Januvia

Pharmacologic class: dipeptidyl peptidase-4 (DPP-4) enzyme inhibitor
Pregnancy risk category B

AVAILABLE FORMS
Tablets: 25 mg, 50 mg, 100 mg

INDICATIONS & DOSAGES
➤ To improve glycemic control in type 2 diabetes, alone or with metformin or a thiazolidinedione
Adults: 100 mg P.O. once daily, with or without food.
Adjust-a-dose: For patients with creatinine clearance of 30 to 50 ml/minute, give 50 mg once daily; for patients with clearance less than 30 ml/minute or end stage renal disease with hemodialysis or peritoneal dialysis, give 25 mg once daily. Drug may be taken without regard to timing of dialysis session.

ACTION
Inhibits DPP-4, an enzyme that rapidly inactivates incretin hormones, which play a part in the body's regulation of glucose. By increasing and prolonging active incretin levels, the drug helps to increase insulin release and decrease circulating glucose.

Route	Onset	Peak	Duration
P.O.	Rapid	1–4 hr	Unknown

Half-life: 12½ hours.

ADVERSE REACTIONS
CNS: headache.
EENT: nasopharyngitis.
GI: abdominal pain, nausea, diarrhea.
Metabolic: hypoglycemia.
Respiratory: upper respiratory tract infection.

INTERACTIONS
None significant.

EFFECTS ON LAB TEST RESULTS
- May increase creatinine level.
- May increase WBC count.

CONTRAINDICATIONS & CAUTIONS
- Contraindicated in patients with type 1 diabetes or diabetic ketoacidosis.
- Use cautiously in patients with moderate to severe renal insufficiency and in those taking other antidiabetics.

NURSING CONSIDERATIONS
- In elderly patients and those at risk for renal insufficiency, periodically assess renal function.
- Monitor glycosylated hemoglobin level periodically to assess long-term glycemic control.
- Management of type 2 diabetes should include diet control. Because caloric restrictions, weight loss, and exercise help improve insulin sensitivity and help make drug therapy effective, these measure are essential for proper diabetes management.
- Watch for hypoglycemia, especially in patients receiving combination therapy.
- Safety and effectiveness of drug in children haven't been evaluated.

PATIENT TEACHING
- Tell patient that drug isn't a substitute for diet and exercise and that it's important to follow a prescribed dietary and physical activity routine and to monitor his glucose levels.
- Inform patient and family members of the signs and symptoms of hyperglycemia and hypoglycemia and the steps to take if these symptoms occur.
- Provide patient with information on complications associated with diabetes and ways to assess for them.
- Tell patient to notify prescriber during periods of stress, such as fever, infection, or surgery; dosage may need adjustment.
- Tell patient drug may be taken without regard to food or meals.

56 Thyroid hormones

levothyroxine sodium
liothyronine sodium
liotrix
thyroid, desiccated

levothyroxine sodium (T_4 L-thyroxine sodium)

Eltroxin†, Levo-T, Levotec†, Levothroid, Levoxine, Levoxyl✐, Novothyrox, Oroxine‡, Synthroid✐, Thyro-Tabs, Unithroid

Pharmacologic class: thyroid hormone
Pregnancy risk category A

AVAILABLE FORMS

Lyophilized powder for injection: 200-mcg vial, 500-mcg vial
Tablets: 25 mcg, 50 mcg, 75 mcg, 88 mcg, 100 mcg, 112 mcg, 125 mcg, 137 mcg, 150 mcg, 175 mcg, 200 mcg, 300 mcg

INDICATIONS & DOSAGES

➤ **Myxedema coma**
Adults: Give an initial dose of 200 to 500 mcg I.V. An additional dose of 100 to 300 mcg or more may be given on the second day if there hasn't been substantial or progressive improvement. Continue with lower daily I.V. dosages until patient is stable and oral maintenance therapy can begin.

➤ **Thyroid hormone replacement**
Adults : For patients younger than age 50 or those older than age 50 who have been recently treated for hyperthyroidism, or have been hypothyroid for a short time, give 1.7 mcg/kg P.O. once daily. Monitor TSH levels q 6 to 8 weeks, making dosage adjustments in 12.5 to 25 mcg increments until patient is euthyroid and TSH level normalizes.
Adults: For patients age 50 or older or those younger than age 50 with underlying cardiac disease, give 25 to 50 mcg P.O. daily. Adjust dose q 6 to 8 weeks, if needed, until patient is euthyroid and TSH level normalizes.
Children older than age 12: More than 150 mcg or 2 to 3 mcg/kg P.O. daily.
Children ages 6 to 12: Give 100 to 150 mcg or 4 to 5 mcg/kg P.O. daily.
Children ages 1 to 5: Give 75 to 100 mcg or 5 to 6 mcg/kg P.O. daily.
Children ages 6 months to 1 year: 50 to 75 mcg or 6 to 8 mcg/kg P.O. daily.
Children age 3 to 6 months: 25 to 50 mcg or 8 to 10 mcg/kg P.O. daily.
Infants and neonates birth to 3 months: 10 to 15 mcg/kg P.O. daily. In neonates at risk for cardiac failure, use a lower initial dose (such as 25 mcg daily), and increase q 4 to 6 weeks as needed.
Elderly patients with underlying cardiovascular disease: 12.5 to 25 mcg P.O. daily; increase by 12.5 to 25 mcg q 4 to 6 weeks, depending on response.

➤ **Severe, long-standing hypothyroidism**
Adults: 12.5 to 25 mcg P.O. daily. Increase in increments of 25 mcg q 2 to 4 weeks, as needed.
Children: 25 mcg P.O. daily. Increase in increments of 25 mcg q 2 to 4 weeks, as needed.

I.V. ADMINISTRATION

- First I.V. dose is about half the previously established oral dose of tablets.
- Prepare I.V. dose immediately before injection. Dilute Synthroid powder for injection with 5 ml of normal saline solution for injection to 200- or 500-mcg vial; don't use other diluents. Resulting solutions contain 40 or 100 mcg/ml, respectively. Inject into vein over 1 to 2 minutes.
- Monitor blood pressure and heart rate closely. High initial I.V. dosage is usually well tolerated by patients in myxedema coma. Normal T_4 level should occur within 24 hours, followed by a threefold increase in T_3 in 3 days.

INCOMPATIBILITIES

Other I.V. solutions.

ACTION

Not completely defined. Stimulates metabolism of all body tissues by accelerating rate of cellular oxidation.

Route	Onset	Peak	Duration
P.O.	24 hr	Unknown	Unknown
I.V., I.M.	Unknown	Unknown	Unknown

Half-life: 3 to 4 days in hyperthyroidism; 9 to 10 days in hypothyroidism.

ADVERSE REACTIONS

CNS: *nervousness, insomnia, tremor,* headache, fever.
CV: *tachycardia, palpitations,* ***arrhythmias,*** *angina pectoris,* **cardiac arrest.**
GI: diarrhea, vomiting.
GU: menstrual irregularities.
Metabolic: weight loss.
Musculoskeletal: decreased bone density.
Skin: allergic skin reactions, diaphoresis.
Other: heat intolerance.

INTERACTIONS

Drug-drug. *Aminoglutethimide, amiodarone, iodide (including iodine-containing radiographic contrast agents), lithium:* May reduce thyroid hormone secretion. Monitor thyroid function studies if used together.
Beta blockers: May reduce beta blocker effects. Monitor patient.
Cholestyramine, colestipol, sucralfate: May impair levothyroxine absorption. Separate doses by 4 to 5 hours.
Digoxin: May decrease glycoside effects. Monitor patient for clinical effect.
Estrogens: May decrease thyroid levels. Monitor levels after 12 weeks of therapy and adjust levothyroxine dose as needed.
Fosphenytoin, phenytoin: May release free thyroid hormone. Monitor patient for tachycardia.
Insulin, oral antidiabetics: May alter glucose level. Monitor glucose level. Dosage adjustments may be needed.
Sympathomimetics such as epinephrine: May increase risk of coronary insufficiency. Monitor patient closely.
Theophylline: May decrease theophylline clearance in hypothyroidism; clearance may return to normal when euthyroid state is achieved. Monitor theophylline level.
Warfarin: May increase anticoagulant effects. Monitor patient for bleeding and check PT and INR closely. Warfarin dosage adjustment may be needed.
Drug-herb. *Horseradish:* May cause abnormal thyroid function. Discourage use in patients undergoing thyroid function tests.
Lemon balm: May have antithyroid effects; may inhibit thyroid-stimulating hormone. Discourage use together.
Drug-food. *Cottonseed meal, dietary fiber, soybean flour, walnuts:* May decrease absorption of drug. Dosage adjustments may be needed.

EFFECTS ON LAB TEST RESULTS

- May decrease thyroid function test results. May alter results of liothyronine, protein-bound iodine, and radioactive ^{131}I uptake studies.

CONTRAINDICATIONS & CAUTIONS

- Contraindicated in patients hypersensitive to drug and in those with acute MI uncomplicated by hypothyroidism, untreated subclinical or overt thyrotoxicosis, or uncorrected adrenal insufficiency.
- Use cautiously in elderly patients and in those with angina pectoris, hypertension, other CV disorders, renal insufficiency, or ischemia.
- Use cautiously in patients with diabetes mellitus, diabetes insipidus, or myxedema and during rapid replacement in those with arteriosclerosis.

NURSING CONSIDERATIONS

- ***Alert:*** Drug may be given I.V. or I.M. when P.O. use isn't possible for long periods. I.M. use isn't usually recommended because of variable absorption and difficulty regulating dose.
- Patients with diabetes mellitus may need increased antidiabetic doses when starting thyroid hormone replacement.
- Watch for angina, coronary occlusion, or stroke in patients with arteriosclerosis who are receiving rapid replacement.
- In patients with coronary artery disease who must receive thyroid hormone, observe carefully for possible coronary insufficiency.

• Thyroid hormone replacement requirements are about 25% lower in patients older than age 60 than in young adults.
• Patients with adult hypothyroidism are unusually sensitive to thyroid hormone. Start at lowest dosage and adjust to higher dosages according to patient's symptoms and laboratory data until euthyroid state is reached.
• When changing from levothyroxine to liothyronine, stop levothyroxine and begin liothyronine. Increase dosage in small increments after residual effects of levothyroxine have disappeared. When changing from liothyronine to levothyroxine, start levothyroxine several days before withdrawing liothyronine to avoid relapse. Drugs aren't interchangeable.
• Long-term therapy causes bone loss in premenopausal and postmenopausal women. Consider a basal bone density measurement and monitor patient closely for osteoporosis.
• Patients taking levothyroxine who need to have ^{131}I uptake studies performed must stop drug 4 weeks before test.
• Patients taking anticoagulants may need their dosage modified and require careful monitoring of coagulation status.
• Dosage may need to be increased in pregnant patients.
• Drug shouldn't be used for infertility (unless associated with hypothyroidism) or weight loss.
• ***Look alike–sound alike:*** Don't confuse levothyroxine with liothyronine or liotrix.
• Synthroid may contain tartrazine.

PATIENT TEACHING
• Teach patient the importance of compliance. Tell him to take drug at same time each day, preferably ½ to 1 hour before breakfast, to maintain constant hormone levels and help prevent insomnia.
• Make sure patient understands that replacement therapy is usually for life. The drug should never be stopped unless directed by prescriber.
• Warn patient (especially elderly patient) to notify prescriber at once about chest pain, palpitations, sweating, nervousness, shortness of breath, or other signals of overdose or aggravated CV disease.
• Tell caregiver of infant or child who can't swallow tablets to crush tablet and suspend in small amount of formula (except soy formula, which may decrease the absorption), breast milk, or water, and give by spoon or dropper. Crushed tablet can be sprinkled over food, except foods containing large amounts of soybean, fiber, or iron.
• Tell patient to take pill with plenty of water to avoid choking, gagging, or getting the pill stuck in his throat.
• Advise patient who has achieved stable response not to change brands.
• Tell patient to report unusual bleeding and bruising.
• Advise patient not to take OTC or other prescription drugs without first consulting prescriber.
• Advise patient to report pregnancy to prescriber because dosage may need adjustment.
• Advise patient to protect tablets from light and moisture.

liothyronine sodium (T_3)
Cytomel, Tertroxin‡, Triostat

Pharmacologic class: thyroid hormone
Pregnancy risk category A

AVAILABLE FORMS
Injection: 10 mcg/ml in 1-ml vials*
Tablets: 5 mcg, 20 mcg‡, 25 mcg, 50 mcg

INDICATIONS & DOSAGES
➤ Congenital hypothyroidism
Children: 5 mcg P.O. daily; increase by 5 mcg q 3 to 4 days until desired response is achieved.
➤ Myxedema
Adults: Initially, 2.5 to 5 mcg P.O. daily; increase by 5 to 10 mcg q 1 to 2 weeks until daily dose reaches 25 mcg. Then, increase by 12.5 to 25 mcg daily q 1 to 2 weeks. Maintenance dosage is 50 to 100 mcg daily.
➤ Myxedema coma, premyxedema coma
Adults: Initially, 10 to 20 mcg I.V. for patients with CV disease; 25 to 50 mcg I.V. for patients who don't have CV disease. Adjust dosage based on patient's condition and response. Switch patient to oral therapy as soon as possible.

➤ **Simple (nontoxic) goiter**
Adults: Initially, 5 mcg P.O. daily; may increase by 5 to 10 mcg daily q 1 to 2 weeks, until daily dose reaches 25 mcg. Then, increase by 12.5 to 25 mcg daily q 1 to 2 weeks. Usual maintenance dosage is 75 mcg daily.

➤ **Thyroid hormone replacement**
Adults: Initially, 25 mcg P.O. daily; increase by 12.5 to 25 mcg q 1 to 2 weeks until satisfactory response occurs. Usual maintenance dosage is 25 to 50 mcg daily.
Patients older than age 65 and children: 5 mcg daily; increase by 5 mcg daily q 1 to 2 weeks.

➤ **T_3 suppression test to differentiate hyperthyroidism from euthyroidism**
Adults: 75 to 100 mcg P.O. daily for 7 days.

I.V. ADMINISTRATION

- Give repeat doses 4 to 12 hours apart.
- To store, refrigerate vials.

INCOMPATIBILITIES

None reported.

ACTION

Unclear. Enhances oxygen consumption by most tissues of the body; increases the basal metabolic rate and the metabolism of carbohydrates, lipids, and proteins.

Route	Onset	Peak	Duration
P.O.	Unknown	2–3 days	3 days
I.V.	Unknown	Unknown	Unknown

Half-life: Less than or equal to 2½ days.

ADVERSE REACTIONS

CNS: *nervousness, insomnia, tremor,* headache.
CV: *tachycardia,* ***arrhythmias,*** angina, ***cardiac decompensation and collapse.***
GI: diarrhea, vomiting.
GU: menstrual irregularities.
Metabolic: weight loss.
Musculoskeletal: accelerated bone maturation in infants and children.
Skin: skin reactions, diaphoresis.
Other: heat intolerance.

INTERACTIONS

Drug-drug. *Beta blockers:* May reduce beta-blocker effect. Monitor patient for clinical effect.
Aluminum and magnesium antacids, cholestyramine, colestipol, sucralfate: May impair liothyronine absorption. Separate doses by 4 to 5 hours.
Digoxin: May decrease glycoside effect. Monitor patient for clinical effect.
Insulin, oral antidiabetics: First thyroid replacement therapy may increase insulin or oral hypoglycemic requirements. Monitor glucose level. Dosage adjustments may be needed.
Sympathomimetics such as epinephrine: May increase risk of coronary insufficiency. Monitor patient closely.
Theophylline: May decrease theophylline clearance in hypothyroidism; clearance may return to normal when euthyroid state is achieved. Monitor theophylline level.
Warfarin: May increase warfarin effect. Monitor patient for bleeding and check PT and INR closely. Warfarin dosage adjustment may be needed.
Drug-herb. *Lemon balm:* May have antithyroid effects; may inhibit thyroid-stimulating hormone. Discourage use together.
Drug-food. *Cottonseed meal, dietary fiber, soybean flour, walnuts:* May decrease absorption of drug. Dosage adjustments may be needed.

EFFECTS ON LAB TEST RESULTS

- May decrease thyroid function test results. May alter results of liothyronine, protein-bound iodine, and radioactive ^{131}I uptake studies.

CONTRAINDICATIONS & CAUTIONS

- Contraindicated in patients hypersensitive to drug and in those with acute MI uncomplicated by hypothyroidism, untreated thyrotoxicosis, or uncorrected adrenal insufficiency. Also contraindicated with artificial rewarming of patients.
- Use cautiously in elderly patients and in those with angina pectoris, hypertension, other CV disorders, renal insufficiency, or ischemia.
- Use cautiously in patients with diabetes mellitus, diabetes insipidus, or myxedema

and during rapid replacement in those with arteriosclerosis.

NURSING CONSIDERATIONS

- Watch for angina, coronary occlusion, or stroke in patients with arteriosclerosis who are receiving rapid replacement. In patients with coronary artery disease who must receive thyroid hormones, watch for possible coronary insufficiency.
- ***Alert:*** Drug may be used when a rapid-onset or a rapidly reversible drug is desirable, or in patients with impaired peripheral conversion of levothyroxine to liothyronine.
- Long-term therapy causes bone loss in premenopausal and postmenopausal women. Consider a basal bone density measurement, and monitor patient closely for osteoporosis.
- Thyroid hormone replacement requirements are about 25% lower in patients older than age 60 than in young adults.
- Monitor pulse and blood pressure.
- When changing from levothyroxine to this drug, stop levothyroxine and start this drug at a low dosage. Increase dosage in small increments after residual effects of levothyroxine have disappeared. When changing from this drug to levothyroxine, start levothyroxine several days before stopping this drug to avoid relapse.
- When switching from I.V. to P.O. therapy, gradually increase I.V. dose while starting P.O. dose.
- Patients who need ^{131}I uptake studies done must stop drug 7 to 10 days before test.
- In pregnant patients, dosage may need to be increased.
- ***Look alike–sound alike:*** Don't confuse levothyroxine with liothyronine or liotrix. Don't confuse Cytomel with Cytotec.
- ***Alert:*** Don't give injection I.M. or subcutaneously.

PATIENT TEACHING

- Teach patient importance of compliance. Tell him to take thyroid hormones at same time each day, preferably before breakfast, to maintain constant hormone levels and help prevent insomnia.
- Make sure patient understands that replacement therapy is usually for life. Drug should never be stopped unless directed by prescriber.
- Advise patient who has achieved a stable response not to change brands.
- Warn patient (especially elderly patient) to notify prescriber at once about chest pain, palpitations, sweating, nervousness, or other signals of overdose or aggravated CV disease.
- Tell patient to report unusual bleeding and bruising.
- For diabetic patients, advise them to monitor glucose level closely.
- Tell patient not to take OTC or other prescription medications without first consulting his prescriber.
- Advise woman to report pregnancy to prescriber because dosage may need adjustment.

liotrix

Thyrolar

Pharmacologic class: thyroid hormone
Pregnancy risk category A

AVAILABLE FORMS

Tablets: Levothyroxine sodium 12.5 mcg and liothyronine sodium 3.1 mcg (Thyrolar-1/4); levothyroxine sodium 25 mcg and liothyronine sodium 6.25 mcg (Thyrolar-1/2); levothyroxine sodium 50 mcg and liothyronine sodium 12.5 mcg (Thyrolar-1); levothyroxine sodium 100 mcg and liothyronine sodium 25 mcg (Thyrolar-2); levothyroxine sodium 150 mcg and liothyronine sodium 37.5 mcg (Thyrolar-3)

INDICATIONS & DOSAGES

Dosages are expressed in thyroid equivalents and must be individualized to approximate the deficit in patient's thyroid secretion.

➤ Hypothyroidism

Adults: Initially, a single daily dose of Thyrolar-1/2. Adjust dosage by 1 tablet of Thyrolar-1/4 at 2 to 3 week intervals. Maintenance dose is 1 tablet of Thyrolar-1 or Thyrolar-2 daily. Readjust dose within the first 4 weeks of therapy after proper clinical and laboratory evaluations of T_4 and TSH.

Adjust-a-dose: For elderly patients and patients with long-standing myxedema with cardiovascular impairment, initial dose is 1 tablet of Thyrolar-1/4 daily. Reduce dose if angina occurs.

➤ **Congenital hypothyroidism**
Children older than age 12: More than 18.75/75 (T_3/T_4) mcg P.O. daily.
Children ages 6 to 12: 12.5/50 (T_3/T_4) to 18.75/75 mcg (T_3/T_4) P.O. daily.
Children ages 1 to 5: 9.35/37.5 (T_3/T_4) to 12.5/50 (T_3/T_4) mcg P.O. daily.
Children ages 6 to 12 months: 6.25/25 (T_3/T_4) to 9.35/37.5 (T_3/T_4) mcg P.O. daily.
Newborns and infants birth to 6 months: 3.1/12.5 (T_3/T_4) to 6.25/25 (T_3/T_4) mcg P.O. daily.

ACTION

Not clearly defined. Stimulates metabolism of all body tissues by accelerating the rate of cellular oxidation and provides both T_3 and T_4 to the tissues.

Route	Onset	Peak	Duration
P.O.	Unknown	Unknown	Unknown

Half-life: Unknown.

ADVERSE REACTIONS

CNS: *nervousness, insomnia, tremor,* headache.
CV: *tachycardia,* ***arrhythmias,*** angina pectoris, ***cardiac decompensation and collapse.***
GI: diarrhea, vomiting.
GU: menstrual irregularities.
Metabolic: weight loss.
Musculoskeletal: accelerated rate of bone maturation in infants and children.
Skin: allergic skin reactions, diaphoresis.
Other: heat intolerance.

INTERACTIONS

Drug-drug. *Beta blockers:* May reduce beta-blocker effect. Monitor patient for clinical effect.
Cholestyramine, colestipol: May impair liotrix absorption. Separate doses by 4 to 5 hours.
Digoxin: May decrease glycoside effect. Monitor patient for clinical effect.
Estrogens: May decrease thyroid levels. Monitor levels after 12 weeks of therapy and adjust liotrix dose as needed.
Fosphenytoin, phenytoin: May release free thyroid hormone. Monitor patient for tachycardia.
Insulin, oral antidiabetics: May alter glucose level. Monitor glucose level. Dosage adjustments may be needed.
Sympathomimetics such as epinephrine: May increase risk of coronary insufficiency. Monitor patient closely.
Theophylline: May decrease theophylline clearance in hypothyroidism; clearance may return to normal when euthyroid state is achieved. Monitor theophylline level.
Warfarin: May increase anticoagulant effects. Monitor patient for bleeding and check PT and INR closely. Warfarin dosage adjustment may be needed.
Drug-herb. *Lemon balm:* May have antithyroid effects; may inhibit thyroid-stimulating hormone. Discourage use together.

EFFECTS ON LAB TEST RESULTS

- May decrease thyroid function test results. May alter results of liothyronine, protein-bound iodine, and radioactive ^{131}I uptake studies.

CONTRAINDICATIONS & CAUTIONS

- Contraindicated in patients hypersensitive to drug and in those with acute MI uncomplicated by hypothyroidism, untreated thyrotoxicosis, or uncorrected adrenal insufficiency.
- Use cautiously in elderly patients and in those with angina pectoris, hypertension, other CV disorders, renal insufficiency, or ischemia.
- Use cautiously in patients with diabetes mellitus, diabetes insipidus, or myxedema and during rapid replacement in those with arteriosclerosis.

NURSING CONSIDERATIONS

- Watch for angina, coronary occlusion, or stroke in patients with arteriosclerosis who are receiving rapid replacement.
- In patients with coronary artery disease who must receive thyroid hormones, monitor patient for possible coronary insufficiency. Also watch carefully during surgery because arrhythmias may arise.

• Thyroid hormone replacement requirements are about 25% lower in patients older than age 60 than in young adults.
• Dosage may need to be increased in pregnant patients.
• Monitor pulse and blood pressure.
• Long-term therapy causes bone loss in premenopausal and postmenopausal women. Consider a basal bone density measurement and monitor patient closely for osteoporosis.
• Patients taking liotrix must stop drug 7 to 10 days before undergoing ^{131}I uptake studies.
• ***Look alike–sound alike:*** Don't confuse Thyrolar with thyroid or Synthroid; don't confuse liotrix with levothyroxine or liothyronine.

PATIENT TEACHING
• Teach patient importance of compliance. He should take thyroid hormones at same time each day, preferably before breakfast, to maintain constant hormone levels and help prevent insomnia.
• Tell patient that drug should never be stopped unless directed by prescriber.
• Warn patient (especially elderly patient) to notify prescriber at once about chest pain, palpitations, sweating, nervousness, or other signs of overdose or aggravated CV disease.
• Tell patient to report unusual bleeding and bruising.
• Advise patient not to take other drugs (OTC or prescription) without first consulting his prescriber.
• Advise patient to report pregnancy to prescriber because dosage may need adjustment.

thyroid, desiccated
Armour Thyroid

Pharmacologic class: thyroid hormone
Pregnancy risk category A

AVAILABLE FORMS
Tablets: 15 mg, 30 mg, 60 mg, 90 mg, 120 mg, 180 mg, 240 mg, 300 mg

INDICATIONS & DOSAGES
➤ **Mild hypothyroidism**
Adults: Initially, 60 mg P.O. daily, increased by 60 mg q 30 days until desired response occurs. Usual maintenance dose is 60 to 120 mg daily as single dose.
Elderly patients: Start at lower dose.
➤ **Severe hypothyroidism**
Adults: Initially, 15 mg P.O. daily; increased by 30 mg daily after 2 weeks, and 2 weeks later increased to 60 mg daily. After 2 months, increase to 120 mg daily if response is still inadequate. May further increase to 180 mg if response remains inadequate. Usual maintenance dose is 60 to 180 mg daily.
Patients older than age 65: Give 7.5 to 15 mg daily. May double dose q 6 to 8 weeks until desired result is obtained.
➤ **Congenital or severe hypothyroidism in children**
Children older than age 12: Give more than 90 mg or 1.2 to 1.8 mg/kg P.O. daily.
Children ages 6 to 12: Give 60 to 90 mg or 2.4 to 3 mg/kg P.O. daily.
Children ages 1 to 5: Give 45 to 60 mg or 3 to 3.6 mg/kg P.O. daily.
Children ages 6 months to 1 year: 30 to 45 mg or 3.6 to 4.8 mg/kg P.O. daily.
Neonates and infants younger than age 6 months: 7.5 to 30 mg or 2.4 to 6 mg/kg P.O. daily.
Adjust-a-dose: In patients with long-term disease, other endocrine diseases, severe hypothyroidism, or CV disease, start at lower dose.

ACTION
Not clearly defined. Stimulates metabolism of all body tissues by accelerating the rate of cellular oxidation.

Route	Onset	Peak	Duration
P.O.	Unknown	Unknown	Unknown

Half-life: T_4, 7 days; T_3, 2 days.

ADVERSE REACTIONS
CNS: *nervousness, insomnia,* tremor, headache.
CV: *tachycardia,* ***arrhythmias,*** angina pectoris, ***cardiac decompensation and collapse.***
GI: diarrhea, vomiting.
GU: menstrual irregularities.

Metabolic: weight loss.
Musculoskeletal: accelerated rate of bone maturation in infants and children.
Skin: allergic skin reactions, diaphoresis.
Other: heat intolerance.

INTERACTIONS

Drug-drug. *Beta blockers:* May reduce beta-blocker effect. Monitor patient for clinical effect.
Cholestyramine: May impair thyroid absorption. Separate doses by 4 to 5 hours.
Digoxin: May decrease glycoside effect. Monitor patient for effect.
Estrogens: May decrease thyroid levels. Monitor levels after 12 weeks of therapy and adjust thyroid dose, as needed.
Insulin, oral antidiabetics: May alter glucose level. Monitor glucose level, and adjust dosage as needed.
Sympathomimetics such as epinephrine: May increase risk of coronary insufficiency. Monitor patient closely.
Theophylline: May decrease theophylline clearance in hypothyroidism; clearance may return to normal when euthyroid state is achieved. Monitor theophylline level.
Warfarin: May increase warfarin's effect. Monitor patient for bleeding and check PT and INR closely. Warfarin dosage adjustment may be needed.
Drug-herb. *Lemon balm:* May have antithyroid effects; may inhibit thyroid-stimulating hormone. Discourage use together.

EFFECTS ON LAB TEST RESULTS

- May decrease thyroid function test results. May alter results of liothyronine, protein-bound iodine, and radioactive ^{131}I uptake studies.

CONTRAINDICATIONS & CAUTIONS

- Contraindicated in patients hypersensitive to drug and in those with acute MI uncomplicated by hypothyroidism, untreated thyrotoxicosis, or uncorrected adrenal insufficiency.
- Use cautiously in elderly patients and in those with angina pectoris, hypertension, other CV disorders, renal insufficiency, or ischemia.
- Use cautiously in patients with myxedema, diabetes mellitus, or diabetes insipidus.

NURSING CONSIDERATIONS

- Check for coronary insufficiency in patients with coronary artery disease.
- Thyroid hormone replacement requirements are about 25% lower in patients older than age 60 than in young adults.
- Dosage may need to be increased in pregnant women.
- Monitor pulse and blood pressure.
- Reduce dose if angina occurs.
- Long-term therapy causes bone loss in premenopausal and postmenopausal women. Consider a basal bone density measurement, and monitor patient closely for osteoporosis.
- In children, treatment is guided by sleeping pulse rate and basal morning temperature.
- Patient must stop thyroid hormones 7 to 10 days before undergoing ^{131}I studies.
- ***Look alike–sound alike:*** Don't confuse thyroid with Thyrolar.

PATIENT TEACHING

- Tell patient to take thyroid hormones at same time each day, preferably before breakfast, to maintain constant hormone levels and help prevent insomnia.
- Tell patient the drug should never be stopped unless directed by prescriber.
- Advise patient who has achieved stable response not to change brands.
- Warn patient (especially elderly patient) to notify prescriber at once about chest pain, palpitations, or other signs of overdose or aggravated CV disease.
- Tell patient to report unusual bleeding and bruising.
- Advise patient not to take other drugs (OTC or prescription) without first consulting his prescriber.
- Advise patient to report pregnancy to prescriber, because dosage may need adjustment.

57
Thyroid hormone antagonists

methimazole
potassium iodide
propylthiouracil
radioactive iodine

methimazole
Tapazole

Pharmacologic class: thyroid hormone antagonist
Pregnancy risk category D

AVAILABLE FORMS
Tablets: 5 mg, 10 mg

INDICATIONS & DOSAGES
➤ **Hyperthyroidism**
Adults: If mild, 15 mg P.O. daily. If moderately severe, 30 to 40 mg daily. If severe, 60 mg daily. Daily amount is divided into three equal doses and given at 8-hour intervals. Maintenance dosage is 5 to 30 mg daily.
Children: 0.4 mg/kg P.O. in three divided doses daily. Maintenance dosage is 0.2 mg/kg in divided doses daily.

ACTION
Inhibits oxidation of iodine in thyroid gland, blocking ability of iodine to combine with tyrosine to form T_4. Also may prevent coupling of monoiodotyrosine and diiodotyrosine to form T_4 and T_3.

Route	Onset	Peak	Duration
P.O.	Rapid	30–60 min	Unknown

Half-life: 5 to 13 hours.

ADVERSE REACTIONS
CNS: headache, drowsiness, vertigo, paresthesia, neuritis, neuropathies, CNS stimulation, depression, fever.
GI: diarrhea, nausea, vomiting, salivary gland enlargement, loss of taste, epigastric distress.
GU: nephritis.
Hematologic: ***agranulocytosis, leukopenia, thrombocytopenia, aplastic anemia.***
Hepatic: jaundice, hepatic dysfunction, ***hepatitis.***
Metabolic: hypothyroidism.
Musculoskeletal: arthralgia, myalgia.
Skin: rash, urticaria, discoloration, pruritus, erythema nodosum, exfoliative dermatitis, lupuslike syndrome, abnormal hair loss.
Other: lymphadenopathy.

INTERACTIONS
Drug-drug. *Aminophylline, theophylline:* May decrease clearance of these drugs. Dosage may need to be adjusted.
Beta blockers: Hyperthyroidism may increase beta-blocker clearance. May need to reduce dosage of beta blocker when patient becomes euthyroid.
Cardiac glycosides: May increase cardiac glycoside level. Cardiac glycoside dosage may need to be reduced.
Potassium iodide: May decrease response to drug. Methimazole dosage may need to be increased.
Warfarin: May alter dosage requirements. Monitor PT, PTT, and INR.

EFFECTS ON LAB TEST RESULTS
- May decrease hemoglobin level.
- May decrease granulocyte, WBC, and platelet counts.
- May alter ^{123}I or ^{131}I uptake by the thyroid.

CONTRAINDICATIONS & CAUTIONS
- Contraindicated in patients hypersensitive to drug and in breast-feeding women.
- Use cautiously in pregnant patients.

NURSING CONSIDERATIONS
- Pregnant women may need less drug as pregnancy progresses. Monitor thyroid function studies closely. Thyroid hormone may be added to regimen. Drug may be stopped during last few weeks of pregnancy.
- Monitor CBC periodically to detect impending leukopenia, thrombocytopenia, and agranulocytosis; also monitor hepatic

function. Stop drug if liver abnormality occurs.
- ***Alert:*** Doses higher than 30 mg daily increase risk of agranulocytosis.
- ***Alert:*** Patients older than age 40 may have an increased risk of drug-induced agranulocytosis.
- Watch for evidence of hypothyroidism (mental depression, cold intolerance, hard, nonpitting edema); notify prescriber because patient may need dosage adjustment.
- ***Alert:*** Stop drug and notify prescriber if severe rash or enlarged cervical lymph nodes develop.
- ***Look alike–sound alike:*** Don't confuse methimazole with mebendazole or methazolamide.

PATIENT TEACHING

- Tell patient to take drug with meals to reduce adverse GI reactions.
- Warn patient to report fever, sore throat, mouth sores, skin eruptions, anorexia, itching, right upper quadrant pain, yellow skin or eyes.
- Tell patient to ask prescriber about using iodized salt and eating shellfish because the iodine in these foods may make the drug less effective.
- Warn patient that drug may cause drowsiness; advise patient to use caution when operating machinery or a vehicle.
- Instruct patient to store drug in light-resistant container.
- Teach patient to watch for evidence of hypothyroidism (unexplained weight gain, fatigue, cold intolerance) and to notify prescriber if it arises.
- Tell woman not to use drug while breast-feeding.

potassium iodide

saturated solution (SSKI), strong iodine solution (Lugol solution), ThyroSafe, ThyroShield

Pharmacologic class: salt of stable iodine
Pregnancy risk category D

AVAILABLE FORMS

Oral solution (Lugol solution): iodine 5% and potassium iodide 10%
Oral solution (SSKI): 1 g/ml
Oral solution (ThyroShield): 65 mg/ml
Tablets: 65 mg, 130 mg

INDICATIONS & DOSAGES

➤ To prepare for thyroidectomy
Adults and children: 3 to 5 drops strong iodine solution P.O. t.i.d.; or 1 to 5 drops SSKI in water P.O. t.i.d. after meals for 10 days before surgery.

➤ Thyrotoxic crisis
Adults and children: 500 mg P.O. q 4 hours (about 10 drops of SSKI); or 1 ml of strong iodine solution t.i.d. Give at least 1 hour after the first dose of propylthiouracil or methimazole.

➤ Radiation protectant for thyroid gland
Adults: 130 mg P.O. daily until risk of substantial exposure to radioiodines no longer exists. Start no later than 3 or 4 hours after acute exposure. Avoid repeat doses in pregnant or breast-feeding women.
Children ages 3 to 18: Give 65 mg P.O. daily until risk of substantial exposure to radioiodines no longer exists. Start no later than 3 or 4 hours after acute exposure.
Children age 1 month to 3 years: 32 mg P.O. daily until risk of substantial exposure to radioiodines no longer exists. Start no later than 3 or 4 hours after acute exposure.
Infants age 1 month or younger: 16 mg P.O. Avoid repeat dosing, if possible.

ACTION

Inhibits thyroid hormone formation, limits iodide transport into the thyroid gland, and blocks thyroid hormone release.

Route	Onset	Peak	Duration
P.O.	< 24 hr	10–15 days	Unknown

Half-life: Unknown.

ADVERSE REACTIONS

CNS: fever.
EENT: periorbital edema.
GI: nausea, vomiting, diarrhea, inflammation of salivary glands, burning mouth and throat, sore teeth and gums, *metallic taste.*
Metabolic: ***potassium toxicity.***
Skin: acneiform rash.
Other: hypersensitivity reactions.

INTERACTIONS

Drug-drug. *ACE inhibitors, potassium-sparing diuretics:* May cause hyperkalemia. Avoid using together.
Antithyroid drugs: May increase hypothyroid or goitrogenic effects. Monitor patient closely.
Lithium carbonate: May cause hypothyroidism. Use together cautiously.
Drug-food. *Iodized salt, shellfish:* May alter drug's effectiveness. Urge caution.

EFFECTS ON LAB TEST RESULTS

- May increase potassium level.
- May alter thyroid function test results.

CONTRAINDICATIONS & CAUTIONS

- Contraindicated in patients with tuberculosis, acute bronchitis, iodide hypersensitivity, or hyperkalemia. Some formulations contain sulfites, which may cause allergic reactions in hypersensitive patients.
- Use cautiously in patients with hypocomplementemic vasculitis, goiter, or autoimmune thyroid disease.

NURSING CONSIDERATIONS

- The FDA doesn't recommend prophylaxis with potassium iodide for a radiation emergency in adults over 40 years of age unless a large internal radiation dose is anticipated.
- For thyrotoxicosis, first iodine dose is given at least 1 hour after first dose of propylthiouracil and methimazole.
- Dilute oral solution in water, milk, or fruit juice, and give after meals to prevent gastric irritation, hydrate patient, and mask salty taste.
- Give iodides through straw to avoid tooth discoloration.
- ***Alert:*** Earliest signs of delayed hypersensitivity reactions caused by iodides are irritation and swollen eyelids.
- Signs of an iodide hypersensitivity reaction include angioedema, cutaneous and mucosal hemorrhage, fever, arthralgia, lymph node enlargement, and eosinophilia.
- Monitor patient for iodism, which can cause metallic taste, burning in mouth and throat, sore teeth and gums, increased salivation, coryza, sneezing, eye irritation with swelling of eyelids, severe headache, productive cough, GI irritation, diarrhea, rash, or soreness of the pharynx, larynx, and tonsils.
- Store in light-resistant container.

PATIENT TEACHING

- Show patient how to mask salty taste of oral solution. Tell him to take all forms of drug after meals.
- ***Alert:*** Warn patient that sudden withdrawal may precipitate thyroid crisis.
- ***Alert:*** Teach patient signs and symptoms of potassium toxicity, including confusion, irregular heartbeat, numbness, tingling, pain or weakness of hands or feet, and tiredness.
- Tell patient to ask prescriber about using iodized salt and eating shellfish. These foods contain iodine and may alter drug's effectiveness.
- Tell patient not to increase the amount of potassium through diet.
- Tell patient to stop drug and notify prescriber if epigastric pain, rash, metallic taste, nausea, or vomiting occurs.

propylthiouracil (PTU)

Propyl-Thyracil†

Pharmacologic class: thyroid hormone antagonist
Pregnancy risk category D

AVAILABLE FORMS

Tablets: 50 mg, 100 mg†

INDICATIONS & DOSAGES

➤ Hyperthyroidism

Adults: 300 to 450 mg P.O. daily in divided doses. Patients with severe hyperthyroidism or very large goiters may need initial doses of 600 to 1,200 mg daily. Continue until patient is euthyroid; then start maintenance dose of 100 mg to 150 mg P.O. daily.
Children older than age 10: Initially, 150 to 300 mg or 150 mg/m^2 P.O. daily in divided doses. Continue until patient is euthyroid. Individualize maintenance dose.
Children ages 6 to 10: Initially, 50 to 150 mg P.O. daily in divided doses q 8 hours. Continue until patient is euthyroid. Individualize maintenance dose.

Neonates: 5 to 10 mg/kg P.O. daily in divided doses t.i.d.

➤ **Thyrotoxic crisis**

Adults: 200 mg P.O. q 4 to 6 hours on first day; once symptoms are fully controlled, gradually reduce dosage to usual maintenance levels.

ACTION

Inhibits oxidation of iodine in thyroid gland, blocking ability of iodine to combine with tyrosine to form T_4, and may prevent coupling of monoiodotyrosine and diiodotyrosine to form T_4 and T_3.

Route	Onset	Peak	Duration
P.O.	Unknown	60–90 min	Unknown

Half-life: 1 to 2 hours.

ADVERSE REACTIONS

CNS: headache, drowsiness, vertigo, paresthesia, neuritis, neuropathies, CNS stimulation, depression, fever.
CV: vasculitis.
EENT: visual disturbances, loss of taste.
GI: diarrhea, *nausea, vomiting,* epigastric distress, salivary gland enlargement.
GU: nephritis.
Hematologic: ***agranulocytosis, leukopenia, thrombocytopenia, aplastic anemia.***
Hepatic: jaundice, ***hepatotoxicity.***
Metabolic: dose-related hypothyroidism.
Musculoskeletal: arthralgia, myalgia.
Skin: rash, urticaria, skin discoloration, pruritus, erythema nodosum, exfoliative dermatitis, lupuslike syndrome.
Other: lymphadenopathy.

INTERACTIONS

Drug-drug. *Aminophylline, oxtriphylline, theophylline:* May decrease clearance of these drugs. Dosage may need to be adjusted.
Cardiac glycosides: May increase glycoside level. Dosage may need to be reduced.
Potassium iodide: May decrease response to drug. Dosage of antithyroid drug may need to be increased.
Warfarin: May increase anticoagulation. Monitor PT and INR.
Drug-food. *Iodized salt, shellfish:* May alter drug's effectiveness. Urge caution.

EFFECTS ON LAB TEST RESULTS

- May decrease hemoglobin level.
- May decrease granulocyte, WBC, and platelet counts and liothyronine uptake.

CONTRAINDICATIONS & CAUTIONS

- Contraindicated in patients hypersensitive to drug and in breast-feeding women.
- Use cautiously in pregnant patients.

NURSING CONSIDERATIONS

- Pregnant women may need less drug as pregnancy progresses. Monitor thyroid function studies closely. Thyroid hormone may be added to regimen. Drug may be stopped during last few weeks of pregnancy.
- ***Alert:*** Patients older than age 40 may have an increased risk of agranulocytosis.
- Give drug with meals to reduce adverse GI reactions.
- Watch for hypothyroidism (mental depression, cold intolerance, and hard, nonpitting edema); adjust dosage.
- Monitor CBC periodically to detect impending leukopenia, thrombocytopenia, and agranulocytosis.
- ***Alert:*** Stop drug and notify prescriber if severe rash develops or cervical lymph nodes enlarge.
- Monitor hepatic function. Stop drug if transaminase levels are greater than three times the upper limit of normal.
- Store drug in light-resistant container.

PATIENT TEACHING

- Instruct patient to take drug with meals.
- Warn patient to report fever, sore throat, mouth sores, and skin eruptions.
- Tell patient to report unusual bleeding or bruising.
- Tell patient to ask prescriber about using iodized salt and eating shellfish. These foods contain iodine and may alter effectiveness of drug.
- Teach patient to watch for signs and symptoms of hypothyroidism (unexplained weight gain, fatigue, cold intolerance) and to notify prescriber if they occur.

SAFETY ALERT!

radioactive iodine (sodium iodide ^{131}I)

Iodotope, Sodium Iodide ^{131}I Therapeutic

Pharmacologic class: thyroid hormone antagonist
Pregnancy risk category X

AVAILABLE FORMS

All radioactivity concentrations are determined at time of calibration.
Iodotope
Capsules: Radioactivity range 8 to 100 millicuries (mCi)/capsule
Oral solution: Radioactivity concentration 7.05 mCi/ml
Sodium Iodide ^{131}I Therapeutic
Capsules: Radioactivity range 0.75 to 100 mCi/capsule
Oral solution: Radioactivity range 3.5 to 150 mCi/vial

INDICATIONS & DOSAGES

➤ **Hyperthyroidism**
Adults: Usual dosage is 4 to 10 mCi P.O. Dosage is based on estimated weight of thyroid gland and thyroid uptake. Repeat treatment after 6 weeks, based on T_4 level.
➤ **Thyroid cancer**
Adults: Initially, 50 to 100 mCi P.O., with subsequent doses of 100 to 150 mCi. Dosage is based on estimated malignant thyroid tissue and metastatic tissue as determined by total body scan. Repeat treatment according to clinical status.

ACTION

Limits thyroid hormone secretion by destroying thyroid tissue. Affinity of thyroid tissue for radioactive iodine facilitates uptake of drug by cancerous thyroid tissue that has metastasized to other sites in the body.

Route	Onset	Peak	Duration
P.O.	Unknown	60–90 min	Unknown

Half-life: Unknown.

ADVERSE REACTIONS

CV: chest pain, tachycardia.
EENT: *fullness in neck,* pain on swallowing, sore throat.
GI: nausea, vomiting.
Hematologic: anemia, blood dyscrasia, ***leukopenia, thrombocytopenia.***
Metabolic: hypothyroidism, radiation-induced thyroiditis.
Respiratory: cough.
Skin: rash, pruritus, urticaria, temporary thinning of hair.
Other: radiation sickness, allergic-type reactions.

INTERACTIONS

Drug-drug. *Lithium carbonate:* May cause hypothyroidism. Use together cautiously.

These drugs may interfere with the action of ^{131}I and should be withheld for the specified time before the ^{131}I dose is given:
Adrenocorticoids: 1 week.
Benzodiazepines: 1 month.
Cholecystographic drugs: 6 to 9 months.
Contrast media that contain iodine: 1 to 2 months.
Products containing iodine, including topical drugs, and vitamins: 2 weeks.
Salicylates: 1 to 2 weeks.

EFFECTS ON LAB TEST RESULTS

- May decrease hemoglobin, T_4, and thyroid-stimulating hormone levels. May increase or decrease protein-bound iodine level.
- May decrease platelet and WBC counts. May alter ^{131}I thyroid uptake.

CONTRAINDICATIONS & CAUTIONS

- Contraindicated in women who are or may become pregnant or are breast-feeding. Also contraindicated in a patient who is vomiting or has diarrhea.

NURSING CONSIDERATIONS

- All antithyroid drugs and thyroid preparations must be stopped 1 week before ^{131}I dose. If this isn't possible, patient may receive thyroid-stimulating hormone for 3 days before ^{131}I dose.
- Measure the dose by a radioactivity calibration system immediately before administration.

- Sodium iodide ^{131} I is not typically used for treatment of hyperthyroidism in patients younger than age 30.
- When treating women of childbearing age, give dose during menstruation or within 7 days afterward.
- After therapy for hyperthyroidism, patient shouldn't resume antithyroid drugs but should continue propranolol or other drugs used to treat symptoms of hyperthyroidism until onset of full ^{131}I effect (usually 6 weeks).
- Monitor thyroid function by T_4 and thyroid-stimulating hormone levels.
- Institute full radiation precautions. Have patient use proper disposal methods when coughing and expectorating. After dose for hyperthyroidism, patient's urine and saliva are slightly radioactive for 24 hours; vomitus is highly radioactive for 6 to 8 hours.
- After dose for thyroid cancer, patient's urine, saliva, and perspiration are radioactive for 3 days. Isolate patient and observe these precautions: Don't allow pregnant personnel to care for patient; provide disposable eating utensils and linens; instruct patient to save urine in lead container for 24 to 48 hours; limit contact with patient to 30 minutes per shift per person on day 1, and increase time, as needed, to 1 hour on day 2 and longer on day 3.

PATIENT TEACHING

- Tell patient to fast overnight before therapy and to drink as much fluid as possible for 48 hours afterward.
- Instruct patient about appropriate radiation exposure precautions to use after receiving drug.
- Warn patient who is discharged fewer than 7 days after ^{131}I dose for thyroid cancer to avoid close contact with small children and not to sleep in same room with another person for 7 days after treatment.
- Teach patient the signs and symptoms of hypothyroidism (unexplained weight gain, fatigue, cold intolerance) and instruct him to notify prescriber if they occur.

58
Pituitary hormones

desmopressin acetate
leuprolide acetate
(See Chapter 70, ANTINEOPLASTICS THAT ALTER HORMONE BALANCE.)
somatropin
vasopressin

desmopressin acetate
DDAVP, Minirin‡, Octostim‡, Stimate

Pharmacologic class: posterior pituitary hormone
Pregnancy risk category B

AVAILABLE FORMS
Injection: 4 mcg/ml, 15 mcg/ml
Nasal solution: 0.1 mg/ml, 1.5 mg/ml
Tablets: 0.1 mg, 0.2 mg

INDICATIONS & DOSAGES
➤Nonnephrogenic diabetes insipidus, temporary polyuria, and polydipsia related to pituitary trauma
Adults and children older than age 12: Give 0.1 to 0.4 ml intranasally daily in one to three doses. Most adults need 0.2 ml daily in two divided doses. Or, give 0.5 to 1 ml I.V. or subcutaneously daily, usually in two divided doses. Or, give 0.05 mg P.O. b.i.d.; adjust dosage to patient response. If patient previously received the drug intranasally, begin oral therapy 12 hours after last intranasal dose.
Children ages 3 months to 12 years: 0.05 to 0.3 ml intranasally daily in one or two doses.
➤Hemophilia A and von Willebrand disease
Adults and children: 0.3 mcg/kg diluted in normal saline solution and infused I.V. over 15 to 30 minutes. Repeat dose, if needed, as indicated by laboratory response and patient's condition. Or, 300 mcg (one spray in each nostril) of solution containing 1.5 mcg/ml. Dose of 150 mcg (one spray of solution containing 1.5 mg/ml into a single nostril) may be adequate for patients weighing less than 50 kg (110 lb). Give drug 2 hours before surgery.
➤Primary nocturnal enuresis
Children age 6 and older: Initially, 20 mcg (0.2 ml) intranasally at bedtime. (10 mcg in each nostril). Adjust dosage based on response; maximum recommended dosage is 40 mcg daily. Or, initially 0.2 mg P.O. at bedtime, and adjust dose up to 0.6 mg to achieve desired response. For patients previously on intranasal DDAVP therapy, start tablet 24 hours after last intranasal dose in the nighttime.

I.V. ADMINISTRATION
- For adults and children who weigh more than 10 kg (22 lb), dilute with 50 ml sterile physiologic saline solution. For children who weigh 10 kg or less, 10 ml of diluent is recommended.
- Inspect drug for particulates and discoloration before infusing.
- Monitor blood pressure and pulse during infusion.

INCOMPATIBILITIES
None reported.

ACTION
Increases the permeability of renal tubular epithelium to adenosine monophosphate and water, enabling the epithelium to promote reabsorption of water and produce a concentrated urine. Also increases factor VIII activity by releasing endogenous factor VIII from plasma storage sites.

Route	Onset	Peak	Duration
P.O.	1 hr	1–1½ hr	8–12 hr
I.V.	15–30 min	Unknown	4–12 hr
Intranasal	1 hr	1–5 hr	8–12 hr

Half-life: Fast phase, about 8 minutes; slow phase, 114 hours.

ADVERSE REACTIONS
CNS: headache.
CV: flushing, slight rise in blood pressure.
EENT: rhinitis, epistaxis, sore throat.

GI: nausea, abdominal cramps.
GU: vulval pain.
Respiratory: cough.
Skin: local erythema, swelling, or burning after injection.

INTERACTIONS

Drug-drug. *Carbamazepine, chlorpropamide:* May increase ADH; may increase desmopressin effect. Avoid using together.
Clofibrate: May enhance and prolong effects of desmopressin. Monitor patient closely.
Demeclocycline, epinephrine, heparin, lithium: May increase risk of adverse effects. Monitor patient closely.
Pressor agents: May enhance pressor effects with large doses of desmopressin. Monitor patient closely.
Drug-lifestyle. *Alcohol use:* May increase risk of adverse effects. Discourage use together.

EFFECTS ON LAB TEST RESULTS

None reported.

CONTRAINDICATIONS & CAUTIONS

- Contraindicated in patients hypersensitive to drug and in those with type IIB von Willebrand disease.
- Use cautiously in patients with coronary artery insufficiency, hypertensive CV disease, and conditions linked to fluid and electrolyte imbalances, such as cystic fibrosis, because these patients are susceptible to hyponatremia.
- Use cautiously in breast-feeding women; it's unknown if drug appears in breast milk.

NURSING CONSIDERATIONS

- Morning and evening doses are adjusted separately for adequate diurnal rhythm of water turnover.
- Don't give injection to patients with hemophilia A with factor VIII of up to 5% or with severe von Willebrand disease.
- Ensure nasal passages are intact, clean, and free of obstruction before giving intranasally.
- Intranasal use can cause changes in the nasal mucosa, resulting in erratic, unreliable absorption. Report worsening condition to prescriber, who may recommend injectable DDAVP.
- Adjust fluid intake to reduce risk of water intoxication and sodium depletion, especially in children or elderly patients.
- ***Alert:*** Overdose may cause oxytocic or vasopressor activity. Withhold drug and notify prescriber. If fluid retention is excessive, give furosemide.
- ***Look alike–sound alike:*** Don't confuse desmopressin with vasopressin.
- Nasal spray pump only delivers doses of 10 mcg DDAVP or 150 mcg Stimate. If doses other than those are required, use the nasal tube delivery system or injection.

PATIENT TEACHING

- Some patients may have trouble measuring and inhaling drug into nostrils. Teach patient and caregivers correct administration method.
- Instruct patient to clear nasal passages before giving drug.
- Instruct patient to press down four times to prime pump. Tell him to discard the bottle after 25 (150 mcg/spray) or 50 doses (10 mcg/spray), depending on the strength, because the amount left may be less than desired dose.
- Advise patient to report nasal congestion, allergic rhinitis, or upper respiratory tract infection to prescriber; dosage adjustment may be needed.
- Teach patient using subcutaneous drug to rotate injection sites to prevent tissue damage.
- Warn patient to drink only enough water to satisfy thirst.
- Inform patient with hemophilia A or von Willebrand disease that taking desmopressin may prevent hazards of using blood products.
- Advise patient to carry medical identification indicating use of drug.

somatropin

Genotropin, Genotropin MiniQuick, Humatrope, Norditropin, Nutropin, Nutropin AQ, Saizen, Serostim, Tev-Tropin

Pharmacologic class: anterior pituitary hormone
Pregnancy risk category C; B (Serostim)

AVAILABLE FORMS

Genotropin injection: 1.5 mg (about 4.5 international units/vial), 5.8 mg (about 17.4 international units/vial), 13.8 mg (about 41.4 international units/vial)
Genotropin MiniQuick injection: 0.2 mg/vial, 0.4 mg/vial, 0.6 mg/vial, 0.8 mg/vial, 1 mg/vial, 1.2 mg/vial, 1.4 mg/vial, 1.6 mg/vial, 1.8 mg/vial, 2 mg/vial
Humatrope injection: 2 mg (about 6 international units/vial)†, 5 mg (about 15 international units/vial), 6 mg (18 international units/cartridge), 12 mg (36 international units/cartridge), 24 mg (72 international units/cartridge)
Norditropin injection: 4 mg (about 12 international units/ml), 8 mg (about 24 international units/ml), 5 mg/1.5 ml cartridges, 10 mg/1.5 ml cartridges, 15 mg/1.5 ml cartridges
Nutropin AQ injection: 10 mg (about 30 international units/vial)
Nutropin injection: 5 mg (about 15 international units/vial), 10 mg (about 30 international units/vial)
Saizen injection: 5 mg (about 15 international units/vial)
Serostim injection: 4 mg (about 12 international units/vial), 5 mg (about 15 international units/vial), 6 mg (about 18 international units/vial)
Tev-Tropin injection: 5 mg (15 international units/vial)

INDICATIONS & DOSAGES

➤ **Long-term treatment of growth failure in children with inadequate secretion of endogenous growth hormone (GH)**
Children: 0.18 mg/kg Humatrope I.M. or subcutaneously weekly, divided equally and given on 3 alternate days, six times weekly or once daily. Or, 0.3 mg/kg Nutropin or Nutropin AQ subcutaneously weekly in daily divided doses; in pubertal patients, a weekly dosage of 0.7 mg/kg (Nutropin or Nutropin AQ) in daily divided doses may be used. Or, 0.06 mg/kg Saizen I.M. or subcutaneously three times weekly. Or, 0.024 to 0.034 mg/kg Norditropin subcutaneously six to seven times weekly. Or, 0.16 to 0.24 mg/kg Genotropin subcutaneously weekly, divided into five to seven doses. Or, up to 0.1 mg/kg Tev-Tropin subcutaneously three times weekly.

➤ **Growth failure from chronic renal insufficiency up to time of renal transplantation**
Children: Up to 0.35 mg/kg weekly Nutropin or Nutropin AQ subcutaneously divided into daily doses.

➤ **Long-term treatment of short stature from Turner syndrome**
Children: Up to 0.375 mg/kg/week Humatrope, Nutropin, or Nutropin AQ subcutaneously divided into equal doses given three to seven times weekly.

➤ **Long-term treatment of growth failure in children with Prader-Willi syndrome diagnosed by genetic testing**
Children: 0.24 mg/kg Genotropin subcutaneously weekly, divided into six to seven doses.

➤ **Replacement of endogenous GH in adult patients with GH deficiency**
Adults: Initially, not more than 0.006 mg/kg Genotropin, Humatrope, Nutropin, or Nutropin AQ subcutaneously daily. May be increased to maximum of 0.0125 mg/kg Humatrope daily.

Nutropin or Nutropin AQ dosages may be increased to maximum of 0.025 mg/kg daily in patients younger than age 35 or 0.0125 mg/kg daily in patients older than age 35. Or, starting dosages not exceeding 0.04 mg/kg Genotropin subcutaneously weekly, divided into six to seven doses, may be increased at 4- to 8-week intervals to a maximum dose of 0.08 mg/kg subcutaneously weekly, divided into six to seven doses.

➤ **Replacement of endogenous GH in adult patients with GH deficiency**
Adults: Initially, not more than 0.005 mg/kg Saizen daily. May increase after 4 weeks to a maximum dose of

0.01 mg/kg daily based on patient tolerance and clinical response.

➤AIDS wasting or cachexia

Adults and children who weigh more than 55 kg (121 lb): 6 mg Serostim subcutaneously at bedtime.

Adults and children who weigh 45 to 55 kg (99 to 121 lb): 5 mg Serostim subcutaneously at bedtime.

Adults and children who weigh 35 to 45 kg (77 to 99 lb): 4 mg Serostim subcutaneously at bedtime.

Adults and children who weigh less than 35 kg: 0.1 mg/kg/day Serostim subcutaneously at bedtime.

➤Long-term treatment of growth failure in children born small for gestational age (SGA) who don't catch up by age 2

Children: 0.48 mg/kg Genotropin subcutaneously weekly, divided into five to seven doses.

➤Idiopathic short stature

Children: Up to 0.37 mg/kg Humatrope subcutaneously weekly, divided into six to seven equal doses.

ACTION

Purified GH of recombinant DNA origin that stimulates skeletal, linear, muscle, and organ growth.

Route	Onset	Peak	Duration
I.M., SubQ	Unknown	3–5 hr	12–48 hr

Half-life: 20 to 30 minutes.

ADVERSE REACTIONS

CNS: headache, weakness.
CV: mild, transient edema.
Hematologic: ***leukemia.***
Metabolic: mild hyperglycemia, hypothyroidism.
Musculoskeletal: localized muscle pain.
Skin: injection site pain.
Other: antibodies to GH.

INTERACTIONS

Drug-drug. *Corticotropin, corticosteroids:* Long-term use may inhibit growth response to GH. Monitor patient for lack of effect.

EFFECTS ON LAB TEST RESULTS

- May increase glucose, inorganic phosphorus, alkaline phosphatase, and parathyroid hormone levels.

CONTRAINDICATIONS & CAUTIONS

- Don't begin therapy in patients with acute critical illness from complications following open heart or abdominal surgery, trauma, or acute respiratory failure. Contraindicated in patients with closed epiphyses, active malignancy, or an active underlying intracranial lesion. For patients hypersensitive to either Metacresol or glycerin, don't use supplied diluent to reconstitute Humatrope. Genotropin is also contraindicated in patients with Prader-Willi syndrome who are severely obese or have severe respiratory impairment.
- Use cautiously in children with hypothyroidism and in those whose GH deficiency is caused by an intracranial lesion.

NURSING CONSIDERATIONS

- Frequently examine children with hypothyroidism and those whose GH deficiency is caused by an intracranial lesion for progression or recurrence of underlying disease.
- To prepare solution, inject supplied diluent into vial containing drug by aiming stream of liquid against wall of glass vial. Then swirl vial gently until contents are completely dissolved. Don't shake vial.
- After reconstitution, make sure solution is clear. Don't inject solution if it's cloudy or contains particles.
- For patients on hemodialysis, give drug before bedtime or 3 to 4 hours after dialysis. For long-term cycling peritoneal dialysis, give drug in the morning after completion of dialysis. For long-term ambulatory peritoneal dialysis, give drug in the evening at the time of the overnight exchange.
- Store reconstituted drug in refrigerator; use within 14 days.
- If patient develops sensitivity to diluent, reconstitute drug with sterile water for injection. When drug is reconstituted in this way, use only one reconstituted dose per vial, refrigerate solution if it isn't used immediately after reconstitution, use recon-

stituted dose within 24 hours, and discard unused portion.

- ***Alert:*** In patients with Prader-Willi syndrome who are morbidly obese and in those with a history of respiratory impairment, sleep apnea, or unidentified respiratory infection, therapy may be life-threatening. Assess patients with Prader-Willi syndrome for sleep apnea and upper airway obstruction before treatment. Interrupt treatment if signs of upper airway obstruction occur.
- Monitor patient with Prader-Willi syndrome for signs of respiratory infection.
- Monitor child's height regularly. Regular checkups, including monitoring of blood and radiologic studies, are also needed.
- Monitor patient's glucose level regularly because GH may induce a state of insulin resistance.
- Excessive glucocorticoid therapy inhibits somatropin's growth-promoting effect. Patients with coexisting corticotropin deficiency should have their glucocorticoid replacement dosage carefully adjusted to avoid growth inhibition.
- Watch for slipped capital femoral epiphysis or progression of scoliosis in patients with rapid growth.
- Monitor results of periodic thyroid function tests for hypothyroidism; condition may need thyroid hormone treatment. Laboratory measurements of thyroid hormone may change.
- Patient should have ophthalmic exams to monitor for intracranial hypertension before therapy (to establish baseline) and periodically thereafter.
- ***Look alike–sound alike:*** Don't confuse somatropin with somatrem or sumatriptan.
- Only adults with GH deficiency alone or together with multiple hormone deficiencies from pituitary or hypothalamic disease, surgery, radiation, or trauma or those who were GH deficient as children and have been confirmed GH deficient as adults can take Saizen.

PATIENT TEACHING

- Inform parents that child with endocrine disorders (including GH deficiency) may have an increased risk of slipped capital epiphyses. Tell parents to notify prescriber if they notice their child limping.
- Instruct patients with diabetes to monitor glucose level closely and report changes to prescriber.
- Stress importance of close follow-up care.

vasopressin (ADH)

Pitressin

Pharmacologic class: posterior pituitary hormone
Pregnancy risk category C

AVAILABLE FORMS

Injection: 20 units/ml

INDICATIONS & DOSAGES

➤ Nonnephrogenic, nonpsychogenic diabetes insipidus

Adults: 5 to 10 units I.M. or subcutaneously b.i.d. to q.i.d., p.r.n. Or, intranasally (aqueous solution used as spray or applied to cotton balls) in individualized dosages, based on response.
Children: 2.5 to 10 units I.M. or subcutaneously b.i.d. to q.i.d., p.r.n. Or, intranasally (aqueous solution used as spray or applied to cotton balls) in individualized doses.

➤ To prevent and treat abdominal distention

Adults: Initially, 5 units I.M.; give subsequent injections q 3 to 4 hours, increasing to 10 units if needed. Children may receive reduced dosages. Or, for adults, aqueous vasopressin 5 to 15 units subcutaneously at 2 hours before and again at 30 minutes before abdominal radiography or kidney biopsy.

➤ Abdominal roentgenography

Adults: 2 injections of 10 units each I.M. or subcutaneously, given at 2 hours and at 30 minutes before abdominal radiography.

➤ GI bleeding ♦

Adults: Initially, 0.2 to 0.4 units/minute I.V.; increase to 0.9 units/minute as needed. For intra-arterial infusion, 0.1 to 0.5 units/minute. Aqueous vasopressin is diluted in normal saline solution or D_5W to a concentration of 0.1 to 1 unit/ml.

ACTION

Increases permeability of the renal tubular epithelium to adenosine monophosphate and water; the epithelium promotes reabsorption of water and produces a concentrated urine.

Route	Onset	Peak	Duration
I.M., SubQ, intranasal	Unknown	Unknown	2–8 hr

Half-life: 10 to 20 minutes.

ADVERSE REACTIONS
CNS: tremor, headache, vertigo.
CV: vasoconstriction, ***arrhythmias, cardiac arrest,*** myocardial ischemia, circumoral pallor, decreased cardiac output, angina in patients with vascular disease.
GI: abdominal cramps, nausea, vomiting, flatulence.
GU: uterine cramps.
Respiratory: ***bronchoconstriction.***
Skin: diaphoresis, cutaneous gangrene, urticaria.
Other: water intoxication, ***hypersensitivity reactions.***

INTERACTIONS
Drug-drug. *Carbamazepine, chlorpropamide, clofibrate, fludrocortisone, tricyclic antidepressant, urea:* May increase antidiuretic response. Use together cautiously.
Demeclocycline, heparin, lithium, norepinephrine: May reduce antidiuretic activity. Use together cautiously.
Drug-lifestyle. *Alcohol use:* May reduce antidiuretic activity. Discourage use together.

EFFECTS ON LAB TEST RESULTS
None reported.

CONTRAINDICATIONS & CAUTIONS
- Contraindicated in patients allergic to vasopressin or any of its components and in those with chronic nephritis and nitrogen retention.
- Use cautiously in children; elderly patients; pregnant women; patients with preoperative or postoperative polyuria; and those with seizure disorders, migraines, asthma, CV disease, heart failure, renal disease, goiter with cardiac complications, arteriosclerosis, or fluid overload.

NURSING CONSIDERATIONS
- Monitor patient for hypersensitivity reactions, including urticaria, angioedema, bronchoconstriction, and anaphylaxis.
- Synthetic desmopressin is sometimes preferred because of its longer duration of action and less frequent adverse reactions. Desmopressin also is available commercially as a nasal solution.
- Drug may be used for transient polyuria from ADH deficiency in neurosurgery or head injury.
- Use minimum effective dose to reduce adverse reactions.
- Give with 1 or 2 glasses of water to reduce adverse reactions and improve therapeutic response.
- Warm the vial in your hands, and mix until the hormone is distributed throughout the solution before administration.
- Monitor urine specific gravity and fluid intake and output to aid evaluation of drug effectiveness.
- Monitor ECG and fluid or electrolyte status at periodic intervals.
- To prevent possible seizures, coma, and death, observe patient closely for early evidence of water intoxication, including drowsiness, listlessness, headache, confusion, and weight gain.
- Water intoxication may be treated with water restriction and temporary withdrawal of drug until polyuria occurs. Severe water intoxication may require osmotic diuresis with mannitol, hypertonic dextrose, or urea, alone or with furosemide.
- Monitor blood pressure of patient taking vasopressin twice daily. Watch for excessively elevated blood pressure or lack of response to drug, which may be indicated by hypotension. Also, monitor weight daily.
- ***Look alike–sound alike:*** Don't confuse vasopressin with desmopressin.

PATIENT TEACHING
- Instruct patient to rotate injection sites to prevent tissue damage.
- Tell patient to report adverse reactions, drowsiness, listlessness, and headache to prescriber promptly.
- Tell patient to avoid alcohol and OTC drugs unless approved by prescriber.
- Tell patient to restrict water intake.

59
Parathyroid-like drugs

alendronate sodium
calcitonin
calcitriol
cinacalcet hydrochloride
ibandronate sodium
pamidronate disodium
risedronate sodium
teriparatide
zoledronic acid

alendronate sodium
Fosamax, Fosamax Plus D

Pharmacologic class: bisphosphonate
Pregnancy risk category C

AVAILABLE FORMS
Tablets: 5 mg, 10 mg, 35 mg, 40 mg, 70 mg, 70 mg plus 2,800 international units vitamin D_3
Oral solution: 70 mg/75 ml

INDICATIONS & DOSAGES
➤ **Osteoporosis in postmenopausal women; to increase bone mass in men with osteoporosis**
Adults: 10 mg P.O. daily or 70-mg tablet or solution P.O. once weekly.
➤ **Paget disease of bone**
Adults: 40 mg P.O. daily for 6 months.
➤ **To prevent osteoporosis in postmenopausal women**
Adults: 5 mg P.O. daily or 35-mg tablet P.O. once weekly.
➤ **Glucocorticoid-induced osteoporosis in patients receiving glucocorticoids in a daily dose equivalent to 7.5 mg or more of prednisone and who have low bone mineral density**
Adults: 5 mg P.O. daily. For postmenopausal women not receiving estrogen, recommended dose is 10 mg P.O. daily.

ACTION
Suppresses osteoclast activity on newly formed resorption surfaces, which reduces bone turnover. Bone formation exceeds resorption at remodeling sites, leading to progressive gains in bone mass.

Route	Onset	Peak	Duration
P.O.	Unknown	Unknown	Unknown

Half-life: More than 10 years.

ADVERSE REACTIONS
CNS: headache.
GI: abdominal pain, nausea, dyspepsia, constipation, diarrhea, flatulence, acid regurgitation, esophageal ulcer, vomiting, dysphagia, abdominal distention, gastritis, taste perversion.
Musculoskeletal: musculoskeletal pain.

INTERACTIONS
Drug-drug. *Antacids, calcium supplements, many oral drugs:* May interfere with absorption of alendronate. Instruct patient to wait at least 30 minutes after taking alendronate before taking other drug orally.
Aspirin, NSAIDs: May increase risk of upper GI adverse reactions with drug doses greater than 10 mg daily. Monitor patient closely.
Ranitidine (I.V. form): May increase availability of alendronate. Reduce dosage, as needed.
Drug-food. *Any food:* May decrease absorption of drug. Advise patient to take with full glass of water at least 30 minutes before food, beverages, or ingestion of other drugs.

EFFECTS ON LAB TEST RESULTS
- May decrease calcium and phosphate levels.

CONTRAINDICATIONS & CAUTIONS
- Contraindicated in patients hypersensitive to drug and in those with hypocalcemia, severe renal insufficiency, or abnormalities of the esophagus that delay esophageal emptying.
- Use cautiously in patients with active upper GI problems (dysphagia, symptomatic esophageal diseases, gastritis, duo-

denitis, ulcers) or mild to moderate renal insufficiency.

NURSING CONSIDERATIONS

- Correct hypocalcemia and other disturbances of mineral metabolism (such as vitamin D deficiency) before therapy begins.
- When used to treat osteoporosis, disease may be confirmed by findings of low bone mass on diagnostic studies or by history of osteoporotic fracture.
- The recommended daily intake of vitamin D is 400 to 800 international units. Fosamax Plus D provides 400 international units daily when taken once weekly. Patients at risk for vitamin D deficiency, such as those who are chronically ill, nursing home bound, who have a GI malabsorption syndrome, or who are older than age 70, may require additional supplementation.
- In Paget disease, drug is indicated for patients with alkaline phosphatase level at least two times upper limit of normal, for those who are symptomatic, and for those at risk for future complications from the disease.
- ***Alert:*** Give drug with 6 to 8 ounces of water at least 30 minutes before patient's first food or drink of the day to facilitate delivery to the stomach. Don't allow patient to lie down for 30 minutes after taking drug.
- Monitor patient's calcium and phosphate levels throughout therapy.
- ***Look alike–sound alike:*** Don't confuse Fosamax with Flomax.

PATIENT TEACHING

- Stress importance of taking tablet only with 6 to 8 ounces of water at least 30 minutes before ingesting anything else, including food, beverages, and other drugs. Tell patient that waiting longer than 30 minutes improves absorption.
- Warn patient not to lie down for at least 30 minutes after taking drug to facilitate delivery to stomach and to reduce risk of esophageal irritation.
- Advise patient to report adverse effects immediately, especially chest pain or difficulty swallowing.
- Advise patient to take supplemental calcium and vitamin D if dietary intake is inadequate.
- Tell patient about benefits of weightbearing exercises in increasing bone mass. If applicable, explain importance of reducing or eliminating cigarette smoking and alcohol use.

calcitonin

Fortical, Miacalcin

Pharmacologic class: polypeptide hormone
Pregnancy risk category C

AVAILABLE FORMS

Injection: 200 units/ml in 2-ml ampules
Nasal spray: 200 units/activation

INDICATIONS & DOSAGES

➤Paget disease of bone (osteitis deformans)

Adults: Initially, 100 units daily I.M. or subcutaneously. Maintenance dosage is 50 to 100 units daily I.M. or subcutaneously, every other day, or three times weekly.

➤Hypercalcemia

Adults: 4 units/kg q 12 hours I.M. or subcutaneously. If response is inadequate after 1 or 2 days, increase dosage to 8 units/kg I.M. q 12 hours. If response remains unsatisfactory after 2 additional days, increase dosage to maximum of 8 units/kg I.M. q 6 hours.

➤Postmenopausal osteoporosis

Adults: 200 units (one activation) daily intranasally, alternating nostrils daily. Or, 100 units I.M. or subcutaneously every other day. Patient should receive adequate vitamin D and calcium supplements (1.5 g calcium carbonate and 400 units of vitamin D) daily.

ACTION

Decreases osteoclastic activity by inhibiting osteocytic osteolysis; decreases mineral release and matrix or collagen breakdown in bone.

Route	Onset	Peak	Duration
I.M., SubQ	15 min	4 hr	8–24 hr
Intranasal	Rapid	30 min	1 hr

Half-life: 43 to 60 minutes.

ADVERSE REACTIONS
CNS: headache, weakness, dizziness, paresthesia.
CV: chest pressure, *facial flushing.*
EENT: eye pain, *nasal congestion, rhinitis.*
GI: *transient nausea,* unusual taste, diarrhea, anorexia, *vomiting,* epigastric discomfort, abdominal pain.
GU: *increased urinary frequency,* nocturia.
Respiratory: shortness of breath.
Skin: rash, pruritus of ear lobes, *inflammation at injection site.*
Other: hypersensitivity reactions, ***anaphylaxis,*** edema of feet, chills, tender palms and soles.

INTERACTIONS
None significant.

EFFECTS ON LAB TEST RESULTS
None reported.

CONTRAINDICATIONS & CAUTIONS
- Contraindicated in patients hypersensitive to drug.

NURSING CONSIDERATIONS
- Skin test is usually done in patients with suspected drug sensitivity before therapy.
- ***Alert:*** Systemic allergic reactions are possible because hormone is protein. Keep epinephrine nearby.
- Give at bedtime, when possible, to minimize nausea and vomiting.
- I.M. route is preferred if volume of dose to be given exceeds 2 ml.
- Use freshly reconstituted solution within 2 hours.
- ***Alert:*** Observe patient for signs of hypocalcemic tetany during therapy (muscle twitching, tetanic spasms, and seizures when hypocalcemia is severe).
- Monitor calcium level closely. Watch for symptoms of hypercalcemia relapse: bone pain, renal calculi, polyuria, anorexia, nausea, vomiting, thirst, constipation, lethargy, bradycardia, muscle hypotonicity, pathologic fracture, psychosis, and coma.
- Periodic examinations of urine sediment are recommended.
- Monitor periodic alkaline phosphatase and 24-hour urine hydroxyproline levels to evaluate drug effect.
- In Paget disease, maximum reductions of alkaline phosphatase and urinary hydroxyproline excretion may take 6 to 24 months of continuous treatment.
- In patients with good first response to drug who have a relapse, expect to evaluate antibody response to the hormone protein.
- If symptoms have been relieved after 6 months, treatment may be stopped until symptoms or radiologic signs recur.
- Refrigerate drug at 36° to 46° F (2° to 8° C).
- ***Look alike–sound alike:*** Don't confuse calcitonin with calcifediol or calcitriol.

PATIENT TEACHING
- When drug is given for postmenopausal osteoporosis, remind patient to take adequate calcium and vitamin D supplements.
- Show home care patient and family member how to give drug. Tell them to do so at bedtime if only one dose is needed daily. If nasal spray is prescribed, tell patient to alternate nostrils daily.
- Advise patient to notify prescriber if significant nasal irritation or evidence of an allergic response occurs.
- Inform patient that facial flushing and warmth occur in 20% to 30% of patients within minutes of injection and usually last about 1 hour.
- Tell patient that nausea and vomiting may occur at the onset of therapy.
- Tell patient to inform prescriber promptly if signs and symptoms of hypercalcemia occur. Inform patient that, if drug loses its hypocalcemic activity, other drugs or increased dosages won't help.

calcitriol (1,25-dihydroxycholecalciferol)
Calcijex, Rocaltrol

Pharmacologic class: vitamin D analog
Pregnancy risk category C

AVAILABLE FORMS
Capsules: 0.25 mcg, 0.5 mcg
Injection: 1 mcg/ml, 2 mcg/ml
Oral solution: 1 mcg/ml

INDICATIONS & DOSAGES

➤Hypocalcemia in patients undergoing long-term dialysis
Adults: Initially, 0.25 mcg P.O. daily; may increase by 0.25 mcg daily at 4- to 8-week intervals. Maintenance dosage is 0.5 to 1 mcg daily. Or, 0.5 mcg I.V. three times weekly about q other day. If response to first dosage is inadequate, may increase by 0.25 to 0.5 mcg at 2- to 4-week intervals. Maintenance dosage is 0.5 to 3 mcg I.V. three times weekly.

➤Hypoparathyroidism, pseudohypoparathyroidism
Adults and children age 6 and older: Initially, 0.25 mcg P.O. daily in the morning. Dosage may be increased at 2- to 4-week intervals. Maintenance dosage is 0.25 to 2 mcg P.O. daily.

➤Hypoparathyroidism
Children ages 1 to 5: Give 0.25 to 0.75 mcg P.O. daily.

➤To manage secondary hyperparathyroidism and resulting metabolic bone disease in predialysis patients (with creatinine clearance of 15 to 55 ml/minute)
Adults and children age 3 and older: Initially, 0.25 mcg P.O. daily. Dosage may be increased to 0.5 mcg/day if needed.
Children younger than age 3: Initially, 0.01 to 0.015 mcg/kg P.O. daily.

I.V. ADMINISTRATION

- For hypocalcemia in patient undergoing hemodialysis, give drug by rapid injection through catheter at end of hemodialysis session.

INCOMPATIBILITIES

None reported.

ACTION

Stimulates calcium absorption from the GI tract and promotes movement of calcium from bone to blood.

Route	Onset	Peak	Duration
P.O.	2–6 hr	3–6 hr	3–5 days
I.V.	Immediate	Unknown	3–5 days

Half-life: 3 to 6 hours.

ADVERSE REACTIONS

CNS: headache, somnolence, weakness, irritability.
CV: hypertension, ***arrhythmias.***
EENT: conjunctivitis, photophobia, rhinorrhea.
GI: nausea, vomiting, constipation, polydipsia, ***pancreatitis,*** metallic taste, dry mouth, anorexia.
GU: polyuria, nocturia.
Metabolic: weight loss.
Musculoskeletal: bone and muscle pain.
Skin: pruritus.
Other: hyperthermia, nephrocalcinosis, decreased libido.

INTERACTIONS

Drug-drug. *Cardiac glycosides:* May increase risk of arrhythmias. Use together cautiously.
Cholestyramine, colestipol, excessive use of mineral oil: May decrease absorption of oral vitamin D analogues. Avoid using together.
Corticosteroids: May counteract vitamin D analogue effects. Avoid using together.
Magnesium-containing antacids: May cause hypermagnesemia, especially in patients with chronic renal failure. Avoid using together.
Phenytoin, phenobarbital: May inhibit calcitriol synthesis. Dose may need to be increased.
Thiazides: May cause hypercalcemia. Use together cautiously.

EFFECTS ON LAB TEST RESULTS

None reported.

CONTRAINDICATIONS & CAUTIONS

- Contraindicated in patients with hypercalcemia or vitamin D toxicity. Withhold all preparations containing vitamin D.
- Use cautiously in patients receiving cardiac glycosides and in those with sarcoidosis or hyperparathyroidism.

NURSING CONSIDERATIONS

- Monitor calcium level; this level times the phosphate level shouldn't exceed 70. During dose adjustment, determine calcium level twice weekly. If hypercalcemia occurs, stop drug and notify prescriber, but resume after calcium level returns to normal. Patient should receive adequate

daily intake of calcium. Observe for hypocalcemia, bone pain, and weakness before and during therapy.
- Monitor phosphorous level, especially in hypoparathyroid patients and dialysis patients.
- Reduce dose as parathyroid hormone levels decrease in response to therapy.
- The symptoms of vitamin D intoxication include headache, somnolence, weakness, irritability, hypertension, arrhythmias, conjunctivitis, photophobia, rhinorrhea, nausea, vomiting, constipation, polydipsia, pancreatitis, metallic taste, dry mouth, anorexia, nephrocalcinosis, polyuria, nocturia, weight loss, bone and muscle pain, pruritus, hyperthermia, and decreased libido.
- Protect drug from heat and light.
- ***Look alike–sound alike:*** Don't confuse calcitriol with calcifediol or calcitonin.

PATIENT TEACHING

- Tell patient to immediately report early symptoms of vitamin D intoxication: weakness, nausea, vomiting, dry mouth, constipation, muscle or bone pain, or metallic taste.
- Instruct patient to adhere to diet and calcium supplementation and to avoid unapproved OTC drugs and antacids that contain magnesium.
- ***Alert:*** Tell patient that drug is the most potent form of vitamin D available and shouldn't be taken by anyone else.

cinacalcet hydrochloride
Sensipar

Pharmacologic class: calcimimetic
Pregnancy risk category C

AVAILABLE FORMS

Tablets: 30 mg, 60 mg, 90 mg

INDICATIONS & DOSAGES

➤ **Secondary hyperparathyroidism in patients with chronic kidney disease undergoing dialysis**
Adults: Initially, 30 mg P.O. once daily; adjust no more than q 2 to 4 weeks through sequential doses of 60 mg, 90 mg, 120 mg, and 180 mg P.O. once daily to reach target range of 150 to 300 picograms (pg)/ml for intact parathyroid hormone (PTH).

➤ **Hypercalcemia in patients with parathyroid carcinoma**
Adults: Initially, 30 mg P.O. b.i.d.; adjust q 2 to 4 weeks through sequential doses of 30 mg, 60 mg, and 90 mg P.O. b.i.d., and 90 mg P.O. t.i.d. or q.i.d. daily if needed to normalize calcium level.

ACTION

Increases sensitivity of calcium-sensing receptor to extracellular calcium, letting calcium be absorbed despite decreased PTH.

Route	Onset	Peak	Duration
P.O.	Unknown	2–6 hr	Unknown

Half-life: 2 hours.

ADVERSE REACTIONS

CNS: *dizziness,* asthenia.
CV: chest pain, hypertension.
GI: *diarrhea, nausea, vomiting,* anorexia.
Musculoskeletal: *myalgia.*
Other: access infection.

INTERACTIONS

Drug-drug. *Amitriptyline:* Amitriptyline and nortriptyline exposure increases by 20% in patients who are CYP2D6 extensive metabolizers. Avoid using together, if possible.
Drugs metabolized mainly by CYP2D6 with a narrow therapeutic index (such as flecainide, thioridazine, most tricyclic antidepressants, vinblastine): May strongly inhibit CYP2D6, decreasing metabolism and increasing levels of these drugs. Adjust dosage of other drugs, as needed.
Drugs that strongly inhibit CYP3A4 (such as erythromycin, itraconazole, ketoconazole): May increase cinacalcet level. Use together cautiously, monitoring PTH and calcium level closely and adjusting cinacalcet dosage, as needed.

EFFECTS ON LAB TEST RESULTS

- May decrease calcium, phosphorus, and testosterone levels.

CONTRAINDICATIONS & CAUTIONS

- Contraindicated in patients hypersensitive to drug or its components and in patients with calcium level less than 8.4 mg/dl.

- Use cautiously in patients with history of seizures and in those with moderate to severe hepatic impairment.

NURSING CONSIDERATIONS

- ***Alert:*** Monitor calcium level closely, especially if patient has a history of seizures, because decreased calcium level lowers seizure threshold.
- Patients with moderate to severe hepatic impairment may need dosage adjustment based on PTH and calcium level. Monitor these patients closely.
- Give drug alone or with vitamin D sterols, phosphate binders, or both.
- Measure calcium level within 1 week after starting therapy or adjusting dosage. Once maintenance dose is established, measure calcium level monthly for patients with chronic kidney disease receiving dialysis and every 2 months for those with parathyroid carcinoma.
- Watch carefully for evidence of hypocalcemia: paresthesias, myalgias, cramping, tetany, and seizures.
- If calcium level is 7.5 to 8.4 mg/dl or patient develops symptoms of hypocalcemia, give calcium-containing phosphate binders, vitamin D sterols, or both, to raise calcium level. If calcium level is below 7.5 mg/dl or hypocalcemia symptoms persist and the vitamin D dose can't be increased, withhold drug until calcium level reaches 8.0 mg/dl, hypocalcemia symptoms resolve, or both. Resume therapy with the next lowest dose.
- Measure intact PTH level 1 to 4 weeks after therapy starts or dosage changes. Once the maintenance dose is established, monitor PTH level every 1 to 3 months. Levels in patients with chronic kidney disease receiving dialysis should be 150 to 300 pg/ml.
- Adynamic bone disease may develop if intact PTH levels are suppressed below 100 pg/ml. If this occurs, notify prescriber. The dosage of cinacalcet or vitamin D sterols may need to be reduced or stopped.
- ***Alert:*** Don't use drug in patients with chronic kidney disease who aren't receiving dialysis because they have an increased risk of hypocalcemia.

PATIENT TEACHING

- Tell patient not to divide tablets but to take them whole, with food or shortly after a meal.
- Advise patient to report to prescriber adverse reactions and signs of hypocalcemia, which include paresthesias, muscle weakness, muscle cramping, and muscle spasm.

ibandronate sodium

Boniva

Pharmacologic class: bisphosphonate
Pregnancy risk category C

AVAILABLE FORMS

Injection: 3 mg/3 ml prefilled syringe
Tablets: 2.5 mg, 150 mg

INDICATIONS & DOSAGES

➤ To treat or prevent postmenopausal osteoporosis

Women: 2.5 mg P.O. daily or 150 mg P.O. once monthly, taken first thing in the morning, with a large glass of plain water, 1 hour before any food or other drugs. Or, for treatment, 3 mg I.V. bolus once every 3 months.

I.V. ADMINISTRATION

- Prefilled syringes are for single-use only.
- Give undiluted using needle provided with the syringe.
- Give by I.V. bolus over 15 to 30 seconds.
- Don't use if drug contains particulate matter or is discolored.
- Store at room temperature.

INCOMPATIBILITIES

Calcium-containing solutions and other I.V. drugs.

ACTION

Inhibits bone breakdown and removal to reduce bone loss and increase bone mass.

Route	Onset	Peak	Duration
P.O.	Unknown	½–2 hr	Unknown
I.V.	Rapid	Unknown	Unknown

Half-life: 1½ to 6½ days for the 150-mg dose.

ADVERSE REACTIONS

CNS: asthenia, dizziness, headache, insomnia, nerve root lesion, vertigo.
CV: hypertension.
EENT: nasopharyngitis, pharyngitis.
GI: *dyspepsia,* abdominal pain, constipation, diarrhea, gastritis, nausea, vomiting.
GU: UTI.
Musculoskeletal: *back pain,* arthralgia, arthritis, joint disorder, limb pain, localized osteoarthritis, muscle cramps, myalgia.
Respiratory: *bronchitis, upper respiratory tract infection,* pneumonia.
Skin: rash.
Other: allergic reaction, infection, influenza, tooth disorder.

INTERACTIONS

Drug-drug. *Aspirin, NSAIDs:* May increase GI irritation. Use together cautiously.
Products containing aluminum, calcium, magnesium, or iron: May decrease ibandronate absorption. Give oral ibandronate 1 hour before vitamins, minerals, or antacids.
Drug-food. *Food, milk, beverages (except water):* May decrease drug absorption. Give oral drug on an empty stomach with plain water.
Drug-lifestyle. *Alcohol use:* May decrease drug absorption and increase risk of esophageal irritation. Discourage use together.

EFFECTS ON LAB TEST RESULTS

- May increase cholesterol level. May decrease total alkaline phosphatase level.
- May interfere with bone-imaging agents.

CONTRAINDICATIONS & CAUTIONS

- Contraindicated in patients hypersensitive to drug and in those with uncorrected hypocalcemia. Oral form is contraindicated in those who can't stand or sit upright for 60 minutes.
- Don't give to patients with severe renal impairment.
- Use cautiously in patients with a history of GI disorders.

NURSING CONSIDERATIONS

- Correct hypocalcemia or other disturbances of bone and mineral metabolism before therapy.
- Make sure patient has adequate intake of calcium and vitamin D.
- Watch for signs or symptoms of esophageal irritation, including dysphagia, painful swallowing, retrosternal pain, and heartburn.
- Monitor patient for bone, joint, and muscle pain, which may be severe and incapacitating.
- Watch for signs and symptoms of uveitis and scleritis.
- ***Alert:*** Drug may lead to osteonecrosis, mainly in the jaw. Dental surgery may worsen condition. Consider stopping drug if patient needs a dental procedure.
- Use during pregnancy only if benefit outweighs risk to fetus.
- Use cautiously in breast-feeding women.

PATIENT TEACHING

- Tell patient receiving I.V. form, if she misses a dose, reschedule the missed dose as soon as possible. Subsequent injections should be rescheduled once every 3 months from that dose. She shouldn't receive more than one dose in a 3-month time frame.
- Tell patient taking monthly dose to take it on same date each month and to wait at least 7 days between doses if she misses a scheduled dose.
- Tell patient taking daily dose not to take a missed dose later in the day. She should skip the missed dose and resume her normal schedule the next day.
- Instruct patient to take oral drug first thing in the morning 1 hour before eating or drinking and before any other drugs, including OTC drugs, such as calcium, antacids, and vitamins.
- Advise patient to swallow drug whole with a full glass of plain water while standing or sitting and to remain upright for at least 1 hour after taking drug.
- Caution patient to take only with plain water and no other beverage.
- Instruct patient not to chew or suck on the tablet.
- Advise patient to take calcium and vitamin D supplements as directed by prescriber.

• Tell patient to report any bone, joint, or muscle pain.
• Advise patient to stop drug and immediately report to prescriber signs and symptoms of esophageal irritation, such as dysphagia, painful swallowing, retrosternal pain, or heartburn.

pamidronate disodium

Aredia

Pharmacologic class: bisphosphonate
Pregnancy risk category D

AVAILABLE FORMS

Powder for injection: 30-mg/vial, 90-mg/vial
Solution for injection: 3 mg/ml, 6 mg/ml, 9 mg/ml, in 10-ml vials

INDICATIONS & DOSAGES

➤ Moderate to severe hypercalcemia from cancer (with or without bone metastases)
Adults: Dosage depends on severity of hypercalcemia. Correct calcium level for albumin. Corrected calcium (CCa) level is calculated using this formula:

$$\text{CCa (mg/dl)} = \text{serum calcium (mg/dl)} + 0.8\,(4 - \text{serum albumin (g/dl)})$$

Patients with CCa levels of 12 to 13.5 mg/dl may receive 60 to 90 mg by I.V. infusion as a single dose over 2 to 24 hours. Patients with CCa levels greater than 13.5 mg/dl may receive 90 mg by I.V. infusion over 2 to 24 hours. Allow at least 7 days before retreatment to permit full response to first dose.
➤ Moderate to severe Paget disease
Adults: 30 mg I.V. as a 4-hour infusion on 3 consecutive days for total dose of 90 mg. Repeat cycle, p.r.n.
➤ Osteolytic bone metastases of breast cancer with standard antineoplastic therapy
Adults: 90 mg I.V. infusion over 2 hours q 3 to 4 weeks.
➤ Osteolytic bone lesions of multiple myeloma
Adults: 90 mg I.V. over 4 hours once monthly.

I.V. ADMINISTRATION

• Reconstitute drug with 10 ml of sterile water for injection. After drug is completely dissolved, add to 250 ml (2-hour infusion), 500 ml (4-hour infusion), or 1,000 ml (up to 24-hour infusion) of half-normal or normal saline solution for injection or D_5W.
• Inspect solution for precipitate before use.
• Give drug only by I.V. infusion. Injecting a bolus may cause nephropathy.
• Infusions longer than 2 hours may reduce the risk for renal toxicity, particularly in patients with preexisting renal insufficiency.
• Solution is stable for 24 hours at room temperature.
• Store reconstituted drug at 36° to 46° F (2° to 8° C).

INCOMPATIBILITIES

Calcium-containing infusion solutions, such as Ringer injection or lactated Ringer solution.

ACTION

An antihypercalcemic that inhibits resorption of bone but apparently not bone formation. Adsorbs to hydroxyapatite crystals in bone and may directly block calcium phosphate dissolution and mature osteoclast formation.

Route	Onset	Peak	Duration
I.V.	Unknown	Unknown	Unknown

Half-life: Alpha, 1½ hours; beta, 27¼ hours.

ADVERSE REACTIONS

CNS: ***seizures,*** *fatigue,* somnolence, syncope, fever.
CV: ***atrial fibrillation,*** tachycardia, *hypertension, fluid overload.*
GI: *abdominal pain, anorexia, constipation, nausea, vomiting,* ***GI hemorrhage.***
GU: renal dysfunction, *urinary tract infection,* ***renal failure.***
Hematologic: ***leukopenia, thrombocytopenia,*** *anemia.*

Metabolic: hypophosphatemia, hypokalemia, hypomagnesemia, hypocalcemia.
Musculoskeletal: osteonecrosis of the jaw.
Skin: *infusion-site reaction, pain at infusion site.*

INTERACTIONS

None significant.

EFFECTS ON LAB TEST RESULTS

- May increase creatinine level. May decrease phosphate, potassium, magnesium, calcium, and hemoglobin levels.
- May decrease WBC and platelet counts.

CONTRAINDICATIONS & CAUTIONS

- Contraindicated in patients hypersensitive to drug or other bisphosphonates such as etidronate.
- Use with caution, considering risks versus benefits, in patients with renal impairment.

NURSING CONSIDERATIONS

- Assess hydration before treatment. Use drug only after patient has been vigorously hydrated with normal saline solution. In patients with mild to moderate hypercalcemia, hydration alone may be sufficient.
- Because drug can cause electrolyte disturbances, carefully monitor electrolyte levels, especially calcium, phosphate, and magnesium. Short-term use of calcium may be needed in patients with severe hypocalcemia. Also monitor CBC and differential count, creatinine and hemoglobin levels, and hematocrit.
- Carefully monitor patients with anemia, leukopenia, or thrombocytopenia during first 2 weeks of therapy.
- Monitor patient's temperature. Patient may experience a slight elevation for 24 to 48 hours after therapy.
- ***Alert:*** Because renal dysfunction may lead to renal failure, single doses shouldn't exceed 90 mg.
- Monitor creatinine level before each treatment.
- In patients treated for bone metastases who have renal dysfunction, withhold dose until renal function returns to baseline. Treating bone metastases in patients with severe renal impairment isn't recommended. For other indications, determine whether the potential benefit outweighs the potential risk.
- ***Alert:*** Patients should have a dental examination with appropriate preventive dentistry before taking drug, especially those with risk factors, including cancer, chemotherapy or corticosteroid therapy, and poor oral hygiene.
- Use cautiously in breast-feeding women; it's unknown if drug appears in breast milk.

PATIENT TEACHING

- Explain use and administration of drug to patient and family.
- Instruct patient to report adverse reactions promptly.
- Advise woman to alert her health care provider if she is pregnant or breast-feeding.

risedronate sodium

Actonel✐

Pharmacologic class: bisphosphonate
Pregnancy risk category C

AVAILABLE FORMS

Tablets: 5 mg, 30 mg, 35 mg

INDICATIONS & DOSAGES

➤ **To prevent and treat postmenopausal osteoporosis**
Women: 5-mg tablet P.O. once daily, or 35-mg tablet once weekly.
✱***NEW INDICATION:*** **To increase bone mass with osteoporosis**
Men: One 35-mg tablet P.O. once weekly.
➤ **Glucocorticoid-induced osteoporosis in patients taking 7.5 mg or more of prednisone or equivalent glucocorticoid daily**
Adults: 5 mg P.O. daily.
➤ **Paget disease**
Adults: 30 mg P.O. daily for 2 months. If relapse occurs or alkaline phosphatase level doesn't normalize, may repeat treatment course 2 months or more after completing first treatment course.
Adjust-a-dose: Don't use if creatinine clearance is less than 30 ml/minute.

ACTION

Reverses the loss of bone mineral densi-tyby reducing bone turnover and bone resorption. In patients with Paget disease, drug causes bone turnover to return to normal.

Route	Onset	Peak	Duration
P.O.	1 hr	Unknown	Unknown

Half-life: 1½ hours to 20 days.

ADVERSE REACTIONS

CNS: asthenia, *headache,* depression, dizziness, insomnia, anxiety, neuralgia, vertigo, hypertonia, paresthesia, *pain.*
CV: *hypertension,* CV disorder, angina pectoris, chest pain, peripheral edema.
EENT: pharyngitis, rhinitis, sinusitis, cataract, conjunctivitis, otitis media, amblyopia, tinnitus.
GI: *nausea, diarrhea, abdominal pain,* flatulence, gastritis, rectal disorder, constipation.
GU: *UTI,* cystitis.
Hematologic: ecchymosis, anemia.
Musculoskeletal: *arthralgia,* neck pain, *back pain,* myalgia, bone pain, leg cramps, bursitis, tendon disorder.
Respiratory: dyspnea, pneumonia, bronchitis.
Skin: *rash,* pruritus, skin carcinoma.
Other: *infection,* tooth disorder.

INTERACTIONS

Drug-drug. *Calcium supplements, antacids that contain calcium, magnesium, or aluminum:* May interfere with risedronate absorption. Advise patient to separate dosing times.
Drug-food. *Any food:* May interfere with absorption of drug. Advise patient to take drug at least 30 minutes before first food or drink of the day (other than water).

EFFECTS ON LAB TEST RESULTS

- May decrease calcium and phosphorus levels.

CONTRAINDICATIONS & CAUTIONS

- Contraindicated in patients hypersensitive to any component of the product, in hypocalcemic patients, in patients with creatinine clearance less than 30 ml/minute, and in those who can't stand or sit upright for 30 minutes after administration.
- Use cautiously in patients with upper GI disorders, such as dysphagia, esophagitis, and esophageal or gastric ulcers.

NURSING CONSIDERATIONS

- Risk factors for the development of osteoporosis include family history, previous fracture, smoking, a decrease in bone mineral density below the premenopausal mean, a thin body frame, White or Asian race, and early menopause.
- ***Alert:*** Drug may cause dysphagia, esophagitis, and esophageal or gastric ulcers. Monitor patient for symptoms of esophageal disease.
- Give supplemental calcium and vitamin D if dietary intake is inadequate. Because calcium supplements and drugs containing calcium, aluminum, or magnesium may interfere with risedronate absorption, separate dosing times.
- Bisphosphonates can interfere with bone-imaging agents.

PATIENT TEACHING

- Explain that drug may reverse bone loss by stopping more bone loss and increasing bone strength.
- Caution patient about the importance of adhering to special dosing instructions.
- Tell patient to take drug at least 30 minutes before the first food or drink of the day other than water. Urge patient to take the drug with 6 to 8 ounces of water while sitting or standing. Warn patient against lying down for 30 minutes after taking.
- Tell patient not to chew or suck the tablet because doing so may irritate his mouth.
- Advise patient to contact prescriber immediately if he develops GI discomfort (such as difficulty or pain when swallowing, retrosternal pain, or severe heartburn).
- Advise patient to take calcium and vitamin D if dietary intake is inadequate, but to take them at a different time than risedronate.
- Advise patient to stop smoking and drinking alcohol, as appropriate. Also, advise patient to perform weightbearing exercise.

• Tell patient to store drug in a cool, dry place, at room temperature, and away from children.
• Urge patient to read the Patient Information Guide before starting therapy.
• Tell patient if he misses a dose of the 35-mg tablet, he should take 1 tablet on the morning after he remembers and return to taking 1 tablet once a week, as originally scheduled on his chosen day. Patient shouldn't take 2 tablets on the same day.

teriparatide (rDNA origin)

Forteo

Pharmacologic class: recombinant human parathyroid hormone (PTH)
Pregnancy risk category C

AVAILABLE FORMS

Injection: 750 mcg/3 ml in a prefilled pen

INDICATIONS & DOSAGES

➤ **Osteoporosis in postmenopausal women at high risk for fracture; primary or hypogonadal osteoporosis in men at high risk for fracture**
Adults: 20 mcg subcutaneously in thigh or abdominal wall once daily.

ACTION

Promotes new bone formation, skeletal bone mass, and bone strength by regulating calcium and phosphorus metabolism in bones and kidneys.

Route	Onset	Peak	Duration
SubQ	Rapid	30 min	3 hr

Half-life: 1 hour.

ADVERSE REACTIONS

CNS: asthenia, depression, dizziness, headache, insomnia, syncope, vertigo.
CV: angina pectoris, hypertension, orthostatic hypotension.
EENT: pharyngitis, rhinitis.
GI: constipation, diarrhea, dyspepsia, nausea, tooth disorder, vomiting.
Metabolic: hypercalcemia.
Musculoskeletal: *arthralgia,* leg cramps, neck pain.
Respiratory: dyspnea, increased cough, pneumonia.
Skin: rash, sweating.
Other: *pain.*

INTERACTIONS

Drug-drug. *Calcium supplements:* May increase urinary calcium excretion. Dosage may need adjustment.
Digoxin: May predispose hypercalcemic patient to digitalis toxicity. Use together cautiously.

EFFECTS ON LAB TEST RESULTS

• May increase calcium and uric acid levels. May decrease phosphorus level.
• May increase urinary calcium and phosphorus excretion.

CONTRAINDICATIONS & CAUTIONS

• Contraindicated in patients hypersensitive to teriparatide or its components.
• Contraindicated in patients at increased risk for osteosarcoma, such as those with Paget disease or unexplained alkaline phosphatase elevations, children, and patients who have had skeletal radiation; in patients with bone metastases, a history of skeletal malignancies, hypercalcemia, or metabolic bone diseases other than osteoporosis; and in patients with hypercalcemia.
• Use cautiously in patients with active or recent urolithiasis or hepatic, renal, or cardiac disease.

NURSING CONSIDERATIONS

• ***Alert:*** Because of the risk of osteosarcoma, give drug only to patients for whom benefits outweigh risk.
• Inspect solution before giving; drug is a colorless, clear liquid. Don't use if solid particles are present or if the solution is cloudy or colored.
• Treatment may last for up to 2 years.
• If patient may have urolithiasis or hypercalciuria, measure urinary calcium excretion before treatment.
• Monitor patient for orthostatic hypotension, which may occur within 4 hours of dosing.
• Monitor calcium level. If persistent hypercalcemia develops, stop drug and evaluate possible cause.

PATIENT TEACHING

- Instruct patient on proper use and disposal of prefilled pen.
- Tell patient not to share pen with others.
- Advise patient to sit or lie down if drug causes a fast heartbeat, light-headedness, or dizziness. Tell patient to report persistent or worsening symptoms.
- Urge patient to report persistent symptoms of hypercalcemia, which include nausea, vomiting, constipation, lethargy, and muscle weakness.

zoledronic acid

Zometa

Pharmacologic class: bisphosphonate
Pregnancy risk category D

AVAILABLE FORMS

Injection: 4 mg/vial

INDICATIONS & DOSAGES

➤ **Hypercalcemia caused by malignancy**
Adults: 4 mg by I.V. infusion over at least 15 minutes. If albumin-corrected calcium level doesn't return to normal, may repeat 4 mg. Let at least 7 days pass before retreatment to allow a full response to the first dose.

➤ **Multiple myeloma and bone metastases of solid tumors in conjunction with standard antineoplastics**
Adults: 4 mg I.V. infused over at least 15 minutes q 3 to 4 weeks. Treatment duration depends on type of cancer. Use for prostate cancer only after it has progressed after treatment with at least one course of hormonal therapy.

Adjust-a-dose: For patients with creatinine clearance of 50 to 60 ml/minute, give 3.5 mg. If 40 to 49 ml/minute, give 3.3 mg. If 30 to 39 ml/minute, give 3 mg. For patients with normal baseline creatinine level but an increase of 0.5 mg/dl and in those with abnormal baseline creatinine level who have an increase of 1 mg/dl, withhold drug. Resume treatment only when creatinine level has returned to within 10% of baseline value.

I.V. ADMINISTRATION

- Reconstitute by adding 5 ml of sterile water to each vial. Inspect solution to make sure that drug is dissolved completely and that there is no particulate matter or discoloration.
- For patient with creatinine clearance greater than 60 ml/minute, withdraw 5 ml to obtain 4 mg of drug and mix in 100 ml of normal saline solution or D_5W. For patient with creatinine clearance of 60 ml/minute or less, withdraw 4.4 ml for the 3.5-mg dose, 4.1 ml for the 3.3-mg dose, or withdraw 3.8 ml for the 3-mg dose.
- Give as I.V. infusion over at least 15 minutes.
- If drug not used immediately after reconstitution, refrigerate solution and give within 24 hours.

INCOMPATIBILITIES

Solutions containing calcium (such as lactated Ringer solution) or other I.V. drugs.

ACTION

Inhibits bone resorption, probably by inhibiting osteoclast activity and osteoclastic resorption of mineralized bone and cartilage. Decreases calcium release induced by the stimulatory factors produced by tumors.

Route	Onset	Peak	Duration
I.V.	Unknown	Unknown	7–28 days

Half-life: Alpha is 0.23 hours; beta is 1.75 hours for early distribution. Terminal half-life is 167 hours.

ADVERSE REACTIONS

Hypercalcemia

CNS: headache, somnolence, *anxiety, confusion*, agitation, *insomnia, fever.*
CV: hypotension.
GI: *nausea, constipation, diarrhea, abdominal pain, vomiting,* anorexia, dysphagia.
GU: ***decreased creatinine level,*** *urinary infection, candidiasis.*
Hematologic: ANEMIA, ***granulocytopenia, thrombocytopenia, thrombocytopenia.***
Metabolic: *decreased calcium, phosphate, and magnesium levels,* dehydration.

Musculoskeletal: *skeletal pain,* arthralgia.
Respiratory: *dyspnea, cough,* pleural effusion.
Other: *progression of cancer,* infection.
Bone metastases
CNS: *headache,* anxiety, *insomnia, depression, paresthesia, hypoesthesia, fatigue, weakness, dizziness, fever.*
CV: *hypotension, leg edema.*
GI: *nausea, constipation, diarrhea, abdominal pain, vomiting, anorexia, increased appetite.*
GU: ***decreased creatinine level,*** *urinary infection.*
Hematologic: *anemia,* ***neutropenia.***
Metabolic: *decreased calcium, phosphate, and magnesium levels, dehydration, weight decrease.*
Musculoskeletal: *skeletal pain, arthralgia, myalgia, back pain,* osteonecrosis of the jaw.
Respiratory: *dyspnea, cough.*
Skin: alopecia, dermatitis.
Other: **PROGRESSION OF CANCER,** *rigors,* infection.

INTERACTIONS

Drug-drug. *Aminoglycosides, loop diuretics:* May have additive effects that lower calcium level. Use together cautiously, and monitor calcium level.
Thalidomide: May increase risk of renal dysfunction in patients with multiple myeloma. Use together cautiously.

EFFECTS ON LAB TEST RESULTS

- May increase creatinine level. May decrease calcium, phosphorus, magnesium, potassium, and hemoglobin levels and hematocrit.
- May decrease RBC, WBC, and platelet counts.

CONTRAINDICATIONS & CAUTIONS

- Contraindicated in patients hypersensitive to drug, other bisphosphonates, or any of its ingredients, in patients with hypercalcemia of malignancy whose creatinine level is more than 4.5 mg/dl, in patients with bone metastases and a creatinine level of more than 3 mg/dl, and in breast-feeding women.
- Use cautiously in elderly patients and those with aspirin-sensitive asthma because other bisphosphonates have been linked to bronchoconstriction in aspirin-sensitive patients with asthma.

NURSING CONSIDERATIONS

- Hydrate patient adequately before giving; urine output should be about 2 L daily.
- Each vial contains 220 mg mannitol and 24 mg sodium citrate.
- ***Alert:*** Because of the risk of decreased renal function progressing to renal failure, don't exceed 4 mg as a single dose and always infuse over at least 15 minutes.
- Monitor calcium, phosphate, magnesium, and creatinine levels carefully. Correct decreased calcium, phosphorus, and magnesium levels using I.V. calcium gluconate, potassium and sodium phosphate, and magnesium sulfate.
- Monitor renal function closely. Patients with renal impairment may be at a greater risk for adverse reactions.
- ***Alert:*** Patients—especially those who have cancer or poor oral hygiene or who are receiving chemotherapy or corticosteroids—should have a dental exam with appropriate preventive dentistry before therapy.
- Give patients an oral calcium supplement of 500 mg and a multiple vitamin containing 400 international units of vitamin D daily.

PATIENT TEACHING

- Review the use and administration of drug with patient and family.
- Instruct patient to report adverse effects promptly.
- Explain the importance of periodic laboratory tests to monitor therapy and renal function.
- If a woman becomes pregnant or is breast-feeding, advise her to alert prescriber.

60
Diuretics

acetazolamide
acetazolamide sodium
bumetanide
furosemide
hydrochlorothiazide
indapamide
mannitol
metolazone
spironolactone
torsemide
triamterene

acetazolamide
Acetazolam†, Apo-Acetazolamide†, Diamox Sequels

acetazolamide sodium

Pharmacologic class: carbonic anhydrase inhibitor
Pregnancy risk category C

AVAILABLE FORMS
acetazolamide
Capsules (extended-release): 500 mg
Tablets: 125 mg, 250 mg
acetazolamide sodium
Powder for injection: 500-mg vial

INDICATIONS & DOSAGES
➤ **Secondary glaucoma; preoperative treatment of acute angle-closure glaucoma**
Adults: 250 mg P.O. q 4 hours or 250 mg P.O. b.i.d. for short-term therapy. In acute cases, 500 mg P.O.; then 125 to 250 mg P.O. q 4 hours. To rapidly lower intraocular pressure (IOP), initially, 500 mg I.V.; may repeat in 2 to 4 hours, if needed, followed by 125 to 250 mg P.O. q 4 hours.
Children: 10 to 15 mg/kg P.O. daily in divided doses q 6 to 8 hours. For acute angle-closure glaucoma, 5 to 10 mg/kg I.M. or I.V. q 6 hours.
➤ **Chronic open-angle glaucoma**
Adults: 250 mg to 1 g P.O. daily in divided doses q.i.d., or 500 mg extended-release P.O. b.i.d.
➤ **To prevent or treat acute mountain sickness**
Adults: 500 mg to 1 g (regular or extended-release) P.O. daily in divided doses q 12 hours. Start 24 to 48 hours before ascent and continue for 48 hours while at high altitude. When rapid ascent is required, start with 1,000 mg P.O. daily.
➤ **Adjunct for epilepsy and myoclonic, refractory, generalized tonic-clonic, absence, or mixed seizures**
Adults and children: 8 to 30 mg/kg P.O. daily in divided doses. For adults, 375 mg to 1 g daily is ideal. If given with other anticonvulsants, start at 250 mg P.O. once daily, and increase to 375 mg to 1 g daily.
➤ **Edema caused by heart failure; drug-induced edema**
Adults: 250 mg to 375 mg (5 mg/kg) P.O. daily in the morning. For best results, use q other day or 2 days on followed by 1 to 2 days off.
Children: 5 mg/kg or 150 mg/m^2 P.O. or I.V. daily in the morning.

I.V. ADMINISTRATION
- Reconstitute drug in 500-mg vial with at least 5 ml of sterile water for injection. Use within 12 hours of reconstitution.
- Inject 100 to 500 mg/minute into a large vein using a 21G or 23G needle.
- Direct I.V. injection is the preferred route.
- Intermittent and continuous infusions aren't recommended.

INCOMPATIBILITIES
Multivitamins.

ACTION
Promotes renal excretion of sodium, potassium, bicarbonate, and water. As anticonvulsant, drug normalizes neuronal discharge. In mountain sickness, drug stimulates ventilation and increases cerebral blood flow; also reduces IOP.

Route	Onset	Peak	Duration
P.O.	60–90 min	1–4 hr	8–12 hr
P.O. (extended-release)	2 hr	3–6 hr	18–24 hr
I.V.	2 min	15 min	4–5 hr

Half-life: 10 to 15 hours.

ADVERSE REACTIONS

CNS: ***seizures,*** drowsiness, paresthesia, confusion, depression, weakness, ataxia.
EENT: transient myopia, hearing dysfunction, tinnitus.
GI: nausea, vomiting, anorexia, metallic taste, diarrhea, black tarry stools, constipation.
GU: polyuria, hematuria, crystalluria, glycosuria, phosphaturia, renal calculus.
Hematologic: ***aplastic anemia, leukopenia,*** hemolytic anemia.
Metabolic: hypokalemia, asymptomatic hyperuricemia, hyperchloremic acidosis.
Skin: *pain at injection site,* ***Stevens-Johnson syndrome,*** rash, urticaria.
Other: sterile abscesses.

INTERACTIONS

Drug-drug. *Amphetamines, anticholinergics, mecamylamine, procainamide, quinidine:* May decrease renal clearance of these drugs, increasing toxicity. Monitor patient for toxicity.
Cyclosporine: May increase cyclosporine level, causing nephrotoxicity and neurotoxicity. Monitor patient for toxicity.
Diflunisal: May increase acetazolamide adverse effects; may significantly decrease intracranial pressure. Use together cautiously.
Lithium: May increase lithium excretion, decreasing its effect. Monitor lithium level.
Methenamine: May reduce methenamine effect. Avoid using together.
Primidone: May decrease serum and urine primidone levels. Monitor patient closely.
Salicylates: May cause accumulation and toxicity of acetazolamide, including CNS depression and metabolic acidosis. Monitor patient for toxicity.
Drug-lifestyle. *Sun exposure:* May increase risk of photosensitivity reactions. Advise patient to avoid excessive sunlight exposure.

EFFECTS ON LAB TEST RESULTS

- May increase uric acid level. May decrease potassium and hemoglobin levels.
- May decrease WBC count and iodine uptake by the thyroid.
- May cause false-positive urine protein test result.

CONTRAINDICATIONS & CAUTIONS

- Contraindicated in patients hypersensitive to drug and in those with hyponatremia or hypokalemia, renal or hepatic disease or dysfunction, renal calculi, adrenal gland failure, hyperchloremic acidosis, or severe pulmonary obstruction.
- Contraindicated in those receiving long-term treatment for chronic noncongestive angle-closure glaucoma.
- Use cautiously in patients receiving other diuretics and in those with respiratory acidosis or COPD.

NURSING CONSIDERATIONS

- Cross-sensitivity between antibacterial sulfonamides and sulfonamide-derivative diuretics such as acetazolamide has been reported.
- If patient can't swallow oral form, pharmacist may make a suspension using crushed tablets in a highly flavored syrup, such as cherry, raspberry, or chocolate. Although concentrations up to 500 mg/5 ml are possible, concentrations of 250 mg/5 ml are more palatable. Refrigeration improves palatability but doesn't improve stability. Suspensions are stable for 1 week.
- Capsules shouldn't be crushed or chewed.
- I.M. injection is painful because of the highly alkaline pH. Don't use I.M.
- Monitor fluid intake and output, glucose, and electrolytes, especially potassium, bicarbonate, and chloride. When drug is used in diuretic therapy, consult prescriber and dietitian about providing a high-potassium diet.
- Monitor elderly patients closely because they are especially susceptible to excessive diuresis.
- Weigh patient daily. Rapid or excessive fluid loss may cause weight loss and hypotension.

- Diuretic effect decreases when acidosis occurs but can be reestablished by withdrawing drug for several days and then restarting or by using intermittent administration schedules.
- Monitor patient for signs of hemolytic anemia (pallor, weakness, and palpitations).
- Drug may increase glucose level and cause glycosuria.
- ***Look alike–sound alike:*** Don't confuse acetazolamide with acetaminophen or acyclovir.

PATIENT TEACHING

- Tell patient to take oral form with food to minimize GI upset.
- Caution patient not to perform hazardous activities if adverse CNS reactions occur.
- Instruct patient to avoid prolonged exposure to sunlight because drug may cause phototoxicity.
- Instruct patient to notify prescriber of any unusual bleeding, bruising, tingling, or tremors.

bumetanide

Bumex, Burinex‡

Pharmacologic class: loop diuretic
Pregnancy risk category C

AVAILABLE FORMS

Injection: 0.25 mg/ml
Tablets: 0.5 mg, 1 mg, 2 mg

INDICATIONS & DOSAGES

➤ **Edema caused by heart failure or hepatic or renal disease**

Adults: 0.5 to 2 mg P.O. once daily. If diuretic response isn't adequate, a second or third dose may be given at 4- to 5-hour intervals. Maximum dose is 10 mg daily. May be given parenterally if oral route isn't possible. Usual first dose is 0.5 to 1 mg given I.V. or I.M. If response isn't adequate, a second or third dose may be given at 2- to 3-hour intervals. Maximum, 10 mg daily.

I.V. ADMINISTRATION

- For direct injection, give drug over 1 to 2 minutes using a 21G or 23G needle.
- For intermittent infusion, give diluted drug through an intermittent infusion device or piggyback into an I.V. line containing a free-flowing, compatible solution.
- In patients with severe chronic renal insufficiency, a continuous infusion of 12 mg over 12 hours may be more effective and less toxic than intermittent bolus therapy.

INCOMPATIBILITIES

Dobutamine, fenoldopam, midazolam.

ACTION

A potent drug that inhibits sodium and chloride reabsorption at the ascending loop of Henle.

Route	Onset	Peak	Duration
P.O.	30–60 min	1–2 hr	4–6 hr
I.V.	Within min	15–30 min	30–60 min
I.M.	40 min	Unknown	5–6 hr

Half-life: 1 to 1½ hours.

ADVERSE REACTIONS

CNS: *weakness,* dizziness, headache, vertigo, pain.
CV: orthostatic hypotension, ECG changes, chest pain.
EENT: transient deafness, tinnitus.
GI: nausea, vomiting, upset stomach, dry mouth, diarrhea.
GU: premature ejaculation, difficulty maintaining erection, oliguria.
Hematologic: ***thrombocytopenia,*** azotemia.
Metabolic: volume depletion and dehydration, hypokalemia, hypochloremic alkalosis, hypomagnesemia, asymptomatic hyperuricemia.
Musculoskeletal: arthritic pain, muscle cramps and pain.
Skin: rash, pruritus, diaphoresis.

INTERACTIONS

Drug-drug. *Aminoglycoside antibiotics:* May increase ototoxicity. Avoid using together if possible.
Antidiabetics: May decrease hypoglycemic effects. Monitor glucose level.
Antihypertensives: May increase risk of hypotension. Use together cautiously.

Cardiac glycosides: May increase risk of digoxin toxicity from bumetanide-induced hypokalemia. Monitor potassium and digoxin levels.
Chlorothiazide, chlorthalidone, hydrochlorothiazide, indapamide, metolazone: May cause excessive diuretic response, causing serious electrolyte abnormalities or dehydration. Adjust doses carefully, and monitor patient closely for signs and symptoms of excessive diuretic response.
Cisplatin: May increase risk of ototoxicity. Monitor patient closely.
Lithium: May decrease lithium clearance, increasing risk of lithium toxicity. Monitor lithium level.
Neuromuscular blockers: May prolong neuromuscular blockade. Monitor patient closely.
NSAIDs, probenecid: May inhibit diuretic response. Use together cautiously.
Other potassium-wasting drugs (such as amphotericin B, corticosteroids): May increase risk of hypokalemia. Use together cautiously.
Warfarin: May increase anticoagulant effect. Use together cautiously.
Drug-herb. *Dandelion:* May interfere with drug activity. Discourage use together.
Licorice: May cause unexpected, rapid potassium loss. Discourage use together.

EFFECTS ON LAB TEST RESULTS
- May increase alkaline phosphatase, ALT, AST, bilirubin, cholesterol, creatinine, glucose, LDH, and urine urea levels. May decrease calcium, magnesium, potassium, sodium, and chloride levels.
- May decrease platelet count. May increase or decrease WBC count.

CONTRAINDICATIONS & CAUTIONS
- Contraindicated in patients hypersensitive to drug or sulfonamides (possible cross-sensitivity) and in patients with anuria, hepatic coma, or severe electrolyte depletion.
- Use cautiously in patients with hepatic cirrhosis and ascites, in elderly patients, and in those with depressed renal function.

NURSING CONSIDERATIONS
- To prevent nocturia, give drug in the morning. If second dose is needed, give in early afternoon.
- Safest and most effective dosage schedule is alternate days or 3 or 4 consecutive days with 1 or 2 days off between cycles.
- Monitor fluid intake and output, weight, and electrolyte, BUN, creatinine, and carbon dioxide levels frequently.
- Watch for evidence of hypokalemia, such as muscle weakness and cramps. Instruct patient to report these symptoms.
- Consult prescriber and dietitian about a high-potassium diet. Foods rich in potassium include citrus fruits, tomatoes, bananas, dates, and apricots.
- Monitor glucose level in diabetic patients.
- Monitor uric acid level, especially in patients with history of gout.
- Monitor blood pressure and pulse rate during rapid diuresis. Profound water and electrolyte depletion may occur.
- If oliguria or azotemia develops or increases, prescriber may stop drug.
- Drug can be safely used in patients allergic to furosemide; 1 mg of bumetanide equals about 40 mg of furosemide.
- ***Look alike–sound alike:*** Don't confuse Bumex with Buprenex.

PATIENT TEACHING
- Instruct patient to take drug with food to minimize GI upset.
- Advise patient to take drug in morning to avoid need to urinate at night; if patient needs second dose, have him take it in early afternoon.
- Advise patient to avoid sudden posture changes and to rise slowly to avoid dizziness upon standing quickly.
- Instruct patient to notify prescriber about extreme thirst, muscle weakness, cramps, nausea, or dizziness.
- Instruct patient to weigh himself daily to monitor fluid status.

furosemide (frusemide†)

Apo-Furosemide†, Furosemide Special IV†, Furoside†, Lasix*✐, Novo-semide†, Uritol†

Pharmacologic class: loop diuretic
Pregnancy risk category C

AVAILABLE FORMS

Injection: 10 mg/ml
Oral solution: 10 mg/ml, 40 mg/5 ml
Tablets: 20 mg, 40 mg, 80 mg, 500 mg†

INDICATIONS & DOSAGES

➤ **Acute pulmonary edema**
Adults: 40 mg I.V. injected slowly over 1 to 2 minutes; then 80 mg I.V. in 60 to 90 minutes if needed.

➤ **Edema**
Adults: 20 to 80 mg P.O. daily in the morning. If response is inadequate, give a second dose, and each succeeding dose, q 6 to 8 hours. Carefully increase dose in 20- to 40-mg increments up to 600 mg daily. Once effective dose is attained, may give once or twice daily. Or, 20 to 40 mg I.V. or I.M., increased by 20 mg q 2 hours until desired effect achieved.
Infants and children: 2 mg/kg P.O. daily, increased by 1 to 2 mg/kg in 6 to 8 hours if needed; carefully adjusted up to 6 mg/kg daily if needed.

➤ **Hypertension**
Adults: 40 mg P.O. b.i.d. Dosage adjusted based on response. May be used as adjunct to other antihypertensives if needed.
Children♦*:* 0.5 to 2 mg/kg P.O. once or twice daily. Increase dose as needed up to 6 mg/kg daily.

I.V. ADMINISTRATION

- If discolored yellow, don't use.
- For direct injection, give over 1 to 2 minutes.
- For infusion, dilute with D_5W, normal saline solution, or lactated Ringer solution.
- To avoid ototoxicity, infuse no more than 4 mg/minute.
- Use prepared infusion solution within 24 hours.

INCOMPATIBILITIES

Acidic solutions, aminoglycosides, amiodarone, ascorbic acid, azithromycin, bleomycin, buprenorphine, chlorpromazine, ciprofloxacin, diazepam, diltiazem, dobutamine, doxapram, doxorubicin, droperidol, epinephrine, erythromycin, esmolol, filgrastim, fluconazole, fructose 10% in water, gentamicin, hydralazine, idarubicin, invert sugar 10% in electrolyte #2, isoproterenol, levofloxacin, mannitol, meperidine, methocarbamol, metoclopramide, midazolam, milrinone, morphine, netilmicin, norepinephrine, ondansetron, oxytetracycline, prochlorperazine, promethazine, protamine, quinidine, tetracycline, thiamine, vinblastine, vincristine, vitamins B and C.

ACTION

A potent drug that inhibits sodium and chloride reabsorption at the proximal and distal tubules and the ascending loop of Henle.

Route	Onset	Peak	Duration
P.O.	20–60 min	1–2 hr	6–8 hr
I.V.	5 min	30 min	2 hr

Half-life: 30 minutes.

ADVERSE REACTIONS

CNS: vertigo, headache, dizziness, paresthesia, weakness, restlessness, fever.
CV: orthostatic hypotension, thrombophlebitis with I.V. administration.
EENT: transient deafness, blurred or yellowed vision, tinnitus.
GI: abdominal discomfort and pain, diarrhea, anorexia, nausea, vomiting, constipation, ***pancreatitis.***
GU: nocturia, polyuria, frequent urination, oliguria.
Hematologic: ***agranulocytosis, aplastic anemia, leukopenia, thrombocytopenia,*** azotemia, anemia.
Hepatic: hepatic dysfunction, jaundice.
Metabolic: volume depletion and dehydration, asymptomatic hyperuricemia, impaired glucose tolerance, hypokalemia, hypochloremic alkalosis, hyperglycemia, dilutional hyponatremia, hypocalcemia, hypomagnesemia.
Musculoskeletal: muscle spasm.

Skin: dermatitis, purpura, photosensitivity reactions, transient pain at I.M. injection site.
Other: gout.

INTERACTIONS

Drug-drug. *Aminoglycoside antibiotics, cisplatin:* May increase ototoxicity. Use together cautiously.
Amphotericin B, corticosteroids, corticotropin, metolazone: May increase risk of hypokalemia. Monitor potassium level closely.
Antidiabetics: May decrease hypoglycemic effects. Monitor glucose level.
Antihypertensives: May increase risk of hypotension. Use together cautiously. Decrease antihypertensive dose if needed.
Cardiac glycosides, neuromuscular blockers: May increase toxicity of these drugs from furosemide-induced hypokalemia. Monitor potassium level.
Chlorothiazide, chlorthalidone, hydrochlorothiazide, indapamide, metolazone: May cause excessive diuretic response, causing serious electrolyte abnormalities or dehydration. Adjust doses carefully, and monitor patient closely for signs and symptoms of excessive diuretic response.
Ethacrynic acid: May increase risk of ototoxicity. Avoid using together.
Lithium: May decrease lithium excretion, resulting in lithium toxicity. Monitor lithium level.
NSAIDs: May inhibit diuretic response. Use together cautiously.
Phenytoin: May decrease diuretic effects of furosemide. Use together cautiously.
Propranolol: May increase propranolol level. Monitor patient closely.
Salicylates: May cause salicylate toxicity. Use together cautiously.
Sucralfate: May reduce diuretic and antihypertensive effect. Separate doses by 2 hours.
Drug-herb. *Aloe:* May increase drug effect. Discourage use together.
Dandelion: May interfere with drug activity. Discourage use together.
Ginseng: May decrease drug effect. Discourage use together.
Licorice: May cause unexpected rapid potassium loss. Discourage use together.
Drug-lifestyle. *Sun exposure:* May increase risk for photosensitivity reactions. Advise patient to avoid excessive sunlight exposure.

EFFECTS ON LAB TEST RESULTS

- May increase cholesterol, glucose, BUN, creatinine, and uric acid levels. May decrease calcium, hemoglobin, magnesium, potassium, and sodium levels.
- May decrease granulocyte, platelet, and WBC counts.

CONTRAINDICATIONS & CAUTIONS

- Contraindicated in patients hypersensitive to drug and in those with anuria.
- Use cautiously in patients with hepatic cirrhosis and in those allergic to sulfonamides. Use during pregnancy only if potential benefits to mother clearly outweigh risks to fetus.

NURSING CONSIDERATIONS

- To prevent nocturia, give P.O. and I.M. preparations in the morning. Give second dose in early afternoon.
- ***Alert:*** Monitor weight, blood pressure, and pulse rate routinely with long-term use and during rapid diuresis. Use can lead to profound water and electrolyte depletion.
- If oliguria or azotemia develops or increases, drug may need to be stopped.
- Monitor fluid intake and output and electrolyte, BUN, and carbon dioxide levels frequently.
- Watch for signs of hypokalemia, such as muscle weakness and cramps.
- Consult prescriber and dietitian about a high-potassium diet or potassium supplements. Foods rich in potassium include citrus fruits, tomatoes, bananas, dates, and apricots.
- Monitor glucose level in diabetic patients.
- Drug may not be well absorbed orally in patient with severe heart failure. Drug may need to be given I.V. even if patient is taking other oral drugs.
- Monitor uric acid level, especially in patients with a history of gout.
- Monitor elderly patients, who are especially susceptible to excessive diuresis, because circulatory collapse and thromboembolic complications are possible.
- Store tablets in light-resistant container to prevent discoloration (doesn't affect po-

tency). Refrigerate oral solution to ensure drug stability.

• ***Look alike–sound alike:*** Don't confuse furosemide with torsemide or Lasix with Lonox, Lidex, or Luvox.

PATIENT TEACHING

• Advise patient to take drug with food to prevent GI upset, and to take drug in morning to prevent need to urinate at night. If patient needs second dose, tell him to take it in early afternoon, 6 to 8 hours after morning dose.

• Inform patient of possible need for potassium or magnesium supplements.

• Instruct patient to stand slowly to prevent dizziness and to limit alcohol intake and strenuous exercise in hot weather to avoid worsening dizziness upon standing quickly.

• Advise patient to immediately report ringing in ears, severe abdominal pain, or sore throat and fever; these symptoms may indicate toxicity.

• ***Alert:*** Discourage patient from storing different types of drugs in the same container, increasing the risk of drug errors. The most popular strengths of this drug and digoxin are white tablets about equal in size.

• Tell patient to check with prescriber or pharmacist before taking OTC drugs.

• Teach patient to avoid direct sunlight and to use protective clothing and a sunblock because of risk of photosensitivity reactions.

hydrochlorothiazide

Apo-Hydro†, Dichlotride‡, Diuchlor H†, Esidrix, Ezide, HydroDIURIL, Hydro-Par, Microzide, Neo-Codema†, Novo-Hydrazide†, Oretic, Urozide†

Pharmacologic class: thiazide diuretic
Pregnancy risk category D

AVAILABLE FORMS

Capsules: 12.5 mg
Oral solution: 50 mg/5 ml
Tablets: 25 mg, 50 mg, 100 mg

INDICATIONS & DOSAGES

➤ **Edema**

Adults: 25 to 100 mg P.O. daily as a single or divided dose; patient may respond to intermittent therapy on alternate days or 3 to 5 days/week.

➤ **Hypertension**

Adults: 12.5 to 50 mg P.O. once daily. Increase or decrease daily dose based on blood pressure.

Children ages 2 to 12: Give 2.2 mg/kg or 60 mg/m² daily in two divided doses. Usual dosage range is 37.5 to 100 mg daily.

Children ages 6 months to 2 years: 2.2 mg/kg or 60 mg/m² daily in two divided doses. Usual dosage range is 12.5 to 37.5 mg daily.

Children younger than age 6 months: Up to 3.3 mg/kg P.O. daily in two divided doses.

ACTION

Increases sodium and water excretion by inhibiting sodium and chloride reabsorption in distal segment of the nephron.

Route	Onset	Peak	Duration
P.O.	2 hr	4–6 hr	6–12 hr

Half-life: 5½ to 15 hours.

ADVERSE REACTIONS

CNS: dizziness, vertigo, headache, paresthesia, weakness, restlessness.
CV: orthostatic hypotension, allergic myocarditis, vasculitis.
GI: ***pancreatitis,*** anorexia, nausea, epigastric distress, vomiting, abdominal pain, diarrhea, constipation.
GU: ***renal failure,*** polyuria, frequent urination, interstitial nephritis.
Hematologic: ***aplastic anemia, agranulocytosis, leukopenia, thrombocytopenia,*** hemolytic anemia.
Hepatic: jaundice.
Metabolic: asymptomatic hyperuricemia, hypokalemia, hyperglycemia and impaired glucose tolerance, fluid and electrolyte imbalances, including dilutional hyponatremia and hypochloremia, metabolic alkalosis, hypercalcemia, volume depletion and dehydration.
Musculoskeletal: muscle cramps.

Respiratory: ***respiratory distress,*** pneumonitis.
Skin: dermatitis, photosensitivity reactions, rash, purpura, alopecia.
Other: ***anaphylactic reactions,*** hypersensitivity reactions, gout.

INTERACTIONS

Drug-drug. *Amphotericin B, corticosteroids:* May increase risk of hypokalemia. Monitor potassium level closely.
Antidiabetics: May decrease hypoglycemic effects. Adjust dosage if needed. Monitor glucose level.
Antihypertensives: May have additive antihypertensive effect. Use together cautiously.
Barbiturates, opioids: May increase orthostatic hypotensive effect. Monitor patient closely.
Bumetanide, ethacrynic acid, furosemide, torsemide: May cause excessive diuretic response, causing serious electrolyte abnormalities or dehydration. Adjust doses carefully, and monitor patient closely for signs and symptoms of excessive diuretic response.
Cardiac glycosides: May increase risk of digoxin toxicity from diuretic-induced hypokalemia. Monitor potassium and digoxin levels.
Cholestyramine, colestipol: May decrease intestinal absorption of thiazides. Separate doses by 2 hours.
Diazoxide: May increase antihypertensive, hyperglycemic, and hyperuricemic effects. Use together cautiously.
Lithium: May decrease lithium excretion, increasing risk of lithium toxicity. Monitor lithium level.
NSAIDs: May increase risk of renal failure. Monitor renal function closely.
Drug-herb. *Dandelion:* May interfere with diuretic activity. Discourage use together.
Licorice: May cause unexpected rapid potassium loss. Discourage use together.
Drug-lifestyle. *Alcohol use:* May increase orthostatic hypotensive effect. Discourage use together.

EFFECTS ON LAB TEST RESULTS

- May increase glucose, cholesterol, triglyceride, calcium, and uric acid levels. May decrease potassium, sodium, chloride, and hemoglobin levels.
- May decrease granulocyte, WBC, and platelet counts.

CONTRAINDICATIONS & CAUTIONS

- Contraindicated in patients with anuria and patients hypersensitive to other thiazides or other sulfonamide derivatives.
- Use cautiously in children and in patients with severe renal disease, impaired hepatic function, or progressive hepatic disease.

NURSING CONSIDERATIONS

- To prevent nocturia, give drug in the morning.
- Monitor fluid intake and output, weight, blood pressure, and electrolyte levels.
- Watch for signs and symptoms of hypokalemia, such as muscle weakness and cramps.
- Drug may be used with potassium-sparing diuretic to prevent potassium loss.
- Consult prescriber and dietitian about a high-potassium diet or potassium supplement. Foods rich in potassium include citrus fruits, tomatoes, bananas, dates, and apricots.
- Monitor creatinine and BUN levels regularly. Cumulative effects of drug may occur with impaired renal function.
- Monitor uric acid level, especially in patients with history of gout.
- Monitor glucose level, especially in diabetic patients.
- Monitor elderly patients, who are especially susceptible to excessive diuresis.
- Stop thiazides and thiazide-like diuretics before parathyroid function tests.
- In patients with hypertension, therapeutic response may be delayed several weeks.

PATIENT TEACHING

- Instruct patient to take drug with food to minimize GI upset.
- Advise patient to take drug in morning to avoid need to urinate at night; if patient needs second dose, have him take it in early afternoon.
- Advise patient to avoid sudden posture changes and to rise slowly to avoid dizziness upon standing quickly.

• Encourage patient to use a sunblock to prevent photosensitivity reactions.
• Tell patient to check with prescriber or pharmacist before using OTC drugs.

indapamide
Lozide†, Lozol, Natrilix‡

Pharmacologic class: thiazide-like diuretic
Pregnancy risk category B

AVAILABLE FORMS
Tablets: 1.25 mg, 2.5 mg

INDICATIONS & DOSAGES
➤ Edema
Adults: Initially, 2.5 mg P.O. daily in the morning. Increased to 5 mg daily after 1 week, if needed.
➤ Hypertension
Adults: Initially, 1.25 mg P.O. daily in the morning. Increased to 2.5 mg daily after 4 weeks, if needed. Increased to 5 mg daily after 4 more weeks, if needed. If response is inadequate, a second antihypertensive, given at 50% of the usual starting dose, may be needed.

ACTION
Probably inhibits sodium reabsorption in distal segment of nephron. Also has a direct vasodilating effect, possibly resulting from calcium channel-blocking action.

Route	Onset	Peak	Duration
P.O.	1–2 hr	2–5 hr	18 hr

Half-life: About 14 hours.

ADVERSE REACTIONS
CNS: headache, nervousness, dizziness, light-headedness, weakness, vertigo, restlessness, drowsiness, fatigue, anxiety, depression, numbness of limbs, irritability, agitation, lethargy.
CV: orthostatic hypotension, palpitations, PVCs, irregular heartbeat, vasculitis, flushing.
EENT: rhinorrhea, blurred vision.
GI: anorexia, nausea, epigastric distress, vomiting, abdominal pain or cramps, diarrhea, constipation.
GU: nocturia, polyuria, frequent urination, impotence.
Metabolic: asymptomatic hyperuricemia, fluid and electrolyte imbalances, including dilutional hyponatremia, hypochloremia, metabolic alkalosis, and hypokalemia, weight loss, volume depletion and dehydration, hyperglycemia.
Musculoskeletal: muscle cramps and spasms.
Skin: rash, pruritus, urticaria.
Other: gout.

INTERACTIONS
Drug-drug. *Amphotericin B, corticosteroids:* May increase risk of hypokalemia. Monitor potassium level closely.
Antidiabetics: May decrease hypoglycemic effect of sulfonylureas, causing elevated glucose levels. Adjust dosage, if needed. Monitor glucose level.
Barbiturates, opioids: May increase orthostasis. Monitor patient closely.
Bumetanide, ethacrynic acid, furosemide, torsemide: May cause excessive diuretic response, causing serious electrolyte abnormalities or dehydration. Adjust doses carefully, and monitor patient closely for signs and symptoms of excessive diuretic response.
Cardiac glycosides: May increase risk of digoxin toxicity from indapamide-induced hypokalemia. Monitor potassium and digoxin levels.
Cholestyramine, colestipol: May decrease absorption of thiazides. Separate doses by 2 hours.
Diazoxide: May increase antihypertensive, hyperglycemic, and hyperuricemic effects. Use together cautiously.
Lithium: May decrease lithium clearance that may increase lithium toxicity. Avoid using together.
NSAIDs: May increase risk of NSAID-induced renal failure. Monitor patient for signs and symptoms of renal failure.
Drug-herb. *Dandelion:* May interfere with drug activity. Discourage use together.
Licorice: May cause unexpected rapid potassium loss. Discourage use together.
Drug-lifestyle. *Alcohol use:* May increase orthostatic hypotensive effect. Discourage use together.

EFFECTS ON LAB TEST RESULTS
• May increase BUN, creatinine, glucose, cholesterol, triglyceride, calcium, and uric acid levels. May decrease potassium, sodium, phosphate, and chloride levels.

CONTRAINDICATIONS & CAUTIONS
• Contraindicated in patients hypersensitive to other sulfonamide-derived drugs and in those with anuria.
• Use cautiously in patients with severe renal disease, impaired hepatic function, or progressive hepatic disease.

NURSING CONSIDERATIONS
• To prevent nocturia, give drug in the morning.
• Monitor fluid intake and output, weight, blood pressure, and electrolyte levels.
• Watch for signs of hypokalemia, such as muscle weakness and cramps. Drug may be used with potassium-sparing diuretic to prevent potassium loss.
• Consult prescriber and dietitian about a high-potassium diet or potassium supplement. Foods rich in potassium include citrus fruits, tomatoes, bananas, dates, and apricots.
• Monitor creatinine and BUN levels regularly. Cumulative effects of drug may occur in patients with impaired renal function.
• Monitor uric acid level, especially in patients with history of gout.
• Monitor glucose level, especially in diabetic patients.
• Monitor elderly patients, who are especially susceptible to excessive diuresis.
• Stop thiazides and thiazide-like diuretics before parathyroid function tests.
• Therapeutic response may be delayed several weeks in hypertensive patients.

PATIENT TEACHING
• Instruct patient to take drug in morning to prevent need to urinate at night.
• Tell patient to take drug with food to minimize GI upset.
• Advise patient to avoid sudden posture changes and to rise slowly to avoid dizziness upon standing quickly.

mannitol
Osmitrol

Pharmacologic class: osmotic diuretic
Pregnancy risk category C

AVAILABLE FORMS
Injection: 5%, 10%, 15%, 20%, 25%

INDICATIONS & DOSAGES
➤ **Test dose for marked oliguria or suspected inadequate renal function**
Adults and children older than age 12: 200 mg/kg or 12.5 g as a 15% to 20% I.V. solution over 3 to 5 minutes. Response is adequate if 30 to 50 ml of urine/hour is excreted over 2 to 3 hours; if response is inadequate, a second test dose is given. If still no response after second dose, stop drug.
➤ **Oliguria**
Adults and children older than age 12: 50 to 100 g I.V. as a 15% to 25% solution over 90 minutes to several hours.
➤ **To prevent oliguria or acute renal failure**
Adults and children older than age 12: 50 to 100 g I.V. of a 5% to 25% solution. Determine exact concentration by fluid requirements.
➤ **To reduce intraocular or intracranial pressure**
Adults and children older than age 12: 1.5 to 2 g/kg as a 15% to 20% I.V. solution over 30 to 60 minutes. For maximum intraocular pressure reduction before surgery, give 60 to 90 minutes preoperatively.
➤ **Diuresis in drug intoxication**
Adults and children older than age 12: 5% to 10% solution continuously up to 200 g I.V., while maintaining 100 to 500 ml urine output/hour and a positive fluid balance.
➤ **Irrigating solution during transurethral resection of prostate gland**
Adults: 2.5% to 5% solution, p.r.n.

I.V. ADMINISTRATION
• To redissolve crystallized solution (crystallization occurs at low temperatures or in concentrations higher than 15%), warm bottle or bag in a hot water bath and shake vigorously. Cool to body temperature be-

fore giving. Don't use solution with undissolved crystals.
• Give as intermittent or continuous infusion at prescribed rate, using an inline filter and an infusion pump. Don't give as direct injection.
• Check patency at infusion site before and during administration.
• Monitor patient for signs and symptoms of infiltration; if it occurs, watch for inflammation, edema, and necrosis.

INCOMPATIBILITIES

Blood products, cefepime, doxorubicin liposomal, filgrastim, imipenem-cilastatin, meropenem, potassium chloride, sodium chloride, strongly acidic or alkaline solutions.

ACTION

Increases osmotic pressure of glomerular filtrate, inhibiting tubular reabsorption of water and electrolytes; drug elevates plasma osmolality, increasing water flow into extracellular fluid.

Route	Onset	Peak	Duration
I.V.	30–60 min	1 hr	6–8 hr

Half-life: about 1½ hours.

ADVERSE REACTIONS

CNS: ***seizures,*** dizziness, headache, fever.
CV: edema, thrombophlebitis, hypotension, hypertension, ***heart failure,*** tachycardia, angina-like chest pain, vascular overload.
EENT: blurred vision, rhinitis.
GI: thirst, dry mouth, nausea, vomiting, *diarrhea.*
GU: urine retention.
Metabolic: dehydration.
Skin: local pain, urticaria.
Other: chills.

INTERACTIONS

Drug-drug. *Lithium:* May increase urinary excretion of lithium. Monitor lithium level closely.

EFFECTS ON LAB TEST RESULTS

• May increase or decrease electrolyte levels.
• May interfere with tests for inorganic phosphorus or ethylene glycol level.

CONTRAINDICATIONS & CAUTIONS

• Contraindicated in patients hypersensitive to drug.
• Contraindicated in patients with anuria; severe pulmonary congestion; frank pulmonary edema; active intracranial bleeding (except during craniotomy); severe dehydration; metabolic edema; previous progressive renal disease or dysfunction after starting drug, including increasing azotemia and oliguria; or previous progressive heart failure or pulmonary congestion after drug.

NURSING CONSIDERATIONS

• Monitor vital signs, including central venous pressure and fluid intake and output hourly. Report increasing oliguria. Check weight, renal function, fluid balance, and serum and urine sodium and potassium levels daily.
• In comatose or incontinent patient, use urinary catheter because therapy is based on strict evaluation of fluid intake and output. If patient has urinary catheter, use an hourly urometer collection bag to evaluate output accurately and easily.
• Drug can be used to measure GFR.
• To relieve thirst, give frequent mouth care or fluids.
• Drug is commonly used in chemotherapy regimens to enhance diuresis of renally toxic drugs.
• Don't give electrolyte-free solutions with blood. If blood is given simultaneously, add at least 20 mEq of sodium chloride to each liter of drug solution to avoid pseudoagglutination.

PATIENT TEACHING

• Tell patient that he may feel thirsty or have a dry mouth, and emphasize importance of drinking only the amount of fluids ordered.
• Instruct patient to promptly report adverse reactions and discomfort at I.V. site.

metolazone
Zaroxolyn

Pharmacologic class: thiazide-like diuretic
Pregnancy risk category B

AVAILABLE FORMS
Tablets (extended-release): 2.5 mg, 5 mg, 10 mg

INDICATIONS & DOSAGES
➤ **Edema in heart failure or renal disease**
Adults: 5 to 20 mg P.O. daily.
➤ **Hypertension**
Adults: 2.5 to 5 mg P.O. daily. Base maintenance dosage on blood pressure.

ACTION
Increases sodium and water excretion by inhibiting sodium reabsorption in ascending loop of Henle.

Route	Onset	Peak	Duration
P.O.	1 hr	2–8 hr	12–24 hr

Half-life: About 14 hours.

ADVERSE REACTIONS
CNS: *dizziness,* headache, fatigue, vertigo, paresthesia, weakness, restlessness, drowsiness, anxiety, depression, nervousness, blurred vision.
CV: orthostatic hypotension, palpitations, vasculitis.
GI: ***pancreatitis,*** anorexia, nausea, epigastric distress, vomiting, abdominal pain, diarrhea, constipation, dry mouth.
GU: nocturia, polyuria, impotence.
Hematologic: ***aplastic anemia, agranulocytosis, leukopenia,*** purpura.
Hepatic: jaundice, ***hepatitis.***
Metabolic: hyperglycemia and impaired glucose tolerance, fluid and electrolyte imbalances, including hypokalemia, hypomagnesemia, dilutional hyponatremia and hypochloremia, metabolic alkalosis, and hypercalcemia, volume depletion and dehydration.
Musculoskeletal: muscle cramps.
Skin: dermatitis, photosensitivity reactions, rash, pruritus, urticaria.

INTERACTIONS
Drug-drug. *Amphotericin B, corticosteroids:* May increase risk of hypokalemia. Monitor potassium level closely.
Anticoagulants: May affect hypoprothrombinemic response. Monitor PT and INR.
Antidiabetics: May alter glucose level and require dosage adjustment of antidiabetics. Monitor glucose level.
Barbiturates, opioids: May increase orthostatic hypotensive effect. Monitor patient closely.
Bumetanide, ethacrynic acid, furosemide, torsemide: May cause excessive diuretic response, causing serious electrolyte abnormalities or dehydration. Adjust doses carefully, and monitor patient closely for signs and symptoms of excessive diuretic response.
Cardiac glycosides: May increase risk of digoxin toxicity from metolazone-induced hypokalemia. Monitor potassium and digoxin levels.
Cholestyramine, colestipol: May decrease intestinal absorption of thiazides. Separate doses.
Diazoxide: May increase antihypertensive, hyperglycemic, and hyperuricemic effects. Use together cautiously.
Lithium: May decrease lithium clearance, increasing risk of lithium toxicity. Monitor lithium level.
NSAIDs: May increase risk of NSAID-induced renal failure. Monitor patient for signs of renal failure.
Other antihypertensives: May have additive effects. Use together cautiously.
Drug-herb. *Dandelion:* May interfere with diuretic activity. Discourage use together.
Licorice: May cause unexpected rapid potassium loss. Discourage use together.
Drug-lifestyle. *Alcohol use:* May increase orthostatic hypotensive effect. Discourage use together.
Sun exposure: May increase risk for photosensitivity reaction. Advise patient to avoid excessive sunlight exposure.

EFFECTS ON LAB TEST RESULTS
- May increase glucose, calcium, cholesterol, and triglyceride levels. May decrease potassium, sodium, magnesium, chloride, and hemoglobin levels.

• May decrease granulocyte and WBC counts.

CONTRAINDICATIONS & CAUTIONS
• Contraindicated in patients hypersensitive to thiazides or other sulfonamide-derived drugs and in those with anuria, hepatic coma, or precoma.
• Use cautiously in patients with impaired renal or hepatic function.

NURSING CONSIDERATIONS
• To prevent nocturia, give drug in the morning.
• Monitor fluid intake and output, weight, blood pressure, and electrolyte levels.
• Watch for signs and symptoms of hypokalemia, such as muscle weakness and cramps. Drug may be used with potassium-sparing diuretic to prevent potassium loss.
• Consult prescriber and dietitian about a high-potassium diet. Foods rich in potassium include citrus fruits, tomatoes, bananas, dates, and apricots.
• Monitor glucose level, especially in diabetic patients.
• Monitor uric acid level, especially in patients with history of gout.
• Monitor elderly patients, who are especially susceptible to excessive diuresis.
• In hypertensive patients, therapeutic response may be delayed several weeks.
• Monitor blood pressure. If response is inadequate, another antihypertensive may be added.
• Metolazone and furosemide may be used together to enhance diuretic effect.
• Unlike thiazide diuretics, metolazone is effective in patients with decreased renal function.
• Stop thiazides and thiazide-like diuretics before parathyroid function tests.
• ***Look alike–sound alike:*** Don't confuse Zaroxolyn with Zarontin.

PATIENT TEACHING
• Tell patient to take drug in morning to prevent need to urinate at night.
• Advise patient to avoid sudden posture changes and to rise slowly to avoid effects of dizziness upon standing quickly.
• Instruct patient to use a sunblock to prevent photosensitivity reactions.

spironolactone
Aldactone, Novospiroton†, Spiractin‡

Pharmacologic class: potassium-sparing diuretic
Pregnancy risk category D

AVAILABLE FORMS
Tablets: 25 mg, 50 mg, 100 mg

INDICATIONS & DOSAGES
➤ **Edema**
Adults: Initially, 100 mg P.O. daily given as a single dose or in divided doses. Usual range is 25 to 200 mg P.O. daily.
Children: Give 3.3 mg/kg P.O. daily or in divided doses.
➤ **Hypertension**
Adults: 50 to 100 mg P.O. daily or in divided doses. Some practitioners use a lower dose range of 25 to 50 mg daily and add another antihypertensive to the regimen, rather than continually increasing this drug.
Children ♦: Give 1 to 3.3 mg/kg P.O. (up to 100 mg daily) as a single dose or divided b.i.d.
➤ **Diuretic-induced hypokalemia**
Adults: 25 to 100 mg P.O. daily.
➤ **To detect primary hyperaldosteronism**
Adults: 400 mg P.O. daily for 4 days (short test) or 3 to 4 weeks (long test). If hypokalemia and hypertension are corrected, a presumptive diagnosis of primary hyperaldosteronism is made.
➤ **To manage primary hyperaldosteronism**
Adults: 100 to 400 mg P.O. daily. Use lowest effective dose.
➤ **Heart failure, as adjunct to ACE inhibitor or loop diuretic, with or without cardiac glycoside)** ♦
Adults: 12.5 to 25 mg P.O. daily. May increase to 50 mg daily after 8 weeks.
➤ **Hirsutism** ♦
Women: 50 to 200 mg P.O. daily. Or, 50 mg P.O. b.i.d. days 4 to 21 of menstrual cycle.
➤ **Premenstrual syndrome** ♦
Adults: 25 mg P.O. q.i.d. starting on day 14 of the menstrual cycle.
➤ **Acne vulgaris** ♦
Adults: 100 mg P.O. daily.

➤ **Familial male precocious puberty**♦
Boys: 2 mg/kg P.O. daily with 20 to 40 mg/kg testolactone P.O. daily for at least 6 months.

ACTION
Antagonizes aldosterone in the distal tubules, increasing sodium and water excretion.

Route	Onset	Peak	Duration
P.O.	1–2 days	2–3 days	2–3 days

Half-life: 1¼ to 2 hours.

ADVERSE REACTIONS
CNS: headache, drowsiness, lethargy, confusion, ataxia.
GI: diarrhea, gastric bleeding, ulceration, cramping, gastritis, vomiting.
GU: inability to maintain erection, menstrual disturbances.
Hematologic: ***agranulocytosis.***
Metabolic: ***hyperkalemia,*** dehydration, hyponatremia, mild acidosis.
Skin: urticaria, hirsutism, maculopapular eruptions.
Other: ***anaphylaxis,*** gynecomastia, breast soreness, drug fever.

INTERACTIONS
Drug-drug. *ACE inhibitors, indomethacin, other potassium-sparing diuretics, potassium supplements:* May increase risk of hyperkalemia. Use together cautiously, especially in patients with renal impairment.Monitor potassium level.
Anticoagulants: May decrease anticoagulant effects. Monitor PT and INR.
Aspirin and other salicylates: May block diuretic effect of spironolactone. Watch for diminished spironolactone response.
Digoxin: May alter digoxin clearance, increasing risk of toxicity. Monitor digoxin level.
Drug-herb. *Licorice:* May block ulcer-healing and aldosterone-like effects of herb; may increase risk of hypokalemia. Discourage use together.
Drug-food. *Potassium-rich foods, such as citrus fruits and tomatoes, salt substitutes containing potassium:* May increase risk of hyperkalemia. Urge caution.

EFFECTS ON LAB TEST RESULTS
- May increase BUN and potassium levels. May decrease sodium level.
- May decrease granulocyte count.
- May alter fluorometric determinations of plasma and urinary 17-hydroxycorticosteroid levels.

CONTRAINDICATIONS & CAUTIONS
- Contraindicated in patients hypersensitive to drug and in those with anuria, acute or progressive renal insufficiency, or hyperkalemia.
- Use cautiously in patients with fluid or electrolyte imbalances, impaired renal function, or hepatic disease, or in pregnant women.

NURSING CONSIDERATIONS
- To enhance absorption, give drug with meals.
- Protect drug from light.
- Monitor electrolyte levels, fluid intake and output, weight, and blood pressure.
- Monitor elderly patients closely, who are more susceptible to excessive diuresis.
- Inform laboratory that patient is taking spironolactone because drug may interfere with tests that measure digoxin level.
- Drug is less potent than thiazide and loop diuretics and is useful as an adjunct to other diuretic therapy. Diuretic effect is delayed 2 to 3 days when used alone.
- Maximum antihypertensive response may be delayed for up to 2 weeks.
- Watch for hyperchloremic metabolic acidosis, especially in patients with hepatic cirrhosis.
- Breast cancer may occur, but a causal relationship hasn't been established.
- ***Look alike–sound alike:*** Don't confuse Aldactone with Aldactazide.

PATIENT TEACHING
- Instruct patient to take drug in morning to prevent need to urinate at night. If second dose is needed, tell him to take it with food in early afternoon.
- ***Alert:*** To prevent serious hyperkalemia, warn patient to avoid excessive ingestion of potassium-rich foods (such as citrus fruits, tomatoes, bananas, dates, and apricots), salt substitutes containing potassium, and potassium supplements.

• Caution patient not to perform hazardous activities if adverse CNS reactions occur.
• Advise men about possible breast tenderness or enlargement.

torsemide
Demadex

Pharmacologic class: loop diuretic
Pregnancy risk category B

AVAILABLE FORMS
Injection: 10 mg/ml
Tablets: 5 mg, 10 mg, 20 mg, 100 mg

INDICATIONS & DOSAGES
➤ **Diuresis in patients with heart failure**
Adults: Initially, 10 to 20 mg P.O. or I.V. once daily. If response is inadequate, double dose until desired effect is achieved. Maximum, 200 mg daily.
➤ **Diuresis in patients with chronic renal failure**
Adults: Initially, 20 mg P.O. or I.V. once daily. If response is inadequate, double dose until response is obtained. Maximum, 200 mg daily.
➤ **Diuresis in patients with hepatic cirrhosis**
Adults: Initially, 5 to 10 mg P.O. or I.V. once daily with an aldosterone antagonist or a potassium-sparing diuretic. If response is inadequate, double dose until desired effect is achieved. Maximum, 40 mg daily.
➤ **Hypertension**
Adults: Initially, 5 mg P.O. daily. Increased to 10 mg if needed and tolerated. Add another antihypertensive if response is still inadequate.

I.V. ADMINISTRATION
• Inspect ampules for precipitate or discoloration before use.
• Give by direct injection over at least 2 minutes. Rapid injection may cause ototoxicity. Don't give more than 200 mg at a time.

INCOMPATIBILITIES
None reported.

ACTION
Enhances excretion of sodium, chloride, and water by acting on the ascending loop of Henle.

Route	Onset	Peak	Duration
P.O.	1 hr	1–2 hr	6–8 hr
I.V.	10 min	1 hr	6–8 hr

Half-life: 3½ hours.

ADVERSE REACTIONS
CNS: asthenia, dizziness, headache, nervousness, insomnia, syncope.
CV: ECG abnormalities, chest pain, edema, orthostatic hypotension.
EENT: rhinitis, sore throat.
GI: *excessive thirst,* ***hemorrhage,*** diarrhea, constipation, nausea, dyspepsia.
GU: excessive urination, impotence.
Metabolic: *electrolyte imbalances including hypokalemia and hypomagnesemia,* ***dehydration,*** hypochloremic alkalosis, hyperuricemia, hypercholesterolemia.
Musculoskeletal: arthralgia, myalgia.
Respiratory: cough.
Skin: rash.

INTERACTIONS
Drug-drug. *Aminoglycoside antibiotics, cisplatin:* May increase ototoxicity. Use together cautiously.
Amphotericin B, corticosteroids, metolazone: May increase risk of hypokalemia. Monitor potassium level.
Anticoagulants: May enhance anticoagulant activity. Use together cautiously.
Antidiabetics: May decrease hypoglycemic effect, resulting in higher glucose level. Monitor glucose level.
Chlorothiazide, chlorthalidone, hydrochlorothiazide, indapamide, metolazone: May cause excessive diuretic response, resulting in serious electrolyte abnormalities or dehydration. Adjust doses carefully, and monitor patient closely for signs and symptoms of excessive diuretic response.
Cholestyramine: May decrease absorption of torsemide. Separate doses by at least 3 hours.
Digoxin: Electrolyte imbalance caused by diuretic may lead to digitalis-induced arrhythmia. Use together cautiously.

Indomethacin: May decrease diuretic effect in sodium-restricted patients. Avoid using together.
Lithium: May increase lithium level and cause toxicity. Use together cautiously and monitor lithium level.
NSAIDs: May decrease effects of loop diuretics. Use together cautiously.
Probenecid: May decrease diuretic effect. Avoid using together.
Salicylates: May decrease excretion, possibly leading to salicylate toxicity. Avoid using together.
Spironolactone: May decrease renal clearance of spironolactone. Use together cautiously.
Drug-herb. *Dandelion:* May interfere with drug activity. Discourage use together.
Licorice: May cause unexpected rapid potassium loss. Discourage use together.
Drug-lifestyle. *Sun exposure:* May cause photosensitivity. Advise patient to take precautions.

EFFECTS ON LAB TEST RESULTS

- May increase BUN, creatinine, cholesterol, glucose, and uric acid levels. May decrease potassium and magnesium levels.

CONTRAINDICATIONS & CAUTIONS

- Contraindicated in patients hypersensitive to drug or other sulfonamide derivatives and in those with anuria.
- Use cautiously in patients with hepatic disease and related cirrhosis and ascites; sudden changes in fluid and electrolyte balance may precipitate hepatic coma in these patients.

NURSING CONSIDERATIONS

- To prevent nocturia, give drug in the morning.
- Monitor fluid intake and output, electrolyte levels, blood pressure, weight, and pulse rate during rapid diuresis and routinely with long-term use. Drug can cause profound diuresis and water and electrolyte depletion.
- Watch for signs of hypokalemia, such as muscle weakness and cramps.
- Consult prescriber and dietitian about providing a high-potassium diet or potassium supplement. Foods rich in potassium include citrus fruits, tomatoes, bananas, dates, and apricots.
- Monitor elderly patients, who are especially susceptible to excessive diuresis with potential for circulatory collapse and thromboembolic complications.
- ***Look alike–sound alike:*** Don't confuse torsemide with furosemide.

PATIENT TEACHING

- Tell patient to take drug in morning to prevent the need to urinate at night.
- Advise patient to change positions slowly to prevent dizziness and to limit alcohol intake and strenuous exercise in hot weather to prevent dizziness.
- Advise patient to immediately report ringing in ears because it may indicate toxicity.
- Tell patient to report weakness, cramping, nausea, and dizziness.
- Tell patient to check with prescriber or pharmacist before taking OTC drugs.
- Advise patient that drug may cause photosensitivity, and tell him to take precautions with sun exposure.

triamterene

Dyrenium

Pharmacologic class: potassium-sparing diuretic
Pregnancy risk category C

AVAILABLE FORMS

Capsules: 50 mg, 100 mg

INDICATIONS & DOSAGES

➤ Edema

Adults: Initially, 100 mg P.O. b.i.d. after meals. Maximum, 300 mg daily.

ACTION

Inhibits sodium reabsorption and potassium and hydrogen excretion by direct action on the distal tubules.

Route	Onset	Peak	Duration
P.O.	2–4 hr	6–8 hr	12–16 hr

Half-life: 1½ to 2½ hours.

ADVERSE REACTIONS

CNS: dizziness, weakness, fatigue, headache.
CV: hypotension.

GI: dry mouth, nausea, vomiting, diarrhea.
GU: interstitial nephritis, nephrolithiasis.
Hematologic: ***thrombocytopenia, agranulocytosis,*** megaloblastic anemia from low folic acid level.
Hepatic: jaundice.
Metabolic: ***hyperkalemia,*** azotemia, hypokalemia, hyponatremia, hyperglycemia, acidosis.
Musculoskeletal: muscle cramps.
Skin: photosensitivity reactions, rash.
Other: ***anaphylaxis.***

INTERACTIONS

Drug-drug. *ACE inhibitors, potassium supplements:* May increase risk of hyperkalemia. If used together, monitor potassium level.
Amantadine: May increase risk of amantadine toxicity. Avoid using together.
Chlorpropamide: May increase risk of hyponatremia. Monitor sodium level.
Cimetidine: May increase bioavailability and decrease renal clearance of triamterene. Monitor potassium level and blood pressure closely.
Lithium: May decrease lithium clearance, increasing risk of lithium toxicity. Monitor lithium level.
NSAIDs: May enhance risk of nephrotoxicity. Use together cautiously.
Quinidine: May interfere with some laboratory tests that measure quinidine level. Inform laboratory that patient is taking triamterene.
Drug-herb. *Licorice:* May increase risk of hypokalemia. Discourage use together.
Drug-food. *Potassium-containing salt substitutes, potassium-rich foods:* May increase risk of hyperkalemia. Urge caution, and monitor potassium level.
Drug-lifestyle. *Sun exposure:* May increase risk for photosensitivity reactions. Advise patient to avoid excessive sunlight exposure.

EFFECTS ON LAB TEST RESULTS

- May increase BUN, creatinine, glucose, and uric acid levels. May decrease sodium and hemoglobin levels. May increase or decrease potassium level.
- May decrease granulocyte and platelet counts. May increase liver function test values.
- May interfere with enzyme assays that use fluorometry, such as quinidine determinations.

CONTRAINDICATIONS & CAUTIONS

- Contraindicated in patients hypersensitive to drug and in those with anuria, severe or progressive renal disease or dysfunction, severe hepatic disease, or hyperkalemia.
- Use cautiously in elderly or debilitated patients and in those with hepatic impairment or diabetes mellitus.

NURSING CONSIDERATIONS

- To minimize nausea, give drug after meals.
- Monitor blood pressure, uric acid, CBC, and glucose, BUN, and electrolyte levels.
- Monitor potassium levels frequently, especially with dosage changes or with illness that may affect renal function.
- Obtain an ECG if hyperkalemia is present or suspected.
- Stop potassium supplements when therapy starts.
- Watch for blood dyscrasia.
- To minimize excessive rebound potassium excretion, withdraw drug gradually.
- Drug is less potent than thiazides and loop diuretics and is useful as an adjunct to other diuretic therapy. It's usually used with potassium-wasting diuretics; full effect is delayed 2 to 3 days when used alone.
- ***Look alike–sound alike:*** Don't confuse triamterene with trimipramine.

PATIENT TEACHING

- Tell patient to take drug after meals to minimize nausea.
- If a single daily dose is prescribed, instruct patient to take it in the morning to prevent need to urinate at night.
- ***Alert:*** Warn patient that to prevent serious hyperkalemia, he should avoid excessive ingestion of potassium-rich foods (such as citrus fruits, tomatoes, bananas, dates, and apricots), potassium-containing salt substitutes, and potassium supplements.
- Teach patient to avoid direct sunlight, wear protective clothing, and use sunblock to prevent photosensitivity reactions.
- Tell patient that urine may turn blue.

61

Electrolytes and replacement solutions

calcium acetate
calcium chloride
calcium citrate
calcium glubionate
calcium gluconate
calcium lactate
calcium phosphate, dibasic
calcium phosphate, tribasic
magnesium chloride
magnesium sulfate
potassium acetate
potassium bicarbonate
potassium chloride
potassium gluconate
sodium chloride

calcium acetate
PhosLo

calcium chloride

calcium citrate ◇
Citracal ◇, Citracal Liquitab† ◇

calcium glubionate
Calciquid

calcium gluconate

calcium lactate ◇
Cal-Lac ◇

calcium phosphate, dibasic ◇

calcium phosphate, tribasic
Posture ◇

Pharmacologic class: calcium salts
Pregnancy risk category C

AVAILABLE FORMS
calcium acetate
Contains 253 mg or 12.7 mEq of elemental calcium/g
Capsules: 333.5 mg, 667 mg
Gelcaps: 667 mg
Tablets: 667 mg
calcium chloride
Contains 270 mg or 13.5 mEq of elemental calcium/g
Injection: 10% solution in 10-ml ampules, vials, and syringes
calcium citrate
Contains 211 mg or 10.6 mEq of elemental calcium/g
Tablets: 250 mg, 950 mg ◇
Tablets (effervescent): 500 mg of elemental calcium ◇
calcium glubionate
Contains 64 mg or 3.2 mEq elemental calcium/g
Syrup: 1.8 g/5 ml
calcium gluconate
Contains 90 mg or 4.5 mEq of elemental calcium/g
Injection: 10% solution in 10-ml ampules and vials, 10-ml or 50-ml vials
Powder for oral suspension: 3,756 mg/15 ml
Tablets: 500 mg ◇, 650 mg ◇, 1 g ◇
calcium lactate
Contains 130 mg or 6.5 mEq of elemental calcium/g
Capsules: 500 mg (96 mg elemental calcium)
Tablets: 100 mg, 650 mg (84.5 mg elemental calcium)
calcium phosphate, dibasic
Contains 230 mg or 11.5 mEq of elemental calcium/g
Tablets: 500 mg ◇
calcium phosphate, tribasic
Contains 400 mg or 20 mEq of elemental calcium/g
Tablets: 300 mg ◇, 600 mg ◇

INDICATIONS & DOSAGES
➤ **Hypocalcemic emergency**
Adults: 7 mEq to 14 mEq calcium I.V. May give as a 10% calcium gluconate solution, 2% to 10% calcium chloride solution.
Children: 1 mEq to 7 mEq calcium I.V.
Infants: Up to 1 mEq calcium I.V.
➤ **Hypocalcemic tetany**
Adults: 4.5 mEq to 16 mEq calcium I.V. Repeat until tetany is controlled.

Children: 0.5 to 0.7 mEq/kg calcium I.V. t.i.d. to q.i.d. until tetany is controlled.
Neonates: 2.4 mEq/kg calcium I.V. daily in divided doses.

➤ **Adjunctive treatment of magnesium intoxication**
Adults: Initially, 7 mEq I.V. Base subsequent doses on patient's response.

➤ **During exchange transfusions**
Adults: 1.35 mEq I.V. with each 100 ml citrated blood.
Neonates: 0.45 mEq I.V. after each 100 ml citrated blood.

➤ **Hyperphosphatemia**
Adults: 1,334 to 2,000 mg P.O. calcium acetate or 2 to 5.2 g calcium ion t.i.d. with meals. Most dialysis patients need 3 to 4 tablets with each meal.

➤ **Dietary supplement**
Adults: 500 mg to 2 g P.O. daily.

➤ **Hyperkalemia with secondary cardiac toxicity**
Adults: 2.25 mEq to 14 mEq I.V. Repeat dose after 1 to 2 minutes if needed.

I.V. ADMINISTRATION

- Calcium salts aren't interchangeable; verify preparation before use.
- Give calcium chloride only by I.V. route. When adding to parenteral solutions that contain other additives (especially phosphorus or phosphate), watch for precipitate. Use an in-line filter.
- When giving calcium gluconate as injection, give only by I.V. route.
- Monitor ECG when giving calcium I.V. Stop drug and notify prescriber if patient complains of discomfort.
- Extravasation may cause severe necrosis and tissue sloughing. Calcium gluconate is less irritating to veins and tissues than calcium chloride.

Direct injection

- Don't use scalp veins in children.
- Warm solution to body temperature before giving it.
- For calcium chloride, give at 1 ml/minute (1.5 mEq/minute); for calcium gluconate, 2 ml/minute.
- Give slowly through a small needle into a large vein or through an I.V. line containing a free-flowing, compatible solution.
- After injection, keep patient recumbent for 15 minutes.

Intermittent infusion

- Infuse diluted solution through an I.V. line containing a compatible solution.
- For calcium gluconate, don't exceed 200 mg/minute.

INCOMPATIBILITIES

Drug will precipitate if given with sodium bicarbonate or other alkaline drugs.
Calcium chloride: amphotericin B, chlorpheniramine, dobutamine.
Calcium gluconate: amphotericin B, dobutamine, fluconazole, indomethacin sodium trihydrate, methylprednisolone sodium succinate, prochlorperazine edisylate.

ACTION

Replaces calcium and maintains calcium level.

Route	Onset	Peak	Duration
P.O.	Unknown	Unknown	Unknown
I.V., I.M.	Immediate	Immediate	30 min–2 hr

Half-life: Unknown.

ADVERSE REACTIONS

CNS: tingling sensations, sense of oppression or heat waves with I.V. use, syncope with rapid I.V. use.
CV: ***bradycardia, arrhythmias, cardiac arrest with rapid I.V. use,*** mild drop in blood pressure, vasodilation.
GI: *constipation,* irritation, chalky taste, hemorrhage, nausea, vomiting, thirst, abdominal pain.
GU: polyuria, renal calculi.
Metabolic: hypercalcemia.
Skin: local reactions, including burning, necrosis, tissue sloughing, cellulitis, soft-tissue calcification with I.M. use, pain, irritation at subcutaneous injection site.

INTERACTIONS

Drug-drug. *Atenolol, tetracyclines:* May decrease bioavailability of these drugs and calcium when oral preparations are taken together. Separate dosing times.
Cardiac glycosides: May increase digoxin toxicity. Give calcium cautiously, if at all, to digitalized patients.
Ciprofloxacin, levofloxacin, lomefloxacin, moxifloxacin, norfloxacin, ofloxacin: May decrease effects of quinolone. Give cal-

cium carbonate at least 6 hours before or 2 hours after the quinolone.
Fosphenytoin, phenytoin: Use together may decrease absorption of both drugs. Avoid using together, or monitor levels carefully.
Sodium polystyrene sulfonate: May cause metabolic acidosis in patients with renal disease. Avoid using together.
Thiazide diuretics: May cause hypercalcemia. Avoid using together.
Verapamil: May reduce effects and toxicity of verapamil. Monitor patient closely.
Drug-food. *Foods containing oxalic acid (rhubarb, spinach), phytic acid (bran, whole-grain cereals), phosphorus (dairy products, milk):* May interfere with calcium absorption. Discourage use together.

EFFECTS ON LAB TEST RESULTS

- May increase calcium level.

CONTRAINDICATIONS & CAUTIONS

- Contraindicated in cancer patients with bone metastases and in those with ventricular fibrillation, hypercalcemia, hypophosphatemia, or renal calculi.

NURSING CONSIDERATIONS

- Use all calcium products with extreme caution in digitalized patients and patients with sarcoidosis and renal or cardiac disease. Use calcium chloride cautiously in patients with cor pulmonale, respiratory acidosis, or respiratory failure.
- Give I.M. in gluteals in adults and in side of the thigh in infants. Use I.M. only in emergencies when no I.V. route is available because of irritation of tissue by calcium salts.
- ***Alert:*** Double-check that you are giving the correct form of calcium; resuscitation cart may contain both calcium gluconate and calcium chloride.
- Monitor calcium levels frequently. Maintain calcium level of 9 to 10.4 mg/dl. Don't allow level to exceed 12 mg/dl. Hypercalcemia may result after large doses in chronic renal failure. Report abnormalities.
- Signs and symptoms of severe hypercalcemia may include stupor, confusion, delirium, and coma. Signs and symptoms of mild hypercalcemia may include anorexia, nausea, and vomiting.
- ***Look alike–sound alike:*** Don't confuse calcium with calcitriol, calcium gluconate with calcium glubionate, or calcium chloride with calcium gluconate.

PATIENT TEACHING

- Tell patient to take oral calcium 1 to 1½ hours after meals if GI upset occurs.
- Tell patient to take oral calcium with a full glass of water.
- Tell patient to report anorexia, nausea, vomiting, constipation, abdominal pain, dry mouth, thirst, or polyuria.
- Warn patient that, in the meal before he takes calcium, he shouldn't have rhubarb, spinach, bran and whole-grain cereals, or dairy products; these foods may interfere with calcium absorption.
- Inform patient that some products may contain phenylalanine or tartrazine.

magnesium chloride

Slow-Mag ◇

magnesium sulfate

Pharmacologic class: magnesium salt
Pregnancy risk category D

AVAILABLE FORMS

magnesium chloride
Injection: 20% in 50-ml vials
Tablets (delayed-release): 64 mg
magnesium sulfate
Injectable solutions: 10%, 12.5%, 50% in 2-, 5-, 10-, 20-, and 30-ml ampules, vials, and prefilled syringes

INDICATIONS & DOSAGES

➤ Mild hypomagnesemia
Adults: 1 g I.V. by piggyback or I.M. q 6 hours for four doses, depending on magnesium level. Or, 3 g P.O. q 6 hours for four doses.

➤ Symptomatic severe hypomagnesemia, with magnesium 0.8 mEq/L or less
Adults: 2 to 5 g I.V. in 1 L of solution over 3 hours. Base subsequent doses on magnesium level.

➤ Magnesium supplementation
Adults: 64 mg (one tablet) P.O. t.i.d.

➤**Magnesium supplementation in total parenteral nutrition (TPN)**
Adults and children: 4 to 24 mEq I.V. daily added to TPN solution.
Infants: 2 to 10 mEq I.V. daily added to TPN solution. Each 2 ml of 50% solution contains 1 g, or 8.12 mEq, magnesium sulfate.
➤**Seizures**
Adults: 4 to 5 g magnesium sulfate 50% solution I.M. q 4 hours, p.r.n. Or 4 g of 10% to 20% magnesium sulfate solution I.V. at no more than 1.5 ml/minute of 10% solution. Or, for I.V. infusion, 4 to 5 g in 250 ml of D_5W or sodium chloride, not exceeding 3 ml/minute.
Children: 20 to 40 mg/kg I.M. in a 20% solution. Repeat as needed.

I.V. ADMINISTRATION
- Inject bolus dose slowly at a rate not exceeding 150 mg/minute, or use infusion pump for continuous infusion to avoid respiratory or cardiac arrest. Maximum infusion rate is 150 mg/minute. Rapid drip causes feeling of heat.
- For severe hypomagnesemia, watch for respiratory depression and evidence of heart block. Respirations should exceed 16 breaths/minute before dose is given.

INCOMPATIBILITIES
Alcohol (in high concentrations), alkali carbonates and bicarbonates, amiodarone, amphotericin B, calcium chloride, calcium gluconate, cefepime, ciprofloxacin, clindamycin, cyclosporine, dobutamine, drotrecogin alfa, heavy metals, hydralazine, hydrocortisone sodium succinate, I.V. fat emulsion 10%, phytonadione, polymyxin B, procaine, quinolones, salicylates, sodium bicarbonate, soluble phosphates, vitamin B complex.

ACTION
Replaces magnesium and maintains magnesium level; as an anticonvulsant, reduces muscle contractions by interfering with release of acetylcholine at myoneural junction.

Route	Onset	Peak	Duration
P.O.	Unknown	4 hr	4–6 hr
I.V.	Immediate	Unknown	30 min
I.M.	1 hr	Unknown	3–4 hr

Half-life: Unknown.

ADVERSE REACTIONS
CNS: toxicity, *weak or absent deep tendon reflexes,* flaccid paralysis, drowsiness, stupor.
CV: slow, weak pulse, ***arrhythmias,*** *hypotension,* ***circulatory collapse,*** flushing.
GI: diarrhea.
Metabolic: hypocalcemia.
Respiratory: ***respiratory paralysis.***
Skin: diaphoresis.
Other: hypothermia.

INTERACTIONS
Drug-drug. *Alendronate, fluoroquinolones, nitrofurantoin, penicillamine, sodium polystyrene sulfonate, tetracyclines:* May decrease bioavailability with oral magnesium supplements. Separate doses by 2 to 3 hours.
Cardiac glycosides: May cause serious cardiac conduction changes. Use together with caution.
CNS depressants: May have additive effect. Use together cautiously.
Neuromuscular blockers: May cause increased neuromuscular blockage. Use together cautiously.

EFFECTS ON LAB TEST RESULTS
- May increase magnesium level. May decrease calcium level.

CONTRAINDICATIONS & CAUTIONS
- Contraindicated in patients with myocardial damage or heart block, coma, and in pregnant women in actively progressing labor.
- Use parenteral magnesium with caution in patients with impaired renal function.

NURSING CONSIDERATIONS
- Undiluted 50% solutions may be given by deep I.M. injection to adults. Dilute solutions to 20% or less for use in children.
- Keep I.V. calcium available to reverse magnesium intoxication.

• Test knee-jerk and patellar reflexes before each additional dose. If absent, notify prescriber and give no more magnesium until reflexes return; otherwise, patient may develop temporary respiratory failure and need cardiopulmonary resuscitation or I.V. administration of calcium.
• Check magnesium level after repeated doses.
• Monitor fluid intake and output. Output should be 100 ml or more during 4-hour period before dose.
• Monitor renal function.
• After giving to toxemic pregnant woman within 24 hours before delivery, watch neonate for signs and symptoms of magnesium toxicity, including neuromuscular and respiratory depression.
• ***Look alike–sound alike:*** Don't confuse magnesium chloride with magnesium sulfate.

PATIENT TEACHING

• Explain use and administration of drug to patient and family.
• Tell patient to report adverse effects.

potassium acetate

Pharmacologic class: potassium salt
Pregnancy risk category C

AVAILABLE FORMS

Injection: 2 mEq/ml in 20-, 50-, and 100-ml vials, 4 mEq/ml in 50-ml vial

INDICATIONS & DOSAGES

➤ **Hypokalemia**
Adults: No more than 20 mEq/hour in concentration of 40 mEq/L or less. Total 24-hour dose shouldn't exceed 150 mEq (3 mEq/kg in children).
➤ **To prevent hypokalemia**
Adults: Dosage is individualized to patient's needs, not to exceed 150 mEq daily. Give as an additive to I.V. infusions. Usual dose is 20 mEq/L, infused at no more than 20 mEq/hour.
Children: Individualize dose; don't exceed 3 mEq/kg daily. Give as an additive to I.V. infusions.

I.V. ADMINISTRATION

• Use only in life-threatening hypokalemia or when oral replacement isn't feasible.
• Don't give undiluted potassium. Maximum concentration is 80 mEq/L.
• Don't add potassium to a hanging bag. Mix well to avoid layering.
• To prevent pain, use largest peripheral vein and a well-placed small-bore needle.
• Give only by infusion, never I.V. push or I.M. Watch for pain and redness at infusion site.
• Give slowly as diluted solution; rapid infusion may cause fatal hyperkalemia.

INCOMPATIBILITIES

None reported.

ACTION

Replaces potassium and maintains potassium level.

Route	Onset	Peak	Duration
I.V.	Immediate	Immediate	Unknown

Half-life: Unknown.

ADVERSE REACTIONS

CNS: paresthesia of limbs, listlessness, mental confusion, weakness or heaviness of legs, flaccid paralysis, pain, fever.
CV: ***arrhythmias, cardiac arrest, heart block,*** ECG changes, hypotension.
GI: nausea, vomiting, abdominal pain, diarrhea.
Metabolic: ***hyperkalemia.***
Respiratory: ***respiratory paralysis.***
Skin: redness at infusion site.

INTERACTIONS

Drug-drug. *ACE inhibitors, digoxin, potassium-sparing diuretics:* May increase risk of hyperkalemia. Use together with caution.
Digoxin: May cause digoxin toxicity, from hypokalemia. Stop potassium cautiously if patient is on digoxin.

EFFECTS ON LAB TEST RESULTS

• May increase potassium level.

CONTRAINDICATIONS & CAUTIONS

- Contraindicated in patients with severe renal impairment with oliguria, anuria, or azotemia.
- Contraindicated in those with untreated Addison disease, acute dehydration, heat cramps, hyperkalemia, hyperkalemic form of familial periodic paralysis, or conditions linked to extensive tissue breakdown.
- Use cautiously in patients with cardiac disease or renal impairment.

NURSING CONSIDERATIONS

- During therapy, monitor ECG, renal function, fluid intake and output, and potassium, creatinine, and BUN levels. Never give potassium postoperatively until urine flow is established.
- Many adverse reactions may reflect hyperkalemia.
- ***Look alike–sound alike:*** Potassium preparations aren't interchangeable; verify preparation before use.

PATIENT TEACHING

- Explain use and administration to patient and family.
- Tell patient to report adverse effects, especially pain at insertion site.

potassium bicarbonate

K+ Care ET, K-Lyte, Klor-Con/EF

Pharmacologic class: potassium salt
Pregnancy risk category C

AVAILABLE FORMS

Tablets (effervescent): 25 mEq, 50 mEq

INDICATIONS & DOSAGES

➤ To prevent hypokalemia

Adults and children: Initially, 25 mEq P.O. daily, in divided doses. Adjust dosage, as needed.

➤ Hypokalemia

Adults and children: 50 to 100 mEq P.O. divided into two to four daily doses. Use I.V. potassium chloride when oral replacement isn't feasible. Don't exceed 150 mEq P.O. daily in adults and 3 mEq/kg daily P.O. in children.

ACTION

Replaces potassium and maintains potassium level.

Route	Onset	Peak	Duration
P.O.	Unknown	4 hr	Unknown

Half-life: Unknown.

ADVERSE REACTIONS

CNS: paresthesia of limbs, listlessness, confusion, weakness or heaviness of legs, flaccid paralysis.
CV: ***arrhythmias,*** ECG changes, hypotension, ***heart block, cardiac arrest.***
GI: *nausea, vomiting, abdominal pain,* diarrhea.

INTERACTIONS

Drug-drug. *ACE inhibitors, digoxin, potassium-sparing diuretics:* May cause hyperkalemia. Use with extreme caution. Monitor potassium levels.

EFFECTS ON LAB TEST RESULTS

- May increase potassium level.

CONTRAINDICATIONS & CAUTIONS

- Contraindicated in patients with severe renal impairment with oliguria, anuria, or azotemia; untreated Addison disease; or acute dehydration, heat cramps, hyperkalemia, hyperkalemic form of familial periodic paralysis, or other conditions linked to extensive tissue breakdown.
- Use cautiously in patients with cardiac disease or renal impairment.

NURSING CONSIDERATIONS

- Dissolve tablets completely in 4 to 8 ounces of cold water.
- Ask patient's flavor preference: lime, fruit punch, citrus, or orange.
- Don't give potassium supplements postoperatively until urine flow has been established.
- ***Alert:*** Potassium preparations aren't interchangeable; verify preparation before use. Never switch potassium products without prescriber's order. Potassium chloride can't be given instead of potassium bicarbonate.
- Monitor fluid intake and output and BUN, potassium, and creatinine levels.

PATIENT TEACHING

- Tell patient to take drug with meals and sip slowly over 5 to 10 minutes.
- Tell patient to report adverse effects.
- Warn patient not to use salt substitutes at the same time, except with prescriber's permission.

SAFETY ALERT!

potassium chloride

Apo-K*†, Cena-K, Gen-K, K-8, K+ 10, Kalium Durules†, Kaochlor, Kaochlor S-F, Kaon-Cl, Kaon-Cl-10, Kaon-Cl 20%, Kay Ciel, K+ Care, K-Dur 20🖉, K-Lease, K-Lor, Klor-Con, Klor-Con 8, Klor-Con 10, Klor-Con/25, Klor-Con M10, Klor-Con M15, Klor-Con M20, Klorvess, Klotrix, K-Lyte/Cl, K-Norm, K-Tab, Micro-K, Micro-K 10, Micro-K LS, Potasalan, Rum-K, Slow-K, Ten-K

Pharmacologic class: potassium salt
Pregnancy risk category C

AVAILABLE FORMS

Capsules (controlled-release): 8 mEq, 10 mEq
Injection concentrate: 1.5 mEq/ml, 2 mEq/ml
Injection for I.V. infusion: 0.1 mEq/ml, 0.2 mEq/ml, 0.3 mEq/ml, 0.4 mEq/ml
Oral liquid: 20 mEq/15 ml, 30 mEq/15 ml, 40 mEq/15 ml
Powder for oral administration: 15 mEq/packet, 20 mEq/packet, 25 mEq/packet
Tablets (controlled-release): 6.7 mEq, 8 mEq, 10 mEq, 20 mEq
Tablets (extended-release): 8 mEq, 10 mEq, 15 mEq, 20 mEq

INDICATIONS & DOSAGES

➤ To prevent hypokalemia
Adults and children: Initially, 20 mEq of potassium supplement P.O. daily, in divided doses. Adjust dosage, as needed, based on potassium levels.

➤ Hypokalemia
Adults and children: 40 to 100 mEq P.O. in two to four divided doses daily. Maximum dose of diluted I.V. potassium chloride is 40 mEq/L at 10 mEq/hour. Don't exceed 150 mEq daily in adults and 3 mEq/kg daily in children. Further doses are based on potassium levels and blood pH. Give I.V. potassium replacement only with monitoring of ECG and potassium level.

➤ Severe hypokalemia
Adults and children: Dilute potassium chloride in a suitable I.V. solution of less than 80 mEq/L, and give at no more than 40 mEq/hour.

Further doses are based on potassium level. Don't exceed 150 mEq I.V. daily in adults and 3 mEq/kg I.V. daily or 40 mEq/m^2 daily in children. Give I.V. potassium replacement only with monitoring of ECG and potassium level.

➤ Acute MI♦
Adults: For high dose, 80 mEq/L at 1.5 ml/kg/hour for 24 hours with an I.V. infusion of 25% dextrose and 50 units/L regular insulin. For low dose, 40 mEq/L at 1 ml/kg/hour for 24 hours, with an I.V. infusion of 10% dextrose and 20 units/L regular insulin.

I.V. ADMINISTRATION

- Use only when oral replacement isn't feasible or when hypokalemia is life-threatening.
- Give by infusion only, never I.V. push or I.M. Give slowly as dilute solution; rapid infusion may cause fatal hyperkalemia.
- If burning occurs during infusion, decrease rate.

INCOMPATIBILITIES

Amikacin, amoxicillin, amphotericin B, azithromycin, diazepam, dobutamine, ergotamine, etoposide with cisplatin and mannitol, fat emulsion 10%, methylprednisolone, penicillin G, phenytoin, promethazine.

ACTION

Replaces potassium and maintains potassium level.

Route	Onset	Peak	Duration
P.O.	Unknown	Unknown	Unknown
I.V.	Immediate	Immediate	Unknown

Half-life: Unknown.

ADVERSE REACTIONS

CNS: paresthesia of limbs, listlessness, confusion, weakness or heaviness of limbs, flaccid paralysis.
CV: *postinfusion phlebitis,* ***arrhythmias, heart block, cardiac arrest,*** ECG changes, hypotension.
GI: nausea, vomiting, abdominal pain, diarrhea.
Metabolic: ***hyperkalemia.***
Respiratory: ***respiratory paralysis.***

INTERACTIONS

Drug-drug. *ACE inhibitors, digoxin, potassium-sparing diuretics:* May cause hyperkalemia. Use together with extreme caution. Monitor potassium level.

EFFECTS ON LAB TEST RESULTS

- May increase potassium level.

CONTRAINDICATIONS & CAUTIONS

- Contraindicated in patients with severe renal impairment with oliguria, anuria, or azotemia; with untreated Addison disease; or with acute dehydration, heat cramps, hyperkalemia, hyperkalemic form of familial periodic paralysis, or other conditions linked to extensive tissue breakdown.
- Use cautiously in patients with cardiac disease or renal impairment.

NURSING CONSIDERATIONS

- ***Look alike–sound alike:*** Potassium preparations aren't interchangeable; verify preparation before use and don't switch products.
- Make sure powders are completely dissolved before giving.
- Enteric-coated tablets aren't recommended because of increased risk of GI bleeding and small-bowel ulcerations.
- Patients at an increased risk of GI lesions include those with scleroderma, diabetes, mitral valve replacement, cardiomegaly, or esophageal strictures, and in elderly or immobile patients.
- Tablets in wax matrix sometimes lodge in the esophagus and cause ulceration in cardiac patients with esophageal compression from an enlarged left atrium. Use sugar-free liquid form (Kaochlor S-F) in such patients and in those with esophageal stasis or obstruction. Have patient sip slowly to minimize GI irritation.
- Drug is commonly used orally with potassium-wasting diuretics to maintain potassium levels.
- Don't crush sustained-release potassium products.
- Monitor ECG and electrolyte levels during therapy.
- Monitor renal function. After surgery, don't give drug until urine flow is established.
- Many adverse reactions may reflect hyperkalemia.
- Patient may be sensitive to tartrazine in some of these products,

PATIENT TEACHING

- Teach patient how to prepare powders and how to take drug. Tell patient to take with or after meals with full glass of water or fruit juice to lessen GI distress.
- Teach patient signs and symptoms of hyperkalemia, and tell patient to notify prescriber if they occur.
- Tell patient to report discomfort at I.V. insertion site.
- Warn patient not to use salt substitutes concurrently, except with prescriber's permission.
- ***Alert:*** Tell patient not to be concerned if wax matrix appears in stool because the drug has already been absorbed.

---

potassium gluconate

Kaon, Kaylixir*, K-G Elixir*, Potassium-Rougier†

Pharmacologic class: potassium salt
Pregnancy risk category C

AVAILABLE FORMS

Elixir: 20 mEq/15 ml*
Tablets: 500 mg (83 mg potassium), 595 mg (99 mg potassium)

INDICATIONS & DOSAGES

➤ To prevent hypokalemia
Adults and children: Initially, 20 mEq of potassium supplement P.O. daily, in divided doses. Adjust dosage, as needed, based on potassium level.

➤ **Hypokalemia**
Adults and children: 40 to 100 mEq P.O. divided into two to four daily doses. Use I.V. potassium chloride when oral replacement isn't feasible. Don't exceed 150 mEq P.O. daily in adults and 3 mEq/kg daily P.O. in children.

ACTION
Replaces potassium and maintains intracellular and extracellular potassium levels.

Route	Onset	Peak	Duration
P.O.	Unknown	Unknown	4 hr

Half-life: Unknown.

ADVERSE REACTIONS
CNS: paresthesia of limbs, listlessness, confusion, weakness or heaviness of legs, flaccid paralysis.
CV: ***arrhythmias,*** ECG changes.
GI: *nausea, vomiting, abdominal pain,* diarrhea.

INTERACTIONS
Drug-drug. *ACE inhibitors, digoxin, potassium-sparing diuretics:* May cause hyperkalemia. Use with caution. Monitor potassium level.

EFFECTS ON LAB TEST RESULTS
- May increase potassium level.

CONTRAINDICATIONS & CAUTIONS
- Contraindicated in patients with severe renal impairment with oliguria, anuria, or azotemia; untreated Addison disease; or acute dehydration, heat cramps, hyperkalemia, hyperkalemic form of familial periodic paralysis, or other conditions linked to extensive tissue breakdown.
- Use cautiously in patients with cardiac disease or renal impairment.

NURSING CONSIDERATIONS
- ***Alert:*** Give oral potassium supplements with caution because different forms deliver varying amounts of potassium. Never switch products without prescriber's order.
- Don't give potassium supplements postoperatively until urine flow has been established.
- Monitor ECG, fluid intake and output, and BUN, potassium, and creatinine levels.

PATIENT TEACHING
- Advise patient to sip liquid potassium slowly to minimize GI irritation. Also tell him to take drug with meals, with a full glass of water or fruit juice.
- Warn patient not to use potassium gluconate with a salt substitute, except with prescriber's permission.
- Teach patient signs and symptoms of hyperkalemia, and tell patient to notify prescriber if they occur.

SAFETY ALERT!

sodium chloride
Slo-Salt, Slo-Salt-K, Sustain

Pharmacologic class: sodium salt
Pregnancy risk category C

AVAILABLE FORMS
Injection: Half-normal saline solution 25 ml, 50 ml, 150 ml, 250 ml, 500 ml, 1,000 ml; normal saline solution 2 ml, 3 ml, 5 ml, 10 ml, 20 ml, 25 ml, 30 ml, 50 ml, 100 ml, 150 ml, 250 ml, 500 ml, 1,000 ml; 3% sodium chloride solution 500 ml; 5% sodium chloride solution 500 ml; 14.6% sodium chloride solution 20 ml, 40 ml, 200 ml; 23.4% sodium chloride solution 30 ml, 50 ml, 100 ml, 200 ml
Tablets: 220 mg (with 18 mg calcium carbonate and 15 mg potassium chloride), 650 mg, 1 g, 2.25 g
Tablets (slow-release): 410 mg (with 150 mg potassium chloride), 600 mg

INDICATIONS & DOSAGES
➤ **Fluid and electrolyte replacement in hyponatremia caused by electrolyte loss or in severe salt depletion**
Adults: Dosage is individualized. Use 3% or 5% solution only with frequent electrolyte level determination and only slow I.V. For 0.45% solution, 3% to 8% of body weight, according to deficiencies, over 18 to 24 hours. For 0.9% solution, 2% to 6% of body weight, according to deficiencies, over 18 to 24 hours.

➤ **Heat cramp caused by excessive perspiration**
Adults: 1 g P.O. with each glass of water.

I.V. ADMINISTRATION

- Don't confuse 14.6% form with 23.4% form when adding to parenteral nutrient solutions with normal saline solution for injection, and never give without diluting. Read label carefully
- Infuse 3% and 5% solutions slowly and cautiously to avoid pulmonary edema. Use only for critical situations, and observe patient continually. Infuse through central line, if possible.
- In neonates, never use the bacteriostatic injection.
- If infusing peripherally, infuse into the largest vein possible, using a well-placed small-bore needle to prevent pain. Infuse slowly.

INCOMPATIBILITIES

Amphotericin B, chlordiazepoxide, diazepam, fat emulsion, mannitol, methylprednisolone sodium succinate, phenytoin sodium.

ACTION

Replaces sodium and chloride and maintains levels.

Route	Onset	Peak	Duration
P.O.	Unknown	Unknown	Unknown
I.V.	Immediate	Immediate	Unknown

Half-life: Unknown.

ADVERSE REACTIONS

CV: ***aggravation of heart failure,*** thrombophlebitis, edema when given too rapidly or in excess.
Metabolic: hypernatremia, aggravation of existing metabolic acidosis with excessive infusion.
Respiratory: ***pulmonary edema.***
Skin: local tenderness, tissue necrosis at injection site.
Other: abscess.

INTERACTIONS

None significant.

EFFECTS ON LAB TEST RESULTS

- May increase sodium level. May decrease potassium level.
- May cause electrolyte imbalance.

CONTRAINDICATIONS & CAUTIONS

- Contraindicated in patients with conditions in which sodium and chloride administration is detrimental.
- Sodium chloride 3% and 5% injections contraindicated in patients with increased, normal, or only slightly decreased electrolyte levels.
- Use cautiously in elderly or postoperative patients and in patients with heart failure, circulatory insufficiency, renal dysfunction, or hypoproteinemia.

NURSING CONSIDERATIONS

- Monitor electrolyte levels.

PATIENT TEACHING

- Explain use and administration of drug to patient and family.
- Tell patient to report adverse reactions promptly.
- Tell patient that wax matrix may appear in stool.

62 Alkalinizers

sodium bicarbonate
sodium lactate
tromethamine

sodium bicarbonate

Arm & Hammer Baking Soda ◇, Bell/ans ◇, Neut, Soda Mint ◇

Pharmacologic class: alkalinizer
Pregnancy risk category C

AVAILABLE FORMS

Injection: 4% (2.4 mEq/5 ml), 4.2% (5 mEq/10 ml), 5% (297.5 mEq/500 ml), 7.5% (8.92 mEq/10 ml and 44.6 mEq/ 50 ml), 8.4% (10 mEq/10 ml and 50 mEq/ 50 ml)
Tablets ◇: 325 mg, 650 mg

INDICATIONS & DOSAGES

➤ Metabolic acidosis
Adults and children: Dosage depends on blood carbon dioxide content, pH, and patient's condition; usually, 2 to 5 mEq/kg I.V. infused over 4- to 8-hour period.

➤ Systemic or urinary alkalinization
Adults: Initially, 4 g P.O.; then 1 to 2 g q 6 hours.
Children: 84 to 840 mg/kg P.O. daily.

➤ Antacid
Adults: 300 mg to 2 g P.O. up to q.i.d. taken with glass of water.

➤ Cardiac arrest
Adults: 1 mEq/kg I.V. of 7.5% or 8.4% solution; then 0.5 mEq/kg I.V. q 10 minutes, depending on arterial blood gas (ABG) level. Base further dosages on results of ABG analysis. If ABG level is unavailable, use 0.5 mEq/kg I.V. q 10 minutes until spontaneous circulation returns.
Infants and children: 1 mEq/kg (1 ml/kg of 8.4% solution) I.V. slowly followed by 1 mEq/kg q 10 minutes of arrest. Don't give more than 8 mEq/kg I.V. total; a 4.2% solution may be preferred.

I.V. ADMINISTRATION

- Drug isn't routinely used in cardiac arrest because it may produce a paradoxical acidosis from carbon dioxide production. It shouldn't be routinely given during the early stages of resuscitation unless acidosis is clearly present.
- The 4% form is usually used for neutralizing I.V. drugs such as erythromycin. Consult pharmacist before use.
- Flush I.V. line thoroughly between medications.

INCOMPATIBILITIES

Alcohol 5% in dextrose 5%; allopurinol; amino acids; amiodarone; amobarbital; amphotericin B; ascorbic acid injection; atropine; bupivacaine; calcium salts; carbenicillin; carboplatin; carmustine; cefotaxime; chlorpromazine; ciprofloxacin; cisatracurium; cisplatin; codeine; corticotropin; dextrose 5% in lactated Ringer injection; diazepam; diltiazem; dobutamine; dopamine; doxapram; doxorubicin liposomal; doxycycline; epinephrine hydrochloride; fat emulsion 10%; fenoldopam; glycopyrrolate; hetastarch; hydromorphone; idarubicin; imipenem-cilastatin sodium; inamrinone; Ionosol B, D, or G with invert sugar 10%; isoproterenol; labetalol; lactated Ringer injection; levorphanol; leucovorin calcium; lidocaine; magnesium sulfate; meperidine; meropenem; metaraminol; methylprednisolone sodium succinate; metoclopramide; midazolam; morphine sulfate; MVI-12 multivitamin; nafcillin; nalbuphine; nitrofurantoin; norepinephrine bitartrate; ondansetron; oxacillin; penicillin G potassium; pentazocine lactate; pentobarbital sodium; procaine; Ringer injection; sargramostim; 1/6 M sodium lactate; streptomycin; succinylcholine; thiopental; ticarcillin disodium and clavulanate potassium; vancomycin; verapamil; vinca alkaloids; vitamin B complex with vitamin C.
Drug inactivates catecholamines, such as norepinephrine, dobutamine, and dopamine, and it forms precipitate with cal-

cium. Don't mix with these drugs, and flush line thoroughly.

ACTION
Restores buffering capacity of the body and neutralizes excess acid.

Route	Onset	Peak	Duration
P.O.	Unknown	Unknown	Unknown
I.V.	Immediate	Immediate	Unknown

Half-life: Unknown.

ADVERSE REACTIONS
CNS: tetany.
CV: edema.
GI: gastric distention, belching, flatulence.
Metabolic: hypokalemia, ***metabolic alkalosis,*** hypernatremia, hyperosmolarity with overdose.
Skin: pain and irritation at injection site.

INTERACTIONS
Drug-drug. *Anorexiants, flecainide, mecamylamine, methenamine, quinidine, sympathomimetics:* May decrease renal clearance of these drugs and increase risk of toxicity. Monitor patient closely for toxicity.
Chlorpropamide, lithium, methotrexate, salicylates, tetracycline: May increase urine alkalinization, increase renal clearance of these drugs, and decrease their effect. Monitor patient closely for drug's effect.
Enteric-coated drugs: May be released prematurely in stomach. Avoid using together.
Ketoconazole: May decrease ketoconazole absorption. Separate use by at least 2 hours.

EFFECTS ON LAB TEST RESULTS
- May increase sodium and lactate levels. May decrease potassium level.

CONTRAINDICATIONS & CAUTIONS
- Contraindicated in patients with metabolic or respiratory alkalosis and in those with hypocalcemia in which alkalosis may produce tetany, hypertension, seizures, or heart failure.
- Contraindicated in patients losing chloride because of vomiting or continuous GI suction and in those receiving diuretics that produce hypochloremic alkalosis. Oral drug is contraindicated for acute ingestion of strong mineral acids.
- Use with caution in patients with renal insufficiency, heart failure, or other edematous or sodium-retaining condition.

NURSING CONSIDERATIONS
- To avoid risk of alkalosis, obtain blood pH, partial pressure of arterial oxygen, partial pressure of arterial carbon dioxide, and electrolyte levels. Tell prescriber laboratory results.
- Oral products may contain 27% sodium.

PATIENT TEACHING
- Tell patient not to take drug with milk because doing so may cause high levels of calcium in the blood, abnormally high alkalinity in tissues and fluids, or kidney stones.

sodium lactate

Pharmacologic class: alkalinizer
Pregnancy risk category NR

AVAILABLE FORMS
Injection: 1/6 M solution (167 mEq/L)

INDICATIONS & DOSAGES
➤ To alkalinize urine
Adults: 30 ml/kg (1/6 M solution) I.V. daily, in divided doses.
➤ Metabolic acidosis
Adults: Dosage of 1/6 M solution depends on degree of bicarbonate deficit, according to this formula:

$$(60 - \text{plasma } CO_2) \times (0.8 \times \text{body weight in pounds}) = \text{Dose in ml}$$

I.V. ADMINISTRATION
- Add to other solutions or give as an isotonic 1/6 M solution. Drug is compatible with most common solutions.
- Don't exceed infusion rate of 300 ml/hour.

INCOMPATIBILITIES
Sodium bicarbonate.

ACTION
Metabolizes to sodium bicarbonate, producing buffering effect.

Route	Onset	Peak	Duration
I.V.	Immediate	1–2 hr	Unknown

Half-life: Unknown.

ADVERSE REACTIONS
CNS: fever.
CV: thrombophlebitis at injection site, edema.
Metabolic: ***metabolic alkalosis,*** hypernatremia, hyperosmolarity with overdose, hypervolemia.
Other: infection.

INTERACTIONS
None significant.

EFFECTS ON LAB TEST RESULTS
• May increase sodium level.

CONTRAINDICATIONS & CAUTIONS
• Contraindicated in patients with hypernatremia, severe acidosis, lactic acidosis, or conditions in which sodium administration is detrimental, such as heart failure or during corticosteroid administration.
• Use cautiously in patients with metabolic or respiratory alkalosis, severe hepatic or renal disease, heart failure, shock, hypoxia, or beriberi.

NURSING CONSIDERATIONS
• Monitor electrolyte levels to avoid alkalosis.
• ***Look alike–sound alike:*** Don't confuse sodium lactate with sodium bicarbonate.

PATIENT TEACHING
• Explain use and administration of drug to patient and family.
• Tell patient to report adverse reactions to prescriber.

tromethamine
Tham

Pharmacologic class: alkalinizer
Pregnancy risk category C

AVAILABLE FORMS
Injection: 18 g/500 ml

INDICATIONS & DOSAGES
➤ Metabolic acidosis during cardiac bypass surgery or cardiac arrest
Adults: Dosage depends on bicarbonate deficit. Calculate as follows:

$$\begin{array}{c}\text{Each ml}\\ \text{of 0.3 M}\\ \text{tromethamine}\\ \text{solution}\\ \text{needed}\end{array} = \begin{array}{c}\text{weight}\\ \text{in kg}\end{array} \times \begin{array}{c}\text{bicarbonate}\\ \text{deficit}\\ \text{(mEq/L)}\end{array} \times 1.1$$

Base additional therapy on serial bicarbonate deficit determinations. Give over at least 1 hour; don't exceed 500 mg/kg per dose.
➤ Acidosis during bypass surgery
Adults: Average dose of 9 ml/kg (2.7 mEq/kg or 0.32 g/kg); total single dose of 500 ml (150 mEq or 18 g) is adequate for most adults. Don't exceed 500 mg/kg and don't give over less than 1 hour.
➤ Acidosis associated with cardiac arrest
Adults: If chest is open, inject 2 to 6 g (62 to 185 ml) directly into the ventricular cavity. Don't inject into cardiac muscle. If chest isn't open, inject 3.6 to 10.8 g (111 to 333 ml) into a large peripheral vein. More doses may be needed after arrest is reversed.

I.V. ADMINISTRATION
• Give slowly either through 18G to 20G needle into largest antecubital vein or through indwelling I.V. catheter.
• If extravasation occurs, infiltrate area with 1% procaine.
• Highly alkaline solution may erode glass. Discard solutions 24 hours after reconstituting.

INCOMPATIBILITIES
None reported.

ACTION
Combines with hydrogen ions and associated acid anions; resulting salts are excreted. Also has osmotic diuretic effect.

Route	Onset	Peak	Duration
I.V.	Immediate	Immediate	Unknown

Half-life: Unknown.

ADVERSE REACTIONS
CNS: fever.
Hepatic: ***hemorrhagic hepatic necrosis in neonates.***
Metabolic: ***hypoglycemia, hyperkalemia with decreased urine output.***
Respiratory: ***respiratory depression.***
Other: venospasm, I.V. thrombosis, inflammation, necrosis, sloughing if extravasation occurs.

INTERACTIONS
None significant.

EFFECTS ON LAB TEST RESULTS
- May increase potassium level. May decrease glucose level.

CONTRAINDICATIONS & CAUTIONS
- Contraindicated in patients with anuria, uremia, or chronic respiratory acidosis; also contraindicated during pregnancy (except in acute, life-threatening situations).
- Use cautiously in patients with renal disease and poor urine output. Monitor ECG and potassium level.

NURSING CONSIDERATIONS
- Determine blood pH, carbon dioxide tension, and bicarbonate, glucose, and electrolyte levels before, during, and after therapy.
- Have mechanical ventilation available for patients with respiratory acidosis.
- To prevent blood pH from rising above normal, adjust dosage carefully. Correct only the existing acidosis.
- Monitor ECG and potassium level in renally impaired patients.
- Don't give for more than 1 day except in life-threatening situations.

PATIENT TEACHING
- Explain use of drug to patient and family.
- Tell patient to report adverse reactions to prescriber.

63
Hematinics

ferrous fumarate
ferrous gluconate
ferrous sulfate
ferrous sulfate, dried
iron dextran
iron sucrose injection
sodium ferric gluconate complex

ferrous fumarate

Femiron ◊, Feostat ◊, Hemocyte ◊, Ircon ◊, Nephro-Fer ◊, Novofumar†, Palafer†, Palafer Pediatric Drops†, Vitron-C

Pharmacologic class: hematinic
Pregnancy risk category A

AVAILABLE FORMS

Each 100 mg of ferrous fumarate provides 33 mg of elemental iron.
Drops: 45 mg/0.6 ml ◊
Oral suspension: 100 mg/5 ml ◊
Tablets: 63 mg ◊, 200 mg ◊, 324 mg ◊, 325 mg ◊, 350 mg ◊
Tablets (chewable): 100 mg ◊

INDICATIONS & DOSAGES

➤Iron deficiency
Adults: 150 to 300 mg P.O. elemental iron daily in three divided doses.
Children: Give 3 to 6 mg/kg P.O. daily in three divided doses.
➤As a supplement during pregnancy
Women: 15 to 30 mg elemental iron P.O. daily during last two trimesters.

ACTION

Provides elemental iron, an essential component in the formation of hemoglobin.

Route	Onset	Peak	Duration
P.O.	4 days	7–10 days	2–4 mo

Half-life: Unknown.

ADVERSE REACTIONS

GI: *nausea,* epigastric pain, vomiting, *constipation,* diarrhea, *black stools,* anorexia.
Other: temporarily stained teeth from suspension and drops.

INTERACTIONS

Drug-drug. *Antacids, cholestyramine resin, cimetidine:* May decrease iron absorption. Separate doses by at least 2 hours.
Chloramphenicol: May delay response to iron therapy. Monitor patient.
Fluoroquinolones, penicillamine, tetracyclines: May decrease GI absorption of these drugs, possibly causing decreased levels or effect. Separate doses by 2 to 4 hours.
Levodopa, methyldopa: May decrease absorption and effectiveness of levodopa and methyldopa. Watch for decreased effect of these drugs.
L-Thyroxine: May decrease L-thyroxine absorption. Separate doses by at least 2 hours. Monitor thyroid function.
Vitamin C: May increase iron absorption. Use together for therapeutic effect.
Drug-herb. *Black cohosh, chamomile, feverfew, gossypol, hawthorn, nettle, plantain, St. John's wort:* May decrease iron absorption. Discourage use together.
Oregano: May decrease iron absorption. Tell patient to separate ingestion of herb from ingestion of food containing iron or iron supplement by at least 2 hours.
Drug-food. *Cereals, cheese, coffee, eggs, milk, tea, whole-grain breads, yogurt:* May decrease iron absorption. Discourage use together.

EFFECTS ON LAB TEST RESULTS

- May yield false-positive guaiac test results. May decrease uptake of technetium-99m and interfere with skeletal imaging.

CONTRAINDICATIONS & CAUTIONS

- Contraindicated in patients with primary hemochromatosis or hemosiderosis, hemolytic anemia (unless patient also has iron deficiency anemia), peptic ulcer disease, regional enteritis, or ulcerative colitis.

• Contraindicated in those receiving repeated blood transfusions.
• Use cautiously on long-term basis.

NURSING CONSIDERATIONS

• GI upset may be related to dose.
• Between-meal doses are preferable, but drug can be given with some foods, although absorption may be decreased.
• Enteric-coated products reduce GI upset but also reduce amount of iron absorbed.
• Check for constipation; record color and amount of stools.
• ***Alert:*** Oral iron may turn stools black. Although this unabsorbed iron is harmless, it could mask presence of melena.
• Monitor hemoglobin level, hematocrit, and reticulocyte count during therapy.
• Combination products such as Ferro-Sequels contain stool softeners, which help prevent constipation—a common adverse reaction.

PATIENT TEACHING

• Tell patient to take tablets with juice (preferably orange juice) or water but not with milk or antacids.
• Tell patient to take suspension with straw and place drops at back of throat to avoid staining teeth.
• Caution patient not to crush tablets or chew extended-release forms.
• Advise patient not to substitute one iron salt for another; the amount of elemental iron may vary.
• ***Alert:*** Inform parents that as few as 5 or 6 tablets of a high-potency form can cause fatal poisoning in children.
• Advise patient to report constipation and change in stool color or consistency.

ferrous gluconate

Fergon ◇, Fertinic†, Novoferrogluc†

Pharmacologic class: hematinic
Pregnancy risk category A

AVAILABLE FORMS

Each 100 mg of ferrous gluconate provides 11.6 mg of elemental iron.
Tablets: 240 mg ◇, 325 mg ◇

INDICATIONS & DOSAGES

➤ Iron deficiency

Adults: 150 to 300 mg P.O. elemental iron daily in three divided doses.
Children: Give 3 to 6 mg/kg P.O. daily in three divided doses.

➤ As a supplement during pregnancy

Adults: 15 to 30 mg elemental iron P.O. daily during last two trimesters.

ACTION

Provides elemental iron, an essential component in the formation of hemoglobin.

Route	Onset	Peak	Duration
P.O.	4 days	7–10 days	2–4 mo

Half-life: Unknown.

ADVERSE REACTIONS

GI: *nausea,* epigastric pain, vomiting, *constipation,* diarrhea, *black stools,* anorexia.

INTERACTIONS

Drug-drug. *Antacids, cholestyramine resin, cimetidine:* May decrease iron absorption. Separate doses by at least 2 hours.
Chloramphenicol: Delays response to iron therapy. Monitor patient.
Fluoroquinolones, penicillamine, tetracyclines: May decrease GI absorption of these drugs, possibly causing decreased level or effect. Separate doses by 2 to 4 hours.
Levodopa, methyldopa: May decrease levodopa and methyldopa absorption and effect. Watch for decreased effect of these drugs.
L-Thyroxine: May decrease L-thyroxine absorption. Separate doses by at least 2 hours. Monitor thyroid function.
Penicillamine: May decrease absorption and effect of penicillamine. Separate doses by 2 hours.
Vitamin C: May increase iron absorption. Use together for therapeutic effect.
Drug-herb. *Black cohosh, chamomile, feverfew, gossypol, hawthorn, nettle, plantain, St. John's wort:* May decrease iron absorption. Discourage use together.
Oregano: May decrease iron absorption. Tell patient to separate ingestion of herb

from ingestion of food containing iron or iron supplement by at least 2 hours.
Drug-food. *Cereals, cheese, coffee, eggs, milk, tea, whole-grain breads, yogurt:* May decrease iron absorption. Discourage using together.

EFFECTS ON LAB TEST RESULTS

- May yield false-positive guaiac test results. May decrease uptake of technetium-99m and interfere with skeletal imaging.

CONTRAINDICATIONS & CAUTIONS

- Contraindicated in patients with peptic ulceration, regional enteritis, ulcerative colitis, hemosiderosis, primary hemochromatosis, or hemolytic anemia (unless patient also has iron deficiency anemia) and in those receiving repeated blood transfusions.
- Use cautiously on long-term basis.

NURSING CONSIDERATIONS

- GI upset may be related to dose.
- Between-meal doses are preferable, but drug can be given with some foods, although absorption may be decreased.
- Enteric-coated products reduce GI upset but also reduce amount of iron absorbed.
- Check for constipation; record color and amount of stools.
- ***Alert:*** Oral iron may turn stools black. Although this unabsorbed iron is harmless, it could mask melena.
- Monitor hemoglobin level, hematocrit, and reticulocyte count during therapy.

PATIENT TEACHING

- Tell patient to take tablets with juice (preferably orange juice) or water, but not with milk or antacids.
- ***Alert:*** Inform parents that as few as 5 or 6 high-potency tablets can cause fatal poisoning in children.
- Caution patient not to substitute one iron salt for another because the amounts of elemental iron vary.
- Advise patient to report constipation and change in stool color or consistency.

ferrous sulfate

Apo-Ferrous Sulfate†, ED-IN-SOL, Feosol* ◊, Fer-gen-sol* ◊, Fer-In-Sol* ◊, Fer-Iron* ◊

ferrous sulfate, dried

Fe50 ◊, Feosol ◊, Feratab ◊, Novoferrosulfate†, PMS-Ferrous Sulfate†, Slow FE ◊

Pharmacologic class: hematinic
Pregnancy risk category A

AVAILABLE FORMS

Each 100 mg of ferrous sulfate provides 20 mg of elemental iron, about 30 mg of elemental iron in ferrous sulfate dried products.
Caplets (extended-release) ◊*:* 160 mg (dried)
Drops ◊*:* 125 mg/ml
Elixir ◊*:* 220 mg/5 ml* ◊
Syrup ◊*:* 90 mg/5 ml
Tablets ◊*:* 187 mg (dried), 200 mg (dried), 324 mg, 325 mg
Tablets (slow-release) ◊*:* 160 mg (dried)

INDICATIONS & DOSAGES

➤ **Iron deficiency**
Adults: 150 to 300 mg P.O. elemental iron daily in three divided doses.
Children: 3 to 6 mg/kg P.O. daily in three divided doses.
➤ **As a supplement during pregnancy**
Adults: 15 to 30 mg elemental iron P.O. daily during last two trimesters.

ACTION

Provides elemental iron, an essential component in the formation of hemoglobin.

Route	Onset	Peak	Duration
P.O.	4 days	7–10 days	2–4 mo

Half-life: Unknown.

ADVERSE REACTIONS

GI: *nausea,* epigastric pain, vomiting, *constipation, black stools,* diarrhea, anorexia.
Other: temporarily stained teeth from liquid forms.

INTERACTIONS

Drug-drug. *Antacids, cholestyramine resin, cimetidine:* May decrease iron absorption. Separate doses if possible.
Chloramphenicol: May delay response to iron therapy. Monitor patient.
Fluoroquinolones, penicillamine, tetracyclines: May decrease GI absorption of these drugs, possibly resulting in decreased levels or effect. Separate doses by 2 to 4 hours.
Levodopa, methyldopa: May decrease absorption and effect of levodopa and methyldopa. Watch for decreased effect of these drugs.
L-Thyroxine: May decrease L-thyroxine absorption. Separate doses by at least 2 hours. Monitor thyroid function.
Penicillamine: May decrease absorption and effect of penicillamine. Separate doses by 2 hours.
Vitamin C: May increase iron absorption. Use together for therapeutic effect.
Drug-herb. *Black cohosh, chamomile, feverfew, gossypol, hawthorn, nettle, plantain, St. John's wort:* May decrease iron absorption. Discourage use together.
Oregano: May decrease iron absorption. Tell patient to separate ingestion of herb from ingestion of food containing iron or iron supplement by at least 2 hours.
Drug-food. *Cereals, cheese, coffee, eggs, milk, tea, whole-grain breads, yogurt:* May decrease iron absorption. Discourage use together.

EFFECTS ON LAB TEST RESULTS

- May yield false-positive guaiac test results. May decrease uptake of technetium-99m and interfere with skeletal imaging.

CONTRAINDICATIONS & CAUTIONS

- Contraindicated in patients with hemosiderosis, primary hemochromatosis, hemolytic anemia (unless patient also has iron deficiency anemia), peptic ulceration, ulcerative colitis, or regional enteritis and in those receiving repeated blood transfusions.
- Use cautiously on long-term basis.

NURSING CONSIDERATIONS

- GI upset may be related to dose.
- Between-meal doses are preferable. Drug can be given with some foods, although absorption may be decreased.
- Enteric-coated products reduce GI upset but also reduce amount of iron absorbed.
- ***Alert:*** Oral iron may turn stools black. Although this unabsorbed iron is harmless, it could mask melena.
- Monitor hemoglobin level, hematocrit, and reticulocyte count during therapy.
- ***Look alike–sound alike:*** Don't confuse different iron salts; elemental content may vary.

PATIENT TEACHING

- Tell patient to take tablets with juice (preferably orange juice) or water, but not with milk or antacids.
- Instruct patient not to crush or chew extended-release forms.
- ***Alert:*** Inform parents that as few as 5 to 6 high-potency tablets can cause fatal poisoning in a child.
- Caution patient not to substitute one iron salt for another because amounts of elemental iron vary.
- Advise patient to report constipation and change in stool color or consistency.

iron dextran

DexFerrum, InFeD

Pharmacologic class: hematinic
Pregnancy risk category C

AVAILABLE FORMS

1 ml iron dextran provides 50 mg elemental iron.
Injection: 50 mg elemental iron/ml in 2-ml single-dose vials

INDICATIONS & DOSAGES

➤ Iron deficiency anemia

Adults and children: I.V. or I.M. test dose is required. Total dose is calculated using the following formula:

$$\text{Dose (ml)} = 0.0442\ (\text{desired Hb} - \text{observed Hb}) \times \text{Weight in kg} + (0.26 \times \text{Weight in kg})$$

I.V.

Inject 0.5-ml test dose over 30 seconds. If no reaction occurs in 1 hour, give remainder of therapeutic I.V. dose. Repeat therapeutic I.V. dose daily. Single daily dose shouldn't exceed 100 mg. Give slowly (1 ml/minute).

I.M. (by Z-track method)

Inject 0.5-ml test dose. If no reaction occurs in 1 hour, give remainder of dose. Daily dose should ordinarily not exceed 0.5 ml (25 mg) for infants who weigh less than 5 kg (11 lb); 1 ml (50 mg) for those who weigh less than 10 kg (22 lb); and 2 ml (100 mg) for heavier children and adults. Don't give drug in the first 4 months of life.

I.V. ADMINISTRATION

- Check hospital policy before giving I.V.
- After completing I.V. dose, flush the vein with 10 ml of normal saline solution.
- Patient should rest for 15 to 30 minutes after I.V. administration.

INCOMPATIBILITIES

Other I.V. drugs, parenteral nutrition solutions for I.V. infusion.

ACTION

Provides elemental iron, an essential component in the formation of hemoglobin.

Route	Onset	Peak	Duration
I.V.	Unknown	Unknown	Unknown
I.M.	72 hr	Unknown	3–4 wk

Half-life: 6 hours.

ADVERSE REACTIONS

CNS: headache, transitory paresthesia, dizziness, malaise, fever, chills.
CV: chest pain, tachycardia, ***bradycardia,*** *hypotensive reaction, peripheral vascular flushing.*
GI: nausea, anorexia.
Musculoskeletal: arthralgia, myalgia.
Respiratory: ***bronchospasm,*** dyspnea.
Skin: rash, urticaria, *soreness, inflammation, brown skin discoloration at I.M. injection site, local phlebitis at I.V. injection site,* sterile abscess, necrosis, atrophy.
Other: fibrosis, ***anaphylaxis, delayed sensitivity reactions.***

INTERACTIONS

Drug-drug. *Chloramphenicol:* May increase iron level. Monitor patient closely.

EFFECTS ON LAB TEST RESULTS

- May cause false increase in bilirubin level and false decrease in calcium level. Use of more than 250 mg iron may color the serum brown. Drug may alter measurement of iron level and total iron-binding capacity for up to 3 weeks; I.M. injection may cause dense areas of activity for 1 to 6 days on bone scans using technetium-99m diphosphonate.

CONTRAINDICATIONS & CAUTIONS

- Contraindicated in patients hypersensitive to drug, in those with acute infectious renal disease, and in those with any anemia except iron deficiency anemia.
- Use cautiously in patients who have serious hepatic impairment, rheumatoid arthritis, or other inflammatory diseases because these patients may be at higher risk for certain delays and reactions.
- Use cautiously in patients with history of significant allergies or asthma.

NURSING CONSIDERATIONS

- Have epinephrine immediately available in event of acute hypersensitivity reaction.
- Don't give iron dextran with oral iron preparations.
- I.V. or I.M. injections of iron are advisable only for patients in whom oral administration is impossible or ineffective.
- Inject I.M. deep into upper outer quadrant of buttock—never into the arm or other exposed area—with a 2- to 3-inch 19G or 20G needle. Use Z-track method to avoid leakage into subcutaneous tissue and staining of skin. After drawing up drug, use a new sterile needle to give injection.
- Monitor hemoglobin level, hematocrit, and reticulocyte count.

PATIENT TEACHING

- Teach patient signs and symptoms of hypersensitivity and iron toxicity, and tell him to report them to prescriber.
- Inform patient that drug may stain skin.

iron sucrose injection
Venofer

Pharmacologic class: hematinic
Pregnancy risk category B

AVAILABLE FORMS
Injection: 20 mg/ml of elemental iron in 5-ml single-dose vials

INDICATIONS & DOSAGES
➤ **Iron deficiency anemia in patients who are hemodialysis dependent**
Adults: 100 mg (5 ml) of elemental iron I.V. directly in the dialysis line, either by slow injection over 2 to 5 minutes or by infusion over 15 minutes during the dialysis session one to three times a week to a total of 1,000 mg in 10 doses; repeat as needed.
➤ **Iron deficiency anemia in chronic kidney disease patients not on dialysis**
Adults: 200 mg by undiluted slow I.V. injection over 2 to 5 minutes on 5 separate occasions in a 14-day period to a total cumulative dose of 1,000 mg.
➤ **Iron deficiency anemia in peritoneal dialysis-dependent chronic kidney disease patients**
Adults: 300 mg I.V. infusion over 90 minutes on 2 separate occasions 14 days apart, followed by one 400-mg infusion over 2½ hours 14 days later.

I.V. ADMINISTRATION
- Inspect drug for particulate matter and discoloration before giving.
- For slow injection, give drug at rate of 1 ml (20 mg elemental iron) undiluted solution per minute, not exceeding 1 vial (100 mg elemental iron) per injection.
- For infusion, dilute 100 mg elemental iron in a maximum of 100 ml normal saline solution immediately before infusion and infuse over at least 15 minutes. Dilute dose 300 mg or greater in a maximum of 250 ml normal saline solution.

INCOMPATIBILITIES
Other I.V. drugs, parenteral nutrition solutions.

ACTION
Exogenous source of iron that replenishes depleted body iron stores and is essential for hemoglobin synthesis.

Route	Onset	Peak	Duration
I.V.	Unknown	Unknown	Variable

Half-life: 6 hours.

ADVERSE REACTIONS
CNS: headache, asthenia, malaise, dizziness, fever.
CV: ***heart failure,*** *hypotension,* chest pain, hypertension, fluid retention.
GI: nausea, vomiting, diarrhea, abdominal pain, taste perversion.
Musculoskeletal: *leg cramps,* bone and muscle pain.
Respiratory: dyspnea, wheezing, pneumonia, cough.
Skin: rash, pruritus, application site reaction.
Other: accidental injury, pain, ***sepsis, hypersensitivity reactions.***

INTERACTIONS
Drug-drug. *Oral iron preparations:* May reduce absorption of oral iron preparations. Avoid using together.

EFFECTS ON LAB TEST RESULTS
- May increase liver enzyme levels.

CONTRAINDICATIONS & CAUTIONS
- Contraindicated in patients with hypersensitivity to drug or its components, evidence of iron overload, or anemia not caused by iron deficiency.
- Use cautiously in breast-feeding women.

NURSING CONSIDERATIONS
- ***Alert:*** Rare but fatal hypersensitivity reactions, characterized by anaphylactic shock, loss of consciousness, collapse, hypotension, dyspnea, or seizures, may occur. Have epinephrine readily available.
- Mild to moderate hypersensitivity reactions, with wheezing, dyspnea, hypotension, rash, or pruritus, may occur.
- Giving drug by infusion may reduce the risk of hypotension.
- Transferrin saturation level increases rapidly after I.V. administration of drug. Obtain iron level 48 hours after I.V. use.

• Monitor ferritin, transferrin saturation, and hemoglobin levels, and hematocrit.
• Withhold dose in patient with signs and symptoms of iron overload.
• Keep dose selection in elderly patients conservative because of decreased hepatic, renal, or cardiac function; other disease; and other drug therapy.

PATIENT TEACHING
• Instruct patient to notify prescriber if symptoms of overdose (headache, nausea, dizziness, joint aches, tingling, or abdominal and muscle pain) or of allergic reaction (labored breathing, collapse, or loss of consciousness) occur.

sodium ferric gluconate complex
Ferrlecit

Pharmacologic class: macromolecular iron complex; hematinic
Pregnancy risk category B

AVAILABLE FORMS
Injection: 62.5 mg elemental iron (12.5 mg/ml) in 5-ml ampules

INDICATIONS & DOSAGES
➤ **Iron deficiency anemia in patients receiving long-term hemodialysis and supplemental erythropoietin**
Adults: 10 ml (125 mg elemental iron) I.V. over 1 hour. Most patients need minimum cumulative dose of 1 g elemental iron given over more than eight sequential dialysis treatments to achieve a favorable hemoglobin or hematocrit response.
Children age 6 and older: 1.5 mg/kg (maximum 125 mg) I.V. over 1 hour during 8 consecutive hemodialysis treatments.

I.V. ADMINISTRATION
• Contains benzyl alcohol. Don't use in neonates.
• For adults, dilute in 100 ml normal saline solution; for children, dilute in 25 ml normal saline solution. Give immediately over 1 hour.
• May also give undiluted at a rate not to exceed 1 ml/minute (12.5 mg/minute) at the end of dialysis.
• Life-threatening hypersensitivity reactions, such as CV collapse, cardiac arrest, bronchospasm, oral or pharyngeal edema, dyspnea, angioedema, urticaria, and pruritus, that are sometimes linked to pain and muscle spasm of chest or back, may occur during infusion. Have adequate supportive measures readily available. Monitor patient closely during infusion.
• After rapid administration, profound hypotension with flushing, lightheadedness, malaise, fatigue, weakness, or severe chest, back, flank, or groin pain may occur; these symptoms aren't hypersensitivity reactions. Don't exceed 2.1 mg/minute. Monitor patient closely during infusion.

INCOMPATIBILITIES
Other I.V. drugs. Don't add drug to parenteral nutrition solutions for infusion.

ACTION
Restores total body iron content, which is critical for normal hemoglobin synthesis and oxygen transport.

Route	Onset	Peak	Duration
I.V.	Unknown	Unknown	Unknown

Half-life: 1 hour in healthy, iron-deficient people.

ADVERSE REACTIONS
CNS: asthenia, headache, fatigue, malaise, *dizziness,* paresthesia, agitation, insomnia, somnolence, syncope, pain, chills, fever.
CV: *hypotension, hypertension,* tachycardia, ***bradycardia,*** angina, chest pain, ***MI,*** edema, flushing.
EENT: conjunctivitis, abnormal vision, rhinitis.
GI: *nausea, vomiting, diarrhea,* rectal disorder, dyspepsia, eructation, flatulence, melena, abdominal pain.
GU: urinary tract infection.
Hematologic: anemia.
Metabolic: ***hyperkalemia, hypoglycemia,*** hypokalemia, hypervolemia.
Musculoskeletal: myalgia, arthralgia, back pain, arm pain, *cramps.*

Respiratory: *dyspnea,* coughing, upper respiratory tract infection, pneumonia, pulmonary edema.
Skin: pruritus, increased sweating, rash, *injection site reaction.*
Other: infection, rigors, flu syndrome, ***sepsis, carcinoma,*** hypersensitivity reactions, lymphadenopathy.

INTERACTIONS

Drug-Drug. *ACE inhibitors:* May cause sensitivity reactions. Stop I.V. iron if sensitivity reactions occur.

EFFECTS ON LAB TEST RESULTS

- May decrease glucose and hemoglobin levels. May increase or decrease potassium level.

CONTRAINDICATIONS & CAUTIONS

- Contraindicated in patients hypersensitive to drug or its components (such as benzyl alcohol) and in those with iron overload or anemias not related to iron deficiency.
- Don't use in patients with ferritin levels greater than 1,000 nanograms/ml.
- Use cautiously in elderly patients.

NURSING CONSIDERATIONS

- ***Alert:*** Dosage is expressed in milligrams of elemental iron.
- Don't give to patients with iron overload, which often occurs in hemoglobinopathies and other refractory anemias.
- Monitor ferritin, iron saturation, and hemoglobin levels and hematocrit.
- In hemodialysis patients, adverse reactions may be related to dialysis itself or to chronic renal failure.
- Check with patient about other potential sources of iron, such as OTC iron preparations and iron-containing multiple vitamins with minerals.

PATIENT TEACHING

- Abdominal pain, diarrhea, vomiting, drowsiness, and rapid breathing may indicate iron poisoning. Urge patient to notify prescriber immediately.

64 Anticoagulants

argatroban
bivalirudin
dalteparin sodium
desirudin
enoxaparin sodium
fondaparinux sodium
heparin sodium
tinzaparin sodium
warfarin sodium

argatroban

Pharmacologic class: direct thrombin inhibitor
Pregnancy risk category B

AVAILABLE FORMS
Injection: 100 mg/ml

INDICATIONS & DOSAGES
➤ **To prevent or treat thrombosis in patients with heparin-induced thrombocytopenia**
Adults: 2 mcg/kg/minute, given as a continuous I.V. infusion; adjust dose until the steady-state activated PTT is 1½ to 3 times the initial baseline value, not to exceed 100 seconds; maximum dose 10 mcg/kg/minute.
Adjust-a-dose: For patients with moderate hepatic impairment, reduce first dose to 0.5 mcg/kg/minute, given as a continuous infusion. Monitor PTT closely and adjust dosage as needed.
➤ **Anticoagulation in patients with or at risk for heparin-induced thrombocytopenia during percutaneous coronary intervention (PCI)**
Adults: 350 mcg/kg I.V. bolus over 3 to 5 minutes. Start a continuous I.V. infusion at 25 mcg/kg/minute. Check activated clotting time (ACT) 5 to 10 minutes after the bolus dose is completed.
Adjust-a-dose: Use the following table to adjust the dosage.

Activated clotting time	Additional I.V. bolus	Continuous I.V. infusion
< 300 sec	150 mcg/kg	30 mcg/kg/min*
300–450 sec	None needed	25 mcg/kg/min
> 450 sec	None needed	15 mcg/kg/min*

*Check ACT again after 5 to 10 minutes.

In case of dissection, impending abrupt closure, thrombus formation during the procedure, or inability to achieve or maintain an ACT exceeding 300 seconds, give an additional bolus of 150 mcg/kg and increase infusion rate to 40 mcg/kg/minute. Check ACT again after 5 to 10 minutes.

I.V. ADMINISTRATION
- Dilute in normal saline solution, D_5W, or lactated Ringer injection to a final concentration of 1 mg/ml.
- Dilute each 2.5-ml vial 100-fold by mixing it with 250 ml of diluent.
- Mix the solution by repeated inversion of the diluent bag for 10 minutes.
- Don't expose solution to direct sunlight.
- Prepared solutions are stable for up to 24 hours at 77° F (25° C).

INCOMPATIBILITIES
Other I.V. drugs.

ACTION
Reversibly binds to the thrombin-active site and inhibits thrombin-catalyzed or -induced reactions: fibrin formation, coagulation factor V, VIII, and XIII activation, protein C activation, and platelet aggregation. May inhibit the action of free and clot-associated thrombin.

Route	Onset	Peak	Duration
I.V.	Rapid	1–3 hr	Duration of infusion

Half-life: 39 to 51 minutes.

ADVERSE REACTIONS
CNS: ***cerebrovascular disorder, hemorrhage,*** fever, pain.

CV: ***atrial fibrillation, cardiac arrest,*** hypotension, ***ventricular tachycardia.***
GI: abdominal pain, diarrhea, ***GI bleeding,*** nausea, vomiting.
GU: abnormal renal function, groin bleeding, *hematuria,* UTI.
Respiratory: cough, dyspnea, pneumonia, hemoptysis.
Other: allergic reactions, brachial bleeding, infection, ***sepsis.***

INTERACTIONS

Drug-drug. *Antiplatelet drugs, heparin, thrombolytics:* May increase risk of intracranial bleeding. Avoid using together.
Oral anticoagulants: May prolong PT and INR and may increase risk of bleeding. Monitor patient closely.

EFFECTS ON LAB TEST RESULTS

- May decrease hemoglobin level and hematocrit.

CONTRAINDICATIONS & CAUTIONS

- Contraindicated in patients who have overt major bleeding who are hypersensitive to drug or any of its components.
- Use cautiously in patients with hepatic disease or conditions that increase the risk of hemorrhage, such as severe hypertension.
- Use cautiously in patients who have just had lumbar puncture, spinal anesthesia, or major surgery, especially of the brain, spinal cord, or eye; patients with hematologic conditions causing increased bleeding tendencies, such as congenital or acquired bleeding disorders; and patients with GI ulcers or other lesions.

NURSING CONSIDERATIONS

- Stop all parenteral anticoagulants before giving drug. Giving with antiplatelets, thrombolytics, and other anticoagulants may increase risk of bleeding.
- Get results of baseline coagulation tests, platelet count, hemoglobin level, and hematocrit before starting therapy, and report any abnormalities to the prescriber.
- Check activated PTT 2 hours after giving drug; dose adjustments may be required to get a targeted activated PTT of 1.5 to 3 times the baseline, no longer than 100 seconds. Steady state is achieved 1 to 3 hours after starting drug.
- Draw blood for additional ACT about every 20 to 30 minutes during prolonged PCI.
- Patients can hemorrhage from any site in the body. Any unexplained decrease in hematocrit or blood pressure or any other unexplained symptoms may signify a hemorrhagic event.
- To convert to oral anticoagulant therapy, give warfarin P.O. with argatroban at up to 2 mcg/kg/minute until the INR exceeds 4 on combined therapy. After argatroban is stopped, repeat the INR in 4 to 6 hours. If the repeat INR is less than the desired therapeutic range, resume the I.V. argatroban infusion. Repeat the procedure daily until the desired therapeutic range on warfarin alone is reached.
- Use cautiously in breast-feeding women; it's unknown if drug appears in breast milk.
- ***Look alike–sound alike:*** Don't confuse argatroban with Aggrastat.

PATIENT TEACHING

- Tell patient that this drug can cause bleeding, and ask him to report any unusual bruising or bleeding (nosebleeds, bleeding gums) or tarry stools to the prescriber immediately.
- Advise patient to avoid activities that carry a risk of injury, and to use a soft toothbrush and an electric razor during therapy.
- Instruct patient to notify prescriber if he has wheezing, trouble breathing, or skin rash.
- Instruct woman who is pregnant, has recently delivered, or is breast-feeding to notify her prescriber.
- Tell patient to notify prescriber if he has GI ulcers or liver disease, or has had recent surgery, radiation treatment, falling episodes, or injury.

bivalirudin
Angiomax

Pharmacologic class: direct thrombin inhibitor
Pregnancy risk category B

AVAILABLE FORMS

Injection: 250-mg vial

INDICATIONS & DOSAGES

➤ **Anticoagulation in patients with unstable angina undergoing percutaneous transluminal coronary angioplasty (PTCA); anticoagulation in patients with unstable angina undergoing percutaneous coronary intervention (PCI), with provisional use of a platelet glycoprotein IIb/IIIa inhibitor (GPI)**

Adults: Give 0.75 mg/kg I.V. bolus followed by a continuous infusion of 1.75 mg/kg/hour during the procedure. Check activated clotting time 5 minutes after bolus dose is given. May give additional 0.3 mg/kg bolus dose if needed. Infusion may continue for up to 4 hours after procedure. After 4-hour infusion, may give an additional infusion of 0.2 mg/kg/hour for up to 20 hours, if needed. Use with 300 to 325 mg aspirin.

➤ **Patients undergoing PCI who have or are at risk for heparin-induced thrombocytopenia (HIT) or heparin-induced thrombocytopenia and thrombosis syndrome (HITTS)**

Adults: 0.75 mg/kg I.V. bolus, followed by a continuous infusion of 1.75 mg/kg/hour throughout the procedure. Consult prescriber about continuing the infusion after PCI.

Adjust-a-dose: For patients with creatinine clearance of 30 ml/minute or less, decrease infusion rate to 1 mg/kg/hour. For patients on hemodialysis, reduce infusion rate to 0.25 mg/kg/hour. No reduction of bolus dose is needed.

I.V. ADMINISTRATION

- Reconstitute each 250-mg vial with 5 ml of sterile water for injection.
- Dilute each reconstituted vial in 50 ml D_5W or normal saline solution to yield a final concentration of 5 mg/ml.
- To prepare low-rate infusion, further dilute each reconstituted vial in 500 ml D_5W or normal saline solution to yield a final concentration of 0.5 mg/ml.
- Solutions with concentrations of 0.5 to 5 mg/ml are stable at room temperature for 24 hours.

INCOMPATIBILITIES

Alteplase, amiodarone, amphotericin B, chlorpromazine, diazepam, prochlorperazine, reteplase, streptokinase, vancomycin.

ACTION

Drug binds specifically and rapidly to thrombin to produce an anticoagulant effect.

Route	Onset	Peak	Duration
I.V.	Rapid	Immediate	1–2 hr

Half-life: 25 minutes in patients with normal renal function.

ADVERSE REACTIONS

CNS: anxiety, *headache,* insomnia, nervousness, fever, *pain.*
CV: ***bradycardia,*** hypertension, *hypotension.*
GI: abdominal pain, dyspepsia, *nausea,* vomiting.
GU: urine retention.
Hematologic: ***severe, spontaneous bleeding (cerebral, retroperitoneal, GU, GI).***
Musculoskeletal: *back pain,* pelvic pain.
Skin: pain at injection site.

INTERACTIONS

Drug-drug. *Heparin, warfarin, other oral anticoagulants:* May increase risk of hemorrhage. Use together cautiously.

EFFECTS ON LAB TEST RESULTS

None reported.

CONTRAINDICATIONS & CAUTIONS

- Contraindicated in patients hypersensitive to drug or its components and in those with active major bleeding. Avoid using in patients with unstable angina who aren't undergoing PTCA or PCI or in patients with other acute coronary syndromes.
- Use cautiously in patients with HIT or HITTS, and in patients with diseases linked to increased risk of bleeding.
- Use cautiously in breast-feeding women; it's unknown if drug appears in breast milk.

NURSING CONSIDERATIONS

- Circumstances for provisional use of a GPI during PCI include decreased thrombolysis-in-MI, or TIMI, flow; slow reflow; dissection with decreased flow; new or suspected thrombus; persistent residual stenosis; distal embolization; unplanned stent; suboptimal stenting; side-branch closure; abrupt closure; instability; and prolonged ischemia.

- Monitor coagulation test results, hemoglobin level, and hematocrit before starting therapy and periodically thereafter.
- Hemorrhage can occur at any site in the body. If patient has unexplained decrease in hematocrit, decrease in blood pressure, or other unexplained symptoms, suspect hemorrhage.
- Monitor venipuncture sites for bleeding, hematoma, or inflammation.
- Puncture-site hemorrhage and catheterization-site hematoma may occur in patients age 65 and older more often than in younger patients.
- Don't give I.M.

PATIENT TEACHING

- Advise patient that drug can cause bleeding and tell him to report unusual bruising or bleeding (nosebleeds, bleeding gums) or tarry stools immediately.
- Counsel patient that drug is given with aspirin and caution him to avoid other aspirin-containing drugs or NSAIDs while receiving this drug.
- Advise patient to avoid activities that carry a risk of injury and instruct him to use a soft toothbrush and electric razor while on drug.

SAFETY ALERT!

dalteparin sodium
Fragmin

Pharmacologic class:
low–molecular-weight heparin
Pregnancy risk category B

AVAILABLE FORMS

Injection: 2,500 antifactor Xa international units/0.2 ml syringe, 5,000 antifactor Xa international units/0.2 ml syringe, 7,500 antifactor Xa international units/0.3 ml syringe, 10,000 antifactor Xa international units/ml syringe, 10,000 antifactor Xa international units/ml in 9.5-ml vial, 25,000 antifactor Xa international units/ml in 3.8-ml vial.

INDICATIONS & DOSAGES

➤ **To prevent deep vein thrombosis (DVT) in patients undergoing abdominal surgery who are at moderate to high risk for thromboembolic complications**

Adults: 2,500 international units subcutaneously daily, starting 1 to 2 hours before surgery and repeated once daily for 5 to 10 days postoperatively. Or, for patients at high risk, give 5,000 international units subcutaneously 8 to 12 hours before surgery, then once daily postoperatively for 5 to 10 days.

➤ **To prevent DVT in patients undergoing hip replacement surgery**

Adults: 2,500 international units subcutaneously within 2 hours before surgery and second dose 2,500 international units subcutaneously in the evening after surgery (at least 6 hours after first dose). If surgery is performed in the evening, omit second dose on day of surgery. Starting on first postoperative day, give 5,000 international units subcutaneously once daily for 5 to 10 days. Or, give 5,000 international units subcutaneously on the evening before surgery; then 5,000 international units subcutaneously once daily starting in the evening of surgery for 5 to 10 days postoperatively.

➤ **Unstable angina non–ST-elevation MI**

Adults: 120 international units/kg subcutaneously every 12 hours with aspirin P.O., unless contraindicated. Maximum dose, 10,000 international units. Treatment usually lasts 5 to 8 days.

➤ **To prevent DVT in patients at risk for thromboembolic complications because of severely restricted mobility during acute illness**

Adults: 5,000 international units subcutaneously once daily for 12 to 14 days.

ACTION

A low–molecular-weight heparin derivative that enhances inhibition of factor Xa and thrombin by antithrombin.

Route	Onset	Peak	Duration
SubQ	Unknown	4 hr	Unknown

Half-life: 3 to 5 hours.

ADVERSE REACTIONS

CNS: fever.
Hematologic: ***thrombocytopenia, hemorrhage,*** ecchymoses, bleeding complications.
Skin: pruritus, rash, *hematoma at injection site,* injection site pain.
Other: ***anaphylaxis.***

INTERACTIONS

Drug-drug. *Antiplatelet drugs, oral anticoagulants, thrombolytics:* May increase risk of bleeding. Use together cautiously.

EFFECTS ON LAB TEST RESULTS

- May increase ALT and AST levels.
- May decrease platelet count.

CONTRAINDICATIONS & CAUTIONS

- Contraindicated in patients hypersensitive to drug, heparin, or pork products; in those with active major bleeding; and in those with thrombocytopenia and antiplatelet antibodies in presence of drug.
- Use with caution in patients with history of heparin-induced thrombocytopenia and in patients at increased risk for hemorrhage, such as those with severe uncontrolled hypertension, bacterial endocarditis, congenital or acquired bleeding disorders, active ulceration, angiodysplastic GI disease, or hemorrhagic stroke; also use with caution shortly after brain, spinal, or ophthalmic surgery. Monitor vital signs.
- Use with caution in patients with bleeding diathesis, thrombocytopenia, platelet defects, severe hepatic or renal insufficiency, hypertensive or diabetic retinopathy, or recent GI bleeding.

NURSING CONSIDERATIONS

- ***Alert:*** Patients who have received epidural or spinal anesthesia are at increased risk for developing an epidural or spinal hematoma, which may result in long-term or permanent paralysis. Monitor these patients closely for neurologic impairment.
- DVT is a risk factor in patients who are candidates for therapy, including those older than age 40, those who are obese, those undergoing surgery under general anesthesia lasting longer than 30 minutes, and those who have additional risk factors (such as malignancy or history of DVT or pulmonary embolism).
- Have patient sit or lie supine when giving drug. Give subcutaneous injection deeply. Injection sites include a U-shaped area around the navel, upper outer side of thigh, and upper outer quadrangle of buttock. Rotate sites daily. When area around the navel or thigh is used, use thumb and forefinger to lift up a fold of skin while giving injection. Insert the entire length of needle at a 45- to 90-degree angle.
- Never give drug I.M.
- Don't mix with other injections or infusions unless specific compatibility data support such mixing.
- Multidose vial shouldn't be used in pregnant women.
- ***Alert:*** Drug isn't interchangeable (unit for unit) with unfractionated heparin or other low–molecular-weight heparin.
- Periodic, routine CBC and fecal occult blood tests are recommended during therapy. Patients don't need regular monitoring of PT or activated PTT.
- Monitor patient closely for thrombocytopenia.
- Stop drug if a thromboembolic event occurs despite dalteparin prophylaxis. May use alternative therapy, or may have been inadequate dose.

PATIENT TEACHING

- Instruct patient and family to watch for and report signs of bleeding (bruising and blood in stools).
- Tell patient to avoid OTC drugs containing aspirin or other salicylates unless ordered by prescriber.
- Tell patient to use a soft toothbrush and electric razor during treatment.

desirudin

Iprivask

Pharmacologic class: thrombin inhibitor
Pregnancy risk category C

AVAILABLE FORMS

Injection: 15.75 mg desirudin lyophilized powder and 0.6 ml mannitol (3%) diluent

INDICATIONS & DOSAGES

➤ To prevent deep vein thrombosis in patients undergoing hip replacement surgery

Adults: 15 mg subcutaneously every 12 hours for 9 to 12 days. Give first injection 5 to 15 minutes before surgery, after induction of regional block anesthesia, if used.

Adjust-a-dose: If creatinine clearance is 31 to 60 ml/minute, give 5 mg subcutaneously q 12 hours. If creatinine clearance is less than 31 ml/minute, give 1.7 mg subcutaneously q 12 hours. Check activated PTT and creatinine daily. If activated PTT exceeds two times control, stop therapy until it's within two times control; then resume at a reduced dose.

ACTION

Selectively inhibits free and clot-bound thrombin, which prolongs plasma clotting time.

Route	Onset	Peak	Duration
SubQ	30 min	60–90 min	Unknown

Half-life: 2 to 3 hours.

ADVERSE REACTIONS

CNS: cerebrovascular disorder, dizziness, fever.
CV: ***thrombosis,*** deep thrombophlebitis, hypotension.
EENT: epistaxis.
GI: ***hematemesis,*** nausea, vomiting.
GU: hematuria.
Hematologic: ***hemorrhage,*** anemia.
Other: ***anaphylaxis,*** impaired healing, injection site mass, leg edema, leg pain, wound seeping.

INTERACTIONS

Drug-drug. *Abciximab, acetylsalicylic acid, clopidogrel, dipyridamole, glycoprotein IIb/IIIa antagonists, ketorolac, salicylates, sulfinpyrazone, ticlopidine:* May increase the risk of bleeding. Use together cautiously.

Anticoagulants, dextran 40, glucocorticoids, thrombolytics: May increase the risk of bleeding. Avoid using together.

Epidural or spinal anesthesia: May increase risk of neuraxial hematoma and paralysis. Catheter may be placed before desirudin is started and removed when anticoagulant effect is low.

Drug-herb. *Alfalfa, anise:* May increase the risk of bleeding because of coumarin components. Discourage use together.

Black currant, cat's claw, evening primrose oil: May inhibit platelet function and prolong bleeding time. Discourage use together.

EFFECTS ON LAB TEST RESULTS

- May decrease hemoglobin level and hematocrit.

CONTRAINDICATIONS & CAUTIONS

- Contraindicated in patients hypersensitive to natural or recombinant hirudins and in patients with active bleeding or irreversible coagulation disorders.
- Use cautiously in patients with a creatinine clearance less than 60 ml/minute; patients undergoing spinal or epidural anesthesia; patients with hepatic insufficiency or injury; patients with GI or pulmonary bleeding within 3 months; patients with severe uncontrolled hypertension, bacterial endocarditis, or a hemostatic disorder; and patients with an increased risk of bleeding, such as those with recent major surgery, organ biopsy, puncture of a noncompressible vessel (within 1 month), intracranial or intraocular bleeding, or hemorrhagic or ischemic stroke.

NURSING CONSIDERATIONS

- Reconstitute each 15-mg vial with 0.5 ml of provided diluent (mannitol 3%).
- Shake vial gently until powder is dissolved. Once reconstituted, each 0.5 ml contains 15.75 mg of desirudin.
- Inspect vial. If solution contains visible particles, don't use it.
- Use reconstituted solutions immediately or store them at room temperature for up to 24 hours protected from light.
- Use a syringe with a ½-inch 26G or 27G needle to withdraw all the reconstituted solution.
- With the patient lying down, inject entire contents of syringe by deep subcutaneous injection. Insert entire length of needle into a skinfold held between thumb and forefinger.

• Rotate sites between the right and left thigh or right and left anterolateral and posterolateral abdominal walls.
• Don't give this drug I.M.
• Don't mix other drugs with desirudin before or during administration.
• ***Alert:*** If the patient has either an unexplained decline in hematocrit or blood pressure or other unexplained symptoms, consider the possibility of hemorrhage.
• Monitor coagulation tests, hemoglobin level, hematocrit, and renal function throughout therapy.
• Watch venipuncture sites for bleeding, hematoma, or inflammation.
• ***Alert:*** Patients who receive epidural or spinal anesthesia are at increased risk of an epidural or spinal hematoma, which may result in long-term or permanent paralysis. Monitor these patients closely for neurologic impairment.

PATIENT TEACHING

• Advise patient that this drug can cause bleeding. Stress the need to report unusual bruising or bleeding (nosebleeds, blood in urine, tarry stools) immediately.
• Caution patient not to take any other drugs that increase the risk of bleeding, such as aspirin or NSAIDs, while receiving desirudin.
• Advise against activities that risk injury.
• Tell patient to use a soft toothbrush and electric razor during therapy.

SAFETY ALERT!

enoxaparin sodium

Lovenox

Pharmacologic class:
low—molecular-weight heparin
Pregnancy risk category B

AVAILABLE FORMS

Ampules: 30 mg/0.3 ml
Syringes (prefilled): 30 mg/0.3 ml, 40 mg/0.4 ml
Syringes (graduated prefilled): 60 mg/0.6 ml, 80 mg/0.8 ml, 100 mg/ml, 120 mg/ 0.8 ml, 150 mg/ml
Vial (multidose): 300 mg/3 ml (contains 15 mg/ml of benzyl alcohol)

INDICATIONS & DOSAGES

➤ To prevent pulmonary embolism and deep vein thrombosis (DVT) after hip or knee replacement surgery
Adults: 30 mg subcutaneously every 12 hours for 7 to 10 days. Give initial dose between 12 and 24 hours postoperatively, as long as hemostasis has been established. Continue treatment during postoperative period until risk of DVT has diminished. Hip replacement patients may receive 40 mg subcutaneously given 12 hours preoperatively. After initial phase of therapy, hip replacement patients should continue with 40 mg subcutaneously daily for 3 weeks.

➤ To prevent pulmonary embolism and DVT after abdominal surgery
Adults: 40 mg subcutaneously daily with initial dose 2 hours before surgery. Give subsequent dose, as long as hemostasis has been established, 24 hours after initial preoperative dose and continue once daily for 7 to 10 days. Continue treatment during postoperative period until risk of DVT has diminished.

➤ To prevent pulmonary embolism and DVT in patients with acute illness who are at increased risk because of decreased mobility
Adults: 40 mg once daily subcutaneously for 6 to 11 days. Treatment for up to 14 days has been well tolerated.
Adjust-a-dose: In patients with creatinine clearance less than 30 ml/minute receiving drug as prophylaxis after abdominal surgery or hip or knee replacement surgery, and in medical patients for prophylaxis during acute illness, give 30 mg subcutaneously once daily.

➤ To prevent ischemic complications of unstable angina and non–ST-elevation MI with oral aspirin therapy
Adults: 1 mg/kg subcutaneously every 12 hours until clinical stabilization (minimum 2 days) with aspirin 100 to 325 mg P.O. once daily.

➤ Inpatient treatment of acute DVT with and without pulmonary embolism when given with warfarin sodium
Adults: 1 mg/kg subcutaneously q 12 hours. Or, 1.5 mg/kg subcutaneously

once daily (at same time daily) for 5 to 7 days until therapeutic oral anticoagulant effect (INR 2 to 3) is achieved. Warfarin sodium therapy is usually started within 72 hours of enoxaparin injection.

➤Outpatient treatment of acute DVT without pulmonary embolism when given with warfarin sodium

Adults: 1 mg/kg subcutaneously q 12 hours for 5 to 7 days until therapeutic oral anticoagulant effect (INR 2 to 3) is achieved. Warfarin sodium therapy is usually started within 72 hours of enoxaparin injection.

Adjust-a-dose: In patients with creatinine clearance less than 30 ml/minute receiving drug for acute DVT or prophylaxis of ischemic complications of unstable angina and non–ST-elevation MI, give 1 mg/kg subcutaneously once daily.

ACTION

A low–molecular-weight heparin derivative that accelerates formation of antithrombin III–thrombin complex and deactivates thrombin, preventing conversion of fibrinogen to fibrin. Has a higher antifactor-Xa-to-antifactor-IIa activity ratio than heparin.

Route	Onset	Peak	Duration
SubQ	Unknown	4 hr	Unknown

Half-life: 4½ hours.

ADVERSE REACTIONS

CNS: fever, pain.
CV: edema, peripheral edema.
GI: nausea.
Hematologic: ***thrombocytopenia, hemorrhage,*** ecchymoses, bleeding complications, hypochromic anemia.
Skin: irritation, pain, hematoma, and erythema at injection site, *rash, urticaria.*
Other: ***angioedema, anaphylaxis.***

INTERACTIONS

Drug-drug. *Anticoagulants, antiplatelet drugs, NSAIDs:* May increase risk of bleeding. Use together cautiously. Monitor PT and INR.

EFFECTS ON LAB TEST RESULTS

- May increase ALT and AST levels. May decrease hemoglobin level.

CONTRAINDICATIONS & CAUTIONS

- Contraindicated in patients hypersensitive to drug, heparin, or pork products; in those with active major bleeding; and in those with thrombocytopenia and antiplatelet antibodies in presence of drug.
- Use cautiously in patients with history of heparin-induced thrombocytopenia, aneurysms, cerebrovascular hemorrhage, spinal or epidural punctures (as with anesthesia), uncontrolled hypertension, or threatened abortion.
- Use cautiously in elderly patients and in those with conditions that place them at increased risk for hemorrhage, such as bacterial endocarditis, congenital or acquired bleeding disorders, ulcer disease, angiodysplastic GI disease, hemorrhagic stroke, or recent spinal, eye, or brain surgery.
- Use cautiously in patients with prosthetic heart valves, with regional or lumbar block anesthesia, blood dyscrasias, recent childbirth, pericarditis or pericardial effusion, renal insufficiency, or severe CNS trauma.

NURSING CONSIDERATIONS

- The vascular access sheath for instrumentation should remain in place for 6 to 8 hours after a dose; give next dose no sooner than 6 to 8 hours after sheath removal. Monitor vital signs.
- Monitor pregnant women closely. Warn pregnant women and women of childbearing age about the potential risk of therapy to her and the fetus .
- Monitor anti-X_a levels in pregnant women with mechanical heart valves.
- ***Alert:*** Patients who receive epidural or spinal anesthesia during therapy are at increased risk for developing an epidural or spinal hematoma, which may result in long-term or permanent paralysis. Monitor these patients closely for neurologic impairment.
- Draw blood to establish baseline coagulation parameters before therapy.
- Never give drug I.M.
- ***Alert:*** Don't try to expel the air bubble from the 30- or 40-mg prefilled syringes. This may lead to loss of drug and an incorrect dose.
- With patient lying down, give by deep subcutaneous injection, alternating doses

between left and right anterolateral and posterolateral abdominal walls.

- Don't massage after subcutaneous injection. Watch for signs of bleeding at site. Rotate sites and keep record.
- Avoid I.M. injections of other drugs to prevent or minimize hematoma.
- Monitor platelet counts regularly. Patients with normal coagulation won't need close monitoring of PT or PTT.
- Regularly inspect patient for bleeding gums, bruises on arms or legs, petechiae, nosebleeds, melena, tarry stools, hematuria, hematemesis.
- To treat severe overdose, give protamine sulfate (a heparin antagonist) by slow I.V. infusion at concentration of 1% to equal dose of drug injected.
- ***Alert:*** Drug isn't interchangeable with heparin or other low–molecular-weight heparins.

PATIENT TEACHING

- Instruct patient and family to watch for signs of bleeding or abnormal bruising and to notify prescriber immediately if any occur.
- Tell patient to avoid OTC drugs containing aspirin or other salicylates unless ordered by prescriber.

fondaparinux sodium

Arixtra

Pharmacologic class: activated factor X inhibitor
Pregnancy risk category B

AVAILABLE FORMS

Injection: 2.5 mg/0.5 ml, 5 mg/0.4 ml, 7.5 mg/0.6 ml, 10 mg/0.8 ml single-dose prefilled syringe

INDICATIONS & DOSAGES

➤ **To prevent DVT, which may lead to pulmonary embolism, in patients undergoing surgery for hip fracture, hip replacement, knee replacement, or abdominal surgery**

Adults who weigh 50 kg (110 lb) or more: 2.5 mg subcutaneously once daily for 5 to 9 days. Give first dose after hemostasis is established, 6 to 8 hours after surgery. Giving the dose earlier than 6 hours after surgery increases the risk of major bleeding. Patients undergoing hip fracture surgery should receive an extended prophylaxis course of up to 24 additional days; a total of 32 days (perioperative and extended prophylaxis) has been tolerated.

➤ **Acute DVT (with warfarin); acute pulmonary embolism (with warfarin) when treatment is started in the hospital**

Adults who weigh more than 100 kg (220 lb): Give 10 mg subcutaneously daily for 5 to 9 days, and until INR level is 2 to 3. Begin warfarin therapy as soon as possible, usually within 72 hours.
Adults who weigh 50 to 100 kg: Give 7.5 mg subcutaneously daily for 5 to 9 days, and until INR level is 2 to 3. Begin warfarin therapy as soon as possible, usually within 72 hours.
Adults who weigh less than 50 kg: Give 5 mg subcutaneously daily for 5 to 9 days, and until INR level is 2 to 3. Begin warfarin therapy as soon as possible, usually within 72 hours.

ACTION

Binds to antithrombin III (AT-III) and potentiates the neutralization of factor Xa by AT-III, which interrupts coagulation and inhibits formation of thrombin and blood clots.

Route	Onset	Peak	Duration
SubQ	Unknown	2–3 hr	Unknown

Half-life: 17 to 21 hours.

ADVERSE REACTIONS

CNS: *fever,* insomnia, dizziness, confusion, headache, pain.
CV: hypotension, edema.
GI: *nausea,* constipation, vomiting, diarrhea, dyspepsia.
GU: UTI, urine retention.
Hematologic: ***hemorrhage,*** *anemia,* hematoma, ***postoperative hemorrhage, thrombocytopenia.***
Metabolic: hypokalemia.
Skin: mild local irritation (injection site bleeding, rash, pruritus), bullous eruption, purpura, rash, increased wound drainage.

INTERACTIONS

Drug-drug. *Drugs that increase risk of bleeding (NSAIDs, platelet inhibitors, anticoagulants):* May increase risk of hemorrhage. Stop these drugs before starting fondaparinux. If use together is unavoidable, monitor patient closely.

EFFECTS ON LAB TEST RESULTS

- May increase AST, ALT, and bilirubin levels. May decrease potassium and hemoglobin levels and hematocrit.
- May decrease platelet count.

CONTRAINDICATIONS & CAUTIONS

- Contraindicated in patients with creatinine clearance less than 30 ml/minute and in those who are hypersensitive to the drug.
- Contraindicated for prophylaxis in patients who weigh less than 50 kg who are undergoing hip fracture, hip replacement, knee replacement, or abdominal surgery.
- Contraindicated in patients with active major bleeding, bacterial endocarditis, or thrombocytopenia with a positive test result for antiplatelet antibody after taking fondaparinux.
- Use cautiously in patients being treated with platelet inhibitors; in those at increased risk for bleeding, such as congenital or acquired bleeding disorders; in those with active ulcerative and angiodysplastic GI disease; in those with hemorrhagic stroke; and in patients shortly after brain, spinal, or ophthalmologic surgery.
- Use cautiously in patients who have had epidural or spinal anesthesia or spinal puncture; they are at increased risk for developing an epidural or spinal hematoma (which may cause paralysis).
- Use cautiously in elderly patients, in patients with creatinine clearance of 30 to 50 ml/minute, and in those with a history of heparin-induced thrombocytopenia, a bleeding diathesis, uncontrolled arterial hypertension, or a history of recent GI ulceration, diabetic retinopathy, or hemorrhage.

NURSING CONSIDERATIONS

- Give subcutaneously only, never I.M. Inspect the single-dose, prefilled syringe for particulate matter and discoloration before administration.
- Don't mix with other injections or infusions.
- Don't use interchangeably with heparin, low–molecular-weight heparins, or heparinoids.
- ***Alert:*** To avoid loss of drug, don't expel air bubble from the syringe.
- Give the drug subcutaneously in fatty tissue, rotating injection sites. If the drug has been properly injected, the needle will pull back into the syringe security sleeve and the white safety indicator will appear above the blue upper body. A soft click may be heard or felt when the syringe plunger is fully released. After injection of the syringe contents, the plunger automatically rises while the needle withdraws from the skin and retracts into the security sleeve. Don't recap the needle.
- ***Alert:*** Patients who receive epidural or spinal anesthesia are at increased risk for developing an epidural or spinal hematoma, which may result in long-term or permanent paralysis. Monitor these patients closely for neurologic impairment.
- Monitor renal function periodically and stop drug in patients who develop unstable renal function or severe renal impairment while receiving therapy.
- Routinely assess patient for signs and symptoms of bleeding, and regularly monitor CBC, platelet count, creatinine level, and stool occult blood test results. Stop use if platelet count is less than 100,000/mm^3.
- Anticoagulant effects may last for 2 to 4 days after stopping drug in patients with normal renal function.
- PT and activated PTT aren't suitable monitoring tests to measure fondaparinux activity. If coagulation parameters change unexpectedly or patient develops major bleeding, stop drug.

PATIENT TEACHING

- Tell patient to report signs and symptoms of bleeding.
- Instruct patient to avoid OTC products that contain aspirin or other salicylates.
- Teach patient the correct technique for subcutaneous use, if needed.

SAFETY ALERT!

heparin sodium

Hepalean†, Heparin Leo†, Heparin Lock Flush Solution (with Tubex), Heparin Sodium Injection, Hep-Lock, Hep-Pak, Uniparin‡

Pharmacologic class: anticoagulant
Pregnancy risk category C

AVAILABLE FORMS

Products are derived from beef lung or pork intestinal mucosa.

heparin sodium
Carpuject: 5,000 units/ml
Premixed I.V. solutions: 1,000 units in 500 ml of normal saline solution; 2,000 units in 1,000 ml of normal saline solution; 12,500 units in 250 ml of half-normal saline solution; 25,000 units in 250 ml of half-normal saline solution; 25,000 units in 500 ml of half-normal saline solution; 10,000 units in 100 ml of D_5W; 12,500 units in 250 ml of D_5W; 20,000 units in 500 ml of D_5W; 25,000 units in 250 ml D_5W; 25,000 units in 500 ml D_5W
Syringes: 1,000 units/ml, 2,500 units/ml, 5,000 units/ml, 7,500 units/ml, 10,000 units/ml, 20,000 units/ml
Unit-dose vials: 1,000 units/ml, 5,000 units/ml, 10,000 units/ml, 20,000 units/ml, 40,000 units/ml
Vials: 1,000 units/ml, 2,000 units/ml, 2,500 units/ml, 5,000 units/ml, 7,500 units/ml, 10,000 units/ml, 20,000 units/ml, 40,000 units/ml

heparin sodium flush
Syringes: 10 units/ml, 100 units/ml
Vials: 10 units/ml, 100 units/ml

INDICATIONS & DOSAGES

➤ Full-dose continuous I.V. infusion therapy for DVT, MI, pulmonary embolism
Adults: Initially, 5,000 units by I.V. bolus; then 750 to 1,500 units/hour by I.V. infusion with pump. Titrate hourly rate based on PTT results (q 4 to 6 hours in the early stages of treatment).
Children: Initially, 50 units/kg I.V.; then 25 units/kg/hour or 20,000 units/m^2 daily by I.V. infusion pump. Titrate dosage based on PTT.

➤ Full-dose subcutaneous therapy for DVT, MI, pulmonary embolism
Adults: Initially, 5,000 units I.V. bolus and 10,000 to 20,000 units in a concentrated solution subcutaneously; then 8,000 to 10,000 units subcutaneously q 8 hours or 15,000 to 20,000 units in a concentrated solution q 12 hours.

➤ Full-dose intermittent I.V. therapy for DVT, MI, pulmonary embolism
Adults: Initially, 10,000 units by I.V. bolus; then titrated according to PTT, and 5,000 to 10,000 units I.V. q 4 to 6 hours.
Children: Initially, 100 units/kg by I.V. bolus; then 50 to 100 units/kg q 4 hours.

➤ Fixed low-dose therapy for prevention of venous thrombosis, pulmonary embolism, embolism associated with atrial fibrillation, and postoperative DVT
Adults: 5,000 units subcutaneously q 12 hours. In surgical patients, give first dose 1 to 2 hours before procedure; then 5,000 units subcutaneously q 8 to 12 hours for 5 to 7 days or until patient can walk.

➤ Consumptive coagulopathy (such as disseminated intravascular coagulation)
Adults: 50 to 100 units/kg by I.V. bolus or continuous I.V. infusion q 4 hours.
Children: 25 to 50 units/kg by I.V. bolus or continuous I.V. infusion every 4 hours. If no improvement within 4 to 8 hours, stop heparin.

➤ Open-heart surgery
Adults: For total body perfusion, 150 to 400 units/kg continuous I.V. infusion.

➤ Patency maintenance of I.V. indwelling catheters
Adults: 10 to 100 units I.V. flush. Use sufficient volume to fill device. Not intended for therapeutic use.

I.V. ADMINISTRATION

- Use an infusion pump to provide maximum safety. Check constant infusions regularly, even when pumps are in good working order, to ensure correct dosing. Place notice above patient's bed to caution I.V. team or laboratory personnel to apply pressure dressings after taking blood.
- During intermittent infusion, always draw blood 30 minutes before next scheduled dose to avoid falsely elevated PTT.

Blood for PTT may be drawn 4 hours after continuous I.V. heparin therapy starts. Blood for PTT should never be drawn from the tubing of the heparin infusion or from the infused vein, because falsely elevated PTT will result. Always draw blood from the opposite arm.

- Don't skip a dose or "catch up" with a solution containing heparin. If solution runs out, restart it as soon as possible, and reschedule bolus dose immediately. Monitor PTT.
- Concentrated heparin solutions (more than 100 units/ml) can irritate blood vessels.
- Never piggyback other drugs into an infusion line while heparin infusion is running. Never mix another drug and heparin in same syringe when giving a bolus.

INCOMPATIBILITIES

Alteplase; amikacin; amiodarone; ampicillin sodium; atracurium; chlorpromazine; ciprofloxacin; codeine phosphate; cytarabine; dacarbazine; daunorubicin; dextrose 4.3% in sodium chloride solution 0.18%; diazepam; diltiazem; dobutamine; doxorubicin; doxycycline hyclate; droperidol; ergotamine; erythromycin gluceptate or lactobionate; filgrastim; gentamicin; haloperidol lactate; hydrocortisone sodium succinate; hydroxyzine hydrochloride; idarubicin; kanamycin; labetalol; levorphanol; meperidine; methadone; methylprednisolone sodium succinate; morphine sulfate; netilmicin; nicardipine; penicillin G potassium; penicillin G sodium; pentazocine lactate; phenytoin sodium; polymyxin B sulfate; prochlorperazine edisylate; promethazine hydrochloride; quinidine gluconate; 1/6 M sodium lactate; solutions containing a phosphate buffer, sodium carbonate, or sodium oxalate; streptomycin; tobramycin sulfate; trifluoperazine; triflupromazine; vancomycin; vinblastine; warfarin.

ACTION

Accelerates formation of antithrombin III-thrombin complex and deactivates thrombin, preventing conversion of fibrinogen to fibrin.

Route	Onset	Peak	Duration
I.V.	Immediate	Unknown	Variable
SubQ	20–60 min	2–4 hr	Variable

Half-life: 1 to 2 hours. Half-life is dose-dependent and nonlinear and may be disproportionately prolonged at higher doses.

ADVERSE REACTIONS

CNS: fever.
EENT: rhinitis.
Hematologic: ***hemorrhage, overly prolonged clotting time, thrombocytopenia.***
Skin: irritation, mild pain, hematoma, ulceration, cutaneous or subcutaneous necrosis, pruritus, urticaria.
Other: ***white clot syndrome,*** hypersensitivity reactions, including chills, ***anaphylactoid reactions.***

INTERACTIONS

Drug-drug. *Other antiplatelet drugs, Salicylates:* May increase anticoagulant effect. Use together cautiously. Monitor coagulation studies and patient closely.
Cephalosporins , penicillins: May increase risk of bleeding. Monitor patient closely.
Nitroglycerin: May decrease effects of heparin. Monitor patient closely.
Oral anticoagulants: May increase additive anticoagulation. Monitor PT, INR, and PTT.
Thrombolytics: May increase risk of hemorrhage. Monitor patient closely.
Drug-herb. *Garlic, ginkgo, motherwort, red clover, white willow:* May increase risk of bleeding. Discourage herb use.

EFFECTS ON LAB TEST RESULTS

- May increase ALT and AST levels.
- May increase INR, PT, and PTT. May decrease platelet count.
- Drug may cause false elevations in some tests for thyroxine level.

CONTRAINDICATIONS & CAUTIONS

- Contraindicated in patients hypersensitive to drug. Conditionally contraindicated in patients with active bleeding, blood dyscrasia, or bleeding tendencies, such as hemophilia, thrombocytopenia, or hepatic disease with hypoprothrombinemia; suspected intracranial hemorrhage; suppurative thrombophlebitis; inaccessible ulcera-

tive lesions (especially of GI tract) and open ulcerative wounds; extensive denudation of skin; ascorbic acid deficiency and other conditions that cause increased capillary permeability.
• Conditionally contraindicated during or after brain, eye, or spinal cord surgery; during spinal tap or spinal anesthesia; during continuous tube drainage of stomach or small intestine; and in subacute bacterial endocarditis, shock, advanced renal disease, threatened abortion, or severe hypertension.
• Use cautiously in women during menses or after childbirth and in patients with mild hepatic or renal disease, alcoholism, occupations with high risk of physical injury, or history of allergies, asthma, or GI ulcerations.

NURSING CONSIDERATIONS

• Although heparin use is clearly hazardous in certain conditions, its risks and benefits must be evaluated.
• Draw blood to establish baseline coagulation parameters before therapy.
• If a woman needs anticoagulation during pregnancy, most prescribers use heparin.
• Some commercially available heparin injections contain benzyl alcohol. Avoid using these products in neonates and pregnant women if possible.
• Drug requirements are higher in early phases of thrombogenic diseases and febrile states; they are lower when patient's condition stabilizes.
• Elderly patients should usually start at lower dosage.
• Check order and vial carefully; heparin comes in various concentrations.
• ***Alert:*** USP and international units aren't equivalent for heparin.
• ***Alert:*** Heparin, low–molecular-weight heparins, and danaparoid aren't interchangeable.
• ***Alert:*** Don't change concentrations of infusions unless absolutely necessary. This is a common source of dosage errors.
• Give low-dose injections sequentially between iliac crests in lower abdomen deep into subcutaneous fat. Inject drug subcutaneously slowly into fat pad. Don't massage, and watch for signs of bleeding at injection site. Alternate sites every 12 hours—right for morning, left for evening.
• Draw blood for PTT 4 to 6 hours after dose given subcutaneously.
• Avoid I.M. injections of other drugs to prevent or minimize hematoma. .
• Measure PTT carefully and regularly. Anticoagulation is present when PTT values are 1½ to 2 times the control values.
• Monitor platelet count regularly.
• ***Alert:*** If heparin-induced thrombocytopenia (HIT) occurs, stop heparin. HIT and thrombosis may occur within several weeks after stopping drug.
• Regularly inspect patient for bleeding gums, bruises on arms or legs, petechiae, nosebleeds, melena, tarry stools, hematuria, and hematemesis.
• ***Alert:*** To treat severe overdose, use protamine sulfate, a heparin antagonist. Dosage is based on the dose of heparin, its route of administration, and the time since it was given. Generally, 1 to 1.5 mg of protamine per 100 units of heparin is given if only a few minutes have elapsed; 0.5 to 0.75 mg protamine per 100 units heparin, if 30 to 60 minutes have elapsed; and 0.25 to 0.375 mg protamine per 100 units heparin, if 2 hours or more have elapsed. Don't give more than 50 mg protamine in a 10-minute period.
• Abrupt withdrawal may cause increased coagulability; warfarin therapy usually overlaps heparin therapy for continuation of prophylaxis or treatment.
• ***Look alike–sound alike:*** Don't confuse heparin with Hespan.

PATIENT TEACHING

• Instruct patient and family to watch for signs of bleeding or bruising and to notify prescriber immediately if any occur.
• Tell patient to avoid OTC drugs containing aspirin, other salicylates, or drugs that may interact with heparin unless ordered by prescriber.

SAFETY ALERT!

tinzaparin sodium
Innohep

Pharmacologic class: low–molecular-weight heparin
Pregnancy risk category B

AVAILABLE FORMS
Injection: 20,000 anti-factor Xa international units/ml in 2-ml vials

INDICATIONS & DOSAGES
➤ **Symptomatic DVT with or without pulmonary embolism**
Adults: 175 anti-factor Xa international units/kg of body weight subcutaneously once daily for at least 6 days and until patient is adequately anticoagulated with warfarin sodium (INR of at least 2) for 2 consecutive days. Start warfarin sodium therapy when appropriate, usually within 1 to 3 days of tinzaparin initiation. Volume of dose to be given may be calculated as follows:

Patient weight in kg × 0.00875 ml/kg = Volume to be given in ml

ACTION
Inhibits reactions that lead to blood clotting, including formation of fibrin clots. Also a potent co-inhibitor of several activated coagulation factors, especially factors Xa and IIa (thrombin). Drug binds antithrombin, thereby increasing ability to inactivate coagulation enzymes factor Xa and thrombin. Drug also induces release of tissue factor pathway inhibitor, which may contribute to the antithrombotic effect.

Route	Onset	Peak	Duration
SubQ	2–3 hr	4–5 hr	18–24 hr

Half-life: 3 to 4 hours.

ADVERSE REACTIONS
CNS: ***cerebral or intracranial bleeding,*** headache, dizziness, insomnia, confusion, fever, pain.
CV: ***arrhythmias, MI, thromboembolism,*** chest pain, hypotension, hypertension, tachycardia, dependent edema, angina pectoris.
EENT: epistaxis, ocular hemorrhage.
GI: ***GI hemorrhage,*** anorectal bleeding, constipation, flatulence, hematemesis, nausea, vomiting, dyspepsia, retroperitoneal or intra-abdominal bleeding, melena.
GU: ***vaginal hemorrhage,*** dysuria, hematuria, UTI, urine retention.
Hematologic: ***granulocytopenia, thrombocytopenia, agranulocytosis, pancytopenia, hemorrhage,*** anemia.
Musculoskeletal: back pain, hemarthrosis.
Respiratory: ***pulmonary embolism,*** pneumonia, respiratory disorder, dyspnea.
Skin: bullous eruption, cellulitis, *injection site hematoma,* pruritus, purpura, rash, skin necrosis, wound hematoma, bullous eruption.
Other: ***allergic reaction, fetal death, spinal or epidural hematoma,*** hypersensitivity reaction, infection, impaired healing, congenital anomaly, fetal distress.

INTERACTIONS
Drug-drug. *Oral anticoagulants, platelet inhibitors (such as dextran, dipyridamole, NSAIDs, salicylates, sulfinpyrazone), thrombolytics:* May increase risk of bleeding. Use together cautiously. If drugs must be given together, monitor patient.

EFFECTS ON LAB TEST RESULTS
- May increase AST and ALT levels. May decrease hemoglobin level.
- May decrease granulocyte, platelet, RBC, and WBC counts.

CONTRAINDICATIONS & CAUTIONS
- Contraindicated in patients hypersensitive to tinzaparin sodium or other low–molecular-weight heparins, heparin, sulfites, benzyl alcohol, or pork products. Also contraindicated in patients with active major bleeding and in those with history of heparin-induced thrombocytopenia.
- Use cautiously in patients with increased risk of hemorrhage, such as those with bacterial endocarditis; uncontrolled hypertension; diabetic retinopathy; congenital or acquired bleeding disorders, including hepatic failure and amyloidosis; GI ulceration; or hemorrhagic stroke. Also use

cautiously in patients who have recently undergone brain, spinal, or ophthalmologic surgery, and in patients being treated with platelet inhibitors. Elderly patients and patients with renal insufficiency may show reduced elimination of drug. Use drug with care in these patients.
• Use cautiously in breast-feeding women; it's unknown if drug appears in breast milk.

NURSING CONSIDERATIONS
• Drug isn't intended for I.M. or I.V. administration, nor should it be mixed with other injections or infusions.
• Don't interchange drug (unit to unit) with heparin or other low–molecular-weight heparins.
• When giving drug, have patient lie or sit down. Give by deep subcutaneous injection into abdominal wall. Introduce whole length of needle into skinfold held between thumb and forefinger. Make sure to hold skinfold throughout injection. Rotate injection sites between right and left anterolateral and posterolateral abdominal wall. To minimize bruising, don't rub injection site after administration.
• Use an appropriate calibrated syringe to ensure correct withdrawal of volume of drug from vials.
• Monitor platelet count during therapy. Stop drug if platelet count goes below $100,000/mm^3$.
• Periodically monitor CBC count and stool tests for occult blood during treatment.
• Drug may affect PT and INR levels. Patient also receiving warfarin should have blood for PT and INR drawn just before next scheduled dose of tinzaparin.
• Drug contains sodium metabisulfite, which may cause allergic reactions in susceptible people.
• ***Alert:*** Patients who receive epidural or spinal anesthesia are at increased risk of epidural or spinal hematoma, which may result in long-term or permanent paralysis. Monitor these patients closely for neurologic impairment.
• If woman becomes pregnant while taking drug, warn her of potential risks to the fetus. Cases of gasping syndrome may occur in premature infants when large amounts of benzyl alcohol are given.
• Store drug at room temperature.

PATIENT TEACHING
• Explain to patient importance of laboratory monitoring to ensure effectiveness of drug while maintaining safety.
• Teach patient warning signs of bleeding and instruct him to report these signs immediately.
• Caution patient to use soft toothbrush and electric razor to prevent cuts and bruises.
• Instruct patient that warfarin will be started when appropriate, within 1 to 3 days of therapy. Explain importance of warfarin and the monitoring for safety and effectiveness.

SAFETY ALERT!

warfarin sodium
Coumadin✐, Warfilone†, Jantoven

Pharmacologic class: coumarin derivative
Pregnancy risk category X

AVAILABLE FORMS
Powder for injection: 5-mg vial
Tablets: 1 mg, 2 mg, 2.5 mg, 3 mg, 4 mg, 5 mg, 6 mg, 7.5 mg, 10 mg

INDICATIONS & DOSAGES
➤ **Pulmonary embolism, DVT, MI, rheumatic heart disease with heart valve damage, prosthetic heart valves, chronic atrial fibrillation**
Adults: 2 to 5 mg P.O. or I.V. daily for 2 to 4 days; then dosage based on daily PT and INR. Usual maintenance dosage is 2 to 10 mg P.O. or I.V. daily.

I.V. ADMINISTRATION
• I.V. form may be ordered in rare instances when oral therapy can't be given.
• Reconstitute powder with 2.7 ml sterile water, or as instructed in manufacturer guidelines.
• Give as a slow bolus injection over 1 to 2 minutes into a peripheral vein.
• Because onset of action is delayed, heparin sodium is often given during the first few days of treatment of embolic disease. Blood for PT and INR may be drawn at

any time during continuous heparin infusion.

INCOMPATIBILITIES
Aminophylline, ammonium chloride, bretylium tosylate, ceftazidime, cimetidine, ciprofloxacin, dobutamine, esmolol, gentamicin, heparin sodium, labetalol, lactated Ringer injection, metronidazole, promazine, Ringer injection, vancomycin.

ACTION
Inhibits vitamin K-dependent activation of clotting factors II, VII, IX, and X, formed in the liver.

Route	Onset	Peak	Duration
P.O.	Within 24 hr	4 hr	2–5 days
I.V.	Within 24 hr	< 4 hr	2–5 days

Half-life: 20 to 60 hours.

ADVERSE REACTIONS
CNS: *fever,* headache.
GI: *diarrhea,* anorexia, nausea, vomiting, cramps, mouth ulcerations, sore mouth, melena.
GU: hematuria, excessive menstrual bleeding.
Hematologic: ***hemorrhage.***
Hepatic: ***hepatitis,*** jaundice.
Skin: dermatitis, urticaria, necrosis, gangrene, alopecia, *rash.*
Other: enhanced uric acid excretion.

INTERACTIONS
Drug-drug. *Acetaminophen:* May increase bleeding with long-term therapy (more than 2 weeks) at high doses (more than 2 g/day) of acetaminophen. Monitor patient very carefully.
Allopurinol, ***amiodarone, anabolic steroids,*** *antidepressants,* ***azole antifungals,*** *aspirin, celecoxib, cephalosporins, chloramphenicol, cimetidine,* ***danazol,*** *diazoxide, diflunisal, disulfiram, erythromycin, ethacrynic acid,* ***fibric acids, fluoxymesterone, fluoroquinolones,*** *furosemide, glucagon, heparin, influenza virus vaccine, isoniazid,* ***lansoprazole,*** *meclofenamate, methimazole, methyldopa, methylphenidate,* ***methyltestosterone, metronidazole, nalidixic acid,*** *neomycin (oral),* ***NSAIDs,*** *omeprazole,* ***oxandrolone,*** *pentoxifylline, propafenone, propoxyphene, propylthiouracil, quinidine,* ***salicylates,*** *SSRIs,* ***sulfinpyrazone, sulfonamides,*** *tamoxifen, tetracyclines, thiazides, thrombolytics,* ***thyroid drugs,*** *ticlopidine, tramadol, vitamin E, valproic acid, zafirlukast:* May increase anticoagulant effect. Monitor patient carefully for bleeding. Reduce anticoagulant dosage as directed.
Anticonvulsants: May increase levels of phenytoin and phenobarbital. Monitor drug levels closely.
Ascorbic acid, ***barbiturates,*** *carbamazepine, clozapine, corticosteroids, corticotropin, cyclosporine, dicloxacillin, ethchlorvynol, griseofulvin, haloperidol, meprobamate, mercaptopurine, nafcillin, oral contraceptives containing estrogen, rifampin, spironolactone, sucralfate, thiazide diuretics, trazodone, vitamin K:* May decrease PT and INR with reduced anticoagulant effect. Monitor PT and INR carefully. Increase warfarin dosage, p.r.n.
Chloral hydrate, cyclophosphamide, hypolipidemics, phenytoin, propylthiouracil, ranitidine: May increase or decrease PT and INR. Monitor PT and INR carefully.
Cholestyramine: May decrease response when given too closely together. Give 6 hours after oral anticoagulants.
Sulfonylureas (oral antidiabetics): May increase hypoglycemic response. Monitor glucose levels.
Drug-herb. *Angelica:* May significantly prolong PT and INR. Discourage use together.
Anise, arnica flower, asafoetida, bogbean, bromelain, celery, chamomile, clove, dandelion, danshen, devil's claw, dong quai, fenugreek, feverfew, garlic, ginger, ***ginkgo, ginseng,*** *horse chestnut, licorice, meadowsweet, motherwort, onion, papain, parsley, passion flower, quassia, red clover, Reishi mushroom, rue, sweet clover, turmeric, white willow:* May increase risk of bleeding. Discourage use together.
Coenzyme Q10, ginseng, St. John's wort: May reduce action of drug. Ask patient about use of herbal remedies, and advise caution.
Green tea: May decrease anticoagulant effect caused by vitamin K content of green tea. Advise patient to minimize variable consumption of green tea and other foods or nutritional supplements containing vitamin K.

Drug-food. *Foods, multivitamins, and other enteral products containing vitamin K:* May impair anticoagulation. Tell patient to maintain consistent daily intake of foods containing vitamin K.
Cranberry juice: My increase risk of severe bleeding. Avoid using together.
Drug-lifestyle. *Alcohol use:* May enhance anticoagulant effects. Tell patient to avoid large amounts of alcohol.

EFFECTS ON LAB TEST RESULTS

- May increase ALT and AST levels.
- May increase INR, PT, and PTT.
- May falsely decrease theophylline level.

CONTRAINDICATIONS & CAUTIONS

- Contraindicated in patients hypersensitive to drug and in those with bleeding from the GI, GU, or respiratory tract; aneurysm; cerebrovascular hemorrhage; severe or malignant hypertension; severe renal or hepatic disease; subacute bacterial endocarditis, pericarditis, or pericardial effusion; or blood dyscrasias or hemorrhagic tendencies.
- Contraindicated during pregnancy, threatened abortion, eclampsia, or preeclampsia, and after recent surgery involving large open areas, eye, brain, or spinal cord; recent prostatectomy; major regional lumbar block anesthesia, spinal puncture, or diagnostic or therapeutic invasive procedures.
- Avoid using in patients with a history of warfarin-induced necrosis; in unsupervised patients with senility, alcoholism, or psychosis; or in situations in which there are inadequate laboratory facilities for coagulation testing.
- Use cautiously in patients with diverticulitis, colitis, mild or moderate hypertension, or mild or moderate hepatic or renal disease; with drainage tubes in any orifice; with regional or lumbar block anesthesia; or in conditions that increase risk of hemorrhage.
- Use cautiously in breast-feeding women.

NURSING CONSIDERATIONS

- Draw blood to establish baseline coagulation parameters before therapy. PT and INR determinations are essential for proper control. INR range for chronic atrial fibrillation is usually 2 to 3.
- Give drug at same time daily.
- Avoid all I.M. injections.
- Regularly inspect patient for bleeding gums, bruises on arms or legs, petechiae, nosebleeds, melena, tarry stools, hematuria, and hematemesis. Check for unexpected bleeding in breast-fed infants of women on drug.
- ***Alert:*** Withhold drug and call prescriber at once in the event of fever or rash (signs of severe adverse reactions).
- Effect can be neutralized by oral or parenteral vitamin K.
- Elderly patients and patients with renal or hepatic failure are especially sensitive to drug's effect.

PATIENT TEACHING

- Stress importance of complying with prescribed dosage and follow-up appointments. Tell patient to carry a card that identifies his increased risk of bleeding.
- Tell patient and family to watch for signs of bleeding or abnormal bruising and to call prescriber at once if they occur.
- Warn patient to avoid OTC products containing aspirin, other salicylates, or drugs that may interact with warfarin unless ordered by prescriber.
- Tell patient to consult a prescriber before using miconazole vaginal cream or suppositories. Abnormal bleeding and bruising have occurred.
- Instruct woman to notify prescriber if menstruation is heavier than usual; she may need dosage adjustment.
- Tell patient to use electric razor when shaving, and to use a soft toothbrush.
- Tell patient to read food labels. Food, nutritional supplements, and multivitamins that contain vitamin K may impair anticoagulation.
- Tell patient to eat a daily, consistent diet of food and drinks containing vitamin K, because eating varied amounts may alter anticoagulant effects.

65

Blood derivatives

albumin 5%
albumin 25%
antihemophilic factor
anti-inhibitor coagulant complex
factor IX complex
factor IX (human)
factor IX (recombinant)
plasma protein fractions

albumin 5%

Albumarc, Albuminar-5, Albunex, Albutein 5%, Buminate 5%, Plasbumin-5

albumin 25%

Albuminar-25, Albutein 25%, Buminate 25%, Plasbumin-25

Pharmacologic class: blood derivative
Pregnancy risk category C

AVAILABLE FORMS

albumin 5%
Injection: 50 mg/ml in 5-ml, 10-ml, 20-ml, 50-ml, 250-ml, 500-ml, 1,000-ml vials
albumin 25%
Injection: 250 mg/ml in 20-ml, 50-ml, 100-ml vials

INDICATIONS & DOSAGES

➤Hypovolemic shock
Adults: Initially, 500 to 750 ml of 5% solution by I.V. infusion, repeated q 30 minutes, p.r.n. As plasma volume approaches normal, rate of infusion of 5% solution shouldn't exceed 2 to 4 ml/minute. Or, 100 to 200 ml I.V. of 25% solution, repeated after 10 to 30 minutes, if needed. Dosage varies with patient's condition and response. As plasma volume approaches normal, rate of infusion of 25% solution shouldn't exceed 1 ml/minute.
Children: Give 12 to 20 ml of 5% solution/kg by I.V. infusion, repeated in 15 to 30 minutes if response is inadequate. Or, 2.5 to 5 ml I.V. of 25% solution/kg, repeated after 10 to 30 minutes, if needed.

➤Hypoproteinemia
Adults: 200 to 300 ml of 25% albumin. Dosage varies with patient's condition and response. Rate of infusion shouldn't exceed 2 to 3 ml/minute.

➤Hyperbilirubinemia
Infants: Give 1 g albumin (4 ml of 25%) per kg 1 to 2 hours before exchange transfusion; or 50 ml of 25% albumin substituted for 50 ml of donor plasma.

I.V. ADMINISTRATION

- Make sure patient is properly hydrated before infusion.
- Minimize waste when preparing and giving drug. This product is expensive, and supply shortages are common.
- Albumin 5% is infused undiluted; albumin 25% may be infused undiluted or diluted with normal saline solution or D_5W injection.
- Avoid rapid I.V. infusion. Specific rate is based on patient's age, condition, and diagnosis.
- Don't give more than 250 g in 48 hours.
- Use solution promptly. Discard unused solution.
- Make sure solution is a clear amber color. Don't use cloudy or sediment-filled solutions.
- Follow storage instructions on bottle. Freezing may cause bottle to break.

INCOMPATIBILITIES

Verapamil hydrochloride.

ACTION

Albumin 5% supplies colloid to the blood and expands plasma volume. Albumin 25% provides intravascular oncotic pressure in a 5:1 ratio, shifting fluid from interstitial spaces to the circulation and slightly increasing plasma protein level.

Route	Onset	Peak	Duration
I.V.	< 15 min	< 15 min	Several hr

Half-life: 15 to 20 days.

ADVERSE REACTIONS
CNS: headache, fever.
CV: ***vascular overload after rapid infusion,*** hypotension, tachycardia.
GI: increased salivation, nausea, vomiting.
Musculoskeletal: back pain.
Respiratory: altered respiration, dyspnea, pulmonary edema.
Skin: urticaria, rash.
Other: chills.

INTERACTIONS
Drug-drug. *ACE inhibitors:* May increase risk of atypical reactions, such as flushing and hypotension. Withhold ACE inhibitors 24 hours before giving albumin, if possible.

EFFECTS ON LAB TEST RESULTS
- May increase albumin level.

CONTRAINDICATIONS & CAUTIONS
- Contraindicated in patients hypersensitive to drug and in those with severe anemia, pulmonary edema, or cardiac failure.
- Use with extreme caution in patients with hypertension, low cardiac reserve, hypervolemia, pulmonary edema, or hypoalbuminemia with peripheral edema.

NURSING CONSIDERATIONS
- Watch for hemorrhage or shock after surgery or injury. Rapid increase in blood pressure may cause bleeding from sites that aren't apparent at lower pressures.
- Monitor vital signs carefully.
- Watch for signs of vascular overload (heart failure or pulmonary edema).
- Monitor fluid intake and output; protein, electrolyte, and hemoglobin levels; and hematocrit during therapy.

PATIENT TEACHING
- Explain use and administration to patient and family.
- Tell patient to report adverse reactions promptly.

antihemophilic factor (AHF, Factor VIII)

Advate, Alphanate, Bioclate, Helixate FS, Hemofil M, Hyate:C, Koate-DVI, Kogenate FS, Monarc-M, Monoclate-P, Recombinate, ReFacto

Pharmacologic class: plasma protein
Pregnancy risk category C

AVAILABLE FORMS
Injection: Vials, with diluent; units specified on label

INDICATIONS & DOSAGES
Drug provides hemostasis in factor VIII deficiency, hemophilia A. The specific dosage depends on the patient's weight, severity of hemorrhage, and presence of inhibitors. Mild bleeding episodes require a circulating factor VIII level 20% to 40% of normal; moderate to major bleeding episodes and minor surgery, a level 30% to 60% of normal; severe bleeding or major surgery, a level 60% to 100% of normal. The following dosages provide guidelines. Refer to specific brand for actual dosage.
The dose (international units/kg) can be calculated by dividing the desired level (as a percent of normal) by 2. For example, if a peak level of 50% is the goal, divide 50 by 2 to get 25 international units/kg.

➤ **Mild bleeding in patients with hemophilia**
Adults and children: 10 to 20 international units/kg daily.

➤ **Moderate bleeding and minor surgery in patients with hemophilia**
Adults and children: Initially, 15 to 30 international units/kg, then repeat one dose at 12 to 24 hours if needed.

➤ **Severe bleeding and bleeding near vital organs in patients with hemophilia**
Adults and children: Initially, 40 to 50 international units/kg, then 20 to 25 international units/kg q 8 to 12 hours, p.r.n.

➤ **Major surgery in patients with hemophilia**
Adults and children: 50 international units/kg 1 hour before surgery, then repeat p.r.n. 6 to 12 hours after first dose.

Maintain circulating factor levels at 30% to 60% of normal for 10 to 14 days after surgery.

I.V. ADMINISTRATION

- Refrigerate concentrate until ready to use.
- Kogenate FS (formulated with sucrose) may be refrigerated or stored at room temperature (for up to 3 months). Product stored at room temperature shouldn't be returned to refrigeration.
- Warm concentrate and diluent bottles to room temperature before reconstituting.
- Follow manufacturer's instructions for reconstituting.
- To mix drug, gently roll vial between hands. Don't shake.
- Use reconstituted solution within 3 hours.
- Filter solution before giving it.
- Use plastic syringe; drug may bind to glass syringe.
- Take baseline pulse rate before administration.
- Give at 2 ml/minute; may be given up to 10 ml/minute, depending on the preparation being used.
- If pulse rate increases significantly, reduce flow rate or stop administration.
- Store reconstituted drug away from heat, and don't refrigerate. Refrigeration after reconstitution may cause active ingredient to precipitate.

INCOMPATIBILITIES

Protein precipitants or other I.V. solutions.

ACTION

Directly replaces deficient clotting factor.

Route	Onset	Peak	Duration
I.V.	Immediate	1–2 hr	Unknown

Half-life: 10 to 18 hours.

ADVERSE REACTIONS

CNS: headache, somnolence, lethargy, dizziness, tingling asthenia, *fever.*
CV: tightness in chest, ***thrombosis.***
GI: nausea.
Hematologic: ***hemolytic anemia, thrombocytopenia.***
Hepatic: ***risk of hepatitis B, risk of hepatitis C.***
Respiratory: wheezing.
Skin: ***urticaria,*** stinging at injection site.
Other: *chills,* hypersensitivity reactions, ***anaphylaxis, risk of HIV infection.***

INTERACTIONS

None significant.

EFFECTS ON LAB TEST RESULTS

- May decrease hemoglobin level.
- May decrease platelet count.

CONTRAINDICATIONS & CAUTIONS

- For AHF that is monoclonally prepared, contraindicated in patients hypersensitive to drug or murine (mouse) protein.
- Use cautiously in neonates, infants, and patients with hepatic disease because of their susceptibility to hepatitis, which may be transmitted in AHF.

NURSING CONSIDERATIONS

- Monitor coagulation studies before therapy.
- Monitor patients with blood types A, B, and AB for possible hemolysis.
- Orange or red urine discoloration may signify a hemolytic reaction.
- Give hepatitis B vaccine before giving AHF.
- Don't give drug I.M. or subcutaneously.
- Monitor vital signs regularly.
- Monitor coagulation studies and platelets frequently during therapy.
- Monitor patient for allergic reactions.
- Patient may develop inhibitors to factor VIII, resulting in decreased response to drug.
- Risk of hepatitis must be weighed against risk of patient not receiving drug.
- Because of manufacturing process, risk of HIV transmission is extremely low.

PATIENT TEACHING

- Explain use and administration of AHF to patient and family.
- Advise patient to report adverse reactions promptly.
- Advise patient to carry medical identification.
- Tell patient to notify prescriber if drug seems less effective; a change may signify the development of antibodies.

anti-inhibitor coagulant complex
Autoplex T, Feiba VH Immuno

Pharmacologic class: plasma protein
Pregnancy risk category C

AVAILABLE FORMS
Injection: Number of units of factor VIII correctional activity indicated on label of vial

INDICATIONS & DOSAGES
➤ **To prevent or control hemorrhagic episodes in some patients with hemophilia A in whom inhibitor antibodies to antihemophilic factor have developed; to manage bleeding in patients with acquired hemophilia who have spontaneously acquired inhibitors to factor VIII**

Drug controls hemorrhage in hemophilia A patients who have a factor VIII inhibitor level above 10 Bethesda units. Patients with a level of 2 to 10 Bethesda units may receive the drug if they have severe hemorrhage or respond poorly to factor VIII infusion.

Dosage is highly individualized and varies among manufacturers. For Autoplex T, give 25 to 100 units/kg I.V. depending on the severity of hemorrhage. If no hemostatic improvement occurs within 6 hours after first administration, repeat dosage. For Feiba VH Immuno, give 50 to 100 units/kg I.V. q 6 or 12 hours until patient shows signs of improvement. Maximum daily dose of Feiba VH Immuno is 200 units/kg.

➤ **Joint hemorrhage**
Adults and children: Give 50 to 100 units/kg Feiba VH Immuno q 12 hours until patient's condition improves.

➤ **Mucous membrane hemorrhage**
Adults and children: Give 50 units/kg Feiba VH Immuno q 6 hours, increasing to 100 units/kg q 6 hours if hemorrhage continues. Maximum daily dose, 200 units/kg.

➤ **Soft-tissue hemorrhage**
Adults and children: Give 100 units/kg Feiba VH Immuno q 12 hours. Maximum daily dose, 200 units/kg.

➤ **Other severe hemorrhage**
Adults and children: Give 100 units/kg Feiba VH Immuno q 12 hours (occasionally, q 6 hours).

I.V. ADMINISTRATION
- Dosages of the two available products aren't equivalent.
- Warm drug and diluent to room temperature before reconstitution. Reconstitute according to manufacturer's directions. Give drug as soon as possible.
- Use filter needle provided by manufacturer to withdraw reconstituted solution from vial into syringe; then replace filter needle with a sterile injection needle for administration.
- For infusion, use administration set with filter.
- Individualize rate of administration based on patient's response. Autoplex T infusion may start at 2 ml/minute; if well tolerated, increase gradually to 10 ml/minute. Feiba VH Immuno infusion shouldn't exceed 2 units/kg/minute.
- Complete Autoplex T infusion within 1 hour after reconstitution; complete Feiba VH Immuno infusion within 3 hours.
- If flushing, lethargy, headache, transient chest discomfort, or changes in blood pressure or pulse rate develop because of a rapid infusion, stop drug and notify prescriber. These problems usually disappear when infusion stops. Resume at a slower rate.

INCOMPATIBILITIES
Other I.V. drugs or solutions.

ACTION
May be related to presence of activated factors, which leads to more complete factor X activation with tissue factor, phospholipid, and ionic calcium and allows the coagulation process to proceed beyond those stages in which factor VIII is needed.

Route	Onset	Peak	Duration
I.V.	10–30 min	Unknown	Unknown

Half-life: Unknown.

ADVERSE REACTIONS
CNS: headache, lethargy, fever.

CV: changes in blood pressure, flushing, ***acute MI, thromboembolic events.***
GI: nausea, vomiting.
Hematologic: ***DIC.***
Hepatic: ***hepatitis C infection.***
Skin: rash, urticaria.
Other: chills, hypersensitivity reactions, ***anaphylaxis, HIV infection.***

INTERACTIONS

Drug-drug. *Antifibrinolytic drugs:* May alter effects of anti-inhibitor coagulant complex. Avoid using together.

EFFECTS ON LAB TEST RESULTS

None reported.

CONTRAINDICATIONS & CAUTIONS

- Contraindicated in patients hypersensitive to drug, in those with DIC or a normal coagulation mechanism, and in those showing signs of fibrinolysis.
- Feiba VH Immuno is contraindicated in neonates.
- Use cautiously in patients with hepatic disease.
- Use Autoplex T cautiously in neonates.

NURSING CONSIDERATIONS

- Give hepatitis B vaccine before giving drug.
- Keep epinephrine available to treat anaphylaxis. Monitor patient closely for hypersensitivity reactions.
- Monitor vital signs regularly, and report significant changes to prescriber.
- Observe patient closely for signs of thromboembolic events.
- Reassure patient that, because of manufacturing process, risk of HIV transmission is extremely low.

PATIENT TEACHING

- Explain use and administration of anti-inhibitor coagulant complex to patient and family.
- Tell patient to report adverse reactions promptly.

factor IX complex

Bebulin VH, Profilnine SD, Proplex T

factor IX (human)

AlphaNine SD, Mononine

factor IX (recombinant)

BeneFix

Pharmacologic class: plasma protein
Pregnancy risk category C

AVAILABLE FORMS

Injection: Vials, with diluent; International units specified on label

INDICATIONS & DOSAGES

➤ Factor IX deficiency (also called hemophilia B or Christmas disease), anticoagulant overdosage; factor VII deficiency (Proplex T only)
Adults and children: To calculate international units of factor IX needed, use the following equations:

Human product

$$\frac{1 \text{ international unit}}{\text{kg}} \times \text{body weight in kg} \times \text{percentage of desired increase of factor IX level}$$

Recombinant product

$$\frac{1.21 \text{ international unit}}{\text{kg}} \times \text{body weight in kg} \times \text{percentage of desired increase of factor IX level}$$

Proplex T

$$\frac{0.5 \text{ international unit}}{\text{kg}} \times \text{body weight in kg} \times \text{percentage of desired increase of factor VII level}$$

➤ Factor IX deficiency, anticoagulant overdosage
Adults and children: Infusion rates vary with product and patient comfort. Dosage is highly individualized, depending on degree of deficiency, level of factor VII or IX desired, patient weight, and severity of bleeding.

I.V. ADMINISTRATION
- Warm to room temperature before reconstituting.
- Reconstitute each vial of lyophilized drug with sterile water for injection according to manufacturer's directions.
- Don't shake, refrigerate, or mix with other solutions.
- Use factor IX (human) within 3 hours after reconstitution. Factor IX complex is stable 12 hours after reconstitution, although delivery should start within 3 hours of reconstitution.
- Filter drug before giving.
- Avoid rapid infusion. If tingling sensation, fever, chills, or headache develop, decrease flow rate and notify prescriber.
- Store away from heat.

INCOMPATIBILITIES
All I.V. drugs and solutions, except normal saline solution.

ACTION
Directly replaces deficient clotting factor.

Route	Onset	Peak	Duration
I.V.	Immediate	10–30 min	Unknown

Half-life: 20 to 25 hours.

ADVERSE REACTIONS
CNS: headache, *transient fever, chills.*
CV: ***thromboembolic reactions, MI, DIC, pulmonary embolism,*** changes in blood pressure, *flushing.*
GI: nausea, vomiting.
Skin: urticaria.
Other: *tingling.*

INTERACTIONS
Drug-drug. *Aminocaproic acid:* May increase risk of thrombosis. Avoid using together.

EFFECTS ON LAB TEST RESULTS
None reported.

CONTRAINDICATIONS & CAUTIONS
- Mononine is contraindicated in patients hypersensitive to murine (mouse) protein.
- Use cautiously in neonates and infants because of susceptibility to hepatitis, which may be transmitted with factor.

NURSING CONSIDERATIONS
- Give hepatitis A and B vaccines before giving factor.
- Observe patient for allergic reactions and monitor vital signs regularly.
- Observe patient closely for signs and symptoms of thromboembolic events.
- Risk of hepatitis must be weighed against risk of not receiving drug.
- Risk of HIV transmission is extremely low because of manufacturing process.

PATIENT TEACHING
- Explain use and administration of factor to patient and family.
- Tell patient to report adverse reactions promptly and to stop using drug if they occur.
- Advise patient to report chest tightness, wheezing, respiratory distress, cough, or low blood pressure.

plasma protein fractions
Plasmanate, Plasma-Plex, Plasmatein, Protenate

Pharmacologic class: plasma protein
Pregnancy risk category C

AVAILABLE FORMS
Injection: 5%(50 mg/ml) solution in 50-ml, 250-ml, 500-ml vials

INDICATIONS & DOSAGES
➤ Shock
Adults: Varies with patient's condition and response, but usual dose is 250 to 500 ml I.V. (12.5 to 25 g protein), usually no faster than 10 ml/minute.
Infants and children: 6.6 to 33 ml/kg (0.33 to 1.65 g/kg of protein) I.V., 5 to 10 ml/minute.
➤ Hypoproteinemia
Adults: 1,000 to 1,500 ml I.V. daily. Maximum infusion rate is 5 to 8 ml/minute.

I.V. ADMINISTRATION
- Check expiration date before using. Don't use solutions that are cloudy, contain sediment, or have been frozen. Discard solutions in containers that have been open for longer than 4 hours because solution contains no preservatives.

• Don't give more than 250 g or 5,000 ml in 48 hours.
• If patient is dehydrated, give additional fluids either P.O. or I.V.

INCOMPATIBILITIES
Protein hydrolysates, solutions containing alcohol, norepinephrine bitartrate.

ACTION
Supplies colloid to the blood and expands plasma volume. Primary constituent is albumin.

Route	Onset	Peak	Duration
I.V.	Immediate	Immediate	Unknown

Half-life: Unknown.

ADVERSE REACTIONS
CNS: headache, fever.
CV: hypotension, ***vascular overload,*** tachycardia, flushing.
GI: nausea, vomiting, hypersalivation.
Musculoskeletal: back pain.
Respiratory: dyspnea, ***pulmonary edema.***
Skin: rash, erythema.
Other: chills.

INTERACTIONS
None significant.

EFFECTS ON LAB TEST RESULTS
None reported.

CONTRAINDICATIONS & CAUTIONS
• Contraindicated in patients with severe anemia or heart failure and in those undergoing cardiac bypass.
• Use cautiously in patients with hepatic or renal failure, low cardiac reserve, or restricted sodium intake.

NURSING CONSIDERATIONS
• Hypotension risk is greater when infusion rate exceeds 10 ml/minute.
• Monitor blood pressure. Be prepared to slow or stop infusion if hypotension suddenly occurs. Vital signs should return to normal gradually; assess them hourly.
• Watch for signs of vascular overload (heart failure or pulmonary edema).
• ***Alert:*** Watch for hemorrhage or shock after surgery or injury. A rapid increase in blood pressure may cause bleeding that isn't apparent at lower pressures.
• Report decreased urine output.
• Drug contains 130 to 160 mEq of sodium per liter.

PATIENT TEACHING
• Explain use of drug to patient and family.
• Tell patient to report adverse reactions promptly.

66

Thrombolytic enzymes

alteplase
drotrecogin alfa
reteplase, recombinant
streptokinase
tenecteplase
urokinase

SAFETY ALERT!

alteplase (tissue plasminogen activator, recombinant; t-PA)

Actilyse‡, Activase, Cathflo Activase

Pharmacologic class: enzyme
Pregnancy risk category C

AVAILABLE FORMS

Cathflo Activase injection: 2-mg single-patient vials
Injection: 50-mg (29 million international units), 100-mg (58 million international units) vials

INDICATIONS & DOSAGES

➤ **Lysis of thrombi obstructing coronary arteries in acute MI**
3-hour infusion
Adults who weigh 65 kg (143 lb) or more: 100 mg by I.V. infusion over 3 hours, as follows: 60 mg in first hour, 6 to 10 mg of which is given as a bolus over first 1 to 2 minutes. Then 20 mg/hour infused for 2 hours.
Adults who weigh less than 65 kg: Give 1.25 mg/kg in a similar fashion (60% in first hour, 10% of which is given as a bolus; then 20% of total dose per hour for 2 hours.
Accelerated infusion
Adults who weigh more than 67 kg (147 lb): 100 mg total dose. Give 15 mg I.V. bolus over 1 to 2 minutes, followed by 50 mg infused over the next 30 minutes; then 35 mg infused over the next hour.
Adults who weigh 67 kg or less: 15 mg I.V. bolus over 1 to 2 minutes, followed by 0.75 mg/kg (not to exceed 50 mg) infused over the next 30 minutes; then 0.5 mg/kg (not to exceed 35 mg) infused over the next hour.

➤ **To manage acute massive pulmonary embolism**
Adults: 100 mg by I.V. infusion over 2 hours. Begin heparin at end of infusion when PTT or thrombin time returns to twice normal or less. Don't exceed 100-mg dose. Higher doses may increase risk of intracranial bleeding.

➤ **Acute ischemic stroke**
Adults: 0.9 mg/kg by I.V. infusion over 1 hour with 10% of total dose given as an initial I.V. bolus over 1 minute. Maximum total dose is 90 mg.

➤ **To restore function to central venous access devices**
Cathflo Activase
Adults and children older than age 2: For patients who weigh more than 30 kg (66 lb), instill 2 mg in 2 ml sterile water into catheter. For patients who weigh 10 kg (22 lb) to 30 kg, instill 110% of the internal lumen volume of the catheter, not to exceed 2 mg in 2 ml sterile water. After 30 minutes of dwell time, assess catheter function by aspirating blood. If function is restored, aspirate 4 to 5 ml of blood to remove drug and residual clot, and gently irrigate the catheter with normal saline solution. If catheter function isn't restored after 120 minutes, instill a second dose.

➤ **Lysis of arterial occlusion in a peripheral vessel or bypass graft♦**
Adults: 0.05 to 0.1 mg/kg/hour infused intra-arterially for 1 to 8 hours.

I.V. ADMINISTRATION

- Immediately before use, reconstitute solution with unpreserved sterile water for injection. Check manufacturer's labeling for specific information.
- Don't use 50-mg vial if vacuum isn't present; 100-mg vials don't have a vacuum.
- Using an 18G needle, direct stream of sterile water at lyophilized cake. Don't shake.

- Slight foaming is common. Let it settle before giving drug. Solution should be colorless or pale yellow.
- Drug may be given reconstituted (at 1 mg/ml) or diluted with an equal volume of normal saline solution or D_5W to yield 0.5 mg/ml.
- Don't add other drugs to the infusion.
- Give drug using a controlled infusion device.
- Discard any unused drug after 8 hours.

Cathflo Activase

- Assess the cause of catheter dysfunction before using drug. Possible causes of occlusion include catheter malposition, mechanical failure, constriction by a suture, and lipid deposits or drug precipitates in the catheter lumen. Don't try to suction the catheter because you risk damaging the vessel wall or collapsing a soft-walled catheter.
- Reconstitute Cathflo Activase with 2.2 ml sterile water to yield 1 mg/ml. Dissolve completely to produce a colorless to pale yellow solution.
- Don't use excessive pressure while instilling drug into catheter; doing so could rupture the catheter or expel a clot into circulation.
- Solution is stable up to 8 hours at room temperature.

INCOMPATIBILITIES

None reported, but don't mix with other drugs.

ACTION

Binds to fibrin in a thrombus and locally converts plasminogen to plasmin, which starts local fibrinolysis.

Route	Onset	Peak	Duration
I.V.	Unknown	Unknown	Unknown

Half-life: Less than 10 minutes.

ADVERSE REACTIONS

CNS: ***cerebral hemorrhage,*** fever.
CV: ***arrhythmias, venous thrombosis,*** hypotension, edema.
GI: ***GI bleeding (Cathflo Activase),*** nausea, vomiting.
Hematologic: ***spontaneous bleeding.***
Other: ***cholesterol embolization, anaphylaxis, sepsis (Cathflo Activase),*** bleeding at puncture sites, hypersensitivity reactions.

INTERACTIONS

Drug-drug. *Aspirin,* ***clopidogrel,*** *dipyridamole, drugs affecting platelet activity (abciximab), heparin, warfarin anticoagulants:* May increase risk of bleeding. Monitor patient carefully.
Nitroglycerin: May decrease alteplase antigen level. Avoid using together. If use together is unavoidable, use the lowest effective dose of nitroglycerin.

EFFECTS ON LAB TEST RESULTS

- May alter coagulation and fibrinolytic test results.

CONTRAINDICATIONS & CAUTIONS

- Contraindicated in patients with active internal bleeding, intracranial neoplasm, arteriovenous malformation, aneurysm, severe uncontrolled hypertension, or history or current evidence of intracranial hemorrhage, suspicion of subarachnoid hemorrhage, or seizure at onset of stroke when used for acute ischemic stroke.
- Contraindicated in patients with history of stroke, intraspinal or intracranial trauma or surgery within 2 months, or known bleeding diathesis.
- Use cautiously in patients having major surgery within 10 days (when bleeding is difficult to control because of its location); organ biopsy; trauma (including cardiopulmonary resuscitation); GI or GU bleeding; cerebrovascular disease; systolic pressure of 180 mm Hg or higher or diastolic pressure of 110 mm Hg or higher; mitral stenosis, atrial fibrillation, or other conditions that may lead to left heart thrombus; acute pericarditis or subacute bacterial endocarditis; hemostatic defects caused by hepatic or renal impairment; septic thrombophlebitis; or diabetic hemorrhagic retinopathy.
- Use cautiously in patients receiving anticoagulants, in patients age 75 and older, and during pregnancy and the first 10 days postpartum.

NURSING CONSIDERATIONS

- ***Alert:*** When used for acute ischemic stroke, give drug within 3 hours after

symptoms occur and only when intracranial bleeding has been ruled out.
- Drug may be given to menstruating women.
- To recanalize occluded coronary arteries and to improve heart function, begin treatment as soon as possible after symptoms start.
- Anticoagulant and antiplatelet therapy is commonly started during or after treatment, to decrease risk of another thrombosis.
- Monitor vital signs and neurologic status carefully. Keep patient on strict bed rest.
- Coronary thrombolysis is linked with arrhythmias caused by reperfusion of ischemic myocardium. Such arrhythmias don't differ from those commonly linked with MI. Have antiarrhythmics readily available, and carefully monitor ECG.
- Avoid invasive procedures during thrombolytic therapy. Closely monitor patient for signs of internal bleeding, and frequently check all puncture sites. Bleeding is the most common adverse effect and may occur internally and at external puncture sites.
- If uncontrollable bleeding occurs, stop infusion (and heparin) and notify prescriber.
- Avoid I.M. injections.

PATIENT TEACHING
- Explain use and administration of drug to patient and family.
- Tell patient to report adverse reactions promptly.

drotrecogin alfa (activated)
Xigris

Pharmacologic class: recombinant human activated protein C
Pregnancy risk category C

AVAILABLE FORMS
Injection: 5-mg vial, 20-mg vial

INDICATIONS & DOSAGES
➤ **To reduce the risk of death in patients with severe sepsis from acute organ dysfunction**
Adults: 24 mcg/kg/hour I.V. infusion for a total of 96 hours.

I.V. ADMINISTRATION
- Avoid exposing drug to heat or direct sunlight.
- Use aseptic technique during preparation.
- Reconstitute 5-mg vial with 2.5 ml or 20-mg vial with 10 ml sterile water for injection. Swirl vial gently until powder is completely dissolved. Don't invert or shake vial.
- Use reconstituted solution immediately.
- Dilute with sterile normal saline for injection by adding drug to infusion bag. Direct the stream to the side of the bag to avoid agitating solution.
- When using an infusion pump, dilute drug to between 100 mcg/ml and 200 mcg/ml.
- When using a syringe pump, dilute drug to between 100 mcg/ml and 1,000 mcg/ml.
- Gently invert the infusion bag to mix.
- Don't transport the infusion bag between locations using a mechanical delivery system.
- Inspect solution for particulates and discoloration before giving drug.
- If drug is diluted to less than 200 mcg/ml and flow rate is less than 5 ml/hour, prime the infusion set for about 15 minutes at 5 ml/hour.
- Give through a dedicated I.V. line or lumen of a multilumen central venous catheter. The only other solutions that can be given through the same line are normal saline solution, lactated Ringer's injection, D_5W, or dextrose in saline mixtures.
- If the infusion is interrupted, restart at the 24-mcg/kg/hour infusion rate.
- Complete infusion within 12 hours after preparing solution.
- Store in refrigerator at 35° to 46° F (2° to 8° C). Don't freeze.
- If needed, reconstituted vial may be stored at 59° to 86° F (15° to 30° C) for up to 3 hours.

INCOMPATIBILITIES
Other I.V. drugs.

ACTION
May produce dose-dependent reductions in D-dimer and interleukin (IL)-6. Activated protein C exerts an antithrombotic effect by inhibiting factors Va and VIIIa.

Route	Onset	Peak	Duration
I.V.	Immediate	Unknown	Unknown

Half-life: Unknown.

ADVERSE REACTIONS
Hematologic: ***hemorrhage.***

INTERACTIONS
Drug-drug. *Drugs that affect hemostasis:* May increase risk of bleeding. Use together cautiously.

EFFECTS ON LAB TEST RESULTS
- May prolong PT and PTT.

CONTRAINDICATIONS & CAUTIONS
- Contraindicated in patients hypersensitive to drug or any of its components, those with active internal bleeding, and those who have had hemorrhagic stroke in the past 3 months or intracranial or intraspinal surgery in the past 2 months.
- Contraindicated in patients with severe head trauma, trauma with increased risk of life-threatening bleeding, an epidural catheter, intracranial neoplasm or mass lesion, or cerebral herniation.
- ***Alert:*** Use only after assessing the risk versus benefit in patients with single organ dysfunction and recent surgery because these patients may not be at a high risk of death.
- Use cautiously in patients taking other drugs that affect hemostasis such as heparin (at least 15 units/kg/hour) and in those with a platelet count less than 30,000 × 10^6/L (even if the platelet count is increased after transfusions) or an INR greater than 3.
- Use cautiously in patients who have had GI bleeding in the past 6 weeks; thrombolytic therapy in the past 3 days; oral anticoagulants, glycoprotein IIb/IIIa inhibitors, or aspirin (more than 650 mg/day) or other platelet inhibitors in the past week; ischemic stroke in the past 3 months; or intracranial arteriovenous malformation or aneurysm, bleeding diathesis, chronic severe hepatic disease, or any condition in which bleeding poses a significant hazard or would be difficult to manage because of its location.

NURSING CONSIDERATIONS
- Monitor patient closely for bleeding. Notify prescriber if bleeding occurs.
- Stop drug 2 hours before an invasive surgical procedure. After hemostasis has been achieved, drug may be restarted 12 hours after major invasive procedure or immediately after uncomplicated less invasive procedure.
- Because drug has minimal effect on the PT, this value can be used to monitor the patient's coagulopathy status.

PATIENT TEACHING
- Inform patient of the potential adverse reactions.
- Instruct patient to promptly report signs of bleeding.
- Advise patient that bleeding may occur for up to 28 days after treatment.

SAFETY ALERT!

reteplase, recombinant
Retavase

Pharmacologic class: tissue plasminogen activator
Pregnancy risk category C

AVAILABLE FORMS
Injection: 10.4 units (18.1 mg)/vial. Supplied in a kit with components for reconstitution for two single-use vials

INDICATIONS & DOSAGES
➤ To manage acute MI
Adults: Double-bolus injection of 10 + 10 units. Give each bolus I.V. over 2 minutes. If complications, such as serious bleeding or anaphylactoid reaction, don't occur after first bolus, give second bolus 30 minutes after start of first.

I.V. ADMINISTRATION
- Reconstitute drug according to manufacturer's instructions using items provided

in kit and sterile water for injection, without preservatives. Make sure reconstituted solution is colorless; resulting concentration is 1 unit/ml. If foaming occurs, let vial stand for several minutes. Inspect for precipitation. Use within 4 hours of reconstitution; discard unused portions.
• Drug is given I.V. as a double-bolus injection. If bleeding or anaphylactoid reaction occurs after first bolus, notify prescriber; second bolus may be withheld.

INCOMPATIBILITIES
Other I.V. drugs.

ACTION
Enhances cleavage of plasminogen to generate plasmin, which leads to fibrinolysis.

Route	Onset	Peak	Duration
I.V.	Unknown	Unknown	Unknown

Half-life: 13 to 16 minutes.

ADVERSE REACTIONS
CNS: ***intracranial hemorrhage.***
CV: ***arrhythmias, cholesterol embolization, hemorrhage.***
GI: ***hemorrhage.***
GU: hematuria.
Hematologic: ***bleeding tendency,*** anemia.
Other: bleeding at puncture sites, ***hypersensitivity reaction.***

INTERACTIONS
Drug-drug. *Heparin, oral anticoagulants, platelet inhibitors (abciximab, aspirin, dipyridamole, eptifibatide, tirofiban):* May increase risk of bleeding. Use together cautiously.

EFFECTS ON LAB TEST RESULTS
• May increase PT, PTT, and INR.
• May alter coagulation study results.

CONTRAINDICATIONS & CAUTIONS
• Contraindicated in patients with active internal bleeding, known bleeding diathesis, history of stroke, recent intracranial or intraspinal surgery or trauma, severe uncontrolled hypertension, intracranial neoplasm, arteriovenous malformation, or aneurysm.
• Use cautiously in patients with previous puncture of noncompressible vessels; in those with recent (within 10 days) major surgery, obstetric delivery, organ biopsy, GI or GU bleeding, or trauma; in those with cerebrovascular disease, systolic blood pressure 180 mm Hg or higher or diastolic pressure 110 mm Hg or higher, and conditions that may lead to left heart thrombus, including mitral stenosis, acute pericarditis, subacute bacterial endocarditis, and hemostatic defects.
• Use cautiously in those with diabetic hemorrhagic retinopathy, septic thrombophlebitis, and other conditions in which bleeding would be difficult to manage.
• Use cautiously in patients age 75 and older and in breast-feeding women.

NURSING CONSIDERATIONS
• Drug remains active in vitro and can lead to degradation of fibrinogen in sample, changing coagulation study results. Collect blood samples with chloromethylketone at 2-micromolar concentrations.
• Drug may be given to menstruating women.
• Carefully monitor ECG during treatment. Coronary thrombolysis may cause arrhythmias linked with reperfusion. Be prepared to treat bradycardia or ventricular irritability.
• Closely monitor patient for bleeding. Avoid I.M. injections, invasive procedures, and nonessential handling of patient. Bleeding is the most common adverse reaction and may occur internally or at external puncture sites. If local measures don't control serious bleeding, stop anticoagulant and notify prescriber. Withhold second bolus of reteplase.
• Potency is expressed in units specific to reteplase and isn't comparable with other thrombolytics.
• Avoid use of noncompressible pressure sites during therapy. If an arterial puncture is needed, use an arm vessel that can be compressed manually. Apply pressure for at least 30 minutes; then apply a pressure dressing. Check site frequently.

PATIENT TEACHING
• Explain use and administration of drug to patient and family.

• Tell patient to report adverse reactions immediately.

SAFETY ALERT!

streptokinase
Streptase

Pharmacologic class: plasminogen activator
Pregnancy risk category C

AVAILABLE FORMS
Injection: 250,000 international units; 750,000 international units; 1.5 million international units in vials for reconstitution

INDICATIONS & DOSAGES
➤ Arteriovenous-cannula occlusion
Adults: 250,000 international units in 2 ml I.V. solution by I.V. pump infusion into each occluded limb of the cannula over 25 to 35 minutes. Clamp off cannula for 2 hours. Then aspirate contents of cannula, flush with normal saline solution, and reconnect.
➤ Venous thrombosis, pulmonary embolism, arterial thrombosis, and embolism
Adults: Loading dose is 250,000 international units by I.V. infusion over 30 minutes. Sustaining dose is 100,000 international units/hour I.V. infusion for 72 hours for deep vein thrombosis and 100,000 international units/hour over 24 to 72 hours by I.V. infusion pump for pulmonary embolism and arterial thrombosis or embolism.
➤ Lysis of coronary artery thrombi following acute MI
Adults: Infuse 1.5 million international units I.V. over 30 to 60 minutes.

I.V. ADMINISTRATION
• Reconstitute drug in each vial with 5 ml of normal saline solution for injection or D_5W solution. Further dilute to 45 ml (if needed, total volume may be increased to 500 ml in a glass or 50 ml in a plastic container). Don't shake; roll gently to mix. Solution may precipitate after reconstituting; discard if large amounts are present.
• Filter solution with 0.8-micron or larger filter.
• Refrigerate and use within 8 hours.
• Use an infusion pump to start a continuous infusion of heparin 1 to 4 hours after stopping streptokinase. Starting heparin 12 hours after intracoronary streptokinase may minimize bleeding risk.
• Store powder at room temperature.

INCOMPATIBILITIES
Dextrans. Don't mix with other drugs or give other drugs through the same I.V. line.

ACTION
Activates plasminogen in two steps. Plasminogen and streptokinase form a complex that exposes the plasminogen-activating site; plasminogen is then converted to plasmin by cleavage of the peptide bond, which leads to fibrinolysis.

Route	Onset	Peak	Duration
I.V.	Immediate	20 min–2 hr	4–24 hr

Half-life: First phase, 18 minutes; second phase, 83 minutes.

ADVERSE REACTIONS
CNS: polyradiculoneuropathy, headache, *fever.*
CV: ***reperfusion arrhythmias,*** *hypotension,* vasculitis, flushing.
EENT: periorbital edema.
GI: nausea.
Hematologic: ***bleeding,*** moderately decreased hematocrit.
Respiratory: minor breathing difficulty, ***bronchospasm, pulmonary edema.***
Skin: urticaria, pruritus.
Other: phlebitis at injection site, hypersensitivity reactions, ***anaphylaxis,*** delayed hypersensitivity reactions, ***angioedema.***

INTERACTIONS
Drug-drug. *Anticoagulants:* May increase risk of bleeding. Monitor patient closely.
Antifibrinolytic drugs (such as aminocaproic acid): May inhibit and reverse streptokinase activity. Avoid using together.
Aspirin, dipyridamole, drugs affecting platelet activity (abciximab, eptifibatide, tirofiban), indomethacin, NSAIDs, phenylbutazone: May increase risk of bleeding. Monitor patient closely.

EFFECTS ON LAB TEST RESULTS

- May decrease hematocrit.
- May increase PT, PTT, and INR.

CONTRAINDICATIONS & CAUTIONS

- Contraindicated in patients with ulcerative wounds, active internal bleeding, recent stroke, recent trauma with possible internal injuries, visceral or intracranial malignant neoplasms, ulcerative colitis, diverticulitis, severe hypertension, acute or chronic hepatic or renal insufficiency, uncontrolled hypocoagulation, chronic pulmonary disease with cavitation, subacute bacterial endocarditis or rheumatic valvular disease, previous severe allergic reaction to streptokinase, or recent cerebral embolism, thrombosis, or hemorrhage.
- Contraindicated within 10 days after intra-arterial diagnostic procedure or any surgery, including liver or kidney biopsy, lumbar puncture, thoracentesis, paracentesis, or extensive or multiple cutdowns.
- Contraindicated with I.M. injections and other invasive procedures.
- Use cautiously when treating arterial embolism that originates from left side of heart because of danger of cerebral infarction.

NURSING CONSIDERATIONS

- Drug may be given to menstruating women.
- Only prescribers with experience managing thrombotic disease should give drug and only where clinical and laboratory monitoring can be performed.
- Before using drug to clear an occluded AV cannula, try flushing with heparinized saline solution.
- Keep aminocaproic acid available to treat bleeding and corticosteroids to treat allergic reactions.
- Before starting therapy, draw blood for coagulation studies, hematocrit, platelet count, and type and cross-matching. Rate of infusion depends on thrombin time and drug resistance.
- To check for hypersensitivity in acutely ill patients or patients with known allergies, give 100 international units I.D.; a wheal-and-flare response within 20 minutes means patient is probably allergic. Monitor vital signs frequently.
- For patient who has had a streptococcal infection or has been treated with streptokinase or anistreplase in the last 2 years, use a different thrombolytic.
- Combined therapy with low-dose aspirin (162.5 mg) or dipyridamole has improved short- and long-term results.
- Monitor patient for excessive bleeding every 15 minutes for first hour, every 30 minutes for second through eighth hours, and then every 4 hours. If bleeding is evident, stop therapy and notify prescriber. Pretreatment with heparin or drugs that affect platelets causes high risk of bleeding but may improve long-term results.
- Monitor pulse, color, and sensation of arms and legs every hour.
- Keep involved limb in straight alignment to prevent bleeding from infusion site.
- Monitor blood pressure closely.
- Avoid unnecessary handling of patient; pad side rails. Bruising is more likely during therapy.
- Keep a laboratory flow sheet on patient's chart to monitor PTT, PT, thrombin time, hemoglobin level, and hematocrit. Monitor vital signs and neurologic status.
- Avoid I.M. injection. Keep venipuncture sites to a minimum; use pressure dressing on puncture sites for at least 15 minutes.
- ***Alert:*** Watch for signs of hypersensitivity and notify prescriber immediately if any occur. Antihistamines or corticosteroids may be used for mild allergic reactions. If a severe reaction occurs, stop infusion immediately and notify prescriber.
- Thrombolytic therapy in patients with acute MI may decrease infarct size, improve ventricular function, and decrease risk of heart failure. For optimal effect, streptokinase must be given within 6 hours after symptoms start.

PATIENT TEACHING

- Explain use and administration of drug to patient and family.
- Tell patient to promptly report adverse reactions, such as bleeding and bruising.

SAFETY ALERT!

tenecteplase
TNKase

Pharmacologic class: recombinant tissue plasminogen activator
Pregnancy risk category C

AVAILABLE FORMS
Injection: 50 mg

INDICATIONS & DOSAGES
➤To reduce risk of death from an acute MI
Adults who weigh 90 kg (198 lb) or more: 50 mg (10 ml) by I.V. bolus over 5 seconds.
Adults who weigh 80 to 89 kg (176 to 196 lb): 45 mg (9 ml) by I.V. bolus over 5 seconds.
Adults who weigh 70 to 79 kg (154 to 174 lb): 40 mg (8 ml) by I.V. bolus over 5 seconds.
Adults who weigh 60 to 69 kg (132 to 152 lb): 35 mg (7 ml) by I.V. bolus over 5 seconds.
Adults who weigh less than 60 kg (132 lb): 30 mg (6 ml) by I.V. bolus over 5 seconds.

I.V. ADMINISTRATION
- Use syringe prefilled with sterile water for injection, and inject the entire contents into drug vial. Gently swirl solution once mixed. Don't shake. Visually inspect product for particulate matter before administration.
- Draw up the appropriate dose needed from the reconstituted vial with the syringe and discard any unused portion. Give drug immediately, or refrigerate and use within 8 hours.
- Give drug in a designated line. Flush dextrose-containing lines with normal saline solution before administration.
- Give the drug rapidly over 5 seconds.

INCOMPATIBILITIES
Solutions containing dextrose.

ACTION
A human tissue plasminogen activator that binds to fibrin and converts plasminogen to plasmin. The specificity to fibrin decreases systemic activation of plasminogen and the resulting breakdown of circulating fibrinogen.

Route	Onset	Peak	Duration
I.V.	Immediate	Immediate	Unknown

Half-life: 20 minutes to 2 hours.

ADVERSE REACTIONS
CNS: ***stroke, intracranial hemorrhage.***
CV: ***arrhythmias, cardiogenic shock, myocardial reinfarction, thrombosis, embolism.***
EENT: pharyngeal bleeding, epistaxis.
GI: ***GI bleeding.***
GU: hematuria.
Respiratory: ***pulmonary edema.***
Skin: *hematoma.*
Other: bleeding at puncture site, ***hypersensitivity reactions.***

INTERACTIONS
Drug-drug. *Anticoagulants (heparin, vitamin K antagonists), drugs that alter platelet function (acetylsalicylic acid, dipyridamole, glycoprotein IIb/IIIa inhibitors, NSAIDs):* May increase risk of bleeding when used before, during, or after tenecteplase use. Use together cautiously.

EFFECTS ON LAB TEST RESULTS
- May increase PT, PTT, and INR.

CONTRAINDICATIONS & CAUTIONS
- Contraindicated in patients with active internal bleeding; history of stroke; intracranial or intraspinal surgery or trauma during previous 2 months; intracranial neoplasm, aneurysm, or arteriovenous malformation; severe uncontrolled hypertension; or bleeding diathesis.
- Use cautiously in patients who have had recent major surgery (such as coronary artery bypass graft), organ biopsy, obstetric delivery, or previous puncture of noncompressible vessels.
- Use cautiously in pregnant women, patients age 75 and older, and patients with recent trauma, recent GI or GU bleeding, high risk of left ventricular thrombus, acute pericarditis, systolic blood pressure 180 mm Hg or higher or diastolic pressure 110 mm Hg or higher, severe hepatic dysfunction, hemostatic defects, subacute

bacterial endocarditis, septic thrombophlebitis, diabetic hemorrhagic retinopathy, or cerebrovascular disease.

NURSING CONSIDERATIONS
- Begin therapy as soon as possible after onset of MI symptoms.
- Avoid noncompressible arterial punctures and internal jugular and subclavian venous punctures. Minimize all arterial and venous punctures during treatment.
- Avoid I.M. use.
- Give heparin but not in the same I.V. line.
- Monitor patient for bleeding. If serious bleeding occurs, stop heparin and antiplatelet drugs immediately.
- ***Alert:*** Use exact patient weight for dosage. An overestimation in patient weight can lead to significant increase in bleeding or intracerebral hemorrhage.
- Monitor ECG for reperfusion arrhythmias.
- A life-threatening cholesterol embolism is rarely caused by thrombolytics. Signs and symptoms may include livedo reticularis (blue toe syndrome), acute renal failure, gangrenous digits, hypertension, pancreatitis, MI, cerebral infarction, spinal cord infarction, retinal artery occlusion, bowel infarction, and rhabdomyolysis.

PATIENT TEACHING
- Advise patient about proper dental care to avoid excessive gum bleeding.
- Tell patient to report any adverse effects or excessive bleeding immediately.
- Explain to patient and family about the use of drug.

SAFETY ALERT!

urokinase
Abbokinase

Pharmacologic class: enzyme
Pregnancy risk category B

AVAILABLE FORMS
Injection: 250,000 international units/vial

INDICATIONS & DOSAGES
➤ Lysis of acute massive pulmonary embolism and of pulmonary embolism with unstable hemodynamics

Adults: For I.V. infusion only by constant infusion pump. For priming dose, give 4,400 international units/kg with normal saline solution or D_5 W solution, over 10 minutes, followed by 4,400 international units/kg/hour for 12 hours. Then give continuous I.V. infusion of heparin and oral anticoagulants.

➤ Lysis of coronary artery thrombi following an acute MI♦

Adults: After bolus dose of heparin ranging from 2,500 to 10,000 units, infuse 6,000 international units/minute urokinase into occluded artery for up to 2 hours. Average total dose is 500,000 international units. Start drug within 6 hours after symptoms start.

➤ Venous catheter occlusion♦

Adults: Instill 5,000 international units into occluded line.

I.V. ADMINISTRATION
- Reconstitute according to manufacturer's directions using sterile water for injection. Gently roll vial; don't shake. Don't use bacteriostatic water for injection to reconstitute; it contains preservatives. Dilute further with normal saline solution or D_5W solution before infusion. Filter urokinase solutions through a 0.45-micron or smaller cellulose-membrane filter before administration. Discard unused solution. Total volume of fluid given by I.V. infusion shouldn't exceed 200 ml.
- Heparin by continuous infusion may be started concurrently or within 3 to 4 hours after urokinase has been stopped to prevent recurrent thrombosis.

INCOMPATIBILITIES
Other I.V. drugs. Give through separate I.V. line.

ACTION
Activates plasminogen to plasmin by directly cleaving peptide bonds at two different sites, causing fibrinolysis.

Route	Onset	Peak	Duration
I.V.	Immediate	20 min–4 hr	12–24 hr

Half-life: 10 to 20 minutes.

ADVERSE REACTIONS

CNS: fever.
CV: ***reperfusion arrhythmias,*** tachycardia, transient hypotension or hypertension.
GI: nausea, vomiting.
Hematologic: ***bleeding.***
Respiratory: bronchospasm, minor breathing difficulties.
Skin: phlebitis at injection site, rash.
Other: anaphylaxis, chills.

INTERACTIONS

Drug-drug. *Anticoagulants, aspirin, dipyridamole, indomethacin, NSAIDs, phenylbutazone, other drugs affecting platelet activity:* May increase risk of bleeding. Monitor patient.

EFFECTS ON LAB TEST RESULTS

- May decrease hematocrit.
- May increase PT, PTT, and INR.

CONTRAINDICATIONS & CAUTIONS

- Contraindicated in patients with active internal bleeding, history of stroke, aneurysm, arteriovenous malformation, known bleeding diathesis, recent trauma with possible internal injuries, visceral or intracranial malignancy, ulcerative colitis, diverticulitis, severe hypertension, hemostatic defects including those secondary to severe hepatic or renal insufficiency, uncontrolled hypocoagulation, chronic pulmonary disease with cavitation, subacute bacterial endocarditis or rheumatic valvular disease, and recent cerebral embolism, thrombosis, or hemorrhage.
- Contraindicated within 10 days after intra-arterial diagnostic procedure or surgery (liver or kidney biopsy, lumbar puncture, thoracentesis, paracentesis, or extensive or multiple cutdowns) or within 2 months after intracranial or intraspinal surgery.
- Contraindicated during pregnancy and first 10 days postpartum.
- I.M. injections and other invasive procedures are contraindicated during urokinase therapy.

NURSING CONSIDERATIONS

- Have aminocaproic acid and cross-matched and -typed RBCs, whole blood, plasma expanders (other than dextran) available for bleeding. Keep corticosteroids, epinephrine, and antihistamines available for allergic reactions.
- Drug may be given to menstruating women.
- Only prescribers with extensive experience in thrombotic disease management should use drug. and only in facilities where clinical and laboratory monitoring can be performed.
- Monitor patient for excessive bleeding every 15 minutes for first hour; every 30 minutes for second through eighth hours; then once every 4 hours. Pretreatment with drugs affecting platelets places patient at high risk of bleeding.
- Monitor pulse, color, and sensation of arms and legs every hour.
- Although risk of hypersensitivity reactions is low, monitor patient.
- Keep a laboratory flow sheet on patient's chart to monitor PTT, PT, thrombin time, hemoglobin level, and hematocrit.
- Monitor vital signs and neurologic status. Don't take blood pressure in legs because doing so could dislodge a clot.
- Keep venipuncture sites to a minimum; use pressure dressing on puncture sites for at least 15 minutes.
- Avoid I.M. injections.
- Keep involved limb in straight alignment to prevent bleeding from infusion site.
- Because bruising is more likely during therapy, avoid unnecessary handling of patient, and pad side rails.
- Rarely, orolingual edema, urticaria, cholesterol embolization, and infusion reactions causing hypoxia, cyanosis, acidosis, and back pain may occur.

PATIENT TEACHING

- Explain use and administration of drug to patient and family.
- Instruct patient to report adverse reactions promptly.

67
Alkylating drugs

busulfan
carboplatin
carmustine
chlorambucil
cisplatin
cyclophosphamide
ifosfamide
lomustine
mechlorethamine hydrochloride
melphalan
melphalan hydrochloride
oxaliplatin
thiotepa

SAFETY ALERT!

busulfan
Busulfex, Myleran

Pharmacologic class: alkyl sulfonate
Pregnancy risk category D

AVAILABLE FORMS
Injection: 6 mg/ml
Tablets: 2 mg

INDICATIONS & DOSAGES
➤Chronic myelocytic (granulocytic) leukemia
Adults: Give 4 to 8 mg P.O. daily until WBC count falls to 15,000/mm^3; stop drug until WBC count rises to 50,000/mm^3, and then resume dosage as before. Or, 4 to 8 mg P.O. daily until WBC count falls to 10,000 to 20,000/mm^3; then reduce daily dose, as needed, to maintain WBC count at this level. Dosage is highly variable; range is 2 mg weekly to 4 mg daily.
Children: Give 0.06 to 0.12 mg/kg daily or 1.8 to 4.6 mg/m^2 daily P.O.; adjust dosage to maintain WBC count at 20,000/mm^3 but never below 10,000/mm^3.
➤Allogenic hematopoietic stem cell transplantation in patients with chronic myelogenous leukemia
Adults: Give 0.8 mg/kg I.V. q 6 hours for 4 days (a total of 16 doses). Give cyclophosphamide 60 mg/kg I.V. over 1 hour daily for 2 days beginning 6 hours after the 16th dose of busulfan injection.
Children who weigh more than 12 kg (26 lbs): Give 0.8 mg/kg I.V. with cyclophosphamide.
Children who weigh 12 kg or less: Give 1.1 mg/kg I.V. with cyclophosphamide.

I.V. ADMINISTRATION
- Follow facility policy when preparing and handling drug. Label as a hazardous drug.
- Dilute drug in either D_5W or normal saline solution to at least 0.5 mg/ml.
- Use the 5-micron nylon filter to withdraw the calculated volume from the ampule. Then use a new needle to inject the drug into the I.V. bag or syringe.
- Invert several times to ensure mixing.
- A central venous catheter must be used.
- Flush the catheter line with 5 ml of D_5W or normal saline solution before and after each infusion.
- Infuse over 2 hours through a central venous catheter using a controlled-infusion device.
- Busulfan solutions are stable 8 hours at room temperature or 12 hours when diluted in normal saline solution and refrigerated. Infusions must be completed within these times.

INCOMPATIBILITIES
Don't mix or give with other I.V. solutions of unknown compatibility.

ACTION
Unknown. Thought to cross-link strands of cellular DNA and interfere with RNA transcription, causing an imbalance of growth that leads to cell death. Not specific to cell cycle.

Route	Onset	Peak	Duration
P.O.	1–2 wk	Unknown	Unknown
I.V.	Unknown	Unknown	Unknown

Half-life: About 2½ hours.

ADVERSE REACTIONS
CNS: *confusion, fever, headache, asthenia, pain, insomnia, anxiety, dizziness, de-*

pression, ***encephalopathy, seizures,*** delirium, agitation, hallucination, lethargy, somnolence.
CV: *edema, chest pain, tachycardia, hypertension, hypotension, vasodilation, heart rhythm abnormalities,* ***heart failure, pericardial effusion, thrombosis,*** cardiomegaly, ECG abnormalities.
EENT: *rhinitis, epistaxis, pharyngitis,* sinusitis, ear disorder, cataracts.
GI: *cheilosis (P.O.), nausea, stomatitis, mucositis, vomiting, anorexia, diarrhea, abdominal pain and enlargement, dyspepsia, constipation, dry mouth, rectal disorder,* ***pancreatitis.***
GU: *oliguria,* dysuria, hematuria, hemorrhagic cystitis.
Hematologic: **GRANULOCYTOPENIA, THROMBOCYTOPENIA, LEUKOPENIA,** *anemia.*
Hepatic: *jaundice,* ***hepatic necrosis,*** hepatomegaly.
Metabolic: *hypomagnesemia, hyperglycemia, hypokalemia, hypocalcemia, hypervolemia, weight gain, hypophosphatemia,* hyponatremia.
Musculoskeletal: *back pain, myalgia, arthralgia.*
Respiratory: *lung disorder, cough, dyspnea,* ***irreversible pulmonary fibrosis, alveolar hemorrhage,*** asthma, atelectasis, pleural effusion hypoxia, hemoptysis.
Skin: *hyperpigmentation, inflammation at injection site, rash, pruritus, alopecia,* exfoliative dermatitis, erythema nodosum, acne, skin discoloration, anhidrosis.
Other: *chills, allergic reaction, hiccup,* ***infection,*** Addison-like wasting syndrome, gynecomastia (P.O.).

INTERACTIONS

Drug-drug. *Acetaminophen, itraconazole:* May decrease busulfan clearance. Use together cautiously.
Anticoagulants, aspirin: May increase risk of bleeding. Avoid using together.
Cyclophosphamide: May increase risk of cardiac tamponade in patients with thalassemia. Monitor patient.
Metronidazole: May increase busulfan toxicity. Avoid using together.
Myelosuppressives: May increase myelosuppression. Monitor patient.
Other cytotoxic agents causing pulmonary injury: May cause additive pulmonary toxicity. Avoid using together.
Phenytoin: May decrease busulfan level. Monitor busulfan level.
Thioguanine: May cause hepatotoxicity, esophageal varices, or portal hypertension. Use together cautiously.

EFFECTS ON LAB TEST RESULTS

- May increase alkaline phosphatase, ALT, bilirubin, BUN, creatinine, and glucose levels. May decrease calcium, hemoglobin, magnesium, phosphorus, potassium, and sodium levels.
- May decrease WBC and platelet counts.

CONTRAINDICATIONS & CAUTIONS

- Contraindicated in patients with chronic myelogenous leukemia resistant to drug and in those with chronic lymphocytic or acute leukemia or in the blastic crisis of chronic myelogenous leukemia.
- Use cautiously in patients recently given other myelosuppressives or radiation treatment and in those with depressed neutrophil or platelet count.
- Use cautiously in patients with history of head trauma or seizures and in those receiving other drugs that lower the seizure threshold because high-dose therapy has been linked to seizures.

NURSING CONSIDERATIONS

- Give antiemetic before first dose of busulfan injection and then on a fixed schedule during therapy; give phenytoin to prevent seizures.
- Therapeutic effects are commonly accompanied by toxicity.
- To prevent bleeding, avoid all I.M. injections when platelet count is less than $50{,}000/mm^3$.
- Monitor patient response (increased appetite and sense of well-being, decreased total WBC count, reduced size of spleen), which usually begins in 1 to 2 weeks.
- Monitor for jaundice and liver function abnormalities in patients receiving high-dose busulfan.
- Anticipate possible blood transfusion during treatment because of cumulative anemia. Patients may receive injections of RBC colony-stimulating factor to pro-

mote RBC production and decrease the need for blood transfusions.

• ***Alert:*** Pulmonary fibrosis may occur as late as 8 months to 10 years after therapy. (Average length of therapy is 4 years.)

PATIENT TEACHING

• Advise patient to watch for signs of infection (fever, sore throat, fatigue) and bleeding (easy bruising, nosebleeds, bleeding gums, tarry stools). Tell patient to take temperature daily.
• Instruct patient to report signs and symptoms of toxicity so dosage can be adjusted. Persistent cough and progressive labored breathing with liquid in the lungs, suggestive of pneumonia, may be caused by drug toxicity.
• Instruct patient to avoid OTC products containing aspirin and NSAIDs.
• Inform patient that drug may cause skin darkening.
• Advise woman of childbearing age to avoid becoming pregnant during therapy. Recommend that she consult prescriber before becoming pregnant.
• Advise patient not to breast-feed during therapy because of risk of toxicity to infant.
• Instruct patient to take drug on empty stomach to decrease nausea and vomiting.
• Because of risk of impotence and sterility, advise men who want to father a child about sperm banking before therapy.

SAFETY ALERT!

carboplatin

Paraplatin, Paraplatin-AQ†

Pharmacologic class: platinum coordination complex
Pregnancy risk category D

AVAILABLE FORMS

Aqueous solution for injection: 50 mg/5 ml, 150 mg/15 ml, 450 mg/45 ml, 600 mg/60 ml
Lyophilized powder for injection: 50-mg, 150-mg, 450-mg vials

INDICATIONS & DOSAGES

➤ **Advanced ovarian cancer**
Adults: 360 mg/m^2 I.V. on day 1 q 4 weeks or 300 mg/m^2 when used with other chemotherapy drugs; doses shouldn't be repeated until platelet count exceeds 100,000/mm^3 and neutrophil count exceeds 2,000/mm^3. Subsequent doses are based on blood counts. Or, refer to package for formula dosing.
Adjust-a-dose: If creatinine clearance is 41 to 59 ml/minute, first dose is 250 mg/m^2. If creatinine clearance is 16 to 40 ml/minute, first dose is 200 mg/m^2. Drug isn't recommended for patients with creatinine clearance of 15 ml/minute or less.

I.V. ADMINISTRATION

• Keep epinephrine, corticosteroids, and antihistamines available when giving carboplatin because anaphylaxis may occur within minutes of administration.
• Preparing and giving parenteral form of drug may be mutagenic, teratogenic, or carcinogenic. Follow facility policy to reduce risks.
• Don't use aluminum needles or I.V. administration sets because drug may precipitate or lose potency.
• For premixed aqueous solution of 10 mg/ml, dilute for infusion with normal saline solution or D_5W to a concentration as low as 0.5 mg/ml.
• For vials of lyophilized powder, reconstitute with sterile water for injection, D_5W, or normal saline. For 50-mg vial, use 5 ml solution; for 150-mg vial, use 15 ml solution; for 450-mg vial, use 45 ml solution to yield a concentration of 10 mg/ml.
• Give drug by continuous or intermittent infusion over at least 15 minutes.
• Store unopened vials at room temperature.
• Once reconstituted and diluted as directed, drug is stable at room temperature for 8 hours.
• Because drug contains no preservatives, discard after 8 hours.

INCOMPATIBILITIES

Amphotericin B cholesteryl sulfate complex, fluorouracil, mesna, sodium bicarbonate.

ACTION

May cross-link strands of cellular DNA and interfere with RNA transcription, causing an imbalance of growth that leads to cell death. Not specific to cell cycle.

Route	Onset	Peak	Duration
I.V.	Unknown	Unknown	Unknown

Half-life: 5 hours.

ADVERSE REACTIONS

CNS: *asthenia,* dizziness, confusion, ***stroke,*** peripheral neuropathy, central neurotoxicity, paresthesia.
CV: ***heart failure, embolism.***
EENT: ototoxicity, visual disturbances.
GI: constipation, diarrhea, *nausea, vomiting,* mucositis, change in taste, stomatitis.
Hematologic: **THROMBOCYTOPENIA,** ***leukopenia,*** **NEUTROPENIA,** anemia, **BONE MARROW SUPPRESSION.**
Skin: alopecia.
Other: hypersensitivity reactions, *pain,* ***anaphylaxis.***

INTERACTIONS

Drug-drug. *Aspirin, NSAIDs:* May increase risk of bleeding. Avoid using together.
Bone marrow suppressants, including radiation therapy: May increase hematologic toxicity. Monitor CBC with differential closely.
Nephrotoxic drugs, especially aminoglycosides and amphotericin B: May enhance nephrotoxicity of carboplatin. Use together cautiously.

EFFECTS ON LAB TEST RESULTS

- May increase alkaline phosphatase, AST, BUN, and creatinine levels. May decrease electrolyte and hemoglobin levels and hematocrit.
- May decrease neutrophil, platelet, RBC, and WBC counts.

CONTRAINDICATIONS & CAUTIONS

- Contraindicated in patients with severe bone marrow suppression or bleeding or with history of hypersensitivity to cisplatin, platinum-containing compounds, or mannitol.

NURSING CONSIDERATIONS

- Determine electrolyte, creatinine, and BUN levels; CBC; and creatinine clearance before first infusion and before each course of treatment.
- Monitor CBC and platelet count frequently during therapy and, when indicated, until recovery. Lowest WBC and platelet counts usually occur by day 21. Levels usually return to baseline by day 28. Don't repeat unless platelet count exceeds 100,000/mm^3.
- Bone marrow suppression may be more severe in patients with creatinine clearance below 60 ml/minute; adjust dosage.
- ***Alert:*** Carefully check ordered dose against laboratory test results. Only one increase in dosage is recommended. Subsequent doses shouldn't exceed 125% of starting dose.
- Therapeutic effects are commonly accompanied by toxicity.
- Drug has less nephrotoxicity and neurotoxicity than cisplatin, but it causes more severe myelosuppression.
- To prevent bleeding, avoid all I.M. injections when platelet count is below 50,000/mm^3.
- Monitor vital signs during infusion.
- Give antiemetic to reduce nausea and vomiting.
- Anticipate blood transfusions during treatment because of cumulative anemia. Patient may receive injections of RBC colony–stimulating factor to promote cell production.
- Patients older than age 65 are at greater risk for neurotoxicity.
- ***Look alike–sound alike:*** Don't confuse carboplatin with cisplatin.

PATIENT TEACHING

- Advise patient of most common adverse reactions: nausea, vomiting, bone marrow suppression, anemia, and reduction in blood platelets.
- Advise patient to watch for signs of infection (fever, sore throat, fatigue) and bleeding (easy bruising, nosebleeds, bleeding gums, tarry stools). Tell patient to take temperature daily.
- Instruct patient to avoid OTC products containing aspirin and NSAIDs.
- Advise women to stop breast-feeding during therapy because of risk of toxicity to infant.
- Because of risk of impotence, sterility, and menstruation cessation, counsel both

men and women of childbearing age before starting therapy. Also recommend that women consult prescriber before becoming pregnant.

SAFETY ALERT!

carmustine (BCNU)
BiCNU, Gliadel Wafer

Pharmacologic class: nitrosourea
Pregnancy risk category D

AVAILABLE FORMS
Injection: 100-mg vial (lyophilized), with a 3-ml vial of absolute alcohol supplied as a diluent
Wafer: 7.7 mg, for intracavitary use

INDICATIONS & DOSAGES
➤ **Brain tumor, Hodgkin lymphoma, malignant lymphoma, multiple myeloma**
Adults: 150 to 200 mg/m^2 I.V. by slow infusion q 6 weeks; may be divided into daily injections of 75 to 100 mg/m^2 on 2 successive days; repeat dose q 6 weeks if platelet count is greater than 100,000/mm^3 and WBC count is greater than 4,000/mm^3.
Adjust-a-dose: Dosage is reduced by 30% when WBC nadir is 2,000 to 2,999/mm^3 and platelet nadir is 25,000 to 74,999/mm^3. Dosage is reduced by 50% when WBC nadir is less than 2,000/mm^3 and platelet nadir is less than 25,000/mm^3.
➤ **Adjunct to surgery to prolong survival in patients with recurrent glioblastoma multiforme for whom surgical resection is indicated**
Adults: 8 wafers placed in the resection cavity if size and shape of cavity allow. If 8 wafers can't be accommodated, use maximum number of wafers allowed. Or, 150 to 200 mg/m^2 I.V. by slow infusion as single dose, repeated q 6 to 8 weeks.
➤ **Cutaneous T-cell lymphoma (mycosis fungoides)** ♦
Adults: Apply 0.05% to 0.4% topical solution or ointment once or twice daily. Usual dose is 10 mg daily applied topically for 6 to 8 weeks. If response is inadequate, after a 6-week rest period, apply 20 mg daily topically for 30 days. For persistent papules or small nodules, give intralesionally at a concentration of 0.1% to 0.2%.
➤ **Adjunct to surgery and radiation in patients with newly diagnosed high-grade malignant glioma**
Adults: 8 wafers placed in the resection cavity if size and shape of cavity allow. If 8 wafers can't be accommodated, use maximum number of wafers allowed.

I.V. ADMINISTRATION
- Preparing and giving parenteral form of drug may be mutagenic, teratogenic, or carcinogenic. Follow facility policy to reduce risks. Wear gloves when handling any form of drug.
- Prepare drug only in glass containers. Solution is unstable in plastic I.V. bags.
- If powder liquefies or appears oily, discard drug because decomposition has occurred.
- To reconstitute, dissolve 100 mg of drug in 3 ml of absolute alcohol provided by manufacturer.
- Dilute solution with 27 ml of sterile water for injection. Resulting solution contains 3.3 mg of carmustine/ml in 10% alcohol.
- For infusion, dilute in normal saline solution or D_5W.
- Don't mix with other drugs during administration.
- Give at least 250 ml over 1 to 2 hours.
- To reduce pain on infusion, dilute further or slow infusion rate.
- Solution may be stored in refrigerator for 24 hours or at room temperature for 8 hours. It may decompose at temperatures above 80° F (27° C).

INCOMPATIBILITIES
Sodium bicarbonate.

ACTION
Inhibits enzymatic reactions involved with DNA synthesis, cross-links strands of cellular DNA, and interferes with RNA transcription, causing an imbalance of growth that leads to cell death. Not specific to cell cycle.

Route	Onset	Peak	Duration
I.V., intracavitary	Unknown	Unknown	Unknown

Half-life: 15 to 30 minutes.

ADVERSE REACTIONS

CNS: ataxia, drowsiness, ***brain edema, seizures.***
EENT: ocular toxicities.
GI: *nausea, vomiting, stomatitis.*
GU: ***nephrotoxicity,*** azotemia, ***renal failure.***
Hematologic: ***cumulative bone marrow suppression, leukopenia, thrombocytopenia, acute leukemia or bone marrow dysplasia,*** anemia.
Hepatic: ***hepatotoxicity.***
Respiratory: ***pulmonary fibrosis.***
Skin: facial flushing, hyperpigmentation.
Other: *intense pain at infusion site from venous spasm,* ***secondary malignancies.***

INTERACTIONS

Drug-drug. *Anticoagulants, aspirin, NSAIDs:* May increase risk of bleeding. Avoid using together.
Cimetidine: May increase carmustine's bone marrow toxicity. Avoid using together.
Digoxin, phenytoin: May decrease levels of these drugs. Monitor patient.
Mitomycin: May increase corneal and conjunctival damage with high doses. Monitor patient.
Myelosuppressives: May increase myelosuppression. Monitor patient.

EFFECTS ON LAB TEST RESULTS

- May increase alkaline phosphatase, AST, bilirubin, hemoglobin, and urine urea levels.
- May decrease platelet and WBC counts.

CONTRAINDICATIONS & CAUTIONS

- Contraindicated in patients hypersensitive to drug.

NURSING CONSIDERATIONS

- Pulmonary toxicity appears to be dose related and may occur 9 days to 15 years after treatment. Obtain pulmonary function tests before and during therapy.
- Bone marrow suppression is delayed with carmustine. Drug shouldn't be given more often than every 6 weeks.
- Give antiemetic before drug to reduce nausea.
- If drug touches skin, wash off thoroughly. Avoid contact with skin because drug will stain skin brown.
- Perform liver, renal function, and pulmonary function tests periodically.
- Monitor CBC with differential. The absolute neutrophil count may be used to better calculate the patient's immunosuppressive state.
- Monitor uric acid level. To prevent hyperuricemia with resulting uric acid nephropathy, allopurinol may be used with adequate hydration.
- Therapeutic levels are commonly toxic.
- Acute leukemia or bone marrow dysplasia may occur after long-term use.
- To prevent bleeding, avoid using I.M. when platelet count is less than 50,000/mm^3.
- Anticipate blood transfusions during treatment because of cumulative anemia. Patient may receive injections of RBC colony-stimulating factor to promote cell production.
- Unopened foil pouches of wafer may be kept at room temperature for a maximum of 6 hours.
- Wafers broken in half may be used; however, discard wafers broken into more than two pieces.

PATIENT TEACHING

- Advise patient about common adverse reactions to drug.
- Tell patient to watch for signs and symptoms of infection (fever, sore throat, fatigue) and bleeding (easy bruising, nosebleeds, bleeding gums, tarry stools). Tell him to take temperature daily.
- Instruct patient to avoid OTC products containing aspirin and NSAIDs.
- Advise women to stop breast-feeding during therapy because of possible risk of toxicity to infant.
- Caution woman of childbearing age to avoid becoming pregnant during therapy. Recommend that she consult prescriber before becoming pregnant.

SAFETY ALERT!

chlorambucil
Leukeran

Pharmacologic class: nitrogen mustard
Pregnancy risk category D

AVAILABLE FORMS
Tablets: 2 mg

INDICATIONS & DOSAGES
➤Chronic lymphocytic leukemia; malignant lymphomas, including lymphosarcoma, giant follicular lymphoma, and Hodgkin lymphoma
Adults: 0.1 to 0.2 mg/kg P.O. daily for 3 to 6 weeks, then adjust for maintenance (usually 4 to 10 mg daily); or, 3 to 6 mg/m^2 P.O. daily.
Children: 0.1 to 0.2 mg/kg P.O. or 4.5 mg/m^2 P.O. daily for 3 to 6 weeks.
Adjust-a-dose: Reduce first dose if given within 4 weeks after a full course of radiation therapy or myelosuppressive drugs, or if pretreatment leukocyte or platelet counts are depressed from bone marrow disease.
➤Macroglobulinemia ♦
Adults: 2 to 10 mg P.O. daily for up to 9 years. Or, 8 mg/m^2 P.O. daily with prednisone for 10 days; repeat q 6 to 8 weeks p.r.n.
➤Nephrotic syndrome ♦
Children: 0.1 to 0.2 mg/kg P.O. daily with prednisone for 8 to 12 weeks.
➤Intractable idiopathic uveitis, Behçet syndrome ♦
Adults: 6 to 12 mg or 0.1 to 0.2 mg/kg P.O. daily for at least 1 year.

ACTION
Cross-links strands of cellular DNA and interferes with RNA transcription, causing an imbalance of growth that leads to cell death. Not specific to cell cycle.

Route	Onset	Peak	Duration
P.O.	Unknown	1 hr	Unknown

Half-life: 2 hours for parent compound; 2½ hours for phenylacetic acid metabolite.

ADVERSE REACTIONS
CNS: ***seizures,*** peripheral neuropathy, tremor, muscle twitching, confusion, agitation, ataxia, flaccid paresis.
GI: *nausea, vomiting,* stomatitis, diarrhea.
GU: *azoospermia, infertility,* sterile cystitis.
Hematologic: ***neutropenia, bone marrow suppression, thrombocytopenia,*** anemia, ***myelosuppression.***
Hepatic: ***hepatotoxicity.***
Respiratory: interstitial pneumonitis, ***pulmonary fibrosis.***
Skin: rash, ***erythema multiforme,*** epidermal necrolysis, ***Stevens-Johnson syndrome.***
Other: drug fever, hypersensitivity reactions, ***secondary malignancies.***

INTERACTIONS
Drug-drug. *Anticoagulants, aspirin:* May increase risk of bleeding. Avoid using together.
Myelosuppressives: May increase myelosuppression. Monitor patient.

EFFECTS ON LAB TEST RESULTS
- May increase alkaline phosphatase, AST, and blood and urine uric acid levels. May decrease hemoglobin level.
- May decrease granulocyte, neutrophil, platelet, RBC, and WBC counts.

CONTRAINDICATIONS & CAUTIONS
- Contraindicated in patients with hypersensitivity or resistance to previous therapy. Patients hypersensitive to other alkylating drugs may also be hypersensitive to this drug.
- Use cautiously in patients with history of head trauma or seizures and in patients receiving other drugs that lower the seizure threshold.
- Use cautiously within 4 weeks of a full course of radiation or chemotherapy.

NURSING CONSIDERATIONS
- Monitor CBC with differential.
- Monitor patient for neutropenia, which may not appear until after the third week of treatment. The absolute neutrophil count (ANC) may continue to decrease for up to 10 days after treatment ends.

- Use the ANC to calculate the patient's immunosuppression.
- Monitor uric acid level. To prevent hyperuricemia with resulting uric acid nephropathy, allopurinol may be used with adequate hydration.
- If WBC count falls below 2,000/mm^3 or granulocyte count falls below 1,000/mm^3, follow institutional policy for infection control in immunocompromised patients. Patients may receive injections of WBC colony-stimulating factor to increase WBC count recovery. Severe neutropenia is reversible up to cumulative dose of 6.5 mg/kg in a single course.
- Therapeutic effects are frequently accompanied by toxicity.
- To prevent bleeding, avoid all I.M. injections when platelet count is below 50,000/mm^3.
- Anticipate blood transfusions during treatment because of cumulative anemia. Patient may receive injections of RBC colony-stimulating factor to promote RBC production and decrease need for blood transfusions.

PATIENT TEACHING

- Advise patient to watch for signs of infection (fever, sore throat, fatigue) and bleeding (easy bruising, nosebleeds, bleeding gums, tarry stools). Tell patient to take temperature daily.
- Instruct patient to avoid OTC products containing aspirin and NSAIDs.
- Advise women to stop breast-feeding during therapy because of risk of toxicity to infant.
- Advise women of childbearing age to avoid becoming pregnant during therapy and to notify prescriber immediately if pregnancy is suspected.

SAFETY ALERT!

cisplatin (CDDP, cisplatinum†)

Platinol AQ

Pharmacologic class: platinum coordination complex
Pregnancy risk category D

AVAILABLE FORMS

Injection: 0.5 mg/ml†, 1 mg/ml

INDICATIONS & DOSAGES

➤ **Adjunctive therapy in metastatic testicular cancer**
Adults: 20 mg/m^2 I.V. daily for 5 days. Repeat q 3 weeks for three or four cycles.

➤ **Adjunctive therapy in metastatic ovarian cancer**
Adults: 100 mg/m^2 I.V.; repeat q 4 weeks. Or, 75 to 100 mg/m^2 I.V. once q 4 weeks with cyclophosphamide.

➤ **Advanced bladder cancer**
Adults: 50 to 70 mg/m^2 I.V. q 3 to 4 weeks. Give 50 mg/m^2 q 4 weeks in patients who have received other antineoplastics or radiation therapy.

➤ **Cervical cancer**
Adults: 40 to 75 mg/m^2 I.V. weekly or daily as monotherapy, in combination therapy, or with radiation therapy.

➤ **Non–small-cell lung cancer**
Adults: 75 to 100 mg/m^2 I.V. q 3 to 4 weeks in combination therapy.

➤ **Osteogenic sarcoma or neuroblastoma**
Children: 90 mg/m^2 I.V. q 3 weeks, or 30 mg/m^2 I.V. once weekly.

➤ **Recurrent brain tumor**
Children: 60 mg/m^2 I.V. daily for 2 consecutive days q 3 to 4 weeks.

➤ **Head and neck cancer ♦**
Adults: 80 to 120 mg/m^2 I.V. q 3 weeks or 50 mg/m^2 I.V. on days 1 and 8 q 4 weeks. Doses of 50 to 120 mg/m^2 I.V. may be used in combination therapy.

I.V. ADMINISTRATION

- Preparing and giving parenteral form of drug may be mutagenic, teratogenic, or carcinogenic. Follow facility policy to reduce risks.
- Hydrate patient with normal saline solution before giving drug. Maintain urine output of at least 100 ml/hour for 4 consecutive hours before therapy and for 24 hours after therapy.
- Reconstitute powder using sterile water for injection. Add 10 ml to 10-mg vial or 50 ml to 50-mg vial to make a solution containing 1 mg/ml.
- Infusions are most stable in solutions containing chloride (such as normal or half-normal saline solution and 0.22% sodium chloride). Don't use D_5W alone.
- Further dilute with dextrose 5% in 0.3% sodium chloride injection or dextrose 5%

in half-normal saline solution for injection.
- Give mannitol or furosemide boluses or infusions before and during cisplatin infusion to maintain diuresis of 100 to 400 ml/hour during and for 24 hours after therapy.
- Add potassium chloride (10 to 20 mEq/L) to I.V. fluids before and after cisplatin therapy to prevent hypokalemia. Add magnesium sulfate to I.V. fluids before and after therapy to prevent hypomagnesemia.
- Give drug as an I.V. infusion in 2 L of dextrose 5% in half-normal saline solution or dextrose 5% in 0.33% sodium chloride solution with 37.5 g of mannitol over 6 to 8 hours.
- Solutions are stable for 20 hours at room temperature. Don't refrigerate.

INCOMPATIBILITIES

Aluminum administration sets, amifostine, amphotericin B cholesteryl sulfate complex, cefepime, D_5W, etoposide with mannitol and potassium chloride, fluorouracil, mesna, 0.1% sodium chloride solution, paclitaxel, piperacillin sodium with tazobactam sodium, sodium bicarbonate, sodium bisulfate, sodium thiosulfate, solutions with a chloride content less than 2%, thiotepa.

ACTION

May cross-link strands of cellular DNA and interfere with RNA transcription, causing an imbalance of growth that leads to cell death. Not specific to cell cycle.

Route	Onset	Peak	Duration
I.V.	Unknown	Unknown	Several days

Half-life: Initial phase, 25 to 79 minutes; terminal phase, 58 to 78 hours.

ADVERSE REACTIONS

CNS: *peripheral neuritis,* ***seizures.***
EENT: *tinnitus, hearing loss, ototoxicity,* vestibular toxicity, optic neuritis, papilledema, cerebral blindness, blurred vision.
GI: loss of taste, *nausea, vomiting.*
GU: **PROLONGED RENAL TOXICITY WITH REPEATED COURSES OF THERAPY.**
Hematologic: **MYELOSUPPRESSION,** ***leukopenia, thrombocytopenia,*** anemia.
Metabolic: *hypomagnesemia,* hypokalemia, hypocalcemia, hyponatremia, hypophosphatemia, hyperuricemia.
Other: ***anaphylactoid reaction.***

INTERACTIONS

Drug-drug. *Aminoglycosides:* May increase nephrotoxicity. Carefully monitor renal function study results.
Aminoglycosides, bumetanide, ethacrynic acid, furosemide, torsemide: May increase ototoxicity. Avoid using together, if possible.
Aspirin, NSAIDs: May increase risk of bleeding. Avoid using together.
Fosphenytoin, phenytoin: May decrease phenytoin and fosphenytoin levels. Monitor levels.
Myelosuppressives: May increase myelosuppression. Monitor patient.

EFFECTS ON LAB TEST RESULTS

- May increase uric acid level. May decrease calcium, hemoglobin, magnesium, phosphate, potassium, and sodium levels.
- May decrease platelet and WBC counts.

CONTRAINDICATIONS & CAUTIONS

- Contraindicated in patients hypersensitive to drug or other platinum-containing compounds and in those with severe renal disease, hearing impairment, or myelosuppression.
- Use cautiously in patients previously treated with radiation or cytotoxic drugs and in those with peripheral neuropathies; also use cautiously with other ototoxic and nephrotoxic drugs.

NURSING CONSIDERATIONS

- Monitor CBC, electrolyte levels (especially potassium and magnesium), platelet count, and renal function studies before initial and subsequent doses.
- To detect hearing loss, obtain audiometry tests before initial and subsequent doses.
- Prehydration and mannitol diuresis may significantly reduce renal toxicity and ototoxicity.
- Therapeutic effects are frequently accompanied by toxicity.
- Some prescribers use I.V. sodium thiosulfate or amifostine to minimize toxicity. Check current protocol.

• Patients may experience vomiting 3 to 5 days after treatment, requiring prolonged antiemetic treatment. Some prescribers combine metoclopramide with dexamethasone and antihistamines, or ondansetron or granisetron with dexamethasone to control vomiting. Monitor intake and output. Continue I.V. hydration until patient can tolerate adequate oral intake.
• Renal toxicity is cumulative; don't give next dose until renal function returns to normal.
• Don't repeat dose unless platelet count exceeds 100,000/mm^3, WBC count exceeds 4,000/mm^3, creatinine level is below 1.5 mg/dl, creatinine clearance is 50 ml/minute or more, and BUN level is below 25 mg/dl.
• To prevent bleeding, avoid all I.M. injections when platelet count is less than 50,000/mm^3.
• Anticipate need for blood transfusions during treatment because of cumulative anemia.
• ***Alert:*** Immediately give epinephrine, corticosteroids, or antihistamines for anaphylactoid reactions.
• Safety of drug in children hasn't been established.
• ***Look alike–sound alike:*** Don't confuse cisplatin with carboplatin; they aren't interchangeable.

PATIENT TEACHING

• Advise patient to watch for signs and symptoms of infection (fever, sore throat, fatigue) and bleeding (easy bruising, nosebleeds, bleeding gums, tarry stools). Tell patient to take temperature daily.
• Tell patient to immediately report ringing in the ears or numbness in hands or feet.
• Instruct patient to avoid OTC products containing aspirin.
• Advise women to stop breast-feeding during therapy because of risk of toxicity to infant.
• Advise women of childbearing age to consult prescriber before becoming pregnant.

SAFETY ALERT!

cyclophosphamide

Cycloblastin‡, Cytoxan, Cytoxan Lyophilized, Endoxan‡, Neosar, Procytox†

Pharmacologic class: nitrogen mustard
Pregnancy risk category D

AVAILABLE FORMS

Injection: 100-mg, 200-mg, 500-mg, 1-g, 2-g vials
Tablets: 25 mg, 50 mg

INDICATIONS & DOSAGES

➤ **Breast or ovarian cancer, Hodgkin lymphoma, chronic lymphocytic leukemia, chronic myelocytic leukemia, acute lymphoblastic leukemia, acute myelocytic and monocytic leukemia, neuroblastoma, retinoblastoma, malignant lymphoma, multiple myeloma, mycosis fungoides, sarcoma**

Adults: Initially for induction, 40 to 50 mg/kg I.V. in divided doses over 2 to 5 days. Or, 10 to 15 mg/kg I.V. q 7 to 10 days, 3 to 5 mg/kg I.V. twice weekly, or 1 to 5 mg/kg P.O. daily, based on patient tolerance.
Children: Initially for induction, 2 to 8 mg/kg or 60 to 250 mg/m^2 P.O. or I.V. daily. Maintenance dose is 2 to 5 mg/kg P.O. or 50 to 150 mg/m^2 P.O. twice weekly.

Adjust subsequent doses according to evidence of antitumor activity or leukopenia.

➤ **Minimal-change nephrotic syndrome**

Children: 2 to 3 mg/kg P.O. daily for 60 to 90 days.

I.V. ADMINISTRATION

• Preparing and giving parenteral form of drug may be mutagenic, teratogenic, or carcinogenic. Follow facility policy to reduce risks.
• Reconstitute powder using sterile water for injection or bacteriostatic water for injection containing only parabens.
• For the nonlyophilized product, add 5 ml to 100-mg vial, 10 ml to 200-mg vial,

25 ml to 500-mg vial, 50 ml to 1-g vial, or 100 ml to 2-g vial to produce a solution containing 20 mg/ml. Shake vigorously to dissolve. If powder doesn't dissolve completely, let vial stand for a few minutes.
• Lyophilized product is much easier to reconstitute; check package insert for amount of diluent needed.
• Check reconstituted solution for small particles. Filter solution if needed.
• Give by direct I.V. injection or infusion.
• For infusion, further dilute with D_5W, dextrose 5% in normal saline solution for injection, dextrose 5% in Ringer injection, lactated Ringer injection, sodium lactate injection, or half-normal saline solution for injection.
• Reconstituted solution is stable 6 days if refrigerated or 24 hours at room temperature, but use stored solutions cautiously because drug contains no preservatives.

INCOMPATIBILITIES
Amphotericin B cholesteryl sulfate complex.

ACTION
Cross-links strands of cellular DNA and interferes with RNA transcription, causing an imbalance of growth that leads to cell death. Not specific to cell cycle.

Route	Onset	Peak	Duration
P.O.	Unknown	Unknown	Unknown
I.V.	Unknown	2–3 hr	Unknown

Half-life: 3 to 12 hours.

ADVERSE REACTIONS
CV: ***cardiotoxicity with very high doses and with doxorubicin,*** flushing.
GI: *nausea and vomiting,* anorexia, abdominal pain, stomatitis, mucositis.
GU: HEMORRHAGIC CYSTITIS, impaired fertility.
Hematologic: ***leukopenia, thrombocytopenia,*** anemia.
Hepatic: ***hepatotoxicity.***
Metabolic: hyperuricemia, SIADH.
Respiratory: ***pulmonary fibrosis with high doses.***
Skin: *reversible alopecia,* rash, pigmentation, nail changes, itching.
Other: ***secondary malignant disease, anaphylaxis,*** hypersensitivity reactions.

INTERACTIONS
Drug-drug. *Allopurinol, myelosuppressives:* May increase myelosuppression. Monitor patient for toxicity.
Anticoagulants: May increase anticoagulant effect. Monitor patient for bleeding.
Aspirin, NSAIDs: May increase risk of bleeding. Avoid using together.
Barbiturates: May enhance cyclophosphamide toxicity. Monitor patient closely.
Cardiotoxic drugs: May increase adverse cardiac effects. Monitor patient for toxicity.
Chloramphenicol, corticosteroids: May reduce activity of cyclophosphamide. Use together cautiously.
Ciprofloxacin: May decrease antimicrobial effect. Monitor patient for effect.
Digoxin: May decrease digoxin level. Monitor level closely.
Succinylcholine: May prolong neuromuscular blockade. Avoid using together.

EFFECTS ON LAB TEST RESULTS
• May increase uric acid level. May decrease hemoglobin and pseudocholinesterase levels.
• May decrease platelet, RBC, and WBC counts.
• May suppress positive reaction to *Candida*, mumps, *Trichophyton*, and tuberculin skin test results. May cause a false-positive Papanicolaou test result.

CONTRAINDICATIONS & CAUTIONS
• Contraindicated in patients hypersensitive to drug and in those with severe bone marrow suppression.
• Use cautiously in patients with leukopenia, thrombocytopenia, malignant cell infiltration of bone marrow, or hepatic or renal disease and in those who have recently undergone radiation therapy or chemotherapy.

NURSING CONSIDERATIONS
• Don't give drug at bedtime; infrequent urination during the night may increase possibility of cystitis. If cystitis occurs, stop drug and notify prescriber. Cystitis can occur months after therapy ends. Mesna may be given to reduce frequency and

severity of bladder toxicity. Test urine for blood.
- Adequately hydrate patients before and after dose to decrease risk of cystitis.
- Use caution to ensure correct dose to decrease risk of cardiac toxicity.
- Monitor CBC and renal and liver function test results.
- Monitor patient closely for leukopenia (nadir between days 8 and 15, recovery in 17 to 28 days).
- Monitor uric acid level. To prevent hyperuricemia with resulting uric acid nephropathy, allopurinol may be used with adequate hydration.
- To prevent bleeding, avoid all I.M. injections when platelet count is less than 50,000/mm^3.
- Anticipate blood transfusions because of cumulative anemia. Patients may receive injections of RBC colony-stimulating factor to promote RBC production and decrease need for blood transfusions.
- Therapeutic effects are often accompanied by toxicity.
- In boys, using drug for nephrotic syndrome for more than 60 days increases the incidence of oligospermia and azoospermia. Use for more than 90 days increases the risk of sterility.
- Drug may be used to treat nononcologic disorders, such as lupus, nephritis, and rheumatoid arthritis.

PATIENT TEACHING
- Warn patient that hair loss is likely to occur but is reversible.
- Advise patient to watch for signs and symptoms of infection (fever, sore throat, fatigue) and bleeding (easy bruising, nosebleeds, bleeding gums, tarry stools). Tell patient to take temperature daily.
- Instruct patient to avoid OTC products that contain aspirin.
- To minimize risk of hemorrhagic cystitis, encourage patient to urinate every 1 to 2 hours while awake and to drink at least 3 L of fluid daily.
- If patient is taking tablets, tell him not to take it at bedtime because infrequent urination increases risk of cystitis.
- Advise both men and women to practice contraception during therapy and for 4 months afterward; drug may cause birth defects.
- Advise women to stop breast-feeding during therapy because of risk of toxicity to infant.
- Drug can cause irreversible sterility in both men and women. Before therapy, counsel patients who are considering parenthood. Also recommend that women consult prescriber before becoming pregnant.

SAFETY ALERT!

ifosfamide
Holoxan‡, Ifex

Pharmacologic class: nitrogen mustard
Pregnancy risk category D

AVAILABLE FORMS
Powder for injection: 1 g, 2 g†‡, 3 g

INDICATIONS & DOSAGES
➤ Testicular cancer
Adults: 1.2 g/m^2 daily I.V. for 5 consecutive days. Repeat treatment q 3 weeks or after patient recovers from hematologic toxicity Don't repeat doses until WBC count exceeds 4,000/mm^3 and platelet count exceeds 100,000/mm^3.
➤ Sarcomas; small-cell lung, cervical, ovarian, and uterine cancer ♦
Adults: 1.2 to 2.5 g/m^2 I.V. daily for 3 to 5 days. Repeat cycle as needed, based on patient response.

I.V. ADMINISTRATION
- Preparing and giving may be mutagenic, teratogenic, or carcinogenic. Follow institutional policy to reduce risks.
- Give a protective drug such as mesna to prevent hemorrhagic cystitis. Ifosfamide and mesna are physically compatible and may be mixed in the same I.V. solution.
- Obtain urinalysis before each dose. If microscopic hematuria occurs, notify prescriber. Adjust dosage of mesna if needed. Adequate fluid intake (2 L daily, either P.O. or I.V.) is essential before, and 72 hours after, therapy.
- Reconstitute each gram of drug with 20 ml of diluent to yield a solution of 50 mg/ml. Use sterile water for injection

or bacteriostatic water for injection. Solutions may then be further diluted with sterile water, dextrose 2.5% or 5% in water, half-normal or normal saline solution for injection, dextrose 5% and normal saline solution for injection, or lactated Ringer injection.

- Infuse each dose over at least 30 minutes.
- Reconstituted solution is stable for 1 week at room temperature or 6 weeks if refrigerated. However, use solution within 6 hours if drug was reconstituted with sterile water without a preservative (such as benzyl alcohol or parabens).

INCOMPATIBILITIES

Cefepime, mesna with epirubicin, methotrexate sodium.

ACTION

Cross-links strands of cellular DNA and interferes with RNA transcription, causing an imbalance of growth that leads to cell death. Not specific to cell cycle.

Route	Onset	Peak	Duration
I.V.	Unknown	Unknown	Unknown

Half-life: About 14 hours.

ADVERSE REACTIONS

CNS: *somnolence, confusion,* ***coma, seizures,*** ataxia, hallucinations, depressive psychosis, dizziness, disorientation, cranial nerve dysfunction.
GI: *nausea, vomiting,* diarrhea.
GU: *hemorrhagic cystitis, hematuria,* ***nephrotoxicity,*** Fanconi syndrome.
Hematologic: ***leukopenia, thrombocytopenia, myelosuppression.***
Hepatic: ***hepatotoxicity.***
Metabolic: ***metabolic acidosis.***
Skin: *alopecia.*
Other: infection, phlebitis.

INTERACTIONS

Drug-drug. *Anticoagulants, aspirin, NSAIDs:* May increase risk of bleeding. Avoid using together.
Barbiturates, chloral hydrate, fosphenytoin, phenytoin: May increase ifosfamide toxicity. Monitor patient closely.
Corticosteroids: May inhibit hepatic enzymes, reducing ifosfamide's effect. Monitor patient for increased ifosfamide toxicity if corticosteroid dosage is suddenly reduced or stopped.
Cyclophosphamide: May increase risk of cardiac tamponade in patients with thalassemia. Monitor patient closely.
Myelosuppressives: May enhance hematologic toxicity. Dosage adjustment may be needed.

EFFECTS ON LAB TEST RESULTS

- May increase liver enzyme levels.
- May decrease WBC and platelet counts.

CONTRAINDICATIONS & CAUTIONS

- Contraindicated in patients hypersensitive to drug and in those with severe bone marrow suppression.
- Use cautiously in patients with renal impairment or compromised bone marrow reserve as indicated by leukopenia, granulocytopenia, extensive bone marrow metastases, previous radiation therapy, or previous therapy with cytotoxic drugs.

NURSING CONSIDERATIONS

- Give antiemetic before drug, to reduce nausea.
- Ensure that patient is adequately hydrated during therapy.
- Don't give drug at bedtime; infrequent urination during the night may increase possibility of cystitis. If cystitis develops, stop drug and notify prescriber.
- Bladder irrigation with normal saline solution may be done to treat cystitis.
- Monitor CBC and renal and liver function tests.
- To prevent bleeding, avoid all I.M. injections when platelet count is less than 50,000/mm^3.
- Anticipate blood transfusions because of cumulative anemia. Patients may receive injections of RBC colony-stimulating factor to promote RBC production and decrease need for blood transfusions.
- Assess patient for mental status changes; dosage may have to be decreased.
- ***Look alike–sound alike:*** Don't confuse ifosfamide with cyclophosphamide.

PATIENT TEACHING

- Remind patient to urinate frequently to minimize contact of drug and its metabolites with the lining of the bladder.
- Advise patient to watch for signs and symptoms of infection (fever, sore throat, fatigue) and bleeding (easy bruising, nosebleeds, bleeding gums, tarry stools). Tell patient to take temperature daily.
- Instruct patient to avoid OTC products that contain aspirin.
- Advise women to stop breast-feeding during therapy because of possible risk of toxicity to infant.
- Caution woman of childbearing age to avoid becoming pregnant during therapy. Recommend that she consult prescriber before becoming pregnant.

SAFETY ALERT!

lomustine (CCNU)

CeeNU

Pharmacologic class: nitrosourea
Pregnancy risk category D

AVAILABLE FORMS

Capsules: 10 mg, 40 mg, 100 mg, dose pack (two 10-mg, two 40-mg, two 100-mg capsules)

INDICATIONS & DOSAGES

➤ **Brain tumor, Hodgkin lymphoma**
Adults and children: 100 to 130 mg/m^2 P.O. as single dose q 6 weeks. Repeat doses shouldn't be given until WBC count exceeds 4,000/mm^3 and platelet count is greater than 100,000/mm^3.
Adjust-a-dose: Reduce dosage according to degree of bone marrow suppression or when used with other myelosuppressive drugs. Reduce dosage by 30% for WBC count nadir 2,000 to 2,999/mm^3 and platelet count nadir 25,000 to 74,999/mm^3; by 50% for WBC count nadir less than 2,000/mm^3 and platelet count nadir less than 25,000/mm^3.

ACTION

Cross-links strands of cellular DNA and interferes with RNA transcription, causing an imbalance of growth that leads to cell death. Not specific to cell cycle.

Route	Onset	Peak	Duration
P.O.	Unknown	Unknown	Unknown

Half-life: 1 to 2 days.

ADVERSE REACTIONS

CNS: disorientation, lethargy, ataxia.
GI: *nausea, vomiting,* stomatitis.
GU: ***nephrotoxicity,*** progressive azotemia, ***renal failure,*** amenorrhea, azoospermia.
Hematologic: *anemia,* ***leukopenia, thrombocytopenia, bone marrow suppression.***
Hepatic: ***hepatotoxicity.***
Respiratory: ***pulmonary fibrosis.***
Skin: alopecia.
Other: ***secondary malignant disease.***

INTERACTIONS

Drug-drug. *Anticoagulants, aspirin, NSAIDs:* May increase risk of bleeding. Avoid using together.
Myelosuppressives: May increase myelosuppression. Monitor patient.

EFFECTS ON LAB TEST RESULTS

- May increase urine urea level. May decrease hemoglobin level.
- May decrease WBC, RBC, and platelet counts.

CONTRAINDICATIONS & CAUTIONS

- Contraindicated in patients hypersensitive to drug.
- Use cautiously in patients with decreased platelet, WBC, or RBC counts and in those receiving other myelosuppressives.

NURSING CONSIDERATIONS

- Give antiemetic before drug, to reduce nausea.
- Give 2 to 4 hours after meals; drug will be more completely absorbed if taken when stomach is empty.
- Monitor CBC weekly. Usually not given more often than every 6 weeks; bone marrow toxicity is cumulative and delayed, usually occurring 4 to 6 weeks after drug administration.
- Periodically monitor liver function test results.

• To prevent bleeding, avoid all I.M. injections when platelet count is less than 50,000/mm³.
• Anticipate blood transfusions because of cumulative anemia. Patients may receive RBC colony-stimulating factor to promote RBC production and decrease need for blood transfusions.
• Therapeutic effects come with toxicity.
• Store capsules at room temperature. Avoid exposure to moisture, and protect from temperatures greater than 104° F (40° C).

PATIENT TEACHING
• Advise patient to take capsules on an empty stomach, if possible.
• Advise patient to watch for signs and symptoms of infection (fever, sore throat, fatigue) and bleeding (easy bruising, nosebleeds, bleeding gums, tarry stools). Tell patient to take temperature daily.
• Instruct patient to avoid OTC products that contain aspirin or NSAIDs.
• Advise women to stop breast-feeding during therapy because of possible risk of toxicity to infant.
• Caution woman of childbearing age to avoid becoming pregnant during therapy. Recommend that she consult prescriber before becoming pregnant.

SAFETY ALERT!

mechlorethamine hydrochloride (nitrogen mustard)
Mustargen

Pharmacologic class: nitrogen mustard
Pregnancy risk category D

AVAILABLE FORMS
Powder for injection: 10-mg vials

INDICATIONS & DOSAGES
Dosage is based on patient response and degree of toxicity.
➤ **Hodgkin lymphoma**
Adults and children: 6 mg/m² daily on days 1 and 8 of 28-day cycle in combination with other antineoplastics, such as mechlorethamine-vincristine-procarbazine-prednisone (MOPP) regimen. Repeat dosage for six cycles.
Adjust-a-dose: Subsequent doses reduced by 50% in MOPP regimen when WBC count is 3,000 to 3,999/mm³ and by 75% when WBC count is 1,000 to 2,999/mm³ or platelet count is 50,000 to 100,000/mm³.
➤ **Polycythemia vera, chronic lymphocytic leukemia, chronic myelocytic leukemia, bronchogenic cancer**
Adults and children: 0.4 mg/kg as single dose or 0.1 to 0.2 mg/kg divided in two or four successive daily doses during each course of therapy.
➤ **Malignant effusions (pericardial, peritoneal, pleural)**
Adults: 0.4 mg/kg intracavitarily, although 0.2 mg/kg (10 to 20 mg) has been used intrapericardially.

I.V. ADMINISTRATION
• Preparing and giving drug may be mutagenic, teratogenic, or carcinogenic. Follow institutional policy to reduce risks.
• Reconstitute drug using 10 ml of sterile water for injection or normal saline solution for injection. Resulting solution contains 1 mg/ml of drug. Give by direct injection into a vein or into tubing of a free-flowing I.V. solution.
• Prepare immediately before infusion. Solution is very unstable. Visually inspect before using; make sure solution is colorless. Use within 15 minutes, and discard unused solution.
• Dispose of equipment used in preparation and administration of mechlorethamine properly and according to institutional policy. Neutralize unused solution with an equal volume of 5% sodium bicarbonate and 5% sodium thiosulfate for 45 minutes.
• Drug is a potent vesicant. If extravasation occurs, apply cold compresses for 6 to 12 hours, and infiltrate area with isotonic sodium thiosulfate.

INCOMPATIBILITIES
Allopurinol, cefepime, D_5W, methohexital, normal saline solution.

ACTION
Cross-links strands of cellular DNA and interferes with RNA transcription, caus-

ing an imbalance of growth that leads to cell death. Not specific to cell cycle.

Route	Onset	Peak	Duration
I.V., intracavitary	Few sec– few min	Unknown	Unknown

Half-life: Unknown.

ADVERSE REACTIONS

CNS: weakness, vertigo, neurotoxicity.
CV: *thrombophlebitis.*
EENT: tinnitus, deafness with high doses.
GI: *nausea, vomiting, anorexia,* diarrhea, metallic taste.
GU: menstrual irregularities, impaired spermatogenesis.
Hematologic: ***agranulocytosis, thrombocytopenia,*** lymphocytopenia, mild anemia beginning in 2 to 3 weeks.
Hepatic: jaundice.
Metabolic: hyperuricemia.
Skin: *alopecia,* rash, sloughing, severe skin irritation with extravasation or contact.
Other: ***anaphylaxis, secondary malignant disease,*** precipitation of herpes zoster.

INTERACTIONS

Drug-drug. *Anticoagulants, aspirin, NSAIDs:* May increase risk of bleeding. Avoid using together.
Myelosuppressives: May increase myelosuppression. Monitor patient.

EFFECTS ON LAB TEST RESULTS

- May increase urine urea level. May decrease hemoglobin level.
- May decrease granulocyte, lymphocyte, RBC, and platelet counts.

CONTRAINDICATIONS & CAUTIONS

- Contraindicated in patients hypersensitive to drug and in those with infectious diseases.
- Use cautiously in patients with severe anemia or depressed neutrophil or platelet count and in those who have recently undergone radiation therapy or chemotherapy.

NURSING CONSIDERATIONS

- When given intracavitarily for sclerosing effect, dilute using up to 100 ml of normal saline solution for injection. Turn patient from side to side every 5 to 10 minutes for 1 hour to distribute drug.
- Monitor uric acid level. To prevent hyperuricemia with resulting uric acid or nephropathy, make sure patient is adequately hydrated. Alkalinizing the urine and using allopurinol may also be helpful.
- Therapeutic effects are commonly accompanied by toxicity.
- Neurotoxicity increases with dosage and patient age.
- To prevent bleeding, avoid all I.M. injections when platelet count is less than $50,000/mm^3$.
- Monitor patient closely for bone marrow suppression (nadir of myelosuppression occurring between days 4 and 10 and lasting 10 to 21 days).
- Give blood transfusions for cumulative anemia. Patients may receive RBC colony-stimulating factor to promote RBC cell production and decrease need for blood transfusions.

PATIENT TEACHING

- Advise patient to report any pain or burning at site of injection during or after administration.
- Advise patient to watch for signs and symptoms of infection (fever, sore throat, fatigue) and bleeding (easy bruising, nosebleeds, bleeding gums, tarry stools). Tell patient to take temperature daily.
- Tell patient that severe nausea and vomiting can occur.
- Instruct patient to avoid OTC products that contain aspirin or NSAIDs.
- Advise women to stop breast-feeding during therapy because of risk of toxicity to infant.
- Advise women of childbearing age to consult prescriber before becoming pregnant.
- Tell patient about the risk of sterility.

SAFETY ALERT!

melphalan (L-PAM, phenylalanine mustard)
Alkeran

melphalan hydrochloride
Alkeran

Pharmacologic class: nitrogen mustard
Pregnancy risk category D

AVAILABLE FORMS
Lyophilized powder for injection: 50 mg
Tablets (scored): 2 mg

INDICATIONS & DOSAGES
➤ Multiple myeloma
Adults: Initially, 6 mg P.O. daily for 2 to 3 weeks; then stop drug for up to 4 weeks or until WBC and platelet counts stop dropping and begin to rise again; maintenance dose is 2 mg daily. Or, 0.15 mg/kg P.O. daily for 7 days, or 0.25 mg/kg for 4 days; repeat q 4 to 6 weeks.

Or, give I.V. to patients who can't tolerate oral therapy, 16 mg/m^2 given by infusion over 15 to 20 minutes at 2-week intervals for four doses. After patient has recovered from toxicity, give drug at 4-week intervals.
Adjust-a-dose: For patients with renal insufficiency, reduce dosage by up to 50%.
➤ Nonresectable advanced ovarian cancer
Adults: 0.2 mg/kg P.O. daily for 5 days. Repeat q 4 to 6 weeks, depending on bone marrow recovery.

I.V. ADMINISTRATION
• Preparing and giving this form may be mutagenic, teratogenic, or carcinogenic. Follow institutional policy to reduce risks.
• Because drug isn't stable in solution, reconstitute immediately before giving with the 10 ml of sterile diluent supplied by manufacturer. Shake vigorously until solution is clear. The resulting solution will contain 5 mg/ml of melphalan. Immediately dilute required dose in normal saline solution for injection to no more than 0.45 mg/ml. Give infusion over 15 to 20 minutes.
• Monitor infusion carefully. Extravasation causes painful inflammation.
• Reconstituted product begins to degrade within 30 minutes. After final dilution, nearly 1% of drug degrades every 10 minutes. Administration must be completed within 60 minutes of reconstitution.
• Don't refrigerate reconstituted product because precipitate will form.

INCOMPATIBILITIES
Amphotericin B, chlorpromazine, D_5W, lactated Ringer injection. Compatibility with normal saline injection depends on the concentration; don't prepare solutions with a concentration exceeding 0.45 mg/ml.

ACTION
Cross-links strands of cellular DNA and interferes with RNA transcription, causing an imbalance of growth that leads to cell death. Not specific to cell cycle.

Route	Onset	Peak	Duration
P.O., I.V.	Unknown	Unknown	Unknown

Half-life: 2 hours.

ADVERSE REACTIONS
CV: hypotension, tachycardia, edema.
GI: nausea, vomiting, diarrhea, oral ulceration, stomatitis.
Hematologic: ***thrombocytopenia, leukopenia, bone marrow suppression,*** hemolytic anemia.
Hepatic: ***hepatotoxicity.***
Metabolic: hyperuricemia.
Respiratory: ***pneumonitis, pulmonary fibrosis,*** dyspnea, ***bronchospasm.***
Skin: pruritus, alopecia, urticaria, ulceration at injection site.
Other: ***anaphylaxis,*** hypersensitivity reactions.

INTERACTIONS
Drug-drug (I.V. melphalan only). *Anticoagulants, aspirin, NSAIDs:* May increase risk of bleeding. Avoid using together.
Carmustine: May decrease threshold for pulmonary toxicity. Use together cautiously.
Cimetidine: May decrease melphalan level. Monitor patient closely.

Cisplatin: May increase renal impairment, decreasing melphalan clearance. Monitor patient closely.
Cyclosporine: May cause severe renal impairment. Monitor renal function closely.
Interferon alfa: May increase melphalan elimination. Monitor patient closely.
Myelosuppressives: May increase myelosuppression. Monitor patient.
Vaccines: May decrease effectiveness of killed virus vaccines and increase risk of toxicity from live virus vaccines. Postpone routine immunization for at least 3 months after last dose of melphalan.
Drug-food. *Any food:* May decrease oral drug absorption. Advise patient to take drug on empty stomach.

EFFECTS ON LAB TEST RESULTS
- May increase urine urea level. May decrease hemoglobin level.
- May decrease RBC, WBC, and platelet counts.
- May cause a false-positive direct Coombs' test.

CONTRAINDICATIONS & CAUTIONS
- Contraindicated in patients hypersensitive to drug and in those with disease resistant to drug. Patients hypersensitive to chlorambucil may have cross-sensitivity to this drug.
- Contraindicated in patients with severe leukopenia, thrombocytopenia, or anemia and in those with chronic lymphocytic leukemia.
- Use cautiously in patients receiving radiation and chemotherapy.
- Safe use in children hasn't been established.

NURSING CONSIDERATIONS
- Dosage may need to be reduced in patients with renal impairment.
- Melphalan is drug of choice with prednisone in patients with multiple myeloma.
- Give oral form on empty stomach because food decreases drug absorption.
- Monitor uric acid level and CBC.
- To prevent bleeding, avoid all I.M. injections when platelet count is less than 50,000/mm^3.
- Give blood transfusions for cumulative anemia. Patients may receive RBC colony-stimulating factor to promote RBC production and decrease need for blood transfusions.
- Anaphylaxis may occur. Keep antihistamines and steroids readily available to give if needed.
- ***Look alike–sound alike:*** Don't confuse melphalan with Mephyton.

PATIENT TEACHING
- Advise patient to take tablets on empty stomach.
- Advise patient to report pain or redness at I.V. site.
- Advise patient to watch for signs and symptoms of infection (fever, sore throat, fatigue) and bleeding (easy bruising, nosebleeds, bleeding gums, tarry stools). Tell patient to take temperature daily.
- Instruct patient to avoid OTC products that contain aspirin or NSAIDs.
- Advise women to stop breast-feeding during therapy because of risk of toxicity to infant.
- Advise women of childbearing age to consult prescriber before becoming pregnant.

SAFETY ALERT!

oxaliplatin
Eloxatin

Pharmacologic class: platinum coordination complex
Pregnancy risk category D

AVAILABLE FORMS
Injection: 50- or 100-mg vials
Solution for injection: 5 mg/ml in 50- or 100-mg vials

INDICATIONS & DOSAGES
➤ **First-line treatment of advanced colorectal cancer with 5-fluorouracil and leucovorin (5-FU/LV)**
Adults: On day 1, give 85 mg/m^2 oxaliplatin I.V. in 250 to 500 ml D_5W and leucovorin 200 mg/m^2 I.V. in D_5W simultaneously over 120 minutes, in separate bags using a Y-line, followed by 5-FU 400 mg/m^2 I.V. bolus over 2 to 4 minutes, followed by 600 mg/m^2 5-FU I.V. infusion in 500 ml D_5W over 22 hours.

On day 2, give 200 mg/m^2 leucovorin I.V. infusion over 120 minutes, followed by 400 mg/m^2 5-FU I.V. bolus over 2 to 4 minutes, followed by 600 mg/m^2 5-FU I.V. infusion in 500 ml D_5W over 22 hours.

Repeat cycle q 2 weeks.

Adjust-a-dose: In patients with unresolved and persistent grade 2 neurosensory events, reduce oxaliplatin to 65 mg/m^2. In those with persistent grade 3 neurosensory events, consider stopping drug. In patients recovering from grade 3 or 4 GI or hematologic events, reduce dose to 65 mg/m^2 and reduce dose of 5-FU by 20%.

➤ **With 5-FU/LV for the adjuvant treatment of stage III colon cancer in patients who have had complete resection of the primary tumor**

Adults: On day 1, give oxaliplatin, 85 mg/m^2 I.V. in 250 to 500 ml D_5W and 200 mg/m^2 leucovorin I.V. infusion in D_5W, both over 120 minutes at the same time, in separate bags, using a Y-line. Follow with 5-FU 400 mg/m^2 I.V. bolus over 2 to 4 minutes, then 600 mg/m^2 5-FU in 500 ml D_5W as a 22-hour continuous infusion.

On day 2, give leucovorin, 200 mg/m^2 I.V. infused over 120 minutes followed by 5-FU 400 mg/m^2 as an I.V. bolus over 2 to 4 minutes, then, 600 mg/m^2 5-FU in 500 ml D_5W as a 22-hour infusion.

Repeat cycle q 2 weeks for a total of 6 months. Premedicate with antiemetics, with or without dexamethasone.

Adjust-a-dose: For patients with persistent grade 2 neurotoxicity, consider an oxaliplatin dose reduction to 75 mg/m^2. For patients who recovered from grade 4 neutropenia, grade 3 or 4 thrombocytopenia, or a grade 3 or 4 GI event, reduce oxaliplatin to 75 mg/m^2 and 5-FU to a 300 mg/m^2 bolus and 500 mg/m^2 22-hour infusion. Delay dose until neutrophils are 1.5×10^9/L or more and platelets are 75×10^9/L or more.

I.V. ADMINISTRATION

- Preparation and administration of parenteral form of drug may be mutagenic, teratogenic, or carcinogenic to staff. Follow institutional policy to reduce risks.
- Reconstitute powder using sterile water for injection or D_5W. Add 10 ml to a 50-mg vial or 20 ml to a 100-mg vial, for a yield of 5 mg/ml. Never reconstitute with sodium chloride solution or other solution containing chloride.
- Reconstituted solutions must be further diluted in an infusion solution of 250 to 500 ml of D_5W.
- Inspect bag for particulate matter and discoloration before administration, and discard if present.
- Don't use needles or I.V. administration sets that contain aluminum because it displaces the platinum, causing it to lose potency and form a black precipitate.
- Give oxaliplatin and leucovorin over 2 hours at the same time in separate bags, using a Y-line. Extend the infusion time to 6 hours to decrease acute toxicities.
- Store unopened vials at room temperature. Reconstituted solutions are stable if refrigerated (36° to 46° F [2° to 8° C]) for up to 24 hours. After final dilution, solutions are stable for 6 hours at room temperature and up to 24 hours under refrigeration.

INCOMPATIBILITIES

Alkaline solutions or drugs such as 5-FU. Flush infusion line with D_5W before giving any other drugs simultaneously.

ACTION

Probably inhibits cell replication and transcription by forming platinum complexes that cross-link with DNA molecules. Not specific to cell cycle.

Route	Onset	Peak	Duration
I.V.	Unknown	Unknown	Unknown

Half-life: Unknown.

ADVERSE REACTIONS

CNS: *pain, peripheral neuropathy, fatigue, headache,* dizziness, *insomnia, fever.*
CV: chest pain, ***thromboembolism,*** *edema, flushing, peripheral edema.*
EENT: *rhinitis,* pharyngolaryngeal dysesthesias, pharyngitis, epistaxis, abnormal lacrimation.
GI: *nausea, vomiting, diarrhea, stomatitis, abdominal pain, anorexia, constipation, dyspepsia, taste perversion,* gastroesophageal reflux, flatulence, mucositis, veno-occlusive disease.

GU: dysuria, hematuria.
Hematologic: FEBRILE NEUTROPENIA, *anemia,* LEUKOPENIA, THROMBOCYTOPENIA.
Metabolic: hypokalemia, dehydration.
Musculoskeletal: *back pain, arthralgia.*
Respiratory: *dyspnea, cough, upper respiratory tract infection,* hiccups, ***pulmonary toxicity.***
Skin: *injection site reaction,* rash, alopecia.
Other: ***anaphylaxis,*** *hand-foot syndrome, allergic reaction,* rigors.

INTERACTIONS

Drug-drug. *Nephrotoxic drugs (such as gentamicin):* May decrease elimination of nephrotoxic drugs and increase gentamicin levels. Monitor patient for signs and symptoms of toxicity.

EFFECTS ON LAB TEST RESULTS

- May increase creatinine, bilirubin, AST, and ALT levels. May decrease potassium and hemoglobin levels.
- May decrease neutrophil, WBC, and platelet counts.

CONTRAINDICATIONS & CAUTIONS

- Contraindicated in patients allergic to drug or other platinum-containing compounds and in pregnant or breast-feeding patients.
- Use cautiously in patients with renal impairment or peripheral sensory neuropathy.

NURSING CONSIDERATIONS

- Drug doesn't require patient prehydration.
- Give antiemetic with or without dexamethasone before drug to reduce nausea.
- Drug clearance is reduced in patients with renal impairment. Dosage adjustment for patients with renal impairment hasn't been established.
- Monitor CBC, platelet count, and liver and kidney function before each chemotherapy cycle.
- Monitor patient for hypersensitivity reactions, which may occur within minutes of administration.
- Monitor patient for injection site reaction; extravasation may occur.
- Monitor patient for neuropathy and pulmonary toxicity. Peripheral neuropathy may be acute or persistent. Acute neuropathy is reversible; it occurs within 2 days of dosing and resolves within 14 days. Persistent peripheral neuropathy occurs more than 14 days after dosing and causes paresthesias, dysesthesias, hypoesthesias, and other neurologic impairment that can interfere with daily activities (such as walking or swallowing).
- Avoid ice and cold exposure during infusion of drug because cold temperatures can worsen acute neurologic symptoms. Cover patient with a blanket during infusion.
- Diarrhea, dehydration, hypokalemia, and fatigue may occur more frequently in elderly patients.

PATIENT TEACHING

- Inform patient of potential adverse reactions.
- Tell patient to avoid exposure to cold or cold objects (such as cold drinks or ice cubes), which can bring on or worsen acute symptoms of peripheral neuropathy. Advise patient to drink warm drinks, wear warm clothing, and cover any exposed skin (hands, face, and head). Have patient warm the air going into his lungs by wearing a scarf or ski mask. Have him wear gloves when touching cold objects (such as frozen foods, door knobs, or mailboxes).
- Tell patient to contact prescriber immediately if he has trouble breathing or experiences signs and symptoms of an allergic reaction, such as rash, hives, swelling of lips or tongue, or sudden cough.
- Tell patient to contact prescriber if fever, signs and symptoms of an infection, persistent vomiting, diarrhea, or signs and symptoms of dehydration (thirst, dry mouth, light-headedness, and decreased urination) occur.

SAFETY ALERT!

thiotepa (TESPA, triethylenethiophosphoramide, TSPA)

Thioplex

Pharmacologic class: alkylating drug
Pregnancy risk category D

AVAILABLE FORMS

Injection: 15- and 30-mg vials

INDICATIONS & DOSAGES

➤ **Breast and ovarian cancers, lymphoma, Hodgkin lymphoma**
Adults and children older than age 12: Give 0.3 to 0.4 mg/kg I.V. q 1 to 4 weeks or 0.2 mg/kg for 4 to 5 days at intervals of 2 to 4 weeks.

➤ **Bladder tumor**
Adults and children older than age 12: Give 30 to 60 mg in 30 to 60 ml of normal saline solution instilled in bladder for 2 hours once weekly for 4 weeks.

➤ **Neoplastic effusions**
Adults and children older than age 12: Give 0.6 to 0.8 mg/kg intracavitarily q 1 to 4 weeks.

I.V. ADMINISTRATION

- Preparation and administration of parenteral form of drug may be mutagenic, teratogenic, or carcinogenic to staff. Follow institutional policy to reduce risks.
- Reconstitute with 1.5 ml of sterile water for injection in 15-mg vial or 3 ml in 30-mg vial to yield 10 mg/ml. Don't reconstitute with other solutions.
- Further dilute with normal saline solution for injection. If larger volume is desired, further dilute with sodium chloride solution, D_5W, dextrose 5% in normal saline solution for injection, Ringer injection, or lactated Ringer injection.
- If solution appears grossly opaque or has a precipitate, discard it. Make sure solutions are clear to slightly opaque. To eliminate haze, filter solutions through a 0.22-micron filter before use.
- If pain occurs at insertion site, dilute drug further or use a local anesthetic to reduce pain. Make sure drug doesn't infiltrate.
- Use solutions within 8 hours.
- Refrigerate and protect dry powder from direct sunlight to avoid possible drug breakdown.

INCOMPATIBILITIES

Cisplatin, filgrastim, minocycline, vinorelbine.

ACTION

Cross-links strands of cellular DNA and interferes with RNA transcription, causing an imbalance of growth that leads to cell death. Not specific to cell cycle.

Route	Onset	Peak	Duration
I.V., intracavitary	Unknown	Unknown	Unknown

Half-life: 2¼ hours.

ADVERSE REACTIONS

CNS: headache, dizziness, fatigue, weakness, fever.
EENT: blurred vision, conjunctivitis.
GI: *nausea, vomiting,* abdominal pain, anorexia, stomatitis.
GU: amenorrhea, decreased spermatogenesis, dysuria, increased urine levels of uric acid, urine retention, hemorrhagic cystitis (with intravesical administration).
Hematologic: ***leukopenia, thrombocytopenia, neutropenia,*** anemia.
Metabolic: hyperuricemia.
Skin: dermatitis, alopecia, pain at injection site.
Other: hypersensitivity reactions (including, ***anaphylaxis, laryngeal edema,*** urticaria, rash.

INTERACTIONS

Drug-drug. *Anticoagulants, aspirin, NSAIDs:* May increase risk of bleeding. Avoid using together.
Myelosuppressives: May increase myelosuppression. Monitor patient.
Neuromuscular blockers: May prolong muscular paralysis. Monitor patient.
Other alkylating drugs, irradiation therapy: May intensify toxicity rather than enhance therapeutic response. Avoid using together.

EFFECTS ON LAB TEST RESULTS

- May increase uric acid level. May decrease pseudocholinesterase and hemoglobin levels.
- May decrease lymphocyte, platelet, WBC, RBC, and neutrophil counts.

CONTRAINDICATIONS & CAUTIONS

- Contraindicated in patients hypersensitive to drug, in breast-feeding patients, and in those with severe bone marrow, hepatic, or renal dysfunction.
- Use in pregnant women only when benefits to mother outweigh risk of teratogenicity.
- Use cautiously in patients with mild bone marrow suppression and renal or hepatic dysfunction.

NURSING CONSIDERATIONS

- For bladder instillation, dehydrate patient 8 to 10 hours before therapy. Instill drug into bladder by catheter; ask patient to retain solution for 2 hours. If discomfort is too great with 60 ml, reduce volume to 30 ml. Reposition patient every 15 minutes for maximum area contact.
- Monitor CBC weekly for at least 3 weeks after last dose.
- If patient's WBC count drops below 3,000/mm^3 or if platelet count falls below 150,000/mm^3, stop drug and notify prescriber. If WBC count falls below 2,000/mm^3 or granulocyte count falls below 1,000/mm^3, follow institutional policy for infection control in immunocompromised patients.
- Monitor uric acid level. To prevent hyperuricemia with resulting uric acid nephropathy, give allopurinol along with adequate hydration.
- Therapeutic effects are commonly accompanied by toxicity.
- To prevent bleeding, avoid all I.M. injections when platelet count is below 50,000/mm^3.
- Give blood transfusions for cumulative anemia. Inject RBC colony-stimulating factor to promote RBC production and decrease need for transfusions.

PATIENT TEACHING

- Advise patient to watch for signs and symptoms of infection (fever, sore throat, fatigue) and bleeding (easy bruising, nosebleeds, bleeding gums, tarry stools). Tell patient to take temperature daily. Tell patient to report even mild infections.
- Instruct patient to avoid OTC products containing aspirin or NSAIDs.
- Advise woman to stop breast-feeding during therapy because of risk of toxicity to infant.
- Caution woman of childbearing age to consult prescriber before becoming pregnant.

68

Antimetabolites

capecitabine
cytarabine
fludarabine phosphate
fluorouracil
gemcitabine hydrochloride
hydroxyurea
mercaptopurine
methotrexate
methotrexate sodium
pemetrexed

SAFETY ALERT!

capecitabine

Xeloda

Pharmacologic class: pyrimidine analog

Pregnancy risk category D

AVAILABLE FORMS

Tablets: 150 mg, 500 mg

INDICATIONS & DOSAGES

➤ **With docetaxel or alone, metastatic breast cancer resistant to both paclitaxel and an anthracycline-containing chemotherapy regimen or resistant to paclitaxel in patients for whom further anthracycline therapy isn't indicated; first-line treatment of metastatic colorectal cancer when fluoropyrimidine therapy alone is preferred; Dukes C colon cancer after complete resection of primary tumor when fluoropyrimidine alone is preferred**

Adults: 2,500 mg/m^2 daily P.O., in two divided doses, about 12 hours apart and after a meal, for 2 weeks, followed by a 1-week rest period; repeat q 3 weeks. Adjuvant treatment in patients with Dukes C colon cancer is recommended for a total of 6 months.

Adjust-a-dose: Follow National Cancer Institute of Canada (NCIC) common toxicity criteria when adjusting dosage. Toxicity criteria relate to degrees of severity of diarrhea, nausea, vomiting, stomatitis, and hand-and-foot syndrome. Refer to drug package insert for specific toxicity definitions.

NCIC grade 1: Maintain dose level.

NCIC grade 2: At first appearance, stop treatment until resolved to grade 0 to 1; then restart at 100% of starting dose for next cycle. At second appearance, stop treatment until resolved to grade 0 to 1 and use 75% of starting dose for next cycle. At third appearance, stop treatment until resolved to grade 0 to 1 and use 50% of starting dose for next cycle. At fourth appearance, stop treatment permanently.

NCIC grade 3: At first appearance, stop treatment until resolved to grade 0 to 1 and use 75% of starting dose for next cycle. At second appearance, stop treatment until resolved to grade 0 to 1 and use 50% of starting dose for next cycle. At third appearance, stop treatment permanently.

NCIC grade 4: At first appearance, stop treatment permanently or until resolved to grade 0 to 1, and use 50% of starting dose for next cycle.

Reduce starting dose for patients with creatinine clearance 30 to 50 ml/minute to 75% of the starting dose.

ACTION

Converted to active 5-fluorouracil (5-FU), which causes cellular injury by interfering with DNA synthesis to inhibit cell division and with RNA processing and protein synthesis.

Route	Onset	Peak	Duration
P.O.	Unknown	90–120 min	Unknown

Half-life: About 45 minutes.

ADVERSE REACTIONS

CNS: dizziness, *fatigue,* headache, insomnia, *paresthesia, pyrexia.*
CV: edema, chest pain.
EENT: eye irritation, vision abnormality.
GI: *diarrhea, nausea, vomiting, stomatitis, abdominal pain, constipation, anorexia,* ***intestinal obstruction,*** *dyspepsia,* taste perversion.

Hematologic: NEUTROPENIA, THROMBOCYTOPENIA, *anemia, lymphopenia.*
Metabolic: dehydration.
Musculoskeletal: myalgia, limb pain, back pain.
Respiratory: *dyspnea.*
Skin: *hand-and-foot syndrome, dermatitis,* nail disorder, alopecia.

INTERACTIONS

Drug-drug. *Antacids containing aluminum hydroxide and magnesium hydroxide:* May increase exposure to capecitabine and its metabolites. Monitor patient.
Leucovorin: May increase cytotoxic effects of 5-FU with enhanced toxicity. Monitor patient carefully.
Phenytoin: May increase toxicity or phenytoin effect. Monitor phenytoin level.
Warfarin: May decrease clearance of warfarin. Monitor PT and INR.

EFFECTS ON LAB TEST RESULTS

- May increase bilirubin level. May decrease hemoglobin level.
- May decrease neutrophil, platelet, and WBC counts.

CONTRAINDICATIONS & CAUTIONS

- Contraindicated in patients hypersensitive to 5-FU and in those with severe renal impairment.
- Use cautiously in elderly patients and patients with history of coronary artery disease, mild to moderate hepatic dysfunction from liver metastases, hyperbilirubinemia, and renal insufficiency.
- Safety and efficacy of drug in patients age 18 or younger haven't been established.

NURSING CONSIDERATIONS

- Patients older than age 80 may have a greater risk of adverse GI effects.
- Assess patient for severe diarrhea, and notify prescriber if it occurs. Give fluid and electrolyte replacement if patient becomes dehydrated. Drug may need to be immediately interrupted until diarrhea resolves or becomes less intense.
- Monitor patient for hand-and-foot syndrome (numbness, paresthesia, painless or painful swelling, erythema, desquamation, blistering, and severe pain of hands or feet), hyperbilirubinemia, and severe nausea. Drug therapy must be immediately adjusted. Hand-and-foot syndrome is staged from 1 to 4; drug may be stopped if severe or recurrent episodes occur.
- Hyperbilirubinemia may require stopping drug.
- ***Alert:*** Monitor patient carefully for toxicity, which may be managed by symptomatic treatment, dose interruptions, and dosage adjustments.

PATIENT TEACHING

- Tell patient how to take drug. Drug is usually taken for 14 days, followed by 7-day rest period (no drug), as a 21-day cycle. Prescriber determines number of treatment cycles.
- Instruct patient to take drug with water within 30 minutes after end of breakfast and dinner.
- If a combination of tablets is prescribed, teach patient importance of correctly identifying the tablets to avoid possible dosing error.
- For missed doses, instruct patient not to take the missed dose and not to double the next one. Instead, he should continue with regular dosing schedule and check with prescriber.
- Instruct patient to inform prescriber if he's taking folic acid.
- Inform patient and caregiver about expected adverse effects of drug, especially nausea, vomiting, diarrhea, and hand-and-foot syndrome (pain, swelling or redness of hands or feet). Tell him that patient-specific dose adaptations during therapy are expected and needed.
- ***Alert:*** Instruct patient to stop taking drug and contact prescriber immediately if he develops diarrhea (more than four bowel movements daily or diarrhea at night), vomiting (two to five episodes in 24 hours), nausea, appetite loss or decrease in amount of food eaten each day, stomatitis (pain, redness, swelling or sores in mouth), hand-and-foot syndrome, temperature of 100.5° F (38° C) or higher, or other evidence of infection.
- Tell patient that most adverse effects improve within 2 to 3 days after stopping drug. If patient doesn't improve, tell him to contact prescriber.
- Advise woman of childbearing age to avoid becoming pregnant during therapy.

- Advise breast-feeding woman to stop breast-feeding during therapy.

SAFETY ALERT!

cytarabine (ara-C, cytosine arabinoside)

Cytosar†, Cytosar-U, Tarabine PFS

Pharmacologic class: pyrimidine analog
Pregnancy risk category D

AVAILABLE FORMS

Injection: 20 mg/ml
Powder for injection: 100-mg, 500-mg, 1-g, 2-g vials

INDICATIONS & DOSAGES

➤ **Acute nonlymphocytic leukemia, acute lymphocytic leukemia**
Adults and children: For single-agent therapy, 200 mg/m^2 daily by continuous I.V. infusion for 5 days at 2-week intervals. For combination therapy, 100 to 200 mg/m^2 I.V. daily by continuous I.V. infusion or in two or three divided doses by rapid I.V. injection or I.V. infusion for 5 to 10 days in a course of therapy or daily until remission is attained. For maintenance, 1 to 1.5 mg/kg I.M. or subcutaneously q 1 to 4 weeks.

➤ **Refractory acute leukemia; refractory non-Hodgkin lymphoma** ♦
Adults: 3 g/m^2 I.V. over 1 to 3 hours q 12 hours for 4 to 12 doses. Repeat at 2- to 3-week intervals or after patient recovers from toxicity.

➤ **Meningeal leukemia**
Adults and children: Varies from 5 to 75 mg/m^2 intrathecally. Frequency varies from once daily for 4 days to once q 2 to 7 days. The most frequently used dose is 30 mg/m^2 q 4 days until CSF fluid is normal; then one additional dose.

I.V. ADMINISTRATION

- Preparing and giving parenteral form of drug may be mutagenic, teratogenic, or carcinogenic. Follow facility policy to reduce risks.
- To reduce nausea, give antiemetic before drug. Nausea and vomiting are more likely with large doses given by I.V. push. Dizziness may occur with rapid infusion.
- Except for neonates or intrathecal use, reconstitute drug using the provided diluent, which is bacteriostatic water for injection containing benzyl alcohol.
- Reconstitute 100-mg vial with 5 ml of diluent or 500-mg vial with 10 ml of diluent.
- Discard cloudy reconstituted solution.
- For I.V. infusion, further dilute using normal saline solution for injection or D_5W.
- Reconstituted solution is stable for 48 hours.

INCOMPATIBILITIES

Allopurinol sodium, amphotericin B cholesteryl sulfate complex, fluorouracil, ganciclovir sodium, heparin sodium, hydrocortisone sodium succinate, insulin, methylprednisolone sodium succinate, nafcillin, oxacillin, penicillin.

ACTION

Inhibits DNA synthesis.

Route	Onset	Peak	Duration
I.V., I.M., intrathecal	Unknown	Unknown	Unknown
SubQ	Unknown	20–60 min	Unknown

Half-life: Initial, 8 minutes; terminal, 1 to 3 hours; in CSF, 2 hours.

ADVERSE REACTIONS

CNS: neurotoxicity, malaise, dizziness, headache, cerebellar syndrome, *fever.*
CV: *thrombophlebitis,* edema.
EENT: conjunctivitis.
GI: *nausea, vomiting, diarrhea, anorexia, anal ulceration,* abdominal pain, oral ulcers in 5 to 10 days, projectile vomiting, bowel necrosis with high doses given by rapid I.V.
GU: urine retention, renal dysfunction.
Hematologic: ***leukopenia,*** anemia, reticulocytopenia, ***thrombocytopenia,*** *megaloblastosis.*
Hepatic: ***hepatotoxicity,*** jaundice.
Metabolic: hyperuricemia.
Musculoskeletal: myalgia, bone pain.
Respiratory: ***pulmonary edema,*** shortness of breath, pulmonary hypersensitivity.
Skin: *rash,* pruritus, alopecia, freckling.

Other: flulike syndrome, infection, ***anaphylaxis.***

INTERACTIONS

Drug-drug. *Digoxin, except oral liquid and liquid-filled capsules:* May decrease oral digoxin absorption. Monitor digoxin level closely.
Flucytosine: May decrease flucytosine activity. Avoid using together.
Gentamicin: May decrease activity against *Klebsiella pneumoniae..* Avoid using together.

EFFECTS ON LAB TEST RESULTS

- May increase bilirubin, phosphorus, potassium, and uric acid levels. May decrease hemoglobin level.
- May increase megaloblast count. May decrease platelet, RBC, reticulocyte, and WBC counts.

CONTRAINDICATIONS & CAUTIONS

- Contraindicated in patients hypersensitive to drug.
- Use cautiously in patients with hepatic or renal compromise, gout, or myelosuppression.

NURSING CONSIDERATIONS

- For intrathecal administration, use preservative-free normal saline solution. Add 5 ml to 100-mg vial or 10 ml to 500-mg vial. Use immediately after reconstitution. Discard unused drug.
- Monitor fluid intake and output carefully. Maintain high fluid intake and give allopurinol to avoid urate nephropathy in leukemia-induction therapy. Monitor uric acid level.
- Monitor hepatic and renal function studies and CBC.
- Therapy may be modified or stopped if granulocyte count is below 1,000/mm^3 or platelet count is below 50,000/mm^3.
- Corticosteroid eyedrops help prevent drug-induced conjunctivitis.
- Provide diligent mouth care to help prevent stomatitis.
- ***Alert:*** Assess patient receiving high doses for neurotoxicity, which may first appear as nystagmus but can progress to ataxia and cerebellar dysfunction.
- To prevent bleeding, avoid all I.M. injections when platelet count is below 50,000/mm^3.
- Anticipate blood transfusions because of cumulative anemia. Patient may receive RBC colony–stimulating factors to promote RBC production and decrease need for blood transfusions.
- Therapeutic effects frequently occur with toxicity.
- In leukopenia, initial WBC count nadir occurs 7 to 9 days after drug is stopped. A second, more severe nadir occurs 15 to 24 days after drug is stopped. In thrombocytopenia, platelet count nadir occurs on days 12 to 15.

PATIENT TEACHING

- Instruct patient to watch for signs and symptoms of infection (fever, sore throat, fatigue) and bleeding (easy bruising, nosebleeds, bleeding gums, tarry stools). Tell patient to take temperature daily.
- Advise patient to report visual changes, blurred vision, or eye pain to prescriber.
- Advise breast-feeding woman to stop breast-feeding during therapy because of risk of toxicity to infant.
- Caution woman of childbearing age to consult prescriber before becoming pregnant because drug may harm fetus.

SAFETY ALERT!

fludarabine phosphate

Fludara

Pharmacologic class: purine analog
Pregnancy risk category D

AVAILABLE FORMS

Powder for injection: 50 mg
Liquid for injection: 50 mg/2 ml

INDICATIONS & DOSAGES

➤ **B-cell chronic lymphocytic leukemia in patients with no or inadequate response to at least one standard alkylating drug regimen**
Adults: 25 mg/m^2 I.V. daily over 30 minutes for 5 consecutive days. Repeat cycle q 28 days.
Adjust-a-dose: In patients with creatinine clearance of 30 to 70 ml/minute, decrease

dose by 20%. Don't use drug in patients with clearance less than 30 ml/minute.

I.V. ADMINISTRATION

- Preparing and giving parenteral drug may be mutagenic, teratogenic, or carcinogenic. Follow facility policy to reduce risks.
- To prepare, add 2 ml of sterile water for injection to the vial. If using the powder for injection, dissolution should occur within 15 seconds.
- Each milliliter contains 25 mg of drug.
- Dilute further in 100 or 125 ml of D_5W or normal saline solution for injection.
- Use within 8 hours of reconstitution.
- Store drug in refrigerator at 36° to 46° F (2° to 8° C).

INCOMPATIBILITIES

Acyclovir sodium, amphotericin B, chlorpromazine, daunorubicin, ganciclovir, hydroxyzine hydrochloride, prochlorperazine edisylate.

ACTION

Unknown. After conversion to its active metabolite, drug interferes with DNA synthesis by inhibiting DNA polymerase alpha, ribonucleotide reductase, and DNA primase.

Route	Onset	Peak	Duration
I.V.	7–21 wk	Unknown	Unknown

Half-life: About 10 hours.

ADVERSE REACTIONS

CNS: *fatigue, malaise, weakness, paresthesia,* peripheral neuropathy, ***stroke,*** headache, sleep disorder, depression, cerebellar syndrome, ***transient ischemic attack,*** agitation, *confusion, fever,* ***coma.***
CV: *edema,* angina, phlebitis, ***arrhythmias, heart failure, MI,*** supraventricular tachycardia, ***deep vein thrombosis, aneurysm, hemorrhage.***
EENT: *visual disturbances,* hearing loss, delayed blindness, sinusitis, pharyngitis, epistaxis.
GI: *nausea, vomiting, diarrhea,* constipation, *anorexia,* stomatitis, ***GI bleeding,*** esophagitis, mucositis.
GU: dysuria, *UTI,* urinary hesitancy, proteinuria, hematuria, ***renal failure.***
Hematologic: ***hemolytic anemia,*** **MYELOSUPPRESSION.**
Hepatic: ***liver failure,*** cholelithiasis.
Metabolic: hypocalcemia, hyperkalemia, hyperglycemia, dehydration, hyperuricemia, hyperphosphatemia.
Musculoskeletal: *myalgia.*
Respiratory: *cough, pneumonia, dyspnea, upper respiratory tract infection,* allergic pneumonitis, hemoptysis, hypoxia, bronchitis.
Skin: *rash,* pruritus, alopecia, seborrhea, diaphoresis.
Other: *chills, pain,* tumor lysis syndrome, **INFECTION,** ***anaphylaxis.***

INTERACTIONS

Drug-drug. *Cytarabine:* May decrease metabolism of subsequently given fludarabine and inhibition of fludarabine activity. Monitor patient closely.
Myelosuppressives: May increase toxicity. Avoid using together, if possible.
Pentostatin: May increase risk of pulmonary toxicity, which can be fatal. Avoid using together.

EFFECTS ON LAB TEST RESULTS

- May increase glucose, phosphate, potassium, and uric acid levels. May decrease calcium and hemoglobin levels.
- May decrease platelet, RBC, and WBC counts.

CONTRAINDICATIONS & CAUTIONS

- Contraindicated in patients hypersensitive to drug or its components and in those with creatinine clearance less than 30 ml/minute.
- Use cautiously in patients with renal insufficiency.

NURSING CONSIDERATIONS

- ***Alert:*** Monitor patient closely and expect modified dosage based on toxicity. Most toxic effects are dose-dependent. Advanced age, renal insufficiency, and bone marrow impairment may predispose patients to increased or excessive toxicity.
- ***Alert:*** Careful hematologic monitoring is needed, especially of neutrophil and

platelet counts. Bone marrow suppression can be severe.
- Severe and fatal neurotoxicity may occur.
- To prevent bleeding, avoid all I.M. injections when platelet count is below 50,000/mm^3.
- Give blood transfusions because of cumulative anemia. Patients may receive RBC colony-stimulating factors to promote RBC production and decrease need for blood transfusions.
- Hyperuricemia, hypocalcemia, hyperkalemia, and renal failure may result from rapid lysis of tumor cells. Take preventative measures against tumor lysis syndrome, such as I.V. hydration, alkalinization of urine, and treatment with allopurinol as appropriate.
- ***Look alike–sound alike:*** Don't confuse fludarabine with floxuridine, fluorouracil, or flucytosine.

PATIENT TEACHING
- Instruct patient to watch for signs and symptoms of infection (fever, sore throat, fatigue) and bleeding (easy bruising, nosebleeds, bleeding gums, tarry stools). Tell patient to take temperature daily.
- Advise woman to consult prescriber before becoming pregnant.
- Caution woman to stop breast-feeding during therapy because of risk of toxicity to infant.

SAFETY ALERT!

fluorouracil (5-fluorouracil, 5-FU)
Adrucil, Carac, Efudex, Fluoroplex

Pharmacologic class: pyrimidine analog
Pregnancy risk category D (injection); X (topical form)

AVAILABLE FORMS
Cream: 1%, 5%
Injection: 50 mg/ml
Topical solution: 1%, 2%, 5%

INDICATIONS & DOSAGES
➤ **Colon, rectal, breast, stomach, and pancreatic cancers**
Adults: Initially, 12 mg/kg I.V. daily for 4 days; if no toxicity, give 6 mg/kg on days 6, 8, 10, and 12; then give a single weekly maintenance dose of 10 to 15 mg/kg I.V. begun after toxicity (if any) from first course has subsided. (Recommended dosages are based on actual body weight unless patient is obese or retaining fluid.) .
➤ **Palliative treatment of advanced colorectal cancer**
Adults: 425 mg/m^2 I.V. daily for 5 consecutive days. Give with 20 mg/m^2 of leucovorin I.V. Repeat at 4-week intervals for two additional courses; then repeat at 4- to 5-week intervals if tolerated.
➤ **Early breast cancer**
Adults: 600 mg/m^2 I.V. on days 1 and 8 of each cycle, combined with cyclophosphamide 100 mg/m^2 on days 1 through 14 of each cycle and methotrexate 40 mg/m^2 on days 1 and 8 of each cycle. Repeat monthly for 6 to 12 months, allowing for a 2-week rest period between cycles. In adults older than age 60, first fluorouracil dose is 400 mg/m^2 and methotrexate dose is 30 mg/m^2.
➤ **Multiple actinic (solar) keratoses**
Adults: Apply Carac cream once daily for up to 4 weeks. Or, apply Efudex or Fluoroplex cream or topical solution b.i.d. for 2 to 6 weeks.
➤ **Superficial basal cell carcinoma**
Adults: Apply 5% Efudex cream or topical solution b.i.d. usually for 3 to 6 weeks, maximum, 12 weeks.

I.V. ADMINISTRATION
- Preparing and giving parenteral drug may be mutagenic, teratogenic, or carcinogenic. Follow facility policy to reduce risks.
- To reduce nausea, give antiemetic before fluorouracil.
- Don't use cloudy solution. If crystals form, redissolve by warming.
- Drug may be given by direct injection without dilution.
- For infusion, drug may be diluted with D_5W, sterile water for injection, or normal saline solution for injection.

- For continuous infusion, use plastic I.V. containers. Solution is more stable in plastic than in glass bottles.
- Don't refrigerate. Protect drug from sunlight.
- Discard unused portion of vial after 1 hour.

INCOMPATIBILITIES
Aldesleukin, amphotericin B cholesterol complex, carboplatin, cisplatin, cytarabine, diazepam, doxorubicin, droperidol, epirubicin, fentanyl citrate, filgrastim, gallium nitrate, leucovorin calcium, metoclopramide, morphine sulfate, ondansetron, topotecan, vinorelbine tartrate.

ACTION
May inhibit DNA and RNA synthesis.

Route	Onset	Peak	Duration
I.V., topical	Unknown	Unknown	Unknown

Half-life: 20 minutes.

ADVERSE REACTIONS
CNS: acute cerebellar syndrome, confusion, disorientation, euphoria, ataxia, headache, *weakness, malaise.*
CV: ***myocardial ischemia,*** angina, thrombophlebitis.
EENT: epistaxis, photophobia, lacrimation, lacrimal duct stenosis, nystagmus, visual changes, eye irritation.
GI: *stomatitis, GI ulcer, nausea, vomiting, diarrhea, anorexia,* ***GI bleeding.***
Hematologic: ***leukopenia, thrombocytopenia, agranulocytosis,*** *anemia.*
Skin: *dermatitis, erythema, scaling, pruritus,* nail changes, pigmented palmar creases, erythematous contact dermatitis, desquamative rash of hands and feet, hand-and-foot syndrome with long-term use, photosensitivity, *reversible alopecia, pain, burning,* soreness, suppuration, *swelling, dryness, erosion with topical use.*
Other: ***anaphylaxis.***

INTERACTIONS
Drug-drug. *Leucovorin calcium:* May increase cytotoxicity and toxicity of fluorouracil. Monitor patient closely.
Drug-lifestyle. *Sun exposure:* May cause photosensitivity reactions. Advise patient to avoid excessive sunlight exposure.

EFFECTS ON LAB TEST RESULTS
- May increase alkaline phosphatase, AST, ALT, bilirubin, 5-hydroxyindoleacetic acid (in urine), and LDH levels. May decrease hemoglobin and plasma albumin levels.
- May decrease granulocyte, platelet, RBC, and WBC counts.

CONTRAINDICATIONS & CAUTIONS
- Contraindicated in patients hypersensitive to drug and in those with bone marrow suppression (WBC counts of 5,000/mm^3 or less or platelet counts of 100,000/mm^3 or less) or potentially serious infections.
- Contraindicated in patients in a poor nutritional state and those who have had major surgery within previous month.
- Topical formulations contraindicated in pregnant women.
- Use cautiously in patients who have received high-dose pelvic radiation or alkylating drugs and in those with impaired hepatic or renal function or widespread neoplastic infiltration of bone marrow.

NURSING CONSIDERATIONS
- Apply topical form cautiously near patient's eyes, nose, and mouth.
- Avoid occlusive dressings with topical form because they increase risk of inflammatory reactions in adjacent normal skin.
- Apply topical form with a nonmetal applicator or suitable gloves. Wash hands immediately after handling topical form.
- The 1% topical strength is used on patient's face. Higher strengths, such as 5%, are used for thicker-skinned areas or resistant lesions, such as superficial basal cell carcinoma.
- Ingestion and systemic absorption of topical form may cause leukopenia, thrombocytopenia, stomatitis, diarrhea, or GI ulceration, bleeding, and hemorrhage. Application to large ulcerated areas may cause systemic toxicity.
- Watch for stomatitis or diarrhea (signs of toxicity). Consider using topical oral

anesthetic to soothe lesions. Stop drug and notify prescriber if diarrhea occurs.
- Encourage diligent oral hygiene to prevent superinfection of denuded mucosa.
- Monitor WBC and platelet counts daily. Watch for ecchymoses, petechiae, easy bruising, and anemia.
- Monitor fluid intake and output, CBC, and renal and hepatic function tests.
- Long-term use may cause erythematous, desquamative rash of the hands and feet, which may be treated with pyridoxine 50 to 150 mg P.O. daily for 5 to 7 days.
- Dermatologic adverse effects are reversible when drug is stopped.
- To prevent bleeding, avoid I.M. injections when platelet count is below 50,000/mm^3.
- Anticipate blood transfusions because of cumulative anemia. Patient may receive injections of RBC colony-stimulating factors to promote RBC production and decrease need for blood transfusions.
- ***Alert:*** Toxicity may be delayed for 1 to 3 weeks.
- The WBC count nadir occurs 9 to 14 days after first dose; the platelet count nadir occurs in 7 to 14 days.
- ***Look alike–sound alike:*** Drug may be ordered as "5-fluorouracil" or "5-FU." The numeral "5" is part of the drug name and shouldn't be confused with dosage units.
- ***Look alike–sound alike:*** Don't confuse fluorouracil with floxuridine, fludarabine, or flucytosine.

PATIENT TEACHING
- Warn patient that hair loss may occur but is reversible.
- Caution patient to avoid prolonged exposure to sunlight or ultraviolet light when topical form is used.
- Tell patient to use highly protective sunblock to avoid inflammatory skin irritation.
- Warn patient that topically treated area may be unsightly during therapy and for several weeks afterward. Complete healing may take 1 or 2 months.
- Caution woman of childbearing age to consult prescriber before becoming pregnant.
- Advise woman to stop breast-feeding during therapy because of risk of toxicity to infant.

SAFETY ALERT!

gemcitabine hydrochloride
Gemzar

Pharmacologic class: pyrimidine analog
Pregnancy risk category D

AVAILABLE FORMS
Powder for injection: 200-mg, 1-g vials

INDICATIONS & DOSAGES
➤ Locally advanced or metastatic adenocarcinoma of pancreas
Adults: 1,000 mg/m^2 I.V. over 30 minutes once weekly for up to 7 weeks, unless toxicity occurs. Monitor CBC with differential and platelet count before giving each dose.
Adjust-a-dose: If bone marrow suppression is detected, adjust therapy. If absolute granulocyte count (AGC) is 1,000/mm^3 or more and platelet count is 100,000/mm^3 or more, give full dose. If AGC is 500 to 999/mm^3 or platelet count is 50,000 to 99,999/mm^3, give 75% of dose. If AGC is below 500/mm^3 or platelet count is below 50,000/mm^3, withhold dose. Course of 7 weeks is followed by 1 week of rest. Subsequent dosage cycles consist of one infusion weekly for 3 of 4 consecutive weeks. Dosage adjustments for subsequent cycles are based on AGC and platelet count nadirs and degree of nonhematologic toxicity.
➤ With cisplatin, first-line treatment of inoperable, locally advanced, or metastatic non–small-cell lung cancer
Adults: For 4-week schedule, 1,000 mg/m^2 I.V. over 30 minutes on days 1, 8, and 15 of each 28-day cycle. 100 mg/m^2 cisplatin on day 1 after gemcitabine infusion.

For 3-week schedule, 1,250 mg/m^2 I.V. over 30 minutes on days 1 and 8 of each 21-day cycle. 100 mg/m^2 cisplatin on day 1 after gemcitabine infusion.
✱ NEW INDICATION: **With carboplatin, for treatment of advanced ovarian**

cancer that relapsed at least 6 months after platinum-based therapy
Adults: 1,000 mg/m² I.V. over 30 minutes on days 1 and 8 of each 21-day cycle. Give carboplatin AUC 4 I.V. on day 1 after gemcitabine. Check CBC with differential and platelet count before each dose. The absolute granulocyte count (AGC) should be 1,500/mm³ or higher and platelet count 100,000/mm³ or higher before each cycle.
Adjust-a-dose: Base adjustment on AGC and platelet count results on day 8 of cycle. If AGC is 1,000 to 1,499/mm³, give 50% of dose. If AGC is below 1,000/mm³ or platelet count is below 75,000/mm³, hold dose. Adjustments for subsequent cycles based on observed toxicities.
➤ **With paclitaxel, first-line therapy for metastatic breast cancer after failure of other adjuvant chemotherapy with an anthracycline**
Adults: 1,250 mg/m² I.V. over 30 minutes on days 1 and 8 of each 21-day cycle, with 175 mg/m² paclitaxel I.V. as a 3-hour infusion given before gemcitabine dose on day 1 of the cycle. Adjust dosage based on total AGC and platelet counts taken on day 8 of the cycle.
Adjust-a-dose: If AGC is 1,000 to 1,199/mm³ or platelet count is 50,000 to 75,000/mm³, give 75% of dose. If AGC is 700 to 999/mm³ and platelet count is 50,000/mm³ or above, give 50% of dose. If AGC is below 700/mm³ or platelet count is below 50,000/mm³, withhold dose.

I.V. ADMINISTRATION
- Preparing and giving parenteral drug may be mutagenic, teratogenic, or carcinogenic. Follow facility policy to reduce risks.
- To prepare solution, add 5 ml of unpreserved normal saline solution for injection to 200-mg vial or 25 ml to 1-g vial. Shake to dissolve.
- Resulting concentration is 40 mg/ml; reconstitution at higher concentrations isn't recommended.
- If needed, consider diluting to as little as 0.1 mg/ml by adding normal saline solution for injection.
- Make sure solution is clear to light straw-colored and free of particles.
- Don't extend infusion time beyond 60 minutes or give drug more often than once weekly; doing so may increase toxicity.
- Drug is stable 24 hours at room temperature.
- Don't refrigerate reconstituted drug because it may crystallize.

INCOMPATIBILITIES
Acyclovir, amphotericin B, cefoperazone, cefotaxime, furosemide, ganciclovir, imipenem and cilastatin, irinotecan, methotrexate, methylprednisolone, mitomycin, piperacillin, piperacillin and tazobactam sodium, prochlorperazine, sodium succinate.

ACTION
Cytotoxic and specific to cell cycle; inhibits DNA synthesis and blocks progression of cells.

Route	Onset	Peak	Duration
I.V.	Unknown	Unknown	Unknown

Half-life: About 2 to 19½ hours

ADVERSE REACTIONS
CNS: *somnolence, paresthesia, pain, fever.*
CV: *edema, peripheral edema.*
GI: *stomatitis, nausea, vomiting, constipation, diarrhea.*
GU: *proteinuria, hematuria.*
Hematologic: *anemia,* ***leukopenia, neutropenia, thrombocytopenia.***
Hepatic: ***hepatotoxicity.***
Respiratory: *dyspnea,* ***bronchospasm, pneumonitis.***
Skin: *alopecia, rash,* pain at injection site.
Other: *flulike syndrome, infection.*

INTERACTIONS
None significant.

EFFECTS ON LAB TEST RESULTS
- May increase ALT, AST, BUN, and creatinine levels. May decrease hemoglobin level.
- May decrease neutrophil, platelet, and WBC counts.

CONTRAINDICATIONS & CAUTIONS

- Contraindicated in patients hypersensitive to drug and in pregnant or breast-feeding women.
- Use cautiously in patients with renal or hepatic impairment.
- In children, safety and effectiveness haven't been determined.

NURSING CONSIDERATIONS

- Monitor patient closely. Expect dosage modification according to toxicity and degree of myelosuppression. Age, gender, and presence of renal impairment may predispose patient to toxicity.
- Carefully monitor hematologic values, especially of neutrophil and platelet counts.
- Obtain baseline and periodic renal and hepatic laboratory tests.

PATIENT TEACHING

- Advise patient to watch for evidence of infection (fever, sore throat, fatigue) and bleeding (easy bruising, nosebleeds, bleeding gums, tarry stools). Tell patient to take temperature daily.
- Advise patient to promptly report flu-like symptoms or breathing problems.
- Tell patient that adverse effects may continue after treatment ends.
- Caution woman to avoid pregnancy or breast-feeding during therapy.

SAFETY ALERT!

hydroxyurea

Droxia, Hydrea

Pharmacologic class: antimetabolite
Pregnancy risk category D

AVAILABLE FORMS

Capsules: 200 mg, 250 mg, 300 mg, 400 mg, 500 mg

INDICATIONS & DOSAGES

➤ **Melanoma; resistant chronic myelocytic leukemia; recurrent, metastatic, or inoperable ovarian cancer; head and neck cancers**
Adults: 80 mg/kg Hydrea P.O. as single dose q 3 days; or 20 to 30 mg/kg P.O. as single daily dose.

➤ **To reduce frequency of painful crises and need for blood transfusions in adult patients with sickle cell anemia with recurrent moderate to severe painful crises**
Adults: 15 mg/kg Droxia P.O. once daily. If blood counts are in acceptable range, dose may be increased by 5 mg/kg daily q 12 weeks until maximum tolerated dose or 35 mg/kg daily has been reached. If blood counts are considered toxic, withhold drug until counts recover. Resume treatment after reducing dose by 2.5 mg/kg daily. Every 12 weeks, drug may then be adjusted up or down in 2.5-mg/kg daily increments until patient is at a stable, nontoxic dose for 24 weeks.

➤ **To reduce platelet count and prevent thrombosis in patients with essential thrombocythemia ♦**
Adults: 15 mg/kg Hydrea P.O. daily.

➤ **Refractory psoriasis ♦**
Adults: 0.5 to 1.5 g Hydrea P.O. daily.

ACTION

May inhibit DNA synthesis.

Route	Onset	Peak	Duration
P.O.	Unknown	2 hr	24 hr

Half-life: 3 to 4 hours.

ADVERSE REACTIONS

CNS: ***seizures,*** hallucinations, headache, dizziness, disorientation, malaise, fever.
GI: *anorexia, nausea, vomiting, diarrhea,* stomatitis, constipation.
Hematologic: ***leukopenia, thrombocytopenia,*** *anemia, megaloblastosis,* ***bone marrow suppression.***
Metabolic: hyperuricemia, weight gain.
Skin: rash, itching, alopecia.
Other: chills.

INTERACTIONS

Drug-drug. *Cytotoxic drugs, radiation therapy:* May enhance toxicity of hydroxyurea. Use together cautiously.

EFFECTS ON LAB TEST RESULTS

- May increase BUN, creatinine, hepatic enzyme, and uric acid levels. May decrease hemoglobin level.
- May decrease WBC, RBC, and platelet counts.

CONTRAINDICATIONS & CAUTIONS
• Contraindicated in patients hypersensitive to drug and in those with WBC count less than 2,500/mm³, platelet count less than 100,000/mm³, or severe anemia.
• Use cautiously in patients with renal dysfunction and in the elderly.

NURSING CONSIDERATIONS
• Routinely measure BUN, uric acid, liver enzyme, and creatinine levels; monitor blood counts every 2 weeks.
• Acceptable blood counts during dosage adjustment are neutrophil count of 2,500/mm³ or more, platelet count of 95,000/mm³ or more, hemoglobin level more than 5.3 g/dl, and reticulocyte count (if hemoglobin level is below 9 g/dl) more than 95,000/mm³. Toxic levels are neutrophil count less than 2,000/mm³, platelet count less than 80,000/mm³, hemoglobin level less than 4.5 g/dl, and reticulocyte count (if hemoglobin level is below 9 g/dl) less than 80,000/mm³.
• Hydroxyurea may dramatically lower WBC count in 24 to 48 hours.
• ***Alert:*** Patients who have received or are currently receiving interferon may be at a greater risk of developing cutaneous vasculitic toxicities. Monitor closely.
• Monitor fluid intake and output; keep patient hydrated.
• Allopurinol is used to treat or prevent tumor lysis syndrome.
• To prevent bleeding, avoid all I.M. injections when platelet count is less than 50,000/mm³.
• Give blood transfusions for cumulative anemia. Patient may receive injections of RBC colony-stimulating factors to promote RBC production and decrease need for blood transfusions.
• Dosage change may be needed after chemotherapy or radiation therapy.
• Auditory and visual hallucinations and hematologic toxicity increase when renal function decreases.
• Drug crosses blood-brain barrier.
• Radiation therapy may increase risk or severity of GI distress or stomatitis.

PATIENT TEACHING
• Tell patient and caregiver to wear gloves when handling drug or its container and to wash their hands before and after contact with the bottle or capsule. If powder from capsule is spilled, wipe it up immediately with a damp towel and dispose of the towel in a closed container, such as a plastic bag.
• Tell patient who can't swallow capsules that he may empty contents into water, drink immediately, and rinse mouth with water afterward. Inform patient that some inert material may not dissolve.
• Advise patient to watch for signs and symptoms of infection (fever, sore throat, fatigue) and bleeding (easy bruising, nosebleeds, bleeding gums, tarry stools). He also should take his temperature daily.
• Caution woman of childbearing age to consult prescriber before becoming pregnant.

SAFETY ALERT!

mercaptopurine (6-mercaptopurine, 6-MP)
Purinethol

Pharmacologic class: purine analogue
Pregnancy risk category D

AVAILABLE FORMS
Tablets (scored): 50 mg

INDICATIONS & DOSAGES
➤ **Acute lymphoblastic leukemia, acute myeloblastic leukemia**
Adults and children: 2.5 mg/kg P.O. once daily (rounded to nearest 25 mg). May increase to 5 mg/kg daily after 4 weeks if no improvement.

After remission is attained, usual maintenance dose for adults and children is 1.5 to 2.5 mg/kg once daily.

ACTION
Inhibits RNA and DNA synthesis.

Route	Onset	Peak	Duration
P.O.	Unknown	Unknown	Unknown

Half-life: Unknown.

ADVERSE REACTIONS
GI: nausea, vomiting, anorexia, painful oral ulcers, diarrhea, ***pancreatitis,*** GI ulceration.

Hematologic: ***leukopenia, thrombocytopenia,*** *anemia.*
Hepatic: *jaundice,* ***hepatotoxicity.***
Metabolic: hyperuricemia.
Skin: rash, hyperpigmentation.

INTERACTIONS

Drug-drug. ***Allopurinol:*** Slows inactivation of mercaptopurine. Decrease mercaptopurine to 25% or 33% of normal dose.
Co-trimoxazole: May enhance bone marrow suppression. Monitor CBC with differential carefully.
Hepatotoxic drugs: May enhance hepatotoxicity of mercaptopurine. Monitor patient for hepatotoxicity.
Nondepolarizing neuromuscular blockers: May antagonize muscle relaxant effect. Notify anesthesiologist that patient is receiving mercaptopurine.
Warfarin: May decrease or increase anticoagulant effect. Monitor PT and INR.

EFFECTS ON LAB TEST RESULTS

- May increase uric acid, transaminase, alkaline phosphatase, and bilirubin levels. May decrease hemoglobin level.
- May decrease WBC, RBC, and platelet counts.

CONTRAINDICATIONS & CAUTIONS

- Contraindicated in patients resistant or hypersensitive to drug.

NURSING CONSIDERATIONS

- Consider modifying dosage after chemotherapy or radiation therapy in patients who have depressed neutrophil or platelet counts or impaired hepatic or renal function.
- ***Alert:*** Drug may be ordered as "6-mercaptopurine" or as "6-MP." The numeral 6 is part of drug name and doesn't refer to dosage.
- Monitor CBC and transaminase, alkaline phosphatase, and bilirubin levels weekly during induction and monthly during maintenance.
- Leukopenia, thrombocytopenia, or anemia may persist for several days after drug is stopped.
- Watch for signs of bleeding and infection.
- Monitor fluid intake and output. Encourage 3 L fluid intake daily.
- ***Alert:*** Watch for jaundice, clay-colored stools, and frothy, dark urine. Hepatic dysfunction is reversible when drug is stopped. If right-sided abdominal tenderness occurs, stop drug and notify prescriber.
- Monitor uric acid level. Use allopurinol cautiously.
- To prevent bleeding, avoid all I.M. injections when platelet count is below 100,000/mm^3.
- Anticipate need for blood transfusions because of cumulative anemia. Patient may receive injections of RBC colony-stimulating factors to promote RBC production and decrease need for blood transfusions.
- GI adverse reactions are less common in children than in adults.

PATIENT TEACHING

- Instruct patient to watch for signs and symptoms of infection (fever, sore throat, fatigue) and bleeding (easy bruising, nosebleeds, bleeding gums, tarry stools). Tell patient to take temperature daily.
- Caution woman of childbearing age to consult prescriber before becoming pregnant.
- Advise woman to stop breast-feeding during therapy because of risk of toxicity to infant.

SAFETY ALERT!

methotrexate (amethopterin, MTX)

methotrexate sodium

Ledertrexate‡, Methoblastin‡, Methotrexate LPF, Rheumatrex, Trexall

Pharmacologic class: folic acid antagonist
Pregnancy risk category X

AVAILABLE FORMS

Injection: 25 mg/ml in 2-ml, 4-ml, 8-ml, 10-ml, 20-ml, and 40-ml preservative-free single use vials; 25 mg/ml in 2-ml and 10-ml vials containing benzyl alcohol
Lyophilized powder: 20-mg, 1,000-mg vials, preservative-free; 2.5-mg/ml, 25-mg/ml vials

Tablets (scored): 2.5 mg, 5 mg, 7.5 mg, 10 mg‡, 15 mg

INDICATIONS & DOSAGES

➤ **Trophoblastic tumors (choriocarcinoma, hydatidiform mole)**
Adults: Give 15 to 30 mg P.O. or I.M. daily for 5 days. Repeat after 1 or more weeks, based on response or toxicity. Number of courses is three to maximum of five.

➤ **Acute lymphocytic leukemia**
Adults and children: Give 3.3 mg/m^2 daily P.O., I.V., or I.M. with 40 to 60 mg/m^2 prednisone daily for 4 to 6 weeks or until remission occurs; then 20 to 30 mg/m^2 P.O. or I.M. weekly in two divided doses or 2.5 mg/kg I.V. q 14 days.

➤ **Meningeal leukemia**
Adults and children: Give 12 mg/m^2 or less (maximum 15 mg) intrathecally q 2 to 5 days until CSF is normal; then one additional dose. Or, for children, use dosages based on age.
Children age 3 and older: Give 12 mg intrathecally q 2 to 5 days.
Children ages 2 to 3: Give 10 mg intrathecally q 2 to 5 days.
Children ages 1 to 2: Give 8 mg intrathecally q 2 to 5 days.
Children younger than age 1: Give 6 mg intrathecally q 2 to 5 days.

➤ **Burkitt lymphoma (stage I, II, or III)**
Adults: 10 to 25 mg P.O. daily for 4 to 8 days, with 1-week rest intervals.

➤ **Lymphosarcoma (stage III)**
Adults: 0.625 to 2.5 mg/kg daily P.O., I.M., or I.V.

➤ **Osteosarcoma**
Adults: Initially, 12 g/m^2 I.V. as 4-hour infusion. Give subsequent doses 15 g/m^2 I.V. as 4-hour I.V. infusion at postoperative weeks 4, 5, 6, 7, 11, 12, 15, 16, 29, 30, 44, and 45. Give with leucovorin, 15 mg P.O. q 6 hours for 10 doses, beginning 24 hours after start of methotrexate infusion.

➤ **Breast cancer**
Adults: 40 mg/m^2 I.V. on days 1 and 8 of each cycle, combined with cyclophosphamide and fluorouracil.
Adjust-a-dose: In patients older than age 60, give 30 mg/m^2.

➤ **Mycosis fungoides**
Adults: 2.5 to 10 mg P.O. daily; or 50 mg I.M. weekly; or 25 mg I.M. twice weekly.

➤ **Psoriasis**
Adults: 10 to 25 mg P.O., I.M., or I.V. as single weekly dose; or 2.5 to 5 mg P.O. q 12 hours for three doses weekly. Dosage shouldn't exceed 30 mg per week.

➤ **Rheumatoid arthritis**
Adults: Initially, 7.5 mg P.O. weekly, either in single dose or divided as 2.5 mg P.O. q 12 hours for three doses once weekly. Dosage may be gradually increased to maximum of 20 mg weekly.

I.V. ADMINISTRATION

- Preparation and administration of parenteral form of drug may be mutagenic, teratogenic, or carcinogenic to staff. Follow institutional policy to reduce risks.
- Dilution of drug depends on product, and infusion guidelines vary, depending on dose.
- Reconstitute 20-mg vial to a concentration no greater than 25 mg/ml. Reconstitute 1-g vial to a concentration of 50 mg/ml.
- If giving infusion, dilute total dose in D_5W.
- Reconstitute solutions without preservatives with normal saline solution or D_5W immediately before use, and discard unused drug.

INCOMPATIBILITIES

Bleomycin, chlorpromazine, droperidol, gemcitabine, idarubicin, ifosfamide, midazolam, nalbuphine, promethazine, propofol.

ACTION

Reversibly binds to dihydrofolate reductase, blocking reduction of folic acid to tetrahydrofolate, a cofactor necessary for purine, protein, and DNA synthesis.

Route	Onset	Peak	Duration
P.O.	Unknown	1–2 hr	Unknown
I.V.	Immediate	Immediate	Unknown
I.M.	Unknown	30 min–1 hr	Unknown
Intrathecal	Unknown	Unknown	Unknown

Half-life: For doses below 30 mg/m^2, about 3 to 10 hours; for doses of 30 mg/m^2 and above, 8 to 15 hours.

ADVERSE REACTIONS

CNS: ***arachnoiditis within hours of intrathecal use, leukoencephalopathy, seizures,*** subacute neurotoxicity possibly beginning a few weeks later, demyelination, malaise, fatigue, dizziness, headache, aphasia, hemiparesis, fever, drowsiness.
EENT: pharyngitis, blurred vision.
GI: gingivitis, *stomatitis, diarrhea,* abdominal distress, anorexia, GI ulceration and bleeding, enteritis, *nausea, vomiting.*
GU: nephropathy, *tubular necrosis,* ***renal failure,*** hematuria, menstrual dysfunction, defective spermatogenesis, infertility, abortion, cystitis.
Hematologic: *anemia,* ***leukopenia, thrombocytopenia.***
Hepatic: ***acute toxicity, chronic toxicity,*** including cirrhosis and, ***hepatic fibrosis.***
Metabolic: diabetes, hyperuricemia.
Musculoskeletal: arthralgia, myalgia, osteoporosis in children on long-term therapy.
Respiratory: ***pulmonary fibrosis, pulmonary interstitial infiltrates,*** pneumonitis, dry, nonproductive cough.
Skin: *urticaria,* pruritus, hyperpigmentation, erythematous rashes, ecchymoses, rash, photosensitivity, alopecia, acne, psoriatic lesions aggravated by exposure to sun.
Other: chills, reduced resistance to infection, septicemia, ***sudden death.***

INTERACTIONS

Drug-drug. ***Acitretin:*** May increase the risk of hepatitis. Avoid using together.
Acyclovir: Use with intrathecal methotrexate may cause neurologic abnormalities. Monitor patient closely.
Digoxin: May decrease digoxin level. Monitor digoxin level closely.
Folic acid derivatives: Antagonizes methotrexate effect. Avoid using together, except for leucovorin rescue with high-dose methotrexate therapy.
Fosphenytoin, phenytoin: May decrease phenytoin and fosphenytoin levels. Monitor drug levels closely.
Hepatotoxic drugs: May increase risk of hepatotoxicity. Monitor patient closely.
NSAIDs, *phenylbutazone, salicylates:* May increase methotrexate toxicity. Avoid using together.
Oral antibiotics: May decrease absorption of methotrexate. Monitor patient closely.
Penicillins, ***sulfonamides, trimethoprim:*** May increase methotrexate level. Monitor patient for methotrexate toxicity.
Probenecid: May impair excretion of methotrexate, causing increased level, effect, and toxicity of methotrexate. Monitor methotrexate level closely and adjust dosage accordingly.
Procarbazine: May increase risk of nephrotoxicity. Monitor patient closely.
Theophylline: May increase theophylline level. Monitor theophylline level closely.
Thiopurines: May increase thiopurine level. Monitor patient closely.
Vaccines: May make immunizations ineffective; may cause risk of disseminated infection with live virus vaccines. Postpone immunization, if possible.
Drug-food. *Any food:* May delay absorption and reduce peak level of methotrexate. Instruct patient to take drug on an empty stomach.
Drug-lifestyle. *Alcohol use:* May increase hepatotoxicity. Discourage alcohol use.
Sun exposure: May cause photosensitivity reactions. Advise patient to avoid excessive sunlight exposure.

EFFECTS ON LAB TEST RESULTS

- May increase uric acid level. May decrease hemoglobin level.
- May decrease WBC, RBC, and platelet counts.
- May alter results of laboratory assay for folate, which interferes with detection of folic acid deficiency.

CONTRAINDICATIONS & CAUTIONS

- Contraindicated in patients hypersensitive to drug and in those with psoriasis or rheumatoid arthritis who also have alcoholism, alcoholic liver, chronic liver disease, immunodeficiency syndromes, or blood dyscrasias.
- Contraindicated in pregnant or breast-feeding women.
- Use cautiously and at modified dosage in patients with impaired hepatic or renal

function, bone marrow suppression, aplasia, leukopenia, thrombocytopenia, or anemia.
- Use cautiously in very young, elderly, or debilitated patients and in those with infection, peptic ulceration, or ulcerative colitis.

NURSING CONSIDERATIONS
- ***Alert:*** Drug may be given daily or once weekly, depending on the disease. To avoid administration errors, know your patient's dosing schedule.
- Monitor pulmonary function tests periodically and fluid intake and output daily. Encourage fluid intake of 2 to 3 L daily.
- Monitor uric acid level.
- Drug distributes readily into pleural effusions and other third-space compartments, such as ascites, leading to prolonged systemic level and risk of toxicity. Use drug cautiously in these patients.
- Tablets may contain lactose. If needed, give OTC lactose enzyme supplement.
- ***Alert:*** Alkalinize urine by giving sodium bicarbonate tablets or fluids to prevent precipitation of drug, especially at high doses. Maintain urine pH above 7. If BUN level is 20 to 30 mg/dl or creatinine level is 1.2 to 2 mg/dl, reduce dosage. If BUN level exceeds 30 mg/dl or creatinine level is higher than 2 mg/dl, stop drug and notify prescriber.
- For intrathecal administration, use preservative-free form.
- Watch for increases in AST, ALT, and alkaline phosphatase levels, which may signal hepatic dysfunction.
- Watch for signs and symptoms of bleeding (especially GI) and infection.
- To prevent bleeding, avoid all I.M. injections when platelet count is below 50,000/mm^3.
- Give blood transfusions for cumulative anemia. Patient may receive injections of RBC colony-stimulating factors to promote RBC production and decrease need for blood transfusions.
- Leucovorin rescue is needed with doses of more than 100 mg and starts 24 hours after therapy starts. Leucovorin is continued until methotrexate level falls below 5×10^{-8} M. Consult specialized references for specific recommendations for leucovorin dosage. Monitor methotrexate level and adjust leucovorin dose.
- The WBC and platelet count nadirs usually occur on day 7.

PATIENT TEACHING
- Advise patient to watch for signs and symptoms of infection (fever, sore throat, fatigue) and bleeding (easy bruising, nosebleeds, bleeding gums, tarry stools). Tell patient to take temperature daily.
- Teach and encourage diligent mouth care to reduce risk of superinfection in the mouth.
- Instruct patient how to take leucovorin. Stress the importance of taking as prescribed until instructed by prescriber to stop.
- Tell patient to use highly protective sunblock when exposed to sunlight.
- Warn both men and women to avoid conception during and for at least 12 weeks after therapy because of risk of abortion, birth defects, or fetal death.
- Advise woman to stop breast-feeding during therapy.

SAFETY ALERT!

pemetrexed
Alimta

Pharmacologic class: folate antagonist
Pregnancy risk category D

AVAILABLE FORMS
Injection: 500 mg in single-use vials

INDICATIONS & DOSAGES
➤ **Malignant pleural mesothelioma, with cisplatin, in patients whose disease is unresectable or who aren't candidates for surgery**
Adults: 500 mg/m^2 I.V. over 10 minutes on day 1 of each 21-day cycle. Starting 30 minutes after pemetrexed infusion ends, give cisplatin 75 mg/m^2 I.V. over 2 hours.
➤ **Locally advanced or metastatic non–small-cell lung cancer after chemotherapy**
Adults: 500 mg/m^2 I.V. over 10 minutes on day 1 of each 21-day cycle.

Adjust-a-dose: In patients who develop toxic reactions, adjust dosage according to the table.

Toxic reaction	Dosage change
– Grade 3 (severe or undesirable) or grade 4 (life-threatening or disabling) diarrhea – Diarrhea that warrants hospitalization – Any grade 3 toxicity (except mucositis and increased transaminase levels) – Any grade 4 toxicity (except mucositis) – Platelet count ≥ 50,000/mm³ and absolute neutrophil count < 500/mm³	Give 75% of previous pemetrexed and cisplatin doses.
Platelet count < 50,000/mm³	Give 50% of previous pemetrexed and cisplatin doses.
Grade 3 or 4 mucositis	Give 50% of previous pemetrexed dose and 100% of previous cisplatin dose.
Grade 2 (moderate) neurotoxicity	Give 100% of previous pemetrexed dose and 50% of previous cisplatin dose.
– Grade 3 or 4 neurotoxicity – Any grade 3 or 4 toxicity (except increased transaminase levels) present after two dose reductions	Stop therapy.

I.V. ADMINISTRATION

- Reconstitute 500-mg vial with 20 ml of preservative-free normal saline solution to yield 25 mg/ml.
- Swirl the vial gently until powder is completely dissolved. The solution should be clear and colorless to yellow or yellow-green.
- Calculate the appropriate dose, and further dilute with 100 ml normal saline solution.
- Give over 10 minutes.
- Reconstituted solution and dilution are stable for 24 hours refrigerated or at room temperature.

INCOMPATIBILITIES

Calcium-containing diluents including Ringer or lactated Ringer for injection; other drugs or diluents.

ACTION

Disturbs cell replication by inhibiting several folate-dependent enzymes involved in nucleotide synthesis. When given with other antineoplastics, drug inhibits growth of mesothelioma cell lines.

Route	Onset	Peak	Duration
I.V.	Unknown	Unknown	Unknown

Half-life: 3½ hours.

ADVERSE REACTIONS

CNS: *depression, fatigue, fever, neuropathy.*
CV: cardiac ischemia, *chest pain, edema,* ***emboli,*** thrombosis.
EENT: *pharyngitis.*
GI: *anorexia, constipation, diarrhea, nausea, stomatitis, vomiting,* esophagitis, painful, difficult swallowing.
GU: ***renal failure.***
Hematologic: **ANEMIA, LEUKOPENIA, NEUTROPENIA, THROMBOCYTOPENIA.**
Metabolic: dehydration.
Musculoskeletal: arthralgia, *myalgia.*
Respiratory: *dyspnea.*
Skin: *alopecia, rash.*
Other: allergic reaction, *infection.*

INTERACTIONS

Drug-drug. *Nephrotoxic drugs, probenecid:* May delay pemetrexed clearance. Monitor patient.
NSAIDs: May decrease pemetrexed clearance in patients with mild to moderate renal insufficiency. For NSAIDs with short half-lives, avoid use for 2 days before, during, and 2 days after pemetrexed therapy. For NSAIDs with long half-lives, avoid use for 5 days before, during, and 2 days after pemetrexed therapy.

EFFECTS ON LAB TEST RESULTS

- May increase ALT, AST, and creatinine levels. May decrease hemoglobin level and hematocrit.
- May decrease absolute neutrophil, platelet, and WBC counts.

CONTRAINDICATIONS & CAUTIONS

- Contraindicated in patients with a history of severe hypersensitivity reaction to drug or its ingredients. Don't use in patients with creatinine clearance less than 45 ml/minute.

NURSING CONSIDERATIONS

- Patient shouldn't start a new cycle of treatment unless absolute neutrophil count is 1,500 cells/mm^3 or more, platelet count is 100,000 cells/mm^3 or more, and creatinine clearance is 45 ml/minute or more.
- Patients with pleural effusion and ascites may need to have effusion drained before therapy.
- Monitor renal function, CBC, platelet count, hemoglobin level, hematocrit, and liver function test values.
- Assess patient for neurotoxicity, mucositis, and diarrhea. Severe symptoms may warrant dosage adjustment.
- ***Alert:*** To reduce the occurrence and severity of cutaneous reactions, give a corticosteroid, such as dexamethasone 4 mg P.O. b.i.d., the day before, the day of, and the day after giving this drug.
- ***Alert:*** To reduce toxicity, patient should take 350 to 1,000 mcg of folic acid daily, 5 days before therapy until 21 days after therapy.
- ***Alert:*** Give vitamin B_{12} 1,000 mcg I.M. once during the week before the first dose and every three cycles thereafter. After the first cycle, vitamin injections may be given on the first day of the cycle.

PATIENT TEACHING

- Inform patient that he may receive corticosteroids and vitamins before pemetrexed to help minimize its adverse effects.
- Tell patient to avoid NSAIDs for several days before, during, and after treatment.
- Urge patient to report adverse effects, especially fever, sore throat, infection, diarrhea, fatigue, and limb pain.
- It isn't known if drug appears in breast milk. Advise patient to stop breast-feeding during treatment.

69

Antibiotic antineoplastics

bleomycin sulfate
daunorubicin citrate liposomal
daunorubicin hydrochloride
doxorubicin hydrochloride
doxorubicin hydrochloride liposomal
epirubicin hydrochloride
idarubicin hydrochloride
mitomycin

SAFETY ALERT!

bleomycin sulfate

Blenoxane

Pharmacologic class: cytotoxic glycopeptide antibiotic
Pregnancy risk category D

AVAILABLE FORMS

Injection: 15-unit vials, 30-unit vials

INDICATIONS & DOSAGES

➤ Squamous cell carcinoma (head, neck, skin, penis, cervix, and vulva), non-Hodgkin lymphoma, testicular carcinoma
Adults: 10 to 20 units/m^2 I.V., I.M., or subcutaneously once or twice weekly to total of 400 units.

➤ Hodgkin lymphoma
Adults: 10 to 20 units/m^2 I.V., I.M., or subcutaneously one or two times weekly. After 50% response, maintenance dose is 1 unit I.V. or I.M. daily or 5 units I.V. or I.M. weekly. Total cumulative dose is 400 units.

➤ Malignant pleural effusion
Adults: 60 units given as single-dose bolus intrapleural injection.

I.V. ADMINISTRATION

- Preparing and giving parenteral form of drug may be mutagenic, teratogenic, and carcinogenic. Follow facility policy to reduce risks.
- Drug may adsorb to plastic I.V. bags. For prolonged infusions, use glass containers.
- Reconstitute drug with 5 or 10 ml of normal saline solution for injection to equal 3 units/ml solution.
- Use reconstituted solution within 24 hours.
- Refrigerate unopened vials containing dry powder.

INCOMPATIBILITIES

Amino acids; aminophylline; ascorbic acid injection; cefazolin; diazepam; drugs containing sulfhydryl groups; fluids containing dextrose; furosemide; hydrocortisone; methotrexate; mitomycin; nafcillin; penicillin G; riboflavin; solutions containing divalent and trivalent cations, especially calcium salts and copper; terbutaline sulfate.

ACTION

May inhibit DNA synthesis and cause scission of single- and double-stranded DNA; also inhibits RNA and protein synthesis.

Route	Onset	Peak	Duration
I.V., SubQ	Unknown	Unknown	Unknown
I.M.	Unknown	30–60 min	Unknown

Half-life: 2 hours.

ADVERSE REACTIONS

CNS: fever.
GI: *stomatitis, anorexia, nausea, vomiting,* diarrhea.
Metabolic: weight loss, hyperuricemia.
Respiratory: PNEUMONITIS, ***pulmonary fibrosis.***
Skin: *erythema, hyperpigmentation, acne, rash, striae, skin tenderness, pruritus, reversible alopecia,* hyperkeratosis, nail changes.
Other: *chills,* ***anaphylactoid reactions.***

INTERACTIONS

Drug-drug. *Anesthesia:* May increase oxygen requirements. Monitor patient closely.
Cardiac glycosides: May decrease digoxin level. Monitor digoxin level closely.
Fosphenytoin, phenytoin: May decrease phenytoin and fosphenytoin levels. Monitor drug levels closely.

EFFECTS ON LAB TEST RESULTS

- May increase uric acid level.

CONTRAINDICATIONS & CAUTIONS

- Contraindicated in patients hypersensitive to drug.
- Use cautiously in patients with renal or pulmonary impairment.

NURSING CONSIDERATIONS

- Obtain pulmonary function tests. If tests show a marked decline, stop drug.
- ***Alert:*** Pulmonary toxicity appears to be dose-related, with an increase when total dose is more than 400 units. Give total doses of more than 400 units with caution.
- For intrapleural use, dilute 60 units of drug in 50 to 100 ml normal saline solution for injection; drug is given through a thoracotomy tube.
- For I.M. use, dilute drug in 1 to 5 ml of sterile water for injection, bacteriostatic water for injection, or normal saline solution for injection.
- Monitor injection site for irritation.
- ***Alert:*** Adverse pulmonary reactions are more common in patients older than age 70. Pulmonary fibrosis is fatal in 1% of patients, especially when cumulative dosage exceeds 400 units. Also, in patients receiving radiation therapy, patients with lung disease, and patients who need oxygen therapy, pulmonary toxic adverse effects may be increased.
- Monitor chest X-ray and listen to lungs regularly.
- Obtain pulmonary function tests and chest X-rays before each course of therapy.
- If patient's condition requires sclerosis, drug may be instilled when chest tube drainage is 100 to 300 ml/24 hours; ideally, drainage should be less than 100 ml. After instillation, thoracotomy tube is clamped and patient is moved from his back to his left then right side for the next 4 hours. The clamp is removed and suction reestablished. Amount of time chest tube is left in place after sclerosis depends on patient's condition.
- Watch for fever, which may be treated with antipyretics. Fever usually occurs within 3 to 6 hours of administration.
- Watch for hypersensitivity reactions, which may be delayed for several hours, especially in patients with lymphoma. (Give test dose of 1 to 2 units before first two doses in these patients. If no reaction occurs, follow regular dosage.)
- Don't use adhesive dressings.

PATIENT TEACHING

- Warn patient that hair loss may occur but is usually reversible.
- Tell patient to report adverse reactions promptly and to take infection-control and bleeding precautions.
- For patient who is to receive anesthesia, tell him to inform anesthesiologist that he has taken this drug. High oxygen levels inhaled during surgery may enhance pulmonary toxicity of drug.

SAFETY ALERT!

daunorubicin citrate liposomal

DaunoXome

Pharmacologic class: anthracycline glycoside antibiotic
Pregnancy risk category D

AVAILABLE FORMS

Injection: 2 mg/ml (equivalent to 50 mg daunorubicin base)

INDICATIONS & DOSAGES

➤ **First-line cytotoxic therapy for advanced HIV-related Kaposi sarcoma**

Adults: 40 mg/m^2 I.V. over 60 minutes once q 2 weeks. Continue treatment until progressive disease becomes evident or until other complications of HIV infection preclude continuation of therapy.

Adjust-a-dose: For patients with impaired hepatic and renal function, if bilirubin level is 1.2 to 3 mg/dl, give three-fourths normal dose; if bilirubin or creatinine level exceeds 3 mg/dl, give one-half normal dose.

I.V. ADMINISTRATION

- Preparing and giving drug may be mutagenic, teratogenic, or carcinogenic. Follow facility policy to reduce risks.
- To dilute, withdraw calculated volume of drug from vial and transfer into an equal amount of D_5W. Recommended concentration after dilution is 1 mg/ml.

• Use immediately after dilution.
• Don't use an in-line filter.
• Give over 60 minutes.
• Back pain, flushing, and chest tightness may develop during first 5 minutes of infusion. These symptoms subside after infusion stops and usually don't recur when drug is infused more slowly.
• Monitor I.V. site closely; watch for irritation and infiltration, which can cause tissue damage and necrosis. If it occurs, stop infusion, apply ice, and notify prescriber.
• If needed, drug may be refrigerated at 36° to 46° F (2° to 8° C) for up to 6 hours.

INCOMPATIBILITIES

Bacteriostatic agents, other I.V. drugs, saline and other solutions.

ACTION

Maximizes selectivity of daunorubicin for solid tumors in situ. After penetrating tumor, drug is released over time to exert antineoplastic activity by inhibiting DNA synthesis and DNA-dependent RNA synthesis.

Route	Onset	Peak	Duration
I.V.	Unknown	Unknown	Unknown

Half-life: 4½ hours.

ADVERSE REACTIONS

CNS: *headache, neuropathy,* depression, dizziness, syncope, insomnia, amnesia, anxiety, ataxia, confusion, ***seizures,*** hallucination, tremor, hypertonia, ***meningitis,*** *fatigue,* malaise, emotional lability, abnormal gait, hyperkinesia, somnolence, abnormal thinking, *fever.*
CV: ***dose-related cardiomyopathy,*** chest pain, hypertension, palpitations, ***arrhythmias, pericardial effusion, pericardial tamponade, cardiac arrest,*** angina pectoris, ***pulmonary hypertension,*** flushing, edema, tachycardia, ***MI.***
EENT: *rhinitis,* stomatitis, sinusitis, abnormal vision, conjunctivitis, tinnitus, eye pain, deafness, earache.
GI: taste disturbances, dry mouth, gingival bleeding, *nausea, diarrhea, abdominal pain, vomiting, anorexia,* constipation, thirst, ***GI hemorrhage,*** gastritis, dysphagia, stomatitis, increased appetite, melena, hemorrhoids, tenesmus.
GU: dysuria, nocturia, polyuria.
Hematologic: NEUTROPENIA, THROMBOCYTOPENIA.
Hepatic: hepatomegaly.
Metabolic: dehydration.
Musculoskeletal: *rigors, back pain,* arthralgia, myalgia.
Respiratory: *cough, dyspnea,* hemoptysis, hiccups, pulmonary infiltration, increased sputum.
Skin: alopecia, pruritus, *increased sweating,* dry skin, seborrhea, folliculitis, injection site inflammation.
Other: splenomegaly, lymphadenopathy, tooth caries, *opportunistic infections,* allergic reactions, flulike symptoms.

INTERACTIONS

None significant.

EFFECTS ON LAB TEST RESULTS

• May decrease neutrophil and platelet counts.

CONTRAINDICATIONS & CAUTIONS

• Contraindicated in patients who have experienced severe hypersensitivity reaction to drug or its components.
• Use cautiously in patients with myelosuppression, cardiac disease, previous radiotherapy encompassing the heart, previous anthracycline use (doxorubicin cumulative dose is 300 mg/m² or above), or hepatic or renal dysfunction.

NURSING CONSIDERATIONS

• Drug causes less nausea, vomiting, alopecia, neutropenia, thrombocytopenia, and potentially less cardiotoxicity than conventional daunorubicin.
• Give only under supervision of prescriber specializing in chemotherapy.
• Monitor cardiac function regularly. Assess patient before giving each dose because of risk of cardiac toxicity and heart failure. Determine left ventricular ejection fraction at total cumulative doses of 320 mg/m² and every 160 mg/m² thereafter. Total cumulative doses generally shouldn't exceed 550 mg/m².
• Provide careful hematologic monitoring because severe myelosuppression may occur. Repeat blood counts and evaluate before giving each dose. If absolute granu-

locyte count is below 750/mm³, withhold drug.
- Monitor patient closely for signs and symptoms of opportunistic infection, especially because patients with HIV infection are immunocompromised.
- ***Look alike–sound alike:*** Don't confuse daunorubicin citrate liposomal with daunorubicin hydrochloride.

PATIENT TEACHING
- Inform patient that hair loss may occur, but that it's usually reversible.
- Instruct patient to call prescriber if sore throat, fever, or other signs or symptoms of infection occur. Tell patient to avoid exposure to people with infections.
- Advise woman to report suspected or confirmed pregnancy during therapy.
- Tell patient to report back pain, flushing, or chest tightness during infusion.

SAFETY ALERT!

daunorubicin hydrochloride
Cerubidine

Pharmacologic class: anthracycline glycoside antibiotic
Pregnancy risk category D

AVAILABLE FORMS
Injection: 20-mg and 50-mg vials

INDICATIONS & DOSAGES
Dosages vary. Check treatment protocol with prescriber.

➤ **To induce remission in acute nonlymphocytic (myelogenous, monocytic, erythroid) leukemia**
Adults age 60 and older: In combination, 30 mg/m² per day I.V. on days 1, 2, and 3 of first course and on days 1 and 2 of subsequent courses with cytarabine infusions.
Adults younger than age 60: In combination, 45 mg/m² per day I.V. on days 1, 2, and 3 of first course and on days 1 and 2 of subsequent courses with cytarabine infusions.

➤ **To induce remission in acute lymphocytic leukemia (with combination therapy)**
Adults: 45 mg/m² per day I.V. on days 1, 2, and 3 of first course.
Children age 2 and older: 25 mg/m² I.V. on day 1 q week for up to 6 weeks, if needed.
Children younger than age 2 or with body surface area less than 0.5 m²: Dose based on body weight, not surface area.
Adjust-a-dose: For patients with impaired hepatic and renal function, reduce dosage as follows: If bilirubin level is 1.2 to 3 mg/dl, give three-fourths normal dose; if bilirubin or creatinine level exceeds 3 mg/dl, give one-half normal dose.

I.V. ADMINISTRATION
- Preparing and giving parenteral drug may be mutagenic, teratogenic, or carcinogenic. Follow facility policy to reduce risks.
- Reconstitute with 4 ml sterile water for injection to yield 5 mg/ml.
- Withdraw desired dose into syringe containing 10 to 15 ml of normal saline solution for injection.
- Inject as a slow I.V. push over 2 to 3 minutes into tubing of a free-flowing I.V. solution of D_5W or normal saline solution for injection.
- If extravasation occurs, stop infusion immediately, apply ice to area for 24 to 48 hours, and notify prescriber. Because drug is a vesicant, extravasation could cause severe tissue necrosis.
- If possible, use within 8 hours of preparation. Reconstituted solution is stable 24 hours at room temperature, 48 hours if refrigerated.

INCOMPATIBILITIES
Other I.V. drugs. If mixed with dexamethasone or heparin, drug may precipitate; don't mix together.

ACTION
May interfere with DNA-dependent RNA synthesis by intercalation.

Route	Onset	Peak	Duration
I.V.	Unknown	Unknown	Unknown

Half-life: Initial, 45 minutes; terminal, 18½ hours.

ADVERSE REACTIONS
CNS: fever.
CV: IRREVERSIBLE CARDIOMYOPATHY, ECG changes.

GI: *nausea, vomiting,* diarrhea, stomatitis.
GU: red urine.
Hematologic: ***bone marrow suppression.***
Hepatic: ***hepatotoxicity.***
Metabolic: hyperuricemia.
Skin: *reversible alopecia, severe cellulitis and tissue sloughing with drug extravasation,* rash, darkening or redness of previously irradiated areas.
Other: ***anaphylactoid reaction,*** chills.

INTERACTIONS

Drug-drug. *Doxorubicin:* May cause additive cardiotoxicity. Monitor patient for toxicity.
Hepatotoxic drugs: May increase risk of additive hepatotoxicity. Monitor hepatic function closely.
Myelosuppressive drugs: May increase risk of myelosuppression. Monitor patient closely.

EFFECTS ON LAB TEST RESULTS

- May increase alkaline phosphatase, AST, bilirubin, and uric acid levels. May decrease hemoglobin level and hematocrit.
- May decrease platelet and WBC counts.

CONTRAINDICATIONS & CAUTIONS

- Contraindicated in patients hypersensitive to the drug.
- Use cautiously in patients with myelosuppression or impaired cardiac, renal, or hepatic function.

NURSING CONSIDERATIONS

- Take preventive measures (including adequate hydration) before starting treatment. Hyperuricemia may result from rapid lysis of leukemic cells. Allopurinol may be ordered.
- Perform cardiac function studies, including ECG and ejection fraction, before treatment and then periodically throughout therapy.
- Never give drug I.M. or subcutaneously.
- ***Alert:*** Cumulative adult dosage is limited to 400 to 550 mg/m^2 (450 mg/m^2 when patient is also receiving or has received cyclophosphamide or radiation therapy to cardiac area).
- Therapeutic effects are commonly accompanied by toxicity.
- Monitor CBC and hepatic function tests; monitor ECG every month during therapy.
- ***Alert:*** If signs of heart failure, cardiomyopathy, or arrhythmia develop, stop drug immediately and notify prescriber.
- Watch for nausea and vomiting, which may last 24 to 48 hours.
- Blood transfusions may be needed to combat anemia. Patient may receive injected RBC colony-stimulating factor to promote RBC production and to decrease need for blood transfusions.
- ***Look alike–sound alike:*** Reddish color of drug is similar to that of doxorubicin; don't confuse the two.
- Lowest blood counts occur 10 to 14 days after dose.
- ***Look alike–sound alike:*** Don't confuse daunorubicin hydrochloride with daunorubicin citrate liposomal.

PATIENT TEACHING

- Advise patient to report any pain or burning at site of injection during or after administration.
- Advise patient to watch for signs and symptoms of infection (fever, sore throat, fatigue) and bleeding (easy bruising, nosebleeds, bleeding gums, tarry stools) and to take temperature daily.
- Inform patient that red urine for 1 to 2 days is normal and doesn't indicate the presence of blood in urine.
- Advise patient that hair loss may occur, but that it's usually reversible.
- Caution woman of childbearing age to avoid becoming pregnant during therapy. Recommend that she consult prescriber before becoming pregnant.

SAFETY ALERT!

doxorubicin hydrochloride

Adriamycin‡, Adriamycin PFS, Adriamycin RDF, Rubex

Pharmacologic class: anthracycline glycoside antibiotic
Pregnancy risk category D

AVAILABLE FORMS

Injection (preservative-free): 2 mg/ml
Powder for injection: 10-mg, 20-mg, 50-mg, 100-mg, 150-mg vials

INDICATIONS & DOSAGES

➤ Bladder, breast, lung, ovarian, stomach, and thyroid cancers; non-Hodgkin lymphoma; Hodgkin lymphoma; acute lymphoblastic and myeloblastic leukemia; Wilms tumor; neuroblastoma; lymphoma; sarcoma

Adults: 60 to 75 mg/m² I.V. as single dose q 3 weeks; or 30 mg/m² I.V. in single daily dose, days 1 to 3 of 4-week cycle.

Or, 20 mg/m² I.V. once weekly. Maximum cumulative dose is 550 mg/m².

Elderly patients: May need reduced dosages.

Adjust-a-dose: Reduce dosage for patients with myelosuppression or impaired cardiac or liver function. Be prepared to decrease dosage if bilirubin level rises: Give 50% of dose when bilirubin level is 1.2 to 3 mg/100 ml; 25% when it's 3.1 to 5 mg/100 ml.

I.V. ADMINISTRATION

- Preparing and giving parenteral drug may be mutagenic, teratogenic, or carcinogenic. Follow facility policy to reduce risks.
- If drug leaks or spills, inactivate it with 5% sodium hypochlorite solution (household bleach).
- Reconstitute with preservative-free normal saline solution for injection to yield 2 mg/ml; add 5 ml to 10-mg vial, 10 ml to 20-mg vial, or 25 ml to 50-mg vial. Shake vial to dissolve drug.
- Don't place I.V. line over joints or in limbs with poor venous or lymphatic drainage.
- Give by direct injection over at least 3 minutes into the tubing of a free-flowing I.V. solution containing D_5W or normal saline solution for injection.
- If vein streaking occurs, slow administration rate. If welts appear, stop drug and notify prescriber.
- Some protocols give doxorubicin as a prolonged infusion, which requires central venous access.
- If extravasation occurs, stop infusion immediately, apply ice to area for 24 to 48 hours, and notify prescriber. Monitor area closely because extravasation may be progressive. Drug is a strong vesicant and may cause tissue necrosis. Early consultation with a plastic surgeon may be advisable.
- Refrigerated, reconstituted solution is stable 48 hours; at room temperature, it's stable 24 hours.

INCOMPATIBILITIES

Allopurinol, aluminum, aminophylline, bacteriostatic diluents, cefepime, dexamethasone sodium phosphate, diazepam, fluorouracil, furosemide, ganciclovir, heparin sodium, hydrocortisone sodium succinate, piperacillin with tazobactam.

ACTION

May interfere with DNA-dependent RNA synthesis by intercalation.

Route	Onset	Peak	Duration
I.V.	Unknown	Unknown	Unknown

Half-life: Initial, 30 minutes; terminal, 16½ hours.

ADVERSE REACTIONS

CV: cardiac depression, ***arrhythmias, acute left ventricular failure, irreversible cardiomyopathy.***
EENT: conjunctivitis.
GI: *nausea, vomiting,* diarrhea, *stomatitis,* esophagitis, anorexia.
GU: transient red urine.
Hematologic: ***leukopenia, thrombocytopenia,*** **MYELOSUPPRESSION.**
Metabolic: hyperuricemia.
Skin: *severe cellulitis and tissue sloughing with drug extravasation,* urticaria, facial flushing, *complete alopecia within 3 to 4 weeks,* hyperpigmentation of nail beds and dermal creases, radiation recall effect.
Other: chills, ***anaphylaxis.***

INTERACTIONS

Drug-drug. *Aminophylline, cephalothin, dexamethasone, fluorouracil, heparin, hydrocortisone:* May form a precipitate. Don't mix together.
Calcium channel blockers: May increase cardiotoxic effects. Monitor patient's ECG closely.
Cyclosporine: May increase doxorubicin concentration. Monitor patient for toxicity.
Digoxin: May decrease digoxin level. Monitor digoxin level closely.
Fosphenytoin, phenytoin: May decrease level of phenytoin or fosphenytoin. Monitor drug level.

Paclitaxel: May decrease doxorubicin clearance. Monitor patient for toxicity.
Phenobarbital: May increase doxorubicin clearance. Monitor patient closely.
Streptozocin: May increase and prolong doxorubicin level. Dosage may have to be adjusted.

EFFECTS ON LAB TEST RESULTS

- May increase uric acid level.
- May decrease platelet and WBC counts.

CONTRAINDICATIONS & CAUTIONS

- Contraindicated in patients with a history of sensitivity reactions to drug or its components.
- Contraindicated in patients with marked myelosuppression induced by previous treatment with other antitumor drugs or radiotherapy and in those who have received a lifetime cumulative dose of 550 mg/m^2 of doxorubicin or daunorubicin.

NURSING CONSIDERATIONS

- Perform cardiac function studies, including ECG and ejection fraction, before treatment and then periodically throughout therapy. Dexrazoxane may be given within 30 minutes of doxorubicin if the accumulated dose of doxorubicin has reached 300 mg/m^2.
- Take preventive measures, including adequate hydration of the patient, before starting treatment. Rapid lysis of leukemic cells may cause hyperuricemia. Allopurinol may be ordered.
- Premedicate with antiemetic to reduce nausea.
- If skin or mucosal contact occurs, immediately wash with soap and water.
- Never give drug I.M. or subcutaneously.
- Dosage modification may be needed in patients with myelosuppression or impaired cardiac or hepatic function, and in elderly patients.
- Monitor CBC with differential and hepatic function tests; monitor ECG monthly during therapy. If WBC count falls below 2,000/mm^3 or granulocyte count falls below 1,000/mm^3, follow institutional policy for infection control in immunocompromised patients.
- Monitor ECG for changes such as sinus tachycardia, T-wave flattening, ST-segment depression, and voltage reduction.
- Leukopenia may occur during days 10 to 15, with recovery by day 21.
- If tachycardia develops, stop drug or slow rate of infusion, and notify prescriber.
- ***Alert:*** If signs of heart failure develop, stop drug and notify prescriber. Heart failure can often be prevented by limiting cumulative dose to 550 mg/m^2 (400 mg/m^2 when patient is also receiving or has received cyclophosphamide or radiation therapy to cardiac area).
- ***Look alike–sound alike:*** Reddish color of drug is similar to that of daunorubicin; don't confuse the two drugs.
- Esophagitis is common in patients who also have received radiation therapy.
- ***Alert:*** If patient has previously received radiation therapy, he is susceptible to radiation recall effect.
- ***Look alike–sound alike:*** Don't confuse doxorubicin with doxorubicin liposomal.

PATIENT TEACHING

- Advise patient to report any pain or burning at site of injection during or after administration.
- Advise patient to watch for signs and symptoms of infection (fever, sore throat, fatigue) and bleeding (easy bruising, nosebleeds, bleeding gums, tarry stools) and to take temperature daily.
- Advise patient that orange to red urine for 1 to 2 days is normal and doesn't indicate presence of blood.
- Inform patient that hair loss may occur, but it's usually reversible. Hair may regrow 2 to 5 months after drug is stopped.

SAFETY ALERT!

doxorubicin hydrochloride liposomal

Doxil

Pharmacologic class: anthracycline glycoside antibiotic
Pregnancy risk category D

AVAILABLE FORMS

Injection: 2 mg/ml in 20-mg and 50-mg vials

INDICATIONS & DOSAGES

➤**Metastatic ovarian carcinoma refractory to both paclitaxel- and platinum-based chemotherapy regimens**

Women: 50 mg/m^2 I.V. initially at 1 mg/minute once q 4 weeks for minimum of four courses. Continue as long as condition doesn't progress, patient shows no evidence of cardiotoxicity, and patient continues to tolerate treatment. If no infusion-related adverse reactions develop, increase infusion rate to complete administration over 1 hour.

➤**AIDS-related Kaposi sarcoma refractory to previous combination chemotherapy and in patients intolerant of such therapy**

Adults: 20 mg/m^2 I.V. over 30 minutes once q 3 weeks. Continue as long as patient responds satisfactorily and tolerates treatment.

Adjust-a-dose: For patients with impaired hepatic function, reduce dosage as follows: If bilirubin level is 1.2 to 3 mg/dl, give one-half normal dose; if bilirubin level is more than 3 mg/dl, give one-fourth normal dose. Dose modifications may be needed for stomatitis, myelosuppression, and hand-foot syndrome, based on toxicity grade.

I.V. ADMINISTRATION

- Follow procedures for proper handling and disposal of antineoplastics.
- Dilute appropriate dose (maximum, 90 mg) in 250 ml D_5W using aseptic technique.
- Carefully check label on I.V. bag before giving drug. Accidentally substituting doxorubicin hydrochloride liposomal for conventional doxorubicin hydrochloride may cause severe adverse reactions. The two products can't be substituted on a milligram-per-milligram basis.
- Don't use an in-line filter.
- Infuse over 30 to 60 minutes, depending on dose. Monitor patient carefully during infusion.
- Acute infusion-related reactions include flushing, shortness of breath, facial swelling, headache, chills, back pain, tightness in chest or throat, and hypotension. They may resolve when infusion rate is slowed, or they may resolve over several hours to a day when infusion is stopped.
- If extravasation occurs, stop infusion immediately. Applying ice at the site for about 30 minutes may help alleviate local reaction. Restart infusion in another vein.
- Refrigerate diluted solution at 36° to 46° F (2° to 8° C) and give within 24 hours.

INCOMPATIBILITIES

Other I.V. drugs.

ACTION

Consists of doxorubicin hydrochloride encapsulated in liposomes. Action may involve drug's ability to bind DNA and inhibit nucleic acid synthesis.

Route	Onset	Peak	Duration
I.V.	Unknown	Unknown	Unknown

Half-life: 5 hours in first phase; 55 hours in second phase with doses of 10 to 20 mg/m^2.

ADVERSE REACTIONS

CNS: *asthenia,* paresthesia, headache, somnolence, dizziness, depression, insomnia, anxiety, malaise, emotional lability, fatigue, fever.
CV: chest pain, hypotension, tachycardia, peripheral edema, ***cardiomyopathy, heart failure, arrhythmias,*** pericardial effusion.
EENT: pharyngitis, rhinitis, conjunctivitis, retinitis, optic neuritis.
GI: *nausea, vomiting, constipation, anorexia, diarrhea,* abdominal pain, dyspepsia, oral candidiasis, enlarged abdomen, esophagitis, dysphagia, *stomatitis,* taste perversion, glossitis.
GU: albuminuria.
Hematologic: **LEUKOPENIA, NEUTROPENIA, THROMBOCYTOPENIA,** *anemia.*
Hepatic: hyperbilirubinemia.
Metabolic: dehydration, weight loss, hypocalcemia, hyperglycemia.
Musculoskeletal: myalgia, back pain.
Respiratory: dyspnea, increased cough, pneumonia.
Skin: *rash, alopecia,* dry skin, pruritus, skin discoloration, skin disorder, exfoliative dermatitis, sweating, *palmar-plantar erythrodysesthesia.*
Other: allergic reaction, chills, *herpes zoster,* infection, infusion-related reactions.

INTERACTIONS

None reported. However, drug may interact with drugs that interact with conventional form of doxorubicin hydrochloride.

EFFECTS ON LAB TEST RESULTS

- May increase bilirubin and glucose levels. May decrease calcium and hemoglobin levels.
- May increase PT and INR. May decrease neutrophil, platelet, and WBC counts.

CONTRAINDICATIONS & CAUTIONS

- Contraindicated in patients hypersensitive to conventional formulation of doxorubicin hydrochloride or any component in the liposomal form.
- Contraindicated in patients with marked myelosuppression and those who have received a lifetime cumulative dose of 550 mg/m^2 (400 mg/m^2 in patients who have received radiotherapy to the mediastinal area or therapy with other cardiotoxic drugs such as cyclophosphamide).
- Use cautiously in patients who have received other anthracyclines.

NURSING CONSIDERATIONS

- Consider previous or current therapy with related compounds such as daunorubicin when calculating total dose of drug to be given. Heart failure and cardiomyopathy may occur after stopping therapy.
- Give drug to patient with history of CV disease only when benefit outweighs risk to patient.
- Don't give I.M. or subcutaneously.
- ***Alert:*** Monitor patient for signs and symptoms of palmar-plantar erythrodysesthesia, hematologic toxicity, or stomatitis. These adverse reactions may be managed with dosage delays and adjustments.
- Evaluate patient's hepatic function before therapy, and adjust dosage accordingly.
- Drug exhibits pharmacokinetic properties different from those of conventional doxorubicin hydrochloride and shouldn't be substituted on a milligram-by-milligram basis.
- Drug may increase toxicity of other antineoplastics.
- Closely monitor cardiac function by endomyocardial biopsy, echocardiography, or gated radionuclide scans. If results indicate possible cardiac injury, the benefit of continued therapy must be weighed against the risk of myocardial injury.
- Monitor CBC, including platelets, before each dose and frequently throughout therapy. Leukopenia is usually transient. Persistent severe myelosuppression may result in superinfection or hemorrhage. Patient may need G-CSF (or GM-CSF) to support blood counts.

PATIENT TEACHING

- Tell patient to notify prescriber if he experiences signs and symptoms of hand-foot syndrome (such as tingling or burning, redness, flaking, bothersome swelling, small blisters, or small sores on palms of hands or soles of feet).
- To reduce the risk of hand-foot syndrome, advise the patient to follow these guidelines at least 1 day before and for 3 to 5 days after treatment:
  - Avoid direct sunlight and use sunblock SPF 15 or higher on all exposed skin.
  - Wear loose clothing and comfortable, well-ventilated, low-heeled shoes.
  - Avoid contact with hot water and take cool, short showers or baths.
  - Don't put pressure on your skin. (Avoid kneeling, leaning on your elbows, wearing tight jewelry or undergarments, and chopping hard foods.)
- Advise patient to report signs and symptoms of mouth inflammation (such as painful redness, swelling, or sores in mouth).
- Warn patient to avoid exposure to people with infections. Tell patient to report temperature of 100.5° F (38° C) or higher.
- Tell patient to report nausea, vomiting, tiredness, weakness, rash, or mild hair loss.
- Advise woman of childbearing age to avoid pregnancy during therapy.

SAFETY ALERT!

epirubicin hydrochloride

Ellence

Pharmacologic class: anthracycline glycoside antibiotic
Pregnancy risk category D

AVAILABLE FORMS

Injection: 2 mg/ml

INDICATIONS & DOSAGES

➤ **Adjuvant therapy in patients with evidence of axillary node tumor involvement after resection of primary breast cancer**

Adults: 100 to 120 mg/m² I.V. infusion over 3 to 5 minutes through a free-flowing I.V. solution on day 1 of each cycle, or divided equally in two doses on days 1 and 8 of each cycle; cycle repeated q 3 to 4 weeks for six cycles; used with regimens containing cyclophosphamide and fluorouracil.

Dosage modification after first cycle is based on toxicity. For patients with platelet count nadir below 50,000/mm³, absolute neutrophil count (ANC) below 250/mm³, neutropenic fever, or grade 3 or 4 nonhematologic toxicity, reduce day 1 dose in subsequent cycles to 75% of day 1 dose given in current cycle. Delay day 1 therapy in subsequent cycles until platelet count is at least 100,000/mm³, ANC is at least 1,500/mm³, and nonhematologic toxicities recover to grade 1.

For patients receiving divided doses (days 1 and 8), day 8 dose should be 75% of day 1 dose if platelet count is 75,000 to 100,000/mm³ and ANC is 1,000 to 1,499/mm³. If day 8 platelet count is below 75,000/mm³, ANC is below 1,000/mm³, or grade 3 or 4 nonhematologic toxicity has occurred, omit day 8 dose.

Adjust-a-dose: For patients with bone marrow dysfunction (heavily pretreated patients, patients with bone marrow depression, or those with neoplastic bone marrow infiltration), start at lower doses of 75 to 90 mg/m². For patients with hepatic dysfunction, if bilirubin is 1.2 to 3 mg/dl or AST is two to four times upper limit of normal, give one-half recommended starting dose. If bilirubin level is above 3 mg/dl or AST is more than four times upper limit of normal, give one-fourth recommended starting dose. For patients with severe renal dysfunction (creatinine level over 5 mg/dl), consider lower doses.

I.V. ADMINISTRATION

- Wear protective clothing (goggles, gown, disposable gloves) when handling drug, which is a vesicant.
- Never give drug I.M. or subcutaneously. Always give it I.V. through free-flowing normal saline solution or D_5W.
- Avoid veins over joints or in limbs with compromised venous or lymphatic drainage.
- Avoid repeated injection into the same vein.
- Give drug over 3 to 5 minutes.
- Facial flushing and erythematous streaking along vein may indicate overly rapid delivery.
- If burning or stinging occurs, stop infusion immediately and restart in another vein.
- After vial has been penetrated, discard unused solution after 24 hours.

INCOMPATIBILITIES

Fluorouracil, heparin, ifosfamide with mesna, other I.V. drugs.

ACTION

May form a complex with DNA by getting between nucleotide base pairs, inhibiting DNA, RNA, and protein synthesis; DNA cleavage occurs, resulting in cytocidal activity. Drug may also interfere with replication and transcription of DNA and may generate cytotoxic free radicals.

Route	Onset	Peak	Duration
I.V.	Unknown	Unknown	Unknown

Half-life: 31 to 35 hours.

ADVERSE REACTIONS

CNS: *lethargy,* fever.
CV: ***cardiomyopathy, heart failure,*** hot flashes.
EENT: *conjunctivitis, keratitis.*
GI: *nausea, vomiting, diarrhea,* anorexia, *mucositis.*
GU: *amenorrhea,* red urine.
Hematologic: LEUKOPENIA, NEUTROPENIA, *febrile neutropenia, anemia,* THROMBOCYTOPENIA.
Skin: *alopecia,* rash, itch, skin changes, local toxicity.
Other: *infection.*

INTERACTIONS

Drug-drug. *Calcium channel blockers, other cardioactive compounds:* May in-

crease risk of heart failure. Monitor cardiac function closely.
Cimetidine: May increase epirubicin level by 50%. Avoid using together.
Cytotoxic drugs: May cause additive toxicities (especially hematologic and GI). Monitor patient closely.

EFFECTS ON LAB TEST RESULTS

- May decrease hemoglobin level.
- May decrease neutrophil, platelet, and WBC counts.

CONTRAINDICATIONS & CAUTIONS

- Contraindicated in patients hypersensitive to drug, other anthracyclines, or anthracenediones, and in patients with baseline neutrophil counts below 1,500/mm^3, severe myocardial insufficiency, recent MI, serious arrhythmias, or severe hepatic dysfunction.
- Contraindicated in patients who have had previous treatment with anthracyclines to total cumulative doses.
- Use cautiously in patients with active or dormant cardiac disease, previous or current radiotherapy to mediastinal and pericardial areas, or previous therapy with other anthracyclines or anthracenediones.
- Use cautiously in patients receiving other cardiotoxic drugs.

NURSING CONSIDERATIONS

- Give drug under supervision of prescriber experienced in cancer chemotherapy. Don't handle drug if you are pregnant.
- For patients taking 120 mg/m^2, give prophylactic co-trimoxazole or fluoroquinolones.
- Give antiemetic before drug to reduce nausea and vomiting.
- Before therapy, obtain total bilirubin, AST, and creatinine levels; CBC including ANC; and left ventricular ejection fraction (LVEF).
- Monitor LVEF regularly during therapy. Stop drug at first sign of impaired cardiac function. Early signs of cardiac toxicity include sinus tachycardia, ECG abnormalities, tachyarrhythmias, bradycardia, AV block, and bundle-branch block.
- Delayed cardiac toxicity may occur 2 to 3 months after treatment ends; indications include reduced LVEF and signs and symptoms of heart failure (tachycardia, dyspnea, pulmonary edema, dependent edema, hepatomegaly, ascites, pleural effusion, and gallop rhythm). Delayed cardiac toxicity depends on cumulative dose of epirubicin. Don't exceed cumulative dose of 900 mg/m^2.
- Obtain total and differential WBC, CBC, platelet counts, and liver function tests before and during each cycle of therapy.
- WBC nadir is usually reached 10 to 14 days after drug administration, and returns to normal by day 21.
- Monitor uric acid, potassium, calcium phosphate, and creatinine levels immediately after initial chemotherapy administration in patients susceptible to tumor lysis syndrome. Hydration, urine alkalinization, and prophylaxis with allopurinol may prevent hyperuricemia and minimize potential complications of tumor lysis syndrome.
- Drug may enhance the effects of radiation therapy or cause an inflammatory cell reaction at irradiation site. Monitor patient closely.

PATIENT TEACHING

- Advise patient to report any pain or burning at site of injection during or after administration.
- Advise patient to report nausea, vomiting, mouth inflammation, dehydration, fever, evidence of infection, or symptoms of heart failure (rapid heartbeat, labored breathing, swelling).
- Tell patient that urine will be reddish-pink for 1 to 2 days after treatment.
- Inform patient of risk of heart damage and treatment-related leukemia with use of drug.
- Advise men to use effective contraception during treatment.
- Advise women that irreversible, premature menopause may occur.
- Tell patient that hair usually regrows within 2 to 3 months after therapy stops.

SAFETY ALERT!

idarubicin hydrochloride
Idamycin PFS

Pharmacologic class: semisynthetic anthracycline
Pregnancy risk category D

AVAILABLE FORMS
Injection: 1 mg/ml in 5-, 10- and 20-ml single-dose vials

INDICATIONS & DOSAGES
Dosages vary. Check treatment protocol with prescriber.

➤ **Acute myeloid leukemia, including French-American-British (FAB) classifications M1 through M7, with other approved antileukemic drugs**
Adults: 12 mg/m^2 daily for 3 days by slow I.V. injection (over 10 to 15 minutes) with 100 mg/m^2 daily of cytarabine for 7 days by continuous I.V. infusion. Or, as a 25-mg/m^2 bolus (cytarabine); then 200 mg/m^2 daily (cytarabine) for 5 days by continuous infusion. A second course may be given, if needed.
Adjust-a-dose: If patient experiences severe mucositis, delay therapy until recovery is complete and reduce dosage by 25%. Reduce dosage in patients with hepatic or renal impairment. Don't give idarubicin if bilirubin level exceeds 5 mg/dl.

I.V. ADMINISTRATION
- Preparation and administration of parenteral form of drug may be mutagenic, teratogenic, or carcinogenic to staff. Follow institutional policy to reduce risks.
- Reconstitute to final concentration of 1 mg/ml using normal saline solution for injection without preservatives. Add 5 ml to 5-mg vial, 10 ml to 10-mg vial, or 20 ml to 20-mg vial. Don't use bacteriostatic saline solution. Vial is under negative pressure.
- Give drug over 10 to 15 minutes into a free-flowing I.V. infusion of normal saline or D_5W solution running into a large vein.
- Drug is a vesicant; tissue necrosis may result. If extravasation occurs, stop infusion immediately and notify prescriber. Treat with intermittent ice packs for one-half hour immediately and then for one-half hour q.i.d. for 4 days.
- Reconstituted solutions are stable for 72 hours at 59° to 86° F (15° to 30° C); 7 days if refrigerated and protected from light. Label unused solutions with chemotherapy hazard label.

INCOMPATIBILITIES
Acyclovir sodium, alkaline solutions, allopurinol, ampicillin sodium with sulbactam, cefazolin, cefepime, ceftazidime, clindamycin phosphate, dexamethasone sodium phosphate, etoposide, furosemide, gentamicin, heparin, hydrocortisone sodium succinate, lorazepam, meperidine, methotrexate sodium, piperacillin sodium with tazobactam, sodium bicarbonate, teniposide, vancomycin, vincristine.

ACTION
Unknown. Probably inhibits nucleic acid synthesis and interacts with the enzyme topoisomerase II. Drug is highly lipophilic, which increases rate of cellular uptake.

Route	Onset	Peak	Duration
I.V.	Unknown	Few min	Unknown

Half-life: 20 to 22 hours.

ADVERSE REACTIONS
CNS: *headache, changed mental status,* peripheral neuropathy, ***seizures, fever.***
CV: **HEMORRHAGE,** ***heart failure, MI, myocardial insufficiency, arrhythmias, myocardial toxicity,*** atrial fibrillation, chest pain, asymptomatic decline in left ventricular ejection fraction.
GI: *nausea, vomiting, cramps, diarrhea, mucositis.*
GU: renal dysfunction, red urine.
Hematologic: ***myelosuppression.***
Hepatic: changes in hepatic function.
Metabolic: hyperuricemia.
Skin: *alopecia, rash, urticaria, bullous erythrodermatous rash on palms and soles,* urticaria, erythema at previously irradiated sites, tissue necrosis if extravasation occurs.
Other: **INFECTION,** ***hypersensitivity reactions.***

INTERACTIONS

Drug-drug. *Alkaline solutions, heparin:* These combinations are incompatible. Don't mix idarubicin with other drugs unless specific compatibility data are known.

EFFECTS ON LAB TEST RESULTS

- May increase uric acid level. May decrease hemoglobin level.
- May decrease WBC, neutrophil, and platelet counts.

CONTRAINDICATIONS & CAUTIONS

- Use cautiously in patients with bone marrow suppression induced by previous drug therapy or radiotherapy, impaired hepatic or renal function, previous treatment with anthracyclines or cardiotoxic drugs, or a cardiac condition.

NURSING CONSIDERATIONS

- Cardiotoxicity is the dose-limiting toxicity of drug.
- Cardiovascular side effects occur with greater frequency in older patients.
- Make sure patient is adequately hydrated before treatment. Hyperuricemia may result from rapid lysis of leukemic cells. Allopurinol may be ordered.
- Assess patient for systemic infection and ensure that it's controlled before therapy begins.
- Give antiemetics to prevent or treat nausea and vomiting.
- Drug must never be given I.M. or subcutaneously.
- Monitor hepatic and renal function tests and CBC frequently.
- To prevent bleeding, avoid all I.M. injections when platelet count is below 50,000/mm^3.
- Anticipate need for blood transfusions for anemia. Patient may receive injections of RBC colony-stimulating factor to promote RBC production and decrease need for blood transfusions.
- Notify prescriber if signs or symptoms of heart failure occur.
- ***Look alike–sound alike:*** Don't confuse idarubicin with daunorubicin or doxorubicin.

PATIENT TEACHING

- Teach patient to recognize signs and symptoms of leakage of drug into surrounding tissue, and tell him to report them if they occur.
- Warn patient to watch for signs and symptoms of infection (fever, sore throat, fatigue) and bleeding (easy bruising, nosebleeds, bleeding gums, tarry stools).
- Advise patient that red urine for several days is normal and doesn't indicate presence of blood.
- Caution woman of childbearing age to avoid becoming pregnant during therapy. Recommend that she consult prescriber before becoming pregnant.

SAFETY ALERT!

mitomycin (mitomycin-C)

Mutamycin

Pharmacologic class: antineoplastic antibiotic
Pregnancy risk category NR

AVAILABLE FORMS

Powder for injection: 5-, 20-, 40-mg vials

INDICATIONS & DOSAGES

Dosage and indications vary. Check treatment protocol with prescriber.

➤ Disseminated adenocarcinoma of stomach or pancreas

Adults: 20 mg/m^2 as an I.V. single dose. Repeat cycle after 6 to 8 weeks when WBC and platelet counts have returned to normal.

Adjust-a-dose: For patients with myelosuppression, if leukocytes are 2,000 to 2,999/mm^3 and platelets are 25,000 to 74,999/mm^3, give 70% of initial dose. If leukocytes are less than 2,000/mm^3 and platelets are less than 25,000/mm^3, give 50% of initial dose.

➤ Bladder cancer ♦

Adults: 20 to 60 mg intravesically once weekly for 8 weeks.

I.V. ADMINISTRATION

- Preparing and giving drug may be mutagenic, teratogenic, or carcinogenic. Follow institutional policy to reduce risks.
- Using sterile water for injection, reconstitute drug in 5-mg vials with 10 ml, 20-mg vials with 40 ml, and 40-mg vials with 80 ml.

- Give drug into the side arm of a free-flowing I.V.
- When reconstituted with sterile water, solution is stable for 14 days under refrigeration and 7 days at room temperature. When diluted, drug is stable in D_5W for 3 hours, normal saline solution for 12 hours, sodium lactate for 24 hours.
- The combination of mitomycin (5 to 15 mg) and heparin (1,000 to 10,000 units) in 30 ml normal saline solution is stable for 48 hours at room temperature.
- Stop infusion immediately and notify prescriber if extravasation occurs because of potential for severe ulceration and necrosis.

INCOMPATIBILITIES

Aztreonam, bleomycin, cefepime, etoposide, filgrastim, gemcitabine, piperacillin sodium-tazobactam sodium, sargramostim, topotecan, vinorelbine.

ACTION

Similar to an alkylating drug, cross-linking strands of DNA and causing an imbalance of cell growth, leading to cell death.

Route	Onset	Peak	Duration
I.V.	Unknown	Unknown	Unknown

Half-life: About 50 minutes.

ADVERSE REACTIONS

CNS: headache, neurologic abnormalities, confusion, drowsiness, fatigue, *fever*.
EENT: blurred vision.
GI: mucositis, *nausea, vomiting, anorexia, diarrhea, stomatitis.*
GU: ***renal toxicity, hemolytic uremic syndrome.***
Hematologic: THROMBOCYTOPENIA, LEUKOPENIA, ***microangiopathic hemolytic anemia.***
Respiratory: ***interstitial pneumonitis,*** pulmonary edema, dyspnea, nonproductive cough, ***adult respiratory distress syndrome.***
Skin: cellulitis, induration, desquamation, pruritus, *pain at injection site, reversible alopecia,* purple bands on nails, rash, sloughing with extravasation.
Other: ***septicemia,*** ulceration, pain.

INTERACTIONS

Drug-drug. *Vinca alkaloids:* May cause acute respiratory distress when given together. Monitor patient closely.

EFFECTS ON LAB TEST RESULTS

- May increase BUN and creatinine levels. May decrease hemoglobin level.
- May decrease WBC and platelet counts.

CONTRAINDICATIONS & CAUTIONS

- Contraindicated in patients hypersensitive to drug and in those with thrombocytopenia, coagulation disorders, or an increased bleeding tendency from other causes.

NURSING CONSIDERATIONS

- Never give drug I.M. or subcutaneously.
- Continue CBC and blood studies at least 8 weeks after therapy stops. Leukopenia and thrombocytopenia are cumulative. If WBC count falls below 2,000/mm^3 or granulocyte count falls below 1,000/mm^3, follow institutional policy for infection control in immunocompromised patients.
- To prevent bleeding, avoid all I.M. injections when platelet count is less than 100,000/mm^3.
- Anticipate need for blood transfusions to combat anemia. Patients may receive injections of RBC colony-stimulating factor to promote RBC production and to decrease need for blood transfusions.
- Monitor patient for dyspnea with nonproductive cough; chest X-ray may show infiltrates.
- Monitor renal function tests.
- Leukopenia may occur up to 8 weeks after therapy and may be cumulative with successive doses.
- Hemolytic uremic syndrome is characterized by microangiopathic hemolytic anemia, thrombocytopenia, and renal failure.

PATIENT TEACHING

- Advise patient to report any pain or burning at site of injection during or after administration.
- Warn patient to watch for signs and symptoms of infection (fever, sore throat, fatigue) and bleeding (easy bruising, nosebleeds, bleeding gums, tarry stools). Tell patient to take temperature daily.
- Inform patient that hair loss may occur, but that it's usually reversible.

70

Antineoplastics that alter hormone balance

anastrozole
estramustine phosphate sodium
exemestane
flutamide
fulvestrant
goserelin acetate
letrozole
leuprolide acetate
megestrol acetate
tamoxifen citrate
testolactone
toremifene citrate

SAFETY ALERT!

anastrozole

Arimidex

Pharmacologic class: aromatase inhibitor

Pregnancy risk category D

AVAILABLE FORMS

Tablets: 1 mg

INDICATIONS & DOSAGES

➤ **First-line treatment of postmenopausal women with hormone receptor–positive or hormone receptor–unknown locally advanced or metastatic breast cancer; advanced breast cancer in postmenopausal women with disease progression after tamoxifen therapy; adjunctive treatment of postmenopausal women with hormone receptor–positive early breast cancer**

Adults: 1 mg P.O. daily.

ACTION

A selective nonsteroidal aromatase inhibitor that significantly lowers estradiol levels, which inhibits breast cancer cell growth in postmenopausal women.

Route	Onset	Peak	Duration
P.O.	< 24 hr	Unknown	< 7 days

Half-life: 50 hours.

ADVERSE REACTIONS

CNS: *headache, asthenia, pain,* dizziness, depression, paresthesia.
CV: *hot flashes,* ***thromboembolic disease,*** chest pain, edema, peripheral edema.
EENT: pharyngitis.
GI: *nausea,* vomiting, diarrhea, constipation, abdominal pain, anorexia, dry mouth.
GU: vaginal hemorrhage, vaginal dryness, pelvic pain.
Metabolic: weight gain.
Musculoskeletal: bone pain, *back pain.*
Respiratory: dyspnea, increased cough.
Skin: alopecia, rash, sweating.

INTERACTIONS

None significant.

EFFECTS ON LAB TEST RESULTS

- May increase liver enzyme levels.

CONTRAINDICATIONS & CAUTIONS

- Don't use in women who are or may be pregnant.
- Use cautiously in breast-feeding women.

NURSING CONSIDERATIONS

- Give drug under supervision of a prescriber experienced in use of antineoplastics.
- Patients with hormone receptor–negative disease and patients who didn't respond to previous tamoxifen therapy rarely respond to anastrozole.
- For patients with advanced breast cancer, continue anastrozole until tumor progresses.

PATIENT TEACHING

- Instruct patient to report adverse reactions, especially difficulty breathing or chest pain.
- Tell patient to take medication at the same time each day.
- Stress need for follow-up care.
- Counsel woman about risks of pregnancy during therapy.

SAFETY ALERT!

estramustine phosphate sodium

Emcyt, Estracyt‡

Pharmacologic class: estrogen and nitrogen mustard
Pregnancy risk category X

AVAILABLE FORMS

Capsules: 140 mg

INDICATIONS & DOSAGES

➤ **Palliative treatment of metastatic or progressive prostate cancer**
Adults: 10 to 16 mg/kg daily P.O. in three or four divided doses. Usual dose is 14 mg/kg daily. Continue therapy for up to 3 months and, if successful, maintain as long as patient responds.

ACTION

Unknown. Uptake into prostate cancer cells is facilitated by the estrogen component. Once intracellular, it may have weak alkylating activity.

Route	Onset	Peak	Duration
P.O.	Unknown	Unknown	Unknown

Half-life: Terminal, 20 hours.

ADVERSE REACTIONS

CNS: lethargy, insomnia, headache, anxiety, ***stroke.***
CV: ***MI,*** *edema,* chest pain, ***thrombophlebitis, heart failure,*** hypertension, flushing.
GI: *nausea, vomiting,* diarrhea, anorexia, flatulence, GI bleeding, thirst.
Hematologic: ***leukopenia, thrombocytopenia, thrombosis.***
Metabolic: sodium and fluid retention.
Musculoskeletal: leg cramps.
Respiratory: ***pulmonary embolism,*** dyspnea.
Skin: rash, pruritus, dry skin, thinning of hair.
Other: decreased libido, *breast tenderness, painful gynecomastia.*

INTERACTIONS

Drug-drug. *Calcium-containing drugs such as antacids:* May impair absorption of estramustine. Avoid using together.

Drug-food. *Calcium-rich foods such as dairy products:* May impair absorption of drug. Discourage use together.

EFFECTS ON LAB TEST RESULTS

- May increase ALT, AST, ceruloplasmin, cortisol, LDH, phospholipid, prolactin, and triglyceride levels. May decrease folate, phosphate, pregnanediol, and pyroxidine levels.
- May increase PT. May decrease glucose tolerance and platelet and WBC counts.

CONTRAINDICATIONS & CAUTIONS

- Contraindicated in patients hypersensitive to estradiol or nitrogen mustard and in those with active thrombophlebitis or thromboembolic disorders, except when actual tumor mass is cause of thromboembolic phenomenon.
- Use cautiously in patients with history of thrombophlebitis, thromboembolic disorders, or cerebrovascular or coronary artery disease.
- Use cautiously in patients with impaired liver function.

NURSING CONSIDERATIONS

- Monitor weight regularly in patients with history of thrombophlebitis, thromboembolic disorders, or cerebrovascular or coronary artery disease. Drug may worsen peripheral edema or heart failure.
- Monitor liver function periodically throughout therapy in patients with impaired liver function.
- Each 140-mg capsule contains 12.5 mg of sodium.
- Drug may increase blood pressure and decrease glucose level. Monitor periodically throughout therapy.
- Drug may be effective in patients who don’t respond to estrogen therapy alone.
- Patient may continue therapy as long as response is favorable. Some patients have taken drug for more than 3 years.
- Drug may increase norepinephrine-induced platelet aggregation and decrease response to the metyrapone test.
- Store capsules in refrigerator.

PATIENT TEACHING

- Tell patient to take drug on an empty stomach (1 hour before or 2 hours after

meals) and to avoid taking within 2 hours of dairy products.
- Because drug may harm fetus, advise woman to use contraception during therapy.
- Instruct patient to store capsules in refrigerator.

SAFETY ALERT!

exemestane
Aromasin

Pharmacologic class: aromatase inhibitor
Pregnancy risk category D

AVAILABLE FORMS
Tablets: 25 mg

INDICATIONS & DOSAGES
➤ **Advanced breast cancer in postmenopausal women whose disease has progressed after treatment with tamoxifen**
Adults: 25 mg P.O. once daily after food.
➤ **To complete 5 consecutive years of adjuvant hormonal therapy in postmenopausal women with estrogen-receptor–positive early-stage breast cancer who have had 2 to 3 years of tamoxifen therapy**
Adults: 25 mg P.O. once daily after food.

ACTION
A highly protein-bound, irreversible, steroidal aromatase inactivator that reduces circulating estrogen levels, which decreases cell growth in estrogen-dependent breast cancer.

Route	Onset	Peak	Duration
P.O.	Unknown	1 hr	24 hr

Half-life: About 24 hours.

ADVERSE REACTIONS
CNS: *fatigue, insomnia, pain,* depression, anxiety, dizziness, headache, paresthesia, generalized weakness, asthenia, confusion, hypoesthesia, fever.
CV: *hot flashes,* hypertension, edema, chest pain.
EENT: sinusitis, rhinitis, pharyngitis.
GI: *nausea,* vomiting, abdominal pain, anorexia, constipation, diarrhea, increased appetite, dyspepsia.
GU: UTI.
Hematologic: *lymphopenia.*
Musculoskeletal: *arthralgia,* pathologic fractures, arthritis, back pain, skeletal pain.
Respiratory: *dyspnea,* bronchitis, cough, upper respiratory tract infection.
Skin: *increased sweating, alopecia,* itching, dermatitis, rash.
Other: infection, flulike syndrome, lymphedema.

INTERACTIONS
Drug-drug. *Drugs containing estrogen:* May interfere with exemestane's action. Avoid using together.
Potent CYP3A4 inducers, such as phenytoin and rifampicin: May increase the metabolism of exemestane, decreasing level. Increase dose of exemestane to 50 mg daily.
Drug-herb. *St. John's wort:* May decrease effectiveness of drug. Discourage use together.

EFFECTS ON LAB TEST RESULTS
- May increase bilirubin, alkaline phosphatase, and creatinine levels.

CONTRAINDICATIONS & CAUTIONS
- Contraindicated in patients hypersensitive to drug or its components.

NURSING CONSIDERATIONS
- Use drug only in postmenopausal women. Pregnancy must be ruled out before starting drug therapy.
- Patients with advanced disease should continue treatment until tumor progression is apparent.
- Patients with early-stage breast cancer who have taken tamoxifen for 2 to 3 years should take this drug to complete a 5-year course, unless cancer recurs or is found in the other breast.

PATIENT TEACHING
- Direct patient to take drug after a meal.
- Stress the importance of maintaining healthy bones by staying active, eating foods containing calcium and vitamin D, minimizing alcohol consumption, and quitting smoking.

• Advise patient to report adverse effects, especially fever or swelling of arms or legs.

SAFETY ALERT!

flutamide
Euflex†

Pharmacologic class: nonsteroidal antiandrogen
Pregnancy risk category D

AVAILABLE FORMS
Capsules: 125 mg, 250 mg†

INDICATIONS & DOSAGES
➤ **Metastatic locally confined prostate cancer (stages B_2, C, D_2), combined with luteinizing hormone-releasing hormone analogues such as leuprolide acetate or goserelin**
Adults: 250 mg P.O. q 8 hours.

ACTION
Inhibits androgen uptake or prevents binding of androgens in nucleus of cells in target tissues.

Route	Onset	Peak	Duration
P.O.	Unknown	2 hr	Unknown

Half-life: For steady-state metabolite, about 6½ hours.

ADVERSE REACTIONS
CNS: drowsiness, ***encephalopathy,*** confusion, depression, anxiety, nervousness, paresthesia.
CV: peripheral edema, hypertension, *hot flashes.*
GI: *diarrhea, nausea, vomiting,* anorexia.
GU: *impotence.*
Hematologic: anemia, ***leukopenia, thrombocytopenia,*** hemolytic anemia.
Hepatic: ***hepatitis.***
Skin: rash, photosensitivity reactions.
Other: *loss of libido,* gynecomastia.

INTERACTIONS
Drug-drug. *Warfarin:* May increase PT. Monitor PT and INR.
Drug-lifestyle. *Sun exposure:* May cause photosensitivity reactions. Advise patient to avoid excessive sunlight exposure.

EFFECTS ON LAB TEST RESULTS
• May increase BUN, creatinine, hemoglobin, and liver enzyme levels.
• May decrease platelet and WBC counts.
• May alter pituitary-gonadal system tests during therapy and for 12 weeks after.

CONTRAINDICATIONS & CAUTIONS
• Contraindicated in patients hypersensitive to drug and in those with severe liver dysfunction.

NURSING CONSIDERATIONS
• Monitor liver function tests and CBC periodically.
• Flutamide must be taken continuously with drug used for medical castration (such as leuprolide) to allow full therapeutic benefit. Leuprolide suppresses testosterone production, whereas flutamide inhibits testosterone action at cellular level; together, they can impair growth of androgen-responsive tumors.

PATIENT TEACHING
• Advise patient not to stop drug without consulting prescriber.
• Instruct patient to report adverse reactions promptly, especially dark yellow or brown urine, vomiting, or yellowing of the eyes or skin.

SAFETY ALERT!

fulvestrant
Faslodex

Pharmacologic class: estrogen antagonist
Pregnancy risk category D

AVAILABLE FORMS
Injection: 50 mg/ml in 2.5-ml and 5-ml prefilled syringes

INDICATIONS & DOSAGES
➤ **Hormone receptor–positive metastatic breast cancer with disease progression after antiestrogen therapy**
Postmenopausal women: 250 mg (one 5-ml syringe or two 2.5-ml syringes) by slow I.M. injection into buttocks once monthly.

ACTION

Competitively binds estrogen receptors and down-regulates estrogen-receptor protein in human breast cancer cells. It's effective in treating estrogen receptor-positive breast tumors.

Route	Onset	Peak	Duration
I.M.	Unknown	7 days	1 mo

Half-life: About 40 days.

ADVERSE REACTIONS

CNS: *asthenia, headache, pain,* dizziness, insomnia, fever, paresthesia, depression, anxiety.
CV: *hot flashes,* chest pain, peripheral edema.
EENT: *pharyngitis.*
GI: *nausea, vomiting, constipation, abdominal pain, diarrhea,* anorexia.
GU: UTI.
Hematologic: anemia.
Musculoskeletal: *bone pain, back pain, pelvic pain,* arthritis.
Respiratory: *dyspnea, cough.*
Skin: *injection site pain,* rash, sweating.
Other: accidental injury, flulike syndrome.

INTERACTIONS

None reported.

EFFECTS ON LAB TEST RESULTS

- May decrease hemoglobin level and hematocrit.

CONTRAINDICATIONS & CAUTIONS

- Contraindicated in pregnant women and in patients allergic to drug or any of its components.
- Use cautiously in patients with moderate or severe hepatic impairment.

NURSING CONSIDERATIONS

- Because drug is given I.M., don't use in patients with bleeding diatheses or thrombocytopenia, or in those taking anticoagulants.
- Make sure woman isn't pregnant before starting drug.
- Expel gas bubble from syringe before administration.
- ***Alert:*** When using the 2.5-ml syringes, both must be given to obtain full dose.

PATIENT TEACHING

- Caution woman to avoid pregnancy and to report suspected pregnancy immediately.
- Inform patient of the most common side effects, including pain at injection site, headache, GI symptoms, back pain, hot flashes, and sore throat.

SAFETY ALERT!

goserelin acetate

Zoladex

Pharmacologic class: gonadotropin-releasing hormone analogue
Pregnancy risk category X (endometriosis and endometrial thinning); D (breast cancer)

AVAILABLE FORMS

Implants: 3.6 mg, 10.8 mg

INDICATIONS & DOSAGES

➤ **Endometriosis, including pain relief and lesion reduction**
Women: 3.6 mg subcutaneously q 28 days into the anterior abdominal wall below the navel. Maximum length of therapy is 6 months.

➤ **Endometrial thinning before endometrial ablation**
Women: 3.6 mg subcutaneously into the anterior abdominal wall below the navel. Give one or two implants, 4 weeks apart.

➤ **Palliative treatment of advanced breast cancer in premenopausal and perimenopausal women**
Women: 3.6 mg subcutaneously q 28 days into the anterior abdominal wall below the navel.

➤ **Palliative treatment of advanced prostate cancer**
Men: 3.6 mg subcutaneously q 28 days or 10.8 mg subcutaneously q 12 weeks into the anterior abdominal wall below the navel.

ACTION

A luteinizing hormone-releasing hormone (LH-RH) analogue that acts on the pituitary gland to decrease the release of follicle-stimulating hormone and LH, dramatically lowering sex hormone levels (estrogen in women and testosterone in men).

Route	Onset	Peak	Duration
SubQ	Rapid	30–60 min	Throughout therapy

Half-life: About 4½ hours.

ADVERSE REACTIONS

CNS: lethargy, pain, dizziness, *insomnia,* anxiety, *depression, headache,* chills, *emotional lability,* ***stroke,*** *asthenia.*
CV: edema, ***heart failure, arrhythmias,*** *peripheral edema,* hypertension, ***MI,*** peripheral vascular disorder, chest pain, *hot flashes.*
GI: nausea, vomiting, diarrhea, constipation, ulcer, anorexia, abdominal pain.
GU: *sexual dysfunction, impotence, lower urinary tract symptoms,* renal insufficiency, urinary obstruction, *vaginitis,* UTI, *amenorrhea.*
Hematologic: anemia.
Metabolic: hypercalcemia, hyperglycemia, weight increase, gout.
Musculoskeletal: back pain, osteoporosis.
Respiratory: COPD, upper respiratory tract infection.
Skin: rash, *diaphoresis, acne, seborrhea,* hirsutism.
Other: *changes in breast size, changes in libido, infection,* breast swelling, pain, and tenderness.

INTERACTIONS

None significant.

EFFECTS ON LAB TEST RESULTS

- May increase calcium and glucose levels. May decrease hemoglobin level.

CONTRAINDICATIONS & CAUTIONS

- Contraindicated in patients hypersensitive to LH-RH, LH-RH agonist analogues, or goserelin acetate.
- Contraindicated in pregnant or breastfeeding women and in patients with obstructive uropathy or vertebral metastases.
- The 10.8-mg implant is contraindicated in women because of insufficient data supporting reliable suppression of estradiol.
- Because drug may cause bone density loss in women, use cautiously in patients with risk factors for osteoporosis, such as family history of osteoporosis, chronic alcohol or tobacco abuse, or use of drugs such as corticosteroids or anticonvulsants that affect bone density.

NURSING CONSIDERATIONS

- Before giving to women, rule out pregnancy.
- Never give by I.V. injection.
- Give drug into the anterior abdominal wall below the navel using aseptic technique. After cleaning area with an alcohol swab and injecting a local anesthetic, stretch patient's skin with one hand while grasping barrel of syringe with the other. Insert needle into the subcutaneous fat; then change direction of needle so that it parallels the abdominal wall. Push needle in until hub touches patient's skin; withdraw about 1 cm (this creates a gap for drug to be injected) before depressing plunger completely.
- To avoid need for a new syringe and injection site, don't aspirate after inserting needle. If needle penetrates a blood vessel, blood will appear in the syringe chamber. Withdraw needle, and inject elsewhere with a new syringe.
- ***Alert:*** Implant comes in a preloaded syringe. If package is damaged, don't use the syringe. Make sure drug is visible in the translucent chamber of the syringe.
- When drug is used for prostate cancer, LH-RH analogues such as goserelin may initially worsen symptoms because drug first increases testosterone level. Some patients may temporarily have increased bone pain. Rarely, disease may get worse (spinal cord compression or ureteral obstruction), although the relationship to therapy is uncertain.
- When drug is used for endometrial thinning, if one implant is given, surgery should be performed 4 weeks later; if two implants are given, surgery should be performed 2 to 4 weeks after patient receives second implant.

PATIENT TEACHING

- Advise patient to return every 28 days for a new implant. A delay of a couple of days is permissible.
- Tell patient that pain may worsen for first 30 days of treatment.

• Tell woman to use a nonhormonal form of contraception during treatment. Caution patient about significant risks to fetus.
• Urge woman to call prescriber if menstruation persists or if breakthrough bleeding occurs. Menstruation should stop during treatment.
• Inform woman that a delayed return of menstruation may occur after therapy ends. Persistent lack of menstruation is rare.

SAFETY ALERT!

letrozole

Femara

Pharmacologic class: aromatase inhibitor
Pregnancy risk category D

AVAILABLE FORMS

Tablets: 2.5 mg

INDICATIONS & DOSAGES

➤ **Metastatic breast cancer with disease progression after antiestrogen therapy (such as tamoxifen)**
Postmenopausal women: 2.5 mg P.O. as single daily dose.
➤ **First-line treatment of hormone receptor–positive or hormone receptor–unknown, locally advanced, or metastatic breast cancer**
Postmenopausal women: 2.5 mg P.O. once daily until tumor progression is evident.
➤ **Adjuvant treatment of hormone-sensitive early breast cancer**
Postmenopausal women: 2.5 mg P.O. daily.
✷ ***NEW INDICATION:*** **Extended adjuvant treatment of early breast cancer following 5 years of adjuvant tamoxifen therapy**
Postmenopausal women: 2.5 mg P.O. once daily for 5 years.

ACTION

Inhibits conversion of androgens to estrogens, which decreases tumor mass or delays progression of tumor growth in some women.

Route	Onset	Peak	Duration
P.O.	Unknown	2 days	Unknown

Half-life: About 2 days.

ADVERSE REACTIONS

CNS: headache, somnolence, dizziness, fatigue, mood changes.
CV: *hot flashes, **MI, thromboembolism,*** chest pain, edema, hypertension.
GI: *nausea,* vomiting, constipation, diarrhea, abdominal pain, anorexia.
Metabolic: hypercholesterolemia, weight gain.
Musculoskeletal: *bone pain, limb pain, back pain,* arthralgia.
Respiratory: dyspnea, cough.
Skin: rash, pruritus.
Other: viral infections, breast pain, alopecia, diaphoresis.

INTERACTIONS

None significant.

EFFECTS ON LAB TEST RESULTS

• May increase cholesterol level.

CONTRAINDICATIONS & CAUTIONS

• Contraindicated in patients hypersensitive to drug or its components.
• Use cautiously in patients with severe liver impairment; dosage adjustment isn't needed in those with mild to moderate liver dysfunction.

NURSING CONSIDERATIONS

• Dosage adjustment isn't needed in patients with creatinine clearance of 10 ml/minute or more.
• Food doesn't affect drug absorption.
• ***Look alike–sound alike:*** Don't confuse Femara with FemHRT.

PATIENT TEACHING

• Instruct patient to take drug exactly as prescribed.
• Tell patient to take drug with or without food.
• Inform patient about potential adverse reactions.

SAFETY ALERT!

leuprolide acetate

Eligard, Lucrin‡, Lupron, Lupron Depot, Lupron Depot-Ped, Lupron Depot–3 Month, Lupron Depot–4 Month, Lupron for Pediatric Use, Viadur

Pharmacologic class: gonadotropin-releasing hormone analogue
Pregnancy risk category X

AVAILABLE FORMS

Depot injection: 3.75 mg, 7.5 mg, 11.25 mg, 15 mg, 22.5 mg, 30 mg, 45 mg
Injection: 5 mg/ml in 2.8-ml multiple-dose vials
Implant: 72 mg

INDICATIONS & DOSAGES

➤ **Advanced prostate cancer**
Adults: 1 mg subcutaneously daily. Or, 7.5 mg I.M. depot injection monthly. Or, 7.5 mg subcutaneous Eligard once monthly. Or, 22.5 mg I.M. depot injection q 3 months. Or, 22.5 mg subcutaneous Eligard q 3 months. Or, 30 mg I.M. depot injection q 4 months. Or, 30 mg subcutaneous Eligard q 4 months. Or, 45 mg subcutaneous Eligard q 6 months. Or, 72-mg Viadur implant inserted subcutaneously q 12 months.

➤ **Endometriosis**
Adults: 3.75 mg I.M. depot injection as single injection once monthly for up to 6 months. Or, 11.25 mg I.M. q 3 months for up to 6 months.

➤ **Central precocious puberty**
Children: Initially, 0.3 mg/kg (minimum 7.5 mg) I.M. depot injection as single injection q 4 weeks. May increase in increments of 3.75 mg q 4 weeks, if needed. Stop drug before girl reaches age 11 or boy reaches age 12.

➤ **Anemia related to uterine fibroids (with iron therapy)**
Adults: 3.75 mg I.M. depot injection once monthly for up to 3 consecutive months. Or 11.25 mg I.M. depot injection for 1 dose.

ACTION

Stimulates and then inhibits release of follicle-stimulating hormone and luteinizing hormone, which suppresses testosterone and estrogen levels.

Route	Onset	Peak	Duration
I.M., SubQ	Variable	1–2 mo	60–90 days
Implant	Unknown	4 hr	12 mo

Half-life: Unknown.

ADVERSE REACTIONS

CNS: *dizziness, depression, headache, pain,* insomnia, paresthesia, *asthenia.*
CV: ***arrhythmias,*** angina, ***MI,*** *peripheral edema, ECG changes,* hypotension, hypertension, murmur, *hot flashes.*
GI: *nausea, vomiting,* anorexia, constipation.
GU: *impotence, vaginitis,* urinary frequency, hematuria, UTI, *amenorrhea.*
Hematologic: anemia.
Metabolic: *weight gain or loss.*
Musculoskeletal: transient bone pain during first week of treatment, joint disorder, myalgia, neuromuscular disorder, bone loss.
Respiratory: dyspnea, sinus congestion, ***pulmonary fibrosis.***
Skin: reactions at injection site, dermatitis, acne.
Other: gynecomastia, androgen-like effects.

INTERACTIONS

None significant.

EFFECTS ON LAB TEST RESULTS

- May increase albumin, alkaline phosphatase, bilirubin, BUN, calcium, creatinine, glucose, LDH, phosphorus, and uric acid levels. May decrease hemoglobin level.
- May alter results of pituitary-gonadal system tests during therapy and for 12 weeks after.

CONTRAINDICATIONS & CAUTIONS

- Contraindicated in patients hypersensitive to drug or other gonadotropin-releasing hormone analogues, in women with undiagnosed vaginal bleeding, and in pregnant or breast-feeding women.
- The 30- and 45-mg depot injections and the Viadur implant are contraindicated in women and children.
- Use cautiously in patients hypersensitive to benzyl alcohol.

NURSING CONSIDERATIONS

- Never give by I.V. injection.
- ***Alert:*** Products have specific mixing and administration instructions. Read manufacturer's directions closely.
- Give depot injections under medical supervision. Use supplied diluent to reconstitute drug (extra diluent is provided; discard remainder). Draw 1 ml into a syringe with a 22G needle. (When preparing Lupron Depot–3 Month 22.5 mg, use a 23G or larger needle. Withdraw 1.5 ml from ampule for the 3-month form.)
- Inject into vial; shake well. Suspension will appear milky. Use immediately.
- When using prefilled dual-chamber syringes, prepare for injection by screwing white plunger into end stopper until stopper begins to turn. Remove and discard tab around base of needle. Hold syringe upright and release diluent by slowly pushing plunger until first stopper is at blue line in middle of barrel. Gently shake syringe to form a uniform milky suspension. If particles adhere to stopper, tap syringe against your finger. Remove needle guard and advance plunger to expel air from syringe. Inject entire contents I.M. as with a normal injection.
- For the two-syringe mixing system, connect the syringes and inject the liquid contents from Syringe A into the powder in Syringe B. Mix product by pushing contents back and forth between syringes for about 45 seconds; shaking the syringes won't mix the contents enough. The suspension will be colorless to pale yellow; the 7.5 mg suspension will be tan. Use immediately. Attach the needle provided in the kit and inject subcutaneously.
- A fractional dose of drug formulated to give every 3, 4, or 6 months isn't equivalent to same dose of once-a-month formulation.
- After starting treatment for central precocious puberty, monitor patient response every 1 to 2 months with a gonadotropin-releasing hormone stimulation test and sex corticosteroid level determinations. Measure bone age for advancement every 6 to 12 months.
- ***Alert:*** During first few weeks of treatment for prostate cancer, signs and symptoms of disease may temporarily worsen or additional signs and symptoms may occur (tumor flare).

PATIENT TEACHING

- Before starting child on treatment for central precocious puberty, make sure parents understand importance of continuous therapy.
- Carefully instruct patient who will give himself subcutaneous injection about the proper technique and advise him to use only the syringes provided by manufacturer.
- Advise patient that, if another syringe must be substituted, a low-dose insulin syringe (U-100, 0.5 ml) may be an appropriate choice but that needle gauge should be no smaller than 22G (except when using Lupron Depot–3 Month 22.5 mg).
- Instruct patient to store leuprolide acetate powder (depot) and diluent at room temperature, to refrigerate unopened vials of leuprolide acetate injection, and to protect leuprolide acetate injection from heat and light.
- Inform patient with history of undesirable effects from other endocrine therapies that leuprolide is easier to tolerate.
- Reassure patient that adverse effects disappear after about 1 week. Explain that symptoms of prostate cancer or central precocious puberty may worsen at first.
- Advise patient to keep implant insertion site clean and dry for 24 hours after procedure and to avoid heavy physical activity until site has healed. Local insertion site reactions such as bruising, burning, itching, and pain may resolve within 2 weeks.
- Advise woman of childbearing age to use a nonhormonal form of contraception during treatment.

SAFETY ALERT!

megestrol acetate

Megace, Megace ES, Megace OS†

Pharmacologic class: progestin
Pregnancy risk category X

AVAILABLE FORMS

Oral suspension: 40 mg/ml
Oral suspension (concentrated): 125 mg/ml
Tablets: 20 mg, 40 mg

INDICATIONS & DOSAGES

➤ **Breast cancer**

Adults: 40 mg P.O. q.i.d.

➤ **Endometrial cancer**

Adults: 40 to 320 mg P.O. daily in divided doses.

➤ **Anorexia, cachexia, or unexplained significant weight loss in patients with AIDS**

Adults: 800 mg P.O. (20 ml regular oral suspension) or 625 mg P.O. (5 ml concentrated oral suspension) once daily.

➤ **Anorexia or cachexia in patients with cancer ♦**

Adults: 480 to 600 mg P.O. daily.

ACTION

A progestin that inhibits hormone-dependent tumor growth by inhibiting pituitary and adrenal steroidogenesis. Drug may also have direct cytotoxicity; its appetite-stimulating mechanism is unknown.

Route	Onset	Peak	Duration
P.O.	Unknown	1–5 hr	Unknown

Half-life: About 10 days.

ADVERSE REACTIONS

CV: thrombophlebitis, ***heart failure,*** hypertension, ***thromboembolism.***
GI: nausea, vomiting, diarrhea, flatulence, constipation, dry mouth, increased appetite.
GU: breakthrough menstrual bleeding, impotence, vaginal bleeding or discharge, UTI.
Metabolic: hyperglycemia, *weight gain.*
Musculoskeletal: carpal tunnel syndrome.
Respiratory: ***pulmonary embolism,*** dyspnea.
Skin: alopecia, rash.
Other: gynecomastia, tumor flare.

INTERACTIONS

None significant.

EFFECTS ON LAB TEST RESULTS

- May increase glucose level.

CONTRAINDICATIONS & CAUTIONS

- Contraindicated in patients hypersensitive to drug.
- Contraindicated as a diagnostic test during pregnancy.
- Use cautiously in patients with history of thrombophlebitis or thromboembolism.

NURSING CONSIDERATIONS

- May increase glucose level in diabetic patients.
- Drug is relatively nontoxic with a low risk of adverse effects.
- Two months is an adequate trial period in patients with cancer.

PATIENT TEACHING

- Inform patient that therapeutic response isn't immediate.
- ***Alert:*** Tell patient that the ES oral suspension is more concentrated than the regular oral suspension so a smaller amount is needed.
- Advise woman to stop breast-feeding during therapy because of risk of toxicity to infant.
- Advise woman of childbearing age to use an effective form of contraception while receiving drug.

SAFETY ALERT!

tamoxifen citrate

Nolvadex-D†‡, Novo-Tamoxifen†, Soltamox*, Tamofen†, Tamone†

Pharmacologic class: nonsteroidal antiestrogen
Pregnancy risk category D

AVAILABLE FORMS

Oral solution: 10 mg/5 ml
Tablets: 10 mg, 20 mg
Tablets (enteric-coated)†: 10 mg, 20 mg

INDICATIONS & DOSAGES

➤ **Advanced breast cancer in women and men**

Adults: 20 mg to 40 mg P.O. daily; divide doses of more than 20 mg per day b.i.d.

➤ **Adjunct treatment of breast cancer**

Women: 20 mg to 40 mg P.O. daily for 5 years; divide doses of more than 20 mg per day b.i.d.

➤ To reduce breast cancer occurrence
High-risk women: 20 mg P.O. daily for 5 years.
➤ Ductal carcinoma in situ (DCIS) after breast surgery and radiation
Adults: 20 mg P.O. daily for 5 years.
➤ McCune-Albright syndrome and precocious puberty ♦
Children ages 2 to 10: Give 20 mg P.O. daily. Treat for up to 12 months.
➤ To stimulate ovulation ♦
Women: 5 to 40 mg P.O. b.i.d. for 4 days.
➤ Mastalgia ♦
Adults: 10 mg P.O. daily for 10 months.

ACTION

Unknown. Drug is selective estrogen receptor modulator.

Route	Onset	Peak	Duration
P.O.	1–Several mo	Unknown	Several wk

Half-life: Distribution phase, 7 to 14 hours; terminal phase, more than 7 days.

ADVERSE REACTIONS

CNS: ***stroke,*** confusion, weakness, sleepiness, headache.
CV: *fluid retention, hot flashes,* ***thromboembolism.***
EENT: corneal changes, cataracts, retinopathy.
GI: *nausea, vomiting, diarrhea.*
GU: *amenorrhea, irregular menses, vaginal discharge,* ***endometrial cancer, uterine sarcoma,*** vaginal bleeding.
Hematologic: ***leukopenia, thrombocytopenia.***
Hepatic: ***hepatic necrosis,*** fatty liver, cholestasis.
Metabolic: *hypercalcemia, weight gain or loss.*
Musculoskeletal: brief worsening of pain from osseous metastases.
Respiratory: ***pulmonary embolism (PE).***
Skin: *skin changes,* rash.
Other: temporary bone or tumor pain, alopecia.

INTERACTIONS

Drug-drug. *Antacids:* May affect absorption of enteric-coated tablet. Separate doses by 2 hours.
Bromocriptine: May elevate tamoxifen level. Monitor patient closely.
Coumarin-type anticoagulants: May significantly increase anticoagulant effect. Monitor patient, PT, and INR closely.
Cytotoxic drugs: May increase risk of thromboembolic events. Monitor patient.
CYP3A4 inducers (such as rifampin): May increase tamoxifen metabolism and may lower drug levels. Monitor patient for clinical effects.

EFFECTS ON LAB TEST RESULTS

- May increase BUN, calcium, T_4, and liver enzyme levels.
- May decrease WBC and platelet counts.

CONTRAINDICATIONS & CAUTIONS

- Contraindicated in patients hypersensitive to drug. Also contraindicated as therapy to reduce risk of breast cancer in high-risk women who also need anticoagulants or in women with history of deep vein thrombosis or pulmonary embolism.
- Use cautiously in patients with leukopenia or thrombocytopenia. Monitor CBC closely.

NURSING CONSIDERATIONS

- Monitor lipid levels during long-term therapy in patients with hyperlipidemia.
- Monitor calcium level. At start of therapy, drug may compound hypercalcemia related to bone metastases.
- Women should have baseline and periodic gynecologic exams because of a slight increased risk of endometrial cancer.
- Rule out pregnancy before therapy.
- Patient may initially experience worsening symptoms.
- Adverse reactions are usually minor and well tolerated.
- In postmenopausal women, karyopyknotic index of vaginal smears and various degrees of estrogen effect of Papanicolaou smears may vary.
- ***Alert:*** Women at high risk for breast cancer or who have DCIS taking drug to reduce risk may experience life-threatening endometrial cancer, uterine sarcoma, stroke, or PE. The benefits of drug outweigh its risks in women already diagnosed with breast cancer.

PATIENT TEACHING

- For enteric-coated Nolvadex-D tablets, tell patient to swallow them whole without crushing or chewing. Tell him not to take antacids within 2 hours of dose.
- Reassure patient that acute worsening of bone pain during therapy usually indicates drug will produce good response. Give analgesics to relieve pain.
- Strongly encourage woman who is taking or has taken drug to have regular gynecologic exams because drug may increase risk of uterine cancer.
- Encourage woman to have annual mammograms and breast exams.
- Advise patient to use a barrier form of contraception because short-term therapy induces ovulation in premenopausal women.
- Instruct patient to report vaginal bleeding or changes in menstrual cycle.
- Caution woman to avoid becoming pregnant during therapy and first 2 months after stopping drug. Advise her to consult prescriber before becoming pregnant.
- Advise patient that breast cancer risk assessment tools are available and that she should discuss her concerns with her prescriber.
- Tell patient to report symptoms of stroke, such as headache, vision changes, confusion, difficulty speaking or walking, and weakness of face, arm, or leg, especially on one side of the body.
- Tell patients to report symptoms of pulmonary embolism, such as chest pain, difficulty breathing, rapid breathing, sweating, and fainting.
- Tell patient to use oral solution within 3 months of opening and not to refrigerate or freeze it.

SAFETY ALERT!

testolactone
Teslac

Pharmacologic class: androgen
Pregnancy risk category C
Controlled substance schedule III

AVAILABLE FORMS

Tablets: 50 mg

INDICATIONS & DOSAGES

➤ **Advanced premenopausal breast cancer in women whose ovarian function has been terminated; advanced postmenopausal breast cancer**
Women: 250 mg P.O. q.i.d for at least 3 months unless disease is actively progressing.

ACTION

Antineoplastic action unknown. Drug may inhibit steroid aromatase activity and decrease estrone synthesis.

Route	Onset	Peak	Duration
P.O.	6–12 wk	Unknown	Unknown

Half-life: Unknown.

ADVERSE REACTIONS

CNS: paresthesia, peripheral neuropathy.
CV: increased blood pressure, edema.
GI: nausea, vomiting, diarrhea, anorexia, glossitis.
Skin: alopecia, erythema, nail changes.

INTERACTIONS

Drug-drug. *Oral anticoagulants:* May increase anticoagulant effects. Monitor patient, PT, and INR carefully.

EFFECTS ON LAB TEST RESULTS

- May increase calcium level.
- May decrease estradiol levels measured by radioimmunoassay.

CONTRAINDICATIONS & CAUTIONS

- Contraindicated in patients hypersensitive to drug and in men with breast cancer.

NURSING CONSIDERATIONS

- Monitor fluid and electrolyte levels, especially calcium level.
- Force fluids to aid calcium excretion and encourage exercise to prevent hypercalcemia. Immobilized patients are susceptible to hypercalcemia.
- While higher doses don't increase likelihood of remission, patients with visceral metastases may benefit from 2 g daily.
- Although similar to testosterone, drug has no androgenic effects.

PATIENT TEACHING
- Inform patient that therapeutic response isn't immediate; 3 months is an adequate trial for drug.
- Tell patient to notify prescriber if numbness or tingling occurs in fingers, toes, or face.
- Advise patient to use contraception during therapy.

SAFETY ALERT!

toremifene citrate
Fareston

Pharmacologic class: nonsteroidal antiestrogen
Pregnancy risk category D

AVAILABLE FORMS
Tablets: 60 mg

INDICATIONS & DOSAGES
➤ **Metastatic breast cancer in postmenopausal women with estrogen receptor–positive or estrogen receptor–unknown tumors**
Adults: 60 mg P.O. once daily. Continue until disease progresses.

ACTION
A nonsteroidal triphenylethylene with antiestrogenic effect. Drug competes with estrogen for binding sites in the tumor, which blocks the tumor's growth-stimulating effects of endogenous estrogen.

Route	Onset	Peak	Duration
P.O.	Unknown	3 hr	Unknown

Half-life: About 5 days.

ADVERSE REACTIONS
CNS: dizziness, fatigue, depression.
CV: *hot flashes,* ***thromboembolism, heart failure, MI,*** edema.
EENT: *cataracts,* visual disturbances, glaucoma, dry eyes.
GI: *nausea,* vomiting.
GU: *vaginal discharge,* vaginal bleeding.
Hepatic: ***hepatotoxicity.***
Metabolic: hypercalcemia.
Respiratory: ***pulmonary embolism.***
Skin: *sweating.*

INTERACTIONS
Drug-drug. *Calcium-elevating drugs such as hydrochlorothiazide:* May increase risk of hypercalcemia. Monitor calcium level closely.
Coumarin-like anticoagulants such as warfarin: May prolong PT and INR. Monitor PT and INR closely.
CYP3A4 enzyme inducers such as carbamazepine, phenobarbital, and phenytoin: May increase toremifene metabolism rate. Monitor patient closely.
CYP3A4-6 enzyme inhibitors such as erythromycin, and ketoconazole: May increase toremifene metabolism rate. Monitor patient closely.

EFFECTS ON LAB TEST RESULTS
- May increase calcium and liver enzyme levels.

CONTRAINDICATIONS & CAUTIONS
- Contraindicated in patients hypersensitive to drug and in those with history of thromboembolic disease.

NURSING CONSIDERATIONS
- Obtain periodic CBC, calcium levels, and liver function tests.
- Monitor calcium level closely during first weeks of treatment in patients with bone metastases because of increased risk of hypercalcemia.

PATIENT TEACHING
- Instruct patient to take drug exactly as prescribed.
- Advise patient that doses may be taken without regard to meals.
- Warn patient not to stop therapy without consulting prescriber.
- Inform patient about vaginal bleeding and other adverse effects; tell her to notify prescriber if bleeding occurs.
- Warn patient that disease flare-up may occur during first weeks of therapy. Reassure her that this doesn't indicate treatment failure.
- Advise patient to report leg or chest pain, severe headache, visual changes, or shortness of breath.
- Counsel woman about risks of becoming pregnant during therapy.

71

Miscellaneous antineoplastics

asparaginase
azacitidine
bevacizumab
bortezomib
cetuximab
clofarabine
dacarbazine
dasatinib
docetaxel
erlotinib
etoposide
etoposide phosphate
gemtuzumab ozogamicin
imatinib mesylate
irinotecan hydrochloride
mitoxantrone hydrochloride
nelarabine
paclitaxel
paclitaxel protein-bound particles
panitumumab
pegaspargase
procarbazine hydrochloride
rituximab
sorafenib
sunitinib malate
teniposide
topotecan hydrochloride
trastuzumab
vinblastine sulfate
vincristine sulfate
vinorelbine tartrate
vorinostat

SAFETY ALERT!

asparaginase

Elspar, Kidrolase†

Pharmacologic class: Escherichia coli–derived enzyme
Pregnancy risk category C

AVAILABLE FORMS

Injection: 10,000-international unit vial

INDICATIONS & DOSAGES

➤ Acute lymphocytic leukemia with other drugs

Adults and children: 1,000 international units/kg I.V. daily for 10 days beginning on day 22 of regimen, injected over 30 minutes. Or, 6,000 international units/m² I.M. at intervals specified in protocol.

➤ Sole induction drug for acute lymphocytic leukemia

Adults and children: 200 international units/kg I.V. daily for 28 days.

I.V. ADMINISTRATION

- Preparing and giving parenteral form of drug may be mutagenic, teratogenic, or carcinogenic. Follow facility policy to reduce risks.
- Reconstitute drug with 5 ml of sterile water for injection or saline solution for injection.
- To avoid foaming, don't shake vial vigorously.
- Use only clear solution.
- Use of a 5-micron filter during infusion removes gelatinous fiber-like particles that occasionally form without reducing drug potency.
- Give injection over 30 minutes through a running infusion of normal saline solution or D_5W.
- Refrigerate unopened dry powder. Reconstituted solution is stable for 8 hours if refrigerated.

INCOMPATIBILITIES

None reported.

ACTION

Leads to death of leukemic cells by destroying the essential amino acid asparagine, which is needed for protein synthesis in acute lymphocytic leukemia.

Route	Onset	Peak	Duration
I.V.	Immediate	Immediate	23–33 days
I.M.	Unknown	14–24 hr	23–33 days

Half-life: 8 to 30 hours.

ADVERSE REACTIONS

CNS: agitation, confusion, drowsiness, depression, fatigue, fever, hallucinations, headache, lethargy, somnolence.

GI: HEMORRHAGIC PANCREATITIS, *anorexia, nausea, vomiting,* cramps, stomatitis.
GU: *azotemia,* ***renal failure,*** glycosuria, polyuria, uric acid nephropathy.
Hematologic: *anemia,* ***DIC, hypofibrinogenemia, leukopenia,*** depression of clotting factor synthesis.
Hepatic: ***hepatotoxicity.***
Metabolic: *hyperglycemia,* hyperammonemia, hyperuricemia, hypocalcemia, weight loss.
Skin: *rash, urticaria.*
Other: ANAPHYLAXIS, chills, hypersensitivity reactions.

INTERACTIONS

Drug-drug. *Methotrexate:* May decrease methotrexate effectiveness. Avoid using together, or give asparaginase after methotrexate.
Prednisone: May cause hyperglycemia. Monitor glucose level.
Vincristine: May increase neuropathy. Give asparaginase after vincristine, and monitor patient closely.

EFFECTS ON LAB TEST RESULTS

- May increase alkaline phosphatase, ammonia, AST, ALT, bilirubin, BUN, glucose, and uric acid levels. May decrease calcium, cholesterol, hemoglobin, and serum albumin levels.
- May decrease thyroid function test values and WBC count.

CONTRAINDICATIONS & CAUTIONS

- Contraindicated in patients hypersensitive to drug (unless desensitized) and in those with pancreatitis or history of pancreatitis.
- Use cautiously in patients with hepatic dysfunction. Drug should first be given in hospital setting under close supervision.

NURSING CONSIDERATIONS

- Monitor blood and urine glucose levels before and during therapy. Watch for signs and symptoms of hyperglycemia.
- Start allopurinol before therapy begins to help prevent uric acid nephropathy.
- ***Alert:*** Risk of hypersensitivity increases with repeated doses. Give 2 international units I.D. before first dose and when 1 week or more has elapsed between doses. Observe site for at least 1 hour for erythema or a wheal, which indicates a positive skin test.
- ***Alert:*** Patient with negative skin test may still develop an allergic reaction; desensitization may be needed before first treatment dose and with retreatment. Give 1 international unit I.V. If no reaction occurs, double dose every 10 minutes until total daily dose is given.
- Drug shouldn't be used alone to induce remission unless combination therapy is inappropriate. Drug isn't recommended for maintenance therapy.
- For I.M. injection, reconstitute with 2 ml normal saline solution to the 10,000-international unit vial. Refrigerate and use within 8 hours.
- Don't give more than 2 ml I.M. at one injection site.
- Don't use cloudy solutions.
- If drug touches skin or mucous membranes, wash with a generous amount of water for at least 15 minutes.
- Keep epinephrine, diphenhydramine, and I.V. corticosteroids available for treating anaphylaxis.
- Monitor CBC and bone marrow function tests.
- Obtain amylase and lipase levels to check pancreatic status. If levels are elevated, stop asparaginase.
- Increase patient's fluid intake to help prevent tumor lysis, which can result in uric acid nephropathy.
- Drug may affect clotting factor synthesis and cause hypofibrinogenemia, leading to thrombosis or, more commonly, severe bleeding. Monitor patient and bleeding studies closely.
- Because of vomiting, give fluids parenterally for 24 hours or until oral fluids are tolerated.
- Patient may become hypersensitive to drug derived from cultures of *Escherichia coli.* Erwinia asparaginase, which is derived from cultures of *E. carotovora,* may be used in these patients without causing cross-sensitivity.
- Drug toxicity is more likely to occur in adults than in children.
- There are several protocols for use of this drug.

PATIENT TEACHING

- Tell patient to watch for signs of infection (fever, sore throat, fatigue) and bleeding (easy bruising, nosebleeds, bleeding gums, tarry stools). Tell patient to take temperature daily.
- Stress importance of maintaining adequate fluid intake to help prevent hyperuricemia. If adverse GI reactions prevent patient from drinking fluids, tell him to notify prescriber.
- Urge patient to immediately report severe headache, stomach pain with nausea or vomiting, or inability to move a limb.
- Advise patient to report signs of a hypersensitivity reaction, including rash, itching, chills, dizziness, chest tightness, or difficulty breathing.

SAFETY ALERT!

azacitidine

Vidaza

Pharmacologic class: pyrimidine nucleoside analog
Pregnancy risk category D

AVAILABLE FORMS

Powder for injection: 100-mg vials

INDICATIONS & DOSAGES

➤ **Myelodysplastic syndrome, including refractory anemia, refractory anemia with ringed sideroblasts (if patient has neutropenia or thrombocytopenia, or needs transfusions), refractory anemia with excess blasts, refractory anemia with excess blasts in transformation, or chronic myelomonocytic leukemia**

Adults: Initially, 75 mg/m^2 subcutaneously daily for 7 days; repeat cycle q 4 weeks. May increase to 100 mg/m^2 if no response after two treatment cycles and nausea and vomiting are the only toxic reactions. At least four treatment cycles are recommended.

Adjust-a-dose: If bicarbonate level is less than 20 mEq/L, reduce next dose by 50%. If BUN or creatinine levels rise during treatment, delay the next cycle until they are normal; then give 50% of previous dose. Adjust further during therapy based on hematologic or renal toxicities.

ACTION

Causes hypomethylation of DNA and is toxic to abnormal hematopoietic cells in bone marrow. Hypomethylation may restore normal function to genes needed for proliferation and differentiation. Drug has little effect on nonproliferating cells.

Route	Onset	Peak	Duration
SubQ	Unknown	30 min	Unknown

Half-life: About 40 minutes.

ADVERSE REACTIONS

CNS: *anxiety, depression, dizziness, fatigue, headache, insomnia, malaise, pain, weakness,* hypoesthesia, lethargy, syncope.
CV: *cardiac murmur, chest pain, edema,* hypotension, peripheral swelling, tachycardia.
EENT: *epistaxis, nasopharyngitis, pharyngitis, rhinorrhea,* nasal congestion, postnasal drip, sinusitis.
GI: *abdominal pain and tenderness, anorexia, constipation, decreased appetite, diarrhea, nausea, vomiting,* abdominal distension, dyspepsia, dysphagia, gingival bleeding, hemorrhoids, loose stools, mouth hemorrhage, oral mucosal petechiae, stomatitis, tongue ulceration.
GU: dysuria, UTI.
Hematologic: *anemia,* FEBRILE NEUTROPENIA, LEUKOPENIA, NEUTROPENIA, THROMBOCYTOPENIA, hematoma, postprocedural hemorrhage.
Metabolic: *decreased weight.*
Musculoskeletal: *arthralgia, back pain, limb pain, myalgia,* muscle cramps.
Respiratory: *atelectasis, cough, crackles, dyspnea, rhonchi, pneumonia, upper respiratory tract infection,* pleural effusion, wheezing.
Skin: *bruising, contusion, ecchymosis, erythema, increased sweating, injection site reaction, pain, pallor, petechiae, pitting edema, rash, skin lesion,* cellulitis, dry skin, granuloma, night sweats, pigmentation, pruritus at injection site, skin nodules, swelling at injection site, urticaria.
Other: *pyrexia, rigors,* herpes simplex, lymphadenopathy.

INTERACTIONS
None reported.

EFFECTS ON LAB TEST RESULTS
• May increase BUN and creatinine levels. May decrease bicarbonate and potassium levels.
• May decrease neutrophil, platelet, and WBC counts.

CONTRAINDICATIONS & CAUTIONS
• Contraindicated in patients hypersensitive to azacitidine or mannitol and in patients with advanced malignant hepatic tumors.
• Use cautiously in patients with hepatic and renal disease.

NURSING CONSIDERATIONS
• Dilute using aseptic and hazardous substances techniques. Reconstitute with 4 ml sterile water for injection. Invert vial two to three times and gently rotate until a uniform suspension forms. The resulting cloudy suspension will be 25 mg/ml. Draw up suspension into syringes for injection (no more than 4 ml per syringe).
• Just before giving drug, resuspend drug by inverting the syringe two to three times and gently rolling between palms for 30 seconds. Divide doses greater than 4 ml into two syringes and inject into two separate sites. Give new injections at least 1 inch from previous site, and never into tender, bruised, red, or hardened skin.
• Check liver function test results and creatinine level before therapy starts.
• Obtain CBC before each cycle or more often.
• Monitor renal function closely in elderly patients and in renally impaired patients receiving drug because renal impairment may increase toxicity.
• Store unreconstituted vials at room temperature (59° to 86° F [15° to 30° C]).
• Reconstituted drug is stable 1 hour at room temperature and 8 hours refrigerated (36° to 46° F [2° to 8° C]). After refrigeration, suspension may be allowed to warm for 30 minutes at room temperature.

PATIENT TEACHING
• Inform patient that blood counts may decrease with febrile neutropenia, thrombocytopenia, and anemia.
• Advise men and women to use birth control during therapy.

SAFETY ALERT!

bevacizumab
Avastin

Pharmacologic class: monoclonal antibody
Pregnancy risk category C

AVAILABLE FORMS
Solution: 25 mg/ml in 4-ml and 16-ml vials

INDICATIONS & DOSAGES
➤ **First- or second-line treatment, with fluorouracil-based chemotherapy, for metastatic colon or rectal cancer**
Adults: If used with bolus irinotecan, fluorouracil, and leucovorin (known as IFL) regimen, give 5 mg/kg I.V. q 14 days. If used with oxaliplatin, fluorouracil, and leucovorin (known as FOLFOX 4) regimen, give 10 mg/kg I.V. q 14 days. Infusion rate varies by patient tolerance and number of infusions.
✱ ***NEW INDICATION:*** **With carboplatin and paclitaxel as first-line treatment of unresectable, locally advanced, recurrent, or metastatic nonsquamous, non-small–cell lung cancer**
Adults: 15 mg/kg I.V. infusion once every 3 weeks.

I.V. ADMINISTRATION
• Don't freeze or shake vials.
• Dilute drug using aseptic technique. Withdraw proper dose and mix in a total volume of 100 ml normal saline solution in an I.V. bag.
• Don't give by I.V. push or bolus.
• Give the first infusion over 90 minutes and, if tolerated, the second infusion over 60 minutes. Later infusions can be given over 30 minutes if previous infusions were tolerated.
• Discard unused portion; drug is preservative-free.
• Drug is stable 8 hours if refrigerated at 36° to 46° F (2° to 8° C) and protected from light.

INCOMPATIBILITIES
Dextrose solutions.

ACTION
A recombinant humanized vascular endothelial growth factor (VEGF) inhibitor. Because VEGF promotes angiogenesis to tumors, it may contribute to metastatic tumor growth.

Route	Onset	Peak	Duration
I.V.	Unknown	Unknown	Unknown

Half-life: About 20 days.

ADVERSE REACTIONS
CNS: *asthenia, dizziness, headache,* abnormal gait, confusion, pain, syncope.
CV: INTRA-ABDOMINAL THROMBOSIS, *hypertension,* ***thromboembolism,*** deep vein thrombosis, heart failure, hypotension.
EENT: *epistaxis,* excess lacrimation, gum bleeding, nasal septum perforation, taste disorder, voice alteration.
GI: *anorexia, constipation, diarrhea, dyspepsia, flatulence, stomatitis, vomiting,* ***GI hemorrhage,*** abdominal pain, colitis, dry mouth, nausea.
GU: ***vaginal hemorrhage,*** proteinuria, urinary urgency.
Hematologic: ***leukopenia, neutropenia, thrombocytopenia.***
Metabolic: *hypokalemia, weight loss,* bilirubinemia.
Musculoskeletal: *myalgia.*
Respiratory: *dyspnea, upper respiratory tract infection,* HEMOPTYSIS.
Skin: *alopecia, dermatitis, discoloration, dry skin, exfoliative dermatitis,* nail disorder, skin ulcer.
Other: decreased wound healing, hypersensitivity.

INTERACTIONS
Drug-drug. *Irinotecan:* May increase level of irinotecan metabolite. Monitor patient.

EFFECTS ON LAB TEST RESULTS
- May increase bilirubin and urine protein levels. May decrease potassium level.
- May decrease neutrophil, platelet, and WBC counts.

CONTRAINDICATIONS & CAUTIONS
- Don't use in patients with recent hemoptysis or within 28 days after major surgery.
- Use cautiously in patients hypersensitive to drug or its components, in those who need surgery, are taking anticoagulants, or have significant CV disease.

NURSING CONSIDERATIONS
- Hypersensitivity reactions can occur during infusion.
- Reversible posterior leukoencephalopathy syndrome (headache, visual disturbances, altered mental status, and seizures) may occur 16 hours to 1 year after starting drug. Monitor patient for these signs.
- In patients who develop nephrotic syndrome, severe hypertension, hypertensive crisis, serious hemorrhage, GI perforation, or wound dehiscence that needs intervention, stop drug.
- Before elective surgery, stop drug, considering drug's half-life is about 20 days. Don't resume therapy until incision is fully healed.
- ***Alert:*** May increase risk of serious arterial thromboembolic events including MI, TIAs, stroke, and angina. Those patients at highest risk are age 65 or older, have a history of arterial thromboembolism, and have taken the drug before. If patient has an arterial thrombotic event, permanently stop drug.
- Monitor urinalysis for worsening proteinuria. Patients with 2+ or greater urine dipstick test should undergo 24-hour urine collection.
- Monitor patient's blood pressure every 2 to 3 weeks.
- It isn't known whether drug appears in breast milk. Women shouldn't breast-feed during and for about 3 weeks after therapy ends.

PATIENT TEACHING
- Tell patient to report adverse reactions immediately, especially abdominal pain, constipation, and vomiting.
- Advise patient that blood pressure and urinalysis will be monitored during treatment.
- Caution woman of childbearing age to avoid pregnancy during treatment.

• Urge patient to alert other health care providers about treatment and to avoid elective surgery during treatment.

SAFETY ALERT!

bortezomib
Velcade

Pharmacologic class: proteosome inhibitor
Pregnancy risk category D

AVAILABLE FORMS
Powder for injection: 3.5 mg

INDICATIONS & DOSAGES
***NEW INDICATION:* Multiple myeloma or mantle cell lymphoma that still progresses after at least one therapy**
Adults: 1.3 mg/m^2 by I.V. bolus twice weekly for 2 weeks (days 1, 4, 8, and 11), followed by a 10-day rest period (days 12 through 21). This 3-week period is a treatment cycle. For therapy longer than 8 cycles, may adjust dosage schedule to once weekly for 4 weeks on days 1, 8, 15, and 22, followed by a rest period on days 23 through 35. Separate consecutive doses of drug by at least 72 hours.
Adjust-a-dose: If grade 3 nonhematologic or grade 4 hematologic toxicity (excluding neuropathy) develops, withhold drug. When toxicity has resolved, restart at a 25% reduced dose. If patient has neuropathic pain, peripheral neuropathy, or both, see the table.

Severity of neuropathy	Dosage
Grade 1 (paresthesias, loss of reflexes, or both) without pain or loss of function	No change.
Grade 1 with pain or grade 2 (function altered but not activities of daily living)	Reduce to 1 mg/m^2.
Grade 2 with pain or grade 3 (interference with activities of daily living)	Hold drug until toxicity resolves; then start at 0.7 mg/m^2 once weekly.
Grade 4 (permanent sensory loss that interferes with function)	Stop drug.

I.V. ADMINISTRATION
• Use caution and aseptic technique when preparing and handling drug. Wear gloves and protective clothing to prevent skin contact.
• Reconstitute with 3.5 ml of normal saline solution and give by I.V. bolus.
• Reconstituted drug may be stored up to 3 hours in a syringe at 59° to 86° F (15° to 30° C), but total storage time must not exceed 8 hours.
• Store unopened vial at a controlled room temperature, in original packaging, protected from light.

INCOMPATIBILITIES
None reported.

ACTION
Disrupts intracellular homeostatic mechanisms by inhibiting the 26S proteosome, which regulates intracellular levels of certain proteins, causing cells to die.

Route	Onset	Peak	Duration
I.V.	Unknown	Unknown	Unknown

Half-life: 9 to 15 hours.

ADVERSE REACTIONS
CNS: *anxiety, asthenia, dizziness, dysesthesia, fever, headache, insomnia, paresthesia, peripheral neuropathy, rigors.*
CV: *edema, hypotension.*
EENT: *blurred vision.*
GI: *abdominal pain, constipation, decreased appetite, diarrhea, dysgeusia, dyspepsia, nausea, vomiting.*
Hematologic: *anemia,* NEUTROPENIA, THROMBOCYTOPENIA.
Musculoskeletal: *arthralgia, back pain, bone pain, limb pain, muscle cramps, myalgia.*
Respiratory: *cough, dyspnea, pneumonia, upper respiratory tract infection.*
Skin: *pruritus,* rash.
Other: *dehydration, herpes zoster, pyrexia.*

INTERACTIONS
Drug-drug. *Antihypertensives:* May cause hypotension. Monitor patient's blood pressure closely.
Drugs linked to peripheral neuropathy, such as amiodarone, antivirals, isoniazid,

nitrofurantoin, statins: May worsen neuropathy. Use together cautiously.
Inhibitors or inducers of CYP3A4: May increase risk of toxicity or may reduce drug's effects. Monitor patient closely.
Oral antidiabetics: May cause hypoglycemia or hyperglycemia. Monitor glucose level closely.

EFFECTS ON LAB TEST RESULTS
- May decrease hemoglobin level.
- May decrease neutrophil and platelet counts.

CONTRAINDICATIONS & CAUTIONS
- Contraindicated in patients hypersensitive to bortezomib, boron, or mannitol.
- Use cautiously in patients with hepatic or renal impairment or with a history of syncope or in those who are dehydrated or receiving other drugs known to cause hypotension.
- Safety and effectiveness haven't been established for pregnant women or children.

NURSING CONSIDERATIONS
- Monitor for evidence of neuropathy, such as a burning sensation, hyperesthesia, hypoesthesia, paresthesia, discomfort, or neuropathic pain.
- Watch carefully for adverse effects, especially in the elderly.
- Be sure patient has an order for an antiemetic, antidiarrheal, or both to treat drug-induced nausea, vomiting, or diarrhea.
- Provide fluid and electrolyte replacement to prevent dehydration.
- To manage orthostatic hypotension, adjust antihypertensive dosage, maintain hydration status, and give mineralocorticoids.
- ***Alert:*** Because thrombocytopenia is common, monitor patient's CBC and platelet counts carefully during treatment, especially on day 11.

PATIENT TEACHING
- Tell patient to notify prescriber about new or worsening peripheral neuropathy.
- Urge women to use effective contraception and not to breast-feed during treatment.
- Teach patient how to avoid dehydration, and stress the need to tell prescriber about dizziness, light-headedness, or fainting spells.
- Tell patient to use caution when driving or performing other hazardous activities because drug may cause fatigue, dizziness, faintness, light-headedness, and doubled or blurred vision.

SAFETY ALERT!

cetuximab
Erbitux

Pharmacologic class: monoclonal antibody
Pregnancy risk category C

AVAILABLE FORMS
Injection: 2 mg/ml in 50-ml vial

INDICATIONS & DOSAGES
✱***NEW INDICATION:*** **Squamous cell carcinoma of the head and neck**
Adults: Give a loading dose of 400 mg/m^2 I.V. over 2 hours (maximum rate, 5 ml/minute) followed by weekly maintenance dose of 250 mg/m^2 I.V. over 1 hour. If used with radiation therapy, begin drug 1 week before radiation course and continue for the duration (6 or 7 weeks). If used as monotherapy for recurrent or metastatic disease, continue until disease progresses or unacceptable toxicity occurs.
➤ **Epidermal growth factor-expressing metastatic colorectal cancer, alone in patients intolerant of irinotecan-based chemotherapy or with irinotecan in patients refractory to irinotecan-based chemotherapy**
Adults: Loading dose, 400 mg/m^2 I.V. over 2 hours (maximum, 5 ml/minute), alone or with irinotecan. Maintenance dosage, 250 mg/m^2 I.V. weekly over 1 hour (maximum, 5 ml/minute).
Adjust-a-dose: If patient develops a grade 1 or 2 infusion reaction, permanently reduce infusion rate by 50%. If patient develops a grade 3 or 4 infusion reaction, stop drug immediately and permanently. If patient develops a severe acneiform rash, follow these guidelines:
- After first occurrence, delay infusion 1 to 2 weeks. If patient improves, continue at 250 mg/m^2. If patient doesn't improve, stop drug.

• After second occurrence, delay infusion 1 to 2 weeks. If patient improves, reduce dose to 200 mg/m². If patient doesn't improve, stop drug.
• After third occurrence, delay infusion 1 to 2 weeks. If patient improves, reduce dose to 150 mg/m². If patient doesn't improve, stop drug.
• After fourth occurrence, stop drug.

I.V. ADMINISTRATION

• Solution should be clear and colorless and may contain a small amount of particulates.
• Don't shake or dilute.
• Drug can be given by infusion pump or syringe pump, piggybacked into the patient's infusion line. Don't give drug by I.V. push or bolus.
• Give drug through a low–protein-binding 0.22-micrometer in-line filter.
• Flush line with normal saline solution at the end of the infusion.
• Store vials at 36° to 46° F (2° to 8° C). Don't freeze.
• Solution in infusion container is stable up to 12 hours at 36° to 46° F (2° to 8° C) and up to 8 hours at 68° to 77° F (20° to 25° C).

INCOMPATIBILITIES

Don't dilute with other solutions.

ACTION

An epidermal growth factor receptor (EGFR) antagonist that binds to the EGFR on normal and tumor cells, inhibiting epidermal growth factor from binding, which interrupts cell growth, induces cell death, and decreases growth factor production.

Route	Onset	Peak	Duration
I.V.	Unknown	Unknown	Unknown

Half-life: 4¾ days.

ADVERSE REACTIONS

CNS: *asthenia, depression, fever, headache, insomnia.*
CV: *edema,* ***cardiopulmonary arrest.***
EENT: *conjunctivitis.*
GI: *abdominal pain, anorexia, constipation, dyspepsia, dysphagia, mucositis, nausea, stomatitis, vomiting, xerostomia.*
GU: ***acute renal failure.***
Hematologic: *anemia,* LEUKOPENIA.
Metabolic: *dehydration, weight loss.*
Musculoskeletal: *back pain.*
Respiratory: *cough, dyspnea,* ***pulmonary embolus.***
Skin: *alopecia, maculopapular rash, nail disorder, pruritus, radiation dermatitis,* ***acneiform rash.***
Other: *infection, pain,* ***infusion reaction, sepsis.***

INTERACTIONS

Drug-lifestyle. *Sun exposure:* May worsen skin reactions. Advise patient to avoid excessive sun exposure.

EFFECTS ON LAB TEST RESULTS

None reported.

CONTRAINDICATIONS & CAUTIONS

• Use cautiously in patients hypersensitive to drug, its components, or murine proteins. If used with radiation, use cautiously in patients with a history of coronary artery disease, arrhythmias, and heart failure.

NURSING CONSIDERATIONS

• Premedicate with 50 mg I.V. diphenhydramine.
• ***Alert:*** Severe infusion reactions, including acute airway obstruction, urticaria, and hypotension, may occur, usually with the first infusion. If a severe infusion reaction occurs, stop drug immediately and give symptomatic treatment.
• Keep epinephrine, corticosteroids, I.V. antihistamines, bronchodilators, and oxygen available for severe infusion reactions.
• Manage mild to moderate infusion reactions by decreasing infusion rate and premedicating with an antihistamine for subsequent infusions.
• Monitor patient for infusion reactions for 1 hour after infusion ends.
• Assess patient for acute onset or worsening of pulmonary symptoms. If interstitial lung disease is confirmed, stop drug.
• Monitor patient for skin toxicity, which starts most often during first 2 weeks of therapy. Treat with topical and oral antibiotics.
• In patients also receiving radiation therapy, closely monitor electrolytes, especially magnesium, potassium, and calcium, during and after therapy.

• It's unknown if drug appears in breast milk. Women shouldn't breast-feed until 60 days after last dose.

PATIENT TEACHING

• Tell patient to promptly report adverse reactions.
• Inform patient that skin reactions may occur, typically during the first 2 weeks of treatment.
• Advise patient to avoid prolonged or unprotected sun exposure during treatment.

SAFETY ALERT!

clofarabine

Clolar

Pharmacologic class: purine nucleoside antimetabolite
Pregnancy risk category D

AVAILABLE FORMS

Injection: 1 mg/ml in 20–ml vials

INDICATIONS & DOSAGES

➤ **Relapsed or refractory acute lymphoblastic leukemia (ALL) after at least two previous regimens**
Children ages 1 to 21: Give 52 mg/m² by I.V. infusion over 2 hours daily for 5 consecutive days. Repeat about q 2 to 6 weeks based on recovery or return to baseline of organ function. May also give 100 mg/m² hydrocortisone I.V. on days 1 through 3 of cycle to help prevent capillary leak syndrome.

I.V. ADMINISTRATION

• Use a 0.2-micron syringe filter and dilute with D_5W or normal saline solution before infusion.
• Infuse drug within 24 hours of preparing it.
• Give over 2 hours with I.V. fluids.
• Store undiluted vials and resulting infusion solution at room temperature.

INCOMPATIBILITIES

Other drugs in the same I.V. line.

ACTION

Inhibits DNA synthesis and repair and disrupts integrity of mitochondrial membranes, leading to programmed cell death.

Route	Onset	Peak	Duration
I.V.	Unknown	Unknown	Unknown

Half-life: About 5¼ hours.

ADVERSE REACTIONS

CNS: *anxiety, depression, dizziness, fatigue, headache, irritability, lethargy, somnolence, tremor.*
CV: *edema, flushing, hypertension, hypotension, left ventricular systolic dysfunction, pericardial effusion, tachycardia.*
EENT: *epistaxis, mucosal inflammation, sore throat.*
GI: *abdominal pain, anorexia, constipation, decreased appetite, decreased weight, diarrhea, gingival bleeding, nausea, oral candidiasis, vomiting.*
GU: *hematuria.*
Hematologic: BONE MARROW SUPPRESSION, FEBRILE NEUTROPENIA, NEUTROPENIA.
Hepatic: *hepatomegaly, jaundice.*
Musculoskeletal: *arthralgia, back pain, limb pain, myalgia.*
Respiratory: *dyspnea, pleural effusion, pneumonia,* RESPIRATORY DISTRESS.
Skin: *contusion, dermatitis, dry skin, erythema, hand-foot syndrome, petechiae, pruritus.*
Other: BACTEREMIA, SEPSIS, *injection site pain, pain, pyrexia, rigors,* ***capillary leak syndrome, systemic inflammatory response syndrome (SIRS),*** cellulitis, herpes simplex infection, staphylococcal infections, transfusion reaction.

INTERACTIONS

Drug-drug. *Blood pressure or cardiac drugs:* May increase risk of adverse effects. Monitor patient closely.
Hepatotoxic drugs: May increase the risk of hepatic toxicity. Avoid using together.
Nephrotoxic drugs: May decrease excretion of clofarabine. Avoid using together.

EFFECTS ON LAB TEST RESULTS

• May increase ALT, AST, bilirubin, creatinine, and hemoglobin levels and hematocrit.
• May decrease platelet and WBC count.

CONTRAINDICATIONS & CAUTIONS

- Use cautiously in patients with hepatic or renal dysfunction.

NURSING CONSIDERATIONS

- Monitor patient for dehydration. Give I.V. fluids continuously during treatment.
- If you suspect hyperuricemia, give allopurinol.
- Monitor patient's respiratory status and blood pressure closely.
- Assess patient for signs and symptoms of tumor lysis syndrome, cytokine release (tachypnea, tachycardia, hypotension, pulmonary edema) that could develop into SIRS, capillary leak syndrome, and organ dysfunction.
- If patient shows signs and symptoms of SIRS or capillary leak syndrome, stop drug immediately.
- Obtain CBC and platelet count and monitor hepatic and renal function regularly.
- If hypotension develops, stop drug. If hypotension resolves without treatment, restart drug at a lower dose.

PATIENT TEACHING

- Tell patient and caregiver that adverse effects are common. Patient will need close monitoring.
- Tell patient and caregiver to immediately report dizziness, light-headedness, fainting, decreased urine output, bruising, flulike symptoms, and infection.
- Urge patient and caregiver to also report yellowing of skin or eyes, darkened urine, and abdominal pain.
- Tell women to avoid breast-feeding or pregnancy during therapy.

SAFETY ALERT!

dacarbazine (DTIC)

DTIC†, DTIC-Dome

Pharmacologic class: triazene
Pregnancy risk category C

AVAILABLE FORMS

Injection: 100-mg, 200-mg vials

INDICATIONS & DOSAGES

➤Metastatic malignant melanoma
Adults: 2 to 4.5 mg/kg I.V. daily for 10 days; repeat q 4 weeks, as tolerated. Or, 250 mg/m^2 I.V. daily for 5 days; repeat q 3 weeks.

➤Hodgkin lymphoma
Adults: 150 mg/m^2 I.V. daily (with other drugs) for 5 days; repeat q 4 weeks. Or, 375 mg/m^2 on first day of combination regimen; repeat q 15 days.

I.V. ADMINISTRATION

- Preparing and giving parenteral drug may be mutagenic, teratogenic, or carcinogenic. Follow facility policy to reduce risks.
- Reconstitute drug using sterile water for injection. Add 9.9 ml to 100-mg vial or 19.7 ml to 200-mg vial to yield a concentration of 10 mg/ml.
- Solution should be colorless to clear yellow. If solution turns pink, it has decomposed. Discard it.
- For infusion, dilute with up to 250 ml of normal saline solution or D_5W.
- Infuse over at least 15 to 30 minutes.
- To decrease pain at insertion site, dilute drug further or decrease infusion rate.
- Watch for irritation and infiltration during infusion; extravasation can cause severe pain, tissue damage, and necrosis. If solution infiltrates, stop immediately, apply ice to area for 24 to 48 hours, and notify prescriber.
- Reconstituted solutions in the vial are stable 8 hours at room temperature and normal lighting conditions, or up to 3 days if refrigerated.
- Diluted solutions are stable 8 hours at normal room temperature and lighting, or up to 24 hours if refrigerated.

INCOMPATIBILITIES

Allopurinol sodium, cefepime, hydrocortisone sodium succinate, piperacillin with tazobactam.

ACTION

May cross-link strands of cellular DNA and interfere with RNA and protein synthesis. Not specific to cell cycle.

Route	Onset	Peak	Duration
I.V.	Unknown	Unknown	Unknown

Half-life: Initial phase, 19 minutes; terminal phase, 5 hours.

ADVERSE REACTIONS
CNS: facial paresthesia.
GI: *anorexia, severe nausea and vomiting,* stomatitis.
Hematologic: ***leukopenia, thrombocytopenia.***
Skin: alopecia, facial flushing, phototoxicity, rash.
Other: *flulike syndrome,* ***anaphylaxis,*** severe pain with infiltration or a too-concentrated solution, tissue damage.

INTERACTIONS
Drug-lifestyle. *Sun exposure:* May cause photosensitivity reaction, especially during first 2 days of therapy. Advise patient to avoid excessive sunlight exposure.

EFFECTS ON LAB TEST RESULTS
- May increase BUN and liver enzyme levels.
- May decrease platelet, RBC, and WBC counts.

CONTRAINDICATIONS & CAUTIONS
- Contraindicated in patients hypersensitive to drug.
- Use cautiously in patients with impaired bone marrow function and those with severe renal or hepatic dysfunction.

NURSING CONSIDERATIONS
- Give antiemetics before giving this drug. Nausea and vomiting may subside after several doses.
- To prevent bleeding, avoid all I.M. injections when platelet count is below 50,000/mm^3.
- Anticipate need for blood transfusions to combat anemia. Patient may receive injections of RBC colony–stimulating factors to promote RBC production and decrease need for blood transfusions.
- Therapeutic effects commonly occur with toxicity. Monitor CBC and platelet count.
- Hepatotoxicity may occur. Monitor liver function tests.
- For Hodgkin lymphoma, drug is usually given with bleomycin, vinblastine, and doxorubicin.
- ***Look alike–sound alike:*** Don't confuse dacarbazine with Dicarbosil or procarbazine.

PATIENT TEACHING
- Tell patient to watch for evidence of infection (fever, sore throat, fatigue) and bleeding (easy bruising, nosebleeds, bleeding gums, tarry stools). Tell him to take temperature daily.
- Tell patient to avoid people with upper respiratory tract infections.
- Instruct patient to avoid OTC products that contain aspirin or NSAIDs.
- Advise patient to avoid sunlight and sunlamps for first 2 days after treatment.
- Reassure patient that fever, malaise, and muscle pain, beginning 7 days after treatment ends and possibly lasting 7 to 21 days, may be treated with mild fever reducers such as acetaminophen.
- Tell patient that restricting food intake for 4 to 6 hours before dose may help to decrease adverse GI effects.
- Reassure patient that hair loss is reversible.
- Advise woman to avoid pregnancy and breast-feeding during therapy.

✷ NEW DRUG

dasatinib
Sprycel

Pharmacologic class: protein-tyrosine kinase inhibitor
Pregnancy risk category D

AVAILABLE FORMS
Tablets: 20 mg, 50 mg, 70 mg

INDICATIONS & DOSAGES
➤ **Chronic, accelerated, myeloid, or lymphoid blast-phase chronic myeloid leukemia with resistance or intolerance to earlier treatment, including imatinib; Philadelphia-chromosome–positive acute lymphoblastic leukemia with resistance or tolerance to prior therapy**
Adults: 70 mg P.O. b.i.d., in the morning and evening with or without food. If patient tolerates this dose but fails to respond to treatment, increase to 90 or 100 mg b.i.d. Continue until disease progresses or intolerable adverse effects occur.
Adjust-a-dose: If patient has hematologic toxicity, consider reducing dose or inter-

rupting or stopping therapy. If patient has severe, nonhematologic toxicity, hold dose until condition resolves; then resume at previous or reduced dose.

ACTION

Reduces leukemic cell growth by inhibiting a tyrosine kinase enzyme. As a result, bone marrow can resume production of normal RBCs, WBCs, and platelets.

Route	Onset	Peak	Duration
P.O.	Unknown	½–6 hr	Unknown

Half-life: 3 to 5 hours.

ADVERSE REACTIONS

CNS: *asthenia, chills, dizziness, fatigue, headache, neuropathy,* ***bleeding, pyrexia, seizures,*** anxiety, confusion, depression, insomnia, malaise, somnolence, syncope, tremor, vertigo.
CV: *arrhythmias, chest pain, edema,* ***cardiac dysfunction, heart failure, hemorrhage,*** hypertension, hypotension, pericardial effusion.
EENT: *mucositis, stomatitis,* conjunctivitis, dry eyes, dysgeusia, tinnitus.
GI: *abdominal distention and pain, anorexia, constipation, diarrhea, nausea, vomiting,* ***bleeding,*** anal fissure, colitis, dyspepsia, dysphagia.
GU: ***renal failure,*** urinary frequency.
Hematologic: *anemia,* ***febrile neutropenia, pancytopenia, thrombocytopenia.***
Hepatic: ***hepatitis,*** cholecystitis, cholestasis.
Metabolic: *weight loss or gain* , hyperuricemia.
Musculoskeletal: *arthralgia, myalgia, pain,* inflammation, muscle stiffness.
Respiratory: *cough, dyspnea, upper respiratory tract infection,* ***pleural effusion, pneumonia,*** asthma, ***pulmonary edema and hypertension.***
Skin: *pruritus, rash,* acne, alopecia, dry skin, nail or pigment disorders, sweating.
Other: *infection,* ***tumor lysis syndrome,*** ascites, gynecomastia, herpes infection.

INTERACTIONS

Drug-drug. *Antacids:* May decrease dasatinib absorption. Give antacid 2 hours before or 2 hours after dasatinib.
CYP 3A4 inducers (carbamazepine, dexamethasone, phenobarbital, phenytoin, rifampicin): May decrease dasatinib level. Avoid using together, or increase dasatinib dose in 20-mg increments.
CYP 3A4 inhibitors (atazanavir, clarithromycin, erythromycin, indinavir, itraconazole, ketoconazole, nefazodone, nelfinavir, ritonavir, saquinavir, telithromycin): May increase dasatinib level and toxicity. Avoid using together; if use together can't be avoided, monitor patient closely and consider decreasing dasatinib dose to 20 to 40 mg daily.
CYP 3A4 substrates (cyclosporine, ergot alkaloids, fentanyl, pimozide, quinidine, sirolimus, tacrolimus): May alter levels of these drugs. Use cautiously together, and monitor patient.
H_2-blockers, proton pump inhibitors: May decrease dasatinib level because of gastric acid suppression. Avoid using together. Consider antacids as an alternative.
Drug-herb. *St. John's wort:* May decrease drug level. Discourage use together.

EFFECTS ON LAB TEST RESULTS

- May increase uric acid, bilirubin, creatinine, AST, ALT, CK, and troponin levels. May decrease phosphate and calcium levels.
- May decrease RBC, platelet, and neutrophil counts.

CONTRAINDICATIONS & CAUTIONS

- No known contraindications.
- Use cautiously in patients receiving antiarrhythmics, antiplatelets, or anticoagulants; patients receiving cumulative high-dose anthracycline therapy; patients with a prolonged QT interval or risk of prolonged QT interval (those with hypokalemia, hypomagnesemia, or current use of drugs that prolong the QT interval); patients with liver impairment; and patients who are lactose intolerant.

NURSING CONSIDERATIONS

- Monitor CBC weekly for the first 2 months of treatment, then monthly thereafter, or as indicated.
- Correct electrolyte imbalances, especially of potassium and magnesium, before treatment.

• ***Alert:*** Don't crush or cut tablets. If tablet is crushed or broken, wear chemotherapy gloves to dispose of it. Pregnant women shouldn't handle broken tablets.
• Obtain patient's baseline weight, and check regularly for swelling or weight gain.
• Notify prescriber if patient develops dyspnea or a dry cough. A chest X-ray, oxygen, diuretics, or steroids may be indicated.
• Drug contains lactose.

PATIENT TEACHING
• Tell patient to take the tablets at about the same time every day.
• Caution patient not to crush or cut the tablets.
• Warn women of childbearing age to use reliable contraception during treatment. Men who take drug should use condoms to avoid impregnating their partners.
• Tell patient to report weight gain, swelling, and shortness of breath.
• Advise patient to notify prescriber immediately about easy or unusual bruising.

SAFETY ALERT!

docetaxel
Taxotere

Pharmacologic class: taxoid
Pregnancy risk category D

AVAILABLE FORMS
Injection: 20 mg, 80 mg, in single-dose vials

INDICATIONS & DOSAGES
➤ **Locally advanced or metastatic breast cancer after failure of previous chemotherapy**
Adults: 60 to 100 mg/m^2 I.V. over 1 hour q 3 weeks.
Adjust-a-dose: In patients receiving 100 mg/m^2 who experience febrile neutropenia, neutrophil count of less than 500/mm^3 for longer than 1 week, severe or cumulative cutaneous reactions, or severe peripheral neuropathy, reduce subsequent dose by 25%, to 75 mg/m^2. In patients who continue to experience reactions with decreased dose, either decrease it further to 55 mg/m^2 or stop drug.

➤ **Adjuvant postsurgery treatment of operable, node-positive breast cancer**
Adults: 75 mg/m^2 I.V. as a 1-hour infusion given 1 hour after doxorubicin 50 mg/m^2 and cyclophosphamide 500 mg/m^2 q 3 weeks for six cycles. Patient's neutrophil count should be 1,500/mm^3 or higher.
Adjust-a-dose: Patients who experience febrile neutropenia should receive granulocyte colony-stimulating factor (G-CSF) in all subsequent cycles. If febrile neutropenia doesn't resolve, continue G-CSF and reduce docetaxel dose to 60 mg/m^2. For patients who experience severe or cumulative cutaneous reactions or moderate neurosensory signs and symptoms, reduce dose to 60 mg/m^2. If these reactions persist at the reduced dosage, stop treatment.

➤ **Locally advanced or metastatic non–small-cell lung cancer after failure of previous cisplatin-based chemotherapy**
Adults: 75 mg/m^2 I.V. over 1 hour q 3 weeks.
Adjust-a-dose: In patients who experience febrile neutropenia, neutrophil count of less than 500/mm^3 for longer than 1 week, severe or cumulative cutaneous reactions, or severe peripheral neuropathy, withhold drug until toxicity resolves; then restart at 55 mg/m^2. In patients in whom grade 3 peripheral neuropathy or above develops, stop drug.

➤ **With cisplatin, unresectable, locally advanced, or metastatic non–small-cell lung cancer not previously treated with chemotherapy**
Adults: 75 mg/m^2 docetaxel I.V. over 1 hour, immediately followed by cisplatin 75 mg/m^2 I.V. over 30 to 60 minutes q 3 weeks.
Adjust-a-dose: In patients whose lowest platelet count during the previous course of therapy was less than 25,000/mm^3, and those with febrile neutropenia or serious nonhematologic toxicities, decrease docetaxel dosage to 65 mg/m^2. For patients who require a further dosage reduction, a dosage of 50 mg/m^2 is recommended. For cisplatin dosage adjustments, see manufacturers' prescribing information.

➤**Androgen-independent metastatic prostate cancer, with prednisone**
Adults: 75 mg/m² I.V., as a 1-hour infusion q 3 weeks, given with 5 mg prednisone P.O. b.i.d. continuously. Premedicate with dexamethasone 8 mg P.O. at 12 hours, 3 hours, and 1 hour before docetaxel infusion.
Adjust-a-dose: In patients who experience febrile neutropenia, neutrophil count less than 500/mm³ for more than 1 week, severe or cumulative cutaneous reactions, or moderate neurosensory signs or symptoms, reduce subsequent dose to 60 mg/m². In patients who continue to experience reactions with the decreased dose, stop treatment.
✱***NEW INDICATION:*** **Advanced gastric adenocarcinoma, in combination with cisplatin and fluorouracil (5-FU)**
Adults: Premedicate with antiemetics and hydration per cisplatin recommendations. Give 75 mg/m² docetaxel I.V. over 1 hour, followed by cisplatin 75 mg/m² I.V. over 1 to 3 hours both on day 1 only, then, fluorouracil 750 mg/m² I.V. daily as a 24-hour continuous infusion for 5 days beginning at the end of cisplatin infusion. Repeat cycle every 3 weeks.
Adjust-a-dose: Patients who experience febrile neutropenia should receive G-CSF in subsequent cycles. If episode recurs, reduce dose to 60 mg/m². If subsequent episodes of complicated neutropenia occur, reduce dose to 45 mg/m². In patients who experience grade 4 thrombocytopenia, reduce dosage to 60 mg/m². Don't retreat until neutrophils are greater than 1,500/mm³ and platelets are greater than 100,000/mm³. Stop treatment if toxicity persists.

For patients who experience diarrhea, adjust dosage as follows: for 1st episode of grade 3 diarrhea, reduce 5-FU dose by 20%; for 2nd episode, reduce docetaxel dose by 20%; for 1st episode of grade 4 diarrhea, reduce docetaxel and 5-FU doses by 20%; for 2nd episode, stop drug. For patients who experience stomatitis, adjust dosage as follows: For 1st episode of grade 3, reduce 5-FU dose by 20%; 2nd episode, stop 5-FU in subsequent cycles; 3rd episode, reduce docetaxel dose by 20%. For 1st episode of grade 4, stop 5-FU in subsequent cycles; 2nd episode, reduce docetaxel dose by 20%. For patients who experience liver dysfunction, reduce docetaxel dose by 20%. If AST or ALT is greater than five times upper limit of normal (ULN) or alkaline phosphatase is greater than five times ULN, stop treatment.
✱***NEW INDICATION:*** **Induction treatment of inoperable locally advanced squamous cell cancer of the head and neck, with cisplatin and 5-FU**
Adults: 75 mg/m² I.V. infusion over 1 hour, followed by cisplatin 75 mg/m² I.V. infusion over 1 hour, on day one, followed by 5-FU 750 mg/m² daily as a continuous I.V infusion for 5 days. Repeat this regimen every 3 weeks for four cycles. After chemotherapy, patients should receive radiotherapy. Premedicate with antiemetics and appropriate hydration before and after giving cisplatin.
Adjust-a-dose: Use the same dosage adjustment schedule as for advanced gastric adenocarcinoma.

I.V. ADMINISTRATION

- Wear gloves to prepare and give drug. If solution contacts skin, wash immediately and thoroughly with soap and water. If it contacts mucous membranes, flush thoroughly with water.
- Dilute using supplied diluent. Let drug and diluent stand at room temperature for 5 minutes before mixing. After adding all the diluent to drug vial, gently rotate vial for about 15 seconds. Let solution stand for a few minutes so foam dissipates. All foam need not dissipate before preparing infusion solution.
- Prepare infusion solution by withdrawing needed amount of premixed solution from vial and injecting it into 250 ml normal saline solution or D_5W to yield 0.3 to 0.74 mg/ml. Doses exceeding 200 mg need a larger volume to stay below 0.74 mg/ml of drug. Mix infusion thoroughly by manual rotation.
- Prepare and store infusion solution in bottles (glass or polypropylene) or plastic bags, and give through polyethylene-lined administration sets.

- Contact between undiluted concentrate and polyvinyl chloride equipment or devices isn't recommended.
- If solution isn't clear or if it contains precipitates, discard it.
- The first dilution is stable for 8 hours. Use infusion solution within 4 hours.
- Infuse over 1 hour.
- Store unopened vials in refrigerator.
- Mark all waste materials with CHEMOTHERAPY HAZARD labels.

INCOMPATIBILITIES

None reported.

ACTION

Promotes formation and stabilization of nonfunctional microtubules. This prevents mitosis and leads to cell death.

Route	Onset	Peak	Duration
I.V.	Rapid	Unknown	Unknown

Half-life: Alpha phase, 4 minutes; beta phase, 36 minutes; terminal phase, 11 hours.

ADVERSE REACTIONS

CNS: *asthenia,* paresthesia, peripheral neuropathy.
CV: *fluid retention, peripheral edema,* arrhythmias, chest tightness, flushing, hypotension.
EENT: altered hearing, tearing.
GI: *anorexia, diarrhea, dysphagia, esophagitis, nausea, stomatitis, vomiting.*
Hematologic: **FEBRILE NEUTROPENIA, LEUKOPENIA, MYELOSUPPRESSION, NEUTROPENIA, THROMBOCYTOPENIA,** *anemia.*
Hepatic: ***hepatotoxicity.***
Musculoskeletal: *myalgia,* arthralgia, back pain.
Respiratory: dyspnea, ***pulmonary edema.***
Skin: *alopecia,* desquamation, skin eruptions, nail pigmentation alterations, nail pain, rash, reaction at injection site.
Other: *infection,* chills, drug fever, hypersensitivity reactions.

INTERACTIONS

Drug-drug. *Compounds that induce, inhibit, or are metabolized by CYP3A4, such as cyclosporine, erythromycin, ketoconazole, troleandomycin:* May modify metabolism of docetaxel. Use together cautiously.
Ketoconazole or other CYP3A4 inhibitors: May increase docetaxel level and toxicity, including neutropenia. Monitor patient closely.

EFFECTS ON LAB TEST RESULTS

- May increase alkaline phosphatase, ALT, AST, and bilirubin levels. May decrease hemoglobin level.
- May decrease platelet and WBC counts.

CONTRAINDICATIONS & CAUTIONS

- Contraindicated in patients severely hypersensitive to drug or to other forms containing polysorbate 80 and in those with neutrophil count below 1,500/mm^3.
- Patients with severe hepatic impairment shouldn't receive this drug. Don't give drug to patients with bilirubin levels exceeding ULN, those with ALT or AST levels above 1½ times ULN and alkaline phosphatase levels above 2½ times ULN, or those with baseline neutrophil count less than 1,500/mm^3.
- Safety and effectiveness in children haven't been established.

NURSING CONSIDERATIONS

- Give oral corticosteroid such as dexamethasone 16 mg P.O. (8 mg b.i.d.) daily for 3 days, starting 1 day before docetaxel administration, to reduce risk or severity of fluid retention and hypersensitivity reactions.
- Bone marrow toxicity is the most frequent and dose-limiting toxicity. Frequent blood count monitoring is needed during therapy.
- Monitor patient closely for hypersensitivity reactions, especially during first and second infusions.
- Fluid retention is dose related and may be severe. Monitor patient closely.
- ***Look alike–sound alike:*** Don't confuse Taxotere with Taxol.

PATIENT TEACHING

- Caution woman of childbearing age to avoid pregnancy or breast-feeding during therapy.
- Advise patient to report any pain or burning at injection site during or after administration.

• Warn patient that hair loss occurs in almost 80% of patients and reverses when treatment stops.
• Tell patient to promptly report sore throat, fever, or unusual bruising or bleeding, as well as signs and symptoms of fluid retention, such as swelling or shortness of breath.

SAFETY ALERT!

erlotinib
Tarceva

Pharmacologic class: epidermal growth factor receptor inhibitor
Pregnancy risk category D

AVAILABLE FORMS
Tablets: 25 mg, 100 mg, 150 mg

INDICATIONS & DOSAGES
✷*NEW INDICATION:* With gemcitabine, first-line treatment of locally advanced, unresectable, or metastatic pancreatic cancer
Adults: 100 mg P.O. once daily taken at least 1 hour before or 2 hours after meals. Continue until disease progresses or intolerable toxicity occurs.
➤Locally advanced or metastatic non–small-cell lung cancer after failure of at least one chemotherapy regimen
Adults: 150 mg P.O. once daily taken at least 1 hour before or 2 hours after meals. Continue until disease progresses or intolerable toxicity occurs.
Adjust-a-dose: In patients with severe skin reactions or severe diarrhea refractory to loperamide, reduce dose in 50-mg decrements or stop therapy.

ACTION
Probably inhibits tyrosine kinase activity in epidermal growth factor receptors, which are expressed on the surface of normal and cancer cells. Is particularly selective for human epidermal growth factor receptor 1.

Route	Onset	Peak	Duration
P.O.	Unknown	4 hr	Unknown

Half-life: About 36 hours.

ADVERSE REACTIONS
CNS: *fatigue.*
EENT: *conjunctivitis, keratoconjuctivitis sicca.*
GI: *abdominal pain, anorexia, diarrhea, nausea, stomatitis, vomiting.*
Respiratory: *cough, dyspnea,* ***pulmonary toxicity.***
Skin: *dry skin, pruritus, rash.*
Other: *infection.*

INTERACTIONS
Drug-drug. *Anticoagulants, such as warfarin:* May increase risk of bleeding. Monitor PT and INR.
CYP3A4 inducers, such as carbamazepine, phenobarbital, phenytoin, rifabutin, rifampin: May increase erlotinib metabolism. Erlotinib dosage may need to be increased.
Strong CYP3A4 inhibitors, such as atazanavir, clarithromycin, indinavir, itraconazole, ketoconazole, nefazodone, nelfinavir, ritonavir, saquinavir, telithromycin, troleandomycin, voriconazole: May decrease erlotinib metabolism. Use together cautiously, and consider reducing erlotinib dosage.
Drug-herb. *St. John's wort:* May increase drug metabolism. Drug dosage may need to be increased. Discourage use together.

EFFECTS ON LAB TEST RESULTS
• May increase ALT, AST, and bilirubin levels.
• May increase INR and PT.

CONTRAINDICATIONS & CAUTIONS
• None reported.
• Use cautiously in patients with pulmonary disease or liver impairment. Also use cautiously in patients who have received or are receiving chemotherapy because it may worsen adverse pulmonary effects.

NURSING CONSIDERATIONS
• Monitor liver function tests periodically during therapy. Notify prescriber of abnormal findings.
• ***Alert:*** Rarely, serious interstitial lung disease may occur. If patient develops dyspnea, cough, and fever, notify prescriber. Therapy may need to be interrupted or stopped.

- Monitor patient for severe diarrhea, and give loperamide if needed.
- Women shouldn't breast-feed while taking this drug.

PATIENT TEACHING

- ***Alert:*** Tell patient to immediately report new or worsened cough, shortness of breath, eye irritation, or severe or persistent diarrhea, nausea, anorexia, or vomiting.
- Instruct patient to take drug 1 hour before or 2 hours after food.
- Advise women to avoid pregnancy while taking this drug and for 2 weeks after treatment ends. Drug can harm an unborn baby.
- Explain the likelihood of serious interactions with other drugs and herbal supplements and the need to tell prescriber about any change in drugs and supplements taken.

SAFETY ALERT!

etoposide (VP-16, VP-16-213)
Toposar, VePesid

etoposide phosphate
Etopophos

Pharmacologic class: podophyllotoxin derivative
Pregnancy risk category D

AVAILABLE FORMS

etoposide
Capsules: 50 mg
Injection: 20 mg/ml in 5-, 12.5-, and 25-ml vials
etoposide phosphate
Injection: 119.3-mg vials equivalent to 100 mg etoposide

INDICATIONS & DOSAGES

➤Testicular cancer
Adults: 50 to 100 mg/m^2 daily I.V. on five consecutive days q 3 to 4 weeks. Or, 100 mg/m^2 daily I.V. on days 1, 3, and 5 q 3 to 4 weeks for three or four courses of therapy.
➤Small-cell carcinoma of the lung
Adults: 35 mg/m^2 daily I.V. for 4 days. Or, 50 mg/m^2 daily I.V. for 5 days. P.O. dose is two times I.V. dose, rounded to nearest 50 mg.
Adjust-a-dose: For patients with creatinine clearance of 15 to 50 ml/minute, reduce dose by 25%.
➤Kaposi sarcoma♦
Adults: 150 mg/m^2 I.V. daily for 3 days q 4 weeks. Repeat as needed, based on response.

I.V. ADMINISTRATION

- Preparing and giving parenteral drug may be mutagenic, teratogenic, or carcinogenic. Follow facility policy to reduce risks.
- For etoposide infusion, dilute to 0.2 or 0.4 mg/ml in either D_5W or normal saline solution. Higher concentrations may crystallize.
- Give etoposide by slow infusion over at least 30 minutes to prevent severe hypotension.
- For etoposide phosphate, give without further dilution or dilute to as low as 0.1 mg/ml in either D_5W or normal saline solution.
- Give etoposide phosphate over 5 to 210 minutes.
- Check blood pressure every 15 minutes during infusion. Hypotension may occur if infusion is too rapid. If systolic pressure falls below 90 mm Hg, stop infusion and notify prescriber.
- Etoposide diluted to 0.2 mg/ml is stable 96 hours at room temperature in plastic or glass, unprotected from light; at 0.4 mg/ml, it's stable 24 hours under same conditions. Diluted etoposide phosphate solution is stable for same times at room temperature or 24 hours refrigerated.

INCOMPATIBILITIES

Cefepime hydrochloride, filgrastim, gallium nitrate, idarubicin.

ACTION

Inhibits topoisomerase II enzyme, causing inability to repair DNA strand breaks, which leads to cell death. Cell cycle specific to G_2 portion of cell cycle.

Route	Onset	Peak	Duration
P.O., I.V.	Unknown	Unknown	Unknown

Half-life: Initial phase, ½ to 2 hours; terminal phase, 5¼ hours.

ADVERSE REACTIONS

CNS: peripheral neuropathy.
CV: hypotension.
GI: *anorexia, diarrhea, nausea, vomiting,* abdominal pain, stomatitis.
Hematologic: **LEUKOPENIA, NEUTROPENIA, THROMBOCYTOPENIA,** *anemia,* ***myelosuppression.***
Hepatic: ***hepatotoxicity.***
Skin: *reversible alopecia,* rash.
Other: ***anaphylaxis,*** hypersensitivity reactions.

INTERACTIONS

Drug-drug. ***Cyclosporine:*** May increase etoposide level and toxicity. Monitor CBC and adjust etoposide dose.
Phosphatase inhibitors such as levamisole hydrochloride: May decrease etoposide effectiveness. Monitor drug effects.
Warfarin: May further prolong PT. Monitor PT and INR closely.

EFFECTS ON LAB TEST RESULTS

- May decrease hemoglobin level.
- May decrease neutrophil, platelet, RBC, and WBC counts.

CONTRAINDICATIONS & CAUTIONS

- Contraindicated in patients hypersensitive to drug.
- Use cautiously in patients who have had cytotoxic or radiation therapy and in those with hepatic impairment.

NURSING CONSIDERATIONS

- Obtain baseline blood pressure before starting therapy.
- Anticipate need for antiemetics.
- Have diphenhydramine, hydrocortisone, epinephrine, and emergency equipment available to establish an airway in case anaphylaxis occurs.
- Store capsules in refrigerator.
- Monitor CBC. Watch for evidence of bone marrow suppression.
- Observe patient's mouth for signs of ulceration.
- To prevent bleeding, avoid all I.M. injections when platelet count is below 50,000/mm^3.
- Anticipate need for blood transfusions to combat anemia. Patient may receive injections of RBC colony-stimulating factors to promote RBC production and decrease need for blood transfusions.
- Etoposide phosphate dose is expressed as etoposide equivalents; 119.3 mg of etoposide phosphate is equivalent to 100 mg of etoposide.

PATIENT TEACHING

- Tell patient to watch for signs and symptoms of infection (fever, sore throat, fatigue) and bleeding (easy bruising, nosebleeds, bleeding gums, tarry stools). Tell patient to take temperature daily.
- Inform patient of need for frequent blood pressure readings during I.V. administration.
- Caution woman of childbearing age to avoid pregnancy and breast-feeding during therapy.

SAFETY ALERT!

gemtuzumab ozogamicin
Mylotarg

Pharmacologic class: monoclonal antibody

AVAILABLE FORMS

Powder for injection: 5 mg

INDICATIONS & DOSAGES

➤CD33-positive acute myeloid leukemia patients who are in first relapse and aren't candidates for cytotoxic chemotherapy
Adults age 60 and older: 9 mg/m^2 I.V. over 2 hours q 14 days for a total of two doses. Premedicate with diphenhydramine 50 mg P.O. and acetaminophen 650 to 1,000 mg P.O. 1 hour before infusion.

I.V. ADMINISTRATION

- Drug is light sensitive; protect from direct and indirect sunlight and unshielded fluorescent light when preparing and giving.
- Reconstitute powder by adding 5 ml of sterile water for injection to yield 1 mg/ml. Swirl vial gently, and look for particles.
- Drug may be infused by central or peripheral line.
- Use a separate line with a low–protein-binding 1.2-micron terminal filter.

- Don't give drug as push or bolus.
- Give in 100 ml of normal saline solution for injection.
- Place 100-ml I.V. bag into an ultraviolet protectant bag and give solution immediately.
- Reconstituted drug is stable 8 hours if refrigerated.

INCOMPATIBILITIES
None reported.

ACTION
Binds to the CD33 antigen on the surface of leukemic blasts, resulting in the formation of a complex that's internalized by the cell. The cytotoxic antibiotic, a calicheamicin derivative, is then released inside the cell, causing DNA double-strand breaks and cell death.

Route	Onset	Peak	Duration
I.V.	Unknown	Unknown	Unknown

Half-life: Total and unconjugated calicheamicin, 45 and 100 hours, respectively, after the first dose. After the second dose, total calicheamicin, 60 hours.

ADVERSE REACTIONS
CNS: *asthenia, dizziness, fever, headache, insomnia, pain,* depression.
CV: *hypertension, hypotension, tachycardia, peripheral edema.*
EENT: *epistaxis, pharyngitis, rhinitis.*
GI: *abdominal pain, anorexia, constipation, diarrhea, dyspepsia, nausea, stomatitis, vomiting,* enlarged abdomen.
GU: *hematuria,* ***vaginal hemorrhage.***
Hematologic: *anemia,* HEMORRHAGE, LEUKOPENIA, NEUTROPENIA, NEUTROPENIC FEVER, THROMBOCYTOPENIA.
Hepatic: ***hepatotoxicity.***
Metabolic: *hypokalemia, hypomagnesemia,* hyperglycemia.
Musculoskeletal: *back pain,* arthralgia.
Respiratory: *cough, dyspnea, pneumonia,* ***hypoxia.***
Skin: ecchymoses, local reaction, petechiae, rash.
Other: SEPSIS, *chills,* herpes simplex.

INTERACTIONS
None known.

EFFECTS ON LAB TEST RESULTS
- May increase ALT, AST, glucose, and LDH levels. May decrease hemoglobin, magnesium, and potassium levels.
- May decrease neutrophil, platelet, and WBC counts.

CONTRAINDICATIONS & CAUTIONS
- Contraindicated in patients hypersensitive to drug or its components.
- Use cautiously in patients with hepatic impairment.

NURSING CONSIDERATIONS
- Use drug under the supervision of a clinician experienced in the use of cancer chemotherapeutics.
- Premedicate with diphenhydramine and acetaminophen. Give additional doses of acetaminophen 650 to 1,000 mg P.O. q 4 hours, as needed.
- Monitor vital signs during infusion and for 4 hours after infusion.
- Monitor postinfusion symptom complex of chills, fever, hypotension, hypertension, hyperglycemia, hypoxia, and dyspnea that may occur during first 24 hours after administration.
- ***Alert:*** Severe myelosuppression occurs in all patients given recommended dose of drug. Careful hematologic monitoring is required.
- Monitor electrolytes, hepatic function, CBC, and platelet counts during therapy.
- ***Alert:*** Fatal hepatic reno-occlusive disease may occur after treatment with gemtuzumab with subsequent chemotherapy.
- Tumor lysis syndrome may occur. Provide adequate hydration and treat with allopurinol to prevent hyperuricemia.

PATIENT TEACHING
- Advise patient about postinfusion symptoms and instruct him to continue taking 650 to 1,000 mg acetaminophen q 4 hours, as needed.
- Urge patient to watch for fever, sore throat, and fatigue and for easy bruising, nosebleeds, bleeding gums, or tarry stools. Tell him to take temperature daily.
- Tell patient to avoid OTC products that contain aspirin.

SAFETY ALERT!

imatinib mesylate
Gleevec

Pharmacologic class: protein-tyrosine kinase inhibitor
Pregnancy risk category D

AVAILABLE FORMS
Tablets: 100 mg, 400 mg

INDICATIONS & DOSAGES
➤Chronic myeloid leukemia (CML) in blast crisis, in accelerated phase, or in chronic phase after failure of alfa interferon therapy; newly diagnosed Philadelphia-chromosome–positive (Ph+) chronic phase CML
Adults: For chronic-phase CML, 400 mg P.O. daily as single dose with a meal and large glass of water. For accelerated-phase CML or blast crisis, 600 mg P.O. daily as single dose with a meal and large glass of water. Continue treatment as long as patient continues to benefit. May increase daily dose to 600 mg P.O. in chronic phase or to 800 mg P.O. (400 mg P.O. b.i.d.) in accelerated phase or blast crisis.
Children age 2 and older: For newly diagnosed Ph+ chronic-phase CML only, give 340 mg/m² daily P.O. Don't exceed 600 mg.
➤Kit (CD117)-positive unresectable or metastatic malignant GI stromal tumors (GIST)
Adults: 400 or 600 mg P.O. daily.
➤Ph+ chronic phase CML in patients whose disease has recurred after stem cell transplant or who are resistant to interferon alfa therapy
Children age 2 and older: 260 mg/m² daily P.O. as a single dose or divided into two doses. Have patient take with meal and large glass of water. May increase dosage to 340 mg/m² daily.
Adjust-a-dose: Withhold treatment or reduce dosage based on bilirubin or liver transaminase levels, severity of fluid retention, or hematologic toxicities.

ACTION
Inhibits the abnormal tyrosine kinase created by the Philadelphia chromosome abnormality in CML; it inhibits tumor growth of murine myeloid cells and leukemia lines from CML patients in blast crisis.

Route	Onset	Peak	Duration
P.O.	Unknown	2–4 hr	Unknown

Half-life: Within 7 days.

ADVERSE REACTIONS
CNS: CEREBRAL HEMORRHAGE, *fatigue, headache, pyrexia, weakness.*
CV: *edema.*
EENT: *epistaxis,* nasopharyngitis.
GI: GI HEMORRHAGE, *abdominal pain, anorexia, constipation, diarrhea, dyspepsia, nausea, vomiting.*
Hematologic: HEMORRHAGE, NEUTROPENIA, THROMBOCYTOPENIA, *anemia.*
Metabolic: *hypokalemia,* weight increase.
Musculoskeletal: *arthralgia, myalgia, muscle cramps, musculoskeletal pain.*
Respiratory: *cough, dyspnea, pneumonia.*
Skin: *petechiae, rash,* pruritus.
Other: *night sweats.*

INTERACTIONS
Drug-drug. *Acetaminophen:* May increase risk of hepatic toxicity. Monitor patient closely.
CYP3A4 inducers (carbamazepine, dexamethasone, phenobarbital, phenytoin, rifampin): May increase metabolism and decrease imatinib level. Use together cautiously.
CYP3A4 inhibitors (clarithromycin, erythromycin, itraconazole, ketoconazole): May decrease metabolism and increase imatinib level. Monitor patient for toxicity.
Dihydropyridine-calcium channel blockers, certain HMG-CoA reductase inhibitors (simvastatin), cyclosporine, pimozide, triazolo-benzodiazepines: May increase levels of these drugs. Monitor patient for toxicity, and obtain drug levels, if appropriate.
Warfarin: May alter metabolism of warfarin. Avoid using together; use standard heparin or a low–molecular-weight heparin.
Drug-herb. *St. John's wort:* May decrease drug effects. Discourage use together.

EFFECTS ON LAB TEST RESULTS

- May increase creatinine, bilirubin, alkaline phosphatase, AST, and ALT levels. May decrease potassium and hemoglobin levels.
- May decrease neutrophil and platelet counts.

CONTRAINDICATIONS & CAUTIONS

- Contraindicated in patients hypersensitive to drug or its components.
- Use cautiously in elderly patients and in those with hepatic impairment.
- Safety and effectiveness in children younger than age 2 haven't been established.

NURSING CONSIDERATIONS

- Monitor patient closely for possibly severe fluid retention. Elderly patients may have an increased risk of edema.
- Monitor weight daily. Report unexpected, rapid weight gain.
- Monitor CBC weekly for first month; every other week for second month and periodically thereafter.
- For patients unable to swallow tablets, disperse the tablets in water or apple juice (50 ml for 100-mg tablet or 200 ml for 400-mg tablet). Stir and have patient drink immediately.
- Monitor liver function tests carefully because hepatotoxicity (occasionally severe) may occur; decrease dosage as needed.
- May increase dose if no severe adverse reactions or severe non–leukemia-related neutropenia or thrombocytopenia in the following circumstances: disease progression, failure to achieve a satisfactory hematologic response after at least 3 months of treatment, or loss of a previously achieved hematologic response.

PATIENT TEACHING

- Tell patient to take drug with food and a large glass of water.
- Advise patient unable to swallow tablets to mix them in water or apple juice (50 ml for 100-mg tablet or 200 ml for 400-mg tablet). Tell him to stir and drink immediately.
- Advise patient to report to prescriber any adverse effects, such as fluid retention.
- Advise patient to obtain periodic liver and kidney function tests and blood work to determine blood counts.
- Tell patient to avoid or limit the use of acetaminophen in OTC or prescription products because of potential toxic effects on the liver.

SAFETY ALERT!

irinotecan hydrochloride

Camptosar

Pharmacologic class: DNA topoisomerase inhibitor
Pregnancy risk category D

AVAILABLE FORMS

Injection: 20 mg/ml in 2- and 5-ml vials

INDICATIONS & DOSAGES

➤ Metastatic carcinoma of the colon or rectum that has recurred or progressed after fluorouracil (5-FU) therapy

Adults: Initially, 125 mg/m^2 by I.V. infusion over 90 minutes once weekly for 4 weeks; then 2-week rest period. Thereafter, additional courses of treatment may be repeated q 6 weeks with 4 weeks on and 2 weeks off. Subsequent doses may be adjusted to low of 50 mg/m^2 or maximum of 150 mg/m^2 in 25- to 50-mg/m^2 increments based on patient's tolerance. Or, 350 mg/m^2 by I.V. infusion over 90 minutes once q 3 weeks. Additional courses may continue indefinitely in patients who respond favorably and in those whose disease remains stable, provided intolerable toxicity doesn't occur.

Adjust-a-dose: Consider reducing starting dose in patients age 65 and older, in those who have received pelvic or abdominal radiation, or in those who have a performance status of 2 or increased bilirubin level. Give 300 mg/m^2 by I.V. infusion over 90 minutes once q 3 weeks. Or, give 100 mg/m^2 by I.V. infusion over 90 minutes once weekly.

➤ First-line therapy for metastatic colorectal cancer with 5-fluorouracil (5-FU) and leucovorin

Regimen 1

Adults: 125 mg/m^2 I.V. over 90 minutes on days 1, 8, 15, and 22; then leucovorin

20 mg/m² I.V. bolus on days 1, 8, 15, and 22 and 5-FU 500 mg/m² I.V. bolus on days 1, 8, 15, and 22. Courses are repeated q 6 weeks.

Regimen 2

Adults: 180 mg/m² I.V. over 90 minutes on days 1, 15, and 29; then leucovorin 200 mg/m² I.V. over 2 hours on days 1, 2, 15, 16, 29, and 30; then 5-FU 400 mg/m² I.V. bolus on days 1, 2, 15, 16, 29, and 30 and 5-FU 600 mg/m² I.V. infusion over 22 hours on days 1, 2, 15, 16, 29, and 30.

Adjust-a-dose: See manufacturer's package insert for details on dosage adjustment.

I.V. ADMINISTRATION

- Drug is packaged in a plastic blister to protect against inadvertent breakage and leakage. Inspect vial for damage and signs of leakage before removing blister.
- Wear gloves while handling and preparing infusion solutions. If drug contacts skin, wash thoroughly with soap and water. If drug contacts mucous membranes, flush thoroughly with water.
- Dilute drug in D_5W injection (preferred) or normal saline solution for injection before infusion to yield 0.12 to 2.8 mg/ml.
- Solution is stable for up to 24 hours at 77° F (25° C) in ambient fluorescent lighting. Solutions diluted in D_5W, stored at 36° to 46° F (2° to 8° C), and protected from light are stable for 48 hours. However, because microbial contamination may occur during dilution, use admixture within 24 hours if refrigerated or 6 hours if kept at room temperature. Refrigerating admixtures using normal saline solution isn't recommended because of low and sporadic risk of visible particulate. Don't freeze admixture because drug may precipitate.
- Premedicate patient with antiemetic drugs on day of treatment starting at least 30 minutes before giving irinotecan.
- Watch for irritation and infiltration; extravasation can cause tissue damage and necrosis. If extravasation occurs, flush site with sterile water and apply ice. Notify prescriber.
- Store vial at 59° to 86° F (15° to 30° C). Protect from light.

INCOMPATIBILITIES

Other I.V. drugs.

ACTION

Interacts with topoisomerase I, inducing reversible single-strand DNA breaks. Drug binds to the topoisomerase I–DNA complex and prevents relegation of these single-strand breaks.

Route	Onset	Peak	Duration
I.V.	Unknown	1 hr	Unknown

Half-life: About 6 to 12 hours.

ADVERSE REACTIONS

CNS: *asthenia, dizziness, fever, headache, insomnia, pain,* akathisia.
CV: *edema, vasodilation,* orthostatic hypotension.
EENT: *rhinitis.*
GI: ***diarrhea,*** *abdominal cramping, pain, and enlargement, anorexia, constipation, dyspepsia, flatulence, nausea, stomatitis, vomiting.*
Hematologic: *anemia,* ***leukopenia, neutropenia, thrombocytopenia.***
Metabolic: *dehydration, weight loss.*
Musculoskeletal: *back pain.*
Respiratory: *dyspnea, increased cough.*
Skin: *alopecia, rash, sweating.*
Other: *chills, infection.*

INTERACTIONS

Drug-drug. *Dexamethasone:* May increase risk of irinotecan-induced lymphocytopenia. Monitor patient closely.
Diuretics: May increase risk of dehydration and electrolyte imbalance. Consider stopping diuretic during active periods of nausea and vomiting.
Laxatives: May increase risk of diarrhea. Avoid using together.
Prochlorperazine: May increase risk of akathisia. Monitor patient closely.
Other antineoplastics: May cause additive adverse effects, such as myelosuppression and diarrhea. Monitor patient closely.
Drug-herb. ***St. John's wort:*** May decrease drug levels by about 40%. Discourage use together.

EFFECTS ON LAB TEST RESULTS

- May increase alkaline phosphatase, AST, and bilirubin levels. May decrease hemoglobin level.

- May decrease WBC and neutrophil counts.

CONTRAINDICATIONS & CAUTIONS

- Contraindicated in patients hypersensitive to drug.
- Safety and effectiveness of drug in children haven't been established.
- Use cautiously in elderly patients.

NURSING CONSIDERATIONS

- Pelvic or abdominal irradiation may increase risk of severe myelosuppression. Avoid use of drug in patients undergoing irradiation.
- Drug can cause severe diarrhea. Treat diarrhea occurring within 24 hours of drug administration with 0.25 to 1 mg atropine I.V., unless contraindicated.
- Treat late diarrhea (more than 24 hours after irinotecan administration) promptly with loperamide. Monitor patient for dehydration, electrolyte imbalance, or sepsis, and treat appropriately.
- Delay subsequent doses until normal bowel function returns for at least 24 hours without antidiarrheal. If grade 2, 3, or 4 late diarrhea occurs, decrease subsequent doses within the current cycle.
- To decrease risk of dehydration, withhold diuretic during treatment and periods of active vomiting or diarrhea.
- If neutropenic fever occurs or if absolute neutrophil count drops below 500/mm^3, temporarily stop therapy. Reduce dosage, especially if WBC count is below 2,000/mm^3, neutrophil count is below 1,000/mm^3, hemoglobin level is below 8 g/dl, or platelet count is below 100,000/mm^3.
- A colony-stimulating factor may be helpful in patients with significant neutropenia.
- Monitor WBC count with differential, hemoglobin level, and platelet count before each dose.
- ***Look alike–sound alike:*** Don't confuse irinotecan with topotecan.

PATIENT TEACHING

- Inform patient about risk of diarrhea and methods to treat it; tell him to avoid laxatives.
- Instruct patient to contact prescriber if any of the following occur: diarrhea for the first time during treatment; black or bloody stools; symptoms of dehydration such as light-headedness, dizziness, or faintness; inability to drink fluids due to nausea or vomiting; inability to control diarrhea within 24 hours; or fever or infection.
- Warn patient that hair loss may occur.
- Caution women to avoid pregnancy or breast-feeding during therapy.

SAFETY ALERT!

mitoxantrone hydrochloride
Novantrone

Pharmacologic class: DNA-reactive agent
Pregnancy risk category D

AVAILABLE FORMS

Injection: 2 mg/ml in 10-ml, 12.5-ml, 15-ml vials

INDICATIONS & DOSAGES

➤ **Combination initial therapy for acute nonlymphocytic leukemia**
Adults: Induction begins with 12 mg/m^2 I.V. daily on days 1 to 3, with 100 mg/m^2 daily of cytarabine on days 1 to 7. A second induction may be given if response isn't adequate. Maintenance therapy is 12 mg/m^2 on days 1 and 2, with cytarabine 100 mg/m^2 on days 1 to 5.

➤ **To reduce neurologic disability and frequency of relapse in chronic progressive, progressive relapsing, or worsening relapsing–remitting multiple sclerosis**
Adults: 12 mg/m^2 I.V. over 5 to 15 minutes q 3 months.

➤ **Advanced hormone-refractory prostate cancer**
Men: 12 to 14 mg/m^2 as a short I.V. infusion q 21 days. Drug is given as an adjunct to corticosteroid therapy.

I.V. ADMINISTRATION

- Preparing and giving drug may be mutagenic, teratogenic, or carcinogenic. Follow institutional policy to reduce risks.
- Dilute dose in at least 50 ml of normal saline solution for injection or D_5W injec-

tion. Give by direct injection into free-flowing I.V. line of normal saline solution or D_5W injection over at least 3 minutes, usually 15 to 30 minutes. Don't mix with other drugs.

- If extravasation occurs, stop infusion immediately and notify prescriber.
- Once vial is penetrated, undiluted solution may be stored for 7 days at room temperature or 14 days in refrigerator. Don't freeze.

INCOMPATIBILITIES

Amphotericin B, aztreonam, cefepime, doxorubicin liposomal, heparin sodium, hydrocortisone, other I.V. drugs, paclitaxel, piperacillin sodium and tazobactam sodium, propofol, sargramostim.

ACTION

Reacts with DNA, producing cytotoxic effect. Probably not specific to cell cycle.

Route	Onset	Peak	Duration
I.V.	Unknown	Unknown	Unknown

Half-life: Unknown.

ADVERSE REACTIONS

CNS: *fever, headache,* ***seizures.***
CV: ***arrhythmias,*** ECG abnormalities, heart failure, tachycardia.
EENT: conjunctivitis, sinusitis.
GI: *abdominal pain, bleeding, constipation, diarrhea, mucositis, nausea, stomatitis, vomiting.*
GU: *amenorrhea, menstrual disorder, UTI,* ***renal failure.***
Hematologic: ***myelosuppression,*** anemia.
Hepatic: jaundice.
Metabolic: hyperuricemia.
Musculoskeletal: back pain.
Respiratory: *cough, dyspnea, upper respiratory tract infection,* pneumonia.
Skin: *alopecia,* ecchymoses, local irritation or phlebitis, petechiae.
Other: *fungal infections,* ***sepsis.***

INTERACTIONS

None significant.

EFFECTS ON LAB TEST RESULTS

- May increase ALT, AST, bilirubin, GGT, and uric acid levels. May decrease hemoglobin level and hematocrit.
- May decrease leukocyte and granulocyte counts.

CONTRAINDICATIONS & CAUTIONS

- Contraindicated in patients hypersensitive to drug.
- Use cautiously in patients with previous exposure to anthracyclines or other cardiotoxic drugs, previous radiation therapy to mediastinal area, or heart disease. Significantly myelosuppressed patients shouldn't receive drug unless benefits outweigh risks.

NURSING CONSIDERATIONS

- Give allopurinol. Hydrate patient before and during therapy to avoid uric acid nephropathy.
- Closely monitor hematologic and laboratory chemistry parameters.
- Avoid all I.M. injections if platelet count falls below 50,000/mm^3.
- Give blood transfusion for anemia. RBC colony–stimulating factors may promote RBC production and decrease need for blood transfusions, and WBC colony–stimulating factors will promote cell growth and decrease risk of infection.
- Monitor left ventricular ejection fraction; risk of cardiotoxicity increases with cumulative dose of 140 mg/m^2, although toxicities may occur at any dose.
- If severe nonhematologic toxicity occurs during first course, delay second course until patient recovers.

PATIENT TEACHING

- Advise patient to report any pain or burning at site of injection during or after administration.
- Tell patient that urine may appear blue-green within 24 hours after receiving drug and that the whites of his eyes may turn blue. These effects aren't harmful but may persist during therapy.
- Advise patient to watch for signs and symptoms of bleeding and infection.
- Recommend that women consult prescriber before becoming pregnant.

SAFETY ALERT!

nelarabine

Arranon

Pharmacologic class: prodrug of cytotoxic deoxyguanosine
Pregnancy risk category D

AVAILABLE FORMS

Injection: 5 mg/ml in 50-ml vial

INDICATIONS & DOSAGES

➤ **T-cell acute lymphoblastic leukemia and T-cell lymphoblastic lymphoma in patients whose disease hasn't responded to or has relapsed after treatment with at least two chemotherapy regimens**

Adults: 1,500 mg/m^2 I.V. over 2 hours on days 1, 3, and 5. Repeat every 21 days.
Children: 650 mg/m^2 I.V. over 1 hour daily for 5 consecutive days. Repeat every 21 days.

I.V. ADMINISTRATION

- Wear gloves and protective clothing when preparing drug, and avoid skin contact.
- Transfer undiluted dose to a polyvinylchloride infusion bag or glass container.
- Once prepared, drug may be stored for 8 hours at 86° F (30° C).
- For adults, infuse dose over 2 hours; for children, infuse over 1 hour.
- Dispose of drug according to facility's protocol for hazardous waste.

INCOMPATIBILITIES

None reported.

ACTION

Probably accumulates in leukemic cells, inhibiting DNA synthesis and causing cell death.

Route	Onset	Peak	Duration
I.V.	Immediate	2 hr	3–25 hr

Half-life: Parent drug, 30 minutes; active metabolite, 3 hours.

ADVERSE REACTIONS

CNS: *dizziness, fatigue, fever, headache, hypoesthesia, paresthesias, peripheral neuropathy, rigors, somnolence,* ***demyelination peripheral neuropathies, seizures,*** abnormal gait, asthenia, ataxia, confusion, decreased level of consciousness, depression, insomnia.
CV: *edema, petechiae,* chest pain, hypotension, sinus tachycardia.
EENT: blurred vision, epistaxis, sinusitis.
GI: *constipation, diarrhea, nausea, vomiting,* abdominal distention, abdominal pain, anorexia, stomatitis.
Hematologic: FEBRILE NEUTROPENIA, LEUKOPENIA, NEUTROPENIA, THROMBOCYTOPENIA, *anemia.*
Metabolic: ***hypoglycemia,*** dehydration, hyperglycemia, hypocalcemia, hypokalemia, hypomagnesemia.
Musculoskeletal: *myalgia,* arthralgia, back pain, limb pain, muscle weakness.
Respiratory: *cough, dyspnea, pleural effusion,* wheezing.
Other: infection, pain, weakness.

INTERACTIONS

None known.

EFFECTS ON LAB TEST RESULTS

- May increase creatinine, transaminase, bilirubin, glucose, and AST levels. May decrease potassium, calcium, glucose, magnesium, albumin, and hemoglobin levels and hematocrit.
- May decrease WBC, platelet, and neutrophil counts.

CONTRAINDICATIONS & CAUTIONS

- Contraindicated in pregnant or breastfeeding women and in patients hypersensitive to drug or any of its components.
- Use cautiously if patient is receiving or has received intrathecal chemotherapy and in patients with severe renal or hepatic impairment.

NURSING CONSIDERATIONS

- ***Alert:*** Drug should be given only by staff trained in giving chemotherapy.
- Monitor CBC at baseline and regularly throughout treatment.
- ***Alert:*** Monitor patient for signs of severe neurotoxicity, including ataxia, coma, confusion, excessive somnolence, Guillain-Barré–like symptoms, peripheral neuropathy, and seizures. For NCI Com-

mon Toxicity Criteria grade 2 or higher, stop treatment. Patient may not fully recover even after drug is stopped.
• Take steps to prevent hyperuricemia caused by tumor lysis syndrome. Appropriate care includes hydration, alkalinization of body fluids, and allopurinol.

PATIENT TEACHING
• ***Alert:*** Tell patient to immediately report tingling or numbness in hands or feet, problems with fine motor skills, unsteadiness when walking, weakness when getting out of a chair or climbing stairs, tripping while walking, or seizures. These may be signs of serious adverse effects.
• Explain the importance of regular blood tests to evaluate drug effectiveness and detect adverse effects.
• Tell patient to report being more tired or paler than usual, trouble breathing, unusual bruising or bleeding, or fever.
• Advise care when driving or operating hazardous machinery because drug may cause sleepiness or dizziness.
• Urge patient to avoid live-virus vaccines while taking this drug.

SAFETY ALERT!

paclitaxel
Onxol, Taxol

Pharmacologic class: taxoid
Pregnancy risk category D

AVAILABLE FORMS
Injection: 6 mg/ml in 5-, 16.7-, 25-, 50-ml vials

INDICATIONS & DOSAGES
➤ **Second-line treatment of AIDS-related Kaposi sarcoma**
Adults: 135 mg/m² Taxol I.V. over 3 hours q 3 weeks, or 100 mg/m² I.V. over 3 hours q 2 weeks.
Adjust-a-dose: Don't give drug if baseline or subsequent neutrophil counts are less than 1,000/mm³. Reduce subsequent doses of Taxol by 20% for patients who experience severe neutropenia (neutrophil count 500/mm³ for 1 week or longer). Patient also may need reduction in dexamethasone premedication dose (10 mg P.O. instead of 20 mg P.O.) and start of a hematopoietic growth factor.
➤ **First-line and subsequent therapy for advanced ovarian cancer**
Adults (previously untreated): 175 mg/m² over 3 hours q 3 weeks, followed by cisplatin 75 mg/m²; or, 135 mg/m² over 24 hours, followed by cisplatin 75 mg/m², q 3 weeks.
Adults (previously treated): 135 or 175 mg/m² I.V. over 3 hours q 3 weeks.
➤ **Breast cancer after failure of combination chemotherapy for metastatic disease or relapse within 6 months of adjuvant chemotherapy (previous therapy should have included an anthracycline unless contraindicated); adjuvant therapy for node-positive breast cancer given sequentially to standard doxorubicin-containing combination chemotherapy**
Adults: 175 mg/m² I.V. over 3 hours q 3 weeks.
➤ **First treatment of advanced non–small-cell lung cancer for patients who aren't candidates for curative surgery or radiation**
Adults: 135 mg/m² I.V. Taxol infusion over 24 hours, followed by cisplatin 75 mg/m². Repeat cycle q 3 weeks.
Adjust-a-dose: Subsequent courses shouldn't be repeated until neutrophil count is at least 1,500/mm³ and platelet count is at least 100,000/mm³. Reduce subsequent doses of Taxol by 20% for patients who experience severe neutropenia (neutrophil count less than 500/mm³ for a week or longer) or severe peripheral neuropathy. For patients with hepatic impairment, adjust doses for the first courses of therapy as follows: For 24-hour infusion of Taxol if transaminase levels are less than 2 times the upper limit of normal (ULN) and bilirubin levels are 1.5 mg/dl or less, give 135 mg/m². If transaminase levels are 2 to less than 10 times ULN and bilirubin levels are 1.5 mg/dl or less, give 100 mg/m². If transaminase levels are less than 10 × ULN and bilirubin levels are 1.6 to 7.5 mg/dl, give 50 mg/m². If transaminase levels are 10 times ULN or more or bilirubin levels are more than 7.5 mg/dl, don't use drug. For 3-hour infusion of

Taxol, if transaminase levels are less than 10 times ULN and bilirubin levels are 1.25 times ULN or less, give 175 mg/m^2. If transaminase levels are less than 10 times ULN and bilirubin levels are 1.26 to 2 × ULN, give 135 mg/m^2. If transaminase levels are less than 10 times ULN and bilirubin levels are 2.01 to 5 times ULN, give 90 mg/m^2. If transaminase levels are 10 times ULN or more or bilirubin levels are more than 5 times ULN, don't use drug. For subsequent courses, base dosage adjustment on individual tolerance.

I.V. ADMINISTRATION

- Preparing and giving drug may be mutagenic, teratogenic, or carcinogenic. Follow institutional policy to reduce risks. Mark all waste materials with CHEMOTHERAPY HAZARD labels.
- Prepare and store infusion solutions in glass containers. Undiluted concentrate shouldn't contact polyvinyl chloride I.V. bags or tubing.
- Dilute concentrate before infusion. Compatible solutions include normal saline solution for injection, D_5W, 5% dextrose in normal saline solution for injection, and 5% dextrose in Ringer lactate injection. Dilute to yield 0.3 to 1.2 mg/ml. Diluted solutions are stable for 24 hours at room temperature. Prepared solution may appear hazy.
- Give through polyethylene-lined administration sets, and use an in-line 0.22-micron filter.
- Watch for irritation and infiltration; extravasation can cause tissue damage and necrosis.
- Closely monitor patient and vital signs during infusion, especially during the first hour.
- Store diluted solution in glass or polypropylene bottles, or use polypropylene or polyolefin bags.

INCOMPATIBILITIES

Amphotericin B, chlorpromazine, cisplatin, doxorubicin liposomal, hydroxyzine hydrochloride, methylprednisolone sodium succinate, mitoxantrone.

ACTION

Prevents depolymerization of cellular microtubules, inhibiting normal reorganization of microtubule network needed for mitosis and other vital cellular functions.

Route	Onset	Peak	Duration
I.V.	Unknown	Unknown	Unknown

Half-life: After 6- to 12-hour infusion, distribution and elimination half-lives average about 30 minutes and 6 hours, respectively. For 3-hour infusion, distribution and elimination half-lives average about 30 minutes and 2½ hours, respectively.

ADVERSE REACTIONS

CNS: *peripheral neuropathy, asthenia.*
CV: ***bradycardia,*** *hypotension, abnormal ECG.*
GI: *nausea, vomiting, diarrhea, mucositis.*
Hematologic: **NEUTROPENIA, LEUKOPENIA, THROMBOCYTOPENIA,** *anemia, bleeding.*
Musculoskeletal: *myalgia, arthralgia.*
Skin: *alopecia, cellulitis and phlebitis at injection site.*
Other: hypersensitivity reactions, ***anaphylaxis,*** *infections.*

INTERACTIONS

Drug-drug. *Carbamazepine, phenobarbital:* May increase metabolism and may decrease paclitaxel levels. Use together cautiously.
Cisplatin: May cause additive myelosuppressive effects. Give paclitaxel before cisplatin.
Doxorubicin: May increase plasma levels of doxorubicin and its active metabolite, doxorubicinol. Use together cautiously.
Drugs that inhibit cytochrome P-450, such as cyclosporine, dexamethasone, diazepam, etoposide, ***ketoconazole,*** *quinidine, retinoic acid, teniposide, testosterone, verapamil, vincristine:* May increase paclitaxel level. Monitor patient for toxicity.

EFFECTS ON LAB TEST RESULTS

- May increase alkaline phosphatase, AST, and triglyceride levels. May decrease hemoglobin level.
- May decrease neutrophil, WBC, and platelet counts.

CONTRAINDICATIONS & CAUTIONS

- Contraindicated in patients hypersensitive to drug or polyoxyethylated castor oil (a vehicle used in drug solution) and in those with baseline neutrophil counts below 1,500/mm^3 and platelet counts below 100,000/mm^3, or AIDS-related Kaposi sarcoma with baseline neutrophil counts below 1,000/mm^3.
- Use cautiously in patients with hepatic impairment.

NURSING CONSIDERATIONS

- Patient may experience peripheral neuropathies, which may be cumulative and dose related. Patients with severe symptoms may need dosage reduction.
- To reduce risk or severity of hypersensitivity, patients must receive pretreatment with corticosteroids, such as dexamethasone, and antihistamines. Both H_1-receptor antagonists, such as diphenhydramine, and H_2-receptor antagonists, such as cimetidine or ranitidine, may be used.
- Monitor blood counts often during therapy. Bone marrow toxicity is the most common and dose-limiting toxicity. Packed RBC or platelet transfusions may be needed in severe cases. Institute bleeding precautions, as indicated.
- RBC colony-stimulating factors may promote RBC production and decrease need for blood transfusions.
- Avoid all I.M. injections when platelet count is below 50,000/mm^3.
- If patient develops significant cardiac conduction abnormalities, use indicated therapy and continuous cardiac monitoring during therapy and subsequent infusions.
- ***Look alike–sound alike:*** Don't confuse paclitaxel with paroxetine; don't confuse Taxol with Paxil or Taxotere.

PATIENT TEACHING

- Advise patient to report any pain or burning at site of injection during or after administration.
- Urge patient to watch for fever, sore throat, and fatigue and for easy bruising, nosebleeds, bleeding gums, or tarry stools. Tell patient to take temperature daily.
- Teach patient symptoms of peripheral neuropathy, such as a tingling or burning sensation or numbness in limbs, and to report these symptoms immediately.
- Warn patient that reversible hair loss will probably occur.
- Caution woman of childbearing age to avoid becoming pregnant during therapy. Recommend that she consult prescriber before becoming pregnant.

SAFETY ALERT!

paclitaxel protein-bound particles
Abraxane

Pharmacologic class: taxoid
Pregnancy risk category D

AVAILABLE FORMS

Lyophilized powder for injection: 100 mg in single-use vials

INDICATIONS & DOSAGES

➤ **Metastatic breast cancer after failure of combination chemotherapy or relapse within 6 months of adjuvant chemotherapy (previous therapy should have included an anthracycline unless clinically contraindicated at the time)**

Adults: 260 mg/m^2 I.V. over 30 minutes q 3 weeks.

Adjust-a-dose: For patients with severe sensory neuropathy or a neutrophil count less than 500/mm^3 for a week or longer, reduce dose to 220 mg/m^2. For recurring severe sensory neuropathy or severe neutropenia, reduce dose to 180 mg/m^2. For grade 3 (severe) sensory neuropathy, stop drug until condition improves to a grade 1 or 2 (mild to moderate); then restart at a reduced dose for the rest of treatment.

I.V. ADMINISTRATION

- Because of drug's cytotoxicity, handle it cautiously and wear gloves. If drug contacts skin, wash area thoroughly with soap and water. If drug contacts mucous membranes, flush them thoroughly with water.
- Reconstitute the vial with 20 ml of normal saline solution to yield 5 mg/ml of drug. Direct the stream slowly, over at least 1 minute, onto the inside wall of the

vial to avoid foaming. Let the vial sit for 5 minutes to ensure proper wetting of the powder. Gently swirl or turn the vial for at least 2 minutes until completely dissolved. If foaming occurs, let the solution stand for 15 minutes for the foam to subside. If particles are visible, gently invert the vial again to ensure complete resuspension. The solution should appear milky and uniform. Inject the correct dose into an empty polyvinyl chloride-type I.V. bag and use immediately.
• Give drug over 30 minutes.
• The suspension for infusion, when prepared in an infusion bag, is stable at room temperature and normal lighting for up to 8 hours.
• Store unopened vials at room temperature in the original package. Store reconstituted vials at 36° to 46° F (2° to 8° C) for up to 8 hours, protected from light.

INCOMPATIBILITIES
None known.

ACTION
Prevents depolymerization of cellular microtubules, inhibiting reorganization of the microtubule network and disrupting mitosis and other vital cell functions.

Route	Onset	Peak	Duration
I.V.	Unknown	Unknown	Unknown

Half-life: 27 hours.

ADVERSE REACTIONS
CNS: *asthenia, sensory neuropathy.*
CV: *abnormal ECG, edema,* ***cardiac arrest, chest pain, supraventricular tachycardia, thromboembolism, thrombosis,*** hypertension, hypotension.
EENT: *visual disturbances.*
GI: *diarrhea, nausea, oral candidiasis, vomiting,* ***intestinal obstruction, ischemic colitis, pancreatitis, perforation,*** mucositis.
Hematologic: *anemia,* NEUTROPENIA, ***thrombocytopenia,*** bleeding.
Hepatic: ***hepatic encephalopathy, hepatic necrosis.***
Musculoskeletal: *arthralgia, myalgia.*
Respiratory: ***pulmonary embolism,*** *cough, dyspnea, pneumonia, respiratory tract infection.*
Skin: *alopecia,* injection site reactions.
Other: *infections,* hypersensitivity reactions.

INTERACTIONS
Drug-drug. *Cytochrome P-450 inhibitors:* May decrease paclitaxel metabolism. Use together cautiously.

EFFECTS ON LAB TEST RESULTS
• May increase alkaline phosphatase, AST, bilirubin, creatinine, and GGT levels. May decrease hemoglobin level.
• May decrease neutrophil and platelet counts.

CONTRAINDICATIONS & CAUTIONS
• Contraindicated in patients with baseline neutrophil counts of under 1,500/mm^3.
• Don't retreat until neutrophil counts recover to more than 1,500/mm^3 and platelet count recovers to more than 100,000/mm^3.
• In patients with creatinine level over 2 mg/dl or bilirubin level over 1.5 mg/dl, use hasn't been studied.

NURSING CONSIDERATIONS
• Give only under supervision of practitioner experienced in using chemotherapy in a facility that can manage complications of therapy.
• ***Alert:*** Don't substitute Abraxane for other forms of paclitaxel.
• Because drug contains human albumin, a remote risk exists of transmitting viruses and Creutzfeldt-Jakob disease.
• Assess patient for symptoms of sensory neuropathy and severe neutropenia.
• Monitor liver and kidney function test results.
• Monitor infusion site closely.

PATIENT TEACHING
• Warn patient that alopecia commonly occurs but is reversible after therapy.
• Teach patient to recognize signs of neuropathy, such as tingling, burning, and numbness in arms and legs.
• Tell patient to report fever or other signs of infection, severe abdominal pain, or severe diarrhea.
• Advise patient to contact prescriber if nausea and vomiting persist or interfere

with adequate nutrition. Reassure patient that an antiemetic can be prescribed.
- Explain that many patients experience weakness and fatigue, so it's important to rest. Tiredness, paleness, and shortness of breath may result from low blood counts, and patient may need a transfusion.
- To reduce or prevent mouth sores, remind patient to perform proper oral hygiene.
- Tell women to avoid becoming pregnant or breast-feeding and men to avoid fathering a child during therapy.

✱ NEW DRUG

panitumumab
Vectibix

Pharmacologic class: monoclonal antibody
Pregnancy risk category C

AVAILABLE FORMS
Solution for infusion: 20 mg/ml in 5-ml, 10-ml, and 20-ml vials

INDICATIONS & DOSAGES
➤ **Human epidermal growth factor receptor (EGFR)-expressing metastatic colorectal cancer with disease progression during or following fluoropyrimidine-, oxaliplatin-, and irinotecan-containing regimens**
Adults: 6 mg/kg I.V. infusion over 60 minutes q 14 days. For doses greater than 1,000 mg, infuse over 90 minutes.
Adjust-a-dose: For patients with mild or moderate (grade 1 or 2) infusion reactions, reduce infusion rate by 50%. For patients with severe (grade 3 or 4) infusion reactions, stop drug permanently.

For skin toxicities grade 3 or greater, or if considered intolerable, stop drug. If toxicity doesn't improve to grade 2 or less within 1 month, permanently stop therapy. If toxicity improves to grade 2 or less, and patient is symptomatically improved after withholding 2 or fewer doses, restart treatment at 50% of original dose. If toxicity recurs, permanently stop drug. If toxicity doesn't recur, increase subsequent doses in increments of 25% of original dose until a 6 mg/kg dose is reached.

I.V. ADMINISTRATION
- Dilute drug using aseptic technique. The solution should be colorless but may contain white or translucent particles which will be filtered out during infusion. Don't shake vials.
- Withdraw drug and dilute to a total volume of 100 ml with normal saline solution. For doses higher than 1,000 mg, dilute to 150 ml. Final concentration shouldn't exceed 10 mg/ml. Use within 6 hours if stored at room temperature or within 24 hours if refrigerated. Dispose of any unused drug.
- Give by I.V. infusion using a pump with a low-protein binding 0.2 or 0.22 micrometer in-line filter. Don't give by I.V. push or bolus.
- Flush I.V. line with normal saline solution before and after giving drug.
- Refrigerate vials, don't freeze. Protect from sunlight.

INCOMPATIBILITIES
Other I.V. drugs and solutions.

ACTION
Inhibits actions between proteins and cell surface receptors that would normally allow proliferation of cells and new blood vessel growth.

Route	Onset	Peak	Duration
I.V.	Immediate	Unknown	Unknown

Half-life: 7½ days.

ADVERSE REACTIONS
CNS: *chills, fatigue, fever.*
CV: *peripheral edema,* ***hypotension.***
EENT: *eyelash growth, ocular toxicities, oral mucositis.*
GI: *abdominal pain, constipation, diarrhea, nausea, vomiting,* mucosal inflammation, stomatitis.
Metabolic: *hypomagnesemia.*
Respiratory: *cough,* ***pulmonary fibrosis, pulmonary toxicity.***
Skin: *acne, acneiform dermatitis, dry skin, fissures, nail infection, pruritus, rash, redness,* ***skin exfoliation, skin toxicity.***
Other: ***anaphylaxis, severe infusion reaction,*** *general deterioration.*

INTERACTIONS
None known.

EFFECTS ON LAB TEST RESULTS
• May decrease calcium and magnesium levels.

CONTRAINDICATIONS & CAUTIONS
• There are no known contraindications.
• Use cautiously in patients with skin conditions, or preexisting lung or ocular disease.

NURSING CONSIDERATIONS
• ***Alert:*** Drug may cause severe infusion reactions including anaphylaxis, bronchospasm, fever, chills, and hypotension. Monitor patient closely. Keep emergency treatment immediately available to treat severe infusion reactions.
• Notify prescriber if patient develops severe skin, eye, or pulmonary toxicities. The drug may need to be stopped or the dose lowered.
• Drug-induced diarrhea can be especially severe when combined with other chemotherapy drugs. Monitor patient for dehydration. Using with the irinotecan, bolus 5-fluorouracil, leucovorin (IFL) regimen isn't recommended.
• Monitor patient's electrolytes, especially calcium and magnesium, periodically during and for 8 weeks after treatment. Supplementation may be needed.

PATIENT TEACHING
• Warn patient that drug can cause photosensitivity reactions and instruct him to wear a hat, sunscreen, and protective clothing and to limit sun exposure.
• Warn patient about the risk of severe skin, eye, infusion-related, and pulmonary reactions. Advise him to report any skin changes, eye problems, or difficulty breathing to his prescriber.
• Diarrhea may be severe, especially if more than one chemotherapy drug is used. Remind patient to stay well hydrated.
• Tell women of childbearing age that contraception must be used during and for 6 months following treatment.
• Advise mothers to stop breast-feeding during and for 2 months after treatment ends.

SAFETY ALERT!

pegaspargase (PEG-L-asparaginase)
Oncaspar

Pharmacologic class: modified L-asparaginase
Pregnancy risk category C

AVAILABLE FORMS
Injection: 750 international units/ml

INDICATIONS & DOSAGES
➤ **Acute lymphoblastic leukemia, as part of a multidrug chemotherapy regimen**
Adults and children with body surface area (BSA) of at least 0.6 m^2: Give 2,500 international units/m^2 I.V. or I.M. q 14 days.
Children with BSA below 0.6 m^2: Give 82.5 international units/kg I.V. or I.M. q 14 days.

I.V. ADMINISTRATION
• Drug may be a contact irritant, and solution must be handled and given with care. Wear gloves. Avoid inhalation of vapors and contact with skin or mucous membranes, especially in the eyes. If contact occurs, wash with generous amounts of water for at least 15 minutes.
• Don't use if cloudy or contains precipitate. Avoid excessive agitation of drug; don't shake.
• Don't freeze or use drug that has been frozen because freezing destroys drug's effectiveness.
• Give over 1 to 2 hours in 100 ml of normal saline solution or D_5W injection through an infusion that is already running.
• Discard unused portions. Use only one dose per vial; don't reenter vial.
• Don't use if stored at room temperature for longer than 48 hours. Keep refrigerated at 36° to 46° F (2° to 8° C).

INCOMPATIBILITIES
None reported, but don't mix with other I.V. drugs.

ACTION
A modified version of the enzyme L-asparaginase that exerts cytotoxic effects by inactivating the amino acid aspar-

agine, which tumor cells need to synthesize proteins.

Route	Onset	Peak	Duration
I.V., I.M.	Unknown	Unknown	Unknown

Half-life: Unknown.

ADVERSE REACTIONS

CNS: ***coma, seizures, status epilepticus,*** confusion, disorientation, dizziness, emotional lability, fatigue, headache, malaise, mental status changes, mood changes, paresthesia, parkinsonism, somnolence.
CV: chest pain, hypertension, hypotension, peripheral edema, subacute bacterial endocarditis, tachycardia.
EENT: epistaxis.
GI: ***pancreatitis,*** abdominal pain, anorexia, constipation, diarrhea, indigestion, flatulence, mouth tenderness, mucositis, nausea, severe colitis, vomiting.
GU: ***renal failure,*** hematuria, increased urinary frequency, proteinuria, renal dysfunction, severe hemorrhagic cystitis.
Hematologic: ***agranulocytosis, disseminated intravascular coagulation, hemorrhage, leukopenia, pancytopenia, thrombocytopenia, thrombosis,*** easy bruising, hemolytic anemia.
Hepatic: ***liver failure,*** ascites, fatty changes in liver, hypoalbuminemia, jaundice.
Metabolic: ***hypoglycemia,*** hyperglycemia, hyperuricemia, hyponatremia, hypoproteinemia, metabolic acidosis, uric acid nephropathy, weight loss.
Musculoskeletal: arthralgia, cramps, joint stiffness, myalgia, musculoskeletal pain, pain in limbs.
Respiratory: ***bronchospasm,*** cough, upper respiratory tract infection.
Skin: alopecia, ecchymoses, erythema, erythema simplex, fever blister, fungal changes, hand whiteness, injection pain or reaction, itching, localized edema, nail whiteness and ridging, petechial rash, purpura, rash, urticaria.
Other: ***anaphylaxis, sepsis, septic shock,*** hypersensitivity reactions, infection, night sweats.

INTERACTIONS

Drug-drug. *Aspirin, dipyridamole, heparin, NSAIDs, warfarin:* May cause imbalances in coagulation factors, predisposing patient to bleeding or thrombosis. Use together cautiously.
Methotrexate: May interfere with action of methotrexate. Check patient for decreased effectiveness.
Protein-bound drugs: May increase toxicity of other drugs that bind to proteins and may interfere with enzymatic detoxification of other drugs, especially in the liver. Check for toxicity, and use together cautiously.

EFFECTS ON LAB TEST RESULTS

- May increase BUN, creatinine, amylase, lipase, bilirubin, ALT, AST, uric acid, and ammonia levels. May decrease hemoglobin, sodium, and protein levels. May increase or decrease glucose level.
- May increase PT, INR, APTT, and thromboplastin. May decrease antithrombin III, WBC, RBC, platelet, and granulocyte counts.

CONTRAINDICATIONS & CAUTIONS

- Contraindicated in patients with pancreatitis or history of pancreatitis, in those who have had significant hemorrhagic events related to previous treatment with L-asparaginase, and in those with history of serious allergic reactions to drug, such as generalized urticaria, bronchospasm, laryngeal edema, hypotension, or other unacceptable adverse reactions.
- Use cautiously in patients with liver dysfunction; use only when clearly indicated in pregnant women.

NURSING CONSIDERATIONS

- Take preventive measures (including adequate hydration) before starting treatment. Hyperuricemia may result from rapid lysis of leukemic cells. Allopurinol may be ordered.
- I.M. use is preferred because it has the lowest risk of hepatotoxicity, coagulopathy, and GI and renal disorders.
- When giving I.M., limit volume given at a single injection site to 2 ml. If volume to be given exceeds 2 ml, use multiple injection sites.
- ***Alert:*** Monitor patient closely for hypersensitivity (including life-threatening anaphylaxis), especially those hypersensitive to other forms of L-asparaginase. Observe patient for 1 hour after giving drug and

have emergency equipment and other drugs needed to treat anaphylaxis readily available. Moderate to life-threatening hypersensitivity requires stopping L-asparaginase.
- To assess effects of therapy, monitor patient's peripheral blood count and bone marrow. A drop in circulating lymphoblasts is often noted after therapy starts, sometimes accompanied by a marked rise in uric acid level.
- Obtain frequent amylase and lipase determinations to detect pancreatitis. Monitor patient's glucose level during therapy to detect hyperglycemia.
- Monitor patient for liver dysfunction when drug is used with hepatotoxic chemotherapeutic drugs.
- Drug may affect several plasma proteins; monitoring of fibrinogen, PT, INR, and PTT may be indicated.

PATIENT TEACHING
- Inform patient of risk of hypersensitivity reactions and importance of reporting them immediately.
- Tell patient not to take other drugs, including OTC preparations, until approved by prescriber because risk of bleeding is higher when pegaspargase is given with drugs such as aspirin. Drug may also increase toxicity of other drugs.
- Urge patient to report signs and symptoms of infection (fever, chills, and malaise); drug may suppress the immune system.
- Caution woman of childbearing age to avoid pregnancy and breast-feeding during therapy.

SAFETY ALERT!

procarbazine hydrochloride
Matulane, Natulan†

Pharmacologic class: methylhydrazine derivative
Pregnancy risk category D

AVAILABLE FORMS
Capsules: 50 mg

INDICATIONS & DOSAGES
➤ **Adjunct treatment of Hodgkin lymphoma (stages III and IV), other cancers using nitrogen mustard, vincristine, procarbazine, prednisone (known as MOPP) regimen**
Adults: 2 to 4 mg/kg P.O. daily in single dose or divided doses for first week. Then, 4 to 6 mg/kg daily until WBC count falls below 4,000/mm^3, platelet count falls below 100,000/mm^3, or maximum response is obtained. Maintenance dose is 1 to 2 mg/kg daily after bone marrow recovery. For MOPP regimen, 100 mg/m^2 daily P.O. for 14 days of 28-day cycle.
Children: 50 mg/m^2 P.O. daily for first week; then 100 mg/m^2 until response or toxicity occurs. Maintenance dose is 50 mg/m^2 P.O. daily after bone marrow recovery.

ACTION
Unknown. Thought to inhibit DNA, RNA, and protein synthesis.

Route	Onset	Peak	Duration
P.O.	Unknown	Unknown	Unknown

Half-life: 10 minutes.

ADVERSE REACTIONS
CNS: *hallucinations,* ***coma,*** confusion, depression, dizziness, headache, insomnia, nervousness, neuropathy, nightmares, paresthesia, syncope.
CV: flushing, hypotension, tachycardia.
EENT: nystagmus, photophobia, retinal hemorrhage.
GI: *nausea, vomiting,* abdominal pain, anorexia, constipation, diarrhea, dry mouth, dysphagia, hematemesis, melena, stomatitis.
GU: hematuria, nocturia, urinary frequency.
Hematologic: ***anemia, bleeding tendency, leukopenia, thrombocytopenia,*** eosinophilia, hemolytic anemia.
Hepatic: ***hepatotoxicity,*** jaundice.
Respiratory: *pleural effusion,* cough, pneumonitis.
Skin: dermatitis, hyperpigmentation, pruritus, rash, reversible alopecia.
Other: ***secondary malignancies,*** allergic reaction, gynecomastia, herpes outbreak.

INTERACTIONS
Drug-drug. *CNS depressants:* May cause additive depressant effects. Avoid using together.

Digoxin: May decrease digoxin level. Monitor digoxin level closely.
Drugs high in tyramine, local anesthetics, MAO inhibitors, sympathomimetics, tricyclic antidepressants: May cause tremor, palpitations, increased blood pressure. Monitor patient closely.
Levodopa: May cause sudden hypertensive crisis. Don't give within 2 to 4 weeks of procarbazine.
Drug-food. *Caffeine:* May result in arrhythmias and severe hypertension. Discourage caffeine intake.
Foods high in tyramine (cheese, Chianti): May cause tremor, palpitations, and increased blood pressure. Monitor patient closely; advise him to avoid or limit intake.
Drug-lifestyle. *Alcohol use:* Mild disulfiram-like reaction may cause flushing, headache, nausea, and hypotension. Warn patient to avoid alcoholic beverages.

EFFECTS ON LAB TEST RESULTS

- May decrease hemoglobin level.
- May increase eosinophil count. May decrease platelet, RBC, and WBC counts.

CONTRAINDICATIONS & CAUTIONS

- Contraindicated in patients hypersensitive to drug and in those with inadequate bone marrow reserve as shown by bone marrow aspiration.
- Use cautiously in patients with impaired hepatic or renal function.

NURSING CONSIDERATIONS

- Monitor CBC and platelet counts.
- Bone marrow depression begins 2 to 8 weeks after the start of treatment.
- Avoid all I.M. injections when platelet count is below $50,000/mm^3$.
- RBC colony-stimulating factors may promote RBC production and decrease need for blood transfusions.
- Stop drug and notify prescriber if patient becomes confused or develops paresthesia or other neuropathy.
- The manufacturer recommends that if radiation or chemotherapeutic agents with bone marrow depressant activity have been used, give patient a 1-month interval without such therapy before beginning procarbazine therapy.

PATIENT TEACHING

- To decrease nausea and vomiting, advise patient to take drug at bedtime and in divided doses.
- Tell patient to watch for fever, sore throat, fatigue and for easy bruising, nosebleeds, bleeding gums, or tarry stools. Tell patient to take temperature daily.
- Warn patient to avoid alcohol during therapy. Urge him to stop drug and check with prescriber immediately if, after drinking alcohol, he experiences chest pain, rapid or irregular heartbeat, severe headache, or stiff neck.
- Instruct patient to avoid OTC medications that contain sympathomimetics and to avoid foods and drinks high in tyramine, such as wine, tea, coffee, cola, cheese, and bananas.
- Warn patient to avoid hazardous activities that require alertness and good motor coordination until CNS effects of drug are known.
- Caution woman of childbearing age to avoid becoming pregnant during therapy and to consult prescriber before becoming pregnant.

SAFETY ALERT!

rituximab

Rituxan

Pharmacologic class: monoclonal antibody
Pregnancy risk category C

AVAILABLE FORMS

Injection: 10 mg/ml; 10-ml, 50-ml single-use, sterile vials

INDICATIONS & DOSAGES

✷*NEW INDICATION:* **Previously untreated, follicular CD20-positive, B-cell non-Hodgkin lymphoma (NHL) with cyclophosphamide, vincristine, and prednisolone (CVP) chemotherapy regimen**
Adults: 375 mg/m^2 I.V. given on day 1 of each CVP cycle, for up to eight doses.
✷*NEW INDICATION:* **Previously untreated low-grade, CD20-positive,**

B-cell NHL following first-line treatment with CVP chemotherapy
Adults: For patients who fail to progress after six to eight cycles of CVP chemotherapy, give 375 mg/m² I.V. once weekly for four doses q 6 months for up to 16 doses.

➤**Relapsed or refractory low-grade or follicular, CD20-positive, B-cell NHL**
Adults: Initially, 375 mg/m² I.V. once weekly for four or eight doses. Retreatment for patients with progressive disease, 375 mg/m² I.V. infusion once weekly for four doses.

✷***NEW INDICATION:*** **With methotrexate to reduce the signs and symptoms of moderate to severely active rheumatoid arthritis in patients who have had an inadequate response to one or more tumor necrosis factor antagonists**
Adults: Give two 1,000 mg I.V. infusions 2 weeks apart. To reduce the incidence and severity of infusion reactions, give methylprednisolone 100 mg I.V., or its equivalent, 30 minutes before each infusion.

✷***NEW INDICATION:*** **Diffuse large B-cell, CD20-positive, non-Hodgkin lymphoma, given with cyclophosphamide–Adriamycin–Oncovin–prednisone, known as CHOP, or other anthracycline-based chemotherapy regimens**
Adults: 375 mg/m² I.V. given on day 1 of each chemotherapy cycle for up to eight infusions.

I.V. ADMINISTRATION

- Protect vials from direct sunlight.
- Give as an infusion; don't give as I.V. push or bolus.
- Begin infusion at rate of 50 mg/hour. If no hypersensitivity or infusion-related events occur, increase rate by 50 mg/hour q 30 minutes, to maximum of 400 mg/hour. Start subsequent infusions at 100 mg/hour and increase by 100 mg/hour q 30 minutes, to maximum of 400 mg/hour as tolerated.
- Dilute to yield 1 to 4 mg/ml in bag of D_5W or normal saline solution. Gently invert bag to mix solution.
- Discard unused portion left in vial.
- Diluted solutions are stable for 24 hours if refrigerated and for 12 hours at room temperature.

INCOMPATIBILITIES

Other I.V. drugs.

ACTION

A murine and human monoclonal antibody directed against CD20 antigen found on the surface of normal and malignant B lymphocytes. Binding to this antigen mediates the lysis of the B cells.

Route	Onset	Peak	Duration
I.V.	Variable	Variable	6–12 mo

Half-life: Varies widely, possibly because of differences in tumor burden among patients and changes in CD-positive B-cell populations upon repeated therapy.

ADVERSE REACTIONS

CNS: *asthenia, fever, headache,* agitation, dizziness, fatigue, hypesthesia, hypertonia, insomnia, malaise, nervousness, pain, paresthesia, somnolence, vertigo.
CV: *hypotension,* ***arrhythmias, bradycardia,*** chest pain, edema, flushing, hypertension, peripheral edema, tachycardia.
EENT: conjunctivitis, lacrimation disorder, rhinitis, sinusitis, sore throat.
GI: *nausea,* abdominal pain or enlargement, anorexia, diarrhea, dyspepsia, taste perversion, vomiting.
GU: ***acute renal failure.***
Hematologic: **LEUKOPENIA,** ***neutropenia, thrombocytopenia,*** anemia.
Metabolic: hyperglycemia, hypocalcemia, weight decrease.
Musculoskeletal: arthritis, back pain, myalgia.
Respiratory: ***bronchospasm,*** bronchitis, cough increase, dyspnea.
Skin: *pruritus, rash, severe mucocutaneous reactions,* pain at injection site, urticaria.
Other: *chills, rigors,* **ANGIOEDEMA,** ***infusion reaction,*** infection, tumor lysis syndrome, tumor pain.

INTERACTIONS

Drug-drug. *Cisplatin:* May cause renal toxicity. Monitor renal function tests.

EFFECTS ON LAB TEST RESULTS
- May increase glucose and LDH levels. May decrease calcium and hemoglobin levels.
- May decrease WBC, platelet, and neutrophil counts.

CONTRAINDICATIONS & CAUTIONS
- Contraindicated in patients with type I hypersensitivity or anaphylactic reactions to murine proteins or components of drug.

NURSING CONSIDERATIONS
- Monitor patient closely for signs and symptoms of hypersensitivity. Have drugs, such as epinephrine, antihistamines, and corticosteroids available to immediately treat such a reaction. Premedicate with acetaminophen and diphenhydramine before each infusion.
- Monitor patient's blood pressure closely during infusion. If hypotension, bronchospasm, or angioedema occurs, stop infusion and restart at half the rate when symptoms resolve.
- Withhold antihypertensives 12 hours before infusion because transient hypotension may occur.
- If serious or life-threatening arrhythmias occur, stop infusion.
- Severe mucocutaneous reactions (including toxic epidermal necrolysis, Stevens-Johnson syndrome, paraneoplastic pemphigus, and lichenoid or vesiculobullous dermatitis) may occur 1 to 13 weeks after administration. Avoid further infusions and promptly start treatment of the skin reaction.
- Infusion-related reactions are most severe with the first infusion. Subsequent infusions are generally well tolerated.
- Obtain CBC at regular intervals and more frequently in patients in whom cytopenias develop.
- ***Alert:*** Drug may cause progressive multifocal leukoencephalopathy up to 12 months after stopping. If neurologic status changes, suspect this disorder.

PATIENT TEACHING
- Tell patient to report symptoms of hypersensitivity, such as itching, rash, chills, or rigor, during and after infusion.
- Urge patient to watch for fever, sore throat, fatigue, easy bruising, nosebleeds, bleeding gums, or tarry stools. Tell him to take temperature daily.
- Advise breast-feeding women to stop breast-feeding until drug levels are undetectable.

✱ NEW DRUG

sorafenib
Nexavar

Pharmacologic class: multi-kinase inhibitor
Pregnancy risk category D

AVAILABLE FORMS
Tablets: 200 mg

INDICATIONS & DOSAGES
➤ Advanced renal cell carcinoma
Adults: Give 400 mg P.O. b.i.d. at least 1 hour before or 2 hours after eating. Continue until disease progresses or unacceptable toxicity occurs.
Adjust-a-dose: If grade 2 skin toxicity (pain and swelling with normal activities) develops, continue treatment and use topical drugs to relieve symptoms. If symptoms don't improve in 1 week or if they occur a second or third time, stop treatment until toxicity resolves to grade 0 or 1 (able to perform daily activities). Resume treatment at 400 mg daily or every other day. At fourth occurrence of grade 2 toxicity, stop treatment. If grade 3 skin toxicity (ulceration, blistering, severe, debilitating pain of hands and feet) or a second occurrence develops, stop treatment until toxicity resolves to grade 0 or 1. Resume treatment at 400 mg daily or every other day. At third occurrence of grade 3 toxicity, stop treatment.

ACTION
Decreases tumor cell proliferation by interacting with multiple intracellular and cell-surface kinases that may influence growth of new blood vessels into a tumor.

Route	Onset	Peak	Duration
P.O.	Unknown	3 hr	Unknown

Half-life: 1 to 2 days

ADVERSE REACTIONS

CNS: *asthenia, fatigue, headache, neuropathy,* depression.
CV: *hypertension.*
EENT: *hoarseness.*
GI: *abdominal pain, anorexia, constipation, diarrhea, nausea, vomiting,* dyspepsia, dysphagia, mucositis, stomatitis.
GU: erectile dysfunction.
Hematologic: *bleeding,* ***hemorrhage, leukopenia, lymphopenia, neutropenia, thrombocytopenia,*** anemia.
Metabolic: *weight loss,* hypothyroidism.
Musculoskeletal: *joint pain,* arthralgia, myalgia.
Respiratory: *cough, dyspnea.*
Skin: *alopecia, dry skin, erythema, hand-foot reaction, pruritus, rash,* acne, exfoliative dermatitis, flushing.
Other: flulike illness, pyrexia.

INTERACTIONS

Drug-drug. *CYP2B6 or CYP2C8 substrates:* May increase levels of these drugs. Use cautiously together.
CYP3A4 inducers (such as carbamazepine, dexamethasone, phenobarbital, phenytoin, rifampin): May increase sorafenib metabolism and decrease its effects. Monitor patient.
Doxorubicin, drugs metabolized by the UGT1A1 pathway (such as irinotecan): May increase levels of these drugs. Use cautiously together.
Warfarin: May increase the risk of bleeding. Monitor PT, INR, and patient for bleeding.
Drug-herb. *St. John's wort:* May decrease drug effects. Discourage use together.

EFFECTS ON LAB TEST RESULTS

- May increase TSH, lipase, amylase, transaminase, and bilirubin levels. May decrease phosphate levels.
- May decrease RBC, WBC, and platelet counts.

CONTRAINDICATIONS & CAUTIONS

- Contraindicated in patients severely hypersensitive to drug or its components.
- Use cautiously in patients with bleeding disorders, healing wounds, current or previous hand-foot skin reactions, or liver, renal, or cardiac disease, such as hypertension, cardiac ischemia, or a history of MI.

NURSING CONSIDERATIONS

- To avoid serious drug interactions, take a careful drug history.
- Monitor patient closely for hand-foot skin reaction, especially during the first 6 weeks of treatment.
- Measure blood pressure weekly during the first 6 weeks of treatment to check for hypertension.
- If patient is scheduled for major surgery, inform the surgeon that patient is taking this drug; therapy should be stopped. Monitor incision for adequate healing before restarting.
- Monitor patient for symptoms of cardiac ischemia.
- Assess patient for unusual bruising or bleeding.
- Provide patient with contact information for cancer support groups and instructions for managing adverse effects.
- ***Alert:*** Warn women to avoid pregnancy during and for 2 weeks following treatment.

PATIENT TEACHING

- Tell patient to swallow tablet whole, 1 hour before or 2 hours after a meal, with water.
- Remind patient to have his blood pressure checked weekly for the first 6 weeks of treatment and as needed throughout therapy.
- Explain that hair loss, nausea, vomiting, diarrhea, and fatigue are common.
- Inform patient that mild to moderate skin reactions are common. Tell him to notify prescriber if they occur. If they're severe, treatment may have to be stopped or dosage reduced. Urge patient to report pain, redness, blisters, or skin ulceration to prescriber immediately.
- Tell patient to report bleeding episodes right away.
- Tell patient to notify prescriber if chest pain or other serious heart problems develop.
- ***Alert:*** Drug may cause serious birth defects or fetal death. Advise women not to become pregnant during treatment and for at least 2 weeks after. Men should also avoid fathering children at this time.
- Tell patient to keep an up-to-date list of all drugs he takes and to tell all health care

providers, including dentists, that he takes this drug.

✱ NEW DRUG

sunitinib malate

Sutent

Pharmacologic class: multikinase inhibitor

Pregnancy risk category D

AVAILABLE FORMS

Capsules: 12.5 mg, 25 mg, 50 mg

INDICATIONS & DOSAGES

➤**GI stromal tumor that's progressing despite imatinib therapy or because patient is intolerant of imatinib; advanced renal cell carcinoma**

Adults: 50 mg P.O. once daily for 4 weeks, followed by 2 weeks off the drug. Repeat cycle.

Adjust-a-dose: Increase or decrease dosage in 12.5-mg increments based on individual safety and tolerability.

ACTION

A multikinase inhibitor targeting several receptor tyrosine kinases (RTKs), which are involved in tumor growth, pathologic angiogenesis, and metastatic progression of cancer.

Route	Onset	Peak	Duration
P.O.	Rapid	6–12 hr	Unknown

Half-life: 40 to 60 hours; primary metabolite, 80 to 110 hours.

ADVERSE REACTIONS

CNS: *asthenia, dizziness, fatigue, fever, headache, peripheral neuropathy..*

CV: ***decreased left ventricular ejection fraction, thromboembolic events,*** hypertension, peripheral edema.

EENT: increased lacrimation, periorbital edema.

GI: ***GI perforation, pancreatitis,*** abdominal pain, altered taste, anorexia, appetite disturbance, burning sensation in mouth, constipation, diarrhea, dyspepsia, flatulence, mucositis, nausea, oral pain, stomatitis, vomiting.

Hematologic: *bleeding, leukopenia, lymphopenia,* **NEUTROPENIA, THROMBOCYTOPENIA,** anemia.

Metabolic: *dehydration, hypernatremia, hyperuricemia, hypokalemia,* hyperkalemia, hyponatremia, hypophosphatemia, hypothyroidism.

Musculoskeletal: *arthralgia, back pain, limb pain, myalgia.*

Respiratory: *cough, dyspnea.*

Skin: *alopecia, dry skin, hair color changes, hand-foot syndrome, rash, skin discoloration,* skin blistering.

Other: adrenal insufficiency, hypothyroidism.

INTERACTIONS

Drug-drug. *CYP3A4 inducers (such as carbamazepine, dexamethasone, phenobarbital, phenytoin, rifabutin, rifampin, rifapentine):* May decrease sunitinib level and effects. If use together can't be avoided, increase sunitinib dosage to 87.5 mg daily.

Strong CYP3A4 inhibitors (such as atazanavir, clarithromycin, indinavir, itraconazole, ketoconazole, nefazodone, nelfinavir, ritonavir, saquinavir, telithromycin, voriconazole): May increase sunitinib level and toxicity. If use together can't be avoided, decrease sunitinib dosage to 37.5 mg daily.

Drug-herb. *St. John's wort:* May cause an unpredictable decrease in drug level. Discourage use together.

Drug-food. *Grapefruit:* May increase drug level. Tell patient to avoid grapefruit.

EFFECTS ON LAB TEST RESULTS

- May increase AST, ALT, alkaline phosphatase, total and indirect bilirubin, amylase, lipase, creatinine, uric acid, and TSH levels. May decrease phosphorus and hemoglobin levels and hematocrit. May increase or decrease potassium and sodium levels.
- May decrease RBC, neutrophil, lymphocyte, leukocyte, and platelet counts.

CONTRAINDICATIONS & CAUTIONS

- Contraindicated in patients hypersensitive to drug or any of its components. Don't use in patients with non–small-cell lung cancer.

• Use cautiously in patients with a history of hypertension, MI, angina, coronary artery bypass graft, symptomatic heart failure, stroke, TIA, or pulmonary embolism.

NURSING CONSIDERATIONS
• Obtain CBC with platelet count and serum chemistries, including phosphate level, before each treatment cycle.
• Obtain baseline evaluation of ejection fraction in all patients before treatment. If patient had a cardiac event in the year before treatment, check ejection fraction periodically.
• Interrupt therapy or decrease dose in patients with an ejection fraction less than 50% and more than 20% below baseline.
• Monitor patient's blood pressure closely. If severe hypertension occurs, notify prescriber. Treatment may need to be held until blood pressure is controlled.
• Monitor patient for signs and symptoms of heart failure, especially if he has a history of heart disease. Notify prescriber if signs or symptoms of heart failure develop.
• If patient has seizures, he may have reversible posterior leukoencephalopathy syndrome. Signs and symptoms include hypertension, headache, decreased alertness, altered mental functioning, and vision loss. Stop treatment temporarily.
• If patient will be undergoing surgery or suffers trauma or severe infection, assess him for adrenal insufficiency (muscle weakness, weight loss, depression, salt craving, low blood pressure).
• Provide antiemetics or antidiarrheals as needed for adverse GI effects.

PATIENT TEACHING
• Advise patient to keep appointments for blood tests and periodic heart function evaluations.
• Tell patient about common adverse effects, such as diarrhea, nausea, vomiting, fatigue, mouth pain, and taste disturbance.
• Inform patient about changes that may occur in skin and hair, including color changes and dry, red, blistering skin of the hands and feet.
• Urge patient to tell health care provider about all prescribed and OTC drugs or herbal supplements.
• Warn patient not to consume grapefruit during therapy.
• Tell patient to notify his prescriber about unusual bleeding, trouble breathing, wheezing, severe or prolonged diarrhea or vomiting, or swelling of the hands or lower legs.

SAFETY ALERT!

teniposide (VM-26)
Vumon

Pharmacologic class: podophyllotoxin
Pregnancy risk category D

AVAILABLE FORMS
Injection: 10 mg/ml

INDICATIONS & DOSAGES
➤ **Refractory childhood acute lymphoblastic leukemia**
Children: Optimum dosage hasn't been established. Dosages ranging from 165 to 250 mg/m² I.V. once or twice weekly for 4 to 8 weeks have been used. Usually given with other chemotherapy.
Adjust-a-dose: Patients with both Down syndrome and leukemia are at higher risk for myelosuppression. Give first course of treatment at half the recommended dosage.

I.V. ADMINISTRATION
• Contains benzyl alcohol. Avoid use in neonates.
• Preparation and administration of parenteral form of drug may be mutagenic, teratogenic, or carcinogenic. Follow institutional policy to reduce risks.
• Use containers and tubing that don't contain DEHP.
• Dilute drug in either D_5W or normal saline solution for injection to 0.1, 0.2, 0.4, or 1 mg/ml. Don't agitate vigorously; precipitation may occur. Discard cloudy solutions. Prepare and store drug in glass containers.
• Flush administration apparatus and catheters with D_5W or normal saline solution before and after infusion of drug.
• Infuse over at least 30 to 60 minutes to prevent hypotension.
• Ensure correct placement of I.V. catheter. Extravasation can cause local tissue necrosis or sloughing.

- Occlusion of catheters can occur (including those centrally placed), particularly during 24-hour infusions at 0.1 to 0.2 mg/ml. Monitor catheters carefully.
- Don't use a membrane-type in-line filter because diluent may dissolve it.
- Monitor blood pressure every 30 minutes during infusion. If systolic blood pressure falls below 90 mm Hg, stop infusion and notify prescriber.
- In normal saline solution or D_5W, concentrations of 0.1 to 0.4 mg/ml in glass containers are chemically stable for up to 24 hours at room temperature. Give solutions with a concentration of 1 mg/ml within 4 hours to reduce possible precipitation. Refrigeration isn't recommended.

INCOMPATIBILITIES
Idarubicin. Heparin sodium may cause precipitation.

ACTION
A phase-specific cytotoxic drug that acts in the late S or early G_2 phase of the cell cycle, thus preventing cells from entering mitosis.

Route	Onset	Peak	Duration
I.V.	Unknown	Unknown	Unknown

Half-life: 5 hours.

ADVERSE REACTIONS
CNS: fever.
CV: hypotension.
GI: *diarrhea, mucositis, nausea, vomiting.*
Hematologic: LEUKOPENIA, MYELOSUPPRESSION, NEUTROPENIA, THROMBOCYTOPENIA, *anemia.*
Skin: *extravasation at injection site,* alopecia, rash.
Other: *infection, phlebitis,* ***anaphylaxis,*** bleeding, hypersensitivity reactions.

INTERACTIONS
Drug-drug. *Methotrexate:* May increase clearance and intracellular levels of methotrexate. Avoid using together.
Sodium salicylate, sulfamethizole, tolbutamide: May displace teniposide from protein-binding sites and increase toxicity. Avoid using together.

EFFECTS ON LAB TEST RESULTS
- May decrease hemoglobin level.
- May decrease WBC, platelet, and neutrophil counts.

CONTRAINDICATIONS & CAUTIONS
- Contraindicated in patients hypersensitive to drug or to polyoxyethylated castor oil, an injection vehicle.

NURSING CONSIDERATIONS
- Drug may be prescribed despite patient's history of hypersensitivity. Treat such patients with antihistamines and corticosteroids before infusion begins, and observe continuously for first hour of infusion and at frequent intervals thereafter.
- Obtain baseline blood counts and renal and hepatic function tests and monitor regularly.
- Monitor blood pressure before and during therapy. Hypotension can occur from rapid infusion.
- Have on hand diphenhydramine, hydrocortisone, epinephrine, and emergency equipment to establish an airway in case of anaphylaxis. Signs of hypersensitivity include chills, fever, urticaria, tachycardia, bronchospasm, dyspnea, hypotension, and flushing.

PATIENT TEACHING
- Advise patient to report any pain or burning at site of injection during or after administration.
- Tell patient to report signs and symptoms of infection (fever, sore throat, fatigue) and bleeding (easy bruising, nosebleeds, bleeding gums, tarry stools). Tell patient to take temperature daily.
- Caution woman to avoid becoming pregnant during therapy and to consult prescriber before becoming pregnant.

SAFETY ALERT!

topotecan hydrochloride
Hycamtin

Pharmacologic class: DNA topoisomerase inhibitor
Pregnancy risk category D

AVAILABLE FORMS
Injection: 4-mg single-dose vial

INDICATIONS & DOSAGES

✷*NEW INDICATION:* **With cisplatin, stage-IVB, recurrent or persistent cervical cancer unresponsive to surgery or radiation**

Adults: Give 0.75 mg/m² by I.V. infusion over 30 minutes on days 1, 2, and 3, followed by 50 mg/m² cisplatin by I.V. infusion on day 1. Repeat cycle q 21 days. Adjust subsequent doses of each drug based on hematologic toxicities.

➤ **Metastatic carcinoma of the ovary after failure of first or subsequent chemotherapy; small-cell lung cancer-sensitive disease after failure of first-line chemotherapy**

Adults: 1.5 mg/m² I.V. infusion given over 30 minutes daily for 5 consecutive days, starting on day 1 of a 21-day cycle. Give a minimum of four cycles.

Adjust-a-dose: For patients with creatinine clearance of 20 to 39 ml/minute, decrease dosage to 0.75 mg/m². If severe neutropenia occurs, decrease dosage by 0.25 mg/m² for subsequent courses. Or, if severe neutropenia occurs, give granulocyte colony-stimulating factor after subsequent course (before resorting to dosage reduction) starting from day 6 of course (24 hours after completion of topotecan administration).

I.V. ADMINISTRATION

- Protect unopened vials from light.
- Reconstitute each 4-mg vial with 4 ml sterile water for injection. Dilute appropriate volume of reconstituted solution in either normal saline solution or D_5W before giving.
- Lyophilized form contains no antibacterial preservative; use reconstituted product immediately.
- Monitor insertion site during infusion. Extravasation has been linked to mild local reactions, such as erythema and bruising.
- If stored at 68° to 77° F (20° to 25° C) and exposed to normal lighting, reconstituted drug is stable for 24 hours.

INCOMPATIBILITIES

Dexamethasone, fluorouracil, mitomycin, ticarcillin disodium and clavulanate potassium.

ACTION

Interacts with topoisomerase I, inducing reversible single-strand DNA breaks. Drug binds to the topoisomerase I–DNA complex and prevents relegation of these single-strand breaks.

Route	Onset	Peak	Duration
I.V.	Unknown	Unknown	Unknown

Half-life: 2 to 3 hours.

ADVERSE REACTIONS

CNS: *asthenia, fatigue, fever, headache.*
GI: *abdominal pain, anorexia, constipation, diarrhea, nausea, stomatitis, vomiting.*
Hematologic: *anemia,* **LEUKOPENIA, NEUTROPENIA, THROMBOCYTOPENIA.**
Hepatic: ***hepatotoxicity.***
Musculoskeletal: *back and skeletal pain.*
Respiratory: *coughing, dyspnea.*
Skin: *alopecia,* rash.
Other: ***sepsis.***

INTERACTIONS

Drug-drug. *Cisplatin:* May increase severity of myelosuppression. Use together with extreme caution.

Granulocyte colony-stimulating factor: May prolong duration of neutropenia. If granulocyte colony-stimulating factor is to be used, don't start it until day 6 of the course, 24 hours after completion of topotecan treatment.

EFFECTS ON LAB TEST RESULTS

- May increase ALT, AST, and bilirubin levels. May decrease hemoglobin level.
- May decrease WBC, platelet, and neutrophil counts.

CONTRAINDICATIONS & CAUTIONS

- Contraindicated in patients hypersensitive to drug or its components and in those with severe bone marrow depression.
- Contraindicated in pregnant or breast-feeding women.
- Safety and effectiveness of drug in children haven't been established.

NURSING CONSIDERATIONS

- ***Alert:*** Before first course of therapy is started, patient must have baseline neutro-

phil count more than 1,500/mm^3 and platelet count more than 100,000/mm^3.
- Monitor peripheral blood counts frequently. Don't give subsequent courses until neutrophil count recovers to more than 1,000 cells/mm^3, platelet count recovers to more than 100,000/mm^3, and hemoglobin level recovers to more than 9 mg/dl (with transfusion, if needed).
- Prepare drug under vertical laminar flow hood; wear gloves and protective clothing. If drug solution contacts skin, wash immediately and thoroughly with soap and water. If mucous membranes are affected, flush areas thoroughly with water.
- Bone marrow suppression indicates toxic levels of topotecan. The nadir occurs at about 11 days. Neutropenia isn't cumulative over time.
- Duration of thrombocytopenia is about 5 days, with nadir at 15 days. The nadir for anemia is 15 days. Blood or platelet transfusions may be needed.
- WBC colony-stimulating factors may promote cell growth and decrease risk for infection.

PATIENT TEACHING
- Urge patient to report promptly sore throat, fever, chills, or unusual bleeding or bruising.
- Caution women to avoid pregnancy or breast-feeding during therapy.
- Teach patient and family about drug's adverse reactions and need for frequent monitoring of blood counts.

SAFETY ALERT!

trastuzumab
Herceptin

Pharmacologic class: monoclonal antibody
Pregnancy risk category B

AVAILABLE FORMS
Lyophilized powder for injection: 440 mg/vial

INDICATIONS & DOSAGES
➤Metastatic breast cancer in patients whose tumors overexpress the human epidermal growth factor receptor 2 (HER2) protein
Adults: Give loading dose of 4 mg/kg I.V. over 90 minutes. If tolerated, continue with 2 mg/kg I.V. weekly as 30-minute infusion. If patient hasn't previously received one or more chemotherapy regimens for their metastatic disease, drug is given with paclitaxel.

I.V. ADMINISTRATION
- Reconstitute drug in each vial with 20 ml of bacteriostatic water for injection, 1.1% benzyl alcohol preserved, as supplied, to yield a multidose solution containing 21 mg/ml. Don't shake vial during reconstitution. Make sure reconstituted preparation is colorless to pale yellow and free of particulates. Immediately after reconstitution, label vial with expiration 28 days from date of reconstitution.
- If patient is hypersensitive to benzyl alcohol, reconstitute drug with sterile water for injection, use immediately, and discard unused portion. Avoid use of other reconstitution diluents.
- Determine dose based on loading dose of 4 mg/kg or maintenance dose of 2 mg/kg. Calculate volume of 21-mg/ml solution and withdraw this amount from vial and add it to an infusion bag containing 250 ml of normal saline solution. Don't use D_5W or dextrose-containing solutions. Gently invert bag to mix solution.
- Don't give as I.V. push or bolus.
- Infuse loading dose over 90 minutes. If well tolerated, infuse maintenance doses over 30 minutes.
- Vials are stable at 36° to 46° F (2° to 8° C). Discard reconstituted solution after 28 days. Don't freeze drug that has been reconstituted. Store solution of drug diluted in normal saline solution for injection at 36° to 46° F (2° to 8° C) before use; it's stable for up to 24 hours.

INCOMPATIBILITIES
Other I.V. drugs or dextrose solutions.

ACTION
A recombinant DNA-derived monoclonal antibody that selectively binds to HER2, inhibiting proliferation of tumor cells that overexpress HER2.

Route	Onset	Peak	Duration
I.V.	Unknown	Unknown	Unknown

Half-life: Range, 1 to 32 days; mean, 5¾ days.

ADVERSE REACTIONS
CNS: *asthenia, dizziness, fever, headache, insomnia, pain,* depression, neuropathy, paresthesia, peripheral neuritis.
CV: *peripheral edema,* ***heart failure,*** hypotension, tachycardia.
EENT: *pharyngitis, rhinitis,* sinusitis.
GI: *abdominal pain, anorexia, diarrhea, nausea, vomiting.*
GU: UTI.
Hematologic: ***leukopenia,*** anemia.
Musculoskeletal: *back pain,* arthralgia, bone pain.
Respiratory: *dyspnea, increased cough.*
Skin: *rash,* acne.
Other: **ANAPHYLAXIS,** *chills, flulike syndrome, infection,* allergic reaction, herpes simplex.

INTERACTIONS
Drug-drug. *Anthracyclines, cyclophosphamide:* May increase cardiotoxicity. Use together very cautiously.

EFFECTS ON LAB TEST RESULTS
- May decrease hemoglobin level.
- May decrease WBC count.

CONTRAINDICATIONS & CAUTIONS
- Contraindicated in patients hypersensitive to the drug.
- Use cautiously in elderly patients, in patients hypersensitive to drug or its components, and in those with cardiac dysfunction.
- Give drug with extreme caution in patients with pulmonary compromise, symptomatic intrinsic pulmonary disease (such as asthma, COPD), or extensive tumor involvement of the lungs.
- Safety and effectiveness of drug in children haven't been established.

NURSING CONSIDERATIONS
- Before beginning therapy, patient should undergo thorough baseline cardiac assessment, including history and physical examination and methods to identify risk of cardiotoxicity.
- Assess patient for signs and symptoms of cardiac dysfunction, especially if he is receiving drug with anthracyclines and cyclophosphamide.
- Check for dyspnea, increased cough, paroxysmal nocturnal dyspnea, peripheral edema, or S_3 gallop. Treatment may be stopped in patients who develop a significant decrease in left ventricular function.
- Monitor patient receiving both drug and chemotherapy closely for cardiac dysfunction or failure, anemia, leukopenia, diarrhea, and infection.
- Drug is only for patients with metastatic breast cancer whose tumors have HER2 protein overexpression.
- Check for first-infusion symptom complex, commonly consisting of chills or fever. Give acetaminophen, diphenhydramine, and meperidine (with or without reducing rate of infusion). Other signs or symptoms include nausea, vomiting, pain, rigors, headache, dizziness, dyspnea, hypotension, rash, and asthenia and occur infrequently with subsequent infusions.

PATIENT TEACHING
- Tell patient about risk of first-dose infusion-related adverse reactions.
- Urge patient to notify prescriber immediately if signs or symptoms of heart problems occur, such as shortness of breath, increased cough, or swelling in arms or legs. Tell patient that these effects can occur after infusion is complete.
- Instruct patient to report adverse effects to prescriber.
- Advise woman to stop breast-feeding during drug therapy and for 6 months after last dose of drug.

SAFETY ALERT!

vinblastine sulfate (VLB)
Velban, Velbe†‡

Pharmacologic class: vinca alkaloid
Pregnancy risk category D

AVAILABLE FORMS
Injection: 10-mg vials (lyophilized powder), 1 mg/ml in 10-ml and 25-ml vials

INDICATIONS & DOSAGES

➤ **Breast or testicular cancer, Hodgkin and malignant lymphoma, choriocarcinoma, lymphosarcoma, mycosis fungoides, Kaposi sarcoma, histiocytosis**

Adults: 3.7 mg/m^2 I.V. weekly. May increase to maximum dose of 18.5 mg/m^2 I.V. weekly based on response. Don't repeat dose if WBC count is below 4,000/mm^3. Increase dosage at weekly intervals in increments of 1.8 mg/m^2 until desired therapeutic response is obtained, leukocyte count decreases to 3,000/mm^3, or maximum weekly dose of 18.5 mg/m^2 is reached.

Children: First dose is 2.5 mg/m^2 I.V. weekly. Increase dosage by 1.25 mg/m^2 weekly until WBC count is below 3,000/mm^3 or tumor response is seen. Maximum dose is 12.5 mg/m^2 I.V. weekly.

Adjust-a-dose: For patients with direct bilirubin over 3 mg/dl, reduce dose by 50%. For patients with recent exposure to radiation therapy or chemotherapy, single doses usually don't exceed 5.5 mg/m^2. Once a dose is determined to produce a WBC count below 3,000/mm^3, give maintenance doses of one increment less than this amount at weekly intervals.

I.V. ADMINISTRATION

- Preparing and giving drug may be mutagenic, teratogenic, or carcinogenic. Follow institutional policy to reduce risks.
- Drug is fatal if given intrathecally; it's for I.V. use only.
- Reconstitute drug in 10-mg vial with 10 ml of bacteriostatic saline solution for injection. Don't use other diluents. This yields 1 mg/ml. Protect solution from light.
- Inject drug directly into vein or tubing of running I.V. line over 1 minute. Drug is a vesicant; if extravasation occurs, stop infusion immediately and notify prescriber. The manufacturer recommends that moderate heat be applied to area of leakage. Local injection of hyaluronidase may help disperse drug. Moderate heat may be applied on and off every 2 hours for 24 hours, with local injection of hydrocortisone or normal saline solution.
- Drug reconstituted with diluent containing preservatives is stable for 28 days if refrigerated. Immediately discard any unused portion of solution reconstituted with diluent that doesn't contain preservatives.

INCOMPATIBILITIES

Cefepime, doxorubicin, furosemide, heparin.

ACTION

Arrests mitosis in metaphase, blocking cell division.

Route	Onset	Peak	Duration
I.V.	Unknown	Unknown	Unknown

Half-life: Initial phase, 3 minutes; second phase, 1½ hours; terminal phase, 25 hours.

ADVERSE REACTIONS

CNS: *numbness, paresthesia, peripheral neuropathy and neuritis,* ***seizures, stroke,*** depression, headache.
CV: ***MI,*** hypertension.
EENT: pharyngitis.
GI: *anorexia, constipation, ileus, nausea, stomatitis, vomiting,* abdominal pain, bleeding ulcer, diarrhea.
Hematologic: *anemia,* ***leukopenia, thrombocytopenia.***
Metabolic: *weight loss,* hyperuricemia, SIADH.
Musculoskeletal: *loss of deep tendon reflexes, muscle pain and weakness,* jaw pain.
Respiratory: ***acute bronchospasm,*** shortness of breath.
Skin: *irritation, phlebitis,* cellulitis, reversible alopecia, vesiculation and necrosis with extravasation.

INTERACTIONS

Drug-drug. *Azole antifungals, erythromycin,* *other drugs that inhibit cytochrome P-450 pathway:* May increase toxicity of vinblastine. Monitor patient closely for toxicity.
Mitomycin: May increase risk of bronchospasm and shortness of breath. Monitor patient's respiratory status.
Ototoxic drugs such as platinum-containing antineoplastics: May cause temporary or permanent hearing impairment. Monitor hearing function.
Phenytoin: May decrease plasma phenytoin level. Monitor phenytoin level closely.

EFFECTS ON LAB TEST RESULTS
- May increase uric acid and bilirubin levels. May decrease hemoglobin level.
- May decrease WBC and platelet counts.

CONTRAINDICATIONS & CAUTIONS
- Contraindicated in patients with severe leukopenia or bacterial infection or in patients hypersensitive to the drug.
- Use cautiously in patients with hepatic dysfunction.

NURSING CONSIDERATIONS
- To reduce nausea, give antiemetic before drug.
- Don't give drug into a limb with compromised circulation.
- ***Alert:*** After giving drug, check for development of life-threatening acute bronchospasm. If this occurs, notify prescriber immediately. Reaction is most likely to occur in patients who are also receiving mitomycin.
- Monitor patient for stomatitis. If stomatitis occurs, stop drug and notify prescriber.
- Assess bowel activity. Give laxatives as indicated. Stool softeners may be used prophylactically.
- Don't repeat dosage more frequently than every 7 days or severe leukopenia will occur. Nadir occurs on days 4 to 10 and lasts another 7 to 14 days.
- Assess patient for numbness and tingling in hands and feet. Assess gait for early evidence of footdrop.
- Drug is less neurotoxic than vincristine.
- Stop drugs known to cause urine retention for first few days after therapy, particularly in elderly patients.
- ***Look alike–sound alike:*** Don't confuse vinblastine with vincristine or vinorelbine.

PATIENT TEACHING
- Tell patient to report evidence of infection (fever, sore throat, fatigue) and bleeding (easy bruising, nosebleeds, bleeding gums, tarry stools). Tell patient to take temperature daily.
- Urge patient to report pain, swelling, burning, or any unusual feeling at injection site during infusion.
- Warn patient that hair loss may occur but that it's usually temporary.
- Caution woman to avoid pregnancy during therapy.
- Tell patient that pain may occur in jaw and in the organ with the tumor.

SAFETY ALERT!

vincristine sulfate (VCR)
Oncovin, Vincasar PFS

Pharmacologic class: vinca alkaloid
Pregnancy risk category D

AVAILABLE FORMS
Injection: 1 mg/ml in 1-ml, 2-ml, 5-ml multidose vials; 1 mg/ml in 1-ml, 2-ml, 5-ml preservative-free vials

INDICATIONS & DOSAGES
➤ **Acute lymphoblastic and other leukemias, Hodgkin lymphoma, malignant lymphoma, neuroblastoma, rhabdomyosarcoma, Wilms tumor**
Adults: 1.4 mg/m^2 I.V. weekly. Maximum weekly dose is 2 mg.
Children who weigh more than 10 kg (22 lb): Give 1.5 to 2 mg/m^2 I.V. weekly.
Children who weigh 10 kg and less or with body surface area less than 1 m^2: Initially, 0.05 mg/kg I.V. weekly.
Adjust-a-dose: For patients with direct bilirubin over 3 mg/dl, reduce dose by 50%.

I.V. ADMINISTRATION
- Preparing and giving drug may be mutagenic, teratogenic, or carcinogenic. Follow institutional policy to reduce risks.
- Inject directly into vein or tubing of running I.V. line, slowly over 1 minute. Drug is a vesicant; if it extravasates, stop infusion immediately and notify prescriber. Apply heat on and off every 2 hours for 24 hours.
- If protocol requires a continuous infusion, use a central line.
- All vials contain 1 mg/ml solution; refrigerate them.

INCOMPATIBILITIES
Cefepime, furosemide, idarubicin, sodium bicarbonate.

ACTION

Arrests mitosis in metaphase, blocking cell division.

Route	Onset	Peak	Duration
I.V.	Unknown	Unknown	Unknown

Half-life: Initial phase, 4 minutes; second phase, 2¼ hours; terminal phase, 3½ days.

ADVERSE REACTIONS

CNS: *loss of deep tendon reflexes, paresthesia, peripheral neuropathy,* ***coma, seizures,*** ataxia, cranial nerve palsies, fever, headache, sensory loss.
CV: hypertension, hypotension.
EENT: blindness, diplopia, hoarseness, optic and extraocular neuropathy, photophobia, ptosis, visual disturbances, vocal cord paralysis.
GI: *constipation, cramps, nausea, stomatitis, vomiting,* ***intestinal necrosis,*** anorexia, diarrhea, dysphagia, ileus that mimics surgical abdomen, paralytic ileus.
GU: dysuria, polyuria, SIADH, urine retention.
Hematologic: ***leukopenia, thrombocytopenia,*** anemia.
Metabolic: hyponatremia, weight loss.
Musculoskeletal: *cramps, jaw pain, muscle weakness.*
Respiratory: ***acute bronchospasm,*** dyspnea.
Skin: *phlebitis,* cellulitis at injection site, rash, reversible alopecia, severe local reaction following extravasation.

INTERACTIONS

Drug-drug. *Asparaginase:* May decrease hepatic clearance of vincristine. Use together also may result in additive neurotoxicity. Monitor patient for toxicity.
Digoxin: May decrease digoxin's effects. Monitor digoxin level.
Mitomycin: May increase frequency of bronchospasm and acute pulmonary reactions. Monitor patient's respiratory status.
Ototoxic drugs: May potentiate loss of hearing. Use together with caution.
Phenytoin: May reduce phenytoin level. Monitor phenytoin level closely.

EFFECTS ON LAB TEST RESULTS

- May decrease sodium and hemoglobin levels. May increase uric acid level.
- May decrease WBC and platelet counts.

CONTRAINDICATIONS & CAUTIONS

- Contraindicated in patients hypersensitive to drug and in those with demyelinating form of Charcot-Marie-Tooth syndrome.
- Don't give to patients who are receiving radiation therapy through ports that include the liver.
- Use cautiously in patients with hepatic dysfunction, neuromuscular disease, or infection.

NURSING CONSIDERATIONS

- Don't use the 5-mg vials for single doses.
- ***Alert:*** Patient also taking mitomycin has a higher risk of life-threatening bronchospasm. Monitor him after dose, and notify prescriber immediately if it occurs.
- Watch for hyperuricemia, especially in patients with leukemia or lymphoma. Maintain hydration and give allopurinol to prevent uric acid nephropathy. Watch for toxicity.
- If SIADH develops, fluid restriction may be needed. Monitor fluid intake and output.
- Because of risk of neurotoxicity, don't give drug more often than once weekly. Children are more resistant to neurotoxicity than adults. Neurotoxicity is dose related and usually reversible.
- Elderly patients and those with underlying neurologic disease may be more susceptible to neurotoxic effects.
- Monitor patient for Achilles tendon reflex depression, numbness, tingling, footdrop or wristdrop, difficulty walking, ataxia, and slapping gait. Monitor his ability to walk on heels. Support him while walking.
- Monitor bowel function. Give stool softener, laxative, or water before giving dose. Constipation may be an early sign of neurotoxicity.
- Stop drugs known to cause urine retention, particularly in elderly patients, for first few days after therapy.
- ***Alert:*** Drug is fatal if given intrathecally; it's for I.V. use only.

• ***Look alike–sound alike:*** Don't confuse vincristine with vinblastine or vinorelbine.

PATIENT TEACHING

• Advise patient to report any pain or burning at site of injection during or after administration.
• Tell patient to report evidence of infection (fever, sore throat, fatigue) and bleeding (easy bruising, nosebleeds, bleeding gums, tarry stools). Tell patient to take temperature daily.
• Warn patient that hair loss may occur, but explain that it's usually temporary.
• Caution woman to avoid becoming pregnant during therapy and to consult prescriber before becoming pregnant.

SAFETY ALERT!

vinorelbine tartrate

Navelbine

Pharmacologic class: semisynthetic vinca alkaloid
Pregnancy risk category D

AVAILABLE FORMS

Injection: 10 mg/ml, 50 mg/5 ml

INDICATIONS & DOSAGES

➤ **Alone or as adjunct therapy with cisplatin for first-line treatment of ambulatory patients with nonresectable advanced non–small-cell lung cancer (NSCLC); alone or with cisplatin in stage IV of NSCLC; with cisplatin in stage III of NSCLC**
Adults: 30 mg/m^2 I.V. weekly. In combination treatment, same dosage with 120 mg/m^2 of cisplatin given on days 1 and 29, and then q 6 weeks.
Adjust-a-dose: If granulocyte count is 1,000/mm^3 to 1,499/mm^3, give 50% of dose. If less than 1,000/mm^3, dose is withheld. If total bilirubin is 2.1 to 3 mg/dl, reduce dose by 50%; if more than 3 mg/dl, give 25% of dose.
➤ **Breast cancer ♦**
Adults: 20 to 30 mg/m^2 I.V. once weekly.

I.V. ADMINISTRATION

• Drug may be a contact irritant; handle and give with care. Wear gloves. Avoid inhaling vapors and allowing contact with skin or mucous membranes, especially those of the eyes. In case of contact, wash with generous amounts of water for at least 15 minutes.
• Dilute drug before use to 1.5 to 3 mg/ml with D_5W or normal saline solution in a syringe. Or, dilute to 0.5 to 2 mg/ml in an I.V. bag.
• Give drug I.V. over 6 to 10 minutes into side port of a free-flowing I.V. line that is closest to I.V. bag; then flush with 75 to 125 ml or more of D_5W or normal saline solution.
• Monitor site for irritation and infiltration because drug can cause localized tissue damage and necrosis and thrombophlebitis. If extravasation occurs, stop drug immediately and inject remaining dose into a different vein; notify prescriber.
• Drug may be stored for up to 24 hours at room temperature.

INCOMPATIBILITIES

Acyclovir, allopurinol, aminophylline, amphotericin B, ampicillin sodium, cefazolin, cefoperazone, ceftriaxone, cefuroxime, fluorouracil, furosemide, ganciclovir, methylprednisolone, mitomycin, piperacillin, sodium bicarbonate, thiotepa, trimethoprim-sulfamethoxazole.

ACTION

A semisynthetic vinca alkaloid that exerts its primary antineoplastic effect by disrupting microtubule assembly, which in turn disrupts spindle formation and prevents mitosis.

Route	Onset	Peak	Duration
I.V.	Unknown	Unknown	Unknown

Half-life: About 27 to 43½ hours.

ADVERSE REACTIONS

CNS: *asthenia, fatigue, peripheral neuropathy.*
CV: chest pain.
GI: *anorexia, constipation, diarrhea, nausea, stomatitis, vomiting.*
Hematologic: *anemia,* ***agranulocytosis, bone marrow suppression, granulocytopenia, thrombocytopenia,*** LEUKOPENIA.
Hepatic: hyperbilirubinemia.

Musculoskeletal: arthralgia, jaw pain, loss of deep tendon reflexes, myalgia.
Respiratory: dyspnea, shortness of breath.
Skin: *alopecia, injection pain or reaction,* rash.

INTERACTIONS

Drug-drug. *Cisplatin:* May increase risk of bone marrow suppression when used with cisplatin. Monitor hematologic status closely.
Cytochrome P-450 inhibitors: May decrease metabolism of vinorelbine. Watch for increased adverse effects.
Mitomycin: May cause pulmonary reactions. Monitor respiratory status closely.
Paclitaxel: May increase risk of neuropathy. Monitor patient closely.

EFFECTS ON LAB TEST RESULTS

- May increase bilirubin level. May decrease hemoglobin level.
- May increase liver function test values. May decrease granulocyte, WBC, and platelet counts.

CONTRAINDICATIONS & CAUTIONS

- Contraindicated in patients with pretreatment granulocyte count below 1,000/mm^3 and in patients hypersensitive to the drug.
- Use with caution in patients whose bone marrow may have been compromised by previous exposure to radiation therapy or chemotherapy or whose bone marrow is still recovering from chemotherapy.
- Use with caution in patients with hepatic impairment.
- Safety and effectiveness in children haven't been established.

NURSING CONSIDERATIONS

- Check patient's granulocyte count before administration; make sure count is 1,000/mm^3 or higher before giving drug. If count is lower, withhold drug and notify prescriber. Granulocyte count nadir occurs between days 7 and 10.
- ***Alert:*** Drug is fatal if given intrathecally; it's for I.V. use only.
- Adjust dosage by hematologic toxicity or hepatic insufficiency, whichever results in the lower dosage. If granulocyte count falls below 1,500/mm^3 but is greater than 1,000/mm^3, reduce dosage by 50%. If three consecutive doses are skipped because of agranulocytosis, don't resume therapy.
- In patients with hepatic impairment, monitor liver enzyme levels.
- Patient may receive injections of WBC colony-stimulating factors to promote cell growth and decrease risk of infection.
- ***Alert:*** Monitor deep tendon reflexes; loss may represent cumulative toxicity.
- Monitor patient closely for hypersensitivity.
- As a guide to the effects of therapy, monitor patient's peripheral blood count and bone marrow.
- ***Look alike–sound alike:*** Don't confuse vinorelbine with vinblastine or vincristine.

PATIENT TEACHING

- Advise patient to report any pain or burning at site of injection.
- Instruct patient not to take other drugs, including OTC preparations, until approved by prescriber.
- Tell patient to report evidence of infection (fever, sore throat, fatigue) and bleeding (easy bruising, nosebleeds, bleeding gums, tarry stools). Tell him to take temperature daily.
- Advise patient to report increased shortness of breath, cough, abdominal pain, or constipation.
- Caution woman to avoid becoming pregnant during therapy.

✷ NEW DRUG

vorinostat

Zolinza

Pharmacologic class: histone deacetylase (HDAC) inhibitor
Pregnancy risk category D

AVAILABLE FORMS

Capsules: 100 mg

INDICATIONS & DOSAGES

➤ **Cutaneous T-cell lymphoma in patients who have progressive, persistent or recurrent disease on or following two systemic therapies**
Adults: 400 mg P.O. once daily with food. If patient doesn't tolerate drug, decrease

dose to 300 mg once daily. If necessary, may then reduce frequency to 5 consecutive days per week. Continue until there is evidence of disease progression or unacceptable toxicity.

ACTION

Drug inhibits enzymatic activity of HDAC, inducing cell cycle arrest and programmed cell death of some transformed cells.

Route	Onset	Peak	Duration
P.O.	Unknown	2–10 hr	Unknown

Half-life: 2 hours for drug and one metabolite; 11 hours for the other metabolite.

ADVERSE REACTIONS

CNS: *fatigue, fever, chills, dizziness, headache.*
CV: ***deep vein thrombosis, prolonged QT interval.***
GI: *diarrhea, nausea, dysgeusia, dry mouth, vomiting, constipation.*
Hematologic: *anemia,* ***thrombocytopenia.***
Metabolic: *anorexia, weight loss, hyperglycemia.*
Musculoskeletal: *muscle spasms.*
Respiratory: ***pulmonary embolism (PE),*** *cough, upper respiratory infection.*
Skin: ***squamous cell carcinoma,*** *alopecia, pruritus.*
Other: *peripheral edema.*

INTERACTIONS

Drug-drug. *Warfarin:* May prolong PT and INR and increase the risk of bleeding. Carefully monitor PT/INR.
Other HDAC inhibitors (such as valproic acid): May cause severe thrombocytopenia and GI bleeding. Monitor platelet count every 2 weeks for the first 2 months of therapy and then monthly thereafter.

EFFECTS ON LAB TEST RESULTS

- May increase glucose and serum creatinine levels.
- May decrease RBC and platelet counts.
- May cause proteinuria.

CONTRAINDICATIONS & CAUTIONS

- No known contraindications.
- Use cautiously in patients with a history of thromboembolism, or in those with thrombocytopenia, anemia, diabetes or high glucose level; prolonged QT interval; hepatic or renal insufficiency; or in women who may become pregnant.

NURSING CONSIDERATIONS

- If hemoglobin or platelet counts decrease, notify prescriber; dose may need to be changed or therapy interrupted.
- Provide fluids, antidiarrheals, and antiemetics as needed.
- Monitor blood counts, creatinine, and electrolytes every 2 weeks for first 2 months and monthly thereafter.
- Correct electrolyte imbalances, especially in potassium, magnesium and calcium, before therapy.
- Obtain a baseline and periodic ECG to check for prolonged QTc.
- Monitor glucose level carefully in patients with diabetes or high glucose levels. Provide nutritional counseling, as appropriate.
- Be alert for symptoms of deep vein thrombosis or PE.
- Monitor patient for unusual or easy bruising.

PATIENT TEACHING

- Remind patient to take drug exactly as prescribed; tell him to swallow each capsule whole and take with food.
- Caution patient to not let any of the dry powder within the capsule come in contact with his skin or mucous membranes.
- Advise patient to drink at least eight 8-ounce glasses of water daily to avoid dehydration.
- Explain the importance of regular blood tests to monitor effects of drug.
- Inform patient to tell the prescriber of any history of blood clots, high glucose level or diabetes, nausea, vomiting, diarrhea, or heart problems.
- Advise women to avoid pregnancy because of the risk of fetal harm.

72

Immunosuppressants

✱ NEW DRUG

abatacept

Orencia

Pharmacologic class: immunomodulator
Pregnancy risk category C

AVAILABLE FORMS

Lyophilized powder for injection: 250 mg/15-ml single-use vial

INDICATIONS & DOSAGES

➤ **To reduce signs and symptoms and structural damage and improve physical function in patients with moderate to severe rheumatoid arthritis whose response to one or more disease-modifying drugs has been inadequate. Used alone or with other disease-modifying drugs (except tumor necrosis factor [TNF] antagonists and anakinra)**

Adults weighing more than 100 kg (220 lb): 1 g I.V. over 30 minutes. Repeat 2 and 4 weeks after initial infusion and then every 4 weeks thereafter.

Adults weighing 60 to 100 kg (132 to 220 lb): 750 mg I.V. over 30 minutes. Repeat 2 and 4 weeks after initial infusion and then every 4 weeks thereafter.

Adults weighing less than 60 kg: 500 mg I.V. over 30 minutes. Repeat 2 and 4 weeks after initial infusion and then every 4 weeks thereafter.

I.V. ADMINISTRATION

- Reconstitute vial with 10 ml of sterile water for injection, using only the silicone-free disposable syringe provided, to yield 25 mg/ml.
- Gently swirl contents until completely dissolved. Avoid vigorous shaking.
- Vent the vial with a needle to clear away foam.
- The solution should be clear and colorless to pale yellow.
- Further dilute the solution to 100 ml with normal saline solution. Infuse over 30 minutes using an infusion set and a sterile, nonpyrogenic, low–protein-binding filter.
- Store diluted solution at room temperature or refrigerate at 36° to 46° F (2° to 8° C). Complete infusion within 24 hours of reconstituting.

INCOMPATIBILITIES

Don't infuse in the same line with other I.V. drugs.

ACTION

Inhibits T-cell activation, decreases T-cell proliferation, and inhibits production of TNF-alpha, interferon-gamma, and interleukin-2.

Route	Onset	Peak	Duration
I.V.	Unknown	Unknown	Unknown

Half-life: 13 days.

ADVERSE REACTIONS

CNS: *headache,* dizziness.
CV: hypertension.
EENT: *nasopharyngitis,* rhinitis, sinusitis.

GI: *nausea,* diverticulitis, dyspepsia.
GU: acute pyelonephritis, UTI.
Musculoskeletal: back pain, limb pain.
Respiratory: *upper respiratory tract infection,* bronchitis, cough, pneumonia.
Skin: cellulitis, rash.
Other: *infections,* ***malignancies,*** herpes simplex, influenza, infusion reactions.

INTERACTIONS
Drug-drug. *Anakinra, TNF antagonists:* May increase risk of infection. Don't use together.
Live-virus vaccines: May decrease effectiveness of vaccine. Avoid giving vaccines during or for 3 months after abatacept therapy.

EFFECTS ON LAB TEST RESULTS
None reported.

CONTRAINDICATIONS & CAUTIONS
- Contraindicated in patients hypersensitive to drug or its components. Don't use in patients taking a TNF antagonist or anakinra.
- Use cautiously in patients with active infection, history of chronic infections, scheduled elective surgery, or COPD. Patients who test positive for tuberculosis should be treated before receiving drug.

NURSING CONSIDERATIONS
- Make sure patient has been screened for tuberculosis before giving.
- Monitor patient, especially an older adult. carefully for infections and malignancies.
- If patient develops a severe infection, notify prescriber; therapy may need to be stopped.
- If patient has COPD, watch for worsening.
- Drug may cause serious adverse reactions in a breast-fed infant and may affect his developing immune system.

PATIENT TEACHING
- Urge patient to have tuberculosis screening before therapy.
- Tell patient to continue taking prescribed arthritis drugs. Caution against taking TNF antagonists, such as Enbrel, Remicade, and Humira, or anakinra.
- Tell patient to avoid exposure to infections.
- Tell patient to immediately report signs and symptoms of infection, swollen face or tongue, and difficulty breathing.
- Tell patient with COPD to report worsening signs and symptoms.
- Advise patient to avoid live-virus vaccines during and for 3 months after therapy.
- Advise woman to consult prescriber if she becomes pregnant or plans to breastfeed.
- Advise patient to contact prescriber before taking any other drugs or herbal supplements.
- Remind patient to contact prescriber before scheduling surgery.

adalimumab
Humira

Pharmacologic class: tumor necrosis factor (TNF)-alpha blocker
Pregnancy risk category B

AVAILABLE FORMS
Injection: 40 mg/0.8 ml as prefilled syringes or pens

INDICATIONS & DOSAGES
➤ **Rheumatoid arthritis (RA); psoriatic arthritis; ankylosing spondylitis**
Adults: 40 mg subcutaneously q other week. Patient may continue to take methotrexate, steroids, NSAIDs, salicylates, analgesics or other disease-modifying antirheumatic drugs (known as DMARDs) during therapy. Patients with RA who aren't also taking methotrexate may have the dose increased to 40 mg weekly, if needed.
✷ ***NEW INDICATION:*** **Moderate to severe Crohn disease when response to conventional therapy is inadequate or when patient loses response to or can't tolerate infliximab**
Adults: Initially, 160 mg subcutaneously q.i.d. on day 1 or divided b.i.d. on days 1 and 2; then 80 mg at week 2, followed by a maintenance dose of 40 mg q other week starting at week 4.

ACTION
A recombinant human immunoglobulin G_1 monoclonal antibody that blocks human TNF-alpha. TNF-alpha participates in normal inflammatory and immune responses and in the inflammation and joint destruction of RA.

Route	Onset	Peak	Duration
SubQ	Variable	Variable	Unknown

Half-life: 10 to 20 days.

ADVERSE REACTIONS
CNS: headache.
CV: hypertension.
EENT: *sinusitis.*
GI: abdominal pain, nausea.
GU: hematuria, UTI.
Hematologic: ***leukopenia, pancytopenia, thrombocytopenia.***
Metabolic: hypercholesterolemia, hyperlipidemia.
Musculoskeletal: back pain.
Respiratory: *upper respiratory tract infection,* bronchitis.
Skin: *rash.*
Other: *accidental injury, hemorrhage, injection site reactions (erythema, itching, pain, swelling),* ***anaphylaxis, malignancy,*** allergic reactions, flulike syndrome.

INTERACTIONS
Drug-drug. *Live-virus vaccines:* No data are available on secondary transmission of infection from live-virus vaccines. Avoid using together.
Methotrexate: May decrease clearance of adalimumab. Dosage adjustment isn't necessary.

EFFECTS ON LAB TEST RESULTS
- May increase alkaline phosphatase and cholesterol levels.

CONTRAINDICATIONS & CAUTIONS
- Contraindicated in patients hypersensitive to drug or its components, in immunosuppressed patients, and those with an active chronic or localized infection.
- Use cautiously in patients with demyelinating disorders, a history of recurrent infection, those with underlying conditions that predispose them to infections, and those who have lived in areas where tuberculosis and histoplasmosis are endemic, and in the elderly.
- Don't give to pregnant women unless benefits outweigh risks. Because of the risk of serious adverse reactions, the patient should stop breast-feeding or stop using the drug.
- Safety and effectiveness in children haven't been established.

NURSING CONSIDERATIONS
- Give first dose under supervision of prescriber.
- Patient should be evaluated, and treated if necessary for latent tuberculosis before starting adalimumab therapy.
- ***Alert:*** Serious infections and sepsis, including tuberculosis and invasive fungal infections, may occur. If patient develops new infection during treatment, monitor him closely, and if infection becomes serious, stop drug. Avoid using anakinra during treatment because this increases the risk.
- Drug may increase the risk for malignancy. Patients with highly active RA may be at an increased risk for lymphoma.
- If patient develops anaphylaxis, a severe infection, other serious allergic reaction, or evidence of a lupuslike syndrome, stop drug.
- ***Alert:*** The needle cover contains latex and shouldn't be handled by those with latex sensitivity.

PATIENT TEACHING
- Tell patient to report evidence of tuberculosis or infection.
- Teach patient or caregiver how to give drug.
- ***Alert:*** Warn patient to seek immediate medical attention for symptoms of blood dyscrasias or infection, including fever, bruising, bleeding, and pallor.
- Tell patient to rotate injection sites and to avoid tender, bruised, red, or hard skin.
- Teach patient to dispose of used vials, needles, and syringes properly and not in the household trash or recyclables.
- Tell patient to refrigerate drug in its original container before use.

alefacept
Amevive

Pharmacologic class: immunosuppressant
Pregnancy risk category B

AVAILABLE FORMS
Powder for injection: 15-mg single-dose vial

INDICATIONS & DOSAGES
➤ **Moderate to severe chronic plaque psoriasis in candidates for systemic therapy or phototherapy**
Adults: 15 mg I.M. once weekly for 12 weeks. Another 12-week course may be given if CD4+ T lymphocyte count is normal and at least 12 weeks have passed since the previous treatment.
Adjust-a-dose: Withhold dose if CD4+ T lymphocyte count is below 250 cells/mm^3. Stop drug if CD4+ count remains below 250 cells/mm^3 for 1 month.

ACTION
An immunosuppressive protein that interferes with lymphocyte activation and reduces subsets of CD2+ T lymphocytes, which reduces circulating total CD4+ and CD8+ T lymphocyte counts.

Route	Onset	Peak	Duration
I.M.	Unknown	Unknown	Unknown

Half-life: About 11 days.

ADVERSE REACTIONS
CNS: dizziness.
CV: ***coronary artery disorder, MI.***
EENT: pharyngitis.
GI: nausea.
Hematologic: **LYMPHOPENIA.**
Musculoskeletal: myalgia.
Respiratory: cough.
Skin: pruritus, *injection site pain, inflammation,* bleeding, edema, or mass.
Other: ***infection,*** chills, ***malignancy, hypersensitivity reaction,*** accidental injury, antibody formation.

INTERACTIONS
Drug-drug. *Immunosuppressants, phototherapy:* May increase risk of excessive immunosuppression. Avoid using together.

EFFECTS ON LAB TEST RESULTS
- May decrease CD4+ and CD8+ T lymphocyte counts.

CONTRAINDICATIONS & CAUTIONS
- Contraindicated in patients hypersensitive to drug or its components, in breast-feeding women, and in patients with HIV, a history of systemic malignancy, or important infection.
- Use cautiously in patients at high risk for malignancy, patients with chronic or recurrent infections, and pregnant women. Give drug cautiously to elderly patients because of their increased rate of infection and malignancies.
- Safety and effectiveness in children haven't been established.

NURSING CONSIDERATIONS
- Ensure that CD4+ T lymphocyte count is normal before therapy. Monitor CD4+ T lymphocyte count weekly for the 12-week course.
- Monitor patient carefully for evidence of infection or malignancy, and stop drug if it appears.
- For I.M. administration, reconstitute 15-mg vial of alefacept with 0.6 ml of supplied diluent.
- Rotate I.M. injection sites so that the new injection is given at least 1 inch away from the old site, and not in an area that is bruised, tender, or hard.
- Because effects on fetal development aren't known, give drug only if clearly needed. Enroll pregnant women receiving alefacept into the Biogen pregnancy registry at 1-800-811-0104.

PATIENT TEACHING
- Tell patient about potential adverse reactions.
- Urge patient to report evidence of infection immediately.
- Tell patient that blood tests will be done regularly to monitor WBC counts.
- Tell patient to notify prescriber if she is or could be pregnant within 8 weeks of receiving drug.

• Advise patient to either stop breast-feeding or stop using the drug because of the risk of serious adverse reactions in the infant.

anakinra
Kineret

Pharmacologic class: interleukin-1 receptor antagonist
Pregnancy risk category B

AVAILABLE FORMS
Injection: 100 mg/ml in a prefilled glass syringe

INDICATIONS & DOSAGES
➤ **To reduce signs and symptoms and slow progression of structural damage in moderately to severely active rheumatoid arthritis (RA) after one or more failures with disease-modifying antirheumatic drugs (DMARDs), alone or combined with DMARDs other than tumor necrosis factor (TNF)-blocking drugs**
Adults: 100 mg subcutaneously daily.

ACTION
A recombinant, nonglycosylated form of the human interleukin-1 receptor antagonist (IL-1Ra). The level of naturally occurring IL-1Ra in synovium and synovial fluid from patients with RA isn't enough to compete with the elevated level of locally produced IL-1. Anakinra blocks the biologic activity of IL-1 by competitively inhibiting IL-1 from binding to the interleukin-1 type receptor, which is expressed in various tissues and organs.

Route	Onset	Peak	Duration
SubQ	Unknown	3–7 hr	Unknown

Half-life: 4 to 6 hours.

ADVERSE REACTIONS
CNS: *headache.*
EENT: sinusitis.
GI: abdominal pain, diarrhea, nausea.
Hematologic: ***neutropenia,*** eosinophilia.
Respiratory: *upper respiratory tract infection.*
Skin: *ecchymosis, injection site reactions (erythema, inflammation, pain).*
Other: *infection (cellulitis, pneumonia, bone and joint),* flulike symptoms.

INTERACTIONS
Drug-drug. *Etanercept, other TNF-blocking drugs:* May increase risk of severe infection. Use together with caution.
Vaccines: May decrease effectiveness of vaccines or may increase risk of secondary transmission of infection with live vaccines. Avoid using together.

EFFECTS ON LAB TEST RESULTS
• May increase eosinophil count. May decrease neutrophil, platelet, and WBC counts.

CONTRAINDICATIONS & CAUTIONS
• Contraindicated in patients hypersensitive to *Escherichia coli*–derived proteins or any components of the product, or in patients with active infections.
• Use drug cautiously in immunosuppressed patients, those with a chronic infection, the elderly, and breast-feeding women.
• Safety and effectiveness in patients with juvenile RA haven't been established.

NURSING CONSIDERATIONS
• Don't start treatment if patient has active infection.
• Obtain neutrophil count before treatment, monthly for the first 3 months of treatment, and then quarterly for up to 1 year.
• Inject entire contents of prefilled syringe.
• Monitor patient for infections and injection site reactions.
• Stop drug if a serious infection develops.
• Monitor patient for possible anaphylactic reaction.
• Store drug in the refrigerator at 35° to 46° F (2° to 8° C). Don't freeze or shake.
• Protect drug from light.
• ***Look alike–sound alike:*** Don't confuse anakinra with amikacin.

PATIENT TEACHING
• Tell patient to store drug in refrigerator and not to freeze or expose to excessive heat. Advise letting drug come to room temperature before giving dose.

- Teach patient proper dosage and administration.
- Urge patient to rotate injection sites.
- Teach proper disposal of syringes in a puncture-resistant container. Also, caution patient not to reuse needles.
- Review signs and symptoms of allergic and other adverse reactions, especially signs of serious infections. Urge patient to contact prescriber if they arise.
- Inform patient that injection site reactions are common, usually mild, and typically last 14 to 28 days.
- Tell patient to avoid live-virus vaccines during therapy.

azathioprine

Azasan, Imuran, Thioprine‡

Pharmacologic class: purine antagonist
Pregnancy risk category D

AVAILABLE FORMS

Powder for injection: 100 mg
Tablets: 25 mg, 50 mg, 75 mg, 100 mg

INDICATIONS & DOSAGES

➤ Immunosuppression in kidney transplantation
Adults: Initially, 3 to 5 mg/kg P.O. or I.V. daily, usually beginning on day of transplantation. Maintained at 1 to 3 mg/kg daily based on patient response and tolerance.
Adjust-a-dose: Give drug in lower doses to patients with oliguria in the posttransplant period and in those with impaired renal function. In patients receiving allopurinol, decrease azathioprine dose to one-fourth to one-third of the usual dose.

➤ Severe, refractory rheumatoid arthritis
Adults: Initially, 1 mg/kg P.O. as single dose or divided into two doses. Usual dose is 50 to 100 mg. If patient response isn't satisfactory after 6 to 8 weeks, dosage may be increased by 0.5 mg/kg daily to maximum of 2.5 mg/kg daily at 4-week intervals. Maintenance therapy should be at lowest effective dose. Attempt gradual dose reduction once the patient is stable. Reduce dosage by 0.5 mg/kg (about 25 mg daily) q 4 weeks.

I.V. ADMINISTRATION

- Use only in patients who can't tolerate oral drugs.
- Reconstitute drug in 100-mg vial with 10 ml of sterile water for injection.
- Inspect for particles before use.
- Give by direct I.V. injection, or further dilute in normal saline solution for injection or D_5W solution and infuse over 30 to 60 minutes.

INCOMPATIBILITIES

None reported.

ACTION

May cause variable alterations in antibody production.

Route	Onset	Peak	Duration
P.O., I.V.	Unknown	Unknown	Unknown

Half-life: About 5 hours.

ADVERSE REACTIONS

CNS: fever.
GI: *nausea, vomiting,* anorexia, ***pancreatitis,*** steatorrhea, diarrhea, abdominal pain.
Hematologic: **LEUKOPENIA,** ***myelosuppression,*** macrocytic anemia, anemia, ***pancytopenia,*** **THROMBOCYTOPENIA,** ***immunosuppression.***
Hepatic: ***hepatotoxicity,*** jaundice.
Musculoskeletal: arthralgia, myalgia.
Skin: rash, alopecia.
Other: ***infections, increased risk of neoplasia.***

INTERACTIONS

Drug-drug. *ACE inhibitors:* May cause severe leukopenia. Monitor patient closely.
Allopurinol: May impair inactivation of azathioprine. Avoid using if possible; decrease azathioprine to one-third to one-fourth usual dose.
Co-trimoxazole and other drugs that interfere with myelopoiesis: May cause severe leukopenia, especially in renal transplant patients. Use cautiously together.
Cyclosporine: May decrease cyclosporine level. Monitor cyclosporine level closely.
Warfarin: May decrease action of warfarin. Monitor patient closely.

EFFECTS ON LAB TEST RESULTS
- May increase alkaline phosphatase, ALT, AST, and bilirubin levels. May decrease hemoglobin and uric acid levels.
- May decrease platelet, RBC, and WBC counts.

CONTRAINDICATIONS & CAUTIONS
- Contraindicated in patients hypersensitive to drug or its components.
- Use cautiously in patients with hepatic or renal dysfunction.
- Benefits must be weighed against risk when giving to patient with systemic viral infection, such as chickenpox or herpes zoster.
- Patients with rheumatoid arthritis previously treated with alkylating drugs, such as cyclophosphamide, chlorambucil, or melphalan, may be at risk for tumor development if treated with this drug.

NURSING CONSIDERATIONS
- Give drug after meals to minimize adverse GI effects.
- To prevent bleeding, avoid all I.M. injections when platelet count is below 100,000/mm^3.
- Monitor CBC and platelet counts weekly for 1 month and then twice monthly. Notify prescriber if counts drop suddenly or become dangerously low. Drug may need to be temporarily withheld.
- Watch for early signs and symptoms of hepatotoxicity (such as clay-colored stools, dark urine, pruritus, and yellow skin and sclera) and for increased alkaline phosphatase, bilirubin, AST, and ALT levels.
- Therapeutic response usually occurs within 8 weeks. Patients not improved after 12 weeks can be considered refractory to treatment.
- ***Look alike–sound alike:*** Don't confuse azathioprine with Azulfidine or azatadine. Don't confuse Imuran with Inderal.

PATIENT TEACHING
- Warn patient to report even mild infections (colds, fever, sore throat, malaise), because drug is a potent immunosuppressant.
- Instruct patient to avoid conception during therapy and for 4 months after therapy stops.
- Warn patient that some hair thinning is possible.
- Tell patient taking drug for refractory rheumatoid arthritis that it may take up to 12 weeks to be effective.
- Advise patient to report unusual bleeding or bruising.
- Tell patient that drug may be taken with food to decrease nausea.
- Advise patient to use soft toothbrush and perform oral care cautiously.

basiliximab
Simulect

Pharmacologic class: monoclonal antibody
Pregnancy risk category B

AVAILABLE FORMS
Injection: 20-mg vials

INDICATIONS & DOSAGES
➤ To prevent acute organ rejection in patients receiving renal transplantation when used as part of an immunosuppressive regimen that includes cyclosporine and corticosteroids
Adults and children weighing 35 kg (77 lb) or more: 20 mg I.V. given within 2 hours before transplant surgery and 20 mg I.V. given 4 days after transplantation.
Children weighing less than 35 kg: 10 mg I.V. given within 2 hours before transplant surgery and 10 mg I.V. given 4 days after transplantation.

I.V. ADMINISTRATION
- Reconstitute with 5 ml sterile water for injection. Shake vial gently to dissolve powder.
- Use reconstituted solution immediately.
- Dilute reconstituted solution to 50 ml with normal saline solution or D_5W for infusion.
- When mixing solution, invert bag gently to avoid foaming. Don't shake.
- Infuse over 20 to 30 minutes.
- Drug may be given as a bolus injection, but doing so may cause nausea, vomiting, pain, and local reactions.
- Reconstituted solution may be refrigerated at 36° to 46° F (2° to 8° C) for up to

24 hours or kept at room temperature for 4 hours.

INCOMPATIBILITIES

Don't add or infuse other drugs simultaneously through same I.V. line.

ACTION

Binds specifically to and blocks the interleukin (IL)-2 receptor alpha chain on the surface of activated T lymphocytes, inhibiting IL-2–mediated activation of lymphocytes, a critical pathway in the cellular immune response involved in allograft rejection.

Route	Onset	Peak	Duration
I.V.	Unknown	Immediate	Unknown

Half-life: About 7¼ days in adults, 9½ days in children, 9 days in adolescents.

ADVERSE REACTIONS

CNS: *fever, headache, insomnia, tremor,* agitation, anxiety, asthenia, depression, dizziness, hypoesthesia, neuropathy, paresthesia, fatigue.
CV: *hypertension, leg or peripheral edema,* ***arrhythmias, heart failure,*** angina pectoris, atrial fibrillation, chest pain, abnormal heart sounds, aggravated hypertension, hypotension, tachycardia, generalized edema.
EENT: *pharyngitis, rhinitis,* abnormal vision, cataract, conjunctivitis, sinusitis.
GI: *abdominal pain, candidiasis, constipation, diarrhea, dyspepsia, nausea, vomiting,* ***GI hemorrhage,*** esophagitis, enlarged abdomen, flatulence, gastroenteritis, GI disorder, gum hyperplasia, melena, ulcerative stomatitis.
GU: *UTI,* abnormal renal function, albuminuria, bladder disorder, dysuria, frequent micturition, genital edema, hematuria, increased nonprotein nitrogen, oliguria, renal tubular necrosis, ureteral disorder, urinary retention, impotence.
Hematologic: *anemia,* ***hemorrhage, thrombocytopenia,*** hematoma, polycythemia, purpura, thrombosis.
Metabolic: *hypercholesterolemia, hyperglycemia, hyperkalemia, hyperuricemia, hypokalemia, hypophosphatemia,* acidosis, dehydration, diabetes mellitus, fluid overload, hypercalcemia, hyperlipemia, hypertriglyceridemia, hypocalcemia, hypomagnesemia, hypoproteinemia, weight gain.
Musculoskeletal: arthralgia, arthropathy, back pain, bone fracture, cramps, hernia, leg pain, myalgia.
Respiratory: *dyspnea, upper respiratory tract infection,* ***bronchospasm, pulmonary edema,*** abnormal chest sounds, bronchitis, cough, pneumonia, pulmonary disorder.
Skin: *acne,* cyst, hypertrichosis, pruritus, rash, skin disorder or ulceration.
Other: *surgical wound complications, viral infection,* ***hypersensitivity reactions, sepsis,*** accidental trauma, infection, herpes zoster, herpes simplex.

INTERACTIONS

None significant.

EFFECTS ON LAB TEST RESULTS

- May increase calcium, cholesterol, glucose, lipid, and uric acid levels. May decrease hemoglobin, magnesium, phosphorus, and protein levels. May increase or decrease potassium level.
- May increase RBC count. May decrease platelet count.

CONTRAINDICATIONS & CAUTIONS

- Contraindicated in patients hypersensitive to drug or its components.
- Use cautiously and only under supervision of prescriber qualified and experienced in immunosuppressive therapy and organ transplantation.
- Use cautiously in elderly patients.

NURSING CONSIDERATIONS

- Severe acute hypersensitivity reactions can occur within 24 hours after administration. Make sure drugs for treating hypersensitivity reactions are readily available; withhold second dose if hypersensitivity reactions occur.
- Check for electrolyte imbalances and acidosis during drug therapy.
- Monitor patient's intake and output, vital signs, hemoglobin level, and hematocrit during therapy.
- Be alert for signs and symptoms of opportunistic infections during drug therapy.

PATIENT TEACHING
- Inform patient of potential benefits of and risks related to immunosuppressive therapy, including decreased risk of graft loss or acute rejection.
- Advise patient that immunosuppressive therapy increases risk of developing infection. Tell him to report signs and symptoms of infection promptly.
- Inform woman of childbearing age to use effective contraception before therapy starts and for 4 months after therapy ends.
- Instruct patient to report adverse effects immediately.
- Explain that drug is used with cyclosporine and corticosteroids.

cyclosporine
Sandimmune, Sandimmun‡

cyclosporine, modified
Gengraf, Neoral

Pharmacologic class: polypeptide antibiotic
Pregnancy risk category C

AVAILABLE FORMS
Capsules: 25 mg, 50 mg, 100 mg
Capsules for microemulsion: 25 mg, 50 mg, 100 mg
Injection: 50 mg/ml
Oral solution: 100 mg/ml

INDICATIONS & DOSAGES
➤ **To prevent organ rejection in renal, hepatic, or cardiac transplantation**
Adults and children: 15 mg/kg P.O. 4 to 12 hours before transplantation and continue daily for 1 to 2 weeks postoperatively. Then reduce dosage by 5% each week to maintenance level of 5 to 10 mg/kg daily. Or, 5 to 6 mg/kg I.V. concentrate 4 to 12 hours before transplantation as a continuous infusion. Postoperatively, repeat dose daily until patient can tolerate P.O. forms.

For conversion from Sandimmune to Gengraf or Neoral, use same daily dose as previously used for Sandimmune. Monitor blood levels q 4 to 7 days after conversion, and monitor blood pressure and creatinine level q 2 weeks during the first 2 months.

➤ **Severe, active rheumatoid arthritis (RA) that hasn't adequately responded to methotrexate**
Adults: 2.5 mg/kg Gengraf or Neoral daily P.O., taken b.i.d. as divided doses. Dosage may be increased by 0.5 to 0.75 mg/kg daily after 8 weeks and again after 12 weeks to a maximum of 4 mg/kg daily. If no response is seen after 16 weeks, stop therapy.

➤ **Psoriasis**
Adults: 1.25 mg/kg Gengraf or Neoral daily P.O. b.i.d. for at least 4 weeks. Increase dosage by 0.5 mg/kg daily once q 2 weeks as needed to a maximum of 4 mg/kg daily.
Adjust-a-dose: For patients with adverse effects such as hypertension, creatinine level 30% above pretreatment level, or abnormal CBC count or liver function test results, decrease dosage by 25% to 50%.

I.V. ADMINISTRATION
- Immediately before use, dilute each milliliter of concentrate in 20 to 100 ml of D_5W or normal saline solution for injection. Give at one-third the oral dose.
- Infuse over 2 to 6 hours.
- Protect diluted drug from light.

INCOMPATIBILITIES
Amphotericin B cholesteryl sulfate complex, magnesium sulfate.

ACTION
May inhibit proliferation and function of T lymphocytes and inhibit production and release of lymphokines.

Route	Onset	Peak	Duration
P.O.	Unknown	90 min–3 hr	Unknown
I.V.	Unknown	Unknown	Unknown

Half-life: Initial phase, about 1 hour; terminal phase, 8½ to 27 hours.

ADVERSE REACTIONS
CNS: *tremor, headache,* confusion, paresthesia.
CV: *hypertension,* flushing.
EENT: *gum hyperplasia,* sinusitis.
GI: *nausea, vomiting,* diarrhea, oral thrush, abdominal discomfort.

GU: NEPHROTOXICITY.
Hematologic: anemia, ***leukopenia, thrombocytopenia.***
Hepatic: ***hepatotoxicity.***
Metabolic: hyperglycemia.
Skin: *hirsutism,* acne.
Other: ***infections, anaphylaxis,*** gynecomastia.

INTERACTIONS

Drug-drug. *Acyclovir, aminoglycosides, amphotericin B, cimetidine, co-trimoxazole, diclofenac, gentamicin, ketoconazole, melphalan, NSAIDs, ranitidine, sulfamethoxazole and trimethoprim, tacrolimus, tobramycin, vancomycin:* May increase risk of nephrotoxicity. Avoid using together.
Allopurinol, ***azole antifungals,*** *bromocriptine,* ***caspofungin,*** *cimetidine, clarithromycin, danazol, diltiazem, erythromycin, imipenem and cilastatin, methylprednisolone, metoclopramide,* ***micafungin,*** *nicardipine, prednisolone, verapamil:* May increase cyclosporine level. Monitor patient for increased toxicity.
Azathioprine, corticosteroids, cyclophosphamide, verapamil: May increase immunosuppression. Monitor patient closely.
Carbamazepine, isoniazid, nafcillin, octreotide, ***orlistat,*** *phenobarbital,* ***phenytoin, rifabutin, rifampin,*** *ticlopidine:* May decrease immunosuppressant effect from low cyclosporine level. Cyclosporine dosage may need to be increased.
Digoxin, lovastatin, prednisolone: May decrease clearance of these drugs. Use together cautiously.
Mycophenolate mofetil: May decrease mycophenolate level. Monitor patient closely when cyclosporine is added to or removed from therapy.
Potassium-sparing diuretics: May induce hyperkalemia. Monitor patient closely.
Sirolimus: May increase sirolimus level. Take sirolimus at least 4 hours after cyclosporine dose. If separating doses isn't possible, monitor patient for increased adverse effects.
Vaccines: May decrease immune response. Delay routine immunization.
Drug-herb. *Astragalus, echinacea, licorice:* May interfere with drug's effect. Discourage use together.
St. John's wort: May reduce drug level, resulting in transplant failure. Discourage use together.
Drug-food. *Alfalfa sprouts:* May interfere with drug's effect. Discourage use together.
Grapefruit and grapefruit juices: May increase drug level and cause toxicity. Advise patient to avoid grapefruit or grapefruit juice.
Drug-lifestyle. *Sunlight:* May increase risk of sensitivity to sunlight. Advise patient to avoid excessive sunlight exposure.

EFFECTS ON LAB TEST RESULTS

- May increase ALT, AST, bilirubin, BUN, creatinine, glucose, and LDL levels. May decrease hemoglobin and magnesium levels.
- May decrease platelet and WBC counts.

CONTRAINDICATIONS & CAUTIONS

- Contraindicated in patients hypersensitive to drug or polyoxyethylated castor oil (found in injectable form).
- Contraindicated in patients with RA or psoriasis with abnormal renal function, uncontrolled hypertension, or malignancies (Neoral or Gengraf).
- Psoriasis patients shouldn't receive psoralen plus ultraviolet A, or PUVA, or ultraviolet B, or UVB, therapy; methotrexate; other immunosuppressants; coal tar; or radiation (Neoral or Gengraf).

NURSING CONSIDERATIONS

- Drug can cause nephrotoxicity and hepatotoxicity.
- Measure oral solution doses carefully in an oral syringe. To improve the taste of Sandimmune oral solution, mix it with milk, chocolate milk, or orange juice. Gengraf or Neoral oral solution may be mixed with orange or apple juice (not grapefruit juice); it is less palatable when mixed with milk. Use a glass container to mix, and have patient drink at once. Don't rinse dosing syringe with water. If syringe is cleaned, it must be completely dry before reuse.
- Monitor elderly patient for renal impairment and hypertension.
- Monitor drug level at regular intervals. Absorption of oral solution can be erratic.

• ***Look alike–sound alike:*** Don't confuse cyclosporine with cyclophosphamide or cycloserine. Don't confuse Sandimmune with Sandoglobulin or Sandostatin.
• Neoral and Gengraf have greater bioavailability than Sandimmune. A lower dose of Neoral or Gengraf may be needed to provide blood level similar to that achieved with Sandimmune. Monitor blood level when switching patients between these two brands.
• Gengraf is bioequivalent to and interchangeable with Neoral capsules.
• Always give with corticosteroids; however, don't give Sandimmune with other immunosuppressants.
• Use Neoral or Gengraf to treat RA or psoriasis.

RA

• Before starting treatment, measure blood pressure at least twice and obtain two creatinine levels to estimate baseline.
• Evaluate blood pressure and creatinine level every 2 weeks during first 3 months and then monthly if patient is stable.
• Monitor blood pressure and creatinine level after an increase in NSAID dosage or introduction of a new NSAID. Monitor CBC and liver function tests monthly if patient also receives methotrexate.
• If hypertension occurs, decrease dosage of Gengraf or Neoral by 25% to 50%. If hypertension persists, decrease dosage further or control blood pressure with antihypertensives.

Psoriasis

• Measure blood pressure at least twice to determine a baseline.
• Evaluate patient for occult infection and tumors initially and throughout treatment.
• Obtain baseline creatinine level (on two occasions), CBC, and BUN, magnesium, uric acid, potassium, and lipid levels.
• Evaluate creatinine and BUN levels every 2 weeks during first 3 months and then monthly thereafter if patient is stable.
• If creatinine level is 25% above pretreatment levels, repeat creatinine level measurement within 2 weeks. If creatinine level stays 25% to 50% above baseline, reduce dosage by 25% to 50%. If creatinine level is ever 50% above baseline, reduce dosage by 25% to 50%. Stop therapy if creatinine level isn't reversed after two dosage modifications.
• Monitor creatinine level after increasing NSAID dose or starting a new NSAID.
• Evaluate blood pressure, CBC, and uric acid, potassium, lipid, and magnesium levels every 2 weeks for the first 3 months and then monthly if patient is stable, or more frequently if a dosage is adjusted.
• If an adverse reaction occurs, reduce dosage by 25% to 50%.
• Improvement in psoriasis takes 12 to 16 weeks of therapy.

PATIENT TEACHING

• Encourage patient to take drug at same time each day and to be consistent with relation to meals.
• Teach patient how to measure dosage and mask taste of oral solution. Tell him not to take drug with grapefruit juice.
• Instruct patient to fill glass with water after dose and drink it to make sure he consumes all of drug.
• Advise patient to take drug with meals if nausea occurs.
• Advise patient to take Neoral or Gengraf on an empty stomach.
• Tell patient being treated for psoriasis that improvement may not occur until after 12 to 16 weeks of therapy.
• Stress that drug shouldn't be stopped without prescriber's approval.
• Explain to patient the importance of frequent laboratory monitoring while receiving therapy.
• Tell patient to avoid people with infections because drug lowers resistance to infection.
• Advise patient to perform careful oral care and to see a dentist regularly because drug can cause gum disease.
• Advise woman to use barrier contraception, not hormonal contraceptives, during therapy. Advise her of the potential risk during pregnancy and the increased risk of tumors, high blood pressure, and renal problems.
• Warn patient to wear protection in the sun and to avoid excessive sun exposure.

daclizumab
Zenapax

Pharmacologic class: interleukin-2 receptor antagonist
Pregnancy risk category C

AVAILABLE FORMS
Injection: 25 mg/5 ml

INDICATIONS & DOSAGES
➤ **To prevent acute organ rejection in patients receiving renal transplants with an immunosuppressive regimen that includes cyclosporine and corticosteroids**
Adults: 1 mg/kg I.V. Standard course of therapy is five doses. Give first dose no more than 24 hours before transplantation; remaining four doses are given at 14-day intervals.

I.V. ADMINISTRATION
- Dilute in 50 ml of sterile normal saline solution. To avoid foaming, don't shake.
- If drug contains particulates or is discolored, don't use.
- Give over 15 minutes via a central or peripheral line.
- Drug may be refrigerated at 36° to 46° F (2° to 8° C) for 24 hours and is stable at room temperature for 4 hours.
- Discard unused solution after 24 hours.

INCOMPATIBILITIES
Other drugs infused through same I.V. line.

ACTION
An interleukin (IL)-2 receptor antagonist that inhibits IL-2 binding to prevent IL-2–mediated activation of lymphocytes, a critical pathway in the cellular immune response against allografts. Once in circulation, drug impairs response of immune system to antigenic challenges.

Route	Onset	Peak	Duration
I.V.	Unknown	Unknown	Unknown

Half-life: 20 days.

ADVERSE REACTIONS
CNS: anxiety, depression, dizziness, fatigue, fever, generalized weakness, headache, insomnia, prickly sensation, tremor.
CV: aggravated hypertension, edema, chest pain, hypertension, hypotension, tachycardia.
EENT: blurred vision, pharyngitis, rhinitis.
GI: abdominal distention, abdominal pain, constipation, diarrhea, dyspepsia, epigastric pain, flatulence, gastritis, hemorrhoids, nausea, pyrosis, vomiting.
GU: ***oliguria, renal tubular necrosis,*** dysuria, hydronephrosis, renal damage, renal insufficiency, urinary tract bleeding, urinary tract disorder, urine retention.
Hematologic: bleeding and clotting disorders, lymphocele, platelet.
Metabolic: dehydration, diabetes mellitus, fluid overload.
Musculoskeletal: arthralgia, leg cramps, musculoskeletal or back pain, myalgia.
Respiratory: ***hypoxia, pulmonary edema,*** abnormal breath sounds, atelectasis, congestion, coughing, crackles, dyspnea, pleural effusion.
Skin: acne, hirsutism, impaired wound healing without infection, increased sweating, night sweats, pruritus, rash.
Other: limb edema, pain, shivering.

INTERACTIONS
Drug-drug. *Corticosteroids, cyclosporine, mycophenolate mofetil:* May increase mortality, especially in patients taking antilymphocyte antibody therapy, and in those in whom severe infections develop. Monitor patient closely.

EFFECTS ON LAB TEST RESULTS
None reported.

CONTRAINDICATIONS & CAUTIONS
- Contraindicated in patients hypersensitive to drug or its components.
- Use cautiously and only under supervision of prescriber experienced in immunosuppressive therapy and management of organ transplantation.

NURSING CONSIDERATIONS
- Protect undiluted solution from direct light.

• ***Alert:*** Using cyclosporine, mycophenolate mofetil, and corticosteroids with this drug may be life-threatening. Monitor patients for increased risk of lymphoproliferative disorders and opportunistic infections.
• ***Alert:*** Monitor patient for severe, acute hypersensitivity reactions when giving each dose. Reactions may include anaphylaxis, hypotension, bronchospasm, loss of consciousness, injection site reactions, edema, and arrhythmias. If a severe reaction occurs, stop drug. Keep drugs for anaphylactic reactions immediately available.

PATIENT TEACHING
• Tell patient to consult prescriber before taking other drugs during therapy.
• Advise patient to practice infection prevention precautions.
• Inform patient that neither he nor any household member should receive vaccinations unless medically approved.
• Urge patient to immediately report wounds that fail to heal, unusual bruising or bleeding, fever, or any sign of allergic reaction.
• Advise patient to drink plenty of fluids during drug therapy and to report painful urination, bloody urine, or decreased urine volume.
• Instruct woman of childbearing age to use effective contraception before therapy starts and to continue for 4 months after therapy stops.

efalizumab
Raptiva

Pharmacologic class: immunosuppressant
Pregnancy risk category C

AVAILABLE FORMS
Injection: 125-mg single-use vial

INDICATIONS & DOSAGES
➤ **Chronic moderate to severe plaque psoriasis when systemic therapy or phototherapy is appropriate**
Adults: A single dose of 0.7 mg/kg subcutaneously followed by weekly doses of 1 mg/kg subcutaneously, beginning 1 week after first dose. Maximum single dose, 200 mg.

ACTION
An immunosuppressant that binds to a leukocyte function antigen and decreases its expression, thus inhibiting the action of T lymphocytes at sites of inflammation, including psoriatic skin.

Route	Onset	Peak	Duration
SubQ	1–2 days	Unknown	25 days

Half-life: Unknown.

ADVERSE REACTIONS
CNS: ***stroke,*** fever, *headache, pain.*
GI: *nausea.*
Musculoskeletal: back pain, myalgia.
Skin: acne.
Other: *chills,* flulike syndrome, ***hypersensitivity reaction,*** *infection.*

INTERACTIONS
Drug-drug. *Other immunosuppressants:* May increase risk of infection and malignancy. Avoid using together.
Vaccines: May decrease or negate immune response to vaccine. Avoid using together.

EFFECTS ON LAB TEST RESULTS
• May increase alkaline phosphatase level.
• May increase leukocyte and lymphocyte counts. May decrease platelet count.

CONTRAINDICATIONS & CAUTIONS
• Contraindicated in patients hypersensitive to drug or its components and in patients with significant infection.
• Use cautiously in patients with chronic infection or history of recurrent infection and in those with history of or high risk for malignancy.

NURSING CONSIDERATIONS
• Reconstitute the drug immediately before use.
• To reconstitute, inject 1.3 ml of sterile water for injection into the vial. Swirl gently to dissolve the powder, which takes less than 5 minutes. Don't shake the vial.
• Use only sterile water as the diluent, and use a vial only once.

• Solution should be colorless to pale yellow and free of particulates. If not used immediately, store at room temperature for up to 8 hours.
• Don't add other drugs to solution.
• Rotate injection sites.
• Notify prescriber if patient develops a severe infection or malignancy is suspected.
• Watch for evidence of thrombocytopenia. Check patient's platelet count monthly during initial treatment and then every 3 months.
• Monitor patient for worsening of psoriasis during or after therapy.
• Keep powder refrigerated, and protect vials from light.

PATIENT TEACHING
• Tell patient to take the drug exactly as prescribed.
• Explain that platelet counts will be monitored during therapy.
• Urge patient to immediately report evidence of severe thrombocytopenia, such as bleeding gums, bruising, or petechiae.
• Tell patient to report weight changes because dose may need to be changed.
• Advise patient to report any infection or worsening psoriasis.
• Advise patient to hold off receiving vaccines during therapy because the immune response may be inadequate.
• Caution patient to immediately report pregnancy or suspected pregnancy.

etanercept
Enbrel

Pharmacologic class: tumor necrosis factor (TNF) blocker
Pregnancy risk category B

AVAILABLE FORMS
Injection: 25-mg multi-use vial
Prefilled syringe: 50 mg/ml

INDICATIONS & DOSAGES
➤ **To reduce signs and symptoms of moderately to severely active polyarticular-course juvenile rheumatoid arthritis (RA) in patients whose response to one or more disease-modifying antirheumatic drugs has been inadequate**
Children ages 4 to 17: Give 0.8 mg/kg subcutaneously weekly (maximum 50 mg/week). For children weighing 63 kg (138 lb) or more, give weekly dose using the prefilled syringe. For children weighing 31 to 62 kg (68 to 136 lb), give total weekly dose as two subcutaneous injections, either on the same day or 3 or 4 days apart using the multi-use vial. For children weighing less than 31 kg (68 lb), give weekly dose as single subcutaneous injection using the correct volume from the multi-use vial. Glucocorticoids, NSAIDs, or analgesics may be continued during treatment. Use with methotrexate hasn't been studied in pediatric patients.
➤ **RA, psoriatic arthritis, ankylosing spondylitis**
Adults: 50 mg subcutaneously once weekly using the 50-mg/ml single-use prefilled syringe. Methotrexate, glucocorticoids, salicylates, NSAIDs, or analgesics may be continued during treatment.
➤ **Chronic moderate to severe plaque psoriasis in patients who are candidates for systemic therapy or phototherapy**
Adults: 50 mg subcutaneously twice weekly, 3 to 4 days apart for 3 months. Then, reduce dose to 50 mg subcutaneously once weekly. Give dose using 50-mg/ml single-use prefilled syringes.

ACTION
Binds specifically to TNF and blocks its action with cell surface TNF receptors, reducing inflammatory and immune responses found in RA.

Route	Onset	Peak	Duration
SubQ	Unknown	72 hr	Unknown

Half-life: About 5 days.

ADVERSE REACTIONS
CNS: *headache,* asthenia, dizziness.
EENT: *rhinitis,* pharyngitis, sinusitis.
GI: abdominal pain, dyspepsia.
Respiratory: *upper respiratory tract infections,* cough, respiratory disorder.
Skin: *injection site reaction,* rash.
Other: *infections,* malignancies.

INTERACTIONS

Drug-drug. *Vaccines:* May affect normal immune response. Postpone live-virus vaccine until therapy stops.

EFFECTS ON LAB TEST RESULTS

None reported.

CONTRAINDICATIONS & CAUTIONS

- Contraindicated in patients hypersensitive to drug or its components, in those with sepsis, and in those receiving a live vaccine.
- Drug isn't indicated for use in children younger than age 4.
- Use cautiously in patients with underlying diseases that predispose them to infection, such as diabetes, heart failure, or history of active or chronic infections. Also use cautiously in RA patients with preexisting or recent onset of demyelinating disorders, including multiple sclerosis, myelitis, and optic neuritis.

NURSING CONSIDERATIONS

- Methotrexate, glucocorticoids, salicylates, NSAIDs, or analgesics may be continued during treatment in adults.
- ***Alert:*** Anti-TNF therapies that include drug, may affect defenses against infection. If serious infection occurs, stop therapy and notify prescriber.
- ***Alert:*** Don't give live vaccines during therapy.
- If possible, bring patients with juvenile RA up-to-date with all immunizations before starting treatment.
- ***Alert:*** Give a 50-mg dose as one subcutaneous injection using a 50-mg/ml single-use prefilled syringe or as two 25-mg subcutaneous injections using multiple-use vial. Give the two 25-mg injections on the same day or 3 to 4 days apart.
- Store prefilled syringe at 36° to 46° F (2° to 8° C), but let it reach room temperature (15 to 30 minutes) before use. Don't remove the needle shield while syringe is being allowed to reach room temperature.
- Reconstitute multiple-use vial aseptically with 1 ml of supplied sterile bacteriostatic water for injection (0.9% benzyl alcohol). Use a 25G needle rather than the supplied vial adapter if the vial will be used for multiple doses. Don't filter reconstituted solution when preparing or giving drug. Inject diluent slowly into vial. Refrigerate in vial for up to 14 days at 36° to 46° F (2° to 8° C).
- Minimize foaming by gently swirling during dissolution rather than shaking. Dissolution takes less than 10 minutes.
- Don't use solution if it's discolored or cloudy, or if it contains particulate matter.
- Don't add other drugs or diluents to solution.
- Separate injection sites by at least 1 inch, rotate regularly, and never use areas where skin is tender, bruised, red, or hard. Use sites on the thigh, abdomen, and upper arm.
- ***Alert:*** Needle covers of diluent syringe and prefilled syringe contain latex and shouldn't be handled by persons sensitive to latex.

PATIENT TEACHING

- If patient will be self-administering drug, advise him about mixing and injection techniques, including rotation of injection sites.
- Instruct patient to use puncture-resistant container for disposal of needles and syringes.
- Tell patient that injection site reactions generally occur within first month of therapy and decrease thereafter.
- Inform patient of importance of avoiding live vaccine administration during therapy.
- Stress importance of alerting other health care providers of etanercept use.
- Instruct patient to promptly report signs and symptoms of infection to prescriber.
- Advise woman to stop breast-feeding during therapy.

infliximab

Remicade

Pharmacologic class: monoclonal antibody immunoglobulin G1k
Pregnancy risk category B

AVAILABLE FORMS

Lyophilized powder for injection: 100-mg vial

INDICATIONS & DOSAGES

➤ **Moderately to severely active Crohn disease; reduction in the number of draining enterocutaneous and rectovaginal fistulas and maintenance of fistula closure in patients with fistulizing Crohn disease**
Adults: 5 mg/kg I.V. infusion over at least 2 hours. Repeat at 2 and 6 weeks, then q 8 weeks thereafter. For patients who respond and then lose their response, consider 10 mg/kg. Patients who don't respond by week 14 are unlikely to respond with continued therapy. In those patients, consider stopping drug.
Children age 6 to 17: For Crohn disease, 5 mg/kg I.V. infusion over at least 2 hours. Repeat at 2 and 6 weeks, then q 8 weeks thereafter.

➤ **Moderately to severely active rheumatoid arthritis**
Adults: 3 mg/kg I.V. infusion over at least 2 hours. Repeat at 2 and 6 weeks after first infusion and q 8 weeks thereafter. Dose may be increased up to 10 mg/kg, or doses may be given q 4 weeks if response is inadequate. Use with methotrexate.

➤ **Moderate to severe ulcerative colitis**
Adults: Induction dose, 5 mg/kg I.V. over at least 2 hours. Repeat at 2 and 6 weeks, then q 8 weeks thereafter.

➤ **Ankylosing spondylitis**
Adults: 5 mg/kg I.V. infusion over at least 2 hours. Repeat at 2 and 6 weeks, then q 6 weeks thereafter.

➤ **Psoriatic arthritis, with or without methotrexate**
Adults: 5 mg/kg I.V. infusion over at least 2 hours. Repeat at 2 and 6 weeks after first infusion, then q 8 weeks thereafter.

✷ ***NEW INDICATION:*** **Chronic severe plaque psoriasis**
Adults: 5 mg/kg I.V. infusion over at least 2 hours. Repeat dose in 2 and 6 weeks, then give 5 mg/kg q 8 weeks thereafter.

I.V. ADMINISTRATION

- Reconstitute with 10 ml sterile water for injection, using syringe with 21G or smaller needle. Don't shake; gently swirl to dissolve powder. Solution should be colorless to light yellow and opalescent. It may also develop a few translucent particles; don't use if other types of particles develop or discoloration occurs.
- Dilute total volume of reconstituted drug to 250 ml with normal saline solution for injection. Infusion concentration range is 0.4 to 4 mg/ml.
- Use an in-line, sterile, nonpyrogenic, low–protein-binding filter with a pore size less than 1.2 micrometer.
- Begin infusion within 3 hours of preparation and give over at least 2 hours.

INCOMPATIBILITIES

Other I.V. drugs.

ACTION

Binds to human tumor necrosis factor (TNF)-alpha to neutralize its activity and inhibit its binding with receptors, thereby reducing the infiltration of inflammatory cells and TNF-alpha production in inflamed areas of the intestine.

Route	Onset	Peak	Duration
I.V.	Unknown	Unknown	Unknown

Half-life: 9½ days.

ADVERSE REACTIONS

CNS: *fatigue, fever, headache,* dizziness, depression, insomnia, malaise, pain, systemic and cutaneous vasculitis.
CV: *hypertension,* chest pain, flushing, hypotension, pericardial effusion, tachycardia.
EENT: *pharyngitis, rhinitis, sinusitis,* conjunctivitis.
GI: *abdominal pain, diarrhea, dyspepsia, nausea,* ***intestinal obstruction,*** constipation, flatulence, oral pain, ulcerative stomatitis, vomiting.
GU: *UTI,* dysuria, increased urinary frequency.
Hematologic: ***leukopenia, neutropenia, pancytopenia, thrombocytopenia,*** anemia, hematoma.
Musculoskeletal: *arthralgia, back pain,* arthritis, myalgia.
Respiratory: *coughing, upper respiratory tract infections,* bronchitis, dyspnea, respiratory tract allergic reaction.
Skin: *rash,* acne, alopecia, candidiasis, dry skin, eczema, erythema, erythema-

tous rash, increased sweating, maculopapular rash, papular rash, urticaria.
Other: abscess, chills, ecchymosis, flu-like syndrome, hot flashes, peripheral edema, toothache.

INTERACTIONS

Drug-drug. *Anakinra:* May increase the risk of serious infections and neutropenia. Avoid use together.
Vaccines: May affect normal immune response. Postpone live-virus vaccine until therapy stops.

EFFECTS ON LAB TEST RESULTS

- May increase liver enzyme level. May decrease hemoglobin level and hematocrit.
- May decrease WBC and platelet counts.
- May cause false-positive antinuclear antibody test result.

CONTRAINDICATIONS & CAUTIONS

- Contraindicated in patients hypersensitive to murine proteins or other components of drug. Doses greater than 5 mg/kg are contraindicated in patients with moderate to severe heart failure.
- Use cautiously in elderly patients and in patients with active infection, history of chronic or recurrent infections, a history of hematologic abnormalities, or preexisting or recent onset of CNS demyelinating or seizure disorders; or in those who have lived in regions where histoplasmosis is endemic.

NURSING CONSIDERATIONS

- ***Alert:*** Watch for infusion-related reactions, including fever, chills, pruritus, urticaria, dyspnea, hypotension, hypertension, and chest pain during administration and for 2 hours afterward. If an infusion-related reaction occurs, stop drug, notify prescriber, and give acetaminophen, antihistamines, corticosteroids, and epinephrine.
- Give for Crohn disease and ulcerative colitis only after patient has an inadequate response to conventional therapy.
- Consider stopping treatment in patient who develops significant hematologic abnormalities or CNS adverse reactions.
- Notify prescriber for symptoms of new or worsening heart failure.
- Watch for development of lymphoma and infection. A patient with chronic Crohn disease and long-term exposure to immunosuppressants is more likely to develop lymphoma and infection.
- Drug may affect normal immune responses. Patient may develop autoimmune antibodies and lupus-like syndrome; stop drug if this happens. Symptoms should resolve.
- ***Alert:*** Drug may cause disseminated or extrapulmonary tuberculosis and fatal opportunistic infections.
- Evaluate patient for latent tuberculosis infection with a tuberculin skin test. Treat latent tuberculosis infection before therapy.
- ***Look alike–sound alike:*** Don't confuse Remicade with Renacidin.

PATIENT TEACHING

- Tell patient about infusion-reaction symptoms and adverse effects and the need to report them promptly.
- Advise patient to seek immediate medical attention for signs and symptoms of infection or unusual bleeding or bruising
- Tell woman to stop breast-feeding during therapy.
- Tell patient that before he receives vaccines, he should alert prescriber to therapy.
- Advise parent to get child up-to-date for all vaccines before therapy.

lymphocyte immune globulin (antithymocyte globulin [equine], ATG, LIG)

Atgam

Pharmacologic class: immunoglobulin
Pregnancy risk category C

AVAILABLE FORMS

Injection: 50 mg of equine IgG/ml in 5-ml ampules

INDICATIONS & DOSAGES

➤ To prevent acute renal allograft rejection
Adults and children: 15 mg/kg I.V. daily for 14 days; then alternate-day therapy for

14 days. Give first dose within 24 hours of transplantation.

➤ **Acute renal allograft rejection**

Adults and children: 10 to 15 mg/kg I.V. daily for 14 days. Additional alternate-day therapy to total of 21 doses can be given. Start therapy when rejection is diagnosed.

➤ **Aplastic anemia**

Adults: 10 to 20 mg/kg I.V. daily for 8 to 14 days. Additional alternate-day therapy to total of 21 doses can be given.

I.V. ADMINISTRATION

- Don't use solutions that are older than 12 hours, including actual infusion time.
- Dilute concentrated drug for injection before giving. Dilute required dose in 250 to 1,000 ml of half-normal or normal saline solution. Final concentration of drug shouldn't exceed 4 mg/ml.
- Allow diluted drug to reach room temperature before infusion.
- When adding drug to infusion solution, make sure container is inverted so drug doesn't contact air inside container. Gently rotate or swirl container to mix contents; don't shake because this may cause excessive foaming or denature the drug protein.
- Infuse with an in-line filter with a pore size of 0.2 to 1 micron over at least 4 hours (most institutions use 4 to 8 hours) into a vascular shunt, arterial venous fistula, or high-flow central vein.
- Refrigerate at 35° to 47° F (2° to 8° C). Concentrate is heat sensitive. Don't freeze.

INCOMPATIBILITIES

Don't dilute with dextrose solutions or solutions with a low salt concentration because a precipitate may form. Proteins in drug can be denatured by air. Drug is unstable in acidic solutions.

ACTION

Unknown. Inhibits cell-mediated immune responses either by altering T-cell function or eliminating antigen-reactive T cells.

Route	Onset	Peak	Duration
I.V.	Immediate	5 days	Unknown

Half-life: About 6 days.

ADVERSE REACTIONS

CNS: ***seizures,*** headache, malaise.
CV: *chest pain, hypotension,* edema, iliac vein obstruction, tachycardia, thrombophlebitis.
EENT: ***laryngospasm.***
GI: *diarrhea, nausea, vomiting,* abdominal distention, epigastric pain, hiccups, stomatitis.
GU: renal artery stenosis.
Hematologic: **LEUKOPENIA, THROMBOCYTOPENIA,** ***aplastic anemia,*** hemolysis.
Metabolic: hyperglycemia.
Musculoskeletal: *arthralgia, myalgia.*
Respiratory: *dyspnea,* ***pulmonary edema.***
Skin: *pruritus, rash, urticaria.*
Other: ***anaphylaxis,*** chills, febrile reactions, hypersensitivity reactions, infections, lymphadenopathy, night sweats, serum sickness.

INTERACTIONS

None significant.

EFFECTS ON LAB TEST RESULTS

- May increase liver enzyme and glucose levels. May decrease hemoglobin level.
- May decrease WBC and platelet counts.

CONTRAINDICATIONS & CAUTIONS

- Contraindicated in patients hypersensitive to drug.
- Use cautiously in patients receiving additional immunosuppressive therapy (such as corticosteroids or azathioprine) because of increased risk of infection.

NURSING CONSIDERATIONS

- ***Alert:*** Do an I.D. skin test at least 1 hour before first dose. Give an I.D. dose of 0.1 ml of a 1:1,000 lymphocyte immune globulin along with a contralateral normal saline control. Marked local swelling or erythema larger than 10 mm indicates increased risk of severe systemic reaction such as anaphylaxis. Severe reactions to skin test, such as hypotension, tachycardia, dyspnea, generalized rash, or anaphylaxis, usually preclude further use of drug. Anaphylaxis may still occur in patients with negative skin tests.
- Monitor patient for hypotension, respiratory distress, and chest, flank, or back

pain, which may indicate anaphylaxis or hemolysis.
- Keep airway adjuncts and anaphylaxis drugs at bedside during administration.
- Watch for signs and symptoms of infection, such as fever, sore throat, malaise.

PATIENT TEACHING
- Instruct patient to report adverse drug reactions promptly, especially signs and symptoms of infection (fever, sore throat, fatigue).
- Tell patient to immediately report discomfort at I.V. insertion site because drug can cause a chemical phlebitis.
- Advise woman to avoid pregnancy during therapy.

muromonab-CD3
Orthoclone OKT3

Pharmacologic class: monoclonal antibody
Pregnancy risk category C

AVAILABLE FORMS
Injection: 1 mg/1 ml in 5-ml ampules

INDICATIONS & DOSAGES
➤ **Acute allograft rejection in renal transplant patients; steroid-resistant hepatic or cardiac allograft rejection**
Adults: 5 mg I.V. daily for 10 to 14 days.
Children: Initially, 2.5 mg/day (if 30 kg or less) or 5 mg/day (if more than 30 kg) I.V. as a single bolus over less than 1 minute for 10 to 14 days. Daily dosage may need 2.5-mg increment increases to decrease CD3+ cells.

I.V. ADMINISTRATION
- Draw solution into syringe through low–protein-binding 0.2- or 0.22-micron filter. Discard filter and attach needle for I.V. bolus injection.
- Give bolus over less than 1 minute.
- Don't shake or freeze.

INCOMPATIBILITIES
Other I.V. drugs.

ACTION
A murine monoclonal antibody that reacts in the T lymphocyte membrane with CD3, needed for antigen recognition. Depletes blood of CD3+ T cells, restoring allograft function and reversing rejection.

Route	Onset	Peak	Duration
I.V.	Immediate	Unknown	1 wk

Half-life: Unknown.

ADVERSE REACTIONS
CNS: *asthenia, fever, headache, tremor,* ***meningitis, seizures,*** confusion, depression, dizziness, fatigue, lethargy, malaise, nervousness, somnolence.
CV: *edema, hypertension, hypotension, tachycardia,* ***arrhythmia, bradycardia, cardiac arrest, heart failure, shock,*** chest pain, vascular occlusion, vasodilation.
EENT: photophobia, tinnitus.
GI: *diarrhea, nausea, vomiting,* abdominal pain, anorexia, GI pain.
GU: ***renal dysfunction.***
Hematologic: anemia, ***leukocytosis, leukopenia, thrombocytopenia.***
Musculoskeletal: arthralgia, myalgia.
Respiratory: *dyspnea,* ***acute respiratory distress syndrome,*** hyperventilation, hypoxia, pneumonia, pulmonary edema, respiratory congestion, wheezing.
Skin: diaphoresis, pruritus, *rash.*
Other: *chills,* ***cytokine release syndrome, hypersensitivity reactions,*** pain in trunk area.

INTERACTIONS
Drug-drug. *Immunosuppressants:* May increase risk of infection. Consider reducing immunosuppressant dosage. Use together cautiously.
Indomethacin: May increase muromonab-CD3 level, causing encephalopathy and other CNS effects. Monitor patient closely.
Live-virus vaccines: May increase replication and effects of vaccine. Use together cautiously.

EFFECTS ON LAB TEST RESULTS
- May increase BUN and creatinine levels.
- May cause abnormal urine cytologic study results.

CONTRAINDICATIONS & CAUTIONS

- Contraindicated in patients hypersensitive to drug or other products of murine (mouse) origin, in those who have history of seizures or are predisposed to seizures, in pregnant or breast-feeding women, and in patients with uncontrolled hypertension.
- Contraindicated in those with antimurine antibody titers of 1:1,000 or more or fluid overload, as evidenced by chest X-ray or weight gain greater than 3% the week before treatment.

NURSING CONSIDERATIONS

- Never give I.M.
- Obtain chest X-ray within 24 hours before starting drug treatment.
- Assess patient for signs and symptoms of fluid overload before treatment.
- Give therapy in facility equipped and staffed for cardiopulmonary resuscitation, where patient can be monitored closely.
- Most adverse reactions develop within 30 minutes to 6 hours after first dose.
- Before giving drug, pretreat patient with an antipyretic to reduce risk of pyrexia and chills. Treat temperature over 100° F (38° C) with antipyretics before giving drug, and evaluate risk of infection.
- ***Alert:*** Give methylprednisolone 1 to 4 hours before first dose to reduce the severity of infusion reaction.
- Patients may develop antibodies to drug, which can lead to loss of effectiveness and more severe adverse reactions if a second course is attempted.

PATIENT TEACHING

- Inform patient of expected adverse reactions.
- Reassure patient that reactions will diminish as treatment progresses.
- Tell patient to avoid people with infections because drug lowers resistance to infection.
- Advise woman to avoid pregnancy during therapy.

mycophenolate mofetil
CellCept, Myfortic

mycophenolate mofetil hydrochloride
CellCept Intravenous

mycophenolic acid
Myfortic

Pharmacologic class: mycophenolic acid derivative
Pregnancy risk category C

AVAILABLE FORMS

mycophenolate mofetil
Capsules: 250 mg
Powder for oral suspension: 200 mg/ml
Tablets: 500 mg
mycophenolate mofetil hydrochloride
Injection: 500 mg/vial
mycophenolic acid
Tablets (extended-release): 180 mg, 360 mg

INDICATIONS & DOSAGES

➤ **To prevent organ rejection in patients receiving allogenic renal transplants**

Adults: 1 g I.V. or P.O. (regular-release) b.i.d. with corticosteroids and cyclosporine. Or, 720 mg extended-release tablets P.O. b.i.d. 1 hour before or 2 hours after food.

Children with a body surface area (BSA) greater than 1.19 m^2: 400 mg/m^2 extended-release tablets b.i.d. up to a maximum of 720 mg b.i.d. Children with a BSA of 1.19 to 1.58 m^2 may be dosed with either three 180-mg tablets b.i.d. or one 180-mg tablet plus one 360-mg tablet b.i.d. for a total daily dosage of 1,080 mg. Children with a BSA greater than 1.58 m^2 can receive either four 180-mg tablets b.i.d. or two 360-mg tablets b.i.d. for a total daily dosage of 1,440 mg.

Adjust-a-dose: For patients with severe chronic renal impairment outside of immediate posttransplant period, avoid doses above 1 g b.i.d. If neutropenia develops, interrupt or reduce dosage.

➤ **To prevent organ rejection in patients receiving allogenic cardiac transplant**
Adults: 1.5 g P.O. or I.V. b.i.d. with cyclosporine and corticosteroids.
➤ **To prevent organ rejection in patients receiving allogenic hepatic transplants**
Adults: 1 g I.V. b.i.d. over no less than 2 hours or 1.5 g P.O. b.i.d. with cyclosporine and corticosteroids.
Adjust-a-dose: If neutropenia develops, stop or reduce dosage.

I.V. ADMINISTRATION
- Reconstitute and dilute to 6 mg/ml using 14 ml of D_5W.
- Never give by rapid or bolus I.V. injection. Infuse drug over at least 2 hours.
- Use within 4 hours of reconstitution and dilution.

INCOMPATIBILITIES
Other I.V. drugs or solutions.

ACTION
Inhibits proliferative response of T and B lymphocytes, suppresses antibody formation by B lymphocytes, and may inhibit recruitment of leukocytes into sites of inflammation and graft rejection.

Route	Onset	Peak	Duration
P.O.	Unknown	30–75 min	7–18 hr
P.O. (extended-release)	Unknown	1½–2¾ hr	8–17 hr
I.V.	Unknown	Unknown	10–17 hr

Half-life: About 18 hours.

ADVERSE REACTIONS
CNS: *asthenia, fever, headache, tremor,* dizziness, insomnia.
CV: *chest pain, edema, hypertension.*
EENT: pharyngitis.
GI: *abdominal pain, constipation, diarrhea, dyspepsia, nausea, oral candidiasis, vomiting,* ***hemorrhage.***
GU: *hematuria, UTI,* renal tubular necrosis.
Hematologic: *anemia,* **LEUKOPENIA, THROMBOCYTOPENIA,** hypochromic anemia, leukocytosis.
Metabolic: *hypercholesterolemia, hyperglycemia, hyperkalemia, hypokalemia, hypophosphatemia.*
Musculoskeletal: *back pain.*
Respiratory: *cough, dyspnea, infection,* bronchitis, pneumonia.
Skin: *acne,* rash.
Other: *pain, infection, peripheral edema,* ***sepsis.***

INTERACTIONS
Drug-drug. *Acyclovir, ganciclovir, other drugs that undergo renal tubular secretion:* May increase risk of toxicity for both drugs. Monitor patient closely.
Antacids with magnesium and aluminum hydroxides: May decrease mycophenolate absorption. Separate dosing times.
Azathioprine: Inhibits purine metabolism. Don't give together.
Cholestyramine: May interfere with enterohepatic recirculation, reducing mycophenolate bioavailability. Avoid using together.
Phenytoin, theophylline: May increase both drug levels. Monitor drug levels closely.
Probenecid, salicylates: May increase mycophenolate level. Monitor patient closely.
Vaccines, live: May decrease vaccine's effectiveness. Avoid using together.
Drug-herb. *Cat's claw, echinacea:* May increase immunostimulation. Discourage use together.
Drug-food. *Food:* May delay absorption of extended-release form. Give Myfortic on an empty stomach.

EFFECTS ON LAB TEST RESULTS
- May increase cholesterol and glucose levels. May decrease phosphorus and hemoglobin levels. May increase or decrease potassium level.
- May decrease platelet count. May increase or decrease WBC count.

CONTRAINDICATIONS & CAUTIONS
- Contraindicated in patients hypersensitive to drug, its ingredients, or mycophenolic acid and in patients sensitive to polysorbate 80.
- Safety and effectiveness of drug in children haven't been established.
- Use cautiously in patients with GI disorders.

NURSING CONSIDERATIONS

- Start drug therapy within 24 hours after transplantation. Use I.V. form in patients unable to take oral forms.
- I.V. form can be given for up to 14 days; switch patient to capsules or tablets as soon as oral drugs can be tolerated.
- ***Alert:*** The extended-release tablets aren't interchangeable with other forms.
- Because drug can cause birth defects, don't open or crush capsule. Avoid inhaling powder in capsule or having it contact skin or mucous membranes. If contact occurs, wash skin thoroughly with soap and water, and rinse eyes with water.

PATIENT TEACHING

- Warn patient not to open or crush capsules or to cut, crush, or chew extended-release tablets but to swallow them whole on an empty stomach.
- Stress importance of following treatment as prescribed.
- Inform patient of the importance of follow-up visits and ongoing lab tests during therapy.
- Tell woman to have a pregnancy test 1 week before therapy begins.
- Instruct woman to use two forms of contraception during therapy and for 6 weeks afterward, even if she has a history of infertility. Tell her to notify prescriber immediately if she suspects pregnancy.
- Warn patient of the increased risk of lymphoma and other malignancies.

sirolimus

Rapamune

Pharmacologic class: macrocyclic lactone
Pregnancy risk category C

AVAILABLE FORMS

Oral solution: 1 mg/ml
Tablet: 1 mg, 2 mg

INDICATIONS & DOSAGES

➤ **With cyclosporine and corticosteroids, to prevent organ rejection in patients receiving renal transplants**

Adults and adolescents: Initially, 6 mg P.O. as one-time dose as soon as possible after transplantation; then maintenance dose of 2 mg P.O. once daily.
Children age 13 and older who weigh less than 40 kg (88 lb): First dose is 3 mg/m^2 P.O. as one-time dose after transplantation; then 1 mg/m^2 P.O. once daily.
Adjust-a-dose: For patients with mild to moderate hepatic impairment, reduce maintenance dose by about one-third. It isn't necessary to reduce loading dose. Two to 4 months after transplant in patients with low to moderate risk of graft rejection, taper off cyclosporine over 4 to 8 weeks. During the taper, adjust sirolimus dose q 1 to 2 weeks to obtain levels between 12 and 24 nanograms/ml. Base dosage adjustments on clinical status, tissue biopsies, and laboratory findings.

Maximum daily dose shouldn't exceed 40 mg. If a daily dose exceeds 40 mg due to a loading dose, give the loading dose over 2 days. Monitor trough concentrations at least 3 to 4 days after a loading dose.

ACTION

An immunosuppressant that inhibits T cell activation and proliferation that occurs in response to antigenic and cytokine stimulation. Also inhibits antibody formation.

Route	Onset	Peak	Duration
P.O.	Unknown	1–3 hr	Unknown

Half-life: About 62 hours.

ADVERSE REACTIONS

CNS: *anxiety, asthenia, depression, fever, headache, insomnia, tremor,* confusion, dizziness, emotional lability, hypertonia, hypesthesia, hypotonia, malaise, neuropathy, paresthesia, somnolence, syncope.
CV: *chest pain, edema, hypertension, peripheral edema,* ***heart failure, hemorrhage,*** atrial fibrillation, hypotension, palpitations, peripheral vascular disorder, tachycardia, thrombophlebitis, thrombosis, vasodilatation.
EENT: *pharyngitis,* abnormal vision, epistaxis, cataract, conjunctivitis, deafness, ear pain, otitis media, rhinitis, sinusitis, tinnitus.
GI: *abdominal pain, constipation, diarrhea, dyspepsia, nausea, vomiting,* ano-

rexia, ascites, dysphagia, enlarged abdomen, eructation, esophagitis, flatulence, gastritis, gastroenteritis, gingivitis, gum hyperplasia, hernia, ileus, peritonitis, mouth ulceration, oral candidiasis, stomatitis.

GU: *UTI, **kidney tubular necrosis, toxic nephropathy,*** albuminuria, bladder pain, dysuria, glycosuria, hematuria, hydronephrosis, impotence, kidney pain, nocturia, oliguria, pelvic pain, pyuria, scrotal edema, testis disorder, urinary frequency, urinary incontinence, urine retention.

Hematologic: *anemia,* **THROMBOCYTOPENIA,** ***leukopenia, thrombotic thrombocytopenia purpura,*** ecchymosis, leukocytosis, polycythemia.

Hepatic: ***hepatic artery thrombosis, hepatotoxicity.***

Metabolic: *hypercholesteremia, hyperkalemia, hyperlipidemia, hypokalemia, hypophosphatemia, weight gain,* ***hypoglycemia,*** acidosis, Cushing syndrome, diabetes mellitus, dehydration, hypercalcemia, hyperglycemia, hyperphosphatemia, hypervolemia, hypocalcemia, hypomagnesemia, hyponatremia, weight loss.

Musculoskeletal: *arthralgia, back pain,* arthrosis, bone necrosis, leg cramps, myalgia, osteoporosis, tetany.

Respiratory: *atelectasis, cough, dyspnea, upper respiratory tract infection,* ***interstitial lung disease,*** asthma, bronchitis, hypoxia, lung edema, pleural effusion, pneumonia.

Skin: *acne, rash,* fungal dermatitis, hirsutism, pruritus, skin hypertrophy, skin ulcer, sweating.

Other: *pain,* ***sepsis,*** abnormal healing, including fascial dehiscence and anastomotic disruption (wound, vascular, airway, ureteral, biliary), abscess, cellulitis, chills, facial edema, flu syndrome, infection, lymphadenopathy, lymphocele.

INTERACTIONS

Drug-drug. *Aminoglycosides, amphotericin B, other nephrotoxic drugs:* May increase risk of nephrotoxicity. Use with caution.

Bromocriptine, cimetidine, clarithromycin, clotrimazole, danazol, erythromycin, fluconazole, indinavir, itraconazole, metoclopramide, nicardipine, ritonavir, verapamil, other drugs that inhibit CYP3A4: May increase blood levels of sirolimus. Monitor sirolimus levels closely.

Carbamazepine, phenobarbital, phenytoin, rifabutin, rifapentine, other drugs that induce CYP3A4: May decrease blood levels of sirolimus. Monitor patient closely.

Cyclosporine: May increase sirolimus level and toxicity. Give sirolimus 4 hours after cyclosporine; monitor levels and adjust dose, as needed.

Diltiazem: May increase sirolimus levels. Monitor sirolimus level, as needed.

HMG-CoA reductase inhibitors or fibrates: May increase risk of rhabdomyolysis with the combination of sirolimus and cyclosporine. Monitor patient closely.

Ketoconazole: May increase rate and extent of sirolimus absorption. Avoid using together.

Live-virus vaccines: May reduce vaccine effectiveness. Avoid using together.

Rifampin: May decrease sirolimus level. Alternative therapy to rifampin may be prescribed.

Drug-food. *Grapefruit juice:* May decrease drug metabolism. Discourage using together.

Drug-lifestyle. *Sun exposure:* May increase risk of skin cancer. Tell patient to take precautions.

EFFECTS ON LAB TEST RESULTS

- May increase BUN, creatinine, liver enzyme, cholesterol, and lipid levels. May decrease sodium, magnesium, and hemoglobin levels. May increase or decrease phosphate, potassium, glucose, and calcium levels.
- May increase RBC count. May decrease platelet count. May increase or decrease WBC count.

CONTRAINDICATIONS & CAUTIONS

- Contraindicated in patients hypersensitive to active drug, its derivatives, or components of product.
- Use cautiously in patients with hyperlipidemia and impaired liver or renal function.
- Safety and effectiveness of sirolimus as immunosuppressive therapy haven't been established in liver or lung transplant patients.

NURSING CONSIDERATIONS

• *Alert:* Using this drug with tacrolimus or cyclosporine may cause hepatic artery thrombosis, leading to graft loss and death.
• Only those experienced in immunosuppressive therapy and management of renal transplant patients should prescribe drug.
• Use drug in regimen with cyclosporine and corticosteroids; have patient take drug 4 hours after cyclosporine dose.
• Cyclosporine withdrawal in patients with high risk of graft rejection isn't recommended. This includes patients with Banff grade III acute rejection or vascular rejection before cyclosporine withdrawal, those who are dialysis dependent, those with serum creatinine level greater than 4.5 mg/dl, black patients, patients with retransplants or multiorgan transplants, and patients with high panel of reactive antibodies.
• Patient should take drug consistently either with or without food.
• Dilute oral solution before use. After dilution, use immediately and discard oral solution syringe.
• When diluting oral solution, empty correct amount into glass or plastic (not Styrofoam) container holding at least ¼ cup (60 ml) of either water or orange juice. Don't use grapefruit juice or any other liquid. Stir vigorously and have patient drink immediately. Refill container with at least ½ cup (120 ml) of water or orange juice, stir again, and have patient drink all contents.
• After transplantation, give antimicrobial prophylaxis for *Pneumocystis jiroveci (carinii)* for 1 year and for cytomegalovirus for 3 months.
• *Alert:* Patients taking drug are more susceptible to infection and lymphoma.
• Monitor renal function tests, because use with cyclosporine may cause creatinine level to increase. Adjustment of immunosuppressive regimen may be needed.
• Monitor cholesterol and triglyceride levels. Treatment with lipid-lowering drugs during therapy isn't uncommon. If hyperlipidemia is detected, additional interventions, such as diet and exercise, should begin.
• Check for rhabdomyolysis.
• Monitor drug levels in patients age 13 and older who weigh less than 40 kg (88 lb), patients with hepatic impairment, those also receiving drugs that induce or inhibit CYP3A4, and patients in whom cyclosporine dosing is markedly reduced or stopped.
• A slight haze may develop during refrigeration. This doesn't affect potency of drug. If haze develops, bring to room temperature and shake until haze disappears.
• Store away from light, and refrigerate at 36° to 46° F (2° to 8° C). After opening bottle, use contents within 1 month. If needed, store bottles and pouches at room temperature (up to 77° F [25° C]) for several days. Drug may be kept in oral syringe for 24 hours at room temperature.

PATIENT TEACHING

• Tell patient how to properly store, dilute, and give drug.
• Advise woman about risks during pregnancy. Tell her to use effective contraception before and during therapy and for 12 weeks after stopping therapy.
• Tell patient to take drug consistently with or without food to minimize absorption variability.
• Tell patient to take drug 4 hours after cyclosporine to avoid drug interactions.
• Advise patient to wash area with soap and water if drug solution touches skin or mucous membranes.

tacrolimus (FK506)
Prograf

Pharmacologic class: macrolide
Pregnancy risk category C

AVAILABLE FORMS

Capsules: 0.5 mg, 1 mg, 5 mg
Injection: 5 mg/ml

INDICATIONS & DOSAGES

➤ **To prevent organ rejection in allogenic liver, kidney, or heart transplant**

Adults: For patients who can't take drug orally, give 0.03 to 0.05 mg/kg/day (liver or kidney) or 0.01 mg/kg/day (heart) I.V. as continuous infusion at least 6 hours after transplant. Switch to oral therapy as soon as possible, with first dose 8 to 12 hours after stopping I.V. infusion. For renal transplant, give oral dose within 24 hours of transplantation after renal function has recovered. Initial P.O. dosages: For liver transplant, give 0.1 to 0.15 mg/kg daily in two divided doses q 12 hours; for kidney transplant, give 0.2 mg/kg daily in two divided doses q 12 hours; for heart transplant, give 0.075 mg/kg daily in two divided doses q 12 hours. Adjust dosages based on patient response.

Children (liver transplant only): Initially, 0.03 to 0.05 mg/kg daily I.V.; then 0.15 to 0.2 mg/kg daily P.O. on schedule similar to that of adults, adjusted as needed.

Adjust-a-dose: Give lowest recommended P.O. and I.V. dosages to patients with renal or hepatic impairment.

I.V. ADMINISTRATION

- Dilute drug with normal saline solution for injection or D_5W injection to 0.004 to 0.02 mg/ml before use.
- Monitor patient continuously during first 30 minutes and frequently thereafter for signs and symptoms of anaphylaxis.
- Store diluted infusion solution for up to 24 hours in glass or polyethylene containers. Don't store drug in a polyvinyl chloride container because of decreased stability and potential for extraction of phthalates.

INCOMPATIBILITIES

Solutions or I.V. drugs with a pH above 9, such as acyclovir and ganciclovir.

ACTION

Exact mechanism unknown. Inhibits T cell activation, which results in immunosuppression.

Route	Onset	Peak	Duration
P.O., I.V.	Unknown	1½–3 hr	Unknown

Half-life: 33 to 56 hours.

ADVERSE REACTIONS

CNS: *asthenia, delirium, fever, headache, insomnia, pain, paresthesia, tremor,* ***coma.***
CV: *peripheral edema,* hypertension.
GI: *abdominal pain, anorexia, ascites, constipation, diarrhea, nausea, vomiting.*
GU: *abnormal renal function, oliguria, UTI.*
Hematologic: THROMBOCYTOPENIA, *anemia, leukocytosis.*
Metabolic: *hyperglycemia, hyperkalemia, hypokalemia, hypomagnesemia.*
Musculoskeletal: *back pain.*
Respiratory: *atelectasis, dyspnea, pleural effusion.*
Skin: *burning, photosensitivity, pruritus, rash,* alopecia.

INTERACTIONS

Drug-drug. *Azole antifungals,* *Bromocriptine, cimetidine, clarithromycin, cyclosporine, danazol, diltiazem, erythromycin, methylprednisolone, metoclopramide, nicardipine, verapamil:* May increase tacrolimus level. Watch for adverse effects.
Carbamazepine, phenobarbital, phenytoin, ***rifamycins:*** May decrease tacrolimus level. Monitor effectiveness of tacrolimus.
Cyclosporine: May increase risk of excess nephrotoxicity. Avoid using together.
Immunosuppressants (except adrenal corticosteroids): May oversuppress immune system. Monitor patient closely, especially during times of stress.
Inducers of cytochrome P-450 enzyme system: May increase tacrolimus metabolism and decrease blood levels. Dosage adjustment may be needed.
Inhibitors of cytochrome P-450 enzyme system (phenobarbital, phenytoin, rifampin): May decrease tacrolimus metabolism and increase blood level. Dosage adjustment may be needed.
Live-virus vaccines: May interfere with immune response to live-virus vaccines. Postpone routine immunizations.
Nephrotoxic drugs, such as aminoglycosides, amphotericin B, cisplatin, cyclosporine: May cause additive or synergistic effects. Monitor patient closely.
Drug-herb. *St. John's Wort:* May decrease drug level. Discourage use together.
Drug-food. *Any food:* May inhibit drug absorption. Urge patient to take drug on empty stomach.
Grapefruit juice: May increase drug level. Discourage patient from taking together.

EFFECTS ON LAB TEST RESULTS

- May increase BUN, creatinine, and glucose levels. May decrease magnesium and

hemoglobin levels. May increase or decrease potassium level and cause abnormal liver function test values.
- May decrease WBC and platelet counts.

CONTRAINDICATIONS & CAUTIONS
- Contraindicated in patients hypersensitive to drug.
- I.V. form is contraindicated in patients hypersensitive to castor oil derivatives.

NURSING CONSIDERATIONS
- ***Alert:*** Patient has increased risk for infections, lymphomas, and other malignant diseases. Use only after other treatments have failed.
- ***Alert:*** Because of risk of anaphylaxis, use injection only in patients who can't take oral form. Keep epinephrine 1:1,000 and oxygen available.
- Children with normal renal and hepatic function may need higher dosages than adults.
- Patients with hepatic or renal dysfunction should receive lowest dosage possible.
- Use with adrenal corticosteroids for all indications. For heart transplant patients, also use with azathioprine or mycophenolate mofetil.
- ***Alert:*** The use of sirolimus with tacrolimus may increase the risk of wound healing complications, renal impairment, and insulin-dependent posttransplant diabetes mellitus in heart transplant patients. Don't use together.
- Monitor patient for signs and symptoms of neurotoxicity and nephrotoxicity, especially if patient is receiving a high dose or has renal or hepatic dysfunction.
- Monitor patient for signs and symptoms of hyperkalemia, such as palpitations and muscle weakness or cramping. Obtain potassium levels regularly. Avoid potassium-sparing diuretics during drug therapy.
- Monitor patient's glucose level regularly. Also monitor patient for signs and symptoms of hyperglycemia, such as dizziness, confusion, and frequent urination. Treatment of hyperglycemia may be needed. Insulin-dependent posttransplant diabetes may occur; in some cases, it's reversible.

PATIENT TEACHING
- Advise patient to check with prescriber before taking other drugs during therapy.
- Urge patient to report adverse reactions promptly.
- Tell diabetic patient that glucose levels may increase.

73

Vaccines and toxoids

diphtheria and tetanus toxoids and acellular pertussis vaccine adsorbed (DTaP)

Daptacel, Infanrix, TRIPACEL†, Tripedia

tetanus toxoid and reduced diphtheria toxoid and acellular pertussis vaccine adsorbed (Tdap)

ADACEL, Boostrix

Pharmacologic class: vaccine/toxoid
Pregnancy risk category C

AVAILABLE FORMS

DTap

Daptacel

Injection: 15 limit flocculation (Lf) units diphtheria toxoid, 5 Lf units tetanus toxoid, 23 mcg acellular pertussis vaccine adsorbed per 0.5 ml

Infanrix

Injection: 25 Lf units diphtheria toxoid, 10 Lf units tetanus toxoid, 58 mcg acellular pertussis vaccine adsorbed per 0.5 ml

Tripedia

Injection: 6.7 Lf units diphtheria toxoid, 5 Lf units tetanus toxoid, 46.8 mcg acellular pertussis vaccine adsorbed per 0.5 ml

Tdap

Adacel

Injection: 5 Lf units tetanus toxoid, 2 Lf units diphtheria toxoid, 15.5 mcg acellular pertussis vaccine adsorbed per 0.5 ml

Boostrix

Injection: 5 Lf units tetanus toxoid, 2.5 Lf units diphtheria toxoid, 18.5 mcg acellular pertussis vaccine adsorbed per 0.5 ml

INDICATIONS & DOSAGES

➤Primary immunization (Daptacel, Infanrix, Tripedia)

Children ages 6 weeks to 7 years: Give 0.5 ml I.M. 4 to 8 weeks apart for three doses (6 to 8 weeks for Daptacel) and a fourth dose at least 6 months after the third dose.

➤**Booster immunization**

Children ages 6 weeks to 7 years: Daptacel may be given to complete the immunization series in children who have received at least one dose of whole-cell DTP vaccine.

Infanrix is indicated as a fifth dose in children ages 4 to 6 before entering school in those who received at least one dose of whole-cell DTP vaccine, unless the fourth dose was given after the fourth birthday.

If Tripedia was used for the first four doses, a fifth dose is recommended at age 4 to 6 before entering school. If the fourth dose was given after age 4, a fifth dose isn't needed.

Adults and children age 11 to 64 (Adacel): 0.5 ml I.M. as a single dose at least 5 years after the last DTaP vaccination.

Children and adolescents age 10 to 18 (Boostrix): 0.5 ml I.M. as a single dose at least 5 years after the last DTaP vaccination.

ACTION

Promotes active immunity to DTP by inducing production of antitoxins and antibodies.

Route	Onset	Peak	Duration
I.M.	2 wk after last dose	Unknown	10 yr

Half-life: Unknown.

ADVERSE REACTIONS

CNS: ***seizures,*** *drowsiness, fever.*

GI: *anorexia,* vomiting.

Skin: *redness and swelling at injection site, tenderness.*

Other: *fretfulness, hypersensitivity reactions,* crying longer than 1 hour, irritability.

INTERACTIONS

Drug-drug. *Immunosuppressants:* May reduce response to DTP vaccine. Avoid using together.

EFFECTS ON LAB TEST RESULTS

None reported.

CONTRAINDICATIONS & CAUTIONS

- Contraindicated in adults or children older than age 7 (except Adacel and Boostrix), immunosuppressed patients, those on corticosteroid therapy, and those with history of seizures.
- Pertussis component of vaccine is contraindicated in children who have neurologic disorders or who exhibited neurologic signs after previous injection. Give these children diphtheria and tetanus toxoids (DT) vaccine instead. Postpone vaccination in patients with acute febrile illness.

NURSING CONSIDERATIONS

- Children whose seizures are well controlled or who had an explainable, single-episode seizure may receive the acellular vaccine.
- Obtain history of allergies and reaction to immunization, especially to pertussis vaccine.
- Keep epinephrine 1:1,000 available to treat anaphylaxis.
- If an immediate allergic reaction occurs after giving the vaccine, withhold subsequent vaccination and refer patient to an allergist for evaluation. Documentation of a specific allergy may warrant desensitization to tetanus toxoid.
- Give only by deep I.M. injection, preferably in thigh or deltoid muscle. Don't give subcutaneously.
- In infants, give I.M. injection in the anterolateral thigh.
- Vaccine may be given at same time as polio vaccine; *Haemophilus influenzae* type b; measles, mumps, and rubella; hepatitis A and B; influenza; meningococcal disease; pneumococcal disease; and varicella.
- Acellular vaccine may be linked to a lower risk of local pain and fever.
- ***Alert:*** DTP preparations usually aren't interchangeable. It's recommended to use the vaccine from the same manufacturer, if possible, for at least the first three doses.

PATIENT TEACHING

- Explain risks and benefits of vaccine to parents before it's given.
- Tell parents to report systemic reactions promptly; remind them that local reactions are common. Acetaminophen in age-

appropriate doses will decrease occurrence of postvaccination fever in children susceptible to febrile seizure activity.
- Stress importance of keeping scheduled appointments for subsequent doses. Full immunization requires a series of injections.

diphtheria and tetanus toxoids, acellular pertussis adsorbed, hepatitis B (recombinant), and inactivated poliovirus vaccine combined
Pediarix

Pharmacologic class: vaccine/toxoid
Pregnancy risk category C

AVAILABLE FORMS
Injection: 0.5-ml single-dose vials and disposable, prefilled Tip-Lok syringes

INDICATIONS & DOSAGES
➤ **Active immunization**
Children ages 6 weeks to 7 years: Primary series is three 0.5-ml doses I.M. at 6- to 8-week intervals (preferably 8), usually starting at age 2 months; may start at age 6 weeks.

ACTION
Promotes active immunity to hepatitis B; poliomyelitis types 1, 2, and 3; diphtheria; tetanus; and pertussis by inducing antitoxin and antibody production.

Route	Onset	Peak	Duration
I.M.	Unknown	Unknown	Unknown

Half-life: Unknown.

ADVERSE REACTIONS
CNS: *fever, fussiness, increased sleeping, restlessness, unusual cry.*
GI: *anorexia.*
Skin: *injection site reactions (pain, redness, swelling).*

INTERACTIONS
Drug-drug. *Immunosuppressive therapies, such as alkylating agents, antimetabolites, corticosteroids, cytotoxic drugs, radiation:* May reduce immune response to the vaccine. If immunosuppressive therapy will end soon, postpone immunization until 3 months after immunosuppressive therapy; otherwise, vaccinate patient during immunosuppressive therapy, but expect inadequate response.

EFFECTS ON LAB TEST RESULTS
None reported.

CONTRAINDICATIONS & CAUTIONS
- Contraindicated in patients hypersensitive to any component of vaccine, including yeast, neomycin, and polymyxin B.
- Contraindicated if a previous dose of vaccine or its components caused a serious allergic reaction.
- Contraindicated in patient with progressive neurologic disorder, including infantile spasms, uncontrolled epilepsy, progressive encephalopathy, or encephalopathy within 7 days of a previous dose of pertussis-containing vaccine that can't be attributed to another cause.
- Use cautiously in children with bleeding disorders, such as hemophilia or thrombocytopenia, and take steps to reduce the risk of hematoma after injection.
- Avoid giving drug to an infant younger than 6 weeks, to a child age 7 or older, or to a child receiving anticoagulant therapy, unless the potential benefit outweighs the risk.
- Drug isn't indicated for adults.

NURSING CONSIDERATIONS
- Inject vaccine into the anterolateral aspect of the thigh or the deltoid muscle of the upper arm. Don't inject in the gluteal area or any area that may contain a major nerve trunk.
- ***Alert:*** The tip cap and plunger of the needleless prefilled syringe contain latex and may cause allergic reactions in sensitive persons.
- Combined vaccine is more likely to cause fever than vaccines given separately.
- For children at high risk of seizures, give an antipyretic with vaccination and for 24 hours afterward to reduce risk of fever.
- Postpone vaccination if patient has a moderate or severe illness with or without fever.
- If patient has seizures within 3 days after being vaccinated, a temperature higher than 105° F (40.50° C), collapse or

shocklike state, or persistent, inconsolable crying lasting 3 hours or more within 48 hours of the vaccine, postpone future doses of this drug or any vaccine containing pertussis until potential benefits and possible risks are reviewed.

• Interrupting the recommended schedule doesn't alter final immunity. The series need not be started over, regardless of the time elapsed between doses.

• Don't give drug as a booster dose after the main three-dose series. Instead, give a diphtheria and tetanus toxoids, acellular pertussis adsorbed vaccine at age 15 to 18 months (Infanrix because its pertussis antigen components match those in Pediarix) and inactivated polio vaccine at age 4 to 6.

PATIENT TEACHING

• Tell parent to expect some redness, soreness, swelling, and hardness at the injection site.

• Tell parent that a nodule may form at the injection site and may persist for several weeks.

• Recommend acetaminophen to relieve discomfort.

• Stress the importance of keeping scheduled appointments for subsequent doses.

Haemophilus b conjugate vaccines

Haemophilus b conjugate vaccine, diphtheria CRM 197 protein conjugate (HbOC)
HibTITER

Haemophilus b conjugate vaccine, diphtheria toxoid conjugate (PRP-D)
Prohibit

Haemophilus b conjugate vaccine, hepatitis B
Comvax

Haemophilus b conjugate vaccine, meningococcal protein conjugate (PRP-OMP)
Pedvaxhib

Haemophilus b conjugate, tetanus toxoid conjugate (PRP-T)
ActHIB

Pharmacologic class: vaccine
Pregnancy risk category C

AVAILABLE FORMS

***Haemophilus influenzae type b* (HIB) conjugate vaccine, diphtheria CRM 197 protein conjugate**
Injection: 10 mcg of purified HIB saccharide and about 25 mcg CRM 197 protein per 0.5 ml

HIB conjugate vaccine, diphtheria toxoid conjugate
Injection: 25 mcg of HIB capsular polysaccharide and 18 mcg of diphtheria toxoid protein per 0.5 ml

HIB conjugate vaccine, hepatitis B
Injection: 7.5 mcg of HIB capsular polysaccharide, 125 mcg *Neisseria meningitidis* OMPC and 5 mcg hepatitis B surface antigen per 0.5 ml

HIB conjugate vaccine, meningococcal protein conjugate
Injection: 7.5 mcg of HIB PRP and 125 mcg *Neisseria meningitidis* OMPC per 0.5 ml

HIB conjugate vaccine, tetanus toxoid conjugate
Injection: 10 mcg HIB capsular polysaccharide, 24 mcg tetanus toxoid

INDICATIONS & DOSAGES

➤Immunization against HIB infection

Conjugate vaccine, diphtheria CRM_{197} protein conjugate
Infants: 0.5 ml I.M. at age 2 months. Repeat at 4 months and 6 months. Give booster dose at age 15 months.
Previously unvaccinated children ages 15 months to 6 years: 0.5 ml I.M. Booster dose isn't needed.
Previously unvaccinated infants ages 12 to 14 months: 0.5 ml I.M. Give booster dose at age 15 months (but no sooner than 2 months after first vaccination).
Previously unvaccinated infants ages 7 to 11 months: 0.5 ml I.M. Repeat in 2 months, for a total of two doses. Give booster dose at age 15 months (but no sooner than 2 months after last vaccination).

Previously unvaccinated infants ages 2 to 6 months: 0.5 ml I.M. Repeat in 2 months and again in 4 months for total of three doses. Give booster at age 15 months.
Conjugate vaccine, diphtheria toxoid conjugate
Previously unvaccinated children ages 15 to 71 months: 0.5 ml I.M. Booster dose isn't needed.
Conjugate vaccine, hepatitis B
Infants born to HBsAg negative mothers: 0.5 ml I.M. at 2, 4, and 12 to 15 months of age for a total of three doses. Infants who received a dose of hepatitis B vaccine at or shortly after birth can still receive the full 3-dose series of Comvax.
Conjugate vaccine, meningococcal protein conjugate
Infants: 0.5 ml I.M. at age 2 months; repeat at age 4 months. Give booster dose at age 12 months.
Previously unvaccinated children ages 15 months to 6 years: 0.5 ml I.M. Booster dose isn't needed.

Premature infants follow same schedule as full-term infants.
Previously unvaccinated infants ages 12 to 14 months: 0.5 ml I.M. Give booster dose at age 15 months (but no sooner than 2 months after first vaccination).
Previously unvaccinated infants ages 7 to 11 months: 0.5 ml I.M.; repeat in 2 months. Give booster dose at age 15 months (but no sooner than 2 months after last vaccination).
Previously unvaccinated infants ages 2 to 6 months: 0.5 ml I.M.; repeat in 2 months. Give booster dose at age 12 months.
Conjugate vaccine, tetanus toxoid conjugate
Infants: 0.5 ml I.M. at age 2 months. Repeat at ages 4 months and 6 months. Give booster doses at ages 15 to 18 months.
Previously unvaccinated infants ages 7 to 11 months: 0.5 ml I.M. Repeat in 2 months, for a total of two doses. Give booster doses at ages 15 to 18 months.
Previously unvaccinated infants ages 12 to 14 months: 0.5 ml I.M. Repeat in 2 months, for a total of two doses.

ACTION

Promotes active immunity to HIB; is a polymer of ribose, ribitol, and phosphate (PRP); and is linked by covalent bonds to highly antigenic substances, enabling the vaccine to promote an immune response in infants.

Route	Onset	Peak	Duration
I.M.	2 wk after last dose	Unknown	Several yr

Half-life: Unknown.

ADVERSE REACTIONS

CNS: fever.
GI: diarrhea, vomiting.
Skin: *erythema, pain at injection site.*
Other: ***anaphylaxis,*** crying.

INTERACTIONS

Drug-drug. *Immunosuppressants:* May suppress antibody response to HIB vaccine. Postpone immunization.

EFFECTS ON LAB TEST RESULTS

None reported.

CONTRAINDICATIONS & CAUTIONS

- Contraindicated in patients hypersensitive to vaccine or its components and in those with acute illness.

NURSING CONSIDERATIONS

- HIB is an important cause of meningitis in infants and preschool children.
- Immunization against HIB infection is recommended for children with HIV infections. Follow usual immunization schedule.
- Diphtheria toxoid conjugate vaccine (Prohibit) isn't recommended in children younger than age 15 months.
- Vaccine isn't routinely given to adults or children older than age 5 unless they're at high risk for infection (including patients with chronic conditions, such as functional asplenia, splenectomy, Hodgkin lymphoma, or sickle cell anemia).
- Keep epinephrine 1:1,000 available to treat anaphylaxis.
- Don't give vaccine I.D. or I.V.; give it only I.M.
- ***Alert:*** Don't give to febrile children.
- Give vaccine into anterolateral aspect of upper thigh in small children. Injections may be made into deltoid muscle of larger children if sufficient muscle is present.

• Drug may interfere with interpretation of antigen detection tests used to diagnose systemic HIB disease.

PATIENT TEACHING

• Warn patient or parents that pain may occur at injection site.

• Tell patient or parents to notify prescriber if adverse reactions persist or become severe.

hepatitis A vaccine, inactivated

Havrix, Vaqta

Pharmacologic class: vaccine
Pregnancy risk category C

AVAILABLE FORMS

Havrix

Injection: 720 enzyme-linked immunosorbent assay (ELISA) units (ELU)/0.5 ml; 1,440 ELU/ml

Vaqta

Injection: 25 units/0.5 ml, 50 units/ml

INDICATIONS & DOSAGES

➤ **Active immunization against hepatitis A virus; with immune globulin, to prevent hepatitis A in those exposed to virus or who travel to endemic areas**

Adults: 1,440 ELU Havrix or 50 units Vaqta I.M. as single dose. For booster dose, give 1,440 ELU Havrix 6 to 12 months after first dose or 50 units Vaqta I.M. 6 to 18 months after first dose. Booster is recommended for prolonged immunity.

Children ages 12 months to 18 years: 720 ELU Havrix or 25 units Vaqta I.M. as single dose. Then, give booster dose of 720 ELU Havrix 6 to 12 months after first dose or 25 units Vaqta I.M. 6 to 18 months after first dose. Booster is recommended for prolonged immunity.

ACTION

Promotes active immunity to hepatitis A virus.

Route	Onset	Peak	Duration
I.M.	1–15 days	Unknown	6 mo

Half-life: Unknown.

ADVERSE REACTIONS

CNS: *fatigue, fever, headache, malaise,* ***seizures,*** dizziness, encephalopathy, hypertonia, insomnia, vertigo.

EENT: pharyngitis, photophobia.

GI: *anorexia, nausea,* abdominal pain, diarrhea, dysgeusia, vomiting.

GU: menstrual disorders.

Musculoskeletal: arthralgia, myalgia.

Respiratory: upper respiratory tract infections.

Skin: *induration, injection site soreness, redness, swelling,* hematoma, jaundice, pruritus, rash, urticaria.

Other: ***anaphylaxis,*** lymphadenopathy.

INTERACTIONS

Drug-drug. *Anticoagulants:* May increase risk of bleeding. Give I.M. injection cautiously.

Immunosuppressants: May suppress antibody response in patients receiving immunosuppressive therapy. Monitor patient.

EFFECTS ON LAB TEST RESULTS

• May increase CK level.

CONTRAINDICATIONS & CAUTIONS

• Contraindicated in patients hypersensitive to vaccine's components.

• Use cautiously in patients with thrombocytopenia or bleeding disorders and in those who are taking an anticoagulant because bleeding may occur after an I.M. injection.

NURSING CONSIDERATIONS

• Shake vial or syringe well before drawing up. After vaccine has been agitated thoroughly, it's an opaque white suspension. If it's not, discard it. No dilution or reconstitution is needed.

• Inject into the deltoid region in adults. Don't give in gluteal region; such injections may result in suboptimal response. Never inject I.V., subcutaneously, or I.D.

• As with other vaccines, postpone hepatitis A vaccination, if possible, in patient with febrile illness.

• Keep epinephrine 1:1,000 available to treat anaphylaxis.

• If vaccine is given to immunosuppressed persons or those receiving immunosuppressants, expected immune response may not occur.

• Persons who should receive vaccine include people traveling to or living in areas endemic for hepatitis A (Africa, Asia [except Japan], the Mediterranean basin, Eastern Europe, the Middle East, Central and South America, Mexico, and parts of the Caribbean), military personnel, Native Americans and Alaskans, persons engaging in high-risk sexual activity, and users of illegal injectable drugs. Certain institutional workers, employees of child day-care centers, laboratory workers who handle live hepatitis A virus, and primate handlers also may benefit.

PATIENT TEACHING

• Inform patient that vaccine won't prevent hepatitis caused by other drugs or pathogens known to infect the liver.
• Warn patient about local adverse reactions. Tell him to report persistent or severe reactions promptly.
• Alert travelers to dangers of eating raw or undercooked shellfish or consuming food or drink in countries with poor hygienic conditions.
• Remind patient to return for booster injection.

hepatitis B vaccine, recombinant

Engerix-B, Recombivax HB, Recombivax HB Dialysis Formulation

Pharmacologic class: vaccine
Pregnancy risk category C

AVAILABLE FORMS

Injection: 5 mcg HBsAg/0.5 ml (Recombivax HB, pediatric and adolescent form with or without preservative); 10 mcg HBsAg/0.5 ml (Engerix-B, pediatric and adolescent form); 10 mcg HBsAg/ml (Recombivax HB, adult form); 20 mcg HBsAg/ml (Engerix-B, adult form); 40 mcg HBsAg/ml (Recombivax HB dialysis form)

INDICATIONS & DOSAGES

➤ **Immunization against infection from all known subtypes of hepatitis B virus (HBV), primary preexposure prophylaxis against HBV, post-exposure prophylaxis when given with hepatitis B immune globulin (HBIG)**

Engerix-B

Adults age 20 and older: Initially, 20 mcg I.M.; then second dose of 20 mcg I.M. after 30 days. A third dose of 20 mcg I.M. is given 6 months after the first dose.

Adjust-a-dose: For adults undergoing dialysis or receiving immunosuppressants, initially, 40 mcg I.M. (divided into two 20-mcg doses and given at different sites). Then second dose of 40 mcg I.M. in 30 days, a third dose after 2 months, and final dose of 40 mcg I.M. 6 months after first dose.

Adolescents ages 11 to 19: Initially, 10 mcg (pediatric and adolescent form) I.M.; then second dose of 10 mcg I.M. 30 days later. Give third dose of 10 mcg I.M. 6 months after first dose. Or, 20 mcg (adult form) I.M.; then second dose of 20 mcg I.M. 30 days later. Give third dose of 20 mcg I.M. 6 months after first dose.

Neonates and children up to age 10: Initially, 10 mcg I.M.; then second dose of 10 mcg I.M. 30 days later. Give third dose of 10 mcg I.M. 6 months after first dose.

Recombivax HB

Adults age 20 and older: Initially, 10 mcg I.M.; then second dose of 10 mcg I.M. after 30 days. Give third dose of 10 mcg I.M. 6 months after first dose.

For adults undergoing dialysis, initially, 40 mcg I.M. (use dialysis form, which contains 40 mcg/ml); then second dose of 40 mcg I.M. in 30 days, and final dose of 40 mcg I.M. 6 months after first dose. A booster or revaccination may be indicated if anti-HBs level is below 10 mIU/ml 1 to 2 months after third dose.

Infants, children, and adolescents age 19 or younger: Initially, 5 mcg I.M.; then second dose of 5 mcg I.M. after 30 days. Give third dose of 5 mcg I.M. 6 months after first dose. Or, in adolescents ages 11 to 15, give 10 mcg (1 ml adult form) I.M.; then second dose of 10 mcg 4 to 6 months later.

Infants born of HBsAg-positive mothers or mothers of unknown HbsAg status: Initially, 5 mcg I.M.; then second dose of 5 mcg I.M. after 30 days. Give third dose of 5 mcg I.M. 6 months after first dose.

Infants born of HBsAg-negative mothers: Initially, 5 mcg I.M.; then second dose of 5 mcg I.M. after 30 days. Give third dose of 5 mcg I.M. 6 months after first dose *Note*: If the mother is found to be HbsAg-positive within 7 days of delivery, also give the infant a dose of HBIG (0.5 ml) in the opposite anterolateral thigh.

➤**Chronic hepatitis C infection**

Engerix-B

Adults: Initially, 20 mcg I.M.; then second dose of 20 mcg I.M. after 30 days. Give third dose of 20 mcg I.M. 6 months after first dose.

ACTION

Promotes active immunity to hepatitis B.

Route	Onset	Peak	Duration
I.M.	2 wk after last dose	Unknown	Years

Half-life: Unknown.

ADVERSE REACTIONS

CNS: dizziness, fever, headache, insomnia, neuropathy, paresthesia, transient malaise.
EENT: pharyngitis.
GI: anorexia, diarrhea, nausea, vomiting.
Musculoskeletal: arthralgia, myalgia, neck stiffness.
Skin: *soreness at injection site,* local inflammation, pruritus.
Other: ***anaphylaxis,*** slight flulike syndrome.

INTERACTIONS

Drug-drug. *Immunosuppressants:* May decrease circulating antibody level. Increase doses of hepatitis B vaccine (recombinant).

EFFECTS ON LAB TEST RESULTS

None reported.

CONTRAINDICATIONS & CAUTIONS

- Contraindicated in patients hypersensitive to yeast or components of vaccine; recombinant vaccines are derived from yeast cultures.
- Use cautiously in patients with serious, active infections or compromised cardiac or pulmonary status and in those for whom a febrile or systemic reaction could pose a risk.

NURSING CONSIDERATIONS

- The American Academy of Pediatrics recommends hepatitis B vaccination for all neonates and encourages immunization for adolescents when resources allow.
- The Recombivax HB vaccine pediatric and adolescent form without preservatives may be used for persons for whom a thimerosal-free vaccine is recommended (such as infants up to age 6 months who may receive other vaccines containing thimerosal).
- Certain populations (neonates born to infected mothers, persons recently exposed to virus, and travelers to high-risk areas) may receive a four-dose regimen using Engerix-B, with the fourth dose given 12 months after the first dose.
- Certain people are at increased risk for infection and should be considered for vaccine, including health care personnel (especially those working with dialysis patients, with high-risk patients and patient contacts who may be infected, in blood banks, in emergency medicine, or among populations in which infection is endemic [Indo-Chinese, native peoples of Alaska, and Haitian refugees]), certain military personnel, morticians and embalmers, sexually active homosexual men, prostitutes, prisoners, and users of illegal injectable drugs.
- Although anaphylaxis hasn't been reported, always keep epinephrine available when giving vaccine to counteract possible reaction.
- Thoroughly agitate vial just before giving to restore suspension.
- Inspect product for particulates or discoloration before giving. Make sure product is a slightly opaque white suspension. Discard if it appears otherwise.
- Give vaccine in deltoid muscle for adults and adolescents; give in anterolateral aspect of thigh for infants and young children. Never give I.V.
- Give subcutaneously in patients at risk for hemorrhage, such as hemophiliacs. Otherwise, don't use this route; it may lead to an increased occurrence or severity of local reactions.

• Recombinant HBV vaccine isn't made with human plasma products.

PATIENT TEACHING

• Warn patient or parents about local adverse reactions such as swelling or redness at injection site. Tell patient to report persistent or severe reactions promptly.
• Review immunization schedule with patient or parents; stress importance of completing series.

✱ NEW DRUG

human papillomavirus recombinant vaccine, quadrivalent

Gardasil

Pharmacologic class: virus antigen
Pregnancy risk category B

AVAILABLE FORMS

Injection: 0.5 ml single-dose vial

INDICATIONS & DOSAGES

➤ **To prevent cervical cancer, genital warts, cervical adenocarcinoma in situ, and cervical, vulval, and vaginal intraepithelial neoplasias caused by human papillomavirus (HPV) types 6, 11, 16, and 18**
Women and girls ages 9 to 26 years: Three separate I.M. injections of 0.5 ml each. Give second injection 2 months after first, then give third injection 6 months after the first.

ACTION

Provides active immunity against HPV types 6, 11, 16, and 18 which cause nearly 70% of cervical cancers and 90% of genital warts.

Route	Onset	Peak	Duration
I.M.	1 mo after 3rd dose	Unknown	Unknown

Half-life: Unknown.

ADVERSE REACTIONS

CNS: dizziness, insomnia, *fever,* malaise.
EENT: nasal congestion, nasopharyngitis.
GI: diarrhea, nausea, vomiting.
Skin: *injection site reaction.*
Musculoskeletal: arthralgia, myalgia.
Respiratory: ***bronchospasm,*** cough, upper respiratory tract infection.
Other: toothache.

INTERACTIONS

Drug-drug. *Immunosuppressants, including antineoplastics and corticosteroids:* May decrease immune response to vaccine. Use cautiously.

EFFECTS ON LAB TEST RESULTS

None reported.

CONTRAINDICATIONS & CAUTIONS

• Contraindicated in patients hypersensitive to any component of the vaccine. Patients experiencing signs or symptoms of hypersensitivity after the first or second dose shouldn't complete the series. Don't use in patients with bleeding disorders, such as hemophilia or thrombocytopenia, or those on anticoagulants unless benefits outweigh the risks.
• Use cautiously in patients with fever, signs of infection, or those who are immunosuppressed.

NURSING CONSIDERATIONS

• Have appropriate medical treatment readily available in case of an anaphylactic reaction.
• Consider deferring vaccine if patient has or recently had a febrile illness. A low-grade fever or mild upper respiratory infection isn't a contraindication to the vaccine.
• Give I.M. in the deltoid or outer thigh.
• Avoid intradermal, subcutaneous, or intravascular administration.
• Give vaccine as supplied without any dilution or reconstitution.
• Shake vigorously to form a uniformly white, cloudy liquid; use immediately.
• Use the needle supplied with the drug. If a different needle is used, it should fit securely on the syringe and be no longer than 1 inch.
• Store refrigerated at 2° to 8° C (36° to 46° F); protect from light.
• Giving the HPV vaccine with the hepatitis B vaccine during the same visit, using separate injection sites, doesn't affect the immune response to either vaccine.

PATIENT TEACHING

- Advise patient or parent that vaccine isn't a substitute for routine cervical cancer screening.
- Tell patient or parent to read the vaccination information sheet before each vaccine is given.
- Inform patient or parent of the importance of completing the full immunization series, unless otherwise advised by the prescriber.
- Tell patient or parent the most common side effects include redness, itching, swelling or pain at the injection site; nausea; dizziness; or fever and to report any symptoms which are unusual or severe.
- Inform patient that vaccination may not protect all those who receive it.
- Tell patient that vaccination is used to prevent--not treat--active genital warts or cervical, vaginal, or vulval cancer and won't protect against diseases that are not caused by the specific HPV types contained in the vaccine.

influenza virus vaccine live, intranasal

FluMist

Pharmacologic class: vaccine
Pregnancy risk category C

AVAILABLE FORMS

Intranasal spray: 0.5 ml

INDICATIONS & DOSAGES

➤Active immunization to prevent disease caused by influenza A and B viruses

Adults younger than age 50 and children older than age 9: Give 0.5-ml intranasal dose (0.25 ml in each nostril) once each season.

Children ages 5 through 8 not previously vaccinated with FluMist: Two intranasal doses of 0.5 ml (0.25 ml in each nostril) 60 days apart for the first season.

Children ages 5 through 8 previously vaccinated with FluMist: 0.5-ml intranasal dose (0.25 ml in each nostril) once each season.

ACTION

Induces antibodies to specific influenza strains, which may help prevent infection, speed recovery, or both.

Route	Onset	Peak	Duration
Intranasal	Unknown	Unknown	Unknown

Half-life: Unknown.

ADVERSE REACTIONS

CNS: *headache, irritability, tiredness, weakness,* fever.
EENT: *nasal congestion, rhinitis, sore throat,* otitis media, sinusitis.
GI: abdominal pain, diarrhea, vomiting.
Musculoskeletal: muscle aches.
Respiratory: *cough.*
Other: *decreased activity,* chills.

INTERACTIONS

Drug-drug. *Antivirals active against influenza A virus, B virus, or both:* May interfere with vaccine. Wait at least 48 hours after antiviral therapy ends before giving vaccine. Wait at least 2 weeks after giving vaccine before starting antiviral therapy.
Aspirin: May cause Reye syndrome in children and adolescents ages 5 to 17 when given with influenza vaccine. Discourage aspirin use in children.
Immunosuppressants, such as alkylating drugs, antimetabolites, corticosteroids, and radiation: May increase risk of getting the flu. Avoid combining vaccine with immunosuppressants.

EFFECTS ON LAB TEST RESULTS

- May cause nasopharyngeal secretions or swabs to be falsely positive for flu virus up to 3 weeks after vaccination.

CONTRAINDICATIONS & CAUTIONS

- Contraindicated in patients hypersensitive to drug or its ingredients, including eggs or egg products, in children ages 5 to 17 who receive aspirin or products that contain aspirin because of the risk of Reye syndrome, and in patients who may be immunosuppressed.
- Contraindicated in those with history of Guillain-Barré syndrome, asthma, or reactive airway disease.

- Safety and effectiveness in children younger than age 5 and adults age 50 and older haven't been established.

NURSING CONSIDERATIONS

- *Alert:* Review patient's history for possible sensitivity to influenza vaccine components, including eggs and egg products.
- Have epinephrine injection (1:1,000) or compatible treatment readily available in case of acute anaphylactic reaction.
- Wait at least 72 hours after patient recovers from a febrile or respiratory illness before giving vaccine.
- Give vaccine before exposure to the influenza virus. Usually, influenza activity peaks in the United States between late December and early March.
- Annual revaccination may increase the likelihood of protection.
- Don't give vaccine with other vaccines.

PATIENT TEACHING

- Inform parent that a child age 5 to 8 who hasn't received the vaccine before will need two doses about 60 days apart.
- Tell patient to avoid close (household) contact with immunocompromised or sick people for at least 21 days after vaccination.
- Urge patient or parent to report adverse effects to prescriber.
- Inform patient or parent that annual revaccination may increase the likelihood of protection.

measles, mumps, and rubella virus vaccine, live

M-M-R II

Pharmacologic class: vaccine
Pregnancy risk category C

AVAILABLE FORMS

Injection: Single-dose vial containing at least 1,000 tissue culture infective doses ($TCID_{50}$), 20,000 $TCID_{50}$ of mumps strain, and 1,000 $TCID_{50}$ rubella virus per 0.5-ml dose.

INDICATIONS & DOSAGES

➤ **Routine immunization**

Adults: 0.5 ml subcutaneously. Patients born after 1957 should receive two doses at least 1 month apart.

Children: 0.5 ml subcutaneously. A two-dose schedule is recommended, with first dose given between 12 to 15 months (6 to 12 months in high-risk areas) and second dose given either at ages 4 to 6 or 11 to 12.

ACTION

Promotes immunity to measles, mumps, and rubella virus by inducing production of antibodies.

Route	Onset	Peak	Duration
SubQ	Unknown	Unknown	< 11 yr

Half-life: Unknown.

ADVERSE REACTIONS

GI: diarrhea.
Musculoskeletal: arthralgia, arthritis.
Skin: erythema at injection site, rash, urticaria.
Other: ***anaphylaxis,*** regional lymphadenopathy.

INTERACTIONS

Drug-drug. *Immune serum globulin, plasma, whole blood:* Antibodies in serum may interfere with immune response. Don't use vaccine within 3 to 11 months of these products, depending on dose of antibody or blood given.
Immunosuppressants: May decrease immune response to vaccine. Postpone immunization until immunosuppressant is stopped.

EFFECTS ON LAB TEST RESULTS

- May temporarily decrease response to tuberculin skin testing.

CONTRAINDICATIONS & CAUTIONS

- Contraindicated in immunosuppressed patients; in those with cancer, blood dyscrasia, gamma globulin disorders, fever, active untreated tuberculosis, or anaphylactic or anaphylactoid reactions to neomycin or eggs; in those receiving corticosteroid or radiation therapy; and in pregnant women.

NURSING CONSIDERATIONS

- Obtain history of allergies, especially anaphylactic reactions to antibiotics, or reaction to immunization.

- Keep epinephrine 1:1,000 available to treat anaphylaxis.
- If skin test is needed, give it either before or simultaneously with vaccine.
- Use only diluent supplied. Discard vaccine 8 hours after reconstituting.
- Inject into outer aspect of upper arm with a 25G ⅝-inch needle. Don't give I.V.
- Refrigerate vaccine; protect from light. Solution may be used if red, pink, or yellow but must be clear.
- Risk of adverse effects is low (0.5% to 4%).
- Treat fever with antipyretics such as acetaminophen.
- Presence of maternal antibodies may prevent response in children younger than age 12 months.
- The Immunization Practices Advisory Committee recommends that colleges, other post-high school educational institutions, and medical institutions obtain documentation of receipt of two doses of vaccine after age 1 (or other evidence of immunity, such as infection, documented by prescriber). Combined measles, mumps, and rubella vaccine is preferred.
- ***Alert:*** The Centers for Disease Control and Prevention recommend that, during a measles outbreak in a health care facility, susceptible personnel exposed to measles virus (whether they received measles vaccine or immunoglobulin) avoid patient contact for days 5 through 21 after such exposure. If personnel become ill, they should avoid patient contact for at least 7 days after developing rash.

PATIENT TEACHING

- Warn patient or parents about adverse reactions linked to vaccine.
- Review immunization schedule with parents, and stress importance of receiving second injection at the appropriate time to maintain immunization.
- Tell woman of childbearing age to use contraceptive measures until 3 months after immunization.
- Febrile seizures have rarely occurred in children after vaccination. Tell parents to treat and promptly report fever, especially in patient with family history of seizures.

measles virus vaccine, live attenuated

Attenuvax

Pharmacologic class: vaccine
Pregnancy risk category C

AVAILABLE FORMS

Injection: Single-dose vial containing not less than 1,000 tissue culture infective doses ($TCID_{50}$) of measles virus derived from the more attenuated line of Enders attenuated Edmonston strain (grown in chick embryo culture); available in 10- and 50-dose vials

INDICATIONS & DOSAGES

➤Immunization

Adults and children age 15 months and older: 0.5 ml (1,000 units) subcutaneously. A two-dose schedule is recommended, with first dose given at 15 months (12 months in high-risk areas) and second dose given at ages 4 to 6 or 11 to 12.

➤Measles outbreak control

Adults: Revaccinate school personnel born in or after 1957 if they lack evidence of measles immunity. If outbreak is in a medical facility, revaccinate all workers born in or after 1957 if they lack evidence of immunity.

Children: If cases occur in children younger than age 1, vaccinate children as young as age 6 months. Revaccinate all students and siblings if they lack documentation of measles immunity.

ACTION

Promotes immunity to measles virus by inducing production of antibodies.

Route	Onset	Peak	Duration
SubQ	Few days	Unknown	> 13 yr

Half-life: Unknown.

ADVERSE REACTIONS

CNS: ***febrile seizures in susceptible children,*** fever.
GI: anorexia.
Hematologic: ***leukopenia, thrombocytopenia.***
Skin: erythema, rash, swelling, tenderness at injection site.

Other: ***anaphylaxis,*** lymphadenopathy.

INTERACTIONS

Drug-drug. *Immune serum globulin, plasma, whole blood:* Antibodies in serum may interfere with immune response. Don't use vaccine for at least 3 months after giving these products.

EFFECTS ON LAB TEST RESULTS

- May decrease WBC and platelet counts.
- May temporarily decrease response to tuberculin skin testing.

CONTRAINDICATIONS & CAUTIONS

- Contraindicated in pregnant women; in immunosuppressed patients; in patients with cancer, blood dyscrasia, gamma globulin disorders, fever, active untreated tuberculosis, or anaphylactic or anaphylactoid reactions to neomycin or eggs; and in patients receiving corticosteroid or radiation therapy.
- Don't give vaccine within 3 months of receiving blood or plasma transfusion or human immune serum globulin.

NURSING CONSIDERATIONS

- Obtain history of allergies, especially anaphylactic reactions to antibiotics, or reaction to immunization. Postpone immunization in patients with acute illness or after giving blood or plasma.
- Keep epinephrine 1:1,000 available to treat anaphylaxis.
- If skin test is needed, give it either before or simultaneously with vaccine.
- Use only diluent supplied. Discard vaccine 8 hours after reconstituting.
- Don't give vaccine I.V.
- The Immunization Practices Advisory Committee recommends that colleges, other adult educational institutions, and medical institutions obtain documentation of receipt of two doses of vaccine after age 1 (or other evidence of immunity, such as infection, documented by prescriber). Combined measles, mumps, and rubella vaccine is preferred.
- ***Alert:*** The Centers for Disease Control and Prevention recommends that during a health care facility measles outbreak, susceptible personnel exposed to the measles virus (whether they received measles vaccine or immune globulin) avoid patient contact for days 5 through 21 after exposure. If personnel become ill, they should avoid patient contact for at least 7 days after developing rash.
- Attenuated measles vaccine given immediately after exposure to the disease may provide some protection. This level of protection is significantly increased if vaccine is given even a few days before exposure.

PATIENT TEACHING

- Warn patient or parents about adverse reactions linked to vaccine.
- Review immunization schedule with patient or parents and stress importance of receiving second injection at appropriate time.
- Stress importance of avoiding pregnancy for 3 months after vaccination. Provide contraception information, if needed.

meningococcal (groups A, C, Y, and W-135) polysaccharide diphtheria toxoid conjugate vaccine

Menactra

Pharmacologic class: vaccine
Pregnancy risk category C

AVAILABLE FORMS

Injection: 0.5 ml single-dose vials

INDICATIONS & DOSAGES

➤ **Active immunization for the prevention of invasive meningococcal disease caused by *Neisseria meningitidis* serogroups A, C, Y, W-135**

Adults and children ages 11 to 55: Give 0.5 ml I.M. as a single dose, preferably in the deltoid muscle.

ACTION

Promotes active immunity against invasive meningococcal disease.

Route	Onset	Peak	Duration
I.M.	Unknown	Unknown	Unknown

Half-life: Unknown.

ADVERSE REACTIONS

CNS: *fatigue, headache, malaise,* fever.
GI: *diarrhea,* vomiting.

Musculoskeletal: *arthralgia.*
Skin: *induration, redness, swelling,* rash.
Other: *pain.*

INTERACTIONS
Drug-drug. *Alkylating drugs, antimetabolites, corticosteroids (high-dose therapy), cytotoxic drugs, immunosuppressants, irradiation:* May reduce immune response of vaccine. Use caution together.

EFFECTS ON LAB TEST RESULTS
None reported.

CONTRAINDICATIONS & CAUTIONS
- Contraindicated in patients hypersensitive to diphtheria toxoid or dry natural rubber latex, patients with a history of Guillain-Barré syndrome, and those with a previous life-threatening reaction to a vaccine containing similar components.
- Don't use in a patient with a history of bleeding disorder (such as hemophilia, thrombocytopenia) unless benefit outweighs risk.
- Follow CDC guidelines for use in patients with recent or acute illness.

NURSING CONSIDERATIONS
- Review patient's medical and immunization history before giving vaccine to detect contraindications or possible sensitivity.
- If the vaccine needs to be given to a patient with a bleeding disorder, take precautions to avoid hematoma or bleeding following injection.
- Have epinephrine 1:1000 and other appropriate drugs and equipment readily available in case of anaphylaxis.
- Vials are for single use only.
- Don't mix with any other drugs or vaccines in same syringe.
- Aspirate after insertion to make sure needle hasn't entered a blood vessel.
- Avoid subcutaneous administration.
- Document date of vaccination and lot number and manufacturer of vaccine in patient record.
- Keep vials refrigerated, don't freeze.

PATIENT TEACHING
- Inform patients, parents, and guardians about benefits and risks of vaccine. Tell them to report any adverse reaction to their health care provider.
- Inform patient or parent that the most common reactions are headache, malaise, joint pain, and fatigue.
- Tell woman about the registry to monitor fetal outcomes if she is pregnant or discovers she was pregnant at the time of vaccination.

mumps virus vaccine, live
Mumpsvax

Pharmacologic class: vaccine
Pregnancy risk category C

AVAILABLE FORMS
Injection: Single-dose vial containing at least 20,000 tissue culture infective doses ($TCID_{50}$) of attenuated mumps virus derived from Jeryl Lynn mumps strain (grown in chick embryo culture) per 0.5 ml and vial of diluent; single-dose vial containing at least 5,000 $TCID_{50}$ of the U.S. Reference Mumps Virus in each 0.5 ml

INDICATIONS & DOSAGES
➤ **Immunization**
Adults and children age 1 and older: 0.5 ml (20,000 units) subcutaneously. Not recommended in children younger than age 12 months; revaccinate children vaccinated before age 12 months.

ACTION
Promotes active immunity to mumps.

Route	Onset	Peak	Duration
SubQ	Unknown	Unknown	> 15 yr

Half-life: Unknown.

ADVERSE REACTIONS
CNS: *slight fever,* malaise.
GI: diarrhea.
Skin: injection site reaction, rash.
Other: ***anaphylaxis,*** mild allergic reactions, mild lymphadenopathy.

INTERACTIONS
Drug-drug. *Immune serum globulin, plasma, whole blood:* Antibodies in serum may interfere with immune response. Don't use vaccine for at least 3 months after giving these products.

EFFECTS ON LAB TEST RESULTS

- May temporarily decrease response to tuberculin skin test.

CONTRAINDICATIONS & CAUTIONS

- Contraindicated in immunosuppressed patients; in those with cancer, blood dyscrasia, gamma globulin disorders, fever, untreated active tuberculosis, or anaphylactic or anaphylactoid reactions to neomycin or eggs; in those receiving corticosteroid or radiation therapy; and in pregnant women.
- Vaccine isn't recommended for infants younger than age 12 months because retained maternal mumps antibodies may interfere with immune response.
- Postpone use in patients with acute or febrile illness and for at least 3 months after transfusions or treatment with immune serum globulin.
- Don't give vaccine less than 1 month before or after immunization with other live-virus vaccines.

NURSING CONSIDERATIONS

- Obtain history of allergies, especially anaphylactic reactions to antibiotics, and reaction to immunization.
- Keep epinephrine 1:1,000 available to treat anaphylaxis.
- If skin test is needed, give it either before or simultaneously with vaccine.
- Use only diluent supplied. Discard vaccine 8 hours after reconstituting.
- Use a 25G ⅝-inch needle to inject.
- Don't give vaccine I.V.
- Refrigerate and protect from light. Reconstituted solution is clear yellow; don't use if discolored.
- Give to asymptomatic HIV-infected children.
- Don't use for delayed hypersensitivity (allergy) skin testing. Use mumps skin-test antigen, a killed viral product.

PATIENT TEACHING

- Warn patient or parents about adverse reactions linked to vaccine.
- Stress importance of avoiding pregnancy for 3 months after vaccination. Provide contraception information, if needed.
- Tell patient to treat fever with fever-reducing drugs.

pneumococcal vaccine, polyvalent

Pneumovax 23

Pharmacologic class: vaccine
Pregnancy risk category C

AVAILABLE FORMS

Injection: 25 mcg each of 23 polysaccharide isolates/0.5 ml

INDICATIONS & DOSAGES

➤ Pneumococcal immunization
Adults and children age 2 and older: 0.5 ml I.M. or subcutaneously.

ACTION

Promotes active immunity to infections caused by *Streptococcus pneumoniae.*

Route	Onset	Peak	Duration
I.M., SubQ	2–3 wk	Unknown	5 yr

Half-life: Unknown.

ADVERSE REACTIONS

CNS: slight fever.
Musculoskeletal: arthralgia, myalgia.
Skin: *injection site soreness,* injection site rash, severe local reaction caused by revaccination within 3 years.
Other: ***anaphylaxis.***

INTERACTIONS

Drug-drug. *Immunosuppressants:* May reduce immune response to vaccine. Postpone immunization until 3 months after immunosuppressant therapy is stopped.

EFFECTS ON LAB TEST RESULTS

None reported.

CONTRAINDICATIONS & CAUTIONS

- Contraindicated in patients hypersensitive to drug or its components (phenol) and in those with Hodgkin lymphoma who have received extensive chemotherapy or nodal irradiation.
- Postpone use in patients with acute respiratory distress syndrome.
- Vaccine isn't recommended for children younger than age 2.

NURSING CONSIDERATIONS

- Vaccine is recommended for all adults older than age 65.
- Check immunization history to avoid re-vaccination within 3 years.
- Obtain history of allergies and reaction to immunization. Eggs and egg protein aren't used during the manufacture of vaccine; contains phenol as a preservative.
- Keep epinephrine 1:1,000 available to treat anaphylaxis.
- Inject in deltoid or midlateral thigh. Don't inject I.V. or I.D.
- When splenectomy is being considered, give vaccine at least 2 weeks before procedure to ensure adequate antibody response. Vaccine may be less effective in splenectomized patients.
- Vaccine protects against 23 pneumococcal types, accounting for 90% of pneumococcal disease.
- Vaccine may be given to children age 2 and older to prevent pneumococcal otitis media, although the Centers for Disease Control and Prevention doesn't recommend otitis media as an indication for vaccine.
- Administration with influenza virus vaccine is safe and effective.

PATIENT TEACHING

- Warn patient about adverse reactions linked to vaccine.
- Tell patient to treat fever with mild fever-reducing drugs and local site reaction with cold compresses.
- Warn patient with a skin rash related to low levels of platelets from unknown cause that there is a possibility of relapse 2 to 14 days after vaccination.

poliovirus vaccine, inactivated (IPV)

IPOL

Pharmacologic class: vaccine
Pregnancy risk category C

AVAILABLE FORMS

0.5-ml prefilled syringe: Mixture of three types of poliovirus (types 1, 2, and 3) grown in tissue culture

INDICATIONS & DOSAGES

➤ Poliovirus immunization

Adults: 0.5 ml subcutaneously; give second dose 4 to 8 weeks later. Give third dose 6 to 12 months later.
Children: 0.5 ml subcutaneously at ages 2 months and 4 months. Give third dose at ages 6 to 18 months. Give a reinforcing dose of 0.5 ml subcutaneously before entry into school at ages 4 to 6.

ACTION

Promotes immunity to poliomyelitis by inducing humoral antibodies and antibodies in the lymphatic tissue.

Route	Onset	Peak	Duration
SubQ	Unknown	Unknown	Several yr

Half-life: Unknown.

ADVERSE REACTIONS

CNS: *fever,* sleepiness.
GI: decreased appetite.
Skin: *pain,* induration, injection site erythema.
Other: crying, hypersensitivity reaction.

INTERACTIONS

Drug-drug. *Immune serum globulin, plasma, whole blood:* Antibodies in serum may interfere with immune response. Don't use vaccine within 3 months of transfusion.
Immunosuppressants: May reduce immune response to vaccine. Postpone immunization until immunosuppressant is stopped.

EFFECTS ON LAB TEST RESULTS

None reported.

CONTRAINDICATIONS & CAUTIONS

- Contraindicated in patients hypersensitive to neomycin, streptomycin, or polymyxin B and in neonates younger than age 6 weeks.

NURSING CONSIDERATIONS

- Vaccine isn't effective in modifying or preventing existing or incubating poliomyelitis.
- Obtain history of allergies and reaction to immunization.

- If skin test is needed, give it either before or with vaccine.
- Keep epinephrine 1:1,000 available to treat anaphylaxis.
- Adults at high risk for exposure who have completed a primary course may receive another dose.
- Document manufacturer, lot number, date given, and name, address, and title of person giving vaccine on patient's record or log.
- Vaccine may temporarily decrease response to tuberculin skin test.

PATIENT TEACHING
- Inform patient or parents about risks and benefits of vaccine before administration.
- Warn patient or parents about adverse reactions linked to vaccine.

rabies vaccine, human diploid cell (HDCV)

Imovax Rabies, Imovax Rabies I.D. Vaccine, RabAvert

Pharmacologic class: vaccine
Pregnancy risk category C

AVAILABLE FORMS
I.D. injection: 0.25 international unit rabies antigen/dose
I.M. injection: 2.5 international units rabies antigen/ml, in single-dose vial with diluent

INDICATIONS & DOSAGES

➤ Postexposure antirabies immunization
Adults and children: Five 1-ml doses of HDCV I.M. Give first dose as soon as possible after exposure; give additional doses on days 3, 7, 14, and 28 after first dose. If no antibody response occurs after this primary series, booster dose is recommended.

➤ Preexposure preventive immunization for persons in high-risk groups
Adults and children: Three 1-ml injections I.M. Give first dose on day 0 (first day of therapy), second dose on day 7, and third dose on day 21 or 28. Or, 0.1 ml I.D. on same dosage schedule.

ACTION
Promotes active immunity to rabies.

Route	Onset	Peak	Duration
I.M., I.D.	1 wk	1–2 mo	> 2 yr

Half-life: Unknown.

ADVERSE REACTIONS
CNS: *fatigue, fever, headache,* dizziness.
GI: *nausea,* abdominal pain, diarrhea.
Musculoskeletal: muscle aches.
Skin: *erythema, injection site pain, itching, swelling.*
Other: *serum sickness,* ***anaphylaxis.***

INTERACTIONS
Drug-drug. *Antimalarials, corticosteroids, immunosuppressants:* May decrease response to rabies vaccine. Avoid using together.

EFFECTS ON LAB TEST RESULTS
None reported.

CONTRAINDICATIONS & CAUTIONS
- No contraindications reported for persons after exposure. An acute febrile illness contraindicates use of vaccine for persons previously exposed.
- Use cautiously in hypersensitive patients.

NURSING CONSIDERATIONS
- Keep epinephrine 1:1,000 available to treat anaphylaxis.
- Use vaccine immediately after reconstitution.
- ***Alert:*** Don't use I.D. for postexposure rabies vaccination.
- Alternative regimen of 0.1-ml doses given I.D. is only for preexposure prophylaxis.
- Stop corticosteroid therapy during immunizing period unless therapy is essential for treatment of other conditions.
- Some patients who receive booster doses experience serum sickness–like hypersensitivity. These reactions usually respond to antihistamines.
- Report all serious reactions to the State Department of Health.
- ***Alert:*** Don't confuse vaccine with rabies immune globulin. Both drugs may be given in some situations.

PATIENT TEACHING

- Inform patient about adverse reactions linked to vaccine. Tell patient to report persistent or severe reactions.
- Stress importance of receiving booster, if appropriate for patient.
- Tell patient to treat mild reaction with appropriate doses of anti-inflammatory or fever-reducing drug.

rubella and mumps virus vaccine, live

Biavax II

Pharmacologic class: vaccine
Pregnancy risk category C

AVAILABLE FORMS

Injection: Single-dose vial containing not less than 1,000 tissue culture infective doses ($TCID_{50}$) of Wistar RA 27/3 rubella virus (propagated in human diploid cell culture) and not less than 20,000 $TCID_{50}$ of Jeryl Lynn mumps strain (grown in chick embryo cell culture)

INDICATIONS & DOSAGES

➤ **Rubella and mumps immunization**
Adults and children age 1 and older: 0.5 ml subcutaneously.

ACTION

Promotes immunity to rubella and mumps by inducing antibody production.

Route	Onset	Peak	Duration
SubQ	Unknown	Unknown	10½ yr

Half-life: Unknown.

ADVERSE REACTIONS

CNS: fever, polyneuritis.
GI: diarrhea.
Musculoskeletal: *arthritis, arthralgia.*
Skin: ***thrombocytopenic purpura,*** rash, pain, erythema, and induration at injection site, urticaria.
Other: ***anaphylaxis,*** lymphadenopathy.

INTERACTIONS

Drug-drug. *Immune serum globulin, plasma, whole blood:* Antibodies in serum may interfere with immune response. Don't give vaccine for at least 3 months after use of these products.
Immunosuppressants: May reduce immune response to vaccine. Postpone immunization until immunosuppressant is stopped.

EFFECTS ON LAB TEST RESULTS

- May temporarily decrease response to tuberculin skin test.

CONTRAINDICATIONS & CAUTIONS

- Contraindicated in immunosuppressed patients; in those with cancer, blood dyscrasia, gamma globulin disorders, fever, active untreated tuberculosis, or history of anaphylaxis or anaphylactoid reactions to neomycin or eggs; in those receiving corticosteroid (except those receiving corticosteroids as replacement therapy) or radiation therapy; and in pregnant women.
- Postpone vaccination in patients with acute illness and after giving immune serum globulin, blood, or plasma.

NURSING CONSIDERATIONS

- Obtain history of allergies, especially anaphylactic reaction to antibiotics, and reaction to immunization.
- Keep epinephrine 1:1,000 available to treat anaphylaxis.
- If skin test is needed, give it either before or with vaccine.
- Use only diluent supplied. Discard vaccine 8 hours after reconstituting.
- Inject into outer upper arm. Don't inject I.V.
- Document drug manufacturer, lot number, date, and name, address, and title of person giving dose on patient record or log.
- Consider patients born before 1956 to have acquired natural immunity.

PATIENT TEACHING

- Inform patient about adverse reactions linked to vaccine.
- Stress importance of avoiding pregnancy for 3 months after vaccination. Provide contraception information, if needed.
- Inform women and girls older than age 12 about risk of self-limited joint pain or arthritis 2 to 4 weeks after vaccination.

rubella virus vaccine, live attenuated (RA 27/3)

Meruvax II

Pharmacologic class: vaccine
Pregnancy risk category C

AVAILABLE FORMS

Injection: Single-dose vial containing not less than 1,000 tissue culture infective doses ($TCID_{50}$) of Wistar RA 27/3 strain of rubella virus (propagated in human diploid cell culture)

INDICATIONS & DOSAGES

➤ **Rubella immunization**

Adults and children age 1 and older: 0.5 ml or 1,000 units subcutaneously.

ACTION

Promotes immunity to rubella by inducing production of antibodies.

Route	Onset	Peak	Duration
SubQ	2–6 wk	Unknown	> 10 yr

Half-life: Unknown.

ADVERSE REACTIONS

CNS: fever, headache, malaise, polyneuritis.
EENT: sore throat.
Musculoskeletal: arthralgia, arthritis.
Skin: ***thrombocytopenic purpura,*** rash, pain, erythema, and induration at injection site, urticaria.
Other: ***anaphylaxis,*** lymphadenopathy.

INTERACTIONS

Drug-drug. *Immune serum globulin, plasma, whole blood:* Antibodies in serum may interfere with immune response. Don't give vaccine for at least 3 months after use of these products.
Immunosuppressants, interferon: May reduce immune response to vaccine. Postpone vaccine until immunosuppressant is stopped.

EFFECTS ON LAB TEST RESULTS

- May temporarily decrease response to tuberculin skin test.

CONTRAINDICATIONS & CAUTIONS

- Contraindicated in immunosuppressed patients; in patients with cancer, blood dyscrasia, gamma globulin disorders, fever, or active untreated tuberculosis; in patients hypersensitive to neomycin; in patients receiving corticosteroids (except those receiving corticosteroids as replacement therapy) or radiation therapy; in pregnant women; and in those with AIDS or symptomatic HIV infection.
- Postpone immunization in patients with acute illness and after administration of human immune serum globulin, blood, or plasma.

NURSING CONSIDERATIONS

- Obtain history of allergies and reaction to immunization.
- Keep epinephrine 1:1,000 available to treat anaphylaxis.
- If skin test is needed, give either before or with vaccine.
- Use only diluent supplied. Discard vaccine 8 hours after reconstituting. Protect from light.
- Inject into outer upper arm. Don't inject vaccine I.V.
- Document drug manufacturer, lot number, date, and name, address, and title of person giving dose on patient record or log.

PATIENT TEACHING

- Inform patient about adverse reactions linked to vaccine.
- Stress importance of avoiding pregnancy for 3 months after vaccination. Provide contraception information, if needed.
- Tell patient to use correct dose of fever-reducing drug for treating fever.

smallpox vaccine, dried

Dryvax

Pharmacologic class: vaccine
Pregnancy risk category C

AVAILABLE FORMS

Injection: About 100 million pock-forming units (pfu) per ml

INDICATIONS & DOSAGES

➤ **Active immunization to prevent smallpox disease**

Adults and children: One drop of vaccine deposited over the deltoid or triceps muscle, followed by a multiple-puncture technique into the superficial layers of skin (two or three needle punctures for primary vaccination and 15 for revaccination).

ACTION

Prevents smallpox by inducing production of antibodies to vaccinia virus.

Route	Onset	Peak	Duration
Multiple-puncture scarification	Unknown	Unknown	Unknown

Half-life: Unknown.

ADVERSE REACTIONS

CNS: *fever.*
Skin: rash.
Other: accidental spread of smallpox to another part of the body or to another person.

INTERACTIONS

None reported.

EFFECTS ON LAB TEST RESULTS

None reported.

CONTRAINDICATIONS & CAUTIONS

Nonemergency situations

- Contraindicated in infants younger than age 1 and in patients allergic to any component of the vaccine, including polymyxin B sulfate, dihydrostreptomycin sulfate, chlortetracycline hydrochloride, and neomycin sulfate.
- Contraindicated in patients who have or those whose household members haveeczema, history of eczema, or other exfoliative skin conditions; congenital or acquired immune system deficiencies, including HIV, leukemia, lymphomas, malignancy, organ transplantation, stem cell transplantation, agammaglobulinemia, and other malignant neoplasms affecting the bone marrow or lymphatic systems; of those receiving systemic corticosteroids, immunosuppressive drugs, or radiation; of women who are or may be pregnant, breast-feeding women, and elderly people.
- Contraindicated in patients with heart disease (such as cardiomyopathy, heart failure, previous MI, history of angina, or evidence of coronary artery disease).
- Contraindicated in those who have three or more of these risk factors: hypertension, hypercholesterolemia, diabetes mellitus or hyperglycemia, smoking, or a first-degree relative with a heart condition before age 50.

Emergency situations

- For patients at high risk of exposure to smallpox, no contraindications exist for vaccination.

NURSING CONSIDERATIONS

- Don't give I.M., I.V., or subcutaneously.
- ***Alert:*** The vial stopper contains latex, which may cause hypersensitivity in patients with latex allergy.
- Give vaccination in the deltoid or posterior aspect of the arm over the triceps muscle.
- ***Alert:*** Rapidly make punctures into skin, and allow 15 to 20 seconds for blood to appear. After vaccination, blot off any vaccine remaining on skin at vaccination site with clean, dry gauze or cotton.
- Burn, boil, or autoclave all items that come in contact with the vaccine before their disposal.
- Inspect the site 6 to 8 days after vaccination to determine whether a major or equivocal reaction has occurred.
- Contact transmission of the virus can occur until the scab separates from the skin lesion, usually 14 to 21 days after vaccination.
- Accidental inoculation of other sites is a common complication of the vaccine. The face, eyelid, nose, mouth, genitalia, and rectum are most frequently involved. Autoinoculation of the eye may cause blindness.
- Recently vaccinated health care workers should avoid contact with patients until the scab has separated from the skin at the vaccination site. If continued contact is essential and unavoidable, cover the vaccination site and maintain good hand-washing technique.
- Cardiac complications such as myopericarditis have occurred within 2 weeks of patients being vaccinated.

- The Centers for Disease Control and Prevention (CDC) can help diagnose and manage patients with suspected complications.
- Contact the Advisory Committee on Immunization Practices (ACIP), the Armed Forces, and the CDC for the most updated information and recommendations for use of the smallpox vaccine.

PATIENT TEACHING

- Tell patient that although he should keep the vaccination site dry, he can still bathe the rest of the body.
- Advise patient that smallpox may be spread to another part of the body or to another person until the scab separates from the skin lesion (14 to 21 days after vaccination). Hand washing is essential for preventing inadvertent contact transmission of the virus.
- Tell patient to leave vaccination site uncovered or to cover it with a porous bandage, such as gauze, until the scab has separated and the underlying skin has healed. He shouldn't routinely use an occlusive bandage.
- Warn patient not to use salves or ointments on vaccination site.
- Instruct patient to seek immediate medical attention if he has chest pain, dyspnea, or other symptoms of cardiac disease in the first 2 weeks after vaccination.
- Instruct patient to place contaminated bandages in sealed plastic bags before trash disposal.

tetanus toxoid, adsorbed

tetanus toxoid, fluid

Pharmacologic class: vaccine
Pregnancy risk category C

AVAILABLE FORMS

tetanus toxoid, adsorbed
Injection: 5 to 10 limit flocculation (Lf) units inactivated tetanus/0.5-ml dose, in 0.5-ml syringes and 5-ml vials
tetanus toxoid, fluid
Injection: 4 to 5 Lf units inactivated tetanus/0.5-ml dose, in 0.5-ml syringes and 7.5-ml vials

INDICATIONS & DOSAGES

➤Primary immunization to prevent tetanus
Adults and children age 7 and older: 0.5 ml (adsorbed) I.M. 4 to 8 weeks apart for two doses; then give third dose 6 to 12 months after second.
Children ages 6 weeks to 6 years: Although use isn't recommended in children younger than age 7, the following dosage schedule may be used: 0.5 ml (adsorbed) I.M. for two doses, each 4 to 8 weeks apart, followed by a third dose 6 to 12 months after the second dose. Diphtheria and tetanus toxoids and acellular pertussis vaccine adsorbed (DTaP) is recommended for active immunization in children younger than age 7.
➤Booster dose to prevent tetanus
Adults and children age 7 and older: 0.5 ml I.M. at 10-year intervals.
➤Postexposure prevention of tetanus
Adults: For a clean, minor wound, give emergency booster dose if more than 10 years have elapsed since last dose. For all other wounds, give booster dose if more than 5 years have elapsed since last dose.

ACTION

Promotes immunity to tetanus by inducing antitoxin production.

Route	Onset	Peak	Duration
I.M., SubQ	After 2 doses	Unknown	> 10 yr

Half-life: Unknown.

ADVERSE REACTIONS

CNS: *seizures,* slight fever, headache, malaise, encephalopathy.
CV: tachycardia, hypotension, flushing.
Musculoskeletal: aches, pains.
Skin: erythema, induration, nodule at injection site, urticaria, pruritus.
Other: ***anaphylaxis,*** chills.

INTERACTIONS

Drug-drug. *Chloramphenicol:* May interfere with response to tetanus toxoid. Monitor patient for effect.
Immunosuppressants, tetanus immune globulin: May reduce immune response

to vaccine. Postpone vaccine until 1 month after immunosuppressant is stopped.

EFFECTS ON LAB TEST RESULTS
None reported.

CONTRAINDICATIONS & CAUTIONS
- Contraindicated in immunosuppressed patients, in those with immunoglobulin abnormalities, and in those with severe hypersensitivity or neurologic reactions to toxoid or its ingredients. Contraindicated in patients with thrombocytopenia or other coagulation disorders that would contraindicate I.M. injection unless benefits outweigh risks.
- Use adsorbed form cautiously in infants or children with cerebral damage, neurologic disorders, or history of febrile seizures.
- Postpone vaccination in patients with acute illness and during polio outbreaks, except in emergencies.

NURSING CONSIDERATIONS
- Obtain history of allergies and reaction to immunization.
- Determine date of last tetanus immunization.
- Keep epinephrine 1:1,000 available to treat anaphylaxis.
- Adsorbed form produces longer immunity. Fluid form provides quicker booster effect in patients actively immunized previously.
- Document manufacturer, lot number, date, and name, address, and title of person giving dose on patient record or log.
- ***Alert:*** Don't confuse drug with tetanus immune globulin, human. Both drugs may be given in some situations.

PATIENT TEACHING
- Advise patient to avoid using hot or cold compresses at injection site; this may increase severity of local reaction.
- Instruct patient to report persistent or severe adverse reactions.
- Advise patient of proper fever-reducing drug dose for fever reaction.
- Tell patient that nodule at injection site may be present for a few weeks.

varicella virus vaccine
Varivax

Pharmacologic class: vaccine
Pregnancy risk category C

AVAILABLE FORMS
Injection: Single-dose vial containing 1,350 plague-forming units of Oka/Merck varicella virus (live)

INDICATIONS & DOSAGES
➤ **To prevent varicella zoster (chickenpox) infections**
Adults and children age 13 and older: 0.5 ml subcutaneously; then, second 0.5-ml dose 4 to 8 weeks later.
Children ages 1 to 12: Give 0.5 ml subcutaneously.

ACTION
Prevents chickenpox by inducing production of antibodies to varicella zoster virus.

Route	Onset	Peak	Duration
SubQ	4–6 wk	Unknown	> 2 yr

Half-life: Unknown.

ADVERSE REACTIONS
CNS: *fever.*
Skin: swelling, redness, pain, rash, varicella-like rash at injection site.
Other: ***anaphylaxis,*** herpes zoster, stiffness.

INTERACTIONS
Drug-drug. *Blood products, immune globulin:* May inactivate vaccine. Don't give vaccine until at least 5 months after blood or plasma transfusions or administration of immune globulin or varicella zoster immune globulin.
Immunosuppressants: May cause severe reactions to live-virus vaccines. Postpone routine vaccination.
Salicylates: May cause Reye syndrome after natural varicella infection. Avoid using salicylates for 6 weeks after varicella immunization.

EFFECTS ON LAB TEST RESULTS
None reported.

CONTRAINDICATIONS & CAUTIONS

- Contraindicated in patients hypersensitive to drug; in those with history of anaphylactoid reaction to neomycin; and in those with blood dyscrasia, leukemia, lymphomas, neoplasms affecting bone marrow or lymphatic system, or primary and acquired immunosuppressive states; and in those receiving immunosuppressants.
- Contraindicated in those with active untreated tuberculosis or any febrile illness or infection.
- Contraindicated in pregnant women.

NURSING CONSIDERATIONS

- To reconstitute vaccine, first withdraw 0.7 ml of diluent into syringe to be used for reconstitution. Inject all diluent in syringe into vial of lyophilized vaccine and gently agitate to mix thoroughly. Give immediately after reconstitution. Discard if not used within 30 minutes.
- Keep epinephrine available to treat anaphylaxis.
- Vaccine has been used safely and effectively with measles, mumps, and rubella vaccine.
- Document manufacturer, lot number, date, and name, address, and title of person giving dose on patient record or log.
- Store vaccine frozen. Store diluent separately at room temperature or refrigerated.
- ***Alert:*** Vaccine contains live, attenuated virus. Vaccinated patients who develop rash may be able to transmit virus.

PATIENT TEACHING

- Inform patient or parents about adverse reactions linked to vaccine.
- Caution woman to report suspected pregnancy before giving.
- Instruct patient to avoid salicylates for 6 weeks after vaccination to prevent Reye syndrome.
- Tell woman to avoid pregnancy for 3 months after vaccination.
- Warn patient to be careful to avoid close contact with susceptible high-risk people (such as pregnant women or the immunocompromised).

✱ NEW DRUG

zoster vaccine, live

Zostavax

Pharmacologic class: vaccine, live attenuated
Pregnancy risk category C

AVAILABLE FORMS

Injection: Lyophilized vaccine in a single-dose vial with supplied diluent

INDICATIONS & DOSAGES

➤Prevention of herpes zoster (shingles)
Adults age 60 and older: One reconstituted vial subcutaneously as a single dose.

ACTION

Stimulates active immunity to varicella-zoster virus, thus protecting against herpes zoster.

Route	Onset	Peak	Duration
SubQ	6 wk	Unknown	about 4 yr

Half-life: Unknown.

ADVERSE REACTIONS

CNS: asthenia, fever, headache.
EENT: rhinitis.
GI: diarrhea.
Musculoskeletal: polymyalgia rheumatica.
Respiratory: ***asthma exacerbation,*** respiratory disorder, respiratory infection.
Skin: *injection site reactions (redness, pain, tenderness, swelling),* hematoma, pruritus, skin disorder, warmth.
Other: flulike symptoms.

INTERACTIONS

Drug-drug. *Immunosuppressants, including corticosteroids:* May decrease immune response. Using together is contraindicated.

EFFECTS ON LAB TEST RESULTS

None reported.

CONTRAINDICATIONS & CAUTIONS

- Contraindicated in patients with a history of anaphylactic or anaphylactoid reactions to gelatin, neomycin, or any component of the vaccine; patients with

primary or acquired immunodeficiency; patients taking immunosuppressive therapy or corticosteroids; patients with active, untreated tuberculosis; and pregnant women.
- Use cautiously in women who are breast-feeding.

NURSING CONSIDERATIONS
- ***Alert:*** Drug is given only by subcutaneous injection; don't give by I.V. route.
- Check patients temperature before giving injection. Vaccine should be deferred if patient has acute illness or a fever higher than 101.3° F (38.5° C).
- Ask if patient has ever had a reaction to a vaccine. Keep epinephrine 1:1,000 available for immediate use for anaphylaxis.
- Inject diluent into the vial of lyophilized vaccine and gently agitate to mix thoroughly.
- Inject the total volume subcutaneously, immediately after reconstitution, into outer aspect of upper arm.
- If reconstituted vaccine isn't used within 30 minutes, discard it.
- Store frozen at 5° F (–15° C) or colder until ready to use.
- The effect of giving other drugs or antivirals that kill varicella at the same time as Zostavax isn't known.
- Zostavax shouldn't be used in children. It can't be substituted for Varivax.

PATIENT TEACHING
- Explain to patient the benefits and risks of the vaccine.
- Inform patient that injection site reactions are common and may include redness, pain, swelling, itching, and bruising.

74

Antivenins

black widow spider antivenin
***Crotalidae* antivenin, polyvalent**
***Micrurus fulvius* antivenin**

black widow spider antivenin

Antivenin *(Latrodectus mactans)*

Pharmacologic class: antivenin
Pregnancy risk category C

AVAILABLE FORMS

Injection: Combination package—one vial of antivenin (6,000-unit vial), one 2.5-ml vial of diluent (sterile water for injection), and one 1-ml vial of normal equine serum (1:10 dilution) for sensitivity testing

INDICATIONS & DOSAGES

➤**Black widow spider bite**

Adults and children: 2.5 ml I.M. in anterolateral thigh; a second dose may be needed.

I.V. ADMINISTRATION

- Reconstitute antivenin with 2.5 ml of diluent.
- Further dilute reconstituted solution in 10 to 50 ml normal saline solution for injection.
- Use reconstituted solutions within 48 hours; diluted solutions, within 12 hours.
- Infuse over 15 minutes.

INCOMPATIBILITIES

None reported.

ACTION

Unknown.

Route	Onset	Peak	Duration
I.V.	Immediate	Unknown	Unknown
I.M.	Unknown	2–3 days	Unknown

Half-life: Less than 15 days.

ADVERSE REACTIONS

CNS: ***neurotoxicity.***

Other: hypersensitivity reactions, ***anaphylaxis, serum sickness.***

INTERACTIONS

Drug-drug. *Antihistamines:* May interfere with sensitivity test results. Avoid using together.

EFFECTS ON LAB TEST RESULTS

None reported.

CONTRAINDICATIONS & CAUTIONS

- Contraindicated in patients hypersensitive to drug or its components (horse serum) when desensitization isn't feasible.

NURSING CONSIDERATIONS

- Immobilize patient; splint the bitten limb to prevent spread of venom.
- Obtain history of allergies, especially to horses, and reaction to immunization. Have epinephrine 1:1,000 available to treat anaphylaxis.
- For best results, give antivenin as soon as possible.
- Perform a skin or conjunctival test before administration.
- ***Alert:*** Give I.M. injection in the upper outer quadrant of the thigh so that a tourniquet may be applied if a systemic reaction occurs.
- Watch patient for 2 to 3 days. Venom is neurotoxic and may cause respiratory paralysis and seizures.
- Signs and symptoms usually subside in 1 to 3 hours.
- Refrigerate at 36° to 46° F (2° to 8° C).
- Discard if injection is frozen.

PATIENT TEACHING

- Explain to patient and family how drug will be given.
- Instruct patient to report adverse reactions promptly.
- Tell patient that serum sickness (urticaria, pruritus, fever, malaise, arthralgia) can occur 8 to 12 days after administration.

Crotalidae antivenin, polyvalent

Pharmacologic class: antivenin
Pregnancy risk category C

AVAILABLE FORMS
Injection: Combination package: one vial of lyophilized serum, one vial of diluent (10 ml of bacteriostatic water for injection)and , one 1-ml vial of normal horse serum (diluted 1:10) for sensitivity testing

INDICATIONS & DOSAGES
➤ **Crotalid (pit viper) bites**
Adults and children: Initially, 20 to 150 ml I.V., depending on severity of bite and patient response. For minimal envenomation, 20 to 40 ml I.V.; for moderate envenomation, 50 to 90 ml I.V.; for severe envenomation, 100 to 150 ml I.V. For a large amount of venom, more than 150 ml may be given I.V. directly into superficial vein. Subsequent doses are based on patient's response; may need another 10 to 50 ml if swelling progresses, systemic symptoms increase, or new signs and symptoms appear.

Test for sensitivity before giving drug. Give 0.02 to 0.03 ml of 1:10 dilution in normal saline solution I.D. Read results after 5 to 10 minutes. Watch carefully for delayed allergic reaction or relapse.

If sensitivity test result is positive, desensitize; prepare 1:10 and 1:100 dilutions of antivenin in normal saline solution for injection.

Adjust-a-dose: Children who have less resistance and less body fluid to dilute venom may need twice adult dose.

I.V. ADMINISTRATION
- Reconstitute drug by adding 10 ml of supplied diluent. Further dilute to make a 1:1 to 1:10 solution using normal saline solution or D_5W. To avoid foaming, don't shake while mixing.
- Start by infusing 5 to 10 ml of diluted antivenin over 3 to 5 minutes; observe patient carefully. If no signs or symptoms of immediate systemic reaction occur, continue infusion.
- Use reconstituted solution within 48 hours and dilutions within 12 hours.

INCOMPATIBILITIES
None reported.

ACTION
Neutralizes and binds venom of crotalid, including rattlesnakes, water moccasins, and copperheads.

Route	Onset	Peak	Duration
I.V.	Immediate	Unknown	Unknown

Half-life: Less than 15 days.

ADVERSE REACTIONS
Musculoskeletal: arthralgia.
Skin: erythema, urticaria.
Other: *serum sickness,* ***anaphylaxis,*** fever, hypersensitivity reactions, lymphadenopathy, pain.

INTERACTIONS
Drug-drug. *Adrenergic-blocking drugs (including cardioselective beta blockers):* May increase incidence and severity of anaphylaxis. Beta blockers may also alter the effect of epinephrine and other adrenergics. Larger-than-normal doses of these drugs may be required to treat anaphylaxis. *Antihistamines:* May increase toxicity of crotalid venoms. Avoid using together.

EFFECTS ON LAB TEST RESULTS
None reported.

CONTRAINDICATIONS & CAUTIONS
- Contraindicated in patients hypersensitive to drug or its components.
- Use drug cautiously. About 60% of patients treated with antivenin develop hypersensitivity.

NURSING CONSIDERATIONS
- Immobilize patient immediately. Splint bitten limb.
- Obtain history of allergies, especially to horses, and reactions to immunizations. Have epinephrine 1:1,000 available in case of hypersensitivity reaction.
- ***Alert:*** Type and crossmatch blood as soon as possible; hemolysis from venom prevents accurate crossmatching.
- For best results, give antivenin as soon as possible, preferably within 4 hours of bite. In severe cases, can be given even 24 hours after the bite.

• Give corticosteroids as indicated. If many vials are given, patient may develop serum sickness (urticaria, pruritus, fever, malaise, arthralgia) 5 to 24 days after infusion.
• Store antivenin without refrigeration for 60 days, but don't expose it to temperatures above 98.6° F (37° C).

PATIENT TEACHING
• Explain to patient and family that test dose will be given first to check for sensitivity to drug.
• Instruct patient to report adverse reactions promptly.

Micrurus fulvius antivenin

Pharmacologic class: antivenin
Pregnancy risk category C

AVAILABLE FORMS
Injection: Combination package with 10 ml of diluent

INDICATIONS & DOSAGES
➤ **Eastern and Texas coral snake bite**
Adults and children: 30 to 50 ml or three to five vials by slow I.V. injection through running I.V. of normal saline solution. Give 1 to 2 ml over 3 to 5 minutes; monitor patient closely for allergic reaction. If no signs or symptoms of allergic reaction develop, continue injection; 100 ml or more may be needed.

Test for sensitivity before giving drug. If result is positive, prepare to desensitize; prepare 1:10 and 1:100 dilutions of antivenin in normal saline solution for injection.

I.V. ADMINISTRATION
• Reconstitute antivenin powder with diluent.
• Further dilute in normal saline solution to achieve a 1:1 to 1:10 dilution.
• To avoid foaming, swirl solution gently.
• Use reconstituted solution within 48 hours and dilutions within 12 hours.
• Inject first 1 to 2 ml over 3 to 5 minutes into the tubing of an I.V. of normal saline solution while closely monitoring patient. If no immediate systemic response occurs, continue infusion at maximum safe rate for I.V. fluid administration.

INCOMPATIBILITIES
None reported.

ACTION
Neutralizes and binds coral snake venom.

Route	Onset	Peak	Duration
I.V.	Immediate	Unknown	Unknown

Half-life: Unknown.

ADVERSE REACTIONS
CNS: fever.
Musculoskeletal: arthralgia.
Skin: erythema, urticaria.
Other: ***anaphylaxis,*** hypersensitivity reactions, lymphadenopathy, pain.

INTERACTIONS
None significant.

EFFECTS ON LAB TEST RESULTS
None reported.

CONTRAINDICATIONS & CAUTIONS
• Contraindicated in patients hypersensitive to drug or its components.

NURSING CONSIDERATIONS
• ***Alert:*** Drug isn't effective for Sonoran or Arizona coral snake bites.
• Immobilize patient and splint bitten limb to prevent spread of venom.
• Obtain accurate patient history of allergies, especially to horses, and reactions to immunizations. Keep epinephrine 1:1,000 available to treat anaphylaxis.
• Give antivenin as soon as possible (before onset of neurotoxic signs), preferably within 4 hours of bite; treat asymptomatic patients because systemic symptoms usually develop later.
• ***Alert:*** Watch patient carefully for 24 hours. Venom is neurotoxic and may cause respiratory paralysis.
• Antivenin, once reconstituted, can be stored at room temperature for 10 days.

PATIENT TEACHING
• Explain to patient and family that test dose will be given first to check for sensitivity to drug.
• Tell patient to report adverse reactions promptly.

75 Immune serums

cytomegalovirus immune globulin, (human) intravenous
hepatitis B immune globulin, human
immune globulin intramuscular
immune globulin intravenous
rabies immune globulin, human
respiratory syncytial virus immune globulin intravenous, human
Rh_O (D) immune globulin, human
Rh_O (D) immune globulin intravenous, human
tetanus immune globulin, human
varicella zoster immune globulin

CMV immune globulin (human), intravenous (CMV-IGIV)

CytoGam

Pharmacologic class: immune globulin
Pregnancy risk category C

AVAILABLE FORMS

Injection: 2,500 mg ± 500 mg in 50 ml (concentration = 50 ± 10 mg/ml)

INDICATIONS & DOSAGES

➤ **To attenuate primary CMV disease in seronegative kidney transplant recipients who receive a kidney from a CMV-seropositive donor**

Adults: Give an initial dose of 150 mg/kg I.V. within 72 hours after transplant. Then give 100 mg/kg once every 2 weeks at 2, 4, 6, and 8 weeks after transplant, followed by 50 mg/kg given at 12 and 16 weeks after transplant. Maximum dose per infusion is 150 mg/kg.

Give first dose at 15 mg/kg/hour. Increase infusion rate to 30 mg/kg/hour after 30 minutes if no adverse reactions occur, and then to 60 mg/kg/hour after another 30 minutes if no reactions occur. Don't exceed volume of 75 ml/hour. Subsequent doses may be given at 15 mg/kg/hour for 15 minutes, increasing q 15 minutes, stepwise, to 60 mg/kg/hour.

➤ **To prevent CMV disease caused by lung, liver, pancreas, and heart transplantations**

Adults: Give an initial dose of 150 mg/kg I.V. within 72 hours after transplant. Additional doses of 150 mg/kg should be given every 2 weeks at 2, 4, 6, and 8 weeks after transplant, followed by 100 mg/kg given at 12 and 16 weeks after transplant.

Give first dose at 15 mg/kg/hour. If no adverse reactions occur after 30 minutes, increase infusion rate to 30 mg/kg/hour. If no adverse reactions occur after another 30 minutes, increase rate to 60 mg/kg/hour (don't exceed 75 ml/hour). Subsequent doses may be given at 15 mg/kg/hour for 15 minutes, increasing q 15 minutes, stepwise, to maximum rate of 60 mg/kg/hour (don't exceed 75 ml/hour). Monitor patient closely during and after each rate change.

I.V. ADMINISTRATION

- Inspect vial for clarity and particles.
- Remove tab portion of vial cap, and clean rubber stopper with 70% alcohol or equivalent.
- To avoid foaming, don't shake vial.
- If possible, give through a separate I.V. line using an infusion pump. Filters aren't needed.
- If unable to give through separate line, piggyback into line of normal saline solution for injection or into 5%, 10%, 20%, or 25% dextrose in water, with or without sodium chloride. Don't dilute more than 1:2 with any of these solutions.
- Start infusion within 6 hours of entering vial; finish within 12 hours.

INCOMPATIBILITIES

Other I.V. drugs.

ACTION
Provides passive immunity by providing immunoglobulin G antibodies against CMV.

Route	Onset	Peak	Duration
I.V.	Unknown	Unknown	Unknown

Half-life: Immediately after transplantation, 8 days; 60 or more days after transplantation, 13 to 15 days.

ADVERSE REACTIONS
CNS: aseptic meningitis syndrome, fever.
CV: *flushing,* hypotension.
GI: *nausea, vomiting.*
Musculoskeletal: *back pain,* muscle cramps.
Respiratory: *wheezing.*
Other: ***anaphylaxis,*** *chills.*

INTERACTIONS
Drug-drug. *Live-virus vaccines:* May interfere with immune response to live-virus vaccines. Postpone vaccination for at least 3 months.

EFFECTS ON LAB TEST RESULTS
None reported.

CONTRAINDICATIONS & CAUTIONS
- Contraindicated in patients sensitive to other human immunoglobulin preparations or with selective immunoglobulin A deficiency.

NURSING CONSIDERATIONS
- Monitor patient's vital signs closely before, during, and after infusion and before and after infusion rate increases.
- ***Alert:*** If anaphylaxis occurs or blood pressure drops, stop infusion, notify prescriber, and give cardiopulmonary resuscitation and drugs, such as diphenhydramine and epinephrine.
- Refrigerate drug at 36° to 46° F (2° to 8° C).

PATIENT TEACHING
- Review drug therapy regimen with patient, and stress importance of compliance in follow-up visits.
- Instruct patient to report adverse reactions promptly.

hepatitis B immune globulin, human
BayHep B, Nabi-HB

Pharmacologic class: immune serum globulin
Pregnancy risk category C

AVAILABLE FORMS
Injection: 1-ml, 5-ml vials; 0.5-ml neonatal single-dose syringe

INDICATIONS & DOSAGES
➤**Hepatitis B exposure in high-risk patients**
Adults and children: 0.06 ml/kg (usual dose is 3 ml to 5 ml) I.M. within 7 days after exposure. Repeat dose 28 days after exposure if patient doesn't elect to receive the hepatitis B vaccine.
Neonates born to hepatitis B surface antigen (HBsAg)–positive patients: 0.5 ml I.M. within 12 hours of birth.

ACTION
Provides passive immunity to hepatitis B.

Route	Onset	Peak	Duration
I.M.	1–6 days	3–11 days	2 mo

Half-life: Antibodies to HBsAG, 21 days.

ADVERSE REACTIONS
Skin: *pain and tenderness at injection site,* urticaria.
Other: ***anaphylaxis, angioedema.***

INTERACTIONS
Drug-drug. *Live-virus vaccines:* May interfere with response to live-virus vaccines. Postpone routine immunization for 3 months.

EFFECTS ON LAB TEST RESULTS
None reported.

CONTRAINDICATIONS & CAUTIONS
- Contraindicated in patients with history of anaphylactic reactions to immune serum.
- Give to patients with coagulation disorders or thrombocytopenia only if benefit outweighs risk.

NURSING CONSIDERATIONS

- Obtain history of allergies and reactions to immunizations. Keep epinephrine 1:1,000 available.
- Inspect for discoloration or particulates. Make sure drug is clear, slightly amber, and moderately viscous.
- Inject into anterolateral thigh or deltoid muscle in older children and adults; inject into anterolateral thigh in neonates and children younger than age 3.
- For postexposure prophylaxis (such as after needlestick or direct contact), drug should be given with hepatitis B vaccine.
- ***Look alike–sound alike:*** This immune globulin provides passive immunity; don't confuse with hepatitis B vaccine. Both drugs may be given at same time. Don't mix in the same syringe.
- ***Look alike–sound alike:*** Don't confuse HyperHep with Hyperstat or Hyper-Tet.

PATIENT TEACHING

- Inform patient that pain and tenderness may occur at injection site.
- Tell patient to report signs and symptoms of hypersensitivity immediately.

immune globulin intramuscular (gamma globulin, IG, IGIM)

BayGam

immune globulin intravenous (IGIV)

Carimune NF, Flebogamma, Gammagard S/D, Gammar-P I.V, Gamunex, Iveegam EN, Octagam, Panglobulin, Panglobulin NF, Polygam S/D, Venoglobulin-S

Pharmacologic class: immune serum
Pregnancy risk category C

AVAILABLE FORMS

immune globulin intramuscular
Injection: 15% to 18% in 2-ml, 10-ml vials (BayGam)
immune globulin intravenous
Injection: 5% in 10-ml, 50-ml, 100-ml, and 200-ml vials (Flebogamma); 5% in 1-g, 2.5-g, 5-g, 10-g single-use bottles (Octagam);
Powder for injection: 1-g, 3-g, 6-g, 12-g vials (Carimune NF), 50 mg protein/ml in 2.5-g, 5-g, 10-g vials (Gammagard S/D); 1-g, 2.5-g, 5-g, 10-g vials (Gammar-P I.V.); 5-g vials (Iveegam EN); 6-g, 12-g vials (Panglobulin); 1-g, 3-g, 6-g, 12-g vials (Panglobulin NF); 2.5-g, 5-g, 10-g vials (Polygam S/D); 5%, 10% in 5-g, 10-g, 20-g vials (Venoglobulin-S)
Solution for injection: 1-g, 2.5-g, 5-g, 10-g, 20-g vials (Gamunex)

INDICATIONS & DOSAGES

➤ **Primary immunodeficiency (IGIV)**
Carimune NF, Panglobulin NF
Adults and children: 200 mg/kg I.V. once monthly. May increase dose to maximum of 300 mg/kg once monthly or give more often to produce desired effect.
Gammagard S/D
Adults and children: 200 to 400 mg/kg I.V. once monthly; minimum 100 mg/kg once monthly.
Gamunex
Adults and children: 300 to 600 mg/kg I.V. q 3 to 4 weeks.
Iveegam EN
Adults and children: 200 mg/kg I.V. once monthly. May increase dose to maximum of 800 mg/kg, or give more often to produce desired effect.
Octagam
Adults and children: 300 to 600 mg/kg I.V. q 3 to 4 weeks Adjust dose over time to produce desired effect.
Polygam S/D
Adults and children: 200 to 400 mg/kg I.V. once monthly. Minimum dose is 100 mg/kg once monthly.
➤ **Primary defective antibody synthesis such as agammaglobulinemia or hypogammaglobulinemia in patients at increased risk of infection**
Gammar-P I.V.
Adults: 200 to 400 mg/kg I.V. q 3 to 4 weeks.
Adolescents and children: 200 mg/kg I.V. q 3 to 4 weeks. Adjust dosage according to clinical effect and to maintain immunoglobulin G (IgG) at desired level.
Venoglobulin-S
Adults and children: 200 mg/kg I.V. once monthly. May increase dose to 300 to

400 mg/kg, or give more often to maintain IgG at desired level.

➤Idiopathic thrombocytopenic purpura (IGIV)

Carimune NF, Panglobulin NF

Adults and children: 400 mg/kg I.V. daily for 2 to 5 consecutive days; maximum 1 g/kg/day.

Gammagard S/D, Polygam S/D

Adults and children: 1 g/kg I.V. Additional doses depend on response. Up to three doses may be given on alternate days, if needed.

Gamunex

Adults and children: 1 g/kg I.V. daily for 2 consecutive days. If adequate increase in platelet count occurs after first dose, second dose may be withheld. Or, 400 mg/kg I.V. daily for 5 consecutive days. Total dosage is 2 g/kg.

Venoglobulin-S

Adults and children: Maximum of 2 g/kg I.V. divided over up to 5 days. Maintenance dose is 1 g/kg I.V. p.r.n. to maintain platelet counts of 30,000/mm^3 in children and 20,000/mm^3 in adults, or to prevent bleeding episodes.

➤B-cell chronic lymphocytic leukemia (IGIV)

Adults: 400 mg/kg Gammagard S/D or Polygam S/D I.V. q 3 to 4 weeks.

➤To prevent coronary artery aneurysm in patients with Kawasaki syndrome (IGIV)

Adults and children: Combine with high-dose aspirin therapy and start within 10 days of fever.

Iveegam EN, Venoglobulin-S 5% or 10%

Adults and children: 2 g/kg I.V. over 10 to 12 hours; may give another dose.

Gammagard S/D, Polygam S/D

Adults and children: Single 1 g/kg dose Or, 400 mg/kg/day for 4 consecutive days.

➤Hepatitis A exposure (IGIM)

Adults and children: 0.02 ml/kg I.M. as soon as possible after exposure; may give up to 0.06 ml/kg for prolonged or intense exposure.

➤Measles exposure (IGIM)

Adults and children: 0.2 to 0.25 ml/kg I.M. within 6 days after exposure.

Immunocompromised children age 12 months and older: 0.5 ml/kg I.M. within 6 days after exposure (maximum 15 ml).

➤Chickenpox exposure (IGIM)♦

Adults and children: 0.6 to 1.2 ml/kg I.M. as soon as exposed.

I.V. ADMINISTRATION

- Before use, refrigerate Iveegam EN at 36° to 46° F (2° to 8° C). Before reconstitution, store Gammagard S/D, Gammar-P I.V., Polygam S/D, and Venoglobulin-S at room temperature, not to exceed 77° F (25° C). Before reconstitution, store Carimune NF and Panglobulin NF at room temperature, below 86° F (30° C).
- After reconstitution, Gammagard S/D and Polygam S/D contain about 50 mg of protein/ml for 5% solution or 100 mg of protein/ml for 10% solution, and both contain at least 90% IgG. Gammar-P I.V. and Iveegam EN contain 50 mg of IgG/ml; Carimune NF and Panglobulin NF contain at least 96% IgG; Venoglobulin-S contains about 50 mg of protein/ml for 5% solution or 100 mg of protein/ml for 10% solution, and both contain at least 99% IgG; Octagam contains about 50 mg of protein/ml and at least 96% IgG.
- Most adverse reactions are related to a rapid infusion rate. If they occur, decrease infusion rate or stop infusion until reaction subsides. Resume infusion at a rate the patient can tolerate.
- Store Octagam at 36° to 46° F (2° to 8° C) for 24 months or at no higher than 77° F (25° C) for up to 18 months from the date of manufacture.

Carimune NF, Panglobulin NF

- Use 15-micron in-line filter when giving. Reconstitute with normal saline solution, D_5W, or sterile water. Infusion rate is 0.5 to 1 ml/minute for 3% solution. After 15 to 30 minutes, increase rate to 1.5 to 2.5 ml/minute.

Gammagard S/D, Polygam S/D

- Reconstitute according to package directions using sterile water for injection as diluent and the transfer device provided to prepare a solution containing 50 mg of protein per ml for 5% immune globulin solution or 100 mg of protein per ml for 10% immune globulin solution. Warm powder and sterile water for injection to room temperature before reconstitution. Give no more than 2 hours after reconstitution.

• Infuse with administration set provided or with 15-micron in-line filter. Begin infusion at 0.5 ml/kg/hour and increase to maximum of 4 ml/kg/hour. Patients who tolerate 5% concentration at 4 ml/kg/hour can be switched to 10% concentration at 0.5 ml/kg/hour and increased to 8 ml/kg/hour, if tolerated.

Gammar-P I.V.

• Reconstitute with sterile water for injection diluent provided. Warm powder and diluent to room temperature before reconstitution. After adding diluent, keep vial in upright position and undisturbed for 5 minutes. Gently swirl vial after 5 minutes. Don't shake. Dissolution may take up to 20 minutes. Start infusion within 3 hours of reconstituting.

• Use 15-micron in-line filter when giving. Start infusion at 0.01 ml/kg/minute and increase to 0.02 ml/kg/minute after 15 to 30 minutes, if tolerated. Maximum infusion rate is 0.06 ml/kg/minute.

Gamunex

• Incompatible with saline solutions. Compatible with D_5W, if needed.

• Infuse I.V. at a rate of 0.01 ml/kg/minute for first 30 minutes. If no problems, rate can be slowly increased to maximum of 0.08 ml/kg/minute.

• Store vials at 36° to 46° F (2° to 8° C). During first 18 months from the date of manufacture, store vials for up to 5 months at room temperature not exceeding 77° F (25° C); then vials must be used immediately or discarded. Don't freeze vials.

Iveegam EN

• Reconstitute Iveegam with sterile water for injection diluent provided. Use 15-micron in-line filter when giving drug. Infusion rate is 1 to 2 ml/minute for 5% solution.

Venoglobulin-S

• Begin infusion at 0.01 to 0.02 ml/kg/minute for 30 minutes; then increase 5% solutions to a rate less than 0.08 ml/kg/minute and 10% solutions to a rate less than 0.05 ml/kg/minute, if tolerated.

Octagam

• Octagam should be at room temperature during infusion. If using an infusion set (not mandatory), the filter size must be 0.2 to 200 microns. Initially, infuse at 30 mg/kg/hour for the first 30 minutes; if tolerated, infuse at 60 mg/kg/hour for the second 30 minutes; if further tolerated, infuse at 120 mg/kg/hour for the third 30 minutes. If tolerated, infusion can be maintained at less than 200 mg/kg/hour. Adverse reactions usually disappear with slowing or stopping the infusion. For patients at risk for renal dysfunction, reduce infusion time to less than 200 mg/kg/hour.

INCOMPATIBILITIES

Other I.V. drugs.

ACTION

Provides passive immunity by increasing antibody titer. The primary component is IgG. It's unknown how it works for idiopathic thrombocytopenic purpura.

Route	Onset	Peak	Duration
I.V.	Immediate	Immediate	Unknown
I.M.	Unknown	2–5 hr	Unknown

Half-life: 21 to 24 days in immunocompromised patients.

ADVERSE REACTIONS

CNS: ***severe headache requiring hospitalization,*** faintness, fever, headache, malaise.
CV: chest pain, heart failure, MI.
GI: nausea, vomiting.
Musculoskeletal: chest pain, chest tightness, hip pain, muscle stiffness at injection site.
Respiratory: ***pulmonary embolism, transfusion related acute lung injury,*** dyspnea.
Skin: erythema, urticaria, pain.
Other: ***anaphylaxis, angioedema,*** chills.

INTERACTIONS

Drug-drug. *Live-virus vaccines:* Length of time to wait before giving live-virus vaccinations varies with dose of immune globulin given. Check the recommendations of the American Academy of Pediatrics.

EFFECTS ON LAB TEST RESULTS

None reported.

CONTRAINDICATIONS & CAUTIONS

• Contraindicated in patients hypersensitive to drug or its components.

• IGIV administration may be linked to thrombotic events. Use IGIV cautiously in patients with a history of CV disease or thrombotic episodes.
• Use IGIV cautiously in patients with renal dysfunction or a predisposition to renal failure, including patients with preexisting renal insufficiency, diabetes mellitus, volume depletion, sepsis, paraproteinemia, those older than age 65, and those receiving nephrotoxic drugs.

NURSING CONSIDERATIONS
• Obtain history of allergies and reactions to immunizations. Keep epinephrine 1:1,000 available to treat anaphylaxis.
• If patient is at a risk for a thrombotic event, make sure infusion concentration is no more than 5% and start infusion rate no faster than 0.5 ml/kg per hour. Advance rate slowly only if well tolerated, to a maximum rate of 4 ml/kg per hour.
• For I.M. use, give in the gluteal region. Divide doses larger than 10 ml and inject into several muscle sites to reduce pain and discomfort.
• Give drug soon after reconstitution.
• Don't give as prophylaxis against hepatitis A if 6 weeks or more since exposure or onset of symptoms.

PATIENT TEACHING
• Explain to patient and family how drug will be given.
• Tell patient that local reactions may occur at injection site. Instruct him to notify prescriber promptly if adverse reactions persist or become severe.
• Inform patient of possible need for therapy more than once monthly to maintain adequate immunoglobulin G levels.

rabies immune globulin, human
Hyperab, Imogam Rabies-HT

Pharmacologic class: immune serum
Pregnancy risk category C

AVAILABLE FORMS
Injection: 150 international units/ml in 2-ml, 10-ml vials

INDICATIONS & DOSAGES
➤ Rabies exposure
Adults and children: 20 international units/kg I.M. at time of first dose of rabies vaccine. Half of dose is used to infiltrate wound area; remainder is given I.M. in a different site.

ACTION
Provides passive immunity to rabies.

Route	Onset	Peak	Duration
I.M.	24 hr	Unknown	Unknown

Half-life: About 24 days.

ADVERSE REACTIONS
CNS: slight fever.
GU: ***nephrotic syndrome.***
Skin: *rash,* pain, redness, and induration at injection site.
Other: ***anaphylaxis, angioedema.***

INTERACTIONS
Drug-drug. *Live-virus vaccines (measles, mumps, or rubella):* May interfere with response to vaccine. Postpone immunization, if possible.

EFFECTS ON LAB TEST RESULTS
None reported.

CONTRAINDICATIONS & CAUTIONS
• No known contraindications.
• Use with caution in patients hypersensitive to thimerosal or history of systemic allergic reactions to human immunoglobulin preparations; also use cautiously in those with immunoglobulin A deficiency.

NURSING CONSIDERATIONS
• Obtain history of animal bites, allergies, and reactions to immunizations. Have epinephrine 1:1,000 ready to treat anaphylaxis.
• Ask patient when last tetanus immunization was received; many prescribers order a booster at this time.
• Use only with rabies vaccine and immediate local treatment of wound. Don't give rabies vaccine and rabies immune globulin in same syringe or at same site. Give as soon as possible after exposure or through day 7. After day 8, antibody response to culture vaccine has occurred.

• Don't give live-virus vaccines within 3 months of rabies immune globulin.
• Don't give more than 5 ml I.M. at one injection site; divide I.M. doses over 5 ml; give at different sites.
• Give large volumes (5 ml) in adults only. Use upper outer quadrant of gluteal area.
• ***Look alike–sound alike:*** This immune serum provides passive immunity. Don't confuse with rabies vaccine, a suspension of killed microorganisms that confers active immunity. The two drugs are often used together prophylactically after exposure to rabid animals.
• Clean wound thoroughly with soap and water; this is the best prophylaxis against rabies.

PATIENT TEACHING
• Inform patient that local reactions may occur at injection site. Instruct him to notify prescriber promptly if reactions persist or become severe.
• Tell patient that a tetanus shot also may be needed.
• Instruct patient in wound care.

respiratory syncytial virus (RSV) immune globulin intravenous, human (RSV-IGIV)
RespiGam

Pharmacologic class: immune globulin
Pregnancy risk category C

AVAILABLE FORMS
Injection: 50 mg ± 10 mg/ml in 20-ml, 50-ml single-use vial

INDICATIONS & DOSAGES
➤ **To prevent serious lower respiratory tract infections from RSV in children with bronchopulmonary dysplasia (BPD) or who were born prematurely (35 weeks gestation or less)**
Premature infants and children younger than age 2: Single infusion monthly. Give 1.5 ml/kg/hour I.V. for 15 minutes; then, if condition allows higher rate, increase to 3.6 ml/kg/hour until infusion ends. Maximum recommended total dose per monthly infusion is 750 mg/kg.

I.V. ADMINISTRATION
• Don't use turbid solution. Enter single-use vial only once. Don't shake; avoid foaming.
• Drug doesn't contain a preservative. Don't dilute before infusion.
• Use a constant infusion pump and an in-line filter with pore size larger than 15 microns.
• Give separately from other drugs.
• Begin infusion within 6 hours and end within 12 hours after vial is entered.

INCOMPATIBILITIES
Other I.V. drugs.

ACTION
Provides passive immunity to RSV.

Route	Onset	Peak	Duration
I.V.	Unknown	Unknown	> 1 mo

Half-life: 22 to 28 days.

ADVERSE REACTIONS
CNS: anxiety, dizziness, fever.
CV: chest tightness, flushing, hypertension, palpitations, tachycardia.
GI: abdominal cramps, diarrhea, gastroenteritis, vomiting.
Metabolic: fluid overload.
Musculoskeletal: arthralgia, myalgia.
Respiratory: crackles, dyspnea, hypoxia, respiratory distress, tachypnea, wheezing.
Skin: inflammation at injection site, rash, pruritus.
Other: ***angioneurotic edema,*** hypersensitivity reactions (including *anaphylaxis),* overdose effect.

INTERACTIONS
Drug-drug. *Live-virus vaccines (such as mumps, rubella, and especially measles):* May interfere with response. If such vaccines are given during or within 10 months after RSV-IGIV, reimmunization is recommended, if appropriate.

EFFECTS ON LAB TEST RESULTS
None reported.

CONTRAINDICATIONS & CAUTIONS

- Contraindicated in patients severely hypersensitive to drug or other human immunoglobulin and selective immunoglobulin A deficiency.
- Children with fluid overload shouldn't receive drug.

NURSING CONSIDERATIONS

- Give first dose before RSV season (November to April) begins; give subsequent doses monthly throughout RSV season to maintain protection. Children with RSV should continue to receive monthly doses for duration of RSV season.
- Follow infusion rate guidelines; adverse reactions may be related to rate. Slower rates may be indicated especially in ill children with BPD.
- Assess cardiopulmonary status and vital signs before infusion, before each rate increase, and every 30 minutes thereafter until 30 minutes after infusion ends.
- Watch patient closely for signs and symptoms of fluid overload. Children with BPD may be more prone to this condition. Report increases in heart rate, respiratory rate, retractions, or crackles. Keep available a loop diuretic, such as furosemide or bumetanide.
- ***Alert:*** If patient develops hypotension, anaphylaxis, or severe allergic reaction, stop infusion and give epinephrine 1:1,000. Patients with selective immunoglobulin A deficiency can develop antibodies to immunoglobulin A and have anaphylactic or allergic reactions to subsequent administration of blood products containing immunoglobulin A, including RSV-IGIV.

PATIENT TEACHING

- Explain to parents the importance of child receiving drug monthly throughout RSV season, even if he is already infected.
- Teach parents how drug is given and which adverse reactions are related to administration. Tell parents to report all adverse reactions promptly.

Rh_o(D) immune globulin, human (IGIM)

BayRho-D Full Dose, BayRho-D Mini-Dose, MICRhoGAM, RhoGAM

Rh_o(D) immune globulin intravenous, human (IGIV)

WinRho SDF

Pharmacologic class: immune serum
Pregnancy risk category C

AVAILABLE FORMS

IGIM
Injection: 300 mcg of Rh_o(D) immune globulin/vial (standard dose); 50 mcg of Rh_o(D) immune globulin/vial (microdose)
IGIV
Injection: 120 mcg, 300 mcg, 1,000 mcg

INDICATIONS & DOSAGES

➤ **Rh exposure after abortion, miscarriage, ectopic pregnancy, or childbirth**
Adults: Transfusion unit or blood bank determines fetal packed RBC volume entering patient's blood; one vial IGIM is given I.M. if fetal packed RBC volume is less than 15 ml. More than one vial I.M. may be needed if severe fetomaternal hemorrhage occurs; must be given within 72 hours after delivery or miscarriage.

➤ **To prevent Rh antibody formation after abortion or miscarriage**
Adults: Consult transfusion unit or blood bank. One IGIM microdose vial I.M. will suppress immune reaction to 2.5 ml Rh_o(D)-positive RBCs. Ideally, give within 3 hours, but may be given up to 72 hours after abortion or miscarriage.

➤ **Rh exposure after abortion, amniocentesis after 34 weeks' gestation, or other manipulations past 34 weeks' gestation with increased risk of Rh isoimmunization**
Adults: 120 mcg IGIV, given I.V. or I.M. within 72 hours of delivery, miscarriage, or manipulation.

➤ **To suppress Rh isoimmunization during pregnancy**
Adults: 300 mcg I.V. or I.M. at 28 weeks' gestation. If given early in pregnancy, give additional doses at 12-week intervals

to maintain adequate levels of passively acquired anti-Rh antibodies. Then, within 72 hours of delivery, give 120 mcg I.M. or I.V. If 72 hours have elapsed, give drug as soon as possible, up to 28 days.

➤**Incompatible blood transfusion**
Adults: 600 mcg I.V. q 8 hours or 1,200 mcg I.M. q 12 hours until total dose given. Total dose depends on volume of packed RBCs or whole blood infused. Consult blood bank or transfusion unit at once; must be given within 72 hours.

➤**Idiopathic thrombocytopenic purpura in Rh_o(D) antigen-positive adults**
Adults: Initially, 50 mcg/kg I.V. as single dose or divided into two doses on separate days. If hemoglobin level is less than 10 g/dl, reduce first dose to 25 to 40 mcg/kg. Then, give 25 to 60 mcg/kg I.V. p.r.n. to elevate platelet counts with specific individually determined dosage.

I.V. ADMINISTRATION
- Reconstitute vials containing 600 or 1,500 units with 2.5 ml of normal saline solution and vials containing 5,000 units with 8.5 ml of normal saline solution. Only use normal saline solution. Slowly inject normal saline solution onto the wall of vial and gently swirl vial until lyophilized pellet is dissolved. Don't shake vial.
- Give injection over 3 to 5 minutes.

INCOMPATIBILITIES
Other I.V. drugs.

ACTION
Mechanism of action not completely known. Suppresses active antibody response and formation of anti-Rh_o(D) antibodies in Rh_o(D)-negative, D^u-negative persons exposed to Rh-positive blood. Rh_o(D) immune globulin I.V. may block platelet destruction in Rh_o(D) antigen–positive adults.

Route	Onset	Peak	Duration
I.V., I.M.	Unknown	Unknown	Unknown

Half-life: 24 to 30 days.

ADVERSE REACTIONS
CNS: slight fever.
Skin: discomfort at injection site.
Other: ***anaphylaxis.***

INTERACTIONS
Drug-drug. *Live-virus vaccines:* May interfere with response. Postpone immunization for 3 months, if possible.

EFFECTS ON LAB TEST RESULTS
None reported.

CONTRAINDICATIONS & CAUTIONS
- Contraindicated in Rh_o(D)-positive or D^u-positive patients and in those previously immunized to Rh_o(D) blood factor. Contraindicated in patients with anaphylactic or severe systemic reaction to human globulin.
- Use extreme caution when giving drug to patients with immunoglobulin A deficiency.

NURSING CONSIDERATIONS
- Patients with immunoglobulin A deficiency may develop immunoglobulin A antibodies and have anaphylactic reaction; prescriber must weigh benefits of treatment against risk of hypersensitivity reactions before giving.
- Obtain history of allergies and reactions to immunizations. Keep epinephrine 1:1,000 ready to treat anaphylaxis.
- ***Alert:*** Immediately after delivery, send a sample of neonate's cord blood to laboratory for typing and crossmatching. Confirm if mother is Rh_o(D)-negative and D^u-negative. Give drug to mother only if infant is Rh_o(D)- or D^u-positive. Administration must occur within 72 hours of delivery.
- This immune serum provides passive immunity to patient exposed to Rh_o(D)-positive fetal blood during pregnancy and prevents formation of maternal antibodies (active immunity), which would endanger future Rh_o(D)-positive pregnancies.
- Postpone vaccination with live-virus vaccines for 3 months after administration of Rh_o(D) immune globulin.
- Minidose preparations are recommended for patient undergoing abortion or miscarriage up to 12 weeks' gestation unless she

is Rh_o(D)-positive or D^u-positive or has Rh antibodies, or unless the father or fetus is Rh-negative.

PATIENT TEACHING

- Explain how drug protects future Rh_o(D)-positive fetuses if used because of pregnancy, or explain other use, if indicated.
- Warn patient about adverse reactions related to drug.
- Reassure patient receiving this drug that there's no risk of HIV transmission.

tetanus immune globulin, human

BayTet

Pharmacologic class: toxoid
Pregnancy risk category C

AVAILABLE FORMS

Injection: 250-unit vial or syringe

INDICATIONS & DOSAGES

➤ **Postexposure prevention of tetanus after injury, in patients whose immunization is incomplete or unknown**

Adults and children: 250 units deep I.M. injection.

➤ **Tetanus**

Adults and children: Single doses of 3,000 to 6,000 units I.M. have been used. Optimal dosage schedules haven't been established.

ACTION

Provides passive immunity to tetanus.

Route	Onset	Peak	Duration
I.M.	Unknown	2–3 days	4 wk

Half-life: About 28 days.

ADVERSE REACTIONS

CNS: slight fever.
GU: ***nephrotic syndrome.***
Musculoskeletal: stiffness.
Skin: erythema at injection site.
Other: ***anaphylaxis, angioedema,*** hypersensitivity reactions, pain.

INTERACTIONS

Drug-drug. *Live-virus vaccines:* May interfere with response. Postpone administration of live-virus vaccines for 3 months after giving tetanus immune globulin.

EFFECTS ON LAB TEST RESULTS

None reported.

CONTRAINDICATIONS & CAUTIONS

- Contraindicated in patients with thrombocytopenia or other coagulation disorders that would contraindicate I.M. injection unless benefits outweigh risks.
- Use cautiously in patients with history of previous systemic allergic reactions after giving human immunoglobulin preparations and in those allergic to thimerosal.

NURSING CONSIDERATIONS

- Obtain history of injury, tetanus immunizations, last tetanus toxoid injection, allergies, and reactions to immunizations. Keep epinephrine 1:1,000 available to treat hypersensitivity reaction.
- Don't give I.V. or I.D. Don't give in gluteal area.
- Tetanus immune globulin is used only if wound is more than 24 hours old or patient has had fewer than two tetanus toxoid injections.
- Thoroughly clean wound and remove all foreign matter.
- ***Look alike–sound alike:*** Don't confuse drug with tetanus toxoid. Tetanus immune globulin isn't a substitute for tetanus toxoid, which should be given at same time to produce active immunization. Don't give at same site as toxoid.
- Antibodies remain at effective levels for about 4 weeks, several times the duration of equine antitetanus antibodies, thereby protecting patients for incubation period of most tetanus cases.
- Don't give live-virus vaccines for 3 months after giving tetanus immune globulin.
- ***Look alike–sound alike:*** Don't confuse Hyper-Tet with HyperHep or Hyperstat.

PATIENT TEACHING

- Warn patient about local adverse reactions related to drug.
- Instruct patient to report serious adverse reactions promptly.

• Advise patient to complete full series of tetanus immunizations.
• Instruct patient to take acetaminophen to reduce fever and to apply cool compresses at injection site for comfort.

varicella zoster immune globulin (VZIG)

Pharmacologic class: immune serum
Pregnancy risk category C

AVAILABLE FORMS

Injection: 10% to 18% solution of the globulin fraction of human plasma containing 125 units of varicella zoster virus antibody (volume is about 2.5 ml or less)

INDICATIONS & DOSAGES

➤ **Passive immunization of susceptible immunodeficient patients after exposure to varicella (chickenpox or herpes zoster)**
Adults and children who weigh more than 40 kg (88 lb): 625 units I.M.
Children who weigh 30 to 40 kg (66 to 88 lb): 500 units I.M.
Children who weigh 20 to 30 kg (44 to 66 lb): 375 units I.M.
Children who weigh 10 to 20 kg (22 to 44 lb): 250 units I.M.
Children who weigh up to 10 kg (22 lb): 125 units I.M.

ACTION

Provides passive immunity to varicella zoster virus in immunodeficient patients.

Route	Onset	Peak	Duration
I.M.	Unknown	Unknown	1 mo

Half-life: 21 days.

ADVERSE REACTIONS

CNS: headache, malaise.
GI: GI distress.
Respiratory: respiratory distress.
Skin: discomfort at injection site, rash.
Other: ***anaphylaxis.***

INTERACTIONS

Drug-drug. *Live-virus vaccines:* May interfere with response. Postpone vaccination for 3 months after administration of VZIG.

EFFECTS ON LAB TEST RESULTS

None reported.

CONTRAINDICATIONS & CAUTIONS

• Contraindicated in patients with thrombocytopenia or history of severe reaction to human immune serum globulin or thimerosal; also contraindicated during pregnancy.

NURSING CONSIDERATIONS

• Obtain accurate patient history of allergies and reactions to immunizations. Keep epinephrine 1:1,000 ready to treat anaphylaxis.
• For maximum benefit, give as soon as possible after presumed exposure. Drug may be of benefit when given as late as 96 hours after exposure.
• Give only by deep I.M. injection into a large muscle such as gluteal muscle. Never give I.V.
• Don't give in divided doses.
• Although usually restricted to children younger than age 15, VZIG may be given to adolescents and adults, if needed.
• VZIG isn't recommended for patients who aren't immunosuppressed.
• ***Look alike–sound alike:*** VZIG provides passive immunity; don't confuse with varicella vaccine. Don't use these two drugs together.
• Drug isn't commercially distributed and is available only from 20 regional United States distribution centers. These centers will distribute to Canada and overseas. Contact the Massachusetts Public Health Biologic Laboratories or the CDC at (800) 232-2522 for more information.

PATIENT TEACHING

• Warn patient about local adverse reactions caused by the drug.
• Instruct patient to report serious adverse reactions to prescriber promptly.
• Suggest use of acetaminophen to reduce fever and cool compresses at injection site for comfort.

76
Biological response modifiers

darbepoetin alfa
epoetin alfa
filgrastim
glatiramer acetate injection
interferon alfa-2a, recombinant
interferon alfa-2b, recombinant
interferon alfacon-1
interferon beta-1a
interferon beta-1b, recombinant
interferon gamma-1b
leflunomide
oprelvekin
pegfilgrastim
peginterferon alfa-2a
peginterferon alfa-2b
sargramostim

SAFETY ALERT!

darbepoetin alfa
Aranesp

Pharmacologic class: recombinant human erythropoietin
Pregnancy risk category C

AVAILABLE FORMS

Injection (with albumin or polysorbate solution): 25 mcg/ml, 40 mcg/ml, 60 mcg/ml, 100 mcg/ml, 150 mcg/0.75 ml, 200 mcg/ml, 300 mcg/ml, and 500 mcg/ml in single-dose vials
Prefilled syringe or autoinjector (with albumin or polysorbate solution): 25 mcg/0.42 ml, 40 mcg/0.4 ml, 60 mcg/0.3 ml, 100 mcg/0.5 ml, 150 mcg/0.3 ml, 200 mcg/0.4 ml, 300 mcg/0.6 ml, and 500 mcg/ml

INDICATIONS & DOSAGES

➤ **Anemia from chronic renal failure**
Adults: 0.45 mcg/kg I.V. or subcutaneously once weekly. The I.V. route is preferred for patients on dialysis. Adjust dose so hemoglobin level doesn't exceed 12 g/dl. Don't increase dose more often than once a month. In adults and children older than age 1 converting from epoetin alfa, base starting dose on the previous epoetin alfa dose (see table). Don't use as initial treatment of anemia in children with chronic renal failure.

Previous epoetin alfa dose (units/wk)	Darbepoetin alfa dose (mcg/wk) Adults	Darbepoetin alfa dose (mcg/wk) Children
< 1,500	6.25	Unknown
1,500–2,499	6.25	6.25
2,500–4,999	12.5	10
5,000–10,999	25	20
11,000–17,999	40	40
18,000–33,999	60	60
34,000–89,999	100	100
≥ 90,000	200	200

Give darbepoetin alfa less often than epoetin alfa. If patient was receiving epoetin alfa two to three times weekly, give darbepoetin alfa once weekly. If patient was receiving epoetin alfa once weekly, give darbepoetin alfa once q 2 weeks.
Adjust-a-dose: If increasing hemoglobin level approaches 12 g/dl, reduce dose by 25%. If hemoglobin level continues to increase, withhold dose until hemoglobin level begins to decrease; then restart therapy at a dose 25% below the previous dose. If hemoglobin level increases more than 1 g/dl over 2 weeks, decrease dose by 25%. If hemoglobin level increases less than 1 g/dl over 4 weeks and iron stores are adequate, increase dose by 25% of previous dose. Make further increases at 4-week intervals until target hemoglobin level is reached. Patients who don't need dialysis may need lower maintenance doses.

➤ **Anemia from chemotherapy in patients with nonmyeloid malignancies**
Adults: 2.25 mcg/kg subcutaneously once weekly or 500 mcg subcutaneously once every 3 weeks.
Adjust-a-dose: For either dosing schedule, adjust dose to maintain a target hemoglobin below 12 g/dl. If hemoglobin ex-

ceeds 13 g/dl, hold drug until hemoglobin drops to 12 g/dl, then resume at 40% of previous dose. If hemoglobin increases more than 1 g/dl in a 2-week period, or when hemoglobin exceeds 11 g/dl, reduce dose by 40%. For patients receiving the drug on a once-a-week schedule, if hemoglobin level increases less than 1 g/dl after 6 weeks of therapy, increase dose up to 4.5 mcg/kg.

I.V. ADMINISTRATION

- Don't shake. Shaking can denature drug.
- If drug contains particles or is discolored, don't use.
- Give undiluted by I.V. injection.
- Single-dose vials contain no preservatives; don't pool unused portions.

INCOMPATIBILITIES

Other I.V. drugs or solutions.

ACTION

Mimics effects of erythropoietin. Functions as a growth factor and as a differentiating factor, enhancing RBC production.

Route	Onset	Peak	Duration
I.V.	Unknown	Unknown	Unknown
SubQ	Unknown	Unknown	Unknown

Half-life: 21 hours (I.V.); 49 hours (subcutaneous).

ADVERSE REACTIONS

CNS: ***seizures,*** *dizziness, fatigue, fever, headache,* asthenia.
CV: CARDIAC ARREST, CARDIAC ARRHYTHMIA, *edema, hypertension, hypotension, peripheral edema,* ***acute MI, heart failure, stroke, thrombosis,*** angina, chest pain, TIA, vascular access thrombosis.
GI: *abdominal pain, constipation, diarrhea, nausea, vomiting,* ***GI hemorrhage.***
Metabolic: dehydration.
Musculoskeletal: *arthralgia, limb pain, myalgia,* back pain.
Respiratory: *cough, dyspnea, upper respiratory tract infection,* ***pulmonary embolism,*** bronchitis, pneumonia.
Skin: pruritus, rash.
Other: *infection,* ***bacteremia, hemorrhage at access site, peritonitis, sepsis,*** abscess, access infection, fluid overload, flulike symptoms, injection site pain.

INTERACTIONS

None reported

EFFECTS ON LAB TEST RESULTS

None reported.

CONTRAINDICATIONS & CAUTIONS

- Contraindicated in patients hypersensitive to drug or its components and in those with uncontrolled hypertension.
- Safety and effectiveness haven't been established in patients with underlying hematologic disease, such as hemolytic anemia, sickle cell anemia, thalassemia, or porphyria. Use with caution.

NURSING CONSIDERATIONS

- ***Alert:*** Monitor hemoglobin level weekly until stabilized. Don't exceed the target of 12 g/dl.
- Hemoglobin level may not increase until 2 to 6 weeks after starting therapy.
- If patient has a minimal response or lack of response at recommended dose, check for deficiencies in folic acid, iron or vitamin B_{12}. Other contributing factors include infection, malignancy, and occult blood loss.
- ***Alert:*** If patient develops a sudden loss of response with severe anemia and low reticulocyte count, withhold drug and test patient for antierythropoietin antibodies. If antibodies are present, stop treatment. Don't switch to another erythropoietic protein because a cross-reaction is possible.
- ***Alert:*** Give I.V., not subcutaneously, in patients with chronic renal failure on dialysis.
- Drug may increase the risk of CV events. Control blood pressure and monitor it carefully.
- Monitor renal function and electrolytes in predialysis patients.
- Patients who are marginally dialyzed may need adjustments in dialysis prescriptions.
- Serious allergic reactions, including skin rash and urticaria, may occur. If an anaphylactic reaction occurs, stop the drug and give appropriate therapy.

- Store drug in the refrigerator; don't freeze. Protect drug from light and avoid vigorous shaking.

PATIENT TEACHING

- Instruct patients on proper administration and use and disposal of needles.
- Advise patient of possible side effects and allergic reactions.
- Inform patient of the need for frequent monitoring of blood pressure and hemoglobin level; stress compliance with his treatment for high blood pressure.
- Instruct patient how to take drug correctly at home, including how to store drug and dispose of supplies properly.

SAFETY ALERT!

epoetin alfa (erythropoietin)

Epogen, Eprex†, Procrit

Pharmacologic class: recombinant human erythropoietin
Pregnancy risk category C

AVAILABLE FORMS

Injection: 2,000 units/ml, 3,000 units/ml, 4,000 units/ml, 10,000 units/ml; multidose vials of 10,000 units/ml, 20,000 units/ml, 40,000 units/ml

INDICATIONS & DOSAGES

➤ Anemia caused by chronic renal failure

Adults: Dosage is individualized. Starting dose is 50 to 100 units/kg subcutaneously or I.V. three times weekly. Maintenance dosage is highly individualized.
Infants and children ages 1 month to 16 years who are on dialysis: Initially, 50 units/kg I.V. or subcutaneously three times weekly. Maintenance dosage is highly individualized to keep hemoglobin level within target range.
Infants and children ages 3 to 20 months who aren't on dialysis♦*:* 50 to 250 units/kg subcutaneously or I.V once to three times per week.
Adjust-a-dose: Reduce dosage when target hemoglobin level approaches 12 g/dl or if it rises more than 1 g/dl in any 2-week period. Increase dosage if hemoglobin level doesn't increase by 2 g/dl after 8 weeks of therapy and is below the target range.

➤ Anemia from zidovudine therapy in HIV-infected patients

Adults: Initially, 100 units/kg I.V. or subcutaneously three times weekly for 8 weeks or until target hemoglobin level is reached. If response isn't satisfactory after 8 weeks, increase dosage by 50 to 100 units/kg I.V. or subcutaneously three times weekly. After 4 to 8 weeks, further increase dosage in increments of 50 to 100 units/kg three times weekly, up to maximum of 300 units/kg I.V. or subcutaneously three times weekly.
Infants and children ages 8 months to 17 years♦*:* 50 to 400 units/kg subcutaneously or I.V. two to three times per week.

➤ Anemia from chemotherapy

Adults: Initially, 150 units/kg subcutaneously three times weekly for 8 weeks or until target hemoglobin level is reached. If response isn't satisfactory after 8 weeks, increase dosage up to 300 units/kg subcutaneously three times weekly. Or, 40,000 units subcutaneously once weekly. If hemoglobin level hasn't increased by at least 1 g/dl (in the absence of RBC transfusion), increase dose to 60,000 units weekly.
Infants and children ages 6 months to 18 years♦*:* 25 to 300 units/kg subcutaneously or I.V. three to seven times per week.
Adjust-a-dose: Withhold drug if hemoglobin level exceeds 13 g/dl. Reduce dose by 25% and resume therapy when hemoglobin level is less than 12 g/dl. If hemoglobin level increases by more than 1 g/dl in any 2-week period, reduce dose by 25%.

➤ Reduce need for allogenic blood transfusion in anemic patients scheduled to have elective, noncardiac, nonvascular surgery

Adults: 300 units/kg daily subcutaneously daily for 10 days before surgery, on day of surgery, and for 4 days after surgery. Or, 600 units/kg subcutaneously in once-weekly doses (21, 14, and 7 days before surgery), plus a fourth dose on day of surgery.

I.V. ADMINISTRATION

- Don't shake.

• Give by direct injection without dilution.
• If patient is having dialysis, drug may be given into venous return line after dialysis session. To keep drug from adhering to tubing, inject drug with blood still in the line. Then flush with normal saline solution.
• Solution contains no preservatives. Discard unused portion.

INCOMPATIBILITIES
Other I.V. drugs.

ACTION
Mimics effects of erythropoietin. Functions as a growth factor and as a differentiating factor, enhancing RBC production.

Route	Onset	Peak	Duration
I.V.	Immediate	Immediate	Unknown
SubQ	Unknown	5–24 hr	Unknown

Half-life: 4 to 13 hours.

ADVERSE REACTIONS
CNS: *asthenia, dizziness, fatigue, headache, paresthesia,* ***seizures.***
CV: *edema, hypertension,* increased clotting of arteriovenous grafts.
EENT: *pharyngitis.*
GI: *abdominal pain and constipation (in children), diarrhea, nausea, vomiting.*
Metabolic: ***hyperkalemia,*** hyperphosphatemia, hyperuricemia.
Musculoskeletal: *arthralgia.*
Respiratory: *cough, shortness of breath.*
Skin: *injection site reactions, rash,* urticaria.
Other: *pyrexia.*

INTERACTIONS
None significant.

EFFECTS ON LAB TEST RESULTS
• May increase BUN, creatinine, phosphate, potassium, and uric acid levels.

CONTRAINDICATIONS & CAUTIONS
• Contraindicated in patients hypersensitive to products derived from mammal cells or albumin (human) and in those with uncontrolled hypertension.
• Use cautiously in breast-feeding women.

NURSING CONSIDERATIONS
• Before starting therapy, evaluate patient's iron status. Patient should receive adequate iron supplementation beginning no later than when epoetin alfa treatment starts and continuing throughout therapy. Patient also may need vitamin B_{12} and folic acid.
• Monitor blood pressure before therapy. Most patients with chronic renal failure have hypertension. Blood pressure may increase, especially when hematocrit increases in the early part of therapy.
• Institute diet restrictions or drug therapy to control blood pressure.
• Monitor hemoglobin level twice weekly until it stabilizes in the target range (10 to 12 g/dl for most patients) and maintenance dose is established, then continue to monitor at regular intervals. Resume twice weekly testing following any dosage adjustments.
• ***Alert:*** Reduce dosage in patients who have an increase in hemoglobin level of more than 1 g/dl in any 2-week period.
• When used in HIV-infected adults, dosage recommendations are for those with endogenous erythropoietin levels of 500 units/L or less and cumulative zidovudine doses of 4.2 g/week or less.
• Monitor blood counts; elevated hematocrit may cause excessive clotting.
• Patient may need additional heparin to prevent clotting during dialysis treatments.
• ***Alert:*** Evaluate patient who experiences a lack or loss of effect for pure red cell aplasia.
• ***Look alike–sound alike:*** Don't confuse Epogen with Neupogen.

PATIENT TEACHING
• Inform patient that pain or discomfort in limbs (long bones) and pelvis, and coldness and sweating may occur after injection (usually within 2 hours). Symptoms may last for 12 hours and then disappear.
• Advise patient to avoid driving or operating heavy machinery at start of therapy. There may be a relationship between too-rapid increase in hematocrit and seizures.
• Tell patient to monitor blood pressure at home and to adhere to dietary restrictions.

• Advise women that they may resume menstruating after therapy and to consider the need for contraception.

SAFETY ALERT!

filgrastim (G-CSF; granulocyte-colony stimulating factor)
Neupogen

Pharmacologic class: hematopoietic
Pregnancy risk category C

AVAILABLE FORMS
Injection: 300 mcg/ml

INDICATIONS & DOSAGES
➤ **To decrease risk of infection in patients with non-myeloid malignant disease receiving myelosuppressive antineoplastics**
Adults and children: 5 mcg/kg daily I.V. or subcutaneously as single dose given no sooner than 24 hours after cytotoxic chemotherapy. Doses may be increased in increments of 5 mcg/kg for each chemotherapy cycle depending on duration and severity of the nadir of absolute neutrophil count (ANC).
➤ **To decrease risk of infection in patients with non-myeloid malignant disease receiving myelosuppressive antineoplastics followed by bone marrow transplantation**
Adults and children: 10 mcg/kg daily I.V. infusion of 4 or 24 hours or as continuous 24-hour subcutaneous infusion at least 24 hours after cytotoxic chemotherapy and bone marrow infusion. Adjust subsequent dosages based on neutrophil response.
Adjust-a-dose: For patients with ANC over 1,000/mm^3 for 3 consecutive days, reduce dosage to 5 mcg/kg daily; if ANC remains over 1,000/mm^3 for 3 more consecutive days, stop drug. If ANC decreases to below 1,000/mm^3, resume therapy at 5 mcg/kg daily.
➤ **Congenital neutropenia**
Adults: 6 mcg/kg subcutaneously b.i.d. Adjust dosage based on patient response.
Adjust-a-dose: For patients with an ANC persistently above 10,000/mm^3, reduce dosage, as directed.
➤ **Idiopathic or cyclic neutropenia**
Adults: 5 mcg/kg subcutaneously daily. Adjust dosage based on patient response.
➤ **Peripheral blood progenitor cell collection and therapy in cancer patients**
Adults: 10 mcg/kg subcutaneously daily. Give 4 days before leukapheresis and continue until last leukapheresis.
Adjust-a-dose: Patients with WBC count over 100,000/mm^3 may need dosage adjustment.
➤ **To reduce the risk of bacterial infection in patients with HIV ♦**
Adults and adolescents: 5 to 10 mcg/kg subcutaneously once daily for 2 to 4 weeks.

I.V. ADMINISTRATION
• Dilute in 50 to 100 ml of D_5W. Dilution to less than 5 mcg/ml isn't recommended.
• If drug yield is 5 to 15 mcg/ml, add albumin at 2 mg/ml (0.2%) to minimize binding of drug to plastic containers or tubing.
• Give by intermittent infusion over 15 to 60 minutes or by continuous infusion over 24 hours.

INCOMPATIBILITIES
Amphotericin B, cefepime, cefonicid, cefotaxime, cefoxitin, ceftizoxime, ceftriaxone, cefuroxime, clindamycin, dactinomycin, etoposide, fluorouracil, furosemide, heparin sodium, mannitol, methylprednisolone sodium succinate, metronidazole, mitomycin, piperacillin, prochlorperazine edisylate, sodium solutions, thiotepa.
Don't dilute with normal saline solution.

ACTION
A glycoprotein that stimulates proliferation and differentiation of hematopoietic cells. Is specific for neutrophils.

Route	Onset	Peak	Duration
I.V.	5–60 min	24 hr	1–7 days
SubQ	5–60 min	2–8 hr	1–7 days

Half-life: About 3½ hours.

ADVERSE REACTIONS
CNS: *fever,* headache, weakness, *fatigue.*
CV: ***MI, arrhythmias,*** chest pain, hypotension.

GI: *nausea, vomiting, diarrhea, mucositis,* stomatitis, constipation.
Hematologic: ***thrombocytopenia,*** leukocytosis.
Metabolic: hyperuricemia.
Musculoskeletal: *bone pain.*
Respiratory: dyspnea, cough.
Skin: *alopecia,* rash, cutaneous vasculitis.
Other: hypersensitivity reactions.

INTERACTIONS

Drug-drug. *Chemotherapeutic drugs:* Rapidly dividing myeloid cells may be sensitive to cytotoxic drugs. Don't use within 24 hours before or after a dose of one of these drugs.

EFFECTS ON LAB TEST RESULTS

- May increase alkaline phosphatase, creatinine, LDH, and uric acid levels.
- May increase WBC count. May decrease platelet count.

CONTRAINDICATIONS & CAUTIONS

- Contraindicated in patients hypersensitive to drug or its components or to proteins derived from *Escherichia coli.*
- Use cautiously in breast-feeding women.

NURSING CONSIDERATIONS

- Obtain baseline CBC and platelet count before therapy.
- Once a dose is withdrawn, don't reuse vial. Discard unused portion. Vials are for single-dose use and contain no preservatives.
- Obtain CBC and platelet count two to three times weekly during therapy. Patients who receive drug also may receive high doses of chemotherapy, which may increase risk of toxicities.
- A transiently increased neutrophil count is common 1 or 2 days after therapy starts. Give daily for up to 2 weeks or until ANC has returned to 10,000/mm^3 after the expected chemotherapy-induced neutrophil nadir.
- ***Look alike–sound alike:*** Don't confuse Neupogen with Epogen or Neumega.

PATIENT TEACHING

- If patient will give drug, teach him how to do so and how to dispose of used needles, syringes, drug containers, and unused medicine.
- ***Alert:*** Rarely, splenic rupture may occur. Advise patient to immediately report upper left abdominal or shoulder tip pain.
- Instruct patient to report persistent or serious adverse reactions promptly.

SAFETY ALERT!

glatiramer acetate injection

Copaxone

Pharmacologic class: synthetic peptide
Pregnancy risk category B

AVAILABLE FORMS

Injection: 20 mg glatiramer acetate and 40 mg mannitol, USP, in a single-use prefilled syringe

INDICATIONS & DOSAGES

➤ **Reduce frequency of relapse in patients with relapsing-remitting multiple sclerosis**
Adults: 20 mg subcutaneously daily.

ACTION

May modify immune processes responsible for the pathogenesis of multiple sclerosis.

Route	Onset	Peak	Duration
SubQ	Unknown	Unknown	Unknown

Half-life: Unknown.

ADVERSE REACTIONS

CNS: *anxiety, asthenia,* abnormal dreams, agitation, confusion, emotional lability, fever, migraine, nervousness, speech disorder, stupor, syncope, tremor, vertigo.
CV: *chest pain, palpitations, vasodilation,* hypertension, tachycardia.
EENT: *rhinitis,* ear pain, eye disorder, laryngismus, nystagmus.
GI: *diarrhea, nausea,* anorexia, bowel urgency, gastroenteritis, GI disorder, oral candidiasis, salivary gland enlargement, ulcerative stomatitis, vomiting.
GU: *urinary urgency,* ***vaginal hemorrhage,*** abnormal Papanicolaou smear, amenorrhea, dysmenorrhea, hematuria,

impotence, menorrhagia, vaginal candidiasis.
Hematologic: ***lymphadenopathy,*** ecchymosis.
Metabolic: weight gain.
Musculoskeletal: *arthralgia, back pain, hypertonia,* foot drop, neck pain.
Respiratory: *dyspnea,* bronchitis, hyperventilation.
Skin: *diaphoresis, injection site reaction, pruritus, rash,* eczema, erythema or hemorrhage, nodule, skin atrophy, urticaria, warts.
Other: *flulike syndrome, infection, pain,* bacterial infection, chills, cyst, dental caries, herpes simplex and zoster, peripheral and facial edema.

INTERACTIONS
None significant.

EFFECTS ON LAB TEST RESULTS
None reported.

CONTRAINDICATIONS & CAUTIONS
- Contraindicated in patients hypersensitive to drug or mannitol.

NURSING CONSIDERATIONS
- Give drug only subcutaneously.
- Store drug in refrigerator (36° to 46° F [2° to 8° C]); allow drug to warm to room temperature for 20 minutes before use.
- Drug doesn't contain preservatives; discard if solution contains particulate matter.
- ***Alert:*** Don't try to expel the air bubble from the prefilled syringe. This may lead to loss of drug and an incorrect dose.
- Immediate postinjection reactions may occur ; symptoms include flushing, chest pain, palpitations, anxiety, dyspnea, constriction of the throat, and urticaria. They typically are transient and self-limiting and don't need specific treatment. Onset of postinjection reaction may occur several months after treatment starts, and patients may have more than one episode.
- Patient may experience at least one episode of transient chest pain, which usually begins at least 1 month after treatment starts; it isn't accompanied by other signs or symptoms and doesn't appear to be clinically important.
- ***Look alike–sound alike:*** Don't confuse Copaxone with Compazine.

PATIENT TEACHING
- Instruct patient how to self-inject drug. Supervise first injection.
- Explain need for aseptic self-injection techniques and warn patient against reuse of needles and syringes. Periodically review proper disposal of needles, syringes, drug containers, and unused drug.
- Tell patient to notify prescriber about planned, suspected, or known pregnancy.
- Tell woman to notify prescriber if she is breast-feeding.
- Advise patient not to change drug or dosage schedule or to stop drug without medical approval.
- Tell patient to notify prescriber immediately if dizziness, hives, profuse sweating, chest pain, difficulty breathing, or if severe pain occurs after drug injection.

SAFETY ALERT!

interferon alfa-2a, recombinant (rIFN-A)
Roferon-A

Pharmacologic class: antineoplastic, antiviral
Pregnancy risk category C

AVAILABLE FORMS
Injection (single use prefilled syringes): 3, 6, 9 million international units/0.5 ml

INDICATIONS & DOSAGES
➤ Chronic hepatitis C
Adults: 3 million international units three times a week subcutaneously for 12 months (48 to 52 weeks). Or, induction dose of 6 million international units three times weekly for the first 3 months (12 weeks) followed by 3 million international units three times weekly for 9 months (36 weeks). If no response after 3 months, stop therapy. Retreatment with either 3 or 6 million international units three times weekly for 6 to 12 months may be considered for those who relapse.
➤ Hairy cell leukemia
Adults: For induction, 3 million international units subcutaneously daily for 16 to

24 weeks. For maintenance, 3 million international units subcutaneously three times weekly.

➤ **Philadelphia chromosome–positive chronic myelogenous leukemia**

Adults: Initially, 3 million international units subcutaneously daily for 3 days; then 6 million international units for 3 days; then 9 million international units for duration of treatment.

ACTION

Appears to involve direct antiproliferative action against tumor or viral cells to inhibit replication and modulation of host immune response by enhancing phagocytic activity of macrophages and augmenting specific cytotoxicity of lymphocytes for target cells.

Route	Onset	Peak	Duration
SubQ	Unknown	4–8 hr	Unknown

Half-life: 3½ to 8½ hours.

ADVERSE REACTIONS

CNS: *confusion, decreased mental status, depression, dizziness,* ***coma,*** anxiety, apathy, fatigue, forgetfulness, gait disturbances, incoordination, insomnia, irritability, lethargy, nervousness, numbness, paresthesia, sedation, syncope, vertigo.
CV: ***arrhythmias, heart failure, MI,*** chest pain, edema, flushing, hypertension, hypotension, palpitations.
EENT: *dryness or inflammation of the oropharynx,* conjunctivitis, earache, eye irritation, rhinorrhea, sinusitis.
GI: *abdominal pain, anorexia, change in taste, diarrhea, nausea, vomiting,* abdominal fullness, constipation, excessive salivation, flatulence, gastric distress, hypermotility.
GU: transient impotence.
Hematologic: **LEUKOPENIA, THROMBOCYTOPENIA,** *anemia.*
Hepatic: ***hepatitis.***
Metabolic: *weight loss,* hypercalcemia, hyperphosphatemia.
Respiratory: cough, cyanosis, dyspnea.
Skin: *inflammation at injection site, partial alopecia, rash,* diaphoresis, dryness, pruritus, urticaria.
Other: *flulike syndrome,* hot flashes, night sweats.

INTERACTIONS

Drug-drug. *Aminophylline, theophylline:* May reduce theophylline clearance. Monitor theophylline level.
Aspirin: May increase risk of GI bleeding. Avoid using together.
CNS depressants: May increase CNS effects. Avoid using together.
Live-virus vaccines: May increase risk of adverse reactions and may decrease antibody response. Avoid using together.
Drugs with neurotoxic, hematotoxic, or cardiotoxic effects: May increase the toxic effects of these drugs. Monitor patient for increased adverse effects.
Drug-lifestyle. *Alcohol use:* May increase risk of GI bleeding. Discourage patient from use during therapy.

EFFECTS ON LAB TEST RESULTS

- May increase calcium, phosphate, AST, ALT, alkaline phosphatase, LDH, and fasting glucose levels. May decrease hemoglobin level and hematocrit.
- May increase PT, INR, and PTT. May decrease WBC and platelet counts.

CONTRAINDICATIONS & CAUTIONS

- Contraindicated in patients hypersensitive to drug, murine (mouse) immunoglobulin, or other drug components. Also contraindicated in patients with history of autoimmune hepatitis or history of autoimmune disease, severe visceral AIDS-related Kaposi sarcoma, neonates (injection contains benzyl alcohol), immunocompromised transplant patients, and severe depression or suicidal behavior.
- Use cautiously in patients with severe hepatic or renal function impairment, seizure disorders, compromised CNS function, cardiac disease, or myelosuppression.
- ***Alert:*** Neurotoxicity and cardiotoxicity are more common in elderly patients, especially those with underlying CNS or cardiac impairment.

NURSING CONSIDERATIONS

- ***Alert:*** Alpha interferons cause or aggravate fatal or life-threatening neuropsychiatric, autoimmune, ischemic, and infec-

tious disorders. Monitor patient closely with periodic clinical and laboratory evaluations. Withdraw patients with persistently severe or worsening signs or symptoms of these conditions from therapy.
- Obtain allergy history. Drug contains phenol as a preservative and albumin as a stabilizer.
- Give drug at bedtime to minimize daytime drowsiness.
- Ensure patient is well hydrated, especially during first stages of treatment.
- At beginning of therapy, assess patient for flulike signs and symptoms, which tend to diminish with continued therapy. Premedicate patient with acetaminophen to minimize signs and symptoms.
- Monitor patient for CNS adverse reactions, such as decreased mental status and dizziness, during therapy.
- Depression and suicidal behavior have been linked to treatment.
- Monitor CBC with differential, platelet count, blood chemistry and electrolyte studies, and liver function tests. If patient has cardiac disorder or advanced stages of cancer, monitor ECG.
- For patients who develop thrombocytopenia, exercise extreme care in performing invasive procedures; inspect injection site and skin frequently for bruising; test urine, emesis fluid, stool, and secretions for occult blood.
- ***Alert:*** Different brands of interferon may not be equivalent and may need different dosages.
- Severe adverse reactions may require reducing dose by one-half or stopping drug until reactions subside.
- Use with blood dyscrasia-causing drugs, bone marrow suppressant, or radiation therapy may increase bone marrow suppression. Dosage may need to be reduced.
- Keep drug refrigerated. Don't freeze.

PATIENT TEACHING

- Advise patient that laboratory tests will be performed before and periodically during therapy.
- Teach patient proper oral hygiene during treatment because bone marrow suppressant effects may lead to microbial infection, delayed healing, and bleeding gums. Drug also may decrease salivary flow.
- Stress need to follow prescriber's instructions about taking and recording temperature and how and when to take acetaminophen.
- Advise patient to check with prescriber for instructions after missing dose.
- Tell patient that drug may cause temporary, partial hair loss.
- If patient will be giving drug to himself, teach him how to prepare and give it and how to dispose of used needles, syringes, containers, and unused drug.
- Instruct patient not to take aspirin or alcohol because use together increases risk of GI bleeding.
- Instruct patient not to switch brands without consulting prescriber.
- Warn patient against performing tasks that require mental alertness.
- Advise patient to immediately report signs and symptoms of depression.

SAFETY ALERT!

interferon alfa-2b, recombinant (IFN-alpha 2)

Intron A

Pharmacologic class: antineoplastic, antiviral
Pregnancy risk category C

AVAILABLE FORMS

Solution for injection: 3, 5, 10 million international units/dose in multidose pens; 3, 5, 10 million international units/vial; 18 and 25 million international units multidose vials
Powder for injection: 3, 5, 10, 18, 25, 50 million international units/vial with diluent

INDICATIONS & DOSAGES

➤ Hairy cell leukemia

Adults: 2 million international units/m^2 I.M. or subcutaneously, three times weekly for 6 months or more.

➤ Condylomata acuminata (genital or venereal warts)

Adults: 1 million international units for each lesion intralesionally three times weekly for 3 weeks.

➤ **AIDS-related Kaposi sarcoma**
Adults: 30 million international units/m^2 subcutaneously or I.M. three times weekly. Maintain dose unless disease progresses rapidly or intolerance occurs.
➤ **Chronic hepatitis B**
Adults: 30 to 35 million international units weekly I.M. or subcutaneously, given as 5 million international units daily or 10 million international units three times weekly for 16 weeks.
Children ages 1 to 17: Initially, 3 million international units/m^2 subcutaneously three times weekly for first week; then increase to 6 million international units/m^2 subcutaneously three times weekly (maximum is 10 million international units three times weekly) for total of 16 to 24 weeks.
➤ **Chronic hepatitis C**
Adults: 3 million international units I.M. or subcutaneously three times weekly. In patients tolerating therapy with normalization of ALT at 16 weeks of therapy, continue for 18 to 24 months. In patients who haven't normalized the ALT, consider stopping therapy.
➤ **Adjunct to surgical treatment in patients with malignant melanoma who are asymptomatic after surgery but at high risk for systemic recurrence for up to 8 weeks after surgery**
Adults: Initially, 20 million international units/m^2 by I.V. infusion 5 consecutive days weekly for 4 weeks; then maintenance dose of 10 million international units/m^2 subcutaneously three times weekly for 48 weeks. If adverse effects occur, stop therapy until they abate; then resume therapy at 50% of the previous dose. If intolerance persists, stop therapy.
➤ **First treatment of clinically aggressive follicular non-Hodgkin lymphoma with chemotherapy containing anthracycline**
Adults: 5 million international units subcutaneously three times weekly for up to 18 months.

I.V. ADMINISTRATION
- Prepare infusion solution immediately before use.
- Based on desired dose, reconstitute appropriate vial strength of drug with diluent provided. Withdraw dose and inject into a 100-ml bag of normal saline solution. Final yield of drug shouldn't be less than 10 million international units/100 ml.
- Infuse over 20 minutes.
- Store solution in refrigerator. Store powder before and after reconstitution in refrigerator. Use within 24 hours.

INCOMPATIBILITIES
Dextrose solutions.

ACTION
May inhibit tumor or viral cell replication and modulate host immune response by enhancing macrophage action and improving specific lymphocytes' cytotoxicity.

Route	Onset	Peak	Duration
I.V.	Unknown	15–60 min	4 hr
I.M., SubQ	Unknown	3–12 hr	16 hr

Half-life: 3½ to 8½ hours.

ADVERSE REACTIONS
CNS: ***suicidal ideation,*** *amnesia, asthenia, confusion, depression, difficulty in thinking or concentrating, dizziness, fatigue, hypoesthesia, insomnia, malaise, paresthesia, somnolence,* anxiety, lethargy, nervousness, weakness.
CV: *chest pain,* ***arrhythmia, bradycardia, cardiac failure,*** angina, flushing, hypertension, hypotension, tachycardia.
EENT: *nasal congestion, sinusitis,* hearing disorders, pharyngitis, rhinitis, stye, visual disturbances.
GI: *anorexia, diarrhea, dry mouth, dyspepsia, nausea, vomiting,* abdominal pain, constipation, dysgeusia, eructation, gingivitis, loose stools, stomatitis.
GU: transient impotence.
Hematologic: ***leukopenia, thrombocytopenia,*** anemia.
Metabolic: hypercalcemia, hyperphosphatemia.
Musculoskeletal: *arthralgia, back pain.*
Respiratory: *coughing, dyspnea,* ***pulmonary embolism.***
Skin: *alopecia, dryness, increased diaphoresis, pruritus, rash,* candidiasis, dermatitis.
Other: *flulike syndrome, rigors,* gynecomastia.

INTERACTIONS

Drug-drug. *Aminophylline, theophylline:* May reduce theophylline clearance. Monitor theophylline level.
CNS depressants: May increase CNS effects. Avoid using together.
Live-virus vaccines: May increase adverse reactions to vaccine or decrease antibody response. Postpone immunization.
Zidovudine: May cause synergistic adverse effects (higher risk of neutropenia). Carefully monitor WBC count.

EFFECTS ON LAB TEST RESULTS

- May increase calcium, phosphate, AST, ALT, LDH, alkaline phosphatase, and fasting glucose levels. May decrease hemoglobin level.
- May increase PT, INR, and PTT. May decrease WBC and platelet counts.

CONTRAINDICATIONS & CAUTIONS

- Contraindicated in patients hypersensitive to drug or its components.
- Use cautiously in patients with history of CV disease, pulmonary disease, diabetes mellitus, coagulation disorders, and severe myelosuppression.
- Depression and suicidal behavior have been linked to drug use; patients with psychotic disorders, especially depression, shouldn't continue drug treatment.
- ***Alert:*** Neurotoxicity and cardiotoxicity are more common in elderly patients, especially those with underlying CNS or cardiac impairment.

NURSING CONSIDERATIONS

- ***Alert:*** Alpha interferons cause or aggravate fatal or life-threatening neuropsychiatric, autoimmune, ischemic, and infectious disorders. Monitor patients closely with periodic clinical and laboratory evaluations. Withdraw patients with persistently severe or worsening signs or symptoms of these conditions from therapy.
- In patients whose platelet count is below 50,000/mm^3, give subcutaneously.
- Give drug at bedtime to minimize daytime drowsiness.
- For condylomata acuminata, use only 10 million international unit vial because dilution of other strengths for intralesional use results in a hypertonic solution. Don't reconstitute drug in 10 million international unit vial with more than 1 ml of diluent. Use tuberculin or similar syringe and 25G to 30G needle. Don't inject too deeply or superficially. Up to five lesions can be treated at once. To ease discomfort, give in evening with acetaminophen.
- Ensure patient is well hydrated, especially at beginning of treatment.
- At start of treatment, monitor patient for flulike signs and symptoms, which tend to diminish with continued therapy. Premedicate patient with acetaminophen to minimize these symptoms.
- Periodically check for adverse CNS reactions, such as decreased mental status and dizziness, during therapy.
- Monitor CBC with differential, platelet count, blood chemistry and electrolyte studies, and liver function tests. Monitor ECG if patient has cardiac disorder or advanced stages of cancer.
- For patients who develop thrombocytopenia, exercise extreme care in performing invasive procedures; inspect injection site and skin frequently for signs and symptoms of bruising; limit frequency of I.M. injections; test urine, emesis fluid, stool, and secretions for occult blood.
- Severe adverse reactions may need dosage reduction to one-half or stoppage of drug until reactions subside.
- Use with blood dyscrasia-causing drugs, bone marrow suppressants, or radiation therapy may increase bone marrow suppression. Dosage reduction may be needed.
- For condylomata acuminata, maximum response usually occurs in 4 to 8 weeks. If results aren't satisfactory after 12 to 16 weeks, a second course may be started. Patients with 6 to 10 condylomata may receive a second course of treatment; patients with more than 10 condylomata may receive additional courses.

PATIENT TEACHING

- Advise patient to avoid contact with persons with viral illness; patient is at increased risk for infection during therapy.
- Advise patient that laboratory tests will be performed before and periodically during therapy.
- Teach patient proper oral hygiene during treatment because bone marrow suppressant effects of interferon may lead to microbial infection, delayed healing, and

bleeding gums. Drug also may decrease salivary flow.
- Advise patient to check with prescriber for instructions after missing a dose.
- Stress need to follow prescriber's instructions about taking and recording temperature and how and when to take acetaminophen.
- If patient will give drug to himself, teach him how to prepare injection and to use disposable syringe. Give him information on drug stability.
- Tell patient that drug may cause temporary partial hair loss; hair should return after drug is stopped.
- Advise patient to notify prescriber if signs or symptoms of depression occur.

SAFETY ALERT!

interferon alfacon-1

Infergen

Pharmacologic class: biologic response modifier
Pregnancy risk category C

AVAILABLE FORMS

Injection: 9 mcg/0.3-ml, 15 mcg/0.5-ml vials

INDICATIONS & DOSAGES

➤ **Chronic hepatitis C viral infection in patients with compensated liver disease**

Adults: 9 mcg subcutaneously three times weekly for 24 weeks; for patients who don't respond or who relapse, 15 mcg subcutaneously three times weekly for up to 48 weeks.

Adjust-a-dose: For patients intolerant to higher doses, dose may be reduced to 7.5 mcg. Don't give doses below 7.5 mcg because decreased efficacy may result.

ACTION

Induces gene-mediated biological responses that include antiviral, antiproliferative, and immunomodulatory effects and cytokine regulation.

Route	Onset	Peak	Duration
SubQ	Unknown	24–36 hr	Unknown

Half-life: Unknown.

ADVERSE REACTIONS

CNS: *amnesia, anxiety, depression, dizziness, emotional lability, headache, insomnia, malaise, nervousness, paresthesia,* ***suicidal ideation,*** agitation, confusion.
CV: hypertension, palpitations, tachycardia.
EENT: *pharyngitis, retinal hemorrhages, rhinitis, sinusitis,* conjunctivitis, ear pain, epistaxis, loss of visual acuity or visual field, tinnitus.
GI: *abdominal pain, anorexia, diarrhea, dyspepsia, nausea, vomiting,* constipation, decreased saliva, flatulence, hemorrhoids, taste perversion.
GU: dysmenorrhea, vaginitis.
Hematologic: ***granulocytopenia, leukopenia, thrombocytopenia,*** ecchymosis, lymphadenopathy, lymphocytosis.
Metabolic: hypothyroidism.
Respiratory: *congestion, cough, infection,* bronchitis, dyspnea.
Skin: *alopecia, erythema at injection site, pain, pruritus, rash,* dry skin.
Other: *body pain, flulike symptoms,* ***hypersensitivity reactions,*** decreased libido, toothache.

INTERACTIONS

Drug-drug. *Drugs metabolized by cytochrome P-450:* May alter drug levels. Monitor changes in levels of these drugs.
Myelosuppressives: May cause added hematologic toxicities; use cautiously together. Monitor CBC and therapeutic or toxic level of myelosuppressive.

EFFECTS ON LAB TEST RESULTS

- May increase triglyceride and TSH levels. May decrease T_4 levels.
- May increase PT and INR. May decrease granulocyte, WBC, and platelet counts.

CONTRAINDICATIONS & CAUTIONS

- Contraindicated in patients hypersensitive to alpha interferons, to *Escherichia coli*–derived products, or to any component of product; and in patients with history of severe psychiatric disorders, autoimmune hepatitis, or decompensated hepatic disease.
- Use with caution in patients with history of cardiac disease and other autoim-

mune or endocrine disorders, in those with abnormally low peripheral blood cell counts, and in those receiving drugs that causes myelosuppression.

NURSING CONSIDERATIONS

- Depression and suicidal behavior have been linked to drug.
- Obtain the following laboratory tests before therapy, 2 weeks after it starts, and periodically during therapy: CBC with platelet count, and creatinine, albumin, bilirubin, TSH, and T_4 levels.
- ***Alert:*** If hypersensitivity reaction occurs, stop drug immediately and treat. Premedication with acetaminophen or ibuprofen may decrease adverse effects.
- Allow at least 48 hours to elapse between doses.
- Dosages and adverse reactions vary among different subtypes of drug. Don't use different subtypes in a single treatment regimen.
- Store drug in refrigerator at 36° to 46° F (2° to 8° C); don't freeze. Injection may be allowed to reach room temperature just before use. Avoid vigorous shaking. Discard unused portion.

PATIENT TEACHING

- If drug is to be used at home, instruct patient on appropriate use, dosage, and administration. Give the patient information leaflet available from the manufacturer to the patient. Also teach patient proper disposal procedures for needles, syringes, drug containers, and unused drug.
- Instruct patient not to reuse needles or syringes or reenter vial.
- Tell patient to discard all syringes and needles in a puncture-resistant container.
- Urge patient not to use vial that is discolored or contains particulates.
- Tell patient that nonnarcotic analgesics and bedtime administration may be used to prevent or lessen flulike symptoms (headache, fever, malaise, muscle pain) related to therapy.
- Instruct patient to immediately report symptoms of depression.

SAFETY ALERT!

interferon beta-1a

Avonex, Rebif

Pharmacologic class: antiviral, immunoregulator
Pregnancy risk category C

AVAILABLE FORMS

Avonex
Lyophilized powder for injection: 33 mcg (6.6 million international units)
Prefilled syringe: 30 mcg (6 million international units)/0.5 ml
Rebif
Parenteral: 8.8 mcg (2.4 million international units)/0.2 ml, and 22 mcg (6 million international units) and 44 mcg (12 million international units) per 0.5-ml prefilled syringe

INDICATIONS & DOSAGES

➤ To slow accumulation of physical disability and decrease frequency of clinical worsening in patients with relapsing forms of multiple sclerosis (MS)
Adults age 18 and older: 30 mcg Avonex I.M. once weekly. Or, initially, 8.8 mcg Rebif subcutaneously three times weekly for 2 weeks; then increase dose to 22 mcg three times weekly for another 2 weeks. Then increase to a maintenance dose of 44 mcg subcutaneously three times weekly.
Adjust-a-dose: For Rebif, in patients with leukopenia or elevated liver function test values (ALT greater than five times upper limit of normal), reduce dosage by 20% to 50% until toxicity is resolved. Stop treatment if jaundice or other signs of hepatic injury occur.
➤ First MS attack if brain magnetic resonance imaging shows abnormalities consistent with MS
Adults: 30 mcg Avonex I.M. once weekly.

ACTION

Exact mechanism unknown. Interacts with specific cell receptors found on the surface of human cells. Binding of these receptors induces the expression of a number of interferon-induced gene products believed to mediate the biological actions of interferon beta-1a.

Route	Onset	Peak	Duration
SubQ	Unknown	16 hr	Unknown.
I.M.	Unknown	3–15 hr	Unknown.

Half-life: I.M., 10 hours; subcutaneous, 69 hours.

ADVERSE REACTIONS

CNS: *asthenia, dizziness, fatigue, fever, headache, sleep difficulty,* ***depression, seizures, suicidal ideation or attempt, suicidal tendency,*** abnormal coordination, ataxia, hypertonia, malaise, speech disorder, syncope.
CV: chest pain, vasodilation.
EENT: *abnormal vision, sinusitis,* decreased hearing, otitis media.
GI: *abdominal pain, diarrhea, dyspepsia, nausea,* anorexia, dry mouth.
GU: increased urinary frequency, ovarian cyst, urinary incontinence, vaginitis.
Hematologic: *lymphadenopathy,* ***leukopenia, pancytopenia, thrombocytopenia,*** anemia.
Hepatic: abnormal hepatic function, autoimmune hepatitis, bilirubinemia, hepatic injury, ***hepatitis.***
Metabolic: hyperthyroidism, hypothyroidism.
Musculoskeletal: *back pain, muscle ache, skeletal pain,* arthralgia, muscle spasm.
Respiratory: *upper respiratory tract infection,* dyspnea.
Skin: *injection site reaction,* alopecia, ecchymosis at injection site, nevus, urticaria.
Other: *chills, flulike syndrome, infection, pain,* ***hypersensitivity reactions,*** herpes simplex, herpes zoster, neutralizing antibodies.

INTERACTIONS

Drug-lifestyle. *Sun exposure:* May cause photosensitivity reactions. Advise patient to take precautions against sun exposure.

EFFECTS ON LAB TEST RESULTS

- May increase liver enzyme level. May decrease hemoglobin level and hematocrit. May increase or decrease thyroid function test levels.
- May increase eosinophil count. May decrease WBC and platelet counts.

CONTRAINDICATIONS & CAUTIONS

- Contraindicated in patients hypersensitive to natural or recombinant interferon beta, human albumin, or other components of drug.
- Use cautiously in patients with depression, seizure disorders, or severe cardiac conditions.
- It's unknown if drug appears in breast milk; a breast-feeding woman must either stop breast-feeding or stop drug.
- Safety and effectiveness of drug in chronic progressive MS or in children younger than age 18 haven't been established.

NURSING CONSIDERATIONS

- Monitor patient closely for depression and suicidal ideation. It isn't known if these symptoms are related to the underlying neurologic basis of MS or to the drug.
- Monitor WBC count, platelet count, and blood chemistries, including liver function tests. Rare but severe liver injury, including liver failure, may occur in patients taking Avonex.
- To reconstitute drug, inject 1.1 ml of supplied diluent (sterile water for injection) into vial and gently swirl to dissolve drug. Don't shake.
- Use drug as soon as possible but may be used within 6 hours after being reconstituted if stored at 36° to 46° F (2° to 8° C).
- Rotate sites of injection.
- After giving each dose, discard any remaining product in the syringe.
- Give analgesics or antipyretics to decrease flulike symptoms.
- Store Rebif in the refrigerator between 36° to 46° F (2° to 8° C). Don't freeze. Rebif may also be stored at or below 77° F (25° C) for up to 30 days and away from heat and light.
- Store Avonex prefilled syringes in the refrigerator at 36° to 46° F (2° to 8° C). Once removed from refrigerator, warm to room temperature (about 30 minutes) and use within 12 hours. Don't use external heat sources such as hot water to warm syringe, or expose to high temperatures. Don't freeze. Protect from light.

PATIENT TEACHING

- Teach patient and family member how to reconstitute drug and give I.M.
- Caution patient not to change dosage or schedule of administration. If a dose is missed, tell him to take it as soon as he remembers. He may then resume his regular schedule. Tell patient not to take two injections within 2 days of each other.
- Show patient how to store drug.
- Inform patient that flulike signs and symptoms, such as fever, fatigue, muscle aches, headache, chills, and joint pain, aren't uncommon at start of therapy. Acetaminophen 650 mg P.O. may be taken immediately before injection and for another 24 hours after each injection, to lessen severity of flulike signs and symptoms.
- Advise patient to report depression, suicidal thoughts, or other adverse reactions.
- Instruct patient to keep syringes and needles away from children. Also, instruct him not to reuse needles or syringes and to discard them in a syringe-disposal unit.
- Caution woman not to become pregnant during therapy because of the risk of spontaneous abortion. If pregnancy occurs, instruct patient to notify prescriber immediately and to stop drug.
- Advise patient to use sunscreen and avoid sun exposure while taking drug because photosensitivity may occur.
- Tell patient to store Rebif in the refrigerator between 36° to 46° F (2° to 8° C) and not to freeze. Rebif may also be stored at or below 77° F (25° C) for up to 30 days and away from heat and light.

SAFETY ALERT!

interferon beta-1b, recombinant

Betaseron

Pharmacologic class: antiviral, immunoregulator
Pregnancy risk category C

AVAILABLE FORMS

Powder for injection: 9.6 million international units (0.3 mg)

INDICATIONS & DOSAGES

➤ To reduce frequency of exacerbations in relapsing forms of multiple sclerosis

Adults: 0.0625 mg subcutaneously every other day for weeks 1 and 2; then 0.125 mg subcutaneously every other day for weeks 3 and 4; then 0.1875 mg subcutaneously every other day for weeks 5 and 6; then 0.25 mg subcutaneously every other day thereafter.

ACTION

A naturally occurring antiviral and immunoregulatory drug derived from human fibroblasts. Attaches to membrane receptors and causes cellular changes, including increased protein synthesis.

Route	Onset	Peak	Duration
SubQ	Unknown	1–8 hr	Unknown

Half-life: 8 minutes to 4¼ hours.

ADVERSE REACTIONS

CNS: depression, anxiety, emotional lability, depersonalization, ***suicidal tendencies,*** confusion, somnolence, *hypertonia, asthenia, migraine,* ***seizures,*** *headache,* dizziness.
CV: palpitations, hypertension, tachycardia, peripheral vascular disorder.
EENT: laryngitis, *sinusitis, conjunctivitis,* abnormal vision.
GI: *diarrhea, constipation, abdominal pain, vomiting.*
GU: *menstrual bleeding or spotting, early or delayed menses, fewer days of menstrual flow, menorrhagia.*
Hematologic: LEUKOPENIA.
Musculoskeletal: *myasthenia.*
Respiratory: dyspnea.
Skin: *inflammation, pain, necrosis at injection site, diaphoresis,* alopecia.
Other: breast pain, *flulike syndrome, pelvic pain, lymphadenopathy, pain,* generalized edema.

INTERACTIONS

None significant.

EFFECTS ON LAB TEST RESULTS

- May increase ALT and bilirubin levels.
- May decrease WBC and neutrophil counts.

CONTRAINDICATIONS & CAUTIONS

- Contraindicated in patients hypersensitive to interferon beta, human albumin, or components of drug.
- Use cautiously in women of childbearing age. Evidence is inconclusive about teratogenic effects, but drug may be an abortifacient.

NURSING CONSIDERATIONS

- ***Alert:*** Serious liver damage, including hepatic failure requiring transplant, can occur. Monitor liver function at 1, 3, and 6 months after therapy starts and periodically thereafter.
- To reconstitute, inject 1.2 ml of supplied diluent (half normal saline solution for injection) into vial and gently swirl to dissolve drug. Don't shake. Reconstituted solution contains 8 million international units (0.25 mg)/ml. Discard vial that contains particulates or discolored solution.
- Inject immediately after preparation.
- Store new formulation at room temperature. After reconstitution, if not used immediately, drug may be refrigerated for up to 3 hours.
- Rotate injection sites to minimize local reactions and observe site for necrosis.
- Monitor patient for signs of depression.

PATIENT TEACHING

- Warn woman about dangers to fetus. If pregnancy occurs during therapy, tell her to notify prescriber and stop taking drug.
- Teach patient how to perform subcutaneous injections, including solution preparation, aseptic technique, injection site rotation, and equipment disposal. Periodically reevaluate patient's technique.
- Tell patient to take drug at bedtime to minimize mild flulike signs and symptoms that commonly occur.
- Advise patient to report suicidal thoughts or depression.
- Urge patient to immediately report signs or symptoms of tissue death.

SAFETY ALERT!

interferon gamma-1b

Actimmune

Pharmacologic class: biologic response modifier
Pregnancy risk category C

AVAILABLE FORMS

Injection: 100 mcg (2 million international units)/0.5-ml vial

INDICATIONS & DOSAGES

➤ **Chronic granulomatous disease, severe malignant osteopetrosis**
Adults with body surface area (BSA) greater than 0.5 m^2: Give 50 mcg/m^2 (1 million international units/m^2) subcutaneously three times weekly, preferably at bedtime, in deltoid or anterior thigh muscle.
Adults with a BSA 0.5 m^2 or less: 1.5 mcg/kg subcutaneously three times weekly.

ACTION

Interleukin-type lymphokine. Has potent phagocyte-activating properties and increases the oxidative metabolism of tissue macrophages.

Route	Onset	Peak	Duration
SubQ	Unknown	7 hr	Unknown

Half-life: 6 hours.

ADVERSE REACTIONS

CNS: *fatigue,* decreased mental status, dizziness, gait disturbance.
GI: *diarrhea, nausea, vomiting,* abdominal pain.
GU: proteinuria.
Hematologic: ***neutropenia, thrombocytopenia.***
Metabolic: weight loss.
Musculoskeletal: back pain.
Skin: *erythema and tenderness at injection site, rash.*
Other: *flulike syndrome.*

INTERACTIONS

Drug-drug. *Myelosuppressives:* May increase myelosuppression. Monitor patient closely.

Zidovudine: May increase zidovudine level. Adjust dosage when used together.

EFFECTS ON LAB TEST RESULTS

- May increase liver enzyme levels.
- May decrease neutrophil and platelet counts.

CONTRAINDICATIONS & CAUTIONS

- Contraindicated in patients hypersensitive to drug or to genetically engineered products derived from *Escherichia coli.*
- Use cautiously in patients with cardiac disease, including arrhythmias, ischemia, or heart failure. The flulike syndrome commonly seen with high doses of drug can worsen these conditions.
- Use cautiously in patients with compromised CNS function or seizure disorders. CNS adverse reactions that may occur at high doses of drug can worsen these conditions.

NURSING CONSIDERATIONS

- ***Alert:*** The drug's activity is expressed in international units (1 million international units/50 mcg). This is equal to what was previously expressed as units (1.5 million units/50 mcg).
- Use myelosuppressives together with caution.
- Premedicate patient with acetaminophen to minimize signs and symptoms at start of therapy; these tend to diminish with continued therapy.
- Before beginning therapy and at 3-month intervals, monitor CBC, platelet count, renal and hepatic function tests, and urinalysis.
- Discard unused drug. Each vial is for single-dose use only and doesn't contain a preservative.

PATIENT TEACHING

- If patient will give drug to himself, teach him how to give it and how to dispose of used needles, syringes, containers, and unused drug.
- Instruct patient how to manage flulike signs and symptoms (fever, fatigue, muscle aches, headache, chills, joint pain) that commonly occur.
- Advise use of acetaminophen.

SAFETY ALERT!

leflunomide

Arava

Pharmacologic class: pyrimidine synthesis inhibitor
Pregnancy risk category X

AVAILABLE FORMS

Tablets: 10 mg, 20 mg, 100 mg

INDICATIONS & DOSAGES

➤ **To reduce signs and symptoms of active rheumatoid arthritis; to slow structural damage as shown by erosions and joint space narrowing seen on X-ray; to improve physical function**

Adults: 100 mg P.O. q 24 hours for 3 days; then 20 mg (maximum daily dose) P.O. q 24 hours. Dose may be decreased to 10 mg daily if higher dose isn't well tolerated.

ACTION

Inhibits dihydroorotate dehydrogenase, an enzyme involved in pyrimidine synthesis, and that has antiproliferative activity and antiinflammatory effects.

Route	Onset	Peak	Duration
P.O.	Unknown	6–12 hr	Unknown

Half-life: 15 to 18 days.

ADVERSE REACTIONS

CNS: anxiety, asthenia, depression, dizziness, fever, headache, insomnia, malaise, migraine, neuralgia, neuritis, paresthesia, sleep disorder, vertigo.
CV: *hypertension,* angina pectoris, chest pain, palpitations, peripheral edema, tachycardia, varicose veins, vasculitis, vasodilation.
EENT: blurred vision, cataracts, conjunctivitis, epistaxis, eye disorder, pharyngitis, rhinitis, sinusitis.
GI: *diarrhea,* abdominal pain, anorexia, cholelithiasis, colitis, constipation, dry mouth, dyspepsia, enlarged salivary glands, esophagitis, flatulence, gastritis, gastroenteritis, gingivitis, melena, mouth ulcer, nausea, oral candidiasis, stomatitis, taste perversion, vomiting.

GU: albuminuria, cystitis, dysuria, hematuria, menstrual disorder, pelvic pain, prostate disorder, urinary frequency, UTI, vaginal candidiasis.
Hematologic: anemia.
Hepatic: ***hepatotoxicity.***
Metabolic: diabetes mellitus, hyperglycemia, hyperlipidemia, hyperthyroidism, hypokalemia, weight loss.
Musculoskeletal: arthralgia, arthrosis, back pain, bone necrosis, bone pain, bursitis, joint disorder, leg cramps, muscle cramps, myalgia, neck pain, synovitis, tendon rupture, tenosynovitis.
Respiratory: *respiratory infection,* asthma, bronchitis, dyspnea, increased cough, lung disorder, pneumonia.
Skin: *alopecia, rash,* acne, contact dermatitis, dry skin, eczema, fungal dermatitis, hair discoloration, hematoma, maculopapular rash, nail disorder, pruritus, skin discoloration, skin disorder, skin nodule, skin ulcer, subcutaneous nodule.
Other: abscess, allergic reaction, cyst, ecchymoses, flulike syndrome, hernia, herpes simplex, herpes zoster, increased sweating, injury or accident, pain, tooth disorder.

INTERACTIONS

Drug-drug. *Charcoal, cholestyramine:* May decrease leflunomide level. Sometimes used for this effect in overdose.
Methotrexate, other hepatotoxic drugs: May increase risk of hepatotoxicity. Monitor liver enzyme levels.
NSAIDs (diclofenac, ibuprofen): May increase NSAID level. Monitor patient.
Rifampin: May increase active leflunomide metabolite level. Use together cautiously.
Tolbutamide: May increase tolbutamide level. Monitor patient.

EFFECTS ON LAB TEST RESULTS

- May increase AST, ALT, glucose, lipid, and CK levels. May decrease potassium level.

CONTRAINDICATIONS & CAUTIONS

- Contraindicated in patients hypersensitive to drug or its components and in women who are or may become pregnant or who are breast-feeding.
- Drug isn't recommended for patients with significant hepatic impairment, evidence of infection with hepatitis B or C viruses, severe immunodeficiency, bone marrow dysplasia, or severe uncontrolled infections; in patients younger than age 18; or in men attempting to father a child.
- Use cautiously in patients with renal insufficiency.

NURSING CONSIDERATIONS

- Vaccination with live vaccines isn't recommended. Consider the long half-life of drug when contemplating giving a live vaccine after stopping drug treatment.
- ***Alert:*** Men planning to father a child should stop drug therapy and follow recommended leflunomide removal protocol (cholestyramine 8 g, P.O. t.i.d. for 11 days). In addition to cholestyramine, verify drug levels are less than 0.02 mg/L by two separate tests at least 14 days apart. If level is greater than 0.02 mg/L, consider additional cholestyramine treatment.
- Risk of malignancy, particularly lymphoproliferative disorders, is increased with use of some immunosuppressants, including leflunomide.
- ***Alert:*** Monitor ALT levels, platelet and WBC counts, and hemoglobin level or hematocrit at baseline and monthly for 6 months after starting therapy and every 6 to 8 weeks thereafter.
- ***Alert:*** Monitor AST, ALT, and serum albumin levels monthly if treatment includes methotrexate or other potential immunosuppressives.
- Stop drug and start cholestyramine or charcoal therapy if bone marrow suppression occurs.
- Watch for overlapping hematologic toxicity when switching to another antirheumatic.
- ***Alert:*** Rare cases of severe liver injury, including cases with fatal outcome, have occurred during leflunomide therapy. Most cases occur within 6 months of therapy and in a setting of multiple risk factors for hepatotoxicity (liver disease, other hepatotoxins).
- For confirmed ALT elevations between two and three times the upper limit of normal (ULN), reduce dose to 10 mg/day; if elevations persist despite dose reduction

or if ALT elevations of greater than three times ULN are present, stop drug and give cholestyramine or charcoal.
- Carefully monitor patient after dose reduction. Because the active metabolite of leflunomide has a prolonged half-life, it may take several weeks for levels to decline.

PATIENT TEACHING
- Explain need for and frequency of required blood tests and monitoring.
- Instruct patient to use birth control during course of treatment and until it's been determined that drug is no longer active.
- Warn patient to immediately notify prescriber if signs or symptoms of pregnancy occur (such as late menstrual periods or breast tenderness).
- Advise woman to stop breast-feeding during therapy.
- Inform patient he may continue taking aspirin, other NSAIDs, and low-dose corticosteroids during treatment.

SAFETY ALERT!

oprelvekin
Neumega

Pharmacologic class: recombinant human interleukin
Pregnancy risk category C

AVAILABLE FORMS
Injection: 5-mg single-dose vial with diluent

INDICATIONS & DOSAGES
➤ **To prevent severe thrombocytopenia and reduce need for platelet transfusions after myelosuppressive chemotherapy with nonmyeloid malignancies**
Adults: 50 mcg/kg as single daily subcutaneous injection until postnadir platelet count is at least 50,000/mm^3. Treatment beyond 21 days per course isn't recommended.

ACTION
Directly stimulates proliferation of hematopoietic stem cells and megakaryocyte progenitor cells. Also induces megakaryocyte maturation, resulting in increased platelet production.

Route	Onset	Peak	Duration
SubQ	Unknown	3–5 hr	Unknown

Half-life: 7 hours.

ADVERSE REACTIONS
CNS: *asthenia, fever, headache, insomnia, dizziness,* paresthesia, *syncope.*
CV: ATRIAL FLUTTER OR FIBRILLATION, *tachycardia, palpitations, edema.*
EENT: *conjunctival injection,* blurred vision, eye hemorrhage, pharyngitis.
GI: *oral candidiasis, nausea, vomiting, diarrhea.*
Hematologic: anemia.
Metabolic: dehydration, hypocalcemia.
Respiratory: dyspnea, cough, pleural effusions.
Skin: *rash,* skin discoloration, exfoliative dermatitis.

INTERACTIONS
Drug-drug. *Diuretics, ifosfamide:* May cause life-threatening hypokalemia. Avoid using together.

EFFECTS ON LAB TEST RESULTS
- May decrease calcium and hemoglobin levels and hematocrit.

CONTRAINDICATIONS & CAUTIONS
- Contraindicated in patients hypersensitive to drug or its components.
- Use drug cautiously in patients with heart failure because of fluid retention.

NURSING CONSIDERATIONS
- Give subcutaneously in the abdomen, thigh, hip, or upper arm. Don't inject I.D. or intravascularly.
- Dosing should begin 6 to 24 hours after completing chemotherapy and end at least 2 days before starting next cycle of chemotherapy.
- Reconstitute each single-dose vial with 1 ml of supplied diluent. Avoid excessive or vigorous agitation. Discard unused portions.
- Use reconstituted drug within 3 hours.
- Store drug and diluent in refrigerator until ready to use. Don't freeze.

• Closely monitor fluid and electrolyte status in patients receiving long-term diuretic therapy.
• Obtain a CBC before chemotherapy and at regular intervals during drug therapy.
• Fluid retention can be severe; monitor patient closely.

PATIENT TEACHING

• Instruct patient about appropriate preparation and administration of drug if he is going to self-administer.
• Warn patient about potential adverse reactions. Tell him to report any occurrence.
• Tell patient to keep drug refrigerated and not to reconstitute until just before use.
• Urge patient to call prescriber immediately if swelling, rapid heart beat, or difficulty breathing occurs.
• Tell patient to report signs and symptoms of increased bleeding or bruising.

SAFETY ALERT!

pegfilgrastim

Neulasta

Pharmacologic class: hematopoietic
Pregnancy risk category C

AVAILABLE FORMS

Injection: 6-mg/0.6-ml single-use, preservative-free, prefilled syringes

INDICATIONS & DOSAGES

➤ **To reduce frequency of infection in patients with nonmyeloid malignancies receiving myelosuppressive chemotherapy that may cause febrile neutropenia**

Adults: 6 mg subcutaneously once per chemotherapy cycle. Don't give in period between 14 days before and 24 hours after administration of cytotoxic chemotherapy.

ACTION

Binds cell receptors to stimulate proliferation, differentiation, commitment, and end-cell function of neutrophils. Pegfilgrastim and filgrastim have the same mechanism of action. Pegfilgrastim has a reduced renal clearance and a longer half-life than filgrastim.

Route	Onset	Peak	Duration
SubQ	Unknown	Unknown	Unknown

Half-life: 15 to 80 hours.

ADVERSE REACTIONS

CNS: *dizziness, fatigue, fever, headache, insomnia.*
GI: *abdominal pain, anorexia, constipation, diarrhea, dyspepsia, mucositis, nausea, stomatitis, taste perversion, vomiting.*
Hematologic: **GRANULOCYTOPENIA, NEUTROPENIC FEVER.**
Musculoskeletal: *arthralgia, bone pain, generalized weakness, myalgia, skeletal pain.*
Respiratory: ***acute respiratory distress syndrome (ARDS).***
Skin: *alopecia.*
Other: ***splenic rupture,*** *peripheral edema.*

INTERACTIONS

Drug-drug. *Lithium:* May increase the release of neutrophils. Monitor neutrophil counts closely.

EFFECTS ON LAB TEST RESULTS

• May increase LDH, alkaline phosphatase, and uric acid levels.
• May decrease granulocyte count.

CONTRAINDICATIONS & CAUTIONS

• Contraindicated in patients hypersensitive to *Escherichia coli*–derived proteins, filgrastim, or any component of the drug. Don't use for peripheral blood progenitor cell mobilization.
• Use cautiously in patients with sickle cell disease, those receiving chemotherapy causing delayed myelosuppression, or those receiving radiation therapy.
• Infants, children, and adolescents who weigh less than 45 kg (99 lb) shouldn't receive the 6-mg single-use syringe dose. Safety and effectiveness in children haven't been established.

NURSING CONSIDERATIONS

• ***Alert:*** Splenic rupture may occur rarely. Assess patient who experiences signs or

symptoms of left upper abdominal or shoulder pain for an enlarged spleen or splenic rupture.
- Obtain CBC and platelet count before therapy.
- Monitor patient's hemoglobin level, hematocrit, CBC, and platelet count, as well as LDH, alkaline phosphatase, and uric acid levels during therapy.
- Monitor patient for allergic-type reactions, including anaphylaxis, skin rash, and urticaria, which can occur with first or subsequent treatment.
- Evaluate patient with fever, lung infiltrates, or respiratory distress for ARDS. If ARDS develops, notify prescriber.
- Keep patient with sickle cell disease well hydrated, and monitor him for symptoms of sickle cell crisis.
- Pegfilgrastim may act as a growth factor for tumors.

PATIENT TEACHING

- Inform patient of the potential side effects of the drug.
- Tell patient to report signs and symptoms of allergic reactions, fever, or breathing problems.
- ***Alert:*** Rarely, splenic rupture may occur. Advise patient to immediately report upper left abdominal or shoulder tip pain.
- Tell patient with sickle cell disease to keep drinking fluids and report signs or symptoms of sickle cell crisis.
- Instruct patient or caregiver how to give drug if it's to be given at home.

SAFETY ALERT!

peginterferon alfa-2a

Pegasys

Pharmacologic class: biological response modifier
Pregnancy risk category C

AVAILABLE FORMS

Injection: 180 mcg/1 ml single-dose vials; 180 mcg/0.5 ml prefilled syringes

INDICATIONS & DOSAGES

➤Chronic hepatitis C with compensated hepatic disease in patients not previously treated with interferon alfa

Adults: 180 mcg subcutaneously in abdomen or thigh, once weekly for 48 weeks. May be used with 800 to 1,200 mg ribavirin daily, divided b.i.d. depending on viral genotype.

➤Chronic hepatitis C (regardless of genotype) in HIV-infected patients who have not previously been treated with interferon

Adults: 180 mcg subcutaneously in abdomen or thigh, once weekly for 48 weeks. May be used with 800 mg ribavirin P.O. daily divided b.i.d.

➤Chronic hepatitis B who have compensated liver disease and evidence of viral replication and liver inflammation

Adults: 180 mcg subcutaneously in abdomen or thigh, once weekly for 48 weeks.
Adjust-a-dose: For patients who experience moderate adverse reactions, decrease dose to 135 mcg subcutaneously once a week; for severe adverse reactions, decrease to 90 mcg subcutaneously once a week. For patients who experience hematologic reactions, if the absolute neutrophil count (ANC) is less than 750/mm^3, reduce dose to 135 mcg subcutaneously once a week; if the ANC is less than 500/mm^3, stop drug until ANC exceeds 1,000/mm^3 and restart at 90 mcg subcutaneously once a week. If platelet count is less than 50,000/mm^3, reduce dose to 90 mcg subcutaneously once a week; stop drug if platelet count drops below 25,000/mm^3. In patients with end-stage renal disease requiring hemodialysis, decrease dose to 135 mcg subcutaneously once a week. In chronic hepatitis C patients with ALT increases above baseline, decrease dose to 135 mcg subcutaneously once a week. For chronic hepatitis B patients with elevations in ALT more than 5 times the upper limit of normal (ULN), reduce dose to 135 mcg subcutaneously once a week or temporarily stop treatment; if less than 10 times the ULN, consider stopping treatment. For patients also taking ribavirin therapy, if hemoglobin level is less than 10 g/dl in patients with no cardiac disease, reduce ribavirin dose to 600 mg/day. If less than 8.5 g/dl in this population, stop ribavirin. If there is a greater than or equal

to 2 g/dl decrease in hemoglobin level during any 4-week period in patients with history of stable cardiac disease, reduce ribavirin dose to 600 mg daily. If less than 12 g/dl despite 4 weeks at reduced dose, stop ribavirin. Ribavirin shouldn't be used in patients with a creatinine clearance less than 50 ml/minute.

ACTION

Causes reversible decreases in leukocyte and platelet counts, partially through stimulation of production of effector proteins in vitro.

Route	Onset	Peak	Duration
SubQ	Unknown	3–4 days	< 1 wk

Half-life: 80 hours.

ADVERSE REACTIONS

CNS: *depression, dizziness, fatigue, headache, insomnia, irritability,* anxiety, asthenia, concentration impairment, memory impairment.
GI: *abdominal pain, anorexia, diarrhea, nausea,* dry mouth, vomiting.
Hematologic: NEUTROPENIA, ***thrombocytopenia,*** *anemia, lymphopenia.*
Musculoskeletal: *arthralgia, myalgia,* back pain.
Skin: *alopecia, pruritus,* dermatitis, increased sweating, rash.
Other: *injection site reaction, pain, pyrexia, rigors.*

INTERACTIONS

Drug-drug. *Ribavirin:* May cause additive hematologic toxicity. Monitor hematologic function.
Theophylline, other drugs metabolized by CYP1A2: May increase theophylline level and may interact with other drugs metabolized by this enzyme system. Monitor theophylline level and adjust dosage as needed.

EFFECTS ON LAB TEST RESULTS

- May increase ALT level. May decrease hemoglobin level and hematocrit.
- May decrease ANC, WBC, and platelet counts. May increase or decrease thyroid function test values.

CONTRAINDICATIONS & CAUTIONS

- Contraindicated in patients hypersensitive to interferon alfa-2a or any components of formulation.
- Contraindicated in patients with autoimmune hepatitis or decompensated liver disease (with monoinfection or coinfected with HIV) before or during treatment with drug and in neonates and infants.
- Safety and effectiveness haven't been established in patients who have failed to respond to other alfa interferon treatments, in organ transplant recipients, and in patients who are also infected with hepatitis B.
- Use cautiously in patients with a history of depression.
- Use cautiously in patients with baseline neutrophil counts less than 1,500/mm^3, baseline platelet counts less than 90,000/mm^3, or baseline hemoglobin level less than 10 g/dl.
- Use cautiously in patients with creatinine clearance less than 50 ml/minute.
- Use cautiously in patients with cardiac disease or hypertension, thyroid disease, autoimmune disorders, pulmonary disorders, colitis, pancreatitis, and ophthalmologic disorders.
- Use cautiously in elderly patients because they may be at increased risk for adverse reactions.
- ***Alert:*** Drug may cause abortion. Use in pregnant women only if benefit outweighs risk.

NURSING CONSIDERATIONS

- Monitor patient for neuropsychiatric reactions, including depression and suicidal ideation. These symptoms may occur in patients without previous psychiatric illness. If severe depression occurs, stop drug and start psychiatric treatment.
- Obtain CBC before treatment and monitor counts routinely during therapy. Stop drug in patients who develop severe decrease in neutrophil or platelet counts.
- Stop drug if uncontrollable thyroid disease, hyperglycemia, hypoglycemia, or diabetes mellitus occurs during treatment.
- If persistent or unexplained pulmonary infiltrates or pulmonary dysfunction occur, stop drug.
- Stop drug if signs and symptoms of colitis occur, such as abdominal pain, bloody

diarrhea, and fever. Symptoms should resolve within 1 to 3 weeks.
• Stop drug if signs and symptoms of pancreatitis occur, including fever, malaise, and abdominal pain.
• Obtain baseline eye examination and periodically monitor eye exams during treatment. Stop drug if new or worsening eye disorders occur.
• Monitor patient with impaired renal function for interferon toxicity.
• Use in women of childbearing potential only when effective contraception is being used.

PATIENT TEACHING
• Teach patient proper way to give drug and dispose of needles and syringes.
• Tell patient to immediately report depression or suicidal ideation.
• Tell patient to report signs and symptoms of pancreatitis, colitis, eye disorders, or respiratory disorders.
• Advise patient to avoid driving or operating machinery if he feels dizzy, tired, confused, or sleepy.

SAFETY ALERT!

peginterferon alfa-2b
PEG-Intron

Pharmacologic class: biological response modifier
Pregnancy risk category C

AVAILABLE FORMS
Injection: 100 mcg/ml, 160 mcg/ml, 240 mcg/ml, 300 mcg/ml

INDICATIONS & DOSAGES
➤ Chronic hepatitis C in patients not previously treated with interferon alfa
Adults: Give 1 mcg/kg subcutaneously once weekly for up to 1 year, on same day each week. The volume of PEG-Intron to be injected depends on the patient's weight and the vial strength used.
Adults who weigh 137 to 160 kg (302 to 353 lb): 150 mcg (0.5 ml) of 300-mcg/ml strength.
Adults who weigh 107 to 136 kg (236 to 300 lb): 120 mcg (0.5 ml) of 240-mcg/ml strength.
Adults who weigh 89 to 106 kg (196 to 234 lb): 96 mcg (0.4 ml) of 240-mcg/ml strength.
Adults who weigh 73 to 88 kg (161 to 194 lb): 80 mcg (0.5 ml) of 160-mcg/ml strength.
Adults who weigh 57 to 72 kg (126 to 159 lb): 64 mcg (0.4 ml) of 160-mcg/ml strength.
Adults who weigh 46 to 56 kg (101 to 123 lb): 50 mcg (0.5 ml) of 100-mcg/ml strength.
Adults who weigh 45 kg (82 to 99 lb) or less: 40 mcg (0.4 ml) of 100-mcg/ml strength.
➤ Chronic hepatitis C in patients not previously treated with interferon alfa, combined with ribavirin
Adults: Give 1.5 mcg/kg subcutaneously once weekly for 24 to 48 weeks on same day q week. The volume of PEG-Intron to be injected depends on the patient's weight and the vial strength used.
Adults who weigh more than 85 kg (more than 187 lb): 150 mcg (0.5 ml) of 300-mcg/ml strength.
Adults who weigh 76 to 85 kg (167 to 187 lb): 120 mcg (0.5 ml) of 240-mcg/ml strength.
Adults who weigh 61 to 75 kg (134 to 165 lb): 96 mcg (0.4 ml) of 240-mcg/ml strength.
Adults who weigh 51 to 60 kg (112 to 132 lb): 80 mcg (0.5 ml) of 160-mcg/ml strength.
Adults who weigh 40 to 50 kg (88 to 110 lb): 64 mcg (0.4 ml) of 160-mcg/ml strength.
Adults who weigh less than 40 kg (less than 88 lb): 50 mcg (0.5 ml) of 100-mcg/ml strength.
Adjust-a-dose: Decrease peginterferon alfa-2b dose by 50% in patients with WBC count less than 1,500/mm^3, neutrophil count less than 750/mm^3, or platelet count less than 80,000/mm^3. Ribavirin dose can be continued. If hemoglobin level is less than 10 g/dl, reduce ribavirin dose by 200 mg. Stop both drugs if hemoglobin level is less than 8.5 g/dl, WBCs less than 1,000/mm^3, neutrophil countless than 500/mm^3, or platelet count less than 50,000/mm^3. If symptoms improve and remain stable for 4 weeks, continue at present dose or resume previous dose.

If patient develops mild depression, continue peginterferon alfa-2b, but evaluate patient once weekly. In moderate depression, reduce peginterferon alfa-2b dose by 50% for 4 to 8 weeks and evaluate patient q week. In severe depression, stop peginterferon alfa-2b.

For patients with stable CV disease, decrease peginterferon alfa-2b dose by 50% and ribavirin dosage by 200 mg daily if hemoglobin level drops more than 2 g/dl in any 4-week period. Stop both drugs if hemoglobin level goes below 12 g/dl after 4 weeks of reduced dosages.

ACTION

Binds to specific membrane receptors on the cell surface, inducing certain enzymes, suppressing cell proliferation, immunomodulating activities, and inhibiting virus replication in virus-infected cells. Increases levels of effector proteins and body temperature, and decreases leukocyte and platelet counts.

Route	Onset	Peak	Duration
SubQ	Unknown	15–44 hr	Unknown

Half-life: 40 hours.

ADVERSE REACTIONS

CNS: *anxiety, depression, dizziness, emotional lability, fatigue, fever, headache, insomnia, irritability,* ***suicidal behavior,*** hypertonia, malaise.
CV: flushing.
EENT: *pharyngitis,* sinusitis.
GI: *abdominal pain, anorexia, diarrhea, nausea,* dyspepsia, right upper quadrant pain, vomiting.
Hematologic: ***neutropenia, thrombocytopenia.***
Hepatic: hepatomegaly.
Metabolic: *weight loss,* hyperthyroidism, hypothyroidism.
Musculoskeletal: *musculoskeletal pain.*
Respiratory: cough.
Skin: *alopecia, dry skin, increased sweating, injection site inflammation or reaction, pruritus, rash,* injection site pain.
Other: *flulike symptoms, rigors, viral infection.*

INTERACTIONS

None reported.

EFFECTS ON LAB TEST RESULTS

- May increase ALT level. May increase or decrease TSH level.
- May decrease neutrophil and platelet counts.

CONTRAINDICATIONS & CAUTIONS

- Contraindicated in patients hypersensitive to drug or any of its components, in patients with autoimmune hepatitis or decompensated liver disease, in those with diabetes or thyroid disorders that can't be controlled with medication, in patients who have failed to respond to other alfa interferon treatment or have had an organ transplant, and in those with HIV or hepatitis B virus (HBV).
- Use cautiously in patients with psychiatric disorders, diabetes mellitus, CV disease, creatinine clearance less than 50 ml/minute, pulmonary infiltrates, pulmonary function impairment, or autoimmune, ischemic, or infectious disorders.

NURSING CONSIDERATIONS

- Obtain eye examination in patient with diabetes or hypertension before starting drug. Retinal hemorrhages, cotton-wool spots, and retinal artery or vein obstruction may occur.
- ***Alert:*** Drug may cause or aggravate fatal or life-threatening neuropsychiatric, autoimmune, ischemic, and infectious disorders. Monitor patients closely with periodic clinical and laboratory evaluations. In patient with persistently severe or worsening signs or symptoms of these conditions from therapy, withhold drug.
- Drug may cause or aggravate hypothyroidism, hyperthyroidism, or diabetes.
- Perform ECG on patient with history of MI or arrhythmias before starting drug.
- Hydrate patient before therapy.
- Monitor patient with history of MI or arrhythmias closely for hypotension, arrhythmias, tachycardia, cardiomyopathy, and signs and symptoms of MI.
- Monitor patient for depression and other mental health disorders. If symptoms are severe, stop drug.
- Monitor patient for signs and symptoms of colitis, such as abdominal pain, bloody diarrhea, and fever. Stop drug if colitis occurs. Symptoms should resolve 1 to 3 weeks after stopping drug.

- Monitor patient for signs and symptoms of pancreatitis or hypersensitivity reactions, and stop drug if these occur.
- Monitor patient with pulmonary disease for dyspnea, pulmonary infiltrates, pneumonitis, and pneumonia.
- Monitor patient with renal disease for signs and symptoms of toxicity.
- Monitor CBC and platelet count and AST, ALT, bilirubin, and TSH levels before starting drug and periodically during treatment.
- Notify prescriber if severe neutropenia or thrombocytopenia occurs.

PATIENT TEACHING

- Teach patient the appropriate use of the drug and the benefits and risks of treatment. Tell patient that adverse reactions may continue for several months after treatment is stopped.
- Tell patient to immediately report symptoms of depression or suicidal thoughts.
- Instruct patient about proper disposal of needles and syringes and caution him against reuse of old needles and syringes.
- Tell patient that drug won't prevent spread of hepatitis C virus (HCV) to others and may not cure hepatitis C or prevent cirrhosis, liver failure, or liver cancer that may result from HCV infection.
- Advise patient that laboratory tests are needed before starting therapy and periodically thereafter.
- Tell patient to take drug at bedtime and to use fever-reducing drugs to decrease risk of flulike signs and symptoms.
- Tell breast-feeding woman to either stop using drug or stop breast-feeding.

SAFETY ALERT!

sargramostim (GM-CSF; granulocyte macrophage-colony stimulating factor)

Leukine

Pharmacologic class: hematopoietic
Pregnancy risk category C

AVAILABLE FORMS

Powder for injection: 250 mcg
Solution: 500 mcg/ml

INDICATIONS & DOSAGES

➤ **To accelerate hematopoietic reconstitution after autologous or allogenic bone marrow transplantation in patients with malignant lymphoma or acute lymphoblastic leukemia or in patients with Hodgkin lymphoma**

Adults: 250 mcg/m^2 daily given as 2-hour I.V. infusion beginning 2 to 4 hours after bone marrow transplantation Continue until absolute neutrophil count (ANC) is more than 1,500/mm^3 for 3 consecutive days.

➤ **Neutrophil recovery following chemotherapy in acute myelogenous leukemia**

Adults 55 years and older: Initially, 250 mcg/m^2 I.V. once daily over 4 hours beginning day 11 or 4 days following completion of induction therapy; initiate only if bone marrow is hypoplastic with less than 5% blasts on day 10. If a second induction cycle is needed, begin sargramostim 4 days after completing chemotherapy and only if bone marrow is hypoplastic with less than 5% blasts. Continue until the ANC is more than 1,500/mm^3 for 3 consecutive days or for a maximum of 42 days.

➤ **Mobilization of peripheral blood progenitor cells (PBPC)**

Adults: Give 250 mcg/m^2 by continuous I.V. infusion over 24 hours or by subcutaneous injection once daily. Continue through PBPC collection.

➤ **Post-PBPC transplantation**

Adults: Give 250 mcg/m^2 by continuous I.V. infusion over 24 hours or by subcutaneous injection once daily beginning immediately following PBPC infusion; continue until ANC more than 1,500/mm^3 for 3 consecutive days.

➤ **Bone marrow transplantation failure or engraftment delay**

Adults: 250 mcg/m^2 as a 2-hour I.V. infusion daily for 14 days. This course of therapy may be repeated after 7 days of no therapy. If engraftment still hasn't occurred, a third course of 500 mcg/m^2 daily I.V. for 14 days may be attempted after another therapy-free 7 days.

Adjust-a-dose: Stimulation of marrow precursors may result in rapid rise of WBC count. If blast cells appear or increase to

10% or more of WBC count or if the underlying disease progresses, stop therapy. If ANC is above 20,000/mm³ or if platelet count is above 500,000/mm³, temporarily stop drug or reduce dose by 50%.

I.V. ADMINISTRATION

- Reconstitute with 1 ml of sterile water for injection. Direct stream of sterile water against side of vial and gently swirl contents to minimize foaming. Avoid excessive or vigorous agitation or shaking.
- Dilute in normal saline solution. If drug yield is below 10 mcg/ml, add human albumin at final concentration of 0.1% to saline solution before adding sargramostim to prevent adsorption to components of the delivery system. To yield 0.1% human albumin, add 1 mg human albumin to each milliliter of saline solution (dilute 1 ml of 5% human albumin in 50 ml of saline solution).
- Don't use in-line filter.
- Give as soon as possible after mixing and no later than 6 hours after reconstituting.

INCOMPATIBILITIES

Other I.V. drugs, unless specific compatibility data are available.

ACTION

Binds to specific receptors on cell surfaces of target cells.

Route	Onset	Peak	Duration
I.V.	15 min	1–3 hr	Unknown
SubQ	15 min	2–4 hr	Unknown

Half-life: About 1 hour (I.V.); about 3 hours (SubQ)

ADVERSE REACTIONS

CNS: *asthenia, CNS disorders, fever, headache, malaise.*
CV: HEMORRHAGE, *blood dyscrasias, edema, hypertension,* ***supraventricular arrhythmias,*** pericardial effusion.
GI: *anorexia, diarrhea, GI disorders, nausea, stomatitis, vomiting,* ***GI hemorrhage.***
GU: *urinary tract disorder,* abnormal kidney function.
Hepatic: *liver damage.*
Musculoskeletal: *arthralgias.*
Respiratory: *dyspnea, lung disorders,* pleural effusion.
Skin: *alopecia, pruritus, rash.*
Other: SEPSIS, *mucous membrane disorder, peripheral edema.*

INTERACTIONS

Drug-drug. *Corticosteroids, lithium:* May increase myeloproliferative effects of sargramostim. Use cautiously together.

EFFECTS ON LAB TEST RESULTS

- May increase BUN, creatinine, AST, ALT, alkaline phosphatase, bilirubin, glucose, and cholesterol levels. May decrease calcium and albumin levels.

CONTRAINDICATIONS & CAUTIONS

- Contraindicated in patients hypersensitive to drug or its components or to yeast-derived products and in those with excessive leukemic myeloid blasts in bone marrow or peripheral blood.
- Giving within 24 hours of chemotherapy or radiation is contraindicated.
- Use cautiously in patients with cardiac disease, hypoxia, fluid retention, pulmonary infiltrates, heart failure, or impaired renal or hepatic function because these conditions may be worsened.

NURSING CONSIDERATIONS

- If severe adverse reactions occur, reduce dose by 50% or temporarily stop drug and notify prescriber. Resume therapy when reactions decrease.
- Rapidly dividing progenitor cells may be sensitive to cytotoxic therapies, making the drug ineffective; don't give within 24 hours of last dose of chemotherapy or within 12 hours of last dose of radiotherapy.
- If giving as a subcutaneous injection, further dilution of injection or reconstituted solution isn't needed.
- Monitor CBC with differential, including examination for presence of blast cells, biweekly.

PATIENT TEACHING

- Review administration schedule with patient and caregivers, and address their concerns.
- Urge patient to report adverse reactions promptly.

77

Ophthalmic anti-infectives

ciprofloxacin hydrochloride
erythromycin
gatifloxacin
gentamicin sulfate
moxifloxacin hydrochloride
ofloxacin 0.3%
sulfacetamide sodium 10%
sulfacetamide sodium 15%
sulfacetamide sodium 30%
tobramycin

ciprofloxacin hydrochloride

Ciloxan

Pharmacologic class: fluoroquinolone
Pregnancy risk category C

AVAILABLE FORMS

Ophthalmic ointment: 0.3 % (base) in 3.5-g tube
Ophthalmic solution: 0.3% (base) in 2.5-ml and 5-ml containers

INDICATIONS & DOSAGES

➤ **Corneal ulcers caused by *Pseudomonas aeruginosa*, *Staphylococcus aureus*, *S. epidermidis*, *Streptococcus pneumoniae*, and possibly *Serratia marcescens* and *Streptococcus viridans***

Adults and children older than age 12: Two drops in affected eye q 15 minutes for first 6 hours; then two drops q 30 minutes for remainder of first day. On the second day, two drops hourly. On days 3 to 14, two drops q 4 hours.

➤ **Bacterial conjunctivitis caused by *Haemophilus influenzae*, *S. aureus*, *S. epidermidis*, and possibly *S. pneumoniae***

Adults and children older than age 12: One or two drops into conjunctival sac of affected eye q 2 hours while awake for first 2 days. Then, one or two drops q 4 hours while awake for next 5 days. Or ½-inch ribbon into the conjunctival sac t.i.d for the first 2 days, then ½ -inch ribbon b.i.d. for the next 5 days.

ACTION

Inhibits bacterial DNA gyrase, an enzyme needed for bacterial replication.

Route	Onset	Peak	Duration
Ophthalmic	Unknown	Unknown	Unknown

Half-life: 3 to 5 hours.

ADVERSE REACTIONS

EENT: *local burning or discomfort, white crystalline precipitate in superficial portion of corneal defect in patients with corneal ulcers,* allergic reactions, conjunctival hyperemia, foreign body sensation, itching.
GI: bad or bitter taste in mouth.

INTERACTIONS

None significant.

EFFECTS ON LAB TEST RESULTS

None reported.

CONTRAINDICATIONS & CAUTIONS

- Contraindicated in patients hypersensitive to drug or other fluoroquinolones.
- It's unknown if drug appears in breast milk after application to eye; however, drug given systemically appears in breast milk. Use cautiously in breast-feeding women.

NURSING CONSIDERATIONS

- ***Alert:*** Stop drug at first sign of hypersensitivity, such as rash, and notify prescriber. Serious hypersensitivity reactions, including anaphylaxis, may occur in patients receiving systemic drug.
- A topical overdose may be flushed from eyes with warm tap water.
- If corneal epithelium is still compromised after 14 days of treatment, continue therapy.
- Institute appropriate therapy if superinfection occurs. Prolonged use may result in overgrowth of nonsusceptible organisms, including fungi.
- ***Look alike–sound alike:*** Don't confuse Ciloxan with Cytoxan or cinoxacin.

PATIENT TEACHING

- Tell patient to clean eye area of excessive discharge before instilling.
- Teach patient how to instill drops or apply ointment. Advise him to wash hands before and after using drug and not to touch tip of dropper to eye or surrounding tissues.
- Instruct patient to apply light finger pressure on lacrimal sac for 1 minute after drops are instilled.
- Advise patient that drug may cause temporary blurring of vision or stinging after administration. If these symptoms become pronounced or worsen, contact prescriber.
- Tell patient to avoid wearing contacts while treating bacterial conjunctivitis. If approved by prescriber, tell patient to wait at least 15 minutes after instilling drops before inserting contact lenses.
- Tell patient not to share drug, washcloths, or towels with family members and to notify prescriber if anyone develops same signs or symptoms.
- Stress importance of compliance with recommended therapy.

erythromycin
Ilotycin

Pharmacologic class: macrolide
Pregnancy risk category B

AVAILABLE FORMS

Ophthalmic ointment: 0.5%

INDICATIONS & DOSAGES

➤**Acute and chronic conjunctivitis, other eye infections**
Adults and children: Apply a ribbon of ointment about 1 cm long directly to infected eye up to six times daily, depending on severity of infection.

➤**Chlamydial ophthalmic infections (trachoma)**
Adults and children: Apply small amount to each eye b.i.d. for 2 months or b.i.d. on first 5 days of each month for 6 months.

➤**To prevent ophthalmia neonatorum caused by *Neisseria gonorrhoeae* or *Chlamydia trachomatis***
Neonates: Apply a ribbon of ointment about 1 cm long in lower conjunctival sac of each eye shortly after birth.

ACTION

Inhibits protein synthesis; usually bacteriostatic, but may be bactericidal in high concentrations or against highly susceptible organisms.

Route	Onset	Peak	Duration
Ophthalmic	Unknown	Unknown	Unknown

Half-life: Unknown.

ADVERSE REACTIONS

EENT: blurred vision, itching and burning eyes, slowed corneal wound healing.
Skin: dermatitis, urticaria.
Other: overgrowth of nonsusceptible organisms with long-term use.

INTERACTIONS

None significant.

EFFECTS ON LAB TEST RESULTS

- May interfere with fluorometric determinations of urine catecholamines.

CONTRAINDICATIONS & CAUTIONS

- Contraindicated in patients hypersensitive to drug.
- Use cautiously in breast-feeding women.

NURSING CONSIDERATIONS

- To prevent ophthalmia neonatorum, apply ointment no later than 1 hour after birth. Drug is used in neonates born either vaginally or by cesarean section. Gently massage eyelids for 1 minute to spread ointment.
- Use drug only when sensitivity studies show it's effective against infecting organisms; don't use in infections of unknown cause.
- Store drug at room temperature in tightly closed, light-resistant container.

PATIENT TEACHING

- Tell patient to clean eye area of excessive discharge before application.

- Teach patient how to apply drug. Advise him to wash hands before and after applying ointment, and warn him not to touch tip of applicator to eye or surrounding tissue.
- Tell patient that vision may be blurred for a few minutes after applying ointment.
- Advise patient to watch for and report signs and symptoms of sensitivity (itching lids, redness, swelling, or constant burning).
- Tell patient not to share drug, washcloths, or towels with family members and to notify prescriber if anyone develops same signs or symptoms.
- Stress importance of compliance with recommended therapy.

gatifloxacin

Zymar

Pharmacologic class: fluoroquinolone
Pregnancy risk category C

AVAILABLE FORMS

Solution: 0.3% in 2.5-ml and 5-ml bottles

INDICATIONS & DOSAGES

➤ **Bacterial conjunctivitis**
Adults and children age 1 and older: Instill 1 drop into affected eye q 2 hours while patient is awake, up to eight times daily for 2 days. Then instill 1 drop up to q.i.d. for 5 more days.

ACTION

Inhibits DNA gyrase and topoisomerase, preventing cell replication and division.

Route	Onset	Peak	Duration
Ophthalmic	Unknown	Unknown	Unknown

Half-life: Unknown.

ADVERSE REACTIONS

CNS: headache.
EENT: *conjunctival irritation, increased lacrimation, keratitis, papillary conjunctivitis,* chemosis, conjunctival hemorrhage, discharge, dry eyes, eye irritation, eyelid edema, pain, red eyes, reduced visual acuity.
GI: taste disturbance.

INTERACTIONS

None reported.

EFFECTS ON LAB TEST RESULTS

None reported.

CONTRAINDICATIONS & CAUTIONS

- Contraindicated in patients hypersensitive to drug or other quinolones.
- Use cautiously in pregnant or breast-feeding women.

NURSING CONSIDERATIONS

- Don't inject solution subconjunctivally or into the anterior chamber of the eye.
- Systemic drug may cause serious hypersensitivity reactions. If allergic reaction occurs, stop drug and treat symptoms.
- Monitor patient for superinfection.

PATIENT TEACHING

- Urge patient to immediately stop drug and seek medical treatment if evidence of a serious allergic reaction develops, such as itching, rash, swelling of the face or throat, or difficulty breathing.
- Tell patient not to wear contact lenses during treatment.
- Warn patient to avoid touching the applicator tip to anything, including eyes and fingers.
- Teach patient that prolonged use may encourage infections with nonsusceptible bacteria.

gentamicin sulfate

Garamycin, Genoptic, Gentacidin, Gentak

Pharmacologic class: aminoglycoside
Pregnancy risk category C

AVAILABLE FORMS

Ophthalmic ointment: 0.3% (base)
Ophthalmic solution: 0.3% (base)

INDICATIONS & DOSAGES

➤ **External ocular infections (conjunctivitis, keratoconjunctivitis, corneal ulcers, blepharitis, blepharoconjunctivitis, meibomianitis, and dacryocystitis) caused by susceptible organisms, especially *Pseudomonas***

***aeruginosa, Proteus, Klebsiella pneumoniae, Escherichia coli*, and other gram-negative organisms**
Adults and children: 1 to 2 drops in affected eye q 4 hours. In severe infections, up to 2 drops q hour. Or, apply ointment to lower conjunctival sac b.i.d. or t.i.d.

ACTION
Thought to inhibit protein synthesis; usually bactericidal.

Route	Onset	Peak	Duration
Ophthalmic	Unknown	Unknown	Unknown

Half-life: Unknown.

ADVERSE REACTIONS
EENT: burning, stinging, or blurred vision with ointment, conjunctival hyperemia, transient irritation from solution.
Other: overgrowth of nonsusceptible organisms with long-term use.

INTERACTIONS
None significant.

EFFECTS ON LAB TEST RESULTS
None reported.

CONTRAINDICATIONS & CAUTIONS
- Contraindicated in patients hypersensitive to drug.
- Use cautiously in patients with history of sensitivity to aminoglycosides because cross-sensitivity may occur.

NURSING CONSIDERATIONS
- Obtain culture before giving drug. Therapy may begin before culture results are known.
- If ophthalmic gentamicin is given together with systemic gentamicin, monitor gentamicin level.
- Systemic absorption from excessive use may cause toxicities.
- Solution isn't for injection into conjunctiva or anterior chamber of eye.
- Store drug away from heat.

PATIENT TEACHING
- Tell patient to clean eye area of excessive discharge before instilling drug.
- Teach patient how to instill drops or apply ointment. Advise him to wash hands before and after applying ointment or solution and not to touch tip of dropper or tube to eye or surrounding tissues.
- Instruct patient to apply light finger pressure on lacrimal sac for 1 minute after drops are instilled.
- Tell patient to wait at least 10 minutes before instilling other eye drops.
- Instruct patient to stop drug and notify prescriber if signs and symptoms of sensitivity (itching lids, swelling, or constant burning) occur.
- Advise patient not to share drug, washcloths, or towels with family members and to notify prescriber if anyone develops same signs or symptoms.
- Tell patient that vision may be blurred for few minutes after application of ointment.
- ***Alert:*** Stress importance of following recommended therapy. *Pseudomonas* infections can cause complete vision loss within 24 hours if infection isn't controlled.

moxifloxacin hydrochloride
Vigamox

Pharmacologic class: fluoroquinolone
Pregnancy risk category C

AVAILABLE FORMS
Solution: 0.5%

INDICATIONS & DOSAGES
➤ **Bacterial conjunctivitis**
Adults and children age 1 and older: 1 drop into affected eye t.i.d. for 7 days.

ACTION
Antibiotic. Inhibits DNA gyrase and topoisomerase, preventing cell replication and division.

Route	Onset	Peak	Duration
Ophthalmic	Unknown	Unknown	Unknown

Half-life: 13 hours.

ADVERSE REACTIONS
CNS: fever.
EENT: conjunctivitis, dry eyes, increased lacrimation, keratitis, ocular discomfort,

pain, or pruritus, otitis media, pharyngitis, reduced visual acuity, rhinitis, subconjunctival hemorrhage.
Respiratory: increased cough.
Skin: rash.
Other: infection.

INTERACTIONS
None reported.

EFFECTS ON LAB TEST RESULTS
None reported.

CONTRAINDICATIONS & CAUTIONS
- Contraindicated in patients hypersensitive to drug or other fluoroquinolones.
- Use cautiously in pregnant or breast-feeding women.

NURSING CONSIDERATIONS
- Don't inject solution subconjunctivally or into anterior chamber of the eye.
- Systemic drug may cause serious hypersensitivity reactions. If allergic reaction occurs, stop drug and treat symptoms.
- Monitor patient for superinfection.
- ***Look alike–sound alike:*** Don't confuse Vigamox with Avonex.

PATIENT TEACHING
- Tell patient to stop drug and seek medical treatment immediately if evidence of hypersensitivity reaction develops, such as itching, rash, swelling of the face or throat, or difficulty breathing.
- Tell patient not to wear contact lenses during treatment.
- Instruct patient not to touch dropper tip to anything, including eyes and fingers.

ofloxacin 0.3%
Ocuflox

Pharmacologic class: fluoroquinolone
Pregnancy risk category C

AVAILABLE FORMS
Ophthalmic solution: 0.3% in 1-ml, 5-ml, and 10-ml solution

INDICATIONS & DOSAGES
➤ **Conjunctivitis caused by *Staphylococcus aureus, S. epidermidis, Streptococcus pneumoniae, Enterobacter cloacae, Haemophilus influenzae, Proteus mirabilis,* and *Pseudomonas aeruginosa***
Adults and children older than age 1: One or two drops in conjunctival sac q 2 to 4 hours daily while patient is awake, for first 2 days; then q.i.d. for up to 5 additional days.
➤ **Bacterial corneal ulcer caused by *S. aureus, S. epidermidis, S. pneumoniae, P. aeruginosa, Serratia marcescens,* and *Propionibacterium acnes***
Adults and children older than age 1: One or two drops q 30 minutes while patient is awake and one or two drops 4 and 6 hours after patient goes to bed on days 1 and 2. On day 3, one or two drops hourly while patient is awake; continue for 4 to 6 days. Then, one or two drops q.i.d for an additional 3 days or until cured.

ACTION
Bactericidal. Inhibits bacterial DNA gyrase, an enzyme needed for bacterial replication.

Route	Onset	Peak	Duration
Ophthalmic	Unknown	Unknown	Unknown

Half-life: 4 to 8 hours.

ADVERSE REACTIONS
EENT: *transient ocular burning or discomfort,* chemical conjunctivitis or keratitis, eye dryness, eye pain, itching, lacrimation, periocular or facial edema, photophobia, redness, stinging.

INTERACTIONS
None significant.

EFFECTS ON LAB TEST RESULTS
None reported.

CONTRAINDICATIONS & CAUTIONS
- Contraindicated in patients hypersensitive to drug or other fluoroquinolones and in breast-feeding women.

NURSING CONSIDERATIONS
- ***Alert:*** Don't inject drug into conjunctiva or introduce directly into anterior chamber of eye.

- Stop drug if improvement doesn't occur within 7 days. Prolonged use may result in overgrowth of nonsusceptible organisms, including fungi.
- ***Look alike–sound alike:*** Don't confuse Ocuflox with Ocufen.

PATIENT TEACHING

- If an allergic reaction occurs, tell patient to stop drug and notify prescriber. Serious acute hypersensitivity reactions may need emergency treatment.
- Tell patient to clean excessive discharge from eye area before application.
- Teach patient how to instill drops. Advise him to wash hands before and after instilling solution, and warn him not to touch tip of dropper to eye or surrounding tissue.
- Advise patient to apply light finger pressure on lacrimal sac for 1 minute after drug instillation.
- Tell patient not to share drug, washcloths, or towels with family members and to notify prescriber if anyone develops same signs or symptoms.
- Stress importance of compliance with recommended therapy.
- Warn patient not to use leftover drug for new eye infection.
- Remind patient to discard drug when it's no longer needed.

sulfacetamide sodium 10%

AK-Sulf, Bleph-10, Cetamide, OcuSulf-10, Sodium Sulamyd, Storz Sulf, Sulf-10

sulfacetamide sodium 15%

Isopto-Cetamide Ophthalmic

sulfacetamide sodium 30%

Sodium Sulamyd

Pharmacologic class: sulfonamide
Pregnancy risk category C

AVAILABLE FORMS

Ophthalmic ointment: 10%
Ophthalmic solution: 10%, 15%, 30%

INDICATIONS & DOSAGES

➤Inclusion conjunctivitis, corneal ulcers, chlamydial infection

Adults and children: 1 or 2 drops of 10% solution into lower conjunctival sac q 2 to 3 hours during day, less often at night. Or, 1 or 2 drops of 15% solution instilled into lower conjunctival sac q 1 to 2 hours initially. Increase interval as condition responds. Or, instill 1 drop of 30% solution into lower conjunctival sac q 2 hours. Apply 0.5 inch of 10% ointment into conjunctival sac t.i.d. to q.i.d. and at bedtime. Ointment may be used at night along with drops during the day.

➤Trachoma

Adults and children: 2 drops of 30% solution into lower conjunctival sac q 2 hours with systemic sulfonamide or tetracycline.

ACTION

Bacteriostatic, although it may be bactericidal in high concentrations. Prevents uptake of PABA, a metabolite of bacterial folic acid synthesis.

Route	Onset	Peak	Duration
Ophthalmic	Unknown	Unknown	Unknown

Half-life: Unknown.

ADVERSE REACTIONS

EENT: burning, eye itching, headache or brow pain, pain on instillation of drops, periorbital edema, photophobia, slowed corneal wound healing with ointment.
Other: overgrowth of nonsusceptible organisms.

INTERACTIONS

Drug-drug. *Gentamicin (ophthalmic):* May cause in vitro antagonism. Avoid using together.
Local anesthetics (procaine, tetracaine), PABA derivatives: May decrease sulfacetamide sodium action. Wait 30 minutes to 1 hour after instilling anesthetic or PABA derivative before instilling sulfacetamide.
Silver preparations: May cause precipitate formation. Avoid using together.
Drug-lifestyle. *Sun exposure:* May cause photophobia. Advise patient to avoid excessive sunlight exposure.

EFFECTS ON LAB TEST RESULTS
None reported.

CONTRAINDICATIONS & CAUTIONS
- Contraindicated in patients hypersensitive to sulfonamides and children younger than age 2 months.
- Contraindicated in epithelial herpes simplex keratitis, vaccinia, varicella, and many other viral diseases of the cornea and conjunctiva; in mycobacterial or fungal diseases of ocular structures; and after uncomplicated removal of a corneal foreign body (corticosteroid combinations).
- Use cautiously in patients with severe dry eye. Ointment may have a negative effect on corneal epithelial healing.

NURSING CONSIDERATIONS
- Drug is often used with oral tetracycline to treat trachoma and inclusion conjunctivitis.
- Store drug away from heat in tightly closed, light-resistant container.
- ***Look alike–sound alike:*** Don't confuse Bleph-10 (sulfacetamide sodium) with Blephamide (sulfacetamide sodium and prednisolone acetate).

PATIENT TEACHING
- Tell patient to clean excessive discharge from eye area before application.
- Teach patient how to instill drops or apply ointment. Advise him to wash hands before and after applying ointment or solution and not to touch tip of dropper to eye or surrounding tissue.
- Instruct patient to apply light finger pressure on lacrimal sac for 1 minute after drops are instilled.
- Warn patient that eyedrops burn slightly.
- Advise patient to watch for and report signs and symptoms of sensitivity (itching lids, swelling, or constant burning).
- Tell patient to wait at least 5 to 10 minutes before instilling other eyedrops.
- Warn patient that solution may stain clothing.
- Tell patient to minimize sensitivity to sunlight by wearing sunglasses and avoiding prolonged exposure to sunlight.
- Advise patient not to use discolored solution.
- Tell patient not to share drug, washcloths, or towels with family members and to notify prescriber if anyone develops same signs or symptoms.
- Stress importance of compliance with recommended therapy.
- Advise patient to alert prescriber if no improvement occurs.

tobramycin
AKTob, Defy, Tobrex

Pharmacologic class: aminoglycoside
Pregnancy risk category B

AVAILABLE FORMS
Ophthalmic ointment: 0.3%
Ophthalmic solution: 0.3%

INDICATIONS & DOSAGES
➤ External ocular infections by susceptible bacteria
Adults and children: In mild to moderate infections, instill 1 or 2 drops into affected eye q 4 hours, or apply 1-cm strip of ointment q 8 to 12 hours. In severe infections, instill 2 drops into infected eye q 30 to 60 minutes until condition improves; then reduce frequency. Or, apply 1-cm strip of ointment q 3 to 4 hours until condition improves; then reduce frequency to b.i.d. to t.i.d.

ACTION
Thought to inhibit protein synthesis; usually bactericidal.

Route	Onset	Peak	Duration
Ophthalmic	Unknown	Unknown	Unknown

Half-life: 2 to 3 hours.

ADVERSE REACTIONS
EENT: blurred vision with ointment, burning or stinging on instillation, conjunctival erythema, increased lacrimation, lid itching or swelling.

INTERACTIONS
None significant.

EFFECTS ON LAB TEST RESULTS
None reported.

CONTRAINDICATIONS & CAUTIONS

- Contraindicated in patients hypersensitive to drug or other aminoglycosides.

NURSING CONSIDERATIONS

- When two different ophthalmic solutions are used, allow at least 5 minutes between instillations.
- ***Alert:*** Tobramycin ophthalmic solution isn't for injection.
- If topical ocular tobramycin is given with systemic tobramycin, carefully monitor levels.
- Prolonged use may result in overgrowth of nonsusceptible organisms, including fungi.
- ***Look alike–sound alike:*** Don't confuse tobramycin with Trobicin or Tobrex with TobraDex.

PATIENT TEACHING

- Tell patient to clean excessive discharge from eye area before application.
- Teach patient how to instill drops or apply ointment. Advise him to wash hands before and after applying and to avoid touching tip of dropper to eye or surrounding tissue.
- Instruct patient to apply light finger pressure on lacrimal sac for 1 minute after drops are instilled.
- Tell patient to wait at least 10 minutes before instilling other eye drops.
- Advise patient to watch for itching lids, swelling, or constant burning. Tell him to stop drug and notify prescriber if these signs and symptoms develop.
- Tell patient not to share drug, washcloths, or towels with family members and to notify prescriber if anyone develops same signs or symptoms.
- Stress importance of compliance with recommended therapy.

78

Ophthalmic anti-inflammatories

bromfenac
dexamethasone
dexamethasone sodium phosphate
fluorometholone
fluorometholone acetate
ketorolac tromethamine
prednisolone acetate
prednisolone sodium phosphate

bromfenac

Xibrom

Pharmacologic class: NSAID
Pregnancy risk category C

AVAILABLE FORMS

Ophthalmic solution: 0.09%

INDICATIONS & DOSAGES

➤ **Inflammation and pain after cataract surgery**

Adults: Give 1 drop in each eye b.i.d., starting 24 hours after surgery and continuing for 2 weeks.

ACTION

Blocks prostaglandin synthesis by inhibiting cyclooxygenase 1 and 2.

Route	Onset	Peak	Duration
Ophthalmic	Unknown	Unknown	Unknown

Half-life: Unknown.

ADVERSE REACTIONS

CNS: headache.
EENT: abnormal sensation in the eye, burning, conjunctival hyperemia, eye irritation, eye pain, eye pruritus, eye redness, iritis, keratitis, stinging.
Other: ***anaphylaxis,*** hypersensitivity reactions.

INTERACTIONS

Drug-drug. *Drugs that affect coagulation:* May further increase bleeding tendency or prolong bleeding time. Avoid using together, if possible, or monitor patient closely for bleeding.
Topical corticosteroids: May delay healing. Avoid using together, if possible, or monitor healing closely.

EFFECTS ON LAB TEST RESULTS

None reported.

CONTRAINDICATIONS & CAUTIONS

- Contraindicated in patients hypersensitive to drug or its ingredients. Drug contains sulfite, which may cause allergic-type reactions, including anaphylaxis and life-threatening or less severe asthmatic episodes in patients sensitive to sulfites.
- Use cautiously in patients with bleeding tendencies, those taking anticoagulants, and those sensitive to aspirin products, phenylacetic acid derivatives, and other NSAIDs.
- Use cautiously in patients who have had complicated or repeat ocular surgeries or those with corneal denervation, corneal epithelial defects, diabetes mellitus, ocular surface diseases (such as dry-eye syndrome), or rheumatoid arthritis because of the increased risk of corneal adverse effects, which may threaten sight.
- Use in pregnant women only if potential benefit justifies risk; avoid use late in pregnancy because NSAIDs may cause premature closure of the ductus arteriosus, a necessary structure of fetal circulation.
- Use cautiously in breast-feeding women.

NURSING CONSIDERATIONS

- Ask patient if he's sensitive to sulfites, aspirin, or other NSAIDs before treatment. Drug contains sulfite, which may cause allergic-type reactions, including anaphylaxis and life-threatening or less severe asthmatic episodes, in patients sensitive to sulfites.
- Sulfite sensitivity is more common in patients with asthma than in those without asthma. If patient has asthma, monitor closely.
- If patient takes an anticoagulant, watch closely for increased bleeding.

• Begin treatment at least 24 hours after surgery and continue for 2 weeks. Starting treatment less than 24 hours after surgery or giving for longer than 14 days increases risk of ocular adverse effects.

PATIENT TEACHING

• Advise patient not to use while wearing contact lenses.
• Teach patient how to instill the drops.
• Instruct patient to start therapy 24 hours after surgery and to continue for 14 days.
• Tell patient not to use for longer than 2 weeks after surgery or to save unused amount for other conditions.
• Tell patient the signs and symptoms of adverse effects. If bothersome or serious adverse effects occur, advise patient to stop therapy and contact prescriber.
• Tell patient to store drug at room temperature.

dexamethasone

Maxidex

dexamethasone sodium phosphate

AK-Dex, Decadron

Pharmacologic class: corticosteroid
Pregnancy risk category C

AVAILABLE FORMS

Ophthalmic solution: 0.1%

INDICATIONS & DOSAGES

➤ **Uveitis; iridocyclitis; inflammatory conditions of eyelids, conjunctiva, cornea, anterior segment of globe; corneal injury from chemical or thermal burns, or penetration of foreign bodies; allergic conjunctivitis; suppression of graft rejection after keratoplasty**

Adults and children: Give 1 or 2 drops of solution into conjunctival sac. In severe disease, give drops q 1 to 2 hours, tapering as condition improves. In mild conditions, give drops up to four to six times daily t.i.d. or q.i.d. As condition improves, taper dosage to b.i.d.; then once daily. Treatment may extend from a few days to several weeks.

ACTION

Anti-inflammatory; suppresses edema, fibrin deposition, capillary dilation, leukocyte migration, capillary proliferation, and collagen deposition.

Route	Onset	Peak	Duration
Ophthalmic	Unknown	Unknown	Unknown

Half-life: Unknown.

ADVERSE REACTIONS

EENT: burning, stinging, or red eyes, cataracts, corneal ulceration, defects in visual acuity and visual field, discharge, discomfort, dry eyes, foreign body sensation, glaucoma worsening, increased intraocular pressure, increased susceptibility to viral or fungal corneal infection, interference with corneal wound healing, mild blurred vision, optic nerve damage with excessive or long-term use, ocular pain, photophobia, thinning of cornea.
Other: adrenal suppression with excessive or long-term use, systemic effects.

INTERACTIONS

None significant.

EFFECTS ON LAB TEST RESULTS

None reported.

CONTRAINDICATIONS & CAUTIONS

• Contraindicated in patients hypersensitive to any component of drug.
• Contraindicated in those with ocular tuberculosis or acute superficial herpes simplex (dendritic keratitis), vaccinia, varicella, or other fungal or viral diseases of cornea and conjunctiva; in patients with acute, purulent, untreated infections of eye; and in those who have had uncomplicated removal of superficial corneal foreign body.
• Use cautiously in patients with corneal abrasions that may be infected (especially with herpes).
• Use cautiously in patients with glaucoma (any form) because intraocular pressure may increase. Dosage of glaucoma drugs may need to be increased to compensate.
• Safe use in pregnant and breast-feeding women hasn't been established.

NURSING CONSIDERATIONS
- Drug isn't for long-term use.
- Watch for corneal ulceration; which may require stopping drug.
- Corneal viral and fungal infections may be worsened by corticosteroid application.
- ***Look alike–sound alike:*** Don't confuse dexamethasone with desoximetasone. Don't confuse Maxidex with Maxzide.

PATIENT TEACHING
- Tell patient to shake suspension well before use.
- Teach patient how to instill drops. Advise him to wash hands before and after applying solution, and warn him not to touch tip of dropper to eye or surrounding tissue.
- Tell patient to apply light finger pressure on lacrimal sac for 1 minute after instillation.
- Advise patient that he may use eye pad with ointment.
- Warn patient not to use leftover drug for new eye inflammation; doing so may cause serious problems.
- ***Alert:*** Warn patient to call prescriber immediately and to stop drug if visual acuity changes or visual field diminishes.
- Tell patient not to share drug, washcloths, or towels with family members and to notify prescriber if anyone develops same signs or symptoms.
- Stress importance of compliance with recommended therapy.
- Tell patient who wears contact lenses to check with prescriber before using lenses again.

---

fluorometholone
Fluor-Op, FML, FML Forte, FML S.O.P.

fluorometholone acetate
Flarex

Pharmacologic class: corticosteroid
Pregnancy risk category C

AVAILABLE FORMS
fluorometholone
Ophthalmic ointment: 0.1%
Ophthalmic suspension: 0.1%, 0.25%

fluorometholone acetate
Ophthalmic suspension: 0.1%

INDICATIONS & DOSAGES
➤ Inflammatory and allergic conditions of cornea, conjunctiva, sclera, anterior uvea
Adults and children older than 2 (acetate form not for use in children of any age): Give 2 drops of 0.1 or 0.25% suspension q 1 to 2 hours or ½ inch ointment q 4 hours during the first 1 to 2 days in severe cases. For mild to moderate inflammation, or when severe cases respond to treatment, 1 to 2 drops b.i.d. to q.i.d. or ½ inch ointment 1 to 3 times daily. For fluorometholone acetate, 1 to 2 drops q.i.d.; may give 2 drops q 2 hours during the initial 24 to 48 hours of treatment.

ACTION
Anti-inflammatory; suppresses edema, fibrin deposition, capillary dilation, leukocyte migration, capillary proliferation, and collagen deposition.

Route	Onset	Peak	Duration
Ophthalmic	Unknown	Unknown	Unknown

Half-life: Unknown.

ADVERSE REACTIONS
EENT: increased intraocular pressure (IOP), thinning of cornea, interference with corneal wound healing, corneal ulceration, increased susceptibility to viral or fungal corneal infections, glaucoma worsening, discharge, discomfort, ocular pain, foreign body sensation, cataracts, decreased visual acuity, diminished visual field, optic nerve damage with excessive or long-term use.
Other: systemic effects, adrenal suppression with excessive or long-term use.

INTERACTIONS
None significant.

EFFECTS ON LAB TEST RESULTS
None reported.

CONTRAINDICATIONS & CAUTIONS
- Contraindicated in patients with vaccinia, varicella, acute superficial herpes simplex (dendritic keratitis), other fungal

or viral eye diseases, ocular tuberculosis, or acute, purulent, untreated eye infections.
- Use cautiously in patients with corneal abrasions that may be contaminated (especially with herpes).
- Safety and effectiveness of fluorometholone in children younger than age 2 haven't been established. Fluorometholone acetate not for use in children of any age.

NURSING CONSIDERATIONS
- Treatment may last from a few days to several weeks, but avoid long-term use. Monitor IOP.
- Drug is less likely to increase IOP with extended use than other ophthalmic anti-inflammatories (except medrysone).
- In chronic conditions, withdraw treatment by gradually decreasing frequency of applications.

PATIENT TEACHING
- Tell patient to shake container well before use.
- Teach patient how to instill drops or apply ointment. Advise him to wash hands before and after using either form, and warn him not to touch tip of dropper to eye or surrounding tissue.
- Advise patient to apply light finger pressure on lacrimal sac for 1 minute after instillation.
- Tell patient not to use any other eye preparation for at least 10 minutes.
- Urge patient to call prescriber immediately and to stop drug if visual acuity decreases or visual field diminishes.
- Tell patient not to share drug, washcloths, or towels with family members and to notify prescriber if anyone develops same signs or symptoms.
- Warn patient not to use leftover drug for new eye inflammation; it may cause serious problems.
- Advise patient to consult prescriber if condition doesn't improve after 2 days. Don't stop treatment prematurely.
- Tell patient to store drug in tightly covered, light-resistant container.

ketorolac tromethamine
Acular, Acular LS

Pharmacologic class: NSAID
Pregnancy risk category C

AVAILABLE FORMS
Acular
Ophthalmic solution: 0.5%
Acular LS
Ophthalmic solution: 0.4%

INDICATIONS & DOSAGES
➤ **Relief from ocular itching caused by seasonal allergic conjunctivitis**
Adults and children age 3 and older: One drop into conjunctival sac in each eye q.i.d.
➤ **Postoperative inflammation in patients who have had cataract extraction**
Adults and children age 3 and older: One drop to affected eye q.i.d. beginning 24 hours after cataract surgery and continuing through first two weeks of postoperative period.
➤ **Reduce ocular pain, burning, and stinging after corneal refractive surgery (Acular LS)**
Adults and children age 3 and older: One drop q.i.d. to affected eye, p.r.n., for up to four days after surgery.

ACTION
Thought to inhibit the action of cyclooxygenase, an enzyme responsible for prostaglandin synthesis. Prostaglandins mediate the inflammatory response and also cause miosis.

Route	Onset	Peak	Duration
Ophthalmic	Unknown	Unknown	Unknown

Half-life: 4 hours.

ADVERSE REACTIONS
CNS: headache (Acular LS).
EENT: *transient stinging and burning on instillation,* conjunctival hyperemia, corneal edema, corneal infiltrates, iritis, ocular edema and ocular pain (Acular LS), ocular inflammation (Acular), ocular

irritation, ocular pain, superficial keratitis, superficial ocular infections.
Other: hypersensitivity reactions.

INTERACTIONS
None significant.

EFFECTS ON LAB TEST RESULTS
None reported.

CONTRAINDICATIONS & CAUTIONS
- Contraindicated in patients hypersensitive to components of drug and in those wearing soft contact lenses.
- Use cautiously in patients with bleeding disorders or those hypersensitive to other NSAIDs or aspirin. Use cautiously in breast-feeding women.

NURSING CONSIDERATIONS
- Store drug away from heat in a dark, tightly closed container and protect from freezing.
- ***Look alike–sound alike:*** Don't confuse Acular with Acthar.

PATIENT TEACHING
- Teach patient how to instill drops. Advise him to wash hands before and after instilling solution, and warn him not to touch tip of dropper to eye or surrounding tissue.
- Advise patient to apply light finger pressure on lacrimal sac for 1 minute after instillation.
- Stress importance of compliance with recommended therapy.
- Tell patient not to instill drops while wearing contact lenses.
- Advise patient to report excessive bleeding or bruising to prescriber.
- Remind patient to discard drug when it's no longer needed.

prednisolone acetate (suspension)
Econopred Plus , Pred Forte, Pred Mild

prednisolone sodium phosphate (solution)
AK-Pred, Blephamide , Inflamase Forte, Inflamase Mild, Predsol‡

Pharmacologic class: corticosteroid
Pregnancy risk category C

AVAILABLE FORMS
prednisolone acetate
Ophthalmic suspension: 0.12%, 0.125%, 1%
prednisolone sodium phosphate
Ophthalmic solution: 0.125%, 1%

INDICATIONS & DOSAGES
➤ Inflammation of palpebral and bulbar conjunctiva, cornea, and anterior segment of globe
Adults and children: Give 1 or 2 drops into eye. In severe conditions, may be used hourly, tapering as inflammation subsides. In mild or moderate inflammation or when a favorable response is attained in severe conditions, dosage may be reduced to 1 or 2 drops q 3 to 12 hours.

ACTION
Anti-inflammatory; suppresses edema, fibrin deposition, capillary dilation, leukocyte migration, capillary proliferation, and collagen deposition.

Route	Onset	Peak	Duration
Ophthalmic	Unknown	Unknown	Unknown

Half-life: Unknown.

ADVERSE REACTIONS
EENT: cataracts, corneal ulceration, discharge, discomfort, foreign body sensation, glaucoma worsening, increased intraocular pressure (IOP), increased susceptibility to viral or fungal corneal infection, interference with corneal wound healing, optic nerve damage with excessive or long-term use, visual acuity and visual field defects.

Other: adrenal suppression with excessive or long-term use, systemic effects.

INTERACTIONS
None significant.

EFFECTS ON LAB TEST RESULTS
None reported.

CONTRAINDICATIONS & CAUTIONS
• Contraindicated in patients with acute, untreated, purulent ocular infections; acute superficial herpes simplex (dendritic keratitis); vaccinia, varicella, or other viral or fungal eye diseases; or ocular tuberculosis.
• Use cautiously in patients with corneal abrasions that may be contaminated (especially with herpes).

NURSING CONSIDERATIONS
• Shake suspension and check dosage before giving to ensure correct strength. Store in tightly covered container.
• ***Look alike–sound alike:*** Don't confuse prednisolone with prednisone.

PATIENT TEACHING
• Teach patient how to instill drops. Advise him to wash hands before and after instillation, and warn him not to touch tip of dropper to eye or surrounding area.
• Advise patient to apply light finger pressure on lacrimal sac for 1 minute after instillation.
• Tell patient on long-term therapy to have IOP tested frequently.
• Tell patient not to share drug, washcloths, or towels with family members and to notify prescriber if anyone develops same signs or symptoms.
• Stress importance of compliance with recommended therapy.
• Tell patient to notify prescriber if improvement doesn't occur within several days or if pain, itching, or swelling of eye occurs.
• Warn patient not to use leftover drug for new eye inflammation because serious problems may occur.

79

Miotics

acetylcholine chloride
carbachol
pilocarpine hydrochloride
pilocarpine nitrate

acetylcholine chloride

Miochol-E

Pharmacologic class: direct-acting parasympathomimetic, cholinergic
Pregnancy risk category C

AVAILABLE FORMS

Ophthalmic injection: 1%

INDICATIONS & DOSAGES

➤ **Anterior segment surgery**

Adults and children: Before or after suturing, surgeon gently instills 0.5 to 2 ml into anterior chamber.

ACTION

Causes contraction of the sphincter muscles of the iris, resulting in miosis, which produces ciliary spasm, deepening of the anterior chamber, and vasodilation of conjunctival vessels of the outflow tract.

Route	Onset	Peak	Duration
Ophthalmic	Immediate	Unknown	10 min

Half-life: Unknown.

ADVERSE REACTIONS

CV: ***bradycardia,*** flushing, hypotension.
EENT: clouding, corneal edema, decompensation.
Respiratory: breathing difficulties.
Other: diaphoresis.

INTERACTIONS

None significant.
Drug-drug. *Topical NSAIDs:* May negate effect of acetylcholine. Monitor patient for effect.

EFFECTS ON LAB TEST RESULTS

None reported.

CONTRAINDICATIONS & CAUTIONS

- Contraindicated in patients hypersensitive to drug or its components.

NURSING CONSIDERATIONS

- Open under aseptic conditions only. Reconstitute immediately before using, shaking vial gently until clear solution is obtained.
- Discard unused solution.
- Don't gas-sterilize vial. Ethylene oxide may produce formic acid. Watch for signs and symptoms of hypotension and bradycardia if this occurs.
- ***Look alike–sound alike:*** Don't confuse acetylcholine with acetylcysteine.

PATIENT TEACHING

- Inform patient about need for drug during surgical procedure; answer questions and address concerns.
- Instruct patient to immediately report breathing difficulties.

carbachol (intraocular)

Carbastat, Miostat

carbachol (topical)

Carboptic, Isopto Carbachol

Pharmacologic class: direct acting parasympathomimetic
Pregnancy risk category C

AVAILABLE FORMS

Intraocular injection: 0.01%
Topical ophthalmic solution: 0.75%, 1.5%, 2.25%, 3%

INDICATIONS & DOSAGES

➤ **To produce pupillary miosis in ocular surgery**

Adults: Before or after securing sutures, 0.5 ml (intraocular form) instilled gently into anterior chamber.

➤ **Glaucoma**

Adults: One or two drops (topical form) instilled up to t.i.d.

ACTION

A cholinergic that causes contraction of the sphincter muscles of the iris, resulting in miosis. That produces ciliary spasm, deepening of the anterior chamber, and vasodilation of conjunctival vessels of the outflow tract.

Route	Onset	Peak	Duration
Intraocular	Seconds	2–5 min	24–48 hr
Ophthalmic (topical)	10–20 min	Unknown	4–8 hr

Half-life: Unknown.

ADVERSE REACTIONS

CV: ***cardiac arrhythmia,*** flushing, hypotension, syncope.
EENT: *transient stinging and burning,* bullous keratopathy, ciliary and conjunctival injection, conjunctival vasodilation, corneal clouding, eye and brow pain, iritis, retinal detachment, salivation, spasm of eye accommodation.
GI: diarrhea, epigastric distress, GI cramps, vomiting.
GU: frequent urge to urinate, tightness in bladder.
Respiratory: asthma.
Other: diaphoresis.

INTERACTIONS

Drug-drug. *Topical NSAIDs:* May inactivate carbachol. Monitor patient for clinical effect.
Pilocarpine: May cause additive effects. Use together cautiously.

EFFECTS ON LAB TEST RESULTS

None reported.

CONTRAINDICATIONS & CAUTIONS

- Contraindicated in patients hypersensitive to drug and in those with conditions in which cholinergic effects, such as constriction, are undesirable (acute iritis, some forms of secondary glaucoma, pupillary block glaucoma, or acute inflammatory disease of the anterior chamber).
- Use cautiously in patients with acute heart failure, bronchial asthma, peptic ulcer, hyperthyroidism, GI spasm, Parkinson disease, and urinary tract obstruction.

NURSING CONSIDERATIONS

- In case of toxicity, give atropine parenterally.
- Drug is used in open-angle glaucoma, especially when patients are resistant or allergic to pilocarpine hydrochloride or nitrate.
- ***Alert:*** Patients with hazel or brown irises may need stronger solutions or more frequent instillation because eye pigment may absorb drug.
- If tolerance to drug develops, prescriber may switch to another miotic for a short time.
- ***Look alike–sound alike:*** Don't confuse Isopto Carbachol with Isopto Carpine.

PATIENT TEACHING

- Teach patient how to instill drug. Advise him to wash hands before and after instillation and to apply light finger pressure on lacrimal sac for 1 minute after drops are instilled. Warn him not to exceed recommended dosage.
- Warn patient to avoid hazardous activities, such as operating machinery or driving, until temporary blurring subsides. Reassure patient that blurred vision usually diminishes with prolonged use.
- Tell glaucoma patient that long-term use may be needed. Stress compliance. Tell him to remain under medical supervision for periodic tests of intraocular pressure.
- Warn patient to use caution during night driving and while performing other hazardous activities in reduced light.

pilocarpine hydrochloride

Adsorbocarpine, Akarpine, Isopto Carpine, Pilocar, Pilopine HS, Pilopt‡, Pilostat

pilocarpine nitrate

Pilagan Liquifilm

Pharmacologic class: direct acting parasympathomimetic
Pregnancy risk category C

AVAILABLE FORMS

pilocarpine hydrochloride
Ophthalmic gel: 4%
Ophthalmic solution: 0.25%, 0.5%, 1%, 2%, 3%, 4%, 5%, 6%, 8%, 10%

pilocarpine nitrate
Ophthalmic solution: 1%, 2%, 4%

INDICATIONS & DOSAGES

➤ **Primary open-angle glaucoma**
Adults and children: Give 1 or 2 drops of 1 to 4% solution q 4 to 12 hours; adjust concentration and frequency to control IOP. Or apply 1.3-cm (½-inch) ribbon of 4% gel into the lower conjunctival sac once daily at bedtime.

➤ **Emergency treatment of acute angle-closure glaucoma**
Adults and children: Give 1 drop of 2% solution q 5 to 10 minutes for three to six doses; then 1 drop q 1 to 3 hours until pressure is controlled.

➤ **Mydriasis caused by mydriatic or cycloplegic drugs**
Adults and children: Give 1 drop of 1% solution.

ACTION

A cholinergic that causes contraction of iris sphincter muscles, resulting in miosis, and that produces ciliary spasm, deepening of the anterior chamber, and vasodilation of conjunctival vessels of the outflow tract.

Route	Onset	Peak	Duration
Ophthalmic	10–30 min	30–85 min	4–8 hr

Half-life: Unknown.

ADVERSE REACTIONS

CV: hypertension, tachycardia.
EENT: *blurred vision, brow pain, myopia,* changes in visual field, ciliary spasm, conjunctival irritation, keratitis, lacrimation, lens opacity, periorbital or supraorbital headache, retinal detachment, salivation, transient stinging and burning.
GI: diarrhea, nausea, vomiting.
Respiratory: ***pulmonary edema,*** bronchiolar spasm.
Other: diaphoresis.

INTERACTIONS

Drug-drug. *Carbachol, echothiophate:* May cause additive effects. Avoid using together.
Cyclopentolate, ophthalmic belladonna alkaloids such as atropine, scopolamine: May decrease pilocarpine's antiglaucoma effect and block mydriatic effects of these drugs. Avoid using together.
Phenylephrine: May decrease dilation by phenylephrine. Avoid using together.

EFFECTS ON LAB TEST RESULTS

None reported.

CONTRAINDICATIONS & CAUTIONS

- Contraindicated in patients hypersensitive to drug and in conditions in which cholinergic effects, such as constriction, are undesirable (acute iritis, some forms of secondary glaucoma, pupillary block glaucoma, or acute inflammatory disease of the anterior chamber).
- Use cautiously in patients with acute cardiac failure, bronchial asthma, peptic ulcer, hyperthyroidism, GI spasm, urinary tract obstruction, and Parkinson disease.

NURSING CONSIDERATIONS

- Monitor vital signs.
- ***Alert:*** Patients with hazel or brown irises may need stronger solutions or more frequent instillation because eye pigment may absorb drug.
- If both solution and gel are used, the solution should be applied first; the gel is then applied at least 5 minutes later.
- Don't confuse Isopto Carpine with Isopto Carbachol.

PATIENT TEACHING

- Instruct patient to apply gel at bedtime because it will blur vision. Warn him to avoid hazardous activities, such as operating machinery or driving, until temporary blurring subsides.
- Teach patient how to instill drug. Advise him to wash hands before and after instillation and to apply light finger pressure on lacrimal sac for 1 minute after drops are instilled. Warn patient not to touch applicator tip to eye or surrounding tissue.
- Warn patient that transient brow pain and nearsightedness are common at first but usually disappear in 10 to 14 days.
- Advise patient to carry medical identification at all times during therapy.

80 Mydriatics

atropine sulfate
epinephrine hydrochloride
epinephryl borate
phenylephrine hydrochloride
scopolamine hydrobromide

atropine sulfate

Atropine 1, Atropisol, Atropt‡, Isopto Atropine

Pharmacologic class: antimuscarinic
Pregnancy risk category C

AVAILABLE FORMS

Ophthalmic ointment: 1%
Ophthalmic solution: 0.5%, 1%, 2%

INDICATIONS & DOSAGES

➤ Acute iritis, uveitis

Adults: Instill 1 to 2 drops up to q.i.d. or apply small strip of ointment to conjunctival sac up to t.i.d.
Children: Instill 1 to 2 drops of 0.5% solution up to t.i.d. or apply small strip of ointment to conjunctival sac up to t.i.d.

➤ Cycloplegic refraction

Adults: One to two drops of 1% solution 1 hour before refraction Or, apply 0.3 to 0.5 cm of ointment to the conjunctival sac 1 to 3 times daily. Apply ointment several hours before the procedure.
Children: One to two drops of 0.5% solution in each eye b.i.d. for 1 to 3 days before eye examination and 1 hour before refraction Or, 0.3 cm of ointment in the conjunctival sac t.i.d. daily for 1 to 3 days before the procedure. Apply ointment several hours before the procedure.

ACTION

A potent mydriatic and cycloplegic whose anticholinergic action leaves the pupil under unopposed adrenergic influence, causing it to dilate.

Route	Onset	Peak	Duration
Ophthalmic	Unknown	30 min–3 hr	7–10 days

Half-life: Unknown.

ADVERSE REACTIONS

CNS: confusion, headache, somnolence.
CV: tachycardia.
EENT: *blurred vision,* conjunctivitis, contact dermatitis of eye, eye dryness, hyperemia, increased intraocular pressure (IOP), irritation, ocular congestion with long-term use, ocular edema, photophobia, transient stinging and burning.
GI: abdominal distention in infants, dry mouth.
Skin: dryness.

INTERACTIONS

Drug-lifestyle. *Sun exposure:* May cause photophobia. Advise patient to wear sunglasses.

EFFECTS ON LAB TEST RESULTS

None reported.

CONTRAINDICATIONS & CAUTIONS

- Contraindicated in patients hypersensitive to drug or belladonna alkaloids and in those with glaucoma or adhesions between the iris and lens. Don't use atropine in infants age 3 months or younger because of possible link between cycloplegia and development of amblyopia.
- Use cautiously in elderly patients and in others who may have increased IOP. Excessive use in children or in certain susceptible patients, including those with spastic paralysis, brain damage, or Down syndrome, may produce systemic symptoms of atropine poisoning.

NURSING CONSIDERATIONS

- ***Alert:*** Treat drops and ointment as poison (not for internal use); signs of poisoning are disorientation and confusion. Antidote of choice is physostigmine salicylate I.V. or I.M.
- Watch patient for signs and symptoms of glaucoma, including increased IOP, ocular pain, headache, and progressive blurring of vision; notify prescriber if they occur.
- ***Look alike–sound alike:*** Don't confuse Atropisol with Aplisol.

PATIENT TEACHING

- Teach patient how to self-instill drug. Advise him to wash hands before and after instillation and to apply light finger pressure on lacrimal sac for 1 minute after instillation. Warn patient not to touch tip of dropper or tube to eye or surrounding tissue.
- Warn patient to avoid hazardous activities, such as operating machinery or driving, until temporary blurring subsides.
- Advise patient to ease photophobia by wearing dark glasses or staying out of bright light.

epinephrine hydrochloride
Epifrin, Glaucon

epinephryl borate
Epinal

Pharmacologic class: catecholamine
Pregnancy risk category C

AVAILABLE FORMS

epinephrine hydrochloride
Ophthalmic solution: 0.1%, 0.5%, 1%, 2%
epinephryl borate
Ophthalmic solution: 0.5%, 1%

INDICATIONS & DOSAGES

➤ Open-angle glaucoma
Adults: One or two drops of 1% or 2% solution once daily or b.i.d. Adjust dosage based on tonometric readings.

ACTION

An adrenergic that dilates the pupil by contracting the dilator muscle.

Route	Onset	Peak	Duration
Ophthalmic	1 hr	4–8 hr	24 hr

Half-life: Unknown.

ADVERSE REACTIONS

CNS: brow ache, headache, lightheadedness.
CV: ***arrhythmias,*** hypertension, palpitations, tachycardia.
EENT: allergic lid reaction, chemosis, conjunctivitis, corneal edema with long-term use, corneal or conjunctival pigmentation, eye pain, eye stinging, burning, tearing on instillation, follicular hypertrophy, hyperemic conjunctiva, iritis, ocular irritation.
Skin: maculopapular rash.

INTERACTIONS

Drug-drug. *Antihistamines (dexchlorpheniramine, diphenhydramine), tricyclic antidepressants:* May increase cardiac effects of epinephrine. Monitor patient closely.
Beta blockers, osmotic drugs, systemic carbonic anhydrase inhibitors, topical miotics: May cause additive lowering of intraocular pressure. Use together cautiously.
Cardiac glycosides: May increase risk of arrhythmias. Monitor patient closely.
Cyclopropane, halogenated hydrocarbons: May cause arrhythmias, tachycardia. Use together cautiously, if at all.
Local or systemic sympathomimetics: May have additive toxic effects. Avoid using together.
MAO inhibitors: May exaggerate adrenergic effects. Adjust dosage of epinephrine carefully.

EFFECTS ON LAB TEST RESULTS

- May increase BUN and glucose levels.
- May interfere with urine catecholamine test results.

CONTRAINDICATIONS & CAUTIONS

- Contraindicated in patients hypersensitive to drug or sulfites and in those with hypertensive CV disease or coronary artery disease.
- Contraindicated in patients with aphakia, those with angle-closure glaucoma, and those with glaucoma of unknown cause.
- Use cautiously in elderly patients and in those with diabetes mellitus, hypertension, Parkinson disease, hyperthyroidism, cardiac disease, cerebral arteriosclerosis, or bronchial asthma.

NURSING CONSIDERATIONS

- Drug can be injected into anterior chamber to produce rapid mydriasis during cataract removal or can be used to control local bleeding during surgery.

• ***Alert:*** The hydrochloride and borate formulations aren't interchangeable.
• Monitor blood pressure and other vital signs.
• ***Look alike–sound alike:*** Don't confuse epinephrine with ephedrine, or Glaucon with glucagon.

PATIENT TEACHING
• Teach patient how to instill drug. Advise him to wash hands before and after instillation and to apply light finger pressure on lacrimal sac for 1 minute after drops are instilled. Warn him not to touch tip of dropper to eye or surrounding tissue.
• Urge patient to immediately report any decrease in visual acuity.
• Advise patient not to use drug while wearing soft contact lenses because lenses may discolor.
• Tell patient not to use darkened solution.

phenylephrine hydrochloride
AK-Dilate, Ophthalmic ◊, Isopto Frin ◊, Mydfrin, Neo-Synephrine, Phenoptic, Prefrin Liquifilm ◊, Relief ◊

Pharmacologic class: sympathomimetic amine, adrenergic
Pregnancy risk category C

AVAILABLE FORMS
Ophthalmic solution: 0.12%, 2.5%, 10%

INDICATIONS & DOSAGES
➤ **Mydriasis without cycloplegia**
Adults and children: Instill 1 drop of 2.5% or 10% solution before examination. May repeat in 1 hour, p.r.n. May need to apply topical anesthetic before use to prevent stinging and dilution from lacrimation.
➤ **Mydriasis and vasoconstriction**
Adults and adolescents: Give 1 drop of 2.5% or 10% solution.
Children: Give 1 drop of 2.5% solution.
➤ **Chronic mydriasis**
Adults and adolescents: Give 1 drop of 2.5% or 10% solution b.i.d. or t.i.d.
Children: Instill 1 drop of 2.5% solution b.i.d. or t.i.d.
➤ **Posterior synechia (adhesion of iris)**
Adults and children: To prevent or break posterior synechiae in patients with anterior uveitis, instill 1 drop of 10% solution 3 or more times daily in combination with atropine sulfate ophthalmic solution or ointment. To prevent posterior synechiae following iridectomy, instill one drop of 10% solution once or twice daily; administer in combination with atropine sulfate ophthalmic solution or ointment if inflammation is severe. Don't use 10% concentration in children younger than 1.
➤ **Minor eye irritations**
Adults and children: Give 1 or 2 drops of the 0.12% solution in affected eye up to q.i.d., p.r.n.

ACTION
Dilates the pupil by contracting the dilator muscle.

Route	Onset	Peak	Duration
Ophthalmic	Rapid	10–90 min	3–7 hr

Half-life: Unknown.

ADVERSE REACTIONS
CNS: brow ache, headache.
CV: *hypertension with 10% solution,* ***MI,*** palpitations, PVCs, tachycardia.
EENT: allergic conjunctivitis, blurred vision, increased intraocular pressure (IOP), keratitis, lacrimation, reactive hyperemia of eye, rebound miosis, transient eye burning or stinging on instillation.
Skin: dermatitis, diaphoresis, pallor.
Other: trembling.

INTERACTIONS
Drug-drug. *Atropine (topical), cyclopentolate, homatropine, scopolamine:* May increase pupil dilation. Use together cautiously.
Beta blockers, MAO inhibitors: May cause arrhythmias because of increased pressor effect. Use together cautiously.
Guanethidine: May increase mydriatic and pressor effects of phenylephrine. Use together cautiously.
Levodopa: May reduce mydriatic effect of phenylephrine. Use together cautiously.

Tricyclic antidepressants: May increase cardiac effects of epinephrine. Use together cautiously.
Drug-lifestyle. *Sun exposure:* May cause photophobia. Advise patient to wear sunglasses.

EFFECTS ON LAB TEST RESULTS
- May lower IOP in normal eyes or in open-angle glaucoma; may cause false-normal tonometry readings.

CONTRAINDICATIONS & CAUTIONS
- Contraindicated in patients hypersensitive to drug, in those with angle-closure glaucoma, and in those who wear soft contact lenses.
- Use cautiously in patients with marked hypertension, cardiac disorders, advanced arteriosclerotic changes, type 1 diabetes, or hyperthyroidism; in children with low body weight; and in elderly patients.

NURSING CONSIDERATIONS
- Systemic adverse reactions are least likely with 0.12% and 2.5% solutions and most likely with 10% solution.
- ***Look alike–sound alike:*** Don't confuse Mydfrin with Midrin.

PATIENT TEACHING
- Teach patient how to instill drug. Advise him to wash hands before and after instillation and to apply light finger pressure on lacrimal sac for 1 minute after drops are instilled. Warn him not to touch tip of dropper to eye or surrounding tissue.
- Warn patient not to exceed recommended dosage because systemic effects can result. Monitor blood pressure and pulse rate.
- Tell patient not to use brown solution or solution that contains precipitate.
- Warn patient to avoid hazardous activities, such as operating machinery or driving, until temporary blurring subsides.
- Advise patient to contact prescriber if condition persists longer than 12 hours after stopping drug.
- Advise patient to ease photophobia by wearing dark glasses.

scopolamine hydrobromide
Isopto Hyoscine

Pharmacologic class: antimuscarinic, anticholinergic
Pregnancy risk category NR

AVAILABLE FORMS
Ophthalmic solution: 0.25%

INDICATIONS & DOSAGES
➤ Cycloplegic refraction
Adults: Instill 1 or 2 drops of 0.25% solution 1 hour before refraction.
Children: Instill 1 drop of 0.25% solution b.i.d. for 2 days before refraction.
➤ Iritis, uveitis
Adults: Instill 1 or 2 drops of 0.25% solution once daily to q.i.d.
Children: Instill 1 drop of 0.25% solution once daily to q.i.d.

ACTION
Leaves the pupil under unopposed adrenergic influence, causing it to dilate.

Route	Onset	Peak	Duration
Ophthalmic	Rapid	15–45 min	< 1 wk

Half-life: Unknown.

ADVERSE REACTIONS
CNS: acute psychotic reactions, confusion, delirium, hallucinations, headache, somnolence.
CV: edema, tachycardia.
EENT: *blurred vision, photophobia,* conjunctivitis, eye dryness, increased intraocular pressure, ocular congestion with prolonged use, transient stinging and burning.
GI: dry mouth.
Skin: contact dermatitis, dryness.

INTERACTIONS
Drug-lifestyle. *Sun exposure:* May cause photophobia. Advise patient to wear sunglasses.

EFFECTS ON LAB TEST RESULTS
None reported.

CONTRAINDICATIONS & CAUTIONS

- Contraindicated in patients hypersensitive to drug and in those with shallow anterior chamber, angle-closure glaucoma, or adhesions between the iris and lens.
- Contraindicated in children with previous severe systemic reaction to atropine.
- Use cautiously in patients with cardiac disease and in infants, small children, and elderly patients.

NURSING CONSIDERATIONS

- Observe patients closely for adverse CNS effects such as disorientation and delirium.
- Drug may be used in patients sensitive to atropine because it's faster acting and has a shorter duration of action and fewer adverse reactions.

PATIENT TEACHING

- Teach patient how to instill drug. Advise him to wash hands before and after instillation and to apply light finger pressure on lacrimal sac for 1 minute after drops are instilled. Warn him to avoid touching tip of dropper to eye or surrounding tissue.
- Warn patient to avoid hazardous activities, such as operating machinery or driving, until temporary blurring subsides.
- Advise patient to ease sun sensitivity by wearing dark glasses.
- Instruct patient to carry medical identification at all times during therapy.

81

Ophthalmic vasoconstrictors

naphazoline hydrochloride
oxymetazoline hydrochloride
tetrahydrozoline hydrochloride

naphazoline hydrochloride

AK-Con, Albalon Liquifilm, Allerest ◇, Clear Eyes ◇, Comfort Eye Drops ◇, Degest 2, Nafazair, Naphcon ◇, Naphcon Forte, VasoClear ◇, Vasocon Regular, 20/20 Eye Drops ◇

Pharmacologic class: sympathomimetic
Pregnancy risk category C

AVAILABLE FORMS

Ophthalmic solution: 0.012% ◇, 0.02% ◇, 0.03% ◇, 0.1%

INDICATIONS & DOSAGES

➤Ocular congestion, irritation, itching

Adults: Instill 1 drop of 0.1% solution q 3 to 4 hours or 1 drop of 0.012% to 0.03% solution up to q.i.d.

ACTION

Thought to cause vasoconstriction by local adrenergic action on the blood vessels of the conjunctiva.

Route	Onset	Peak	Duration
Ophthalmic	10 min	Unknown	2–6 hr

Half-life: Unknown.

ADVERSE REACTIONS

CNS: dizziness, headache, nervousness, weakness.
EENT: blurred vision, eye irritation, increased intraocular pressure, keratitis, lacrimation, photophobia, pupillary dilation, transient eye stinging.
GI: nausea.
Skin: diaphoresis.

INTERACTIONS

Drug-drug. *Anesthetics:* Cyclopropane and halothane may sensitize the myocardium to sympathomimetics; local anesthetics may increase the absorption of topical drugs. Monitor patient for increased adverse effects.
Beta blockers: May cause more systemic adverse effects. Monitor patient for adverse systemic effects.
MAO inhibitors, maprotiline, tricyclic antidepressants: May cause hypertensive crisis if naphazoline is systemically absorbed. Use together cautiously.

EFFECTS ON LAB TEST RESULTS

None reported.

CONTRAINDICATIONS & CAUTIONS

- Contraindicated in patients hypersensitive to drug's ingredients and in those with acute angle-closure glaucoma.
- Use of 0.1% solution is contraindicated in infants and small children.
- Use cautiously in patients with hyperthyroidism, cardiac disease, hypertension, or diabetes mellitus.

NURSING CONSIDERATIONS

- Drug is most widely used ocular decongestant.
- Store drug in tightly closed container.

PATIENT TEACHING

- Teach patient how to instill drug. Advise him to wash hands before and after instillation and to apply light finger pressure on lacrimal sac for 1 minute after drops are instilled. Warn him not to touch tip of dropper to eye or surrounding tissue.
- Warn patient not to exceed recommended dosage. Rebound congestion and conjunctivitis may occur with frequent or prolonged use.
- Tell patient to notify prescriber if sun sensitivity, blurred vision, pain, or lid swelling develops.
- Instruct patient not to use OTC preparations longer than 72 hours without consulting prescriber.

oxymetazoline hydrochloride

OcuClear ◇, Visine L.R. ◇

Pharmacologic class: direct-acting sympathomimetic amine
Pregnancy risk category C

AVAILABLE FORMS

Ophthalmic solution: 0.025%

INDICATIONS & DOSAGES

➤ **Relief from eye redness caused by minor eye irritation**

Adults and children age 6 and older: Instill 1 to 2 drops in affected eye q 6 hours, p.r.n.

ACTION

Acts on alpha-adrenergic receptors in the arterioles of the conjunctiva to produce vasoconstriction, resulting in decreased conjunctival congestion.

Route	Onset	Peak	Duration
Ophthalmic	5 min	Unknown	6 hr

Half-life: Unknown.

ADVERSE REACTIONS

CNS: headache, insomnia, lightheadedness, nervousness.
CV: irregular heartbeat, palpitations, tachycardia.
EENT: *transient stinging on first instillation,* blurred vision, increased intraocular pressure, keratitis, lacrimation, reactive hyperemia with excessive doses or prolonged use.
Other: trembling.

INTERACTIONS

Drug-drug. *Anesthetics:* Cyclopropane and halothane may sensitize the myocardium to sympathomimetics; local anesthetics may increase the absorption of topical drugs. Monitor patient for increased adverse effects.
Beta blockers: May cause more systemic adverse effects. Monitor patient for adverse systemic effects.
MAO inhibitors, maprotiline, tricyclic antidepressants: If significant systemic absorption of oxymetazoline occurs, use together may increase pressor effect of oxymetazoline. Avoid using together.

EFFECTS ON LAB TEST RESULTS

None reported.

CONTRAINDICATIONS & CAUTIONS

- Contraindicated in patients hypersensitive to drug or its components and in those with angle-closure glaucoma.
- Use cautiously in patients with hyperthyroidism, cardiac disease, hypertension, eye disease, infection, or injury.

NURSING CONSIDERATIONS

- Don't use if solution has become cloudy or changes color.
- ***Alert:*** Don't confuse Visine with Visken.

PATIENT TEACHING

- Teach patient how to instill drops. Advise him to wash hands before and after instillation, and warn him not to touch tip of dropper to eye or surrounding tissue.
- Instruct patient to apply light finger pressure on lacrimal sac for 1 minute after drug instillation.
- Advise patient to stop drug and consult prescriber if eye pain occurs, if vision changes, or if redness or irritation continues, worsens, or lasts for longer than 72 hours.

tetrahydrozoline hydrochloride

Collyrium Fresh ◇, Eyesine ◇, Geneye ◇, Murine Plus ◇, Optigene 3 ◇, Tetrasine ◇, Visine Moisturizing ◇

Pharmacologic class: sympathomimetic
Pregnancy risk category C

AVAILABLE FORMS

Ophthalmic solution: 0.05% ◇

INDICATIONS & DOSAGES

➤ **Conjunctival congestion, irritation, and allergic conditions**

Adults and children older than age 2: Instill 1 to 2 drops of 0.05% solution up to q.i.d. or as directed by prescriber.

ACTION

Thought to cause vasoconstriction by local adrenergic action on the blood vessels of the conjunctiva.

Route	Onset	Peak	Duration
Ophthalmic	Few min	Unknown	1–4 hr

Half-life: Unknown.

ADVERSE REACTIONS

CNS: dizziness, drowsiness, headache, insomnia, tremor.
CV: ***arrhythmias.***
EENT: eye irritation, increased intraocular pressure, keratitis, lacrimation, pupillary dilation, transient eye stinging.

INTERACTIONS

Drug-drug. *Anesthetics:* Cyclopropane and halothane may sensitize the myocardium to sympathomimetics; local anesthetics may increase the absorption of topical drugs. Monitor patient for increased adverse effects.
Beta blockers: May cause more systemic adverse effects. Monitor patient for adverse systemic effects.
Guanethidine, MAO inhibitors, tricyclic antidepressants: May cause hypertensive crisis if tetrahydrozoline is systemically absorbed. Avoid using together.

EFFECTS ON LAB TEST RESULTS

None reported.

CONTRAINDICATIONS & CAUTIONS

- Contraindicated in patients hypersensitive to drug or its components and in those with angle-closure glaucoma or other serious eye disease.
- Use cautiously in patients with hyperthyroidism, heart disease, hypertension, or diabetes mellitus.

NURSING CONSIDERATIONS

- Rebound congestion may occur with frequent or prolonged use.
- ***Alert:*** Don't confuse Visine with Visken.

PATIENT TEACHING

- Teach patient how to instill drug. Advise him to wash hands before and after instillation and to apply light finger pressure on lacrimal sac for 1 minute after drops are instilled. Warn him not to touch tip of dropper to eye or surrounding tissue.
- Warn patient not to exceed recommended dosage.
- Tell patient to stop drug and notify prescriber if redness or irritation persists or increases or if no relief occurs within 2 days.
- Warn patient not to share eye drops.

82
Miscellaneous ophthalmics

azelastine hydrochloride
betaxolol hydrochloride
bimatoprost
brimonidine tartrate
carteolol hydrochloride
dorzolamide hydrochloride
epinastine hydrochloride
ketotifen fumarate
latanoprost
levobunolol hydrochloride
timolol maleate
travoprost

azelastine hydrochloride
Optivar

Pharmacologic class: H_1 receptor antagonist
Pregnancy risk category C

AVAILABLE FORMS
Ophthalmic solution: 0.05%

INDICATIONS & DOSAGES
➤ **Pruritus from allergic conjunctivitis**
Adults and children age 3 and older: Instill 1 drop into affected eye b.i.d.

ACTION
Inhibits the release of histamine and other mediators from cells involved in the allergic response.

Route	Onset	Peak	Duration
Ophthalmic	3 min	Unknown	8 hr

Half-life: 22 hours.

ADVERSE REACTIONS
CNS: *headache,* fatigue.
EENT: *bitter taste, transient eye burning or stinging,* conjunctivitis, eye pain, pharyngitis, rhinitis, temporary blurring.
Respiratory: asthma, dyspnea.
Skin: pruritus.
Other: flulike syndrome.

INTERACTIONS
None reported.

EFFECTS ON LAB TEST RESULTS
None reported.

CONTRAINDICATIONS & CAUTIONS
- Contraindicated in patients hypersensitive to any of drug's components.
- Contraindicated for irritation related to contact lenses.

NURSING CONSIDERATIONS
- Drug is for ophthalmic use only. Don't inject or give orally.

PATIENT TEACHING
- Instruct patient not to touch any surface, eyelid, or surrounding areas with tip of dropper.
- Tell patient to keep bottle tightly closed when not in use.
- Advise patient not to wear contact lens if eye is red.
- Warn patient that soft contact lenses may absorb the preservative benzalkonium.
- Instruct patient who wears soft contact lenses and whose eyes aren't red to wait at least 10 minutes after instilling drug before inserting contact lenses.

betaxolol hydrochloride
Betoptic, Betoptic S

Pharmacologic class: cardioselective beta blocker
Pregnancy risk category C

AVAILABLE FORMS
Ophthalmic solution: 0.5%
Ophthalmic suspension: 0.25%

INDICATIONS & DOSAGES
➤ **Chronic open-angle glaucoma, ocular hypertension**
Adults: Instill 1 or 2 drops of 0.5% solution or 0.25% suspension b.i.d.

ACTION

Unknown. Reduces aqueous formation and may increase outflow of aqueous humor.

Route	Onset	Peak	Duration
Ophthalmic	30–60 min	2 hr	> 12 hr

Half-life: Unknown.

ADVERSE REACTIONS

CNS: ***stroke,*** depressive neurosis, insomnia.
CV: ***arrhythmias, heart block, heart failure,*** palpitations.
EENT: *eye stinging on instillation causing brief discomfort,* erythema, itching, keratitis, occasional tearing, photophobia.
Respiratory: ***bronchospasm,*** asthma.

INTERACTIONS

Drug-drug. *Calcium channel blockers:* May cause AV conduction disturbances, ventricular failure, and hypotension if significant systemic absorption occurs. Monitor patient closely.
Cardiac glycosides: May cause excessive bradycardia if significant systemic absorption occurs. Patient may need ECG monitoring.
Dipivefrin, ophthalmic epinephrine: May produce mydriasis. Use together cautiously.
Inhaled hydrocarbon anesthetics: May prolong severe hypotension if significant systemic absorption occurs. Tell anesthesiologist that patient is receiving ophthalmic betaxolol.
Insulin, oral antidiabetics: May cause hypoglycemia or hyperglycemia if significant systemic absorption occurs. May need to adjust dosage of antidiabetics.
Phenothiazines: May have additive hypotensive effects; may increase risk of adverse effects if significant systemic absorption occurs. Monitor patient closely.
Prazosin: May increase risk of orthostatic hypotension in early phases of use together. Assist patient to stand slowly until effects are known.
Reserpine: May cause excessive beta blockade. Monitor patient closely.
Systemic beta blockers: May have additive effects. Monitor patient closely.
Verapamil: May increase effects of both drugs. Monitor cardiac function closely and decrease dosages as necessary.
Drug-lifestyle. *Cocaine use:* May inhibit betaxolol's effects. Tell patient about this interaction.
Sun exposure: May cause photophobia. Advise patient to wear sunglasses.

EFFECTS ON LAB TEST RESULTS

None reported.

CONTRAINDICATIONS & CAUTIONS

- Contraindicated in patients hypersensitive to drug and in those with sinus bradycardia, greater than first-degree AV block, cardiogenic shock, or overt heart failure.
- Use cautiously in patients with restricted pulmonary function, diabetes mellitus, hyperthyroidism, or history of heart failure.

NURSING CONSIDERATIONS

- Stabilization of intraocular pressure (IOP)–lowering response may take a few weeks. Determine IOP after 4 weeks of treatment.

PATIENT TEACHING

- Teach patient how to instill drug. Advise him to wash hands before and after instillation and to apply light finger pressure on lacrimal sac for 1 minute after instilling drug. Warn him not to touch tip of dropper to eye or surrounding tissue. Tell him to shake suspension well before instilling.
- Encourage patient to comply with twice-daily regimen.
- Tell patient to remove contact lenses before instilling drug. Lenses may be reinserted about 15 minutes after using drops.
- Advise patient to ease sun sensitivity by wearing sunglasses.

bimatoprost

Lumigan

Pharmacologic class: prostaglandin analogue
Pregnancy risk category C

AVAILABLE FORMS

Ophthalmic solution: 0.03%

INDICATIONS & DOSAGES

➤ **Increased intraocular pressure (IOP) in patients with open-angle glaucoma or ocular hypertension**

Adults: Instill 1 drop in conjunctival sac of affected eye once daily in the evening.

ACTION

Has ocular hypotensive activity, which selectively mimics the effects of naturally occurring prostaglandins. Drug may also increase outflow of aqueous humor.

Route	Onset	Peak	Duration
Ophthalmic	4 hr	8–12 hr	Unknown

Half-life: 45 minutes.

ADVERSE REACTIONS

CNS: headache, asthenia.
EENT: *conjunctival hyperemia, growth of eyelashes, ocular pruritus,* allergic conjunctivitis, asthenopia, blepharitis, cataract, conjunctival edema, eye discharge, tearing, and pain, eyelash darkening, eyelid erythema, foreign body sensation, increase in iris pigmentation, ocular burning, dryness, and irritation, photophobia, pigmentation of the periocular skin, superficial punctate keratitis, visual disturbance.
Respiratory: *upper respiratory tract infection.*
Skin: hirsutism.
Other: *infection.*

INTERACTIONS

None known.

EFFECTS ON LAB TEST RESULTS

- May cause abnormal liver function test values.

CONTRAINDICATIONS & CAUTIONS

- Contraindicated in patients hypersensitive to bimatoprost, benzalkonium chloride, or other ingredients in product.
- Contraindicated in patients with angle-closure glaucoma or inflammatory or neovascular glaucoma.
- Use cautiously in patients with renal or hepatic impairment.
- Use cautiously in patients with active intraocular inflammation (iritis, uveitis), aphakic patients, pseudophakic patients with torn posterior lens capsule, and patients at risk for macular edema.

NURSING CONSIDERATIONS

- Temporary or permanent increased pigmentation of iris and eyelid, as well as increased pigmentation and growth of eyelashes, may occur.
- Patient should remove contact lenses before using solution. Lenses may be reinserted 15 minutes after administration.
- If more than one ophthalmic drug is being used, give drugs at least 5 minutes apart.
- Store drug in original container between 59° and 77° F (15° and 25° C).

PATIENT TEACHING

- Tell patient receiving treatment in only one eye about potential for increased brown pigmentation of iris, eyelid skin darkening, and increased length, thickness, pigmentation, or number of lashes in treated eye.
- Teach patient how to instill drops, and advise him to wash hands before and after instilling solution. Warn him not to touch tip of dropper to eye or surrounding tissue.
- If eye trauma or infection occurs or if eye surgery is needed, tell patient to seek medical advice before continuing to use multidose container.
- Advise patient to immediately report eye inflammation or lid reactions.
- Advise patient to apply light pressure on lacrimal sac for 1 minute after instillation to minimize systemic absorption of drug.
- Tell patient to remove contact lenses before using solution and that lenses may be reinserted 15 minutes after administration.
- If patient is using more than one ophthalmic drug, tell him to apply them at least 5 minutes apart.
- Stress importance of compliance with recommended therapy.

brimonidine tartrate
Alphagan P

Pharmacologic class: selective alpha$_2$ agonist
Pregnancy risk category B

AVAILABLE FORMS
Ophthalmic solution: 0.1%, 0.15%

INDICATIONS & DOSAGES
➤**To reduce intraocular pressure (IOP) in open-angle glaucoma or ocular hypertension**
Adults: Give 1 drop in affected eye t.i.d., about 8 hours apart.

ACTION
Reduces aqueous humor production and increases uveoscleral outflow.

Route	Onset	Peak	Duration
Ophthalmic	Unknown	30 min–2½ hr	Unknown

Half-life: 2 hours.

ADVERSE REACTIONS
CNS: asthenia, dizziness, headache.
CV: hypertension, hypotension.
EENT: *allergic conjunctivitis, ocular hyperemia, pruritus,* abnormal vision, allergic reaction, blepharitis, burning, conjunctival edema, hemorrhage, or inflammation, dryness, eyelid edema or erythema, follicular conjunctivitis, foreign body sensation, increased tearing, pain, pharyngitis, photophobia, rhinitis, sinus infection or inflammation, stinging, superficial punctate keratopathy, visual disturbances, visual field defect, vitreous floaters, worsened visual acuity.
GI: dyspepsia, oral dryness.
Respiratory: bronchitis, cough, dyspnea.
Skin: rash.
Other: flulike syndrome.

INTERACTIONS
Drug-drug. *Apraclonidine, dorzolamide, pilocarpine, timolol:* May have additive IOP-lowering effects. Use cautiously together.
Antihypertensives, beta blockers, cardiac glycosides: May further decrease blood pressure or pulse. Monitor vital signs.
CNS depressants: May increase effects. Use cautiously together.
MAO inhibitors: May increase effects. Avoid using together.
Tricyclic antidepressants: May interfere with brimonidine's effect. Use cautiously together.
Drug-lifestyle. *Alcohol use:* May increase CNS-depressant effect. Urge patient to avoid alcohol.

EFFECTS ON LAB TEST RESULTS
None reported.

CONTRAINDICATIONS & CAUTIONS
- Contraindicated in patients hypersensitive to drug or benzalkonium chloride and in those taking MAO inhibitors.
- Use cautiously in patients with CV disease, cerebral or coronary insufficiency, hepatic or renal impairment, depression, Raynaud phenomenon, orthostatic hypotension, or thromboangiitis obliterans.

NURSING CONSIDERATIONS
- Monitor IOP because drug effect may reverse after first month of therapy.

PATIENT TEACHING
- Tell patient to wait at least 15 minutes after instilling drug before wearing soft contact lenses.
- Caution patient to avoid hazardous activities because of risk of decreased mental alertness, fatigue, or drowsiness.
- Advise patient to avoid alcohol.

carteolol hydrochloride
Ocupress

Pharmacologic class: nonselective beta blocker
Pregnancy risk category C

AVAILABLE FORMS
Ophthalmic solution: 1%

INDICATIONS & DOSAGES

➤ **Chronic open-angle glaucoma, intraocular hypertension**

Adults: One drop into conjunctival sac of each affected eye b.i.d.

ACTION

Exact mechanism unknown. Reduces intraocular pressure (IOP) by decreasing aqueous humor production.

Route	Onset	Peak	Duration
Ophthalmic	Unknown	2 hr	12 hr

Half-life: Unknown.

ADVERSE REACTIONS

CNS: asthenia, dizziness, headache, insomnia.
CV: ***arrhythmias, bradycardia,*** hypotension, palpitations.
EENT: *burning, conjunctival hyperemia, edema, ocular tearing, transient eye irritation,* abnormal corneal staining, blepharoconjunctivitis, blurred and cloudy vision, corneal sensitivity, decreased night vision, photophobia, ptosis, sinusitis.
GI: constipation, diarrhea, nausea, taste perversion, vomiting.
Respiratory: ***bronchospasm,*** dyspnea.

INTERACTIONS

Drug-drug. *Aminophylline, theophylline:* May act antagonistically, reducing the effects of one or both drugs. May reduce elimination of theophylline. Monitor theophylline levels and patient closely.
Catecholamine-depleting drugs such as reserpine, oral beta blockers: May cause additive effects and development of hypotension or bradycardia. Monitor patient closely; monitor vital signs.
Clonidine: May cause significant increase in blood pressure when either drug is started or stopped. Monitor blood pressure if used together.
Epinephrine: May cause an initial hypertensive episode followed by bradycardia. Stop beta blocker 3 days before anticipated epinephrine use. Monitor patient closely.
Glucagon: May decrease the effect of glucagon. Monitor for therapeutic effect; consider oral glucose supplement if appropriate.
Insulin: May mask symptoms of hypoglycemia as a result of beta blockade (such as tachycardia). Use together cautiously in patients with diabetes.
Prazosin: May increase risk of orthostatic hypotension in early phases of use together. Assist patient to stand slowly until effects are known.
Verapamil: May increase effects of both drugs. Monitor cardiac function closely and decrease dosages as necessary.
Drug-lifestyle. *Sun exposure:* May cause photophobia. Advise patient to wear sunglasses.

EFFECTS ON LAB TEST RESULTS

None reported.

CONTRAINDICATIONS & CAUTIONS

- Contraindicated in patients hypersensitive to drug or its components and in those with bronchial asthma, severe COPD, sinus bradycardia, second- or third-degree AV block, overt cardiac failure, or cardiogenic shock.
- Use cautiously in patients hypersensitive to other beta blockers; in those with nonallergic bronchospastic disease, diabetes mellitus, hyperthyroidism, or decreased pulmonary function; and in breast-feeding women.

NURSING CONSIDERATIONS

- Monitor vital signs.
- ***Alert:*** Stop drug at first sign of cardiac failure, and notify prescriber.

PATIENT TEACHING

- If patient is using more than one topical ophthalmic drug, tell him to apply them at least 10 minutes apart.
- Teach patient how to instill drops. Advise him to wash hands before and after instillation, and warn him not to touch tip of dropper to eye or surrounding tissue.
- Advise patient to apply light finger pressure on lacrimal sac for 1 minute after drug instillation to minimize systemic absorption.
- Tell patient to remove contact lenses before instilling drug.
- Instruct patient to keep bottle tightly closed when not in use and to protect it from light.

• Tell patient that drug is a beta blocker and, although given topically, may be absorbed systemically, causing adverse effects. Advise patient to monitor heart rate and blood pressure closely, to report slow heart rate to prescriber, and, if signs or symptoms of serious adverse reactions or hypersensitivity occur, to stop drug and notify prescriber immediately.
• Stress importance of compliance with recommended therapy.
• Advise patient to ease sun sensitivity by wearing sunglasses.

dorzolamide hydrochloride
Trusopt

Pharmacologic class: carbonic anhydrase inhibitor, sulfonamide
Pregnancy risk category C

AVAILABLE FORMS
Ophthalmic solution: 2%

INDICATIONS & DOSAGES
➤Increased intraocular pressure (IOP) in patients with ocular hypertension or open-angle glaucoma
Adults and children: One drop into conjunctival sac of each affected eye t.i.d.

ACTION
Decreases aqueous humor secretion, presumably by slowing the formation of bicarbonate ions. This reduces sodium and fluid transport, reducing IOP.

Route	Onset	Peak	Duration
Ophthalmic	1–2 hr	2–3 hr	8 hr

Half-life: 4 months.

ADVERSE REACTIONS
CNS: asthenia, fatigue, headache.
EENT: *blurred vision, dryness, lacrimation, ocular allergic reaction, ocular burning, stinging, and discomfort, photophobia, superficial punctate keratitis,* iridocyclitis.
GI: *bitter taste,* nausea.
GU: urolithiasis.
Skin: rash.

INTERACTIONS
Drug-drug. *Oral carbonic anhydrase inhibitors, salicylates:* May cause additive effects. Avoid using together.

EFFECTS ON LAB TEST RESULTS
None reported.

CONTRAINDICATIONS & CAUTIONS
• Contraindicated in patients hypersensitive to drug or its components.
• Use cautiously in patients with hepatic or renal impairment.

NURSING CONSIDERATIONS
• If more than one topical ophthalmic drug is used, give drugs at least 10 minutes apart.

PATIENT TEACHING
• Teach patient how to instill drops. Advise him to wash hands before and after instillation, and warn him not to touch tip of dropper to eye or surrounding tissue.
• Tell patient that drug is a sulfonamide and, although it's given topically, it can be absorbed systemically. Advise patient to apply light finger pressure on lacrimal sac for 1 minute after drug instillation to minimize systemic absorption.
• Tell patient to stop drug and notify prescriber immediately if signs or symptoms of serious adverse reactions or hypersensitivity occur, including eye inflammation and eyelid reactions.
• Tell patient not to wear soft contact lenses during therapy.
• Stress importance of compliance with recommended therapy.

epinastine hydrochloride
Elestat

Pharmacologic class: H_1 receptor antagonist and mast cell stabilizer
Pregnancy risk category C

AVAILABLE FORMS
Ophthalmic solution: 0.05%

INDICATIONS & DOSAGES

➤ **To prevent pruritus from allergic conjunctivitis**

Adults and children age 3 and older: Instill 1 drop into each eye b.i.d. Continue treatment as long as allergen is present, even if symptoms resolve.

ACTION

Inhibits release of mediators from cells involved in hypersensitivity reactions, temporarily preventing pruritus.

Route	Onset	Peak	Duration
Ophthalmic	Immediate	Unknown	8 hr

Half-life: About 12 hours.

ADVERSE REACTIONS

CNS: headache.
EENT: *cold symptoms,* burning eyes, hyperemia, increased lymph nodes near eyes, pharyngitis, pruritus, rhinitis, sinusitis.
Respiratory: increased cough, *upper respiratory tract infection.*

INTERACTIONS

None reported.

EFFECTS ON LAB TEST RESULTS

None reported.

CONTRAINDICATIONS & CAUTIONS

- Contraindicated in patients hypersensitive to drug or its components.
- Contraindicated for irritation related to contact lenses.
- Use cautiously in pregnant or breast-feeding women.
- Safety and effectiveness haven't been established in children younger than age 3.

NURSING CONSIDERATIONS

- Drug is for ophthalmic use only. Don't inject or give orally.
- Monitor patient for signs and symptoms of infection.
- Soft contact lenses may absorb the preservative benzalkonium.

PATIENT TEACHING

- Teach patient proper instillation technique. Instruct him not to touch any surface, eyelid, or surrounding areas with tip of dropper.
- Caution patient not to use drops to treat contact lens–related eye irritation and not to wear contact lenses if eyes are red.
- Warn patient that soft contact lenses may absorb the preservative benzalkonium.
- Advise patient to report adverse reactions to drug.
- Tell patient to keep bottle tightly closed when not in use.
- Instruct patient who wears soft contact lenses and whose eyes aren't red to wait at least 10 minutes after instilling drug before inserting contact lenses.

ketotifen fumarate

Zaditor

Pharmacologic class: H_1 receptor antagonist and mast cell stabilizer
Pregnancy risk category C

AVAILABLE FORMS

Ophthalmic solution: 0.025%

INDICATIONS & DOSAGES

➤ **To temporarily prevent eye itching from allergic conjunctivitis**

Adults and children age 4 and older: Instill 1 drop in each affected eye q 8 to 12 hours.

ACTION

Stabilizes mast cells to inhibit release of mediators involved in hypersensitivity reactions and blocks action of histamine at the H_1 receptor, temporarily preventing itching of the eye.

Route	Onset	Peak	Duration
Ophthalmic	Within min	Unknown	Unknown

Half-life: Unknown.

ADVERSE REACTIONS

CNS: *headache.*
EENT: *conjunctival infection, rhinitis,* burning or stinging of eyes, conjunctivitis, dry eyes, eye discharge, eye pain, eyelid disorder, itching of eyes, keratitis, lacrimation disorder, mydriasis, ocular allergic reactions, ocular rash, pharyngitis, photophobia.
Other: flulike syndrome.

INTERACTIONS
None significant.

EFFECTS ON LAB TEST RESULTS
None reported.

CONTRAINDICATIONS & CAUTIONS
- Contraindicated in patients hypersensitive to components of drug.
- Contraindicated for irritation related to contact lenses.

NURSING CONSIDERATIONS
- Drug is for ophthalmic use only. Don't inject or give orally.
- Drug isn't indicated for irritation related to contact lenses.
- Soft contact lenses may absorb the preservative benzalkonium. Contact lenses shouldn't be inserted until 10 minutes after drug is instilled.
- To prevent contaminating dropper tip and solution, don't touch eyelids or surrounding areas with dropper tip of bottle.

PATIENT TEACHING
- Teach patient the proper technique for instilling drops.
- Advise patient not to wear contact lens if eye is red. Warn him not to use drug to treat contact lens–related irritation.
- Instruct patient who wears soft contact lenses and whose eyes aren't red to wait at least 10 minutes after instilling drug before inserting contact lenses.
- Advise patient to report adverse reactions.
- Advise patient to keep bottle tightly closed when not in use.

latanoprost
Xalatan

Pharmacologic class: prostaglandin analogue
Pregnancy risk category C

AVAILABLE FORMS
Ophthalmic solution: 0.005% (50 mcg/ml)

INDICATIONS & DOSAGES
➤ **First-line treatment of increased intraocular pressure (IOP) in patients with ocular hypertension or open-angle glaucoma**
Adults: Instill 1 drop in conjunctival sac of each affected eye once daily at bedtime.

ACTION
A prostaglandin F_2 alpha-analogue believed to increase outflow of aqueous humor, thereby lowering IOP.

Route	Onset	Peak	Duration
Ophthalmic	3–4 hr	8–12 hr	Unknown

Half-life: 3 hours (from aqueous humor).

ADVERSE REACTIONS
CV: angina pectoris.
EENT: *blurred vision, burning, foreign body sensation, increased brown pigmentation of the iris, itching, stinging,* conjunctival hyperemia, dry eye, excessive tearing, eye pain, eyelash changes, lid crusting or edema, lid discomfort, photophobia, punctate epithelial keratopathy.
Musculoskeletal: muscle, joint, or back pain.
Respiratory: upper respiratory tract infection.
Skin: allergic skin reaction, rash.
Other: cold, flulike syndrome.

INTERACTIONS
Drug-drug. *Eyedrops that contain thimerosal:* May cause precipitation of eyedrops. Give at least 5 minutes apart.

EFFECTS ON LAB TEST RESULTS
None reported.

CONTRAINDICATIONS & CAUTIONS
- Contraindicated in patients hypersensitive to drug, benzalkonium chloride, or other components of drug.
- Use cautiously in patients with impaired renal or hepatic function.
- Use cautiously in breast-feeding women; it's unknown if drug appears in breast milk.
- Safety and effectiveness of drug in children haven't been established.

NURSING CONSIDERATIONS
- Don't give drug while patient is wearing contact lenses.

• Giving drug more frequently than recommended may decrease its IOP-lowering effects; don't exceed once-daily dosing.
• Drug may gradually change eye color, increasing amount of brown pigment in iris. This change in iris color occurs slowly and may not be noticeable for months or years. Increased pigmentation may be permanent.
• To avoid ocular infections, don't allow tip of dispenser to contact eye or surrounding tissue. Serious damage to eye and subsequent vision loss may be caused by contaminated solutions.

PATIENT TEACHING
• Inform patient of risk that iris color may change in treated eye.
• Teach patient how to instill drops, and advise him to wash hands before and after instilling solution. Warn him not to touch tip of dropper to eye or surrounding tissue.
• Advise patient to apply light finger pressure on lacrimal sac for 1 minute after instillation to minimize systemic absorption.
• Instruct patient to report reactions in the eye, especially eye inflammation and lid reactions.
• Tell patient who wears contact lenses to remove them before instilling solution and not to reinsert the lenses until 15 minutes have elapsed.
• If patient is using more than one topical ophthalmic drug, tell him to apply them at least 5 minutes apart.
• If patient develops another eye condition (such as trauma or infection) or needs eye surgery, advise him to contact prescriber about continued use of multidose container.
• Stress importance of compliance with recommended therapy.

levobunolol hydrochloride
AKBeta, Betagan

Pharmacologic class: non-selective beta blocker
Pregnancy risk category C

AVAILABLE FORMS
Ophthalmic solution: 0.25%, 0.5%

INDICATIONS & DOSAGES
➤ Chronic open-angle glaucoma, ocular hypertension
Adults: One or two drops once daily (0.5%) or b.i.d. (0.25%).

ACTION
Thought to reduce formation, and possibly increase outflow, of aqueous humor.

Route	Onset	Peak	Duration
Ophthalmic	1 hr	2–6 hr	24 hr

Half-life: Unknown.

ADVERSE REACTIONS
CNS: *syncope,* depression, headache, insomnia.
CV: *hypotension,* ***bradycardia, heart failure,*** slight reduction in resting heart rate.
EENT: *transient eye stinging and burning,* blepharoconjunctivitis, corneal punctate staining, decreased corneal sensitivity, erythema, itching, keratitis, photophobia, tearing.
GI: nausea.
Respiratory: ***bronchospasm.***
Skin: urticaria.

INTERACTIONS
Drug-drug. *Dipivefrin, epinephrine, systemically administered carbonic anhydrase inhibitors, topical miotics:* May further reduce intraocular pressure (IOP). Use together cautiously.
Metoprolol, propranolol, other oral beta blockers: May increase ocular and systemic effects. Use together cautiously.
Reserpine, other catecholamine-depleting drugs: May increase hypotensive and bradycardiac effects. Monitor blood pressure and heart rate closely.
Drug-lifestyle. *Sun exposure:* May cause photophobia. Advise patient to wear sunglasses.

EFFECTS ON LAB TEST RESULTS
None reported.

CONTRAINDICATIONS & CAUTIONS
• Contraindicated in patients hypersensitive to drug and in those with bronchial asthma, sinus bradycardia, second- or third-degree AV block, cardiac failure,

cardiogenic shock, or history of bronchial asthma or severe COPD.
- Use cautiously in patients with chronic bronchitis, emphysema, diabetes mellitus, hyperthyroidism, or myasthenia gravis.
- Safe use in pregnant or breast-feeding women hasn't been established.

NURSING CONSIDERATIONS
- Don't let tip of dropper touch patient's eye or surrounding tissue.

PATIENT TEACHING
- Teach patient how to instill drug. Advise him to wash hands before and after instillation and to apply light finger pressure on lacrimal sac for 1 minute after drops are instilled.
- Warn patient not to touch tip of dropper to eye or surrounding tissue.
- Advise elderly patient to report shortness of breath, chest pain, or heart irregularities to prescriber. Drug may be absorbed systemically and produce signs and symptoms of beta blockade.
- Advise patient to carry medical identification at all times during therapy.

timolol maleate
Betimol, Istalol, Timoptic, Timoptic-XE

Pharmacologic class: beta blocker
Pregnancy risk category C

AVAILABLE FORMS
Ophthalmic gel: 0.25%, 0.5%
Ophthalmic solution: 0.25%, 0.5%

INDICATIONS & DOSAGES
➤ To reduce intraocular pressure (IOP) in ocular hypertension or open-angle glaucoma
Adults: Initially, 1 drop of 0.25% solution in each affected eye b.i.d.; maintenance dosage is 1 drop once daily. If no response, instill 1 drop of 0.5% solution in each affected eye b.i.d. If IOP is controlled, reduce dosage to 1 drop daily. Or, 1 drop of gel in each affected eye once daily. Or, for Istalol, initially 1 drop 0.5% solution in each affected eye once daily in the morning. If response is unsatisfactory, concomitant therapy may be considered.

ACTION
Thought to reduce formation, and possibly increase outflow, of aqueous humor.

Route	Onset	Peak	Duration
Ophthalmic	30 min	1–2 hr	12–24 hr

Half-life: Unknown.

ADVERSE REACTIONS
CNS: *syncope, **stroke,*** confusion, depression, dizziness, fatigue, hallucinations, lethargy.
CV: *hypotension, **arrhythmia, bradycardia, cardiac arrest, heart block, heart failure,*** palpitations, slight reduction in resting heart rate.
EENT: blepharitis, conjunctivitis, decreased corneal sensitivity with long-term use, diplopia, keratitis, minor eye irritation, ptosis, visual disturbances.
Metabolic: hyperglycemia, hyperuricemia.
Respiratory: ***bronchospasm in patients with history of asthma,*** dyspnea, respiratory infection.

INTERACTIONS
Drug-drug. *Aminophylline, theophylline:* May act antagonistically, reducing effects of one or both drugs; may also reduce elimination of theophylline. Monitor theophylline level and patient closely.
Calcium channel blockers, cardiac glycosides, quinidine: May increase risk of adverse cardiac effects if significant amounts of timolol are systemically absorbed. Use together cautiously.
Cimetidine: May increase beta blocker effects. Consider another H_2 agonist or decrease dose of beta blocker.
Epinephrine: May cause a hypertensive episode, followed by bradycardia. Stop beta blocker 3 days before starting epinephrine. Monitor patient closely.
Insulin, Oral antidiabetic agents: May mask symptoms of hypoglycemia (such as tachycardia) as a result of beta blockade. Use together cautiously in patients with diabetes.

Oral beta blockers: May increase ocular and systemic effects. Use together cautiously.
Prazosin: May increase risk of orthostatic hypotension in early phases of use together. Assist patient to stand slowly until effects are known.
Reserpine, other catecholamine-depleting drugs: May increase hypotensive and bradycardia-induced effects. Avoid using together.
Verapamil: May increase effects of both drugs. Monitor cardiac function closely and decrease dosages as necessary.

EFFECTS ON LAB TEST RESULTS

- May increase BUN, potassium, glucose, and uric acid levels.

CONTRAINDICATIONS & CAUTIONS

- Contraindicated in patients hypersensitive to drug and in those with bronchial asthma, sinus bradycardia, second- or third-degree AV block, cardiac failure, cardiogenic shock, or history of bronchial asthma or severe COPD.
- Use cautiously in patients with nonallergic bronchospasm, chronic bronchitis, emphysema, diabetes mellitus, hyperthyroidism, or cerebrovascular insufficiency.

NURSING CONSIDERATIONS

- Give other ophthalmic drugs at least 10 minutes before giving gel form of drug.
- Monitor diabetic patients carefully. Systemic beta-blocking effects can mask some signs and symptoms of hypoglycemia.
- Some patients may need a few weeks of treatment to stabilize pressure-lowering response. Determine IOP after 4 weeks of treatment.
- Drug can be used safely in patients with glaucoma who wear conventional polymethylmethacrylate (abbreviated PMMA) hard contact lenses.
- ***Look alike–sound alike:*** Don't confuse timolol with atenolol, or Timoptic with Viroptic.

PATIENT TEACHING

- Teach patient how to instill drops. Advise him to wash hands before and after instillation and to apply light finger pressure on lacrimal sac for 1 minute after drops are instilled. Warn patient not to touch tip of dropper to eye or surrounding tissue.
- Instruct patient using gel to invert container and shake once before each use. Also tell him to use other ophthalmic drugs at least 10 minutes before applying gel.
- Tell patient to instill drug without contact lenses in place. Lenses may be reinserted about 15 minutes after drug use.
- Drug may be absorbed systemically and produce signs and symptoms of beta blockade. Advise patient to monitor pulse rate and report slow rate to prescriber.
- Tell patient to report difficulty breathing or chest pain to prescriber.

travoprost

Travatan

Pharmacologic class: prostaglandin analogue
Pregnancy risk category C

AVAILABLE FORMS

Ophthalmic solution: 0.004%

INDICATIONS & DOSAGES

➤ **To reduce intraocular pressure (IOP) in patients with open-angle glaucoma or ocular hypertension who can't tolerate or who respond inadequately to other IOP-lowering drugs**
Adults: One drop in conjunctival sac of each affected eye once daily at bedtime.

ACTION

Thought to reduce IOP by increasing uveoscleral outflow.

Route	Onset	Peak	Duration
Ophthalmic	Unknown	30 min	Unknown

Half-life: 45 minutes.

ADVERSE REACTIONS

CNS: anxiety, depression, headache, pain.
CV: ***bradycardia,*** angina pectoris, chest pain, hypertension, hypotension.
EENT: *eye discomfort, eye pain, eye pruritus, decreased visual acuity, foreign*

body sensation, ocular hyperemia, abnormal vision, blepharitis, blurred vision, cataract, conjunctival hyperemia, conjunctivitis, dry eye, eye disorder, iris discoloration, keratitis, lid margin crusting, photophobia, sinusitis, subconjunctival hemorrhage, tearing.
GI: dyspepsia, GI disorder.
GU: prostate disorder, urinary incontinence, UTI.
Metabolic: hypercholesterolemia.
Musculoskeletal: arthritis, back pain.
Respiratory: bronchitis.
Other: accidental injury, cold syndrome, infection.

INTERACTIONS

Drug-herb. *Areca, jaborandi:* May increase effects. Discourage use together.

EFFECTS ON LAB TEST RESULTS

- May increase cholesterol level.

CONTRAINDICATIONS & CAUTIONS

- Contraindicated in patients hypersensitive to drug, benzalkonium chloride, or other drug components; in pregnant women or women trying to become pregnant; and in those with angle-closure, inflammatory, or neovascular glaucoma.
- Use cautiously in patients with renal or hepatic impairment, active intraocular inflammation (iritis, uveitis), or risk factors for macular edema.
- Use cautiously in aphakic patients and pseudophakic patients with a torn posterior lens capsule.

NURSING CONSIDERATIONS

- Temporary or permanent increased pigmentation of the iris and eyelid may occur as well as increased pigmentation and growth of eyelashes.
- Patient should remove contact lenses before instilling drug and reinsert them 15 minutes after administration.
- If using more than one ophthalmic drug, give the drugs at least 5 minutes apart.
- Store drug between 36° and 77° (2° and 25° C).
- If a pregnant woman or a woman attempting to become pregnant accidentally comes in contact with drug, thoroughly cleanse the exposed area with soap and water immediately.

PATIENT TEACHING

- Teach patient how to instill drops, and advise him to wash hands before and after instilling solution. Warn him not to touch tip of dropper to eye or surrounding tissue.
- Advise patient to apply light finger pressure on lacrimal sac for 1 minute after instillation to minimize systemic absorption of drug.
- Tell patient to remove contact lenses before administration and explain that he can reinsert them 15 minutes afterward.
- Tell patient receiving treatment in only one eye about potential for increased iris pigmentation, eyelid darkening, and increased length, thickness, pigmentation, or number of lashes in the treated eye.
- If eye trauma or infection occurs or if eye surgery is needed, advise patient to seek medical advice before continuing to use the multidose container.
- Advise patient to immediately report eye inflammation or lid reactions.
- If patient is using more than one ophthalmic drug, tell him to apply them at least 5 minutes apart.
- Stress importance of compliance with recommended therapy.
- Tell patient to discard container within 6 weeks of removing it from the sealed pouch.
- If a pregnant woman or a woman attempting to become pregnant accidentally comes in contact with drug, tell her to thoroughly cleanse the exposed area with soap and water immediately.

83
Otics

boric acid
chloramphenicol

boric acid

Auro-Dri ◊, Dri/Ear ◊, Ear-Dry ◊

Pharmacologic class: bacteriostatic, fungistatic
Pregnancy risk category NR

AVAILABLE FORMS

Otic solution: 2.75% boric acid in isopropyl alcohol

INDICATIONS & DOSAGES

➤ **External ear canal infection**

Adults and children: 3 to 8 drops into ear canal t.i.d. or q.i.d.; plug with cotton.

ACTION

A weak bacteriostatic that inhibits or destroys bacteria in the ear canal. Also a fungistatic.

Route	Onset	Peak	Duration
Otic	Unknown	Unknown	Unknown

Half-life: Unknown.

ADVERSE REACTIONS

EENT: ear irritation or itching.
Skin: urticaria.
Other: overgrowth of nonsusceptible organisms.

INTERACTIONS

None significant.

EFFECTS ON LAB TEST RESULTS

None reported.

CONTRAINDICATIONS & CAUTIONS

- Contraindicated in patients with perforated eardrum or excoriated membranes.

NURSING CONSIDERATIONS

- Monitor patient for signs and symptoms of superinfection.

PATIENT TEACHING

- Show patient or caregiver how to give drug.
- To prevent reinfection, warn patient not to touch ear with dropper.
- Tell patient to always moisten cotton plug with drug.

chloramphenicol

Chloromycetin Otic

Pharmacologic class: dichloroacetic acid derivative
Pregnancy risk category C

AVAILABLE FORMS

Otic solution: 0.5%

INDICATIONS & DOSAGES

➤ **External ear canal infection**

Adults and children: Give 2 to 3 drops into ear canal t.i.d.

ACTION

Inhibits or destroys bacteria in ear canal.

Route	Onset	Peak	Duration
Otic	Unknown	Unknown	Unknown

Half-life: Unknown.

ADVERSE REACTIONS

EENT: ear itching or burning.
GU: hemoglobinuria.
Hematologic: ***aplastic anemia, bone marrow depression,*** bone marrow hypoplasia.
Metabolic: lactic acidosis.
Skin: pruritus, urticaria.
Other: overgrowth of nonsusceptible organisms.

INTERACTIONS

None significant.

EFFECTS ON LAB TEST RESULTS

- May decrease hemoglobin level.

CONTRAINDICATIONS & CAUTIONS

- Contraindicated in patients hypersensitive to drug or its components and in those with perforated eardrum.

NURSING CONSIDERATIONS

- Obtain history of drug use and reactions.
- Monitor patient for signs and symptoms of superinfection. Avoid prolonged use.
- Reculture persistent drainage.
- Monitor patient for sore throat (early sign of toxicity).
- ***Look alike–sound alike:*** Don't confuse Chloromycetin with chlorambucil.

PATIENT TEACHING

- Show patient or caregiver how to give drug.
- To avoid reinfection, warn patient not to touch ear with dropper.

84

Nasal drugs

beclomethasone dipropionate
budesonide
flunisolide
oxymetazoline hydrochloride
phenylephrine hydrochloride
pseudoephedrine hydrochloride
pseudoephedrine sulfate
tetrahydrozoline hydrochloride
triamcinolone acetonide

beclomethasone dipropionate

Beconase AQ

Pharmacologic class: corticosteroid
Pregnancy risk category C

AVAILABLE FORMS

Nasal aerosol: 42 mcg/metered spray, 50 mcg/metered spray‡
Nasal spray: 42 mcg/metered spray, 50 mcg/metered spray‡

INDICATIONS & DOSAGES

➤ **To relieve symptoms of seasonal or perennial rhinitis, to prevent nasal polyp recurrence after surgical removal**

Adults and children older than age 12: 1 or 2 sprays in each nostril b.i.d., t.i.d., or q.i.d.
Children ages 6 to 12: Give 1 spray into each nostril t.i.d.

ACTION

May reduce nasal inflammation by inhibiting mediators of inflammation.

Route	Onset	Peak	Duration
Nasal	5–7 days	3 wk	Unknown

Half-life: 15 hours.

ADVERSE REACTIONS

CNS: headache, lightheadedness.
EENT: *mild, transient nasal burning and stinging,* dryness, epistaxis, nasal congestion, nasopharyngeal fungal infections, rhinorrhea, sneezing, watery eyes.
GI: nausea.
Metabolic: growth velocity reduction in children and adolescents.

INTERACTIONS

None significant

EFFECTS ON LAB TEST RESULTS

None reported.

CONTRAINDICATIONS & CAUTIONS

- Contraindicated in patients hypersensitive to drug and in those with untreated localized infection involving the nasal mucosa.
- Use cautiously, if at all, in patients with active or quiescent respiratory tract tuberculous infections or untreated fungal, bacterial, or systemic viral or ocular herpes simplex infections.
- Use cautiously in patients who have recently had nasal septal ulcers, nasal surgery, or trauma until wound healing occurs.

NURSING CONSIDERATIONS

- Observe patient for fungal infections.
- Drug isn't effective for acute exacerbations of rhinitis. Decongestants or antihistamines may be needed.

PATIENT TEACHING

- Advise patient to pump nasal spray three or four times before first use.
- To instill, instruct patient to blow nose to clear nasal passages, shake container, tilt head slightly forward, and insert nozzle into nostril, pointing away from septum. Tell him to hold other nostril closed and inhale gently while spraying, hold breath for a few seconds, and exhale through the mouth. Next, have him shake container and repeat in other nostril.
- Tell patient to pump nasal spray once or twice before first use each day. He should clean the cap and nosepiece of the activator in warm water every day, and then allow them to air-dry.
- Advise patient to use drug regularly, as prescribed, because its effectiveness depends on regular use.

- Explain that unlike decongestants, drug doesn't work right away. Most patients notice improvement within a few days, but some may need 2 to 3 weeks.
- Warn patient not to exceed recommended dosage because of risk of hypothalamic-pituitary-adrenal axis suppression.
- Tell patient to notify prescriber if signs and symptoms don't improve within 3 weeks or if nasal irritation persists.
- Teach patient good nasal and oral hygiene.

budesonide
Rhinocort Aqua

Pharmacologic class: corticosteroid
Pregnancy risk category C

AVAILABLE FORMS
Nasal spray: 32 mcg/metered spray

INDICATIONS & DOSAGES
➤ **Symptoms of seasonal or perennial allergic rhinitis**
Adults and children age 6 and older: 1 spray in each nostril once daily. Maximum recommended dose for adults and children 12 and older is 4 sprays per nostril once daily (256 mcg daily). Maximum recommended dose for children ages 6 to 12 is 2 sprays per nostril once daily (128 mcg daily).

ACTION
May reduce nasal inflammation by inhibiting mediators of inflammation.

Route	Onset	Peak	Duration
Nasal	10 hr	2 wk	Unknown

Half-life: Unknown.

ADVERSE REACTIONS
EENT: epistaxis, nasal irritation, pharyngitis.
Respiratory: ***bronchospasm,*** cough.

INTERACTIONS
None significant.

EFFECTS ON LAB TEST RESULTS
None reported.

CONTRAINDICATIONS & CAUTIONS
- Contraindicated in patients hypersensitive to drug or its components and in those who have had recent septal ulcers, nasal surgery, or nasal trauma until total healing has occurred.
- Contraindicated in those with untreated localized nasal mucosa infections.
- Use cautiously in patients with tuberculous infections, ocular herpes simplex, or untreated fungal, bacterial, or systemic viral infections.

NURSING CONSIDERATIONS
- Systemic effects of corticosteroid therapy may occur if recommended daily dose is exceeded.

PATIENT TEACHING
- Tell patient to avoid exposure to chickenpox or measles.
- To instill drug, instruct patient to shake container before use, blow nose to clear nasal passages, and tilt head slightly forward and insert nozzle into nostril, pointing away from septum. Tell him to hold other nostril closed and inhale gently while spraying. Next, have him shake container and repeat in other nostril.
- Advise patient not to freeze, break, incinerate, or store canister in extreme heat; contents are under pressure.
- Advise patient to store canister with valve upward.
- Warn patient not to exceed prescribed dosage or use drug for long periods because of risk of hypothalamic-pituitary-adrenal axis suppression.
- Tell patient to notify prescriber if signs or symptoms don't improve or if they worsen in 3 weeks.
- Teach patient good nasal and oral hygiene.
- Tell patient to use drug within 6 months of opening the protective aluminum pouch.
- Instruct patient not to share drug because this could spread infection.

flunisolide

Nasarel

Pharmacologic class: corticosteroid
Pregnancy risk category C

AVAILABLE FORMS

Nasal spray: 29 mcg/spray

INDICATIONS & DOSAGES

➤ **Symptoms of seasonal or perennial rhinitis**

Adults: Starting dose is 2 sprays (58 mcg) in each nostril b.i.d. Total daily dose is 232 mcg/day. If needed, dosage may be increased to 2 sprays in each nostril t.i.d. Maximum total daily dose is 8 sprays in each nostril (464 mcg daily).
Children ages 6 to 14: Starting dose is 1 spray (29 mcg) in each nostril t.i.d. or 2 sprays (58 mcg) in each nostril b.i.d. Total daily dose is 174 to 232 mcg. Maximum total daily dose is 4 sprays in each nostril (232 mcg daily).

ACTION

Exact mechanism unknown. Decreases nasal inflammation, mainly by stabilizing leukocyte lysosomal membranes.

Route	Onset	Peak	Duration
Nasal	Unknown	Unknown	Unknown

Half-life: 1 to 2 hours.

ADVERSE REACTIONS

CNS: dizziness, headache.
EENT: *mild, transient nasal burning and stinging,* epistaxis, nasal dryness, nasal congestion, pharyngitis, sneezing, watery eyes.
GI: nausea, vomiting.
Respiratory: cough.
Other: *aftertaste,* hypersensitivity reaction, loss of taste and smell.

INTERACTIONS

None significant.

EFFECTS ON LAB TEST RESULTS

None reported.

CONTRAINDICATIONS & CAUTIONS

- Contraindicated in patients hypersensitive to drug and in those with untreated localized infection involving nasal mucosa.
- Use cautiously, if at all, in patients with active or quiescent respiratory tract tuberculous infections or untreated fungal, bacterial, or systemic viral or ocular herpes simplex infections.
- Use cautiously in patients who have recently had nasal septal ulcers, nasal surgery, or nasal trauma.

NURSING CONSIDERATIONS

- Drug isn't effective for acute exacerbations of rhinitis. Decongestants or antihistamines may be needed.
- ***Look alike–sound alike:*** Don't confuse flunisolide with fluocinonide, fluticasone, or Flumadine.

PATIENT TEACHING

- Tell patient to avoid exposure to chickenpox or measles.
- To instill drug, instruct patient to shake container before use, blow nose to clear nasal passages, tilt head slightly forward, and insert nozzle into nostril, pointing away from septum. Tell him to hold other nostril closed and inhale gently while spraying. Have him repeat procedure in other nostril. Tell him to clean nosepiece with warm water daily.
- Explain that drug doesn't work right away. Most patients notice improvement within a few days, but some may need 2 to 3 weeks.
- Advise patient to use drug regularly, as prescribed.
- Warn patient not to exceed recommended dosage to avoid hypothalamic-pituitary-adrenal axis suppression.
- Tell patient to stop drug and notify prescriber if signs and symptoms don't diminish in 3 weeks or if nasal irritation persists.

oxymetazoline hydrochloride

Afrin ◊, Allerest 12 Hour Nasal Spray ◊, Chlorphed-LA ◊, Dristan 12 Hour Nasal ◊, Drixine Nasal‡, Duramist Plus 12 Hour ◊, Duration ◊, Genasal ◊, Neo-Synephrine 12 Hour Spray ◊, Nostrilla ◊, NTZ Long Acting Nasal ◊, Sinarest 12 Hour ◊

Pharmacologic class: sympathomimetic
Pregnancy risk category C

AVAILABLE FORMS

Nasal solution: 0.05% ◊

INDICATIONS & DOSAGES

➤ Nasal congestion
Adults and children age 6 and older: 2 to 3 drops or sprays of 0.05% solution in each nostril b.i.d. Don't exceed 2 doses in a 24-hour period.

ACTION

Thought to cause local vasoconstriction of dilated arterioles, reducing blood flow and nasal congestion.

Route	Onset	Peak	Duration
Nasal	5–10 min	6 hr	< 12 hr

Half-life: Unknown.

ADVERSE REACTIONS

CNS: anxiety, dizziness, headache, insomnia, restlessness.
CV: ***CV collapse,*** hypertension, palpitations.
EENT: dryness of nose and throat, increased nasal discharge, rebound nasal congestion or irritation, sneezing, stinging.
Other: systemic effects in children.

INTERACTIONS

None significant.

EFFECTS ON LAB TEST RESULTS

None reported.

CONTRAINDICATIONS & CAUTIONS

- Contraindicated in patients hypersensitive to drug and in children younger than age 6.
- Use cautiously in patients with hyperthyroidism, cardiac disease, hypertension, or diabetes mellitus.
- Use cautiously in those with difficulty urinating because of an enlarged prostate.

NURSING CONSIDERATIONS

- Monitor patient for rebound congestion or systemic effects.
- Don't give to children who are younger than age 6.

PATIENT TEACHING

- Teach patient how to use drug. Tell him to hold head upright to minimize swallowing of drug and to sniff spray briskly.
- Caution patient not to share drug because this could spread infection.
- Tell patient not to exceed recommended dosage and to use only when needed.
- Inform patient that prolonged use may result in rebound congestion.
- ***Alert:*** Warn patient that excessive use may cause slow or rapid heart rate, high blood pressure, dizziness, and weakness.

phenylephrine hydrochloride

Alconefrin Nasal Drops 12 ◊, Alconefrin Nasal Drops 25 ◊, Alconefrin Nasal Drops 50 ◊, Doktors ◊, Duration ◊, Little Noses Gentle Formula ◊, Neo-Synephrine ◊, Nostril ◊, Rhinall ◊, Rhinall-10 Children's Flavored Nose Drops ◊, Sinex ◊

Pharmacologic class: adrenergic
Pregnancy risk category C

AVAILABLE FORMS

Nasal solution: 0.125%, 0.25%, 0.5%, 1%

INDICATIONS & DOSAGES

➤ Nasal congestion
Adults and children age 12 and older: 2 to 3 drops or 1 to 2 sprays in each nostril q 4 hours, p.r.n. Don't use for longer than 3 to 5 days.
Children ages 6 to 12: Give 2 to 3 drops or 1 to 2 sprays of 0.25% solution in each nostril q 4 hours, p.r.n.
Children ages 2 to 6: Give 2 to 3 drops of 0.125% solution q 4 hours, p.r.n.

ACTION
Causes local vasoconstriction of dilated arterioles, reducing blood flow and nasal congestion.

Route	Onset	Peak	Duration
Nasal	Rapid	Unknown	30 min–4 hr

Half-life: Unknown.

ADVERSE REACTIONS
CNS: dizziness, headache, nervousness, psychological disturbances, restlessness, tremor.
CV: *palpitations, tachycardia,* hypertension, pallor, PVCs.
EENT: dryness of nasal mucosa, rebound nasal congestion, transient burning or stinging.
GI: nausea.
Other: hypersensitivity reactions, sweating.

INTERACTIONS
Drug-drug. *Beta blockers:* May cause hypertension, then bradycardia. Avoid using together.
MAO inhibitors (MAOI), methyldopa, Tricyclic antidepressants: May potentiate the pressor response of phenylephrine. Avoid using within 14 days of an MAOI.

EFFECTS ON LAB TEST RESULTS
None reported.

CONTRAINDICATIONS & CAUTIONS
- Contraindicated in patients hypersensitive to drug.
- Use cautiously in patients with hyperthyroidism, marked hypertension, type 1 diabetes mellitus, cardiac disease, or advanced arteriosclerotic changes; in children with low body weight; and in elderly patients.

NURSING CONSIDERATIONS
- Monitor patient for systemic adverse effects.
- Don't use in children who are younger than age 2.

PATIENT TEACHING
- Teach patient how to use drug. Tell him to hold head upright to minimize swallowing of drug and to sniff spray briskly.
- Caution patient not to share drug because this could spread infection.
- Tell patient not to exceed recommended dosage and to use only when needed.
- Advise patient to contact prescriber if signs and symptoms persist longer than 3 days.
- Inform patient that prolonged use may result in rebound congestion.

pseudoephedrine hydrochloride
Cenafed ◇, Decofed ◇, Dimetapp, Genaphed ◇, PediaCare Infants' Decongestant Drops ◇, Sudafed ◇, Triaminic

pseudoephedrine sulfate
Drixoral Non-Drowsy Formula ◇

Pharmacologic class: adrenergic
Pregnancy risk category C

AVAILABLE FORMS
pseudoephedrine hydrochloride
Capsules: 30 mg ◇, 60 mg ◇
Oral solution: 7.5 mg/0.8 ml ◇, 15 mg/5 ml ◇, 30 mg/5 ml ◇
Tablets: 30 mg ◇, 60 mg ◇
Tablets (chewable): 15 mg ◇
Tablets (extended-release): 120 mg ◇, 240 mg ◇
pseudoephedrine sulfate
Tablets (extended-release): 120 mg (60 mg immediate-release, 60 mg delayed-release) ◇

INDICATIONS & DOSAGES
➤ **To decongest nose and eustachian tube**
Adults and children older than age 12: Give 60 mg P.O. q 4 to 6 hours; or 120 mg P.O. extended-release tablet q 12 hours; or 240 mg P.O. extended-release tablet once daily. Maximum dosage is 240 mg daily.
Children ages 6 to 12: Give 30 mg P.O. q 4 to 6 hours. Maximum dosage is 120 mg daily.
Children ages 2 to 5: Give 15 mg P.O. q 4 to 6 hours. Maximum dosage is 60 mg daily, or 4 mg/kg or 125 mg/m^2 P.O. divided q.i.d.

ACTION
Stimulates alpha receptors in the respiratory tract, constricting blood vessels, shrinking swollen nasal mucous membranes, increasing airway patency, and reducing tissue hyperemia, edema, and nasal congestion.

Route	Onset	Peak	Duration
P.O.	30 min	30–60 min	4–12 hr

Half-life: Unknown.

ADVERSE REACTIONS
CNS: *anxiety, nervousness,* dizziness, headache, insomnia, transient stimulation, tremor.
CV: *palpitations,* ***arrhythmias, CV collapse,*** tachycardia.
GI: anorexia, dry mouth, nausea, vomiting.
GU: difficulty urinating.
Respiratory: respiratory difficulties.
Skin: pallor.
Other: diaphoresis.

INTERACTIONS
Drug-drug. *Antihypertensives:* May inhibit hypotensive effect. Monitor blood pressure closely.
MAO inhibitors (phenelzine, tranylcypromine): May cause severe headache, hypertension, fever, and hypertensive crisis. Avoid using together.
Methyldopa, reserpine: May increase pressor response. Monitor patient closely.

EFFECTS ON LAB TEST RESULTS
None reported.

CONTRAINDICATIONS & CAUTIONS
- Contraindicated in patients with severe hypertension or severe coronary artery disease, in those receiving MAO inhibitors, and in breast-feeding women. Extended-release forms are contraindicated in children younger than age 12.
- Use cautiously in patients with hypertension, cardiac disease, diabetes, glaucoma, hyperthyroidism, and prostatic hyperplasia.

NURSING CONSIDERATIONS
- Elderly patients are more sensitive to drug's effects. Extended-release tablets shouldn't be given to elderly patients until safety with short-acting preparations has been established.

PATIENT TEACHING
- Tell patient not to crush or break extended-release forms.
- Warn against using OTC products containing other sympathomimetics.
- Instruct patient not to take drug within 2 hours of bedtime because it can cause insomnia.
- Tell patient to stop drug and notify prescriber if he becomes unusually restless.

tetrahydrozoline hydrochloride
Tyzine, Tyzine Pediatric

Pharmacologic class: sympathomimetic
Pregnancy risk category C

AVAILABLE FORMS
Nasal solution: 0.05%, 0.1%

INDICATIONS & DOSAGES
➤ **Nasal congestion**
Adults and children older than age 6: Give 2 to 4 drops or 3 to 4 sprays of 0.1% solution in each nostril no more than q 3 hours, p.r.n.
Children ages 2 to 6: Give 2 to 3 drops of 0.05% solution in each nostril no more than q 3 hours, p.r.n.

ACTION
Thought to cause local vasoconstriction of dilated arterioles, reducing blood flow and nasal congestion.

Route	Onset	Peak	Duration
Nasal	Few min	Unknown	4–8 hr

Half-life: Unknown.

ADVERSE REACTIONS
EENT: rebound nasal congestion, sneezing, transient burning or stinging.

INTERACTIONS
Drug-drug. *Bromocriptine, catechol-O-methyltransferase (COMT) inhibitors, such as tolcapone:* May increase the effects of

these drugs. Monitor patient for increased clinical response and adverse effects.
MAO inhibitors (MAOI): May cause headache, hypertension, and hyperpyrexia. Avoid using tetrahydrozoline within 14 days of stopping an MAOI.
Tricyclic antidepressants: May decrease the effects of tetrahydrozoline. Monitor patient for clinical effect.
Drug-herb. *St. John's wort:* May increase adverse effects of herb. Avoid using together.

EFFECTS ON LAB TEST RESULTS
None reported.

CONTRAINDICATIONS & CAUTIONS
- Contraindicated in patients hypersensitive to drug and in children younger than age 2. The 0.1% solution is contraindicated in children younger than age 6.
- Use cautiously in patients with hyperthyroidism, hypertension, or diabetes mellitus.

NURSING CONSIDERATIONS
- Drug should be used for only 3 to 5 days.
- Overdose in young children may cause oversedation.

PATIENT TEACHING
- Teach patient how to use drug. Tell him to hold head upright to minimize swallowing of drug and to sniff spray briskly.
- Caution patient not to share drug because this could spread infection.
- Tell patient not to exceed recommended dosage and to use only as needed for 3 to 5 days.

---

triamcinolone acetonide
Nasacort AQ, Nasacort HFA

Pharmacologic class: corticosteroid
Pregnancy risk category C

AVAILABLE FORMS
Nasal spray pump: 55 mcg/spray
Nasal aerosol: 55 mcg/actuation

INDICATIONS & DOSAGES
➤Treatment of nasal symptoms of seasonal and perennial allergic rhinitis
Adults and children 12 years and older: Give 2 sprays AQ form in each nostril daily; may decrease to 1 spray in each nostril daily for allergic disorders. Or, 2 sprays HFA form into each nostril once daily. May increase to 4 sprays into each nostril once daily. Adjust to minimum effective dosage.
Children ages 6 to 11: Give 1 spray AQ form in each nostril daily. Maximum dosage is 2 sprays in each nostril daily. Or, 2 sprays HFA form into each nostril once daily. Adjust to minimum effective dosage.

ACTION
Unknown. A glucocorticoid with antiinflammatory properties.

Route	Onset	Peak	Duration
Nasal	Unknown	1½–4 hours	Unknown.

Half-life: AQ form, about 3 hours ; HFA form, 5½ hours.

ADVERSE REACTIONS
CNS: *headache.*
EENT: *nasal irritation,* burning, dry mucous membranes, epistaxis, irritation, nasal and sinus congestion, otitis media, pharyngitis, rhinitis, sinusitis, sneezing, stinging, throat discomfort.
GI: dyspepsia, nausea, vomiting.
Respiratory: asthma symptoms, cough.
Other: fever.

INTERACTIONS
None significant.

EFFECTS ON LAB TEST RESULTS
None reported.

CONTRAINDICATIONS & CAUTIONS
- Contraindicated in patients hypersensitive to drug or its components and in those with untreated mucosal infection.
- Use with caution, if at all, in patients with active or quiescent tuberculous infection of respiratory tract and in patients with untreated fungal, bacterial, or sys-

temic viral infection or ocular herpes simplex.
- Use cautiously in patients already receiving systemic corticosteroids because of increased likelihood of hypothalamic-pituitary-adrenal axis suppression.
- Use cautiously in breast-feeding women and in those with recent nasal septal ulcers, nasal surgery, or trauma because drug may inhibit wound healing.

NURSING CONSIDERATIONS

- ***Alert:*** Excessive doses may cause signs and symptoms of hyperadrenocorticism and adrenal axis suppression; stop drug slowly.
- ***Look alike–sound alike:*** Don't confuse triamcinolone with Triaminicin.

PATIENT TEACHING

- Urge patient to read patient instruction sheet contained in each package before using drug for first time.
- To instill, instruct patient to shake container before use, blow nose to clear nasal passages, tilt head slightly forward, and insert nozzle into nostril, pointing away from septum. Tell him to hold other nostril closed and inhale gently while spraying. Next, have patient shake container and repeat procedure in other nostril.
- Instruct patient to avoid getting aerosol in eyes. If this occurs, tell him to rinse with copious amounts of cool tap water.
- Stress importance of using drug on a regular schedule because its effectiveness depends on regular use. Warn patient not to exceed prescribed dosage because serious adverse reactions can occur.
- Tell patient to notify prescriber if signs and symptoms don't diminish or if condition worsens in 2 to 3 weeks.
- Warn patient to avoid exposure to chickenpox or measles and, if exposed, to notify prescriber.
- Instruct patient to watch for and report signs and symptoms of nasal infection. Drug may need to be stopped and appropriate local therapy given.

85

Local anti-infectives

acyclovir
azelaic acid
clindamycin phosphate
clotrimazole
econazole nitrate
erythromycin
gentamicin sulfate
ketoconazole
metronidazole
miconazole nitrate
mupirocin
sertaconazole nitrate
silver sulfadiazine
terbinafine hydrochloride
terconazole

acyclovir

Avirax†, Zovirax

Pharmacologic class: nucleoside analogue
Pregnancy risk category B

AVAILABLE FORMS

Ointment: 5%
Cream: 5% in 2-g tubes

INDICATIONS & DOSAGES

➤**Initial herpes genitalis; limited, non–life-threatening mucocutaneous herpes simplex virus infections in immunocompromised patients**

Adults and children 12 years and older: Cover all lesions q 3 hours six times daily for 7 days. Although dose varies depending on total lesion area, use about ½-inch (1.3-cm) ribbon of ointment on each 4-inch (10-cm) square of surface area.

➤**Recurrent herpes labialis (cold sores)**

Adults and children 12 years and older: Apply cream five times daily for 4 days. Start therapy as early as possible after signs and symptoms start.

ACTION

Inhibits herpes simplex and varicella zoster viral DNA synthesis by inhibiting viral DNA polymerase action.

Route	Onset	Peak	Duration
Topical	Unknown	Unknown	Unknown

Half-life: Unknown.

ADVERSE REACTIONS

Skin: *mild pain, burning or stinging,* eczema, rash, dryness, pruritus, contact dermatitis, application site reactions.
Other: ***angioedema,*** anaphylaxis.

INTERACTIONS

None significant.

EFFECTS ON LAB TEST RESULTS

None reported.

CONTRAINDICATIONS & CAUTIONS

- Contraindicated in patients hypersensitive to drug and patients with chemical intolerance to drug.

NURSING CONSIDERATIONS

- Start therapy as early as possible after signs or symptoms begin.
- Apply drug with a finger cot or rubber glove to prevent autoinoculation of other body sites and transmission of infection to other persons.
- All lesions must be thoroughly covered.
- Drug is for cutaneous use only; don't apply to eye.
- Drug isn't a cure for herpes, but it helps improve signs and symptoms.

PATIENT TEACHING

- Teach patient that virus transmission can occur during treatment.
- Tell patient that there may be some discomfort with application.
- Stress importance of compliance for successful therapy.
- Teach patient that therapy should begin as soon as signs and symptoms appear.

- Tell patient to notify prescriber if adverse reactions occur.
- Instruct patient to store drug in a dry place at 59° to 77° F (15° to 25° C).

azelaic acid

Azelex, Finacea

Pharmacologic class: dicarboxylic acid
Pregnancy risk category B

AVAILABLE FORMS

Cream: 20%
Gel: 15%

INDICATIONS & DOSAGES

➤ Mild to moderate inflammatory acne vulgaris
Adults: Apply thin film and gently but thoroughly massage into affected areas b.i.d., in morning and evening.

➤ Mild to moderate rosacea
Adults: Apply thin film of Finacea and gently but thoroughly massage into affected areas b.i.d., in morning and evening.

ACTION

May inhibit microbial cellular protein synthesis.

Route	Onset	Peak	Duration
Topical	Unknown	Unknown	Unknown

Half-life: 12 hours.

ADVERSE REACTIONS

Skin: pruritus, burning, stinging, tingling, dermatitis, peeling, erythema.
Other: allergic reaction.
Finacea only
Skin: *burning, stinging, tingling,* dermatitis, pruritus, scaling, erythema, irritation, edema, acne.

INTERACTIONS

None significant.

EFFECTS ON LAB TEST RESULTS

None reported.

CONTRAINDICATIONS & CAUTIONS

- Contraindicated in patients hypersensitive to drug or its components.
- Use cautiously in pregnant or breast-feeding women.

NURSING CONSIDERATIONS

- Monitor patient for early signs and symptoms of hypopigmentation, especially patient with dark complexion.
- If sensitivity or severe irritation occurs, notify prescriber, who may stop drug and order appropriate treatment.
- Avoid using occlusive dressings.

PATIENT TEACHING

- Instruct patient to wash and pat dry affected areas before applying drug and to wash hands well after application. Warn him not to apply occlusive dressings or wrappings to affected areas.
- Warn patient that skin irritation may occur, usually at start of therapy, if drug is applied to broken or inflamed skin. Tell him to notify prescriber if irritation persists.
- Advise patient to keep drug away from mouth, eyes, and other mucous membranes. If contact occurs, tell him to rinse thoroughly with water and to notify prescriber if irritation persists.
- Advise patient to report abnormal changes in skin color.
- Urge patient to use drug for full treatment period. In most patients with inflammatory lesions, improvement occurs in 1 to 2 months.
- Warn patients with rosacea to avoid foods and beverages that may cause flushing, such as spicy foods, hot food or drinks, and alcohol.
- Instruct patient to store drug at 59° to 86° F (15° to 30° C) and protect it from freezing.

clindamycin phosphate

Cleocin, Cleocin T, Clinda-Derm, Clindagel, ClindaMax, Clindesse, Clindets, C/T/S, Evoclin

Pharmacologic class: lincomycin derivative
Pregnancy risk category B

AVAILABLE FORMS

Gel: 1%
Foam: 1%
Lotion: 1%

Pledget: 1%*
Topical solution: 1%*
Vaginal cream: 2%
Vaginal suppositories: 100 mg

INDICATIONS & DOSAGES

➤ Inflammatory acne vulgaris
Adults and adolescents: Apply to skin b.i.d., morning and evening or once daily if using Clindagel or Evoclin.

➤ Bacterial vaginosis
Adults: 1 applicatorful intravaginally at bedtime. for 3 to 7 days in nonpregnant women or 7 days in pregnant women, or 1 suppository intravaginally at bedtime for 3 days, or one applicatorful of Clindesse intravaginally as a single dose.

ACTION

Bacteriostatic or bactericidal based on drug level and susceptibility of organism; suppresses growth of susceptible organisms in sebaceous glands by blocking protein synthesis.

Route	Onset	Peak	Duration
Topical, intravaginal	Unknown	Unknown	Unknown

Half-life: 1½ to 2½ hours for topical and vaginal cream; 11 hours for vaginal suppositories

ADVERSE REACTIONS

CNS: *headache.*
EENT: pharyngitis.
GI: GI upset, diarrhea, bloody diarrhea, abdominal pain, constipation, colitis including pseudomembranous colitis.
GU: *cervicitis, vaginitis,* Candida albicans *overgrowth, vulvar irritation,* UTI, vaginal discharge, vaginal moniliasis.
Skin: *dryness, redness,* pruritus, rash, swelling, irritation, contact dermatitis, burning.

INTERACTIONS

Drug-drug. *Erythromycin:* May antagonize clindamycin's effect. Separate doses.
Isotretinoin: May cause cumulative dryness, resulting in excessive skin irritation. Use together cautiously.
Neuromuscular blockers: May increase action of neuromuscular blocker. Use together cautiously.
Drug-lifestyle. *Abrasive or medicated soaps or cleansers, acne products, or other preparations containing peeling drugs (benzoyl peroxide, resorcinol, salicylic acid, sulfur, tretinoin), alcohol-containing products (aftershave, cosmetics, perfumed toiletries, shaving creams or lotions), astringent soaps or cosmetics, medicated cosmetics or cover-ups:* May cause cumulative dryness, resulting in excessive skin irritation. Urge caution.

EFFECTS ON LAB TEST RESULTS

- May increase liver enzyme levels.

CONTRAINDICATIONS & CAUTIONS

- Contraindicated in patients hypersensitive to clindamycin or lincomycin and in those with history of ulcerative colitis, regional enteritis, or antibiotic-related colitis.

NURSING CONSIDERATIONS

- For treating acne, drug may be used with tretinoin or benzoyl peroxide as well as systemic antibiotics.
- Drug can cause excessive dryness.
- Topical solution and pledgets contain an alcohol base which may irritate the eyes.
- Monitor elderly patients for systemic effects.

PATIENT TEACHING

- Tell patient to wash area with warm water and soap, rinse, pat dry, and wait 30 minutes after washing or shaving to apply.
- Warn patient to avoid excessive washing of area. Tell patient to cover entire affected area but to avoid contact with eyes, nose, mouth, and other mucous membranes.
- Instruct patient to use other prescribed acne medicines at a different time.
- Tell patient to use only as prescribed.
- Instruct patient to dab, not roll, applicator-tipped bottle. If tip becomes dry, patient should invert bottle and depress tip several times to moisten.
- Warn patient not to smoke while applying topical solution.
- For intravaginal application, make sure patient knows how to use applicators that come with drug.
- Advise patient that the vaginal form contains mineral oil that can weaken latex or

rubber products, such as condoms and diaphragms, and that she should use another form of birth control within 5 days of therapy.
- Advise patient to avoid sexual intercourse during intravaginal therapy.
- Advise patient to avoid use of tampons or douches during intravaginal treatment.
- Instruct patient to notify prescriber immediately if abdominal pain or diarrhea occurs. Inform patient that an antidiarrheal may worsen condition and should only be used as directed by prescriber.
- Tell patient to remove pledgets from foil before use.
- Advise patient to use pledgets only once and then discard. Also, more than 1 pledget may be used per application.
- Advise patient to complete entire course of therapy.

clotrimazole

Canesten†, Cruex ◊, Desenex ◊, Gyne-Lotrimin ◊, Lotrimin, Lotrimin AF ◊, Mycelex, Mycelex-7 ◊, Mycelex-G

Pharmacologic class: imidazole derivative
Pregnancy risk category B; C (for lozenges)

AVAILABLE FORMS

Combination pack: Vaginal tablets 100 mg and vulvar cream 1% ◊, vaginal tablets 200 mg and vulvar cream 1% ◊
Topical cream: 1%
Topical lotion: 1%
Topical solution: 1%
Troches (lozenges): 10 mg
Vaginal cream: 1% ◊, 2% ◊
Vaginal suppositories: 100 mg ◊, 200 mg ◊

INDICATIONS & DOSAGES

➤Superficial fungal infections (tinea corporis, tinea cruris, tinea pedis, tinea versicolor, candidiasis)
Adults and children age 2 and older: Apply thin film and massage into affected and surrounding area, morning and evening, for 2 to 4 weeks. If improvement doesn't occur after 4 weeks, reevaluate patient.

➤Vulvovaginal candidiasis
Adults: One 100-mg vaginal suppository inserted daily at bedtime for 7 consecutive days. Or, one 200-mg vaginal suppository at bedtime for 3 days. Or, 1 applicatorful of vaginal cream daily at bedtime for 3 days (2%) or 7 days (1%).

➤Oropharyngeal candidiasis
Adults and children age 3 and older: Dissolve lozenge in mouth over 15 to 30 minutes five times daily for 14 consecutive days.

➤To prevent oropharyngeal candidiasis in patients immunocompromised by chemotherapy, radiotherapy, or corticosteroid therapy in the treatment of leukemia, solid tumors, or renal transplantation
Adults: Dissolve lozenge in mouth over 15 to 30 minutes t.i.d. for duration of chemotherapy or until corticosteroid is reduced to maintenance levels.

ACTION

Fungistatic or fungicidal, depending on level. Alters fungal cell-wall permeability and produces osmotic instability.

Route	Onset	Peak	Duration
P.O.	Unknown	Unknown	3 hr
Topical, intravaginal	Unknown	Unknown	Unknown

Half-life: Unknown.

ADVERSE REACTIONS

GI: lower abdominal cramps, nausea and vomiting with lozenges.
GU: *mild vaginal burning or irritation,* urinary frequency.
Skin: blistering, *erythema,* edema, pruritus, burning, stinging, peeling, urticaria, skin fissures, general irritation.

INTERACTIONS

None significant.

EFFECTS ON LAB TEST RESULTS

- May increase liver enzyme levels.

CONTRAINDICATIONS & CAUTIONS

- Contraindicated in patients hypersensitive to drug.
- Contraindicated for ophthalmic use.

NURSING CONSIDERATIONS

- Clean and dry area before applying drug.
- Consult prescriber before using topical preparations in children younger than age 2. Don't use troches in children younger than age 3; don't use vaginal preparations in children younger than age 12.
- Watch for and report irritation or sensitivity; stop if irritation occurs, and notify prescriber.
- Improvement usually occurs within 1 week; if no improvement is seen within 4 weeks, review diagnosis.
- ***Look alike–sound alike:*** Don't confuse clotrimazole with co-trimoxazole.

PATIENT TEACHING

- Reassure patient that hypopigmentation from tinea versicolor will resolve gradually.
- Warn patient not to use occlusive wrappings or dressings.
- Warn patient to avoid drug contact with eyes.
- Caution patient that frequent or persistent yeast infections may suggest a more serious medical problem.
- Tell patient to refrain from sexual intercourse during intravaginal treatment.
- Warn patient that topical preparation may stain clothing.
- Tell patient that using a sanitary napkin protects clothing when using vaginal preparation.
- Stress need to continue use of vaginal preparations, as prescribed, even if menstruation begins.
- Tell patient with athlete's foot to change shoes and cotton socks daily and to dry between the toes after bathing.
- Tell patient to allow lozenges to dissolve in mouth and not to chew, for full benefit.
- Stress need to continue treatment for full course and to notify prescriber if no improvement occurs after 4 weeks.

econazole nitrate

Ecostatin†, Spectazole

Pharmacologic class: imidazole derivative
Pregnancy risk category C

AVAILABLE FORMS

Cream: 1%

INDICATIONS & DOSAGES

➤ **Tinea corporis, tinea cruris, tinea pedis, tinea versicolor**
Adults and children: Rub into affected areas daily for at least 2 weeks.
➤ **Cutaneous candidiasis**
Adults and children: Rub into affected areas b.i.d.

ACTION

Fungistatic, but may be fungicidal depending on level. Appears to alter fungal cell-wall permeability and produce osmotic instability.

Route	Onset	Peak	Duration
Topical	Unknown	Unknown	Unknown

Half-life: Unknown

ADVERSE REACTIONS

Skin: burning, pruritus, stinging, erythema.

INTERACTIONS

Drug-drug. *Corticosteroids:* May inhibit antifungal activity against certain organisms. Monitor patient for effect.

EFFECTS ON LAB TEST RESULTS

None reported.

CONTRAINDICATIONS & CAUTIONS

- Contraindicated in patients hypersensitive to drug or its components.

NURSING CONSIDERATIONS

- Clean and dry affected area before applying.
- Don't use occlusive dressings.

PATIENT TEACHING

- Tell patient to use drug for entire treatment period, even if signs and symptoms

improve. Instruct him to notify prescriber if no improvement occurs after 2 weeks in fungal infection on hairless skin (tinea corporis), jock itch, or fungal skin infection (tinea versicolor), or after 4 weeks for athlete's foot.
- Reassure patient that lack of pigmentation from tinea versicolor resolves gradually.
- Tell patient to stop drug and notify prescriber if condition persists or worsens or if irritation occurs.
- Warn patient that drug may stain clothing.
- Tell patient with athlete's foot to change shoes and cotton socks daily and to dry between toes after bathing.
- Tell patient to keep drug out of eyes.

erythromycin

Akne-mycin, A/T/S, Del-Mycin, Emgel, Erycette, EryDerm, Erygel, Erymax, EryPads, Ery-Sol†, ETS†, Sans-Acne†, Staticin, T-Stat†

Pharmacologic class: macrolide
Pregnancy risk category C (topical solution); B (other topical preparations)

AVAILABLE FORMS

Ointment: 2%
Pledgets: 2%
Topical gel: 2%
Topical solution: 1.5%*, 2%*

INDICATIONS & DOSAGES

➤ **Inflammatory acne vulgaris**
Adults and children: Apply to affected areas b.i.d., morning and evening.

ACTION

Usually bacteriostatic, but may be bactericidal in high concentrations or against highly susceptible organisms. Disrupts protein synthesis in susceptible bacteria.

Route	Onset	Peak	Duration
Topical	Unknown	Unknown	Unknown

Half-life: Unknown.

ADVERSE REACTIONS

Skin: *burning, dryness, pruritus,* sensitivity reactions, erythema, irritation, peeling, oily skin.

INTERACTIONS

Drug-drug. *Clindamycin:* May antagonize clindamycin's effect. Avoid using together.
Isotretinoin: May cause cumulative dryness, resulting in excessive skin irritation. Use together cautiously.
Drug-lifestyle. *Abrasive or medicated soaps or cleansers, acne products, or other preparations containing peeling drugs (benzoyl peroxide, resorcinol, salicylic acid, sulfur, tretinoin), alcohol-containing products (aftershave, cosmetics, perfumed toiletries, shaving creams or lotions), astringent soaps or cosmetics, medicated cosmetics or cover-ups:* May cause cumulative dryness, resulting in excessive skin irritation. Urge caution.

EFFECTS ON LAB TEST RESULTS

- May interfere with fluorometric determinations of urine catecholamines.

CONTRAINDICATIONS & CAUTIONS

- Contraindicated in patients hypersensitive to drug or its components.

NURSING CONSIDERATIONS

- Wash, rinse, and dry affected areas before application.
- Prolonged use may be needed when treating acne vulgaris, which may result in overgrowth of nonsusceptible organisms.

PATIENT TEACHING

- Advise patient to wash, rinse, and dry face thoroughly before each use.
- Advise patient to avoid use near eyes, nose, mouth, or other mucous membranes.
- Tell patient to wash hands after each application.
- Tell patient to stop using drug and notify prescriber if no improvement occurs or if condition worsens in 3 to 12 weeks.
- Advise patient not to share towels or washcloths.
- Instruct patient to use each pledget once, then discard.

• Caution patient to keep drug away from heat and open flame.

gentamicin sulfate

Garamycin, G-Myticin

Pharmacologic class: aminoglycoside
Pregnancy risk category C

AVAILABLE FORMS

Cream: 0.1%
Ointment: 0.1%

INDICATIONS & DOSAGES

➤ **To treat or prevent superficial infections and superficial burns of the skin caused by susceptible bacteria**
Adults and children older than age 1: Rub in small amount gently t.i.d. or q.i.d., with or without gauze dressing.

ACTION

Exact mechanism unknown. An aminoglycoside that disrupts bacterial protein synthesis by binding to ribosomes. Susceptible bacteria include sensitive strains of streptococci and *Staphylococcus aureus* and gram negative bacteria including *Pseudomonas aeruginosa, Aerobacter aerogenes, Escherichia coli, Proteus vulgaris,* and *Klebsiella pneumoniae.*

Route	Onset	Peak	Duration
Topical	Unknown	Unknown	Unknown

Half-life: Unknown

ADVERSE REACTIONS

Skin: minor skin irritation, erythema, photosensitivity, allergic contact dermatitis.

INTERACTIONS

None significant.

EFFECTS ON LAB TEST RESULTS

None reported.

CONTRAINDICATIONS & CAUTIONS

• Contraindicated in patients hypersensitive to drug or its components and in those who may have cross-sensitivity with other aminoglycosides such as neomycin.

NURSING CONSIDERATIONS

• ***Alert:*** Avoid use on large skin lesions or over a wide area because of possible systemic toxic effects.
• Restrict use of drug to selected patients; widespread use may lead to resistant organisms.
• Prolonged use may result in overgrowth of nonsusceptible organisms.

PATIENT TEACHING

• Tell patient to clean affected area and, to remove crusts of impetigo before applying to increase absorption.
• Tell patient to wash hands after each application.
• Instruct patient to store drug in cool place.
• Tell patient to stop using drug and notify prescriber immediately if no improvement occurs or if condition worsens.

ketoconazole

Nizoral, Nizoral A-D◇

Pharmacologic class: imidazole
Pregnancy risk category C

AVAILABLE FORMS

Cream: 2%
Shampoo: 1%◇, 2%

INDICATIONS & DOSAGES

➤ **Tinea corporis, tinea cruris, tinea pedis, tinea versicolor from susceptible organisms; seborrheic dermatitis; cutaneous candidiasis**
Adults: Cover affected and immediate surrounding areas daily for at least 2 weeks. For seborrheic dermatitis, apply b.i.d. for 4 weeks. Patients with tinea pedis need 6 weeks of treatment.

➤ **Scaling caused by dandruff**
Adults: Using shampoo, wet hair, lather, and massage for 1 minute. Leave drug on scalp for 3 minutes; then rinse and repeat. Shampoo twice weekly for 4 weeks, with at least 3 days between shampoos and then intermittently, as needed, to maintain control.

ACTION
Probably inhibits yeast growth by altering the permeability of the cell membrane.

Route	Onset	Peak	Duration
Topical	Unknown	Unknown	Unknown

Half-life: Unknown.

ADVERSE REACTIONS
Skin: severe irritation, pruritus, and stinging with cream, increase in normal hair loss, irritation, abnormal hair texture, scalp pustules, pruritus, oiliness, or dryness of hair and scalp with shampoo use.

INTERACTIONS
Drug-drug. *Topical corticosteroids:* May cause increased absorption of corticosteroid. Avoid using together.

EFFECTS ON LAB TEST RESULTS
None reported.

CONTRAINDICATIONS & CAUTIONS
- Contraindicated in patients hypersensitive to drug or its components.
- Use cautiously in pregnant and breast-feeding women.

NURSING CONSIDERATIONS
- Most patients show improvement soon after treatment begins.
- Treatment of tinea corporis or tinea cruris should continue for at least 2 weeks to reduce possibility of recurrence.
- ***Alert:*** Product contains sodium sulfite anhydrous, which may cause severe or life-threatening allergic reactions, including anaphylaxis, in patients with asthma.

PATIENT TEACHING
- Tell patient to stop drug and notify prescriber if hypersensitivity reaction occurs.
- Advise patient to check with prescriber if condition worsens; drug may have to be stopped and diagnosis reevaluated.
- Tell patient to avoid using shampoo on scalp if skin is broken or inflamed.
- Warn patient that shampoo applied to permanent-waved hair removes curl.
- Warn patient to avoid drug contact with eyes.
- Tell patient to continue drug for intended duration of therapy, even if signs and symptoms improve soon after starting treatment.
- Tell patient not to store drug above room temperature (77° F [25° C]) and to protect from light.

metronidazole
MetroCream, MetroGel, MetroGel Vaginal, MetroLotion, Noritate

Pharmacologic class: nitroimidazole
Pregnancy risk category B

AVAILABLE FORMS
Topical cream: 0.75%, 1%
Topical emulsion: 0.75%
Topical gel: 0.75%, 1%
Topical lotion: 0.75%
Vaginal gel: 0.75%

INDICATIONS & DOSAGES
➤ Inflammatory papules and pustules of acne rosacea
Adults: If using a 0.75% preparation, apply thin film to affected area b.i.d., morning and evening. If using a 1% preparation, apply thin film to affected area once daily. After response is seen (usually within 3 weeks), adjust frequency and duration of therapy.
➤ Bacterial vaginosis
Adults: 1 applicatorful intravaginally daily or b.i.d. for 5 days. For once-daily use, give at bedtime.

ACTION
Unknown. May cause bactericidal effect by interacting with bacterial DNA. Drug is active against many anaerobic gram-negative bacilli, anaerobic gram-positive cocci, *Gardnerella vaginalis,* and *Campylobacter fetus.*

Route	Onset	Peak	Duration
Topical	Unknown	8–12 hr	Unknown
Intravaginal	Unknown	6–12 hr	Unknown

Half-life: Unknown

ADVERSE REACTIONS
Topical forms
EENT: lacrimation if applied around eyes.

Skin: *transient redness, dryness, mild burning, stinging,* pruritus, contact dermatitis, rash.
Vaginal form
GI: cramps, pain, nausea, loose stools, metallic or bad taste in mouth.
GU: *cervicitis, vaginitis,* perineal and vulvovaginal itching, vaginal burning.
Skin: *transient redness, dryness, mild burning, stinging.*
Other: overgrowth of nonsusceptible organisms.

INTERACTIONS
Drug-drug. *Disulfiram:* May cause disulfiram-like reaction when used with vaginal form of metronidazole. Avoid using together, and wait 2 weeks after stopping disulfiram before starting metronidazole vaginal therapy.
Lithium: May increase lithium level. Monitor lithium level.
Oral anticoagulants: May increase anticoagulant effect. Monitor patient for adverse reactions.
Drug-lifestyle. *Alcohol use:* May cause disulfiram-like reaction when used with vaginal form. Discourage use together.

EFFECTS ON LAB TEST RESULTS
- May interfere with AST, ALT, LDH, triglyceride, and glucose levels.
- May increase or decrease WBC count.

CONTRAINDICATIONS & CAUTIONS
- Contraindicated in patients hypersensitive to drug or its ingredients, such as parabens, and other nitroimidazole derivatives.
- Use cautiously in patients with history or evidence of blood dyscrasia and in those with hepatic impairment.
- Use vaginal gel cautiously in patients with history of CNS diseases. Oral form may cause seizures and peripheral neuropathy.

NURSING CONSIDERATIONS
- Topical therapy hasn't been linked to the adverse effects observed with parenteral or oral therapy, but some drug may be absorbed after topical use.
- Don't use vaginal gel in patients who have taken disulfiram within past 2 weeks.

PATIENT TEACHING
- Instruct patient to avoid use of topical gel around eyes.
- Advise patient to clean area thoroughly before use and to wait 15 to 20 minutes after cleaning skin before applying drug to minimize risk of local irritation. Cosmetics may be used after applying drug.
- If local reactions occur, advise patient to apply drug less frequently or stop using it and notify prescriber.
- Advise patient to avoid sexual intercourse while using vaginal preparation.
- Caution patient to avoid alcohol while being treated with vaginal preparation.

miconazole nitrate

Desenex ◇, Lotrimin AF ◇, Micatin ◇, Monistat-Derm, Monistat 3 ◇, Monistat 7 ◇, Ting ◇, Zeasorb-AF ◇

Pharmacologic class: imidazole
Pregnancy risk category C

AVAILABLE FORMS
Aerosol powder: 2% ◇
Aerosol spray: 1%, 2% ◇
Lotion: 2% ◇
Powder: 2% ◇
Topical cream: 2% ◇
Topical ointment: 2% ◇
Topical solution: 2% ◇
Vaginal cream: 2% ◇
Vaginal suppositories: 100 mg ◇, 200 mg ◇, 1,200 mg ◇

INDICATIONS & DOSAGES
➤ **Tinea corporis, tinea cruris, tinea pedis, cutaneous candidiasis, common dermatophyte infections**
Adults and children older than age 1: Apply sparingly b.i.d. for 2 to 4 weeks. Powder or spray can be used liberally over affected area.
➤ **Tinea versicolor**
Adults and children older than age 1: Apply sparingly daily for 2 weeks.
➤ **Vulvovaginal candidiasis**
Adults: 1 applicatorful or 100-mg Monistat 7 suppository intravaginally at bedtime for 7 days; repeat course, if needed. Or, 200-mg Monistat 3 suppository intravaginally at bedtime for 3 days. Or, one

1,200-mg suppository intravaginally at bedtime for 1 day. Or, apply topical cream sparingly to affected area b.i.d. for 7 days.

ACTION

Fungicidal; disrupts fungal cell membrane permeability.

Route	Onset	Peak	Duration
Topical, intravaginal	Unknown	Unknown	Unknown

Half-life: Unknown.

ADVERSE REACTIONS

CNS: headache.
GU: pelvic cramps, vulvovaginal burning, pruritus, and irritation with vaginal cream.
Skin: irritation, burning, maceration, allergic contact dermatitis.

INTERACTIONS

None significant.

EFFECTS ON LAB TEST RESULTS

None reported.

CONTRAINDICATIONS & CAUTIONS

- Contraindicated in patients hypersensitive to drug or its components. Cross-sensitivity to imidazole antifungals may occur.
- Don't use in children younger than age 2.
- Don't use vaginal preparation during the first trimester of pregnancy.
- Use cautiously in breast-feeding women.

NURSING CONSIDERATIONS

- Avoid using within 72 hours of certain intravaginal and latex products, such as condoms or vaginal contraceptive diaphragms because drug causes latex breakdown.
- Don't use occlusive dressings.
- Lotion is preferred in skinfolds.

PATIENT TEACHING

- Advise patient that vaginal form of drug is for perineal or intravaginal use only and to keep drug out of eyes.
- Caution patient that frequent or persistent yeast infections may suggest a more serious medical problem.
- Tell patient to cautiously insert intravaginal form high into the vagina with applicator provided.
- ***Alert:*** Vaginal preparation shouldn't be used during first trimester of pregnancy. Advise patient to use vaginal preparation during pregnancy only if recommended by prescriber.
- Tell patient that drug may stain clothing.
- Warn patient to stop drug if sensitivity or chemical irritation occurs.
- Tell patient to use drug for full treatment period prescribed and to notify prescriber if signs and symptoms persist or worsen at end of therapy.
- Advise patient to avoid tampons and sexual intercourse during vaginal treatment.
- Instruct patient to apply sparingly in skinfolds and rub in well to prevent skin breakdown.
- Tell patient to store vaginal product between 59° and 86° F (15° and 30° C).

mupirocin

Bactroban, Bactroban Cream, Bactroban Nasal, Centany

Pharmacologic class: antibiotic
Pregnancy risk category B

AVAILABLE FORMS

Intranasal ointment: 2%
Topical cream: 2%
Topical ointment: 2%

INDICATIONS & DOSAGES

➤Impetigo

Adults and children: Apply to affected areas t.i.d. for 1 to 2 weeks. Reevaluate patient in 3 to 5 days; may cover affected area with dressing.

➤Traumatic skin lesions infected with *Staphylococcus aureus* or *Streptococcus pyogenes*

Adults and children: Apply thin film t.i.d. for 10 days; may cover with gauze dressing, if needed. Reevaluate patient if improvement doesn't occur in 3 to 5 days.

➤To eradicate nasal colonization by methicillin-resistant *S. aureus* in

adult patients and health care workers
Adults and children age 12 and older: Divide ointment in single-use tube between nostrils (½ tube per nostril) b.i.d. for 5 days. After application, close nostrils by pressing together and releasing sides of nose repeatedly for 1 minute to spread ointment throughout nares.

ACTION
Inhibits bacterial protein synthesis by reversibly and specifically binding to bacterial isoleucyl transfer-RNA synthetase.

Route	Onset	Peak	Duration
Topical	Unknown	Unknown	Unknown

Half-life: Unknown

ADVERSE REACTIONS
CNS: headache.
EENT: rhinitis, pharyngitis, burning or stinging with intranasal use.
GI: taste perversion, nausea, abdominal pain, ulcerative stomatitis.
Respiratory: upper respiratory tract congestion, cough with intranasal use.
Skin: burning, pruritus, stinging, rash, pain, erythema with topical use.

INTERACTIONS
Drug-drug. *Chloramphenicol:* May interfere with the antibacterial action of mupirocin on RNA synthesis. Monitor patient for clinical effect.

EFFECTS ON LAB TEST RESULTS
None reported.

CONTRAINDICATIONS & CAUTIONS
- Contraindicated in patients hypersensitive to drug or its components.
- Use cautiously in patients with burns or large open wounds and in those with impaired renal function because serious renal toxicity may occur.

NURSING CONSIDERATIONS
- Drug isn't for ophthalmic or internal use.
- Prolonged use may cause overgrowth of nonsusceptible bacteria and fungi.
- Local reactions appear to be caused by polyethylene glycol vehicle.
- Patient shouldn't use other nasal products with intranasal ointment.
- ***Look alike–sound alike:*** Don't confuse Bactroban with bacitracin.

PATIENT TEACHING
- Tell patient to notify prescriber immediately if condition doesn't improve or gets worse in 3 to 5 days.
- Tell patient not to use other nasal products with mupirocin.
- Warn patient about local adverse reactions related to drug use.
- Caution patient not to use cosmetics or other skin products on treated area.

sertaconazole nitrate
Ertaczo

Pharmacologic class: imidazole
Pregnancy risk category C

AVAILABLE FORMS
Topical cream: 2%

INDICATIONS & DOSAGES
➤ **Interdigital tinea pedis caused by *Trichophyton rubrum, Trichophyton mentagrophytes,* or *Epidermophyton floccosum* in immunocompetent patients**
Adults and children age 12 and older: Apply cream twice daily to affected areas between toes and healthy surrounding areas for 4 weeks.

ACTION
May inhibit CYP-dependent synthesis of ergosterol. The lack of ergosterol in the cell membrane causes alterations in cell-wall permeability and osmotic instability, leading to fungal cell injury and death.

Route	Onset	Peak	Duration
Topical	Unknown	Unknown	Unknown

Half-life: Unknown.

ADVERSE REACTIONS
Skin: application site reaction, contact dermatitis, erythema, dryness, burning, tenderness, hyperpigmentation.

INTERACTIONS
None known.

EFFECTS ON LAB TEST RESULTS
None reported.

CONTRAINDICATIONS & CAUTIONS
- Contraindicated in patients hypersensitive to drug, its components, or other imidazoles.
- Use cautiously in pregnant or breast-feeding women.

NURSING CONSIDERATIONS
- Before treatment starts, diagnosis should be confirmed by direct microscopic examination of infected tissue in potassium hydroxide solution or by culture on an appropriate medium.
- Drug is for use only on skin and not for ophthalmic, oral, or intravaginal use.
- If condition hasn't improved after 2 weeks, review diagnosis.
- Stop drug if skin irritation or sensitivity develops.

PATIENT TEACHING
- Warn patient to stop using drug if he develops increased irritation, redness, itching, burning, blistering, swelling, or oozing at the site of application.
- Caution patient that drug is for external use on skin only. Discourage contact with eyes, nose, mouth, and other mucous membranes.
- If cream is to be applied after bathing, tell patient to dry affected area thoroughly before application.
- Tell patient to wash hands after applying cream.
- Urge patient to use drug for full duration of treatment, even if symptoms have improved.
- Instruct patient to notify prescriber if condition worsens or fails to improve.
- Caution patient to avoid occlusive coverings unless directed by prescriber.
- Teach patient proper foot hygiene.

silver sulfadiazine

Flamazine†, Silvadene, SSD, SSD AF, Thermazene

Pharmacologic class: broad-spectrum sulfonamide
Pregnancy risk category B

AVAILABLE FORMS
Cream: 1%

INDICATIONS & DOSAGES
➤ **To prevent or treat wound infection in second- and third-degree burns**
Adults: Apply 1/16-inch ribbon of cream to clean, debrided wound daily or b.i.d.

ACTION
Acts on cell membrane and cell wall; it's bactericidal for many gram-positive and gram-negative organisms.

Route	Onset	Peak	Duration
Topical	Unknown	Unknown	Unknown

Half-life: Unknown

ADVERSE REACTIONS
GU: interstitial nephritis.
Hematologic: ***leukopenia.***
Metabolic: altered serum osmolality.
Skin: ***erythema multiforme,*** pain, burning, rash, pruritus, skin necrosis, skin discoloration.

INTERACTIONS
Drug-drug. *Topical proteolytic enzymes:* May inactivate enzymes. Avoid using together.
Drug-lifestyle. *Sun exposure:* May cause photosensitivity. Advise patient to avoid excessive sun exposure.

EFFECTS ON LAB TEST RESULTS
- May decrease WBC count.

CONTRAINDICATIONS & CAUTIONS
- Contraindicated in patients hypersensitive to drug and in those with G6PD deficiency.
- Contraindicated in pregnant women at or near term and in premature or full-term neonates during first 2 months after birth.

Drug may increase possibility of kernicterus.
• ***Alert:*** Use cautiously in patients hypersensitive to sulfonamides.

NURSING CONSIDERATIONS
• Use sterile application technique to prevent wound contamination.
• Use drug only on affected areas. Keep these areas medicated at all times.
• Bathe patient daily, if possible.
• Inspect patient's skin daily, and note any changes. Notify prescriber if burning or excessive pain develops.
• Monitor sulfadiazine levels and renal function, and check urine for sulfa crystals in patients with extensive burns.
• Tell prescriber if hepatic or renal dysfunction occurs; drug may need to be stopped.
• Leukopenia usually resolves without intervention and doesn't always require stopping drug.
• Absorption of propylene glycol (contained in the cream) can interfere with serum osmolality.
• Discard darkened cream because drug is ineffective.

PATIENT TEACHING
• Instruct patient to promptly report adverse reactions, especially burning or excessive pain with application.
• Inform patient of need for frequent blood and urine tests to watch for adverse effects.
• Tell patient that he may develop sensitivity to the sun.
• Tell patient to continue treatment until satisfactory healing occurs or until site is ready for grafting.

terbinafine hydrochloride
Lamisil, Lamisil AT ◇

Pharmacologic class: allylamine derivative
Pregnancy risk category B

AVAILABLE FORMS
Cream: 1% ◇
Spray: 1% ◇

INDICATIONS & DOSAGES
➤ Athlete's foot, tinea versicolor
Adults and children age 12 and older: Apply b.i.d. for at least 1 week, but no longer than 4 weeks.
➤ Jock itch, ringworm
Adults and children age 12 and older: Apply once daily for at least 1 week, but no longer than 4 weeks.

ACTION
Fungicidal; selectively inhibits an early step in synthesis of sterols used by fungi for cell wall synthesis.

Route	Onset	Peak	Duration
Topical	Unknown	Unknown	Unknown

Half-life: About 21 hours

ADVERSE REACTIONS
Skin: irritation, pruritus, skin exfoliation.

INTERACTIONS
None significant.

EFFECTS ON LAB TEST RESULTS
None reported.

CONTRAINDICATIONS & CAUTIONS
• Contraindicated in patients hypersensitive to drug or its components and in breast-feeding women.

NURSING CONSIDERATIONS
• Observe patient for 2 to 6 weeks after therapy is complete to determine whether treatment was successful; review diagnosis if condition persists.
• Drug isn't intended for oral, ophthalmic, or vaginal use.
• ***Look alike–sound alike:*** Don't confuse terbinafine with terbutaline. Don't confuse Lamisil with Lamictal.

PATIENT TEACHING
• Teach patient proper use of drug. Tell him to wash affected area with soap and water and dry completely before applying.
• Advise patient to use only as directed for full recommended course, even if signs and symptoms disappear, and not to apply near eyes, mouth, or mucous membranes or to use occlusive dressings unless so directed.

• Instruct patient with athlete's foot to wear well-fitting, ventilated shoes.
• Tell patient to wash hands after applying.
• Tell patient to stop drug and contact prescriber if irritation or sensitivity develops.
• Tell patient to store drug between 41° and 86° F (5° and 30° C).

terconazole

Terazol 3, Terazol 7

Pharmacologic class: triazole derivative
Pregnancy risk category C

AVAILABLE FORMS

Vaginal cream: 0.4%, 0.8%
Vaginal suppositories: 80 mg

INDICATIONS & DOSAGES

➤ **Vulvovaginal candidiasis**

Adults: 1 applicatorful of cream or 1 suppository inserted into vagina at bedtime.; 0.4% cream used for 7 consecutive days; 0.8% cream or 80-mg suppository for 3 consecutive days. Repeat course, if needed, after reconfirmation by smear or culture.

ACTION

May increase *Candida* cell membrane permeability.

Route	Onset	Peak	Duration
Intravaginal	Unknown	Unknown	Unknown

Half-life: Unknown

ADVERSE REACTIONS

CNS: *headache,* fever.
GI: abdominal pain.
GU: dysmenorrhea, genital pain, vulvovaginal burning.
Skin: *pruritus,* irritation, photosensitivity.
Other: chills, body aches.

INTERACTIONS

None significant.

EFFECTS ON LAB TEST RESULTS

None reported.

CONTRAINDICATIONS & CAUTIONS

• Contraindicated in patients hypersensitive to drug or its inactive ingredients.

NURSING CONSIDERATIONS

• Therapeutic effect of drug is unaffected by menstruation or hormonal contraceptive use.
• ***Look alike–sound alike:*** Don't confuse terconazole with tioconazole.

PATIENT TEACHING

• Advise patient to continue treatment during menstrual period. However, tell her not to use tampons.
• Instruct patient to insert drug high in vagina (except during pregnancy).
• Tell patient to use drug for full treatment period prescribed. Explain how to prevent reinfection.
• Instruct patient to notify prescriber and stop drug if fever, chills, other flulike signs and symptoms, or sensitivity develops.
• Caution patient to refrain from sexual intercourse during treatment.
• Tell patient that drug base may react with latex, causing decreased effectiveness of condoms and diaphragms (for up to 72 hours after treatment is completed).
• Instruct patient to store drug at room temperature.

86
Scabicides and pediculicides

crotamiton
lindane
permethrin
pyrethrins and piperonyl butoxide

crotamiton
Eurax

Pharmacologic class: scabicide
Pregnancy risk category C

AVAILABLE FORMS
Cream: 10%
Lotion: 10%

INDICATIONS & DOSAGES
➤ **Parasitic infestation (scabies)**
Adults: Scrub entire body with soap and water. Remove scales or crusts. Then apply thin layer of cream over entire body, from chin down (with special attention to skinfolds, creases, interdigital spaces, and genital area). Apply second coat in 24 hours. Wait another 48 hours; then wash off. Repeat treatment in 7 to 10 days if mites reappear or new lesions develop.
➤ **Itching**
Adults: Apply locally, massaging gently into affected area until completely absorbed; repeat p.r.n.

ACTION
Unknown.

Route	Onset	Peak	Duration
Topical	Unknown	Unknown	Unknown

Half-life: Unknown.

ADVERSE REACTIONS
Skin: *irritation,* allergic skin sensitivity.

INTERACTIONS
None significant.

EFFECTS ON LAB TEST RESULTS
None reported.

CONTRAINDICATIONS & CAUTIONS
- Contraindicated in patients hypersensitive to drug or its components and in those whose skin is raw or inflamed.

NURSING CONSIDERATIONS
- Estimate amount of cream needed per application; most patients tend to overuse scabicides. For most adults, a single tube of cream is enough for two applications.
- Don't apply drug to acutely inflamed or raw, weeping areas.
- Apply topical corticosteroids, as prescribed, if dermatitis develops from scratching.
- Make sure hospitalized patients are placed in isolation, with special linen handling precautions, until treatment is completed.
- Monthly maintenance treatments may be needed in long-term care facilities where infestation is a problem.
- ***Look alike–sound alike:*** Don't confuse Eurax with Serax or Urex.
- Treat sexual contacts simultaneously.

PATIENT TEACHING
- Tell patient or family member to shake product well before each use.
- Teach patient or family member how to apply drug. Tell patient not to apply to face, eyes, mucous membranes, or urethral opening. If accidental contact with eyes occurs, tell patient to flush with water and notify prescriber.
- Tell patient to stop using drug, wash it off skin, and notify prescriber immediately if skin irritation or hypersensitivity develops.
- Instruct patient to change all clothing and bed linens and launder them in hot cycle of washing machine or dry clean after drug is washed off body.
- Instruct patient to reapply drug if it's washed off during treatment time.
- Tell patient to warn other family members and sexual contacts about infestation.
- Reassure patient that although itching may continue for several weeks, it will

stop; continued itching doesn't indicate that therapy is ineffective.

lindane

GBH†

Pharmacologic class: ectoparasiticide and ovicide
Pregnancy risk category C

AVAILABLE FORMS

Cream: 1%†
Lotion: 1%
Shampoo: 1%

INDICATIONS & DOSAGES

➤ Parasitic infestation (scabies, pediculosis)

Adults and children: Centers for Disease Control and Prevention recommend not bathing before applying on skin. If patient does bathe, let skin dry and cool thoroughly before using drug. For scabies, apply thin layer of cream or lotion over entire skin surface from the neck down (with special attention to skinfolds, creases, interdigital spaces, and genital area) and rub in thoroughly; for pediculosis, apply thin layer of cream or lotion to hairy areas. After 8 to 12 hours, wash drug off. Repeat process in 1 week if mites reappear or new lesions develop.

Apply shampoo undiluted to dry hair and work into lather for 4 to 5 minutes; small amounts of water may increase lathering. Apply 30 ml of shampoo for short hair, 45 ml for medium-length hair, or 60 ml for long hair. Rinse thoroughly and rub dry with towel. Comb with a fine-tooth comb.

Elderly patients: May need to reduce dosage because of increased skin absorption.

ACTION

May inhibit neuronal membrane function in arthropods, causing neuronal hyperactivity, seizures, and death after penetrating the parasite's exoskeleton.

Route	Onset	Peak	Duration
Topical	190 min	Unknown	Unknown

Half-life: About 18 hours.

ADVERSE REACTIONS

CNS: ***seizures,*** dizziness.
Skin: dermatitis, alopecia, pruritus, urticaria.

INTERACTIONS

Drug-drug. *Drugs that lower the seizure threshold (anticholinesterases, antidepressants, antipsychotics, cyclosporine, chloroquine sulfate, imipenem, isoniazid, methocarbamol, meperidine, mofetil, mycophenolate, penicillins, pyrimethamine, quinolones, tacrolimus, theophylline):* May precipitate seizure activity if used together. Monitor patient if used together.

Drug-lifestyle. *Alcohol use:* May lower seizure threshold. Avoid using together.

Oil-based hair products: May increase absorption of drug. If oil-based hair products are used, urge patient to wash and dry hair before using drug.

EFFECTS ON LAB TEST RESULTS

None reported.

CONTRAINDICATIONS & CAUTIONS

- Contraindicated in premature infants, patients hypersensitive to drug or its components, in those with seizure disorders, and in those with inflamed skin.
- ***Alert:*** Use cautiously in infants, children, elderly patients, patients with skin conditions other than lice infestation, and those who weigh less than 110 lb (50 kg); all are at greater risk of CNS toxicity, including seizures and death.

NURSING CONSIDERATIONS

- Use lindane products only as second-line treatment of lice infestation or in patients who can't tolerate treatment with safer medications. Permethrin 1% cream rinse and pyrethrins with piperonyl butoxide are safer than lindane for pubic lice.
- Apply topical corticosteroids or give oral antihistamines, as prescribed, for pruritus.
- Make sure that hospitalized patients are placed in isolation, with special linen-handling precautions, until treatment is completed.
- Intact skin absorbs 6% to 13% of drug. Absorption is increased if applied to face, scalp, axillae, neck, scrotum, or irritated or broken skin.

• Avoid contact of drug with eyes.
• When used correctly, drug is safe and effective. When overused, it can cause adverse reactions. Don't confuse prolonged itching with reinfestation.
• Treat sexual partners simultaneously.

PATIENT TEACHING
• Teach patient or family member how to apply drug: Apply thin layer to cover body only once. Use 1 ounce for children younger than age 6 and 1 to 2 ounces for older children and adults. Don't leave drug on for longer than 12 hours; remove drug by washing thoroughly.
• If patient bathes before application, tell him to let skin dry thoroughly and cool before applying drug.
• Inform patient that drug can be poisonous when misused. Warn patient not to apply to open areas, acutely inflamed skin, or to face, eyes, mucous membranes, or urethral opening. If accidental contact with eyes occurs, advise patient to flush with water and notify prescriber.
• Tell patient to avoid inhaling vapors.
• Advise family member to wear gloves when applying drug.
• Tell patient to wash drug off skin and to notify prescriber immediately if skin irritation or hypersensitivity develops.
• Discourage repeated use, which can lead to skin irritation, systemic toxicity, or seizures. Advise patient to repeat use only if live lice or nits are found after 1 week.
• Warn patient not to use other creams or oils during treatment because of potential for increased absorption.
• Advise breast-feeding woman to avoid a lot of skin-to-skin contact with infant while drug is present. Interrupt breast-feeding with expression and discarding of milk for at least 24 hours following use.
• Instruct patient to change all clothing and bed linens and launder them in hot water or dry clean after drug is washed off body.
• After application for lice infestation, tell patient to use fine-tooth comb or tweezers to remove nits from hairy areas.
• Advise patient to use shampoo form to clean combs or brushes and to wash them thoroughly afterward. Warn patient not to use lindane routinely.
• Warn patient that itching may continue for several weeks after effective treatment, especially for scabies.
• Instruct patient to reapply drug if it's washed off during treatment time.
• Tell patient to warn other family members and sexual partners about infestation.
• Advise patient to use product carefully and follow all directions. Overusing product will cause unwanted side effects. Tell him not to confuse prolonged itching with reinfestation.

permethrin
Acticin, Elimite, Nix ◊

Pharmacologic class: pyrethroid
Pregnancy risk category B

AVAILABLE FORMS
Cream: 5%
Topical liquid (cream rinse): 1%

INDICATIONS & DOSAGES
➤ **Infestation with *Pediculus humanus capitis* (head louse) and its nits**
Adults and children age 2 and older: Use after hair has been washed with shampoo, rinsed with water, and towel-dried. Apply 25 to 50 ml of liquid to saturate hair and scalp. Allow drug to remain on hair for 10 minutes before rinsing off with water. Remove remaining nits with comb. Usually only one application is needed.
➤ **Infestation with *Sarcoptes scabiei***
Adults and children age 2 months and older: Thoroughly massage into the skin from the head to the soles. Treat infants on hairline, neck, scalp, temple, and forehead. Wash cream off after 8 to 14 hours.

ACTION
Acts on parasites' nerve cells to disrupt the sodium channel current, causing parasitic paralysis.

Route	Onset	Peak	Duration
Topical	10–15 min	Unknown	10 days

Half-life: Unknown.

ADVERSE REACTIONS

Skin: *burning, stinging,* edema, tingling, scalp numbness or discomfort, mild erythema, pruritus, scalp rash.

INTERACTIONS

None significant.

EFFECTS ON LAB TEST RESULTS

None reported.

CONTRAINDICATIONS & CAUTIONS

- Contraindicated in patients hypersensitive to pyrethrins, chrysanthemums, or components of drug.

NURSING CONSIDERATIONS

- Usually only one application is needed. Combing of nits isn't needed for effectiveness, but drug package supplies a fine-tooth comb for cosmetic use and to decrease diagnostic confusion that may lead to retreatment.
- Re-treat for lice if they are seen 7 days after first application.
- Treat sexual partners simultaneously.

PATIENT TEACHING

- Explain that treatment may temporarily worsen signs and symptoms of head lice infestation, such as itching, redness, and swelling.
- Tell patient to disinfect headgear, comb and brush, scarves, coats, and bed linens by machine washing with hot water and machine drying for at least 20 minutes, using hot cycle. Tell him to seal nonwashable items in plastic bag for 2 weeks or spray with product designed to eliminate lice and their nits.
- Warn patient not to use drug on eyes, eyelashes, eyebrows, nose, mouth, or mucous membranes.
- Tell patient to warn other family members and sexual contacts about infestation.

pyrethrins and piperonyl butoxide

A-200, Barc ◊, Blue, End Lice, Pronto, Pyrinyl ◊, R & C, RID ◊, Tegrin-LT, Tisit ◊, Triple X

Pharmacologic class: pyrethrin
Pregnancy risk category C

AVAILABLE FORMS

Shampoo: pyrethrins 0.2% and piperonyl butoxide 2%; pyrethrins 0.3% and piperonyl butoxide 3%; pyrethrins 0.33% and piperonyl butoxide 4%
Shampoo and conditioner: pyrethrins 0.33% and piperonyl butoxide technical 3.15%
Topical gel: pyrethrins 0.3% and piperonyl butoxide 3%
Topical solution: pyrethrins 0.18% and piperonyl butoxide 2%; pyrethrins 0.2%, piperonyl butoxide 2%, and deodorized kerosene 0.8%; pyrethrins 0.3% and piperonyl butoxide 3%; pyrethrins 0.3% and piperonyl butoxide 2%

INDICATIONS & DOSAGES

➤ Infestations of head, body, and pubic (crab) lice and their eggs

Adults and children: Apply to hair, scalp, or other infested areas until entirely wet. Allow to remain for 10 minutes but no longer. Wash thoroughly with warm water and soap or shampoo. Remove dead lice and eggs with fine-tooth comb. Repeat treatment in 7 to 10 days to kill newly hatched lice; don't use more than two applications within 24 hours.

ACTION

Acts as contact poison that disrupts parasite's nervous system, causing parasite's paralysis and death.

Route	Onset	Peak	Duration
Topical	Unknown	Unknown	Unknown

Half-life: Unknown

ADVERSE REACTIONS

Skin: *irritation with repeated use,* erythema, pruritus, urticaria, edema, eczema.

INTERACTIONS
None significant.

EFFECTS ON LAB TEST RESULTS
None reported.

CONTRAINDICATIONS & CAUTIONS
- Contraindicated in patients hypersensitive to drug, ragweed, or chrysanthemums.
- Use cautiously in infants and small children.

NURSING CONSIDERATIONS
- Apply topical corticosteroids or give oral antihistamines if dermatitis develops from scratching.
- Discard container by wrapping in several layers of newspaper.
- Inspect all family members daily for at least 2 weeks for infestation.
- Drug isn't effective against scabies.
- Treat sexual contacts simultaneously.

PATIENT TEACHING
- Instruct patient not to apply to open areas, acutely inflamed skin, eyebrows, eyelashes, face, eyes, mucous membranes, or urethral opening. If accidental contact with eyes occurs, advise patient to flush with water and notify prescriber.
- Warn patient not to swallow or inhale vapors from the drug.
- Tell patient to stop using drug, wash it off skin, and notify prescriber immediately if skin irritation develops. All preparations contain petroleum distillates.
- Instruct patient to change and sterilize all clothing and bed linens after drug is washed off body. Tell him to disinfect washable items by machine washing in hot water and drying on hot cycle for at least 20 minutes. Other items can be dry-cleaned and sealed in plastic bags for 2 weeks, or treated with products made for this purpose.
- Teach patient to remove dead parasites with a fine-tooth comb.
- Tell patient to repeat treatment in 7 to 10 days to kill any newly hatched eggs.
- Urge patient to warn other family members and sexual partners about infestation.

87

Topical corticosteroids

betamethasone dipropionate
betamethasone valerate
clobetasol propionate
desoximetasone
dexamethasone
dexamethasone sodium phosphate
fluocinolone acetonide
fluocinonide
fluticasone propionate
hydrocortisone
hydrocortisone acetate
hydrocortisone butyrate
hydrocortisone probutate
hydrocortisone valerate
triamcinolone acetonide

betamethasone dipropionate

Alphatrex, Diprolene, Diprolene AF, Diprosone, Maxivate, Teladar

betamethasone valerate

Betatrex, Beta-Val, Betnovate†‡, Luxiq, Psorion Cream

Pharmacologic class: corticosteroid
Pregnancy risk category C

AVAILABLE FORMS

betamethasone dipropionate
Aerosol: 0.1%
Cream: 0.05%
Gel: 0.05%
Lotion: 0.05%
Ointment: 0.05%

betamethasone valerate
Cream: 0.01%, 0.05%, 0.1%
Foam: 0.12%
Lotion: 0.1%
Ointment: 0.1%

INDICATIONS & DOSAGES

➤ **Inflammation and pruritus from corticosteroid-responsive dermatoses**

Adults and children older than age 12: Clean area; apply cream, ointment, lotion, aerosol spray, or gel sparingly. Give dipropionate products once daily to b.i.d.; give valerate 0.1% solution b.i.d., or valerate 0.1% cream or ointment once daily to t.i.d. Maximum dosage of augmented betamethasone dipropionate 0.05% ointment, cream, gel, or lotion is 45 g, 50 g, 45 g, or 50 ml per week, respectively. Therapy with augmented formulations should not exceed 2 weeks.

➤ **Inflammation and pruritus from corticosteroid-responsive dermatoses of scalp (valerate only)**

Adults: Gently massage small amounts of foam into affected scalp areas b.i.d., morning and evening, until control is achieved. If no improvement is seen in 2 weeks, reassess diagnosis.

ACTION

Unclear. Is diffused across cell membranes to form complexes with receptors. Has anti-inflammatory, antipruritic, vasoconstrictive, and antiproliferative activity. Considered a medium-potency to very high-potency drug (depending on product), according to vasoconstrictive properties.

Route	Onset	Peak	Duration
Topical	Unknown	Unknown	Unknown

Half-life: Unknown.

ADVERSE REACTIONS

GU: glycosuria with dipropionate.
Metabolic: hyperglycemia.
Skin: burning, pruritus, irritation, dryness, erythema, folliculitis, striae, acneiform eruptions, perioral dermatitis, hypopigmentation, hypertrichosis, allergic contact dermatitis, secondary infection, maceration, atrophy, miliaria with occlusive dressings.
Other: ***hypothalamic-pituitary-adrenal axis suppression,*** Cushing syndrome.

INTERACTIONS

None significant.

EFFECTS ON LAB TEST RESULTS

- May increase glucose level.

CONTRAINDICATIONS & CAUTIONS
- Contraindicated in patients hypersensitive to corticosteroids.
- Don't use as monotherapy in primary bacterial infections (impetigo, paronychia, erysipelas, cellulitis, angular cheilitis), rosacea, perioral dermatitis, or acne.
- Don't use augmented betamethasone dipropionate 0.05% ointment, betamethasone dipropionate 0.05% gel, cream, and ointment; betamethasone valerate 0.1% ointment on the face, groin, or axilla.
- Use cautiously in pregnant or breast-feeding women.

NURSING CONSIDERATIONS
- Drug isn't for ophthalmic use.
- Gently wash skin before applying. To prevent skin damage, rub in gently, leaving a thin coat. When treating hairy sites, part hair and apply directly to lesions.
- Dosing frequency can be decreased to once daily following clinical improvement.
- Avoid applying near eyes or mucous membranes or in ear canal, groin area, or axillae.
- Don't dispense foam directly into warm hands because foam will begin to melt upon contact.
- Because of alcohol content of vehicle, gel products may cause mild, transient stinging, especially when used on or near excoriated skin.
- For patients with eczematous dermatitis whose skin may be irritated by adhesive material, hold dressing in place with gauze, elastic bandages, stockings, or stockinette.
- ***Alert:*** Don't use occlusive dressings.
- If antifungal or antibiotic combined with corticosteroid fails to provide prompt improvement, stop corticosteroid until infection is controlled.
- Systemic absorption is likely with prolonged or extensive body surface treatment. Watch for symptoms.
- Avoid using plastic pants or tight-fitting diapers on treated areas in young children. Children may absorb larger amounts of drug and be more susceptible to systemic toxicity.
- Continue drug for a few days after lesions clear.
- ***Alert:*** Diprolene and Diprolene AF may not be replaced with generics because other products have different potencies.

PATIENT TEACHING
- Teach patient how to apply drug.
- Emphasize that drug is for external use only.
- Tell patient to wash hands after application.
- Tell patient to stop drug and report signs of systemic absorption, skin irritation or ulceration, hypersensitivity, or infection.
- Instruct patient not to use occlusive dressings.
- Discuss personal hygiene measures to reduce chance of infection.

clobetasol propionate

Clobex, Cormax, Dermovate†, Embeline, Embeline E, Olux, Temovate, Temovate E

Pharmacologic class: corticosteroid
Pregnancy risk category C

AVAILABLE FORMS
Cream: 0.05%
Foam: 0.05%
Gel: 0.05%
Lotion: 0.05%
Ointment: 0.05%
Scalp application: 0.05%*
Shampoo: 0.05%
Solution: 0.05%

INDICATIONS & DOSAGES

➤ **Inflammation and pruritus from corticosteroid-responsive dermatoses; short-term topical treatment of mild to moderate plaque-type psoriasis of nonscalp regions, excluding the face and intertriginous areas**

Adults: Apply thin layer of Clobex lotion to affected skin areas b.i.d., morning and evening, for maximum of 14 days. For lesions of moderate to severe plaque psoriasis that haven't improved sufficiently, continue treatment for up to 2 more weeks, as long as 10% or less of the body surface area is affected. Total dose shouldn't exceed 50 g (50 ml) of lotion weekly.

➤ Inflammation and pruritus from corticosteroid-responsive dermatoses; short-term topical treatment of mild to moderate plaque-type psoriasis of nonscalp regions, excluding the face and intertriginous areas
Adults and children age 12 and older: Apply thin layer to affected skin areas b.i.d., morning and evening, for maximum of 14 days. Total dose shouldn't exceed 50 g of foam, cream, or ointment or 50 ml of lotion or solution weekly.
➤ Inflammation and pruritus of moderate to severe corticosteroid-responsive dermatoses of the scalp
Adults: Apply to the affected scalp area b.i.d., morning and evening. Gently massage into affected scalp area until the foam disappears. Repeat until entire affected scalp area is treated. Limit treatment to 14 days, with no more than 50 g of foam weekly.
➤ Moderate to severe scalp psoriasis
Adults: Apply Clobex shampoo to affected areas of dry scalp in thin film once daily. Leave in place for 15 minutes before lathering and rinsing. Limit treatment to 4 consecutive weeks.

ACTION
Unclear. Is diffused across cell membranes to form complexes with receptors. Shows anti-inflammatory, antipruritic, vasoconstrictive, and antiproliferative activity. Considered a very high-potency to high-potency drug, according to vasoconstrictive properties.

Route	Onset	Peak	Duration
Topical	Unknown	Unknown	Unknown

Half-life: Unknown.

ADVERSE REACTIONS
GU: glycosuria.
Metabolic: hyperglycemia.
Skin: burning, pruritus, irritation, dryness, erythema, folliculitis, perioral dermatitis, allergic contact dermatitis, hypopigmentation, hypertrichosis, acneiform eruptions, skin atrophy, telangiectasia.
Other: ***hypothalamic-pituitary-adrenal axis suppression,*** Cushing syndrome, finger numbness.

INTERACTIONS
None significant.

EFFECTS ON LAB TEST RESULTS
- May increase glucose level.

CONTRAINDICATIONS & CAUTIONS
- Contraindicated in patients hypersensitive to corticosteroids and in those with primary scalp infections.
- Don't use as monotherapy for primary bacterial infections (impetigo, paronychia, erysipelas, cellulitis, angular cheilitis, erythrasma), rosacea, perioral dermatitis, or acne.
- Don't use very high-potency or high-potency agents on the face, groin, or axilla areas.
- Drug is not for ophthalmic use.
- Use cautiously in children and in pregnant or breast-feeding women.

NURSING CONSIDERATIONS
- Gently wash skin before applying. To prevent skin damage, rub medication in gently and completely. When treating hairy sites, part hair and apply directly to lesions.
- Avoid applying near eyes or mucous membranes or in ear canal.
- ***Alert:*** Don't use occlusive dressings or bandages. Don't cover or wrap treated areas unless directed by prescriber.
- If antifungal or antibiotic combined with corticosteroid fails to provide prompt improvement, stop corticosteroid until infection is controlled.
- Stop drug and notify prescriber if skin infection, striae, or atrophy occurs.
- Hypothalamic-pituitary-adrenal axis suppression occurs at doses as low as 2 g daily.

PATIENT TEACHING
- Teach patient how to apply drug and to avoid contact with eyes.
- Tell patient to wash hands after application.
- Tell patient to stop drug and report signs of systemic absorption, skin irritation or ulceration, hypersensitivity, or infection.
- Warn patient to use drug for no longer than 14 consecutive days.
- Tell patient using the foam to invert can and dispense a small amount of Olux

foam (up to a golf-ball–size dollop) into the cap of the can, onto a saucer or other cool surface, or directly on the lesion, taking care to avoid contact with the eyes. Dispensing directly onto hands isn't recommended because the foam will melt immediately upon contact with warm skin. Tell him to move hair away from affected area of scalp so that foam can be applied to each affected area.
- Tell patient using foam that contents are flammable and under pressure, so he should avoid smoking during and immediately after application and keep can away from flames. Also tell him not to puncture or incinerate container.

desoximetasone

Topicort, Topicort LP

Pharmacologic class: corticosteroid
Pregnancy risk category C

AVAILABLE FORMS

Cream: 0.05%, 0.25%
Gel: 0.05%
Ointment: 0.25%

INDICATIONS & DOSAGES

➤ **Inflammation from corticosteroid-responsive dermatoses**
Adults and children: Clean area; apply sparingly b.i.d.

ACTION

Unclear. Is diffused across cell membranes to form complexes with receptors. Shows anti-inflammatory, antipruritic, vasoconstrictive, and antiproliferative activity. Considered a high-potency drug (0.25% cream and ointment, 0.05% gel) or medium-potency drug (0.05% cream) according to vasoconstrictive properties.

Route	Onset	Peak	Duration
Topical	Unknown	Unknown	Unknown

Half-life: Unknown.

ADVERSE REACTIONS

GU: glycosuria.
Metabolic: hyperglycemia.
Skin: burning, pruritus, irritation, dryness, erythema, folliculitis, hypertrichosis, acneiform eruptions, perioral dermatitis, hypopigmentation, allergic contact dermatitis, *maceration, secondary infection, atrophy, striae, miliaria with occlusive dressings.*
Other: ***hypothalamic-pituitary-adrenal axis suppression,*** Cushing syndrome.

INTERACTIONS

None significant.

EFFECTS ON LAB TEST RESULTS

- May increase glucose level.

CONTRAINDICATIONS & CAUTIONS

- Contraindicated in patients hypersensitive to drug or its components.
- Don't use as monotherapy in primary bacterial infections (impetigo, paronychia, erysipelas, cellulitis, angular cheilitis), treatment of rosacea, perioral dermatitis, or acne.
- Don't use very high-potency or high-potency agents on the face, groin, or axillae.
- Drug is not for ophthalmic use.
- Use cautiously in children and pregnant or breast-feeding women.

NURSING CONSIDERATIONS

- Gently wash skin before applying. To prevent skin damage, rub in gently, leaving thin coat. When treating hairy sites, part hair and apply directly to lesions.
- Avoid applying near eyes, mucous membranes, or in ear canal.
- For patients with eczematous dermatitis whose skin may be irritated by adhesive material, hold dressing in place with gauze, elastic bandages, stockings, or stockinette.
- Change dressing as prescribed. Stop drug and notify prescriber if skin infection, striae, or atrophy occurs.
- If fever develops and occlusive dressing is in place, notify prescriber and remove occlusive dressing.
- If antifungal or antibiotic combined with corticosteroid fails to provide prompt improvement, stop corticosteroid until infection is controlled.
- Systemic absorption is likely with use of occlusive dressings, prolonged treat-

ment, or extensive body surface treatment. Watch for symptoms.

- Avoid using plastic pants or tight-fitting diapers on treated areas in young children. Children may absorb larger amounts of drug and be more susceptible to systemic toxicity.
- Continue drug for a few days after lesions clear.
- Gel contains alcohol and may cause burning or irritation in open lesions.
- ***Look alike–sound alike:*** Don't confuse desoximetasone with dexamethasone.

PATIENT TEACHING

- Teach patient how to apply drug.
- If an occlusive dressing is ordered, advise patient to leave it in place for no longer than 12 hours each day and not to use the dressing on infected or weeping lesions.
- Tell patient to stop drug and report signs of systemic absorption, skin irritation or ulceration, hypersensitivity, or infection.

dexamethasone

Aeroseb-Dex, Decaspray

dexamethasone sodium phosphate

Decadron Phosphate

Pharmacologic class: corticosteroid
Pregnancy risk category C

AVAILABLE FORMS

dexamethasone
Aerosol: 0.01%, 0.04%
dexamethasone sodium phosphate
Cream: 0.1%

INDICATIONS & DOSAGES

➤ Inflammation from corticosteroid-responsive dermatoses

Adults and children: Clean area; apply cream or aerosol sparingly b.i.d. to q.i.d. For aerosol use on scalp, shake can well but gently, and apply to dry scalp after shampooing. Hold can upright or inverted and 6 inches (15 cm) away from area. Spray while moving container to all affected areas, which should take about 2 seconds. Don't massage drug into scalp or spray forehead or near eyes. When result is obtained, reduce dose gradually, then stop use.

ACTION

Unclear. Is diffused across cell membranes to form complexes with cytoplasmic receptors. Shows anti-inflammatory, antipruritic, vasoconstrictive, and antiproliferative activity. Considered a low-potency drug, according to vasoconstrictive properties.

Route	Onset	Peak	Duration
Topical	Unknown	Unknown	Unknown

Half-life: Unknown.

ADVERSE REACTIONS

GU: glycosuria.
Metabolic: hyperglycemia.
Skin: burning, pruritus, irritation, dryness, erythema, folliculitis, hypertrichosis, acneiform eruptions, perioral dermatitis, hypopigmentation, allergic contact dermatitis, *maceration, secondary infection, atrophy, striae, miliaria with occlusive dressings.*
Other: ***hypothalamic-pituitary-adrenal axis suppression,*** Cushing syndrome, altered growth and development in children.

INTERACTIONS

None significant.

EFFECTS ON LAB TEST RESULTS

- May increase glucose level.

CONTRAINDICATIONS & CAUTIONS

- Contraindicated in patients hypersensitive to drug or its components.
- Don't use as monotherapy in primary bacterial infections (impetigo, paronychia, erysipelas, cellulitis, angular cheilitis), treatment of rosacea, perioral dermatitis, or acne.
- Drug is not for ophthalmic use.
- Use cautiously in pregnant or breast-feeding women.

NURSING CONSIDERATIONS

- Gently wash skin before applying. To prevent skin damage, rub cream in gently, leaving a thin coat. When treating hairy sites, part hair and apply directly to lesions.

- Avoid applying near eyes or mucous membranes or in ear canal, groin, or axillae.
- For patients with eczematous dermatitis whose skin may be irritated by adhesive material, hold dressing in place with gauze, stockings, or stockinette.
- Change dressing as prescribed. Stop drug and tell prescriber if skin infection, striae, or atrophy occurs.
- If an occlusive dressing has been applied and a fever develops, notify prescriber and remove dressing.
- When using aerosol around face, cover patient's eyes and warn against inhalation of spray. Aerosol preparation contains alcohol and may cause irritation or burning when used on open lesions. To avoid freezing tissues, don't spray longer than 1 to 2 seconds or from less than 6 inches (15 cm) away.
- If antifungal or antibiotic combined with corticosteroid fails to provide prompt improvement, stop corticosteroid until infection is controlled.
- Systemic absorption is likely with use of occlusive dressings, prolonged treatment, or extensive body surface treatment. Watch for symptoms.
- Avoid using plastic pants or tight-fitting diapers on treated areas in young children. Children may absorb larger amounts of drug and be more susceptible to systemic toxicity.
- Continue treatment for a few days after lesions clear.
- ***Look alike–sound alike:*** Don't confuse dexamethasone with desoximetasone.

PATIENT TEACHING

- Teach patient and family how to apply drug.
- If an occlusive dressing is used, advise patient to leave it in place for no longer than 12 hours each day and not to use dressing on infected or weeping lesions.
- Tell patient to stop drug and report signs of systemic absorption, skin irritation or ulceration, hypersensitivity, or infection.
- Tell patient to avoid scratching.

fluocinolone acetonide

Capex, Derma-Smoothe/FS, Flurosyn, FS Shampoo, Synalar, Synalar-HP, Synemol

Pharmacologic class: corticosteroid
Pregnancy risk category C

AVAILABLE FORMS

Cream: 0.01%, 0.025%
Oil: 0.01%
Ointment: 0.025%
Shampoo: 0.01%
Topical solution: 0.01%

INDICATIONS & DOSAGES

➤ **Inflammation from corticosteroid-responsive dermatoses**

Adults and children: Clean area; apply product sparingly b.i.d. to q.i.d.

➤ **Atopic dermatitis**

Adults: Apply thin film of topical oil t.i.d.
Children 2 years and older: Apply thin film of topical oil b.i.d. for maximum of 4 weeks. Avoid face and diaper area.

➤ **Scalp psoriasis**

Adults: Wet or dampen hair and scalp thoroughly. Apply a thin film of topical oil and massage into scalp. Cover with supplied shower cap overnight or for a minimum of 4 hours before washing thoroughly with regular shampoo and then rinsing thoroughly with water.

➤ **Seborrheic dermatitis of the scalp**

Adults: Apply no more than 30 ml of 0.01% shampoo to the scalp once daily, lather, and rinse thoroughly with water after 5 minutes.

ACTION

Unclear. Is diffused across cell membranes to form complexes with receptors. Shows anti-inflammatory, antipruritic, vasoconstrictive, and antiproliferative activity. Considered a medium-potency drug to low-potency drug, according to vasoconstrictive properties.

Route	Onset	Peak	Duration
Topical	Unknown	Unknown	Unknown

Half-life: Unknown.

ADVERSE REACTIONS

GU: glycosuria.
Metabolic: hyperglycemia.
Skin: burning, pruritus, irritation, dryness, erythema, folliculitis, hypertrichosis, hypopigmentation, acneiform eruptions, perioral dermatitis, allergic contact dermatitis, *maceration, secondary infection, atrophy, striae, miliaria with occlusive dressings.*
Other: ***hypothalamic-pituitary-adrenal axis suppression,*** Cushing syndrome.

INTERACTIONS

None significant.

EFFECTS ON LAB TEST RESULTS

- May increase glucose level.

CONTRAINDICATIONS & CAUTIONS

- Contraindicated in patients hypersensitive to drug or its components.
- Don't use as monotherapy in primary bacterial infections (impetigo, paronychia, erysipelas, cellulitis, angular cheilitis), treatment of rosacea, perioral dermatitis, or acne.
- Drug isn't for ophthalmic use.
- Use cautiously in pregnant or breast-feeding women.

NURSING CONSIDERATIONS

- Gently wash skin before applying. To prevent skin damage, rub in gently, leaving a thin coat. When treating hairy sites, part hair and apply directly to lesions.
- Avoid application near eyes or mucous membranes; in axillae, groin, or rectal area; or in ear canal if eardrum is perforated.
- For patients with eczematous dermatitis whose skin may be irritated by adhesive material, hold dressing in place with gauze, elastic bandages, stockings, or stockinette.
- Change dressing as prescribed. Stop drug and notify prescriber if skin infection, striae, or atrophy occurs.
- If an occlusive dressing has been applied and a fever develops, notify prescriber and remove dressing.
- If antifungal or antibiotic combined with corticosteroid fails to provide prompt improvement, stop corticosteroid until infection is controlled.
- Systemic absorption is likely with use of occlusive dressings, prolonged treatment, or extensive body surface treatment. Watch for symptoms, such as hyperglycemia, glycosuria, hypothalamic-pituitary-adrenal axis suppression or Cushing syndrome.
- Avoid using plastic pants or tight-fitting diapers on treated areas in young children. Children may absorb larger amounts of drug and be more susceptible to systemic toxicity.
- ***Look alike–sound alike:*** Don't confuse fluocinolone with fluocinonide or fluticasone.

PATIENT TEACHING

- Teach patient or family how to apply drug using gloves or sterile applicator.
- Tell patient to wash hands after application.
- If an occlusive dressing is used, advise patient to leave it in place for no longer than 12 hours each day and not to use dressing on infected or weeping lesions.
- Tell patient to stop using solution and notify prescriber if he develops signs of systemic absorption, skin irritation or ulceration, hypersensitivity, or infection.

fluocinonide

Fluonex, Lidex, Lidex-E, Vanos

Pharmacologic class: corticosteroid
Pregnancy risk category C

AVAILABLE FORMS

Cream: 0.05%, 0.1%
Gel: 0.05%
Ointment: 0.05%
Topical solution: 0.05%

INDICATIONS & DOSAGES

➤ Inflammation from corticosteroid-responsive dermatoses
Adults and children: Clean area; apply cream, gel, ointment, or topical solution sparingly t.i.d. or q.i.d. In children, use lowest dosage that promotes healing. If using Vanos 0.1% cream in adults and

children age 12 and older, apply a thin layer once or twice daily for up to 2 weeks. Don't use more than 60 g/week.

ACTION

Unclear. Is diffused across cell membranes to form complexes with cytoplasmic receptors. Shows anti-inflammatory, antipruritic, vasoconstrictive, and antiproliferative activity. Considered a high-potency drug, according to vasoconstrictive properties.

Route	Onset	Peak	Duration
Topical	Unknown	Unknown	Unknown

Half-life: Unknown.

ADVERSE REACTIONS

GU: glycosuria.
Metabolic: hyperglycemia.
Skin: burning, pruritus, irritation, dryness, erythema, folliculitis, hypertrichosis, hypopigmentation, acneiform eruptions, perioral dermatitis, allergic contact dermatitis, *maceration, secondary infection, atrophy, striae, miliaria with occlusive dressings.*
Other: ***hypothalamic-pituitary-adrenal axis suppression,*** Cushing syndrome.

INTERACTIONS

None significant.

EFFECTS ON LAB TEST RESULTS

- May increase glucose level.

CONTRAINDICATIONS & CAUTIONS

- Contraindicated in patients hypersensitive to drug or its components.
- Don't use as monotherapy in primary bacterial infections (impetigo, paronychia, erysipelas, cellulitis, angular cheilitis), treatment of rosacea, perioral dermatitis, or acne.
- Don't use very high-potency or high-potency agents on the face, groin, or axilla areas.
- Drug isn't for ophthalmic use.
- Use cautiously in pregnant or breast-feeding women.

NURSING CONSIDERATIONS

- Gently wash skin before applying. To prevent skin damage, rub in gently, leaving a thin coat. When treating hairy sites, part hair and apply directly to lesion.
- Avoid applying near eyes or mucous membranes or in ear canal.
- Occlusive dressings may be used in severe or resistant dermatoses.
- For patients with eczematous dermatitis whose skin may be irritated by adhesive material, hold dressing in place with gauze, elastic bandages, stockings, or stockinette.
- Change dressing as prescribed. Stop drug and notify prescriber if skin infection, striae, or atrophy occurs.
- If an occlusive dressing has been applied and a fever develops, notify prescriber and remove dressing.
- If antifungal or antibiotic combined with corticosteroid fails to provide prompt improvement, stop corticosteroid until infection is controlled.
- Systemic absorption is likely with use of occlusive dressings, prolonged treatment, or extensive body surface treatment. Watch for symptoms such as hyperglycemia, glycosuria, and hypothalamic-pituitary-adrenal axis suppression.
- Avoid using plastic pants or tight-fitting diapers on treated areas in young children. Children may absorb larger amounts of drug and be more susceptible to systemic toxicity.
- Continue treatment for a few days after lesions clear.
- ***Look alike–sound alike:*** Don't confuse fluocinonide with fluocinolone or fluticasone.

PATIENT TEACHING

- Teach patient and family how to apply drug using careful hand washing and gloves or sterile applicator.
- If an occlusive dressing is ordered, advise patient to leave it in place no more than 12 hours each day and not to use the dressing on infected or weeping lesions.
- Tell patient to stop drug and report signs of systemic absorption, skin irritation or ulceration, hypersensitivity, or infection.

fluticasone propionate
Cutivate

Pharmacologic class: corticosteroid
Pregnancy risk category C

AVAILABLE FORMS
Cream: 0.05%
Ointment: 0.005%
Lotion: 0.05%

INDICATIONS & DOSAGES
➤ **Inflammation and pruritus from dermatoses responsive to corticosteroids**
Adults: Apply sparingly to affected area b.i.d.; rub in gently and completely.
Children age 3 months and older: Apply a thin film of cream (0.05%) to affected areas b.i.d. Rub in gently. Don't use for longer than 4 weeks. If using lotion (0.05%) in adults and children 1 year and older, apply once daily.
➤ **Inflammation and pruritus from atopic dermatitis**
Children age 3 months and older: Apply thin film (0.05%) to affected areas once daily or b.i.d. Rub in gently. Don't use for longer than 4 weeks.

ACTION
Unclear. Is diffused across cell membranes to form complexes with cytoplasmic receptors. Shows anti-inflammatory, antipruritic, vasoconstrictive, and antiproliferative activity. Considered a medium-potency drug, according to vasoconstrictive properties.

Route	Onset	Peak	Duration
Topical	Rapid	Unknown	10 hr

Half-life: Unknown.

ADVERSE REACTIONS
CNS: light-headedness.
GU: glycosuria.
Metabolic: hyperglycemia.
Skin: urticaria, burning, hypertrichosis, pruritus, irritation, erythema, hives, dryness.
Other: ***hypothalamic-pituitary-adrenal axis suppression,*** Cushing syndrome.

INTERACTIONS
None significant.

EFFECTS ON LAB TEST RESULTS
- May increase glucose level.

CONTRAINDICATIONS & CAUTIONS
- Contraindicated in patients hypersensitive to drug or its components.
- Don't use as monotherapy in primary bacterial, viral, fungal, herpetic, or tubercular skin infections; for treatment of rosacea, perioral dermatitis, or acne
- Drug is not for ophthalmic use.
- Use cautiously in pregnant or breast-feeding women.

NURSING CONSIDERATIONS
- Don't mix drug with other bases or vehicles because doing so may affect potency.
- If adverse reactions occur, prescriber may order less potent drug.
- Stop drug if local irritation or systemic infection, absorption, or hypersensitivity occurs.
- Absorption of corticosteroid is increased when drug is applied to inflamed or damaged skin, eyelids, or scrotal area; it's lowest when applied to intact normal skin, palms of hands, or soles of feet.
- Don't use drug with an occlusive dressing or in diaper area.
- ***Look alike–sound alike:*** Don't confuse fluticasone with fluconazole.

PATIENT TEACHING
- Teach patient or family member how to apply drug using gloves, sterile applicator, or after careful hand washing.
- Tell patient to wash hands after application.
- Tell patient to avoid prolonged use and contact with eyes. Warn him not to apply to face, in skin creases, or around eyes, genitals, underarms, or rectum.
- Instruct patient to notify prescriber if condition persists or worsens or if burning or irritation develops.

hydrocortisone

Acticort 100, Aeroseb-HC, Ala-Cort, Ala-Scalp, Alcortin, Anusol-HC, Bactine Hydrocortisone ◇, Cetacort, Cort-Dome, Cortisone-5 ◇, Cortisone-10 ◇, Cortisone-10 Quickshot, Delcort, Dermolate Anti-Itch ◇, Dermtex HC ◇, Eldecort, Hi-Cor 2.5, Hycort, HydroSkin, HydroTex, Hytone, LactiCare-HC, Maximum Strength Cortaid Faststick, Penecort, Procort ◇, Proctocort ◇, Scalpicin ◇, Synacort, Tegrin-HC ◇, Texacort, T/Scalp

hydrocortisone acetate

Anu-Med HC, Anusol HC-1 ◇, Caldecort (Maximum Strength), Cortaid ◇, Cortamed†, Cortef Feminine Itch ◇, Corticaine ◇, Dermol HC, Gynecort ◇, Hemril-HC Uniserts, Lanacort-5 ◇, Lanacort 10 ◇, ProctoCream-HC, ProctoFoam-HC, Tucks, U-cort

hydrocortisone butyrate

Locoid

hydrocortisone probutate

Pandel

hydrocortisone valerate

Westcort

Pharmacologic class: corticosteroid
Pregnancy risk category C

AVAILABLE FORMS

hydrocortisone
Cream: 0.5% ◇, 1% ◇, 2.5%
Gel: 1%, 2%
Lotion: 0.25%, 0.5% ◇, 1% ◇, 1%, 2%, 2.5%
Ointment: 0.5% ◇, 1% ◇, 2.5%
Rectal cream: 1% ◇
Rectal ointment: 1%
Spray: 1% ◇
Stick roll-on: 1%
Topical solution: 1%

hydrocortisone acetate
Cream: 0.5% ◇, 1% ◇, 1%
Ointment: 0.5% ◇, 1% ◇
Rectal foam: 90 mg per application
Suppositories: 25 mg, 30 mg

hydrocortisone butyrate
Cream: 0.1%
Ointment: 0.1%
Solution: 0.1%

hydrocortisone probutate
Cream: 0.1%

hydrocortisone valerate
Cream: 0.2%
Ointment: 0.2%

INDICATIONS & DOSAGES

➤ **Inflammation and pruritus from corticosteroid-responsive dermatoses, adjunctive topical management of seborrheic dermatitis of scalp**

Adults and children: Clean area; apply cream, gel, lotion, ointment, or topical solution sparingly daily to q.i.d. Spray aerosol onto affected area daily to q.i.d. until acute phase is controlled; then reduce dosage to one to three times weekly, p.r.n. Give children lowest dose that provides positive results.

➤ **Inflammation from proctitis**

Adults: 1 applicatorful of rectal foam P.R. daily or b.i.d. for 2 to 3 weeks; then every other day, p.r.n. Give enema once nightly for 21 days or until patient improves; may use every other night for 2 to 3 months. Insert suppository b.i.d. for 2 weeks.

ACTION

Unclear. Is diffused across cell membranes to form complexes with cytoplasmic receptors. Shows anti-inflammatory, antipruritic, vasoconstrictive, and antiproliferative activity. Considered a low-potency (hydrocortisone, hydrocortisone acetate) and a medium-potency (hydrocortisone butyrate, hydrocortisone probutate, hydrocortisone valerate) drug, according to vasoconstrictive properties.

Route	Onset	Peak	Duration
Topical, P.R.	Unknown	Unknown	Unknown

Half-life: Unknown.

ADVERSE REACTIONS

Topical

GU: glycosuria.

Metabolic: hyperglycemia.

Skin: burning, pruritus, irritation, dryness, erythema, folliculitis, hypertrichosis, hypopigmentation, acneiform eruptions, allergic contact dermatitis, *atrophy, maceration, secondary infection, striae, miliaria with occlusive dressings.*

Other: ***hypothalamic-pituitary-adrenal axis suppression,*** Cushing syndrome.

Rectal

CNS: ***seizures, increased intracranial pressure,*** vertigo, headache.

CV: hypertension.

EENT: cataracts, glaucoma.

GI: peptic ulcer, ***pancreatitis,*** abdominal distention.

GU: menstrual irregularities.

Metabolic: fluid or electrolyte disturbances, decreased carbohydrate tolerance.

Musculoskeletal: muscle weakness, osteoporosis, necrosis and fractures in bone.

Skin: impaired wound healing, fragile skin, petechiae, erythema, sweating.

INTERACTIONS

None significant.

EFFECTS ON LAB TEST RESULTS

- May increase glucose level.

CONTRAINDICATIONS & CAUTIONS

- Contraindicated in patients hypersensitive to drug or its components.
- Don't use as monotherapy in primary bacterial infections (impetigo, paronychia, erysipelas, cellulitis, angular cheilitis), treatment of rosacea, perioral dermatitis, or acne.
- Drug isn't for ophthalmic use.
- Use cautiously in pregnant or breast-feeding women.

NURSING CONSIDERATIONS

- Gently wash skin before applying. To prevent skin damage, rub in gently, leaving a thin coat. When treating hairy sites, part hair and apply directly to lesions.
- Check individual products for frequency of administration.
- Avoid applying near eyes or mucous membranes or in ear canal; may be safely used on face, groin, and armpits and under breasts.
- If an occlusive dressing is applied and a fever develops, notify prescriber and remove dressing.
- Change dressing as prescribed. Stop drug and tell prescriber if skin infection, striae, or atrophy occurs.
- When using aerosol near the face, cover patient's eyes and warn against inhaling spray. Aerosol contains alcohol and may cause irritation or burning when used on open lesions. Don't spray longer than 3 seconds or from closer than 6 inches (15 cm) to avoid freezing tissues. If spray is applied to dry scalp after shampooing, drug need not be massaged into scalp.
- If antifungal or antibiotic combined with corticosteroid fails to provide prompt improvement, stop corticosteroid until infection is controlled.
- Systemic absorption is likely with use of occlusive dressings, prolonged treatment, or extensive body surface treatment. Watch for symptoms, such as hyperglycemia, glycosuria, and hypothalamic-pituitary-adrenal axis suppression.
- Avoid using plastic pants or tight-fitting diapers on treated areas in young children. Children may absorb larger amounts of drug and be more susceptible to systemic toxicity.
- Continue treatment for a few days after lesions clear.
- Monitor patient for fluid or electrolyte disturbances (sodium and fluid retention, potassium loss, hypokalemic alkalosis, negative nitrogen balance from catabolism of protein).
- Drug may suppress skin reaction testing.
- ***Look alike–sound alike:*** Don't confuse hydrocortisone with hydroxychloroquine.

PATIENT TEACHING

- Teach patient or family member how to apply drug.
- Tell patient to wash hands after application.
- If an occlusive dressing is ordered, advise patient to leave it in place for no longer than 12 hours each day and not to use the dressing on infected or weeping lesions.

• Tell patient to stop drug and report signs of systemic absorption, skin irritation or ulceration, hypersensitivity, infection, or lack of improvement.
• Instruct patient to insert suppositories blunt end first after removing foil wrapper.
• For perianal application, instruct patient to place small amount of drug on a tissue and gently rub in.
• Tell patient to disassemble applicator or aerosol cap and clean with warm water after each use.

triamcinolone acetonide

Aristocort, Aristocort A, Delta-Tritex, Flutex, Kenalog, Kenalone‡, Kenonel, Triacet, Triderm

Pharmacologic class: corticosteroid
Pregnancy risk category C

AVAILABLE FORMS

Aerosol: 0.2 mg/2-second spray
Cream: 0.02%‡, 0.025%, 0.1%, 0.5%
Lotion: 0.025%, 0.1%
Ointment: 0.02%‡, 0.025%, 0.1%, 0.5%
Paste: 0.1%

INDICATIONS & DOSAGES

➤ **Inflammation and pruritus from corticosteroid-responsive dermatoses**
Adults and children: Clean area; apply aerosol, cream, lotion, or ointment sparingly b.i.d. to q.i.d. Rub in lightly.

➤ **Inflammation from oral lesions**
Adults and children: Apply paste at bedtime and, if needed, b.i.d. or t.i.d., preferably after meals. Apply small amount without rubbing; press to lesion in mouth until thin film develops.

ACTION

Unclear. Is diffused across cell membranes to form complexes with cytoplasmic receptors. Shows anti-inflammatory, antipruritic, vasoconstrictive, and antiproliferative activity. Considered a medium-potency (0.025% and 0.1% cream, ointment, lotion) and high-potency (0.5% cream, ointment) drug, according to vasoconstrictive properties.

Route	Onset	Peak	Duration
Topical	Several hr	Unknown	> 1 wk

Half-life: Unknown.

ADVERSE REACTIONS

CV: syncope.
GI: peptic ulcer.
GU: glycosuria.
Metabolic: hyperglycemia.
Skin: burning, pruritus, irritation, dryness, erythema, folliculitis, hypertrichosis, hypopigmentation, acneiform eruptions, perioral dermatitis, allergic contact dermatitis, *maceration, secondary infection, atrophy, striae, miliaria with occlusive dressings.*
Other: ***hypothalamic-pituitary-adrenal axis suppression,*** Cushing syndrome.

INTERACTIONS

None significant

EFFECTS ON LAB TEST RESULTS

• May increase glucose level.

CONTRAINDICATIONS & CAUTIONS

• Contraindicated in patients hypersensitive to drug or its components.
• Contraindicated in the presence of fungal, viral, or bacterial infections of the mouth or throat (paste).
• Don't use as monotherapy in primary bacterial infections (impetigo, paryonchia, erysipelas, cellulitis, angular cheilitis), treatment of rosacea, perioral dermatitis, or acne.
• Don't use very high-potency or high-potency agents on the face, groin, or axilla areas.
• Drug isn't for ophthalmic use.
• Use cautiously in pregnant or breastfeeding women.

NURSING CONSIDERATIONS

• Gently wash skin before applying. To avoid skin damage, rub in gently, leaving a thin coat. When treating hairy sites, part hair and apply directly to lesions.
• Don't apply near eyes or in ear canal.
• Stop drug and tell prescriber if skin infection, striae, or atrophy occurs.
• When using aerosol near the face, cover patient's eyes and warn against inhaling

spray. Aerosol contains alcohol and may cause irritation or burning when used on open lesions. Don't spray longer than 3 seconds or from closer than 6 inches (15 cm) to avoid freezing tissues.

- If antifungal or antibiotic combined with corticosteroid fails to provide prompt improvement, stop corticosteroid until infection is controlled.
- Occlusive dressings may be used in severe or resistant dermatoses.
- Systemic absorption is likely with the use of occlusive dressings, prolonged treatment, or extensive body surface treatment. Watch for symptoms, such as hyperglycemia, glycosuria, and hypothalamic-pituitary-adrenal axis suppression.
- Avoid using plastic pants or tight-fitting diapers on treated areas in young children. Children may absorb larger amounts of drug and be more susceptible to systemic toxicity.
- ***Look alike–sound alike:*** Don't confuse triamcinolone with Triaminicin or Triaminicol.

PATIENT TEACHING

- Teach patient or family member how to apply drug.
- If an occlusive dressing is ordered, advise patient to leave it in place for no longer than 12 hours each day and not to use the dressing on infected or weeping lesions.
- Tell patient to stop drug and report signs of systemic absorption, skin irritation or ulceration, hypersensitivity, infection, or lack of improvement.

88

Calorics

amino acid infusions, crystalline
amino acid infusions in dextrose
amino acid infusions with electrolytes
amino acid infusions with electrolytes in dextrose
amino acid infusions for hepatic failure
amino acid infusions for high metabolic stress
amino acid infusions for renal failure
dextrose
fat emulsions

SAFETY ALERT!

amino acid infusions, crystalline

Aminosyn, Aminosyn II, Aminosyn-PF, Aminosyn-RF, FreAmine III, Novamine, Premasol, Travasol, TrophAmine

amino acid infusions in dextrose

Aminosyn II with Dextrose, Travasol in Dextrose

amino acid infusions with electrolytes

Aminosyn with Electrolytes, Aminosyn II with Electrolytes, FreAmine III with Electrolytes, ProcalAmine with Electrolytes, Travasol with Electrolytes

amino acid infusions with electrolytes in dextrose

Aminosyn II with Electrolytes in Dextrose, Travasol with Electrolytes in Dextrose

amino acid infusions for hepatic failure

HepatAmine

amino acid infusions for high metabolic stress

Aminosyn-HBC, BranchAmin, FreAmine HBC

amino acid infusions for renal failure

Aminess, Aminosyn-RF, NephrAmine, RenAmin

Pharmacologic class: protein substrate
Pregnancy risk category C

AVAILABLE FORMS

Injection: 250 ml, 500 ml, 1,000 ml, 2,000 ml containing amino acids in various concentrations
amino acid infusions, crystalline
Aminosyn: 3.5%, 5%, 7%, 8.5%, 10%
Aminosyn II: 3.5%, 5%, 7%, 8.5%, 10%, 15%
Aminosyn-PF: 7%, 10%
Aminosyn-RF: 5.2%
FreAmine III: 8.5%, 10%
Novamine: 11.4%, 15%
Premasol: 6%, 10%
Travasol: 5.5%, 8.5%, 10%
TrophAmine: 6%, 10%
amino acid infusions in dextrose
Aminosyn II: 3.5% in 5% dextrose, 3.5% in 25% dextrose, 4.25% in 10% dextrose, 4.25% in 20% dextrose, 4.25% in 25% dextrose, 5% in 25% dextrose
Travasol: 2.75% in 5% dextrose, 2.75% in 10% dextrose, 2.75% in 25% dextrose, 4.25% in 5% dextrose, 4.25% in 10% dextrose, 4.25% in 25% dextrose
amino acid infusions with electrolytes
Aminosyn: 3.5%, 7%, 8.5%
Aminosyn II: 3.5%, 7%, 8.5%, 10%
FreAmine III: 3%, 8.5%
ProcalAmine: 3%
Travasol: 3.5%, 5.5%, 8.5%
amino acid infusions with electrolytes in dextrose
Aminosyn II: 3.5% with electrolytes in 5% dextrose, 3.5% with electrolytes in 25% dextrose, 4.25% with electrolytes in 10% dextrose, 4.25% with electrolytes in

20% dextrose, 4.25% with electrolytes in 25% dextrose
Travasol: 2.75% with electrolytes in 5% dextrose, 2.75% with electrolytes in 10% dextrose, 4.25% with electrolytes in 5% dextrose, 4.25% with electrolytes in 10% dextrose, 4.25% with electrolytes in 25% dextrose
amino acid infusions for hepatic failure
HepatAmine: 8%
amino acid infusions for high metabolic stress
Aminosyn-HBC: 7%
BranchAmin: 4%
FreAmine HBC: 6.9%
amino acid infusions for renal failure
Aminess: 5.2%
Aminosyn-RF: 5.2%
NephrAmine: 5.4%
RenAmin: 6.5%

INDICATIONS & DOSAGES

➤ **Total parenteral nutrition (TPN) in patients who can't or won't eat**
Adults: 1 to 1.7 g/kg I.V. daily.
Children weighing more than 10 kg (22 lb): 20 to 25 g I.V. daily for first 10 kg; then 1 to 1.25 g/kg I.V. daily for each kg over 10 kg.
Children weighing less than 10 kg: 2 to 4 g/kg I.V. daily.

➤ **Nutritional support in patients with cirrhosis, hepatitis, or hepatic encephalopathy**
Adults: 80 to 120 g of amino acids (12 to 18 g of nitrogen) I.V. daily of formulation for hepatic failure.

➤ **Nutritional support in patients with high metabolic stress**
Adults: 1.5 g/kg I.V. daily of formulation for high metabolic stress.

➤ **Nutritional support in patients with renal failure**
Adults: 0.6 to 0.8 g/kg I.V. daily of formulation for renal failure.
Adjust-a-dose: Patients receiving dialysis may need 1 to 1.2 g/kg daily.

I.V. ADMINISTRATION

- Infuse amino acids only in I.V. fluids or TPN solution.
- Limit peripheral infusions to 2.5% amino acids and 10% dextrose.
- Control infusion rate carefully with infusion pump. If infusion rate falls behind, notify prescriber; don't increase rate to catch up.
- Check infusion site often for erythema, inflammation, irritation, tissue sloughing, necrosis, and phlebitis.

INCOMPATIBILITIES

Bleomycin, ganciclovir, and indomethacin. Because of high risk of incompatibility with other substances, add only needed nutritional products.

ACTION

Provides a substrate for protein synthesis or increases conservation of existing body protein.

Route	Onset	Peak	Duration
I.V.	Immediate	Immediate	Unknown

Half-life: Unknown.

ADVERSE REACTIONS

CNS: fever.
CV: thrombophlebitis, edema, thrombosis, flushing.
GI: nausea.
GU: glycosuria, osmotic diuresis.
Metabolic: *rebound hypoglycemia when long-term infusions are abruptly stopped,* ***hyperosmolar hyperglycemic nonketotic syndrome,*** hyperglycemia, metabolic acidosis, alkalosis, hypophosphatemia, hyperammonemia, electrolyte imbalances, weight gain.
Musculoskeletal: osteoporosis.
Other: ***catheter sepsis,*** hypersensitivity reactions, tissue sloughing at infusion site from extravasation.

INTERACTIONS

Drug-drug. *Tetracycline:* May reduce protein-sparing effects of infused amino acids because of its anti-anabolic activity. Monitor patient.

EFFECTS ON LAB TEST RESULTS

- May increase ammonia and liver enzyme levels. May decrease magnesium, phosphate, and potassium levels. May increase or decrease glucose level.

CONTRAINDICATIONS & CAUTIONS

- Contraindicated in patients with anuria and in those with inborn errors of amino

acid metabolism, such as maple syrup urine disease and isovaleric acidemia.
- Standard amino acid formulations are contraindicated in patients with severe renal failure or hepatic disease.
- Use cautiously in children and neonates.
- Use cautiously in patients with renal or hepatic impairment or failure or diabetes.
- Use cautiously in patients with cardiac disease or insufficiency; drug may cause circulatory overload.

NURSING CONSIDERATIONS

- Patients with fluid restriction may tolerate only 1 to 2 L.
- When diabetic patient receives drug, his insulin requirements may increase.
- Some products contain sulfites. Check contents before giving to patients with sulfite sensitivity.
- Obtain baseline electrolyte, glucose, BUN, calcium, and phosphorus levels before therapy; monitor these levels periodically throughout therapy.
- Safe and effective use of parenteral nutrition requires knowledge of nutrition and clinical expertise in recognizing and treating complications. Frequent evaluations of patient and laboratory studies are needed.
- Check fractional urine for glycosuria every 6 hours initially, and then every 12 to 24 hours in stable patients. Abrupt onset of glycosuria may be an early sign of impending sepsis.
- Assess body temperature every 4 hours; elevation may indicate sepsis or infection.
- Watch for extraordinary electrolyte losses that may occur during nasogastric suction, vomiting, diarrhea, or drainage from GI fistula.
- If patient has chills, fever, or other signs of sepsis, replace I.V. tubing and bottle and send tubing and bottle to the laboratory to be cultured.
- ***Look alike–sound alike:*** Don't confuse Aminosyn with amikacin.

PATIENT TEACHING

- Explain need for supplement to patient and family, and answer any questions.
- Tell patient to report adverse reactions promptly.

SAFETY ALERT!

dextrose (d-glucose)

Pharmacologic class: carbohydrate caloric agent
Pregnancy risk category C

AVAILABLE FORMS

Injection: 3-ml ampule (10%); 10 ml (25%); 25 ml (5%); 50 ml (5% and 50% available in vial, ampule, and Bristoject); 70-ml pin-top vial (70% for additive use only); 100 ml (5%); 150 ml (5%); 250 ml (5%, 10%); 500 ml (5%, 10%, 20%, 30%, 40%, 50%, 60%, 70%); 650 ml (38.5%); 1,000 ml (2.5%, 5%, 10%, 20%, 30%, 40%, 50%, 60%, 70%); 2,000 ml (50%, 70%)

INDICATIONS & DOSAGES

➤Fluid replacement and caloric supplementation in patients who can't maintain adequate oral intake or are restricted from doing so

Adults and children: Dosage depends on fluid and caloric requirements. Use peripheral I.V. infusion of 2.5%, 5%, or 10% solution or central I.V. infusion of 20% solution for minimal fluid needs. Use a 10% to 25% solution to treat acute hypoglycemia in neonate or older infant (2 ml/kg). Use a 50% solution to treat insulin-induced hypoglycemia (20 to 50 ml). Solutions of 10%, 20%, 30%, 40%, 50%, 60%, and 70% are diluted in admixtures, usually amino acid solutions, for total parenteral nutrition (TPN) given through a central vein.

I.V. ADMINISTRATION

- Use central vein to infuse dextrose solutions at concentrations above 10%.
- Use infusion pump when giving dextrose solution with amino acids for TPN.
- Never infuse concentrated solution rapidly. Rapid infusion may cause hyperglycemia and fluid shift. Maximum infusion rate is 0.8 g/kg/hour.
- Check injection site often for irritation, tissue sloughing, necrosis, and phlebitis.

INCOMPATIBILITIES

Ampicillin sodium, cisplatin, diazepam, erythromycin lactobionate, 10% and 25% fat emulsion solutions, phenytoin, procainamide, solutions of 10% thiopental and above, whole blood.

ACTION

A simple water-soluble sugar that minimizes glyconeogenesis and promotes anabolism in patients whose oral caloric intake is limited.

Route	Onset	Peak	Duration
I.V.	Immediate	Immediate	Unknown

Half-life: Unknown.

ADVERSE REACTIONS

CNS: ***unconsciousness in hyperosmolar hyperglycemic nonketotic syndrome,*** fever, confusion.
CV: ***worsened hypertension and heart failure with fluid overload in susceptible patients,*** *phlebitis, venous sclerosis,* tissue necrosis with prolonged or concentrated infusions, especially when given peripherally.
GU: glycosuria, osmotic diuresis.
Metabolic: hypovolemia, hypervolemia, hyperglycemia, dehydration, and hyperosmolarity with rapid infusion of concentrated solution or prolonged infusion, hypoglycemia from rebound hyperinsulinemia with rapid termination of long-term infusions.
Respiratory: *pulmonary edema.*
Skin: sloughing and tissue necrosis if extravasation occurs with concentrated solutions.

INTERACTIONS

Drug-drug. *Corticosteroids:* May cause salt and water retention and increase potassium excretion. Monitor glucose, sodium, and potassium levels.

EFFECTS ON LAB TEST RESULTS

- May increase or decrease glucose level.

CONTRAINDICATIONS & CAUTIONS

- Contraindicated in patients with allergy to corn or corn products.
- Contraindicated in patients in diabetic coma while glucose level remains excessively high.
- Use of concentrated solutions is contraindicated in patients with intracranial or intraspinal hemorrhage; in dehydrated patients with delirium tremens; and in patients with severe dehydration, anuria, diabetic coma, or glucose-galactose malabsorption syndrome.
- Use cautiously in patients with cardiac or pulmonary disease, hypertension, renal insufficiency, urinary obstruction, or hypovolemia.

NURSING CONSIDERATIONS

- ***Alert:*** Never stop hypertonic solutions abruptly. Have dextrose 10% in water available to treat hypoglycemia if rebound hyperinsulinemia occurs.
- Don't give concentrated solutions I.M. or subcutaneously.
- Monitor glucose level carefully. Prolonged therapy with D_5W can cause reduction of pancreatic insulin production and secretion.
- Check vital signs frequently. Report adverse reactions promptly.
- Monitor fluid intake and output and weight carefully. Watch closely for signs and symptoms of fluid overload.
- Monitor patient for signs of mental confusion.

PATIENT TEACHING

- Explain need for supplement to patient and family, and answer any questions.
- Tell patient to report adverse reactions promptly.

SAFETY ALERT!

fat emulsions

Intralipid 10%, Intralipid 20%, Liposyn II 10%, Liposyn II 20%, Liposyn III 10%, Liposyn III 20%

Pharmacologic class: lipids
Pregnancy risk category C

AVAILABLE FORMS

Injection: 50 ml (10%, 20%), 100 ml (10%, 20%), 200 ml (10%, 20%), 250 ml (10%, 20%), 500 ml (10%, 20%)

INDICATIONS & DOSAGES

➤ **Adjunct to total parenteral nutrition (TPN) to provide adequate source of calories**

Adults: 1 ml/minute I.V. for 15 to 30 minutes (10% emulsion) or 0.5 ml/minute I.V.

for 15 to 30 minutes (20% emulsion). If no adverse reactions occur, increase rate to deliver 250 ml (20% Liposyn) or 500 ml (10% Liposyn; 10% or 20% Intralipid) over the first day; don't give more than 2.5 g/kg (10%) or 3 g/kg (20%) daily. *Children:* 0.1 ml/minute for 10 to 15 minutes (10% emulsion) or 0.05 ml/minute I.V. for 10 to 15 minutes (20% emulsion). If no adverse reactions occur, increase rate to deliver 1 g/kg over 4 hours; don't give more than 3 g/kg daily. Fat emulsion supplies 60% of daily caloric intake; protein-carbohydrate TPN should supply remaining 40%.

➤ **Fatty acid deficiency**
Adults and children: 8% to 10% of total caloric intake I.V.

➤ **To prevent fatty acid deficiency**
Adults: 500 ml Liposyn (10% emulsion) I.V. twice weekly. Infuse initially at rate of 1 ml/minute for 30 minutes. Don't exceed 500 ml over 4 to 6 hours.
Children: 5 to 10 ml/kg Liposyn (10% emulsion) I.V. daily. Infuse initially at 0.1 ml/minute for 30 minutes. Don't exceed 100 ml/hour.

I.V. ADMINISTRATION

- Don't use if it separates or becomes oily.
- Drug may be mixed in same container with amino acids, dextrose, electrolytes, vitamins, and other nutrients.
- Because lipids support bacterial and fungal growth, change all tubing before each infusion, and check infusion site daily.
- Use an infusion pump to regulate rate. Rapid infusion may cause fluid or fat overload.
- Refrigeration isn't needed unless part of an admixture.

INCOMPATIBILITIES

Acyclovir, albumin, amikacin, aminophylline, amphotericin B, ampicillin sodium, ascorbic acid injection, calcium chloride, calcium gluconate, cyclosporine, dopamine, doxorubicin, doxycycline, droperidol, fluorouracil, ganciclovir, gentamicin, haloperidol, heparin sodium, hydromorphone hydrochloride (HCl), iron dextran, levorphanol tartrate, lorazepam, magnesium chloride, methyldopate HCl, midazolam HCl, minocycline HCl, morphine sulfate, nalbuphine HCl, ondansetron HCl, penicillin G, pentobarbital sodium, phenobarbital sodium, phenytoin sodium, potassium chloride, potassium phosphates, ranitidine HCl, sodium bicarbonate, sodium chloride solution, sodium phosphates, vitamin B complex.

ACTION

Provides neutral triglycerides, predominantly unsaturated fatty acids; acts as a source of calories and prevents fatty acid deficiency. When substituted for dextrose as a source of calories, fat emulsions decrease carbon dioxide production.

Route	Onset	Peak	Duration
I.V.	Immediate	Immediate	Unknown

Half-life: Unknown.

ADVERSE REACTIONS

Early reactions
CNS: headache, sleepiness, dizziness, fever.
CV: chest and back pains, flushing.
EENT: pressure over eyes.
GI: nausea, vomiting.
Hematologic: hypercoagulability.
Respiratory: dyspnea, cyanosis.
Skin: diaphoresis.
Other: hypersensitivity reactions, irritation at infusion site.

Delayed reactions
CNS: ***focal seizures,*** fever.
Hematologic: ***thrombocytopenia, leukopenia,*** leukocytosis.
Hepatic: hepatomegaly.
Other: splenomegaly.

INTERACTIONS

None significant.

EFFECTS ON LAB TEST RESULTS

- May increase bilirubin, lipid, and liver enzyme levels.
- May decrease platelet count. May increase or decrease WBC count.

CONTRAINDICATIONS & CAUTIONS

- Contraindicated in patients with severe egg allergies, hyperlipidemia, lipid nephrosis, or acute pancreatitis with hyperlipidemia.
- Use cautiously in patients with severe hepatic or pulmonary disease, anemia, or

blood coagulation disorders including thrombocytopenia, and in patients at risk for fat embolism.
- Use cautiously in jaundiced or premature infants.

NURSING CONSIDERATIONS
- Watch for adverse reactions, especially during first half of infusion.
- Monitor lipid levels closely when patient is receiving fat emulsion therapy. Lipemia must clear between doses.
- Monitor hepatic function carefully in long-term therapy.
- Check platelet count frequently in neonates.
- Carefully monitor triglyceride levels and free fatty acids in infants, especially premature and jaundiced infants.
- Available products differ mainly by their fatty acid components.

PATIENT TEACHING
- Explain need for fat emulsion therapy, and answer any questions.
- Tell patient to report adverse reactions promptly.

89

Antigout drugs

allopurinol
allopurinol sodium
colchicine
probenecid
sulfinpyrazone

allopurinol

Allorin‡, Apo-Allopurinol†, Capurate‡, Zyloprim

allopurinol sodium

Aloprim

Pharmacologic class: xanthine oxidase inhibitor
Pregnancy risk category C

AVAILABLE FORMS

allopurinol
Capsules: 100 mg, 300 mg‡
Tablets (scored): 100 mg, 200 mg‡, 300 mg
allopurinol sodium
Injection: 500 mg/30 ml vial

INDICATIONS & DOSAGES

➤ **Gout or hyperuricemia**
Adults: Mild gout, 200 to 300 mg P.O. daily; severe gout with large tophi, 400 to 600 mg P.O. daily. Maximum 800 mg daily. Dosage varies with severity of disease; can be given as single dose or divided, but doses greater than 300 mg should be divided.
➤ **Hyperuricemia caused by malignancies**
Adults and children older than age 10: Give 200 to 400 mg/m^2 daily I.V. as a single infusion or in equally divided doses q 6, 8, or 12 hours. Maximum 600 mg daily.
Children age 10 and younger: Initially, 200 mg/m^2 daily I.V. as single infusion or in equally divided doses q 6, 8, or 12 hours. Then titrate according to uric acid levels. For children ages 6 to 10, give 300 mg P.O. daily or divided t.i.d.; for children younger than age 6, give 150 mg P.O. daily.
➤ **To prevent acute gout attacks**
Adults: 100 mg P.O. daily; increase at weekly intervals by 100 mg without exceeding maximum dose (800 mg) until uric acid falls to 6 mg/dl or less.
➤ **To prevent uric acid nephropathy during cancer chemotherapy**
Adults: 600 to 800 mg P.O. daily for 2 to 3 days, with high fluid intake.
➤ **Recurrent calcium oxalate calculi**
Adults: 200 to 300 mg P.O. daily in single or divided doses.
Adjust-a-dose: If creatinine clearance is 10 to 20 ml/minute, give 200 mg P.O. or I.V. daily; if clearance is less than 10 ml/minute, give 100 mg P.O. or I.V. daily; if clearance is less than 3 ml/minute, give 100 mg P.O. or I.V. at extended intervals.

I.V. ADMINISTRATION

- Dissolve contents of each 30-ml vial in 25 ml of sterile water for injection.
- Dilute solution to desired concentration (no greater than 6 mg/ml) with normal saline solution for injection or D_5W.
- See package insert for drugs that are incompatible with allopurinol in solution.
- Store solution at 68° to 77° F (20° to 25° C) and use within 10 hours. Don't use solution if it contains particulates or is discolored.

INCOMPATIBILITIES

Amikacin, amphotericin B, carmustine, cefotaxime, chlorpromazine, cimetidine, clindamycin phosphate, cytarabine, dacarbazine, daunorubicin, diphenhydramine, doxorubicin, doxycycline hyclate, droperidol, floxuridine, gentamicin, haloperidol lactate, hydroxyzine, idarubicin, imipenem and cilastatin sodium, mechlorethamine, meperidine, methylprednisolone sodium succinate, metoclopramide, minocycline, nalbuphine, netilmicin, ondansetron, prochlorperazine edisylate, promethazine, sodium bicarbonate (or solutions containing sodium bicarbonate), streptozocin, tobramycin sulfate, vinorelbine.

ACTION
Reduces uric acid production by inhibiting xanthine oxidase.

Route	Onset	Peak	Duration
P.O.	Unknown	30–120 hr	1–2 wk
I.V.	Unknown	30 min	Unknown

Half-life: Allopurinol, 1 to 2 hours; oxypurinol, about 15 hours.

ADVERSE REACTIONS
CNS: fever, drowsiness, headache, paresthesia, peripheral neuropathy, neuritis.
CV: hypersensitivity vasculitis, necrotizing angiitis.
EENT: epistaxis.
GI: nausea, vomiting, diarrhea, abdominal pain, gastritis, taste loss or perversion, dyspepsia.
GU: ***renal failure,*** uremia.
Hematologic: ***agranulocytosis,*** anemia, ***aplastic anemia, thrombocytopenia, leukopenia,*** leukocytosis, eosinophilia.
Hepatic: ***hepatitis, hepatic necrosis,*** hepatomegaly, cholestatic jaundice.
Musculoskeletal: arthralgia, myopathy.
Skin: ***erythema multiforme, rash, toxic epidermal necrolysis,*** exfoliative, urticarial, and purpuric lesions, severe furunculosis of nose, ichthyosis, alopecia.
Other: ecchymoses, chills.

INTERACTIONS
Drug-drug. *Amoxicillin, ampicillin:* May increase possibility of rash. Avoid using together.
Anticoagulants: May increase anticoagulant effect. Dosage may need to be adjusted.
Antineoplastics: May increase potential for bone marrow suppression. Monitor patient carefully.
Chlorpropamide: May increase hypoglycemic effect. Avoid using together.
Ethacrynic acid, thiazide diuretics: May increase risk of allopurinol toxicity. Reduce allopurinol dosage, and monitor renal function closely.
Uricosurics: May have additive effect. May be used to therapeutic advantage.
Urine-acidifying drugs (ammonium chloride, ascorbic acid, potassium or sodium phosphate): May increase possibility of kidney stone formation. Monitor patient carefully.
Xanthines: May increase theophylline level. Adjust dosage of theophylline, as needed.
Drug-lifestyle. *Alcohol use:* May increase uric acid level. Discourage use together.

EFFECTS ON LAB TEST RESULTS
• May increase alkaline phosphatase, ALT, and AST levels. May decrease hemoglobin level and hematocrit.
• May increase eosinophil count. May decrease granulocyte and platelet counts. May increase or decrease WBC count.

CONTRAINDICATIONS & CAUTIONS
• Contraindicated in patients hypersensitive to drug and in those with idiopathic hemochromatosis.

NURSING CONSIDERATIONS
• Monitor uric acid level to evaluate drug's effectiveness.
• Monitor fluid intake and output; daily urine output of at least 2 L and maintenance of neutral or slightly alkaline urine are desirable.
• Periodically monitor CBC and hepatic and renal function, especially at start of therapy.
• Optimal benefits may need 2 to 6 weeks of therapy. Because acute gout attacks may occur during this time, concurrent use of colchicine may be prescribed prophylactically.
• Don't restart drug in patients who have a severe reaction.
• ***Look alike–sound alike:*** Don't confuse Zyloprim with ZORprin.

PATIENT TEACHING
• To minimize GI adverse reactions, tell patient to take drug with or immediately after meals.
• Encourage patient to drink plenty of fluids while taking drug unless otherwise contraindicated.
• Drug may cause drowsiness; tell patient not to drive or perform hazardous tasks requiring mental alertness until CNS effects of drug are known.
• If patient is taking drug for recurrent calcium oxalate stones, advise him also to reduce his dietary intake of animal pro-

tein, sodium, refined sugars, oxalate-rich foods, and calcium.
- Tell patient to stop drug at first sign of rash, which may precede severe hypersensitivity or other adverse reactions. Rash is more common in patients taking diuretics and in those with renal disorders. Tell patient to report all adverse reactions.
- Advise patient to avoid alcohol during therapy.
- Teach patient importance of continuing drug even if asymptomatic.

SAFETY ALERT!

colchicine
Colgout‡

Pharmacologic class: colchicum autumnale alkaloid
Pregnancy risk category C; D for I.V.

AVAILABLE FORMS
Injection: 1 mg/2 ml
Tablets: 0.5 mg, 0.6 mg as sugar-coated granules

INDICATIONS & DOSAGES
➤ **To prevent acute gout attacks**
Adults: 0.6 mg P.O. daily. Patients who normally have one attack per year or fewer should receive drug only 3 to 4 days weekly; patients who have more than one attack per year should receive drug daily. In severe cases, 1.2 to 1.8 mg P.O. daily.
➤ **To prevent gout attacks in patients undergoing surgery**
Adults: 0.6 mg P.O. t.i.d. 3 days before and 3 days after surgery.
➤ **Acute gout, acute gouty arthritis**
Adults: Initially, 1.2 mg P.O.; then 0.6 mg q 1 hour or 1.2 mg q 2 hours until pain is relieved; nausea, vomiting, or diarrhea ensues; or maximum dose of 8 mg is reached. Wait 3 days before a second oral course to reduce cumulative toxicity. Or, 2 mg I.V.; then 0.5 mg I.V. q 6 hours if needed. (Some prescribers prefer to give a single I.V. injection of 3 mg.) Total I.V. dose over 24 hours (one course of treatment) shouldn't exceed 4 mg. Give no further colchicine (I.V. or P.O.) for at least 7 days.

Adjust-a-dose: If creatinine clearance is 10 to 50 ml/minute, reduce dose by 50%. Don't use in patients with creatinine clearance below 10 ml/minute. In patients with hepatic impairment, reduce dose by 50%.

I.V. ADMINISTRATION
- Give by slow I.V. push over 2 to 5 minutes.
- If lower concentration of colchicine injection is needed, dilute with normal saline solution or sterile water for injection and give over 2 to 5 minutes by direct injection.
- Preferably, inject into the tubing of a free-flowing I.V. solution.
- Don't inject if diluted solution becomes turbid.
- Monitor patient for extravasation because colchicine irritates tissues.

INCOMPATIBILITIES
D_5W, bacteriostatic normal saline injection.

ACTION
As an antigout drug, may decrease WBC motility, phagocytosis, and lactic acid production, decreasing urate crystal deposits and reducing inflammation. As an antiosteolytic drug, may inhibit mitosis of osteoprogenitor cells and decrease osteoclast activity.

Route	Onset	Peak	Duration
P.O.	12 hr	30–120 min	Unknown
I.V.	6–12 hr	Unknown	Unknown

Half-life: 20 minutes in plasma; 60 hours in leukocytes.

ADVERSE REACTIONS
CNS: peripheral neuritis.
GI: *nausea, vomiting, abdominal pain, diarrhea.*
GU: reversible azoospermia.
Hematologic: ***aplastic anemia, thrombocytopenia, agranulocytosis with long-term use,*** nonthrombocytopenic purpura.
Musculoskeletal: myopathy.
Skin: alopecia, urticaria, dermatitis.
Other: severe local irritation if extravasation occurs, hypersensitivity reactions.

INTERACTIONS

Drug-drug. ***Clarithromycin, erythromycin, telithromycin, verapamil:*** May increase the risk of colchicine toxicity. Monitor colchicine levels and adjust dose or stop colchicine as needed.

Cyclosporine: May cause GI, hepatic, renal and neuromuscular toxicity. Use together cautiously.

Vitamin B_{12}: May impair absorption of oral vitamin B_{12}. Avoid using together.

Drug-lifestyle. *Alcohol use:* May impair effectiveness of drug prophylaxis. Discourage use together.

EFFECTS ON LAB TEST RESULTS

- May increase alkaline phosphatase, AST, and ALT levels. May decrease carotene, cholesterol, and hemoglobin levels and hematocrit.
- May decrease platelet and granulocyte counts.
- May cause false-positive urine RBC or urine hemoglobin test results.

CONTRAINDICATIONS & CAUTIONS

- Contraindicated in patients hypersensitive to drug and in those with blood dyscrasia, serious CV disease, renal disease, or GI disorders.
- Use cautiously in elderly or debilitated patients and in those with early signs of CV, renal, or GI disease.

NURSING CONSIDERATIONS

- Obtain baseline laboratory test results, including CBC, before therapy and periodically throughout therapy.
- ***Alert:*** Don't give I.M. or subcutaneously; severe local irritation occurs.
- As maintenance therapy, give drug with meals to reduce GI effects. Drug may be used with uricosurics.
- Monitor fluid intake and output; keep output at 2 L daily.
- ***Alert:*** After full I.V. course (4 mg), don't give it by any route for at least 7 days. It's a toxic drug, and overdose may be fatal.
- First sign of acute overdose may be GI symptoms, followed by vascular damage, muscle weakness, and ascending paralysis. Delirium and seizures may occur without patient losing consciousness.
- Stop drug as soon as gout pain is relieved or at first sign of GI symptoms.

PATIENT TEACHING

- Teach patient how to take drug, and tell him to drink extra fluids.
- Tell patient to report adverse reactions, especially signs of acute overdose (nausea, vomiting, abdominal pain, diarrhea, unusual bleeding, bruising, tiredness, weakness, numbness, or tingling).
- Advise patient to avoid using alcohol while taking drug.
- Tell patient with gout to limit intake of foods high in purine, such as anchovies, liver, sardines, kidneys, sweetbreads, peas, and lentils.

probenecid

Benuryl†

Pharmacologic class: sulfonamide derivative
Pregnancy risk category B

AVAILABLE FORMS

Tablets: 500 mg

INDICATIONS & DOSAGES

➤ **Adjunct to penicillin therapy**

Adults and children weighing more than 50 kg (111 lb): 500 mg P.O. q.i.d.

Children ages 2 to 14 or weighing 50 kg or less: Initially, 25 mg/kg P.O.; then 40 mg/kg/day in divided doses q.i.d.

➤ **Gonorrhea**

Adults: Give 3.5 g ampicillin or 3 g amoxicillin P.O. along with 1 g probenecid P.O. Or, 1 g probenecid P.O. 30 minutes before 4.8 million units of aqueous penicillin G procaine I.M., injected at two different sites.

➤ **Hyperuricemia of gout, gouty arthritis**

Adults: 250 mg P.O. b.i.d. for first week; then 500 mg b.i.d., to maximum of 2 to 3 g daily. Review maintenance dose q 6 months and reduce by increments of 500 mg, if indicated.

ACTION

Blocks renal tubular reabsorption of uric acid, increasing excretion, and inhibits active renal tubular secretion of many weak organic acids, such as penicillins and cephalosporins.

Route	Onset	Peak	Duration
P.O.	Unknown	2–4 hr	Unknown

Half-life: 3 to 8 hours after 500-mg dose; 4 to 17 hours after larger doses.

ADVERSE REACTIONS

CNS: fever, *headache,* dizziness.
CV: flushing.
GI: anorexia, nausea, vomiting, sore gums.
GU: urinary frequency, renal colic, nephrotic syndrome, costovertebral pain.
Hematologic: ***aplastic anemia, hemolytic anemia,*** anemia.
Hepatic: ***hepatic necrosis.***
Skin: dermatitis, pruritus.
Other: worsening of gout, ***hypersensitivity reactions including anaphylaxis.***

INTERACTIONS

Drug-drug. *Acyclovir, cephalosporins, clofibrate, dapsone, ketamine, lorazepam, meclofenamate, penicillin, rifampin, sulfonamides, thiopental:* May increase levels of these drugs. Use together cautiously.
Allopurinol: May increase uric acid–lowering effects. May be used to therapeutic advantage.
Methotrexate: May impair excretion of methotrexate, causing increased level, effects, and toxicity of methotrexate. Monitor methotrexate level closely and adjust dosage accordingly.
Nitrofurantoin: May increase toxicity and reduce effectiveness of nitrofurantoin. Reduce probenecid dose.
NSAIDs: May increase NSAID toxicity. Avoid using together.
Salicylates: May inhibit uricosuric effect of probenecid, causing urate retention. Avoid using together.
Sulfonylureas: May increase hypoglycemic effect. Monitor glucose level closely. Dosage may need to be adjusted.
Zidovudine: May increase zidovudine level and toxicity symptoms. Monitor patient.
Drug-lifestyle. *Alcohol use:* May increase urate level. Discourage use together.

EFFECTS ON LAB TEST RESULTS

- May decrease hemoglobin level and hematocrit.
- May falsely elevate theophylline level.

CONTRAINDICATIONS & CAUTIONS

- Contraindicated in patients hypersensitive to drug and in those with uric acid kidney stones or blood dyscrasias; also contraindicated in patients with an acute gout attack and in children younger than age 2.
- Use cautiously in patients with peptic ulcer or renal impairment.
- Use cautiously in patients with sulfa allergy because probenecid is a sulfonamide derivative.

NURSING CONSIDERATIONS

- To minimize GI distress, give drug with milk, food, or antacids. Continued disturbances might indicate need to reduce dosage.
- Force fluids to maintain minimum daily output of 2 to 3 L. Alkalinize urine with sodium bicarbonate or potassium citrate. These measures prevent hematuria, renal colic, urate stone development, and costovertebral pain.
- Don't start treating gout until acute attack subsides. Drug has no analgesic or anti-inflammatory effects and is of no value during acute gout attacks.
- Monitor BUN and renal function test results periodically in long-term therapy.
- Drug is suitable for long-term use; no cumulative effects or tolerance have been reported.
- Drug is ineffective in patients with glomerular filtration rate below 30 ml/minute.
- Drug may increase frequency, severity, and length of acute gout attacks during first 6 to 12 months of therapy. Colchicine or another anti-inflammatory may be used preventively during first 3 to 6 months.
- ***Look alike–sound alike:*** Don't confuse probenecid with Procanbid.

PATIENT TEACHING

- Instruct patient with gout to take drug regularly to prevent recurrence.
- Tell patient to visit prescriber regularly so that uric acid can be monitored and

dosage adjusted, if needed. Lifelong therapy may be needed in patients with hyperuricemia.
- Advise patient with gout to avoid all drugs that contain aspirin, which may precipitate gout. Acetaminophen may be used for pain.
- Instruct patient to drink at least 6 to 8 glasses of water per day.
- Urge patient with gout to avoid alcohol; it increases urate level.
- Tell patient with gout to limit intake of foods high in purine, such as anchovies, liver, sardines, kidneys, sweetbreads, peas, and lentils. Also tell him to identify and avoid other foods that may trigger gout attacks.
- Because drug may be prescribed with an antibiotic, instruct patient to take all medicine as prescribed.

sulfinpyrazone

Antazone†, Anturane, Apo-Sulfinpyrazone†, Novo-Pyrazone†, Nu-sulfinpyrazone†

Pharmacologic class: pyrazolone derivative
Pregnancy risk category NR

AVAILABLE FORMS

Capsules: 200 mg
Tablets: 100 mg, 200 mg†

INDICATIONS & DOSAGES

➤ **Intermittent or chronic gouty arthritis**
Adults: 200 to 400 mg P.O. daily, divided b.i.d. during the first week; then 400 mg P.O. daily divided b.i.d. Maximum dose is 800 mg daily.

➤ **To decrease the risk of sudden cardiac death 1 to 6 months after an MI ♦**
Adults: 300 mg P.O. q.i.d.

ACTION

Blocks renal tubular reabsorption of uric acid, increasing excretion, and inhibits platelet aggregation.

Route	Onset	Peak	Duration
P.O.	Unknown	1–2 hr	4–6 hr

Half-life: 3 hours.

ADVERSE REACTIONS

GI: *nausea, dyspepsia,* epigastric pain, reactivation of peptic ulcerations.
Hematologic: ***leukopenia, agranulocytosis, thrombocytopenia, aplastic anemia,*** anemia.
Respiratory: ***bronchoconstriction in patients with aspirin-induced asthma.***
Skin: rash.

INTERACTIONS

Drug-drug. *Aspirin, niacin,* **salicylates:** May inhibit uricosuric effect of sulfinpyrazone. Avoid using together.
Oral anticoagulants: May increase anticoagulant effect and risk of bleeding. Use together cautiously.
Oral antidiabetics: May increase effects of these drugs. Monitor glucose level.
Probenecid: May inhibit renal excretion of sulfinpyrazone. Use together cautiously.
Theophylline, verapamil: May increase clearance of these drugs. Use together cautiously.
Drug-lifestyle. *Alcohol use:* May decrease effectiveness. Discourage use together.

EFFECTS ON LAB TEST RESULTS

- May increase BUN and creatinine levels. May decrease hemoglobin level and hematocrit.
- May decrease WBC, granulocyte, and platelet counts.

CONTRAINDICATIONS & CAUTIONS

- Contraindicated in patients hypersensitive to pyrazolones (including oxyphenbutazone and phenylbutazone) and in those with blood dyscrasias, active peptic ulcer, or symptoms of GI inflammation or ulceration.
- Use cautiously in patients with healed peptic ulcer and in pregnant women.

NURSING CONSIDERATIONS

- Monitor BUN, CBC, and renal function studies periodically during long-term use.

• Monitor fluid intake and output closely. Therapy, especially at start, may lead to renal colic and formation of uric acid stones until acid levels are normal (about 6 mg/dl).
• Force fluids to maintain minimum daily output of 2 to 3 L. Alkalinize urine with sodium bicarbonate or other drug.
• Drug has no anti-inflammatory or analgesic effects and is of no value during acute gout attacks.
• Drug may increase frequency, severity, and length of acute gout attacks during first 6 to 12 months of therapy. Colchicine or another anti-inflammatory may be used preventively during first 3 to 6 months.
• Lifelong therapy may be needed in patients with hyperuricemia.
• ***Look alike–sound alike:*** Don't confuse Anturane with Accutane, Artane, or Antabuse.

PATIENT TEACHING
• Instruct patient and family that drug must be taken regularly, even during acute exacerbations.
• Tell patient to take drug with food, milk, or antacids to reduce GI upset.
• Tell patient to visit prescriber regularly so blood levels can be monitored and dosage adjusted, if needed.
• Warn patient with gout not to take aspirin-containing drugs because these may precipitate gout. Acetaminophen may be used for pain.
• Tell patient with gout to avoid foods high in purine, such as anchovies, liver, sardines, kidneys, sweetbreads, peas, and lentils, and to identify and avoid any other foods that may trigger gout attacks.
• Instruct patient to drink at least 10 to 12 glasses of fluid daily.
• Advise patient to avoid alcohol during therapy.
• Instruct patient to report unusual bleeding, bruising, or flulike symptoms.

Oxytocics

carboprost tromethamine
dinoprostone
methylergonovine maleate
oxytocin, synthetic injection

carboprost tromethamine

Hemabate

Pharmacologic class: prostaglandin
Pregnancy risk category C

AVAILABLE FORMS

Injection: 250 mcg/ml

INDICATIONS & DOSAGES

➤ **To terminate pregnancy between weeks 13 and 20 of gestation**

Adults: Initially, 250 mcg deep I.M. Give subsequent doses of 250 mcg at intervals of 1½ to 3½ hours, depending on uterine response. Dosage may be increased in increments to 500 mcg if contractility is inadequate after several 250-mcg doses. Total dose shouldn't exceed 12 mg or continuous administration for more than 2 days.

➤ **Postpartum hemorrhage from uterine atony not managed by conventional methods**

Adults: 250 mcg by deep I.M. injection. Repeat doses q 15 to 90 minutes, p.r.n. Maximum total dose is 2 mg.

ACTION

Produces strong, prompt contractions of uterine smooth muscle, possibly mediated by calcium and cAMP.

Route	Onset	Peak	Duration
I.M.	Unknown	15–60 min	24 hr

Half-life: Unknown.

ADVERSE REACTIONS

CNS: *fever,* headache, anxiety, paresthesia, syncope, weakness.
CV: ***arrhythmias,*** chest pain, flushing.
EENT: blurred vision, eye pain.
GI: *vomiting, diarrhea, nausea.*
GU: ***uterine rupture,*** endometritis, uterine or vaginal pain.
Musculoskeletal: backache, leg cramps.
Respiratory: coughing, wheezing.
Skin: rash, diaphoresis.
Other: breast tenderness, chills, hot flashes.

INTERACTIONS

Drug-drug. *Other oxytocics:* May increase action. Avoid using together.

EFFECTS ON LAB TEST RESULTS

None reported.

CONTRAINDICATIONS & CAUTIONS

- Contraindicated in patients hypersensitive to drug and in those with acute pelvic inflammatory disease or active cardiac, pulmonary, renal, or hepatic disease.
- Use cautiously in patients with history of asthma, hypotension, hypertension, anemia, jaundice, or diabetes; and those with seizure disorders, previous uterine surgery, or CV, adrenal, renal, or hepatic disease.

NURSING CONSIDERATIONS

- Unlike other prostaglandin abortifacients, drug is given by I.M. injection. Injectable form avoids risk of expelling vaginal suppositories if patient has profuse vaginal bleeding.
- Only trained personnel in a hospital setting should give drug.
- Pretreating and giving with antiemetics and antidiarrheals decreases the risk of common GI effects.

PATIENT TEACHING

- Explain use and administration of drug to patient and family.
- Instruct patient to report adverse reactions promptly.

dinoprostone
Cervidil, Prepidil, Prostin E2

Pharmacologic class: prostaglandin
Pregnancy risk category C

AVAILABLE FORMS
Endocervical gel: 0.5 mg/application (2.5-ml syringe)
Vaginal insert: 10 mg
Vaginal suppositories: 20 mg

INDICATIONS & DOSAGES
➤ **To terminate second-trimester pregnancy; to evacuate uterine contents in missed abortion, intrauterine fetal death up to 28 weeks' gestation, or benign hydatidiform mole**
Women: Insert 20-mg suppository high into posterior vaginal fornix; repeat q 3 to 5 hours until abortion is complete; for a maximum of 2 days.
➤ **To ripen an unfavorable cervix in pregnant woman at or near term**
Women: Apply 0.5 mg endocervical gel intravaginally; if cervix remains unfavorable after 6 hours, repeat dose. Don't exceed 1.5 mg (three applications) within 24 hours. Or, place 10-mg vaginal insert transversely in posterior vaginal fornix immediately after removing insert from foil. Take insert out when active labor begins or after 12 hours have passed, whichever occurs first.

ACTION
Produces strong, prompt contractions of uterine smooth muscle, possibly mediated by calcium and cAMP.

Route	Onset	Peak	Duration
Intravaginal (gel)	15–30 min	Unknown	Unknown
Intravaginal (insert)	Unknown	Unknown	Unknown
Intravaginal (suppository)	10 min	Unknown	2–6 hr

Half-life: 2½ to 5 minutes.

ADVERSE REACTIONS
CNS: *fever, headache, dizziness,* anxiety, paresthesia, weakness, syncope.
CV: ***arrhythmias,*** chest pain.
EENT: blurred vision, eye pain.
GI: *nausea, vomiting, diarrhea.*
GU: vaginal pain, vaginitis, endometritis, uterine rupture.
Musculoskeletal: *nocturnal leg cramps,* backache, muscle cramps.
Respiratory: coughing, dyspnea.
Skin: rash, diaphoresis.
Other: *shivering, chills,* breast tenderness, hot flashes.

INTERACTIONS
Drug-drug. *Other oxytocics:* May increase action. Avoid using together.
Drug-lifestyle. *Alcohol use:* May inhibit effectiveness of drug with high doses. Discourage using together.

EFFECTS ON LAB TEST RESULTS
None reported.

CONTRAINDICATIONS & CAUTIONS
- Gel form contraindicated in patients hypersensitive to prostaglandins or constituents of gel; in those for whom prolonged uterine contractions are undesirable; in those with placenta previa or unexplained vaginal bleeding during pregnancy; and in those for whom vaginal delivery isn't indicated (because of vasa previa or active genital herpes).
- Suppository form contraindicated in patients hypersensitive to drug, in those with acute pelvic inflammatory disease, and in those with active cardiac, pulmonary, renal, or hepatic disease.
- Insert form contraindicated in patients hypersensitive to drug and in those with evidence of fetal distress when delivery isn't imminent, with unexplained vaginal bleeding during pregnancy, or with evidence of marked fetal cephalopelvic disproportion; also contraindicated when oxytocics are contraindicated, when prolonged uterine contraction may be detrimental to fetal safety or uterine integrity, when membranes have ruptured, when patient is already receiving an oxytocic, and when patient is multipara with six or more previous term pregnancies.
- Use gel form cautiously in patients with asthma or history of asthma, renal or hepatic dysfunction, ruptured membranes, glaucoma, or increased intraocular pressure.

• Use suppository form cautiously in patients with asthma, seizure disorders, anemia, diabetes, hypertension or hypotension, jaundice, scarred uterus, cervicitis, acute vaginitis, or CV, renal, or hepatic disease.

NURSING CONSIDERATIONS

• Give only when critical care facilities are available.
• For cervical ripening, have patient lie on her back; the cervix is examined using a speculum. A catheter provided with drug is used to insert gel into cervical canal just below level of the internal os.
• Bring gel to room temperature just before giving. Don't force warming with water bath, microwave, or other external heat source.
• When giving gel form, don't try to give small amount of drug remaining in catheter.
• Patient should lie down for 15 to 30 minutes after using gel.
• Bring vaginal suppository to room temperature just before giving. Patient should lie down for 10 minutes following vaginal suppository insertion.
• When using the vaginal insert, a small amount of water-soluble jelly may be used to aid insertion. There is no need to warm the vaginal insert before insertion.
• Patient should lie down for 2 hours after using vaginal insert. Remove insert at onset of active labor or 12 hours after insertion.
• Treat drug-induced fever with water sponging and increased fluid intake, not with aspirin.
• Check vaginal discharge regularly.
• Abortion should be complete within 30 hours when suppository form is used.

PATIENT TEACHING

• Explain use and administration of drug to patient and family.
• Instruct patient to report adverse reactions promptly.

methylergonovine maleate
Methergine

Pharmacologic class: ergot alkaloid
Pregnancy risk category C

AVAILABLE FORMS

Injection: 0.2 mg/ml in 1-ml ampules
Tablets: 0.2 mg

INDICATIONS & DOSAGES

➤ **To prevent and treat postpartum hemorrhage caused by uterine atony or subinvolution**

Adults: 0.2 mg I.M. q 2 to 4 hours to a maximum of 5 doses. For excessive uterine bleeding or other emergencies, 0.2 mg I.V. over 1 minute while monitoring blood pressure and uterine contractions. After first I.M. or I.V. dose, 0.2 mg P.O. q 6 to 8 hours for 2 to 7 days. Decrease dosage if severe cramping occurs.

I.V. ADMINISTRATION

• Don't routinely use this form because of risk of severe hypertension and stroke.
• Dilute to 5 ml with normal saline solution, p.r.n.
• Give slowly over at least 1 minute while carefully monitoring blood pressure.
• Store solution below 46° F (8° C). Daily stock may be kept at room temperature for 60 to 90 days.

INCOMPATIBILITIES

None reported.

ACTION

Increases motor activity of the uterus by direct stimulation of the smooth muscle, shortening the third stage of labor, and reducing blood loss.

Route	Onset	Peak	Duration
P.O.	5–10 min	30 min	3 hr
I.V.	Immediate	Unknown	45 min
I.M.	2–5 min	Unknown	3 hr

Half-life: 1½ to 12¾ hours.

ADVERSE REACTIONS

CNS: ***seizures, stroke with I.V. use,*** dizziness, headache, hallucinations.

CV: hypertension, transient chest pain, palpitations, hypotension, thrombophlebitis.
EENT: tinnitus, nasal congestion.
GI: *nausea, vomiting,* diarrhea, foul taste.
GU: hematuria.
Musculoskeletal: leg cramps.
Respiratory: dyspnea.
Skin: diaphoresis.

INTERACTIONS
Drug-drug. *Dopamine, ergot alkaloids, I.V. oxytocin, regional anesthetics, vasoconstrictors:* May cause excessive vasoconstriction. Use together cautiously.
Clarithromycin, delavirdine, erythromycin, indinavir, itraconazole, ketoconazole, nelfinavir, ritonavir, telithromycin, troleandomycin, voriconazole: May cause vasospasm, leading to ischemia. Avoid using together.
Clotrimazole, fluconazole, fluoxetine, fluvoxamine, nefazodone, saquinavir, zileuton: May increase risk of vasospasm. Use together cautiously.

EFFECTS ON LAB TEST RESULTS
- May decrease prolactin level.

CONTRAINDICATIONS & CAUTIONS
- Contraindicated in pregnant patients, in patients sensitive to ergot preparations, and in patients with hypertension or toxemia.
- Use cautiously in patients with sepsis, obliterative vascular disease, or hepatic or renal disease.
- Use cautiously during last stage of labor.

NURSING CONSIDERATIONS
- Monitor and record blood pressure, pulse rate, and uterine response; report sudden change in vital signs, frequent periods of uterine relaxation, and character and amount of vaginal bleeding.
- Monitor contractions, which may begin immediately. Contractions may continue for up to 45 minutes after I.V. use or for 3 hours or more after P.O. or I.M. use.
- Store tablets in tightly closed, light-resistant container. Discard if discolored.
- ***Look alike–sound alike:*** Don't confuse Methergine with terbutaline

PATIENT TEACHING
- Explain use of drug to patient and family.
- Instruct patient to report adverse reactions promptly.

oxytocin, synthetic injection
Pitocin

Pharmacologic class: exogenous hormone
Pregnancy risk category NR

AVAILABLE FORMS
Injection: 10 units/ml in 1-ml ampule, 1-ml, 3-ml, and 10-ml vials, or syringe

INDICATIONS & DOSAGES
➤ **To induce or stimulate labor**
Adults: Initially, 10 units in 1,000 ml of D_5W injection, lactated Ringer, or normal saline solution I.V. infused at 0.5 to 2 milliunits/minute. Increase rate by 1 to 2 milliunits/minute at 30- to 60-minute intervals until normal contraction pattern is established. Decrease rate when labor is firmly established. Maximum dose is 20 milliunits/minute.
➤ **To reduce postpartum bleeding after expulsion of placenta**
Adults: 10 to 40 units in 1,000 ml of D_5W injection, lactated Ringer, or normal saline solution I.V. infused at rate needed to control bleeding, which is usually 20 to 40 milliunits/minute. Also, 10 units may be given I.M. after delivery of placenta.
➤ **Incomplete or inevitable abortion**
Adults: 10 units I.V. in 500 ml of normal saline solution, lactated Ringer, or dextrose 5% in normal saline solution. Infuse at 10 to 20 milliunits (20 to 40 drops)/minute. Don't exceed 30 units in 12 hours.

I.V. ADMINISTRATION
- To induce or stimulate labor, dilute drug by adding 10 units to 1 L of normal saline, lactated Ringer, or D_5W solution.
- To produce intense uterine contractions and reduce postpartum bleeding, dilute drug by adding 10 units to 500 ml of normal saline, lactated Ringer, or D_5W solution.
- Don't give bolus injection; use an infusion pump. Give drug only by piggyback

infusion so that it may be stopped without interrupting I.V. line.

INCOMPATIBILITIES

Fibrinolysin (human), norepinephrine bitartrate, Normosol-M with dextrose 5%, plasmin, prochlorperazine, sodium bisulfite, warfarin sodium.

ACTION

Causes potent and selective stimulation of uterine and mammary gland smooth muscle.

Route	Onset	Peak	Duration
I.V.	Immediate	Unknown	1 hr
I.M.	3–5 min	Unknown	2–3 hr

Half-life: 3 to 5 minutes.

ADVERSE REACTIONS

Maternal

CNS: ***subarachnoid hemorrhage, seizures, coma.***

CV: ***arrhythmias,*** hypertension, increased heart rate, systemic venous return, and cardiac output.

GI: nausea, vomiting.

GU: ***abruptio placentae,*** tetanic uterine contractions, ***postpartum hemorrhage, uterine rupture,*** impaired uterine blood flow, pelvic hematoma, increased uterine motility.

Hematologic: ***afibrinogenemia, possibly related to postpartum bleeding.***

Other: ***anaphylaxis, death from oxytocin-induced water intoxication,*** hypersensitivity reactions.

Fetal

CNS: ***infant brain damage.***

CV: ***bradycardia, arrhythmias,*** PVCs.

EENT: neonatal retinal hemorrhage.

Hepatic: neonatal jaundice.

Respiratory: ***anoxia, asphyxia.***

Other: ***low Apgar scores at 5 minutes.***

INTERACTIONS

Drug-drug. *Cyclopropane anesthetics:* May cause less pronounced bradycardia and hypotension. Use together cautiously.
Thiopental anesthetics: May delay induction. Use together cautiously.
Vasoconstrictors: May cause severe hypertension if oxytocin is given within 3 to 4 hours of vasoconstrictor in patient receiving caudal block anesthetic. Avoid using together.

EFFECTS ON LAB TEST RESULTS

None reported.

CONTRAINDICATIONS & CAUTIONS

- Contraindicated in patients hypersensitive to drug.
- Contraindicated when vaginal delivery isn't advised (placenta previa, vasa previa, invasive cervical carcinoma, genital herpes), when cephalopelvic disproportion is present, or when delivery requires conversion, as in transverse lie.
- Contraindicated in fetal distress when delivery isn't imminent, in prematurity, in other obstetric emergencies, and in patients with severe toxemia or hypertonic uterine patterns.
- Use cautiously during first and second stages of labor because cervical laceration, uterine rupture, and maternal and fetal death have been reported.
- Use cautiously, if at all, in patients with invasive cervical cancer and in those with previous cervical or uterine surgery (including cesarean section), grand multiparity, uterine sepsis, traumatic delivery, or overdistended uterus.

NURSING CONSIDERATIONS

- Drug isn't recommended for routine I.M. use, but 10 units may be given I.M. after delivery of placenta to control postpartum uterine bleeding.
- Never give drug simultaneously by more than one route.
- Drug is used to induce or reinforce labor only when pelvis is known to be adequate, when vaginal delivery is indicated, when fetal maturity is assured, and when fetal position is favorable. Use drug only in hospital where critical care facilities and prescriber are immediately available.
- Monitor fluid intake and output. Antidiuretic effect may lead to fluid overload, seizures, and coma from water intoxication.
- Monitor and record uterine contractions, heart rate, blood pressure, intrauterine pressure, fetal heart rate, and character of blood loss every 15 minutes.
- Have 20% magnesium sulfate solution available to relax the myometrium.

• If contractions occur less than 2 minutes apart, exceed 50 mm, or last 90 seconds or longer, stop infusion, turn patient on her side, and notify prescriber.
• Drug doesn't cause fetal abnormalities when used as indicated.
• ***Look alike–sound alike:*** Don't confuse Pitocin with Pitressin.

PATIENT TEACHING
• Explain use and administration of drug to patient and family.
• Instruct patient to report adverse reactions promptly.

91
Spasmolytics

darifenacin hydrobromide
flavoxate hydrochloride
oxybutynin chloride
phenazopyridine hydrochloride
solifenacin succinate
tolterodine tartrate
trospium chloride

darifenacin hydrobromide
Enablex

Pharmacologic class: muscarinic receptor antagonist
Pregnancy risk category C

AVAILABLE FORMS
Tablets (extended-release): 7.5 mg, 15 mg

INDICATIONS & DOSAGES
➤ **Urge incontinence, urgency, and frequency from an overactive bladder**
Adults: Initially, 7.5 mg P.O. once daily. After 2 weeks, may increase to 15 mg P.O. once daily if needed.
Adjust-a-dose: If patient has a Child-Pugh score of B or takes a potent CYP3A4 inhibitor, such as clarithromycin, itraconazole, ketoconazole, nefazodone, nelfinavir, ritonavir, don't exceed 7.5 mg P.O. once daily.

ACTION
Antagonizes muscarinic (M3) receptors, increasing bladder capacity and decreasing unstable detrusor contractions.

Route	Onset	Peak	Duration
P.O.	Unknown	7 hr	Unknown

Half-life: 13 to 19 hours.

ADVERSE REACTIONS
CNS: asthenia, dizziness.
CV: hypertension.
EENT: abnormal vision, dry eyes, pharyngitis, rhinitis, sinusitis.
GI: *dry mouth, constipation,* abdominal pain, diarrhea, dyspepsia, nausea, vomiting.
GU: urinary tract disorder, UTI, vaginitis.
Metabolic: weight gain.
Musculoskeletal: arthralgia, back pain.
Respiratory: bronchitis.
Skin: dry skin, pruritus, rash.
Other: accidental injury, flulike syndrome, pain, peripheral edema.

INTERACTIONS
Drug-drug. *Anticholinergics:* May increase anticholinergic effects, such as dry mouth, blurred vision, and constipation. Monitor patient closely.
Digoxin: May increase digoxin level. Monitor digoxin level.
Drugs metabolized by CYP2D6 (such as flecainide, thioridazine, tricyclic antidepressants): May increase levels of these drugs. Use together cautiously.
Midazolam: May increase midazolam level. Monitor patient carefully.
Potent CYP3A4 inhibitors (such as clarithromycin, itraconazole, ketoconazole, nefazodone, nelfinavir, ritonavir): May increase darifenacin level. Maintain dosage no higher than 7.5 mg P.O. daily.
Drug-lifestyle. *Hot weather:* May cause heat prostration from decreased sweating. Urge caution.

EFFECTS ON LAB TEST RESULTS
None reported.

CONTRAINDICATIONS & CAUTIONS
- Contraindicated in patients hypersensitive to drug or its ingredients.
- Contraindicated in patients who have or who are at risk for urine retention, gastric retention, or uncontrolled narrow-angle glaucoma.
- Avoid use in patients with a Child-Pugh score of C.
- Use cautiously in patients with bladder outflow or GI obstruction, ulcerative colitis, myasthenia gravis, severe constipation, controlled narrow-angle glaucoma,

decreased GI motility, or a Child-Pugh score of B.

NURSING CONSIDERATIONS

- Assess bladder function, and monitor drug effects.
- If patient has bladder outlet obstruction, watch for urine retention.
- Assess patient for decreased gastric motility and constipation.
- Use during pregnancy only if maternal benefit outweighs fetal risk.
- It's unknown if drug appears in breast milk.

PATIENT TEACHING

- Tell patient to swallow tablet whole with plenty of liquid; caution against crushing or chewing tablet.
- Inform patient that drug may be taken with or without food.
- Explain that drug may cause blurred vision. Tell patient to use caution, especially when performing hazardous tasks, until drug effects are known.
- Tell patient to report blurred vision, constipation, and urine retention.
- Discourage use of other drugs that may cause dry mouth, constipation, urine retention, or blurred vision.
- Tell patient that drug decreases sweating, and advise cautious use in hot environments and during strenuous activity.

flavoxate hydrochloride

Urispas

Pharmacologic class: flavone derivative

Pregnancy risk category B

AVAILABLE FORMS

Tablets: 100 mg

INDICATIONS & DOSAGES

➤ Symptomatic relief of dysuria, urinary frequency and urgency, nocturia, incontinence, and suprapubic pain from urologic disorders

Adults and children older than age 12: Give 100 to 200 mg P.O. t.i.d. to q.i.d. Reduce dosage when symptoms improve.

ACTION

Produces a direct spasmolytic effect on urinary tract smooth muscles and provides local anesthesia and analgesia.

Route	Onset	Peak	Duration
P.O.	Unknown	2 hr	Unknown

Half-life: Unknown.

ADVERSE REACTIONS

CNS: *confusion,* nervousness, dizziness, headache, drowsiness, vertigo, fever.
CV: tachycardia, palpitations.
EENT: *blurred vision,* disturbed eye accommodation, increased ocular tension.
GI: dry mouth, nausea, vomiting.
GU: dysuria.
Hematologic: ***leukopenia,*** eosinophilia.
Skin: urticaria, dermatoses.

INTERACTIONS

Drug-lifestyle. *Exercise, hot weather:* May cause heatstroke. Advise patient to use with caution in hot weather.

EFFECTS ON LAB TEST RESULTS

- May increase eosinophil count. May decrease WBC count.

CONTRAINDICATIONS & CAUTIONS

- Contraindicated in patients with pyloric or duodenal obstruction, obstructive intestinal lesions or ileus, achalasia, GI hemorrhage, or obstructive uropathies of lower urinary tract.
- Safety and effectiveness of drug in children age 12 and younger are unknown.
- Use cautiously in patients who may have glaucoma and in pregnant or breastfeeding women.

NURSING CONSIDERATIONS

- Check patient history for other drug use before giving drugs with anticholinergic adverse reactions. Such reactions may be intensified by flavoxate.
- ***Look alike–sound alike:*** Don't confuse Urispas with Urised.

PATIENT TEACHING

- Warn patient to avoid hazardous activities, such as operating machinery or driving, until CNS effects of drug are known.

- Tell patient to contact prescriber if adverse reactions occur or if symptoms aren't diminished.
- Caution patient that using drug during very hot weather may cause fever or heatstroke because it suppresses diaphoresis.
- Tell patient drug may cause dry mouth or blurred vision.

oxybutynin chloride

Ditropan, Ditropan XL, Oxytrol

Pharmacologic class: tertiary amine
Pregnancy risk category B

AVAILABLE FORMS

Syrup: 5 g/5 ml
Tablets: 5 mg
Tablets (extended-release): 5 mg, 10 mg, 15 mg
Transdermal patch: 36-mg patch delivering 3.9 mg/day

INDICATIONS & DOSAGES

➤ Uninhibited or reflex neurogenic bladder

Adults: 5 mg P.O. b.i.d. to t.i.d., to maximum of 5 mg q.i.d.
Children age 5 and older: 5 mg P.O. b.i.d., to maximum of 5 mg t.i.d.

➤ Overactive bladder

Adults: Initially, 5 mg P.O. Ditropan XL once daily. Dosage adjustments may be made weekly in 5-mg increments, as needed, to maximum of 30 mg P.O. daily. Or, apply one patch twice weekly to dry, intact skin on the abdomen, hip, or buttock.

ACTION

Produces a direct spasmolytic effect and an antimuscarinic (atropine-like) effect on urinary tract smooth muscles, increasing urinary bladder capacity, and provides some local anesthesia and analgesia.

Route	Onset	Peak	Duration
P.O.	30–60 min	3–4 hr	6–10 hr
P.O. (extended-release)	Unknown	4–6 hr	24 hr
Transdermal	24–48 hr	Varies	96 hr

Half-life: For tablets or oral solution, 2 to 3 hours; for extended release tablets, 12 to 13 hours; for patch, 7 to 8 hours.

ADVERSE REACTIONS

CNS: dizziness, insomnia, restlessness, hallucinations, asthenia, fever.
CV: *palpitations, tachycardia,* vasodilation.
EENT: mydriasis, cycloplegia, decreased lacrimation, amblyopia.
GI: *constipation, dry mouth,* nausea, vomiting, decreased GI motility.
GU: *urinary hesitancy, urine retention,* impotence.
Skin: rash, decreased diaphoresis.
Other: suppression of lactation.

Transdermal patch

CNS: fatigue, somnolence, headache.
CV: flushing.
EENT: abnormal vision.
GI: *dry mouth,* diarrhea, abdominal pain, nausea, flatulence.
GU: dysuria.
Musculoskeletal: back pain.
Skin: *pruritus,* erythema, vesicles, macules, rash, burning at injection site.

INTERACTIONS

Drug-drug. *Anticholinergics:* May increase anticholinergic effects. Use together cautiously.
Atenolol, digoxin: May increase levels of these drugs. Monitor drug levels closely.
CNS depressants: May increase CNS effects. Use together cautiously.
Haloperidol: May decrease haloperidol level. Monitor drug level closely.
Drug-lifestyle. *Alcohol use:* May increase CNS effects. Discourage use together.
Exercise, hot weather: May cause heatstroke. Advise patient to use with caution in hot weather.

EFFECTS ON LAB TEST RESULTS

None reported.

CONTRAINDICATIONS & CAUTIONS

- Contraindicated in patients hypersensitive to drug or its components and in those with myasthenia gravis, GI obstruction, untreated angle-closure glaucoma, megacolon, adynamic ileus, severe colitis, ulcerative colitis with megacolon, urine or gastric retention, or obstructive uropathy.
- Contraindicated in elderly or debilitated patients with intestinal atony and in hemorrhaging patients with unstable CV status.

• Use cautiously in elderly, pregnant, or breast-feeding patients and in those with autonomic neuropathy, reflux esophagitis, or hepatic or renal disease.
• Use extended-release form cautiously in patients with bladder outflow obstruction, gastric obstruction, ulcerative colitis, intestinal atony, myasthenia gravis, or gastroesophageal reflux and in those taking drugs that worsen esophagitis (bisphosphonates).

NURSING CONSIDERATIONS

• Before giving drug, get confirmation of neurogenic bladder by cystometry and rule out partial intestinal obstruction in patients with diarrhea, especially those with colostomy or ileostomy.
• If patient has UTI, treat him with antibiotics.
• Drug may aggravate symptoms of hyperthyroidism, coronary artery disease, heart failure, arrhythmias, tachycardia, hypertension, or prostatic hyperplasia.
• Obtain periodic cystometry as directed to evaluate response to therapy.
• ***Look alike–sound alike:*** Don't confuse Ditropan with diazepam or Dithranol.

PATIENT TEACHING

• Warn patient to avoid hazardous activities, such as operating machinery or driving, until CNS effects of drug are known.
• Caution patient that using drug during very hot weather may cause fever or heatstroke because it suppresses sweating.
• Tell patient to swallow Ditropan XL whole and not to chew or crush it.
• Instruct patient to measure syrup with a teaspoon.
• Advise patient to store drug in tightly closed container at 59° to 86° F (15° to 30° C).
• Instruct patient using transdermal patch to change patch twice a week and to choose a new application site with each new patch to avoid the same site within 7 days. Warn patient to only wear one patch at a time. Tell patient to dispose of old patches carefully in the trash in a manner that prevents accidental application or ingestion by children and pets.
• Advise patient to avoid alcohol while taking drug.
• Tell patient that drug may cause dry mouth.

phenazopyridine hydrochloride

Azo-Standard ◊, Baridium ◊, Geridium, Phenazo†, Prodium ◊, Pyridiate, Pyridium, Urodine, Urogesic, UTI-Relief

Pharmacologic class: azo dye
Pregnancy risk category B

AVAILABLE FORMS

Tablets: 95 mg ◊, 97.2 mg, 100 mg, 150 mg, 200 mg

INDICATIONS & DOSAGES

➤ **Pain with urinary tract irritation or infection**

Adults: 200 mg P.O. t.i.d. after meals for 2 days.
Children ages 6 to 12: Give 12 mg/kg P.O. daily in three equally divided doses after meals for 2 days.

ACTION

Exerts local anesthetic action on urinary mucosa through unknown mechanism.

Route	Onset	Peak	Duration
P.O.	Unknown	Unknown	Unknown

Half-life: Unknown.

ADVERSE REACTIONS

CNS: headache.
EENT: staining of contact lenses.
GI: nausea, GI disturbances.
Hematologic: hemolytic anemia, methemoglobinemia.
Skin: rash, pruritus.
Other: ***anaphylactoid reactions.***

INTERACTIONS

None significant.

EFFECTS ON LAB TEST RESULTS

• May decrease hemoglobin level and hematocrit.
• May alter Diastix or Chemstrip uG results and interfere with urinary ketone tests (Acetest or Ketostix).

CONTRAINDICATIONS & CAUTIONS

- Contraindicated in patients hypersensitive to drug and in those with glomerulonephritis, severe hepatitis, uremia, renal insufficiency, or pyelonephritis during pregnancy.

NURSING CONSIDERATIONS

- When drug is used with an antibacterial, therapy shouldn't extend beyond 2 days.
- ***Look alike–sound alike:*** Don't confuse Pyridium with pyridoxine.

PATIENT TEACHING

- Advise patient that taking drug with meals may minimize GI distress.
- Caution patient to stop drug and notify prescriber immediately if skin or sclera becomes yellow-tinged, which may indicate drug accumulation from impaired renal excretion.
- Inform patient that drug colors urine red or orange and may stain fabrics and contact lenses.
- Tell diabetic patient to use Clinitest for accurate urine glucose test results. Also tell patient that drug may interfere with urinary ketone tests (Acetest or Ketostix).
- Advise patient to notify prescriber if urinary tract pain persists. Tell him that drug shouldn't be used for long-term treatment.

solifenacin succinate

VESIcare

Pharmacologic class: muscarinic receptor antagonist
Pregnancy risk category C

AVAILABLE FORMS

Tablets (film-coated): 5 mg, 10 mg

INDICATIONS & DOSAGES

➤ Overactive bladder with urinary urgency, frequency, and urge incontinence.
Adults: 5 mg P.O. once daily. May increase to 10 mg once daily if 5-mg dose is well tolerated.
Adjust-a-dose: If creatinine clearance is less than 30 ml/minute or the patient has moderate liver impairment (Child-Pugh score B), maintain the dose at 5 mg.

ACTION

Relaxes smooth muscle of the bladder by competitively antagonizing the muscarinic receptors, relieving the symptoms of an overactive bladder.

Route	Onset	Peak	Duration
P.O.	Unknown	3–8 hr	Unknown

Half-life: 2 to 3 days.

ADVERSE REACTIONS

CNS: depression, dizziness, fatigue.
CV: hypertension, leg swelling.
EENT: blurred vision, dry eyes, pharyngitis.
GI: *constipation, dry mouth,* dyspepsia, nausea, upper abdominal pain, vomiting.
GU: urinary retention, UTI.
Respiratory: cough.
Other: influenza.

INTERACTIONS

Drug-drug. *Drugs that prolong the QT interval:* May increase the risk of serious cardiac arrhythmias. Monitor patient and ECG closely.
Potent CYP3A4 inhibitors (such as ketoconazole): May increase solifenacin levels. Don't exceed solifenacin dose of 5 mg daily when used together.

EFFECTS ON LAB TEST RESULTS

None reported.

CONTRAINDICATIONS & CAUTIONS

- Contraindicated in patients hypersensitive to drug or its components and in patients with urine or gastric retention or uncontrolled narrow-angle glaucoma. Don't use in patients with severe hepatic impairment.
- Use cautiously in patients with a history of prolonged QT interval, those being treated for narrow-angle glaucoma, and those with bladder outflow obstruction, decreased GI motility, renal insufficiency, or moderate liver impairment.

NURSING CONSIDERATIONS

- Assess bladder function, and monitor drug effects.

• If patient has bladder outlet obstruction, watch for urine retention.
• Monitor patient for decreased gastric motility and constipation.
• Safety and effectiveness are similar in older and younger adults, but levels and half-life may increased in the elderly.

PATIENT TEACHING
• Explain that drug may cause blurred vision. Tell patient to use caution when performing hazardous activities or tasks that require clear vision until effects of the drug are known.
• Discourage use of other drugs that may cause dry mouth, constipation, urine retention, or blurred vision.
• Urge patient to notify prescriber about abdominal pain or constipation that lasts 3 days or longer.
• Tell patient that drug decreases the ability to sweat normally, and advise cautious use in hot environments or during strenuous activity.
• Tell patient to swallow tablet whole with liquid.
• Inform patient that drug may be taken with or without food.

tolterodine tartrate
Detrol✐, Detrol LA

Pharmacologic class: antimuscarinic
Pregnancy risk category C

AVAILABLE FORMS
Capsules (extended-release): 2 mg, 4 mg
Tablets: 1 mg, 2 mg

INDICATIONS & DOSAGES
➤ **Overactive bladder in patients with symptoms of urinary frequency, urgency, or urge incontinence**
Adults: 2-mg tablet P.O. b.i.d. or 4-mg extended-release capsule P.O. daily. Dose may be reduced to 1-mg tablet P.O. b.i.d. or 2-mg extended-release capsule P.O. daily, based on patient response and tolerance.
Adjust-a-dose: For patients with significantly reduced hepatic or renal function or those taking a potent CYP3A4 inhibitor, 1-mg tablet P.O. b.i.d. or 2-mg extended-release capsule P.O. daily.

ACTION
Competitively antagonizes muscarinic receptors. Both urinary bladder contraction and salivation are mediated via cholinergic muscarinic receptors.

Route	Onset	Peak	Duration
P.O.	Unknown	1–2 hr	Unknown
P.O. (extended-release)	Unknown	2–6 hours	Unknown

Half-life: 2 to 4 hours; about 8 hours with hepatic impairment.

ADVERSE REACTIONS
CNS: *headache,* fatigue, paresthesia, vertigo, dizziness, nervousness, somnolence.
CV: hypertension, chest pain.
EENT: abnormal vision, xerophthalmia, pharyngitis, rhinitis, sinusitis.
GI: *dry mouth,* abdominal pain, constipation, diarrhea, dyspepsia, flatulence, nausea, vomiting.
GU: dysuria, micturition frequency, urine retention, UTI.
Metabolic: weight gain.
Musculoskeletal: arthralgia, back pain.
Respiratory: bronchitis, coughing, upper respiratory tract infection.
Skin: pruritus, rash, erythema, dry skin.
Other: flulike syndrome, accidental injury, fungal infection, infection.

INTERACTIONS
Drug-drug. *Antifungals (itraconazole, ketoconazole, miconazole), CYP3A4 inhibitors (such as clarithromycin and erythromycin):* May increase tolterodine level. Don't give more than 1-mg tablet b.i.d. or 2-mg extended-release capsule daily of tolterodine if used together.
Fluoxetine: May increase tolterodine level. Monitor patient. No dosage adjustment is needed.

EFFECTS ON LAB TEST RESULTS
None reported.

CONTRAINDICATIONS & CAUTIONS
• Contraindicated in patients hypersensitive to drug or its components and in those

with uncontrolled angle-closure glaucoma or urine or gastric retention.
- Use cautiously in patients with significant bladder outflow obstruction, GI obstructive disorders (such as pyloric stenosis), controlled angle-closure glaucoma, and hepatic or renal impairment.

NURSING CONSIDERATIONS
- Assess baseline bladder function and monitor therapeutic effects.

PATIENT TEACHING
- Tell patient that sugarless gum, hard candy, or saliva substitute may help relieve dry mouth.
- Advise patient to avoid driving or other potentially hazardous activities until visual effects of drug are known.
- Advise women to stop breast-feeding during therapy.
- Instruct patient to immediately report signs of infection, urine retention, or GI problems.
- Tell patient taking extended-release form to swallow capsule whole and take with liquids.

trospium chloride
Sanctura

Pharmacologic class: antimuscarinic
Pregnancy risk category C

AVAILABLE FORMS
Tablets: 20 mg

INDICATIONS & DOSAGES
➤ Overactive bladder with symptoms of urinary urge incontinence, urgency, and frequency
Adults younger than age 75: Give 20 mg P.O. b.i.d. taken on an empty stomach or at least 1 hour before a meal.
Adults age 75 and older: Based on patient tolerance, reduce dose to 20 mg once daily.
Adjust-a-dose: If patient's creatinine clearance is less than 30 ml/minute, give 20 mg P.O. once daily at bedtime.

ACTION
Opposes the effect of acetylcholine on muscarinic receptors, which reduces smooth muscle tone in the bladder and increases maximum bladder capacity and volume at first contraction.

Route	Onset	Peak	Duration
P.O.	Unknown	5–6 hr	Unknown

Half-life: About 20 hours.

ADVERSE REACTIONS
CNS: fatigue, headache.
EENT: dry eyes.
GI: *constipation, dry mouth,* abdominal pain, dyspepsia, flatulence.
GU: urine retention.

INTERACTIONS
Drug-drug. *Anticholinergics:* May increase dry mouth, constipation, or other adverse effects. Monitor patient.
Digoxin, metformin, morphine, procainamide, pancuronium, tenofovir, vancomycin: May alter elimination of these drugs or trospium, increasing levels. Monitor patient closely.
Drug-food. *High-fat foods:* May significantly decrease absorption. Give drug at least 1 hour before meals or on an empty stomach.
Drug-lifestyle. *Alcohol use:* May increase drowsiness. Discourage use together.

EFFECTS ON LAB TEST RESULTS
None reported.

CONTRAINDICATIONS & CAUTIONS
- Contraindicated in patients hypersensitive to the drug or any of its ingredients and in patients with or at risk for urine retention, gastric retention, or uncontrolled narrow-angle glaucoma.
- Use cautiously in patients with significant bladder outflow obstruction, obstructive GI disorders, ulcerative colitis, intestinal atony, myasthenia gravis, renal insufficiency, moderate or severe hepatic impairment, or controlled narrow-angle glaucoma.

NURSING CONSIDERATIONS
- Assess patient to determine baseline bladder function, and monitor patient for therapeutic effects.
- If patient has bladder outflow obstruction, watch for evidence of urine retention.

• Monitor patient for decreased gastric motility and constipation.
• Elderly patients typically need a reduced dosage because they have an increased risk of anticholinergic effects.

PATIENT TEACHING
• Tell patient to take drug on an empty stomach or at least 1 hour before meals.
• Discourage use of other drugs that may cause dry mouth, constipation, blurred vision, or urine retention.
• Tell patient that alcohol may increase drowsiness and fatigue. Urge him to avoid excessive alcohol consumption while taking trospium.
• Explain that drug may decrease sweating and increase the risk of heatstroke when used in hot environments or during strenuous activities.
• Urge patient to avoid activities that are hazardous or require mental alertness until he knows how the drug affects him.

92
Gold salts

auranofin
aurothioglucose
gold sodium thiomalate

auranofin
Ridaura

Pharmacologic class: gold compound
Pregnancy risk category C

AVAILABLE FORMS
Capsules: 3 mg

INDICATIONS & DOSAGES
➤ Rheumatoid arthritis
Adults: 3 mg b.i.d. or 6 mg once daily. After 6 months, may increase to 3 mg t.i.d. If response is inadequate after 3 months of 9 mg/day, stop use.
Children: Initially, 0.1 mg/kg daily. Maintenance dose is 0.15 mg/kg daily; maximum dose is 0.2 mg/kg daily.

ACTION
Probably acts by inhibiting sulfhydryl systems, which alters cellular metabolism. May also alter enzyme function and immune response and suppress phagocytic activity.

Route	Onset	Peak	Duration
P.O.	Unknown	2 hr	Unknown

Half-life: About 26 days.

ADVERSE REACTIONS
CNS: ***seizures,*** confusion, hallucinations.
EENT: conjunctivitis.
GI: *diarrhea, abdominal pain, nausea, stomatitis,* glossitis, anorexia, metallic taste, dyspepsia, flatulence, constipation, dysgeusia, ulcerative colitis.
GU: ***acute renal failure,*** proteinuria, hematuria, nephrotic syndrome, glomerulonephritis.
Hematologic: ***thrombocytopenia, aplastic anemia, agranulocytosis, leukopenia,*** eosinophilia, anemia.
Hepatic: jaundice.
Skin: *rash, pruritus, dermatitis,* exfoliative dermatitis, urticaria, erythema, alopecia.

INTERACTIONS
Drug-drug. *Phenytoin:* May increase phenytoin blood levels. Watch for toxicity.

EFFECTS ON LAB TEST RESULTS
- May increase alkaline phosphatase, ALT, and AST levels. May decrease hemoglobin level and hematocrit.
- May increase eosinophil count. May decrease granulocyte, platelet, and WBC counts.

CONTRAINDICATIONS & CAUTIONS
- Contraindicated in patients with history of severe gold toxicity or toxicity from previous exposure to other heavy metals and in those with necrotizing enterocolitis, pulmonary fibrosis, exfoliative dermatitis, bone marrow aplasia, or severe hematologic disorders.
- Contraindicated in patients with urticaria, eczema, colitis, severe debilitation, hemorrhagic conditions, or systemic lupus erythematosus and in patients who have recently received radiation therapy.
- Manufacturer recommends avoiding use during pregnancy.
- Use cautiously with other drugs that cause blood dyscrasias.
- Use cautiously in patients with rash, history of bone marrow depression, or renal, hepatic, or inflammatory bowel disease.

NURSING CONSIDERATIONS
- Monitor patient's platelet count monthly. Stop drug if platelet count falls below 100,000/mm^3, if hemoglobin level drops suddenly, if granulocyte count is less than 1,500/mm^3, or if leukopenia (WBC count less than 4,000/mm^3) or eosinophilia over 5% exists.
- ***Alert:*** Monitor patient's urinalysis results monthly. If proteinuria or hematuria is detected, stop drug because it can cause nephrotic syndrome or glomerulonephritis, and notify prescriber.

• Monitor renal and liver function test results.
• Warn women of childbearing potential about risks of drug therapy during pregnancy.

PATIENT TEACHING
• Encourage patient to take drug as prescribed.
• Tell patient to continue other drug therapies if prescribed.
• Remind patient to see prescriber for monthly platelet counts.
• Suggest that patient have regular urinalysis.
• Tell patient to keep taking drug if mild diarrhea occurs but to immediately report blood in stool. Diarrhea is the most common adverse reaction.
• Advise patient to report rash or other skin problems and to stop drug until reaction subsides. Itching may precede dermatitis; consider itchy skin eruptions during drug therapy to be a reaction until proven otherwise.
• Inform patient that inflammation of the mouth may be preceded by a metallic taste; tell him to notify prescriber if this occurs. Promote careful oral hygiene during therapy.
• Advise patient to report unusual bleeding or bruising.
• Inform patient that beneficial effect may be delayed as long as 3 months. If response is inadequate and maximum dose has been reached, expect prescriber to stop drug.
• Warn patient not to give drug to others. Auranofin is prescribed only for selected patients with rheumatoid arthritis.

aurothioglucose
Solganal

gold sodium thiomalate
Aurolate

Pharmacologic class: gold compound
Pregnancy risk category C

AVAILABLE FORMS
aurothioglucose
Injection (suspension): 50 mg/ml in sesame oil in 10-ml vial
gold sodium thiomalate
Injection: 50 mg/ml with benzyl alcohol in 2-ml and 10-ml vials

INDICATIONS & DOSAGES
➤Rheumatoid arthritis
aurothioglucose
Adults: Initially, 10 mg I.M., followed by 25 mg q week for second and third doses. Then, 50 mg q week to total dose of 800 mg to 1 g. If condition improves and no toxicity occurs, continue 25 to 50 mg q 3 to 4 weeks indefinitely.
Children ages 6 to 12: One-fourth usual adult dose. Don't exceed 25 mg per dose.
gold sodium thiomalate
Adults: Initially, 10 mg I.M., followed by 25 mg in 1 week. Then, 25 to 50 mg q week to total dose of 1 g. If condition improves and no toxicity occurs, give 25 to 50 mg q 2 weeks for 2 to 20 weeks; then, 25 to 50 mg q 3 to 4 weeks as maintenance therapy. If relapse occurs, resume injections at weekly intervals.
Children: Initially, a test dose of 10 mg I.M.; then, 1 mg/kg I.M. weekly, not to exceed 50 mg for a single injection. Follow adult spacing of doses.

ACTION
Probably acts by inhibiting sulfhydryl systems, which alters cellular metabolism. May also alter enzyme function and immune response and suppress phagocytic activity.

Route	Onset	Peak	Duration
I.M.	Unknown	3–6 hr	Unknown

Half-life: 3 to 27 days (single dose); 14 to 40 days (3rd dose); up to 168 days (11th dose).

ADVERSE REACTIONS
CNS: ***seizures,*** confusion, hallucinations.
CV: ***bradycardia,*** hypotension.
EENT: corneal gold deposition, corneal ulcers.
GI: *diarrhea, metallic taste, stomatitis,* anorexia, abdominal cramps, nausea, vomiting, ulcerative enterocolitis.
GU: ***acute renal failure,*** albuminuria, proteinuria, nephrotic syndrome, nephritis, acute tubular necrosis, hematuria.

Hematologic: ***thrombocytopenia, aplastic anemia, agranulocytosis, leukopenia,*** eosinophilia, anemia.
Hepatic: ***hepatitis,*** jaundice.
Skin: *rash, dermatitis,* erythema, exfoliative dermatitis, diaphoresis, photosensitivity reaction.
Other: ***anaphylaxis, angioedema.***

INTERACTIONS

Drug-lifestyle. *Sun or ultraviolet light exposure:* May cause photosensitivity reaction. Advise patient to avoid excessive sunlight exposure.

EFFECTS ON LAB TEST RESULTS

- May increase alkaline phosphatase, ALT, and AST, levels. May decrease hemoglobin level and hematocrit.
- May increase eosinophil count. May decrease granulocyte, platelet, and WBC counts.

CONTRAINDICATIONS & CAUTIONS

- Contraindicated in patients hypersensitive to drug and in those with history of severe toxicity from previous exposure to gold or other heavy metals.
- Contraindicated in those who have recently received radiation therapy and in those with hepatitis, exfoliative dermatitis, severe uncontrollable diabetes, renal disease, hepatic dysfunction, uncontrolled heart failure, systemic lupus erythematosus, colitis, Sjögren syndrome, urticaria, eczema, hemorrhagic conditions, or severe hematologic disorders.
- Use cautiously, if at all, in patients with rash, marked hypertension, compromised cerebral or CV circulation, or history of renal or hepatic disease, drug allergies, or blood dyscrasias.

NURSING CONSIDERATIONS

- Warn women about risks of gold therapy during pregnancy.
- Give drug only under constant supervision of prescriber thoroughly familiar with drug's toxicities and benefits.
- Immerse aurothioglucose vial in warm water; shake vigorously before injecting.
- Drug should be pale yellow; don't use if it darkens.
- Analyze urine for protein and sediment changes before each injection.
- ***Alert:*** Give drug I.M. only, preferably into gluteal muscle.
- When injecting gold sodium thiomalate, have patient lie down for 10 to 20 minutes to minimize hypotension.
- Watch for anaphylactoid reaction for 30 minutes after administration.
- ***Alert:*** Keep dimercaprol available to treat acute toxicity.
- Monitor CBC, including platelet count, before every second injection.
- If adverse reactions are mild, some rheumatologists resume gold therapy after 2 to 3 weeks' rest.
- Monitor platelet counts if patient develops purpura or ecchymoses.

PATIENT TEACHING

- Inform patient that increased joint pain may occur for 1 to 2 days after injection but usually subsides.
- Advise patient to report rash or skin problems immediately and to stop drug until reaction subsides. Itching may precede skin inflammation; consider itchy skin eruptions during gold therapy to be a reaction until proven otherwise.
- Advise patient to report unusual bleeding or bruising.
- Instruct patient to report a metallic taste. Promote careful oral hygiene.
- Urge patient to avoid sunlight and artificial ultraviolet light, which may cause gray-blue skin pigmentation.
- Tell patient that benefits may not appear for 3 to 4 months.
- Stress need for follow-up care.

93

Miscellaneous antagonists and antidotes

acamprosate calcium
activated charcoal
charcoal
deferasirox
digoxin immune Fab
dimercaprol
disulfiram
edetate calcium disodium
edetate disodium
flumazenil
lanthanum carbonate
naloxone hydrochloride
naltrexone
naltrexone hydrochloride
pentetate calcium trisodium
pentetate zinc trisodium
pralidoxime chloride
protamine sulfate
sevelamer hydrochloride
sodium polystyrene sulfonate
succimer

SAFETY ALERT!

acamprosate calcium

Campral✐

Pharmacologic class: synthetic amino acid neurotransmitter analog
Pregnancy risk category C

AVAILABLE FORMS

Tablets (delayed-release): 333 mg

INDICATIONS & DOSAGES

➤ **Adjunct to management of alcohol abstinence**
Adults: 666 mg P.O. t.i.d.
Adjust-a-dose: In patients with creatinine clearance of 30 to 50 ml/minute, give 333 mg t.i.d.

ACTION

Restores the balance of neuronal excitation and inhibition, probably by interacting with glutamate and gamma-aminobutyric acid neurotransmitter systems, thus reducing alcohol dependence.

Route	Onset	Peak	Duration
P.O.	Unknown	3–8 hr	Unknown

Half-life: 20 to 33 hours.

ADVERSE REACTIONS

CNS: abnormal thinking, amnesia, anxiety, asthenia, depression, dizziness, headache, insomnia, paresthesia, somnolence, ***suicidal thoughts,*** syncope, tremor.
CV: hypertension, palpitations, peripheral edema, vasodilation.
EENT: abnormal vision, pharyngitis, rhinitis.
GI: abdominal pain, anorexia, constipation, *diarrhea,* dry mouth, dyspepsia, flatulence, increased appetite, nausea, taste disturbance, vomiting.
GU: impotence.
Metabolic: weight gain.
Musculoskeletal: arthralgia, back pain, chest pain, myalgia.
Respiratory: bronchitis, dyspnea, increased cough.
Skin: increased sweating, pruritus, rash.
Other: accidental injury, chills, decreased libido, flulike symptoms, infection, pain.

INTERACTIONS

None significant.

EFFECTS ON LAB TEST RESULTS

- May increase ALT, AST, bilirubin, blood glucose, and uric acid levels. May decrease hemoglobin level and hematocrit.
- May decrease platelet count.

CONTRAINDICATIONS & CAUTIONS

- Contraindicated in patients allergic to drug or its components and in those whose creatinine clearance is 30 ml/minute or less.
- Use cautiously in pregnant or breast-feeding women, elderly patients, patients with moderate renal impairment, and patients with a history of depression and suicidal thoughts or attempts.

NURSING CONSIDERATIONS

- Use only after the patient successfully becomes abstinent from drinking.
- Drug doesn't eliminate or reduce withdrawal symptoms.
- Monitor patient for development of depression or suicidal thoughts.
- Drug doesn't cause alcohol aversion or a disulfiram-like reaction if used with alcohol.

PATIENT TEACHING

- Tell patient to continue the alcohol abstinence program, including counseling and support.
- Advise patient to notify his prescriber if he develops depression, anxiety, thoughts of suicide, or severe diarrhea.
- Caution patient's family or caregiver to watch for signs of depression or suicidal ideation.
- Tell patient that drug may be taken without regard to meals, but that taking it with meals may help him remember it.
- Tell patient not to crush, break, or chew the tablets but to swallow them whole.
- Advise women to use effective contraception while taking this drug. Tell patient to contact her prescriber if she becomes pregnant or plans to become pregnant.
- Explain that this drug may impair judgment, thinking, or motor skills. Urge patient to use caution when driving or performing hazardous activities until drug's effects are known.
- Tell patient to continue taking acamprosate and to contact his prescriber if he resumes drinking alcohol.

activated charcoal

Actidose ◊, Actidose-Aqua ◊, Actidose with Sorbitol ◊, CharcoAid ◊, CharcoAid 2000 ◊, Liqui-Char ◊

charcoal

Charcoal Plus DS ◊, CharcoCaps ◊

Pharmacologic class: adsorbent
Pregnancy risk category C

AVAILABLE FORMS

activated charcoal
Granules: 15 g ◊
Liquid: 12.5 g ◊, 15 g* ◊, 25 g* ◊, 30 g* ◊, 50 g* ◊
Oral suspension: 15 g ◊, 30 g ◊
Powder: 15 g ◊, 30 g ◊, 40 g ◊, 120 g ◊, 240 g ◊
charcoal
Capsules: 260 mg ◊
Tablets: 250 mg ◊

INDICATIONS & DOSAGES

➤ Flatulence, dyspepsia, diarrhea
Adults: 500 to 520 mg (charcoal) P.O. after meals or at first sign of discomfort. Repeat as needed, up to 5 g daily.
➤ Poisoning
Adults and children: Initially, 1 to 2 g/kg (30 to 100 g) P.O. or 10 times the amount of poison ingested as a suspension in 120 to 240 ml (4 to 8 ounces) of water.

ACTION

Adheres to many drugs and chemicals, inhibiting their absorption from the GI tract. Also reduces volume of intestinal gas and relieves related discomfort.

Route	Onset	Peak	Duration
P.O.	Immediate	Unknown	Unknown

Half-life: Unknown.

ADVERSE REACTIONS

GI: *black stools,* ***intestinal obstruction,*** nausea, constipation.

INTERACTIONS

Drug-drug. *Acetaminophen, barbiturates, carbamazepine, digitoxin, digoxin, furosemide, glutethimide, hydantoins, methotrexate, nizatidine, phenothiazines, phenylbutazone, propoxyphene, salicylates, sulfonamides, sulfonylureas, tetracyclines, theophyllines, tricyclic antidepressants, valproic acid:* May reduce absorption of these drugs. Give charcoal at least 2 hours before or 1 hour after other drugs.
Acetylcysteine, ipecac: May inactivate these drugs. Give charcoal after vomiting has been induced by ipecac; remove charcoal by nasogastric tube before giving acetylcysteine.
Drug-food. *Milk, ice cream, sherbet:* May decrease adsorptive capacity of drug. Discourage use together.

EFFECTS ON LAB TEST RESULTS
None reported.

CONTRAINDICATIONS & CAUTIONS
- No known contraindications.

NURSING CONSIDERATIONS
- Although there are no known contraindications, drug isn't effective for treating all acute poisonings.
- ***Alert:*** Drug is commonly used for treating poisoning or overdose with acetaminophen, aspirin, atropine, barbiturates, dextropropoxyphene, digoxin, poisonous mushrooms, oxalic acid, parathion, phenol, phenytoin, propantheline, propoxyphene, strychnine, or tricyclic antidepressants. Check with poison control center for use in other types of poisonings or overdoses.
- Give after emesis is complete because activated charcoal absorbs and inactivates ipecac syrup.
- For maximal effect, give within 30 minutes after poison ingestion.
- Mix powder (most effective form) with tap water to consistency of thick syrup. Adding a small amount of fruit juice or flavoring makes mix more palatable. Don't mix with ice cream, milk, or sherbet because these decrease adsorptive capacity of activated charcoal.
- ***Alert:*** Don't aspirate or allow patient to aspirate charcoal powder; this may result in death.
- Give by large-bore nasogastric tube after lavage, if needed.
- If patient vomits shortly after administration, be prepared to repeat dose.
- Space doses at least 1 hour apart from other drugs if treatment is for indications other than poisoning.
- Follow treatment with stool softener or laxative to prevent constipation unless sorbitol is part of product ingredients. Preparations made with sorbitol have a laxative effect that lessens risk of severe constipation or fecal impaction.
- If preparation with sorbitol is used, maintain patient's fluid and electrolyte needs.
- Don't use charcoal with sorbitol in fructose-intolerant patients or in children younger than age 1.
- ***Alert:*** Drug is ineffective for poisoning or overdose of cyanide, mineral acids, caustic alkalis, and organic solvents; it's not very effective for overdose of ethanol, lithium, methanol, and iron salts.
- ***Look alike–sound alike:*** Don't confuse Actidose with Actos.

PATIENT TEACHING
- Explain use and administration of drug to patient (if awake) and family.
- Warn patient that stools will be black until all the charcoal has passed through the body.
- Instruct patient to drink 6 to 8 glasses of liquid per day because drug can cause constipation.

deferasirox
Exjade

Pharmacologic class: heavy metal antagonist
Pregnancy risk category B

AVAILABLE FORMS
Tablets for oral suspension: 125 mg, 250 mg, 500 mg

INDICATIONS & DOSAGES
➤ **Chronic iron overload caused by blood transfusions (transfusional hemosiderosis)**
Adults and children age 2 and older: Initially, 20 mg/kg P.O. daily on an empty stomach 30 minutes before eating. Monitor serum ferritin level monthly and adjust dose q 3 to 6 months by 5 or 10 mg/kg based on ferritin trends. Don't exceed 30 mg/kg daily. Consider stopping therapy if serum ferritin level drops below 500 mcg/L.

ACTION
Binds with high affinity to iron, allowing mainly fecal excretion.

Route	Onset	Peak	Duration
P.O.	Unknown	1½–4 hr	Unknown

Half-life: 8 to 16 hours.

ADVERSE REACTIONS
CNS: *fever, headache,* dizziness, fatigue.

EENT: *nasopharyngitis, pharyngolaryngeal pain,* acute tonsillitis, auditory disturbances, ear infection, pharyngitis, rhinitis, visual disturbances.
GI: *abdominal pain, diarrhea, nausea, vomiting.*
Hepatic: ***liver toxicity.***
Musculoskeletal: back pain, joint pain.
Respiratory: *cough,* bronchitis, respiratory tract infection.
Skin: rash, urticaria.
Other: influenza.

INTERACTIONS

Drug-drug. *Aluminum-containing antacids:* May decrease iron chelation. Don't give together.
Other iron chelators: May increase risk of toxic effects. Avoid using together.
Drug-food. *Any food:* May decrease drug effects. Give on an empty stomach at least 30 minutes before eating.

EFFECTS ON LAB TEST RESULTS

- May increase transaminase and creatinine levels.

CONTRAINDICATIONS & CAUTIONS

- Contraindicated in patients hypersensitive to deferasirox or any component of the drug.
- Use cautiously in breast-feeding women and patients with renal impairment, hepatic impairment, hearing loss, or vision disturbances.

NURSING CONSIDERATIONS

- Test liver function monthly.
- Check creatinine level before treatment starts and monthly thereafter. If level increases, notify prescriber. Dose may need adjustment or drug may need to be stopped.
- Periodically evaluate patient for proteinuria.
- Test patient's hearing and visual acuity before starting drug and yearly thereafter.
- Monitor patient for rash. If mild or moderate, treatment may continue. If severe, drug may be stopped or dose reduced. Patient also may need corticosteroids.

PATIENT TEACHING

- Tell patient to take drug at about the same time each day, on an empty stomach, 30 minutes before eating.
- Caution patient not to chew or swallow the tablets.
- Instruct patient to dissolve tablets in water, orange juice, or apple juice; drink the mixture; swirl a small amount of the same liquid in the glass to pick up any remaining drug; and swallow that as well.
- Tell patient not to take aluminum-containing antacids at the same time.
- Inform patient of the need for monthly blood tests to evaluate the effectiveness of therapy and detect possible side effects.
- Tell patient to report changes in hearing or vision, rash, abdominal pain, yellowing of skin or eyes, pale stools, or dark urine.
- Urge patient to avoid driving or operating hazardous equipment if he becomes dizzy.

digoxin immune Fab (ovine)

Digibind, DigiFab

Pharmacologic class: antibody fragment
Pregnancy risk category C

AVAILABLE FORMS

Injection: 38-mg vial (Digibind), 40-mg vial (DigiFab)

INDICATIONS & DOSAGES

➤ Life-threatening digoxin toxicity
Adults and children: Base dosage on ingested amount or level of digoxin. When calculating amount of antidote, round up to the nearest whole number.

For digoxin tablets, calculate number of antidote vials as follows: multiply ingested amount by 0.8; then divide answer by 0.5. For example, if patient takes 25 tablets of 0.25 mg digoxin, the ingested amount is 6.25 mg. Multiply 6.25 mg by 0.8 and divide answer by 0.5 to obtain 10 vials of antidote.

For digoxin capsules, divide the ingested dose in milligrams by 0.5. For example, if patient takes 50 capsules of 0.2 mg, the ingested amount is 10 mg. Divide 10 mg by 0.5 to obtain 20 vials of antidote.

If digoxin level is known, determine the number of antidote vials as follows: multiply the digoxin level in nanograms per milliliter by patient's weight in kilograms; then divide by 100. For example, if digoxin level is 4 nanograms/ml, and patient weighs 60 kg, multiply together to obtain 240. Divide answer by 100 to obtain 2.4 vials; then round up to 3 vials.

➤ **Acute toxicity or if estimated ingested amount or digoxin level is unknown**

Adults and children: Consider giving 10 vials of digoxin immune Fab and observing patient's response. Follow with another 10 vials if indicated. Dosage should be effective in most life-threatening cases in adults and children but may cause volume overload in young children.

I.V. ADMINISTRATION

- Reconstitute drug immediately before use with 4 ml sterile water for injection.
- For children or other patients who need small doses, reconstitute 38-mg vial Digibind with 38 ml of normal saline solution to yield 1 mg/ml; reconstitute 40-mg vial DigiFab with 40 ml of normal saline solution to yield 1 mg/ml.
- If cardiac arrest seems imminent, drug may be given by direct injection.
- For intermittent infusion, further dilute with normal saline solution for injection to an appropriate volume.
- Infuse drug over 30 minutes through a 0.22-micron membrane filter.
- Refrigerate powder for injection. Reconstituted solutions may be refrigerated 4 hours.

INCOMPATIBILITIES

None reported.

ACTION

Binds molecules of unbound digoxin and digitoxin, making them unavailable for binding at site of action on cells.

Route	Onset	Peak	Duration
I.V.	30 min	End of infusion	15–20 hr

Half-life: 15 to 20 hours.

ADVERSE REACTIONS

CV: ***heart failure,*** rapid ventricular rate, worsening low cardiac output.
Metabolic: hypokalemia.
Other: ***anaphylaxis,*** hypersensitivity reactions.

INTERACTIONS

None significant.

EFFECTS ON LAB TEST RESULTS

- May decrease potassium level.
- May interfere with digitalis immunoassay measurements until drug is cleared from the body (about 48 hours).

CONTRAINDICATIONS & CAUTIONS

- Use cautiously in patients allergic to sheep proteins and in those who have previously received antibodies.

NURSING CONSIDERATIONS

- In patients allergic to sheep proteins and in those who have previously received antibodies, skin testing is recommended because drug is derived from digoxin-specific antibody fragments obtained from immunized sheep.
- Drug is used for life-threatening overdose in patients with anaphylaxis, severe hypotension, or cardiac arrest and in those with ventricular arrhythmias (such as ventricular tachycardia or fibrillation), progressive bradycardia (such as severe sinus bradycardia), or second- or third-degree AV block not responsive to atropine.
- Heart failure and rapid ventricular rate may result by reversal of cardiac glycoside's therapeutic effects.
- Monitor potassium level closely.
- In most patients, signs of digitalis toxicity disappear within a few hours.

PATIENT TEACHING

- Explain use and administration of drug to patient and family.
- Instruct patient to report adverse reactions promptly.

dimercaprol

BAL in Oil

Pharmacologic class: heavy metal antagonist
Pregnancy risk category C

AVAILABLE FORMS
Injection: 100 mg/ml

INDICATIONS & DOSAGES
➤ **Severe arsenic or gold poisoning**
Adults and children: 3 mg/kg deep I.M. q 4 hours for 2 days; then q.i.d. on third day; then b.i.d. for 10 days.
➤ **Mild arsenic or gold poisoning**
Adults and children: 2.5 mg/kg deep I.M. q.i.d. for 2 days; then b.i.d. on third day; then once daily for 10 days.
➤ **Mercury poisoning**
Adults and children: Initially, 5 mg/kg deep I.M.; then 2.5 mg/kg daily or b.i.d. for 10 days.
➤ **Acute lead encephalopathy or lead level greater than 100 mcg/ml**
Adults and children: 4 mg/kg deep I.M.; then q 4 hours with edetate calcium disodium for 2 to 7 days. Use separate sites. For less severe poisoning, reduce dose to 3 mg/kg after first dose.

ACTION
Forms complexes with heavy metals to create chelates that are renally excreted.

Route	Onset	Peak	Duration
I.M.	Unknown	30–60 min	4 hr

Half-life: Unknown.

ADVERSE REACTIONS
CNS: *fever,* headache, paresthesia, anxiety.
CV: *transient increase in blood pressure, tachycardia.*
EENT: blepharospasm, conjunctivitis, lacrimation, rhinorrhea.
GI: *nausea, vomiting,* excessive salivation, *abdominal pain, burning sensation in lips, mouth, and throat.*
Musculoskeletal: muscle pain or weakness.
Other: pain or tightness in throat, chest, or hands.

INTERACTIONS
Drug-drug. *Iron:* May cause toxic metal complex. Take iron 24 hours after last dimercaprol dose.

EFFECTS ON LAB TEST RESULTS
• May block thyroid uptake of ^{131}I, decreasing values.

CONTRAINDICATIONS & CAUTIONS
• Contraindicated in patients with hepatic dysfunction (except postarsenical jaundice) or iron, cadmium, or selenium poisoning; also contraindicated in those allergic to peanuts.
• Don't use in pregnant women except for life-threatening acute poisoning.
• Use cautiously in patients with hypertension, G6PD deficiency, or oliguria.

NURSING CONSIDERATIONS
• ***Alert:*** Don't give drug I.V.; give by deep I.M. route only.
• Don't let drug contact skin because it may cause a skin reaction.
• Drug has an unpleasant, garlicky odor.
• Solution with slight sediment is usable.
• Use antihistamine to prevent or relieve mild adverse reactions.
• Keep urine alkaline to prevent renal damage.

PATIENT TEACHING
• Explain use and administration of drug to patient and family.
• Instruct patient to report adverse reactions promptly.

disulfiram

Antabuse

Pharmacologic class: aldehyde dehydrogenase inhibitor
Pregnancy risk category NR

AVAILABLE FORMS
Tablets: 250 mg, 500 mg

INDICATIONS & DOSAGES
➤ **Adjunct to management of alcohol abstinence**
Adults: 250 to 500 mg P.O. as single dose in morning for 1 to 2 weeks or in evening if drowsiness occurs. Maintenance dosage

is 125 to 500 mg P.O. daily (average 250 mg) until permanent self-control is established. Treatment may continue for months or years.

ACTION

Blocks oxidation of alcohol at the acetaldehyde stage. Excess acetaldehyde produces a highly unpleasant reaction in the presence of even small amounts of alcohol.

Route	Onset	Peak	Duration
P.O.	1–2 hr	Unknown	14 days

Half-life: Unknown.

ADVERSE REACTIONS

CNS: drowsiness, headache, fatigue, delirium, depression, neuritis, peripheral neuritis, polyneuritis, restlessness, psychotic reactions.
EENT: optic neuritis.
GI: metallic or garlicky aftertaste.
GU: impotence.
Skin: acneiform or allergic dermatitis, occasional eruptions.
Other: ***disulfiram reaction precipitated by alcohol use.***

INTERACTIONS

Drug-drug. *Barbiturates:* May prolong duration of barbiturate effect. Closely monitor patient.
CNS depressants: May increase CNS depression. Use together cautiously.
Coumarin anticoagulants: May increase anticoagulant effect. Adjust dosage of anticoagulant.
Isoniazid: May cause ataxia or marked change in behavior. Avoid using together.
Metronidazole: May cause psychotic reaction. Avoid using together.
Midazolam: May increase midazolam level. Use together cautiously.
Paraldehyde: May cause toxic level of acetaldehyde. Avoid using together.
Phenytoin: May increase toxic effect of phenytoin. Monitor phenytoin level closely and adjust dose as necessary.
Tricyclic antidepressants, especially amitriptyline: May cause transient delirium. Closely monitor patient.
Drug-herb. *Herbal preparations containing alcohol:* May cause disulfiram reaction. Warn patient against using together. Alcohol reaction may occur as long as 2 weeks after single drug dose.
Drug-food. *Caffeine:* May increase elimination half-life of caffeine. Tell patient to watch for effects.
Drug-lifestyle. *Alcohol use:* May cause drug reaction including flushing, tachycardia, bronchospasm, sweating, nausea and vomiting, or death. Warn patient not to use products containing alcohol, including back rub preparations, cough syrups, liniments, and shaving lotion, or to drink alcoholic beverages.

EFFECTS ON LAB TEST RESULTS

- May increase cholesterol level.

CONTRAINDICATIONS & CAUTIONS

- Contraindicated in patients hypersensitive to drug or other thiram derivatives used in pesticides and rubber vulcanization; in those with psychoses, myocardial disease, or coronary occlusion; in those receiving metronidazole, paraldehyde, alcohol, or alcohol-containing products; and in those experiencing alcohol intoxication or who have ingested alcohol in preceding 12 hours.
- Don't give drug during pregnancy.
- Use with caution in patients also receiving phenytoin therapy and in those with diabetes mellitus, hypothyroidism, seizure disorder, cerebral damage, nephritis, or hepatic cirrhosis or insufficiency.

NURSING CONSIDERATIONS

- Never give until patient has abstained from alcohol for at least 12 hours. He should clearly understand consequences of drug and give permission for its use. Use drug only in patients who are cooperative, well-motivated, and receiving supportive psychiatric therapy.
- Perform complete physical examination and laboratory studies, including CBC, SMA-12, and transaminase level, before therapy and repeat regularly.
- Drug reaction may result from alcohol use, with flushing, throbbing headache, dyspnea, nausea, copious vomiting, diaphoresis, thirst, chest pain, palpitations, hyperventilation, hypotension, syncope, anxiety, weakness, blurred vision, confusion, and arthropathy.

• ***Alert:*** A severe drug reaction can cause respiratory depression, CV collapse, arrhythmias, MI, acute heart failure, seizures, unconsciousness, and death.
• The longer the patient remains on the drug, the more sensitive he becomes to alcohol.
• ***Look alike–sound alike:*** Don't confuse Antabuse with Anturane.

PATIENT TEACHING

• ***Alert:*** Caution patient's family that drug should never be given to patient without his knowledge; severe reaction or death could result if patient drinks alcohol.
• Tell patient to carry medical identification that identifies him as a disulfiram user.
• Mild reactions may occur in sensitive patient with blood alcohol levels of 5 to 10 mg/dl; symptoms are fully developed at 50 mg/dl; unconsciousness typically occurs at 125 to 150 mg/dl level. Reaction may last from 30 minutes to several hours or as long as alcohol remains in blood.
• Reassure patient that drug-induced adverse reactions (unrelated to alcohol use), such as drowsiness, fatigue, impotence, headache, peripheral neuritis, and metallic or garlic taste, subside after about 2 weeks of therapy.
• Advise patient not to drink alcoholic beverages or use products containing alcohol, including topical preparations and mouthwash.
• Have patient verify content of OTC products with pharmacist before use.

edetate calcium disodium

Calcium Disodium Versenate, Calcium EDTA

Pharmacologic class: heavy metal antagonist
Pregnancy risk category B

AVAILABLE FORMS

Injection: 200 mg/ml

INDICATIONS & DOSAGES

➤ Acute lead encephalopathy or lead levels greater than 70 mcg/dl
Adults and children: 1 to 1.5 g/m^2 I.V. or I.M. daily in divided doses at 8- to 12-hour intervals for 5 days, usually with dimercaprol. A second course may be given after at least a 2-day drug-free interval.

➤ Lead poisoning without encephalopathy or asymptomatic with lead levels less than 70 mcg/dl
Children: 1 g/m^2 I.V. or I.M. daily in divided doses for 5 days.

I.V. ADMINISTRATION

• Dilute 5-ml ampule with 500 ml or 250 ml of D_5W or normal saline solution for injection to yield 2 mg/ml to 4 mg/ml, respectively.
• Infuse half of daily dose over 1 hour and remaining infusion at least 12 hours later. Or, give by slow infusion over at least 8 hours.

INCOMPATIBILITIES

Amphotericin B, dextrose 10% in water, hydralazine hydrochloride, invert sugar 10% in normal saline solution, invert sugar 10% in water, lactated Ringer solution, Ringer injection, 1/6 M sodium lactate.

ACTION

Forms stable, soluble complexes with metals, particularly lead.

Route	Onset	Peak	Duration
I.V., I.M.	1 hr	24–48 hr	Unknown

Half-life: 20 minutes to 1¼ hours.

ADVERSE REACTIONS

CNS: fever, tremors, headache, paresthesia, malaise, fatigue.
CV: hypotension, rhythm irregularities.
EENT: histamine-like reactions (including sneezing, congestion, and lacrimation).
GI: cheilosis, nausea, vomiting, anorexia, excessive thirst.
GU: ***nephrotoxicity with renal tubular necrosis, leading to fatal nephrosis,*** proteinuria, hematuria.
Hematologic: ***transient bone marrow suppression,*** anemia.
Metabolic: zinc deficiency, hypercalcemia.
Musculoskeletal: myalgia, arthralgia.
Skin: rash.
Other: pain at I.M. injection site, chills.

INTERACTIONS

Drug-drug. *Insulin:* May interfere with action of insulin by binding with zinc. Adjust insulin dosage as directed.

EFFECTS ON LAB TEST RESULTS

- May increase ALT, AST, and calcium levels. May decrease hemoglobin level and hematocrit.

CONTRAINDICATIONS & CAUTIONS

- Contraindicated in patients with anuria, hepatitis, or acute renal disease.
- Use with caution in patients with mild renal disease. Dosage may be reduced.

NURSING CONSIDERATIONS

- Add procaine hydrochloride to I.M. solution to minimize pain. Watch for local reactions.
- ***Alert:*** Because rapid I.V. use may increase intracranial pressure, I.M. route may be preferred for lead encephalopathy. I.V. infusion is still recommended whenever possible.
- Monitor fluid intake and output, urinalysis, BUN level, and ECG daily.
- To avoid toxicity, use with dimercaprol; don't mix in same syringe.
- ***Look alike–sound alike:*** Don't confuse edetate calcium disodium with edetate disodium.

PATIENT TEACHING

- Explain use of drug to patient and family.
- Tell patients with lead encephalopathy to avoid excess fluids.

edetate disodium

Disodium EDTA, Endrate

Pharmacologic class: heavy metal antagonist
Pregnancy risk category C

AVAILABLE FORMS

Injection: 150 mg/ml

INDICATIONS & DOSAGES

➤ Hypercalcemic crisis

Adults: 50 mg/kg/day by slow I.V. infusion over at least 3 hours. Maximum dose is 3 g/day.

Children♦: 40 mg/kg/day by slow I.V. infusion over at least 3 hours. Maximum dose is 70 mg/kg/day. Or, a dose of 1.5 g/m^2 may be used as a single dose.

I.V. ADMINISTRATION

- Dilute drug in 500 ml of D_5W or normal saline solution.
- Drug isn't recommended for direct or intermittent injection.
- Avoid rapid infusion; profound hypocalcemia may occur, leading to tetany, seizures, arrhythmias, and respiratory arrest.
- Infuse over 3 or more hours.
- Monitor patient for signs of extravasation.
- Record site used, and avoid repeated use of same site because doing so increases likelihood of thrombophlebitis.

INCOMPATIBILITIES

None reported.

ACTION

Chelates with metals such as calcium to form a stable, soluble complex.

Route	Onset	Peak	Duration
I.V.	Unknown	Unknown	Unknown

Half-life: Unknown.

ADVERSE REACTIONS

CNS: circumoral paresthesia, numbness, headache.
CV: hypotension, thrombophlebitis.
EENT: erythema.
GI: nausea, vomiting, diarrhea.
GU: ***nephrotoxicity with urinary urgency, renal failure, tubular necrosis,*** nocturia, dysuria, polyuria, proteinuria, renal insufficiency.
Metabolic: severe hypocalcemia.
Skin: exfoliative dermatitis.
Other: pain at infusion site.

INTERACTIONS

None significant.

EFFECTS ON LAB TEST RESULTS

- May decrease calcium and magnesium levels.

CONTRAINDICATIONS & CAUTIONS

- Contraindicated in patients hypersensitive to drug and in those with anuria, known or suspected hypocalcemia, significant renal disease, active or healed tubercular lesions, or history of seizures or intracranial lesions.
- Use cautiously in patients with limited cardiac reserve, heart failure, or hypokalemia.

NURSING CONSIDERATIONS

- Keep I.V. calcium available to treat hypocalcemia.
- Keep patients in bed for 30 minutes after infusion to avoid effects of orthostatic hypotension. Monitor blood pressure closely.
- Monitor ECG and renal function tests frequently.
- Obtain calcium level after each dose.
- Don't use to treat lead toxicity; use edetate calcium disodium instead.
- ***Look alike–sound alike:*** Don't confuse edetate disodium with edetate calcium disodium.

PATIENT TEACHING

- Explain use of drug to patient and family.
- Instruct patient to report adverse reactions promptly.

---

flumazenil

Romazicon

Pharmacologic class: benzodiazepine antagonist
Pregnancy risk category C

AVAILABLE FORMS

Injection: 0.1 mg/ml in 5- and 10-ml multiple-dose vials

INDICATIONS & DOSAGES

➤Complete or partial reversal of sedative effects of benzodiazepines after anesthesia or conscious sedation

Adults: Initially, 0.2 mg I.V. over 15 seconds. If patient doesn't reach desired level of consciousness after 45 seconds, repeat dose. Repeat at 1-minute intervals, if needed, until cumulative dose of 1 mg has been given (first dose plus four more doses). Most patients respond after 0.6 to 1 mg of drug. In case of resedation, dosage may be repeated after 20 minutes, but never give more than 1 mg at any one time or exceed 3 mg/hour.

Children age 1 year and older: 0.01 mg/kg I.V. over 15 seconds. If patient doesn't reach desired level of consciousness after 45 seconds, repeat dose. Repeat at 1-minute intervals, if needed, until cumulative dose of 0.05 mg/kg or 1 mg, whichever is lower, has been given (first dose plus four more doses).

➤Suspected benzodiazepine overdose

Adults: Initially, 0.2 mg I.V. over 30 seconds. If patient doesn't reach desired level of consciousness after 30 seconds, give 0.3 mg over 30 seconds. If patient still doesn't respond adequately, give 0.5 mg over 30 seconds. Repeat 0.5-mg doses, p.r.n., at 1-minute intervals until cumulative dose of 3 mg has been given. Most patients with benzodiazepine overdose respond to cumulative doses between 1 and 3 mg; rarely, patients who respond partially after 3 mg may need additional doses, up to 5 mg total. If patient doesn't respond in 5 minutes after receiving 5 mg, sedation is unlikely to be caused by benzodiazepines. In case of resedation, dosage may be repeated after 20 minutes, but never give more than 1 mg at any one time or exceed 3 mg/hour.

I.V. ADMINISTRATION

- Store drug in vial until use.
- Make sure airway is secure and patent.
- Compatible solutions include D_5W, lactated Ringer injection, and normal saline solution.
- To minimize pain at injection site, inject drug over 15 to 30 seconds into large vein through free-flowing solution.
- Monitor patient for signs of extravasation.
- Drug is stable in a syringe for 24 hours.

INCOMPATIBILITIES

None reported.

ACTION

Competitively inhibits the actions of benzodiazepines on the GABA–benzodiazepine receptor complex.

Route	Onset	Peak	Duration
I.V.	1–2 min	6–10 min	Variable

Half-life: 54 minutes.

ADVERSE REACTIONS

CNS: *dizziness, abnormal or blurred vision, headache,* ***seizures,*** agitation, emotional lability, tremor, insomnia.
CV: ***arrhythmias,*** cutaneous vasodilation, palpitations.
GI: *nausea, vomiting.*
Respiratory: dyspnea, hyperventilation.
Skin: *diaphoresis.*
Other: *pain at injection site.*

INTERACTIONS

Drug-drug. *Antidepressants, drugs that may cause seizures or arrhythmias:* May increase risk of seizures or arrhythmias. Don't use flumazenil when overdose involves more than one drug, especially when seizures (from any cause) are likely.

EFFECTS ON LAB TEST RESULTS

None reported.

CONTRAINDICATIONS & CAUTIONS

- Contraindicated in patients hypersensitive to flumazenil or benzodiazepines, in those with evidence of serious tricyclic antidepressant overdose, and in those who have received benzodiazepines to treat a potentially life-threatening condition, such as status epilepticus.
- Use cautiously in patients with head injury, psychiatric disorders, or alcohol dependence.
- Use cautiously in patients at high risk for developing seizures and in those who have recently received multiple doses of a parenteral benzodiazepine, who display signs of seizure activity, or who may be at risk for benzodiazepine dependence, such as intensive care unit patients.

NURSING CONSIDERATIONS

- Monitor patient closely for resedation that may occur after reversal of benzodiazepine effects; drug's duration of action is the shortest of all benzodiazepines. Length of monitoring period depends on specific drug being reversed. Monitor patient closely after doses of long-acting benzodiazepines, such as diazepam, or after high doses of short-acting benzodiazepines, such as 10 mg of midazolam. In most cases, severe resedation is unlikely in patients who fail to show signs of resedation 2 hours after a 1-mg dose.

PATIENT TEACHING

- Warn patient not to perform hazardous activities within 24 hours of procedure because of resedation risk.
- Tell patient to avoid alcohol, CNS depressants, and OTC drugs for 24 hours.
- Give family necessary instructions or provide patient with written instructions. Patient won't recall information given after the procedure; drug doesn't reverse amnesic effects of benzodiazepines.

lanthanum carbonate

Fosrenol

Pharmacologic class: non-calcium, non–aluminum phosphate binder
Pregnancy risk category C

AVAILABLE FORMS

Tablets (chewable): 250 mg, 500 mg, 750 mg, 1 g

INDICATIONS & DOSAGES

➤ **To reduce phosphate level in patients with end-stage renal disease (ESRD)**

Adults: Initially, 250 to 500 mg P.O. t.i.d. with meals. Adjust q 2 to 3 weeks by 750 mg daily until reaching desired phosphate level. Reducing phosphate level to less than 6 mg/dl usually requires 1,500 to 3,000 mg daily.

ACTION

Inhibits phosphate absorption by binding to phosphate released during digestion and forming highly insoluble lanthanum-phosphate complexes.

Route	Onset	Peak	Duration
P.O.	Unknown	Unknown	Unknown

Half-life: 53 hours.

ADVERSE REACTIONS
CNS: headache.
CV: *hypotension.*
EENT: rhinitis.
GI: *constipation, diarrhea, nausea, vomiting,* abdominal pain.
Metabolic: hypercalcemia.
Respiratory: bronchitis.
Other: *dialysis graft occlusion or complication.*

INTERACTIONS
None reported.

EFFECTS ON LAB TEST RESULTS
- May increase calcium level.

CONTRAINDICATIONS & CAUTIONS
- No known contraindications.
- Use cautiously in breast-feeding women and patients with acute peptic ulcer, ulcerative colitis, Crohn disease, or bowel obstruction.

NURSING CONSIDERATIONS
- Give drug with or just after a meal.
- Monitor patient for bone pain and skeletal deformities.
- Check serum phosphate levels during dosage adjustment and regularly as needed throughout treatment.
- Drug isn't recommended for children because it's deposited in developing bone, including the growth plate.

PATIENT TEACHING
- Urge patient to follow a low-phosphorus diet. Assist with meal planning as needed.
- Tell patient to take drug with or immediately after meals.
- ***Alert:*** Remind patient to chew tablets completely before swallowing them.
- Instruct patient to avoid taking lanthanum within 2 hours of oral drugs known to interact with antacids.
- Explain that the most common side effects are nausea and vomiting and that they tend to subside over time.

naloxone hydrochloride
Narcan

Pharmacologic class: opioid antagonist
Pregnancy risk category C

AVAILABLE FORMS
Injection: 0.02 mg/ml, 0.4 mg/ml, 1 mg/ml

INDICATIONS & DOSAGES
➤Known or suspected opioid-induced respiratory depression, including that caused by pentazocine and propoxyphene
Adults: 0.4 to 2 mg I.V., I.M., or subcutaneously. Repeat dose q 2 to 3 minutes, p.r.n. If patient doesn't respond after 10 mg have been given, question diagnosis of opioid-induced toxicity.
Children: 0.01 mg/kg I.V.; then, second dose of 0.1 mg/kg I.V., if needed. If I.V. route isn't available, drug may be given I.M. or subcutaneously in divided doses.
Neonates: 0.01 mg/kg I.V., I.M., or subcutaneously. Repeat dose q 2 to 3 minutes, p.r.n.
➤Postoperative opioid depression
Adults: 0.1 to 0.2 mg I.V. q 2 to 3 minutes, p.r.n. Repeat dose within 1 to 2 hours, if needed.
Children: 0.005 to 0.01 mg I.V. repeated q 2 to 3 minutes, p.r.n.
Neonates (asphyxia neonatorum): 0.01 mg/kg I.V. into umbilical vein. May be repeated q 2 to 3 minutes.

I.V. ADMINISTRATION
- Give continuous infusion to control adverse effects of epidural morphine.
- Dilute 2 mg of drug in 500 ml D_5W or normal saline solution to yield a concentration of 0.004 mg/ml.
- Titrate rate to patient's response.
- If 0.02 mg/ml isn't available, adult concentration (0.4 mg) may be diluted by mixing 0.5 ml with 9.5 ml of sterile water for injection to make neonatal concentration (0.02 mg/ml).

INCOMPATIBILITIES
Alkaline solutions, amphotericin B cholesteryl sulfate, preparations containing

bisulfite, sulfite, long-chain or high-molecular-weight anions.

ACTION
May displace opioid analgesics from their receptors (competitive antagonism); drug has no pharmacologic activity of its own.

Route	Onset	Peak	Duration
I.V.	1–2 min	5–15 min	Variable
I.M., SubQ	2–5 min	5–15 min	Variable

Half-life: 30 to 81 minutes in adults; 3 hours in neonates.

ADVERSE REACTIONS
CNS: ***seizures,*** tremors.
CV: ***ventricular fibrillation,*** tachycardia, hypertension with higher-than-recommended doses, hypotension.
GI: nausea, vomiting.
Respiratory: ***pulmonary edema.***
Skin: diaphoresis.
Other: withdrawal symptoms in opioid-dependent patients with higher-than-recommended doses.

INTERACTIONS
None significant.

EFFECTS ON LAB TEST RESULTS
None reported.

CONTRAINDICATIONS & CAUTIONS
- Contraindicated in patients hypersensitive to drug.
- Use cautiously in patients with cardiac irritability or opioid addiction. Abrupt reversal of opioid-induced CNS depression may result in nausea, vomiting, diaphoresis, tachycardia, CNS excitement, and increased blood pressure.

NURSING CONSIDERATIONS
- Duration of action of the opioid may exceed that of naloxone, and patients may relapse into respiratory depression.
- Respiratory rate increases within 1 to 2 minutes.
- ***Alert:*** Drug is only effective for reversing respiratory depression caused by opioids and not for other drug-induced respiratory depression including that caused by benzodiazepines.
- Patients who receive drug to reverse opioid-induced respiratory depression may exhibit tachypnea.
- Monitor respiratory depth and rate. Provide oxygen, ventilation, and other resuscitation measures.
- ***Look alike–sound alike:*** Don't confuse naloxone with naltrexone.

PATIENT TEACHING
- Reassure family that patient will be monitored closely until effects of opioid resolve.

naltrexone
Vivitrol

naltrexone hydrochloride
ReVia

Pharmacologic class: opioid antagonist
Pregnancy risk category C

AVAILABLE FORMS
naltrexone
Injection: 380 mg/vial dose kit
naltrexone hydrochloride
Tablets: 25 mg, 50 mg, 100 mg

INDICATIONS & DOSAGES
➤Adjunct for maintaining opioid-free state in detoxified patients
Adults: Initially, 25 mg P.O. If no withdrawal signs occur within 1 hour, give an additional 25 mg. Once patient has been started on 50 mg q 24 hours, a flexible maintenance schedule may be used. From 50 to 150 mg may be given daily, depending on schedule prescribed.
➤Alcohol dependence
Adults: 50 mg P.O. once daily or 380 mg I.M. in the gluteal muscle once monthly.

ACTION
Probably reversibly blocks the effects of I.V. opioids by competitively occupying opiate receptors in the brain.

Route	Onset	Peak	Duration
P.O.	15–30 min	1 hr	24 hr
I.M.	Unknown	2–3 days	> 30 days

Half-life: About 4 hours.

ADVERSE REACTIONS
CNS: *insomnia, anxiety, nervousness, headache,* ***suicidal ideation,*** depression, dizziness, fatigue, somnolence.
GI: *nausea, vomiting, abdominal pain,* anorexia, constipation, increased thirst.
GU: delayed ejaculation, decreased potency.
Hepatic: ***hepatotoxicity.***
Musculoskeletal: *muscle and joint pain.*
Skin: injection site reaction, rash.
Other: chills.

INTERACTIONS
Drug-drug. *Products that contain opioids:* May decrease effect of opioid. Avoid using together.
Thioridazine: May increase somnolence and lethargy. Monitor patient closely.

EFFECTS ON LAB TEST RESULTS
- May increase AST, ALT, and LDH levels.
- May increase lymphocyte count.

CONTRAINDICATIONS & CAUTIONS
- Contraindicated in patients hypersensitive to drug or dependent on opioids, those receiving opioid analgesics, those who fail the naloxone challenge test or who have a positive urine screen for opioids, those in acute opioid withdrawal, or with acute hepatitis or liver failure.
- Use cautiously in patients with mild hepatic disease or history of recent hepatic disease.

NURSING CONSIDERATIONS
- Don't begin treatment for opioid dependence until patient receives naloxone challenge, a test of opioid dependence. If signs and symptoms of opioid withdrawal persist after naloxone challenge, don't give drug.
- Patient must be completely free from opioids before taking naltrexone or severe withdrawal symptoms may occur. Patients who have been addicted to short-acting opioids, such as heroin and meperidine, must wait at least 7 days after last opioid dose before starting drug. Patients who have been addicted to longer-acting opioids such as methadone should wait at least 10 days.
- In an emergency, patient may be given an opioid analgesic, but dose must be higher than usual to overcome naltrexone's effect. Watch for respiratory depression from the opioid; it may be longer and deeper.
- For patients expected to be noncompliant because of history of opioid dependence, use a flexible maintenance-dose regimen of 100 mg on Monday and Wednesday and 150 mg on Friday.
- Use drug only as part of a comprehensive rehabilitation program.
- Use only the diluent, needles, and other components supplied with the dose kit. Don't substitute.
- ***Look alike–sound alike:*** Don't confuse naltrexone with naloxone.

PATIENT TEACHING
- Advise patient to carry medical identification and to tell medical personnel that he takes naltrexone.
- Tell patient that drug can block the effects of opioids or opioid-like drugs, including heroin, pain medicine, antidiarrheals, or cough medicine.
- ***Alert:*** Warn patient if he uses large doses of heroin or any other opioid, serious injury, coma, or death can occur.
- Advise patient who previously used opioids that he may be more sensitive to lower doses of opioids once naltrexone therapy is stopped.
- Tell patient to report adverse effects, especially those related to liver injury, to prescriber immediately.
- Tell caregiver of alcohol-dependent patient to monitor him closely for signs of depression or suicide ideation and to report this immediately to prescriber.
- Give patient the names of nonopioid drugs that he can continue to take for pain, diarrhea, or cough.

pentetate calcium trisodium (Ca-DTPA)

pentetate zinc trisodium (Zn-DTPA)

Pharmacologic class: chelating drug
Pregnancy risk category C (Ca-DTPA); B (Zn-DTPA)

AVAILABLE FORMS

Injection: 200 mg/ml in 5-ml single-use vials

INDICATIONS & DOSAGES

➤ To increase rate of plutonium, americium, or curium elimination in patients with internal contamination

Adults and children age 12 and older: Initially, 1 g Ca-DTPA by slow I.V. push over 3 to 4 minutes (or diluted in 100 to 250 ml D_5W, Ringer lactate, or normal saline solution and infused over 30 minutes) within the first 24 hours of exposure. Then, 1 g once daily of Zn-DTPA by slow I.V. push over 3 to 4 minutes (or diluted in 100 to 250 ml D_5W, Ringer lactate, or normal saline solution and infused over 30 minutes) until radioactive substances are removed.

Adjust-a-dose: If patient was exposed by inhalation, solution may be given by nebulized inhalation at a rate of 1:1 with sterile water or saline.

Children younger than age 12: Initially, 14 mg/kg Ca-DTPA (maximum dose, 1 g) by slow I.V. push over 3 to 4 minutes within the first 24 hours of exposure. Then, 14 mg/kg once daily of Zn-DTPA by slow I.V. push over 3 to 4 minutes (maximum dose, 1 g) until radioactive substances are removed.

I.V. ADMINISTRATION

- I.V. use is preferred when the route of contamination is unknown or if contamination occurred by multiple routes.
- Use a sterile filter if particles appear after ampule is opened.
- Give by slow I.V. push over 3 to 4 minutes or dilute in 100 to 250 ml of D_5W, lactated Ringer solution, or normal saline solution and infuse over 30 minutes.
- Store at room temperature.

INCOMPATIBILITIES

None reported.

ACTION

Forms stable complexes with metal ions by exchanging calcium or zinc ions for radioactive plutonium, americium, or curium ions. The complex is excreted into urine faster than the unbound radioactive contaminant, thus speeding removal from the body.

Route	Onset	Peak	Duration
I.V., inhalation	Unknown	Unknown	< 24 hr

Half-life: About 7 hours.

ADVERSE REACTIONS

CNS: headache, light-headedness.
CV: chest pain.
GI: diarrhea, metallic taste, nausea.
Skin: dermatitis, injection site reactions.
Other: allergic reaction.

INTERACTIONS

None reported.

EFFECTS ON LAB TEST RESULTS

- May decrease manganese, magnesium, and zinc levels with prolonged therapy.

CONTRAINDICATIONS & CAUTIONS

- No known contraindications.
- Use cautiously in patients with severe hemochromatosis.
- Use inhalation route cautiously in patients with asthma.

NURSING CONSIDERATIONS

- Binding capacity of Ca-DTPA is greatest in first 24 hours after exposure.
- ***Alert:*** If patient needs further therapy after receiving Ca-DTPA, switch to Zn-DTPA to avoid mineral depletion. If Zn-DTPA isn't available, treatment may continue with Ca-DTPA as long as the patient receives supplemental zinc.
- If contamination occurred only by inhalation and within 24 hours, drug may be delivered by nebulized inhalation. It should be diluted 1:1 with sterile water or saline solution.

- Before treatment starts, obtain baseline CBC, serum zinc level, BUN level, serum chemistries and electrolytes, urine analysis, and blood and urine radioassays.
- The elimination rate is based on the quantity of radioactivity taken in.
- During treatment, measure the radioactivity of blood, urine, and feces weekly.
- Monitor CBC, BUN level, serum chemistries and electrolytes, and urine analysis regularly during treatment.
- For pregnant women, start and continue with Zn-DTPA unless she has a high level of internal radioactive contamination. If the level of contamination is high, therapy may start with a single dose of Ca-DTPA and vitamins or mineral supplements that contain zinc .
- Nebulized inhalation isn't indicated for children.

PATIENT TEACHING

- Instruct patient to drink plenty of fluids to cause frequent urination.
- Remind patient that drug enhances elimination of radioactivity in urine, which may make urine highly radioactive and dangerous to others. Instruct patient to flush the toilet several times after each use and to wash hands thoroughly after urinating.
- If the patient is coughing, tell him to dispose of phlegm carefully and not to swallow it, if possible.
- Tell parents of young children to dispose of dirty diapers properly and to avoid handling urine, feces, or phlegm of children receiving treatment.
- Tell woman that radiocontaminants appear in breast milk. Women shouldn't breast-feed during therapy and should take precautions when discarding breast milk.

pralidoxime chloride (2-PAM chloride, 2-pyridine-aldoxime methochloride)

Protopam Chloride

Pharmacologic class: quaternary ammonium oxime
Pregnancy risk category C

AVAILABLE FORMS

Injection: 1 g/20 ml in 20-ml vial

INDICATIONS & DOSAGES

➤ **Antidote for organophosphate poisoning**

Adults: 1 to 2 g in 100 ml of normal saline solution by I.V. infusion over 15 to 30 minutes. Repeat in 1 hour if muscle weakness persists. Additional doses may be given cautiously. I.M. or subcutaneous injection may be used if I.V. isn't feasible.
Children: 20 to 40 mg/kg I.V., given as for adults.

➤ **Cholinergic crisis in myasthenia gravis**

Adults: 1 to 2 g I.V.; then 250 mg I.V. q 5 minutes, p.r.n.

I.V. ADMINISTRATION

- Reconstitute by adding 20 ml of sterile water for injection to vial containing 1 g of drug.
- Dilute by adding 100 ml of normal saline solution.
- Infuse over 15 to 30 minutes. Too-rapid infusion may cause tachycardia, laryngospasm, and muscle rigidity.
- If patient has pulmonary edema, give drug by slow I.V. push over 5 minutes. Don't exceed 200 mg/minute.

INCOMPATIBILITIES

None reported.

ACTION

Reactivates cholinesterase inactivated by organophosphorus pesticides and related compounds, permitting degradation of accumulated acetylcholine and facilitating normal functioning of neuromuscular junctions.

Route	Onset	Peak	Duration
I.V.	Unknown	5–15 min	Unknown
I.M.	Unknown	10–20 min	Unknown
SubQ	Unknown	Unknown	Unknown

Half-life: 1½ hours.

ADVERSE REACTIONS

CNS: dizziness, headache, drowsiness.
CV: tachycardia.
EENT: blurred vision, diplopia, impaired accommodation.
GI: nausea.
Musculoskeletal: muscle weakness.

Respiratory: hyperventilation.
Other: mild to moderate pain at injection site.

INTERACTIONS
Drug-drug. *Barbiturates:* May increase anticholinesterase level. Use together cautiously to treat seizures.

EFFECTS ON LAB TEST RESULTS
• May increase liver enzyme levels.

CONTRAINDICATIONS & CAUTIONS
• Contraindicated in patients hypersensitive to drug.
• Use cautiously in patients with myasthenia gravis (overdose may trigger myasthenic crisis) and in those with impaired renal function.

NURSING CONSIDERATIONS
• Initially, remove secretions, maintain patent airway, and institute mechanical ventilation, if needed. After dermal exposure to organophosphate, remove patient's clothing and wash his skin and hair with sodium bicarbonate, soap, water, and alcohol as soon as possible. A second washing may be needed. When washing patient, wear protective gloves and clothes to avoid exposure.
• Draw blood for cholinesterase level before giving drug.
• Use drug only in hospitalized patients; have respiratory and other supportive measures available. If possible, obtain accurate medical history and chronology of poisoning. Give drug as soon as possible after poisoning; drug is most effective if started within 24 hours after exposure.
• To improve muscarinic effects and block accumulation of acetylcholine from organophosphate poisoning, give atropine 2 to 4 mg I.V. with pralidoxime if cyanosis isn't present; if cyanosis is present, give atropine I.M. Give atropine every 5 to 10 minutes until signs of atropine toxicity (flushing, tachycardia, dry mouth, blurred vision, excitement, delirium, and hallucinations) appear; maintain atropinization for at least 48 hours.
• Observe patient for 48 to 72 hours if he ingested poison. Delayed absorption may occur from lower bowel. It's difficult to distinguish between toxic effects produced by atropine or organophosphate compounds and those resulting from pralidoxime.
• In a patient with myasthenia gravis being treated for overdose of cholinergics, watch for signs of rapid weakening. He can pass quickly from cholinergic crisis to myasthenic crisis and need more cholinergics to treat myasthenia. Keep edrophonium available for differentiating diagnoses.
• Avoid use of aminophylline, morphine, phenothiazinelike tranquilizers, reserpine, succinylcholine, and theophylline in patients with organophosphate poisoning.
• Drug isn't effective against poisoning caused by phosphorus, inorganic phosphates, or organophosphates with no anticholinesterase activity.
• ***Look alike–sound alike:*** Don't confuse pralidoxime with pramoxine or pyridoxine.

PATIENT TEACHING
• Explain use and administration of drug to patient and family.
• Tell patient to report adverse effects.
• Caution patient treated for organophosphate poisoning to avoid contact with insecticides for several weeks.

protamine sulfate

Pharmacologic class: heparin antagonist
Pregnancy risk category C

AVAILABLE FORMS
Injection: 10 mg/ml

INDICATIONS & DOSAGES
➤ **Heparin overdose**
Adults: Base dosage on venous blood coagulation studies, usually 1 mg for each 90 to 115 units of heparin. Give by slow I.V. injection over 10 minutes in doses not to exceed 50 mg.

I.V. ADMINISTRATION
• Have emergency equipment available to treat anaphylaxis or severe hypotension.
• Give slowly by direct injection. Excessively rapid administration may cause

acute hypotension, bradycardia, pulmonary hypertension, dyspnea, transient flushing, and a feeling of warmth.

INCOMPATIBILITIES
Cephalosporins, diatrizoate meglumine 52% and diatrizoate sodium 8%, diatrizoate sodium 60%, ioxaglate meglumine 39.3% and ioxaglate sodium 19.6%, penicillins.

ACTION
Forms a physiologically inert complex with heparin sodium.

Route	Onset	Peak	Duration
I.V.	30–60 sec	Unknown	2 hr

Half-life: Shorter than heparin.

ADVERSE REACTIONS
CNS: lassitude.
CV: ***bradycardia, circulatory collapse,*** hypotension, transient flushing.
GI: nausea, vomiting.
Respiratory: ***acute pulmonary hypertension, pulmonary edema.*** ***dyspnea,***
Other: ***anaphylaxis, anaphylactoid reactions,*** feeling of warmth.

INTERACTIONS
None significant.

EFFECTS ON LAB TEST RESULTS
None reported.

CONTRAINDICATIONS & CAUTIONS
- Contraindicated in patients hypersensitive to drug.

NURSING CONSIDERATIONS
- Base postoperative dose on coagulation studies, and repeat activated PTT time 15 minutes after administration.
- Calculate dosage carefully. One milligram neutralizes 90 to 115 units of heparin, depending on salt (heparin calcium or heparin sodium) and source of heparin (beef or pork).
- Risk of hypersensitivity reaction increases in patients hypersensitive to fish, in vasectomized or infertile men, and in patients taking protamine–insulin products.
- Monitor patient continually.
- Watch for spontaneous bleeding (heparin rebound), especially in dialysis patients and in those who have undergone cardiac surgery.
- Drug may act as an anticoagulant in very high doses.
- ***Look alike–sound alike:*** Don't confuse protamine with Protopam.

PATIENT TEACHING
- Explain use and administration of drug to patient and family.
- Tell patient to report adverse effects.

sevelamer hydrochloride
Renagel

Pharmacologic class: polymeric phosphate binder
Pregnancy risk category C

AVAILABLE FORMS
Tablets (film-coated): 400 mg, 800 mg

INDICATIONS & DOSAGES
➤ **To control phosphorus level in chronic kidney disease patients on dialysis**
Adults not taking a phosphate binder: Initially, 800 to 1,600 mg (one to two 800-mg tablets or two to four 400-mg tablets) with each meal, based on phosphorus level. If phosphorus level is greater than 5.5 and less than 7.5 mg/dl, start with 800 mg t.i.d. with meals. If phosphorus level is greater than or equal to 7.5 and less than 9 mg/dl, start with two 800-mg tablets t.i.d., or three 400-mg tablets t.i.d. with meals. If phosphorus level is greater than or equal to 9 mg/dl, start with 1,600 mg t.i.d. (two 800-mg tablets or four 400-mg tablets) with meals.
Adults switching from calcium acetate: Initially, if taking one 667-mg calcium acetate tablet per meal, start with 800 mg per meal. If taking two 667-mg calcium acetate tablets per meal, start with two 800-mg tablets or three 400-mg tablets per meal. If taking three 667-mg calcium acetate tablets per meal, start with three 800-mg tablets or five 400-mg tablets per meal.
Adjust-a-dose: If phosphorus level is greater than 5.5 mg/dl, increase by 1 tab-

let per meal at 2-week intervals. If phosphorus level is 3.5 to 5.5 mg/dl, maintain current dose. If phosphorus level is less than 3.5 mg/dl, decrease dose by 1 tablet per meal.

ACTION
A phosphate binder that inhibits intestinal phosphate absorption and decrease phosphorus levels.

Route	Onset	Peak	Duration
P.O.	Unknown	Unknown	Unknown

Half-life: Unknown.

ADVERSE REACTIONS
CNS: *headache, pain,* fever.
CV: *hypertension,* ***thrombosis.***
GI: *diarrhea, dyspepsia, vomiting, nausea,* constipation, flatulence.
EENT: *nasopharyngitis.*
Musculoskeletal: *limb pain, arthralgia,* back pain.
Respiratory: *bronchitis, dyspnea,* increased cough, upper respiratory infection.
Skin: *pruritus.*

INTERACTIONS
Drug-drug. *Ciprofloxacin:* May decrease the effectiveness of ciprofloxacin. Give 1 hour before or 3 hours after sevelamer.

EFFECTS ON LAB TEST RESULTS
None reported.

CONTRAINDICATIONS & CAUTIONS
- Contraindicated in patients hypersensitive to drug or its components and in those with hypophosphatemia or bowel obstruction.
- Use cautiously in patient with dysphagia, swallowing disorders, severe GI motility disorders, or major GI tract surgery.

NURSING CONSIDERATIONS
- Monitor calcium, bicarbonate, and chloride levels.
- Don't cut, crush, or allow patient to chew tablets.
- Watch for symptoms of thrombosis (numbness or tingling of limbs, chest pain, shortness of breath), and notify prescriber if they occur.
- Drug may bind to other drugs and decrease their bioavailability. Give other drugs 1 hour before or 3 hours after this drug. Take special precautions when using antiarrhythmics or anticonvulsants with this drug.

PATIENT TEACHING
- Instruct patient to take with meals and to adhere to prescribed diet.
- ***Alert:*** Inform patient that tablets must be taken whole because contents expand in water. Tell him not to cut, crush or chew.
- Tell patient to take other drugs as directed, but they must be taken either 1 hour before or 3 hours after sevelamer.
- Inform patient about common adverse reactions. Teach patient signs and symptoms of thrombosis, such as numbness, tingling in arms or legs, or chest pain, and to report these immediately.

sodium polystyrene sulfonate
Kayexalate, Kionex, SPS

Pharmacologic class: cation-exchange resin
Pregnancy risk category C

AVAILABLE FORMS
Powder: 1-lb jar (3.5 g/tsp)
Suspension: 15 g/60 ml*

INDICATIONS & DOSAGES
➤ **Hyperkalemia**
Adults: 15 g P.O. daily to q.i.d. in water or sorbitol (3 to 4 ml/g of resin). Or, mix powder with appropriate medium—aqueous suspension or diet appropriate for renal failure—and instill through a nasogastric tube. Or, 30 to 50 g/dl of sorbitol q 6 hours as warm emulsion deep into sigmoid colon (20 cm).
Children: 1 g/kg of body weight/dose P.O. q 6 hours, p.r.n.

ACTION
A potassium-removing resin that exchanges sodium ions for potassium ions in the intestine: 1 g of sodium polystyrene sulfonate is exchanged for 0.5 to 1 mEq of potassium. The resin is then eliminated. Much of the exchange capacity is used

for cations other than potassium (calcium and magnesium) and possibly for fats and proteins.

Route	Onset	Peak	Duration
P.O., P.R.	2–12 hr	Unknown	Unknown

Half-life: Unknown.

ADVERSE REACTIONS

GI: *constipation, diarrhea with sorbitol emulsions,* fecal impaction, anorexia, gastric irritation, nausea, vomiting.
Metabolic: hypokalemia, hypocalcemia, hypomagnesemia, sodium retention.

INTERACTIONS

Drug-drug. ***Antacids and laxatives containing magnesium and calcium:*** May cause systemic alkalosis and reduce potassium exchange capability. Avoid using together. If it can't be avoided, separate doses by several hours.

EFFECTS ON LAB TEST RESULTS

- May increase sodium level. May decrease potassium, calcium, and magnesium levels.

CONTRAINDICATIONS & CAUTIONS

- Contraindicated in patients hypersensitive to drug and in those with hypokalemia.
- Use cautiously in patients with severe heart failure, severe hypertension, or marked edema. Drug provides 100 mg of sodium per gram.

NURSING CONSIDERATIONS

- Don't heat resin; this impairs drug's effect. Mix resin only with water or sorbitol for P.O. use. Never mix with orange juice (high potassium content) to disguise taste.
- Chill oral suspension for greater palatability.
- Oral administration is preferred because drug should remain in intestine for at least 30 minutes.
- If sorbitol is given, mix with resin suspension.
- Consider giving in solid form. Resin cookie and candy recipes are available; ask pharmacist or dietitian to supply.
- Premixed forms (SPS and others) are available. If preparing manually, mix polystyrene resin only with water or sorbitol for rectal use. Don't use mineral oil for P.R. administration to prevent impaction; ion exchange needs aqueous medium. Sorbitol content prevents impaction.
- Prepare P.R. dose at room temperature. Stir emulsion gently during administration.
- Use #28 French rubber tube for rectal dose; insert 20 cm into sigmoid colon. Tape tube in place. Or, consider an indwelling urinary catheter with a 30-ml balloon inflated distal to anal sphincter to aid in retention. This is especially helpful for patients with poor sphincter control. Use gravity flow. Drain returns constantly through Y-tube connection. Place patient in knee-chest position or with hips on pillow for a while if back leakage occurs.
- After P.R. administration, flush tubing with 50 to 100 ml of non-sodium fluid to ensure delivery of all drug. Flush rectum to remove resin.
- Prevent fecal impaction in elderly patients by giving resin P.R. Give cleansing enema before P.R. administration. Have patient retain enema for 6 to 10 hours if possible, but 30 to 60 minutes is acceptable.
- Watch for constipation with oral or nasogastric administration. Give 10 to 20 ml of 70% sorbitol syrup every 2 hours, as needed, to produce one or two watery stools daily.
- Monitor potassium level at least once daily. Treatment may result in potassium deficiency and is usually stopped when potassium is reduced to 4 or 5 mEq/L.
- Watch for signs of hypokalemia: irritability, confusion, arrhythmias, ECG changes, severe muscle weakness or even paralysis, and digitalis toxicity in digitalized patients.
- When hyperkalemia is severe, polystyrene resin alone isn't adequate for lowering potassium. Dextrose 50% with regular insulin I.V. push may also be given.
- Watch for symptoms of other electrolyte deficiencies (magnesium, calcium) because drug is nonselective. Monitor calcium level in patients receiving sodium

polystyrene therapy for more than 3 days. Supplementary calcium may be needed.
- Watch for sodium overload. Drug contains about 100 mg sodium per gram. About one-third of resin's sodium is retained.

PATIENT TEACHING
- Explain use and administration of drug to patient.
- Advise patient to report adverse reactions promptly.
- Teach patient about low-potassium diet.

succimer
Chemet

Pharmacologic class: heavy metal
Pregnancy risk category C

AVAILABLE FORMS
Capsules: 100 mg

INDICATIONS & DOSAGES
➤ Lead poisoning in children with lead levels greater than 45 mcg/dl
Children: Initially, 10 mg/kg or 350 mg/m² q 8 hours for 5 days. Because capsules come only in 100 mg, round dose to nearest 100 mg, as appropriate (see table). Then reduce frequency of administration to q 12 hours for another 2 weeks.

Weight in kg (lb)	Dose (mg)
> 45 (> 100)	500
35–44 (76–100)	400
24–34 (56–75)	300
16–23 (36–55)	200
8–15 (18–35)	100

ACTION
A chelating drug that forms water-soluble complexes with lead and increases its excretion in urine.

Route	Onset	Peak	Duration
P.O.	Unknown	1–2 hr	Unknown

Half-life: 48 hours.

ADVERSE REACTIONS
CNS: *drowsiness, dizziness, sensorimotor neuropathy, sleepiness, paresthesia, headache.*
CV: ***arrhythmias.***
EENT: plugged ears, cloudy film in eyes, otitis media, watery eyes, sore throat, rhinorrhea, nasal congestion.
GI: *nausea, vomiting, diarrhea, anorexia, abdominal cramps, hemorrhoidal symptoms, metallic taste in mouth, loose stools.*
GU: decreased urination, difficult urination, proteinuria.
Hematologic: ***neutropenia,*** increased platelet count, intermittent eosinophilia.
Musculoskeletal: *leg, kneecap, back, stomach, rib, or flank pain.*
Respiratory: cough, head cold.
Skin: papular rash, herpetic rash, mucocutaneous eruptions, pruritus.
Other: *flulike syndrome,* candidiasis.

INTERACTIONS
Drug-drug. *Other chelating drugs (such as edetate calcium disodium):* May cause unknown adverse effects. Separate administration times by 4 weeks.

EFFECTS ON LAB TEST RESULTS
- May increase AST, ALT, alkaline phosphatase, and cholesterol levels.
- May increase eosinophil and platelet counts.
- May cause false-positive urine ketone results.

CONTRAINDICATIONS & CAUTIONS
- Contraindicated in patients hypersensitive to drug.
- Use cautiously in patients with compromised renal function.

NURSING CONSIDERATIONS
- Measure severity of poisoning by initial lead level and by rate and degree of rebound of lead level. Use severity as a guide for more frequent lead monitoring.
- Monitor patient at least once weekly for rebound lead levels. Elevated levels and associated symptoms may return rapidly after drug is stopped because of redistribution of lead from bone to soft tissues and blood.

- Monitor transaminase levels before and at least weekly during therapy. Transient mild elevations may occur.
- Course of treatment lasts 19 days and may be repeated if indicated by weekly monitoring of lead levels.
- Minimum of 2 weeks between courses is recommended unless high lead levels indicate need for immediate therapy.
- Don't give with other chelating drugs. Patient who has received edetate calcium disodium with or without dimercaprol may use succimer after a 4-week interval.

PATIENT TEACHING

- Explain drug use and administration to parents and child. Stress importance of complying with frequent blood tests.
- Tell parents of young child who can't swallow capsules that capsule can be opened and its contents sprinkled on a small amount of soft food. Or, beads from capsule may be poured on a spoon and followed with flavored beverage.
- Tell parents to give child adequate fluids.
- Assist parents with identifying and removing sources of lead in child's environment. Chelation therapy isn't a substitute for preventing further exposure.
- Tell parents to notify prescriber if rash occurs. Tell them allergic or other mucocutaneous reactions may occur each time drug is used.

94

Uncategorized drugs

alfuzosin hydrochloride
alprostadil
amifostine
clomiphene citrate
conivaptan hydrochloride
diclofenac sodium
dutasteride
finasteride
high–molecular-weight hyaluronan
imiquimod
isotretinoin
mecasermin rinfabate
mesna
minoxidil (topical)
nimodipine
orlistat
palifermin
pimecrolimus
pregabalin
raloxifene hydrochloride
riluzole
sildenafil citrate
tacrolimus (topical)
tadalafil
tamsulosin hydrochloride
tretinoin
vardenafil hydrochloride
varenicline

alfuzosin hydrochloride

UroXatral

Pharmacologic class: alpha$_1$ blocker
Pregnancy risk category B

AVAILABLE FORMS

Tablets (extended-release): 10 mg

INDICATIONS & DOSAGES

➤ **BPH**

Men: 10 mg P.O. immediately after same meal each day.

ACTION

Selectively blocks alpha receptors in the prostate, which relaxes the smooth muscles in the bladder neck and prostate, improving urine flow and reducing symptoms of BPH.

Route	Onset	Peak	Duration
P.O.	Unknown	8 hr	Unknown

Half-life: 10 hours.

ADVERSE REACTIONS

CNS: dizziness, fatigue, headache, pain.
EENT: pharyngitis, sinusitis.
GI: abdominal pain, constipation, dyspepsia, nausea.
GU: impotence.
Respiratory: bronchitis, upper respiratory tract infection.

INTERACTIONS

Drug-drug. *Antihypertensives (diltiazem):* May cause hypotension. Monitor blood pressure and use together cautiously.
Atenolol: May cause hypotension and reduce heart rate. Monitor blood pressure and heart rate for these effects.
Cimetidine: May increase alfuzosin level. Use together cautiously.
Potent CYP3A4 inhibitors (itraconazole, ketoconazole, ritonavir): May inhibit hepatic metabolism of alfuzosin. Use together is contraindicated.

EFFECTS ON LAB TEST RESULTS

None reported.

CONTRAINDICATIONS & CAUTIONS

- Contraindicated in patients with Child-Pugh categories B and C and those hypersensitive to alfuzosin or its ingredients.
- Use cautiously in patients with severe renal insufficiency, congenital or acquired QT-interval prolongation, or symptomatic hypotension and hypotensive responses to other drugs.

NURSING CONSIDERATIONS

- Don't use drug to treat hypertension.
- Asymptomatic orthostatic hypotension may develop within a few hours.

- Symptoms of BPH and prostate cancer are similar; rule out prostate cancer before therapy.
- If angina pectoris develops or worsens, stop drug.
- Current or previous use of an alpha blocker may predispose the patient to intraoperative floppy iris syndrome during cataract surgery.

PATIENT TEACHING

- Tell patient to take drug just after the same meal each day.
- At start of therapy, warn patient about possible hypotension and explain that it may cause dizziness. Caution patient against performing hazardous activities until he knows how the drug affects him.
- Tell patient to avoid situations in which he could be injured if he became lightheaded or fainted.
- Warn patient not to crush or chew the tablets.
- Advise patient planning cataract surgery to alert his ophthalmologist about this drug and current or previous alpha blocker therapy.

alprostadil

Caverject, Edex, Muse

Pharmacologic class: prostaglandin
Pregnancy risk category NR

AVAILABLE FORMS

Injection: 5 mcg/ml, 10 mcg/ml, 20 mcg/ml, 40 mcg/ml after reconstitution
Urogenital suppository: 125 mcg, 250 mcg, 500 mcg, 1,000 mcg

INDICATIONS & DOSAGES

➤ **Erectile dysfunction of vasculogenic, psychogenic, or mixed causes**

Injection

Men: Dosages are highly individualized; initially, inject 2.5 mcg intracavernosally. If partial response occurs, give second dose of 2.5 mcg; then increase in increments of 5 to 10 mcg until patient achieves erection suitable for intercourse and lasting no longer than 1 hour. If patient doesn't respond to first dose, increase second dose to 7.5 mcg within 1 hour, and then increase further in increments of 5 to 10 mcg until patient achieves suitable erection. Patient must remain in prescriber's office until complete detumescence occurs. Don't repeat procedure for at least 24 hours.

Urogenital suppository

Men: Initially, 125 to 250 mcg, under supervision of prescriber. Adjust dosage as needed until response is sufficient for sexual intercourse. Maximum of two administrations in 24 hours; maximum dose is 1,000 mcg.

➤ **Erectile dysfunction of neurogenic cause (spinal cord injury)**

Men: Dosages are highly individualized; initially, inject 1.25 mcg intracavernously. If partial response occurs, give second dose of 1.25 mcg. Increase in increments of 2.5 mcg, to dose of 5 mcg; then increase in increments of 5 mcg until patient achieves erection suitable for intercourse and lasting no longer than 1 hour. If patient doesn't respond to first dose, give next higher dose within 1 hour. Patient must remain in prescriber's office until complete detumescence occurs. If there is a response, don't repeat procedure for at least 24 hours.

ACTION

A prostaglandin derivative that induces erection by relaxing trabecular smooth muscle and dilating cavernosal arteries. This leads to expansion of lacunar spaces and entrapment of blood by compressing venules against the tunica albuginea, a process referred to as the corporal venoocclusive mechanism.

Route	Onset	Peak	Duration
Intracavernous	5–20 min	5–20 min	1–6 hr
Urogenital	10 min	16 min	1 hr

Half-life: About 5 to 10 minutes.

ADVERSE REACTIONS

CNS: headache, dizziness.
CV: hypertension, hypotension.
EENT: sinusitis, nasal congestion.
GU: *penile pain,* prolonged erection, penile fibrosis, rash, or edema, prostatic disorder.
Musculoskeletal: back pain.
Respiratory: upper respiratory tract infection, cough.

Skin: injection site hematoma or ecchymosis.
Other: localized trauma or pain, flulike syndrome.

INTERACTIONS

Drug-drug. *Anticoagulants:* May increase risk of bleeding from intracavernosal injection site. Monitor patient closely.
Cyclosporine: May decrease cyclosporine level. Monitor cyclosporine level closely.
Vasoactive drugs: Safety and effectiveness haven't been studied. Avoid using together.

EFFECTS ON LAB TEST RESULTS

None reported.

CONTRAINDICATIONS & CAUTIONS

- Contraindicated in patients hypersensitive to drug, in those with conditions predisposing them to priapism (sickle cell anemia or trait, multiple myeloma, leukemia) or penile deformation (angulation, cavernosal fibrosis, Peyronie disease), in men with penile implants or for whom sexual activity is inadvisable or contraindicated, in women or children, and in sexual partners of pregnant women unless condoms are used.

NURSING CONSIDERATIONS

- Stop drug in patients who develop penile angulation, cavernosal fibrosis, or Peyronie disease.

PATIENT TEACHING

- Teach patient how to prepare and give drug before he begins treatment at home. Stress importance of reading and following patient instructions in each package insert. Tell him to store unopened suppositories in refrigerator (36° to 46° F [2° to 8° C]) and store injection at or below room temperature (77° F [25° C]).
- Tell patient not to shake contents of reconstituted vial, and remind him that vial is designed for a single use. Tell him to discard vial if solution is discolored or contains precipitate.
- Instruct patient to urinate before inserting suppository because moisture makes it easier to insert drug in penis and will help dissolve it.
- Review administration and aseptic technique.
- Inform patient that he can expect an erection 5 to 20 minutes after administration, with a preferable duration of no more than 1 hour. If his erection lasts more than 6 hours, tell him to seek medical attention immediately.
- Remind patient to take drug as instructed (generally, no more than three times weekly, with at least 24 hours between each use). Warn him not to change dosage without consulting prescriber.
- Caution patient to use a condom if his sexual partner could be pregnant.
- Review possible adverse reactions. Tell patient to inspect his penis daily and to report redness, swelling, tenderness, curvature, excessive erection (priapism), unusual pain, nodules, or hard tissue.
- Urge patient not to reuse or share needles, syringes, or drug.
- Warn patient that drug doesn't protect against sexually transmitted diseases. Also, caution him that bleeding at injection site can increase risk of transmitting blood-borne diseases to his partner.
- Remind patient to keep regular follow-up appointments so prescriber can evaluate drug effectiveness and safety.

amifostine

Ethyol

Pharmacologic class: organic thiophosphate
Pregnancy risk category C

AVAILABLE FORMS

Injection: 500 mg anhydrous base and 500 mg mannitol in 10-ml vial

INDICATIONS & DOSAGES

➤ **To reduce cumulative renal toxicity of repeated cisplatin therapy in patients with advanced ovarian cancer**
Women: 910 mg/m² daily as a 15-minute I.V. infusion, starting 30 minutes before chemotherapy. If hypotension occurs and blood pressure doesn't return to normal within 5 minutes, give 740 mg/m² in later cycles.

➤ **To reduce moderate to severe xerostomia in patients undergoing postoperative radiation treatment for head and neck cancer**
Adults: 200 mg/m^2 daily as 3-minute I.V. infusion, starting 15 to 30 minutes before standard fraction radiation therapy.

I.V. ADMINISTRATION
- Inspect vial for particulates and discoloration; discard drug if it's cloudy or precipitated.
- Reconstitute each single-dose vial with 9.7 ml of sterile normal saline injection. Other solutions aren't recommended.
- Don't infuse for longer than 15 minutes; longer infusion increases the risk of adverse reactions.
- Keep patient supine during infusion. Monitor blood pressure every 5 minutes.
- If hypotension occurs and drug must be stopped, notify prescriber, keep patient supine with legs elevated, and infuse normal saline solution in a separate I.V. line. If blood pressure returns to normal within 5 minutes and patient is asymptomatic, restart infusion and give full dose. If full dose can't be given, limit later doses to 740 mg/m^2.
- Reconstituted solution (500 mg/10 ml) is chemically stable for 5 hours at room temperature (about 77° F [25° C]) or 24 hours if refrigerated (36° to 46° F [2° to 8° C]).
- Drug can be prepared in polyvinyl chloride bags in concentrations of 5 to 40 mg/ml; stability is the same as when reconstituted in single-use vial.

INCOMPATIBILITIES
Acyclovir sodium, amphotericin B, cefoperazone, chlorpromazine, cisplatin, ganciclovir, hydroxyzine, minocycline, prochlorperazine.

ACTION
Dephosphorylated by alkaline phosphatase in tissue to a pharmacologically active free thiol metabolite. Free thiol in normal tissues binds and detoxifies reactive metabolites of cisplatin, reducing the toxic effects of cisplatin on renal tissue. Free thiol can also act as a scavenger of free radicals in tissues exposed to cisplatin.

Route	Onset	Peak	Duration
I.V.	5–8 min	Unknown	Unknown

Half-life: About 8 minutes.

ADVERSE REACTIONS
CNS: dizziness, somnolence.
CV: *hypotension.*
GI: *nausea, vomiting.*
Metabolic: hypocalcemia.
Respiratory: hiccups, sneezing.
Other: ***allergic reactions, ranging from rash to rigors,*** flushing or feeling of warmth, chills or feeling of coldness.

INTERACTIONS
Drug-drug. *Antihypertensives, other drugs that could increase hypotension:* May cause profound hypotension. Monitor patient closely.

EFFECTS ON LAB TEST RESULTS
- May decrease calcium level.

CONTRAINDICATIONS & CAUTIONS
- Contraindicated in patients hypersensitive to aminothiol compounds or mannitol.
- Contraindicated in patients who are hypotensive, dehydrated, or receiving antihypertensives that can't be stopped 24 hours before therapy
- Drug shouldn't be used in patients receiving chemotherapy for potentially curable malignancies (including certain malignancies of germ-cell origin), or in patients receiving definitive radiotherapy, except for patients involved in clinical studies.
- Use cautiously in elderly patients and in patients with ischemic heart disease, arrhythmias, heart failure, or history of stroke or transient ischemic attacks.
- Use cautiously in patients for whom common adverse effects of nausea, vomiting, and hypotension may have serious consequences.

NURSING CONSIDERATIONS
- If possible, stop antihypertensive therapy 24 hours before therapy.
- Make sure patient is adequately hydrated before giving drug. Monitor patient's blood pressure before and immediately af-

ter infusion and periodically thereafter as indicated.
- Give antiemetics, including 20 mg I.V. dexamethasone and a serotonin 5-HT_3–receptor antagonist, before and with this drug. Additional antiemetics may be needed, based on the chemotherapy.
- If drug is used with highly emetogenic chemotherapy, monitor patient's fluid balance .
- Monitor calcium level in patients at risk for hypocalcemia such as those with nephrotic syndrome. If needed, give calcium supplements.
- Safety and effectiveness of drug in children haven't been established.

PATIENT TEACHING
- Instruct patient to lie down throughout infusion.
- Advise woman not to breast-feed; it's unknown if drug appears in breast milk.

clomiphene citrate
Clomid, Milophene, Serophene

Pharmacologic class: chlorotrianisene derivative
Pregnancy risk category X

AVAILABLE FORMS
Tablets: 50 mg

INDICATIONS & DOSAGES
➤ To induce ovulation
Women: 50 mg P.O. daily for 5 days, starting on day 5 of menstrual cycle (first day of menstrual flow is day 1) if bleeding occurs, or at any time if patient hasn't had recent uterine bleeding. If ovulation doesn't occur, may increase dose to 100 mg P.O. daily for 5 days as soon as 30 days after previous course. Repeat until conception occurs or until three courses of therapy are completed.

ACTION
Appears to stimulate release of follicle-stimulating hormone, luteinizing hormone, and pituitary gonadotropins, resulting in maturation of the ovarian follicle, ovulation, and development of the corpus luteum.

Route	Onset	Peak	Duration
Topical	Unknown	Unknown	Unknown

Half-life: 5 days.

ADVERSE REACTIONS
CNS: headache, restlessness, insomnia, dizziness, light-headedness, depression, fatigue.
EENT: blurred vision, diplopia, scotoma, photophobia.
GI: nausea, vomiting, bloating, distention.
GU: *ovarian enlargement,* urinary frequency and polyuria, abnormal uterine bleeding, ovarian cyst that regresses spontaneously when drug is stopped.
Metabolic: weight gain.
Skin: reversible alopecia, urticaria, rash, dermatitis.
Other: *hot flashes, breast discomfort.*

INTERACTIONS
None significant.

EFFECTS ON LAB TEST RESULTS
None reported.

CONTRAINDICATIONS & CAUTIONS
- Contraindicated in pregnant women and in those with undiagnosed abnormal genital bleeding, ovarian cyst not related to polycystic ovarian syndrome, hepatic disease or dysfunction, uncontrolled thyroid or adrenal dysfunction, or organic intracranial lesion (such as a pituitary tumor).

NURSING CONSIDERATIONS
- Monitor patient closely because of potentially serious adverse reactions.
- Long-term cyclic therapy isn't recommended.
- ***Look alike–sound alike:*** Don't confuse clomiphene with clomipramine or clonidine. Don't confuse Serophene with Sarafem.

PATIENT TEACHING
- Tell patient about the risk of multiple births, which increases with higher doses.
- Teach patient to take and chart basal body temperature to ascertain if ovulation has occurred.
- Reinforce importance of compliance with drug regimen.

- Reassure patient that ovulation typically occurs after first course of therapy. If pregnancy doesn't occur, therapy may be repeated twice.
- Advise patient to stop drug and contact prescriber immediately if pregnancy is suspected because drug may have teratogenic effect.
- ***Alert:*** Advise patient to stop drug and contact prescriber immediately if abdominal symptoms or pain occur; these symptoms may indicate ovarian enlargement or ovarian cyst. Also tell patient to immediately notify prescriber if signs and symptoms of impending visual toxicity occur, such as blurred vision, double vision, vision defect in one part of the eye (scotoma), or sensitivity to the sun.
- Warn patient to avoid hazardous activities, such as driving or operating machinery, until CNS effects are known. Drug may cause dizziness and visual disturbances.

✷ NEW DRUG

conivaptan hydrochloride

Vaprisol

Pharmacologic class: arginine vasopressin receptor antagonist
Pregnancy risk category C

AVAILABLE FORMS

Injection: 20 mg/4 ml

INDICATIONS & DOSAGES

➤ **Euvolemic hyponatremia (as from SIADH, hypothyroidism, adrenal insufficiency, pulmonary disorders) in hospitalized patients**

Adults: Loading dose of 20 mg I.V. over 30 minutes; then 20 mg I.V. by continuous infusion over 24 hours for 1 to 3 days. If sodium level isn't rising at desired rate, increase to 40 mg/day by continuous infusion. Don't give for more than 4 days after loading dose.

Adjust-a-dose: If sodium level rises more than 12 mEq/L in 24 hours, stop infusion. If hyponatremia persists or recurs and the patient has had no adverse neurologic effects from the rapid rise in sodium level, restart infusion at a reduced dose. If patient develops hypotension or hypovolemia, stop infusion. Monitor vital signs and volume status often. If hyponatremia persists once the patient is no longer hypotensive and volume returns to normal, restart infusion at a reduced dose.

I.V. ADMINISTRATION

- Dilute only with D_5W. For the loading dose, add 20 mg to 100 ml of D_5W. Gently invert bag to ensure complete mixing. Infuse over 30 minutes. For continuous infusion, add 40 mg to 250 ml of D_5W. Gently invert bag to ensure complete mixing. Infuse over 24 hours.
- Give via a large vein, and change infusion site q 24 hours.
- Solution is stable for 24 hours at room temperature.

INCOMPATIBILITIES

Lactated Ringer solution, normal saline solution. Don't mix or infuse with other I.V. drugs.

ACTION

Increases the amount of free water eliminated by the kidneys by antagonizing V1A and V2 receptors in renal collecting ducts, inhibiting inappropriate or excessive arginine vasopressin (antidiuretic hormone) secretion. Typically, this causes increased net fluid loss, increased urine output, and decreased urine osmolality.

Route	Onset	Peak	Duration
I.V.	Unknown	2–4 hr	12 hr

Half-life: 5 hours.

ADVERSE REACTIONS

CNS: *headache,* confusion, fever, insomnia.
CV: atrial fibrillation, hypertension, hypotension, orthostatic hypotension.
GI: constipation, diarrhea, dry mouth, nausea, oral candidiasis, *vomiting.*
GU: hematuria, pollakiuria, polyuria, UTI.
Hematologic: anemia.
Metabolic: ***hypoglycemia, hypokalemia,*** dehydration, hyperglycemia, hypomagnesemia, hyponatremia.
Respiratory: pneumonia.

Skin: erythema.
Other: *infusion site reactions, thirst.*

INTERACTIONS
Drug-drug. *Amlodipine:* May increase amlodipine level and half-life. Monitor blood pressure.
Digoxin: May increase digoxin level. Monitor patient, and adjust digoxin dose as needed.
Midazolam: May increase midazolam level. Monitor patient for respiratory depression and hypotension.
Potent CYP3A4 inhibitors (clarithromycin, indinavir, itraconazole, ketoconazole, ritonavir): May seriously increase levels and toxic effects. Use together is contraindicated.
Simvastatin: May increase simvastatin level. Monitor patient for signs of rhabdomyolysis, including muscle pain, weakness, and tenderness.

EFFECTS ON LAB TEST RESULTS
- May decrease potassium, magnesium, sodium, and hemoglobin levels and hematocrit. May increase or decrease blood glucose level.

CONTRAINDICATIONS & CAUTIONS
- Contraindicated in patients with hypovolemic hyponatremia, patients hypersensitive to drug or its components, and patients taking potent CYP3A4 inhibitors, such as clarithromycin, indinavir, itraconazole, ketoconazole, or ritonavir.
- Use cautiously in hyponatremic patients with underlying heart failure and patients with hepatic or renal impairment.

NURSING CONSIDERATIONS
- Monitor sodium level and neurologic status regularly during therapy.
- ***Alert:*** Rapid correction of sodium level may cause osmotic demyelination syndrome. Monitor patient's sodium level and volume status.
- Drug may cause significant infusion site reactions, even with proper dilution and administration. Rotate infusion site every 24 hours to reduce risk of reaction.

PATIENT TEACHING
- Inform patient that he may experience low blood pressure when standing. If he feels dizzy or faint, advise him to sit or lie down.
- Advise patient to promptly report signs and symptoms of hypoglycemia, such as feeling shaky, nervous, tired, sweaty, cold, hungry, confused, irritable, or impatient.
- Emphasize the importance of reporting an unusually fast heartbeat or weakness.
- Tell patient that analgesics and moist heating pads can be used to treat pain and inflammation at the infusion site.
- Inform patient that the infusion will be given for a maximum of 4 days after the loading dose.

diclofenac sodium
Solaraze

Pharmacologic class: NSAID
Pregnancy risk category B

AVAILABLE FORMS
Topical gel: 3% in 25-g and 50-g tubes

INDICATIONS & DOSAGES
➤ Actinic keratosis
Adults: Apply gently to lesion b.i.d. for 60 to 90 days. Use enough gel to cover the lesion; for example, use 0.5 g of gel on a 5-cm × 5-cm lesion.

ACTION
Unknown.

Route	Onset	Peak	Duration
Topical	Unknown	4–12 hr	Unknown

Half-life: 1 to 3 hours.

ADVERSE REACTIONS
CNS: *paresthesia,* headache, pain, asthenia, migraine, hypokinesia.
CV: chest pain, hypertension.
EENT: sinusitis, pharyngitis, rhinitis, conjunctivitis, eye pain.
GI: diarrhea, dyspepsia, abdominal pain.
GU: hematuria, renal impairment.
Hepatic: liver impairment.
Metabolic: hypercholesterolemia, hyperglycemia.

Musculoskeletal: arthralgia, arthrosis, back pain, myalgia, neck pain.
Respiratory: asthma, dyspnea, pneumonia.
Skin: *reaction at application site, contact dermatitis, dry skin, exfoliation, localized pain, pruritus, rash,* localized edema, acne, alopecia, photosensitivity, skin carcinoma, skin ulcer.
Other: ***anaphylaxis,*** *flulike syndrome,* infection, allergic reaction.

INTERACTIONS

Drug-drug. *Oral NSAIDs:* May increase drug effects. Minimize use together.
Drug-lifestyle. *Sun exposure:* May increase risk of photosensitivity reactions. Advise patient to avoid excessive sun exposure.

EFFECTS ON LAB TEST RESULTS

- May increase ALT, AST, cholesterol, creatinine, glucose, and phosphokinase levels.

CONTRAINDICATIONS & CAUTIONS

- Contraindicated in patients hypersensitive to diclofenac, benzyl alcohol, polyethylene glycol monomethyl ether 350, or hyaluronic acid.
- Use cautiously in patients with the aspirin triad; these patients are usually asthmatics who develop rhinitis, with or without nasal polyps, after taking aspirin or other NSAIDs.
- Use cautiously in patients with active GI bleeding or ulceration and in those with severe renal or hepatic impairment.
- Use cautiously in breast-feeding women; it's unknown if drug appears in breast milk. Patient should either stop breast-feeding or stop treatment, taking into account importance of drug to mother.

NURSING CONSIDERATIONS

- Don't apply to open wounds or broken skin.
- Avoid contact with eyes.
- Safety and effectiveness of sunscreens, cosmetics, or other topical medications used with drug are unknown.
- Complete healing or optimal therapeutic effect may not be seen until 30 days after therapy is complete.
- Reevaluate lesions that don't respond to therapy.
- Because of the risk of premature closure of the ductus arteriosus, avoid drug in late pregnancy.

PATIENT TEACHING

- Inform patient about risk of skin reactions (rash, itchiness, pain, irritation) at the application site. Urge patient to seek medical attention if adverse reactions persist or worsen.
- Encourage patient to minimize sun exposure during therapy. Explain that sunscreen may be helpful but that the safety of using sunscreen with drug is unknown.
- Caution patient not to apply gel to open wounds or broken skin.
- Instruct patient to avoid contact with eyes.
- Instruct patient not to apply other topical drugs or cosmetics to affected area while using drug, unless directed.
- Tell woman to notify prescriber if she's pregnant or breast-feeding.

dutasteride

Avodart

Pharmacologic class: 5-alpha-reductase enzyme inhibitor
Pregnancy risk category X

AVAILABLE FORMS

Capsules: 0.5 mg

INDICATIONS & DOSAGES

➤ **To improve the symptoms of BPH, reduce the risk of acute urine retention, and reduce the need for BPH-related surgery**
Men: 0.5 mg P.O. once daily.

ACTION

Inhibits conversion of testosterone to dihydrotestosterone (DHT), the androgen primarily responsible for the initial development and subsequent enlargement of the prostate gland.

Route	Onset	Peak	Duration
P.O.	Unknown	2–3 hr	Unknown

Half-life: About 5 weeks.

ADVERSE REACTIONS

GU: impotence, decreased libido, ejaculation disorder.
Other: gynecomastia.

INTERACTIONS

Drug-drug. *Cytochrome P-450 inhibitors (such as cimetidine, ciprofloxacin, diltiazem, ketoconazole, ritonavir, verapamil):* May increase dutasteride level. Use together cautiously.

EFFECTS ON LAB TEST RESULTS

- May lower prostate-specific antigen (PSA) level.

CONTRAINDICATIONS & CAUTIONS

- Contraindicated in women and children and in patients hypersensitive to dutasteride or its ingredients or to other 5-alpha-reductase inhibitors.
- Use cautiously in patients with hepatic disease and in those taking long-term potent cytochrome P-450 inhibitors.

NURSING CONSIDERATIONS

- Because drug may be absorbed through the skin, women who are or may become pregnant shouldn't handle the drug.
- If contact is made with leaking capsules, wash the contact area immediately with soap and water.
- Carefully monitor patients with a large residual urine volume or severely diminished urine flow, or both, for obstructive uropathy.
- Patients should wait at least 6 months after their last dose before donating blood.
- Establish a new baseline PSA level in men treated for 3 to 6 months and use it to assess potentially cancer-related changes in PSA level.
- To interpret PSA values in men treated for 6 months or more, double the PSA value for comparison with normal values in untreated men.

PATIENT TEACHING

- Tell patient to swallow the capsule whole.
- Inform patient that ejaculate volume may decrease but that sexual function should remain normal.
- Teach women who are pregnant or may become pregnant not to handle drug. A male fetus exposed to drug by the mother's swallowing or absorbing the drug through her skin may be born with abnormal sex organs.
- ***Alert:*** Tell patient not to donate blood for at least 6 months after final dose.
- Tell patient he'll need periodic blood tests to monitor therapeutic effects.

finasteride

Propecia, Proscar

Pharmacologic class: steroid derivative
Pregnancy risk category X

AVAILABLE FORMS

Tablets: 1 mg, 5 mg

INDICATIONS & DOSAGES

➤ **Male pattern hair loss (androgenetic alopecia) in men only**
Men: 1 mg P.O. Propecia daily.
➤ **To improve symptoms of BPH and reduce risk of acute urine retention and need for surgery, including transurethral resection of prostate and prostatectomy**
Men: 5 mg P.O. Proscar daily.
➤ **With doxazosin, to reduce the risk of BPH symptom progression (Proscar)**
Men: 5 mg P.O. daily.

ACTION

Inhibits conversion of testosterone to dihydrotestosterone (DHT), the androgen primarily responsible for the initial development and subsequent enlargement of the prostate gland. In male pattern baldness, the scalp contains miniaturized hair follicles and increased DHT level; drug decreases scalp DHT level in such cases.

Route	Onset	Peak	Duration
P.O.	Unknown	1–2 hr	24 hr

Half-life: Unknown.

ADVERSE REACTIONS

GU: impotence, decreased volume of ejaculate, decreased libido.

INTERACTIONS
None significant.

EFFECTS ON LAB TEST RESULTS
- May decrease prostate-specific antigen (PSA) level.

CONTRAINDICATIONS & CAUTIONS
- Contraindicated in patients hypersensitive to drug or to other 5-alpha-reductase inhibitors, such as dutasteride. Although drug isn't used in women or children, manufacturer indicates pregnancy as a contraindication.
- Use cautiously in patients with liver dysfunction.

NURSING CONSIDERATIONS
- Before therapy, evaluate patient for conditions that mimic BPH, including hypotonic bladder, prostate cancer, infection, or stricture.
- Carefully monitor patients who have a large residual urine volume or severely diminished urine flow.
- Sustained increase in PSA level could indicate noncompliance with therapy.
- A minimum of 6 months of therapy may be needed for treatment of BPH.

PATIENT TEACHING
- Tell patient that drug may be taken without regard to meals.
- Warn woman who is or may become pregnant not to handle crushed tablets because of risk of adverse effects on male fetus.
- Inform patient that signs of improvement may require at least 3 months of daily use when drug is used to treat hair loss or at least 6 months when taken for BPH.
- Reassure patient that drug may decrease volume of ejaculate without impairing normal sexual function.

high–molecular-weight hyaluronan
Orthovisc

Pharmacologic class: viscoelastic hyaluronan
Pregnancy risk category NR

AVAILABLE FORMS
Injection: 30 mg/2 ml

INDICATIONS & DOSAGES
➤ **To reduce pain caused by osteoarthritis of the knee in patients who haven't responded to nondrug therapy or simple analgesics**
Adults: Intra-articular injection (one syringe) into affected knee once weekly for a total of three to four injections.

ACTION
Supplements body's natural supply of hyaluronan, which acts as a shock absorber and lubricant in the joints.

Route	Onset	Peak	Duration
Intra-articular	Unknown	Unknown	Unknown

Half-life: Unknown.

ADVERSE REACTIONS
CNS: *headache,* pain.
Musculoskeletal: *arthralgia,* back pain, bursitis.
Other: injection site pain.

INTERACTIONS
Drug-drug. *Skin preparation disinfectants that contain quaternary ammonium salts:* May cause hyaluronan to precipitate. Avoid using together.

EFFECTS ON LAB TEST RESULTS
None reported.

CONTRAINDICATIONS & CAUTIONS
- Contraindicated in patients allergic to hyaluronate preparations, birds, eggs, feathers, and poultry. Also contraindicated in patients with infection or skin disease in area of injection site or joint.

NURSING CONSIDERATIONS

- Drug should be given by staff trained in intra-articular administration.
- Remove joint effusion before injecting drug.
- Use an 18G to 21G needle. Using strict aseptic technique, inject contents of one syringe into one knee; if needed, use a second syringe for the second knee.
- Pain may not be relieved until after the third injection.
- Don't give less than three injections in a treatment cycle.
- Use of drug for more than one treatment cycle or in joints other than the knee haven't been studied.
- Inflammation may increase briefly in affected knee in patients with inflammatory osteoarthritis.
- Don't use drug if original package is open or damaged. Give drug immediately after opening. Store in original package at room temperature lower than 77° F (25° C); don't freeze. Discard unused drug.

PATIENT TEACHING

- Tell patient that pain and inflammation may increase briefly after the injection.
- Urge patient to avoid strenuous activity or prolonged (more than 1 hour) weight-bearing activity, such as in running or tennis, within 48 hours after the injection.
- Tell patient to report injection site reactions such as pain, swelling, itching, heat, rash, bruising, or redness.
- Inform patient that a treatment cycle includes at least three injections and that pain may not be relieved until after the third injection.
- Caution patient to report planned or suspected pregnancy.

imiquimod

Aldara

Pharmacologic class: immune response modifier
Pregnancy risk category B

AVAILABLE FORMS

Cream: 5% in single-use packets containing 250 mg

INDICATIONS & DOSAGES

➤ External genital and perianal warts

Adults and adolescents age 12 and older: Apply thin layer to affected area three times weekly before normal sleeping hours and leave on skin for 6 to 10 hours. Continue treatment until genital or perianal warts clear completely or maximum of 16 weeks.

➤ Typical, nonhyperkeratotic, nonhypertrophic actinic keratoses on the face or scalp in immunocompetent adults

Adults: Wash area with mild soap and water and dry at least 10 minutes. Apply cream to face or scalp, but not both concurrently, twice weekly at bedtime and wash off after about 8 hours. Treat for 16 weeks.

✱ ***NEW INDICATION:* Superficial basal cell carcinoma**

Adults: Wash area with mild soap and water and allow to dry thoroughly. Apply a thin layer of cream to a 1-cm margin around the biopsy-confirmed area five times a week at bedtime; wash off after about 8 hours. Treat for 6 weeks.

ACTION

Has no direct antiviral activity in cell culture. Drug induces mRNA-encoding cytokines including interferon alfa at the treatment site.

Route	Onset	Peak	Duration
Topical	Unknown	Unknown	Unknown

Half-life: About 20 hours.

ADVERSE REACTIONS

CNS: headache.
Musculoskeletal: myalgia.
Skin: local itching, burning, pain, soreness, erythema, ulceration, edema, erosion, induration, flaking, excoriation.
Other: *fungal infection,* flulike symptoms.

INTERACTIONS

None significant

EFFECTS ON LAB TEST RESULTS

None reported.

CONTRAINDICATIONS & CAUTIONS

- Drug isn't recommended for treatment of urethral, intravaginal, cervical, rectal, or intra-anal human papillomavirus disease.
- Safety of drug in breast-feeding women is unknown.

NURSING CONSIDERATIONS

- Don't use until genital or perianal tissue is healed from previous drug or surgical treatment.
- Patient usually experiences local skin reactions at site of application or surrounding areas. Use nonocclusive dressings, such as cotton gauze, or cotton undergarments in management of skin reactions. Patient's discomfort or severity of the local skin reaction may require a rest period of several days. Resume treatment once reaction subsides.
- Drug isn't a cure; new warts may develop during therapy.
- Maximum tumor diameter of superficial basal cell carcinoma should be 2 cm or smaller. Cream may be applied to neck, trunk, or arms and legs (excluding hands and feet).
- Assess treatment site for clearance 12 weeks posttreatment.

PATIENT TEACHING

- Advise patient that effect of cream on transmission of genital or perianal warts is unknown. New warts may develop during therapy; drug isn't a cure.
- Tell patient to use cream only as directed and to avoid contact with eyes, lips, or nostrils.
- Tell patient to wash hands before and after applying cream.
- Tell patient to wash the area with mild soap and water and dry completely before applying cream.
- Advise patient to apply cream in thin layer over affected area and rub in until cream isn't visible. Advise patient to avoid excessive use of cream. Tell him not to occlude area after applying cream and to wash with mild soap and water 6 to 10 hours after application of cream.
- Advise patient that mild local skin reactions, such as redness, erosion, excoriation, flaking, and swelling at site of application or surrounding areas, are common. Tell him that most skin reactions are mild to moderate. Advise him to report severe skin reactions promptly.
- Instruct uncircumcised man being treated for warts under the foreskin to retract foreskin and clean area daily.
- Advise patient that drug can weaken condoms and vaginal diaphragms and that use together isn't recommended.
- Advise patient to avoid sexual contact while cream is on the skin.
- Advise patient to minimize or avoid exposure to sunlight and other UV light; encourage sunscreen use.
- Tell patient to store drug at temperatures below 86° F (30° C) and to avoid freezing.
- Tell patient to discard partially used packets and not to reuse.

isotretinoin

Accutane, Amnesteem, Claravis, Roaccutane‡, Sotret

Pharmacologic class: retinoic acid derivative
Pregnancy risk category X

AVAILABLE FORMS

Capsules: 10 mg, 20 mg, 30 mg, 40 mg

INDICATIONS & DOSAGES

➤ **Severe nodular acne that's unresponsive to conventional therapy**
Adults and adolescents: 0.5 to 2 mg/kg P.O. daily in two divided doses with food for 15 to 20 weeks.

ACTION

May normalize keratinization, reversibly decrease size of sebaceous glands, and make sebum less viscous and less likely to plug follicles.

Route	Onset	Peak	Duration
P.O.	Unknown	3 hr	Unknown

Half-life: 30 minutes to 39 hours.

ADVERSE REACTIONS

CNS: *pseudotumor cerebri,* ***depression, psychosis, suicidal ideation or attempts, suicide, aggressive and violent behavior,*** emotional instability, headache, fatigue.

EENT: *conjunctivitis, epistaxis, drying of mucous membranes, dry nose,* corneal deposits, dry eyes, hearing impairment (sometimes irreversible), decreased night vision, visual disturbances.
GI: nonspecific GI symptoms, *nausea, vomiting, abdominal pain, dry mouth,* anorexia, gum bleeding and inflammation, ***acute pancreatitis,*** inflammatory bowel disease.
Hematologic: *increased erythrocyte sedimentation rate,* anemia, thrombocytosis.
Hepatic: ***hepatitis.***
Metabolic: *hypertriglyceridemia,* hyperglycemia.
Musculoskeletal: ***rhabdomyolysis,*** skeletal hyperostosis, tendon and ligament calcification, premature epiphyseal closure, decreased bone mineral density and other bone abnormalities, back pain, arthralgia, arthritis, tendinitis.
Skin: *cheilitis, cheilosis, fragility, rash, dry skin, facial skin desquamation, petechiae, pruritus, nail brittleness,* thinning of hair, skin infection, peeling of palms and toes, photosensitivity reaction.

INTERACTIONS

Drug-drug. *Corticosteroids:* May increase risk of osteoporosis. Use together cautiously.
Medicated soaps, cleansers, and coverups, preparations containing alcohol, topical resorcinol peeling agents (benzoyl peroxide): May have cumulative drying effect. Use together cautiously.
Micro-dosed progesterone hormonal contraceptives ("minipills") that don't contain estrogen: May decrease effectiveness of contraceptive. Advise patient to use different contraceptive method.
Phenytoin: May increase risk of osteomalacia. Use together cautiously.
Tetracyclines: May increase risk of pseudotumor cerebri. Avoid using together.
Products containing vitamin A, vitamin A: May increase toxic effects of isotretinoin. Avoid using together.
Drug-food. *Any food:* May increase absorption of drug. Advise patient to take drug with milk, a meal, or shortly after a meal.
Drug-lifestyle. *Alcohol use:* May increase risk of hypertriglyceridemia. Discourage use together.
Sun exposure: May increase photosensitivity reaction. Advise patient to avoid excessive sunlight exposure.

EFFECTS ON LAB TEST RESULTS

- May increase AST, ALT, alkaline phosphatase, triglyceride, glucose, and uric acid levels.
- May increase platelet count and erythrocyte sedimentation rate.

CONTRAINDICATIONS & CAUTIONS

- Contraindicated in patients hypersensitive to parabens (used as preservatives), vitamin A, or other retinoids.
- Contraindicated in woman of childbearing potential, unless patient has had two negative pregnancy test results before beginning therapy, will begin drug therapy on second or third day of next menstrual period, and will comply with stringent contraceptive measures for 1 month before therapy, during therapy, and for at least 1 month after therapy.
- Use cautiously in patients with a history of mental illness or a family history of psychiatric disorders, asthma, liver disease, diabetes, heart disease, osteoporosis, genetic predisposition for age-related osteoporosis, history of childhood osteoporosis, weak bones, anorexia nervosa, osteomalacia, or other disorders of bone metabolism.

NURSING CONSIDERATIONS

- Before use, have patient read patient information and sign accompanying consent form.
- Patient must have negative results from two urine or serum pregnancy tests; one is performed in the office when the patient is qualified for therapy, the second during the first 5 days of the next normal menstrual period immediately preceding the beginning of therapy. For patients with amenorrhea, the second test should be done at least 11 days after the last unprotected act of sexual intercourse. A pregnancy test must be repeated every month before the patient receives the prescription.
- Monitor baseline lipid studies, liver function tests, and pregnancy tests before therapy and at monthly intervals.

- Regularly monitor glucose level and CK levels in patients who participate in vigorous physical activity.
- Most adverse reactions occur at doses exceeding 1 mg/kg daily. Reactions are generally reversible when therapy is stopped or dosage is reduced.
- ***Alert:*** If patient experiences headache, nausea and vomiting, or visual disturbances, screen for papilledema. Signs and symptoms of pseudotumor cerebri require stopping the drug immediately and administering neurologic interventions promptly.
- To minimize the risk of fetal exposure, the drug is only available through a restricted FDA-approved distribution program called iPLEDGE.
- A second course of therapy may begin 8 weeks after completion of the first course, if necessary. Improvements may continue after first course is complete.
- Patients may be at increased risk of bone fractures or injury when participating in sports with repetitive impact.
- Spontaneous reports of osteoporosis, osteopenia, bone fractures, and delayed healing of bone fractures have occurred in patients taking drug. To decrease this risk, don't exceed recommended doses and duration.

PATIENT TEACHING

- ***Alert:*** Warn woman of childbearing age that, if this drug is used during pregnancy, severe fetal abnormalities may occur. Advise her to either abstain from sex or use two reliable forms of contraception simultaneously for 1 month before, during, and for 1 month after treatment.
- Advise patient to take drug with or shortly after meals to facilitate absorption.
- Tell patient to immediately report visual disturbances and bone, muscle, or joint pain.
- Warn patient that contact lenses may feel uncomfortable during therapy.
- Warn patient against using abrasives, medicated soaps and cleansers, acne preparations containing peeling drugs, and topical products containing alcohol (including cosmetics, aftershave, cologne) because they may cause cumulative irritation or excessive drying of skin.
- Tell patient to avoid prolonged sun exposure and to use sunblock. Drug may have additive effect if used with other drugs that cause photosensitivity reaction.
- Tell women that manufacturer will supply urine pregnancy tests for monthly testing during therapy.
- Warn patient that transient exacerbations may occur during therapy.
- Warn patient not to donate blood during therapy and for 1 month after stopping drug because drug could harm fetus of a pregnant recipient.
- Tell patient to report adverse reactions immediately, especially depression, suicidal thoughts, persistent headaches, and persistent GI pain.

✱ NEW DRUG

mecasermin rinfabate

Increlex

Pharmacologic class: human insulin growth factor
Pregnancy risk category C

AVAILABLE FORMS

Injection: 36 mg/0.6-ml vial

INDICATIONS & DOSAGES

➤ Growth failure in children with severe primary insulin growth factor-1 (IGF-1) deficiency or children with growth-hormone gene deletion who have developed neutralizing antibodies to growth hormone
Children age 3 and older: Initially, 0.5 mg/kg subcutaneously. Adjust to therapeutic range (1 to 2 mg/kg once daily) based on glucose and IGF-1 levels. Give at about the same time each day, before the morning or evening meal, as long as the child maintains a balanced diet.

ACTION

Promotes growth because synthetic drug is identical to endogenous insulin-like growth factor-binding protein-3 (IGFBP-3) and IGF-1.

Route	Onset	Peak	Duration
SubQ, IGF-1	1 hr	5–17½ hr	Unknown
SubQ, IGFBP-3	1 hr	10½–28½ hr	Unknown

Half-life: About 6 hours.

ADVERSE REACTIONS

CNS: *headache,* dizziness, intracranial hypertension.
EENT: *tonsillar hypertrophy,* otitis media, papilledema.
GI: vomiting.
GU: hematuria, ovarian cysts.
Hematologic: *iron deficiency anemia.*
Metabolic: hyperglycemia, hypoglycemia.
Musculoskeletal: *muscle atrophy,* arthralgia, bone pain, scoliosis.
Other: *enlarged thyroid, pain,* injection site reaction, lymphadenopathy, snoring.

INTERACTIONS

None known.

EFFECTS ON LAB TEST RESULTS

- May increase AST, LDH, and transaminase levels. May increase or decrease glucose level.

CONTRAINDICATIONS & CAUTIONS

- Contraindicated in patients with closed epiphyses, active or suspected cancer, or allergy to drug or its components. I.V. use is also contraindicated. Don't use in place of growth hormone or for other causes of growth failure.
- Use cautiously in pregnant or breast-feeding women.

NURSING CONSIDERATIONS

- Make sure patient has had a baseline ophthalmic examination before therapy.
- Give drug at the same time each day. Because of its insulin-like effects, withhold dose if patient can't or won't eat.
- Monitor glucose level carefully, especially in small children, whose oral intake can be inconsistent.
- Check patient regularly for adenotonsillar enlargement. Ask parent or caregiver if the child has developed snoring, sleep apnea, or reduced hearing.
- Monitor patient for changes typical of acromegaly.
- Monitor child experiencing rapid growth closely for development of a limp, hip or knee pain or progression of scoliosis (if present).
- Safety and effectiveness in children younger than age 3 isn't known.

PATIENT TEACHING

- Explain that drug must be kept frozen until ready to use. Tell parent or caregiver to discard unused drug after 2 months, even if it has remained frozen.
- Instruct parent to let drug thaw at room temperature for about 45 minutes before giving it and to give it within 1 hour of thawing. Explain that drug must be discarded if not used within 2 hours of thawing because it may be ineffective.
- Warn parent not to use drug if it's cloudy.
- Tell parent to give drug before the same meal daily and to withhold dose if the child can't or won't eat.
- Teach parent how to inject drug and dispose of syringes properly.
- Tell parent to inject drug subcutaneously into child's upper arm, upper thigh, stomach area, or buttocks. Caution against injecting it into a muscle or vein.
- To decrease injection site reactions, advise parent to rotate the injection site for each dose.
- Tell parent to regularly monitor the child's glucose level. Review signs and symptoms of hypoglycemia, including dizziness, tiredness, hunger, irritability, sweating, nausea, and a fast or irregular heartbeat.
- Advise parent and child to keep a quick source of sugar (such as orange juice, glucose gel, or candy) readily available in case hypoglycemia occurs.
- Explain that child should avoid hazardous activities while the dose is being adjusted. Hypoglycemia can cause unconsciousness, seizures, or death.
- Advise parent to have the child's tonsils checked regularly and to monitor child for enlarged tonsils and snoring or sleep apnea.
- Tell parent to notify prescriber if child develops nausea and vomiting with headache, hypoglycemic episodes, limping, hip or knee pain, snoring, trouble swallowing, earaches, or breathing problems.

mesna
Mesnex

Pharmacologic class: thiol derivative
Pregnancy risk category B

AVAILABLE FORMS
Injection: 100 mg/ml in 10-ml vials
Tablets: 400 mg

INDICATIONS & DOSAGES
➤ To prevent hemorrhagic cystitis in patients receiving ifosfamide
Adults: Dosage varies with amount of ifosfamide given; calculated as 20% of ifosfamide dose at time of ifosfamide administration. Usual dose is 240 mg/m^2 as an I.V. bolus with administration of ifosfamide; repeated at 4 and 8 hours after administration of ifosfamide. Or, calculate daily dose as 100% of the ifosfamide dose. Give as a single bolus injection (20%), followed by two oral doses (40% each). Protocols that use 1.2 g/m^2 ifosfamide would use 240 mg/m^2 I.V. mesna at 0 hours, and then 480 mg/m^2 P.O. at 2 and 6 hours.

I.V. ADMINISTRATION
- Prepare I.V. solution by diluting commercially available ampules with D_5W, dextrose 5% and normal saline solution for injection, normal saline solution for injection, or lactated Ringer solution to obtain final solution of 20 mg/ml.
- Although diluted solutions are stable for 24 hours at room temperature, they should be refrigerated.
- Mesna and ifosfamide are compatible in same I.V. infusion.

INCOMPATIBILITIES
Amphotericin B, carboplatin, cisplatin, ifosfamide with epirubicin.

ACTION
Prevents ifosfamide-induced hemorrhagic cystitis by reacting with urotoxic ifosfamide metabolites.

Route	Onset	Peak	Duration
P.O.	Rapid	4 hr	Unknown
I.V.	Rapid	Unknown	Unknown

Half-life: 4 to 8 hours.

ADVERSE REACTIONS
CNS: *fatigue, fever, asthenia,* dizziness, headache, somnolence, anxiety, confusion, insomnia.
CV: chest pain, edema, hypotension, tachycardia, flushing.
GI: *nausea, vomiting, constipation, anorexia, abdominal pain,* diarrhea, dyspepsia.
GU: hematuria.
Hematologic: ***leukopenia, thrombocytopenia, anemia, granulocytopenia.***
Metabolic: hypokalemia, dehydration.
Musculoskeletal: back pain.
Respiratory: dyspnea, coughing, pneumonia.
Skin: alopecia, increased sweating, injection site reaction, pallor.
Other: allergy, pain.

INTERACTIONS
None significant.

EFFECTS ON LAB TEST RESULTS
- May decrease potassium and hemoglobin levels and hematocrit.
- May decrease WBC, platelet, and granulocyte counts.

CONTRAINDICATIONS & CAUTIONS
- Contraindicated in patients hypersensitive to drug or compounds containing thiol.

NURSING CONSIDERATIONS
- Drug isn't effective in preventing hematuria from other causes (such as thrombocytopenia).
- Because drug is used with ifosfamide and other chemotherapeutic drugs, it may be difficult to tell which adverse reactions are just from this drug.
- Although made to protect against hemorrhagic cystitis from ifosfamide, drug won't protect against other toxicities from other drugs.

• If patient vomits within 2 hours of taking P.O. drug, give another P.O. dose or give the drug I.V.
• Monitor urine samples for hematuria daily. Monitor BUN and creatinine levels and intake and output.
• Drug contains benzyl alcohol, which has been linked to fatal gasping syndrome in premature infants.

PATIENT TEACHING
• Explain to patient and family or other caregiver why drug is needed and how it's given.
• Advise patient to drink at least 4 cups of liquid each day during treatment.
• Instruct patient to report persistent or severe adverse reactions.
• Advise patient to promptly report blood in urine.

minoxidil (topical)

Rogaine ◇, Rogaine Extra Strength for Men ◇, Rogaine for Women ◇

Pharmacologic class: direct-acting vasodilator
Pregnancy risk category C

AVAILABLE FORMS
Topical solution: 2% ◇, 5% ◇

INDICATIONS & DOSAGES
➤ **Androgenetic alopecia**
Adults: 1 ml of solution applied to affected area b.i.d. Maximum daily dose is 2 ml.

ACTION
Stimulates hair growth, possibly by dilating arterial microcapillaries around hair follicles.

Route	Onset	Peak	Duration
Topical	Unknown	Unknown	Unknown

Half-life: Unknown.

ADVERSE REACTIONS
CNS: headache, dizziness, faintness, light-headedness.
CV: edema, chest pain, hypertension, hypotension, palpitations, increased or decreased pulse rate.
EENT: sinusitis.
GI: diarrhea, nausea, vomiting.
GU: UTI, renal calculi, urethritis.
Metabolic: weight gain.
Musculoskeletal: back pain, tendinitis.
Respiratory: bronchitis, upper respiratory infection.
Skin: *irritant dermatitis, dry skin or scalp, flaking, local erythema, pruritus,* allergic contact dermatitis, eczema, hypertrichosis, worsening of hair loss.

INTERACTIONS
Drug-drug. *Petroleum jelly, topical corticosteroids, topical retinoids, other drugs that may increase skin absorption:* May increase risk of systemic effects of minoxidil. Avoid using together.

EFFECTS ON LAB TEST RESULTS
None reported.

CONTRAINDICATIONS & CAUTIONS
• Contraindicated in patients hypersensitive to drug or components of solution.
• Use cautiously in patients older than age 50 and in those with cardiac, renal, or hepatic disease.

NURSING CONSIDERATIONS
• Patient needs to have normal, healthy scalp before beginning therapy because absorption of drug through irritated skin may cause adverse systemic effects.
• Treatment will most likely succeed in patients with balding area smaller than 4 inches (10 cm) that developed within past 10 years.
• Don't use 5% solution in women.

PATIENT TEACHING
• Teach patient how to apply drug. Tell him to dry hair and scalp thoroughly before application and not to apply drug to other body areas. Tell patient not to use drug on irritated or sunburned scalp or with other drugs on scalp. Tell him to thoroughly wash hands after application.
• Warn patient to avoid inhaling any spray or mist from drug and to avoid spraying around eyes, because solution contains alcohol and may be irritating.

• Inform patient that more frequent applications or using more than 2 ml daily won't increase hair growth but instead may increase adverse reactions. Tell patient not to double the dose for missed applications.
• Teach patient to monitor pulse rate and body weight.
• Advise patient that therapy will be prolonged and will continue for at least 4 months before clinical effects appear. Tell him that drug must be used daily for optimal results. Almost half of patients will experience moderate to dense hair growth.
• Tell patient that stopping drug may cause loss of new hair growth. New hair growth is usually fine and may be colorless but will resemble existing hair after continued treatment.

nimodipine
Nimotop

Pharmacologic class: calcium channel blocker
Pregnancy risk category C

AVAILABLE FORMS
Capsules: 30 mg

INDICATIONS & DOSAGES
➤ **To improve neurologic deficits after subarachnoid hemorrhage from ruptured intracranial berry aneurysm**
Adults: 60 mg P.O. q 4 hours for 21 days. Begin therapy within 96 hours after subarachnoid hemorrhage.
Adjust-a-dose: For patients with hepatic failure, 30 mg P.O. q 4 hours for 21 days.

ACTION
Inhibits calcium ion influx across cardiac and smooth-muscle cells, decreasing myocardial contractility and oxygen demand; also dilates coronary and cerebral arteries and arterioles.

Route	Onset	Peak	Duration
P.O.	Unknown	1 hr	Unknown

Half-life: 8 to 9 hours; may be 1 to 2 hours.

ADVERSE REACTIONS
CNS: headache, psychic disturbances.
CV: hypotension, flushing, edema, tachycardia.
GI: nausea, diarrhea, abdominal discomfort.
Musculoskeletal: muscle cramps.
Respiratory: dyspnea, wheezing.
Skin: dermatitis, rash.

INTERACTIONS
Drug-drug. *Antihypertensives:* May increase hypotensive effect. Monitor blood pressure.
Calcium channel blockers: May increase CV effects. Monitor patient closely.
Cimetidine: May increase nimodipine bioavailability. Monitor patient for adverse effects.
Drug-food. *Any food:* May decrease drug absorption. Advise patient to take drug on empty stomach.

EFFECTS ON LAB TEST RESULTS
None reported.

CONTRAINDICATIONS & CAUTIONS
• No known contraindications.
• Use cautiously in patients with hepatic failure.

NURSING CONSIDERATIONS
• Monitor blood pressure and heart rate in all patients, especially at start of therapy.
• If patient can't swallow capsule, make a hole in each end of capsule with an 18G needle, and extract contents into syringe. Empty syringe into patient's nasogastric tube. Flush tube with 30 ml of normal saline solution.
• ***Alert:*** If using a needle to extract contents of capsule, make sure that drug isn't then given I.V. instead of P.O. Label the syringe "for oral use only" before withdrawing the contents of the capsule.

PATIENT TEACHING
• Explain use of drug and review administration schedule with patient and family. Stress importance of compliance for maximum drug effectiveness.
• Instruct patient to report persistent or severe adverse reactions promptly.

• Tell patient not to drink grapefruit juice while taking this drug.

orlistat

Xenical

Pharmacologic class: lipase inhibitor
Pregnancy risk category B

AVAILABLE FORMS

Capsules: 120 mg

INDICATIONS & DOSAGES

➤ **To manage obesity, including weight loss and weight maintenance with a reduced-calorie diet; to reduce risk of weight gain after previous weight loss**
Adults and children ages 12 to 16: Give 120 mg P.O. t.i.d. with or up to 1 hour after each main meal containing fat.

ACTION

A reversible lipase inhibitor that forms a bond with active site of gastric and pancreatic lipases, inactivating them. As a result, enzymes can't hydrolyze dietary triglycerides into absorbable free fatty acids and monoglycerides. The undigested triglycerides aren't absorbed, resulting in caloric deficit.

Route	Onset	Peak	Duration
P.O.	Unknown	Unknown	Unknown

Half-life: 1 to 2 hours.

ADVERSE REACTIONS

CNS: *headache,* dizziness, fatigue, sleep disorder, anxiety, depression.
CV: pedal edema.
EENT: otitis.
GI: *flatus with discharge, fecal urgency, fatty or oily stool, oily spotting, increased defecation, abdominal pain,* fecal incontinence, nausea, infectious diarrhea, rectal pain, vomiting.
GU: menstrual irregularity, vaginitis, UTI.
Musculoskeletal: *back pain, leg pain,* arthritis, myalgia, joint disorder, tendinitis.
Respiratory: *influenza, upper respiratory tract infection,* lower respiratory tract infection.
Skin: rash, dry skin.
Other: tooth and gingival disorders.

INTERACTIONS

Drug-drug. ***Cyclosporine:*** May decrease cyclosporine levels, risking organ rejection. Avoid use together.
Fat-soluble vitamins (such as vitamins A and E and beta-carotene): May decrease absorption of vitamins. Separate doses by 2 hours.
Pravastatin: May slightly increase pravastatin levels and lipid-lowering effects of drug. Monitor patient.
Warfarin: May change coagulation values. Monitor INR.

EFFECTS ON LAB TEST RESULTS

None reported.

CONTRAINDICATIONS & CAUTIONS

• Contraindicated in patients hypersensitive to drug or its components and in those with chronic malabsorption syndrome or cholestasis.
• Use cautiously in patients with history of hyperoxaluria or calcium oxalate nephrolithiasis or those at risk for anorexia nervosa or bulimia.
• Use cautiously in patients receiving cyclosporine therapy because of potential changes in cyclosporine absorption related to variations in dietary intake.

NURSING CONSIDERATIONS

• Exclude organic causes of obesity, such as hypothyroidism, before starting drug therapy.
• Drug is recommended for use in patients with an initial body mass index (BMI) of 30 or more or those with a BMI of 27 or more and other risk factors (such as hypertension, diabetes, or dyslipidemia).
• In diabetic patients, dosage of oral antidiabetic or insulin may need to be reduced because improved metabolic control may accompany weight loss.
• As with other weight-loss drugs, potential for misuse exists in certain patients (such as those with anorexia nervosa or bulimia).
• ***Look alike–sound alike:*** Don't confuse Xenical with Xeloda.

PATIENT TEACHING

- Advise patient to follow a nutritionally balanced, reduced-calorie diet that derives only 30% of its calories from fat. Tell him to distribute daily intake of fat, carbohydrate, and protein over three main meals. If a meal is occasionally missed or contains no fat, tell patient that dose of drug can be omitted.
- Advise patient to adhere to dietary guidelines. GI effects may increase when patient takes drug with high-fat foods, specifically when more than 30% of total daily calories come from fat.
- Drug reduces absorption of some fat-soluble vitamins and beta-carotene.
- Tell patient with diabetes that weight loss may improve his glycemic control, so dosage of his oral antidiabetic (such as a sulfonylurea or metformin) or insulin may need to be reduced during drug therapy.
- Tell woman of childbearing age to inform prescriber if pregnancy or breast-feeding is planned during therapy.

palifermin

Kepivance

Pharmacologic class: keratinocyte growth factor
Pregnancy risk category C

AVAILABLE FORMS

Lyophilized powder for injection: 6.25-mg vials

INDICATIONS & DOSAGES

➤ **To decrease frequency and duration of severe oral mucositis in patients with hematologic malignancies who are receiving myelotoxic chemotherapy requiring hematopoietic stem cell support**
Adults: 60 mcg/kg/day by I.V. bolus for 3 consecutive days before myelotoxic chemotherapy, with the third dose 24 to 48 hours before myelotoxic chemotherapy starts. Repeat dose for 3 consecutive days after myelotoxic chemotherapy ends, for a total of six doses. Give first dose after myelotoxic therapy ends on the same day as, but after, hematopoietic stem cell infusion and at least 4 days after the most recent palifermin dose.

I.V. ADMINISTRATION

- To reconstitute powder, slowly add 1.2 ml sterile water for injection to vial.
- Swirl vial gently; don't shake or agitate it vigorously.
- The final concentration will be 5 mg/ml, and the solution should be clear and colorless.
- Don't filter drug while preparing or giving it.
- Use drug immediately after preparing it, or refrigerate it for up to 24 hours.
- Give by I.V. bolus; if the I.V. line has been flushed with heparin, flush it with normal saline solution before and after giving.
- Discard reconstituted drug if at room temperature for more than 1 hour.
- Protect reconstituted drug from light.

INCOMPATIBILITIES

Heparin.

ACTION

Increases proliferation of epithelial cells, increasing thickness of tongue tissue, buccal mucosa, and GI tract.

Route	Onset	Peak	Duration
I.V.	Immediate	1–4 hr	Unknown

Half-life: 3¼ to 5¾ hours.

ADVERSE REACTIONS

CNS: *dysesthesia, fever, hyperesthesia, hypoesthesia, pain, paresthesia.*
CV: *edema,* hypertension.
GI: *mouth or tongue thickness or discoloration, taste alteration.*
Musculoskeletal: *arthralgia.*
Skin: *erythema, pruritus, rash.*

INTERACTIONS

Drug-drug. *Heparin:* May bind to palifermin and alter dose. Flush I.V. line with normal saline solution before and after giving palifermin.
Myelotoxic chemotherapy: May increase severity and duration of oral mucositis. Don't give palifermin within 24 hours of chemotherapy.

EFFECTS ON LAB TEST RESULTS

- May increase amylase and lipase levels.

CONTRAINDICATIONS & CAUTIONS

- Contraindicated in patients hypersensitive to *Escherichia coli*–derived proteins or to drug or its components.
- Use cautiously in patients with nonhematologic malignancies.

NURSING CONSIDERATIONS

- ***Alert:*** To avoid increasing severity and duration of oral mucositis, don't give drug within 24 hours of myelotoxic chemotherapy.
- Monitor patient for fever, arthralgia, and adverse mucocutaneous effects.
- Skin-related toxicities are most likely to occur 6 days after the first three consecutive doses.
- Drug may enhance growth of tumor cells.

PATIENT TEACHING

- Tell patient to report to prescriber rash, reddening, swelling, or itching of skin; unpleasant sensation around the mouth; tongue discoloration or thickening; altered taste; fever; and joint pain.
- Explain that drug may stimulate growth of other types of cancer cells.
- Urge patient to keep all scheduled appointments for treatment.

pimecrolimus

Elidel

Pharmacologic class: topical immunomodulator
Pregnancy risk category C

AVAILABLE FORMS

Cream: 1% 30-g, 60-g, and 100-g tubes. Base contains benzyl alcohol, cetyl alcohol, oleyl alcohol, and stearyl alcohol

INDICATIONS & DOSAGES

➤ **Short- and intermittent long-term treatment of mild to moderate atopic dermatitis in nonimmunocompromised patients in whom the use of other conventional therapies is deemed inadvisable, or in patients with inadequate response to or intolerance of conventional therapies**

Adults and children age 2 and older: Apply a thin layer to the affected skin b.i.d. and rub in gently and completely.

ACTION

Unknown. Inhibits T-cell activation and prevents the release of inflammatory cytokines and mediators from mast cells.

Route	Onset	Peak	Duration
Topical	Unknown	Unknown	Unknown

Half-life: Unknown.

ADVERSE REACTIONS

CNS: *headache, fever.*
EENT: *nasopharyngitis,* otitis media, sinusitis, pharyngitis, tonsillitis, eye infection, nasal congestion, rhinorrhea, sinus congestion, rhinitis, epistaxis, conjunctivitis, earache.
GI: gastroenteritis, abdominal pain, vomiting, diarrhea, nausea, constipation, loose stools.
GU: dysmenorrhea.
Musculoskeletal: back pain, arthralgias.
Respiratory: *upper respiratory tract infections, bronchitis, cough,* asthma, pneumonia, wheezing, dyspnea.
Skin: *application site reaction (burning, irritation, erythema, pruritus),* skin infections, impetigo, folliculitis, molluscum contagiosum, herpes simplex, varicella, papilloma, urticaria, acne.
Other: *influenza,* flulike illness, hypersensitivity, toothache, bacterial infection, viral infection.

INTERACTIONS

Drug-drug. *Cytochrome P-450 inhibitors (such as erythromycin, itraconazole, ketoconazole, fluconazole, calcium channel blockers):* May affect metabolism of pimecrolimus. Use together cautiously.
Drug-lifestyle. *Natural or artificial sunlight exposure:* May worsen atopic dermatitis. Avoid or minimize exposure.

EFFECTS ON LAB TEST RESULTS

None reported.

CONTRAINDICATIONS & CAUTIONS

- Contraindicated in patients hypersensitive to drug or its components, in patients with Netherton syndrome, and in immunocompromised patients.
- Contraindicated in patients with active cutaneous viral infections or infected atopic dermatitis.
- Use cautiously in patients with varicella zoster virus infection, herpes simplex virus infection, or eczema herpeticum.
- Safety of use in pregnant women hasn't been established.

NURSING CONSIDERATIONS

- ***Alert:*** Use drug only after other therapies have failed because of the risk of cancer.
- Drug may be used on all skin surfaces, including the head, neck, and intertriginous areas.
- Clear infections at treatment sites before using.
- If symptoms persist longer than 6 weeks, reevaluate the patient.
- Don't use with occlusive dressing.
- May cause local symptoms such as skin burning. Most local reactions start within 1 to 5 days after treatment, are mild to moderately severe, and last no longer than 5 days.
- Monitor patient for lymphadenopathy. If lymphadenopathy occurs and its cause is unknown, or if the patient develops acute infectious mononucleosis, consider stopping drug.
- Drug use may cause papillomas or warts. Consider stopping drug if papillomas worsen or don't respond to conventional treatment.
- It's unknown if drug appears in breast milk. Serious adverse reactions may occur in breast-feeding infants exposed to drug. Patient should either stop breastfeeding or stop treatment.

PATIENT TEACHING

- Inform patient that this drug is for external use only and that he should use it as directed.
- Tell patient to report adverse reactions.
- Tell patient not to use with an occlusive dressing.
- Instruct patient to wash hands after application if hands aren't treated.
- Tell patient to stop therapy after signs and symptoms have resolved. If symptoms persist longer than 6 weeks, tell him to contact his prescriber.
- Tell patient to resume treatment at first signs of recurrence.
- Stress that patient should minimize or avoid exposure to natural or artificial sunlight (including tanning beds and UVA-UVB treatment) while using this drug.
- Tell patient to expect application site reactions but to notify his prescriber if reaction is severe or persists for longer than 1 week.

pregabalin
Lyrica

Pharmacologic class: CNS drug
Pregnancy risk category C
Controlled substance schedule V

AVAILABLE FORMS

Capsules: 25 mg, 50 mg, 75 mg, 100 mg, 150 mg, 200 mg, 225 mg, 300 mg

INDICATIONS & DOSAGES

➤ **Diabetic peripheral neuropathy**
Adults: Initially, 50 mg P.O. t.i.d. May increase to 100 mg P.O. t.i.d. within 1 week.

➤ **Postherpetic neuralgia**
Adults: Initially, 75 mg P.O. b.i.d. or 50 mg P.O. t.i.d. May increase to 300 mg/day in two or three equally divided doses within 1 week. If pain relief insufficient after 2 to 4 weeks, may increase to 300 mg b.i.d. or 200 mg t.i.d.

➤ **Adjunctive treatment of partial onset seizures**
Adults: Initially, 75 mg P.O. b.i.d. or 50 mg P.O. t.i.d. Range, 150 to 600 mg/day.

Adjust-a-dose: If creatinine clearance is 30 to 60 ml/minute, give 75 to 300 mg/day in two or three divided doses. If clearance is 15 to 30 ml/minute, give 25 to 150 mg/day in one dose or divided into two doses. If clearance is less than 15 ml/minute, give 25 to 75 mg/day in one dose. If patient undergoes hemodialysis, give one supplemental dose according to these guidelines. If patient takes 25 mg daily, give 25 or 50 mg. If patient takes 25 to

50 mg daily, give 50 or 75 mg. If patient takes 75 mg daily, give 100 or 150 mg.

ACTION
May contribute to analgesic and anticonvulsant effects by binding to sites in CNS.

Route	Onset	Peak	Duration
P.O.	Unknown	1½ – 3 hr	Unknown

Half-life: 6½ hours.

ADVERSE REACTIONS
CNS: *ataxia, dizziness, somnolence, tremor,* abnormal gait, abnormal thinking, amnesia, anxiety, asthenia, confusion, depersonalization, euphoria, headache, hypesthesia, hypertonia, incoordination, myoclonus, nervousness, nystagmus, paresthesia, stupor, twitching, vertigo.
CV: *edema, **PR interval prolongation.***
EENT: blurred or abnormal vision, conjunctivitis, diplopia, eye disorder, otitis media, tinnitus.
GI: *dry mouth,* abdominal pain, constipation, flatulence, gastroenteritis, vomiting.
GU: anorgasmia, impotence, urinary incontinence, urinary frequency.
Metabolic: HYPOGLYCEMIA, *weight gain,* increased or decreased appetite.
Musculoskeletal: arthralgia, back and chest pain, leg cramps, myalgia, myasthenia, neuropathy.
Respiratory: bronchitis, dyspnea.
Skin: ecchymosis, pruritus.
Other: *accidental injury, infection, **allergic reaction,*** decreased libido, flu syndrome, pain.

INTERACTIONS
Drug-drug. *CNS depressants:* May have additive effects on cognitive and gross motor function. Monitor patient for increased dizziness and somnolence.
Pioglitazone, rosiglitazone: May cause additive fluid retention and weight gain. Monitor patient closely.
Drug-lifestyle. *Alcohol use:* May have additive depressant effects on cognitive and gross motor function. Discourage alcohol use.

EFFECTS ON LAB TEST RESULTS
- May increase CK level.
- May decrease platelet count.

CONTRAINDICATIONS & CAUTIONS
- Contraindicated in patients hypersensitive to drug or its components.
- Use cautiously in patients with New York Heart Association class III or class IV heart failure.

NURSING CONSIDERATIONS
- Monitor patient's weight and fluid status, especially if he has heart failure.
- Check for changes in vision.
- ***Alert:*** Watch for signs of rhabdomyolysis, such as dark, red, or cola-colored urine; muscle tenderness; generalized weakness; or muscle stiffness or aching.
- Don't stop drug abruptly. Instead, taper it gradually over at least 1 week.

PATIENT TEACHING
- Explain that drug may be taken with or without food.
- Warn patient not to stop drug abruptly.
- Caution patient to avoid hazardous activities until drug's effects are known.
- Instruct patient to watch for weight changes and water retention.
- Advise patient to report vision changes and malaise or fever accompanied by muscle pain, tenderness, or weakness.
- Tell women to immediately report planned or suspected pregnancy.
- Tell a man who plans to father a child that he should consult prescriber about possible risks to fetus.
- If patient has diabetes, urge him to inspect his skin closely for ulcer formation.

raloxifene hydrochloride
Evista🖉

Pharmacologic class: selective estrogen receptor modulator
Pregnancy risk category X

AVAILABLE FORMS
Tablets: 60 mg

INDICATIONS & DOSAGES
➤ **To prevent or treat osteoporosis**
Postmenopausal women: 60 mg P.O. once daily.

ACTION

Reduces resorption of bone and decreases overall bone turnover. These effects on bone are manifested as reductions in serum and urine levels of bone turnover markers and increases in bone mineral density.

Route	Onset	Peak	Duration
P.O.	Unknown	Unknown	24 hr

Half-life: 27½ hours.

ADVERSE REACTIONS

CNS: depression, insomnia, fever, migraine.
CV: chest pain.
EENT: *sinusitis,* pharyngitis, laryngitis.
GI: nausea, dyspepsia, vomiting, flatulence, gastroenteritis, abdominal pain.
GU: vaginitis, UTI, cystitis, leukorrhea, endometrial disorder, vaginal bleeding.
Metabolic: weight gain.
Musculoskeletal: *arthralgia,* myalgia, arthritis, leg cramps.
Respiratory: increased cough, pneumonia.
Skin: rash, diaphoresis.
Other: *infection, flulike syndrome, hot flashes,* breast pain, peripheral edema.

INTERACTIONS

Drug-drug. *Cholestyramine:* May cause significant reduction in absorption of raloxifene. Avoid using together.
Highly protein-bound drugs (such as clofibrate, diazepam, diazoxide, ibuprofen, indomethacin, naproxen): May interfere with binding sites. Use together cautiously.
Warfarin: May cause a decrease in PT. Monitor PT and INR closely.

EFFECTS ON LAB TEST RESULTS

- May increase calcium, inorganic phosphate, total protein, albumin, hormone-binding globulin, and apolipoprotein A levels. May decrease total and LDL cholesterol levels and apolipoprotein B levels.

CONTRAINDICATIONS & CAUTIONS

- Contraindicated in women hypersensitive to drug or its components; in those with past or current venous thromboembolic events, including deep vein thrombosis, pulmonary embolism, and retinal vein thrombosis; in women who are pregnant, planning to get pregnant, or breast-feeding; and in children.
- Use cautiously in patients with severe hepatic impairment.
- Safety and efficacy of drug haven't been evaluated in men.

NURSING CONSIDERATIONS

- Watch for signs of blood clots. Greatest risk of thromboembolic events occurs during first 4 months of treatment.
- Stop drug at least 72 hours before prolonged immobilization and resume only after patient is fully mobilized.
- Report unexplained uterine bleeding; drug isn't known to cause endometrial proliferation.
- Watch for breast abnormalities; drug isn't known to cause an increased risk of breast cancer.
- Effect on bone mineral density beyond 2 years of drug treatment isn't known.
- Use with hormone replacement therapy or systemic estrogen hasn't been evaluated and isn't recommended.

PATIENT TEACHING

- Advise patient to avoid long periods of restricted movement (such as during traveling) because of increased risk of venous thromboembolic events.
- Inform patient that hot flashes or flushing may occur and that drug doesn't aid in reducing them.
- Instruct patient to practice other bone loss–prevention measures, including taking supplemental calcium and vitamin D if dietary intake is inadequate, performing weight-bearing exercises, and stopping alcohol consumption and smoking.
- Tell patient that drug may be taken without regard to food.
- Advise patient to report unexplained uterine bleeding or breast abnormalities during therapy.
- Explain adverse reactions and instruct patient to read patient package insert before starting therapy and each time prescription is renewed.

riluzole

Rilutek

Pharmacologic class: benzothiazole
Pregnancy risk category C

AVAILABLE FORMS

Tablets: 50 mg

INDICATIONS & DOSAGES

➤ **Amyotrophic lateral sclerosis**

Adults: 50 mg P.O. q 12 hours, taken on empty stomach 1 hour before or 2 hours after a meal.

ACTION

May protect motor neurons from excitotoxic effects of glutamate by inhibiting glutamate release, inactivating some sodium channels, and interfering with transmitter binding.

Route	Onset	Peak	Duration
P.O.	Unknown	Unknown	Unknown

Half-life: 12 hours with repeated doses.

ADVERSE REACTIONS

CNS: *asthenia,* headache, aggravation reaction, hypertonia, depression, dizziness, insomnia, malaise, somnolence, vertigo, circumoral paresthesia.
CV: hypertension, tachycardia, palpitations, orthostatic hypotension.
EENT: rhinitis, sinusitis.
GI: *nausea,* abdominal pain, vomiting, dyspepsia, anorexia, diarrhea, flatulence, stomatitis, dry mouth, oral candidiasis.
GU: UTI, dysuria.
Metabolic: weight loss.
Musculoskeletal: back pain, arthralgia.
Respiratory: *decreased lung function,* increased cough.
Skin: pruritus, eczema, alopecia, exfoliative dermatitis.
Other: phlebitis, peripheral edema, tooth disorder.

INTERACTIONS

Drug-drug. *Allopurinol, methyldopa, sulfasalazine:* May increase risk of hepatotoxicity. Monitor liver function closely.
Cytochrome P-450 inducers (omeprazole, rifampin): May increase riluzole elimination. Monitor for lack of effect.
Cytochrome P-450 inhibitors (amitriptyline, caffeine, phenacetin, quinolones, theophylline): May decrease riluzole elimination. Watch for adverse effects.
Drug-food. *Any food:* May decrease drug bioavailability. Advise patient to take drug 1 hour before or 2 hours after meals.
Charbroiled foods: May increase elimination of drug. Discourage use together.
Drug-lifestyle. *Alcohol use:* May increase risk of hepatotoxicity. Discourage excessive use.
Smoking: May increase drug elimination. Discourage patient from smoking.

EFFECTS ON LAB TEST RESULTS

- May increase AST, ALT, bilirubin, and GGT levels.

CONTRAINDICATIONS & CAUTIONS

- Contraindicated in patients with history of severe hypersensitivity to drug or its components.
- Use cautiously in patients with hepatic or renal dysfunction, in elderly patients, and in women and Japanese patients who may have lower metabolic capacity to eliminate drug than men and white patients, respectively.

NURSING CONSIDERATIONS

- Elevated baseline liver function studies (especially bilirubin) rule out therapy. Perform liver function studies periodically during therapy. In many patients, drug may increase aminotransferase level; if level exceeds five times upper limit of normal or if clinical jaundice develops, notify prescriber.
- Give drug at least 1 hour before or 2 hours after meals to avoid decreased bioavailability.

PATIENT TEACHING

- Tell patient to take drug at same time each day. If a dose is missed, tell him to take next tablet when planned.
- Instruct patient to take drug on an empty stomach to facilitate full dose absorption.
- Instruct patient to report fever to prescriber, who may order a WBC count.

• Warn patient to avoid hazardous activities until CNS effects of drug are known and to limit alcohol use during therapy.
• Tell patient to store drug at room temperature, protect from bright light, and keep out of children's reach.

sildenafil citrate
Viagra

Pharmacologic class: phosphodiesterase type-5 inhibitor
Pregnancy risk category B

AVAILABLE FORMS
Tablets: 25 mg, 50 mg, 100 mg

INDICATIONS & DOSAGES
➤ **Erectile dysfunction**
Adults younger than age 65: About 1 hour before sexual activity, 50 mg P.O., p.r.n. Dosage range is 25 to 100 mg based on effectiveness and tolerance. Maximum is one dose daily.
Elderly patients (age 65 and older): 25 mg P.O., p.r.n., about 1 hour before sexual activity. Dosage may be adjusted based on patient response. Maximum is one dose daily.
Adjust-a-dose: For adults with hepatic or severe renal impairment, 25 mg P.O. about 1 hour before sexual activity. Dosage may be adjusted based on patient response. Maximum is one dose daily.

ACTION
Increases effect of nitric oxide by inhibiting phosphodiesterase type 5 (PDE_5), which is responsible for degradation of cyclic guanosine monophosphate (cGMP) in the corpus cavernosum. When sexual stimulation causes local release of nitric oxide, inhibition of PDE_5 by sildenafil causes increased levels of cGMP in the corpus cavernosum, resulting in smooth muscle relaxation and inflow of blood to the corpus cavernosum.

Route	Onset	Peak	Duration
P.O.	15–30 min	30–120 min	4 hr

Half-life: 4 hours.

ADVERSE REACTIONS
CNS: *headache,* ***seizures,*** anxiety, dizziness, somnolence, vertigo.
CV: ***MI, sudden cardiac death, ventricular arrhythmias, cerebrovascular hemorrhage, transient ischemic attack,*** hypotension, flushing.
EENT: diplopia, temporary vision loss, ocular redness or bloodshot appearance, increased intraocular pressure, retinal vascular disease, retinal bleeding, vitreous detachment or traction, paramacular edema, photophobia, altered color perception, blurred vision, burning, swelling, pressure, nasal congestion.
GI: *dyspepsia,* diarrhea.
GU: hematuria, prolonged erection, priapism, UTI.
Musculoskeletal: arthralgia, back pain.
Respiratory: respiratory tract infection.
Skin: rash.
Other: flulike syndrome.

INTERACTIONS
Drug-drug. *Beta blockers, loop and potassium-sparing diuretics:* May increase sildenafil metabolite level. Monitor patient.
Cytochrome P-450 inducers, rifampin: May reduce sildenafil level. Monitor effect.
Delavirdine, protease inhibitors: May increase sildenafil level, increasing risk of adverse events, including hypotension, visual changes, and priapism. Reduce initial sildenafil dose to 25 mg.
Hepatic isoenzyme inhibitors (such as cimetidine, erythromycin, itraconazole, ketoconazole): May reduce sildenafil clearance. Avoid using together.
Isosorbide, nitroglycerin: May cause severe hypotension. Use of nitrates in any form with sildenafil is contraindicated.
Drug-food. *High-fat meal:* May reduce absorption rate and peak level of drug. Advise patient to take drug on empty stomach.
Grapefruit: May increase drug level, while delaying absorption. Advise patient to avoid using together.

EFFECTS ON LAB TEST RESULTS
None reported.

CONTRAINDICATIONS & CAUTIONS

- Contraindicated in patients hypersensitive to drug or its components and in those taking organic nitrates.
- Use cautiously in patients age 65 and older; in patients with hepatic or severe renal impairment, retinitis pigmentosa, bleeding disorders, or active peptic ulcer disease; in those who have suffered an MI, a stroke, or life-threatening arrhythmia within last 6 months; in those with history of cardiac failure, coronary artery disease, uncontrolled high or low blood pressure, or anatomic deformation of the penis (such as angulation, cavernosal fibrosis, or Peyronie disease); and in those with conditions that may predispose them to priapism (such as sickle cell anemia, multiple myeloma, or leukemia).

NURSING CONSIDERATIONS

- ***Alert:*** Drug increases risk of cardiac events. Systemic vasodilatory properties cause transient decreases in supine blood pressure and cardiac output (about 2 hours after ingestion). Patients with underlying CV disease are at increased risk for cardiac effects related to sexual activity.
- ***Alert:*** Serious CV events, including MI, sudden cardiac death, ventricular arrhythmias, cerebrovascular hemorrhage, transient ischemic attack, and hypertension, may occur with drug use. Most, but not all, of these incidents involve CV risk factors. Many events occur during or shortly after sexual activity; a few occur shortly after drug use without sexual activity; and others occur hours to days after drug use and sexual activity.
- Drug isn't indicated for use in newborns, children, or women.

PATIENT TEACHING

- Advise patient that drug shouldn't be used with nitrates under any circumstances.
- Advise patient of potential cardiac risk of sexual activity, especially in presence of CV risk factors. Instruct patient to notify prescriber and refrain from further activity if such symptoms as chest pain, dizziness, or nausea occur when starting sexual activity.
- Warn patient that erections lasting longer than 4 hours and priapism (painful erections lasting longer than 6 hours) may occur, and tell him to seek immediate medical attention. Penile tissue damage and permanent loss of potency may result if priapism isn't treated immediately.
- Inform patient that drug doesn't protect against sexually transmitted diseases; advise patient to use protective measures such as condoms.
- Tell patient receiving HIV medications that he's at increased risk for sildenafil adverse events, including low blood pressure, visual changes, and priapism, and that he should promptly report such symptoms to his prescriber. Tell him not to exceed 25 mg of sildenafil in 48 hours.
- Instruct patient to take drug 30 minutes to 4 hours before sexual activity; maximum benefit can be expected less than 2 hours after ingestion.
- Advise patient that drug is most rapidly absorbed if taken on an empty stomach.
- Inform patient that impairment of color discrimination (blue, green) may occur and to avoid hazardous activities that rely on color discrimination.
- Instruct patient to notify prescriber of visual changes.
- Advise patient that drug is effective only in presence of sexual stimulation.
- Caution patient to take drug only as prescribed.

tacrolimus (topical)

Protopic

Pharmacologic class: macrolide
Pregnancy risk category C

AVAILABLE FORMS

Ointment: 0.03%, 0.1%

INDICATIONS & DOSAGES

➤ **Moderate to severe atopic dermatitis in patients unresponsive to other therapies or unable to use other therapies because of potential risks**

Adults: Thin layer of 0.03% or 0.1% strength applied to affected areas b.i.d. and rubbed in completely. Continue for 1 week after affected area clears.

Children age 2 and older: Thin layer of 0.03% strength applied to affected areas b.i.d. and rubbed in completely. Continue for 1 week after affected area clears.

ACTION

Unknown. Probably acts as an immune system modulator in the skin by inhibiting T-lymphocyte activation, which causes immunosuppression. Drug also inhibits the release of mediators from mast cells and basophils in skin.

Route	Onset	Peak	Duration
Topical	Unknown	Unknown	Unknown

Half-life: Unknown.

ADVERSE REACTIONS

CNS: *headache,* hyperesthesia, asthenia, insomnia.
CV: peripheral edema.
EENT: *otitis media, pharyngitis,* rhinitis, sinusitis, conjunctivitis.
GI: diarrhea, vomiting, nausea, abdominal pain, gastroenteritis, dyspepsia.
GU: dysmenorrhea.
Musculoskeletal: back pain, myalgia.
Respiratory: *increased cough, asthma,* pneumonia, bronchitis.
Skin: *burning, pruritus, erythema, infection, herpes simplex,* eczema herpeticum, pustular rash, *folliculitis,* urticaria, maculopapular rash, fungal dermatitis, acne, sunburn, tingling, benign skin neoplasm, vesiculobullous rash, dry skin, varicella zoster, herpes zoster, eczema, exfoliative dermatitis, contact dermatitis.
Other: *flulike symptoms, accidental injury, infection,* facial edema, alcohol intolerance, periodontal abscess, cyst, *allergic reaction, fever,* pain, lymphadenopathy.

INTERACTIONS

Drug-drug. ***Calcium channel blockers, cimetidine, CYP3A4 inhibitors (erythromycin, itraconazole, ketoconazole, fluconazole):*** May interfere with effects of tacrolimus. Use together cautiously.
Drug-lifestyle. *Sun exposure:* May cause phototoxicity. Advise patient to avoid excessive sunlight or artificial ultraviolet light exposure.

EFFECTS ON LAB TEST RESULTS

None reported.

CONTRAINDICATIONS & CAUTIONS

- Contraindicated in patients hypersensitive to drug.
- Don't use in immunocompromised patients or in patients with Netherton syndrome or generalized erythroderma.
- ***Alert:*** Use only after other therapies have failed because of the risk of cancer.

NURSING CONSIDERATIONS

- Use drug only for short-term or intermittent long-term therapy.
- In patients with infected atopic dermatitis, clear infections at treatment site before using drug.
- Don't use with occlusive dressings.
- Use of this drug may increase the risk of varicella zoster, herpes simplex virus, and eczema herpeticum.
- Consider stopping drug in patients with lymphadenopathy if cause is unknown or acute mononucleosis is diagnosed.
- Monitor all cases of lymphadenopathy until resolution.
- Local adverse effects are most common during the first few days of treatment.
- Use only the 0.03% ointment in children ages 2 to 15.

PATIENT TEACHING

- Tell patient to wash hands before and after applying drug and to avoid applying drug to wet skin.
- Urge patient not to use bandages or other occlusive dressings.
- Tell patient not to bathe, shower, or swim immediately after application because doing so could wash the ointment off.
- Tell patient to continue treatment for 1 week after affected area clears.
- Advise patient to avoid or minimize exposure to natural or artificial sunlight.
- Caution patient not to use drug for any disorder other than that for which it was prescribed.
- Encourage patient to report adverse reactions.
- Tell patient to store the ointment at room temperature.

tadalafil

Cialis

Pharmacologic class: phosphodiesterase type-5 inhibitor
Pregnancy risk category B

AVAILABLE FORMS

Tablets (film-coated): 5 mg, 10 mg, 20 mg

INDICATIONS & DOSAGES

➤ **Erectile dysfunction**

Adults: 10 mg P.O. as a single dose, p.r.n., before sexual activity. Range is 5 to 20 mg, based on effectiveness and tolerance. Maximum is one dose daily.
Adjust-a-dose: If creatinine clearance is 31 to 50 ml/minute, starting dosage is 5 mg once daily and maximum is 10 mg once q 48 hours. If clearance is 30 ml/minute or less, maximum is 5 mg once daily. Patients with Child-Pugh category A or B shouldn't exceed 10 mg daily. Patients taking potent cytochrome P-450 inhibitors (such as erythromycin, itraconazole, ketoconazole, and ritonavir) shouldn't exceed one 10-mg dose q 72 hours.

ACTION

By preventing breakdown of cGMP by phosphodiesterase, drug increases cGMP levels, prolongs smooth muscle relaxation, and promotes blood flow into the corpus cavernosum.

Route	Onset	Peak	Duration
P.O.	Immediate	½–6 hr	Unknown

Half-life: 17½ hours.

ADVERSE REACTIONS

CNS: *headache.*
CV: flushing.
EENT: nasal congestion.
GI: *dyspepsia.*
Musculoskeletal: back pain, limb pain, myalgia.

INTERACTIONS

Drug-drug. *Alpha blockers (except 0.4 mg tamsulosin daily), nitrates:* May enhance hypotensive effects. Use together is contraindicated.
Potent cytochrome P-450 inhibitors (such as erythromycin, itraconazole, ketoconazole, ritonavir): May increase tadalafil level. Patient shouldn't exceed a 10-mg dose q 72 hours.
Rifampin and other cytochrome P-450 inducers: May decrease tadalafil level. Monitor patient closely.
Drug-food. *Grapefruit:* May increase drug level. Discourage use together.
Drug-lifestyle. *Alcohol use:* May increase risk of headache, dizziness, orthostatic hypotension, and increased heart rate. Discourage use together.

EFFECTS ON LAB TEST RESULTS

None reported.

CONTRAINDICATIONS & CAUTIONS

- Contraindicated in patients hypersensitive to drug or its components and in those taking nitrates or alpha blockers (other than tamsulosin 0.4 mg once daily).
- Drug isn't recommended for patients with Child-Pugh category C, unstable angina, angina that occurs during sexual intercourse, New York Heart Association class II or greater heart failure within past 6 months, uncontrolled arrhythmias, hypotension (lower than 90/50 mm Hg), uncontrolled hypertension (higher than 170/100 mm Hg), stroke within past 6 months, or an MI within past 90 days.
- Drug isn't recommended for patients whose cardiac status makes sexual activity inadvisable or for those with hereditary degenerative retinal disorders.
- Use cautiously in patients taking potent Cytochrome P-450 inhibitors (such as erythromycin, itraconazole, ketoconazole, and ritonavir) and in patients with bleeding disorders, significant peptic ulceration, or renal or hepatic impairment.
- Use cautiously in patients with conditions predisposing them to priapism (such as sickle cell anemia, multiple myeloma, and leukemia), anatomical penis abnormalities, or left ventricular outflow obstruction.
- Use cautiously in elderly patients, who may be more sensitive to drug effects.

NURSING CONSIDERATIONS

- ***Alert:*** Sexual activity may increase cardiac risk. Evaluate patient's cardiac risk before he starts taking drug.
- Before patient starts drug, assess him for underlying causes of erectile dysfunction.
- Transient decreases in supine blood pressure may occur.
- Prolonged erections and priapism may occur.

PATIENT TEACHING

- Warn patient that taking drug with nitrates could cause a serious drop in blood pressure, which increases the risk of heart attack or stroke.
- Tell patient to seek immediate medical attention if chest pain develops after taking the drug.
- Tell patient that drug doesn't protect against sexually transmitted diseases and that he should use protective measures.
- Urge patient to seek emergency medical care if his erection lasts more than 4 hours.
- Tell patient to take drug about 60 minutes before anticipated sexual activity. Explain that drug has no effect without sexual stimulation.
- Warn patient not to change dosage unless directed by prescriber.
- Caution patient against drinking large amounts of alcohol while taking drug.

tamsulosin hydrochloride

Flomax

Pharmacologic class: alpha blocker
Pregnancy risk category B

AVAILABLE FORMS

Capsules: 0.4 mg

INDICATIONS & DOSAGES

➤ BPH

Adults: 0.4 mg P.O. once daily, given 30 minutes after same meal each day. If no response after 2 to 4 weeks, increase dosage to 0.8 mg P.O. once daily.

ACTION

Selectively blocks alpha receptors in the prostate, leading to relaxation of smooth muscles in the bladder neck and prostate, improving urine flow and reducing symptoms of BPH.

Route	Onset	Peak	Duration
P.O.	Unknown	4–5 hr	9–15 hr

Half-life: 9 to 13 hours.

ADVERSE REACTIONS

CNS: *dizziness, headache,* asthenia, insomnia, somnolence, syncope, vertigo.
CV: chest pain, orthostatic hypotension.
EENT: *rhinitis,* amblyopia, pharyngitis, sinusitis.
GI: diarrhea, nausea.
GU: decreased libido, abnormal ejaculation, priapism.
Musculoskeletal: back pain.
Respiratory: increased cough.
Other: *infection,* tooth disorder.

INTERACTIONS

Drug-drug. *Alpha blockers:* May interact with tamsulosin. Avoid using together.
Cimetidine: May decrease tamsulosin clearance. Use together cautiously.

EFFECTS ON LAB TEST RESULTS

None reported.

CONTRAINDICATIONS & CAUTIONS

- Contraindicated in patients hypersensitive to drug or its components.

NURSING CONSIDERATIONS

- Monitor patient for decreases in blood pressure.
- Symptoms of BPH and prostate cancer are similar; rule out prostate cancer before starting therapy.
- If treatment is interrupted for several days or more, restart therapy at 1 capsule daily.
- ***Look alike–sound alike:*** Don't confuse Flomax with Fosamax or Volmax.

PATIENT TEACHING

- Instruct patient not to crush, chew, or open capsules.
- Tell patient to rise slowly from chair or bed when starting therapy and to avoid situations in which injury could occur as a result of fainting. Advise him that drug may cause sudden drop in blood pressure,

especially after first dose or when changing doses.

- Inform patient about the rare, but serious, possibility of priapism.
- Instruct patient not to drive or perform hazardous tasks for 12 hours after first dose or changes in dose until response can be monitored.
- Tell patient to take drug about 30 minutes after same meal each day.
- Advise patient undergoing cataract surgery to tell the surgeon that he is taking an alpha blocker.

tretinoin (retinoic acid, vitamin A acid)

Avita, Renova, Retin-A, Retin-A Micro, StieVA-A†

Pharmacologic class: retinoid
Pregnancy risk category C

AVAILABLE FORMS

Cream: 0.02%, 0.025%, 0.05%, 0.1%
Gel: 0.01%, 0.025%
Microsphere gel: 0.04%, 0.1%
Solution: 0.05%

INDICATIONS & DOSAGES

➤ Acne vulgaris
Adults and children: Clean affected area and lightly apply once daily at bedtime.

➤ Adjunctive use in the mitigation of fine facial wrinkles in patients who use comprehensive skin care and sunlight avoidance programs
Adults: Apply a small, pearl-sized amount (¼ inch or 5 mm in diameter) to cover affected area lightly, once daily in the evening.

ACTION

Inhibits comedones by increasing epidermal cell mitosis and turnover.

Route	Onset	Peak	Duration
Topical	Unknown	Unknown	Unknown

Half-life: Unknown.

ADVERSE REACTIONS

Skin: *feeling of warmth, slight stinging, local erythema, peeling,* chapping, swelling, blistering, crusting, temporary hyperpigmentation or hypopigmentation.

INTERACTIONS

Drug-drug. *Topical drugs containing benzoyl peroxide, resorcinol, salicylic acid, or sulfur:* May increase risk of skin irritation. Avoid using together.
Topical minoxidil or photosensitizing drugs (fluoroquinolones, phenothiazines, sulfonamides, tetracyclines, thiazides): May increase risk of skin irritation. Avoid using together.
Drug-lifestyle. *Abrasive cleansers, medicated cosmetics, skin preparations containing alcohol:* May increase risk of skin irritation. Discourage use together.
Sun exposure: May increase photosensitivity reaction. Advise patient to avoid excessive sunlight exposure.

EFFECTS ON LAB TEST RESULTS

None reported.

CONTRAINDICATIONS & CAUTIONS

- Contraindicated in patients hypersensitive to drug or its components and in those with sunburn.
- Use cautiously in patients with eczema.

NURSING CONSIDERATIONS

- Initially, drug may be applied every 2 to 3 days using a lower concentration to reduce irritation.
- Relapses typically occur within 3 to 6 weeks after therapy is stopped.
- ***Look alike–sound alike:*** Don't confuse tretinoin with trientine.

PATIENT TEACHING

- Instruct patient to clean area thoroughly before application and to avoid getting drug in eyes, mouth, or mucous membranes.
- Tell patient to wash hands after application.
- Tell patient to wash face with mild soap no more than b.i.d. or t.i.d. Warn patient against using strong or medicated cosmetics, soaps, or other skin cleansers. Also advise him to avoid topical products containing alcohol, astringents, spices, and lime because they may interfere with drug's actions.

- Tell patient using drug for treatment of fine wrinkles to wait 20 minutes after washing face to apply drug, and to avoid washing face or applying another skin product or cosmetic for 1 hour after application.
- Tell patient that normal use of cosmetics is allowed.
- Advise patient not to stop drug if temporary worsening of inflammatory lesions occurs. If severe local irritation develops, advise patient to stop drug temporarily and notify prescriber. Dosage will be readjusted when application is resumed. Some redness and scaling are normal reactions.
- Warn patient that he may experience increased sensitivity to wind or cold temperatures.
- Instruct patient to minimize exposure to sunlight or ultraviolet rays during treatment. If he becomes sunburned, he should delay therapy until sunburn subsides. Tell patient who can't avoid exposure to sunlight to use SPF-15 sunblock and to wear protective clothing.
- Warn patient that he may have a temporary increase in lesions, which will improve in 2 to 3 weeks.

vardenafil hydrochloride

Levitra

Pharmacologic class: phosphodiesterase type-5 inhibitor
Pregnancy risk category B

AVAILABLE FORMS

Tablets (film-coated): 2.5 mg, 5 mg, 10 mg, 20 mg

INDICATIONS & DOSAGES

➤Erectile dysfunction

Adults: 10 mg P.O. as a single dose, p.r.n., 1 hour before sexual activity. Dosage range is 5 to 20 mg, based on effectiveness and tolerance. Maximum, one dose daily.
Elderly patients age 65 and older: Initially 5 mg as a single dose, p.r.n., 1 hour before sexual activity.
Adjust-a-dose: For patients with Child-Pugh category B, first dose is 5 mg daily, p.r.n. Don't exceed 10 mg daily in patients with hepatic impairment.

ACTION

Increases cGMP levels, prolongs smooth muscle relaxation, and promotes blood flow into the corpus cavernosum.

Route	Onset	Peak	Duration
P.O.	Immediate	30–120 min	Unknown

Half-life: 4 to 5 hours.

ADVERSE REACTIONS

CNS: *headache,* dizziness.
CV: *flushing.*
EENT: rhinitis, sinusitis.
GI: dyspepsia, nausea.
Musculoskeletal: back pain.
Other: flulike syndrome.

INTERACTIONS

Drug-drug. *Alpha blockers, nitrates:* May enhance hypotensive effects. Avoid using together.
Antiarrhythmics of class IA (quinidine, procainamide) and class III (amiodarone, sotalol): May prolong QTc interval. Avoid using together.
Erythromycin, indinavir, itraconazole, ketoconazole, ritonavir: May increase vardenafil level. Reduce dose of vardenafil. If taken with ritonavir, reduce and extend dosage interval to once every 72 hours.
Drug-food. *High-fat meals:* May reduce peak level of drug. Discourage use with a high-fat meal.

EFFECTS ON LAB TEST RESULTS

- May increase CK level.

CONTRAINDICATIONS & CAUTIONS

- Contraindicated in patients hypersensitive to drug or its components and in those taking nitrates or alpha blockers.
- Contraindicated in patients with unstable angina, hypotension (systolic less than 90 mm Hg), uncontrolled hypertension (over 170/110 mm Hg), stroke, life-threatening arrhythmia, an MI within past 6 months, severe cardiac failure, Child-Pugh category C, end-stage renal disease requiring dialysis, congenital QTc-interval prolongation, or hereditary degenerative retinal disorders.
- Use cautiously in patients with bleeding disorders or significant peptic ulceration.

• Use cautiously in those with anatomical penis abnormalities or conditions that predispose patient to priapism (such as sickle cell anemia, multiple myeloma, or leukemia).

NURSING CONSIDERATIONS

• ***Alert:*** Sexual activity may increase cardiac risk. Evaluate patient's cardiac risk before he starts taking drug.
• Before patient starts drug, assess for underlying causes of erectile dysfunction.
• Transient decreases in supine blood pressure may occur.
• Prolonged erections and priapism may occur.

PATIENT TEACHING

• Tell patient that drug doesn't protect against sexually transmitted diseases and that he should use protective measures.
• Advise patient that drug is absorbed most rapidly if taken on an empty stomach.
• Tell patient to notify prescriber about visual changes.
• Urge patient to seek immediate medical care if erection lasts more than 4 hours.
• Tell patient to take drug 60 minutes before anticipated sexual activity. Explain that drug has no effect without sexual stimulation.
• Warn patient not to change dosage unless directed by prescriber.

✱ NEW DRUG

varenicline

Chantix✐

Pharmacologic class: nicotinic acetylcholine receptor partial agonist
Pregnancy risk category C

AVAILABLE FORMS

Tablets: 0.5 mg, 1 mg

INDICATIONS & DOSAGES

➤ Smoking cessation

Adults: Starting 1 week before patient stops smoking, give 0.5 mg P.O. once daily on days 1 through 3. Days 4 through 7, give 0.5 mg P.O. b.i.d. Day 8 through the end of week 12, give 1 mg P.O. b.i.d. If patient successfully stops smoking, give an additional 12-week course to help with long-term success.

Adjust-a-dose: In patient with renal impairment, 0.5 mg P.O. once daily. Adjust as needed to maximum of 0.5 mg b.i.d. In patient with end-stage renal disease who is undergoing dialysis, 0.5 mg once daily.

ACTION

Blocks the effects of nicotine by binding at alpha$_4$beta$_2$ neuronal nicotinic acetylcholine receptors. Drug also provides some of nicotine's effects to ease withdrawal.

Route	Onset	Peak	Duration
P.O.	4 days	3–4 hr	24 hr

Half-life: 24 hours.

ADVERSE REACTIONS

CNS: *abnormal dreams, headache, insomnia,* altered attention or emotions, anxiety, asthenia, depression, dizziness, fatigue, irritability, lethargy, malaise, nightmares, restlessness, sensory disturbance, sleep disorder, somnolence.
CV: chest pain, edema, hot flush, hypertension.
EENT: altered taste, epistaxis.
GI: *nausea,* abdominal pain, constipation, diarrhea, dry mouth, dyspepsia, flatulence, gingivitis, vomiting.
GU: menstrual disorder, polyuria.
Metabolic: decreased appetite, increased appetite, thirst.
Musculoskeletal: arthralgia, back pain, muscle cramps, myalgia.
Respiratory: dyspnea, upper respiratory tract disorder.
Skin: rash.
Other: flulike illness.

INTERACTIONS

Drug-drug. *Nicotine-replacement therapy:* May increase nausea, vomiting, dizziness, dyspepsia, and fatigue. Monitor patient closely.

EFFECTS ON LAB TEST RESULTS

• May increase liver function test values.

CONTRAINDICATIONS & CAUTIONS

- Use cautiously in pregnant or breast-feeding women, elderly patients, and patients with severe renal impairment.

NURSING CONSIDERATIONS

- Assess patient's readiness and motivation to stop smoking.
- Notify prescriber if patient develops intolerable nausea; dosage reduction may be needed.
- Temporarily monitor levels of drugs—such as theophylline, warfarin, and insulin—after patient stops smoking to be sure levels are still within therapeutic range.

PATIENT TEACHING

- Provide patient with educational materials and needed counseling.
- Instruct patient to choose a date to stop smoking and to begin treatment 1 week before this date.
- Advise patient to take each dose with a full glass of water after eating.
- Teach patient to gradually increase the dose over the first week to a target of 1 mg in the morning and 1 mg in the evening.
- Explain that nausea and insomnia are common and usually temporary. Urge him to contact the prescriber if adverse effects are persistently troubling; a dosage reduction may help.
- Urge patient to continue trying to abstain from smoking if he has early lapses after successfully quitting.
- Tell patient that dosages of other drugs he takes may need adjustment when he stops smoking.
- If woman plans to become pregnant or to breast-feed, explain the risks of smoking and the risks and benefits of taking drug to aid smoking cessation.

Abbreviations to avoid

The Joint Commission requires every health care facility to develop a list of approved abbreviations for staff use. Certain abbreviations should be avoided because they're easily misunderstood, especially when handwritten. The Joint Commission has identified a minimum list of dangerous abbreviations, acronyms, and symbols. This do-not-use list includes the following items.

Abbreviation	Intended meaning	Misinterpretation	Correction
U or *u*	unit	Frequently misinterpreted as a "0" or a "4," causing a tenfold or greater overdose	Write "unit."
IU	international unit	Frequently misinterpreted as I.V. or 10	Write "international unit."
q.d., q.o.d.	every day, every other day	Mistaken for each other. The period after the "q" has sometimes been misinterpreted as "i," the "o" can be mistaken for "i," and the drug has been given q.i.d. rather than daily.	Write them out.
Trailing zero (5.0 mg)	5 mg	Frequently misinterpreted dosage, such as: 50 mg	Never write a zero by itself after a decimal point and always use a zero before a decimal point if no other number is present.
Lack of leading zero (.5 mg)	0.5 mg	5 mg	
MS, MSO_4, $MgSO_4$	morphine sulfate magnesium sulfate	Confused with each other	Write "morphine sulfate" or "magnesium sulfate."

The Joint Commission, 2007. Reprinted with permission.

(continued)

In addition to the minimum required list, the following items should also be considered when expanding the do-not-use list.

Abbreviation	Intended meaning	Misinterpretation	Correction
MTX	methotrexate	Misinterpreted as Mustargen (mechlorethamine hydrochloride)	Use the complete spelling for drug names.
DIG	digoxin	Misinterpreted as digitoxin	Use the complete spelling for drug names.
HCTZ	hydrochlorothiazide	Misinterpreted as hydrocortisone (HCT)	Use the complete spelling for drug names.
ara-A	vidarabine	Misinterpreted as cytarabine (ara-C)	Use the complete spelling for drug names.
µg	microgram	Frequently misinterpreted as "mg"	Write "mcg."
cc	cubic centimeter	Frequently misinterpreted as U (units)	Write "ml" for milliliters.
A.S., A.D., and AU	Latin abbreviations for left ear, right ear, and both ears, respectfully	Frequently misinterpreted as O.S., O.D., and OU	Write "left ear," "right ear," or "both ears."
OD	once daily	Frequently misinterpreted as "O.D." (*oculus dexter*—right eye)	Don't abbreviate "daily." Write it out.
OJ	orange juice	Frequently misinterpreted as "O.D." (*oculus dexter*—right eye) or "O.S." (*oculus sinister*—left eye) Drugs meant to be diluted in orange juice may be given in the eye.	Write it out.
qn.	nightly or at bedtime	Frequently misinterpreted as "q.h." (every hour)	Write out "nightly" or "at bedtime."
S.C. SQ	subcutaneous	Mistaken as SL for sublingual or "5 every"	Use "SubQ," "subQ," or write out "subcutaneous."
D/C	discharge or discontinue	Frequently misinterpreted	Write "discharge" or "discontinue."
h.s.	half-strength or bedtime	Frequently misinterpreted as the other	Write out "half-strength" or "at bedtime."
T.I.W.	three times per week	Frequently misinterpreted as three times per day or twice weekly	Write it out.

The Joint Commission, 2007. Reprinted with permission.

Quick guide to combination drugs

This guide lists trade names and generic ingredients of common combination drugs.

222†: 375 mg aspirin, 8 mg codeine phosphate, and 30 mg caffeine citrate
282 MEP†: 375 mg aspirin, 15 mg codeine phosphate, and 30 mg caffeine citrate
292†: 375 mg aspirin, 30 mg codeine phosphate, and 30 mg caffeine citrate
692†: 375 mg aspirin, 65 mg codeine phosphate, and 30 mg caffeine citrate
Aceta with Codeine: 300 mg acetaminophen and 30 mg codeine phosphate
Act HIB/DTP: 10 mcg *Haemophilus* b polyribosylribitol phosphate (PRP) conjugated to 24 mcg tetanus toxoid, 6.7 limit flocculation (Lf) units diphtheria toxoid, 5 Lf units tetanus toxoid, and 4 units whole-cell pertussis vaccine per 0.5 ml
Advicor: 1,000 mg niacin and 20 mg lovastatin; 500 mg niacin and 20 mg lovastatin
Advil Cold and Sinus Caplets ◊ : 30 mg pseudoephedrine hydrochloride and 200 mg ibuprofen
AK-Poly-Bac ◊ : 10,000 units polymyxin B sulfate and 500 units bacitracin zinc
Alavert Allergy & Sinus D-12 Hour ◊ : 5 mg loratadine and 120 mg pseudoephedrine sulfate
Alka-Seltzer Gold ◊ : 958 mg sodium bicarbonate, 832 mg citric acid, and 312 mg potassium bicarbonate
Alka-Seltzer Original ◊ : 325 mg aspirin, 1000 mg citric acid, and 9 mg phenylalanine
Allegra-D ◊ : 60 mg fexofenadine hydrochloride and 120 mg pseudoephedrine sulfate
Allerest Maximum Strength Tablets ◊ : 30 mg pseudoephedrine hydrochloride and 2 mg chlorpheniramine maleate
Aludrox ◊ : 307 mg aluminum hydroxide and 103 mg per 5 ml magnesium hydroxide
Apresazide 25/25: 25 mg hydrochlorothiazide and 25 mg hydralazine hydrochloride
Apresazide 50/50: 50 mg hydrochlorothiazide and 50 mg hydralazine hydrochloride
Arthrotec: 50 mg diclofenac sodium and 200 mcg misoprostol; 75 mg diclofenac sodium and 200 mcg misoprostol
Ascriptin ◊ : 325 mg aspirin, 50 mg magnesium hydroxide, 50 mg aluminum hydroxide, and 50 mg calcium carbonate
Ascriptin A/D ◊ : 325 mg aspirin, 75 mg magnesium hydroxide, 75 mg aluminum hydroxide, and 75 mg calcium carbonate
BenzaClin: 1% clindamycin and 5% benzoyl peroxide
Benzamycin: 3% erythromycin and 5% benzoyl peroxide
Bicillin C-R 900/300: Injection—1.2 million units/2 ml; each milliliter contains 450,000 units penicillin G benzathine and 150,000 units penicillin G procaine
Bicillin C-R: Injection—300,000 units/ml, 600,000 units/ml, 1.2 million units/2 ml, and 2.4 million units/4 ml, containing equal volumes of penicillin G benzathine and procaine
Blephamide Sterile Ophthalmic Ointment: 10% sulfacetamide sodium and 0.2% prednisolone acetate
Bronchial Capsules: 150 mg theophylline and 90 mg guaifenesin
Bronkaid Dual Action Tablets: 25 mg ephedrine sulfate and 400 mg guaifenesin
Children's Advil Cold ◊ : 15 mg pseudoephedrine and 100 mg per 5 ml ibuprofen
Children's Advil Cold Suspension ◊ : 100 mg ibuprofen and 15 mg per 5 ml pseudoephedrine
Chlor-Trimeton Allergy-D 12-Hour Relief Tablets ◊ : 8 mg chlorpheniramine maleate and 120 mg pseudoephedrine sulfate
Chlor-Trimeton Allergy-D 4-Hour Tablets ◊ : 4 mg chlorpheniramine maleate and 60 mg pseudoephedrine sulfate
Citracal + D ◊ : 315 mg calcium with 200 units cholecalciferol

†Canada ◊ OTC.

Comvax: 7.5 mcg *Haemophilus* b PRP, 125 mcg *Neisseria meningitidis* OMPC, and 5 mcg hepatitis B surface antigen per 0.5 ml

Contac Severe Cold & Flu Caplets ◊ **:** 500 mg acetaminophen, 15 mg dextromethorphan hydrobromide, 30 mg pseudoephedrine hydrochloride, 2 mg and chlorpheniramine maleate

Coricidin 'D' Cold, Flu, & Sinus ◊ **:** 2 mg chlorpheniramine maleate, 325 mg acetaminophen, and 30 mg pseudoephedrine sulfate

Coricidin HBP Cold & Flu ◊ **:** 2 mg chlorpheniramine maleate and 325 mg acetaminophen

Cortisporin Ophthalmic Suspension: 10,000 units polymyxin B sulfate, 0.35% neomycin sulfate, and 1% hydrocortisone

Cyclomydril Ophthalmic: 0.2% cyclopentolate hydrochloride and 1% phenylephrine hydrochloride

Decadron Phosphate with Xylocaine: 4 mg dexamethasone phosphate and 10 mg per ml lidocaine hydrochloride

Deconamine ◊ **:** 60 mg pseudoephedrine hydrochloride and 4 mg chlorpheniramine maleate

Dical-D ◊ **:** 117 mg calcium (as phosphate tribasic) with 133 units cholecalciferol

Dical-D Wafers ◊ **:** 232 mg calcium (as phosphate tribasic) with 200 units cholecalciferol

Di-Gel Advanced ◊ **:** 128 mg magnesium hydroxide and 280 mg calcium carbonate, and 20 mg simethicone

Donnatal Elixir: atropine sulfate 0.0194 mg/5 ml, scopolamine hydrobromide 0.0065 mg/5 ml, 23% ethanol, hyoscyamine hydrobromide or 0.1037 mg/5 ml sulfate, and 16.2 mg/5 ml phenobarbital

Donnatal Extentabs: 0.0582 mg atropine sulfate, 0.0195 mg scopolamine hydrobromide, 0.3111 mg hyoscyamine sulfate, and 48.6 mg phenobarbital

Donnatal Tablets: 0.0194 mg atropine sulfate, 0.0065 mg scopolamine hydrobromide, 0.1037 mg hyoscyamine hydrobromide or sulfate, and 16.2 mg phenobarbital

Dristan Sinus Caplets ◊ **:** 30 mg pseudoephedrine hydrochloride and 200 mg ibuprofen

Duac: 1% clindamycin and 5% benzoyl peroxide

Dyflex-G Tablets: 200 mg dyphylline and 200 mg guaifenesin

Dyline G.G. Tablets: 200 mg dyphylline and 200 mg guaifenesin

Empirin with Codeine No. 3: 325 mg aspirin and 30 mg codeine phosphate

Empirin with Codeine No. 4: 325 mg aspirin and 60 mg codeine phosphate

Entex PSE: 120 mg pseudoephedrine and 600 mg guaifenesin

Equagesic: 200 mg meprobamate and 325 mg aspirin

Estratest: 1.25 mg esterified estrogens and 2.5 mg methyltestosterone

Estratest H.S.: 0.625 mg esterified estrogens and 1.25 mg methyltestosterone

Excedrin Extra Strength ◊ **:** 250 mg aspirin, 250 mg acetaminophen, and 65 mg caffeine

Excedrin Migraine ◊ **:** 250 mg acetaminophen, 250 mg aspirin, and 65 mg caffeine

Excedrin P.M. ◊ **:** 500 mg acetaminophen and 25 mg diphenhydramine

Extra Strength Alka-Seltzer ◊ **:** 500 mg aspirin, 1000 mg citric acid, and 1985 mg sodium bicarbonate

Ferro-Sequels ◊ **:** 50 mg ferrous fumarate and 100 mg docusate sodium

Gaviscon Tablets: 80 mg aluminum hydroxide and 20 mg magnesium trisilicate

Gelusil Tablets ◊ **:** 200 mg aluminum hydroxide, 200 mg magnesium hydroxide, and 25 mg simethicone

Glyceryl-T Capsules: 150 mg theophylline and 90 mg guaifenesin

Haley's M-O ◊ **:** 3.75 ml mineral oil and 900 mg/15 ml magnesium hydroxide

Inderide LA 80/50: 80 mg propranolol hydrochloride and 50 mg hydrochlorothiazide

Inderide LA 120/50: 120 mg propranolol hydrochloride and 50 mg hydrochlorothiazide

Inderide LA 160/50: 160 mg propranolol hydrochloride and 50 mg hydrochlorothiazide

Kaodene Nonnarcotic ◊ **:** 3.9 g kaolin and 194.4 mg pectin in 30-ml bismuth subsalicylate liquid

Kapectolin ◊ **:** 90 g kaolin and 2 g pectin in 30-ml suspension

†Canada ◊ OTC.

Kolyum: 20 mEq potassium, 3.4 mEq/15 ml chloride (from potassium gluconate and potassium chloride)

Librax: 5 mg chlordiazepoxide hydrochloride and 2.5 mg methscopolamine nitrate

Lotrisone: 1% clotrimazole and 0.05% betamethasone dipropionate

Maalox Extra Strength Suspension ◊ : 500 mg aluminum hydroxide, 450 mg magnesium hydroxide, and 40 mg simethicone

Maalox Suspension ◊ : 225 mg aluminum hydroxide, 200 mg magnesium hydroxide, and 25 mg simethicone

Maalox TC Suspension ◊ : 600 mg aluminum hydroxide and 300 mg/5 ml magnesium hydroxide

Magnaprin ◊ : 325 mg aspirin, 50 mg magnesium hydroxide, 50 mg aluminum hydroxide, and 50 mg calcium carbonate

Magnaprin Arthritis Strength ◊ : 325 mg aspirin, 75 mg magnesium hydroxide, 75 mg aluminum hydroxide, and 75 mg calcium carbonate

Marax: 130 mg theophylline, 25 mg ephedrine sulfate, and 10 mg hydroxyzine hydrochloride

Marax-DF Syrup: 97.5 mg theophylline, 18.75 mg ephedrine sulfate, 7.5 mg hydroxyzine hydrochloride

Maxitrol Ointment/Ophthalmic Suspension: 0.1% dexamethasone, 0.35% neomycin sulfate, and 10,000 units polymyxin B sulfate

Metimyd Ophthalmic Ointment/Suspension: 10% sulfacetamide sodium and 0.5% prednisolone acetate

Midrin: 65 mg isometheptene mucate, 100 mg dichloralphenazone, and 325 mg acetaminophen

Motrin Sinus Headache Tablets: 30 mg pseudoephedrine hydrochloride and 200 mg ibuprofen

Mudrane GG-2 Tablets: 111 mg theophylline and 100 mg guaifenesin

Murocoll-2: 0.3% scopolamine hydrobromide and 10% phenylephrine hydrochloride

Mycolog II: 0.1% triamcinolone acetonide and 100,000 units/g nystatin

Mylanta Liquid ◊ : 200 mg aluminum hydroxide, 200 mg magnesium hydroxide, and 20 mg/5 ml simethicone

Mylanta Tablets ◊ : 200 mg aluminum hydroxide, 200 mg magnesium hydroxide, and 20 mg simethicone

Neosporin G.U. Irrigant: 40 mg neomycin sulfate and 200,000 units polymyxin B sulfate per milliliter

Neosporin Ophthalmic Ointment: 10,000 units polymyxin B sulfate, 3.5 mg neomycin sulfate, and 400 units/g bacitracin zinc

Neosporin Ophthalmic Solution: 10,000 units polymyxin B sulfate, 1.75 mg neomycin sulfate, and 0.025 mg gramicidin

Neosporin Plus Pain Relief Ointment ◊ : 5,000 units polymyxin B sulfate, 400 units bacitracin zinc, and 3.5 mg/g neomycin sulfate

Neutra-phos ◊ : 250 mg phosphorus, 164 mg sodium, 278 mg potassium

Norgesic Forte: 50 mg orphenadrine citrate, 770 mg aspirin, and 60 mg caffeine

Norgesic: 25 mg orphenadrine citrate, 385 mg aspirin, and 30 mg caffeine

Novo-gesic C8 : 300 mg acetaminophen, 8 mg codeine phosphate, and 15 mg caffeine

Opcon-A Ophthalmic Solution ◊ : 0.027% naphazoline hydrochloride and 0.315% pheniramine maleate

Ornex No Drowsiness Caplets ◊ : 325 mg acetaminophen and 30 mg pseudoephedrine hydrochloride

Pepcid Complete ◊ : 800 mg calcium carbonate, 165 mg magnesium hydroxide, and 10 mg famotidine

Polysporin Ophthalmic Ointment: 10,000 units polymyxin B sulfate and 500 units bacitracin zinc

Polytrim Ophthalmic: 1 mg trimethoprim sulfate and 10,000 units/ml polymyxin B sulfate

Posture-D ◊ : 600 mg calcium (as phosphate tribasic) with 125 units cholecalciferol

Pred-G S.O.P.: 0.6% prednisolone acetate and 0.3% gentamicin sulfate equivalent to gentamicin base

Preven: 50 mcg ethinyl estradiol and 0.25 mg levonorgestrel

Primatene Tablets: 12.5 mg ephedrine hydrochloride and 200 mg guaifenesin

Prosed/DS Tablets: 81.6 mg methenamine, 36.2 mg phenyl salicylate, 0.8 mg methylene blue, 9 mg benzoic acid, 0.06 mg atropine sulfate, and 0.06 mg hyoscyamine sulfate

Pyridium Plus: 150 mg phenazopyridine, 15 mg butabarbital, and 0.3 mg hyoscyamine

Quinaretic 10/12.5: 10 mg quinapril hydrochloride and 12.5 mg hydrochlorothiazide

Quinaretic 20/12.5: 20 mg quinapril hydrochloride and 12.5 mg hydrochlorothiazide

Quinaretic 20/25: 20 mg quinapril hydrochloride and 25 mg hydrochlorothiazide

Rauzide: 4 mg bendroflumethiazide and 50 mg powdered *rauwolfia serpentina*

Renese-R: 2 mg polythiazide and 0.25 mg reserpine

Rifamate: 150 mg isoniazid and 300 mg rifampin

Rifater: 50 mg isoniazid, 120 mg rifampin, and 300 mg pyrazinamide

Riopan Plus Chewable Tablets ◊ : 480 mg magaldrate and 20 mg simethicone

Riopan Plus Double Strength Chewable Tablets ◊ : 1080 mg magaldrate and 20 mg simethicone

Semprex-D: 8 mg acrivastine and 60 mg pseudoephedrine hydrochloride

Senokot-S ◊ : 50 mg docusate sodium and 8.6 mg sennosides

Sinus-Relief ◊ : 325 mg acetaminophen and 30 mg pseudoephedrine hydrochloride

Sinutab Maximum Strength Without Drowsiness ◊ : 325 mg acetaminophen and 30 mg pseudoephedrine hydrochloride

Soma Compound: 200 mg carisoprodol and 325 mg aspirin

Soma Compound with Codeine: 200 mg carisoprodol, 325 mg aspirin, and 16 mg codeine phosphate

Synophylate-GG Syrup: 33.3 mg/5 ml guaifenesin and 100 mg/5 ml theophylline sodium glycinate

Terak with Polymyxin B Sulfate Ophthalmic Ointment: 10,000 units polymyxin B sulfate and 5 mg/g oxytetracycline hydrochloride

Theomax DF Syrup: 97.5 mg theophylline, 18.75 mg ephedrine sulfate, 7.5 mg hydroxyzine hydrochloride

Timolide 10-25: 10 mg timolol maleate and 25 mg hydrochlorothiazide

Titralac Plus ◊ : 420 mg calcium carbonate and 21 mg simethicone

TobraDex: 0.1% dexamethasone and 0.3% tobramycin

Triaminic Cold & Allergy ◊ : 15 mg pseudoephedrine hydrochloride and 1 mg chlorpheniramine maleate

Tuinal 100 mg Pulvules: 50 mg amobarbital sodium and 50 mg secobarbital sodium

Tuinal 200 mg Pulvules: 100 mg amobarbital sodium and 100 mg secobarbital sodium

Twinrix: At least 720 ELISA units inactivated hepatitis A and 20 mcg recombinant HBsAg protein per 1 ml

Tylenol PM Extra Strength ◊ : 500 mg acetaminophen, and 25 mg diphenhydramine

Ultracet: 325 mg acetaminophen and 37.5 mg tramadol hydrochloride

Urimax Tablets: 81.6 mg methenamine, 40.8 mg sodium biphosphate, 36.2 mg phenyl salicylate, 10.8 mg methylene blue, and 0.12 mg hyoscyamine sulfate

Urised Tablets: 40.8 mg methenamine, 18.1 mg phenyl salicylate, 5.4 mg methylene blue, 4.5 mg benzoic acid, 0.03 mg atropine sulfate, and 0.03 mg hyoscyamine sulfate

Vanquish ◊ : 227 mg aspirin, 194 mg acetaminophen, 33 mg caffeine, 25 mg aluminum hydroxide, and 50 mg magnesium hydroxide

Vasocidin Ophthalmic Solution: 10% sulfacetamide sodium and 0.25% prednisolone phosphate

Vicoprofen: 7.5 mg hydrocodone bitartrate and 200 mg ibuprofen

Zincfrin ◊ : 0.12% phenylephrine hydrochloride and 0.25% zinc sulfate

Zyrtec-D 12-hour Extended-Release Tablets: 5 mg cetirizine hydrochloride and 120 mg pseudoephedrine hydrochloride

Pregnancy risk categories

The FDA has assigned a pregnancy risk category to each drug based on available clinical and preclinical information. The five categories (A, B, C, D, and X) reflect a drug's potential to cause birth defects. Although drugs should ideally be avoided during pregnancy, sometimes they're needed; this rating system permits rapid assessment of the risk-benefit ratio. Drugs in category A are generally considered safe to use in pregnancy; drugs in category X are generally contraindicated.

- A: Adequate studies in pregnant women have failed to show a risk to the fetus.
- B: Animal studies haven't shown a risk to the fetus, but controlled studies haven't been conducted in pregnant women; or animal studies have shown an adverse effect on the fetus, but adequate studies in pregnant women haven't shown a risk to the fetus.
- C: Animal studies have shown an adverse effect on the fetus, but adequate studies haven't been conducted in humans. The benefits from use in pregnant women may be acceptable despite potential risks.
- D: The drug may cause risk to the fetus, but the potential benefits of use in pregnant women may be acceptable despite the risks (such as in a life-threatening situation or a serious disease for which safer drugs can't be used or are ineffective).
- X: Studies in animals or humans show fetal abnormalities, or adverse reaction reports indicate evidence of fetal risk. The risks involved clearly outweigh potential benefits.
- NR: Not rated.

Controlled substance schedules

Drugs regulated under the jurisdiction of the Controlled Substances Act of 1970 are divided into the following groups or schedules:

- Schedule I (C-I): High abuse potential and no accepted medical use. Examples include heroin, marijuana, and LSD.
- Schedule II (C-II): High abuse potential with severe dependence liability. Examples include opioids, amphetamines, and some barbiturates.
- Schedule III (C-III): Less abuse potential than schedule II drugs and moderate dependence liability. Examples include nonbarbiturate sedatives, nonamphetamine stimulants, anabolic steroids, and limited amounts of certain opioids.
- Schedule IV (C-IV): Less abuse potential than schedule III drugs and limited dependence liability. Examples include some sedatives, anxiolytics, and nonopioid analgesics.
- Schedule V (C-V): Limited abuse potential. This category includes mainly small amounts of opioids, such as codeine, used as antitussives or antidiarrheals. Under federal law, limited quantities of certain C-V drugs may be purchased without a prescription directly from a pharmacist if allowed under specific state statutes. The purchaser must be at least age 18 and must furnish suitable identification. All such transactions must be recorded by the dispensing pharmacist.

Cytochrome P-450 enzymes and common drug interactions

Cytochrome P-450 enzymes, identified by "CYP" followed by numbers and letters identifying the enzyme families and subfamilies, are found throughout the body (primarily in the liver) and are important in the metabolism of many drugs. This table lists common drug-drug interactions based on substrates, inducers, and inhibitors that can influence drug metabolism.

CYP enzyme	Substrates
1A2	acetaminophen, aminophylline, amitriptyline, betaxolol, caffeine, chlordiazepoxide, clomipramine, clozapine, cyclobenzaprine, desipramine, diazepam, doxepin, flutamide, haloperidol, imipramine, mirtazapine, olanzapine, pimozide, ropinirole, tacrine, theophylline, warfarin, zileuton
2C9	alosetron, amiodarone, amitriptyline, bosentan, carvedilol, clomipramine, dapsone, diazepam, diclofenac, flurbiprofen, fluvastatin, glimepiride, glipizide, ibuprofen, imipramine, indomethacin, losartan, mirtazapine, montelukast, naproxen, omeprazole, phenytoin, pioglitazone, piroxicam, ritonavir, sildenafil, tolbutamide, torsemide, vardenafil, voriconazole, warfarin, zafirlukast, zileuton
2C19	amitriptyline, carisoprodol, citalopram, clomipramine, cyclophosphamide, desogestrol, diazepam, doxepin, escitalopram, esomeprazole, imipramine, lansoprazole, mephenytoin, omeprazole, pantoprazole, pentamidine, phenytoin, phenobarbital, rabeprazole, voriconazole, warfarin
2D6	amitriptyline, aripiprazole, atomoxetine, betaxolol, captopril, carvedilol, chlorpheniramine, chlorpromazine, clomipramine, clozapine, codeine, cyclobenzaprine, delavirdine, desipramine, dextromethorphan, donepezil, doxepin, fentanyl, flecainide, fluoxetine, fluphenazine, fluvoxamine, haloperidol, hydrocodone, imipramine, labetalol, loratadine, maprotiline, meperidine, methadone, methamphetamine, metoprolol, mexiletine, mirtazapine, morphine, nefazodone, nortriptyline, oxycodone, paroxetine, perphenazine, procainamide, propafenone, propoxyphene, propranolol, risperidone, thioridazine, timolol, tolterodine, tramadol, trazodone, venlafaxine
3A	albuterol, alfentanil, alprazolam, amiodarone, amitriptyline, amlodipine, amprenavir, aripiprazole, atazanavir, atorvastatin, bosentan, bromocriptine, buspirone, busulfan, carbamazepine, chlordiazepoxide, chlorpheniramine, citalopram, clarithromycin, clomipramine, clonazepam, clorazepate, cocaine, colchicine, corticosteroids, cyclophosphamide, cyclosporine (neural), dapsone, delavirdine, doxorubicin, dexamethasone, diazepam, diltiazem, disopyramide, docetaxel, doxepin, doxycycline, efavirenz, enalapril, eplerenone, ergotamine, erythromycin, escitalopram, esomeprazole, estrogens, ethosuximide, etoposide, felodipine, fentanyl, fexofenadine, finasteride, flurazepam, flutamide, fluvastatin, haloperidol, ifosfamide, imatinib, imipramine, indinavir, isosorbide, isradipine, itraconazole, ketamine, ketoconazole, lansoprazole, lidocaine, loratadine, losartan, lovastatin, midazolam, methadone, methylprednisolone, miconazole, mirtazapine, montelukast, nefazodone, nevirapine, nicardipine, nifedipine, nimodipine, nisoldipine, ondansetron, paclitaxel, pantoprazole, pioglitazone, pravastatin, prednisone, quinidine, quinine, rabeprazole, rifabutin, ritonavir, saquinavir, sertraline, sildenafil, simvastatin, tacrolimus, tamoxifen, teniposide, testosterone, tolterodine, trazodone, triazolam, troleandomycin, vardenafil, verapamil, vinca alkaloids, voriconazole, warfarin, zileuton, zolpidem

Inducers	Inhibitors
carbamazepine, cigarette smoking, phenobarbital, phenytoin, primidone, rifampin, ritonavir	atazanavir, caffeine, cimetidine, ciprofloxacin, clarithromycin, enoxacin, erythromycin, fluvoxamine, grapefruit juice, isoniazid, ketoconazole, levofloxacin, mexiletine, norethindrone, norfloxacin, omeprazole, paroxetine, tacrine, zileuton
carbamazepine, phenobarbital, phenytoin, primidone, rifampin	amiodarone, atazanavir, chloramphenicol, cimetidine, co-trimoxazole, delavirdine, disulfiram, fluconazole, fluoxetine, fluvastatin, fluvoxamine, isoniazid, itraconazole, ketoconazole, metronidazole, omeprazole, ritonavir, sulfinpyrazone, ticlopidine, zafirlukast
carbamazepine, phenytoin, rifampin	delavirdine, esomeprazole, felbamate, fluconazole, fluoxetine, fluvoxamine, lansoprazole, omeprazole, sertraline, ticlopidine
carbamazepine, phenobarbital, phenytoin, primidone	amiodarone, bupropion, chloroquine, chlorpheniramine, cimetidine, cocaine, delavirdine, fluoxetine, fluphenazine, fluvoxamine, haloperidol, methadone, nefazodone, paroxetine, perphenazine, propafenone, propoxyphene, quinidine, quinine, ritonavir, rosiglitazone, sertraline, terbinafine, thioridazine, venlafaxine
barbiturates, carbamazepine, glucocorticoids, griseofulvin, nafcillin, nevirapine, oxcarbazepine, phenytoin, primidone, rifabutin, rifampin	amprenavir, atazanavir, bromocriptine, clarithromycin, cimetidine, cyclosporine (neural), danazol, delavirdine, diltiazem, erythromycin, fluconazole, fluoxetine, fluvoxamine, fosamprenavir, grapefruit juice, imatinib, indinavir, isoniazid, itraconazole, ketoconazole, metronidazole, miconazole, nefazodone, nelfinavir, nicardipine, nifedipine, norfloxacin, omeprazole, prednisone, quinidine, quinine, rifabutin, ritonavir, saquinavir, sertraline, troleandomycin, verapamil, zafirlukast

Drugs that prolong the QTc interval

Changes in a patient's heart rate can affect the QT interval of his ECG. To account for such changes, you can use a formula such as the one below. Such formulas let you determine the corrected QT (QTc) interval.

$$\frac{\text{QT interval}}{\sqrt{\text{R-R internal}}} = \text{QTc interval}$$

For men younger than age 55, a normal QTc interval is 350 to 430 msec; for women younger than age 55, a normal QTc interval is 350 to 450 msec.

A prolonged QTc interval may cause fatal arrhythmias, including ventricular tachycardia and torsades de pointes. The causes of a prolonged QTc interval include disorders such as hypokalemia, hypomagnesemia, renal failure, and heart failure. These drugs may also cause an abnormal QTc interval.

amantadine
amiodarone
arformoterol
aripiprazole
arsenic trioxide
azithromycin
bepridil
chloral hydrate
chloroquine
chlorpromazine
clarithromycin
clozapine
cyclobenzaprine
disopyramide
dofetilide
dolasetron
domperidone
droperidol
erythromycin
felbamate
flecainide
foscarnet
fosphenytoin
gatifloxacin
gemifloxacin
granisetron
halofantrine
haloperidol
halothane
ibutilide
indapamide
isradipine
levofloxacin
levomethadyl
mesoridazine
methadone
moexipril
moxifloxacin
naratriptan
nicardipine
octreotide
palonosetron
pentamidine
pimozide
procainamide
propafenone
quinidine
ranolazine
risperidone
salmeterol
sotalol
sparfloxacin
sumatriptan
tacrolimus
tamoxifen
telithromycin
thioridazine
tizanidine
tricyclic antidepressants
vardenafil
venlafaxine
vorinostat
ziprasidone
zolmitriptan

Herbal supplements

If your patient is taking an herbal supplement, ask him some general questions, such as why he's taking the herb and how long he's been taking it. Find out if the condition he's trying to treat has been diagnosed. If so, is he taking or has he taken prescription or OTC drugs for the condition?

If your patient is taking a prescription or OTC drug and an herbal supplement, explain that drug–herb interactions can occur, and advise him to report any unusual signs or symptoms.

For nursing considerations and patient-teaching information on specific herbal supplements, see the table below.

Herb and reported uses	Nursing considerations	Patient teaching
Aloe • Bowel evacuation • Burns and skin irritation • Cathartic • To ease defecation	• Herb's laxative effects are apparent within 10 hours of ingestion. • Monitor patient for signs of dehydration. Elderly patients are particularly at risk. • Monitor electrolyte levels, especially potassium, after long-term use. • If patient is using herb topically, monitor wound for healing.	• Caution patient that if he delays seeking medical diagnosis and treatment, his condition could worsen. • If patient is taking digoxin or another drug to control his heart rate, a diuretic, or a corticosteroid, warn him not to take herb without consulting his health care provider. • Advise patient not to take herb for longer than 1 to 2 weeks at a time without consulting his health care provider.
Chamomile • Antibacterial, antiviral • Diarrhea, flatulence, stomatitis, motion sickness • Hemorrhagic cystitis • Sedation, relaxation • Skin inflammation, wounds, burns	• **ALERT:** Patients sensitive to ragweed and chrysanthemums or other Compositae family members (arnica, yarrow, feverfew, tansy, artemisia) may be more susceptible to contact allergies and anaphylaxis. Patients with hay fever or bronchial asthma caused by pollens are more susceptible to anaphylactic reactions.	• Advise patient against use during pregnancy. • If patient is taking an anticoagulant, advise him not to use herb because of possible enhanced anticoagulant effects. • Advise patient that herb may enhance an allergic reaction or make existing symptoms worse in susceptible patients. • Instruct parent not to give herb to any child before checking with an experienced practitioner.
Cranberry • Asthma • Fever • Kidney stones • Urinary tract infection (UTI)	• Tinctures may contain up to 45% alcohol. • Herb's ability to prevent bacteria from adhering to the bladder wall seems important in preventing UTIs. • Herb is safe for pregnant and breast-feeding women. • When consumed regularly, herb may be effective in reducing the frequency of bacteriuria with pyuria in women with recurrent UTIs.	• Advise patient that an appropriate antibiotic is usually needed to treat an active UTI. • If patient is using herb to prevent a UTI, advise him to notify his health care provider if signs or symptoms of a UTI appear. • If patient has diabetes, inform him that the juice contains sugar but that sugar-free supplements and juices are available. • Only the unsweetened, unprocessed juice is effective in preventing bacteria from adhering to the bladder wall.

(continued)

Herb and reported uses	Nursing considerations	Patient teaching
Echinacea • Abscesses, burns, eczema, skin ulcers • Immune system stimulant • Prevention of common cold, upper respiratory infections • Upper respiratory tract infection	• Daily dose depends on the preparation and potency but shouldn't exceed 8 weeks. Consult specific manufacturer's instructions for parenteral administration, if applicable. • Herb is considered supportive treatment for infection; it shouldn't be used in place of antibiotic therapy. • Herb is usually taken at the first sign of illness and continued for up to 14 days. Regular prophylactic use isn't recommended. • A liquid preparation is recommended because herb is thought to function in the mouth and should have direct contact with the lymph tissues at the back of the throat.	• Advise patient not to delay seeking appropriate medical evaluation for a prolonged illness. • Advise patient that prolonged use may result in overstimulation of the immune system and possible immune suppression. Herb shouldn't be used longer than 14 days for supportive treatment of infection. • The herb should be stored away from direct light. • Warn patients to keep all herbal products away from children and pets.
Ephedra • Appetite suppressant • Asthma • CV stimulant • Chills, cough, cold, flu, fever, headache, edema, nasal congestion • Respiratory tract diseases, mild bronchospasm	• Compounds containing herb may be linked to several deaths and more than 800 adverse effects, many of which appear to be dose related. • Patients with eating disorders may abuse this herb. • **ALERT:** Pills containing herb have been combined with other stimulants such as caffeine and sold as "natural" stimulants in weight loss products. Death from overstimulation may occur. • Signs and symptoms of toxic reaction include diaphoresis, dilated pupils, muscle spasms, fever, and cardiac and respiratory failure. • If overdose occurs, perform gastric lavage and give activated charcoal. Treat spasms with diazepam, replace electrolytes with I.V. fluids, and prevent acidosis with sodium bicarbonate infusions.	• Advise patient not to use this herb in place of getting the proper medical evaluation for a prolonged illness. • **ALERT:** The FDA has banned the sale of dietary supplements containing this herb because of unreasonable risk of injury or illness. • Advise patient with thyroid disease, hypertension, CV disease, or diabetes to avoid using herb. • Advise patient not to use herb. Dosages that are purported to produce psychoactive or hallucinogenic effects are toxic to the heart. • Advise patient to watch for adverse reactions, particularly chest pain, shortness of breath, palpitations, dizziness, and fainting. • Warn patient to keep all herbal products away from children and pets.
Feverfew • Abortifacient • Asthma • Menstrual cramps • Migraine headache • Mouthwash • Psoriasis • Rheumatoid arthritis • Tranquilizer	• If patient is taking an anticoagulant, monitor appropriate coagulation values, such as INR, PTT, and PT. Also, observe patient for abnormal bleeding. • Rash or contact dermatitis may indicate sensitivity to herb. Patient should stop use immediately. • Abruptly stopping the herb may cause "postfeverfew syndrome," involving tension headaches, insomnia, joint stiffness and pain, and lethargy.	• Use during pregnancy isn't recommended. • Educate patient about the risk of abnormal bleeding when combining herb with an anticoagulant, such as warfarin or heparin, or an antiplatelet, such as aspirin or another NSAID. • Caution patient that a rash or abnormal skin alteration may indicate an allergy to herb. Instruct patient to stop taking the herb if a rash appears.
Flax • Constipation • Diarrhea • Diverticulitis	• When herb is used internally, it should be taken with more than 5 oz of liquid per tablespoon of flaxseed.	• Warn patient not to treat chronic constipation or other GI disturbances or ophthalmic injury with herb before seeking appropriate medical evalua-

Herb and reported uses	Nursing considerations	Patient teaching
Flax *(continued)* • Irritable bowel syndrome • Externally as poultice for skin inflammation	• Cyanogenic glycosides may release cyanide; however, the body only metabolizes these to a certain extent. At therapeutic doses, flax doesn't elevate cyanide ion level. • Although herb may decrease a patient's cholesterol level or increase bleeding time, it isn't necessary to monitor cholesterol level or platelet aggregation.	tion because doing so may delay diagnosis of a potentially serious medical condition. • Discourage use during pregnancy. • Instruct patient to drink plenty of water when taking flaxseed. • Instruct patient not to take any drug for at least 2 hours after taking herb.
Garlic • Atherosclerosis prevention • Cholesterol and triglyceride levels reduction • Colds, coughs, fever, and sore throat • GI tract cancers prevention • HDL cholesterol level increase • MI and stroke prevention	• Herb isn't recommended for patients with diabetes, insomnia, pemphigus, organ transplants, or rheumatoid arthritis or for postsurgical patients. • Consuming excessive amounts of raw garlic increases the risk of adverse reactions. • Monitor patient for signs and symptoms of bleeding. • Herb may lower glucose level. If patient is taking an antidiabetic, watch for signs and symptoms of hypoglycemia, and monitor his glucose level. • **ALERT:** Advise parents not to use oil to treat inner ear infection in children.	• Advise patient not to delay seeking appropriate medical evaluation because doing so may delay diagnosis of a serious medical condition. • Advise patient to consume herb in moderation, to minimize the risk of adverse reactions. • Discourage heavy use of herb before surgery. • If patient is using herb to lower his cholesterol levels, advise him to notify his health care provider and to have his cholesterol levels monitored. • Advise patient that using herb with anticoagulants may increase the risk of bleeding. • If patient is using herb as a topical antiseptic, avoid prolonged exposure to the skin because burns can occur.
Ginger • Antiemetic • Anti-inflammatory, antiarthritic • Antispasmodic • Antitumorigenic • Colic, flatulence, indigestion • Hypercholesterolemia, burns, ulcers, depression, impotence, liver toxicity	• Adverse reactions are uncommon. • Monitor patient for signs and symptoms of bleeding. If patient is taking an anticoagulant, monitor PTT, PT, and INR carefully. • Use in pregnant patients is questionable, although small amounts used in cooking are safe. It's unknown if ginger appears in breast milk. • Herb may interfere with the intended therapeutic effect of conventional drugs. • If overdose occurs, monitor patient for arrhythmias and CNS depression.	• If woman is pregnant, advise her to consult an experienced practitioner before using herb medicinally. • Educate patients to look for signs of bleeding, such as nosebleeds or excessive bruising. • Warn patient to keep all herbal products away from children and pets.
Ginkgo • Cerebral insufficiency, dementia, and circulatory disorders • Headaches, asthma, colitis, impotence, depression, altitude sickness, tinnitus, cochlear deafness, vertigo, pre-	• Extracts are considered standardized if they contain 24% flavonoid glycosides and 6% terpene lactones. • Treatment should continue for at least 6 to 8 weeks, but therapy beyond 3 months isn't recommended. • **ALERT:** Seizures have been reported in children after ingestion of more than 50 seeds.	• If patient is taking the herb for motion sickness, advise him to begin taking it 1 to 2 days before taking the trip and to keep taking it for the duration of his trip. • Inform patient that the therapeutic and toxic components of ginkgo can vary significantly from product to

(continued)

Herb and reported uses	Nursing considerations	Patient teaching
Ginkgo *(continued)* menstrual syndrome, macular degeneration, diabetic retinopathy, and allergies • Pancreatic cancer and schizophrenia adjunct	• Patients must be monitored for possible adverse reactions, such as GI problems, headaches, dizziness, allergic reactions, and serious bleeding. • Toxicity may cause atonia and adynamia.	product. Advise him to obtain herb from a reliable source. • Warn patient to keep all herbal products away from children and pets. • Advise patient to stop use at least 2 weeks before surgery.
Ginseng, Asian • Fatigue and lack of concentration, atherosclerosis, bleeding disorders, colitis, diabetes, depression, and cancer • Health and strength recovery after sickness or weakness	• The German Commission E doesn't recommend using herb for longer than 3 months. • Herb may strengthen the body and increase resistance to disease. • **ALERT:** Reports have circulated of a severe reaction known as the ginseng abuse syndrome in patients taking more than 3 g/day for up to 2 years: Increased motor and cognitive activity with diarrhea, nervousness, insomnia, hypertension, edema, and skin eruptions.	• Inform patient that the therapeutic and toxic components can vary significantly from product to product. Advise him to obtain herb from a reliable source.
Green tea • To prevent cancer, hyperlipidemia, atherosclerosis, dental caries, headaches • Wounds, skin disorders, stomach disorders, and infectious diarrhea • CNS stimulant, mild diuretic, antibacterial, topical astringent	• Daily consumption should be limited to fewer than 5 cups, or the equivalent of 300 mg of caffeine, to avoid the adverse effects of caffeine. • Prolonged high caffeine intake may cause restlessness, irritability, insomnia, palpitations, vertigo, headache, and adverse GI effects. • The adverse GI effects of chlorogenic acid and tannin can be avoided if milk is added to the tea mixture. • The tannin content in tea increases the longer it's left to brew; this increases the antidiarrheal properties of the tea. • The first signs of a toxic reaction are vomiting and abdominal spasm.	• Advise patient that heavy consumption may be associated with esophageal cancer secondary to the tannin content in the mixture. • Tell patient that the first signs of toxic reaction are vomiting and abdominal spasm. • Tell patient that herb interferes with iron absorption from supplements or multivitamins.
Hawthorn • Atherosclerosis • Blood pressure regulation • Cardiotonic and sedative • Mild heart conditions	• High doses may cause hypotension and sedation. Monitor patient for CNS adverse effects, and monitor blood pressure. • Herb may interfere with digoxin's effects or serum monitoring. • Observe patient closely for adverse reactions, especially adverse CNS reactions.	• Advise patient that when he fills a prescription, he should tell the pharmacist of any herb or dietary supplement he's taking. • Advise patient to avoid herb because of toxic adverse effects. • Warn patient to keep all herbal products away from children and pets.
Horse chestnut • Analgesic, anticoagulant, antipyretic, astringent, expectorant, and tonic	• **ALERT:** The nuts, seeds, twigs, sprouts, and leaves of horse chestnut are poisonous and can be lethal. • Standardized formulations remove most of the toxins and standardize the amount of aescin.	• Inform patient that the FDA considers herb unsafe and that death may occur. • Advise patient not to confuse horse chestnut with sweet chestnut, used as a food.

Herb and reported uses	Nursing considerations	Patient teaching
Horse chestnut *(continued)* • Chronic venous insufficiency, varicose veins, leg pain, tiredness, tension, and leg swelling and edema • Lymphedema, hemorrhoids, and enlarged prostate • Skin ulcers, phlebitis, leg cramps, cough, and diarrhea	• Signs and symptoms of toxicity include loss of coordination, salivation, hemolysis, headache, dilated pupils, muscle twitching, seizures, vomiting, diarrhea, depression, paralysis, respiratory and cardiac failure, and death. • Monitor patient for signs of toxicity. • Monitor glucose level in patients taking antidiabetics for hypoglycemia.	• warn patient to keep the herb away from children. Consumption of amounts of leaves, twigs, and seeds equaling 1% of a child's weight may be lethal.
Kava • Nervous anxiety, stress, and restlessness • Skin diseases, including leprosy • Intestinal problems, otitis, and abscesses • Urogenital infections, including chronic cystitis, venereal disease, uterine inflammation, menstrual problems, and vaginal prolapse • Wound healing, headaches, seizure disorders, the common cold, respiratory tract infection, tuberculosis, and rheumatism	• Patient shouldn't use herb with conventional sedative-hypnotics, anxiolytics, MAO inhibitors, other psychopharmacologic drugs, levodopa, or antiplatelet drugs without first consulting a health care provider. • Use for longer than 3 months may be habit-forming. • Herb can cause drowsiness and may impair motor reflexes. • Patients should avoid taking herb with alcohol because of increased risk of CNS depression and liver damage. • Periodic monitoring of liver function tests and CBC may be needed. • Toxic doses can cause progressive ataxia, muscle weakness, and ascending paralysis, all of which resolve when herb is stopped. Extreme use (more than 300 g per week) may increase GGT levels.	• Tell patient oral use is probably safe for 3 months or less, but use for longer than 3 months may be habit forming. • Warn patient to avoid taking herb with alcohol because of increased risk of CNS depression and liver damage. • **ALERT:** Tell patient that the FDA has linked herb to liver problems including cirrhosis, hepatitis, and liver failure. Herb users should immediately contact their health care provider if their skin or eyes begin to yellow, or they experience severe itching, easy bruising, dark urine, or bloody vomit.
Melatonin • Insomnia, jet lag, shift-work disorder, blind entrainment, immune system enhancement, tinnitus, depression, and benzodiazepine withdrawal • Cancer therapy adjunct, antiaging product, and preganancy and cluster headaches preventative • Skin protection against ultraviolet light	• Monitor patient for excessive daytime drowsiness. • May increase human growth hormone levels.	• Warn patient to avoid hazardous activities until full extent of CNS depressant effect is known. • If patient wishes to conceive, tell her that herb may have a contraceptive effect. However, herb shouldn't be used as birth control. • Although no chemical interactions have been reported, tell patient that herb may interfere with therapeutic effects of conventional drugs. • Warn patient about possible additive effects if taken with alcohol. • Advise patient not to use herb for prolonged periods because safety data aren't available.

(continued)

Herb and reported uses	Nursing considerations	Patient teaching
Milk thistle • Dyspepsia, liver damage from chemicals, Amanita mushroom poisoning, supportive therapy for inflammatory liver disease and cirrhosis, loss of appetite, and gall bladder and spleen disorders • Liver protectant	• Mild allergic reactions may occur, especially in people allergic to members of the Astertaceae family, including ragweed, chrysanthemums, marigolds, and daisies. • Don't confuse seeds or fruit with other parts of the plant or with blessed thistle.	• Warn woman not to take this herb while pregnant or breast-feeding. • Tell patient to stay alert for possible allergic reactions, especially if allergic to ragweed, chrysanthemums, marigolds, or daisies. • Warn patient not to take herb for liver inflammation or cirrhosis before seeking appropriate medical evaluation because doing so may delay diagnosis of a potentially serious medical condition.
Passion flower • Sedative, hypnotic, analgesic, antispasmodic, menstrual cramps, pain, migraines • Neuralgia, generalized seizures, hysteria, nervous agitation, and insomnia • Topically for cuts and bruises	• Monitor patient for possible adverse CNS effects. • No adverse effects have been observed with recommended doses. • A disulfiram-like reaction may produce nausea, vomiting, flushing, headache, hypotension, tachycardia, ventricular arrhythmias, and shock leading to death. • Patients with liver disease and alcoholics shouldn't use herbal products that contain alcohol.	• Because sedation is possible, caution patient to avoid hazardous activities. • Warn patient not to take herb for chronic pain or insomnia before seeking medical attention because doing so may delay diagnosis of a potentially serious medical condition. • Caution pregnant patients to avoid this herb.
Saw palmetto • BPH and coughs and congestion from colds, bronchitis, or asthma • Mild diuretic, urinary antiseptic, and astringent	• Herb should be used cautiously for conditions other than BPH because data about its effectiveness in other conditions are lacking. • Obtain a baseline prostate-specific antigen (PSA) value before patient starts taking herb because it may cause a false-negative PSA result. • Saw palmetto may not alter prostate size. • Laboratory values didn't change significantly in clinical trials using dosages of 160 mg to 320 mg daily.	• Warn patient not to take herb for bladder or prostate problems before seeking medical attention because doing so could delay diagnosis of a potentially serious medical condition. • Tell patient to take herb with food to minimize GI effects. • Caution patient to promptly notify health care provider about new or worsened adverse effects. • Warn women to avoid herb if planning pregnancy, if pregnant, or if breast-feeding.
St. John's wort • To moderate depression, anxiety, sciatica, and viral infections, including herpes simplex virus, hepatitis C, influenza virus, murine cytomegalovirus, and poliovirus • Bronchitis, asthma, gallbladder disease, nocturnal enuresis, gout, and rheumatism	• Recommended duration of therapy for depression is 4 to 6 weeks; if no improvement occurs, a different therapy should be considered. • Monitor patient for response to herbal therapy, as evidenced by improved mood and lessened depression. • By using standardized extracts, patient can better control the dosage. Studies have used forms of standardized 0.3% hypericin as well as hyperforin-stabilized version of the extract. • Serotonin syndrome may cause dizziness, nausea, vomiting, headache, epigastric pain, anxiety, confusion, restlessness, and irritability.	• Instruct patient to consult a health care provider for a thorough medical evaluation before using herb. • If patient takes herb for mild to moderate depression, explain that several weeks may pass before effects occur. Tell patient that a new therapy may be needed if no improvement occurs in 4 to 6 weeks. • Inform patient that herb interacts with many other prescription and OTC products and may reduce their effectiveness. • Tell patient that herb may cause increased sensitivity to direct sunlight. Recommend protective clothing, sunscreen, and limited sun exposure.

Herb and reported uses	Nursing considerations	Patient teaching
St. John's wort *(continued)*	• Because herb decreases the effect of certain prescription drugs, watch for signs of drug toxicity if patient stops using the herb. Drug dosage may need to be reduced. • Herb has mutagenic effects on sperm and egg cells. It shouldn't be used by pregnant patients, women planning pregnancy, or men wishing to father a child.	• Inform patient that a sufficient wash-out period is needed after stopping an antidepressant before switching to herb. • Tell patient to report adverse effects to a health care provider. • Warn patient to keep all herbal products away from children and pets.
Tea tree oil • Contusions, inflammation, myalgia, burns, hemorrhoids, and vitiligo • Tonsillitis and lotion for dermatoses	• Because of systemic toxicity, herb shouldn't be used internally. • Essential oil should be used externally only after being diluted. • Herb may cause burns or itching in tender areas and shouldn't be used around nose, eyes, and mouth. • 100% pure essential oil is rarely used and should be used only with close supervision by a health care provider.	• Explain that a few drops are sufficient in mouthwash, shampoo, or sitz bath. • Caution patient not to apply oil to wounds or to skin that's dry or cracked. • Warn patient to keep all herbal products away from children and pets.

(continued)

Adverse reactions misinterpreted as age-related changes

In elderly patients, adverse drug reactions can easily be misinterpreted as the typical signs and symptoms of aging. The table below, which shows possible adverse reactions for common drug classes, can help you avoid such misinterpretations.

	Adverse reactions							
Drug classifications	Agitation	Anxiety	Arrhythmias	Ataxia	Changes in appetite	Confusion	Constipation	Depression
ACE inhibitors						●	●	●
Alpha$_1$ blockers		●					●	●
Antianginals	●	●	●			●		
Antiarrhythmics			●				●	
Anticholinergics	●	●	●			●	●	●
Anticonvulsants	●		●	●	●	●	●	●
Antidepressants, tricyclic	●	●	●	●	●	●	●	
Antidiabetics, oral								
Antihistamines					●	●	●	
Antilipemics							●	
Antiparkinsonians	●	●		●	●	●	●	●
Antipsychotics	●	●	●	●	●	●	●	●
Barbiturates	●	●	●			●		
Benzodiazepines	●			●		●	●	●
Beta blockers		●	●					●
Calcium channel blockers		●	●				●	
Corticosteroids	●					●		●
Diuretics						●		
NSAIDs		●				●	●	●
Opioids	●	●				●	●	●
Skeletal muscle relaxants	●	●		●		●		●
Thyroid hormones			●		●			

Difficulty breathing	Disorientation	Dizziness	Drowsiness	Edema	Fatigue	Hypotension	Insomnia	Memory loss	Muscle weakness	Restlessness	Sexual dysfunction	Tremors	Urinary dysfunction	Visual changes
		●			●	●	●				●			●
		●	●	●	●	●	●				●		●	●
		●		●	●	●	●			●	●		●	●
●		●		●	●									
	●	●	●		●	●		●	●	●			●	●
●		●	●	●	●	●	●					●	●	●
●	●	●	●		●	●	●			●	●	●	●	●
		●			●									
	●	●	●		●							●	●	●
		●					●				●		●	●
	●	●	●		●	●	●		●			●	●	●
		●	●		●	●	●			●	●	●	●	●
●	●		●		●	●				●				
●	●	●	●		●		●	●	●			●	●	●
●		●			●			●			●	●	●	●
●		●		●	●	●	●				●		●	●
				●	●		●		●					●
		●			●	●			●				●	
		●	●		●		●		●					●
●	●	●	●		●	●	●	●		●	●		●	●
		●	●		●	●	●					●		
							●					●		

Infusion flow rates

The infusion flow rates are based on the concentrations shown at the top of each table. Check the label on the drug you're infusing to verify the correct infusion flow rate.

Nitroglycerin infusion rates

Determine the infusion rate in ml/hr using the ordered dose and the concentration of the drug solution.

Dose (mcg/min)	**25 mg/250 ml (100 mcg/ml)**	**50 mg/250 ml (200 mcg/ml)**	**100 mg/250 ml (400 mcg/ml)**
5	3	2	1
10	6	3	2
20	12	6	3
30	18	9	5
40	24	12	6
50	30	15	8
60	36	18	9
70	42	21	10
80	48	24	12
90	54	27	14
100	60	30	15
150	90	45	23
200	120	60	30

Dobutamine infusion rates

Mix 250 mg in 250 ml of D_5W (1,000 mcg/ml). Determine the infusion rate in ml/hr using the ordered dose and the patient's weight in pounds or kilograms.

Dose (mcg/kg/min)	**lb 88**	**99**	**110**	**121**	**132**	**143**	**154**	**165**	**176**	**187**	**198**	**209**	**220**	**231**	**242**
	kg 40	**45**	**50**	**55**	**60**	**65**	**70**	**75**	**80**	**85**	**90**	**95**	**100**	**105**	**110**
2.5	6	7	8	8	9	10	11	11	12	13	14	14	15	16	17
5	12	14	15	17	18	20	21	23	24	26	27	29	30	32	33
7.5	18	20	23	25	27	29	32	34	36	38	41	43	45	47	50
10	24	27	30	33	36	39	42	45	48	51	54	57	60	63	66
12.5	30	34	38	41	45	49	53	56	60	64	68	71	75	79	83
15	36	41	45	50	54	59	63	68	72	77	81	86	90	95	99
20	48	54	60	66	72	78	84	90	96	102	108	114	120	126	132
25	60	68	75	83	90	98	105	113	120	128	135	143	150	158	165
30	72	81	90	99	108	117	126	135	144	153	162	171	180	189	198
35	84	95	105	116	126	137	147	158	168	179	189	200	210	221	231
40	96	108	120	132	144	156	168	180	192	204	216	228	240	252	264

Dopamine infusion rates

Mix 400 mg in 250 ml of D_5W (1,600 mcg/ml). Determine the infusion rate in ml/hr using the ordered dose and the patient's weight in pounds or kilograms.

Dose (mcg/kg/min)	lb 88	99	110	121	132	143	154	165	176	187	198	209	220	231
	kg 40	45	50	55	60	65	70	75	80	85	90	95	100	105
2.5	4	4	5	5	6	6	7	7	8	8	8	9	9	10
5	8	8	9	10	11	12	13	14	15	16	17	18	19	20
7.5	11	13	14	15	17	18	20	21	23	24	25	27	28	30
10	15	17	19	21	23	24	26	28	30	32	34	36	38	39
12.5	19	21	23	26	28	30	33	35	38	40	42	45	47	49
15	23	25	28	31	34	37	39	42	45	48	51	53	56	59
20	30	34	38	41	45	49	53	56	60	64	68	71	75	79
25	38	42	47	52	56	61	66	70	75	80	84	89	94	98
30	45	51	56	62	67	73	79	84	90	96	101	107	113	118
35	53	59	66	72	79	85	92	98	105	112	118	125	131	138
40	60	68	75	83	90	98	105	113	120	128	135	143	150	158
45	68	76	84	93	101	110	118	127	135	143	152	160	169	177
50	75	84	94	103	113	122	131	141	150	159	169	178	188	197

Nitroprusside infusion rates

Mix 50 mg in 250 ml of D_5W (200 mcg/ml). Determine the infusion rate in ml/hr using the ordered dose and the patient's weight in pounds or kilograms.

Dose (mcg/kg/min)	lb 88	99	110	121	132	143	154	165	176	187	198	209	220	231	242
	kg 40	45	50	55	60	65	70	75	80	85	90	95	100	105	110
0.3	4	4	5	5	5	6	6	7	7	8	8	9	9	9	10
0.5	6	7	8	8	9	10	11	11	12	13	14	14	15	16	17
1	12	14	15	17	18	20	21	23	24	26	27	29	30	32	33
1.5	18	20	23	25	27	29	32	34	36	38	41	43	45	47	50
2	24	27	30	33	36	39	42	45	48	51	54	57	60	63	66
3	36	41	45	50	54	59	63	68	72	77	81	86	90	95	99
4	48	54	60	66	72	78	84	90	96	102	108	114	120	126	132
5	60	68	75	83	90	98	105	113	120	128	135	143	150	158	165
6	72	81	90	99	108	117	126	135	144	153	162	171	180	189	198
7	84	95	105	116	126	137	147	158	168	179	189	200	210	221	231
8	96	108	120	132	144	156	168	180	192	204	216	228	240	252	264
9	108	122	135	149	162	176	189	203	216	230	243	257	270	284	297
10	120	135	150	165	180	195	210	225	240	255	270	285	300	315	330

Combination drugs: Indications and dosages

AMPHETAMINES

Adderall
Adderall XL

Controlled Substance Schedule (CSS) II

GENERIC COMPONENTS

Tablets

5 mg: 1.25 mg dextroamphetamine sulfate, 1.25 mg dextroamphetamine saccharate, and 1.25 mg amphetamine aspartate, 1.25 mg amphetamine sulfate
7.5 mg: 1.875 mg dextroamphetamine sulfate, 1.875 mg dextroamphetamine saccharate, 1.875 mg amphetamine aspartate, and 1.875 mg amphetamine sulfate
10 mg: 2.5 mg dextroamphetamine sulfate, 2.5 mg dextroamphetamine saccharate, 2.5 mg amphetamine aspartate, and 2.5 mg amphetamine sulfate
12.5 mg: 3.125 mg dextroamphetamine sulfate, 3.125 mg dextroamphetamine saccharate, 3.125 mg amphetamine aspartate, and 3.125 mg amphetamine sulfate
15 mg: 3.75 mg dextroamphetamine sulfate, 3.75 mg dextroamphetamine saccharate, 3.75 mg amphetamine aspartate, and 3.75 mg amphetamine sulfate
20 mg: 5 mg dextroamphetamine sulfate, 5 mg dextroamphetamine saccharate, 5 mg amphetamine aspartate, and 5 mg amphetamine sulfate
30 mg: 7.5 mg dextroamphetamine sulfate, 7.5 mg dextroamphetamine saccharate, 7.5 mg amphetamine aspartate, and 7.5 mg amphetamine sulfate

Capsules (extended-release)

5 mg: 1.25 mg dextroamphetamine sulfate, 1.25 mg dextroamphetamine saccharate, 1.25 mg amphetamine aspartate, and 1.25 mg amphetamine sulfate
10 mg: 2.5 mg dextroamphetamine sulfate, 2.5 mg dextroamphetamine saccharate, 2.5 mg amphetamine aspartate, and 2.5 mg amphetamine sulfate
15 mg: 3.75 mg dextroamphetamine sulfate, 3.75 mg dextroamphetamine saccharate, 3.75 mg amphetamine aspartate, and 3.75 mg amphetamine sulfate
20 mg: 5 mg dextroamphetamine sulfate, 5 mg dextroamphetamine saccharate, 5 mg amphetamine aspartate, and 5 mg amphetamine sulfate
25 mg: 6.25 mg dextroamphetamine sulfate, 6.25 mg dextroamphetamine saccharate, 6.25 mg amphetamine aspartate, and 6.25 mg amphetamine sulfate
30 mg: 7.5 mg dextroamphetamine sulfate, 7.5 mg dextroamphetamine saccharate, 7.5 mg amphetamine aspartate, and 7.5 mg amphetamine sulfate

DOSAGES

Narcolepsy

Adults and children age 12 and older: Initially, 10 mg immediate-release tablet daily. Increase by 10 mg weekly to maximum dose of 60 mg in 2 or 3 divided doses q 4 to 6 hours.
Children ages 6 to 12: Initially, 5 mg immediate-release tablet P.O. daily. Increase by 5 mg at weekly intervals to maximum dose of 60 mg in divided doses.

Attention deficit hyperactivity disorder

Adults: 20 mg extended-release capsules P.O. daily.
Adolescents ages 13 to 17: Initially, 10 mg extended-release capsule P.O. daily. Increase after 1 week to 20 mg daily if needed.
Children age 6 and older: Initially, 5 mg immediate-release tablet P.O. daily or b.i.d. Increase by 5 mg at weekly intervals until optimal response. Dosage should rarely exceed 40 mg.
Children ages 6 to 12: Give 10 mg extended-release capsule P.O. daily in a.m. Increase by 5 to 10 mg in weekly intervals to a maximum dose of 30 mg.
Children ages 3 to 5: Initially, 2.5 mg immediate-release tablet P.O. daily. Increase by 2.5 mg at weekly intervals until optimal response. Divide total daily dose into 2 or 3 doses and give 4 to 6 hours apart.

ANALGESICS

Alor 5/500
Azdone
Damason-P
Lortab ASA
Panasal 5/500
CSS III

GENERIC COMPONENTS
500 mg aspirin and 5 mg hydrocodone bitartrate

DOSAGES
Moderate to moderately severe pain
Adults: 1 or 2 tablets q 4 hours. Maximum dosage, 8 tablets in 24 hours.

Anexsia 5/325
Norco 5/325
CSS III

GENERIC COMPONENTS
325 mg acetaminophen and 5 mg hydrocodone bitartrate

DOSAGES
Moderate to moderately severe pain
Adults: 1 to 2 tablets q 4 to 6 hours. Maximum dosage, 12 tablets in 24 hours.

Anexsia 5/500
Co-Gesic
Lorcet HD
Lortab 5/500
Panacet 5/500
Vicodin
CSS III

GENERIC COMPONENTS
500 mg acetaminophen and 5 mg hydrocodone bitartrate

DOSAGES
Moderate to moderately severe pain
Adults: 1 to 2 tablets q 4 to 6 hours. Maximum dosage, 8 tablets in 24 hours.

Anexsia 7.5/325
Norco 7.5/325
CSS III

GENERIC COMPONENTS
325 mg acetaminophen and 7.5 mg hydrocodone bitartrate

DOSAGES
Moderate to moderately severe pain
Adults: 1 to 2 tablets q 4 to 6 hours. Maximum dosage, 12 tablets in 24 hours.

Anexsia 7.5/650
Lorcet Plus
CSS III

GENERIC COMPONENTS
650 mg acetaminophen and 7.5 mg hydrocodone bitartrate

DOSAGES
Arthralgia, bone pain, dental pain, headache, migraine, moderate pain
Adults: 1 to 2 tablets q 4 hours. Maximum dosage, 6 tablets in 24 hours.

Anexsia 10/660
Vicodin HP
CSS III

GENERIC COMPONENTS
660 mg acetaminophen and 10 mg hydrocodone bitartrate

DOSAGES
Arthralgia, bone pain, dental pain, headache, migraine, moderate pain
Adults: 1 tablet q 4 to 6 hours. Maximum dosage, 6 tablets in 24 hours.

Capital with Codeine
Tylenol with Codeine Elixir
CSS V

GENERIC COMPONENTS
120 mg acetaminophen and 12 mg codeine phosphate/5 ml

DOSAGES
Mild to moderate pain
Adults: 15 ml q 4 hours.

Darvocet-A500
CSS IV

GENERIC COMPONENTS
500 mg acetaminophen and 100 mg propoxyphene napsylate

DOSAGES
Mild to moderate pain
Adults: 1 tablet q 4 hours. Maximum dosage, 8 tablets in 24 hours.

Darvocet-N50
CSS IV

GENERIC COMPONENTS
325 mg acetaminophen and 50 mg propoxyphene napsylate

DOSAGES
Mild to moderate pain
Adults: 2 tablets q 4 hours. Maximum dosage, 12 tablets in 24 hours.

Darvocet-N100
CSS IV

GENERIC COMPONENTS
650 mg acetaminophen and 100 mg propoxyphene napsylate

DOSAGES
Mild to moderate pain
Adults: 1 tablet q 4 hours. Maximum dosage, 6 tablets in 24 hours.

Empirin with Codeine No. 3
CSS III

GENERIC COMPONENTS
325 mg aspirin and 30 mg codeine phosphate

DOSAGES
Fever and mild to moderate pain
Adults: 1to 2 tablets q 4 hours. Maximum dosage, 12 tablets in 24 hours.

Empirin with Codeine No. 4
CSS III

GENERIC COMPONENTS
325 mg aspirin and 60 mg codeine phosphate

DOSAGES
Fever and mild to moderate pain
Adults: 1 tablet q 4 hours. Maximum dosage, 6 tablets in 24 hours.

Endocet 5/325
Percocet 5/325
Roxicet
CSS II

GENERIC COMPONENTS
325 mg acetaminophen and 5 mg oxycodone hydrochloride

DOSAGES
Moderate to moderately severe pain
Adults: 1 tablet q 6 hours. Maximum dosage, 12 tablets in 24 hours.

Endocet 7.5/325
Percocet 7.5/325
CSS II

GENERIC COMPONENTS
325 mg acetaminophen and 7.5 mg oxycodone hydrochloride

DOSAGES
Moderate to moderately severe pain
Adults: 1 tablet q 6 hours. Maximum dosage, 8 tablets in 24 hours.

Endocet 7.5/500
Percocet 7.5/500
CSS II

GENERIC COMPONENTS
500 mg acetaminophen and 7.5 mg oxycodone hydrochloride

DOSAGES
Moderate to moderately severe pain
Adults: 1 tablet q 6 hours. Maximum dosage, 8 tablets in 24 hours.

Endocet 10/325
Percocet 10/325
CSS II

GENERIC COMPONENTS
325 mg acetaminophen and 10 mg oxycodone hydrochloride

DOSAGES
Moderate to moderately severe pain
Adults: 1 tablet q 6 hours. Maximum dosage, 6 tablets in 24 hours.

Endodan
Percodan
CSS II

GENERIC COMPONENTS
325 mg aspirin, 4.5 mg oxycodone hydrochloride and 0.38 mg oxycodone terephthalate

DOSAGES
Moderate to moderately severe pain
Adults: 1 tablet q 6 hours. Maximum dosage, 12 tablets in 24 hours.

Fioricet with Codeine
CSS III

GENERIC COMPONENTS
325 mg acetaminophen, 50 mg butalbital, 40 mg caffeine, and 30 mg codeine phosphate

DOSAGES
Headache, mild to moderate pain
Adults: 1 to 2 capsules q 4 hours. Maximum dosage, 6 capsules in 24 hours.

Fiorinal with Codeine
CSS III

GENERIC COMPONENTS
325 mg aspirin, 50 mg butalbital, 40 mg caffeine, and 30 mg codeine phosphate

DOSAGES
Headache, mild to moderate pain
Adults: 1 to 2 tablets or capsules q 4 hours. Maximum dosage, 6 tablets or capsules in 24 hours.

Lorcet 10/650
CSS III

GENERIC COMPONENTS
650 mg acetaminophen and 10 mg hydrocodone bitartrate

DOSAGES
Moderate to moderately severe pain
Adults: 1 tablet q 4 to 6 hours. Maximum dosage, 6 tablets in 24 hours.

Lortab 2.5/500
CSS III

GENERIC COMPONENTS
500 mg acetaminophen and 2.5 mg hydrocodone bitartrate

DOSAGES
Moderate to moderately severe pain
Adults: 1 to 2 tablets q 4 to 6 hours. Maximum dosage, 8 tablets in 24 hours.

Lortab 7.5/500
CSS III

GENERIC COMPONENTS
500 mg acetaminophen and 7.5 mg hydrocodone bitartrate

DOSAGES
Moderate to moderately severe pain
Adults: 1 tablet q 4 to 6 hours. Maximum dosage, 8 tablets in 24 hours.

Lortab 10/500
CSS III

GENERIC COMPONENTS
500 mg acetaminophen and 10 mg hydrocodone bitartrate

DOSAGES
Moderate to moderately severe pain
Adults: 1 tablet q 4 to 6 hours. Maximum dosage, 6 tablets in 24 hours.

Lortab Elixir
CSS III

GENERIC COMPONENTS
167 mg acetaminophen and 2.5 mg/5 ml hydrocodone bitartrate

DOSAGES
Moderately severe pain
Adults: 15 ml q 4 to 6 hours. Maximum dosage, 90 ml/day.

Norco 325/10
CSS III

GENERIC COMPONENTS
325 mg acetaminophen and 10 mg hydrocodone bitartrate

DOSAGES
Moderate to moderately severe pain
Adults: 1 tablet q 4 to 6 hours. Maximum dosage, 6 tablets in 24 hours.

Percocet 2.5/325
CSS II

GENERIC COMPONENTS
325 mg acetaminophen and 2.5 mg oxycodone hydrochloride

DOSAGES
Moderate to moderately severe pain
Adults: 1 to 2 tablets q 4 to 6 hours. Maximum dosage, 12 tablets in 24 hours.

Percocet 10/650
CSS II

GENERIC COMPONENTS
650 mg acetaminophen and 10 mg oxycodone hydrochloride

DOSAGES
Moderate to moderately severe pain
Adults: 1 tablet q 4 hours. Maximum dosage, 6 tablets in 24 hours.

Roxicet 5/500
Roxilox
Tylox
CSS II

GENERIC COMPONENTS
500 mg acetaminophen and 5 mg oxycodone hydrochloride

DOSAGES
Moderate to moderately severe pain
Adults: 1 tablet q 6 hours.

Roxicet Oral Solution
CSS II

GENERIC COMPONENTS
325 mg acetaminophen and 5 mg/5 ml oxycodone hydrochloride

DOSAGES
Moderate to moderately severe pain
Adults: 5 ml q 6 hours. Maximum dosage, 60 ml in 24 hours.

Talacen
CSS IV

GENERIC COMPONENTS
650 mg acetaminophen and 25 mg pentazocine hydrochloride

DOSAGES
Mild to moderate pain
Adults: 1 tablet q 4 hours. Maximum dosage, 6 tablets in 24 hours.

Talwin Compound
CSS IV

GENERIC COMPONENTS
325 mg aspirin and 12.5 mg pentazocine hydrochloride

DOSAGES
Moderate pain
Adults: 2 tablets q 6 to 8 hours. Maximum dosage, 8 tablets in 24 hours.

Talwin NX
CSS IV

GENERIC COMPONENTS
0.5 mg naloxone and 50 mg pentazocine hydrochloride

DOSAGES
Moderate to severe pain
Adults: 1 to 2 tablets q 3 to 4 hours. Maximum dosage, 12 tablets daily.

Tylenol with Codeine No. 2
CSS III

GENERIC COMPONENTS
300 mg acetaminophen and 15 mg codeine phosphate

DOSAGES
Fever, mild to moderate pain
Adults: 1 to 2 tablets q 4 hours. Maximum dosage, 12 tablets in 24 hours.

Tylenol with Codeine No. 3
CSS III

GENERIC COMPONENTS
300 mg acetaminophen and 30 mg codeine phosphate

DOSAGES
Fever, mild to moderate pain
Adults: 1 to 2 tablets q 4 hours. Maximum dosage, 12 tablets in 24 hours.

Tylenol with Codeine No. 4
CSS III

GENERIC COMPONENTS
300 mg acetaminophen and 60 mg codeine phosphate

DOSAGES
Fever, mild to moderate pain
Adults: 1 tablet q 4 hours. Maximum dosage, 6 tablets in 24 hours.

Tylox 5/500
CSS II

GENERIC COMPONENTS
500 mg acetaminophen and 5 mg oxycodone hydrochloride

DOSAGES
Moderate to moderately severe pain
Adults: 1 capsule q 6 hours. Maximum dosage, 8 capsules in 24 hours.

Vicodin ES
CSS III

GENERIC COMPONENTS
750 mg acetaminophen and 7.5 mg hydrocodone bitartrate

DOSAGES
Moderate to moderately severe pain
Adults: 1 tablet q 4 to 6 hours. Maximum dosage, 5 tablets in 24 hours.

Wygesic
CSS IV

GENERIC COMPONENTS
650 mg acetaminophen and 65 mg propoxyphene napsylate

DOSAGES
Mild to moderate pain
Adults: 1 tablet q 4 hours. Maximum dosage, 6 tablets in 24 hours.

Zydone 5/400
CSS III

GENERIC COMPONENTS
400 mg acetaminophen and 5 mg hydrocodone bitartrate

DOSAGES
Moderate to moderately severe pain
Adults: 1 to 2 tablets q 4 to 6 hours. Maximum dosage, 8 tablets in 24 hours.

Zydone 7.5/400
CSS III

GENERIC COMPONENTS
400 mg acetaminophen and 7.5 mg hydrocodone bitartrate

DOSAGES
Moderate to moderately severe pain
Adults: 1 tablet q 4 to 6 hours. Maximum dosage, 6 tablets in 24 hours.

Zydone 10/400
CSS III

GENERIC COMPONENTS
400 mg acetaminophen and 10 mg hydrocodone bitartrate

DOSAGES
Moderate to moderately severe pain
Adults: 1 tablet q 4 to 6 hours. Maximum dosage, 6 tablets in 24 hours.

ANTIACNE DRUGS

Estrostep 21
Estrostep Fe

GENERIC COMPONENTS
Tablets
1 mg norethindrone and 20 mcg ethinyl estradiol, 1 mg norethindrone and 30 mcg ethinyl estradiol, or 1 mg norethindrone and 35 mcg ethinyl estradiol and 75 mg ferrous fumarate

DOSAGES
Women older than age 15: 1 tablet P.O. daily.

Ortho Tri-Cyclen

GENERIC COMPONENTS
Tablets
0.18 mg norgestimate and 35 mcg ethinyl estradiol
0.215 mg norgestimate and 35 mcg ethinyl estradiol
0.25 mg norgestimate and 35 mcg ethinyl estradiol

DOSAGES
Women older than age 15: 1 tablet P.O. daily.

ANTIBACTERIALS

Eryzole
Pediazole

GENERIC COMPONENTS
Granules for oral suspension
Erythromycin ethylsuccinate (equivalent of 200 mg erythromycin activity) and 600 mg sulfisoxazole per 5 ml when reconstituted according to manufacturer's directions

DOSAGES
Acute otitis media
Children: 50 mg/kg/day erythromycin and 150 mg/kg/day sulfisoxazole in divided doses q.i.d. for 10 days. Give without regard to meals. Refrigerate after reconstitution; use within 14 days.

ANTIDIABETICS

Avandamet

GENERIC COMPONENTS
Tablets
1 mg rosiglitazone and 500 mg metformin
2 mg rosiglitazone and 500 mg metformin
2 mg rosiglitazone and 1 g metformin
4 mg rosiglitazone and 500 mg metformin
4 mg rosiglitazone and 1 g metformin

DOSAGES
Adults: 4 mg rosiglitazone with 500 mg metformin, once a day or in divided doses. Not for initial therapy; adjust using individual drugs alone then switch to the appropriate dosage of the combination product. See package insert for details on adjusting dosage based on use of other drugs and previous dosage levels.

Glucovance

GENERIC COMPONENTS
Tablets
1.25 mg glyburide and 250 mg metformin
2.5 mg glyburide and 500 mg metformin
5 mg glyburide and 500 mg metformin

DOSAGES
Adults: 1 tablet daily P.O., usually in the morning.
Not for initial therapy; adjust using the individual drugs alone, then switch to the appropriate dosage of the combination product.

Metaglip

GENERIC COMPONENTS
Tablets
2.5 mg glipizide and 250 mg metformin
2.5 mg glipizide and 500 mg metformin
5 mg glipizide and 500 mg metformin

DOSAGES
Adults: 1 tablet per day with a meal; adjust dose based on patient response. Maximum dose, 20 mg glipizide with 2,000 mg metformin daily.

ANTIHYPERTENSIVES

Accuretic

GENERIC COMPONENTS
Tablets
10 mg quinapril and 12.5 mg hydrochlorothiazide
20 mg quinapril and 12.5 mg hydrochlorothiazide
20 mg quinapril and 25 mg hydrochlorothiazide

DOSAGES
Adults: 1 tablet P.O. per day in the morning. Adjust drug using the individual products, then switch to appropriate dosage of the combination product.

Aldoclor

GENERIC COMPONENTS
Tablets
250 mg methyldopa and 150 mg chlorothiazide
250 mg methyldopa and 250 mg chlorothiazide

DOSAGES
Adults: 1 tablet P.O. per day taken in the morning. Adjust dosage using the individual products, then switch to the combination product when patient's adjustment schedule is stable.

Aldoril
Aldoril D

GENERIC COMPONENTS
Tablets
250 mg methyldopa and 15 mg hydrochlorothiazide
250 mg methyldopa and 25 mg hydrochlorothiazide
500 mg methyldopa and 30 mg hydrochlorothiazide
500 mg methyldopa and 50 mg hydrochlorothiazide

DOSAGES
Adults: 1 tablet P.O. daily, in the morning. Adjust dosage using the individual products, then switch to the combination product when patient's adjustment schedule is stable.

Atacand HCT

GENERIC COMPONENTS
Tablets
16 mg candesartan and 12.5 mg hydrochlorothiazide
32 mg candesartan and 12.5 mg hydrochlorothiazide

DOSAGES
Adults: 1 tablet P.O. daily in the morning. Adjust dosage using the individual products, then switch to appropriate dosage.

Avalide

GENERIC COMPONENTS
Tablets
150 mg irbesartan and 12.5 mg hydrochlorothiazide
300 mg irbesartan and 12.5 mg hydrochlorothiazide
300 mg irbesartan and 25 mg hydrochlorothiazide

DOSAGES
Adults: 1 tablet P.O. daily. Adjust dosage with individual products, then switch to combination product when patient's condition is stabilized. Maximum daily dose, 300 mg irbesartan and 25 mg hydrochlorothiazide.

Benicar HCT

GENERIC COMPONENTS
Tablets
20 mg olmesartan and 12.5 mg hydrochlorothiazide
40 mg olmesartan and 12.5 mg hydrochlorothiazide
40 mg olmesartan and 25 mg hydrochlorothiazide

DOSAGES
Adults: 1 tablet P.O. per day in the morning. Adjust dosage using the individual products, then switch to the combination product when patient's adjustment schedule is stable.

Capozide

GENERIC COMPONENTS
Tablets
25 mg captopril and 15 mg hydrochlorothiazide
50 mg captopril and 15 mg hydrochlorothiazide
25 mg captopril and 25 mg hydrochlorothiazide
50 mg captopril and 25 mg hydrochlorothiazide

DOSAGES
Adults: 1 to 2 tablets P.O. daily, in the morning. Adjust dosage using the individual products, then switch to the combination product when patient's adjustment schedule is stable.

Clorpres
Combipres

GENERIC COMPONENTS
Tablets
15 mg chlorthalidone and 0.1 mg clonidine hydrochloride
15 mg chlorthalidone and 0.2 mg clonidine hydrochloride
15 mg chlorthalidone and 0.3 mg clonidine hydrochloride

DOSAGES
Adults: 1 to 2 tablets per day P.O. in the morning. Adjust dosage using the individual products, then switch to the combination product when patient's adjustment schedule is stable.

Corzide

GENERIC COMPONENTS
Tablets
40 mg nadolol and 5 mg bendroflumethiazide
80 mg nadolol and 5 mg bendroflumethiazide

DOSAGES
Adults: 1 tablet P.O. per day in the morning. Adjust dosage using the individual products, then switch to the combination product when patient's adjustment schedule is stable.

Diovan HCT

GENERIC COMPONENTS
Tablets
80 mg valsartan and 12.5 mg hydrochlorothiazide
160 mg valsartan and 12.5 mg hydrochlorothiazide
160 mg valsartan and 25 mg hydrochlorothiazide

DOSAGES
Adults: 1 tablet per day P.O. Not for initial therapy; start using each component first.

Hyzaar

GENERIC COMPONENTS
Tablets
50 mg losartan and 12.5 mg hydrochlorothiazide
100 mg losartan and 25 mg hydrochlorothiazide

DOSAGES
Adults: 1 tablet per day P.O. in the morning. Not for initial therapy; start using each component and if desired effects are obtained, Hyzaar may be used.

Inderide

GENERIC COMPONENTS
Tablets
40 mg propranolol hydrochloride and 25 mg hydrochlorothiazide
80 mg propranolol hydrochloride and 25 mg hydrochlorothiazide

DOSAGES
Adults: 1 tablet P.O. b.i.d. Adjust dosage using the individual products, then switch to the combination product when patient's adjustment schedule is stable. Maximum total daily dose shouldn't exceed 160 mg propranolol and 50 mg hydrochlorothiazide

Lexxel

GENERIC COMPONENTS
Extended-release tablets
5 mg enalapril maleate and 2.5 mg felodipine
5 mg enalapril maleate and 5 mg felodipine

DOSAGES
Adults: 1 tablet per day P.O. Adjust dosage using the individual products, then switch to the combination product when patient's adjustment schedule is stable. Make sure that patient swallows tablet whole. Don't cut, crush, or allow him to chew.

Lopressor HCT

GENERIC COMPONENTS
Tablets
50 mg metoprolol and 25 mg hydrochlorothiazide
100 mg metoprolol and 25 mg hydrochlorothiazide
100 mg metoprolol and 50 mg hydrochlorothiazide

DOSAGES
Adults: 1 tablet P.O. per day. Adjust dosage using the individual products, then switch to the combination product when patient's adjustment schedule is stable.

Lotensin HCT

GENERIC COMPONENTS
Tablets
5 mg benazepril and 6.25 mg hydrochlorothiazide
10 mg benazepril and 12.5 mg hydrochlorothiazide
20 mg benazepril and 12.5 mg hydrochlorothiazide
20 mg benazepril and 25 mg hydrochlorothiazide

DOSAGES
Adults: 1 tablet per day P.O. in the morning. Adjust dosage using the individual products, then switch to the combination product when patient's adjustment schedule is stable.

Lotrel

GENERIC COMPONENTS
Capsules
2.5 mg amlodipine and 10 mg benazepril
5 mg amlodipine and 10 mg benazepril
5 mg amlodipine and 20 mg benazepril
10 mg amlodipine and 20 mg benazepril

DOSAGES
Adults: 1 tablet P.O. daily in the morning. Monitor patient for hypertension and adverse effects closely over first 2 weeks and regularly thereafter.

Micardis HCT

GENERIC COMPONENTS
Tablets
40 mg telmisartan and 12.5 mg hydrochlorothiazide
80 mg telmisartan and 12.5 mg hydrochlorothiazide
80 mg telmisartan and 25 mg hydrochlorothiazide

DOSAGES
Adults: 1 tablet P.O. per day; may be adjusted up to 160 mg telmisartan and 25 mg hydrochlorothiazide, based on patient's response.

Minizide

GENERIC COMPONENTS
Tablets
1 mg prazosin and 0.5 mg polythiazide
2 mg prazosin and 0.5 mg polythiazide
5 mg prazosin and 0.5 mg polythiazide

DOSAGES
Adults: 1 capsule P.O. b.i.d. or t.i.d. Adjust drug using the individual products, then switch to appropriate dosage of the combination product.

Monopril-HCT

GENERIC COMPONENTS
Tablets
10 mg fosinopril and 12.5 mg hydrochlorothiazide
20 mg fosinopril and 12.5 mg hydrochlorothiazide

DOSAGES
Adults: 1 tablet P.O. per day in the morning. Adjust dosage using the individual products, then switch to appropriate dosage of the combination product.

Prinzide
Zestoretic

GENERIC COMPONENTS
Tablets
10 mg lisinopril and 12.5 mg hydrochlorothiazide
20 mg lisinopril and 12.5 mg hydrochlorothiazide

20 mg lisinopril and 25 mg hydrochlorothiazide

DOSAGES
Adults: 1 tablet per day P.O. taken in the morning. Adjust dosage using the individual products, then switch to the combination product when patient's adjustment schedule is stable.

Tarka

GENERIC COMPONENTS
Tablets
1 mg trandolapril and 240 mg verapamil
2 mg trandolapril and 180 mg verapamil
2 mg trandolapril and 240 mg verapamil
4 mg trandolapril and 240 mg verapamil

DOSAGES
Adults: 1 tablet P.O. per day, taken with food. Adjust dosage using the individual products, then switch to the combination product when patient's adjustment schedule is stable. Make sure that patient swallows tablet whole. Don't cut, crush, or allow him to chew.

Teczem

GENERIC COMPONENTS
Extended-release tablets
5 mg enalapril maleate and 180 mg diltiazem hydrochloride

DOSAGES
Adults: 1 to 2 tablets per day P.O. in the morning. Adjust dosage using the individual products, then switch to the combination product when patient's adjustment schedule is stable. Make sure that patient swallows tablet whole. Don't cut, crush, or allow him to chew.

Tenoretic

GENERIC COMPONENTS
Tablets
50 mg atenolol and 25 mg chlorthalidone
100 mg atenolol and 25 mg chlorthalidone

DOSAGES
Adults: 1 tablet P.O. daily in the morning. Adjust dosage using the individual products, then switch to appropriate dosage of the combination product.

Teveten HCT

GENERIC COMPONENTS
Tablets
600 mg eprosartan and 12.5 mg hydrochlorothiazide
600 mg eprosartan and 25 mg hydrochlorothiazide

DOSAGES
Adults: 1 tablet P.O. each day. Establish dosage with each component alone before using the combination product; if blood pressure isn't controlled on 600 mg/25 mg tablet, 300 mg eprosartan may be added each evening.

Uniretic

GENERIC COMPONENTS
Tablets
7.5 mg moexipril and 12.5 mg hydrochlorothiazide
15 mg moexipril and 25 mg hydrochlorothiazide

DOSAGES
Adults: Give ½ to 2 tablets per day. Not for initial therapy. Adjust dose to maintain appropriate blood pressure.

Vaseretic

GENERIC COMPONENTS
Tablets
5 mg enalapril maleate and 12.5 mg hydrochlorothiazide
10 mg enalapril maleate and 25 mg hydrochlorothiazide

DOSAGES
Adults: 1 to 2 tablets per day P.O. in the morning. Adjust dosage using the individual products, then switch to the combination product when patient's adjustment schedule is stable.

Ziac

GENERIC COMPONENTS
Tablets
2.5 mg bisoprolol and 6.25 mg hydrochlorothiazide
5 mg bisoprolol and 6.25 mg hydrochlorothiazide
10 mg bisoprolol and 6.25 mg hydrochlorothiazide

DOSAGES
Adults: 1 tablet daily P.O. in morning. Initial dose is 2.5/6.25 mg tablet P.O. daily. Adjust dosage within 1 week; optimal antihypertensive effect may require 2 to 3 weeks.

ANTIMIGRAINE DRUGS

Cafergot
Cafatine-PB
Ercaf

GENERIC COMPONENTS
Tablets
1 mg ergotamine tartrate and 100 mg caffeine
Suppositories:
2 mg ergotamine tartrate and 100 mg caffeine

DOSAGES
Adults: 2 tablets P.O. at the first sign of attack. Follow with 1 tablet every 30 minutes, if needed. Maximum dose is 6 tablets per attack. Don't exceed 10 tablets per week. Or, 1 suppository P.R. at first sign of attack; follow with second dose after 1 hour, if needed. Maximum dose is 2 suppositories per attack. Don't exceed 5 suppositories per week. Don't combine this drug with ritonavir, nelfinavir, indinavir, erythromycin, clarithromycin, or troleandomycin, as serious vasospasm could occur.

ANTIPLATELET DRUGS

Aggrenox

GENERIC COMPONENTS
Capsules
25 mg aspirin and 200 mg dipyridamole

DOSAGES
Adults: To decrease risk of stroke, 1 capsule P.O. b.i.d. in the morning and evening. Swallow capsule whole; may be taken with or without food.

ANTIULCER DRUGS

Helidac

GENERIC COMPONENTS
Tablets
262.4 mg bismuth subsalicylate, 250 mg metronidazole, and 500 mg tetracycline hydrochloride

DOSAGES
Active duodenal ulcers associated with* Helicobacter pylori *infection.
Adults: 2 chewable bismuth subsalicylate tablets, 1 metronidazole tablet, and 1 tetracycline capsule P.O. q.i.d. for 14 days along with a prescribed H_2 antagonist.

Prevpac

GENERIC COMPONENTS
Daily administration pack
Two 30-mg lansoprazole capsules, four 500-mg amoxicillin capsules, and two 500-mg clarithromycin tablets.

DOSAGES
Adults: Divide pack equally to take twice daily, morning and evening.

ANTIRETROVIRALS

Combivir

GENERIC COMPONENTS
Tablets
150 mg lamivudine and 300 mg zidovudine

DOSAGES
Adults and children age 12 and older who weigh more then 50 kg (110 lb): 1 tablet P.O. b.i.d.

Epzicom

GENERIC COMPONENTS
Tablets
600 mg abacavir with 300 mg lamivudine

DOSAGES
Adults: 1 tablet daily, taken without regard to food and in combination with other antiretrovirals.

Trizivir

GENERIC COMPONENTS
Tablets
300 mg abacavir sulfate, 150 mg lamivudine, and 300 mg zidovudine

DOSAGES
Adults and adolescents who weigh 40 kg (88 lb) or more: 1 tablet P.O. b.i.d., alone or with other antiretrovirals.

Truvada

GENERIC COMPONENTS
Tablets
200 mg emtricitabine with 300 mg tenofovir

DOSAGES
Adults and adolescents weighing more than 40 kg (88 lb): 1 tablet daily, taken without regard to food and in combination with other antiretrovirals.

DIURETICS

Aldactazide

GENERIC COMPONENTS
Tablets
25 mg spironolactone and 25 mg hydrochlorothiazide
50 mg spironolactone and 50 mg hydrochlorothiazide

DOSAGES
Adults: One to eight 25 mg spironolactone and 25 mg hydrochlorothiazide tablets daily. Or, one to four 50 mg spironolactone and 50 mg hydrochlorothiazide tablets daily.

Dyazide

GENERIC COMPONENTS
Capsules
37.5 mg triamterene and 25 mg hydrochlorothiazide

DOSAGES
Adults: 1 to 2 tablets daily.

Maxzide

GENERIC COMPONENTS
Tablets
75 mg triamterene and 50 mg hydrochlorothiazide

DOSAGES
Adults: 1 tablet daily.

Moduretic

GENERIC COMPONENTS
Tablets
5 mg amiloride and 50 mg hydrochlorothiazide

DOSAGES
Adults: 1 to 2 tablets per day with meals.

HEART FAILURE DRUGS

BiDil

GENERIC COMPONENTS
Tablets
20 mg isosorbide dinitrate and 37.5 mg hydralazine

DOSAGES
Adults: 1 to 2 tablets P.O. t.i.d.

IMMUNOMODULATORS

Rebetron

GENERIC COMPONENTS
Capsules
200 mg ribavirin
Injection
3 million international units interferon alfa-2b

DOSAGES
Chronic hepatitis C in patients who relapse after interferon alfa therapy
Adults: 400 mg ribavirin per day P.O. in the morning and 600 mg per day P.O. in the evening with 3 million international units interferon alfa-2b subcutaneously 3 times per week for patients weighing less than 75 kg (165 lb); 600 mg ribavirin per day P.O. in the morning, 600 mg per day P.O. in evening with 3 million international units interferon alfa-2b subcutaneously 3 times per week for patients weighing more than 75 kg.

LIPID-LOWERING DRUGS

Advicor

GENERIC COMPONENTS
Tablets
20 mg lovastatin and 500 mg niacin
20 mg lovastatin and 1,000 mg niacin

DOSAGES
Adults: 1 tablet daily P.O. at night.

Pravigard PAC

GENERIC COMPONENTS
Tablets
20 mg pravastatin packaged with 81 mg buffered aspirin
40 mg pravastatin packaged with 81 mg buffered aspirin
80 mg pravastatin packaged with 81 mg buffered aspirin
20 mg pravastatin packaged with 325 mg buffered aspirin
40 mg pravastatin packaged with 325 mg buffered aspirin
80 mg pravastatin packaged with 325 mg buffered aspirin

DOSAGES
Adults: Initially, 40 mg pravastatin with 81 or 325 mg buffered aspirin; adjust dose to regulate cholesterol levels.

Vytorin

GENERIC COMPONENTS
Tablets
10 mg ezetimibe with 10, 20, 40, or 80 mg simvastatin

DOSAGES
Adults: 1 tablet daily, taken in the evening in combination with a cholesterol-lowering diet and exercise. Dosage of simvastatin in the combination may be adjusted based on patient response. If given with a bile sequestrant, must be given at least 2 hours before or 4 hours after the bile sequestrant.

MENOPAUSE DRUGS

Activella
femHRT

GENERIC COMPONENTS
Tablets
2.5 mcg ethinyl estradiol and 0.5 mg norethindrone acetate (femHRT)
5 mcg ethinyl estradiol and 1 mg norethindrone acetate (femHRT)
1 mg ethinyl estradiol and 0.5 mg norethindrone acetate (Activella)

DOSAGES
Signs and symptoms of menopause; to prevent osteoporosis
Women with intact uterus: 1 tablet P.O. daily.

Prefest

GENERIC COMPONENTS
Tablets
1 mg estradiol and 0.09 mg norgestimate

DOSAGES
Moderate to severe symptoms of menopause; to prevent osteoporosis
Women with intact uterus: 1 tablet/day P.O. (3 days of pink tablets: estradiol alone; followed by 3 days of white tablets: estradiol and norgestimate combination; continue cycle uninterrupted).

Premphase

GENERIC COMPONENTS
Tablets
0.625 mg conjugated estrogens; 0.625 mg conjugated estrogens with 5 mg medroxyprogesterone

DOSAGES
Moderate to severe symptoms of menopause; to prevent osteoporosis
Women with intact uterus: 1 tablet per day P.O. Use estrogen alone on days 1 to 14 and estrogen-medroxyprogesterone tablet on days 15 to 28.

Prempro

GENERIC COMPONENTS
Tablets
0.3 mg conjugated estrogen and 1.5 mg medroxyprogesterone
0.45 mg conjugated estrogen and 1.5 mg medroxyprogesterone
0.625 mg estrogen and 2.5 mg medroxyprogesterone
0.625 mg conjugated estrogen and 5 mg medroxyprogesterone

DOSAGES
Symptoms of menopause; to prevent osteoporosis
Women with intact uterus: One tablet per day P.O.

MISCELLANEOUS CARDIAC DRUGS

Caduet

GENERIC COMPONENTS
Tablets
2.5 mg amlodipine with 10 mg, 20 mg, or 40 mg atorvastatin
5 mg amlodipine with 10 mg, 20 mg, 40 mg, or 80 mg atorvastatin
10 mg amlodipine with 10 mg, 20 mg, 40 mg, or 80 mg atorvastatin

DOSAGES
Adults, boys, and postmenarchal girls age 10 and older: Determine the most effective dose for each component. Then, select the most appropriate combination product.

OPIOID AGONIST

Suboxone
CSS III

GENERIC COMPONENTS
Sublingual tablets
2 mg buprenorphine and 0.5 mg naloxone
8 mg buprenorphine and 2 mg naloxone

DOSAGES
Opioid dependence
Adults: 12 to 16 mg S.L. once daily, after induction with S.L. buprenorphine.

PSYCHOTHERAPEUTICS

Limbitrol
Limbitrol DS

GENERIC COMPONENTS
Tablets
5 mg chlordiazepoxide and 12.5 mg amitriptyline
10 mg chlordiazepoxide and 25 mg amitriptyline

DOSAGES
Adults: 10 mg chlordiazepoxide with 25 mg amitriptyline 3 to 4 times per day up to 6 times daily. For patients who don't tolerate the higher doses, 5 mg chlordiazepoxide with 12.5 mg amitriptyline 3 to 4 times per day. Reduce dosage after initial response.

perphenazine and amitriptyline

GENERIC COMPONENTS
Tablets
2 mg perphenazine and 10 mg amitriptyline
2 mg perphenazine and 25 mg amitriptyline
4 mg perphenazine; 10 mg amitriptyline
4 mg perphenazine and 25 mg amitriptyline
4 mg perphenazine and 50 mg amitriptyline

DOSAGES
Adults: 2 to 4 mg perphenazine with 10 to 50 mg amitriptyline 3 to 4 times daily. Reduce dosage after initial response.

Symbyax

GENERIC COMPONENTS
Capsules
6 mg olanzapine and 25 mg fluoxetine
6 mg olanzapine and 50 mg fluoxetine
12 mg olanzapine and 25 mg fluoxetine
12 mg olanzapine and 50 mg fluoxetine

DOSAGES
Adults: 1 capsule daily in the evening. Begin with 6 mg/25 mg capsule and adjust according to efficacy and tolerability.

RESPIRATORY DRUGS

Claritin-D

GENERIC COMPONENTS
Extended-release tablets
5 mg loratadine and 120 mg pseudoephedrine

DOSAGES
Adults: 1 tablet q 12 hours.

Claritin-D 24 Hour

GENERIC COMPONENTS
Extended-release tablets
10 mg loratadine and 240 mg pseudoephedrine

DOSAGES
Adults: 1 tablet q day.

Combivent

GENERIC COMPONENTS
Metered dose inhaler
18 mcg ipratropium bromide and 90 mcg albuterol

DOSAGES
Bronchospasm with COPD in patients who require more than a single bronchodilator
Adults: Two inhalations q.i.d. Not for use during acute attack. Use caution with known sensitivity to atropine, soy, or peanuts.

Vitamins and minerals: Indications and dosages

vitamin A (retinol)

Aquasol A, Palmitate-A

Pregnancy risk category A if dose is under 800 mcg retinol equivalents; C if dose exceeds 800 mcg retinol equivalents; X for Aquasol

AVAILABLE FORMS

Capsules: 10,000 international units ◊, 15,000 international units ◊, 25,000 international units
Drops: 30 ml with dropper (5,000 international units/ 0.1 ml, 50,000 international units/ml)
Injection: 2-ml vials (50,000 international units/ml with 0.5% chlorobutanol, polysorbate 80, butylated hydroxyanisole, butylated hydroxytoluene)
Tablets: 5,000 international units ◊, 10,000 international units

INDICATIONS AND DOSAGES

➤ RDA

Men and boys older than age 14: Give 900 mcg retinol equivalent (RE) or 3,000 international units.
Women and girls older than age 14: Give 700 mcg RE or 2,330 international units.
Children ages 9 to 13: Give 600 mcg RE or 2,000 international units.
Children ages 4 to 8: Give 400 mcg RE or 1,330 international units.
Children ages 1 to 3: Give 300 mcg RE or 1,000 international units.
Infants ages 7 to 12 months: 500 mcg RE or 1,665 international units.
Neonates and infants younger than age 6 months: 400 mcg RE or 1,330 international units.
Pregnant women ages 14 to 18: Give 750 mcg RE or 2,500 international units.
Pregnant women ages 19 to 50: Give 770 mcg RE or 2,564 international units.
Breast-feeding women ages 14 to 18: Give 1,200 mcg RE or 4,000 international units.
Breast-feeding women ages 19 to 50: Give 1,300 mcg RE or 4,330 international units.

➤ Severe vitamin A deficiency

Adults and children older than age 8: Give 100,000 international units I.M. or 100,000 to 500,000 international units P.O. for 3 days; then 50,000 international units P.O. or I.M. for 2 weeks, followed by 10,000 to 20,000 international units P.O. for 2 months. Follow with adequate dietary nutrition and RE vitamin A supplements.
Children age 8 and younger: 5,000 to 15,000 international units I.M. daily for 10 days.

➤ Maintenance dose to prevent recurrence of vitamin A deficiency

Children ages 1 to 8: Give 5,000 to 10,000 international units P.O. daily for 2 months; then adequate dietary nutrition and RE vitamin A supplements.

vitamin B complex

cyanocobalamin (vitamin B12)

Crystamine, Crysti-12, Cyanoject, Cyomin

hydroxocobalamin (vitamin B12)

Hydro-Cobex, Hydro-Crysti-12, LA-12

Pregnancy risk category A ; C if dose exceeds RDA

AVAILABLE FORMS

cyanocobalamin

Injection: 100 mcg/ml, 1,000 mcg/ml
Intranasal gel: 500 mcg/0.1 ml
Intranasal spray ◊ : 500 mcg/spray

Tablets ◊: 25 mcg ◊, 50 mcg ◊, 100 mcg ◊, 250 mcg ◊, 500 mcg ◊, 1,000 mcg ◊
hydroxocobalamin
Injection: 1,000 mcg/ml

INDICATIONS AND DOSAGES

➤ **RDA for cyanocobalamin**
Adults and children ages 14 and older: 2.4 mcg.
Children ages 9 to 13: Give 1.8 mcg.
Children ages 4 to 8: Give 1.2 mcg.
Children ages 1 to 3: Give 0.9 mcg.
Infants ages 6 months to 1 year: 0.5 mcg.
Neonates and infants younger than age 6 months: 0.4 mcg.
Pregnant women: 2.6 mcg.
Breast-feeding women: 2.8 mcg.

➤ **Vitamin B12 deficiency from inadequate diet, subtotal gastrectomy, or other condition, disorder, or disease, except malabsorption, related to pernicious anemia or other GI disease**
Adults: 30 mcg hydroxocobalamin I.M. daily for 5 to 10 days, depending on severity of deficiency. Maintenance dose is 100 to 200 mcg I.M. once monthly or 500 mcg gel intranasally once weekly. For subsequent prophylaxis, advise adequate nutrition and daily RDA vitamin B12 supplements.
Children: 1 to 5 mg hydroxocobalamin in single doses of 100 mcg I.M. over 2 or more weeks, depending on severity of deficiency. Maintenance dose is 60 mcg/month I.M. For subsequent prophylaxis, advise adequate nutrition and daily RDA vitamin B12 supplements.

➤ **Pernicious anemia or vitamin B12 malabsorption**
Adults: Initially, 100 mcg cyanocobalamin I.M. or subcutaneously daily for 6 to 7 days. If response is observed, 100 mcg I.M. or subcutaneously every other day for 7 doses, then 100 mcg q 3 to 4 days for 2 to 3 weeks; then 100 mcg I.M. or subcutaneously once monthly.
Children: 30 to 50 mcg I.M. or subcutaneously daily over 2 or more weeks; then 100 mcg I.M. or subcutaneously monthly for life.

➤ **Maintenance therapy for remission of pernicious anemia after I.M. vitamin B12 therapy in patients without nervous system involvement; dietary deficiency, malabsorption disorders, and inadequate secretion of intrinsic factor**
Adults: Initially, one spray in one nostril once weekly. Give at least one hour before or after hot foods or liquids.

➤ **Prevention of methylmalonic aciduria**
Mothers and their neonates: 5,000 mcg cyanocobalamin I.M. daily to the mother prepartum, then 1,000 mcg I.M. daily to the neonate for 11 days, with a protein-restricted diet.

➤ **Methylmalonic aciduria**
Neonates: 1,000 mcg cyanocobalamin I.M. daily.

➤ **Schilling test flushing dose**
Adults and children: 1,000 mcg hydroxocobalamin I.M. as single dose.

folic acid (vitamin B9)
Folvite, Novo-Folacid†

Pregnancy risk category A

AVAILABLE FORMS
Injection: 10-ml vials (5 mg/ml with 1.5% benzyl alcohol, 5 mg/ml with 1.5% benzyl alcohol and 0.2% ethylenediaminetetraacetic acid)
Tablets: 0.4 mg, 0.8 mg, 1 mg

INDICATIONS AND DOSAGES

➤ **RDA**
Adults and children age 14 and older: Give 400 mcg.
Children ages 9 to 13: Give 300 mcg.
Children ages 4 to 8: Give 200 mcg.
Children ages 1 to 3: Give 150 mcg.
Infants ages 6 months to 1 year: 80 mcg.
Neonates and infants younger than age 6 months: 65 mcg.
Pregnant women: 600 mcg.
Breast-feeding women: 500 mcg.

†Canada ◊OTC.

➤ **Megaloblastic or macrocytic anemia from folic acid or other nutritional deficiency, hepatic disease, alcoholism, intestinal obstruction, or excessive hemolysis**
Adults and children age 4 and older: 0.4 to 1 mg P.O., I.M., or subcutaneously daily. After anemia caused by folic acid deficiency is corrected, proper diet and RDA supplements are needed to prevent recurrence.
Children younger than age 4: Up to 0.3 mg P.O., I.M., or subcutaneously daily.
Pregnant and breast-feeding women: 0.8 mg P.O., I.M., or subcutaneously daily.
➤ **To prevent fetal neural tube defects during pregnancy**
Adults: 0.4 mg P.O. daily.
➤ **To prevent megaloblastic anemia during pregnancy to prevent fetal damage**
Adults: Up to 1 mg P.O., I.M., or subcutaneously daily throughout pregnancy.
➤ **Test for folic acid deficiency in patients with megaloblastic anemia without masking pernicious anemia**
Adults and children: 0.1 to 0.2 mg P.O. or I.M. for 10 days while maintaining a diet low in folate and vitamin B12.
➤ **Tropical sprue**
Adults: 3 to 15 mg P.O. daily.

leucovorin calcium (citrovorum factor, folinic acid)

Pregnancy risk category C

AVAILABLE FORMS
Injection: 1-ml ampule (3 mg/ml with 0.9% benzyl alcohol); 10 mg/ml in 5-ml vial; 50-mg, 100-mg, 350-mg, 500-mg vials for reconstitution (contains no preservatives)
Tablets: 5 mg, 10 mg, 15 mg, 25 mg

INDICATIONS AND DOSAGES
➤ **Overdose of folic acid antagonist (methotrexate, trimethoprim, or pyrimethamine)**
Adults and children: I.M. or I.V. dose equivalent to weight of antagonist given. For methotrexate overdose, up to 75 mg I.V. infusion within 12 hours, followed by 12 mg I.M. q 6 hours for four doses. For adverse effects after average doses of methotrexate, 6 to 12 mg I.M. q 6 hours for four doses.
➤ **Leucovorin rescue after high methotrexate dose in treatment of malignant disease**
Adults and children: 10 mg/m^2 P.O., I.M., or I.V. q 6 hours until methotrexate level falls below 5×10^{-8} M.
➤ **Megaloblastic anemia from congenital enzyme deficiency**
Adults and children: 3 to 6 mg I.M. daily.
➤ **Folate-deficient megaloblastic anemia**
Adults and children: Up to 1 mg I.M. daily. Duration of treatment depends on hematologic response.
➤ **To prevent hematologic toxicity from pyrimethamine or trimethoprim therapy**
Adults and children: 400 mcg to 5 mg I.M. with each dose of folic acid antagonist. Oral dosages of 10 to 35 mg once daily or 25 mg once weekly may also be used.
➤ **Hematologic toxicity from pyrimethamine or trimethoprim therapy**
Adults and children: 5 to 15 mg I.M. daily.
➤ **Palliative treatment of advanced colorectal cancer**
Adults: 20 mg/m^2 I.V.; then fluorouracil 425 mg/m^2 I.V. or 200 mg/m^2 I.V. (over 3 minutes or longer) followed by fluorouracil 370 mg/m^2 daily for 5 consecutive days. Repeat at 4-week intervals for two additional courses; then at intervals of 4 to 5 weeks, if tolerated.

niacin (nicotinic acid, vitamin B3)

Nia-Bid ◊, Niacor ◊, Niaspan, Nicobid ◊ Nicotinex, Slo-Niacin ◊

niacinamide ◊ (nicotinamide ◊)

Pregnancy risk category A ; C if dose exceeds RDA

AVAILABLE FORMS

niacin

Capsules (timed-release): 125 mg ◊, 250 mg ◊, 300 mg ◊, 400 mg ◊, 500 mg

Elixir: 50 mg/5 ml ◊ *

Tablets: 25 mg ◊, 50 mg ◊, 100 mg ◊, 250 mg ◊, 500 mg

Tablets (extended-release): 250 mg ◊, 375 mg ◊, 500 mg ◊, 750 mg ◊, 1,000 mg ◊

niacinamide

Tablets: 50 mg ◊, 100 mg ◊, 125 mg ◊, 250 mg ◊, 500 mg ◊

INDICATIONS AND DOSAGES

➤ **RDA**

Adult men and boys ages 14 to 18: Give 16 mg

Adult women and girls ages 14 to 18: Give 14 mg.

Children ages 9 to 13: Give 12 mg.

Children ages 4 to 8: Give 8 mg.

Children ages 1 to 3: Give 6 mg.

Infants ages 6 months to 1 year: 4 mg.

Neonates and infants younger than age 6 months: 2 mg.

Pregnant women: 18 mg.

Breast-feeding women: 17 mg.

➤ **Pellagra**

Adults: 300 to 500 mg P.O. daily in divided doses.

Children: 100 to 300 mg P.O. daily in divided doses.

➤ **Hartnup disease**

Adults: 50 to 200 mg P.O. daily.

➤ **Niacin deficiency**

Adults: Up to 100 mg P.O. daily.

➤ **Hyperlipidemias, especially with hypercholesterolemia**

Adults: 250 mg P.O. daily at bedtime. Increase at 4- to 7-day intervals up to 1.5 to 2 g P.O. daily divided b.i.d. to t.i.d. Maximum 6 g daily. Or, 1 to 2 g extended-release tablets P.O. daily at bedtime.

pyridoxine hydrochloride (vitamin B6)

Nestrex ◊, Rodex

Pregnancy risk category A; C if dose exceeds RDA

AVAILABLE FORMS

Injection: 100 mg/ml

Tablets: 10 mg ◊, 25 mg ◊, 32.5 MG ◊, 50 mg ◊, 100 mg ◊, 200 mg ◊, 250 mg ◊, 500 mg ◊

Tablets (enteric-coated): 20 mg ◊

Tablets (extended-release): 100 mg ◊, 200 mg ◊, 500 mg ◊

INDICATIONS AND DOSAGES

➤ **RDA**

Adults ages 19 to 50: Give 1.3 mg.

Men age 51 and older: 1.7 mg.

Women age 51 and older: 1.5 mg.

Boys ages 14 to 19: Give 1.3 mg.

Girls ages 14 to 19: Give 1.2 mg.

Children ages 9 to 13: Give 1 mg.

Children ages 4 to 8: Give 0.6 mg.

Children ages 1 to 3: Give 0.5 mg.

Infants ages 6 months to 1 year: 0.3 mg.

Neonates and infants younger than age 6 months: 0.1 mg.

Pregnant women: 2.2 mg.

Breast-feeding women: 2.1 mg.

➤ **Dietary vitamin B6 deficiency**

Adults: 2.5 to 10 mg P.O., I.V., or I.M. daily for 3 weeks; then 2 to 5 mg daily as supplement to proper diet.

➤ **Seizures related to vitamin B6 deficiency or dependency**

Adults and children: 100 mg I.V. or I.M. in single dose.

➤ **Vitamin B6-responsive anemias or dependency syndrome (inborn errors of metabolism)**

Adults: Up to 500 mg P.O., I.V., or I.M. daily until symptoms subside; then same dosage daily for life.

➤ **To prevent vitamin B6 deficiency during drug therapy with isoniazid or penicillamine**
Adults: 10 to 50 mg P.O. daily.
➤ **To prevent seizures during cycloserine therapy**
Adults: 100 to 300 mg P.O. daily.
➤ **Antidote for isoniazid poisoning**
Adults: 4 g I.V.; then 1 g I.M. q 30 minutes until amount of pyridoxine given equals amount of isoniazid ingested.

thiamine hydrochloride (vitamin B1)

Pregnancy risk category A ; C if dose exceeds RDA

AVAILABLE FORMS
Elixir†: 250 mcg/5 ml
Injection: 100 mg/ml
Tablets: 25 mg ◊, 50 mg ◊, 100 mg ◊, 250 mg ◊, 500 mg
Tablets (enteric-coated): 20 mg

INDICATIONS AND DOSAGES
➤ **RDA**
Adult men: 1.2 mg.
Adult women: 1.1 mg.
Boys ages 14 to 18: Give 1.2 mg.
Girls ages 14 to 18: Give 1 mg.
Children ages 9 to 13: Give 0.9 mg.
Children ages 4 to 8: Give 0.6 mg.
Children ages 1 to 3: Give 0.5 mg.
Infants ages 6 months to 1 year: 0.3 mg.
Neonates and infants younger than age 6 months: 0.2 mg.
Pregnant women: 1.4 mg.
Breast-feeding women: 1.5 mg.
➤ **Beriberi**
Adults: Depending on severity, 5 to 30 mg I.M. t.i.d. for 2 weeks; then dietary correction and multivitamin supplement containing 5 to 30 mg thiamine daily for 1 month.
Children: Depending on severity, 10 to 25 mg I.V. or I.M. daily. For noncritically ill children, 10 to 50 mg P.O. daily in divided doses for several weeks with adequate diet.
➤ **Wet beriberi with myocardial failure**
Adults and children: 10 to 30 mg I.V. t.i.d.
➤ **Wernicke encephalopathy**
Adults: Initially, 100 mg I.V.; then 50 to 100 mg I.V. or I.M. daily until patient is consuming a regular balanced diet.

vitamin C (ascorbic acid)

Ascor L 500, Cecon ◊, Cenolate ◊, Cevi-Bid ◊, Dull-C ◊, Flavorcee ◊, Vicks Vitamin C Drops ◊, Vita-C ◊

Pregnancy risk category A ; C if dose exceeds RDA

AVAILABLE FORMS
Capsules: 500 mg ◊
Capsules (timed-release): 250 mg ◊, 500 mg ◊
Crystals: 1,000 mg/¼ tsp ◊
Injection: 222 mg/ml, 250 mg/ml, 500 mg/ml
Lozenges: 60 mg ◊
Oral solution: 100 mg/ml ◊
Powder: 60 mg/¼ tsp ◊, 1,060 mg/¼ tsp ◊
Tablets: 250 mg ◊, 500 mg ◊, 1,000 mg ◊, 1,500 mg ◊
Tablets (chewable): 100 mg ◊, 250 mg ◊, 500 mg ◊, 1,000 mg ◊
Tablets (timed-release): 500 mg ◊, 1,000 mg ◊

INDICATIONS AND DOSAGES
➤ **RDA**
Men age 19 and older: 90 mg.
Women age 19 and older: 75 mg.
Boys ages 14 to 18: Give 75 mg.
Girls ages 14 to 18: Give 65 mg.
Children ages 9 to 13: Give 45 mg.
Children ages 4 to 8: Give 25 mg.
Children ages 1 to 3: Give 15 mg.
Infants ages 7 months to 1 year: 50 mg.
Neonates and infants up to age 6 months: 40 mg.
Pregnant women: 80 to 85 mg.
Breast-feeding women: 115 to 120 mg.
➤ **Frank and subclinical scurvy**
Adults: Depending on severity, 100 to 250 mg P.O., I.V., I.M., or subcutaneously daily; then 70 to 150 mg daily for maintenance.

†Canada ◊ OTC.

Children: Depending on severity, 100 to 300 mg P.O., I.V., I.M., or subcutaneously daily; then at least 30 mg daily for maintenance.

➤ **Extensive burns, delayed fracture or wound healing, postoperative wound healing, severe febrile or chronic disease states**

Adults: 300 to 500 mg I.V., I.M., or subcutaneously daily for 7 to 10 days; 1 to 2 g daily for extensive burns.

Children: 100 to 200 mg P.O., I.V., I.M, or subcutaneously daily.

➤ **To prevent vitamin C deficiency in patients with poor nutritional habits or increased requirements**

Adults: 70 to 150 mg P.O., I.V., I.M., or subcutaneously daily.

Children: At least 40 mg P.O., I.V., I.M., or subcutaneously daily.

Infants: At least 35 mg P.O., I.V., I.M., or subcutaneously daily.

Pregnant and breast-feeding women: At least 70 to 150 mg P.O., I.V., I.M., or subcutaneously daily.

➤ **To acidify urine**

Adults: 4 to 12 g P.O. daily in divided doses.

➤ **Macular degeneration**

Adults: 500 mg daily in combination with beta carotene, vitamin E, zinc, and copper.

vitamin D

cholecalciferol (vitamin D3)

Delta-D ◊

ergocalciferol (vitamin D2)

Calciferol, Drisdol , Radiostol†

Pregnancy risk category A ; C if dose exceeds RDA

AVAILABLE FORMS

Capsules: 1.25 mg (50,000 international units)

Injection: 12.5 mg (500,000 international units)/ml

Oral liquid: 8,000 international units/ml in 60-ml dropper bottle ◊

Tablets: 1.25 mg (50,000 international units)

INDICATIONS AND DOSAGES

➤ **RDA for cholecalciferol**

Adults older than age 70: Give 600 international units.

Adults ages 51 to 70: Give 400 international units.

Children and adults up to age 50: Give 200 international units.

Pregnant or breast-feeding women: 200 international units.

➤ **Rickets and other vitamin D deficiency diseases, renal osteodystrophy**

Adults: Initially, 10,000 international units P.O. or I.M. daily; expect to increase, based on response, to maximum of 500,000 international units daily.

Children: 1,500 to 5,000 international units P.O. or I.M. daily for 2 to 4 weeks; repeat after 2 weeks, if needed. Or, give single dose of 600,000 international units. After correction of deficiency, maintenance includes adequate diet and RDA supplements.

➤ **Hypoparathyroidism**

Adults and children: 25,000 to 200,000 international units P.O. or I.M. daily, with calcium supplement.

➤ **Familial hypophosphatemia**

Adults: 250 mcg to 1.5 mg P.O. daily with phosphate supplement.

Children: 1 to 2 mg P.O. daily with phosphate supplement, increased in 250- to 500-mcg increments at 3- to 4-month intervals.

vitamin D analogue

doxercalciferol

Hectorol

Pregnancy risk category B

AVAILABLE FORMS

Capsules: 0.5 mcg, 2.5 mcg

Injection: 2 mcg/ml

†Canada ◊ OTC.

INDICATIONS AND DOSAGES

➤ **Secondary hyperparathyroidism in dialysis patients with chronic kidney disease**

Adults: Initially, 10 mcg P.O. three times weekly at dialysis. Adjust dosage as needed to lower intact parathyroid hormone (iPTH) levels to 150 to 300 picograms (pg)/ml. Increase dose by 2.5 mcg at 8-week intervals if iPTH level hasn't decreased by 50% and fails to reach target range. Maximum dose is 20 mcg P.O. three times weekly. If iPTH levels fall below 100 pg/ml, suspend drug for 1 week; then give dose of at least 2.5 mcg less than last dose Or, 4 mcg I.V. bolus 3 times a week at the end of dialysis about q other day. Adjust dose as needed to lower iPTH levels to 150 to 300 pg/ml. Dosage may be increased by 1 to 2 mcg at 8-week intervals if the iPTH level isn't decreased by 50% and fails to reach target range. Maximum dose is 18 mcg weekly. If iPTH levels go below 100 pg/ml, suspend drug for 1 week, then resume at a dose that's at least 1 mcg P.O. lower than the last dose.

➤ **Secondary hyperparathyroidism in predialysis patients with stage 3 or 4 chronic kidney disease**

Adults: 1 mcg P.O. daily. Adjust dosage as needed to lower iPTH levels to 35 to 70 pg/ml for stage 3 or 70 to 110 pg/ml for stage 4. Increase dosage at 2-week intervals by 0.5 mcg if levels are above 70 pg/ml for stage 3 or above 110 pg/ml for stage 4. If level falls below 35 pg/ml for stage 3 or 70 pg/ml for stage 4, suspend treatment for 1 week, then give dose at least 0.5 mcg lower than last dose. Maximum dose, 3.5 mcg daily.

paricalcitol
Zemplar

Pregnancy risk category C

AVAILABLE FORMS

Capsules: 1 mcg, 2 mcg, 4 mcg
Injection: 2 mcg/ml, 5 mcg/ml

INDICATIONS AND DOSAGES

➤ **To prevent or treat secondary hyperparathyroidism in patients with stage 3 or 4 chronic kidney disease**

Adults: Initial dose is based on baseline intact parathyroid hormone (iPTH) levels. If iPTH is less than or equal to 500 picograms (pg)/ml, give 1 mcg P.O. daily or 2 mcg P.O. three times weekly, no more often than every other day. If iPTH is greater than 500 pg/ml, give 2 mcg P.O. daily or 4 mcg P.O. three times weekly, no more often than every other day. Adjust dose at 2- to 4-week intervals, based on iPTH levels.

➤ **To prevent or treat secondary hyperparathyroidism in patients with chronic renal failure**

Adults: 0.04 to 0.1 mcg/kg (2.8 to 7 mcg) I.V. no more frequently than every other day during dialysis. Doses as high as 0.24 mcg/kg (16.8 mcg) may be safely given. If satisfactory response isn't observed, increase dosage by 2 to 4 mcg at 2- to 4-week intervals.

vitamin E (tocopherols)
Aquasol E ◊, Aquavit-E ◊, d-alpha E

Pregnancy risk category A

AVAILABLE FORMS

Capsules: 100 international units ◊, 200 international units ◊, 400 international units ◊, 600 international units ◊, 1,000 international units ◊
Drops: 15 international units/0.3 ml
Liquid: 15 international units/30 ml
Tablets: 100 international units ◊, 200 international units ◊, 400 international units ◊, 500 international units ◊, 600 international units ◊, 800 international units ◊, 1,000 international units ◊

INDICATIONS AND DOSAGES

Note: RDAs for vitamin E have been converted to α-tocopherol equivalents (α-TE). One α-TE equals 1 mg of D-α tocopherol, or 1.49 international units.

➤ **RDA**
Adults and children ages 14 to 18: Give 15 mg.
Children ages 9 to 13: Give 11 mg.
Children ages 4 to 8: Give 7 mg.
Children ages 1 to 3: Give 6 mg.
Infants ages 6 months to 1 year: 5 mg.
Neonates and infants younger than age 6 months: 4 mg.
Pregnant women: 15 mg.
Breast-feeding women: 19 mg.
➤ **Vitamin E deficiency in premature neonates and in patients with impaired fat absorption**
Adults: Depending on severity, 60 to 75 international units P.O. daily.
Children: 1 international unit/kg daily.

vitamin K analogue

phytonadione (vitamin K1)
Mephyton

Pregnancy risk category C

AVAILABLE FORMS
Injection (aqueous colloidal solution): 2 mg/ml, 10 mg/ml
Injection (aqueous dispersion): 2 mg/ml, 10 mg/ml
Tablets: 5 mg

INDICATIONS AND DOSAGES
➤ **RDA**
Men age 19 and older: 120 mcg.
Women age 19 and older, including pregnant and breast-feeding women: 90 mcg.
Children ages 14 to 18: Give 75 mcg.
Children ages 9 to 13: Give 60 mcg.
Children ages 4 to 8: Give 55 mcg.
Children ages 1 to 3: Give 30 mcg.
Infants ages 7 months to 1 year: 2.5 mcg.
Neonates and infants younger than age 6 months: 2 mcg.
➤ **Hypoprothrombinemia caused by vitamin K malabsorption, drug therapy, or excessive vitamin A dosage**
Adults: Depending on severity, 2.5 to 10 mg P.O., I.M., or subcutaneously, repeated and increased up to 50 mg, p.r.n.
Children: 5 to 10 mg P.O. or parenterally.
Infants: 2 mg P.O. or parenterally.
➤ **Hypoprothrombinemia caused by effect of oral anticoagulants**
Adults: 2.5 to 10 mg P.O., I.M., or subcutaneously, based on PT and INR; repeat if needed within 12 to 48 hours after oral dose or within 6 to 8 hours after parenteral dose. In emergency, 10 to 50 mg slow I.V. at rate not to exceed 1 mg/minute, repeated q 4 hours, p.r.n.
➤ **To prevent hemorrhagic disease of newborn**
Neonates: 0.5 to 1 mg I.M. within 1 hour after birth.
➤ **Hemorrhagic disease of newborn**
Neonates: 1 mg subcutaneously or I.M. Higher doses may be needed if mother has bee n receiving oral anticoagulants.

Therapeutic drug monitoring guidelines

Drug	Laboratory test monitored	Therapeutic ranges of test
aminoglycoside antibiotics (amikacin, gentamicin, tobramycin)	Amikacin peak Amikacin trough Creatinine Gentamicin, tobramycin peak Gentamicin, tobramycin trough	20–30 mcg/ml 1–4 mcg/ml 0.6–1.3 mg/dl 4–12 mcg/ml < 2 mcg/ml
amphotericin B	BUN CBC with differential and platelets Creatinine Electrolytes (especially potassium and magnesium) Liver function	5–20 mg/dl ***** 0.6–1.3 mg/dl Potassium: 3.5–5 mEq/L Magnesium: 1.5–2.5 mEq/L Sodium: 135–145 mEq/L Chloride: 98–106 mEq/L *
ACE inhibitors (benazepril, captopril, enalapril, enalaprilat, fosinopril, lisinopril, moexipril, quinapril, ramipril, trandolapril)	Creatinine BUN Potassium WBC with differential	0.6–1.3 mg/dl 5–20 mg/dl 3.5–5 mEq/L *****
antibiotics	Cultures and sensitivities WBC with differential	 *****
biguanides (metformin)	CBC Creatinine Fasting glucose Glycosylated hemoglobin	***** 0.6–1.3 mg/dl 70–110 mg/dl 4%–7% of total hemoglobin
carbamazepine	BUN Carbamazepine CBC with differential Liver function Platelet count	5–20 mg/dl 4–12 mcg/ml ***** * 150–450 × 10^3/mm^3
clozapine	WBC with differential	*****
corticosteroids (cortisone, hydrocortisone, prednisone, prednisolone, triamcinolone, methylprednisolone, dexamethasone, betamethasone	Electrolytes (especially potassium) Fasting glucose	Potassium: 3.5–5 mEq/L Magnesium 1.7–2.1 mEq/L Sodium 135–145 mEq/L Chloride 98–106 mEq/L Calcium 8.6–10 mg/dl 70–110 mg/dl

***** For those areas marked with asterisks, the following values can be used:

Hemoglobin: Women: 12–16 g/dl
Men: 14–18 g/dl
Hematocrit: Women: 37%–48%
Men: 42%–52%
RBCs: 4–5.5 × 10^6/mm^3
WBCs: 5–10 × 10^3/mm^3

Differential: Neutrophils: 45%–74%
Bands: 0%–8%
Lymphocytes: 16%–45%
Monocytes: 4%–10%
Eosinophils: 0%–7%
Basophils: 0%–2%

Monitoring guidelines

Wait until after the third dose is given to check drug levels. Obtain blood for peak level 30 minutes after I.V. infusion ends or 60 minutes after I.M. administration. For trough levels, draw blood just before next dose. Dosage may need to be adjusted accordingly. Recheck after three doses. Monitor creatinine and BUN levels and urine output for signs of decreasing renal function. Monitor urine for increased proteins, cells, and casts.

Monitor creatinine, BUN, and electrolyte levels at least weekly during therapy. Regularly monitor blood counts and liver function test results during therapy.

Monitor WBC with differential before therapy, monthly during the first 3 to 6 months, then periodically for the first year. Monitor renal function and potassium level periodically.

Monitor WBC with differential weekly during therapy. Specimen cultures and sensitivities will determine the cause of the infection and the best treatment.

Check renal function and hematologic values before starting therapy and at least annually thereafter. If the patient has impaired renal function, don't use metformin because it may cause lactic acidosis. Monitor response to therapy by periodically evaluating fasting glucose and glycosylated hemoglobin levels. A patient's home monitoring of glucose levels helps monitor compliance and response.

Monitor blood counts and platelets before therapy, monthly during the first 2 months, then yearly. Liver function, BUN, and urinalysis should be checked before and periodically during therapy.

Before starting, patient must have a basline WBC count of at least 3,500/mm³ and a basline ANC of at least 2,000/mm³. during the first 6 months of therapy, monitor patient weekly. If acceptable WBC and ANC values are maintained, reduce monitoring to every other week. After 6 months of monitoring without leukopenia, monitor every 4 weeks. WBC count and ANC must be monitored weekly for at least 4 weeks after stopping drug.

Monitor electrolyte and glucose levels regularly during long-term therapy.

(continued)

* For those areas marked with one asterisk, the following values can be used:

ALT: 7–56 units/L
AST: 5–40 units/L
Alkaline phosphatase: 17–142 units/L
LDH: 60–220 units/L
GGT: < 40 units/L

Total bilirubin: 0.2–1 mg/dl

Drug	Laboratory test monitored	Therapeutic ranges of test
digoxin	Creatinine	0.6–1.3 mg/dl
	Digoxin	0.8–2 nanograms/ml
	Electrolytes	Potassium: 3.5–5 mEq/L Magnesium: 1.7–2.1 mEq/L Sodium: 135–145 mEq/L Chloride: 98–106 mEq/L Calcium: 8.6–10 mg/dl
erythropoietin	CBC with differential	*****
	Hematocrit	Women: 36%–48% Men: 42%–52%
	Platelet count	150–450 × 10^3/mm^3
	Serum ferritin	10–383 mg/ml
	Transferrin saturation	220–400 mg/dl
ethosuximide	CBC with differential	*****
	Ethosuximide	40–100 mcg/ml
	Liver function	*
gemfibrozil	CBC	*****
	Lipids	Total cholesterol: < 200 mg/dl LDL: < 100 mg/dl HDL: Women: 40–75 mg/dl Men: 37–70 mg/dl Triglycerides: 10–150 mg/dl
	Liver function	*
	Serum glucose	70–100 mg/dl
heparin	Partial thromboplastin time (PTT)	1.5–2.5 times control
	Hematocrit	*****
	Platelet count	150–450 × 10^3/mm^3
HMG-CoA reductase inhibitors (atorvastatin, fluvastatin, lovastatin, pravastatin, simvastatin)	Lipids	Total cholesterol: < 200 mg/dl LDL: < 100 mg/dl HDL: Women: 40–75 mg/dl Men: 37–70 mg/dl Triglycerides: 10–150 mg/dl
	Liver function	*
insulin	Fasting glucose	70–110 mg/dl
	Glycosylated hemoglobin	4%–7% of total hemoglobin
isotretinoin	CBC with differential	*****
	Liver function	*
	Lipids	Total cholesterol: < 200 mg/dl LDL: < 130 mg/dl HDL: Women: 40–75 mg/dl Men: 37–70 mg/dl Triglycerides: 10–160 mg/dl
	Platelet count	150–450 × 10^3/mm^3
	Pregnancy test	Negative

***** For those areas marked with asterisks, the following values can be used:

Hemoglobin: Women: 12–16 g/dl
Men: 14–18 g/dl
Hematocrit: Women: 37%–48%
Men: 42%–52%
RBCs: 4–5.5 × 10^6/mm^3
WBCs: 5–10 × 10^3/mm^3

Differential: Neutrophils: 45%–74%
Bands: 0%–8%
Lymphocytes: 16%–45%
Monocytes: 4%–10%
Eosinophils: 0%–7%
Basophils: 0%–2%

Monitoring guidelines
Check digoxin levels just before the next dose or at least 6 to 8 hours after the last dose. To monitor maintenance therapy, check drug levels at least 1 to 2 weeks after therapy is initiated or changed. Make any adjustments in therapy based on entire clinical picture, not solely on drug levels. Also, check electrolyte levels and renal function periodically during therapy.
After therapy is initiated or changed, monitor the hematocrit twice weekly for 2 to 6 weeks until stabilized in the target range and a maintenance dose determined. Monitor hematocrit regularly thereafter.
Check drug level 8 to 10 days after therapy is initiated or changed. Periodically monitor CBC with differential, liver function tests, and urinalysis.
Therapy is usually withdrawn after 3 months if response is inadequate. Patient must be fasting to measure triglyceride levels. Periodically obtain blood counts during the first 12 months.
When drug is given by continuous I.V. infusion, check PTT every 4 hours in the early stages of therapy, and daily thereafter. When drug is given by deep subcutaneous injection, check PTT 4 to 6 hours after injection, and daily thereafter. Periodically during therapy, check platelet counts and hematocrit and test for occult blood in stool.
Perform liver function tests at baseline, 6 to 12 weeks after therapy is initiated or changed, and about every 6 months thereafter. If adequate response isn't achieved within 6 weeks, consider changing the therapy.
A patient's home monitoring of glucose levels helps measure compliance and response. Glycosylated hemoglobin level is a good measure of long-term control.
Use a serum or urine pregnancy test with a sensitivity of at least 25 milli-international units/ml. Perform one test before therapy and a second test during the first 5 days of the menstrual cycle before therapy begins or at least 11 days after the last unprotected act of sexual intercourse, whichever is later. Repeat pregnancy tests monthly. Obtain baseline liver function tests and lipid levels; repeat every 1 to 2 weeks until a response is established (usually 4 weeks).

(continued)

* For those areas marked with one asterisk, the following values can be used:

ALT: 7–56 units/L
AST: 5–40 units/L
Alkaline phosphatase: 17–142 units/L
LDH: 60–220 units/L
GGT: < 40 units/L
Total bilirubin: 0.2–1 mg/dl

Drug	Laboratory test monitored	Therapeutic ranges of test
linezolid	Amylase	35–118 international units/L
	CBC with differential	*****
	Cultures and sensitivities	
	Liver function	*
	Lipase	10–150 units/L
	Platelet count	150–450 × 10^3/mm^3
lithium	Creatinine	0.6–1.3 mg/dl
	CBC	*****
	Electrolytes (especially potassium and sodium)	Potassium: 3.5–5 mEq/L Magnesium: 1.7–2.1 mEq/L Sodium: 135–145 mEq/L Chloride: 98–106 mEq/L
	Fasting glucose	70–110 mg/dl
	Lithium	0.6–1.2 mEq/L
	Thyroid function tests	TSH: 0.2–5.4 microunits/ml T_3: 80–200 nanogram/dl T_4: 5.4–11.5 mcg/dl
methotrexate	CBC with differential	*****
	Creatinine	0.6–1.3 mg/dl
	Liver function	*
	Methotrexate	Normal elimination: ~ 10 micromol 24 hours postdose ~ 1 micromol 48 hours postdose < 0.2 micromol 72 hours postdose
	Platelet count	150–450 × 10^3/mm^3
nonnucleoside reverse transcriptase inhibitors (nevirapine, delavirdine, efavirenz)	Amylase	35–118 international units/L
	CBC with differential and platelets	*****
	Liver function	*
	Lipids (efavirenz)	Total cholesterol: < 200 mg/dl LDL: < 100 mg/dl HDL: Women: 40–75 mg/dl Men: 37–70 mg/dl Triglycerides: 10–150 mg/dl
phenytoin	CBC	*****
	Phenytoin	10–20 mcg/ml
procainamide	ANA titer	Negative
	CBC	*****
	Liver function	*
	N-acetylprocainamide (NAPA)	10–30 mcg/ml
	Procainamide	3–10 mcg/ml

***** For those areas marked with asterisks, the following values can be used:

Hemoglobin: Women: 12–16 g/dl
Men: 14–18 g/dl
Hematocrit: Women: 37%–48%
Men: 42%–52%
RBCs: 4–5.5 × 10^6/mm^3
WBCs: 5–10 × 10^3/mm^3

Differential: Neutrophils: 45%–74%
Bands: 0%–8%
Lymphocytes: 16%–45%
Monocytes: 4%–10%
Eosinophils: 0%–7%
Basophils: 0%–2%

Monitoring guidelines

Obtain baseline CBC with differential and platelet count. Repeat weekly, especially if more than 2 weeks of therapy are received. Monitor liver function tests and amylase and lipase levels during therapy.

Checking drug levels is crucial to the safe use of the drug. Obtain level immediately before next dose. Monitor level twice weekly until stable. Once at steady state, level should be checked weekly; when the patient is on the appropriate maintenance dose, levels should be checked every 2 or 3 months. Monitor CBC; creatinine, electrolyte, and fasting glucose levels; and thyroid function test results before therapy starts and periodically thereafter.

Monitor drug levels according to dosing protocol. Monitor CBC with differential, platelet count, and liver and renal function test results more frequently when therapy starts or changes and when methotrexate levels may be elevated, such as when the patient is dehydrated.

Obtain baseline liver function tests and monitor closely during the first 12 weeks of therapy. Continue to monitor regularly during therapy. Check CBC with differential and platelet count before therapy and periodically during therapy. Monitor lipid levels during efavirenz therapy. Monitor amylase level during efavirenz and delavirdine therapy.

Monitor drug level immediately before next dose and 7 to 10 days after therapy starts or changes. Obtain a CBC at baseline and monthly early in therapy. Watch for toxic effects at therapeutic levels. Adjust the measured level for hypoalbuminemia or renal impairment, which can increase free drug levels.

Measure drug levels 6 to 12 hours after a continuous infusion is started or immediately before the next oral dose. Combined procainamide and NAPA levels can be used as an index of toxicity when renal impairment exists. Obtain CBC, liver function tests, and ANA titer periodically during longer-term therapy.

(continued)

* For those areas marked with one asterisk, the following values can be used:

ALT: 7–56 units/L
AST: 5–40 units/L
Alkaline phosphatase: 17–142 units/L
LDH: 60–220 units/L
GGT: < 40 units/L
Total bilirubin: 0.2–1 mg/dl

Drug	Laboratory test monitored	Therapeutic ranges of test
quinidine	CBC	*****
	Creatinine	0.6–1.3 mg/dl
	Electrolytes (especially potassium)	Potassium: 3.5–5 mEq/L Magnesium: 1.7–2.1 mEq/L Sodium: 135–145 mEq/L Chloride: 98–106 mEq/L
	Liver function	*
	Quinidine	2–6 mcg/ml
sulfonylureas	Fasting glucose	70–110 mg/dl
	Glycosylated hemoglobin	4%–7% of total hemoglobin
theophylline	Theophylline	10–20 mcg/ml
thiazolidinediones (rosiglitazone, pioglitazone)	Fasting glucose	70–110 mg/dl
	Glycosylated hemoglobin	4%–7% of total hemoglobin
	Liver function	*
thyroid hormones	Thyroid function tests	TSH: 0.2–5.4 microunits/ml T_3: 80–200 nanogram/dl T_4: 5.4–11.5 mcg/dl
valproate sodium, valproic acid, divalproex sodium	Ammonia	15–45 mcg/dl
	BUN	5–20 mg/dl
	CBC with differential	*****
	Creatinine	0.6–1.3 mg/dl
	Liver function	*
	Platelet count	$150–450 \times 10^3/mm^3$
	PTT	10–14 seconds
	Valproic acid	50–100 mcg/ml
vancomycin	Creatinine	0.6–1.3 mg/dl
	Vancomycin	20–40 mcg/ml (peak) 5–15 mcg/ml (trough)
warfarin	INR	For an acute MI, atrial fibrillation, treatment of pulmonary embolism, prevention of systemic embolism, tissue heart valves, valvular heart disease, or prophylaxis or treatment of venous thrombosis: 2–3 For mechanical prosthetic valves or recurrent systemic embolism: 3–4.5

***** For those areas marked with asterisks, the following values can be used:

Hemoglobin: Women: 12–16 g/dl
Men: 14–18 g/dl
Hematocrit: Women: 37%–48%
Men: 42%–52%
RBCs: $4–5.5 \times 10^6/mm^3$
WBCs: $5–10 \times 10^3/mm^3$

Differential: Neutrophils: 45%–74%
Bands: 0%–8%
Lymphocytes: 16%–45%
Monocytes: 4%–10%
Eosinophils: 0%–7%
Basophils: 0%–2%

Monitoring guidelines

Obtain levels immediately before next oral dose and 30 to 35 hours after therapy starts or changes. Periodically obtain blood counts, liver and kidney function test results, and electrolyte levels. With more specific assays, therapeutic levels are < 1 mcg/ml.

Monitor response to therapy by periodically evaluating fasting glucose and glycosylated hemoglobin levels. Patient should monitor glucose levels at home to help measure compliance and response.

Obtain drug levels right before next dose of sustained-release oral product and at least 2 days after therapy starts or changes.

Monitor response by evaluating fasting glucose and hemoglobin A_{1c} levels. Obtain baseline liver function test results, and repeat tests periodically during therapy.

Monitor thyroid function test results every 2 to 3 weeks until appropriate maintenance dose is determined and annually thereafter.

Monitor liver function test results, ammonia level, coagulation test results, renal function test results, CBC, and platelet count at baseline and periodically during therapy. Liver function test results should be closely monitored during the first 6 months.

Drug levels may be checked with the third dose administered, at the earliest. Draw peak levels 1.5 to 2.5 hours after a 1-hour infusion or I.V. infusion is complete. Draw trough levels within 1 hour of the next dose administered. Renal function can be used to adjust dosing and intervals.

Check INR daily, beginning 3 days after therapy starts. Continue checking it until therapeutic goal is achieved, and monitor it periodically thereafter. Also, check level 7 days after change in dose or start of a potentially interacting therapy.

* For those areas marked with one asterisk, the following values can be used:

ALT: 7–56 units/L
AST: 5–40 units/L
Alkaline phosphatase: 17–142 units/L
LDH: 60–220 units/L
GGT: < 40 units/L
Total bilirubin: 0.2–1 mg/dl

Drugs that shouldn't be crushed

Slow-release, enteric-coated, encapsulated-bead, wax-matrix, sublingual, and buccal forms are made to release their active ingredients over a certain period or at preset points after administration. Crushing these drug forms can dramatically affect their absorption rate and increase the risk of adverse reactions.

Other reasons not to crush some drug forms include taste, tissue irritation, and unusual formulation—for example, a capsule within a capsule, a liquid within a capsule, or a multiple-compressed tablet. Some drugs shouldn't be crushed because they're teratogenic. Avoid crushing the following drugs, for the reasons noted beside them.

Accutane (irritant)

Aciphex (delayed release)

Actifed 12-hour (sustained release)

Adalat CC (sustained release)

Advicor (extended release)

Aggrenox (extended release)

Allegra D (extended release)

Allerest 12-hour (sustained release)

Altocor (extended release)

Ambien CR (extended release)

Amnesteem (irritant)

Ansaid (taste)

Aricept ODT (orally disintegrating)

Arthrotec (delayed release)

Asacol (delayed release)

aspirin (enteric coated)

Atrohist (long acting)

Augmentin XR (extended release)

Avinza (extended release)

Avodart (irritant)

Azulfidine EN-tabs (enteric coated)

Biaxin XL (extended release)

Biohist LA (long acting)

Bisacodyl (enteric coated)

Bontril Slow-Release (slow release)

Bromfed (slow release)

Bromfed-PD (slow release)

Bronkodyl SR (slow release)

Calan SR (sustained release)

Carbatrol (extended release)

Cardizem CD, LA (slow release)

Cartia XT (extended release)

Ceclor CD (slow release)

Ceftin (strong, persistent taste)

Cellcept (teratogenic)

Chloral Hydrate (liquid within a capsule, taste)

Chlor-Trimeton Allergy 8-hour and 12-hour (slow release)

Choledyl SA (slow release)

Cipro XR (extended release)

Claritin-D 12-hour (slow release)

Claritin-D 24-hour (slow release)

Cleocin (taste)

Colace (liquid within a capsule)

Colazal (granules within capsules must reach colon intact)

Colestid (protective coating)

Compazine Spansules (slow release)

Concerta (extended release)

Contac 12 Hour, Maximum Strength 12 Hour (slow release)

Cotazym-S (enteric coated)

Covera-HS (extended release)

Creon (enteric coated)

Cytovene (irritant)

Cytoxan (toxic)

Dallergy, Dallergy-Jr (slow release)

Deconamine SR (slow release)

Depakene (slow release, mucous membrane irritant)

Depakote (enteric coated)

Depakote ER (extended release)

Dexedrine Spansule (slow release)

Diamox Sequels (slow release)

Dilacor XR (extended release)

Dilatrate-SR (slow release)

Dilt XR (extended release)

Diltia XT (extended release)

Dimetane Extentabs (extended release)

Dimetapp Extentabs (slow release)

Ditropan XL (slow release)

Dolobid (irritant)
Donnatel Extentabs (extended release)
Doxidan Liquigels (liquid in capsule)
Drisdol (liquid filled)
Dristan (protective coating)
Drixoral (slow release)
Dulcolax (enteric coated)
Dynabac (slow release)
DynaCirc CR (slow release)
Easprin (enteric coated)
Ecotrin (enteric coated)
Ecotrin Maximum Strength (enteric coated)
E.E.S. 400 Filmtab (enteric coated)
Effexor XR (extended release)
Emend (hard gelatin capsule)
E-Mycin (enteric coated)
Entex LA (slow release)
Entex PSE (slow release)
Equanil (extended release)
Ergostat (sublingual)
Eryc (enteric coated)
Ery-Tab (enteric coated)
Erythrocin Stearate (enteric coated)
Erythromycin Base (enteric coated)
Eskalith CR (slow release)
Extendryl JR, SR (slow release)
Feldene (mucous membrane irritant)
Feosol (enteric coated)
Feratab (enteric coated)
Fergon (slow release)
Fero-Folic 500 (slow release)
Fero-Grad-500 (slow release)
Ferro-Sequel (slow release)
Feverall Children's Capsules, Sprinkle (taste)
Flomax (slow release)
Focalin XR (extended release)
Fumatinic (slow release)
Geocillin (taste)
Glucophage XR (extended release)
Glucotrol XL (slow release)
Glumetza (extended release)
Guaifed (slow release)
Guaifed-PD (slow release)
Guaifenex LA (slow release)
Guaifenex PPA (slow release)
Guaifenex PSE (slow release)
Guaimax-D (slow release)

Hytakerol (liquid filled)
Hydergine LC (sublingual)
Iberet (slow release)
ICAPS Plus (slow release)
ICAPS Time Release (slow release)
Ilotycin (enteric coated)
Imdur (slow release)
Inderal LA (slow release)
Indocin SR (slow release)
InnoPran XL (extended release)
Ionamin (slow release)
Isoptin SR (sustained release)
Isordil Sublingual (sublingual)
Isordil Tembids (slow release)
Isosorbide Dinitrate Sublingual (sublingual)
Kadian (extended release)
Kaletra (extended release)
Kaon-Cl (slow release)
K-Dur (slow release)
Klor-Con (slow release)
Klotrix (slow release)
K-Tab (slow release)
Levbid (slow release)
Levsinex Timecaps (slow release)
Lithobid (slow release)
Macrobid (slow release)
Mestinon Timespans (slow release)
Metadate CD, ER (extended release)
Methylin ER (extended release)
Micro-K Extencaps (slow release)
Modane (enteric coated)
Motrin (taste)
MS Contin (slow release)
Mucinex (extended release)
Naprelan (slow release)
Nexium (sustained release)
Niaspan (extended release)
Nicotinic acid (slow release)
Nifedical XL (extended release)
Nitroglyn (slow release)
Nitrostat (sublingual)
Noctec (liquid in capsule)
Norflex (slow release)
Norpace CR (slow release)
Oramorph SR (slow release)
Orapred ODT (orally disintegrating)
Oruvail (extended release)

OxyContin (slow release)
Pancrease (enteric coated)
Pancrease MT (enteric coated)
Paxil CR (controlled release)
PCE (slow release)
Pentasa (controlled release)
Phazyme (slow release)
Phazyme 95 (slow release)
Phenytek (extended release)
Plendil (slow release)
Prelu-2 (slow release)
Prevacid, Prevacid SoluTab (delayed release)
Prilosec (slow release)
Prilosec OTC (delayed release)
Pro-Banthine (taste)
Procanbid (slow release)
Procardia XL (slow release)
Propecia (pregnant women shouldn't handle)
Proscar (pregnant women shouldn't handle)
Protonix (delayed release)
Proventil Repetabs (slow release)
Prozac Weekly (slow release)
Quibron-T/SR (slow release)
Qunaglute Dura-Tabs (extended release)
Quinidex Extentabs (slow release)
Respaire SR (slow release)
Respbid (extended release)
Risperdal (orally disintegrating)
Risperdal M-Tab (delayed release)
Ritalin-LA, -SR (slow release)
Rondec-TR (slow release)
Roxanol SR (sustained release)
Sinemet CR (slow release)
Slo-bid Gyrocaps (slow release)
Slo-Niacin (slow release)
Slo-Phyllin GG, Gyrocaps (slow release)
Slow FE (slow release)
Slow-K (slow release)
Slow-Mag (slow release)
Sorbitrate (sublingual)
Sotret (irritant)
Sudafed 12 Hour (slow release)
Sular (extended release)
Surfac Liquigels (liquid in capsule)
Taztia XT (extended release)
Tegretol-XR (extended release)
Ten-K (slow release)
Tenuate Dospan (slow release)
Tessalon Perles (slow release)
Theochron (slow release)
Theo-24 (slow release)
TheoDur (extended release)
Theoclear LA (slow release)
Thorazine Spansules (slow release)
Tiazac (sustained release)
Topamax (taste)
Toprol XL (extended release)
Trental (slow release)
Tylenol Extended Relief (slow release)
Uniphyl (slow release)
Uroxatral (extended release)
Vantin (taste)
Verelan, Verelan PM (slow release)
Volmax (slow release)
Voltaren (enteric coated)
Voltaren-XR (extended release)
Wellbutrin SR (sustained release)
Xanax XR (extended release)
Zerit XR (extended release)
Zomig-ZMT (delayed release)
ZORprin (slow release)
Zyban (slow release)
Zyrtec-D 12 hour (extended release)

Normal laboratory test values

Normal values may differ from laboratory to laboratory. Standard International units are abbreviated SI.

Hematology

Bleeding time
Template: 3–6 min (SI, 3–6 m)
Ivy: 3–6 min (SI, 3–6 m)
Duke: 1–3 min (SI, 1–3 m)

Fibrinogen level
200–400 mg/dl (SI, 2–4 g/L)

Hematocrit
Men: 42%–52% (SI, 0.42–0.52)
Women: 36%–48% (SI, 0.36–0.48)

Hemoglobin, total
Men: 14–17.4 g/dl (SI, 140–174 g/L)
Women: 12–16 g/dl (SI, 120–160 g/L)

PTT
21–35 sec (SI, 21–35 sec)

Platelet aggregation
3–5 min (SI, 3–5 min)

Platelet count
140,000–400,000/mm^3 (SI, 140–400 × 10^9/L)

PT
10–14 sec (SI, 10–14 sec); INR for patients not receiving warfarin, 1.12–1.46; INR for patients receiving warfarin, 2–3 (SI, 2–3) (those with prosthetic heart valve, 2.5–3.5 [SI, 2.5–3.5])

RBC count
Men: 4.5–5.5 million/mm^3 (SI, 4.5–5.5 × 10^{12}/L) venous blood
Women: 4–5 million/mm^3 (SI, 4–5 × 10^{12}/L) venous blood

RBC index
Mean corpuscular volume: 82–98 femtoliters
Mean corpuscular hemoglobin: 26–34 picograms/cell
Mean corpuscular hemoglobin concentration: 31–37 g/dl

Reticulocyte count
0.5%–1.5% (SI, 0.005–0.025) of total RBC count

WBC count
4,500–10,500 cells/mm^3

WBCdifferential, blood
Neutrophils: 54%–75% (SI, 0.54–0.75)
Lymphocytes: 25%–40% (SI, 0.25–0.4)
Monocytes: 2%–8% (SI, 0.02–0.08)
Eosinophils: up to 4% (SI, up to 0.04)
Basophils: up to 1% (SI, up to 0.01)

Blood chemistry

ALT
Adults: 10–35 units/L (SI, 0.17–0.6 μkat/L)
Newborns: 13–45 units/L (SI, 0.22–0.77 μkat/L)

Amylase, serum
Adults ≥ *age 18:* 30–175 units/L (SI, 0.5–2.83 μkat/L)

Arterial blood gases
pH: 7.35–7.45 (SI, 7.35–7.45)
$Paco_2$: 35–45 mm Hg (SI, 4.7–5.3 kPa)
Pao_2: 80–100 mm Hg (SI, 10.6–13.3 kPa)
HCO_3^-: 22–26 mEq/L (SI, 22–25 mmol/L)
Sao_2: 94%–100% (SI, 0.94–1.00)

AST
Men: 14–20 units/L (SI, 0.23–0.33 μkat/L)
Women: 7–34 units/L (SI, 0.12–0.58 μkat/L)

Bilirubin, serum
Adults, total: 0.2–1 mg/dl (SI, 3.5–17 μmol/L)
Neonates, total: 1–10 mg/dl (SI, 17–170 μmol/L)
Neonates, unconjugated indirect: 0–10 mg/dl (SI, 0–170 μmol/L)

BUN
8–20 mg/dl (SI, 2.9–7.5 mmol/L)

Calcium, serum
Adults: 8.2–10.2 mg/dl (SI, 2.05–2.54 mmol/L)
Children: 8.6–11.2 mg/dl (SI, 2.15–2.79 mmol/L)

Carbon dioxide, total blood
22–26 mEq/L (SI, 22–26 mmol/L)

Cholesterol, total serum
Men: < 205 mg/dl (SI, < 5.30 mmol/L) (desirable)
Women: < 190 mg/dl (SI, < 4.90 mmol/L) (desirable)

CK, isoenzymes
CK–BB: none
CK–MB: 0%–7%
CK–MM: 96%–100%

Creatinine, serum
Adults: 0.6–1.3 mg/dl (SI, 53–115 µmol/L)

Glucose, plasma, fasting
70–110 mg/dl (SI, 3.9–6.1 mmol/L)

Glucose, plasma, 2-hour postprandial
< 145 mg/dl (SI, < 8 mmol/L)

LDH
Total: 71–207 units/L in adults (SI, 1.2–3.52 µkat/L)
LDH1: 14%–26% (SI, 0.14–0.26)
LDH2: 29%–39% (SI, 0.29–0.39)
LDH3: 20%–26% (SI, 0.20–0.26)
LDH4: 8%–16% (SI, 0.08–0.16)
LDH5: 6%–16% (SI, 0.06–0.16)

Lipase
< 160 units/L (SI, < 2.72 µkat/L)

Magnesium, serum
1.8–2.6 mg/dl (SI, 0.74–1.07 mmol/L)

Phosphates, serum
2.7–4.5 mg/dl (SI, 0.87–1.45 mmol/L)

Potassium, serum
3.8–5 mEq/L (SI, 3.5–5 mmol/L)

Protein, serum
Total: 6.3–8.3 g/dl (SI, 64–83 g/L)
Albumin fraction: 3.5–5 g/dl (SI, 35–50 g/L)

Sodium, serum
135–145 mEq/L (SI, 135–145 mmol/L)

Triglycerides, serum
Men > age 20: 40–180 mg/dl (SI, 0.11–2.01 mmol/L)
Women > age 20: 10–190 mg/dl (SI, 0.11–2.21 mmol/L)

Uric acid, serum
Men: 3.4–7 mg/dl (SI, 202–416 µmol/L)
Women: 2.3–6 mg/dl (SI, 143–357 µmol/L)

Dialyzable drugs

The amount of a drug removed by dialysis differs among patients and depends on several factors, including the patient's condition, the drug's properties, length of dialysis and dialysate used, rate of blood flow or dwell time, and purpose of dialysis. This table indicates the effect of conventional hemodialysis on selected drugs.

Drug	Level reduced by hemodialysis
acebutolol	Yes
acetaminophen	Yes (may not influence toxicity)
acetazolamide	No
acetylcysteine	Yes
acyclovir	Yes
albuterol	No
allopurinol	Yes
alprazolam	No
amantadine	No
amikacin	Yes
amiodarone	No
amitriptyline	No
amlodipine	No
amoxicillin	Yes
amoxicillin and clavulanate potassium	Yes
amphotericin B	No
ampicillin	Yes
ampicillin and sulbactam sodium	Yes
aprepitant	No
aresenic trioxide	No
ascorbic acid	Yes
aspirin	Yes
atenolol	Yes
atorvastatin	No
atropine	No
auranofin	No
azathioprine	Yes
aztreonam	Yes
bivalirusin	Yes
bretylium	No
bumetanide	No
bupropion	No
buspirone	No
busulfan	Yes
captopril	Yes
carbamazepine	No
carbenicillin	Yes
carboplatin	Yes
carisoprodol	Yes
carmustine	No
carvedilol	No
cefaclor	Yes
cefadroxil	Yes
cefazolin	Yes
cefepime	Yes
cefoperazone	Yes
cefotaxime	Yes
cefotetan	Yes (only by 20%)
cefoxitin	Yes
cefpodoxime	Yes
ceftazidime	Yes
ceftibuten	Yes
ceftizoxime	Yes
ceftriaxone	No
cefuroxime	Yes
cephalexin	Yes
cephalothin	Yes
cephradine	Yes
chloral hydrate	Yes
chlorambucil	No
chloramphenicol	Yes (very small amount)
chlordiazepoxide	No
chloroquine	No
chlorpheniramine	Yes
chlorpromazine	No

(continued)

Drug	Level reduced by hemodialysis
chlorthalidone	No
cilastatin	Yes
cilaxapril	Yes
cimetidine	Yes
ciprofloxacin	Yes (only by 10%)
cisplatin	No
clavulanic acid	Yes
clindamycin	No
clofibrate	No
clonazepam	No
clonidine	No
clorazepate	No
cloxacillin	No
codeine	No
colchicine	No
cortisone	No
co-trimoxazole	Yes
cyclophosphamide	Yes
deferoxamine	Yes
desloratadine	No
dexamethsone	No
diazepam	No
diazoxide	Yes
diclofenac	No
dicloxacillin	No
didanosine	Yes
digoxin	No
digoxin immune Fab	No
diltiazem	No
diphenhydramine	No
dipyridamole	No
disopyramide	Yes
dopamine	No
doxazosin	No
doxepin	No
doxorubicin	No
doxycycline	No
emtrictabine	Yes
enalapril	Yes
enoxaparin	No
epoetin alfa	No

Drug	Level reduced by hemodialysis
ertapenem	Yes
erythromycin	Yes (only by 20%)
ethacrynic acid	No
ethambutol	Yes (only by 20%)
ethosuximide	Yes
famciclovir	Yes
famotidine	No
fenoprofen	No
filgrastim	No
flecainide	No
fluconazole	Yes
flucytosine	Yes
fluorouracil	No
fluoxetine	No
flurazepam	No
foscarnet	Yes
fosinopril	No
furosemide	No
gabapentin	Yes
ganciclovir	Yes
gemcitabine	Yes
gemfibrozil	No
gemifloxacin	Yes
gentamicin	Yes
glipizide	No
glyburide	No
guanfacine	No
haloperidol	No
heparin	No
hydralazine	No
hydrochlorothiazide	No
hydroxyzine	No
ibuprofen	No
ifosfamide	Yes
imipramine	No
indapamide	No
indomethacin	No
insulin	No
irbesartan	No
iron dextran	No
isoniazid	No

Drug	Level reduced by hemodialysis
isosorbide	Yes
isradipine	No
kanamycin	Yes
ketoconazole	No
labetalol	No
lamivudine	No
lansoprazole	No
levetiracetam	Yes
levofloxacin	No
lidocaine	No
linezolid	Yes
lisinopril	Yes
lithium	Yes
lomefloxacin	No
lomustine	No
loracarbef	Yes
loratadine	No
lorazepam	No
mannitol	No
mechlorethamine	No
mefenamic acid	No
meperidine	No
meprobamate	Yes
mercaptopurine	Yes
meropenem	Yes
mesalamine	Yes
metformin	Yes
methadone	No
methicillin	No
methotrexate	Yes
methyldopa	Yes
methylprednisolone	Yes
metoclopramide	No
metolazone	No
metoprolol	Yes
metronidazole	Yes
mexiletine	Yes
miconazole	No
midazolam	No
minocycline	No
minoxidil	Yes

Drug	Level reduced by hemodialysis
misoprostol	No
morphine	No
nabumetone	No
nadolol	Yes
nafcillin	No
nalmefine	No
naltrexone	No
naproxen	No
nelfinavir	No
nicardipine	No
nifedipine	No
nimodipine	No
nitazoxanide	No
nitrofurantoin	Yes
nitroglycerin	No
nitroprusside	Yes
nizatidine	No
norfloxacin	No
nortriptyline	No
octreotide	yes
ofloxacin	Yes
olanzapine	No
omeprazole	No
oxacillin	No
oxazepam	No
paclitaxel	No
paroxetine	No
penicillin G	Yes
pentamidine	No
pentazocine	Yes
pentobarbital	No
perindopril	Yes
phenobarbital	Yes
phenylbutazone	No
phenytoin	No
piperacillin	Yes
piroxicam	No
prazosin	No
prednisone	No
pregabalin	Yes

(continued)

Drug	Level reduced by hemodialysis
primidone	Yes
procainamide	Yes
promethazine	No
propoxyphene	No
propranolol	No
protriptyline	No
pseudoephedrine	No
pyrazinamide	Yes
pyridoxine	Yes
quinapril	No
quinidine	No
quinine	No
ramipril	No
ranitidine	Yes
rifampin	No
ritodrine	Yes
rituximab	No
rosiglitazone	No
salsalate	Yes
sertraline	No
sotalol	Yes
stavudine	Yes
streptomycin	Yes
sucralfate	No
sulbactam	Yes
sulfamethoxazole	Yes
sulfisoxazole	No
sulindac	No
tazobactam	Yes
temazepam	No
theophylline	Yes
ticarcillin	Yes
ticarcillin and clavulanate	Yes
timolol	No
tirofiban	Yes
tobramycin	Yes
tocainide	Yes
tolbutamide	No
topiramate	Yes
toptecan	Yes
torsemide	No

Drug	Level reduced by hemodialysis
tramadol	No
trandopril	Yes
trazodone	No
triazolam	No
trimethoprim	Yes
valacyclovir	Yes
valganciclovir	Yes
valproic acid	No
valsartan	No
vancomycin	Yes
venlafaxine	No
verapamil	No
vigabatrin	Yes
warfarin	No
zolpidem	No
zonisamide	Yes

English-Spanish drug phrase translator

Medication history

Do you take any medications?	**¿Toma Ud. medicamentos?**
– Prescription?	– ¿De receta?
– Over-the-counter?	– ¿Sin necesidad de receta?
– Other?	– ¿Otro?
Which prescription medications do you take routinely?	**¿Qué medicamentos de receta toma Ud. por rutina?**
Which over-the-counter medications do you take routinely?	**¿Qué medicamentos que no necesitan receta toma Ud. por rutina?**
– How often do you take them?	– ¿Con qué frecuencia los toma?
– Once daily?	– ¿Una vez al día?
– Twice daily?	– ¿Dos veces al día?
– Three times daily?	– ¿Tres veces al día?
– Four times daily?	– ¿Cuátro veces al día?
– More often?	– ¿Con más frecuencia?
Why do you take these medications?	**¿Por qué toma Ud. estos medicamentos?**
What is the dosage for each medication?	**¿Cuál es la dosis para cada uno de los medicamentos?**
Are you allergic to any medications?	**¿Está Ud. alérgico(a) a algúnos medicamentos?**

Medication teaching

Purpose of the medication

This medication will:	**Este medicamento hará que:**
– elevate your blood pressure.	– su presión sanguínea suba.
– improve circulation to your ____.	– la circulación por (la región del cuerpo) mejore.
– lower your blood pressure.	– su presión sanguínea baje.
– lower your blood sugar.	– el nivel de azucar en la sangre baje.
– make your heart rhythm more even.	– el ritmo del corazón sea más uniforme.
– raise your blood sugar.	– su nivel de azucar en la sangre suba.
– reduce or prevent the formation of blood clots.	– se reduzca o evite la formación de coágulos de sangre.
– remove fluid from your body.	– se le quite fluido en el cuerpo.
– remove fluid from your feet, ankles, or legs.	– se le quite fluido de los pies, tobillos o piernas.
– remove fluid from your lungs so that they work better.	– se le quite fluido de los pulmones para que funcionen mejor.
– remove fluid from your pancreas so that it works better.	– se le quite fluido de la páncreas para que funcione mejor.
– kill the bacteria in your ____.	– destruir la bacteria de la ____.
– slow down your heart rate.	– reducir el latir del corazón.
– soften your bowel movements.	– ablandar sus evacuaciones.
– speed up your heart rate.	– acelerar el latir del corazón.

– help your body to use insulin more efficiently.	– le ayudar a su cuerpo a usar la insulina más eficazmente.
This medication will help you to:	**Este medicamento le ayudará a Ud. a:**
– breathe better.	– respirar con mayor facilidad.
– fight infections.	– luchar contra infecciones.
– relax.	– relajarse.
– sleep.	– dormir.
– think more clearly.	– pensar con mayor claridad.
This medication will relieve or reduce:	**Este medicamento le aliviará o disminuirá:**
– the acid production in your stomach.	– la producción de acido en el estómago.
– anxiety.	– la angustia.
– bladder spasms.	– espasmos en la vejiga.
– burning in your stomach or chest.	– sensasión ardiente en el estómago o tórax.
– burning when you urinate.	– sensación ardiente al orinar.
– diarrhea.	– diarrea.
– muscle cramps.	– espasmos en los músculos.
– nausea.	– nausea.
– pain in your _____.	– dolor en la (el) _____.
Medication administration	
I would like to give you:	**Quisiera darle a Ud. un(a):**
– an injection.	– inyección.
– an I.V. medication.	– medicamento por vía intravenosa.
– a liquid medication.	– medicamento en forma líquida.
– a medicated cream or powder.	– medicamento en pomada o polvo.
– a medication through your epidural catheter.	– medicamento por el catéter epidural.
– a medication through your rectum.	– medicamento por el recto.
– a medication through your _____ tube.	– medicamento por su _____ tubo.
– a medication under your tongue.	– medicamento debajo de la lengua.
– some pill(s).	– píldoras.
– a suppository.	– supositorio.
This is how you take this medication.	**Así se toma este medicamento.**
If you can't swallow this pill, I can get it in another form.	**Si Ud. no puede tragarse esta píldora, puede obtenerla en otra forma.**
If you can't swallow a pill, you can crush it and mix it in soft food.	**Si Ud. no se puede tragar la píldora, la puede moler y mezclarla en un alimento blando.**
I need to mix this medication in juice or water.	**Tengo que mezclar este medicamento en jugo (zumo) o agua.**
I need to give you this injection in your:	**Tengo que ponerle esta inyección:**
– abdomen.	– en el abdomen.
– buttocks.	– en las nalgas.
– hip.	– en la cadera.
– outer arm.	– en el brazo.
– thigh.	– en el muslo.

Some medications are coated with a special substance to protect your stomach from getting upset.

Algunos medicamentos están cubiertos con una sustancia especial para protegerle contra un trastorno estomacal.

Do not chew:
- enteric-coated pills.
- long-acting pills.
- capsules.
- sublingual medication.

No masque Ud.:
- píldoras con recubrimientoentérico.
- píldoras de efecto prolongado.
- cápsulas.
- medicamentos sublinguales.

Ask your doctor or pharmacist whether you can:
- mix your medication with food or fluids.
- take your medication with or without food.

Pregúntele Ud. a su doctor o farmacéutico si debiera:
- mezclar su medicamento con un alimento o con líquidos.
- tomar su medicamento con o sin alimento.

You need to take your medication:
- after meals.
- before meals.
- on an empty stomach.
- with meals or food.

Ud. tiene que tomarse el medicamento:
- después de las comidas.
- antes de las comidas.
- con el estómago vacío.
- con las comidas o con un alimento.

Skipping doses

If you skip or miss a dose:
- Take it as soon as you remember it.
- Wait until the next dose.
- Call the doctor if you are not sure.
- Don't take an extra dose.

Si Ud. omite o se salta una dosis:
- Tómesela encuanto se acuerde.
- Espérese hasta la siguiente dosis.
- Llame al doctor si Ud. no está seguro(a).
- No se tome una dosis extra.

Adverse effects

Some common adverse effects of _____ are:
- constipation
- diarrhea
- difficulty sleeping
- dry mouth
- fatigue
- headache
- itching
- light-headedness
- nausea
- poor appetite
- rash
- upset stomach
- weight loss or gain
- frequent urination.

Unos efectos adversos comunes a _____ son:
- estreñimiento
- diarrea
- dificultad en dormir
- boca seca
- fatiga
- dolor de cabeza
- comezón (picazón)
- mareo
- nausea
- poco apetito
- erupción
- trastorno estomacal
- perdida o aumento de peso
- orinar con frecuencia.

These adverse effects:
- will go away after your body gets used to the medication.
- may persist as long as you take the medication.

Estos efectos adversos:
- desaparecerán una vez que su cuerpo se acostumbre al medicamento.
- puede continuar mientras Ud. tome el medicamento.

If you have an adverse reaction to your medication, call your doctor right away.	**Si Ud. tiene una reacción adversa a su medicamento, llame a su doctor inmediatamente.**
Other concerns	
Tell your doctor if you are pregnant or breast-feeding.	**Dígale a su doctor si Ud. está ebarazada o si cría a los pechos.**
While you are taking this medication, ask your doctor if:	**Mientras Ud. tome este medicamento, pregúntele a su doctor si:**
– you can safely take other over-the-counter medications.	– puede tomar otros medicamentos que no necesitan receta.
– you can drink alcoholic beverages.	– puede tomar bebidas alcohólicas.
– your medications interact with each other.	– sus medicamentos interaccionan uno con el otro.
Storing medication	
You should keep your medication:	**Ud. debiera guardar sus medicamentos:**
– in a cool, dry place.	– en un lugar fresco, seco.
– in the refrigerator.	– en el refrigerador.
– at room temperature.	– al tiempo.
– out of direct sunlight.	– fuera de la luz de sol.
– away from heat.	– lejos de la calefacción.
– away from children.	– lejos del alcance de los niños.
Subcutaneous injection	
To give yourself an injection, follow these steps:	**Así es como uno se pone una inyección a sí mismo(a):**
– Draw up the medication.	– Saque el medicamento.
– Replace the cap carefully.	– Coloque de nuevo la tapa con cuidado.
– Decide where you are going to give the injection.	– Decida Ud. donde va a ponerse la inyección.
– Clean the skin area with alcohol.	– Limpie el área de la piel con alcohol.
– Gently pinch up a little skin over the area.	– Suavemente pellizque un poco de piel sobre el área.
– Using a dartlike motion, stab the needle into your skin.	– Con un movimiento rápido, penetre la aguja en su piel.
– Gently pull back on the plunger to see if there is any blood in the syringe.	– Con cuidado retire el émbolo para ver si hay sangre en la jeringa.
– Steadily push the medication into your skin.	– Constantemente empuje el medicamento dentro de su piel.
– Pull the needle out.	– Saque la aguja.
– Apply gentle pressure with the alcohol wipe.	– Ejerza presión suavemente con un limpión de alcohol.
– Dispose of the needle in a proper receptacle.	– Deshagase de la aguja en un recipiente apropiado.
Insulin preparation and administration	
The doctor has ordered insulin for you.	**El doctor ha recetado insulina para Ud.**
To draw up insulin, follow these steps:	**Para extraer la insulina siga las siguientes pasos:**
– Wipe the rubber top of the insulin bottle with alcohol.	– Limpie la tapa de hule (goma) de la botella de la insulina con alcohol.
– Remove the needle cap.	– Quítele el capuchón a la aguja.

– Pull out the plunger until the end of the plunger in the barrel aligns with the number of units of insulin that you need.	– Saque el émbolo hasta el otro extremo del émbolo en la cuba esté al nivel de la dosis de insulina (número de unidades) que Ud. necesita.
– Push the needle through the rubber top of the insulin bottle.	– Empuje la aguja por la tapa de hule (goma) de la botella de insulina.
– Inject the air into the bottle.	– Inyecte el aire dentro de la botella.
– Without removing the needle from the bottle, turn it upside down.	– Sin sacar la aguja de la botella, póngala al revés.
– Withdraw the plunger until the end of the plunger aligns with the number of units you need.	– Retire el émbolo hasta que llegue la insulina al número de unidades que Ud. necesita.
– Gently pull the needle out of the bottle.	– Retire Ud. la aguja de la botella suavemente.
To mix insulin, follow these steps:	**Para mezclar la insulina siga los siguientes pasos:**
– Wipe the rubber tops of the insulin bottles with alcohol.	– Limpie la tapa de hule (goma) de las botellas de insulina con alcohol.
– Gently roll the cloudy insulin between your palms.	– Suavemente mueva la insulina turbia entre las palmas de la mano.
– Remove the needle cap.	– Retire el capuchón de la aguja.
– Pull out the plunger until the end of the plunger in the barrel aligns with the number of units of NPH or Lente insulin that you need.	– Saque el émbolo hasta que el otro extremo del émbolo en el barril esté al nivel con la dosis de insulina turbia (NPH o insulina Lente) (número de unidades) que Ud. necesita.
– Push the needle through the rubber top of the cloudy insulin bottle.	– Empuje la aguja por la tapa de goma (hule) de la botella de insulina turbia.
– Inject the air into the bottle.	– Inyecte el aire dentro de la botella.
– Remove the needle.	– Saque la aguja.
– Pull out the plunger until the end of the plunger in the barrel aligns with the number of units of clear regular insulin that you need.	– Retire el émbolo hasta que el otro extremo del émbolo en el barril esté al nivel con la dosis de insulina clara (regular) (número de unidades) que Ud. necesita.
– Push the needle through the rubber top of the clear insulin bottle.	– Empuje Ud. la aguja por la tapa de goma de la botella de insulna clara.
– Inject the air into the bottle.	– Inyecte el aire dentro de la botella.
– Without removing the needle, turn the bottle upside down.	– Sin sacar la aguja, vuelva la botella al revés.
– Withdraw the plunger until it aligns with the number of units of clear regular insulin that you need.	– Retire el émbolo hasta que llegue a la dosis de insulina (regular) clara (número de unidades) que Ud. necesita.
– Gently pull the needle out of the bottle.	– Suavemente saque Ud. la aguja de la botella.
– Push the needle into the cloudy (NPH or Lente) insulin without injecting it into the bottle.	– Empuje la aguja en la insulina turbia (NPH o insulina Lente) sin inyectarla dentro de la botella.
– Withdraw the plunger until you reach your total dosage of insulin in units (regular combined with NPH or Lente).	– Retire el émbolo hasta que llegue a su dosis total de insulina en unidades (regular y NPH/Lente conbinadas).
– We will practice again.	– Practicaremos juntos(as) otra vez.

Home care phrases

Wash your hands before touching medications.	**Lávese Ud. las manos antes de tocar los medicamentos.**
Check the medication bottle for name, dose, and frequency (how often it's supposed to be taken).	**En el envase del medicamento verifique Ud. el nombre, la dosis y la frecuencia (con que frequencia se debe tomar).**
Check the expiration date on all medications.	**Verifique Ud. la fecha en la que el medicamento expira.**
Store medications according to pharmacy instructions.	**Guarde Ud. los medicamentos según las instrucciones de la farmacia.**
Under adequate lighting, read medication labels carefully before taking doses.	**Bajo luz adequada, lea Ud. la etiqueta del medicamento con mucho cuidado antes de tomar las dosis.**
Don't crush medication without first asking the doctor or pharmacist.	**No machaque Ud. el medicamento sin antes preguntárselo al doctor o al farmacéutico.**
Contact your doctor if a new or unexpected symptom or another problem appears.	**Póngase Ud. en contacto con su doctor si un síntoma nuevo o inesperado u otros problemas aparecen.**
Don't stop taking medication unless instructed by your doctor.	**No deje Ud. de tomar el medicamento sólo que se lo ordene su doctor.**
Discard outdated medications.	**Deshágase Ud. de medicamentos caducos.**
Never take someone else's medications.	**Nunca tome Ud. los medicamentos de otra persona.**
Keep a record of your current medications.	**Apunte Ud. (tome nota de) sus medicamentos actuales.**

General drug therapy phrases

Drug classes

Analgesic	**Analgésico**
Anesthetic	**Anestético**
Antacid	**Antiácido**
Antianginal	**Agente antianginal**
Anxiolytic	**Agente ansiolítico**
Antiarrhythmic	**Agente antiarrítmico**
Antibiotic	**Antibiótico**
Anticancer drug	**Agente anticarcinógeno**
Anticoagulant	**Anticoagulante**
Anticonvulsant	**Anticonvulsivante**
Antidepressant	**Antidepresivo**
Antidiarrheal	**Antidiarreico**
Antifungal	**Agente antifúngico**
Antigout drug	**Agente antigota**

Antihistamine	Antihistamínico
Antihyperlipemic	Agente hiperlipémico
Antihypertensive	Agente antihipertenso
Anti-inflammatory drug	Agente antiinflamatorio
Antimalarial	Agente antimalárico
Antiparkinsonian	Agente antiparkinsoniano
Antipsychotic	Agente antipsicótico
Antipyretic	Antipirético
Antiseptic	Antiséptico
Antispasmodic	Antiespasmódico
Antithyroid drug	Agente antitiroideo
Antituberculosis drug	Agente antituberculoso
Antitussive agent	Agente antitusígeno
Antiviral agent	Agente antiviral
Appetite stimulant	Estimulante para el apetito
Appetite suppressant	Supresor de apetito
Bronchodilator	Broncodilatador
Decongestant	Descongestivo
Digestant	Digestivo (agente que estimula la digestión)
Diuretic	Diurético
Emetic	Emético
Fertility drug	Agente para la fertilidad
Hormonal contraceptive	Anticonceptivo oral
Hypnotic	Hipnótico
Insulin	Insulina
Laxative	Laxante
Muscle relaxant	Relajante de músculos
Oral hypoglycemic	Agente hipoglucémico oral
Sedative	Sedante
Steroid	Esteroide
Thyroid hormone	Hormona de la glándula tiroides
Vaccine	Vacuna
Vasodilator	Vasodilatador
Vitamin	Vitamina
Preparations	
Capsule	Cápsula
Cream	Pomada
Drops	Gotas
Elixir	Elixir
Inhaler	Inhalador

Injection	**Inyección**
Lotion	**Loción**
Lozenge	**Pastilla**
Powder	**Polvo**
Spray	**Atomizador**
Suppository	**Supositorio**
Suspension	**Suspensión**
Syrup	**Jarabe**
Tablet	**Tableta**

Frequency

Once daily	**Una vez al día**
Twice daily	**Dos veces al día**
Three times daily	**Tres veces al día**
Four times daily	**Cuatro veces al día**
In the morning	**Por la mañana**
With meals	**Con las comidas**
Before meals	**Antes de las comidas**
After meals	**Después de las comidas**
Before bedtime	**Antes de acostarse**
When you have_____	**Cuando Ud. tome_____**
Only when you need it	**Sólo cuando lo necesite**
Every four hours	**Cada cuatro horas**
Every six hours	**Cada seis horas**
Every eight hours	**Cada ocho horas**

Acknowledgments

We would like to thank the following companies for granting us permission to include their drugs in the full-color photoguide. We would also like to thank Facts & Comparisons for the use of their resources.

Abbott Laboratories
Biaxin®, Biaxin® XL, Depakote®, Depakote® Sprinkle, E-Mycin®, Ery-Tab®, Hytrin®, Isoptin® SR, Kaletra™, Synthroid®, Vicodin®, Vicodin ES®

AstraZeneca LP
Arimidex®, Crestor®, Nolvadex®, Prilosec®, Tenormin®, Toprol-XL®, Zestril®

Aventis Pharmaceuticals
Allegra®, DiaBeta®, Lasix®, Trental®

Axcan Pharma
Carafate®

Bayer Corporation
Cipro®, Levitra®, Nexavar®

Biovail Pharmaceuticals, Inc.
Cardizem®, Cardizem® CD, Cardizem® LA, Cardizem® SR, Vasotec®

Bristol-Myers Squibb Company
BuSpar®, Capoten®, Cefzil®, Coumadin®, Desyrel®, Monopril®, Pravachol®, Reyataz®, Sprycel®, Sinemet®

CV Therapeutics
Ranexa®

Elan Pharmaceuticals, Inc.
Frova™

Forest Pharmaceuticals, Inc.
Campral®, Celexa®, Lexapro™

Gilead Sciences
Viread®

GlaxoSmithKline
Copyright GlaxoSmithKline. Used with permission.
Avandia®, Ceftin®, Combivir ®, Imitrex®, Lanoxin®, Lotronex®, Retrovir®, Wellbutrin®, Wellbutrin® SR, Zantac®, Zovirax®, Zyban®

Janssen Pharmaceutica, Inc.
Risperdal®, Risperdal M-Tab®

King Pharmaceuticals, Inc.
Levoxyl®

Eli Lilly and Company
Cymbalta®, Evista®, Prozac®, Strattera™
Copyright Eli Lilly and Company. Used with permission 2007. ®Cymbalta and Prozac are registered trademarks of Eli Lilly and Company.

Mallinckrodt, Inc.
Pamelor®, Restoril®

McNeil-PPC, Inc.
Concerta®

MedPointe Pharmaceuticals
Soma®

Merck & Co., Inc.
Used with permission of Merck & Co., Inc.
Cozaar®, Crixivan®, Fosamax®, HydroDIURIL®, Januvia®, Mevacor®, Pepcid®, Prinivil®, Singulair®, Zocor®

Merck Santé
An associate of Merck KGaA, Darmstadt, Germany.
Glucophage®, Glucophage® XR

Merck/Schering-Plough Pharmaceuticals
Used with permission of Merck/Schering-Plough Pharmaceuticals.
Zetia™

Novartis Pharmaceuticals, Inc.
Enablex®, Lescol®, Lotensin®, Ritalin®, Ritalin SR®, Stalevo®

Ortho-McNeil Pharmaceutical
Floxin®, Levaquin®, Tylenol® with Codeine No. 3, Ultracet®

Otsuka Pharmaceutical Company, Ltd.
Abilify®

Pfizer, Inc.
Used with permission of Pfizer, Inc.
Accupril®, Cardura®, Celebrex®, Chantix®, Diflucan®, Dilantin® Kapseals®, Glucotrol®, Glucotrol XL®, Lipitor®, Lopid®, Neurontin®, Nitrostat®, Norvasc®, Procardia XL®, Relpax®, Revatio®, Sutent®, Viagra®, Xanax®, Zithromax®, Zoloft®, Zyrtec®

Pharmacia Corporation
Registered Trademarks of Pharmacia Corporation, a Pfizer, Inc,. corporation. All Rights Reserved. Courtesy of Pfizer, Inc.
Calan®, Demulen®, Detrol®, Medrol®, Micronase®, Motrin, Provera®, Xanax®

Procter and Gamble Pharmaceuticals, Inc.
Actonel®, Macrobid®

Purdue Pharma L.P.
OxyContin®

Roche Laboratories, Inc.
Bumex®, Klonopin®, Naprosyn®, Ticlid®, Valium®

Sanofi-Synthelabo, Inc.
Ambien®, Demerol®, Uroxatral®

Sankyo Pharma
Benicar™

Schering Corporation and Key Pharmaceuticals, Inc.
Clarinex™, K-Dur®

Schwarz Pharma
Verelan®

Sepracor Inc.
Lunesta®

Sucampo Pharmaceuticals, Inc,
Amitiza®

Tap Pharmaceuticals, Inc.
Prevacid®

Teva Pharmaceuticals
Azilect®

TibotecInc.
Prezista®

UCB Pharmaceuticals, Inc.
Lortab®

Warner Chilcott Laboratories, Inc.
Duricef®, Eryc®, Estrace®, Sarafem®

Women First HealthCare, Inc.
Bactrim DS®

Wyeth Pharmaceuticals
The appearance of these tablets and capsules is a trademark of Wyeth Pharmaceuticals, Philadelphia, Pa.
Effexor®, Effexor® XR

The appearance of these tablets and capsules is a registered trademark of Wyeth Pharmaceuticals, Philadelphia, Pa.
Inderal®, Inderal® LA

Index

t refers to a table; **boldface** refers to full-color photographs.

†Canada ‡Australia

B

†Canada ‡Australia

†Canada ‡Australia

t refers to a table; **boldface** refers to full-color photographs.

D

†Canada ‡Australia

† refers to a table; **boldface** refers to full-color photographs.

†Canada ‡Australia

E

† refers to a table; **boldface** refers to full-color photographs.

†Canada ‡Australia

t refers to a table; **boldface** refers to full-color photographs.

†Canada ‡Australia

M

N

t refers to a table; **boldface** refers to full-color photographs.

O

t refers to a table; **boldface** refers to full-color photographs.

†Canada ‡Australia

P

t refers to a table; **boldface** refers to full-color photographs.

†Canada ‡Australia

Q

R

†Canada ‡Australia

S

†Canada ‡Australia

†Canada ‡Australia

U

†Canada ‡Australia

V

†Canada ‡Australia

t refers to a table; **boldface** refers to full-color photographs.

Visit NDHnow.com

The Web site of *Nursing2008 Drug Handbook* gives you:

- updates on recently approved drugs, new indications, and new warnings
- patient-teaching aids on new drugs
- news summaries on recent drug developments
- information on herbs
- links to pharmaceutical companies, government agencies, and nursing organizations
- continuing education tests for *Nursing2008 Drug Handbook*
- career opportunities
- a nursing bookstore.

About NDH2008*Plus!*

NDH2008*Plus!* mini-CD lets you:

- customize and print patient-teaching instructions for 200 of the most commonly prescribed drugs, in regular or large print
- view and print monographs on the same 200 common drugs
- link directly to **NDHnow.com** for drug updates and important drug news

Minimum system requirements

- Windows XP Home Edition
- Pentium 4
- 512 MB RAM
- 40 MB free hard-disk space
- SVGA monitor with high color (16-bit)
- CD-ROM drive and mouse

CAUTION: Don't try to use this mini-CD in a floppy disk drive, Zip drive, certain slot drives, or a car stereo. Don't insert the mini-CD into a CD-ROM drive that requires the mini-CD to be in a vertical position. Placing the CD into such a drive may result in jamming.

Before installing this program, make sure your monitor is set up to display high color (16-bit), your display area is set to 800 x 600, and your display font size is set to "Small fonts" or "Normal." If it isn't, consult your user's manual for instructions about changing the display settings.

To install:

- Place the mini-CD on the inner ring of the CD-ROM drive tray. Close the tray.
- In a few moments, the CD should automatically start. Once it starts, click the "Install NDH2008*Plus!*" button to install on your computer.
- Click "Start" and select "Run" if the CD doesn't start automatically.
- Type **d:\setup** (where **d** is the letter of your CD-ROM drive), and click *OK*. Follow on-screen instructions for installing the CD.